MW00837029

DIAGNOSTIC IMAGING
CHEST
SECOND EDITION

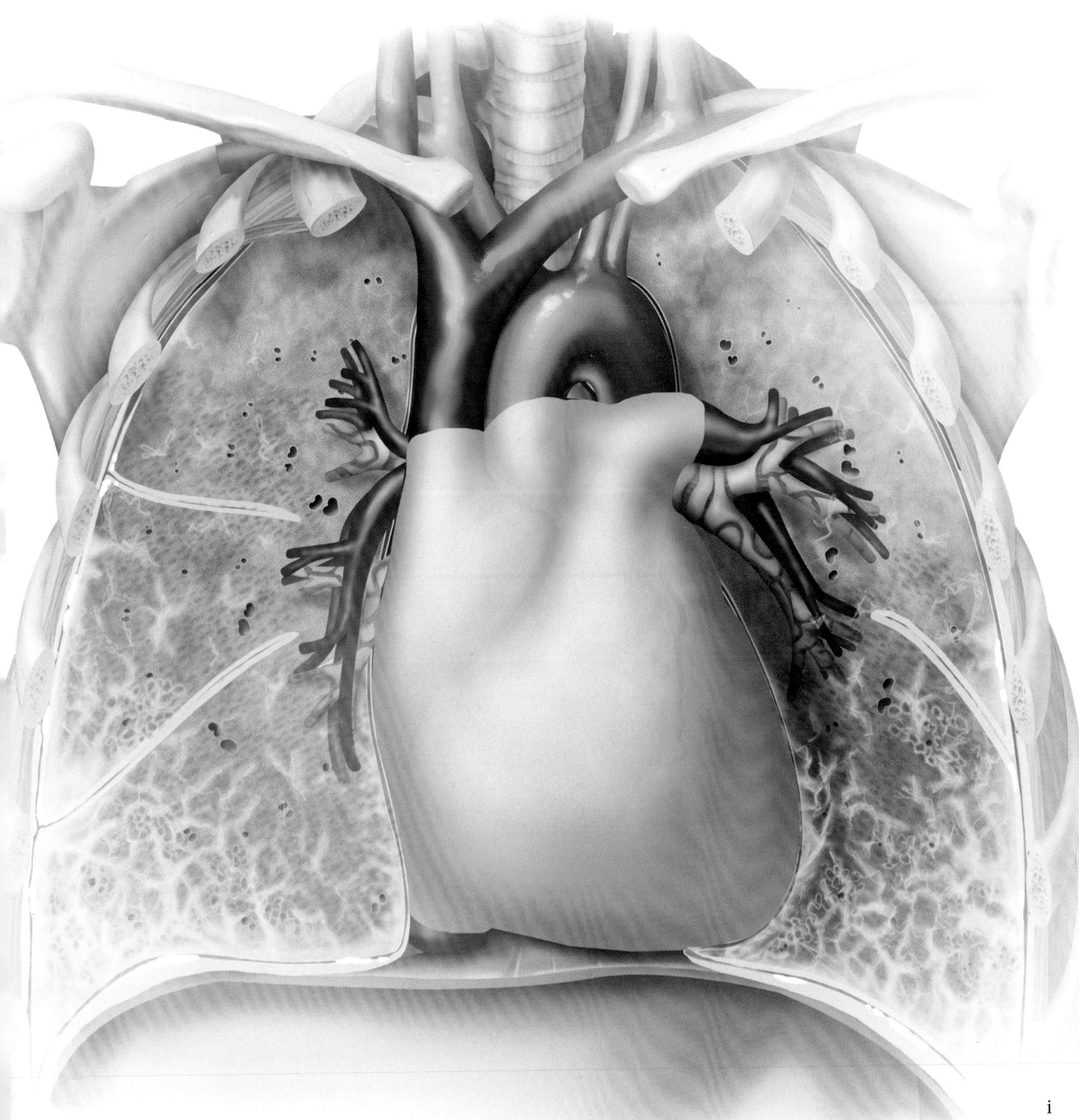

DIAGNOSTIC IMAGING CHEST

SECOND EDITION

Melissa L. Rosado-de-Christenson, MD, FACR
Section Chief, Thoracic Imaging
Saint Luke's Hospital of Kansas City
Professor of Radiology
University of Missouri-Kansas City
Kansas City, Missouri

Gerald F. Abbott, MD
Associate Professor of Radiology
Harvard Medical School
Massachusetts General Hospital
Boston, Massachusetts

Jonathan H. Chung, MD
Assistant Professor of Radiology
National Jewish Health
Denver, Colorado

Santiago Martínez-Jiménez, MD
Associate Professor of Radiology
University of Missouri-Kansas City
Saint Luke's Hospital of Kansas City
Kansas City, Missouri

Carol C. Wu, MD
Instructor of Radiology
Harvard Medical School
Massachusetts General Hospital
Boston, Massachusetts

Terrance T. Healey, MD
Assistant Professor of Diagnostic Imaging
Alpert Medical School
Brown University
Providence, Rhode Island

Brett W. Carter, MD
Director and Section Chief, Thoracic Imaging
Baylor University Medical Center
Dallas, Texas

John P. Lichtenberger III, MD
Chief of Cardiothoracic Imaging
David Grant Medical Center
Travis Air Force Base, California
Assistant Professor of Radiology
Uniformed Services University of the Health Sciences
Bethesda, Maryland

Helen T. Winer-Muram, MD
Professor of Clinical Radiology
Indiana University School of Medicine
Indianapolis, Indiana

Jeffrey P. Kanne, MD
Associate Professor of Thoracic Imaging
Vice Chair of Quality and Safety
Department of Radiology
University of Wisconsin School of Medicine and Public Health
Madison, Wisconsin

Tomás Franquet, MD, PhD
Director of Thoracic Imaging
Hospital de Sant Pau
Associate Professor of Radiology
Universidad Autónoma de Barcelona
Barcelona, Spain

Tyler H. Ternes, MD
Chest Imaging Fellow
Saint Luke's Hospital of Kansas City
University of Missouri-Kansas City
Kansas City, Missouri

Diane C. Strollo, MD, FACR
Clinical Associate Professor
University of Pittsburgh Medical Center
Pittsburgh, Pennsylvania

Megan R. Saettele, MD
Resident Physician
University of Missouri-Kansas City
Kansas City, Missouri

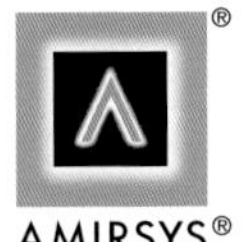

AMIRSYS®

Names you know. Content you trust.®

Second Edition

Printed in Canada by Friesens, Altona, Manitoba, Canada

ISBN: 978-1-931884-75-4

Notice and Disclaimer

The information in this product ("Product") is provided as a reference for use by licensed medical professionals and no others. It does not and should not be construed as any form of medical diagnosis or professional medical advice on any matter. Receipt or use of this Product, in whole or in part, does not constitute or create a doctor-patient, therapist-patient, or other healthcare professional relationship between the copyright holders and any recipient. This Product may not reflect the most current medical developments, and the copyright holders (individually and jointly), make no claims, promises, or guarantees about accuracy, completeness, or adequacy of the information contained in or linked to the Product. The Product is not a substitute for or replacement of professional medical judgment. The copyright holders, and their affiliates, authors, contributors, partners, and sponsors, individually and jointly, disclaim all liability or responsibility for any injury and/or damage to persons or property in respect to actions taken or not taken based on any and all Product information.

In the cases where drugs or other chemicals are prescribed, readers are advised to check the Product information currently provided by the manufacturer of each drug to be administered to verify the recommended dose, the method and duration of administration, and contraindications. It is the responsibility of the treating physician relying on experience and knowledge of the patient to determine dosages and the best treatment for the patient.

To the maximum extent permitted by applicable law, the copyright holders provide the Product AS IS AND WITH ALL FAULTS, AND HEREBY DISCLAIMS ALL WARRANTIES AND CONDITIONS, WHETHER EXPRESS, IMPLIED OR STATUTORY, INCLUDING BUT NOT LIMITED TO, ANY (IF ANY) IMPLIED WARRANTIES OR CONDITIONS OF MERCHANTABILITY, OF FITNESS FOR A PARTICULAR PURPOSE, OF LACK OF VIRUSES, OR ACCURACY OR COMPLETENESS OF RESPONSES, OR RESULTS, AND OF LACK OF NEGLIGENCE OR LACK OF WORKMANLIKE EFFORT. ALSO, THERE IS NO WARRANTY OR CONDITION OF TITLE, QUIET ENJOYMENT, QUIET POSSESSION, CORRESPONDENCE TO DESCRIPTION OR NON-INFRINGEMENT, WITH REGARD TO THE PRODUCT. THE ENTIRE RISK AS TO THE QUALITY OF OR ARISING OUT OF USE OR PERFORMANCE OF THE PRODUCT REMAINS WITH THE READER.

The respective copyright holders, individually and jointly, disclaim all warranties of any kind if the Product was customized, repackaged or altered in any way by any third party.

Library of Congress Cataloging-in-Publication Data

Rosado de Christenson, Melissa L.
Diagnostic imaging. Chest. -- 2nd ed. / Melissa L. Rosado de Christenson.
p. ; cm. -- (Diagnostic imaging)
Chest
Rev. ed. of: Diagnostic imaging. Chest / Jud W. Gurney ... [et al.]. 1st ed. c2006.
Includes bibliographical references and index.
ISBN 978-1-931884-75-4
I. Diagnostic imaging. II. Title. III. Title: Chest. IV. Series: Diagnostic imaging (Salt Lake City, Utah)
[DNLM: 1. Radiography, Thoracic. 2. Thoracic Diseases--radiography. 3. Diagnostic Imaging--methods. WF 975]

617.5'40754--dc23

2011044926

To my dearest husband Dr. Paul J. Christenson, to our beloved daughters Jennifer and Heather, and to the rest of my family for their constant love and support—and particularly for their immense assistance and forbearance during the course of this project.

MRdC

PREFACE

I am immensely grateful to the Amirsys team for the opportunity to serve as lead author of the second edition of *Diagnostic Imaging: Chest*. I am especially humbled to be selected to carry on the legacy of Jud W. Gurney, MD, an outstanding leader, author, and educator, whose untimely passing in early 2009 deprived the thoracic imaging community of one of its brightest stars. Throughout the writing of this book, my coauthors and I endeavored to produce a body of work that Jud would have been proud of.

The second edition is similar to the first in both style and appearance, with a succinct bulleted text style and image-rich depictions of thoracic diseases. However, in response to suggestions from the readers, this edition presents an updated content organization based on both the anatomic location of disease and the type of disease process. The work is further enhanced by a wealth of new material that includes:

- Sixteen new illustrated section introductions that set the stage for the specific diagnoses that follow
- Three new sections that define and illustrate the Fleischner Society glossary of terms for thoracic imaging, classic signs in chest imaging, and the many faces of atelectasis
- A new section on post-treatment changes in the thorax including effects of various surgeries, radiotherapy, chemotherapy, and ablation procedures
- 353 chapters (148 new chapters) supplemented with updated references
- 2,586 images and 1,395 e-book images including radiographic, CT, MR, and PET/CT images
- Updated graphics illustrating the anatomic/pathologic basis of various imaging abnormalities

I was fortunate to recruit a world-class team of authors who delivered meticulously researched content in all areas of thoracic imaging and two outstanding medical editors who scrutinized each chapter for accuracy and clarity. I gratefully acknowledge the tireless work of the Amirsys production staff who sustained me through each step of the work and whose edits and suggestions enhanced each and every chapter. I also want to acknowledge the contribution of our outstanding team of illustrators whose artistry greatly enriched the book. I thank Drs. Gerry Abbott, Santiago Martínez-Jiménez, and Paula Woodward for their wisdom and guidance during my inaugural experience as an Amirsys lead author.

We proudly present the second edition of *Diagnostic Imaging: Chest.*

Melissa L. Rosado-de-Christenson, MD, FACR
Section Chief, Thoracic Imaging
Saint Luke's Hospital of Kansas City
Professor of Radiology
University of Missouri-Kansas City
Kansas City, Missouri

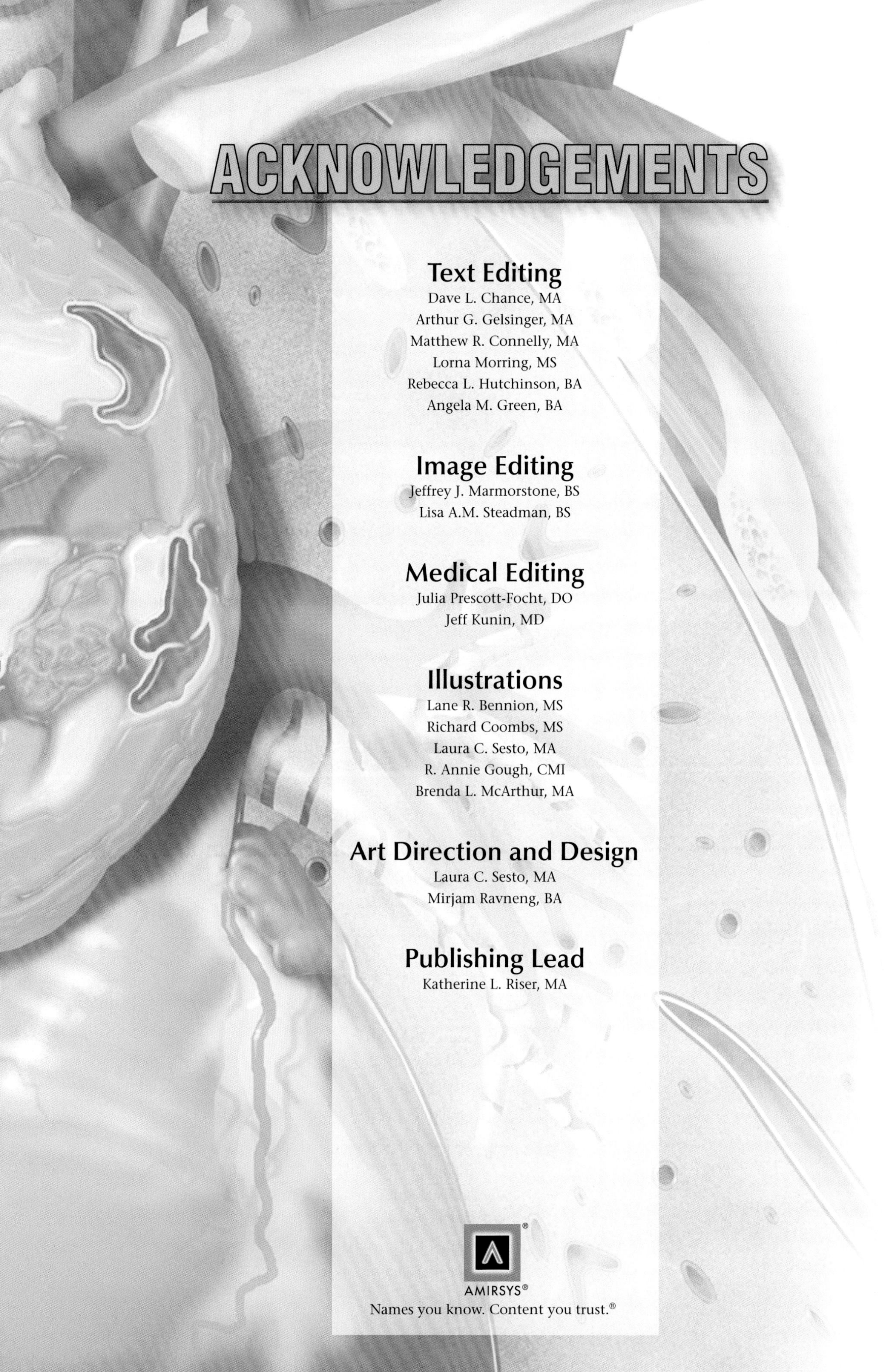

ACKNOWLEDGEMENTS

Text Editing
Dave L. Chance, MA
Arthur G. Gelsinger, MA
Matthew R. Connelly, MA
Lorna Morring, MS
Rebecca L. Hutchinson, BA
Angela M. Green, BA

Image Editing
Jeffrey J. Marmorstone, BS
Lisa A.M. Steadman, BS

Medical Editing
Julia Prescott-Focht, DO
Jeff Kunin, MD

Illustrations
Lane R. Bennion, MS
Richard Coombs, MS
Laura C. Sesto, MA
R. Annie Gough, CMI
Brenda L. McArthur, MA

Art Direction and Design
Laura C. Sesto, MA
Mirjam Ravneng, BA

Publishing Lead
Katherine L. Riser, MA

AMIRSYS®
Names you know. Content you trust.®

TABLE OF CONTENTS

SECTION 1
Overview of Chest Imaging

Introduction and Overview

Illustrated Terminology

Chest Radiographic and CT Signs

Atelectasis and Volume Loss

SECTION 2
Developmental Abnormalities

Introduction and Overview

Airways

Lung

Pulmonary Circulation

Systemic Circulation

Cardiac, Pericardial, and Valvular Defects

Chest Wall & Diaphragm

SECTION 3
Airway Diseases

Introduction and Overview

Benign Neoplasms

Malignant Neoplasms

Airway Narrowing and Wall Thickening

Bronchial Dilatation and Impaction

Emphysema and Small Airway Diseases

SECTION 4 Infections

Introduction and Overview

General

Bacteria

Mycobacteria and Mycoplasma

Viruses

Fungi

Parasites

SECTION 5 Pulmonary Neoplasms

Introduction and Overview

Eosinophilic Lung Disease

Metabolic Diseases and Miscellaneous Conditions

SECTION 7
Connective Tissue Disorders, Immunological Diseases, and Vasculitis

Introduction and Overview

Immunological and Connective Tissue Disorders

Thoracic Complications in Immunocompromised Patients

Pulmonary Hemorrhage and Vasculitis

SECTION 8
Mediastinal Abnormalities

Introduction and Overview

Primary Neoplasms

Pulmonary Edema

Pulmonary Hypertension and Thromboembolic Disease

Diseases of the Heart and Pericardium

Cardiovascular Neoplasms

SECTION 10
Trauma

Introduction and Overview

Airways and Lung

Cardiovascular/Mediastinum

Pleura, Chest Wall, and Diaphragm

SECTION 11
Post-Treatment Chest

Introduction and Overview

Life Support Devices

Surgical Procedures and Complications

Radiation, Chemotherapy, Ablation

SECTION 12
Pleural Diseases

Introduction and Overview

Effusion

Pneumothorax

Pleural Thickening

Neoplasia

SECTION 13
Chest Wall and Diaphragm

Introduction and Overview

Chest Wall

Diaphragm

SECTION 1
Overview of Chest Imaging

Introduction and Overview

Illustrated Terminology

Chest Radiographic and CT Signs

Atelectasis and Volume Loss

Introduction

A wide variety of acute and chronic diseases affect the chest and result from a broad range of etiologies. The three leading causes of death in the United States are heart disease, malignant neoplasms, and chronic lower respiratory diseases. Among the malignant neoplasms, lung cancer remains the leading cause of death of men and women in the United States, although the incidence of this malignancy has recently started to decrease.

Chest diseases can be categorized by anatomic location as affecting the airways, lungs, pleura, mediastinum, chest wall, or diaphragm, and each region may be involved by developmental abnormalities, neoplastic conditions, or infectious processes. Additionally, idiopathic, inflammatory, connective tissue, autoimmune, and lymphoproliferative disorders may also affect the various organs of the chest. The ventilatory and respiratory functions of the lungs and airways provide a portal for exposure to a variety of inhalational diseases, some of which are related to the patient's environment and occupation, such as smoking-related diseases and pneumoconioses, respectively. Thoracic diseases may also be categorized based on their physiological effects as obstructive or restrictive abnormalities. Finally, the various organs and anatomic regions of the chest may be affected by traumatic or iatrogenic conditions, the latter related to various therapies used in the management of both thoracic and systemic disorders.

Clinical Presentation

Patients with chest disease may seek medical attention for symptoms that often include chest pain, dyspnea, and cough. Such symptoms may arise acutely or be chronic. Chest disease may also give rise to systemic complaints including malaise, fatigue, and weight loss. Patients with thoracic malignant neoplasms may present with complaints related to paraneoplastic syndromes, which are systemic effects of the neoplasm unrelated to metastatic disease. In addition, thoracic malignancies may be particularly aggressive and frequently produce systemic metastases, which may produce additional symptoms.

Assessment of Chest Disease

Physicians who care for patients with chest disease have several assessment methods at their disposal. An understanding of the patient's chief complaint and relevant past medical and surgical history is of foremost importance. The history must also include relevant habits, including cigarette smoking and use of illicit drugs, as well as environmental and occupational exposures (e.g., asbestos, silicates). As lung diseases may be related to the use of prescription drugs, the clinician must also ask about the existence of chronic conditions and the specific drugs being used in their treatment. Another important consideration is the determination of the patient's immune status, as individuals with altered immunity are at risk for a variety of infectious, inflammatory, and neoplastic conditions that are not routinely suspected in the immunocompetent subject. The physical exam must include an assessment of vital signs, an external inspection of the thorax, and an "internal" examination that is typically limited to auscultation and percussion. Pulmonary medicine specialists may also rely on pulmonary function tests, bronchoscopic examination of the airways, and bronchoalveolar lavage procedures for the assessment of lung function and the evaluation of the central and peripheral airways.

Imaging plays a pivotal role in the assessment of patients who present with thoracic complaints. In addition, thoracic imaging studies are often obtained in the initial evaluation of systemic disorders that are known to affect the chest. As a result, radiologists are important members of the team of physicians caring for these patients and are able to impact patient management by identifying imaging abnormalities that may direct the clinician to a particular course of action, which may include obtaining additional history or laboratory tests or performing invasive procedures. The radiologist may be the first member of the healthcare team to identify a specific abnormality that may explain the patient's symptoms. In addition, radiologists may identify incidental abnormalities in asymptomatic patients who are imaged for other reasons. In selected cases, the radiologist may offer to perform image-guided biopsy of specific abnormalities or provide treatment with various thoracic interventional procedures (e.g., drainage of thoracic fluid collections, ablation procedures).

Thoracic Imaging

Chest Radiography

The chest radiograph is the initial imaging study obtained on patients who present with chest complaints. Chest radiographs may also be obtained in asymptomatic patients as part of an employment physical exam or in the preoperative evaluation of patients scheduled for elective surgery. The study can be performed expeditiously, is inexpensive, and uses a very small amount of ionizing radiation when compared to many other advanced imaging studies such as computed tomography and angiography.

Chest radiographs allow assessment of the airways, lungs, cardiovascular system, pleura, diaphragm, and chest wall soft tissues. Chest radiographs will occasionally reveal significant cervical or abdominal pathology since the lower neck and upper abdomen are typically included in the image. Chest radiographs are probably the most challenging imaging studies interpreted by radiologists today, because a large number of organs and tissues with a broad range of radiographic densities (air, water, fat, and metal) are superimposed on each other, potentially obscuring subtle abnormalities. Accurate interpretation requires an in-depth knowledge of imaging anatomy, including common normal variants. Thus, the radiologist must work closely with the technical staff to continually evaluate and improve imaging techniques and ensure optimal viewing conditions. This includes paying special attention to control of ambient light and ergonomic issues, and making sure that the environment is free of distractions and conducive to the performance of a systematic assessment of every image submitted for interpretation. Additional challenges are presented by the highly heterogeneous patient population referred for imaging, including patients with large body habitus, those with severe dyspnea, and others who are not able to understand the technologist's directions or cooperate during the performance of the exam.

PA and lateral chest radiography: Symptomatic ambulatory patients are ideally imaged with posteroanterior (PA) and lateral chest radiographs. Imaging assessment with orthogonal views (i.e., at right angles to each other) allows anatomic localization of abnormalities. Ideally, these images are obtained in the upright position, at full inspiration, with no motion or rotation, and with minimal superimposition of the upper extremities, head, neck, or scapulae. The term PA describes the posteroanterior direction of the x-ray beam with the patient positioned so that the heart is closest to the image receptor to avoid magnification. Likewise, the lateral view is a left lateral radiograph obtained with the patient's left side (and heart) closest to the image receptor.

Bedside (portable) chest radiography: Neonates and infants, debilitated and unstable patients, and those who are traumatized, seriously ill, or bed-ridden undergo portable anteroposterior (AP) chest radiographs. The anteroposterior direction of the x-ray beam results in some magnification of the mediastinum and superimposition of anatomic structures such as the scapulae. In spite of its limitations, portable chest radiography is very useful in the assessment of these patients including the mandatory evaluation of each patient's medical life-support devices and possible complications of their use.

Decubitus radiography is only occasionally used today in the evaluation of the pleural space to detect pleural effusion or subtle pneumothorax. Although **apical lordotic** radiography (formerly used to evaluate the apical regions of the lung without superimposition of the clavicles) is rarely used today, many AP portable radiographs display a lordotic projection, and the interpreting radiologist must be familiar with the effects such changes in projection have on the appearance of thoracic structures. Inspiratory and expiratory chest radiography for the assessment of suspected pneumothorax is rarely used today because it has been shown that expiratory radiographs do not improve visualization of small pneumothoraces, yet they effectively double the radiation dose to the patient.

Computed Tomography

Computed tomography (CT) has revolutionized our understanding of thoracic disease and our ability to reach a diagnosis. Chest CT is easily and expeditiously performed and readily demonstrates the specific location and morphologic features of imaging abnormalities. In many cases, CT may be the final step in the patient's evaluation by excluding an abnormality suspected on radiography. In other cases, CT allows optimal assessment of a radiographic abnormality and may detect unexpected associated findings, enabling the radiologist to suggest a diagnosis and a course of management for the affected patient.

It should be noted that since its introduction there has been an explosive growth of the utilization of multidetector CT for medical imaging, and a substantially increased radiation dose to the population. CT is considered an important diagnostic test by Emergency Department physicians as it helps expedite patient throughput and reduce unnecessary hospital stays. Unfortunately, a significant percentage of CT studies performed in the United States are probably not indicated. In addition, it is postulated that up to 2% of all cancers that will occur in future decades will be linked to the current use of CT. In view of these issues, radiologists must actively assess their scanning techniques and protocols and engage in practice quality improvement measures directed at reducing radiation dose. The radiologist must engage in active communication with and education of referring physicians and strive to work with them toward reducing the number of unnecessary studies. Incorporation of an electronic decision support system that uses evidence-based guidelines and appropriateness criteria during the process of ordering imaging studies has been shown to reduce the number of inappropriate examinations as reported by various institutions.

Radiologists can take additional measures to reduce dose by the use of shielding, tube current modulation, and adaptive statistical iterative reconstruction techniques. As it has been shown that the radiation dose during CT imaging is directly proportional to tube current, the reduction of tube current-time product (mAs) can achieve low-dose chest CT studies that preserve satisfactory image quality. Low-dose CT imaging techniques should be used routinely in small patients and in those who will receive serial CT examinations, such as young patients imaged for restaging of malignancy and those imaged for the evaluation of indeterminate lung nodules or diffuse infiltrative pulmonary diseases.

Unenhanced chest CT: Evaluation of the lung parenchyma and airways does not require the administration of intravenous contrast. In fact, the lung is ideally suited for CT imaging without contrast, particularly for the determination of intralesional calcifications, serial evaluation of lung nodules, evaluation of diffuse infiltrative lung diseases, and assessment of airways disease. In some practices, the bulk of thoracic CT is performed without contrast without apparent detriment to diagnostic accuracy.

Contrast-enhanced chest CT: The administration of intravenous contrast is mandatory for vascular imaging and for evaluation of the hilum for lymphadenopathy. Contrast administration is also valuable in the evaluation of thoracic malignancy and may help identify and assess tumors surrounded by atelectasis or consolidation. CT angiography of the chest is mandatory in the setting of traumatic vascular injury and when evaluating for suspected pulmonary thromboembolic disease. In the case of acute aortic syndromes, both unenhanced and enhanced aortic CT must be performed to facilitate the diagnosis of intramural hemorrhage.

Postprocessing: Image reformation in various planes (coronal, sagittal, oblique) is very useful in determining the distribution of pulmonary disease. Because some diseases involve the lung diffusely while others exhibit a predilection for the upper lung zones or lung bases, recognizing the pattern of distribution allows the radiologist to determine the imaging differential diagnosis. For example, lymphangioleiomyomatosis (LAM) and pulmonary Langerhans cell histiocytosis (PLCH) may both manifest with thin-walled pulmonary cysts. However, LAM affects the lung diffusely, while PLCH characteristically spares the lung bases near the costophrenic angles. In addition, since tumor growth may extend in all directions, evaluation of lung neoplasms on multiplanar reformatted images may allow documentation of craniocaudad growth of a tumor that appears stable on axial imaging.

Maximum-intensity projection (MIP) and minimum-intensity projection (MinIP) images: MIP images are particularly useful for detection of subtle lung nodules and evaluation of vascular structures. This method retains the relative maximum value along each ray path and preferentially displays contrast-filled and higher attenuation structures. MinIP images, on the other hand, display the minimum value along the ray paths and are useful for evaluation of emphysema and air-trapping.

Volume and surface rendering: These techniques do not necessarily add value to diagnostic interpretation but are often greatly appreciated by referring physicians. Volume-rendering techniques can provide a three-dimensional image display of vascular anatomy. Surface-rendered displays are ideally suited for depiction of tubular structures, such as airways, and are employed in performing virtual bronchoscopy, which mimics the luminal visualization of the airway achieved on bronchoscopic evaluation.

High-resolution CT (HRCT): HRCT is the modality of choice for evaluating diffuse infiltrative lung disease. It uses a narrow slice width (1-2 mm) and a high spatial resolution image reconstruction algorithm. The ability to analyze diffuse lung involvement in relation to the anatomy of the secondary pulmonary lobule allows accurate and reproducible disease characterization and the formulation of an appropriate differential diagnosis.

Magnetic Resonance Imaging

Magnetic resonance (MR) imaging is routinely employed in evaluating the cardiovascular system and is the imaging modality of choice for assessing a wide range of disorders, including congenital heart disease and cardiac masses. MR is the modality of choice for evaluating myocardial perfusion as well as ventricular and valvular function. In addition, MR may be useful in the evaluation of locally invasive thoracic tumors, particularly to determine whether cardiovascular structures are invaded by the lesion, and in the assessment of the chest wall and brachial plexus in patients with Pancoast tumors. MR has the advantage of imaging the body without using ionizing radiation and allows vascular imaging without the use of contrast material. MR is particularly valuable in the noninvasive evaluation of the abnormal thymus. Use of in-phase and opposed-phase thymic MR, for instance, allows the confident diagnosis of thymic hyperplasia and identification of potentially neoplastic lesions that require tissue sampling.

Positron Emission Tomography

Positron emission tomography (PET) and combined PET/CT are invaluable in evaluating patients with malignancy. In PET/CT, the PET and CT images are obtained in a single imaging session and are fused into a single co-registered image that allows correlation of abnormal metabolic activity with anatomic abnormalities. PET/CT has become the imaging modality of choice for staging and restaging lymphomas and other malignant neoplasms. Residual areas of abnormal metabolic activity following treatment can be localized and targeted for imaging follow-up or tissue sampling. Although PET/CT is extremely useful, the radiologist must be aware of various pitfalls in PET/CT interpretation. Rigorous patient preparation for the study is of utmost importance in order to prevent false-positive areas of increased activity. Normal increased metabolic activity may be seen in certain anatomic regions (e.g., the interatrial septum) corresponding to brown fat deposition. Finally, PET/CT may yield false-positive (infectious or inflammatory process) and false-negative (indolent adenocarcinoma, carcinoid tumor) results in the evaluation of patients with suspected or known malignancy; tissue diagnosis should be pursued if other findings (e.g., morphologic features on CT) are consistent with malignancy.

Ventilation-Perfusion Scintigraphy

Ventilation-perfusion (V/Q) scintigraphy has been largely replaced by CT pulmonary angiography (CTPA) in the evaluation of patients with pulmonary thromboembolic disease, although CTPA and V/Q scintigraphy have similar positive predictive values. CTPA is superior in the evaluation of patients with evidence of lung disease on radiography and has the advantage of demonstrating other potential causes of the patient's symptoms.

However, a growing body of literature supports performing perfusion scintigraphy instead of CTPA in the setting of pregnancy, provided that chest radiographs are normal, and in cases where an alternative diagnosis is not suspected. In this patient population, CTPA may yield indeterminate results due to physiologic hemodilution of contrast and interruption of contrast by unopacified blood from the inferior vena cava. In addition, it should be noted that CTPA delivers a higher radiation dose to the maternal breast when compared to V/Q scintigraphy. In this clinical setting, appropriate measures must be taken (e.g., hydration) to decrease the radiation dose to the fetus.

Approach to Chest Imaging

Chest radiographs are the most frequent imaging studies performed in most practices and are probably the most challenging to interpret. Accurate interpretation requires a substantial knowledge of anatomy, pathology, and related aspects of thoracic disease encountered in internal medicine, pulmonary medicine, thoracic surgery, thoracic oncology, and the infectious disease subspecialty. Detection of an abnormality on chest radiography must be combined with its localization to a specific anatomic compartment in order to narrow the differential diagnosis. Identification of associated findings within the lesion (e.g., calcification, cavitation) or associated with it (e.g., lymphadenopathy, pleural effusion) helps to focus the differential and may facilitate the diagnosis. The process is greatly enhanced by making ample use of the patient's electronic medical record to support the favored prospective diagnosis. Comparison to prior studies is of paramount importance as documentation of stability generally supports a benign diagnosis.

Communication of imaging findings to the referring physician is typically accomplished via the radiologic report. Radiologists must strive to produce concise, clear, and unambiguous reports that "answer the question" for the clinician. The report should include a thorough description of the abnormality, the differential diagnosis, the most likely diagnosis, and recommendations for further management, which may include advanced imaging (e.g., CT, HRCT, MR, scintigraphy, etc.), a course of treatment, tissue sampling, or emergency medical/surgical intervention. Critical and unexpected findings must be verbally communicated to the appropriate member of the healthcare team. In fact, radiologists are uniquely positioned to positively impact the health and well-being of patients with thoracic diseases.

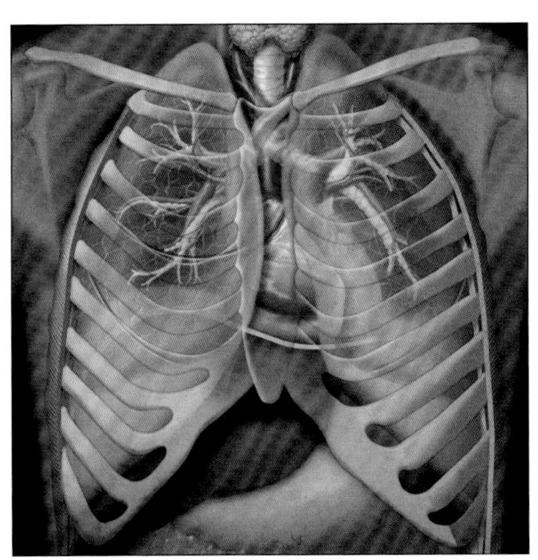

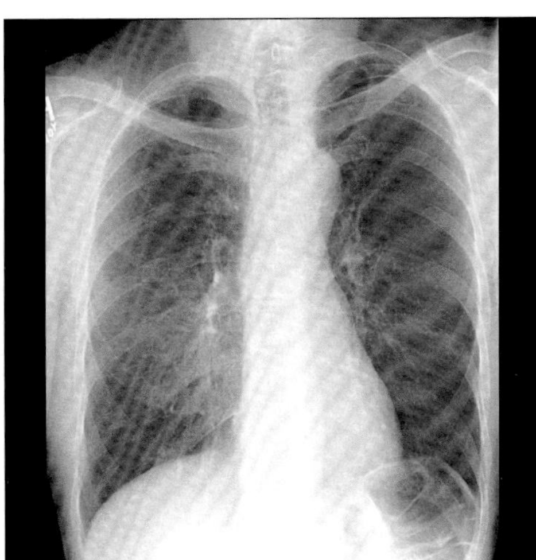

(Left) *Graphic shows the complex and diverse structures and organs in the thorax, including the chest wall skeleton and soft tissues, diaphragm, cardiovascular system, mediastinum, pleura, lungs, and airways. The heterogeneity of tissues imaged contributes to the complexity of chest radiographic images.* ***(Right)*** *PA chest radiograph allows visualization of many aspects of the structures of the thorax and includes the lower neck and upper abdomen. In this case, there is no evidence of thoracic disease.*

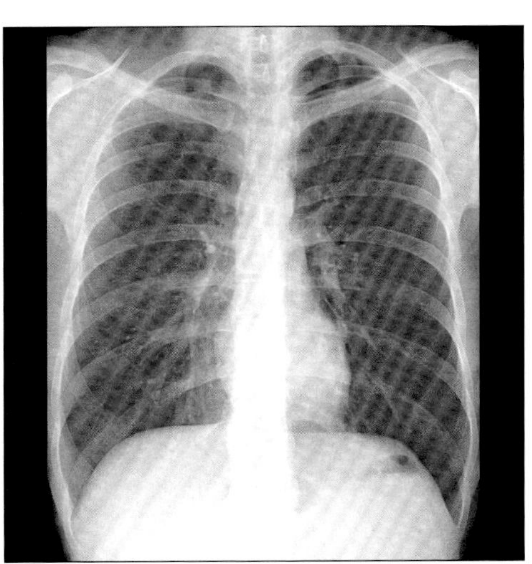

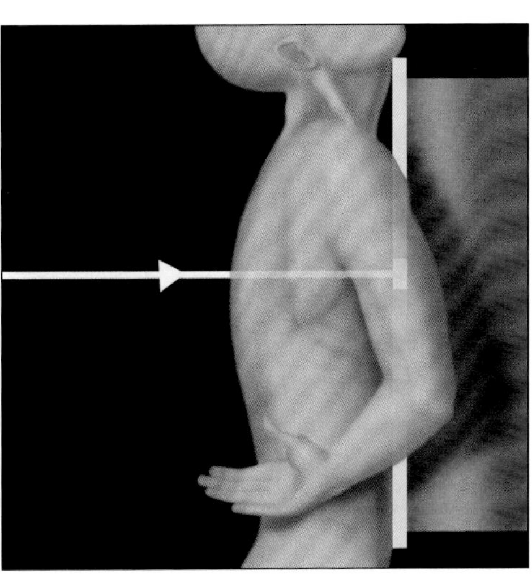

(Left) *PA chest radiograph reflects appropriate positioning and technique. The image is obtained at full inspiration without rotation and includes the upper airway and lung bases.* ***(Right)*** *Graphic shows proper positioning for PA chest imaging. The patient is upright with the anterior chest against the image receptor. The position of the chin and upper extremities prevents superimposition of the head and scapulae over the lungs. The x-ray beam traverses the patient in a posteroanterior direction.*

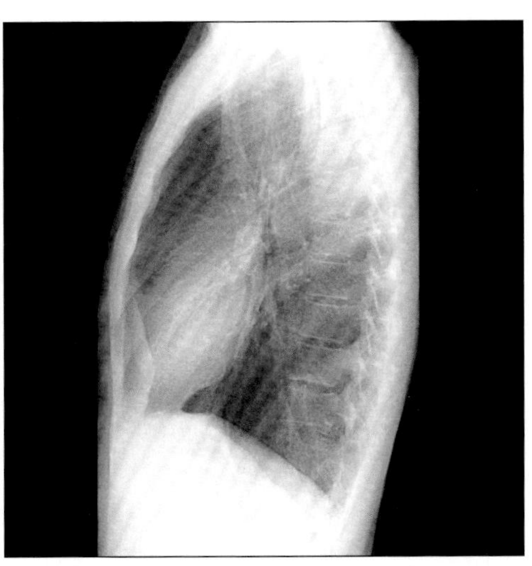

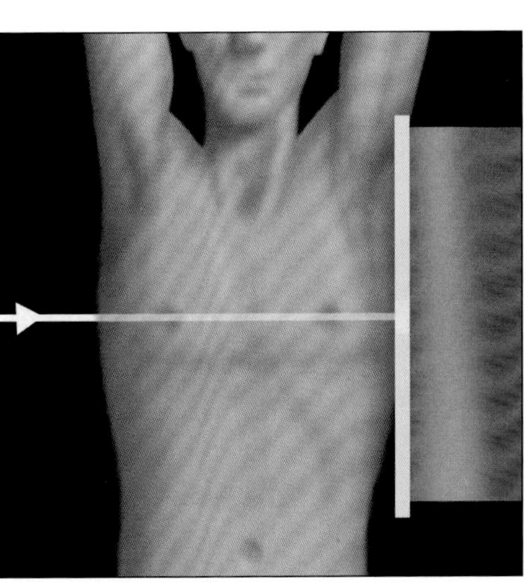

(Left) *Lateral chest radiograph reflects excellent radiographic technique and exposure factors. The image is acquired in the upright position at full inspiration and without rotation.* ***(Right)*** *Graphic shows proper positioning for left lateral chest imaging. The patient is upright with the left lateral chest against the image receptor. Elevation of the upper extremities allows unobstructed imaging of the upper lungs. The x-ray beam traverses the patient from right to left.*

(Left) AP portable chest radiograph of a neonate with respiratory distress shows no abnormality. The scapulae project over the upper lungs. (Right) Graphic shows positioning for supine AP chest radiography. The x-ray beam traverses the patient in an anteroposterior direction. The patient's back is against the cassette with the heart farthest from it, resulting in some magnification. AP chest radiography of critically ill patients often shows superimposed extraneous objects and monitoring devices.

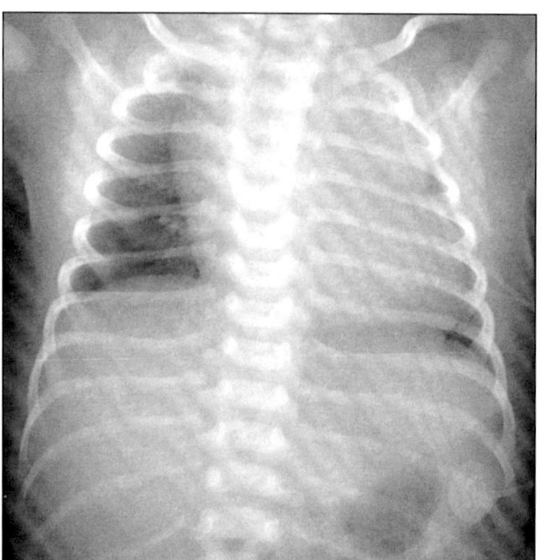

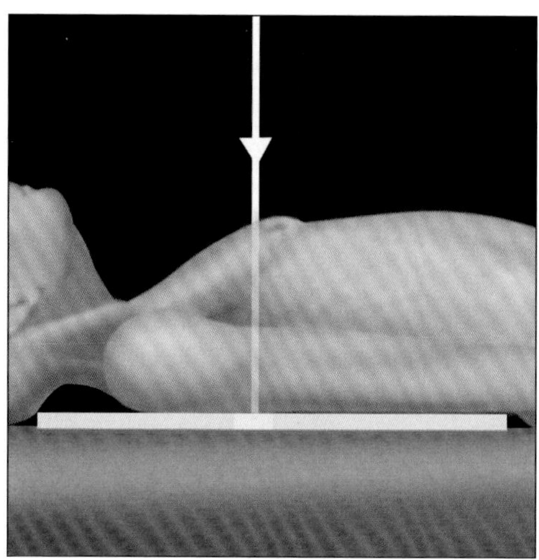

(Left) Axial NECT of a patient with chest pain shows subtle mural high attenuation ➔ in the descending aorta. (Right) Axial CECT of the same patient shows no evidence of aortic dissection, and corresponding mural thickening ➔ is consistent with type B intramural hemorrhage. Although CECT is typically preferred for vascular imaging, NECT is mandatory in the evaluation of acute aortic syndromes. NECT is also preferable for lung nodule follow-up and for assessment of diffuse lung and airway diseases.

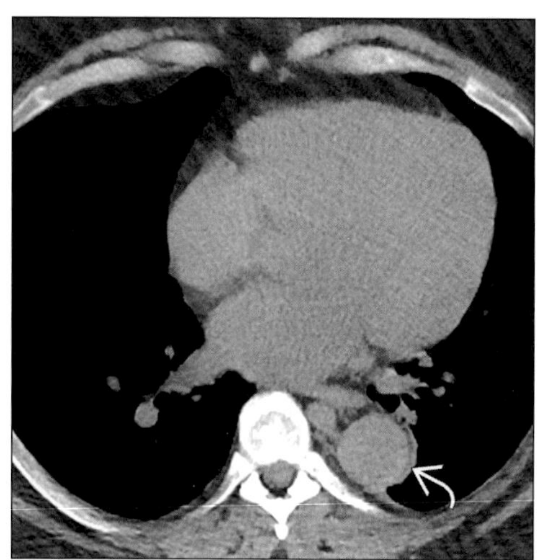

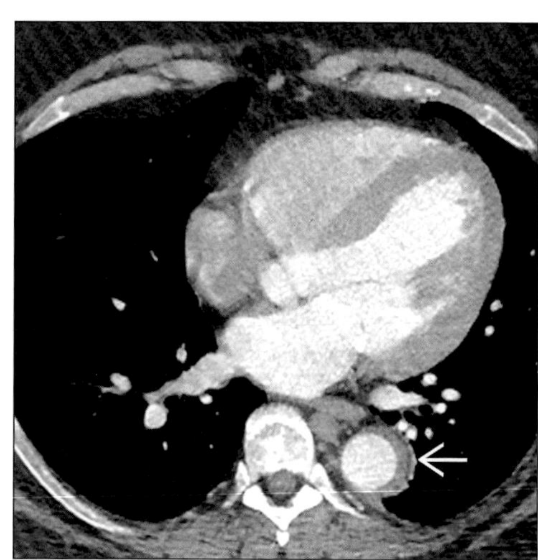

(Left) Axial CECT of a patient evaluated for possible lung abscess shows a loculated right pleural effusion and an apparent cavitary lesion that communicates with the pleural space ➔. (Right) Sagittal NECT shows that an air-filled lesion occupies the right major fissure and is contiguous with the posterior loculated pleural collection resulting in a complicated empyema. In this case, multiplanar reformatted imaging allowed localization of the disease to the pleural space and provided a map for drainage.

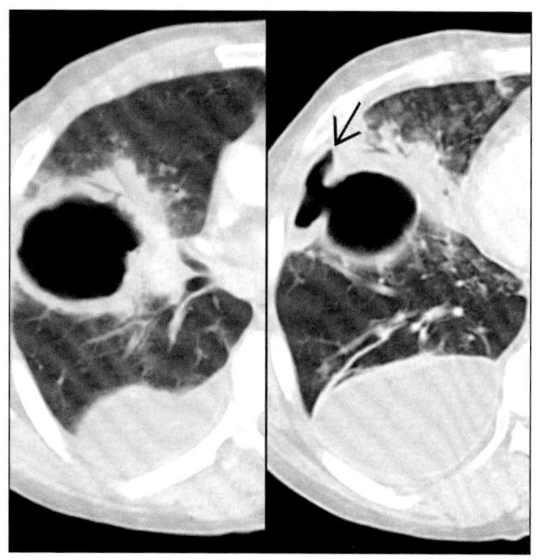

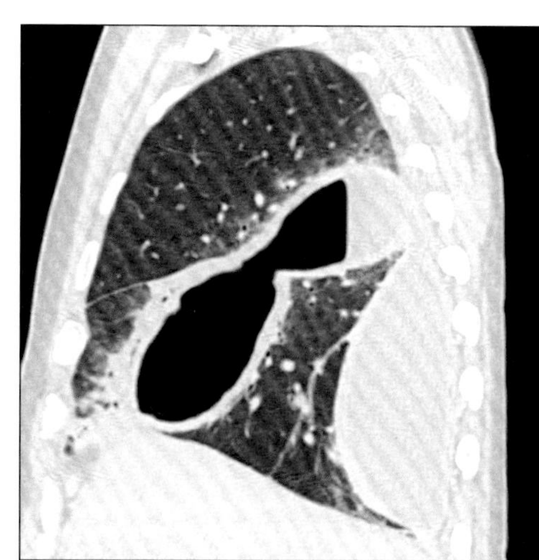

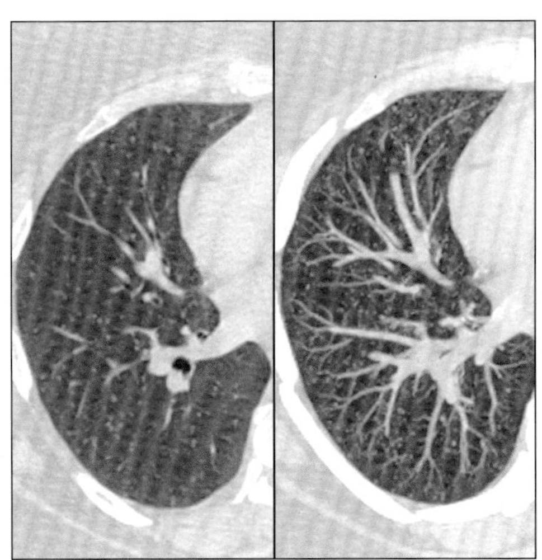

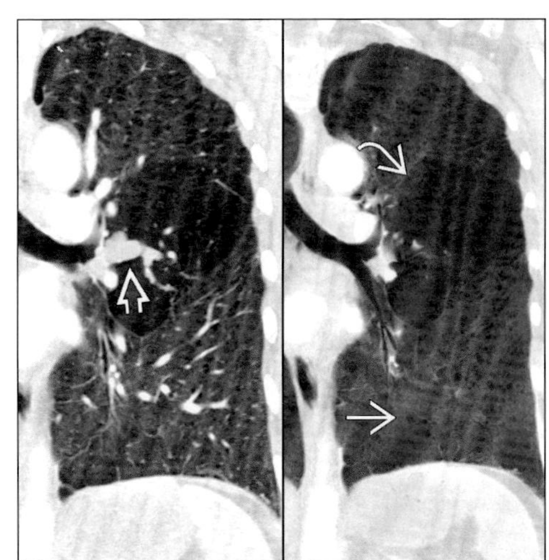

(Left) *Composite image with axial NECT (left) and axial MIP reformation (right) of a patient with miliary histoplasmosis shows subtle tiny nodules on conventional CT that exhibit increased conspicuity on MIP.* ***(Right)*** *Composite image with coronal CECT (left) and coronal MinIP reformation (right) shows bronchial atresia manifesting with a mucocele ➯ surrounded by hyperlucency. On MinIP the mucocele is no longer visible, but emphysema ➔ and lung hyperlucency ➦ are accentuated.*

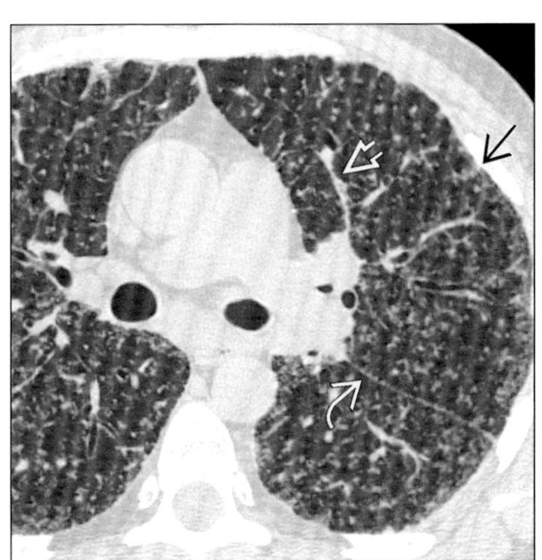

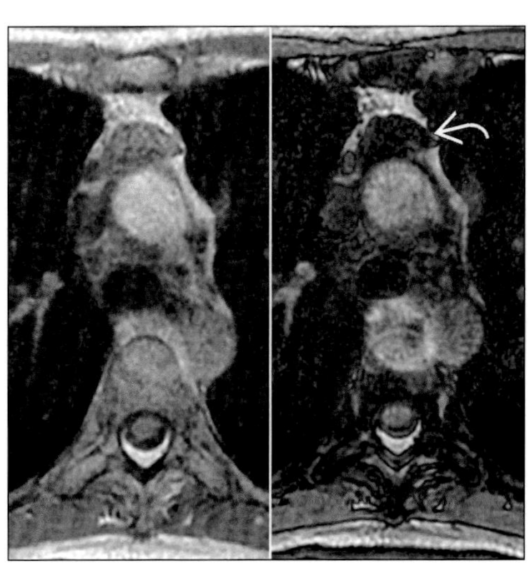

(Left) *Axial HRCT shows bilateral perilymphatic micronodules (subpleural ➦, interlobular septal ➔, and peribronchovascular ➯). The findings support the prospective diagnosis of sarcoidosis in an appropriate clinical setting.* ***(Right)*** *Composite image with in-phase (left) and opposed-phase (right) gradient-echo T1WI MR shows decreased signal of a thymic nodule ➦ on opposed-phase imaging. Determination of chemical shift ratios allowed the confident diagnosis of thymic hyperplasia.*

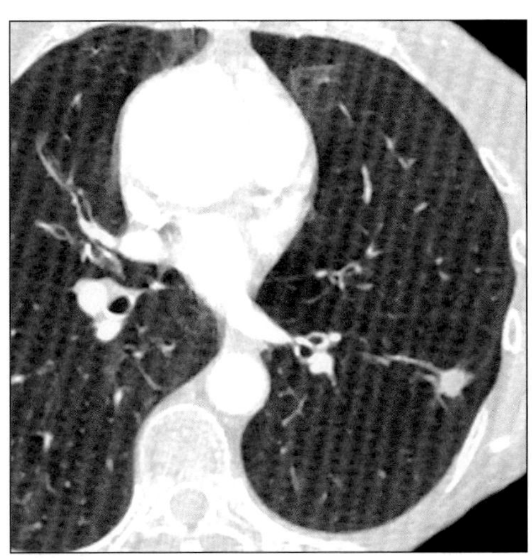

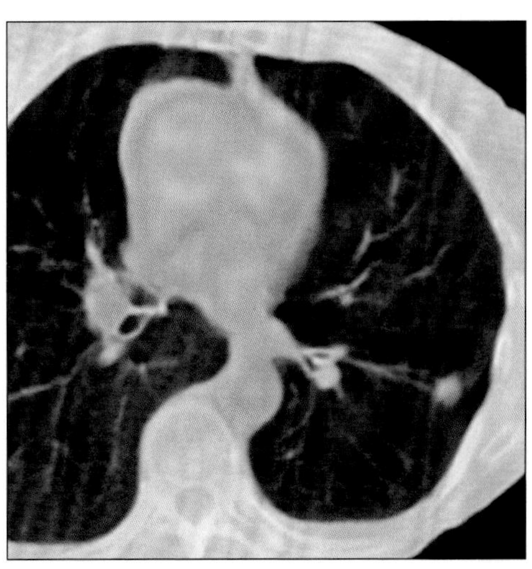

(Left) *Axial CECT of a patient who presented with left spontaneous pneumothorax shows a peripheral left lower lobe nodule with pleural retraction suspicious for lung cancer.* ***(Right)*** *Axial fused FDG PET/CT of the same patient shows minimal metabolic activity in the nodule with a standard uptake value (SUV) of only 1.7. Excision revealed an invasive adenocarcinoma. PET/CT may yield false-negative results in small lesions, indolent lung cancers, and carcinoid tumors.*

APPROACH TO ILLUSTRATED TERMINOLOGY

Introduction

Radiology has undergone substantial technological advances in diagnostic imaging that are not limited to the introduction of advanced imaging equipment, but have also impacted the way radiologists view images and the manner of completing radiologic reports. Picture archiving and communication systems (PACS) permit inexpensive storage of large numbers of images that can be easily accessed by radiologists and referring physicians for interpretation and consultation. Radiologists can readily access prior images and prior reports in order to document change or stability of imaging abnormalities. Speech recognition technology allows radiologists to rapidly generate radiologic reports that can be reviewed for accuracy prior to their release. In addition, the availability of electronic medical records provides access to relevant clinical and laboratory data that enhances interpretation and the formulation of a reasonable differential diagnosis.

The wide availability of viewing stations has also impacted communication between radiologists and clinicians, an interchange that frequently occurs via secure electronic mail or by telephone. In fact, face-to-face communication between clinicians and radiologists has greatly diminished, with the unfortunate consequence of lessening the opportunity to ask for additional medical history that may not be available on the requisition or electronic medical record.

In today's practice, the radiologic report is the principal method used by radiologists to communicate diagnostic imaging findings to referring clinicians. Although unexpected abnormalities should always be verbally communicated to a member of the healthcare team, most abnormalities are communicated via the radiology report. As a result, radiologists must strive to generate concise, clear, and unambiguous reports that not only contain relevant findings, but also include focused differential diagnoses and specific recommendations for further imaging and future management.

The Proper Language

As imaging specialists, we must strive to use proper and correct language in both verbal communications and in the radiology report. For example, the phrase "chest x-ray" may be forever ingrained in colloquial communications in spite of the fact that it is an incorrect descriptor of the imaging study. As x-rays are invisible to the naked eye, a radiologist does not interpret a chest x-ray, but rather a chest radiograph. Likewise, radiologists today rarely review and interpret films or analog images given the ubiquitous nature and broad utilization of PACS systems that allow us to interpret soft copy rather than hard copy images.

Infiltrate is a term formerly used to describe any pulmonary opacity produced by airspace and/or interstitial disease on chest radiography or CT. In medicine, the word "infiltrate" is used to describe the accumulation in tissue of abnormal substances or of an excess of normal substances. The use of this term is controversial, has various meanings, is imprecise in its implications, and is no longer recommended for the description of imaging abnormalities. Instead, the term "opacity" with the addition of appropriate descriptors (airspace, reticular, nodular) is preferred today.

Terminology of Thoracic Imaging

In recent years, thoracic imaging has undergone immense growth and technological advancements. Thoracic computed tomography (CT) and high-resolution computed tomography (HRCT) of the lung are advanced technologies that allow identification and characterization of subtle abnormalities that were previously seen only by anatomists and pathologists. Today, the radiologist can thoroughly analyze pulmonary abnormalities with respect to the underlying units of lung structure, such as the secondary pulmonary lobule and the pulmonary acinus. This requires substantial knowledge and understanding of normal imaging anatomy. The ability to correlate imaging abnormalities with the anatomic portion of the lung affected allows the radiologist to make confident diagnoses of diseases such as pulmonary fibrosis, sarcoidosis, interstitial edema, and emphysema. In fact, thoracic imagers today play an integral role in the multidisciplinary diagnosis of interstitial lung disease and adenocarcinoma of the lung. In addition, the growing field of quantitative lung imaging may allow radiologists to contribute to the noninvasive assessment of the entire lung in the setting of diffuse lung diseases and correlate those findings with abnormalities of pulmonary function.

Thus, advances in thoracic imaging allow us to evaluate a series of complex imaging abnormalities affecting the thorax and to work in conjunction with our clinical colleagues toward an expeditious diagnosis and course of management. The protean and complex findings identified on chest CT and HRCT along with advances in our understanding of lung diseases mandate the consistent use of correct terminology for the description of thoracic abnormalities. In 2008, the Fleischner Society published the latest glossary of terms recommended for thoracic imaging reporting; this lexicon reflects the emergence of new terms and the obsolescence of others.

The Fleischner glossary is not only a list of proper terminology in thoracic imaging, but also includes definitions and illustrations of anatomic locations in the thorax, signs in thoracic imaging, specific disease processes (such as emphysema and rounded atelectasis), and the various idiopathic interstitial pneumonias.

Pneumonia is defined as inflammation of the airspaces and interstitium. The term is predominantly used to denote an infectious process of the lung. The diagnosis may be made clinically or may be proposed by the radiologist based on the clinical history. However, in thoracic imaging, the term "pneumonia" is used for a number of noninfectious pulmonary disorders related to inflammation and fibrosis (e.g., the idiopathic intersitial pneumonias).

Summary

The use of proper terminology facilitates communication with members of the clinical staff and between radiologists. Those who interpret thoracic imaging studies must become familiar with imaging anatomy and the correct descriptors for imaging abnormalities. In many instances, the accurate and correct description of an abnormality allows the radiologist to arrive at the correct diagnosis and to formulate the appropriate next step in patient management.

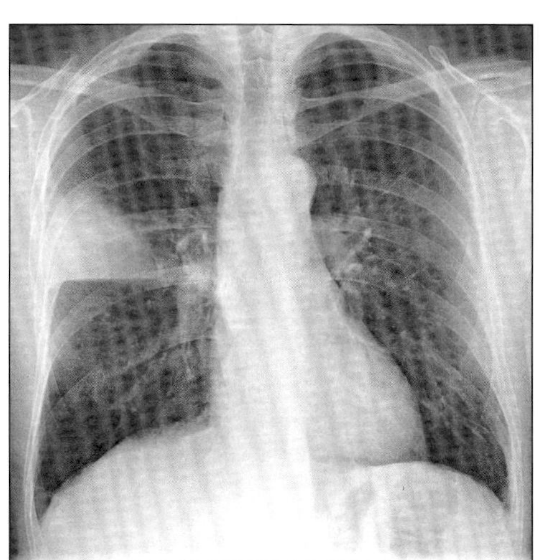

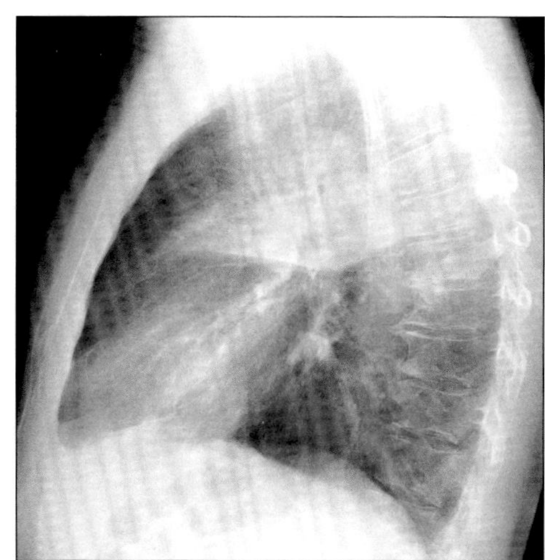

(Left) *PA chest radiograph of a 54-year-old man with cough, fever, and leukocytosis shows a right upper lobe consolidation above the horizontal fissure, therefore involving the anterior segment of the right upper lobe.* ***(Right)*** *Lateral chest radiograph of the same patient shows consolidation in the anterior and posterior segments of the right upper lobe. Based on the radiographic and clinical findings, the diagnosis is most consistent with bacterial pneumonia.*

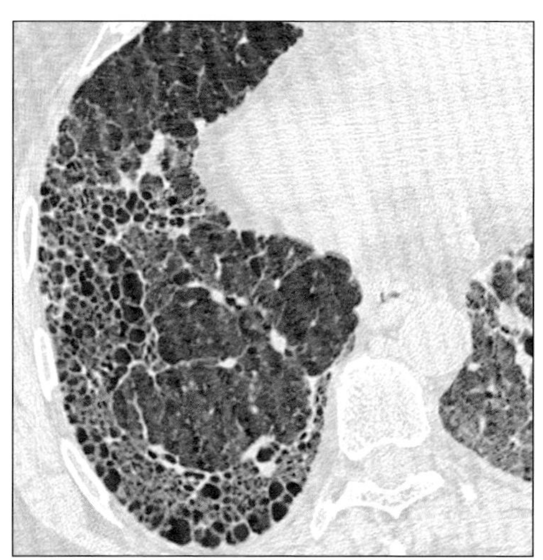

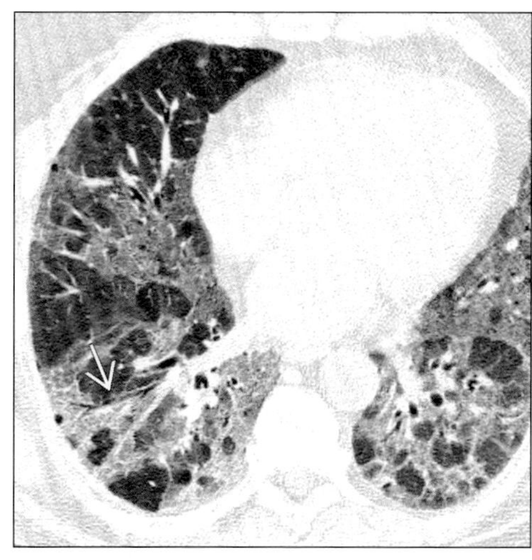

(Left) *Axial HRCT of an 83-year-old woman with idiopathic pulmonary fibrosis shows a usual interstitial pneumonia (UIP) pattern of fibrosis characterized by subpleural honeycomb cysts arrayed in tiers.* ***(Right)*** *Axial NECT of a patient with nonspecific interstitial pneumonia (NSIP) shows patchy, basilar, ground-glass opacities and mild traction bronchiectasis* ➔*. Noninfectious fibrotic lung diseases form part of the spectrum of idiopathic interstitial pneumonias.*

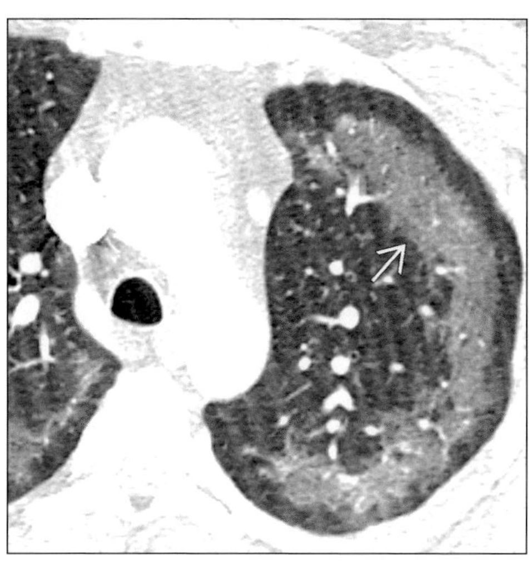

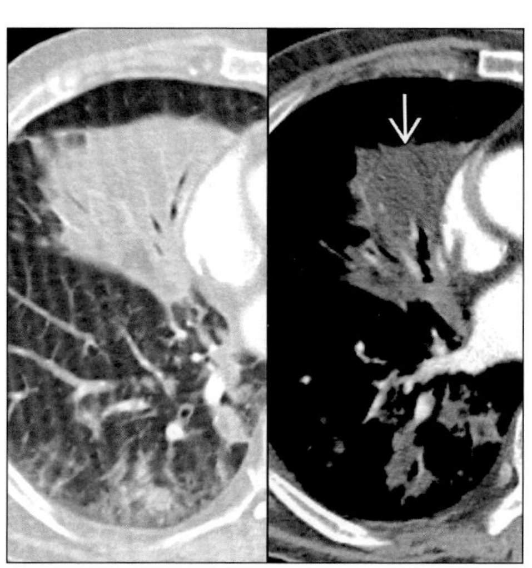

(Left) *Axial NECT of a patient with chronic eosinophilic pneumonia shows peripheral subpleural ground-glass opacities* ➔*. This noninfectious pulmonary disease is characterized by alveolar and interstitial eosinophilic infiltration.* ***(Right)*** *Composite image with axial CECT in lung (left) and soft tissue (right) window shows multifocal parenchymal consolidations with intrinsic fat attenuation* ➔*, representing exogenous lipoid pneumonia secondary to mineral oil aspiration.*

ACINAR NODULES

Key Facts

Terminology

- **Acinus**
  - Structural lung unit distal to terminal bronchiole, supplied by 1st-order respiratory bronchioles
  - Largest structural lung unit in which all airways participate in gas exchange
- **Secondary pulmonary lobule**: 3-24 acini
- **Acinar nodules**: Poorly marginated nodular opacities measuring 5-10 mm, airspace nodules
  - Visible when opacified by fluid, cells, barium

Imaging

- Radiography
  - Poorly defined nodular opacities
  - Multiple "fluffy" nodules measuring 5-10 mm
- CT
  - Nodules with ill-defined borders (5-10 mm)
  - Centrilobular distribution
  - Isolated or adjacent to consolidation

Top Differential Diagnoses

- Alveolar hemorrhage
- Alveolar edema
- Bronchopneumonia, aspiration
- Tuberculosis

Pathology

- Inflammation of terminal & respiratory bronchioles
- Sparing of distal airspaces
- Acinar nodules on imaging tend to be centrilobular or peribronchiolar on pathologic specimens

Diagnostic Checklist

- Consider bronchogenic spread of pulmonary infection in patients with acinar opacities
- Acinar nodules in association with cavitation: Consider active tuberculosis

*(**Left**) PA chest radiograph (coned down to the middle lobe) of a patient who aspirated barium shows rosette-like, high-attenuation nodular opacities representing barium in pulmonary acini. The nodules measure 5-10 mm in size and appear "fluffy." Acinar nodules have also been called airspace nodules. (**Right**) Axial NECT of a patient with active tuberculosis shows multifocal clustered acinar nodules ➡ and scattered tree-in-bud opacities ⇨ due to endobronchial spread of tuberculosis.*

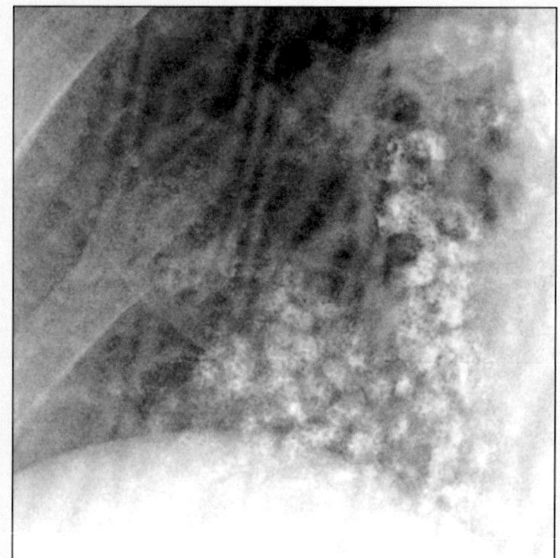

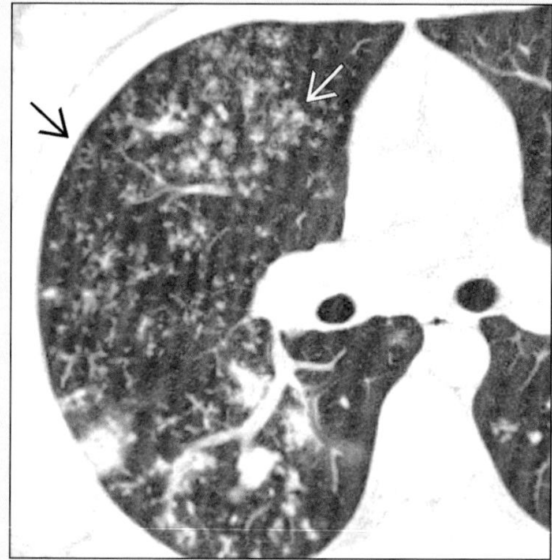

*(**Left**) Axial CECT of a patient with postpartum pulmonary edema shows edema fluid manifesting as multiple acinar nodules ↷ of ground-glass attenuation without associated interlobular septal thickening. Note associated small bilateral pleural effusions. (**Right**) Axial CECT of a patient who presented with hemoptysis and alveolar hemorrhage shows patchy bilateral ground-glass acinar nodules ➡ with ill-defined borders and centrilobular distribution.*

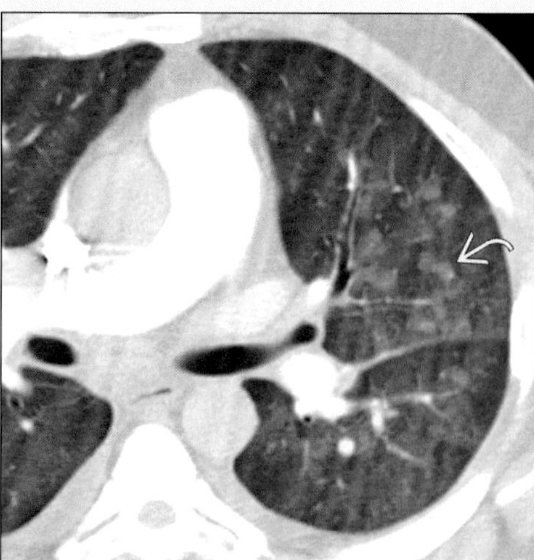

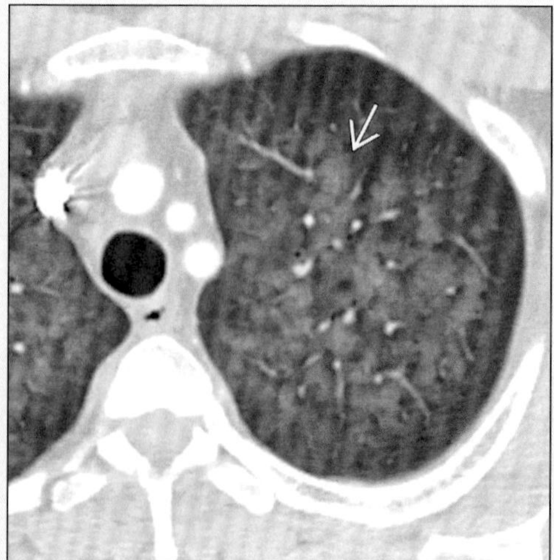

Key Facts

Terminology

- **Air bronchogram**
  - Definition: Visualization of air-filled bronchi within background of opacified lung parenchyma
  - Implies patency of proximal airways
  - Central obstruction is unlikely
  - Also seen in confluent interstitial disease
- Bronchi not normally visible in outer 1/3 of lung

Imaging

- Radiography
  - Air-filled branching lucencies representing patent bronchi
  - Surrounding airspace opacity
- CT
  - Air-filled branching tapering bronchi
  - Surrounded by consolidated lung parenchyma

Top Differential Diagnoses

- Pneumonia: Infectious, lipoid, aspiration
- Neoplasms
  - Lepidic adenocarcinoma
  - Lymphoma
- Alveolar edema, alveolar hemorrhage
- Fibrosis (radiation), sarcoidosis

Pathology

- Alveolar filling with pus, edema fluid, blood, tumor
- Interstitial lymphoproliferative, granulomatous process

Diagnostic Checklist

- Consolidation with air bronchograms in febrile patient is consistent with pneumonia
- Consolidations in adults should be followed to radiographic resolution to exclude underlying malignancy

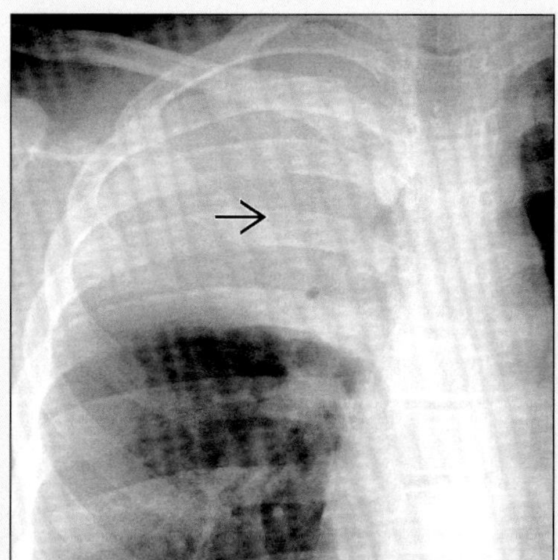

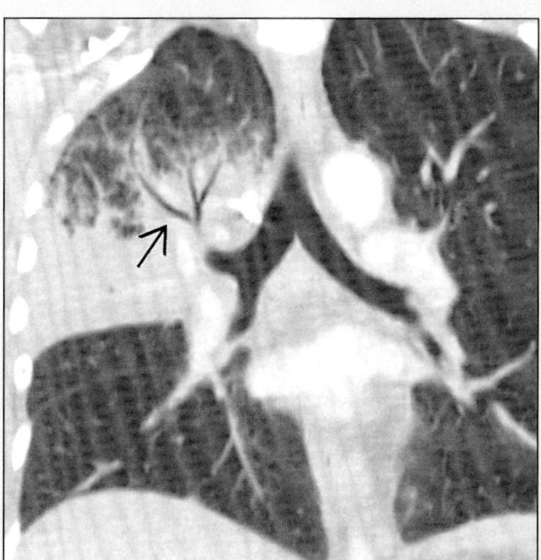

__(Left)__ PA chest radiograph of a patient with right upper lobe pneumonia shows a dense consolidation with an intrinsic air bronchogram →, the presence of which excludes a central obstructing lesion. Nevertheless, consolidations in adults should be followed to complete resolution to exclude underlying malignancy. __(Right)__ Coronal CECT of a patient with pneumonia shows dense right upper lobe consolidation with an intrinsic air bronchogram →.

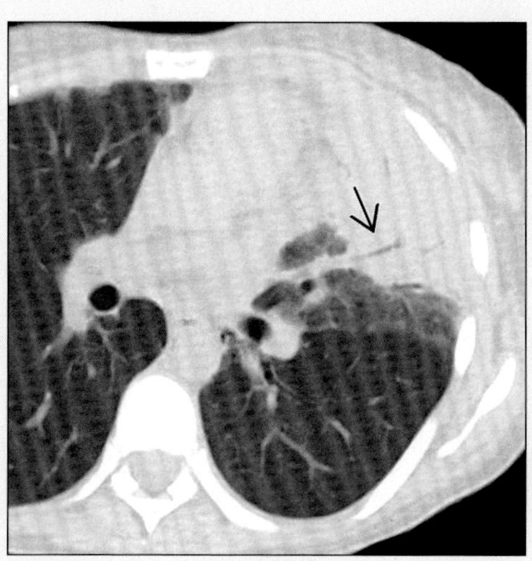

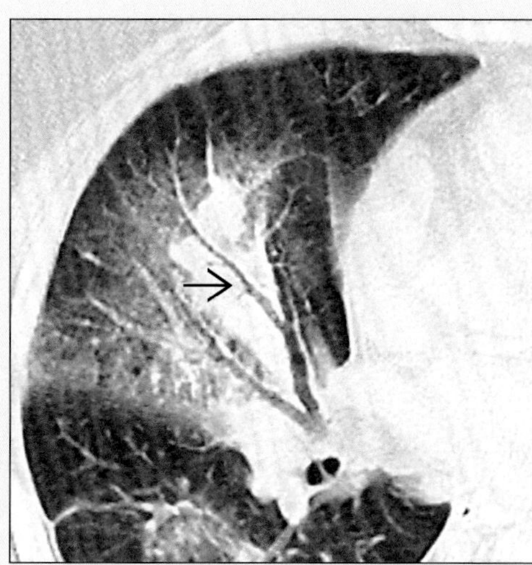

__(Left)__ Axial NECT of a patient with pneumonia shows a lingular consolidation with an intrinsic air bronchogram → manifesting as branching air-filled tubular opacities within surrounding airspace disease. __(Right)__ Axial NECT of a patient with chronic cough and exogenous lipoid pneumonia shows heterogeneous consolidation in the middle and right lower lobes and a middle lobe air bronchogram →. A variety of alveolar filling disease processes may produce air bronchograms.

AIR-TRAPPING

Key Facts

Terminology

- **Air-trapping**
  - Air retention in lung distal to airway obstruction shown on expiratory CT

Imaging

- Inspiratory CT
  - Normal lung is homogeneously lucent
  - Mosaic attenuation may be seen in constrictive bronchiolitis & occlusive vascular disease
- Expiratory CT
  - Normal lung shows increased attenuation
  - Lobular air-trapping involving < 3 adjacent lobules is likely normal
  - Accentuation of subtle or diffuse air-trapping
  - Sharply defined geographic foci of attenuation lower than that of surrounding normal lung; follow outlines of secondary pulmonary lobules
  - Abnormal air-trapping affects > 25% of lung volume & is not limited to lower lobe superior segments or lingular tip

Top Differential Diagnoses

- Constrictive bronchiolitis
  - Infection, chronic rejection in transplantation, connective tissue disease, inhalational lung disease, hypersensitivity pneumonitis
- Chronic pulmonary thromboembolic disease
  - Occlusive vascular disease

Pathology

- Constrictive bronchiolitis: Peribronchiolar fibrosis of membranous & respiratory bronchioles

Diagnostic Checklist

- Consider expiratory HRCT in patients with suspected constrictive bronchiolitis

__(Left)__ Composite image with axial HRCT of a patient with constrictive bronchiolitis obtained in inspiration (top) and expiration (bottom) shows areas of expiratory air-trapping manifesting as focal hyperlucent lung ➔. __(Right)__ Composite image with axial HRCT on inspiration (left) and expiration (right) of a patient with constrictive bronchiolitis shows inspiratory mosaic attenuation and expiratory air-trapping with decreased vascularity. Expiratory imaging accentuates findings of air-trapping.

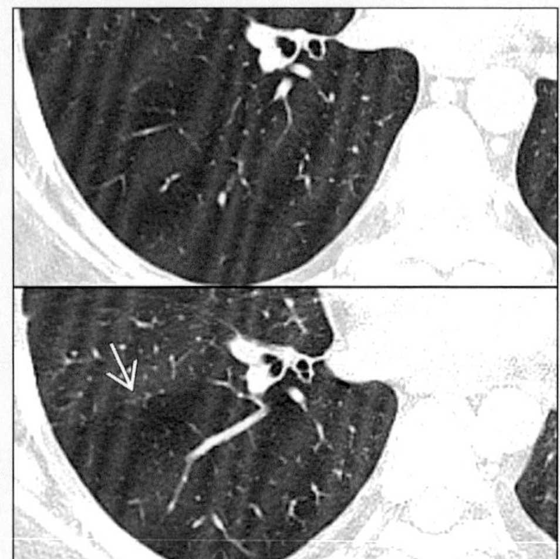

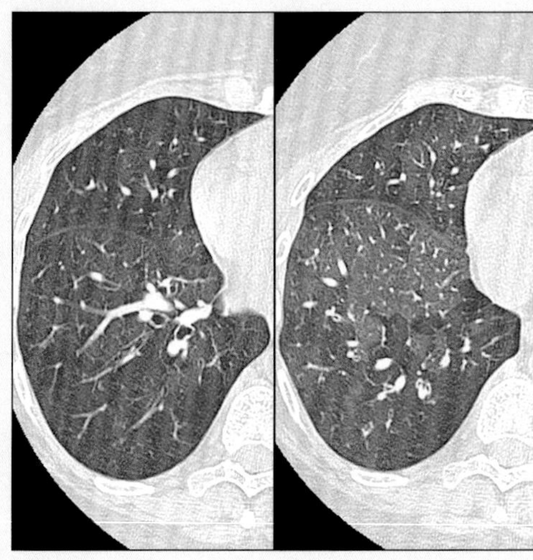

__(Left)__ Axial NECT of a patient with hypersensitivity pneumonitis shows multiple foci of hyperlucent lung ➔ due to air-trapping. In patients with hypersensitivity pneumonitis, areas of air-trapping may be accentuated by surrounding ground-glass opacity. __(Right)__ Axial NECT of a patient with a central partially obstructing carcinoid tumor shows hyperlucency ➔ of the visualized left lower lobe secondary to obstruction by the tumor and resultant air-trapping.

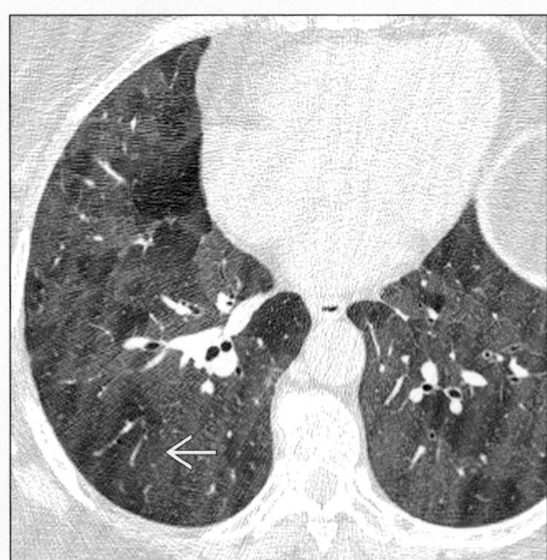

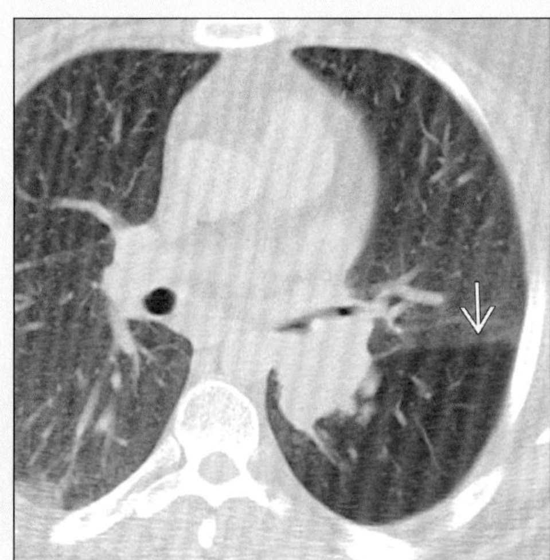

Key Facts

Terminology

- **Airspace**
  - Gas-containing portions of lung
  - Includes respiratory bronchioles, alveolar ducts, alveolar sacs, & alveoli
  - Excludes purely conducting airways
- **Airspace disease**: Increased airspace opacity
  - Atelectasis: Air absorbed & not replaced
  - Consolidation: Air replaced by fluid, purulent material, blood, cells, or other substances

Imaging

- Radiography
  - Airspace consolidation
  - Increased pulmonary opacity that obscures underlying vascular markings
  - May be focal or multifocal
  - Confluent opacity
  - May be heterogeneous
- CT
  - **Airspace consolidation**: Increased pulmonary attenuation with obscuration of underling normal structures
  - **Airspace nodules**: "Fluffy" nodules of increased attenuation in centrilobular distribution

Top Differential Diagnoses

- Pneumonia: Bacterial, viral, fungal
- Aspiration
- Alveolar edema
- Alveolar hemorrhage
- Alveolar proteinosis
- Lepidic adenocarcinoma

Diagnostic Checklist

- Consider differential diagnosis of airspace disease in patients without signs & symptoms of infection

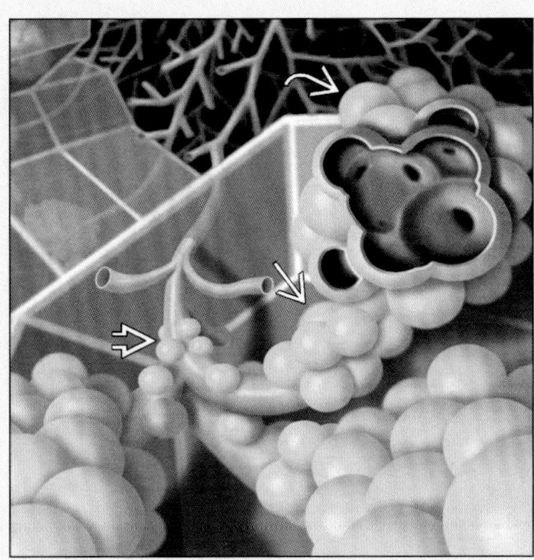

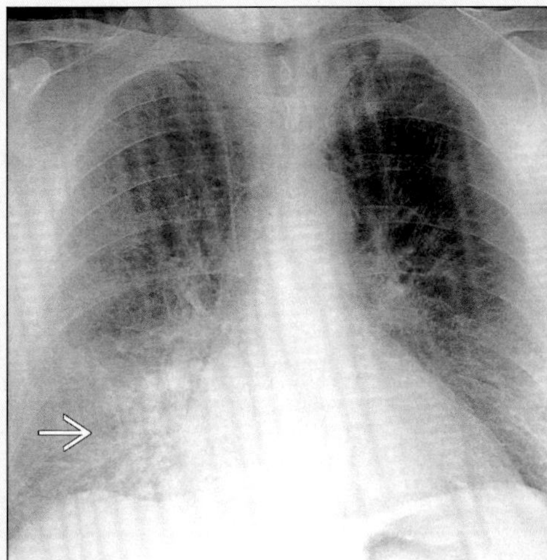

*(**Left**) Graphic demonstrates the airspaces of the lung, which are composed of the small airways that participate in gas exchange (respiratory bronchiole ➡, alveolar duct ➡, and alveolar sac) and the alveoli ➡. (**Right**) PA chest radiograph of a patient with interstitial edema shows interlobular septal thickening, perihilar haze, and focal airspace opacity ➡ in the right lower lobe due to alveolar filling with edema fluid.*

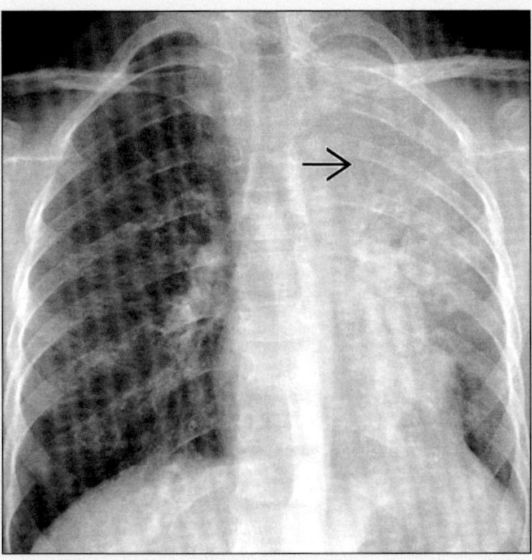

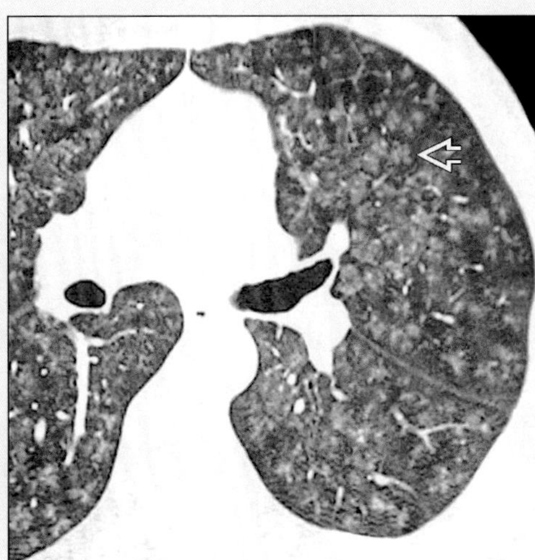

*(**Left**) PA chest radiograph of a patient with fever and cough demonstrates pneumonia manifesting with extensive airspace consolidation in the left upper and lower lobes with intrinsic air bronchograms →, a common manifestation of airspace disease. (**Right**) Axial NECT of a patient with subacute hypersensitivity pneumonitis shows innumerable small airspace nodules ➡ in a centrilobular distribution. This nodular form of airspace disease is also referred to as acinar nodules.*

ARCHITECTURAL DISTORTION

Key Facts

Terminology

- **Architectural distortion**
  - Abnormal displacement of bronchi, vessels, fissures, or septa caused by diffuse or localized retractile fibrotic process
  - Characteristically related to interstitial fibrosis

Imaging

- Radiography
  - Reticular opacities
  - Volume loss with increased opacity
  - Hilar displacement related to volume loss
  - Visualization of associated bronchiectasis
- CT
  - Displacement of pulmonary structures (vessels & bronchi) secondary to pulmonary fibrosis
  - Associated reticular opacities, traction bronchiectasis, honeycombing

Top Differential Diagnoses

- Pulmonary fibrosis
  - Idiopathic pulmonary fibrosis (IPF), fibrotic nonspecific interstitial pneumonia (NSIP)
- End-stage sarcoidosis
- Chronic hypersensitivity pneumonitis
- Radiation fibrosis

Pathology

- Interstitial pulmonary fibrosis

Diagnostic Checklist

- Architectural distortion denotes pulmonary fibrosis, particularly when associated with reticular opacities, traction bronchiectasis, & honeycomb lung
- Architectural distortion is characteristically associated with volume loss

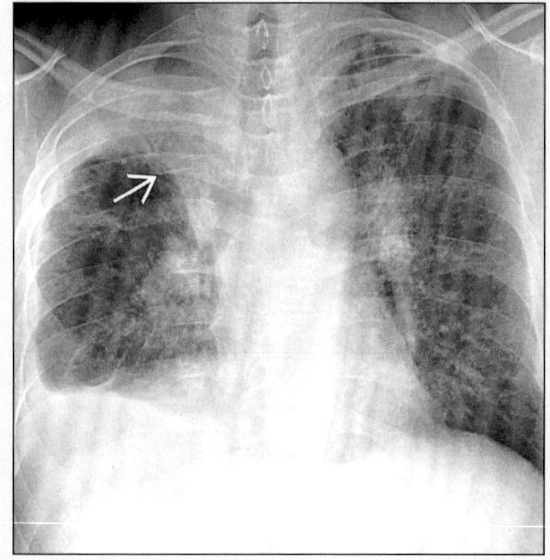

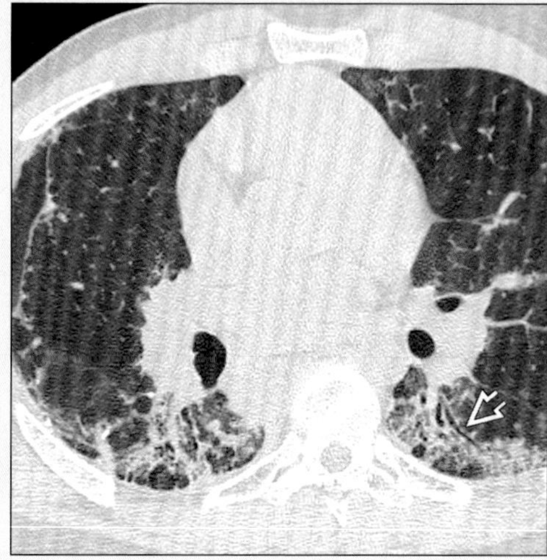

(Left) *PA chest radiograph of a patient with end-stage sarcoidosis shows extensive architectural distortion with perihilar opacities, hilar retraction, and upper lobe volume loss, most pronounced on the right. Note elevation and concavity of the minor fissure* ➡. ***(Right)*** *Axial HRCT of a patient with fibrotic nonspecific interstitial pneumonia (NSIP) shows bilateral lower lobe architectural distortion manifesting as volume loss, reticular opacities, and traction bronchiectasis* ➡ *with posterior hilar retraction.*

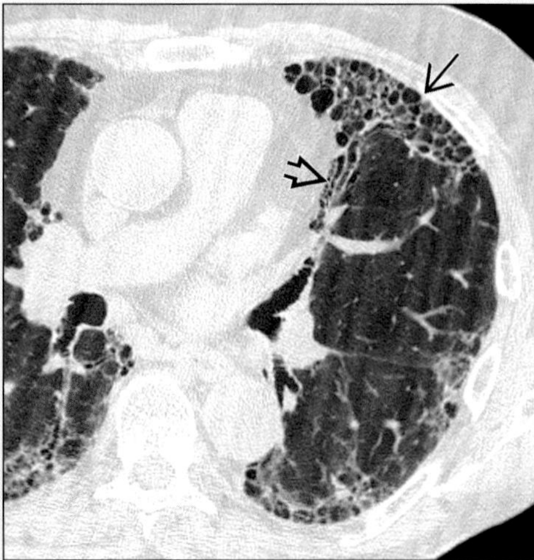

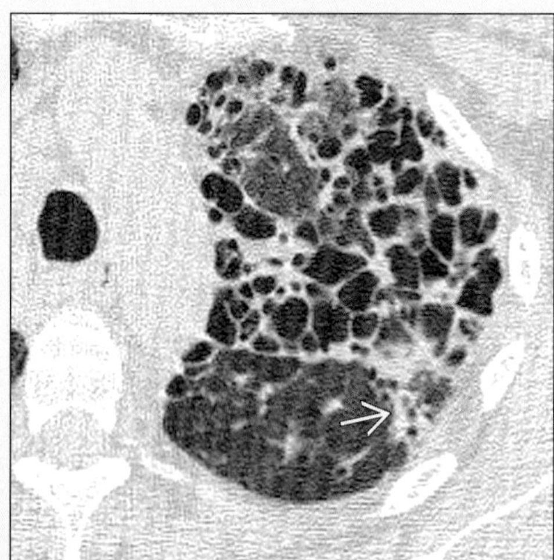

(Left) *Axial HRCT of a patient with idiopathic pulmonary fibrosis (IPF) shows subpleural reticulation and honeycombing* ➡ *with associated left upper lobe architectural distortion and traction bronchiectasis* ➡. ***(Right)*** *Axial HRCT of a patient with end-stage sarcoidosis shows marked architectural distortion in the left lung apex with near complete replacement of the normal lung parenchyma by honeycomb cysts and associated traction bronchiectasis* ➡.

Key Facts

Terminology
- **Bulla**
  - Definition: Air-containing space measuring > 1 cm
  - Surrounded by thin wall < 1 mm thick
  - Subpleural location; largest at lung apex
  - Associated with emphysema: Typically paraseptal but also centrilobular
- **Bleb**
  - Definition: Small gas-containing space within visceral pleural surface measuring < 1 cm
  - Difficult distinction between bleb & bulla as both are peripherally located
  - Term has also been used to describe air-containing space < 1 cm

Imaging
- Radiography
  - Thin-walled apical lucency
  - May mimic solid lesion when fluid-filled
- CT
  - Peripheral subpleural air-filled space
  - Thin walls
  - Typically multifocal
  - Thick walls, intrinsic fluid, air-fluid, or soft tissue should suggest secondary infection but may also relate to hemorrhage or neoplasm

Pathology
- Paraseptal emphysema
  - Bullous disease
- Centrilobular emphysema

Diagnostic Checklist
- Pulmonary bullae are typically manifestations of paraseptal emphysema
- Bullae are a recognized cause of secondary spontaneous pneumothorax

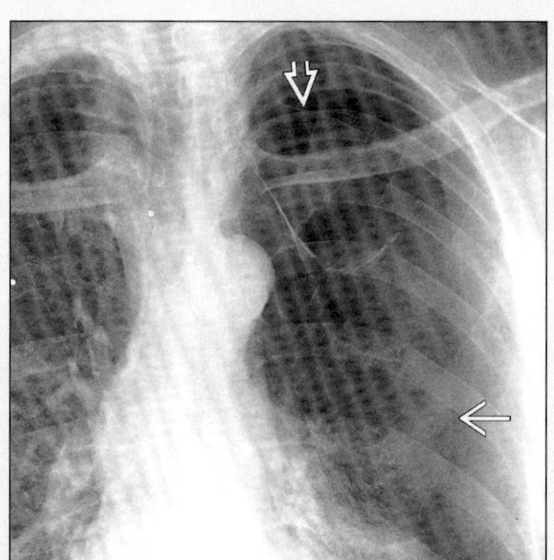

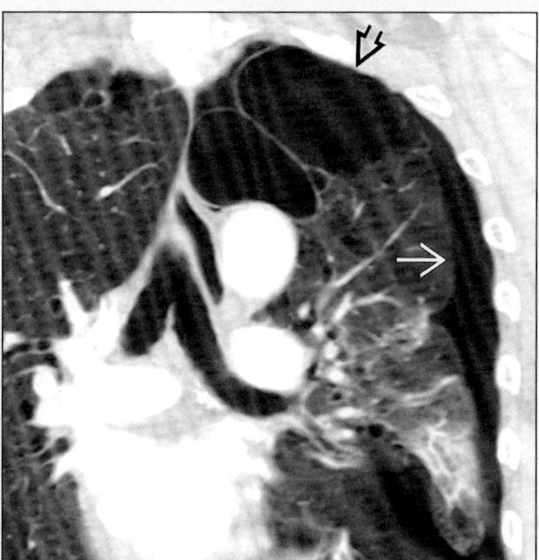

*(**Left**) PA chest radiograph of a patient who presented with acute chest pain and a spontaneous left pneumothorax shows a visible pleural line ➡ and a large bulla ⇨ in the left lung apex, likely responsible for the pneumothorax. (**Right**) Coronal CECT of the same patient shows the left pneumothorax ➡ and a cluster of large left apical bullae ⇨. Paraseptal emphysema with giant bullous disease is one of the causes of secondary spontaneous pneumothorax.*

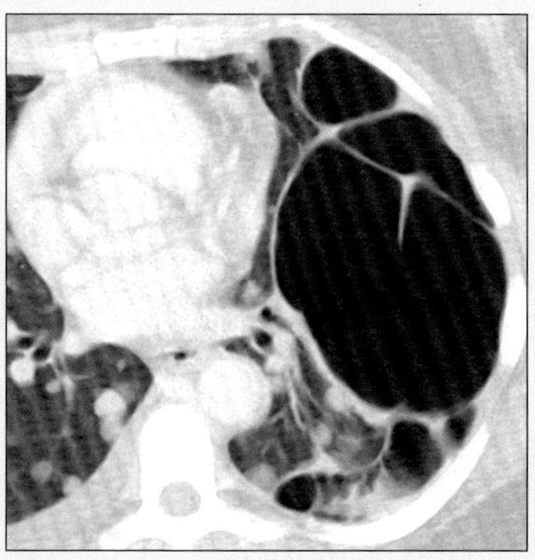

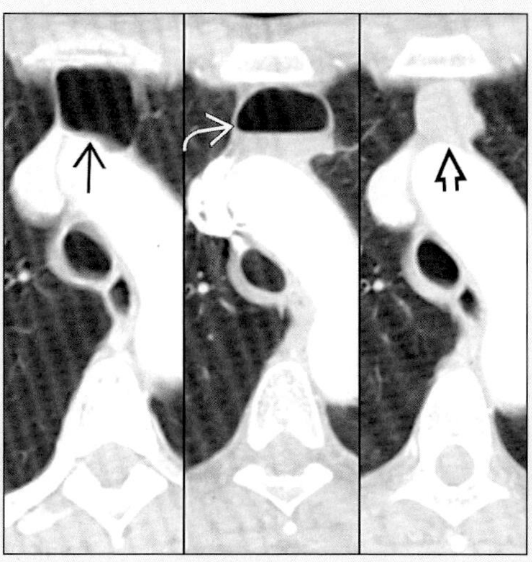

*(**Left**) Axial NECT of a patient with benign metastasizing leiomyoma and left upper lobe giant bullous disease shows a large left apical air-filled space with internal septations. (**Right**) Composite image with axial CECT of a patient with a left upper lobe bulla, which became secondarily infected, shows a thin-walled retrosternal bulla ➡ completely filled with air. Subsequent studies show an internal air-fluid level ➡ within the bulla and eventual complete fluid filling ⇨ secondary to infection.*

CAVITY

Key Facts

Terminology

- **Cavity**
  - Definition: Gas-containing space manifesting as lucency or low attenuation within mass or consolidation
  - Implies pulmonary necrosis with expulsion of necrotic material via communication with tracheobronchial tree

Imaging

- Radiography
  - Lucency within mass or consolidation
  - May exhibit air, air-fluid level
  - Variable cavity wall thickness
  - Cavity wall may be smooth or nodular
- CT
  - Allows optimal assessment of extent of cavitation & areas of involvement
  - Allows optimal evaluation of cavity wall
  - In cases of malignancy, may be initial step in staging neoplasm
  - In cases of infection, associated centrilobular nodules imply bronchogenic dissemination of infection & tuberculosis must be considered in the differential diagnosis

Top Differential Diagnoses

- Infection
  - Necrotizing pneumonia
  - Abscess
  - Septic emboli
- Neoplasia
  - Cavitary lung cancer; squamous cell carcinoma
  - Cavitary metastases
- Vasculitis
  - Wegener granulomatosis
- Pulmonary infarction

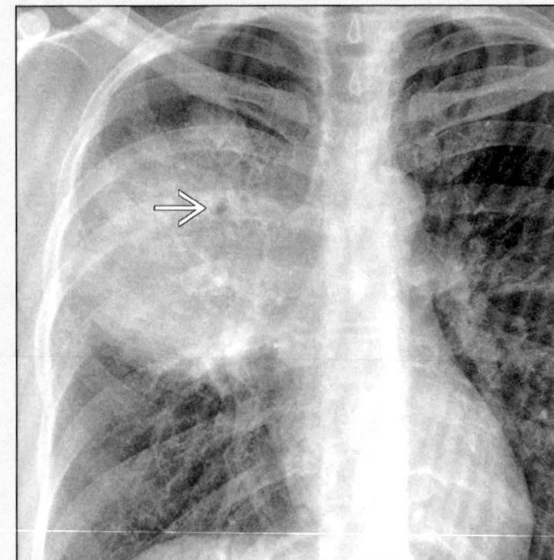
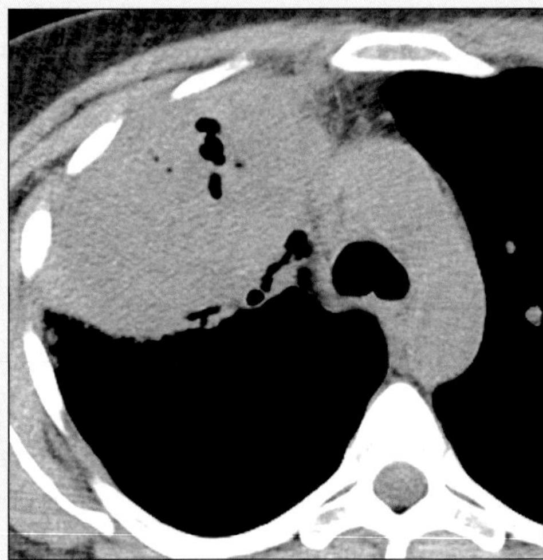

(Left) *PA chest radiograph of a patient with AIDS who presented with cough and fever shows a mass-like consolidation in the right upper lobe with a small focus of internal air ➔, consistent with cavitation.* ***(Right)*** *Axial NECT of the same patient shows a large ovoid right upper lobe mass with central low attenuation and intrinsic air, consistent with tissue necrosis and early cavitation. Although cavitary neoplasm was considered, the patient was diagnosed with necrotizing bacterial pneumonia.*

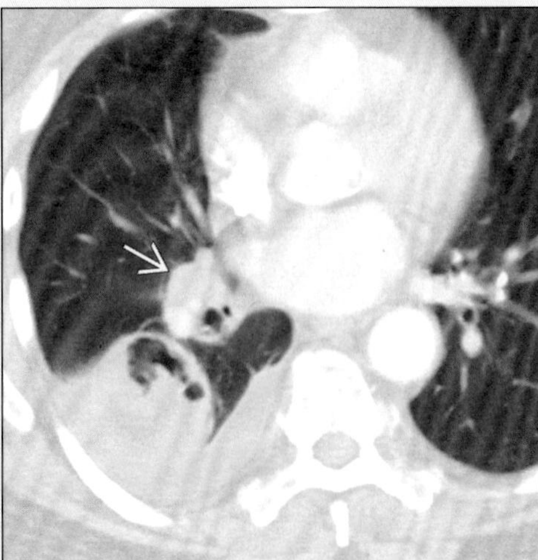
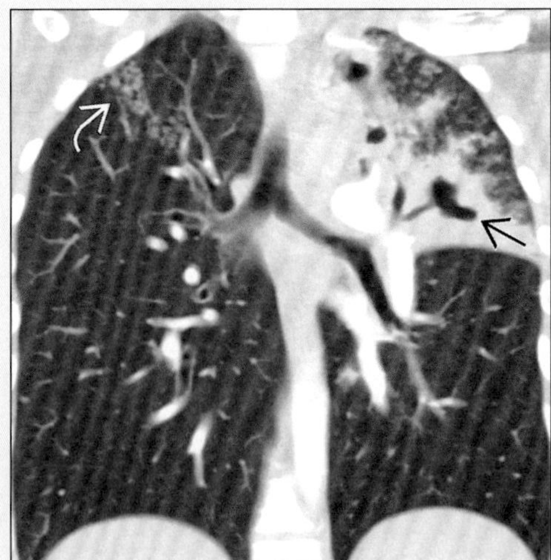

(Left) *Axial CECT of a patient with advanced lung cancer shows a spherical right lower lobe mass with intrinsic cavitation, ipsilateral hilar lymphadenopathy ➔, and a right pleural effusion later proven to be malignant. Primary lung cancer, particularly squamous cell carcinoma, may exhibit cavitation.* ***(Right)*** *Coronal CECT of a patient with active tuberculosis shows a left upper lobe consolidation with cavitation ➔ and scattered tree-in-bud opacities ➔, consistent with endobronchial dissemination of infection.*

Key Facts

Terminology

- **Centrilobular**
  - Definition: Anatomic location in central portion of secondary pulmonary lobule (SPL) that contains lobular artery, bronchiole, & lymphatics
  - Bronchiolar or peribronchiolar abnormalities
  - Nodules: Ground-glass or solid
  - Tree-in-bud opacities
  - Emphysema

Imaging

- **Centrilobular nodule**
  - Solid or ground-glass attenuation
  - Located 5-10 mm from pleural surface
  - Does not abut pleura unless large
- **Centrilobular emphysema**
  - Lung destruction surrounding central lobular artery of SPL
  - Parenchymal lucency with imperceptible walls
  - Central artery often manifests as dot-like structure surrounded by lucency

Top Differential Diagnoses

- **Centrilobular nodules**: Bronchopneumonia, endobronchial spread of tuberculosis, endobronchial or lymphangitic spread of tumor, hypersensitivity pneumonitis, silicosis, histiocytosis
- **Centrilobular emphysema**

Pathology

- Centrilobular nodules constitute cellular bronchiolitis

Diagnostic Checklist

- Consider infection in patient with predominant finding of centrilobular nodules & appropriate clinical history (cough, fever, leukocytosis)

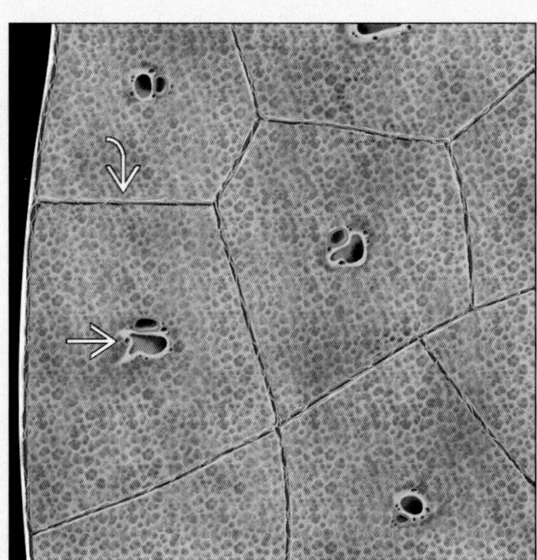

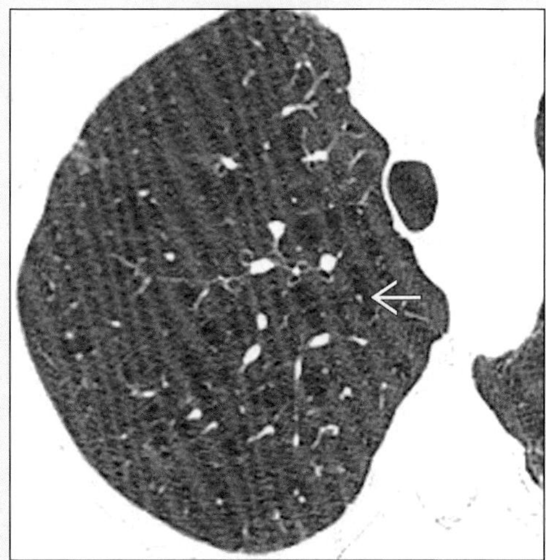

(Left) *Graphic demonstrates the cross-sectional anatomy of the secondary pulmonary lobule bound by the interlobular septa ➡. The central portion of the lobule contains the lobular artery and adjacent bronchiole ➡, surrounded by lymphatics. This lobular core indicates the centrilobular location.* ***(Right)*** *Axial NECT of a patient with centrilobular emphysema shows scattered foci of lung destruction, some of which surround a central dot ➡ corresponding to the central lobular artery.*

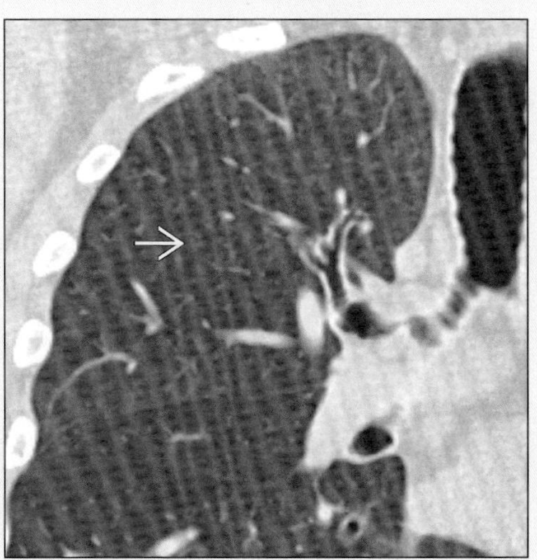

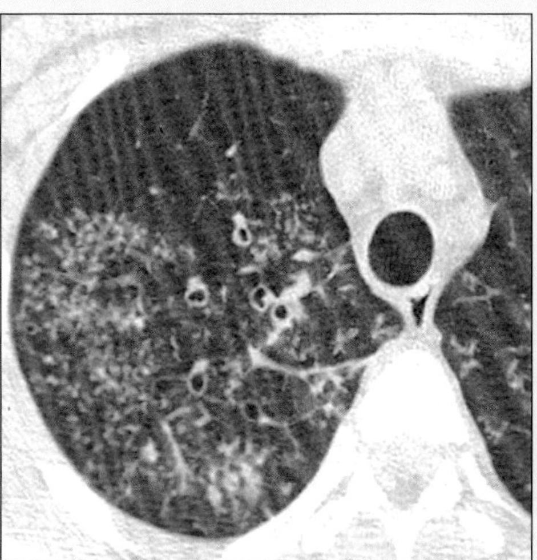

(Left) *Coronal NECT of a patient with respiratory bronchiolitis demonstrates scattered upper lobe ground-glass centrilobular micronodules ➡. Note that the nodules do not extend to the pleural surfaces.* ***(Right)*** *Axial NECT of a patient with active tuberculosis shows multiple clustered centrilobular nodules and tree-in-bud opacities with associated central bronchiectasis and bronchial wall thickening. In this case, the centrilobular nodules are indicative of endobronchial dissemination of pulmonary infection.*

CONSOLIDATION

Key Facts

Terminology

- **Consolidation**
  - Definition: Exudative fluid replacing alveolar air
  - Implies infection
- Synonyms
  - Airspace consolidation
  - Alveolar consolidation
- Consolidation may be focal, patchy, multifocal, or diffuse
- Focal consolidation
  - Nonsegmental, segmental, lobar

Imaging

- Radiography
  - Increased parenchymal density
  - Obscures normal structures (bronchi, vessels)
  - Obscures adjacent structures (silhouette sign)
  - May exhibit air bronchograms
  - May be sublobar, spherical, lobar
- CT
  - Increased lung attenuation
  - Obscures pulmonary architecture (vascular structures)
  - May exhibit air bronchograms
  - May have adjacent acinar nodules
  - Heterogeneous consolidation in emphysema (Swiss cheese appearance)
  - May exhibit fat attenuation: Lipoid pneumonia
  - May exhibit high attenuation: Amiodarone toxicity

Top Differential Diagnoses

- Pulmonary infection
  - Bacterial, viral, fungal
- Pulmonary edema
- Pulmonary hemorrhage
- Eosinophilic lung disease
- Neoplastic
  - Lung cancer, lymphoma

__(Left)__ PA chest radiograph of a patient with fever and leukocytosis shows extensive right lung dense consolidation with surrounding heterogeneous airspace opacity. __(Right)__ Axial NECT of the same patient shows dense right upper lobe consolidation with intrinsic air bronchograms ⇒ and surrounding ground-glass opacity with interlobular septal thickening and intralobular lines ⇗ (the so-called "crazy-paving" pattern). The patient was diagnosed with bacterial pneumonia.

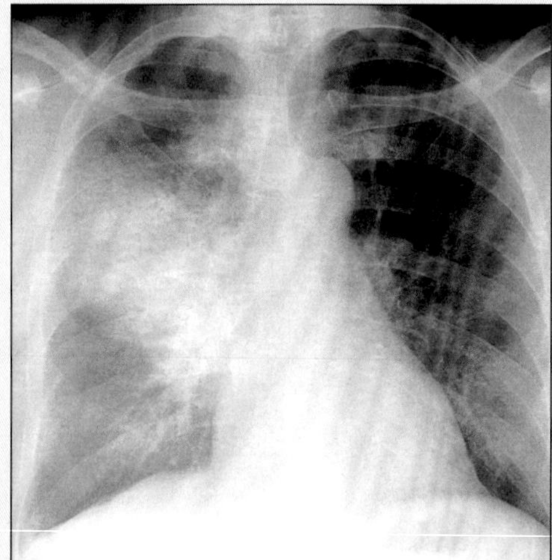

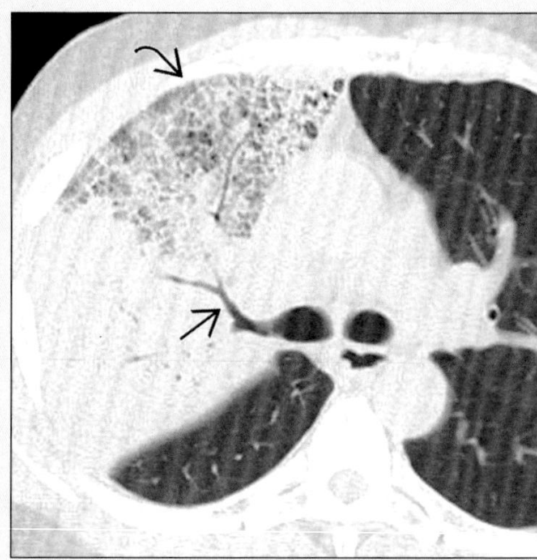

__(Left)__ Axial CECT of a febrile patient with a pulmonary mass on radiography (not shown) shows a dense ovoid mass-like consolidation surrounded by ground-glass opacity ⇗. This round pneumonia resolved with antibiotic treatment. __(Right)__ Axial NECT of a patient with chronic eosinophilic pneumonia demonstrates heterogeneous left upper lobe airspace disease with posterior areas of consolidation ⇒ and anterior ground-glass opacity with associated interlobular septal thickening ⇨.

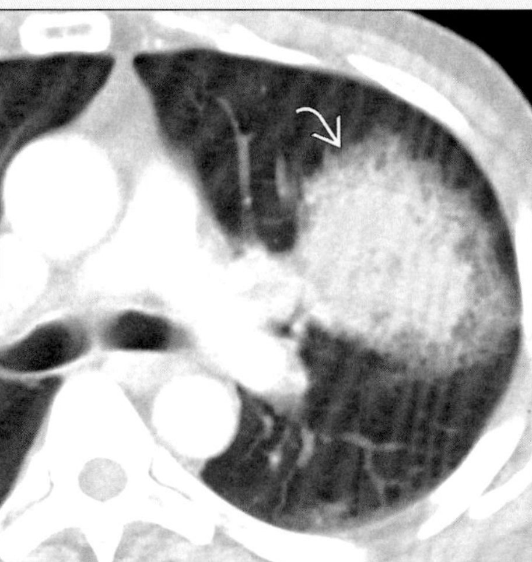

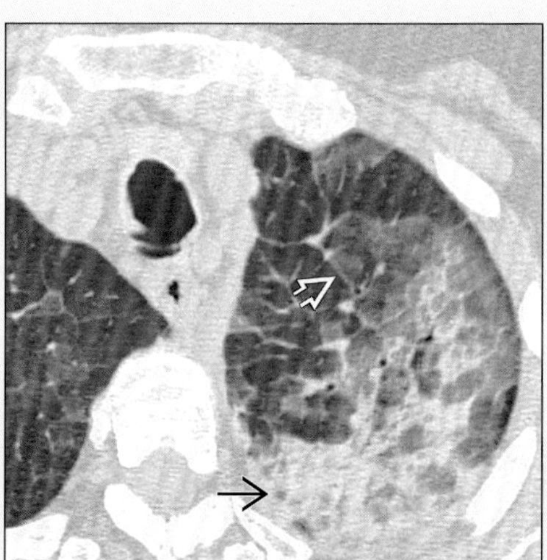

Key Facts

Terminology

- **Cyst**
  - Circumscribed spherical space surrounded by thin fibrous or epithelial wall
  - Cyst wall typically < 2 mm thick
- Term cyst refers to series of conditions characterized by thin-walled air- or fluid-filled spherical spaces
- **Bronchogenic cyst**
  - Congenital anomaly of foregut budding
  - Unilocular cyst
  - Typically occurs in mediastinum
  - Rarely in lung parenchyma

Imaging

- Radiography
  - Small cysts may not be visible
  - Multiple cysts may manifest as reticular opacities
  - Larger cysts may manifest as spherical lucencies with thin walls
- CT
  - Optimal evaluation of size, shape, number, & distribution of pulmonary cysts
  - Variable cyst walls, cyst sizes, & cyst contents
  - Roughly spherical air-filled space with thin peripheral wall

Top Differential Diagnoses

- Indeterminate lung cyst
  - Solitary, thin-walled, uncomplicated
- Congenital: Intrapulmonary bronchogenic cyst, pulmonary airway malformation
- Lymphoproliferative disorder: Lymphoid interstitial pneumonia (LIP)
- Smooth muscle proliferation: Lymphangioleiomyomatosis (LAM)
- Smoking-related bronchiolar disease: Pulmonary Langerhans cell histiocytosis (PLCH)

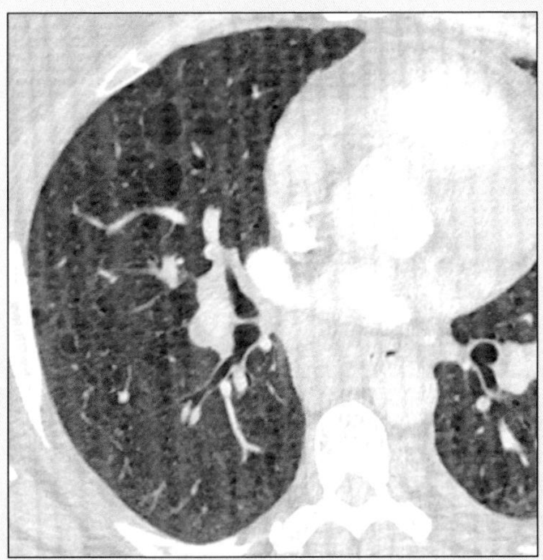

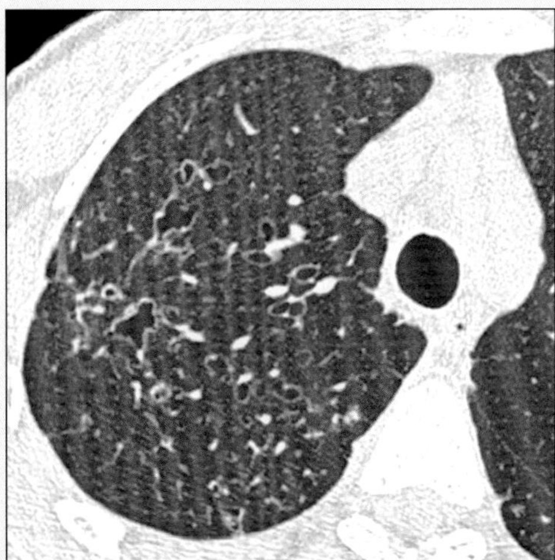

***(Left)** Axial CECT of a patient with lymphangioleiomyomatosis shows multifocal pulmonary cysts of varying size with intervening normal lung parenchyma. The cysts are distributed diffusely throughout both lungs, the cyst walls are thin but perceptible, and there are no associated pulmonary nodules. **(Right)** Axial NECT of a smoker with pulmonary Langerhans cell histiocytosis shows upper lobe predominant pulmonary nodules and pulmonary cysts. The latter exhibit thick nodular walls and bizarre shapes.*

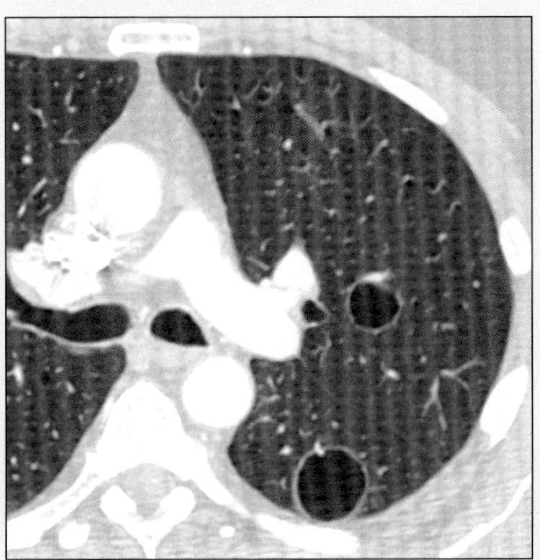

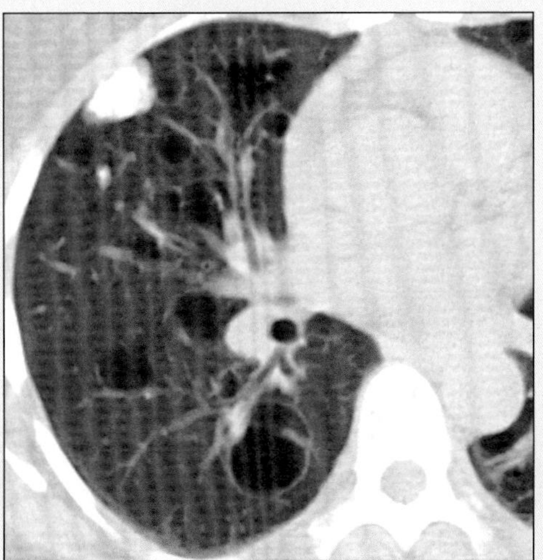

***(Left)** Axial CECT of a patient with lymphocytic interstitial pneumonia shows thin-walled pulmonary cysts in the left lung. **(Right)** Axial NECT of a patient with pulmonary amyloidosis shows a densely calcified middle lobe nodule (amyloidoma) and multifocal thin-walled pulmonary cysts. Lung cysts may occur in a variety of pulmonary disorders. The size, number, and distribution of such cysts and the presence of ancillary findings are helpful in formulating an appropriate differential diagnosis.*

GROUND-GLASS OPACITY

Key Facts

Terminology

- **Ground-glass opacity**
  - Increased lung density or attenuation
  - Does not obscure underlying structures
- Results from
  - Alveolar filling/collapse
  - Interstitial thickening
  - Increased blood volume
  - Combination of above mechanisms

Imaging

- Radiography
  - Hazy increased lung density that does not obscure underlying structures
- CT
  - Increased lung attenuation
  - Does not obscure underlying bronchovascular structures

Top Differential Diagnoses

- Nonspecific finding with broad differential diagnosis
- **Acute**
  - Pneumonia (including *Pneumocystis jiroveci*, viruses, mycoplasma), hemorrhage, edema, acute interstitial pneumonia (AIP), acute respiratory distress syndrome (ARDS), acute eosinophilic pneumonia, radiation pneumonitis
- **Chronic**
  - Idiopathic interstitial pneumonias: Nonspecific interstitial pneumonia, desquamative interstitial pneumonia, respiratory bronchiolitis-associated interstitial lung disease
  - Hypersensitivity pneumonitis, drug reaction, chronic eosinophilic pneumonia, Churg-Strauss syndrome, lipoid pneumonia, adenocarcinoma (preinvasive, minimally invasive, invasive lepidic)

__(Left)__ Axial NECT of a patient with AIDS who presented with several days of dyspnea and fever shows patchy bilateral ground-glass opacities secondary to Pneumocystis jiroveci pneumonia. __(Right)__ Coronal NECT of a patient with mitral valve disease who presented with acute dyspnea shows bilateral ground-glass opacities and acinar nodules ➔ secondary to pulmonary edema. Acute lung diseases that manifest with ground-glass opacity include infection, hemorrhage, and edema.

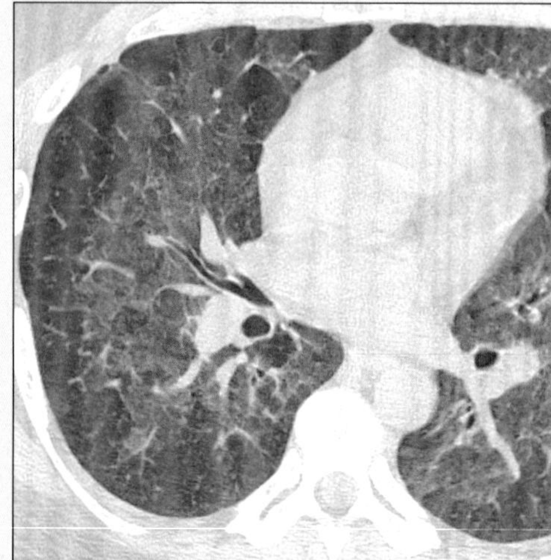

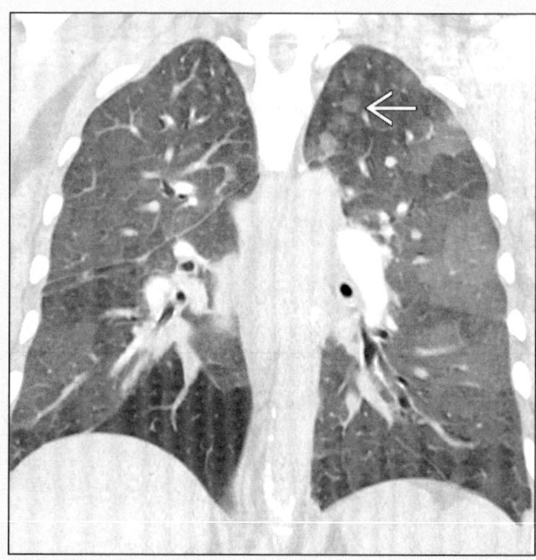

__(Left)__ Axial NECT of a patient with chronic dyspnea and nonspecific interstitial pneumonia shows bilateral lower lobe ground-glass opacities. __(Right)__ Axial NECT of a smoker who presented with dyspnea and cough shows patchy bilateral ground-glass opacities and cystic changes secondary to desquamative interstitial pneumonia. Chronic lung diseases that manifest with ground-glass opacity include idiopathic interstitial pneumonias and chronic eosinophilic pneumonia.

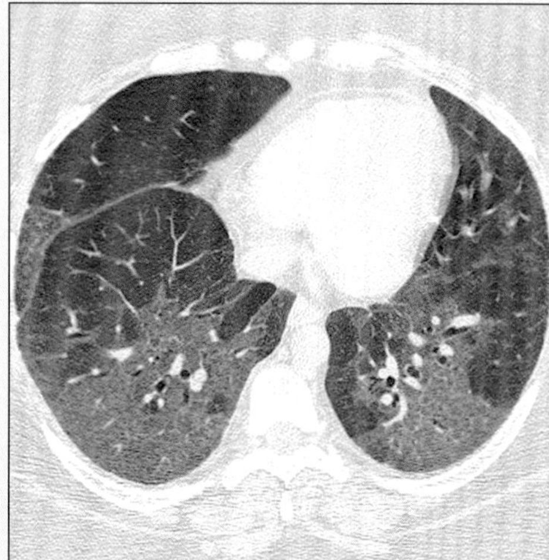

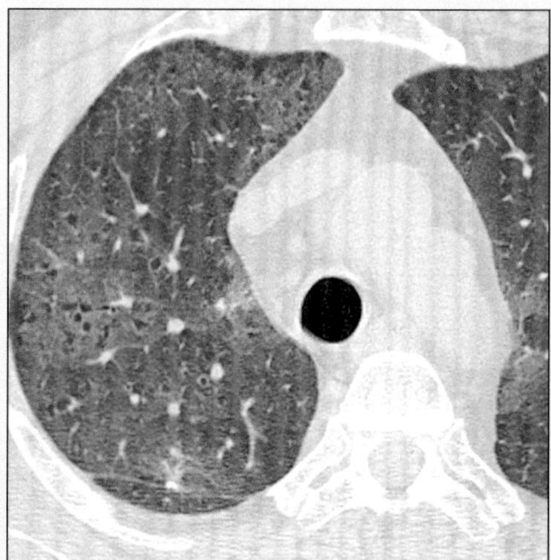

Key Facts

Terminology

- **Honeycombing**: End-stage pulmonary fibrosis
  - Subpleural, clustered cystic spaces that share walls & may occur in several tiers
  - Results from various fibrotic lung diseases

Imaging

- Radiography
  - Peripheral, subpleural, basilar cysts or reticular opacities
  - Volume loss
- CT
  - Peripheral, typically basilar, may be patchy
  - Honeycomb cysts (2-20 mm) with well-defined walls arranged in clusters & tiers
  - Associated findings: Reticular opacities, intralobular lines, traction bronchiectasis, architectural distortion

Top Differential Diagnoses

- Idiopathic pulmonary fibrosis (usual interstitial pneumonia histologic pattern), fibrotic nonspecific interstitial pneumonia
- Fibrotic sarcoidosis
- Chronic hypersensitivity pneumonitis

Pathology

- Reduced lung volume, nodular cobblestone-like pleural surface
- Lower lobe distribution most common
- UIP pattern: Dense fibrosis, honeycomb cysts, fibroblastic lung, interspersed normal lung
  - Microscopy: Temporal heterogeneity

Diagnostic Checklist

- Confident HRCT diagnosis of honeycombing is specific for pulmonary fibrosis, & lung biopsy may be obviated

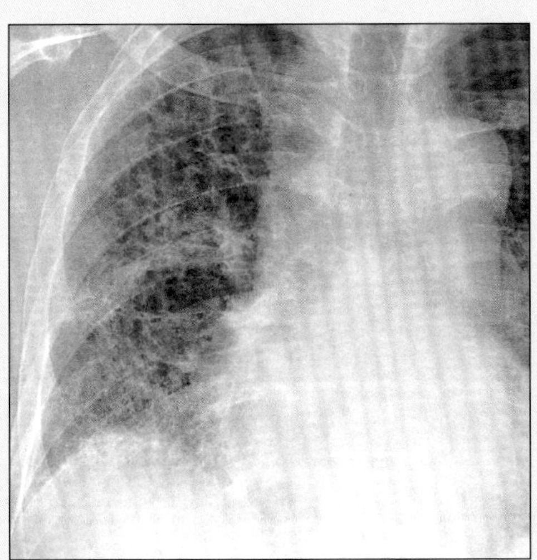

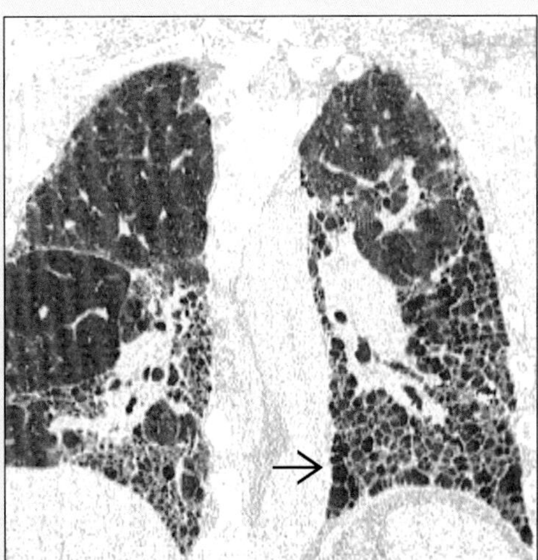

(Left) *PA chest radiograph of a patient with idiopathic pulmonary fibrosis and honeycomb lung shows low lung volumes and a profuse reticular pattern that correlates with findings of honeycomb cysts, traction bronchiectasis, and scattered areas of architectural distortion.* ***(Right)*** *Coronal HRCT of a patient with idiopathic pulmonary fibrosis shows asymmetric honeycombing ➔ predominantly involving the left lower lobe. Several tiers of honeycomb cysts are visible in the subpleural lung.*

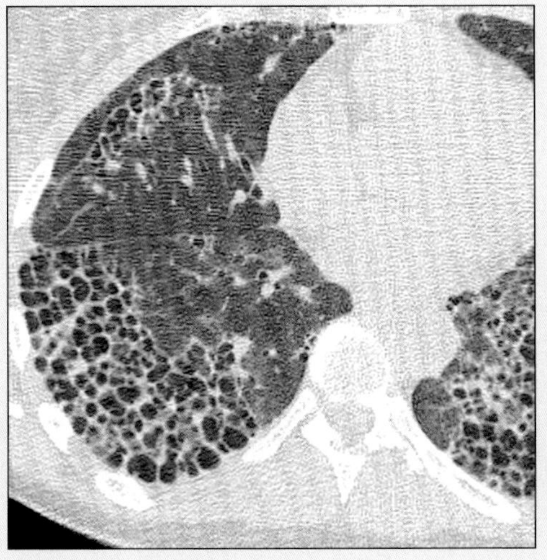

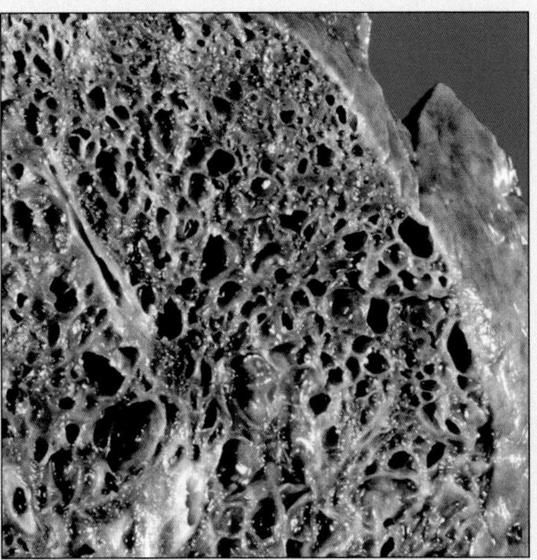

(Left) *Axial NECT of a patient with pulmonary fibrosis shows profuse bilateral subpleural clustered honeycomb cysts arranged in several tiers. The CT appearance is characteristic of honeycombing and consistent with advanced pulmonary fibrosis (end-stage lung).* ***(Right)*** *Cut section of a gross lung specimen shows honeycombing characterized by profuse honeycomb cysts separated by intervening fibrous tissue and associated with a nodular cobblestone-like pleural surface.*

INTERLOBULAR SEPTAL THICKENING

Key Facts

Terminology

- **Interlobular septal thickening**: Thickening of interlobular septa of secondary pulmonary lobule (SPL)
- Normal interlobular septa are not visible

Imaging

- Radiography
  - Thick interlobular septa visible as Kerley lines
  - **Kerley B lines**: Short lines perpendicular to pleura (1.5-2 cm long)
  - **Kerley A lines**: Lines 2-6 cm long in upper lung, directed from hilum toward lung periphery
- CT/HRCT
  - Thick interlobular septa
  - Surround & delineate SPL
  - Smooth or nodular septal thickening
  - Irregular septal thickening in pulmonary fibrosis

Top Differential Diagnoses

- Smooth interlobular septal thickening
  - Interstitial edema
  - Lymphangitic carcinomatosis
  - Alveolar lipoproteinosis: Associated with ground-glass opacity
  - Other interstitial lung diseases
- Nodular interlobular septal thickening
  - Lymphangitic carcinomatosis
  - Lymphoproliferative disorder
  - Sarcoidosis, silicosis & coal workers pneumoconiosis, & amyloidosis
- Irregular interlobular septal thickening
  - Pulmonary fibrosis, end-stage sarcoidosis

Diagnostic Checklist

- Interstitial edema is most common cause of interlobular septal thickening

*(**Left**) PA chest radiograph (coned down to the right lower lobe) of a patient with interstitial edema demonstrates smooth interlobular septal thickening manifesting as Kerley B lines ➡ located in the lung periphery and coursing perpendicular to the adjacent pleura. (**Right**) Coronal CECT of a patient with interstitial edema shows smooth thickening of the interlobular septa ➔. Interstitial edema is the most common cause of interlobular septal thickening.*

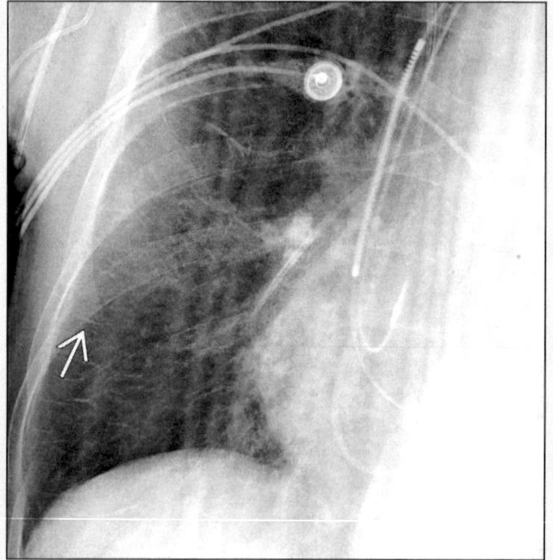

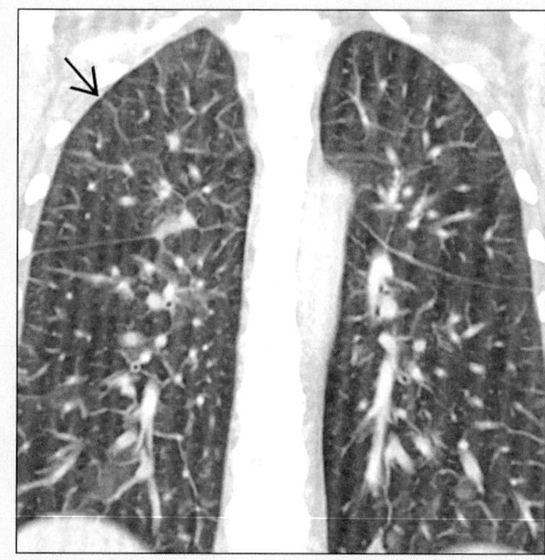

*(**Left**) Axial NECT of a patient with lymphangitic carcinomatosis shows asymmetric lung involvement with profuse right-sided centrilobular micronodules ➔, thick interlobular septa ➡, and extensive thickening of the bronchovascular bundles ➔. (**Right**) Axial NECT of a patient with pulmonary fibrosis shows right basilar reticular opacities secondary to irregular interlobular septal thickening ➔ with intervening intralobular lines.*

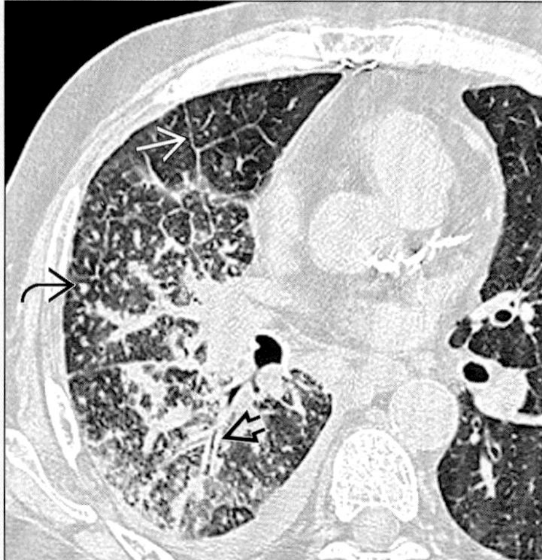

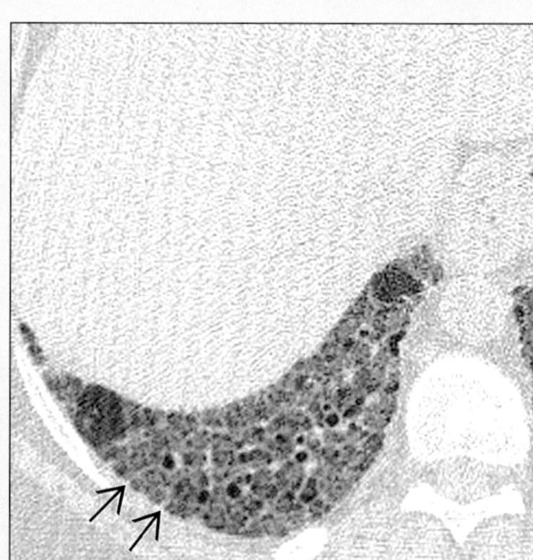

INTRALOBULAR LINES

Key Facts

Terminology
- **Intralobular lines**: Fine linear opacities identified within confines of secondary pulmonary lobule (SPL)
- There are no intralobular septa
  - Term "intralobular septal thickening" is erroneous

Imaging
- Radiography
  - Intralobular lines not visible
- CT/HRCT
  - Fine irregular reticular opacities
  - Separated by only a few millimeters
  - Located within confines of SPL
  - When numerous: Fine reticular pattern

Top Differential Diagnoses
- Idiopathic pulmonary fibrosis (IPF)
- Nonspecific interstitial pneumonia (NSIP)
- Fibrosis associated with collagen vascular disease
- Chronic hypersensitivity pneumonitis
- Sarcoidosis
- Asbestosis
- Alveolar lipoproteinosis

Pathology
- **Parenchymal (intralobular) interstitium**
  - Fine interstitial network of thin connective tissue fibers in alveolar walls
  - Supports structures of SPL
- **Intralobular lines**
  - Thickening of intralobular interstitium
  - Most commonly caused by fibrosis

Diagnostic Checklist
- Visualization of intralobular lines should suggest presence of interstitial fibrosis, & ancillary findings of fibrosis should be sought

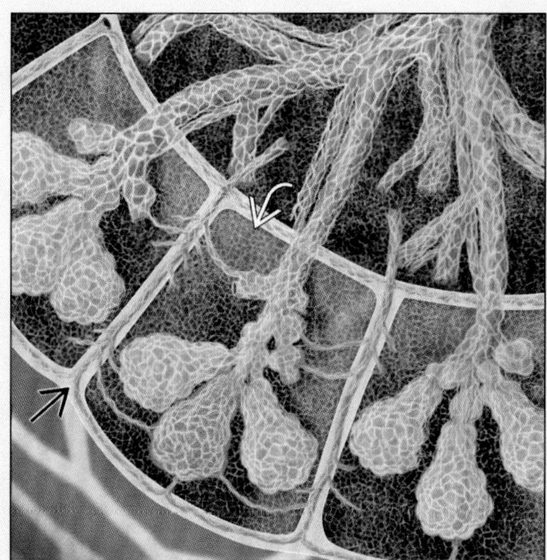

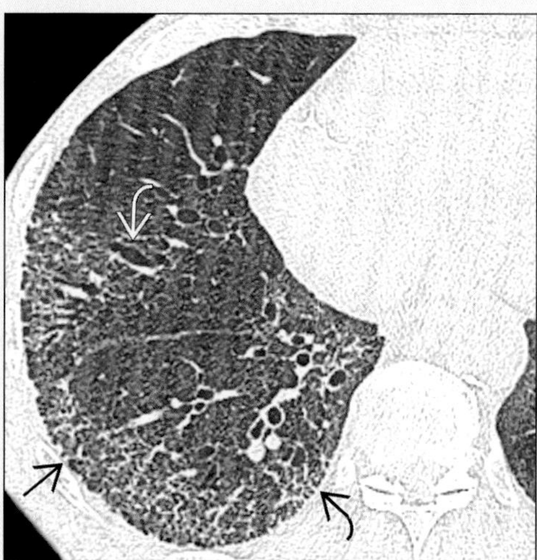

(Left) *Graphic shows the parenchymal and peripheral interstitium of the secondary pulmonary lobule (SPL). The peripheral interstitium extends along the interlobular septa and subpleural regions while the parenchymal interstitium forms a meshwork around alveoli and alveolar sacs within the secondary pulmonary lobule.* ***(Right)*** *Axial HRCT of a patient with scleroderma and fibrotic NSIP shows profuse interlobular septal thickening, intralobular lines, and traction bronchiectasis.*

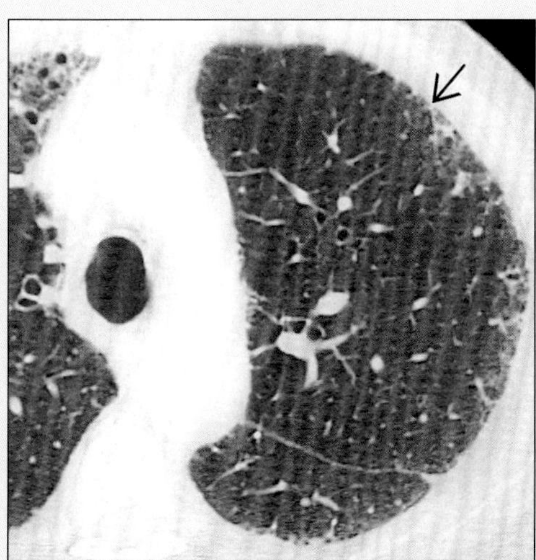

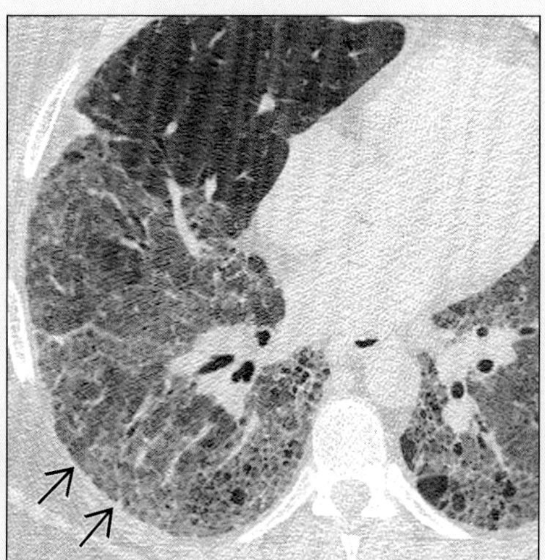

(Left) *Axial HRCT of a patient with early idiopathic pulmonary fibrosis (IPF) shows fine peripheral intralobular lines located within a few mm of each other, indicating early pulmonary fibrosis. Intralobular lines are located within the confines of the SPL.* ***(Right)*** *Axial HRCT of a patient with idiopathic pulmonary fibrosis shows fine linear and ground-glass opacities within the confines of the SPL demarcated by thickened interlobular septa. Note bilateral subtle honeycomb cysts.*

Key Facts

Terminology

- **Mass**: Thoracic lesion measuring > 3 cm in maximal diameter
- Term implies solid lesion, but necrosis & cavitation may occur
- Masses may be located in any anatomic compartment
  - Lung, pleura, mediastinum, chest wall, diaphragm

Imaging

- Radiography
  - Anatomic localization of lesion
  - Lung mass: Surrounded by lung parenchyma, well- or ill-defined, spiculated or lobular borders
  - Pleural mass: May exhibit obtuse angles with pleura & incomplete border sign
  - Mediastinal mass: Localization in mediastinum; focal vs. diffuse; use of lateral radiography for localization in a specific mediastinal compartment
  - Chest wall mass: Incomplete border sign; may exhibit skeletal erosion/destruction
- CT
  - Lung mass: Assessment of morphologic features & clinical staging (lymphadenopathy, metastases)
  - Pleural mass: Focal vs. multifocal; evaluation for local invasion, lymphadenopathy, pleural effusion
  - Chest wall mass: Assessment & characterization of skeletal &/or soft tissue involvement

Top Differential Diagnoses

- Lung: Lung cancer, lung abscess, metastasis
- Pleura: Localized fibrous tumor of pleura, metastasis
- Chest wall: Metastasis, chondrosarcoma, myeloma

Diagnostic Checklist

- Thoracic masses are likely to be malignant
- Exact anatomic origin of very large thoracic masses may be difficult to determine

*(**Left**) PA chest radiograph of an 82-year-old woman who presented with malaise shows a left mid lung zone lesion. Given a size > 3 cm, the lesion is characterized as a mass. The most likely diagnosis is primary lung cancer. (**Right**) PA chest radiograph of an elderly man with myasthenia gravis shows an enormous lobular mediastinal mass that extends to both sides of midline. Lateral chest radiograph (not shown) confirmed location in the anterior mediastinal compartment, consistent with known thymoma.*

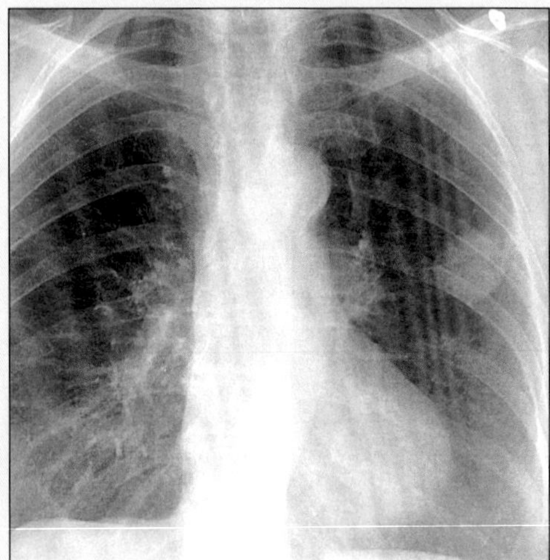

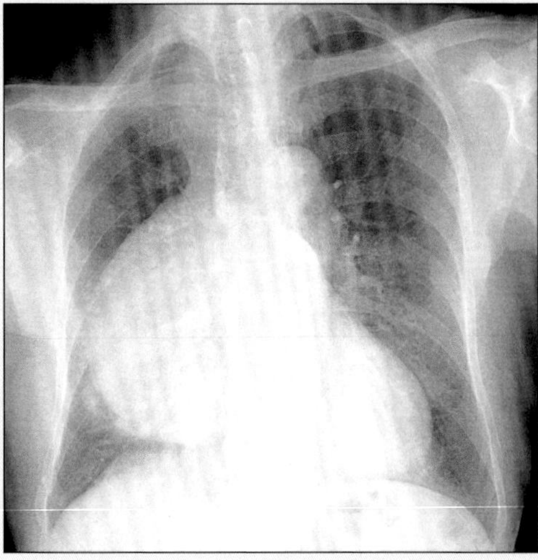

*(**Left**) Composite image with PA (left) and lateral (right) chest radiographs of a patient with a large localized fibrous tumor of the pleura shows a lesion with discrepant margin visualization on these orthogonal images, suggesting an extrapulmonary location. (**Right**) PA chest radiograph of a patient with advanced cancer shows a right chest wall mass that destroys the adjacent right 5th rib ⮫ and mediastinal lymphadenopathy ➡, both consistent with metastases. A mass may occur in any thoracic compartment.*

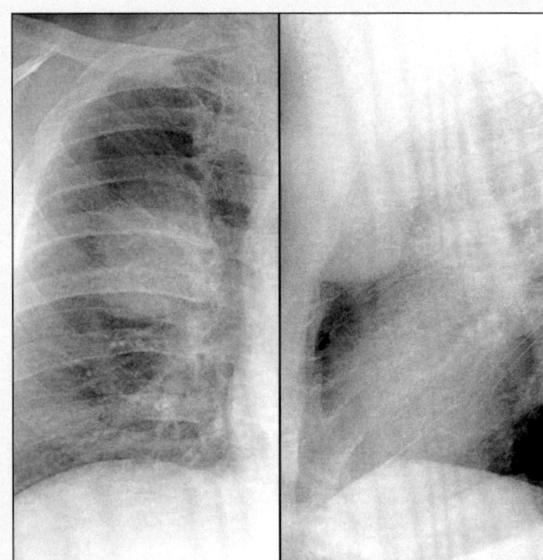

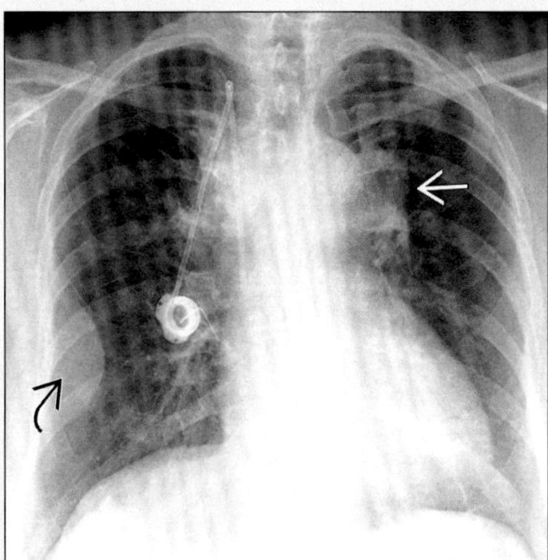

Key Facts

Terminology

- **Miliary pattern**
  - Profuse tiny pulmonary nodules (micronodules)
  - Discrete, round, well defined
  - Size: Uniform, ≤ 3 mm
  - Diffuse distribution in both lungs
- Synonym
  - **Miliary nodules**
- Term "**miliary**"
  - Derived from millet seeds
  - Refers to nodular lesions having size & appearance reminiscent of millet seeds

Imaging

- Radiography
  - Profuse, bilateral, tiny, discrete pulmonary micronodules
  - Diffuse distribution
  - May be subtle
- CT/HRCT
  - Profuse bilateral, discrete, well-defined micronodules
  - **Random** (diffuse & uniform) distribution with no specific relationship to secondary pulmonary lobule

Top Differential Diagnoses

- Hematogenous metastatic disease
- Hematogenous spread of infection, typically in immunocompromised patients
  - Tuberculosis
  - Fungal disease
- Sarcoidosis
  - Atypical sarcoidosis may exhibit miliary pattern

Diagnostic Checklist

- Suggest hematogenous dissemination of disease in patients with miliary pattern on radiography or CT

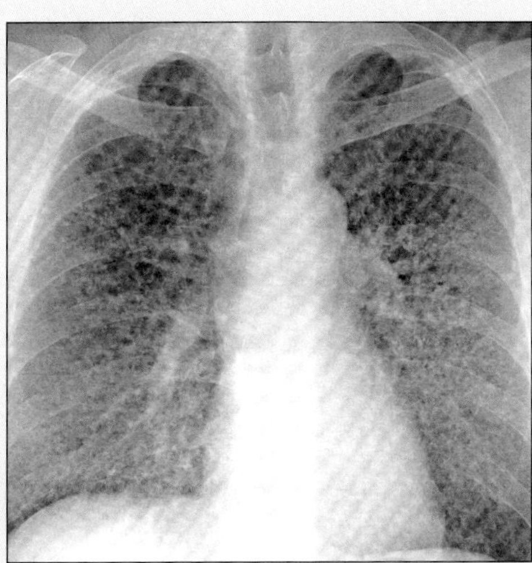

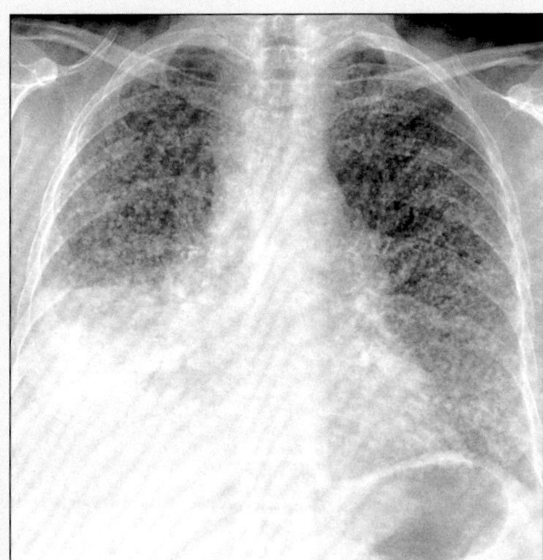

(Left) *PA chest radiograph of a patient with disseminated coccidioidomycosis shows bilateral, profuse, well-defined miliary micronodules, consistent with hematogenous dissemination of disease.* ***(Right)*** *PA chest radiograph of a patient with advanced lung adenocarcinoma shows middle and right lower lobe consolidation and a profuse, bilateral miliary pattern consistent with miliary metastases. The miliary pattern in a patient with known malignancy suggests metastases or opportunistic infection.*

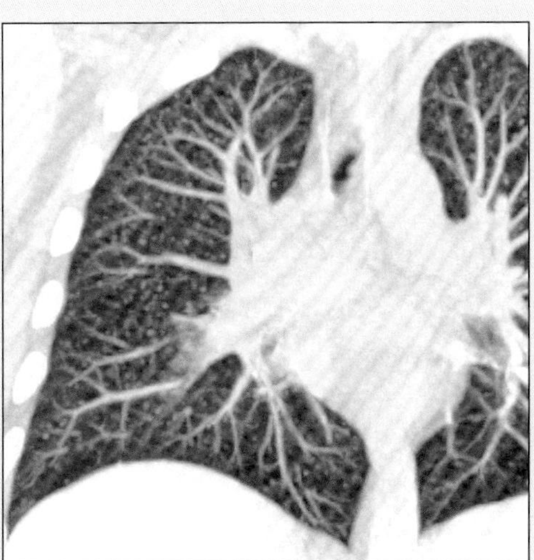

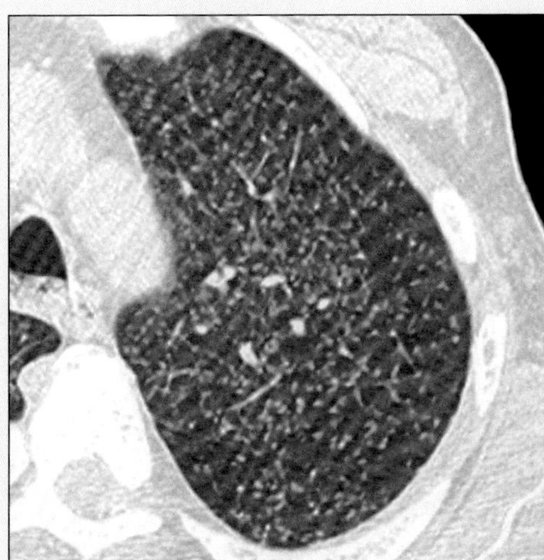

(Left) *Coronal NECT (MIP image) of a patient with rheumatoid arthritis undergoing treatment with adalimumab shows a miliary pattern with profuse tiny bilateral micronodules. Biopsy revealed miliary histoplasmosis.* ***(Right)*** *Axial NECT of a patient with miliary tuberculosis shows profuse pulmonary micronodules producing a miliary pattern. The nodules exhibit a random distribution with respect to the secondary pulmonary lobule. The miliary pattern is consistent with hematogenous dissemination of disease.*

MOSAIC ATTENUATION

Key Facts

Terminology

- **Mosaic attenuation**
  - Heterogeneous lung attenuation with alternating areas of low & high attenuation
- Synonyms
  - Mosaic perfusion
  - Mosaic oligemia
- Mosaic attenuation is more inclusive & the preferred term

Imaging

- Radiography
  - Typically normal chest radiography
  - Identification of associated findings such as bronchiectasis
- CT/HRCT
  - Heterogeneous patchwork-like lung attenuation
  - Areas of low attenuation alternating with areas of higher attenuation
  - May identify reduced vessel caliber in areas of hyperlucency
  - Bronchiectasis, bronchial wall thickening, & mucus plugging suggest airway disease

Top Differential Diagnoses

- Patchy interstitial lung disease
- Cystic fibrosis
- Bronchiectasis
- Constrictive bronchiolitis & air-trapping
- Hypersensitivity pneumonitis
- Occlusive vascular disease
  - Chronic pulmonary thromboembolic disease
  - Pulmonary hypertension

Diagnostic Checklist

- Consider expiratory HRCT for assessment of patients with mosaic attenuation & suspected constrictive bronchiolitis

*(**Left**) Axial NECT of a patient with subacute hypersensitivity pneumonitis shows mild mosaic attenuation of the lung parenchyma without evidence of consolidation. This pattern of mosaic attenuation may be accentuated by expiratory imaging. (**Right**) Axial NECT of a patient with subacute hypersensitivity pneumonitis shows heterogeneous lung attenuation with a patchwork of lower and higher attenuation areas. In this case, heterogeneity may be accentuated by patchy ground-glass opacity.*

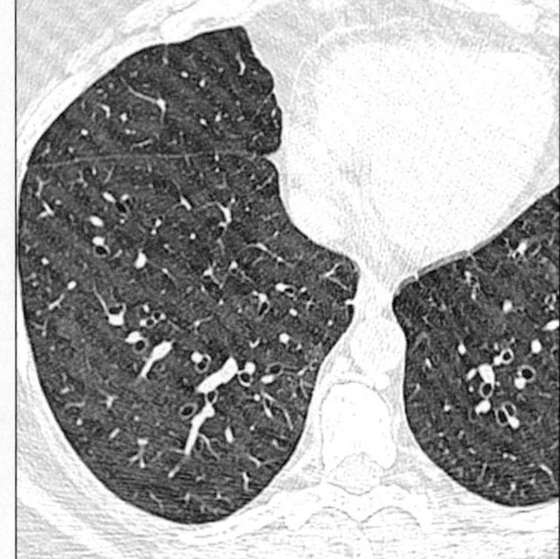

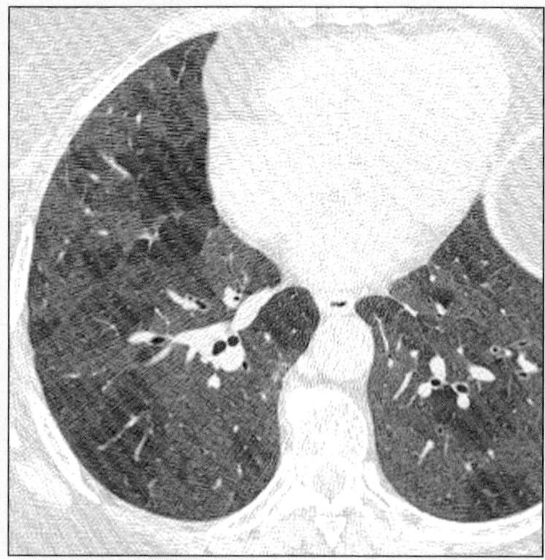

*(**Left**) Axial NECT of a patient with cystic fibrosis shows bilateral mosaic attenuation/ perfusion with areas of low attenuation ↗ alternating with areas of higher attenuation →. Note bronchiectasis and mucus plugs ➡. (**Right**) Coronal CECT of a patient with chronic pulmonary thromboembolic disease shows mosaic attenuation secondary to mosaic perfusion. Note enlarged vascular caliber ➡ in high-attenuation areas. Mosaic attenuation may occur with small airway or vascular disease.*

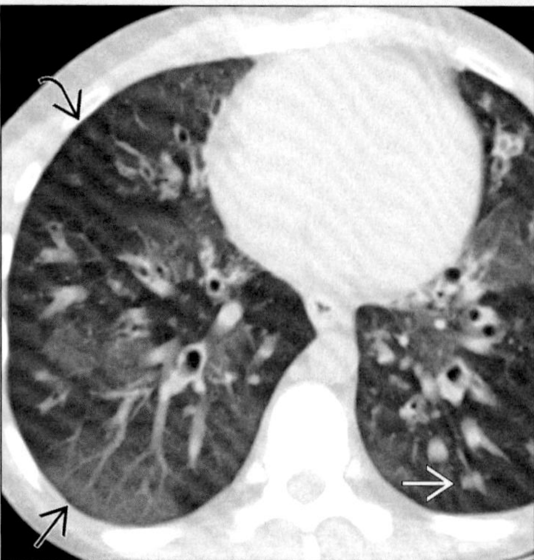

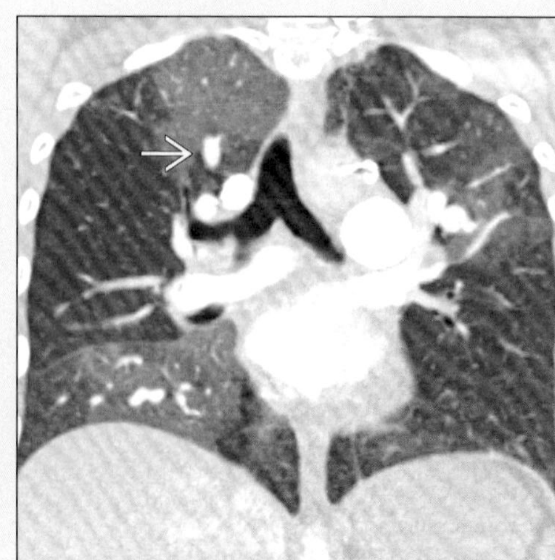

Key Facts

Terminology

- **Nodule**
  - Rounded opacity of variable border characteristics
  - Size: ≤ 3 cm
- **Micronodule**
  - Rounded opacity measuring < 3 mm
- **Pseudonodule**
  - Radiographic nodule mimics: Nipple, rib/skin/ pleural lesion, artifact, summation of markings

Imaging

- Radiography
  - Rounded opacity surrounded by lung ≤ 3 cm
  - May exhibit intrinsic calcification
- CT
  - Rounded opacity of variable borders ≤ 3 cm
  - Nodules characterized as solid or subsolid
  - **Solid** nodules are of soft tissue attenuation
  - **Subsolid** nodules have solid & ground-glass opacity components
  - Subsolid nodules characterized as **nonsolid (ground-glass)** or **part-solid (semisolid)**

Top Differential Diagnoses

- Solitary pulmonary nodule
  - Granuloma, carcinoma, carcinoid, metastasis, hamartoma
  - Pseudonodule must be excluded
- Multiple small nodules
  - Characterization by distribution as centrilobular, perilymphatic, or random

Diagnostic Checklist

- Solitary nodules are characterized as likely benign, possibly malignant, or indeterminate
- Indeterminate nodules require further evaluation with follow-up imaging or tissue sampling

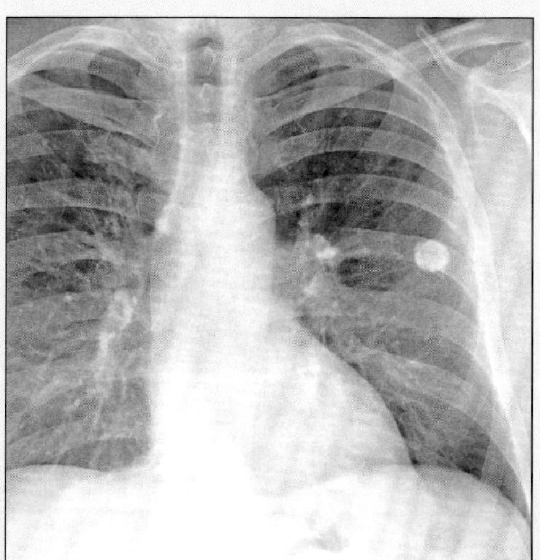

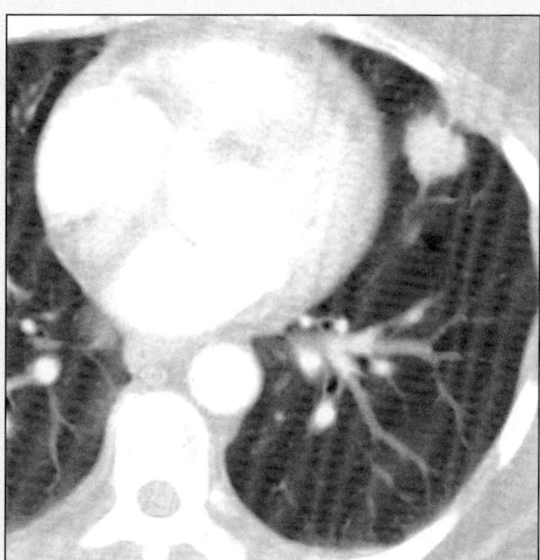

(Left) *PA chest radiograph of an asymptomatic man shows a round, densely calcified pulmonary nodule in the left mid lung and ipsilateral calcified hilar lymph nodes. The findings are consistent with remote granulomatous infection, and no further evaluation is required.* ***(Right)*** *Axial CECT of an asymptomatic smoker shows a solid lingular nodule with spiculated borders and focal pleural retraction. The finding is highly concerning for primary lung cancer. The lesion is accessible to image-guided biopsy.*

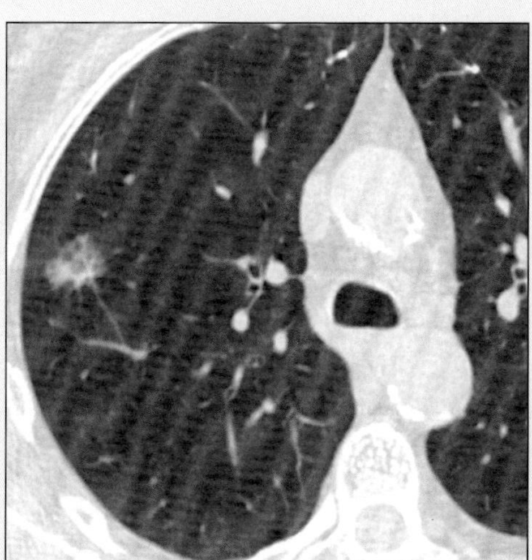

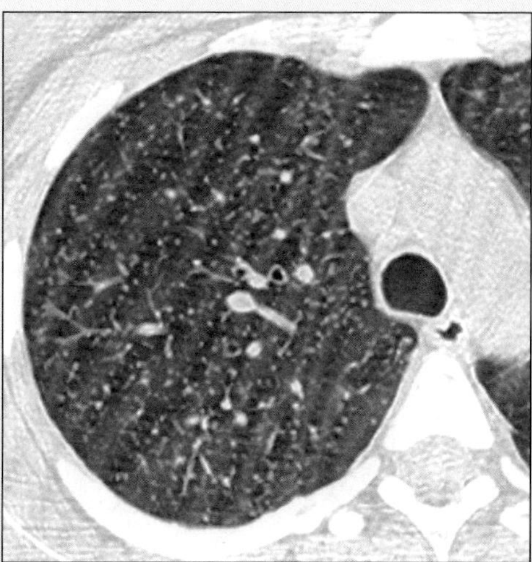

(Left) *Axial NECT of an asymptomatic smoker shows a right upper lobe part-solid nodule on a background of centrilobular emphysema. The nodule was stable for over a year, but likely represents an indolent invasive adenocarcinoma.* ***(Right)*** *Axial NECT of an immunocompromised patient with fever shows profuse miliary micronodules. The nodules exhibit a random distribution with respect to the secondary pulmonary lobule and represent hematogenous dissemination of tuberculosis.*

Key Facts

Terminology

- **Perilymphatic distribution**
  - Distribution of disease process along anatomic location of pulmonary lymphatics
- Lymphatics of secondary pulmonary lobule (SPL)
  - Peribronchovascular lymphatics: Along vessels & airways of lobular core
  - Perilobular lymphatics: Along interlobular septa
  - Visceral pleural lymphatics, including fissures

Imaging

- Radiography
  - May manifest as interlobular septal thickening, reticular opacities or reticulonodular opacities
- CT
  - Peribronchovascular thickening
  - Interlobular septal thickening
  - Subpleural thickening
  - May be smooth or nodular
  - Perilymphatic nodules: Well-defined micronodules, may coalesce into larger nodules

Top Differential Diagnoses

- Sarcoidosis
  - Predominantly peribronchovascular & subpleural micronodules
  - Upper lobe predominant involvement
- Lymphangitic carcinomatosis
  - Predominantly along interlobular septa & peribronchovascular interstitium
  - Smooth or nodular septal thickening
- Silicosis & coal worker's pneumoconiosis
  - Predominant involvement of subpleural & peribronchovascular regions
  - Symmetric posterior upper lobe predominant involvement

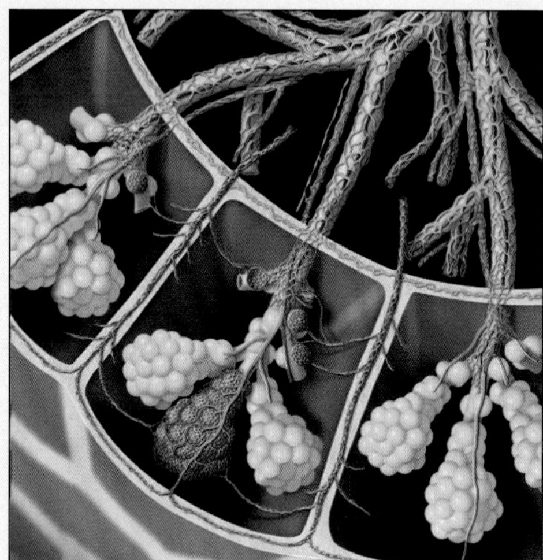

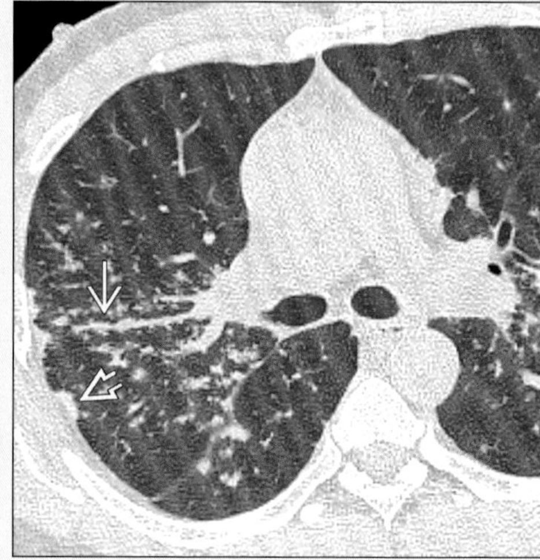

*(**Left**) Graphic shows the complex lymphatic channels of the secondary pulmonary lobule. Peribronchovascular lymphatics course along the airway walls to the level of the respiratory bronchioles. Perilobular lymphatics course in the interlobular septa and anastomose with subpleural lymphatics. (**Right**) Axial HRCT of a patient with sarcoidosis shows perilymphatic nodules and micronodules along bronchovascular structures ➔ and in subpleural regions ⇨.*

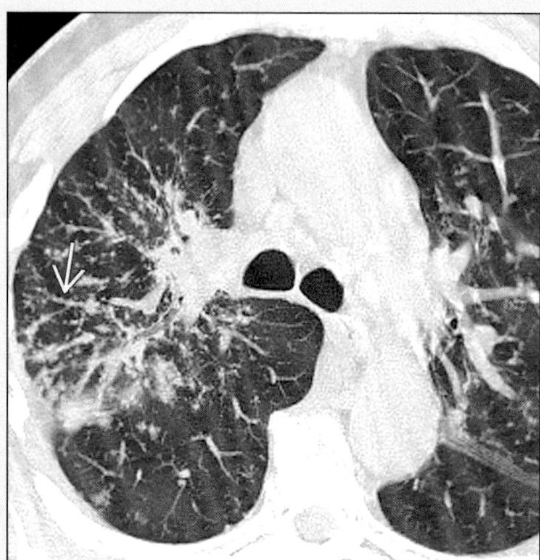

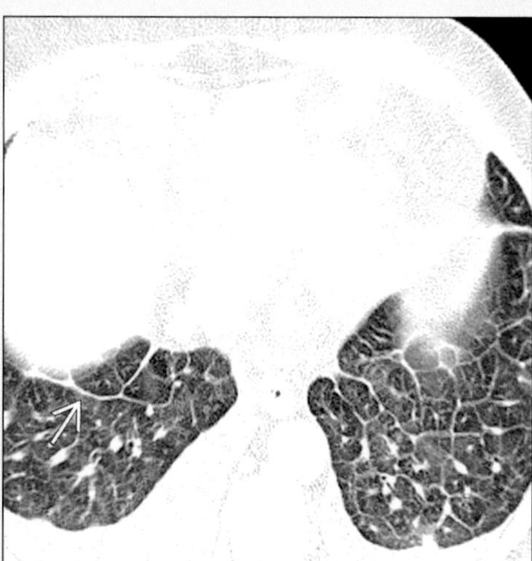

*(**Left**) Axial HRCT of a patient with sarcoidosis shows perilymphatic micronodules ➔ clustered along vessels, bronchi, interlobular septa, and subpleural regions. Perilymphatic nodules follow the distribution of the lymphatics of the SPL. (**Right**) Axial NECT shows lymphangitic carcinomatosis manifesting as smooth interlobular septal thickening ➔ with scattered involvement of the central lobular cores of various SPLs, consistent with tumor and edema in the perilymphatic regions.*

Key Facts

Terminology

- **Pneumatocele**
  - Thin-walled
  - Air-filled
  - Surrounded by lung parenchyma
  - May be multiple
- Etiology
  - "1-way" valve airway obstruction
  - Local necrosis of airway wall
  - Subsequent air dissection into peribronchovascular interstitium
- Natural history
  - Size increase over days to weeks
  - Typically resolves

Imaging

- Radiography
  - Thin-walled cystic structure in lung parenchyma
  - May be multiple
- CT
  - Thin-walled parenchymal cystic structure
  - May be multifocal
  - Identification of associated conditions: Consolidation, ground-glass opacity, pneumothorax
  - May be indistinguishable from cysts or bullae

Top Differential Diagnoses

- Acute pneumonia
  - *Pneumocystis* pneumonia: Immunocompromised patient, surrounding ground-glass opacity, susceptible to secondary spontaneous pneumothorax
  - Staphylococcal pneumonia: Children
- Trauma
  - Must differentiate from pulmonary laceration
- Hydrocarbon aspiration

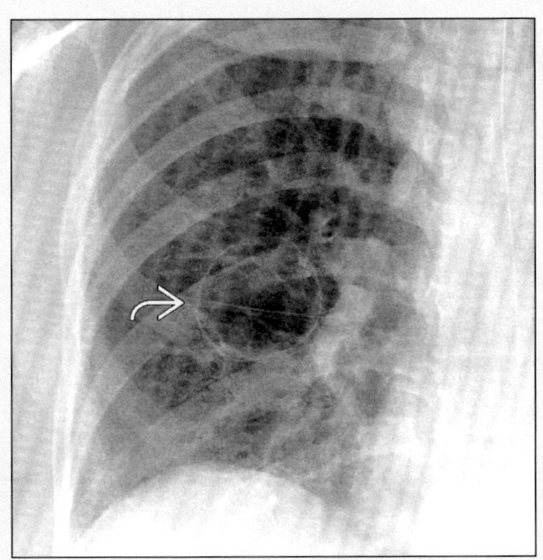

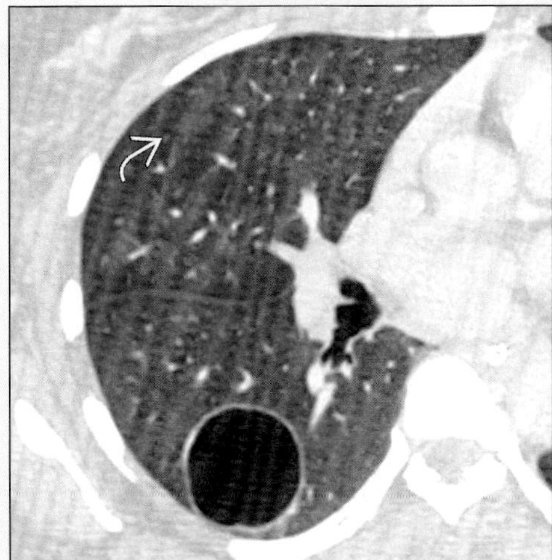

(Left) *PA chest radiograph of an asymptomatic patient evaluated for resolving pulmonary infection shows a well-defined, thin-walled cystic structure ➦ in the right lower lobe. Based on the evolution of the abnormality, the presumptive diagnosis of pneumatocele was made.* ***(Right)*** *Axial NECT of the same patient demonstrates the right lower lobe pneumatocele that exhibits internal air and a thin wall. Note patchy middle lobe centrilobular ground-glass opacities ➦ consistent with resolving infection.*

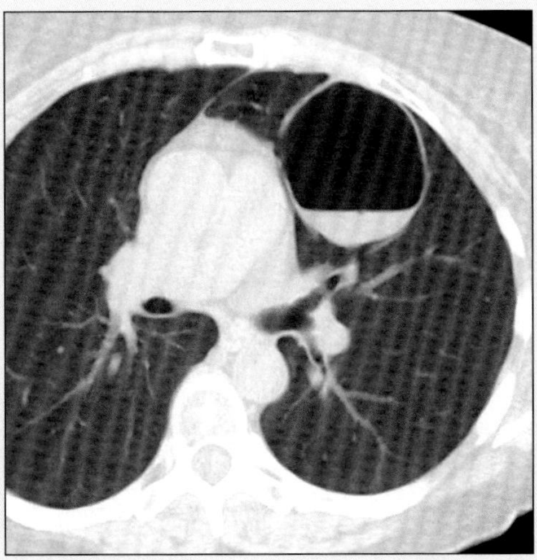

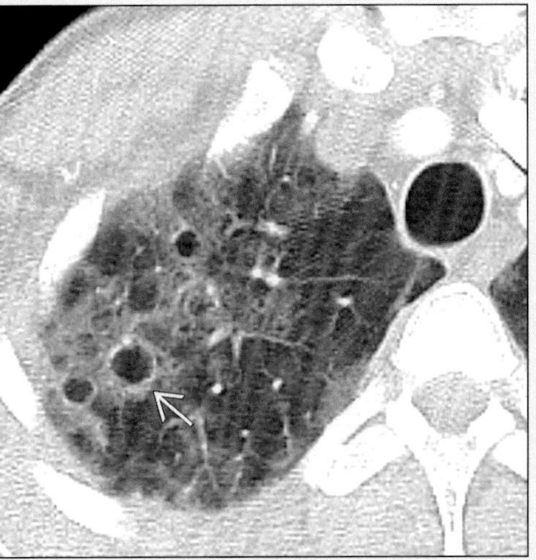

(Left) *Axial NECT shows a left upper lobe pneumatocele manifesting as a large, thin-walled pulmonary cyst containing an air-fluid level. Pneumatoceles are indistinguishable from bullae on imaging but typically resolve with time.* ***(Right)*** *Axial NECT of a patient with HIV-related Pneumocystis pneumonia shows right upper lobe ground-glass opacities and several thin-walled, air-filled cystic structures ➡, consistent with pneumatoceles. Affected patients are at risk for spontaneous pneumothorax.*

RETICULAR PATTERN

Key Facts

Terminology

- **Reticular pattern**
  - Multiple interlacing irregular linear opacities
  - Fine, medium, coarse reticulation
  - Indicative of interstitial lung disease (e.g., fibrosis)

Imaging

- Radiography
  - Multiple irregular linear opacities, resembling fisherman's net
  - Cystic lung disease with summation of cyst walls may result in similar pattern
- CT/HRCT
  - Intralobular lines
  - Irregular interlobular septal thickening
  - Traction bronchiectasis/bronchiolectasis
  - Architectural distortion
  - Honeycomb lung

Top Differential Diagnoses

- Idiopathic pulmonary fibrosis (IPF)
- Nonspecific interstitial pneumonia (NSIP)
- Fibrosis associated with collagen vascular disease
- Chronic hypersensitivity pneumonitis
- Sarcoidosis
- Asbestosis

Pathology

- Indicative of interstitial fibrosis
- Reticular pattern does not indicate honeycombing
- Reticulonodular pattern
  - Summation of reticular & micronodular patterns

Diagnostic Checklist

- HRCT is optimal imaging modality for evaluation of symptomatic patients with reticular pattern on radiography

__(Left)__ PA chest radiograph of an elderly patient with idiopathic pulmonary fibrosis shows fine basilar reticular opacities. __(Right)__ Coronal NECT of the same patient shows that the basilar reticular pattern corresponds to basilar subpleural honeycomb cysts and traction bronchiectasis. Although visualization of a reticular pattern does not necessarily correlate with honeycombing, in this case the reticulations correspond to honeycomb cysts.

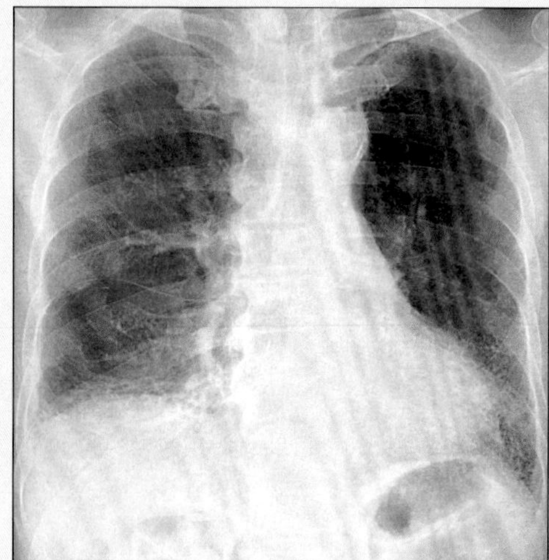

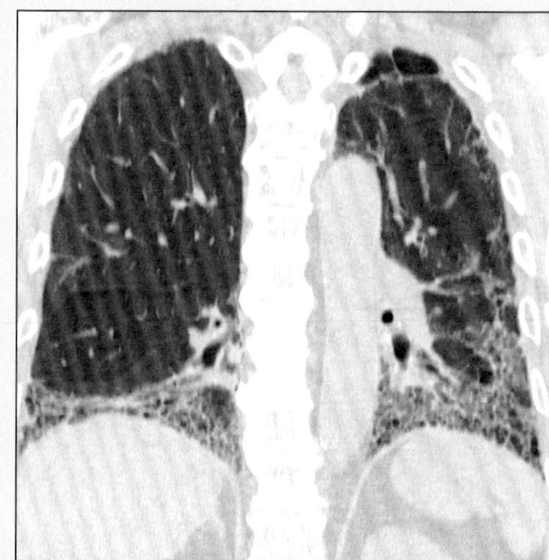

__(Left)__ PA chest radiograph of a patient with end-stage sarcoidosis shows profuse bilateral reticular opacities manifesting as fine interlacing linear opacities. The reticular pattern is consistent with pulmonary fibrosis. __(Right)__ Axial NECT of the same patient shows a reticular pattern characterized by thickening of the interlobular septa ➡ and scattered intralobular lines ⇨. The reticular pattern typically indicates pulmonary fibrosis.

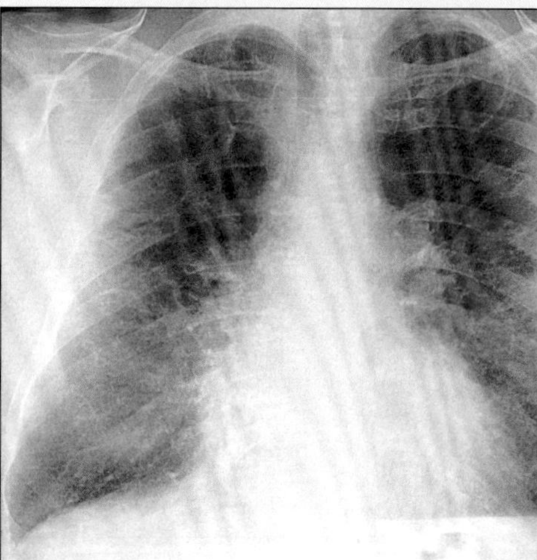

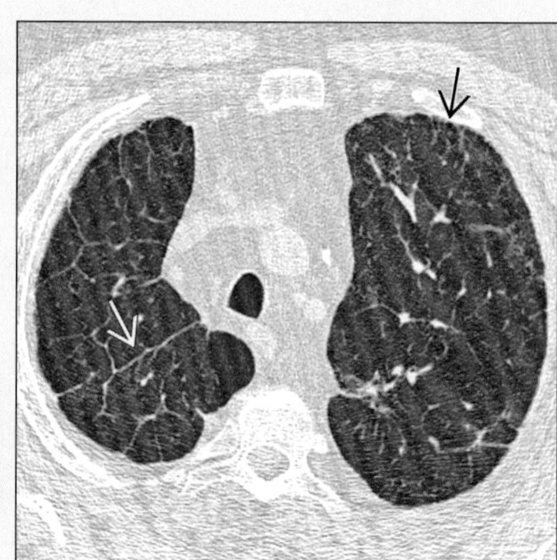

Key Facts

Terminology

- **Secondary pulmonary lobule (SPL)**
  - Smallest discrete unit of lung surrounded by connective tissue & interlobular septa
  - Contains variable number of acini
  - Supplied by lobular bronchiole & branches, lobular artery & branches, & surrounding lymphatics
  - Marginated by interlobular septa containing pulmonary veins & lymphatics
  - Interlobular septa best developed peripherally in anterior, lateral, & paramediastinal regions of upper & middle lobes
- Morphology
  - Irregularly polyhedral
  - Variable shapes
- Size range
  - 1-2.5 cm in diameter
- Synonym: **Lobule**

Imaging

- Radiography: SPL not normally visible
- CT/HRCT
  - SPL not normally visible
  - Occasional identification of interlobular septa
  - Occasional identification of central lobular region (lobular artery)
  - Enhanced visualization of SPLs in disease states

Pathology

- Disease processes described with reference to SPL
- Emphysema
  - Centrilobular, panlobular
- Nodules
  - Centrilobular, perilymphatic

Diagnostic Checklist

- Understanding of SPL anatomy is critical for expert interpretation of HRCT

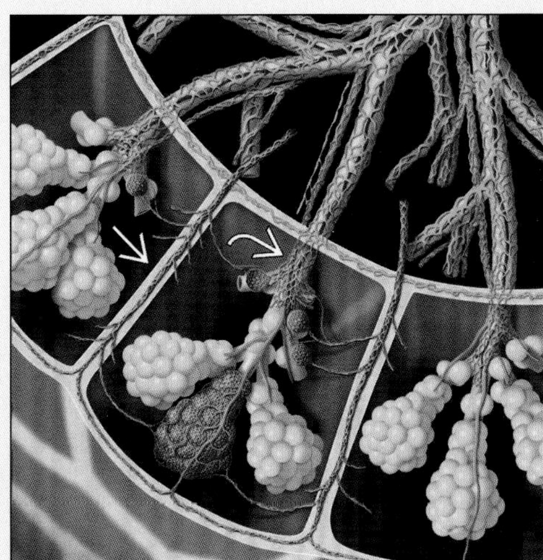

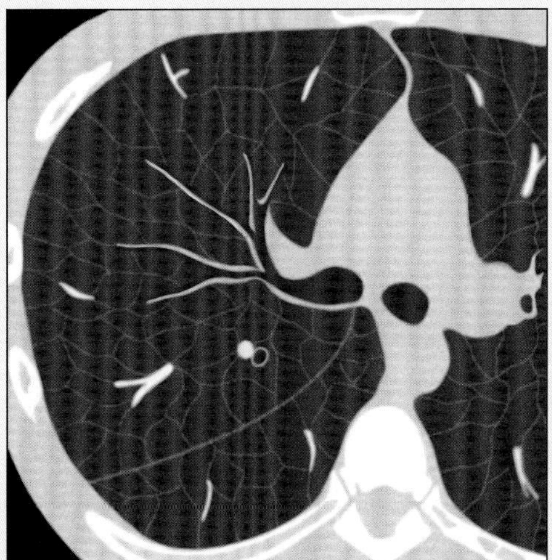

(Left) *Graphic shows the morphology and components of the secondary pulmonary lobule, the smallest structural lung unit surrounded by connective tissue septa. It is supplied by the lobular core (bronchiole and artery) ➩ and surrounded by connective tissue septa ➡ that contain the pulmonary veins and the septal lymphatics.* ***(Right)*** *Graphic depicts a normal HRCT with superimposed lines representing interlobular septa outlining normal secondary pulmonary lobules, which are occasionally visualized on normal HRCT.*

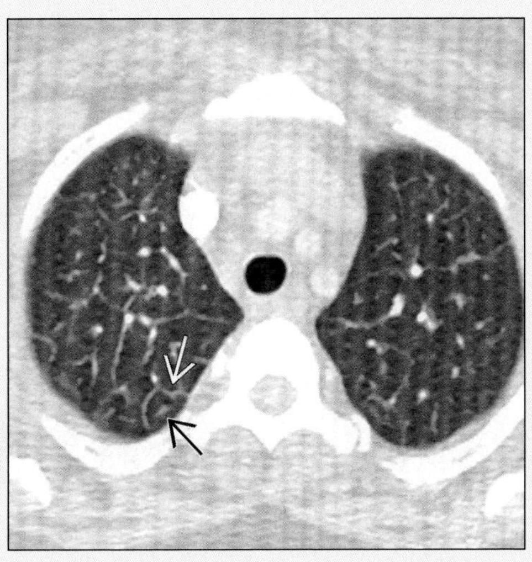

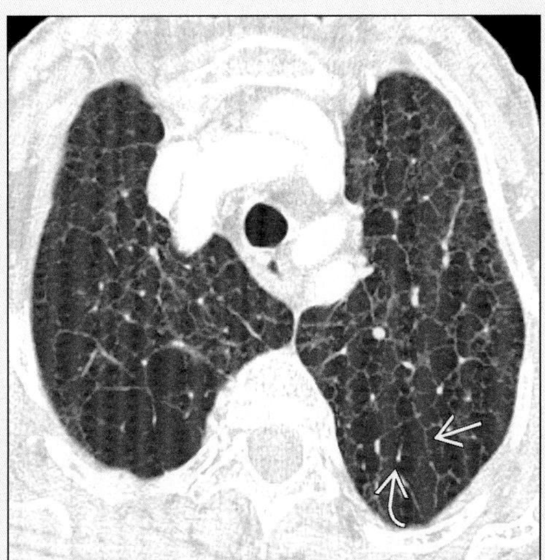

(Left) *Axial NECT of a patient with interstitial edema shows mild smooth thickening of the interlobular septa ➡ bounding the secondary pulmonary lobules and the central lobular artery ⇨ at the lobular core.* ***(Right)*** *Axial CECT shows extensive centrilobular emphysema. The resultant lung destruction outlines several secondary pulmonary lobules identified by visualization of the interlobular septa ➡ and the lobular arteries ➩ manifesting as central dots within the destroyed lung parenchyma.*

TRACTION BRONCHIECTASIS

Key Facts

Terminology

- **Traction bronchiectasis**
  - Bronchial dilatation secondary to fibrosis
- **Traction bronchiolectasis**
  - Bronchiolar dilatation secondary to fibrosis

Imaging

- Radiography
  - Insensitive for diagnosis of bronchiectasis
  - Clustered ring shadows
  - Clustered tram-line opacities
  - Associated architectural distortion
- CT/HRCT
  - Dilated bronchi, may exhibit varicoid morphology
  - Traction bronchiolectasis: Dilated small airways near pleural surface (within 2 cm)
  - Identification & evaluation of surrounding fibrosis
  - Usually seen in association with architectural distortion & honeycomb lung
  - May mimic honeycomb lung on axial imaging
  - Absence of associated infection, bronchiolitis, & mucus plugging

Top Differential Diagnoses

- Idiopathic pulmonary fibrosis (IPF)
- Fibrotic nonspecific interstitial pneumonia (NSIP)
- End-stage sarcoidosis
- Chronic hypersensitivity pneumonitis
- Radiation fibrosis
- Acute respiratory distress syndrome (ARDS)

Pathology

- Radial traction on airway walls by peribronchial/ peribronchiolar retractile fibrosis

Diagnostic Checklist

- Identification of traction bronchiectasis allows diagnosis of fibrosis in absence of honeycombing

*(**Left**) Axial NECT of a patient with scleroderma and fibrotic nonspecific pneumonia (NSIP) shows bibasilar traction bronchiectasis ➡ and bronchiolectasis. Bronchiolectasis ➦ is characterized by dilated airways within 1-2 cm of the pleural surface. In this case, there is surrounding ground-glass opacity. (**Right**) Axial NECT of a patient with scleroderma and fibrotic NSIP demonstrates bibasilar traction bronchiectasis ➡ and bronchiolectasis ➦ with surrounding reticular opacities indicating fibrosis.*

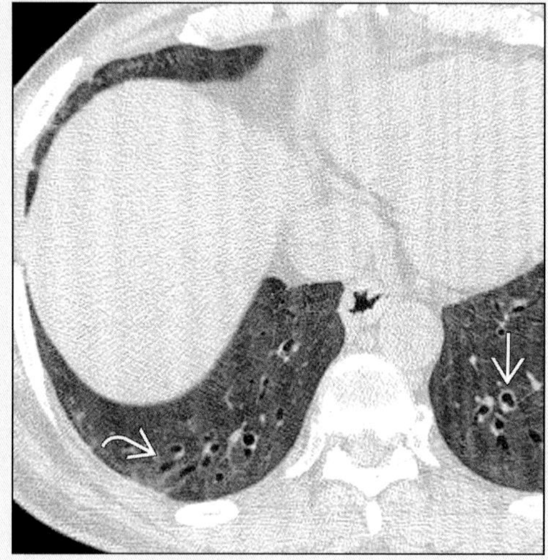

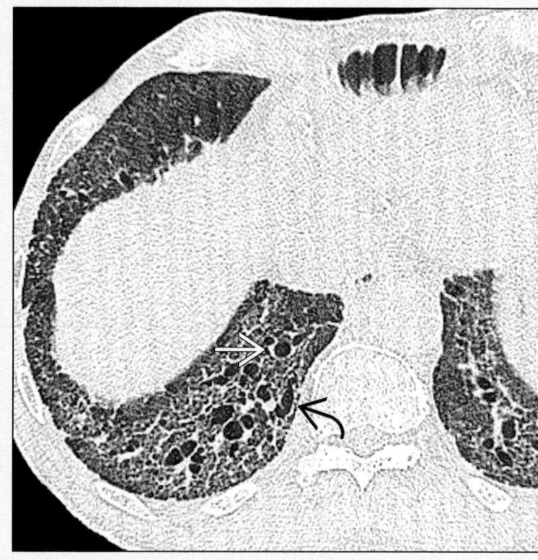

*(**Left**) Coronal NECT of a patient with IPF shows architectural distortion and peripheral honeycomb cysts ➦. Note the varicoid appearance of right mid lung zone bronchiectasis ➡ and basilar traction bronchiolectasis ➡. (**Right**) Coronal NECT MinIP image of a patient with scleroderma and nonspecific interstitial pneumonia shows marked bibasilar traction bronchiectasis and bronchiolectasis. Such findings, when severe, could mimic honeycombing on axial imaging.*

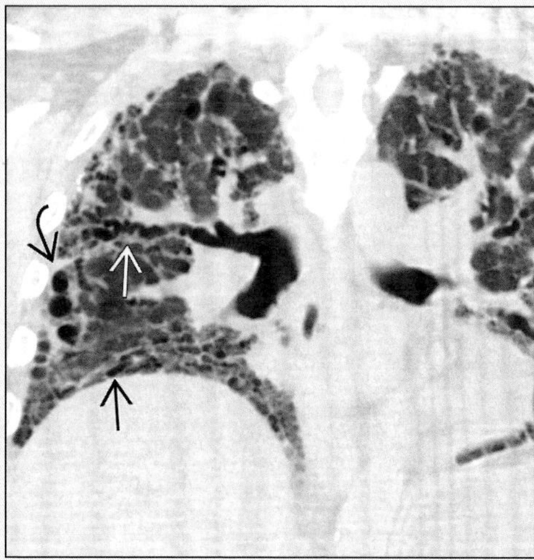

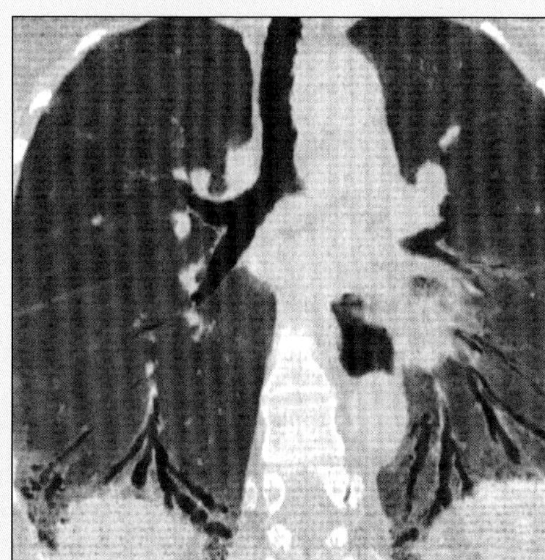

Key Facts

Terminology
- **Tree-in-bud pattern**
  - Centrilobular nodular/linear branching opacities
  - Resembles budding tree
- Synonym: **Tree-in-bud opacities**

Imaging
- Radiography
  - Tree-in-bud opacities not visible
- CT/HRCT
  - Small centrilobular nodules in lung periphery (5-10 cm from pleura); contiguous with short linear or branching opacities
  - Y- or V-shaped
- Correlation of tree-in-bud opacity
  - **Stalks**: Dilated centrilobular bronchioles
  - **Buds**: Peribronchiolar inflammatory tissue

Top Differential Diagnoses
- Infectious bronchiolitis
  - Bacteria, mycobacteria, mycoplasma, viruses, fungi
- Bronchiectasis, cystic fibrosis
- Aspiration
- Diffuse panbronchiolitis
- Microangiopathic arteriolar disease

Pathology
- Dilated fluid-filled centrilobular bronchioles
  - Mucoid impaction, inflammation, fibrosis
  - Arterial lesions less common

Diagnostic Checklist
- Implies high yield for sputum culture &/or bronchoalveolar lavage for diagnosis
- Association with cavitation suggests active tuberculosis

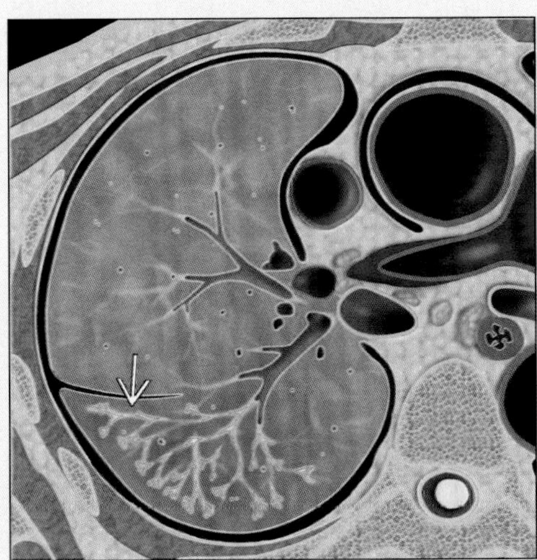
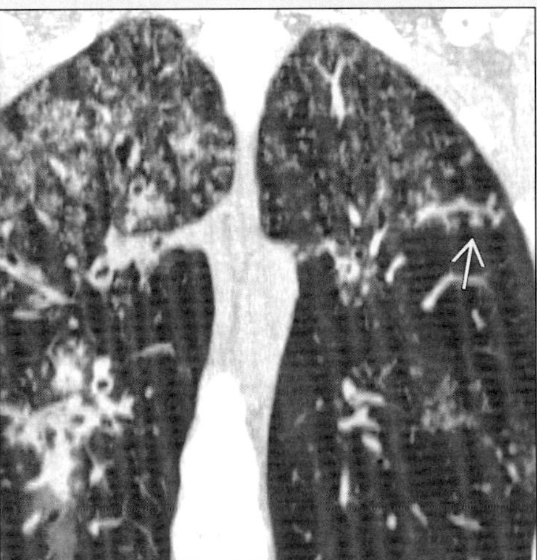

(Left) *Graphic shows the anatomic basis for the tree-in-bud pattern. This finding typically reflects inflamed, dilated fluid-filled centrilobular bronchioles. The stalks ➡ represent dilated centrilobular bronchioles, and the buds represent peribronchiolar inflammation.* ***(Right)*** *Coronal NECT of a patient with tuberculosis shows profuse upper lobe predominant centrilobular micronodules. Tree-in-bud opacities ➡ are consistent with endobronchial dissemination of infection. Sputum analysis showed acid-fast bacilli.*

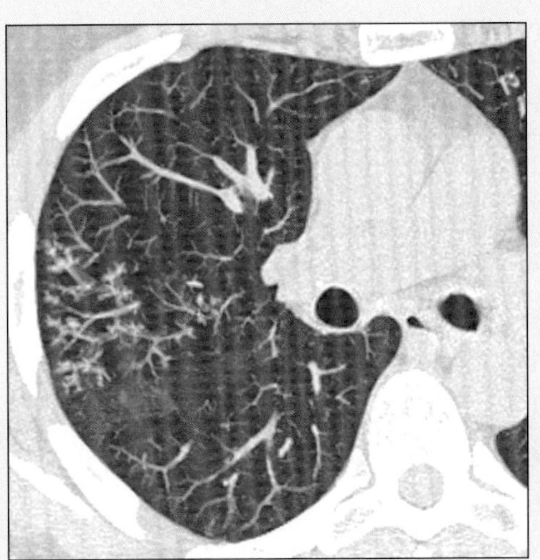
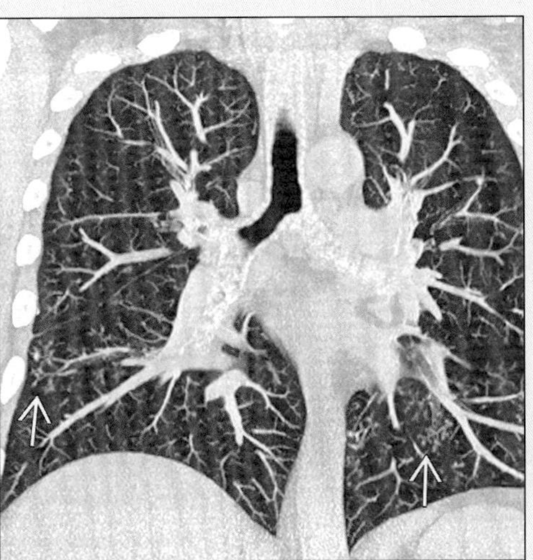

(Left) *Axial NECT (MIP image) of a patient with infectious cellular bronchiolitis shows a cluster of right upper lobe tree-in-bud opacities reflecting associated bronchiolar and peribronchiolar inflammation.* ***(Right)*** *Coronal NECT of the same patient (MIP image) shows multifocal tree-in-bud opacities ➡ in the lower lobes. Patients with the tree-in-bud pattern typically have pulmonary infection and should undergo sputum analysis for identification of the organism. (Courtesy S. Rossi, MD.)*

APPROACH TO CHEST RADIOGRAPHIC AND CT SIGNS

Introduction

The term "Aunt Minnie," coined by Dr. Ed Neuhauser and popularized by Dr. Benjamin Felson, relates to a constellation of radiologic findings that are considered virtually pathognomonic by gestalt (i.e., even Aunt Minnie could make the diagnosis). In psychology, the gestalt theory refers to a holistic perception where the mental whole is greater than the sum of its components. For example, one recognizes an individual's face as a whole rather than as a sum of the eyes, nose, mouth, etc.. The recognition of radiographic and CT signs as characteristic of a given disease process is an excellent example of recognizing an "Aunt Minnie." The perception of such findings by gestalt facilitates a correct imaging diagnosis. Radiologists should gain familiarity with the various imaging signs in order to expedite diagnosis and positively impact patient care.

CT Angiogram Sign

The CT angiogram sign is the visualization of enhancing vessels within a parenchymal opacity on CECT. This sign was originally thought to be specific for adenocarcinoma (formerly bronchioloalveolar carcinoma) but can be seen in a variety of processes (e.g., pneumonia, pulmonary edema, postobstructive pneumonitis, lymphoma, metastases). Absence of the angiogram sign implies derangement of the architecture of the underlying lung parenchyma.

Continuous Diaphragm Sign

The continuous diaphragm sign of pneumomediastinum consists of a continuous linear lucency extending across the midline above the diaphragm, a finding that results from mediastinal air tracking posterior to the heart. It is helpful in differentiating pneumomediastinum from pneumoperitoneum.

Crazy-Paving Sign

Crazy-paving refers to interlobular septal thickening and intralobular lines superimposed on ground-glass opacity on thin-section CT, often exhibiting a geographic distribution demarcated by normal lung. Initially described as characteristic for alveolar proteinosis, this sign can be present in a multitude of other processes, including pulmonary edema, alveolar hemorrhage, infection (e.g., PCP pneumonia), and lipoid pneumonia.

Double Density Sign

The double density sign refers to increased right retrocardiac density with a curving lateral interface as seen through the right heart on frontal chest radiography, representing left atrial enlargement. A distance of > 7 cm between this interface and the left mainstem bronchus is considered confirmatory.

Doughnut Sign

In normal circumstances, the summation of the aortic arch and the right and left pulmonary arteries on the lateral chest radiograph appears as a horseshoe-shaped opacity. When there is subcarinal lymphadenopathy, the horseshoe-shaped opacity is completed inferiorly, resembling the morphology of a doughnut.

Feeding Vessel Sign

The feeding vessel sign refers to a distinct pulmonary vessel leading directly into a nodule or mass and often indicates hematogenous dissemination of disease (e.g., septic embolism, metastases, arteriovenous malformation, and occasionally lung cancer and granuloma).

Fleischner Sign

The Fleischner sign refers to proximal pulmonary artery enlargement on chest radiography in the setting of often massive ipsilateral pulmonary embolism.

Hampton Hump

The Hampton hump refers to a lower lobe triangular or rounded opacity contiguous with the pleura with its apex directed toward the hilum. The finding results from visualization of peripheral pulmonary infarction.

Juxtaphrenic Peak Sign

The juxtaphrenic peak is a finding associated with upper lobe atelectasis and consists of a triangular opacity based on the ipsilateral hemidiaphragm at or near its highest point, with the apex oriented superiorly. It is commonly seen in the presence of an inferior accessory fissure and is thought to relate to superior retraction of that fissure with tethering of the diaphragmatic pleura and subpleural fat.

Split Pleura Sign

The nonfissural pleural surfaces are barely perceptible on CT. Separation of thickened enhancing visceral and parietal pleura by intervening fluid is known as the spilt pleura sign. Visualization of "split pleura" is concerning for empyema, but may be seen in other exudative pleural effusions (e.g., malignant effusion, hemothorax, following surgery, and with other causes of chronic pleural fluid).

Subpleural Curvilinear Line Sign

The subpleural curvilinear line measures 1-3 mm in thickness and lies < 1 cm from and parallel to the pleura. This sign may be a manifestation of dependent atelectasis, pulmonary edema, pulmonary fibrosis, or asbestosis. When isolated, this abnormality should raise suspicion for asbestosis, and a careful search of other findings of asbestos exposure is recommended.

Tree-in-Bud Sign

The tree-in-bud sign refers to solid centrilobular nodules with contiguous short branching lines on HRCT. They typically spare the subpleural and interlobar interstitium. This pattern is very common in bronchiolitis, particularly infectious bronchiolitis. The finding is rarely seen in the setting of arteriolar diseases (e.g., tumor emboli, talc or cellulose-induced granulomatosis, etc.).

Westermark Sign

The Westermark sign refers to unilateral lung hyperlucency on radiography or hypoattenuation on CT corresponding to oligemia distal to an occlusive pulmonary embolus.

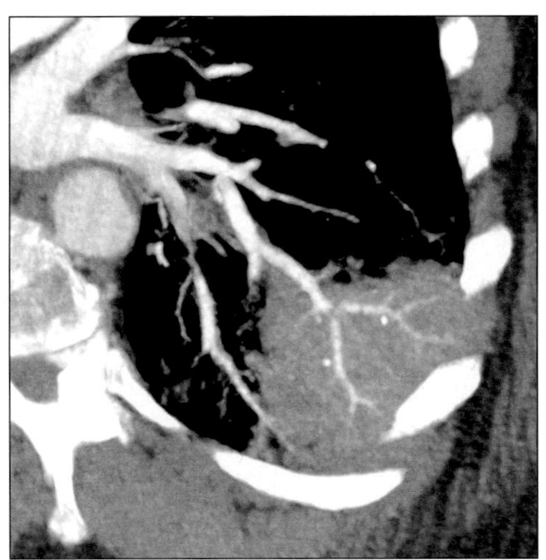

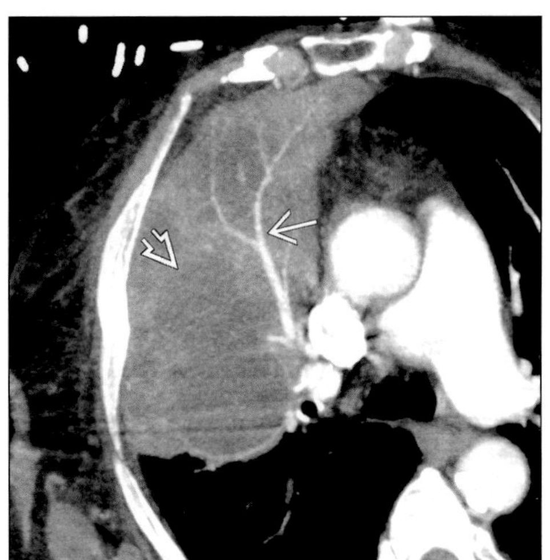

(Left) *Oblique axial CECT of a patient with lung adenocarcinoma shows the CT angiogram sign. Enhancing branching vessels within the parenchymal abnormality indicate preservation of the underlying lung architecture.* ***(Right)*** *Oblique CECT of a patient with Klebsiella pneumonia shows the coexistence of the CT angiogram sign ➔ and its absence in an adjacent area of decreased enhancement and underlying lung necrosis ➲.*

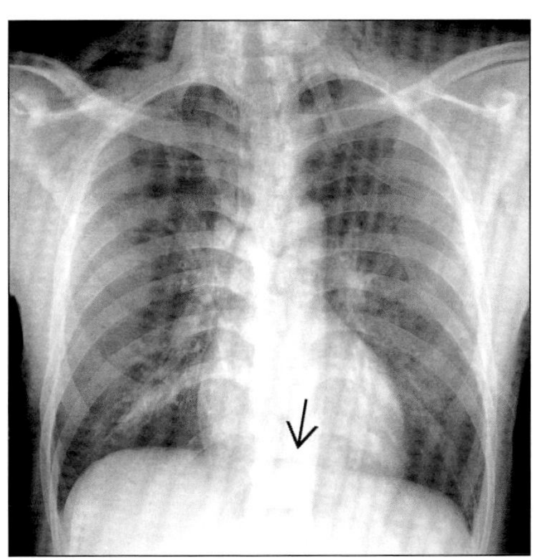

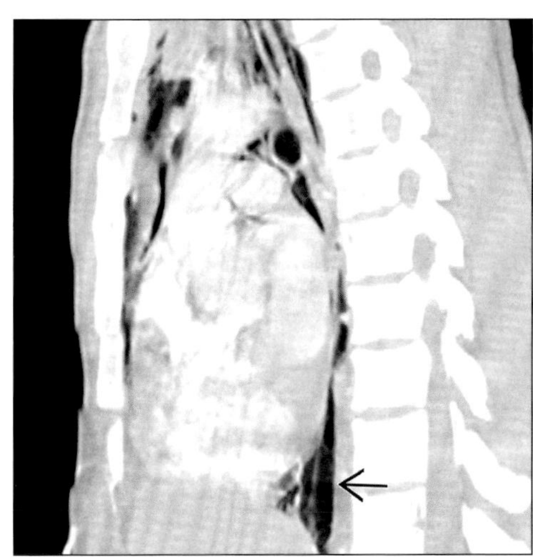

(Left) *PA chest radiograph of a patient with chest pain and pneumomediastinum shows a linear lucency ➔ extending horizontally across the midline, the so-called continuous diaphragm sign. Note bilateral supraclavicular subcutaneous air. This should be differentiated from the cupola sign of pneumoperitoneum that appears as a more arcuate lucency.* ***(Right)*** *Sagittal CECT of the same patient shows extensive pneumomediastinum with retrocardiac extension ➔.*

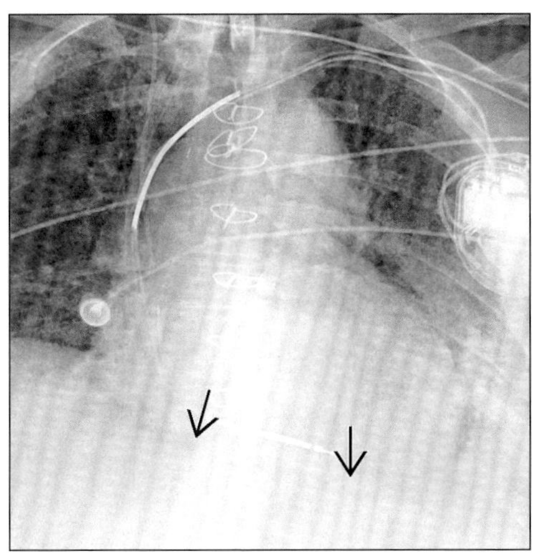

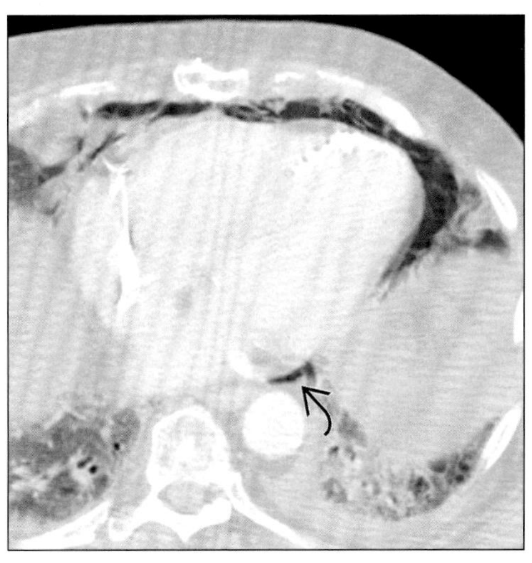

(Left) *AP chest radiograph of a patient involved in a motor vehicle collision shows a pneumomediastinum. Note extensive linear lucency tracking along the heart borders as well as the continuous diaphragm sign ➔.* ***(Right)*** *Axial CECT of the same patient demonstrates an anterior pneumomediastinum corresponding to the lucency that surrounded the heart on radiography. Pneumomediastinum located posterior to the heart ➚ produces the continuous diaphragm sign on radiography.*

*(**Left**) Axial HRCT of a patient with pulmonary alveolar proteinosis shows geographic areas of ground-glass opacity with superimposed interlobular septal thickening and intralobular lines, the so-called crazy-paving sign. (**Right**) Axial HRCT of a patient with exogenous lipoid pneumonia shows geographic ground-glass opacities with superimposed interlobular septal thickening and intralobular lines. While atypical, this pattern may occur in lipoid pneumonia.*

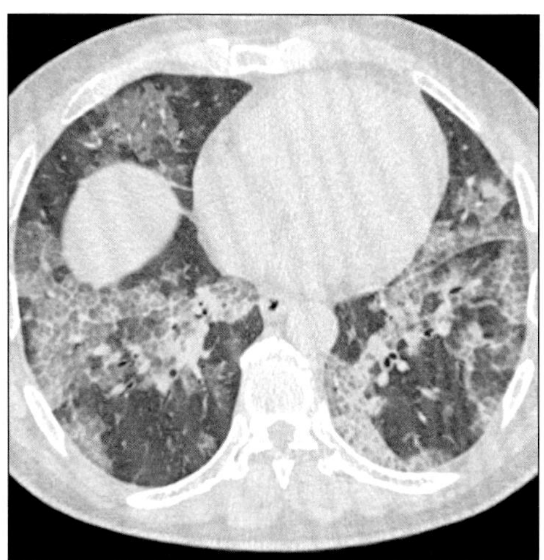

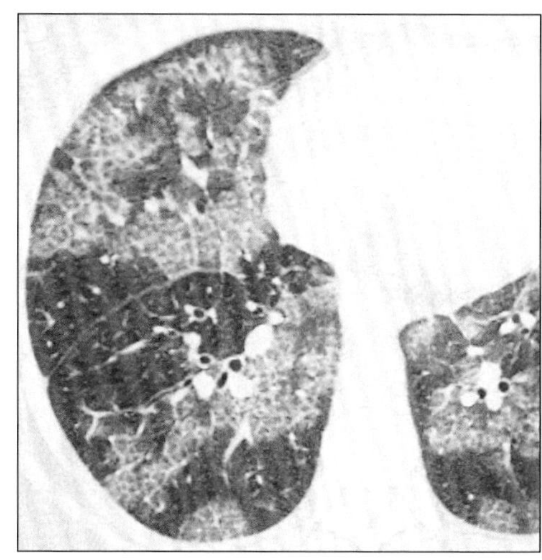

*(**Left**) PA chest radiograph of a patient with severe mitral valve disease shows diffuse cardiomegaly and a double density sign ⮫ when combined with the right heart border ➞, the result of an enlarged left atrium. There is also enlargement of the left atrial appendage ➜ manifesting as an additional convexity along the left heart border. (**Right**) Axial CECT of the same patient shows marked dilatation of the left atrium with its most medial portion ➞ located posterior to the right atrium.*

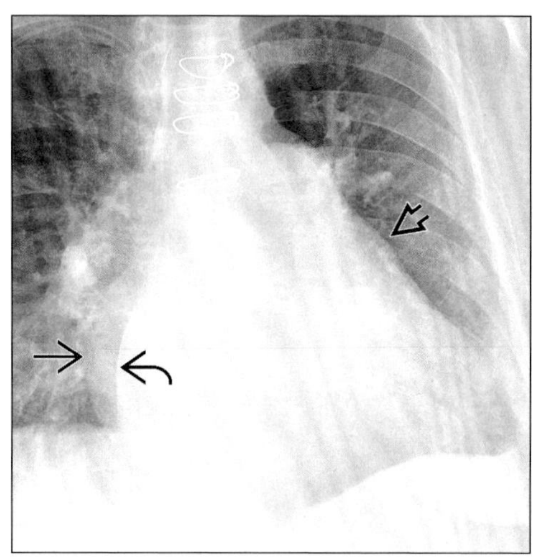

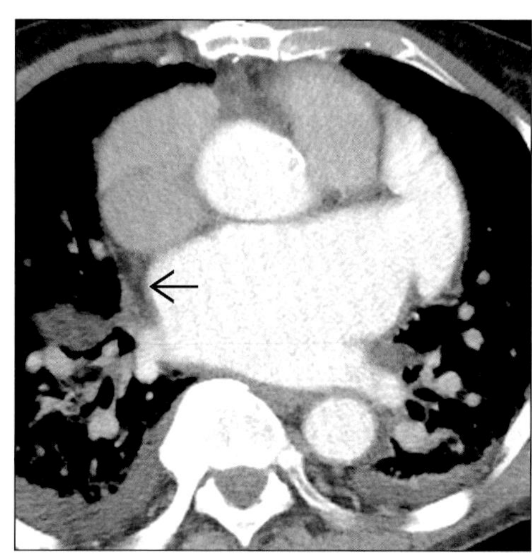

*(**Left**) PA chest radiograph of a patient with sarcoidosis shows extensive bilateral hilar and right paratracheal lymphadenopathy. (**Right**) Lateral chest radiograph of the same patient shows subcarinal lymphadenopathy ⮫ producing the doughnut sign. Anatomically, the doughnut is formed by the aortic arch superiorly, the right and left pulmonary arteries anteriorly and posteriorly (respectively), and the subcarinal lymphadenopathy inferiorly.*

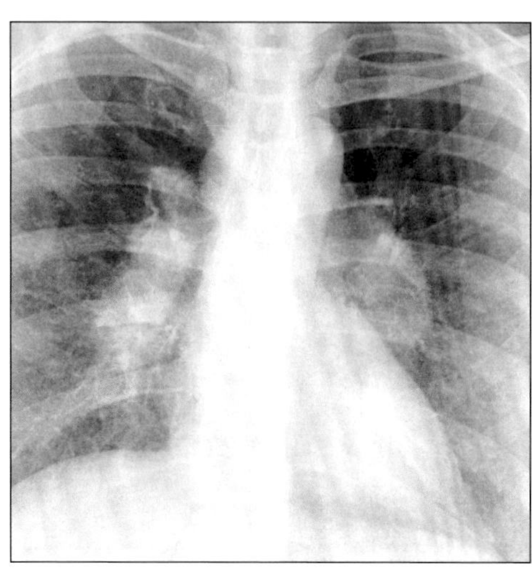

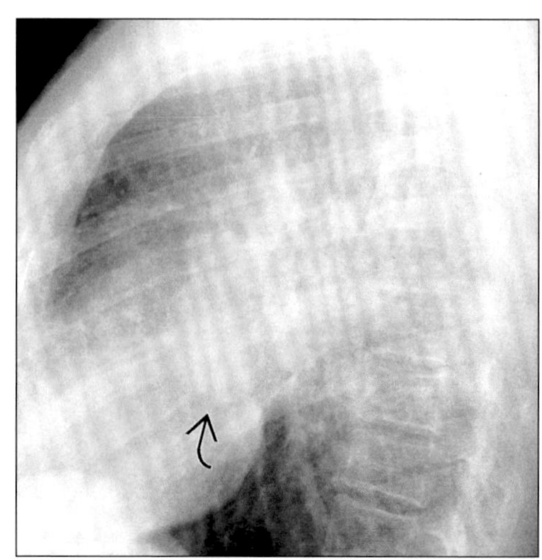

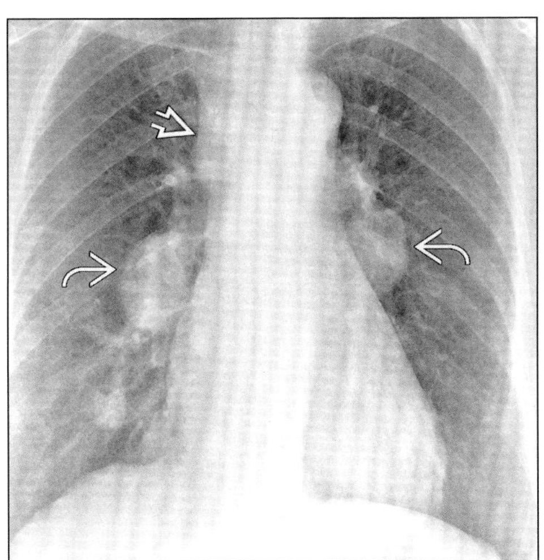

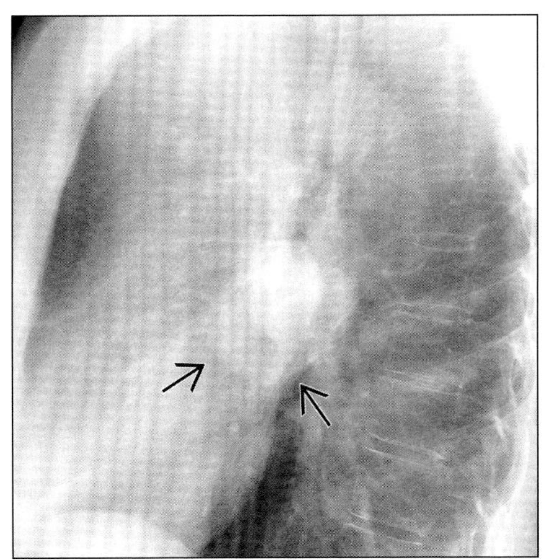

(Left) *PA chest radiograph of a patient with metastatic renal cell carcinoma shows bilateral hilar ➔ and right paratracheal ➔ lymphadenopathy.* ***(Right)*** *Lateral chest radiograph of the same patient shows subcarinal lymphadenopathy ➔ producing the doughnut sign. While nonspecific, mediastinal lymphadenopathy is a common manifestation of metastatic renal cell carcinoma.*

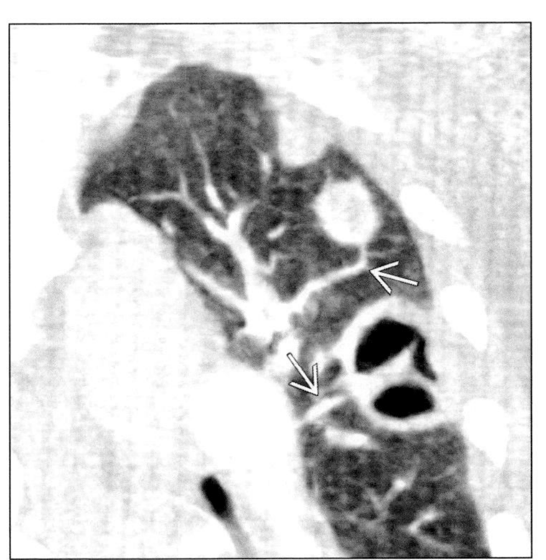

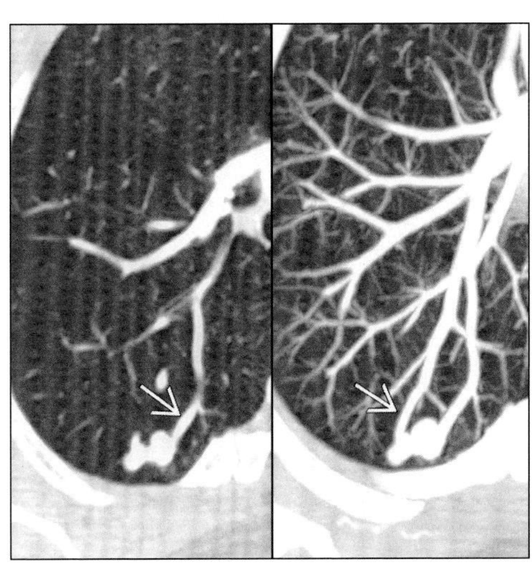

(Left) *Coronal CECT of a patient with septic embolism shows coexistent cavitated and solid nodules. Pulmonary artery branches are directed toward some of these nodules, the so-called feeding vessel sign ➔.* ***(Right)*** *Composite image with axial (left) and MIP image (right) from a CECT of a patient with an arteriovenous malformation shows a right lower lobe nodule that exhibits the feeding vessel sign ➔. MIP image demonstrates afferent and efferent pulmonary vessels, confirming the diagnosis.*

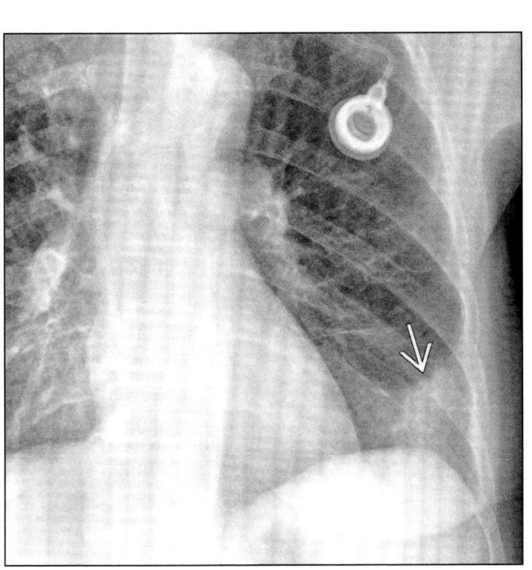

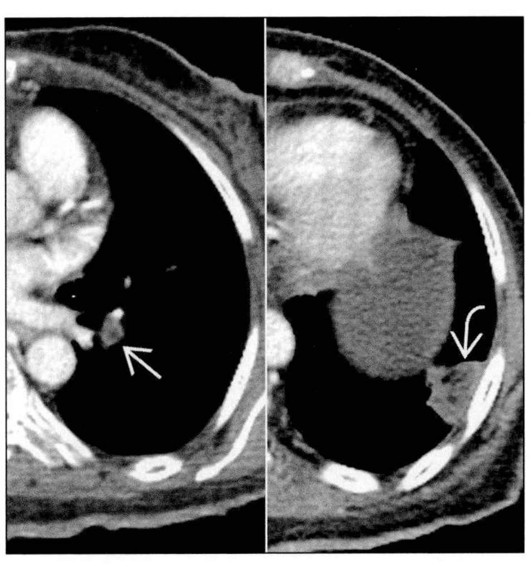

(Left) *PA chest radiograph of a patient with pulmonary thromboembolic disease shows a Hampton hump characterized by a peripheral subpleural opacity ➔.* ***(Right)*** *Composite image with axial CECT of the same patient shows a segmental left lower lobe pulmonary embolus ➔ and a peripheral triangular opacity ➔ (contiguous with the pleura) with its apex oriented toward the hilum. Central lucencies indicate necrosis and are characteristic of a pulmonary infarct.*

(Left) *PA chest radiograph of a patient with complete right upper lobe atelectasis ➡ shows the juxtaphrenic peak sign ➡, believed to result from upward retraction of the inferior accessory fissure, visceral and diaphragmatic pleura, and subpleural fat.* ***(Right)*** *Lateral chest radiograph of the same patient demonstrates anterosuperior shift of the major ➡ and minor fissures, also consistent with right upper lobe atelectasis.*

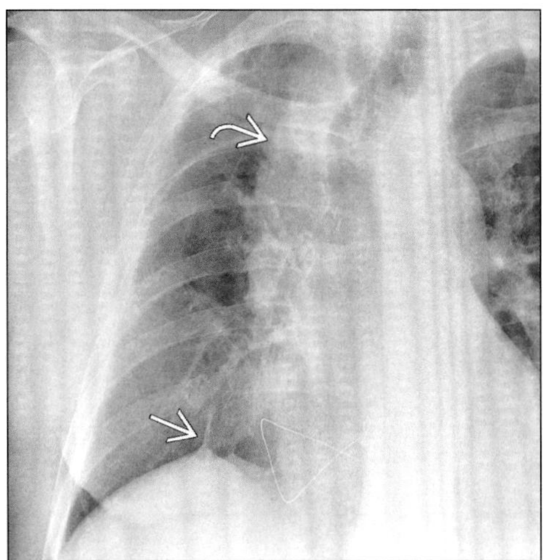

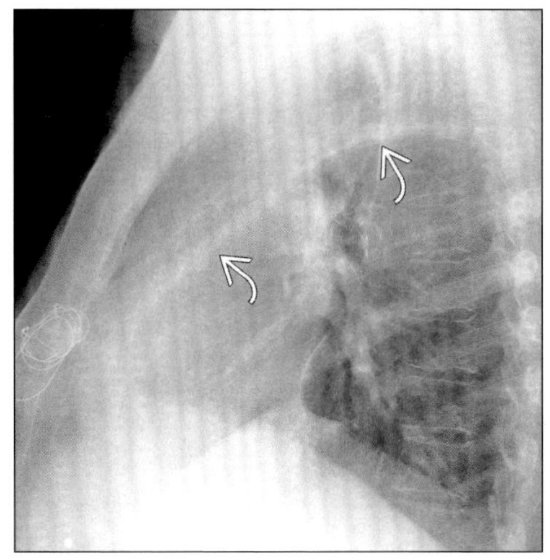

(Left) *PA chest radiograph of a patient with metastatic lung cancer and right upper lobe atelectasis shows the juxtaphrenic peak sign in relation to the right hemidiaphragm ➡. The juxtaphrenic peak sign occurs commonly in right upper lobe atelectasis and can also be seen in middle lobe atelectasis.* ***(Right)*** *Coronal CECT of the same patient shows the morphologic features of the juxtaphrenic peak ➡, widespread metastatic lung nodules, and right upper lobe atelectasis.*

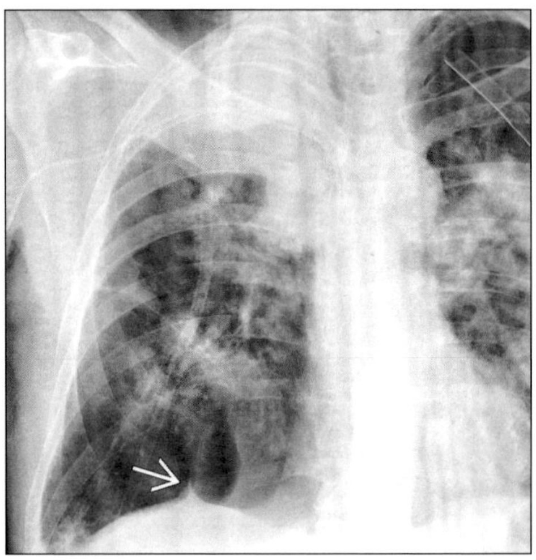

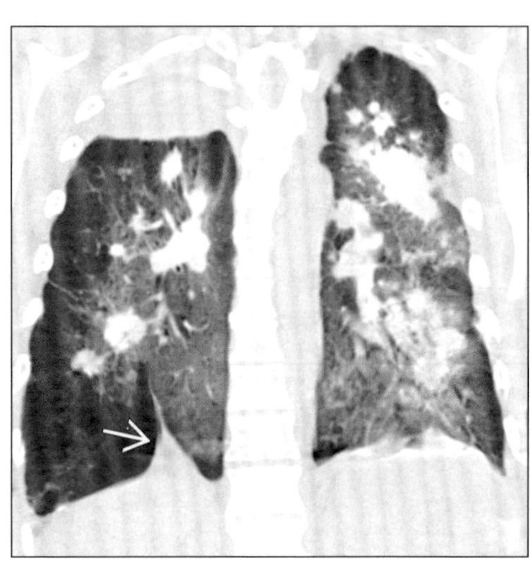

(Left) *Axial NECT of a patient who presented with fever due to empyema shows a loculated pleural fluid collection in the left lower hemithorax with thickening of the visceral ➡ and parietal ➡ pleura, forming the so-called split pleura sign. While this sign is always concerning for empyema, it can also be seen in chronic pleural effusion.* ***(Right)*** *Axial HRCT of a patient with asbestosis shows the curvilinear line sign paralleling the pleural surface ➡ and asbestos-related pleural plaques ➡.*

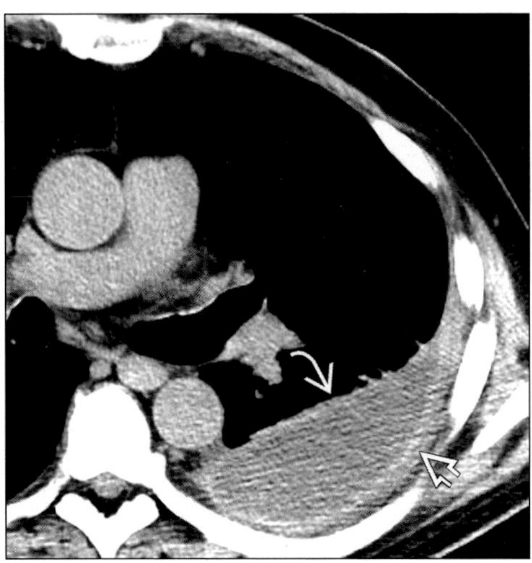

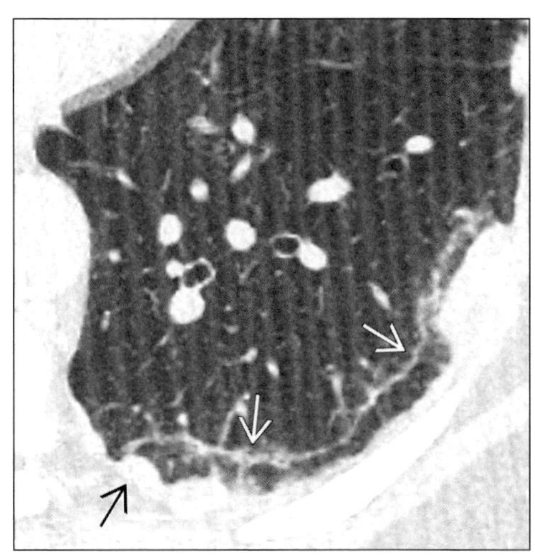

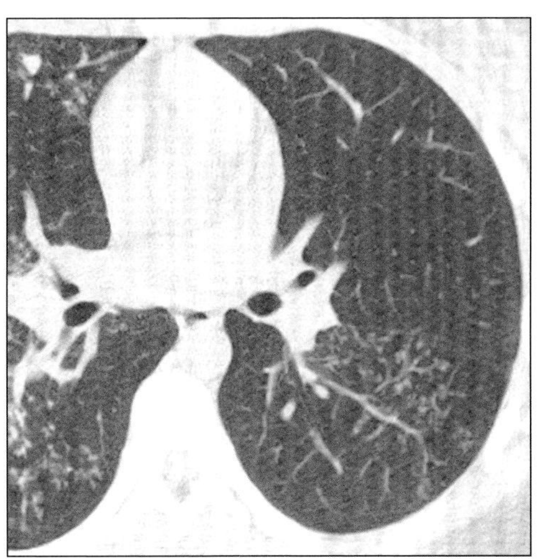

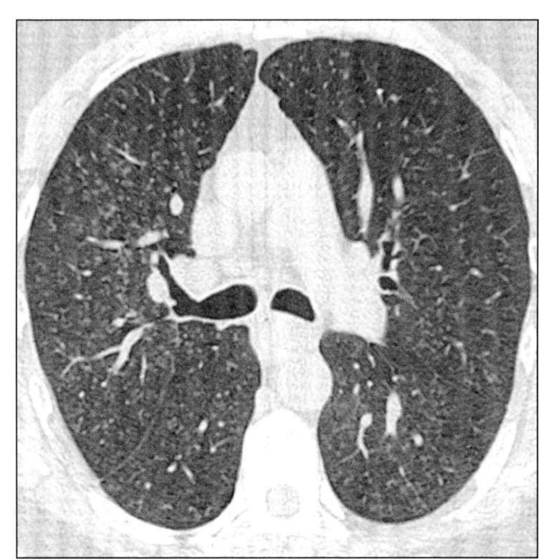

(Left) *Axial HRCT of a patient with active tuberculosis shows clustered solid nodules and branching tree-in-bud opacities in the lower lobes, consistent with endobronchial dissemination of infection. Tree-in-bud opacities are a common CT feature of active tuberculosis.* ***(Right)*** *Axial HRCT of a patient with lentil aspiration bronchiolitis shows extensive centrilobular and tree-in-bud opacities bilaterally, more conspicuous in the right upper lobe.*

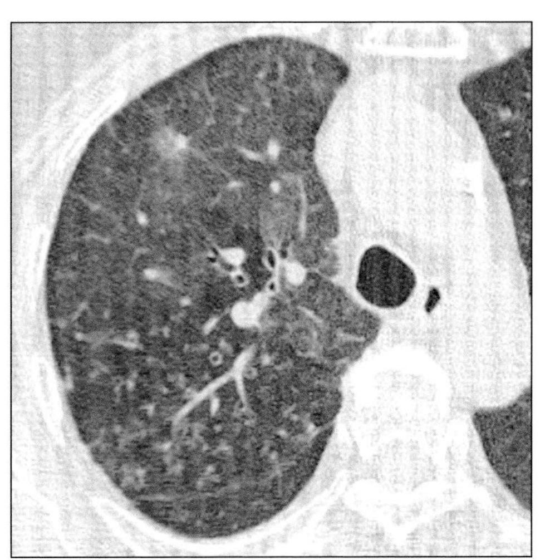

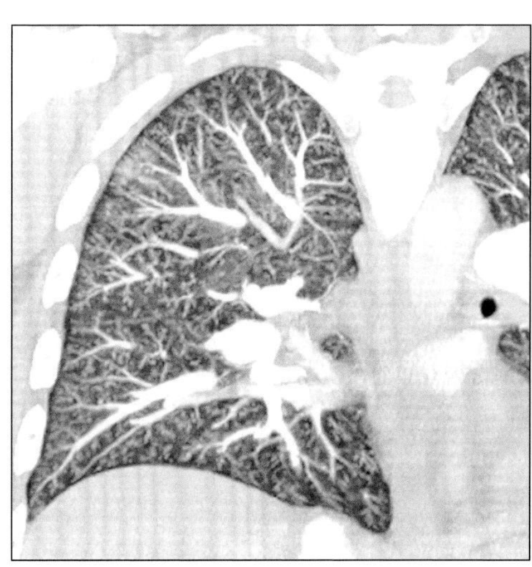

(Left) *Axial HRCT of an Asian patient with panbronchiolitis shows extensive diffuse tree-in-bud opacities, bronchial wall thickening, and mosaic attenuation. Panbronchiolitis typically manifests with diffuse tree-in-bud nodules.* ***(Right)*** *Coronal CECT of a patient with cellulose granulomatosis shows extensive tree-in-bud opacities. Rarely, as in this case, the tree-in-bud sign can be secondary to arteriolar processes.*

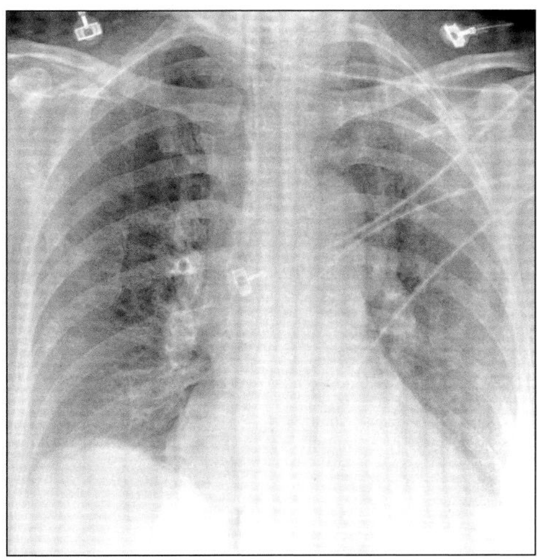

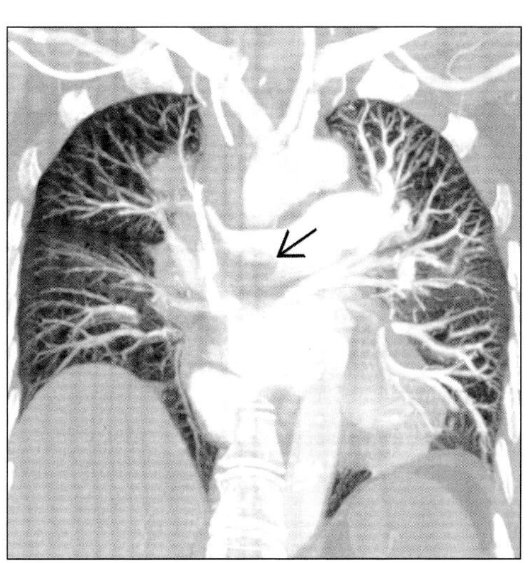

(Left) *PA chest radiograph of a patient with pulmonary embolism who presented with chest pain and dyspnea shows relative hyperlucency of the right hemithorax as compared to the left due to oligemia, the so-called Westermark sign.* ***(Right)*** *Coronal CECT MIP image of the same patient better delineates the right pulmonary oligemia and shows a large embolus ⇒ in the right pulmonary artery. The Westermark sign can be subtle and difficult to detect on radiography.*

AIR CRESCENT SIGN

Key Facts

Terminology

- Definition: Crescent-shaped or circumferential radiolucency surrounding nodule or mass
- Synonyms: Meniscus sign, Monod sign (typically used for fungus ball/mycetoma/aspergilloma)

Imaging

- Chest radiography & CT
  - Mass or nodule surrounded by peripheral crescent-shaped radiolucency
  - Mass or nodule within lung cavity

Top Differential Diagnoses

- Abscess: Often completely air filled or with air-fluid level
- Infarct: May cavitate & exhibit air or air-fluid level
- Infections: Tuberculosis, nocardiosis
- Malignancy: Cavitary necrotic neoplasm

Pathology

- Etiology: Angioinvasive aspergillosis, mycetoma within cavity (e.g., tuberculosis, sarcoidosis, bronchiectasis, lung cancer), hydatid disease
  - Angioinvasive aspergillosis: Arterial thrombosis & lung infarction
  - Preexistent cavity: Saprophytic fungus/fungus ball
  - Hydatid disease: Airway erosion by cyst

Clinical Issues

- Classically described in recovery phase of angioinvasive aspergillosis
- Also described in mycetoma growing within preexistent cavity

Diagnostic Checklist

- Most cases seen in clinical practice are secondary to mycetoma growing in preexistent cavity

(Left) Composite image with PA chest radiograph (left) and axial NECT (right) of a patient with angioinvasive aspergillosis shows a left upper lobe cavity with internal heterogeneous soft tissue surrounded by a crescent of intracavitary air resulting from lung necrosis. (Right) Composite image with PA chest radiograph (left) and axial NECT (right) of a patient with sarcoidosis shows a right upper lobe mycetoma that developed in a preexisting cavity and exhibits the air crescent sign.

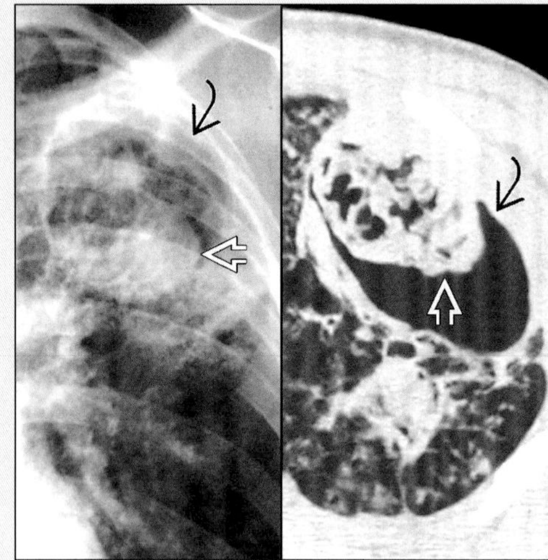

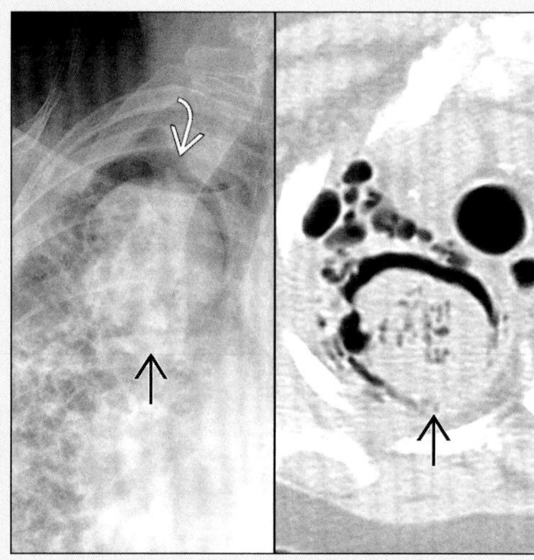

(Left) Composite image with PA chest radiograph (left) and axial NECT (right) of a patient with a cavitary lung cancer shows a mycetoma growing within the cavity that produces the air crescent sign. (Right) Composite image with PA chest radiographs of 2 different patients shows a mycetoma in a cavity from nontuberculous mycobacterial infection (left) and a complicated hydatid cyst with impending rupture. Both lesions exhibit the air crescent sign. (Courtesy P. Boiselle, MD.)

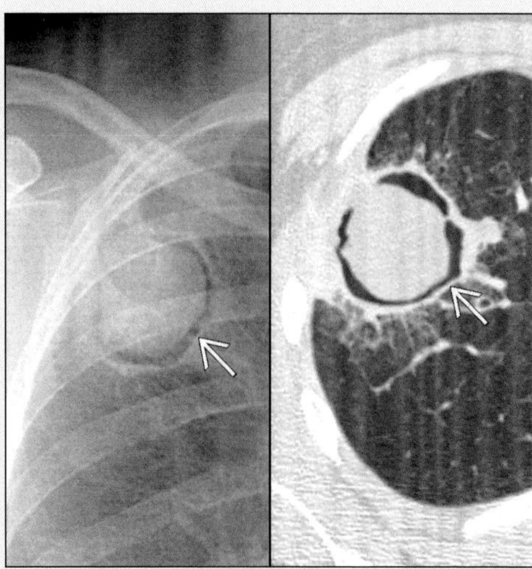

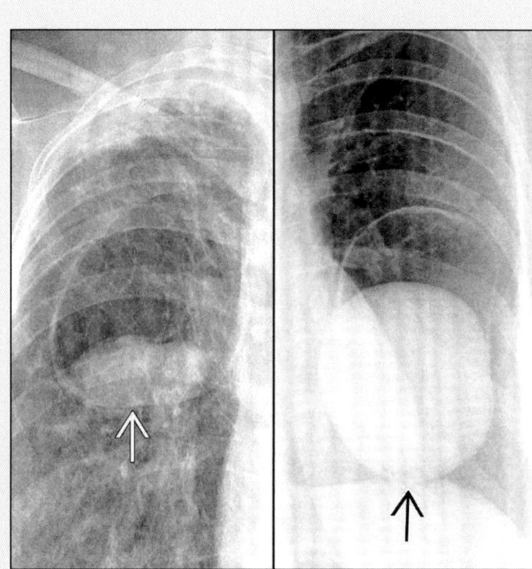

CERVICOTHORACIC SIGN

Key Facts

Terminology

- Definition: Loss of contour of a mediastinal mass as it extends above clavicle
  - Typically masses partially located within thorax with extension into neck

Imaging

- PA chest radiography
  - Fading contour of mass as it extends cephalad above clavicle
- Lateral chest radiography
  - Allows localization of mass within mediastinal compartment
- CT
  - Allows characterization of mediastinal mass
  - Allows localization of mass in specific mediastinal space
  - Identification of extension of mass into neck

Top Differential Diagnoses

- Completely intrathoracic mediastinal masses
  - PA chest radiograph demonstrates well-defined lesion contours above clavicle
  - If cervicothoracic sign is not evident on PA chest radiography, lateral radiography helps confirm mediastinal location of abnormality

Pathology

- Caudal portion of mass outlined by aerated lung
- Cephalad portion of mass obscured by neck soft tissues
- Etiology
  - Intrathoracic thyroid masses
  - Tortuous head/neck vessels
  - Lymphoma
  - Lymphangioma

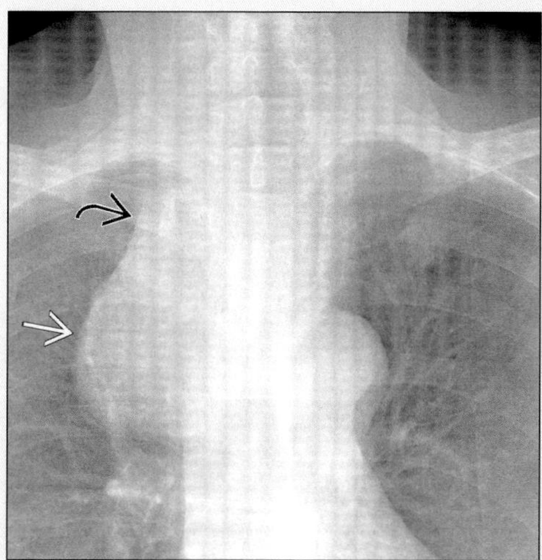

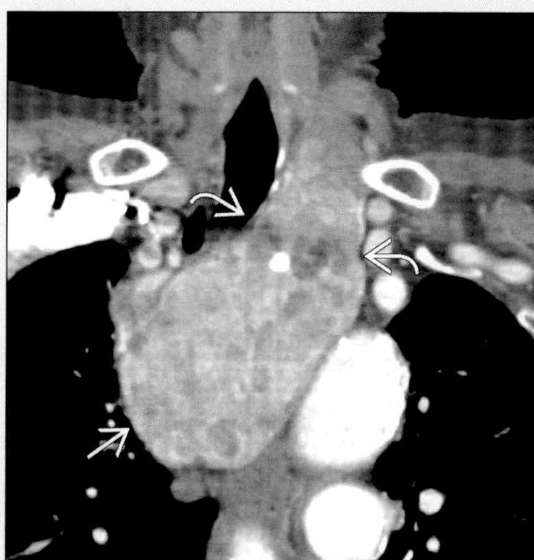

(Left) *PA chest radiograph of a patient with a mediastinal goiter shows a mass with a well-defined contour ➡, which fades when the mass approaches the clavicle ↷ and becomes imperceptible above the clavicle, the so-called cervicothoracic sign.* ***(Right)*** *Coronal CTA of the same patient shows a heterogeneous thyroid mass largely located within the chest ➡ with extension into the left neck ↷. As the mass extends cephalad, it becomes surrounded by neck soft tissues, which obscure its contours on radiography.*

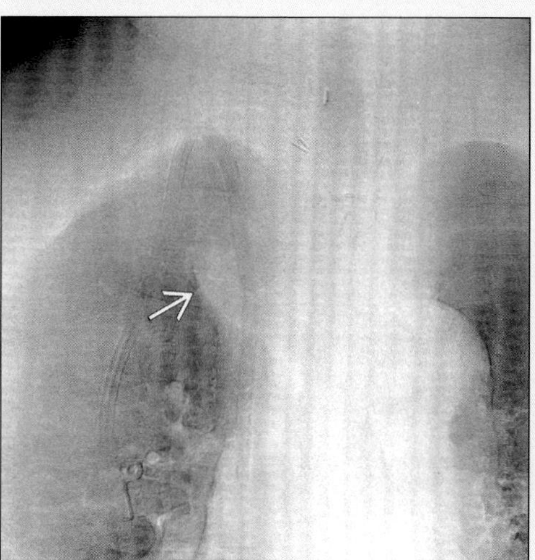

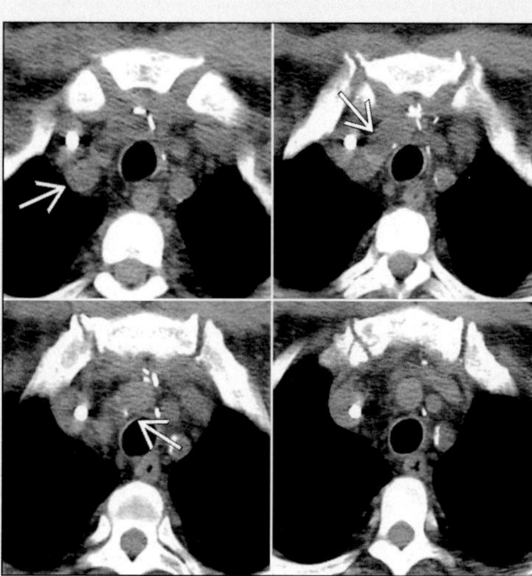

(Left) *PA dual energy chest radiograph shows a tortuous right brachiocephalic trunk ➡ manifesting as a right mediastinal contour abnormality. The vessel borders fade cephalad as the brachiocephalic trunk enters the neck.* ***(Right)*** *Axial NECT of the same patient shows marked tortuosity of the right brachiocephalic trunk ➡ that explains the radiographic findings. As this is a prevalent finding in the elderly, comparison to prior radiographs should be performed to avoid unnecessary CT studies.*

COMET TAIL SIGN

Key Facts

Terminology

- Definition: CT sign characterized by curvilinear opacities extending from peripheral subpleural mass toward hilum
  - Classically described in **rounded atelectasis**

Imaging

- Radiography
  - Primarily CT sign
  - Findings on chest radiography: Peripheral lung mass, adjacent pleural abnormality (e.g., effusion, thickening, plaque)
- CT
  - Criteria for rounded atelectasis: Well-marginated 2-7 cm subpleural spherical or ovoid mass, acute angles with pleura, sharp peripheral margin, poorly defined central margin, comet tail sign
  - **Comet tail sign**: Swirling or curving vessels & bronchi extending from subpleural mass toward ipsilateral hilum
- PET/CT
  - Rounded atelectasis typically not metabolically active
  - PET/CT helpful when no prior studies are available to document stability of mass
  - If uptake is present consider biopsy or resection

Pathology

- Etiology of rounded atelectasis: Chronic pleural reaction including asbestos-related pleural disease, pleural tuberculosis, and chronic pleurisy

Diagnostic Checklist

- Consider rounded atelectasis in subpleural mass with adjacent pleural thickening & comet tail sign on CT

__(Left)__ Composite image with axial NECT of a patient with asbestos-related pleural disease and rounded atelectasis shows curvilinear bronchovascular structures arising from a subpleural mass and coursing toward the ipsilateral hilum, the so-called comet tail sign. __(Right)__ Lateral chest radiograph of a patient with rounded atelectasis shows a subpleural lower lobe mass ➔. Unless prior studies are available for comparison, radiography is often nondiagnostic, and CT is required for further characterization.

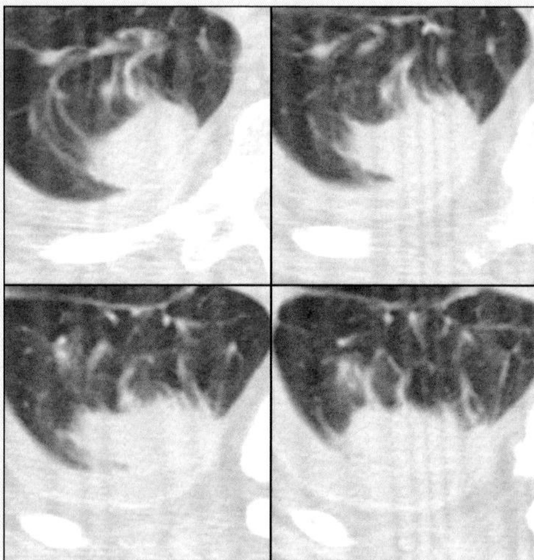

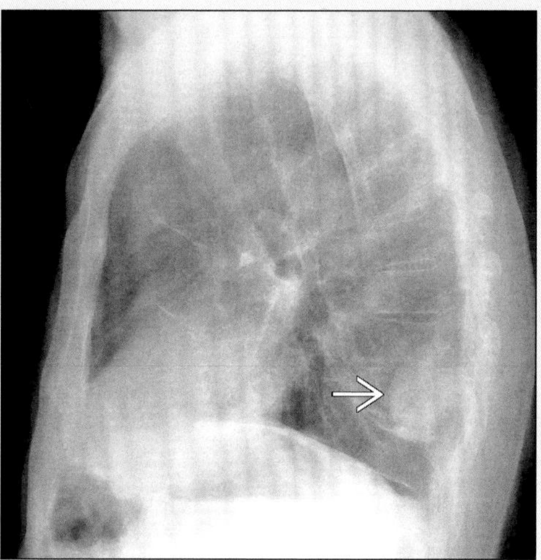

__(Left)__ Composite image with axial NECT (left) and fused PET/CT (right) of a patient with chronic pleurisy shows left lower lobe rounded atelectasis ➔ demonstrating a characteristically low FDG uptake ➔. __(Right)__ Composite image with axial NECT (left) and T1WI MR (right) of a patient with rounded atelectasis shows the comet tail sign ➔ and increased signal ➔ in the lesion. Although often unnecessary, MR with contrast has excellent accuracy for differentiation of rounded atelectasis from neoplasm.

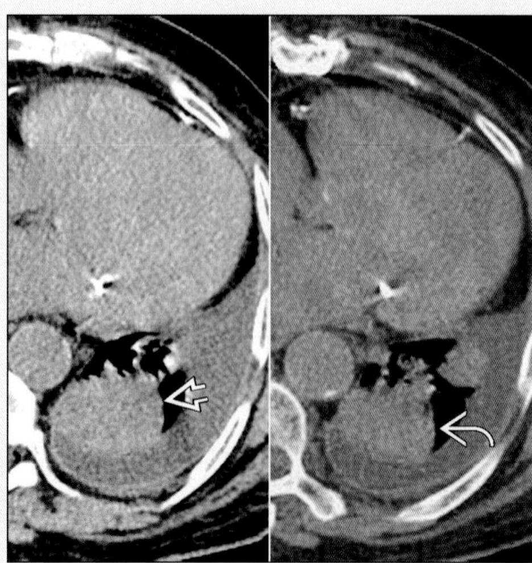

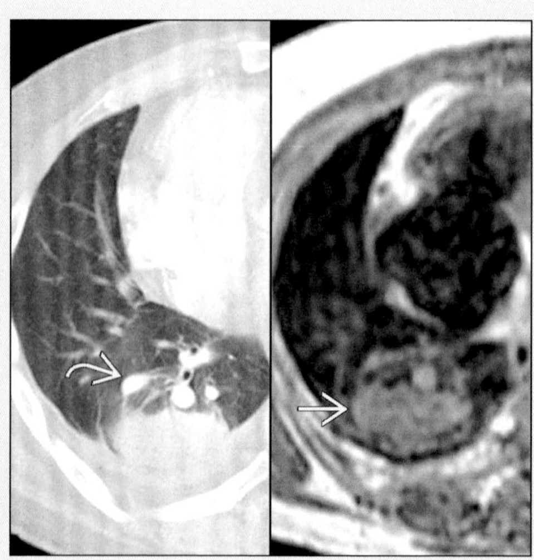

Key Facts

Terminology

- Definition: Zone of ground-glass attenuation surrounding pulmonary soft tissue nodule or mass

Imaging

- CT
  - Soft tissue nodule or mass with varying surrounding ground-glass opacity
  - Ground-glass opacity: Opacity that does not obscure pulmonary vessels
  - Ground-glass opacity is optimally appreciated on thin-section CT

Top Differential Diagnoses

- **Reverse halo sign**
  - Central ground-glass opacity with surrounding crescentic or ring-like consolidation
  - Differential diagnosis: Cryptogenic organizing pneumonia, infection, Wegener granulomatosis, pulmonary infarct, sarcoidosis, radiofrequency ablation, lymphomatoid granulomatosis

Pathology

- Ground-glass opacity classically relates to hemorrhage, but may be inflammation or neoplasm
- Etiology
  - Infectious: Angioinvasive fungus (classically *Aspergillus*, also *Candida, Mucor*, etc.), mycobacteria, rickettsia, virus, & septic embolism
  - Inflammatory: Wegener granulomatosis, eosinophilic pneumonia, cryptogenic organizing pneumonia, endometriosis
  - Neoplastic: Kaposi sarcoma, lung adenocarcinoma (former BAC), vascular metastasis (e.g., angiosarcoma, choriocarcinoma, osteosarcoma)
  - Iatrogenic: Post transbronchial biopsy (e.g., lung transplant patient after surveillance biopsy), catheter-induced pulmonary pseudoaneurysm

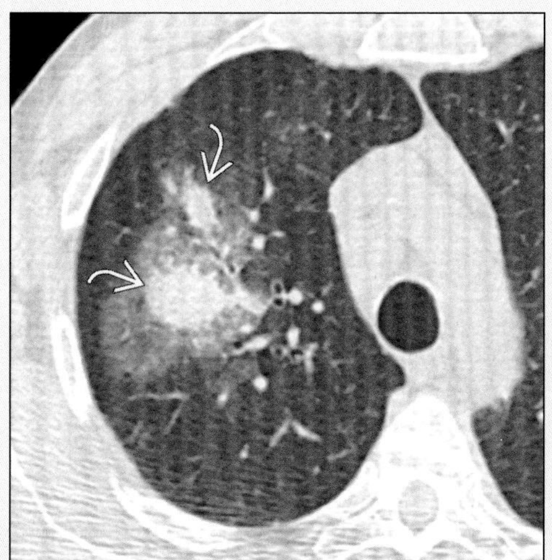
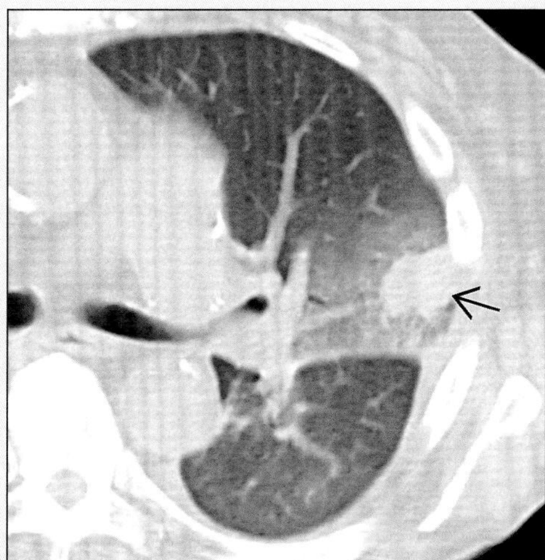

(Left) *Axial NECT of a patient with angioinvasive aspergillosis shows 2 solid nodules surrounded by "halos" of ground-glass opacity, the so-called CT halo sign.* ***(Right)*** *Axial NECT of a patient with CMV pneumonia post bilateral lung transplant shows a solid left upper lobe nodule surrounded by extensive ground-glass opacity. While angioinvasive aspergillosis has been classically associated with this appearance, many other fungal, viral, and bacterial infections can also cause the CT halo sign.*

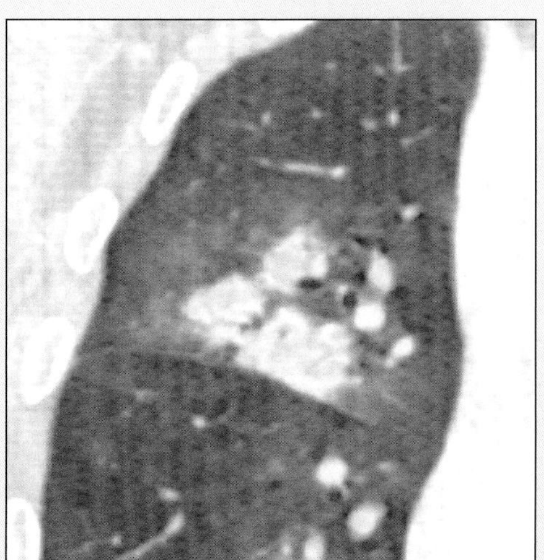
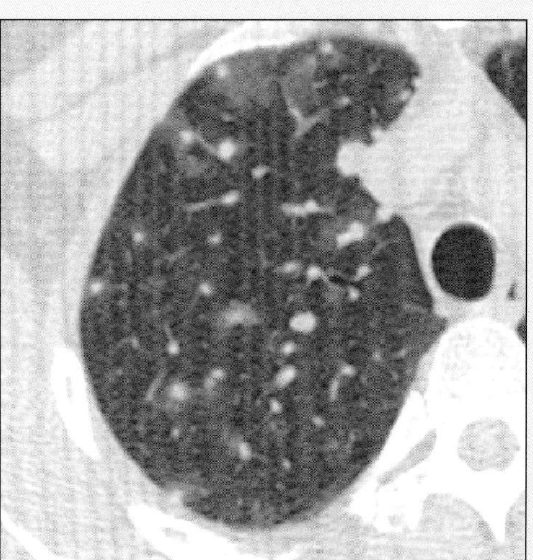

(Left) *Coronal NECT of a patient with Wegener granulomatosis shows multiple soft tissue nodules with surrounding ground-glass opacity. The CT halo sign in this case is secondary to perilesional hemorrhage.* ***(Right)*** *Axial NECT of a patient with right atrial angiosarcoma shows small pulmonary nodules with surrounding ground-glass opacity halos. Highly vascular metastases prone to hemorrhage are often responsible for this finding (e.g., angiosarcoma, choriocarcinoma, osteosarcoma).*

DEEP SULCUS SIGN

Key Facts

Terminology

- Definition: Lucency & deepening of lateral costophrenic angle

Imaging

- Chest radiography
  - Lucency extending from lateral costophrenic angle to hypochondrium
  - Depression of ipsilateral hemidiaphragm compared to contralateral side
  - Ancillary findings: Pleural line occasionally seen & confirmatory of pneumothorax, ↑ sharpness cardiomediastinal silhouette, ↑ sharpness of mediastinal fat, ↑ sharpness of diaphragm, double diaphragm sign
- CT
  - Confirmation of pneumothorax in doubtful cases
  - Helps establish etiology if unclear on radiography

Top Differential Diagnoses

- Pneumoperitoneum
  - Left upper quadrant loculated pneumoperitoneum; confirmation with erect or lateral decubitus chest radiography
- COPD
  - Hyperaeration may deepen lateral costophrenic angle; CT may be required for differentiation

Clinical Issues

- 30% of all pneumothoraces are undetected on supine chest radiography
- Most useful in patients in intensive care unit, after trauma & when pleural adhesions preclude typical configuration of pneumothorax

Diagnostic Checklist

- When deep sulcus sign is present, suspect large ipsilateral pneumothorax

*(**Left**) AP chest radiograph of a patient who sustained recent chest trauma shows a left pneumothorax manifesting with an ipsilateral deep sulcus sign with characteristic deepening of the left costophrenic angle ⊳. (**Right**) Coronal CECT of the same patient shows a large left pneumothorax and a deep costophrenic angle ➔ accentuated by air in the pleural space. This sign is especially helpful in patients imaged in the supine position in whom pneumothorax may not manifest with a visible pleural line.*

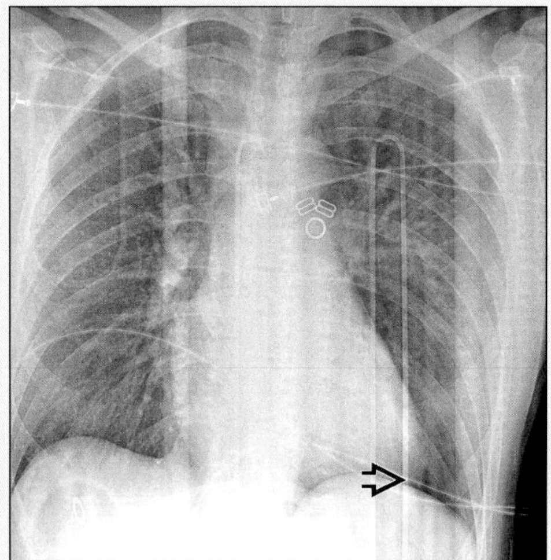

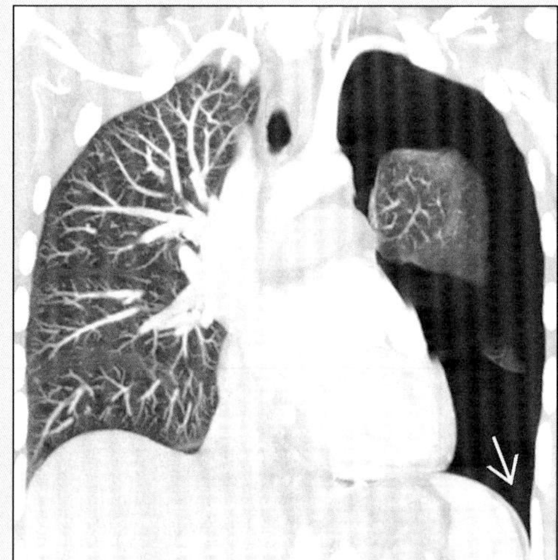

*(**Left**) AP chest radiograph of an ICU patient with a large left pneumothorax due to barotrauma shows marked deepening and lucency of the costophrenic angle ➔. (**Right**) Composite image with AP chest radiograph following thoracotomy (left) and AP chest radiograph after left chest tube reinsertion (right) shows a left deep sulcus sign ➔ that resolves following chest tube removal and reinsertion. The pneumothorax presumably resulted from chest tube malfunction.*

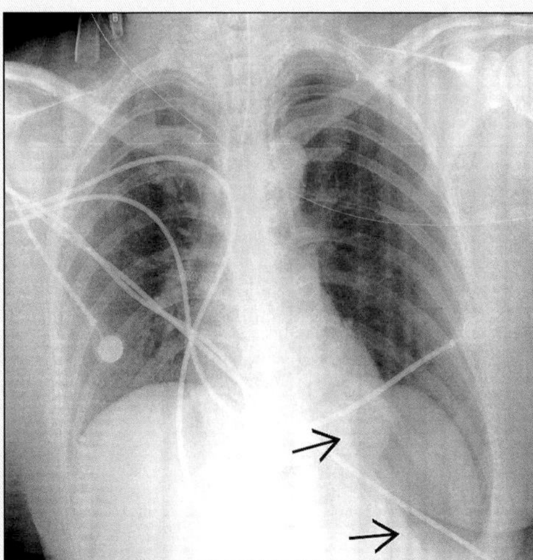

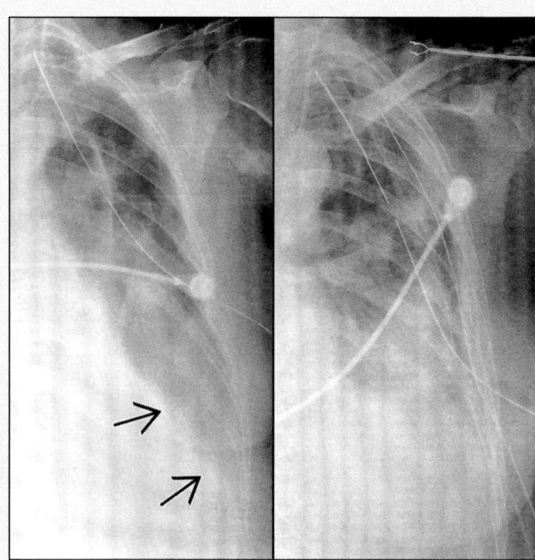

Key Facts

Terminology

- Definition: Soft tissue density (> 2 mm) separating mediastinal & subepicardial fat secondary to pericardial effusion
- Synonyms: Sandwich sign, Oreo cookie sign, bun sign

Imaging

- Chest radiography
  - Retrosternal soft tissue between 2 lucent bands on lateral chest radiography
  - Often more conspicuous if narrow window (more contrast) used to view images
  - May also be seen on PA chest radiography as lucent band subjacent to cardiac border
  - Comparison to prior studies may allow detection of interval enlargement of heart/cardiomediastinal silhouette
- CT
  - Fluid between mediastinal and subepicardial fat

Top Differential Diagnoses

- Pneumomediastinum
  - Linear air collections in retrosternal region without conspicuous soft tissue component
- Morgagni hernia
  - Retrosternal opacity, may exhibit intrinsic lucency & occasionally air-filled bowel loops
- Mediastinal fat
  - Retrosternal opacity, may exhibit intrinsic lucency

Diagnostic Checklist

- High index of suspicion & window manipulation (i.e., narrow window) important to detect this finding
- Consider further evaluation with echocardiography for confirmation or if radiography inconclusive

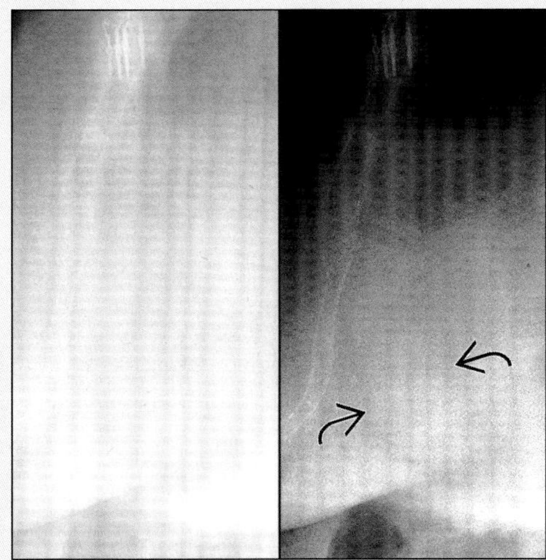

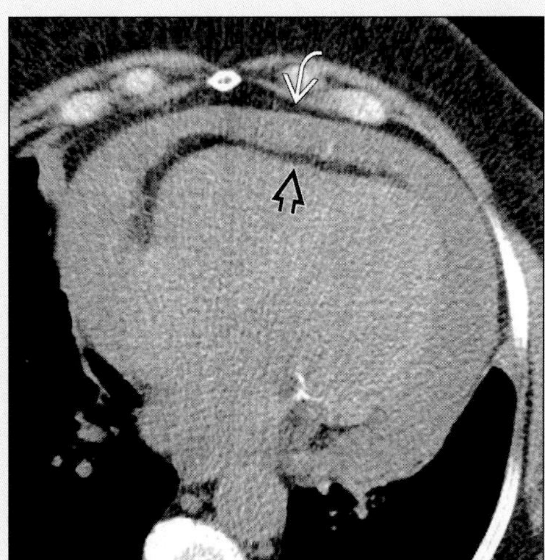

(Left) *Composite image with lateral chest radiographs viewed with routine (left) and narrow window (right) settings shows a large pericardial effusion manifesting with a water density band outlined by anterior and posterior fat density lucent stripes ➢. The abnormality may be difficult to identify if the window is not purposely manipulated.* ***(Right)*** *Axial NECT of the same patient confirms a large pericardial effusion outlined by mediastinal ➢ and subepicardial fat ⊳.*

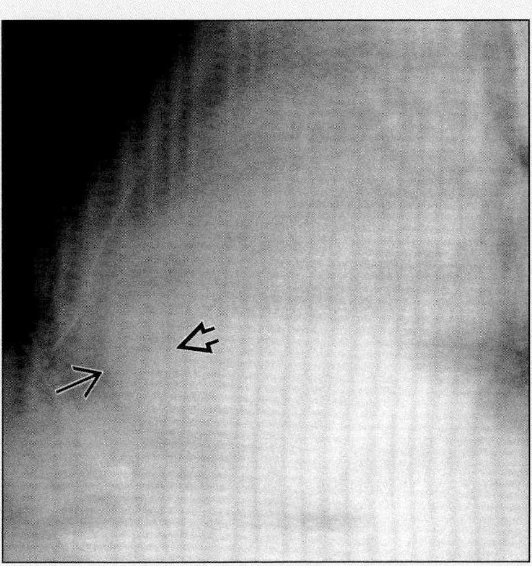

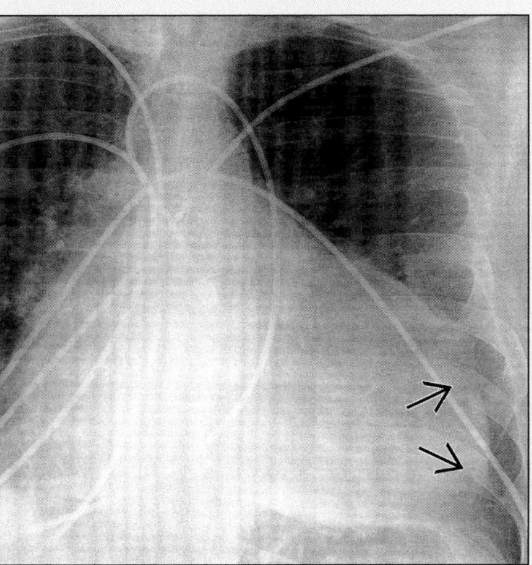

(Left) *Lateral chest radiograph of a patient with a large pericardial effusion shows the fat pad sign. In this case, the window has been manipulated to highlight the mediastinal → and subepicardial fat ⊳.* ***(Right)*** *PA chest radiograph of a patient with a moderate pericardial effusion shows an enlarged cardiac silhouette and a faint lateral lucency → representing the subepicardial fat. While not as frequently visualized as on lateral radiography, the fat pad sign can also be seen on frontal chest radiographs.*

"FINGER IN GLOVE" SIGN

Key Facts

Terminology

- Definition: Tubular or branching opacities resembling fingers (mucus plugs) in glove (dilated bronchi)
- Synonyms: Gloved finger, mucoid impaction

Imaging

- Radiography
  - Described on radiography; can be seen on CT
  - Tubular or branching opacities
- CT
  - Should always be performed to exclude central obstructing lesion
  - Confirmation of bronchiectasis & endoluminal mucus plugs
  - Inspissated low-attenuation mucus plugs
  - High-attenuation mucus plugs suggest ABPA
  - Multiplanar imaging helpful for characterization

Top Differential Diagnoses

- Arteriovenous malformation (AVM) & pulmonary vein varix
  - May appear as branching opacities
  - CT allows determination of whether opacities represent mucus plugs or pulmonary vessels
  - AVM typically exhibits afferent & efferent vessels

Pathology

- Most common etiologies: Allergic bronchopulmonary aspergillosis (ABPA), bronchial atresia, cystic fibrosis, foreign body, malignancy

Diagnostic Checklist

- While "finger in glove" sign is more commonly seen in ABPA and bronchial atresia, malignancy should always be excluded
- CT should be always performed to confirm diagnosis & exclude endoluminal malignancy

*(**Left**) Composite image with PA chest radiograph (left) and axial HRCT (right) of a patient with asthma and ABPA shows a right upper lobe branching opacity ➔ representing inspissated mucus within dilated bronchi. Subsequent HRCT shows persistent bronchiectasis with resolved mucoid impactions. (**Right**) Composite image with PA chest radiograph (left) and coronal NECT MIP image (right) shows bronchial atresia manifesting with branching right upper lobe opacities on both radiography ➔ and CT ➔.*

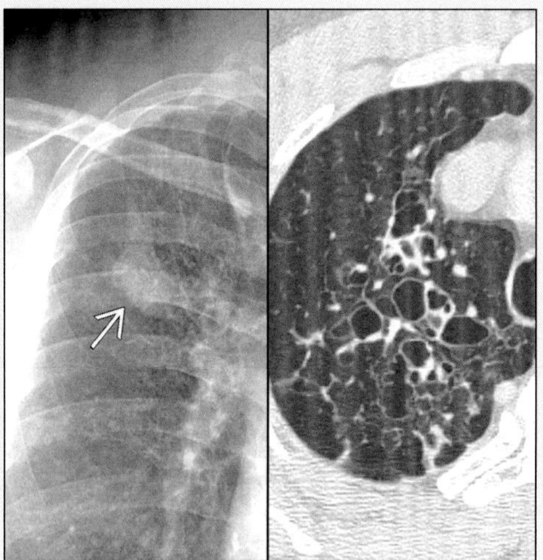

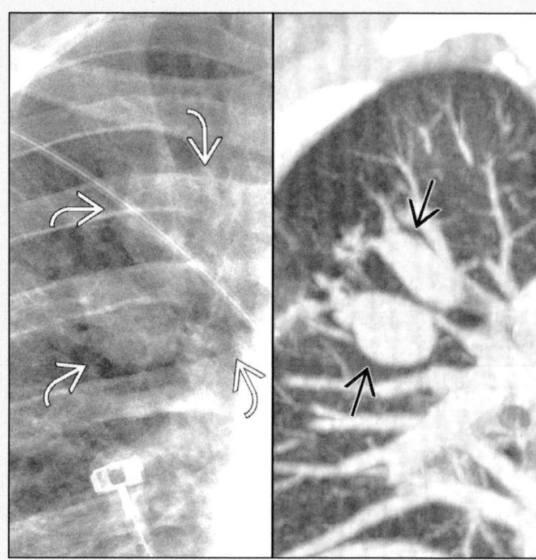

*(**Left**) Composite image with PA chest radiograph (left) and coronal NECT (right) shows the "finger in glove" sign ➔ secondary to a central squamous cell carcinoma. (**Right**) Composite image with PA chest radiograph (left) and axial CECT (right) of a patient with cystic fibrosis shows multiple small nodular opacities in the right lung, some of which exhibit branching ➔. CT confirms mucoid impactions in dilated bronchi ➔. The more distal the impaction, the less conspicuous the "finger in glove" sign.*

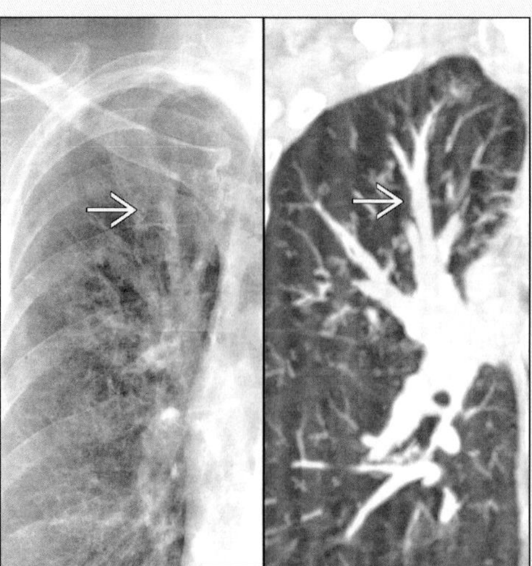

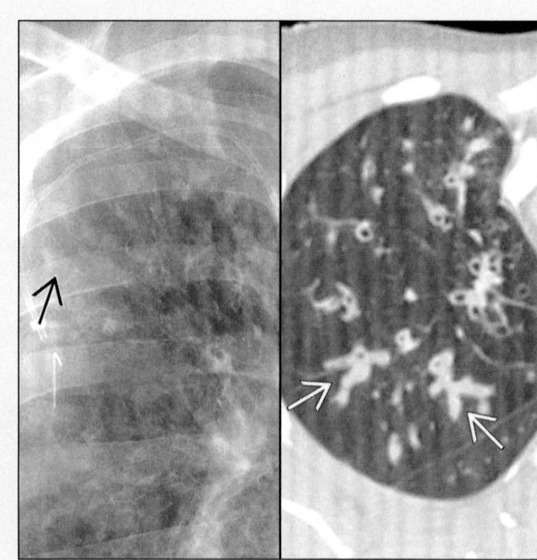

HILUM CONVERGENCE SIGN

Key Facts

Terminology

- Definition: Hilar contour abnormality (convexity) in which pulmonary artery branches arise from lateral margin of convexity

Imaging

- PA chest radiography
  - Right &/or left pulmonary artery arising from hilar convexity
  - **Pulmonary hypertension**: Dilated pulmonary trunk, right & left pulmonary arteries
  - **Pulmonic stenosis**: Dilated pulmonary trunk & left pulmonary artery
- Lateral chest radiography
  - Enlarged pulmonary trunk
  - No anterior or posterior mediastinal mass
- CT
  - Dilated pulmonary trunk (> 3 cm)
  - Pulmonary hypertension: Dilated pulmonary trunk, right & left pulmonary arteries
  - Pulmonic stenosis: Dilated pulmonary trunk & left pulmonary artery

Top Differential Diagnoses

- Hilum overlay sign
  - Pulmonary artery visible through hilar convexity > 1 cm medial to lateral margin of hilar convexity
- Left atrial appendage enlargement
  - Hilar abnormality below level of mainstem bronchus
- Cardiomegaly & pericardial effusion
  - Pulmonary artery remains lateral to hilar convexity

Pathology

- Etiology
  - Pulmonary hypertension
  - Pulmonic stenosis

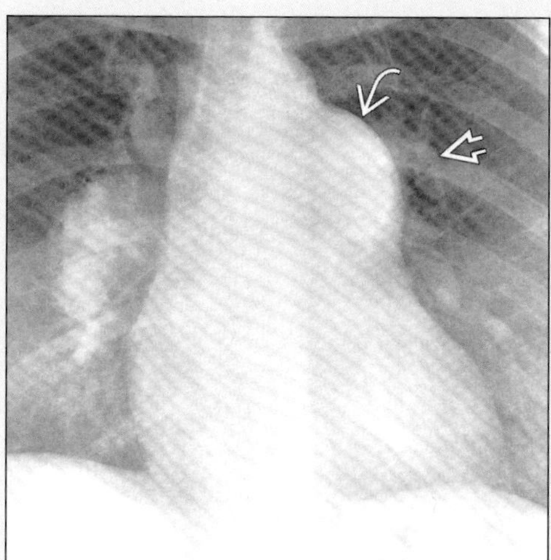

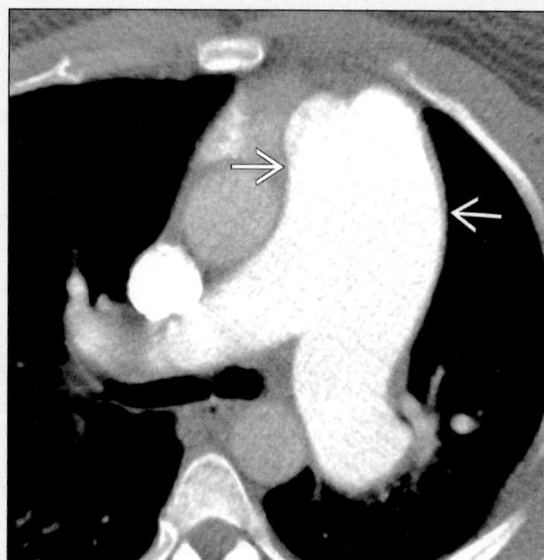

(Left) *PA chest radiograph of a patient with pulmonary hypertension shows the hilum convergence sign, in which left pulmonary artery branches ⇨ arise from the left hilar convexity ➘. In this case, there is also enlargement of the right pulmonary artery.* ***(Right)*** *Axial CTA of the same patient demonstrates a markedly dilated pulmonary trunk ➡, a finding that correlates with the hilar convexity seen on PA chest radiography.*

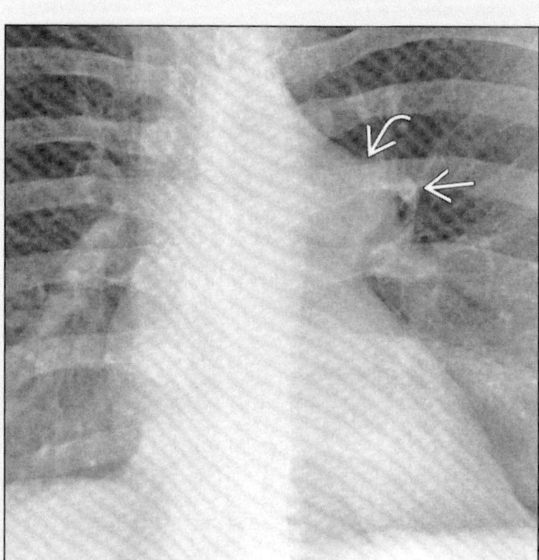

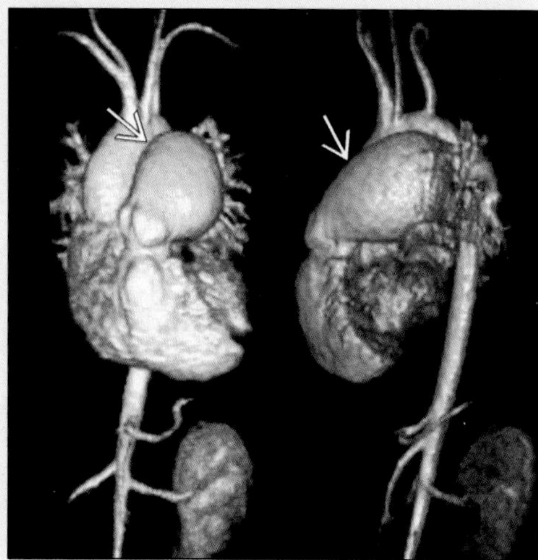

(Left) *PA chest radiograph of a young patient with pulmonic stenosis shows a left hilar convexity ➘. Unlike the hilum overlay sign, the proximal left pulmonary artery ➡ arises from the lateral margin of the convexity rather than being visible through it.* ***(Right)*** *3D MR of the same patient shows fusiform dilatation of the pulmonary trunk ➘. This is thought to be the consequence of a systolic jet generated as blood flows through the stenotic pulmonic valve.*

Key Facts

Terminology

- Definition: Hilar contour abnormality (convexity) through which pulmonary artery is visible

Imaging

- PA chest radiography
  - Pulmonary artery interface > 1 cm medial to hilar convexity interface
  - Peripheral calcifications common in vascular lesions
  - Pitfall: Rotated PA radiograph may simulate hilar convexity
- Lateral chest radiography
  - Determination of anterior or posterior location within the chest
- CT
  - Mass anterior or posterior to pulmonary artery
  - IV contrast useful for establishing vascular etiology

Top Differential Diagnoses

- **Hilum convergence sign**
  - Pulmonary artery branches arising from lateral aspect of hilar convexity
- Left atrial appendage enlargement
  - Hilar abnormality below level of mainstem bronchus
- Cardiomegaly & pericardial effusion
  - Pulmonary artery remains lateral to hilar convexity

Pathology

- Classically described for anterior mediastinal mass; also seen in middle-posterior mediastinal or paravertebral masses
- Etiology
  - Neoplasm: Thymic neoplasm, lymphoma, germ cell tumor, lymphadenopathy
  - Vascular lesion: Pseudoaneurysm, aneurysm

*(**Left**) PA chest radiograph of a patient with an anterior mediastinal thymoma shows a left "hilar" convexity ➡ through which the right pulmonary artery ➡ is identified, the so-called hilum overlay sign. (**Right**) Lateral chest radiograph of the same patient confirms the presence of an anterior mediastinal mass ➡. If the pulmonary artery arises from the hilar convexity, the contour abnormality represents an enlarged pulmonary artery, the so-called hilum convergence sign.*

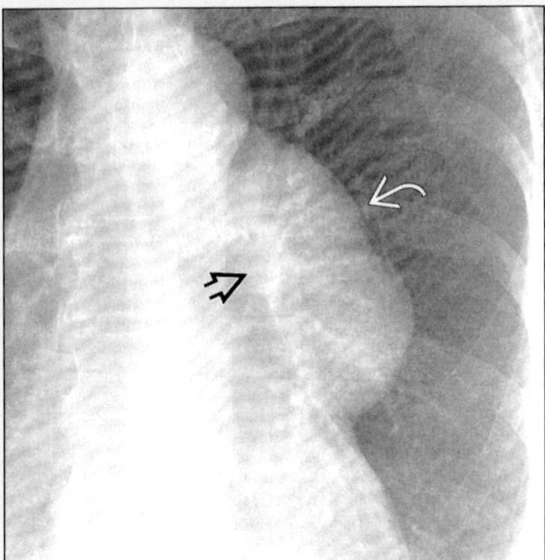

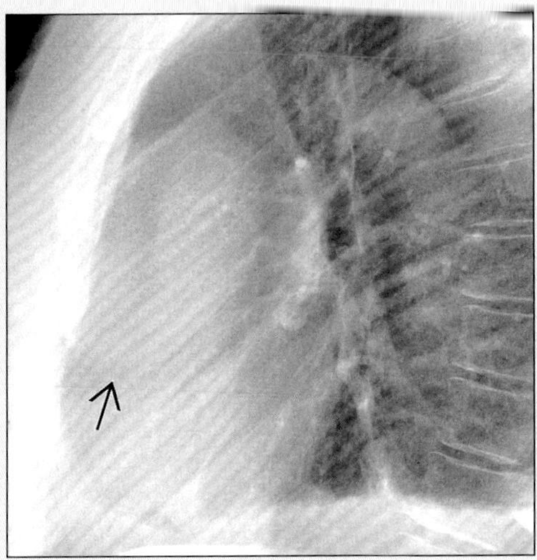

*(**Left**) Composite image with PA chest radiograph (left) and axial CECT (right) of a patient with metastatic disease shows visualization of the right pulmonary artery ➡ through a large anterior mediastinal mass ➡. (**Right**) Composite image with PA chest radiograph (left) and axial CECT (right) of a patient with aortic dissection manifesting with the hilum overlay sign shows visualization of the pulmonary artery ➡ through the enlarged aorta ➡. The hilum overlay sign may also be seen with posterior mediastinal masses.*

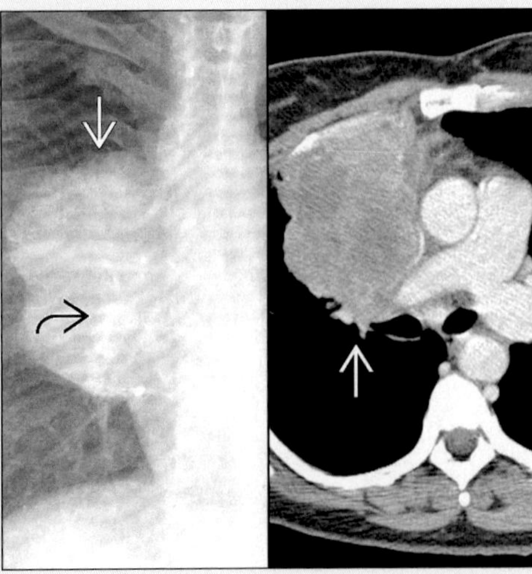

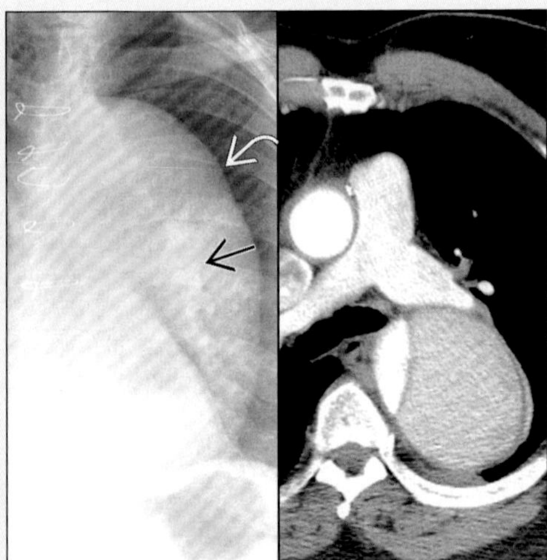

INCOMPLETE BORDER SIGN

Key Facts

Terminology

- Definition: Lesion with both well- & ill-defined borders or discrepancy of border visualization on different views; implies extrapulmonary location

Imaging

- Chest radiography
  - Portion of lesion border appears well defined
  - Portion of lesion border appears obscured
  - Discrepant margins on orthogonal radiographs
  - Allows differentiation of intrapulmonary from extrapulmonary lesions
  - Does not allow differentiation of chest wall from cutaneous lesions
- CT
  - Lesion localization in pleura, chest wall, or skin
  - Allows lesion characterization & formulation of focused differential diagnosis

Top Differential Diagnoses

- Pleural lesions: Loculated effusion, pleural plaque, metastasis, localized fibrous tumor, mesothelioma
- Chest wall lesions: Lipoma, metastasis, plasmacytoma, primary osseous malignancy
- Nipple & skin nodules/tags

Pathology

- Sharp border correlates with tangential imaging of lesion border in contact with air (i.e., lungs, external to patient)
- Ill-defined border correlates with en face imaging of lesion border abutting extrapulmonary tissues
- Obtuse angle at pleural interface loses tangential relationship to x-ray beam

Diagnostic Checklist

- Consider extrapulmonary lesion if incomplete border sign is present on radiography

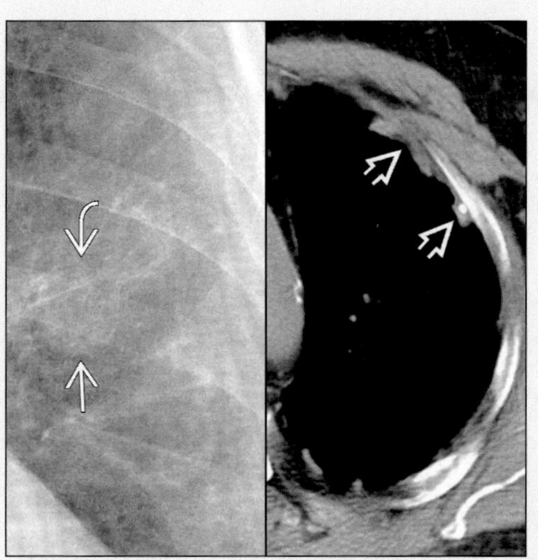

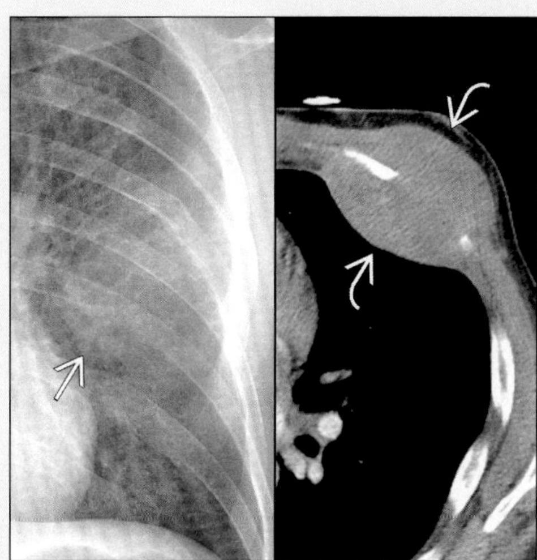

(Left) *Composite image with PA chest radiograph (left) and axial NECT (right) of a patient with pleural plaques shows several nodular opacities with both sharp ➔ and ill-defined ➔ margins. CT confirms multiple partially calcified pleural plaques ➔.* ***(Right)*** *Composite image with PA chest radiograph (left) and axial CECT (right) shows a chest wall metastasis with a well-defined inferomedial border ➔ and an ill-defined superolateral border. CT confirms the chest wall location of the lesion ➔.*

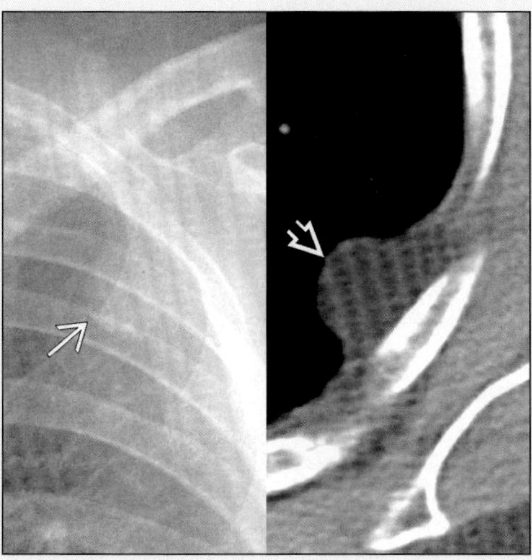

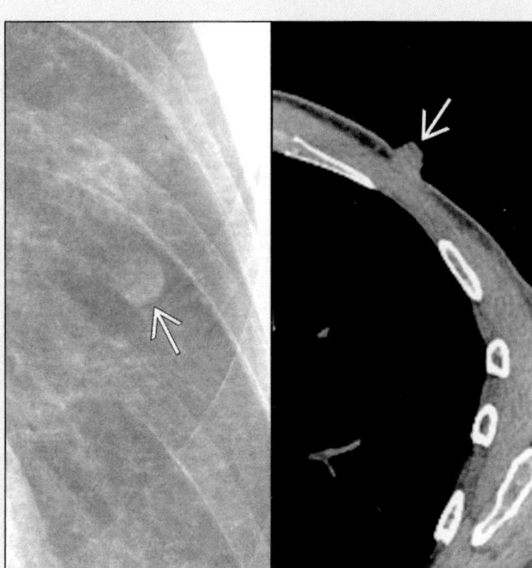

(Left) *Composite image with PA chest radiograph (left) and axial NECT (right) shows a lipoma that exhibits incomplete borders on radiography ➔ and fat attenuation ➔ on CT. The distinct inferomedial border results from tangential imaging of the portion of the lesion in contact with the lung.* ***(Right)*** *Composite image with PA chest radiograph (left) and axial NECT (right) shows a nipple ➔ exhibiting the incomplete border sign. The sharp lateral border results from contact with surrounding room air.*

LUFTSICHEL SIGN

Key Facts

Terminology

- Luftsichel (classic): Left upper lobe atelectasis
- "Luftsichel" from German, air sickle or air crescent

Imaging

- PA chest radiography
  - Sharply marginated left paraaortic crescentic lucency extending anywhere from left apex to left superior pulmonary vein
  - Absence of obscuration of aortic arch
  - Hazy opacity along hilar region that fades superiorly, laterally, & inferiorly
- Lateral chest radiography
  - Anterior displacement of major fissure, paralleling anterior chest wall
- CT
  - Homogeneous lobar opacity & volume loss
  - Extends from anterior chest wall to mediastinum
  - V-shaped posterior margin towards hilum

Top Differential Diagnoses

- Hyperinflation & herniation of right lung across midline
  - Occurs anteriorly behind sternum
  - Leftward displacement of anterior junction line
- Medial pneumothorax
  - Often not associated with other signs of volume loss

Pathology

- Luftsichel sign results from hyperexpanded & displaced left lower lobe superior segment interposed between aortic arch & atelectatic left upper lobe
- Etiology
  - Endobronchial obstructing lesion
  - Typically endobronchial malignancy

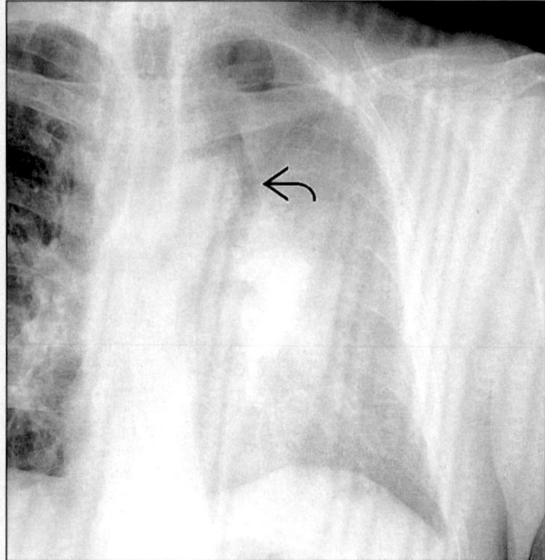

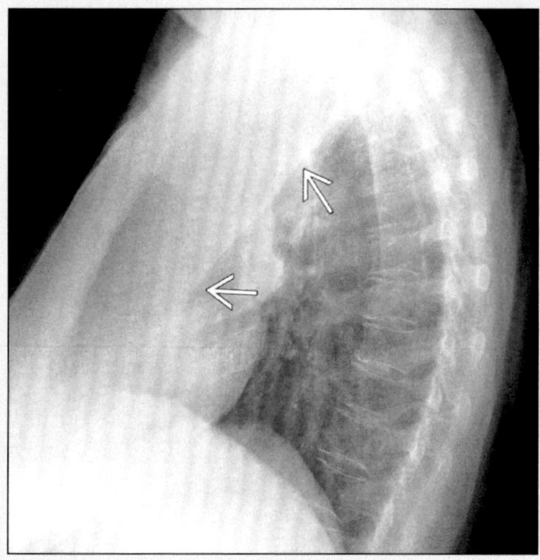

(Left) PA chest radiograph of a patient with a left hilar lung cancer that produced left upper lobe atelectasis shows a sickle-shaped lucency ⇗ outlining the aortic arch, the so-called luftsichel sign. *(Right)* Lateral chest radiograph of the same patient shows anterior displacement of the left major fissure ➡ paralleling the anterior chest wall and accentuated by the atelectatic left upper lobe. The left lower lobe superior segment becomes interposed between the aorta and the atelectatic left upper lobe.

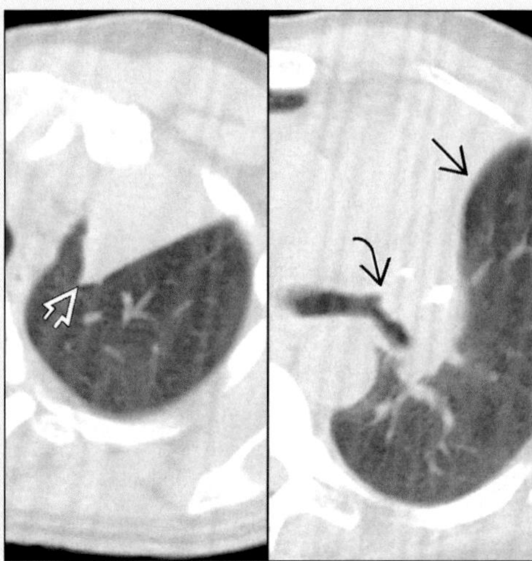

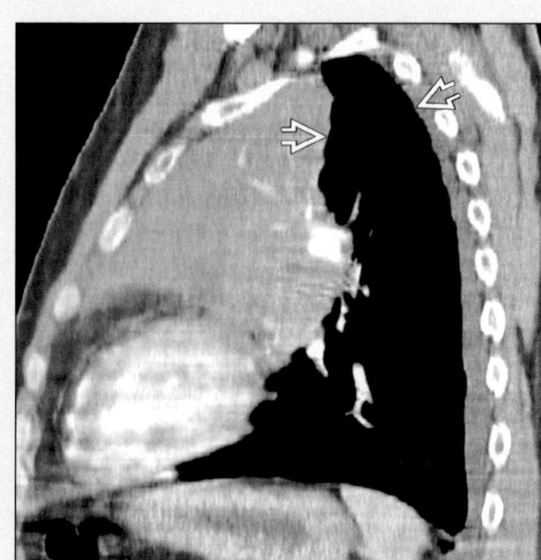

(Left) Composite image with axial NECT shows a left hilar lung cancer with left upper lobe atelectasis. Note obstruction of the left upper lobe bronchus ⇗, displacement of the major fissure ➡, and a V-shaped posterior contour of the atelectatic lobe toward the hilum ⇨. *(Right)* Sagittal CECT shows a left hilar lung cancer with anteriorly located left upper lobe atelectasis. The superior segment of the left lower lobe ⇨ occupies the expected position of the left upper lobe.

Key Facts

Terminology

- Definition: CT sign; central ground-glass opacity with surrounding crescentic consolidation
- Synonym: Atoll sign (atoll = coral island)

Imaging

- CT
  - Optimally visualized on HRCT
  - Central ground-glass opacity with surrounding ring-shaped or crescentic peripheral airspace consolidation
  - Morphology: Nodule or mass; round, oval, or slightly lobulated

Top Differential Diagnoses

- **Halo sign**: Central soft tissue nodule with surrounding ground-glass opacity (e.g., angioinvasive fungal disease, Wegener granulomatosis, hemorrhagic metastasis, etc.)

Pathology

- Initially described in & thought to be specific for cryptogenic organizing pneumonia (COP)
- Other etiologies: Bacterial pneumonia, mucormycosis, paracoccidioidomycosis, tuberculosis, sarcoidosis, radiofrequency ablation, lymphomatoid granulomatosis, Wegener granulomatosis, tumor, infarct
- In setting of COP, central ground-glass opacity corresponds to alveolar septal inflammation & intraalveolar cellular debris; ring-shaped or crescentic peripheral airspace consolidation corresponds to organizing pneumonia

Diagnostic Checklist

- Always consider COP when CT reverse halo sign is present; however, a wide variety of other causes may be associated with this CT sign

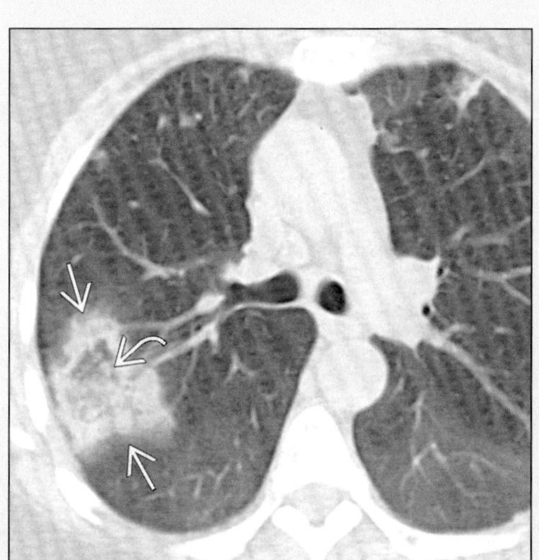

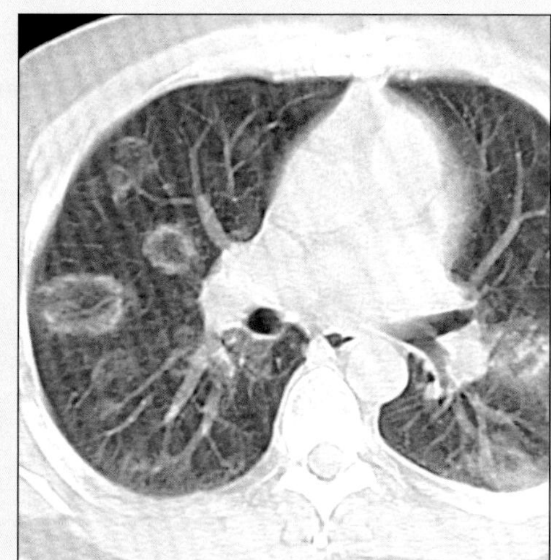

(Left) *Axial NECT of a patient with cryptogenic organizing pneumonia (COP) shows a right lower lobe mass-like consolidation with a ground-glass opacity center ➡ and surrounding crescentic consolidation ➡, the so-called reverse halo sign. The sign is not specific for COP and can be present in other lung diseases.* ***(Right)*** *Axial NECT of a patient with Wegener granulomatosis shows bilateral pulmonary nodular opacities that exhibit the reverse halo sign, an uncommon manifestation of this disease.*

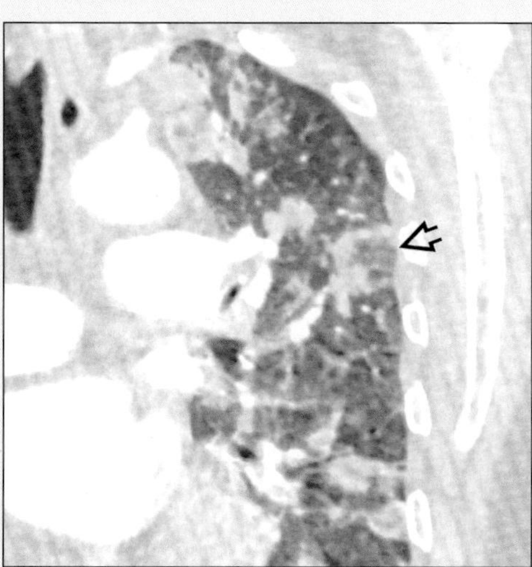

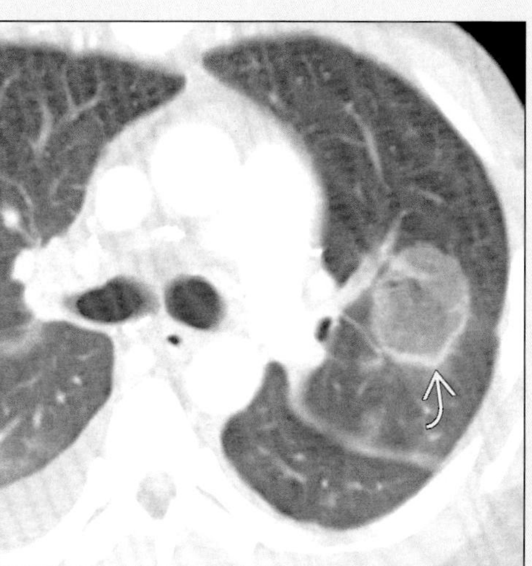

(Left) *Coronal CECT of a patient with septic embolism shows peripheral nodular opacities ⇨ with central ground-glass opacity, consistent with the reverse halo sign.* ***(Right)*** *Axial CECT of a patient with bilateral lung transplant complicated by mucormycosis shows a left upper lobe ground-glass opacity nodule with a crescentic peripheral consolidation ➡, consistent with the reverse halo sign, or, more specifically, an "atoll" sign. Another infection associated with this CT pattern is paracoccidioidomycosis.*

RIGLER SIGN

Key Facts

Terminology

- **Rigler sign**: Pneumoperitoneum outlining both sides of bowel wall
- **Cupola sign**: Pneumoperitoneum accumulated under central tendon of diaphragm

Imaging

- Chest radiography
  - Normally only luminal surface of bowel wall is outlined by gas
  - **Rigler sign**: Discernible bowel wall, outlined by luminal & free peritoneal air
  - **Cupola sign**: Arcuate lucency overlying lower thoracic spine, caudal to heart, with well-defined superior margin & ill-defined inferior border
  - Helpful in supine patients as infradiaphragmatic air may not be evident
  - When in doubt, erect or left lateral decubitus radiography can confirm pneumoperitoneum

Top Differential Diagnoses

- Pneumomediastinum
  - Continuous diaphragm sign may mimic cupola sign
  - Former tends to be straighter and latter more curved
- Normal bowel loops
  - Contiguous bowel loops can be positioned in a way that adjacent luminal walls may simulate Rigler sign
  - Air in transverse colon, in lesser sac, or in pericardium can mimic cupola sign

Diagnostic Checklist

- Diagnosis of pneumoperitoneum can be challenging in supine patients
- Consider erect or left lateral decubitus radiography for confirmation

__(Left)__ Coned-down PA chest radiograph shows a large left upper quadrant pneumoperitoneum. Both sides of the bowel wall are visible ⇒ outlined by intraluminal and extraluminal air. __(Right)__ Coronal NECT of the abdomen of the same patient shows visualization of the walls of multiple bowel loops ➡ due to intraluminal and extraluminal air. Normally only the intraluminal surface of the bowel wall is outlined by air and therefore visible.

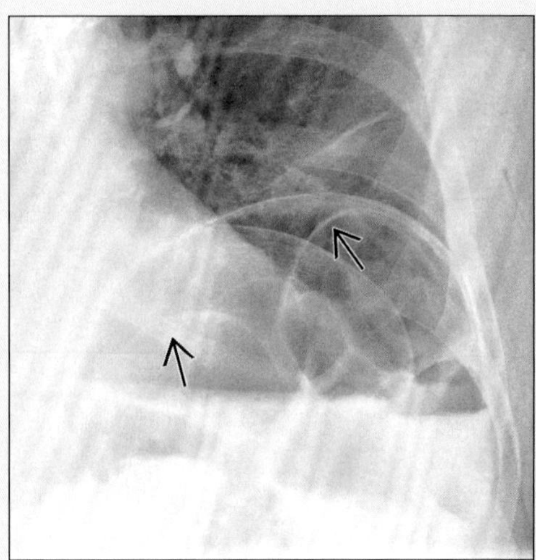

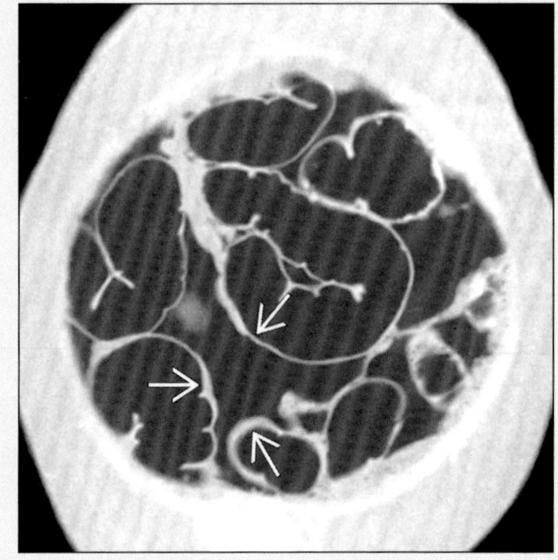

__(Left)__ PA chest radiograph of a patient with pneumoperitoneum shows air underneath the right hemidiaphragm ⇗ forming an arcuate lucency ⇒ near the midline, the so-called cupola sign. __(Right)__ AP chest radiograph of a patient with pneumoperitoneum shows air under the diaphragm. Note the midline infradiaphragmatic air collection, which exhibits a curvilinear morphology ⇒ with a well-defined superior border and an ill-defined inferior border consistent with the cupola sign.

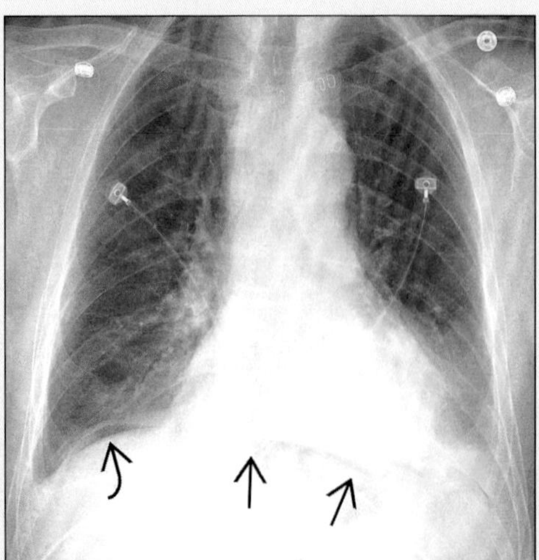

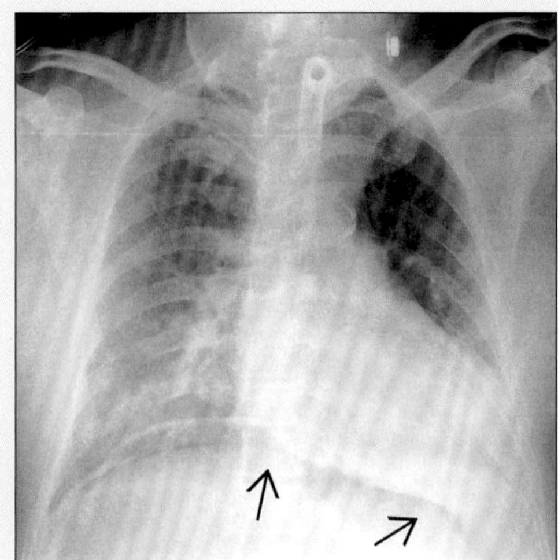

S-SIGN OF GOLDEN

Key Facts

Terminology

- Definition: Coexistence of superomedial displacement of minor fissure & hilar mass in setting of right upper lobe atelectasis

Imaging

- PA chest radiography
  - Superomedial displacement of minor fissure
  - Superior convexity of minor fissure
  - Right hilar mass
- Lateral
  - Anterosuperior displacement of major fissure
- CT
  - Identification & characterization of endobronchial obstructing lesion
  - Staging of malignancy
  - Intravenous contrast rarely necessary, but may help demonstrate central obstructing lesion

Top Differential Diagnoses

- Right upper lobe atelectasis without central mass
  - May exhibit superomedial displacement of minor fissure
  - Lacks convexity from central mass

Pathology

- **S-sign of Golden**
  - Named after Golden, who described characteristic reverse "S" configuration
  - Reverse "S" formed by superomedially displaced minor fissure & hilar convexity from central mass
- Etiology
  - Lung cancer (most common)
  - Lymphadenopathy
  - Mediastinal tumor
  - Endobronchial metastases

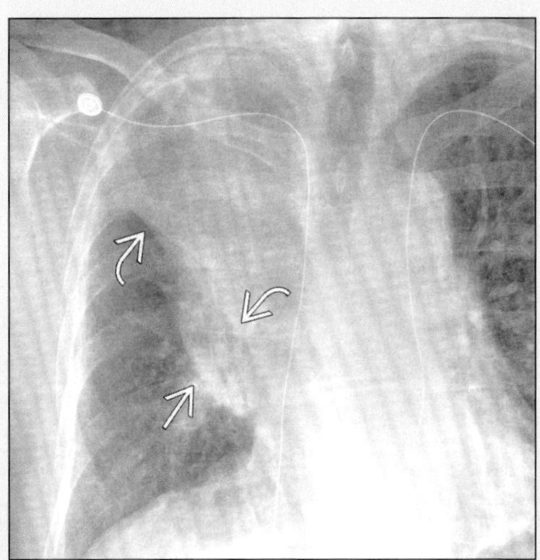

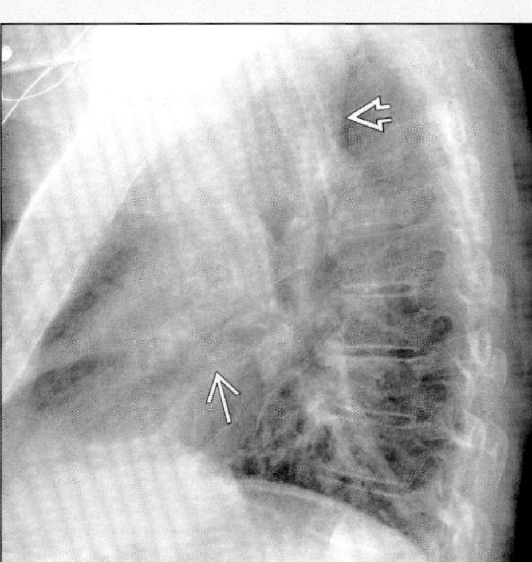

(Left) *PA chest radiograph of a patient with an obstructing right upper lobe lung cancer shows the S-sign of Golden. Note the superomedial displacement of the minor fissure ➡ secondary to volume loss and the convexity produced by a right hilar mass ➡. The minor fissure normally projects over the 4th anterior intercostal space.* ***(Right)*** *Lateral chest radiograph of the same patient demonstrates a large central mass ➡ and anterosuperior displacement of the major fissure ➡.*

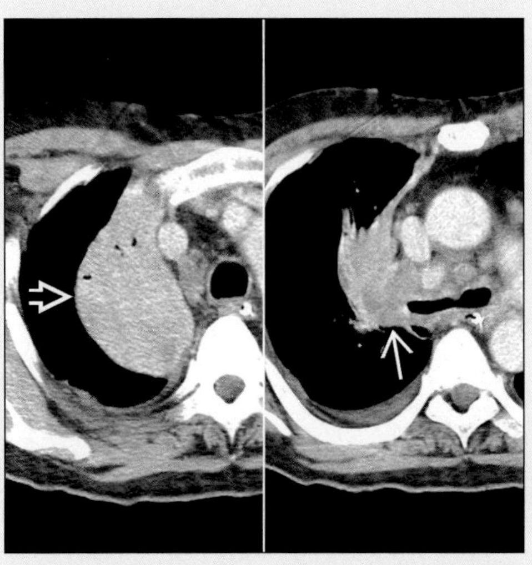

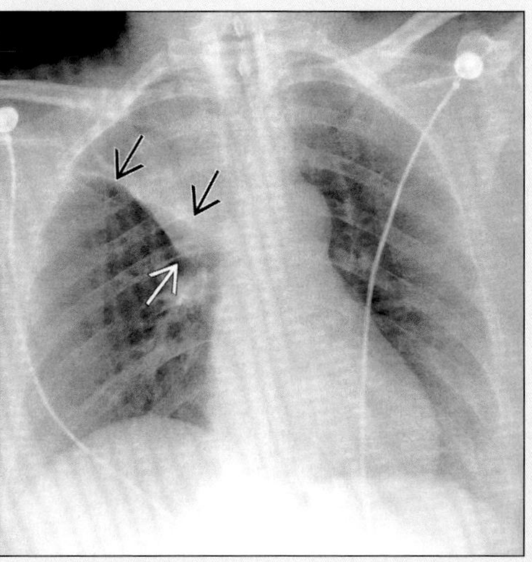

(Left) *Composite image with axial CECT of the same patient shows an enhancing atelectatic right upper lobe ➡ and a relatively hypodense right hilar mass ➡ obstructing the right upper lobe bronchus. While the S-sign of Golden can be seen in a variety of bronchial obstructions, lung cancer is the most common etiology.* ***(Right)*** *PA chest radiograph of a patient with a central lung cancer shows the reverse "S" morphology of the superomedially displaced minor fissure ➡ and the right hilar mass ➡.*

SIGNET RING SIGN

Key Facts

Terminology

- Definition: CT sign; small round soft tissue opacity (artery) abutting air-attenuation ring (bronchus) with ratio exceeding 1:1

Imaging

- HRCT
  - Normally, bronchus appears round when imaged along short axis
  - Normally, accompanying pulmonary artery also appears rounded & has similar diameter (bronchoarterial ratio 1:1)
  - In bronchial dilatation (i.e., bronchiectasis), bronchus appears larger than accompanying artery (bronchoarterial ratio > 1:1)
  - If bronchus imaged along long axis, bronchiectasis appears as nontapering or frankly dilated branching tubular lucencies
  - Ancillary findings: Bronchial wall thickening, visible bronchi within 1 cm of pleura, mosaic attenuation, expiratory air-trapping, mucoid impaction, and air-fluid levels within dilated bronchi

Top Differential Diagnoses

- Mild bronchial dilatation reported in asymptomatic elderly subjects

Pathology

- Etiologies: Cystic fibrosis, humoral immunodeficiencies, post infection, asthma, ABPA, interstitial lung disease, radiation therapy, etc.

Diagnostic Checklist

- Mild bronchiectasis is often overlooked; compare bronchial diameter to that of accompanying artery to identify large airway abnormalities

__(Left)__ Axial HRCT of a patient with a history of inhalational injury shows multiple dilated bronchi in the left lower lobe, some of which exhibit the so-called signet ring sign ➔. Other ancillary findings in this case include mosaic attenuation due to concomitant small airways disease. __(Right)__ Axial HRCT of a patient with a history of lung transplant and bronchiolitis obliterans syndrome shows numerous bronchiectatic airways, some of which demonstrate the signet ring sign ➔.

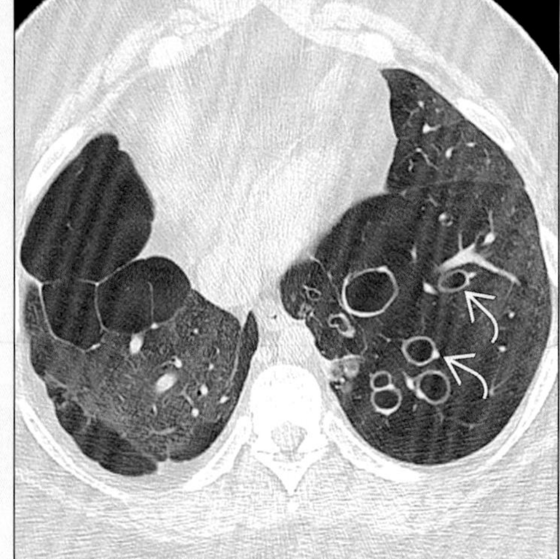

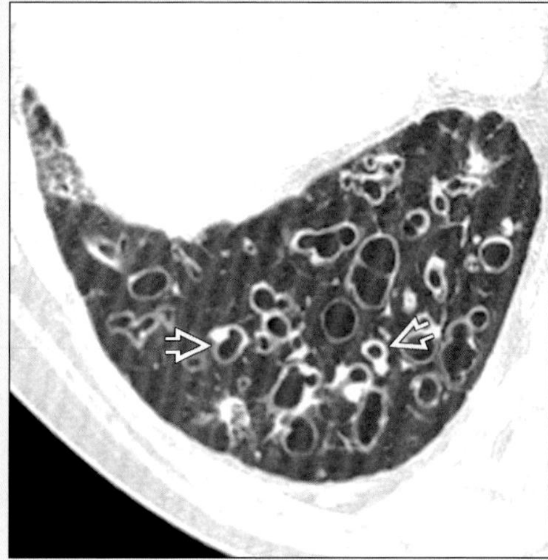

__(Left)__ Axial thin-section NECT of a patient with cystic fibrosis shows bronchiectasis imaged along the long axis of the bronchi. Note absence of bronchial tapering and progressive dilatation ➔ of bronchi as they extend peripherally. __(Right)__ Coronal CECT of a patient with common variable immunodeficiency shows diffuse bronchiectasis and bilateral mosaic attenuation due to air-trapping, a common ancillary finding associated with bronchiectasis.

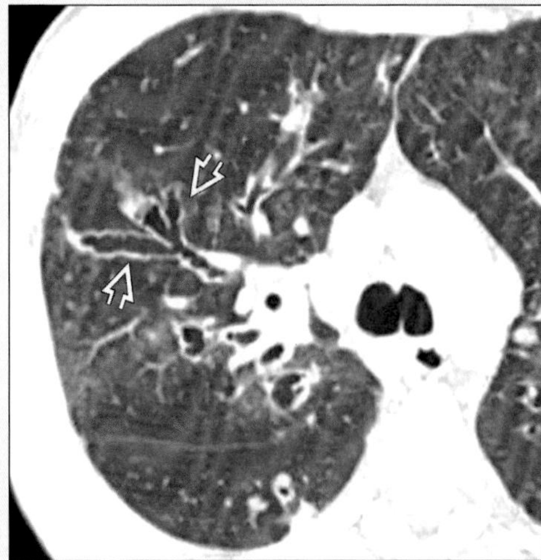

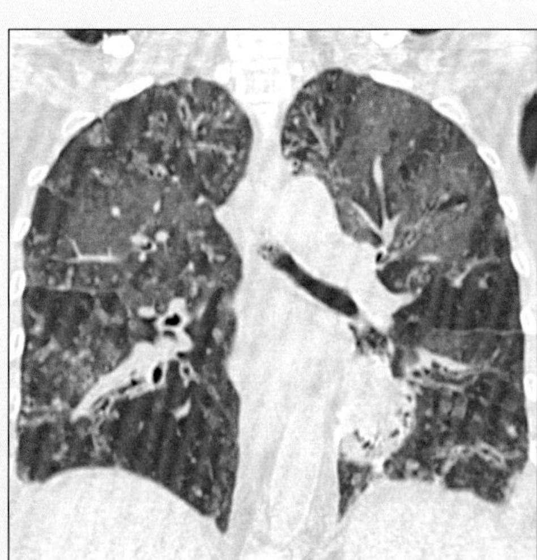

SILHOUETTE SIGN

Key Facts

Terminology

- Definition
  - Obscuration of heart, aorta, or diaphragm interface previously outlined by aerated lung
  - Produced by replacement of alveolar air with water density material

Imaging

- Radiography
  - Middle lobe or right upper lobe anterior segment abnormality obscures right heart border
  - Lingular or left upper lobe anterior segment abnormality obscures left heart border
  - Left upper lobe apicoposterior segment abnormality obscures aortic arch
  - Lower lobe basal segment abnormality obscures ipsilateral hemidiaphragm
  - Pleural effusion obscures ipsilateral hemidiaphragm
  - Margin of mediastinal mass extending into neck is obscured above clavicle due to lack of adjacent aerated lung (**cervicothoracic sign**)
  - Margin of mediastinal mass extending into abdomen is obscured below diaphragm due to lack of adjacent aerated lung (**thoracoabdominal sign**)
- CT
  - Depending on clinical scenario &/or availability of prior radiographs, CT may allow further characterization of lesions producing **sign of silhouette**

Pathology

- Etiology: Atelectasis, consolidation, mass
- Concept may be applicable to other radiographic abnormalities in which interface of a particular anatomic structure is obscured

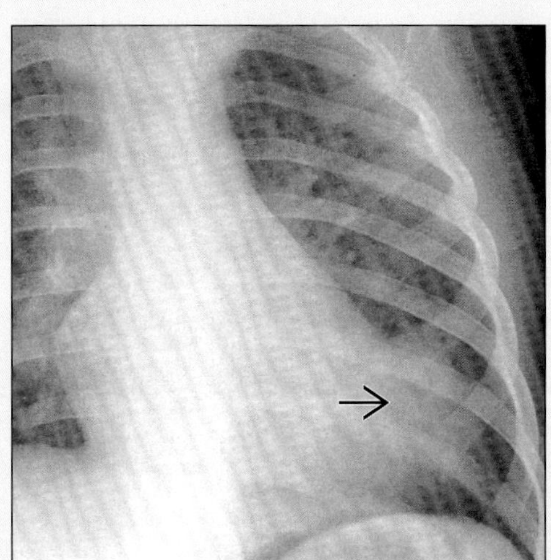

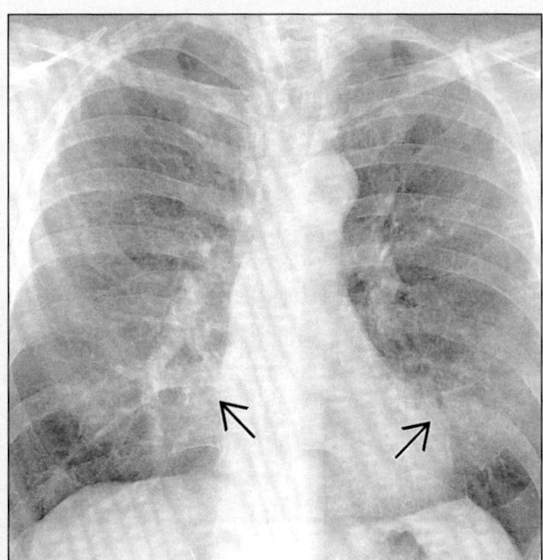

(Left) *PA chest radiograph of a child with lingular pneumonia shows obscuration of the left ventricular convexity ➔. If the consolidation was located in the left lower lobe, it could be in a similar location, but it would not obscure the left heart border.* ***(Right)*** *PA chest radiograph of a patient with atypical mycobacterial infection affecting the right middle lobe and the lingula shows subtle obscuration of the right and left heart borders ➔ by adjacent consolidation or atelectasis.*

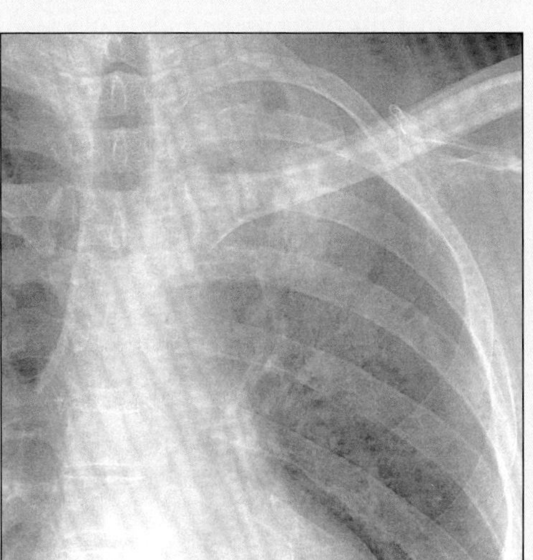

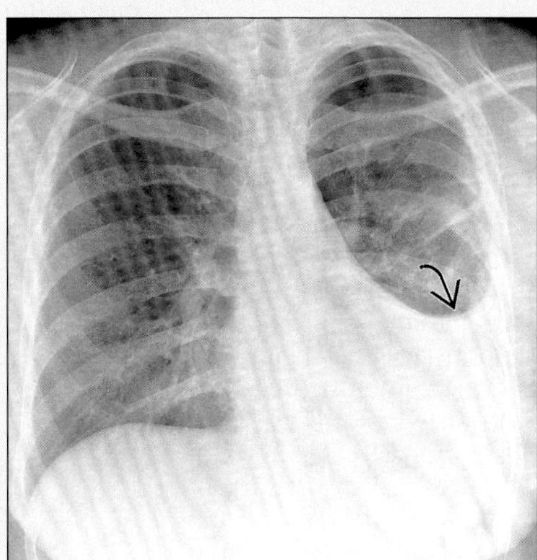

(Left) *PA chest radiograph of a patient with acquired immunodeficiency syndrome and Staphylococcus aureus pneumonia shows a left apical consolidation that obscures the aortic arch and is therefore located in the left upper lobe apicoposterior segment.* ***(Right)*** *PA chest radiograph of a patient with systemic lupus erythematosus shows a moderate left pleural effusion that exhibits a meniscus sign ➔ and obscuration of the left hemidiaphragm due to displacement of adjacent aerated lung.*

APPROACH TO ATELECTASIS AND VOLUME LOSS

Background

When evaluating the lungs on imaging studies, loss of volume (atelectasis) is one of the most common radiographic and CT abnormalities encountered. Radiologists must be familiar with the various imaging manifestations of atelectasis, which range from subsegmental atelectasis (often seen in hospitalized and bedridden patients) to the various patterns of lobar atelectasis that may herald the presence of an underlying obstructive tumor. The term atelectasis is derived from the Greek "ateles" (incomplete) "ektasis" (expansion). When atelectasis is detected on imaging studies, radiologists should consider which of the following mechanisms may be operating.

Mechanisms

The mechanisms that cause atelectasis may be **obstructive** or **nonobstructive** in nature, and each mechanism may operate independently or in combination with the others. Obstructive atelectasis occurs most commonly and involves resorption of air that may result from a variety of endobronchial lesions or by extrinsic bronchial compression. **Endobronchial lesions** that may cause obstructive atelectasis include mucus plugs, malpositioned endotracheal tubes, foreign bodies, endobronchial tumors, airway rupture, and/or areas of bronchial stricture or stenosis from various causes. **Extrinsic bronchial compression** and obstruction is usually caused by lymphadenopathy related to neoplastic disease but may also occur in patients with other diseases that affect hilar lymph nodes (e.g., tuberculosis, histoplasmosis, sarcoidosis).

Nonobstructive atelectasis is related to various mechanisms encountered in the entities of relaxation, adhesive, and cicatrization atelectasis. Relaxation atelectasis may either be caused by a space-occupying process that allows the lung to retract in a passive manner (e.g., pneumothorax) or one that compresses the lung (i.e., a mass or a large pleural effusion).

Adhesive atelectasis is related to surfactant deficiency, whether through an abnormality of the surfactant itself, in its local availability and distribution, or through insufficient surfactant production. The etiologies of adhesive atelectasis include the respiratory distress syndrome encountered in the pediatric population and the more common entity of postoperative atelectasis; the latter is a characteristic finding in patients following coronary artery bypass (CABG) surgery. Other causes include pneumonia, smoke inhalation, prolonged shallow breathing, pulmonary thromboembolism, acute radiation pneumonitis, and acute respiratory distress syndrome (ARDS).

Cicatricial atelectasis is an irreversible process related to underlying fibrosis, typically as a result of an infectious or inflammatory condition. As fibrous tissue within the lung retracts, there is resultant volume loss, and the same retractile forces may act upon airways within the involved parenchyma to produce traction bronchiectasis. Cicatricial atelectasis may be localized or diffuse. On imaging studies, the localized form is characterized by an increase in lung opacity/attenuation within an area of parenchymal distortion, often with associated foci of traction bronchiectasis. Adjacent areas of lung may appear hyperinflated in a compensatory fashion, and associated findings such as diaphragmatic elevation may be encountered. Diffuse cicatricial atelectasis is characterized on imaging studies by diffuse loss of volume in the affected lung, with associated parenchymal distortion and heterogeneous lung density. Interstitial pulmonary fibrosis is a characteristic disease process resulting in diffuse cicatrization atelectasis.

Linear and Rounded Atelectasis

Other forms of volume loss in the lungs include linear and rounded atelectasis. **Linear atelectasis** has also been referred to as discoid, plate-like, or subsegmental atelectasis. In previous decades, findings of linear atelectasis were often referred to as "Fleischner lines" in deference to Dr. Felix Fleischner, one of the first practitioners of chest radiology. Such linear and band-like areas of atelectasis may be horizontal, oblique, or near vertical in their alignment and are most frequently encountered in the mid to lower lung zones.

Rounded atelectasis is a unique form of volume loss that is typically associated with pleural thickening often related to previous asbestos exposure. It is also frequently found in patients with chronic pleural thickening related to other causes including previous thoracic surgery, notably involving the left hemithorax in patients with previous CABG surgery. Rounded atelectasis often mimics lung cancer on imaging studies by its characteristic formation of a subpleural mass, most often in the posterior aspect of either lower lobe. As in all cases of atelectasis, comparison with prior imaging studies is a key step in performing accurate radiologic interpretation.

Imaging Signs of Atelectasis

The imaging signs of atelectasis may be categorized as direct or indirect, which are sometimes described as primary or secondary signs, respectively. The two **direct signs** are: 1) displacement of a fissure or fissures within the involved lung, and 2) crowding of bronchovascular structures. **Indirect signs** of atelectasis include increased lung opacity or attenuation, mediastinal shift toward the affected lung, compensatory hyperinflation of adjacent lung parenchyma, hilar displacement, and elevation of the ipsilateral hemidiaphragm. The anterior mediastinal structures are more prone to shift in response to atelectasis than are the posterior structures, which are relatively tethered to the paraspinal tissues. The superior mediastinum tends to shift with upper lobe atelectasis, whereas the inferior mediastinum is more likely to shift in association with lower lobe loss of volume. Other indirect signs of atelectasis are the juxtaphrenic peak sign (associated primarily with upper lobe atelectasis) and the luftsichel sign (seen in some but not all cases of left upper lobe atelectasis).

The typical radiographic findings in each of the various types of lobar atelectasis are illustrated on the following pages with graphic illustrations and case examples. It should be noted that a displaced fissure (a direct imaging sign of atelectasis) may appear as a linear opacity, but with increasing degrees of atelectasis may instead form a sharp interface or border along the edge of an atelectatic lobe as the involved lung loses volume while increasing in its density and radiographic opacity. Recognition of this finding is often the key to diagnosing lobar atelectasis.

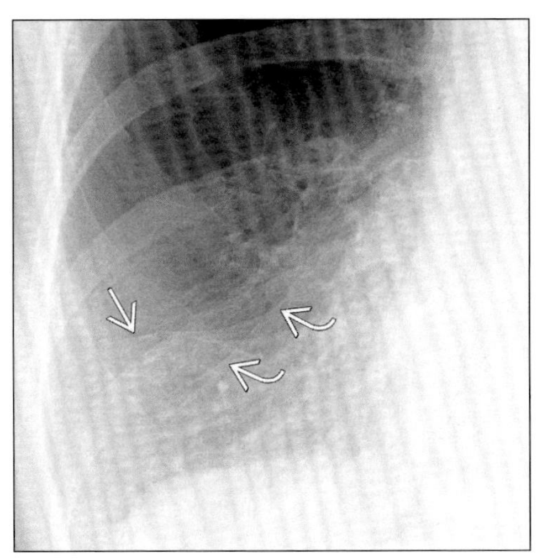

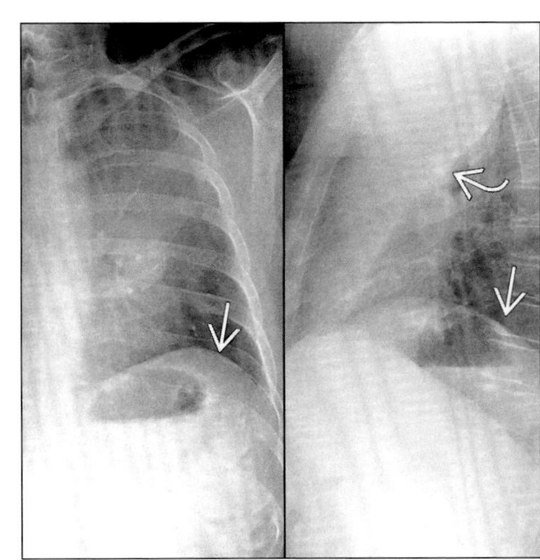

(Left) *PA chest radiograph (coned down to the right base) of a patient with right upper lobe bullae shows compressive middle and right lower lobe atelectasis, crowding of bronchovascular structures, and displacement of the minor and major fissures.* ***(Right)*** *Composite image with PA (left) and lateral (right) chest radiographs shows left upper lobe atelectasis with anterior displacement of the major fissure, an opaque atelectatic left upper lobe, and an elevated left hemidiaphragm.*

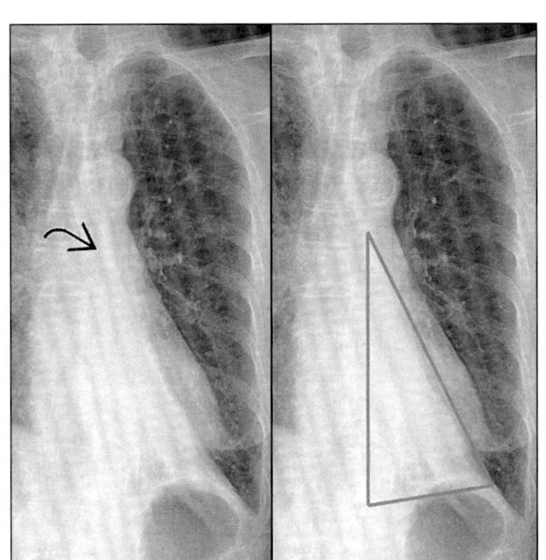

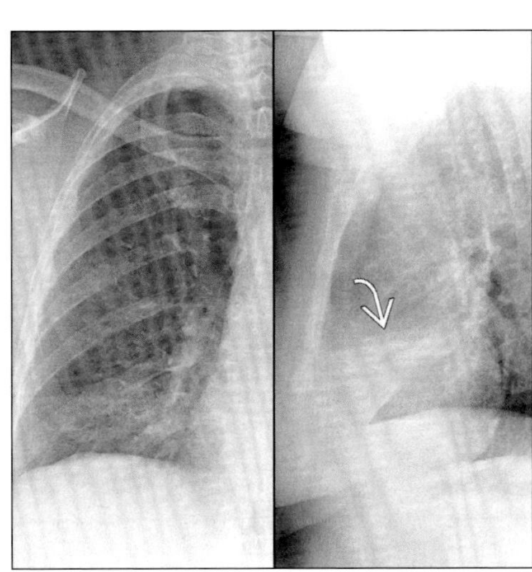

(Left) *Composite image with PA chest radiographs without (left) and with a graphic overlay (right) shows the triangular configuration of an atelectatic left lower lobe with its apex at the hilum and its base along the left hemidiaphragm. Atelectatic lobes often assume a triangular shape in the setting of moderate to marked loss of volume.* ***(Right)*** *Composite image with PA (left) and lateral (right) chest radiographs shows middle lobe atelectasis exhibiting a triangular shape on lateral radiography.*

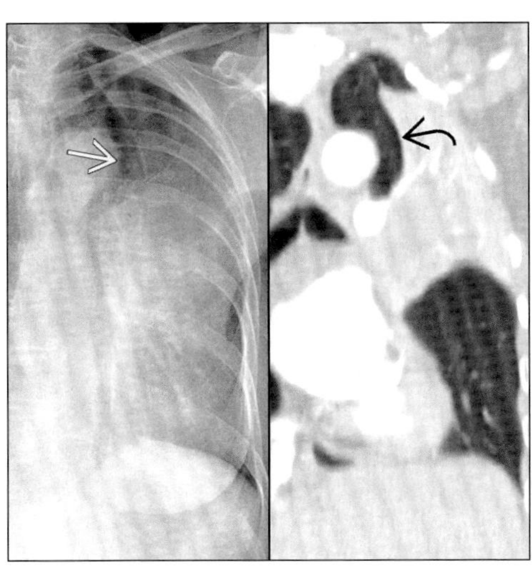

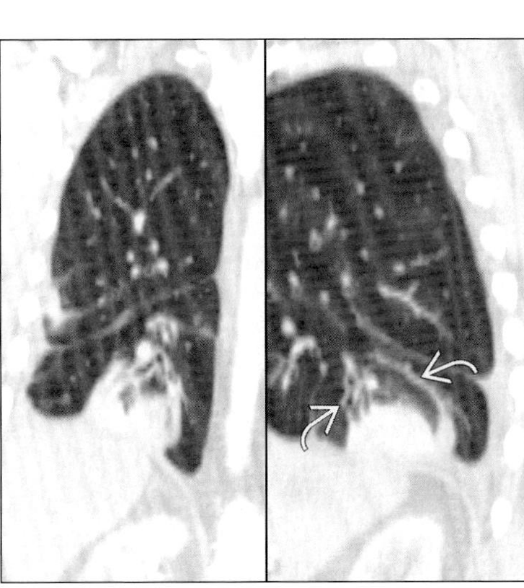

(Left) *Composite image with PA chest radiograph (left) and coronal CECT (right) shows left upper lobe atelectasis with a luftsichel sign formed by the hyperinflated superior segment of the left lower lobe as it insinuates itself between the atelectatic left upper lobe and the adjacent mediastinum. Bronchoscopy revealed lung cancer.* ***(Right)*** *Composite image with coronal (left) and sagittal (right) CECT shows left basilar rounded atelectasis with a characteristic "comet tail" sign.*

APPROACH TO ATELECTASIS AND VOLUME LOSS

*(**Left**) Graphic shows radiographic findings of progressive right upper lobe atelectasis with elevation and medial displacement of the minor fissure on the PA view and upward displacement of the minor and upper portion of the major fissures on the lateral view. There is increasing opacity of the collapsing lobe with progressive loss of volume. (**Right**) Composite with PA (left) and lateral (right) chest radiographs shows the same findings in this patient with a small obstructing right upper lobe cancer.*

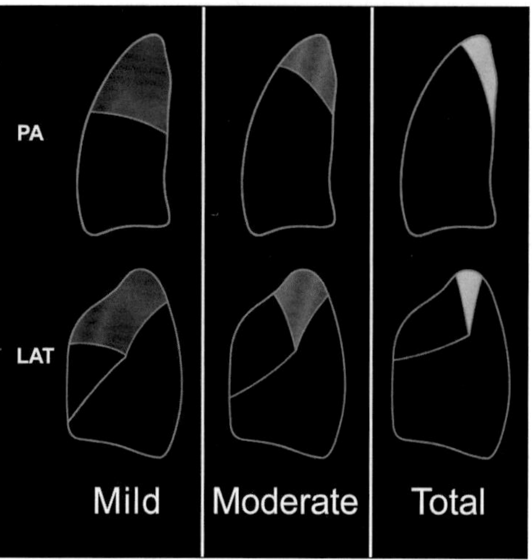

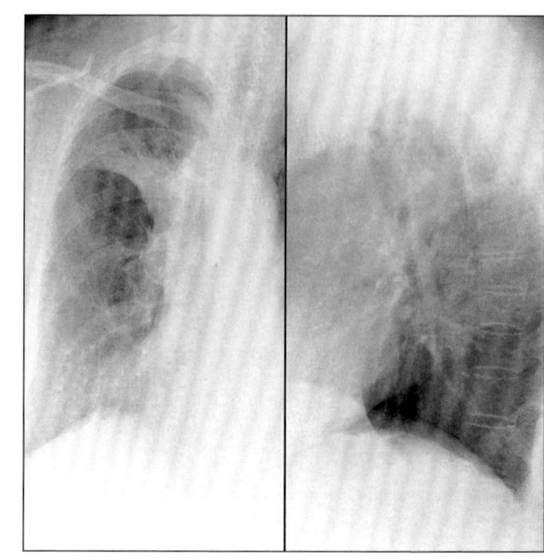

*(**Left**) Graphic shows radiographic findings of progressive middle lobe atelectasis with inferior displacement of the minor fissure and anterior displacement of the inferior major fissure, forming a triangular opacity on the lateral view that tapers to the right hilum. (**Right**) Composite with PA (left) and lateral (right) chest radiographs shows obscuration of the right heart border on the PA view and the triangular-shaped opacity of the atelectatic middle lobe on the lateral view.*

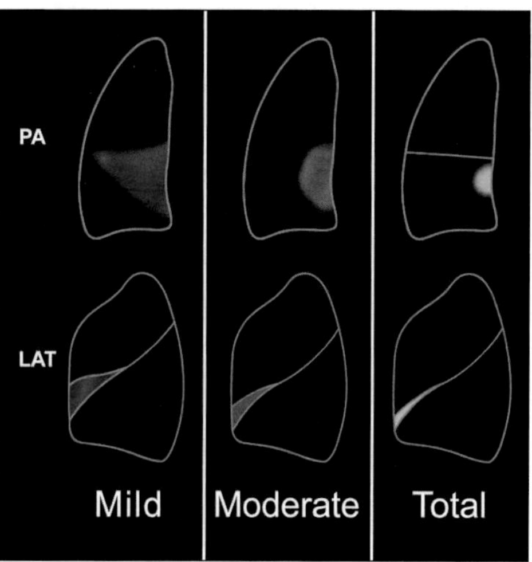

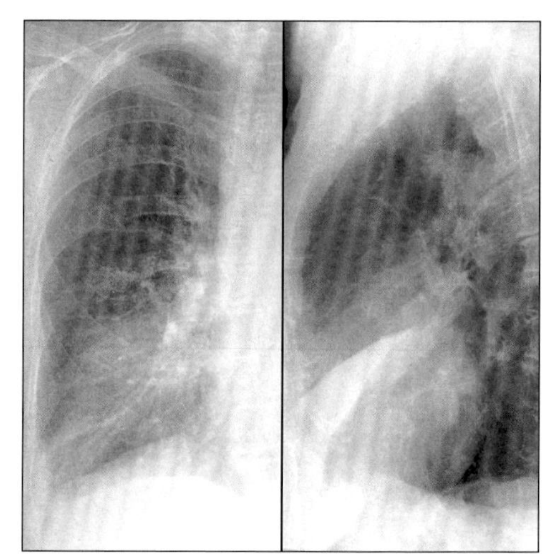

*(**Left**) Graphic shows findings of progressive right lower lobe atelectasis with medial displacement of the major fissure on the PA view, forming a triangular opacity and inferior displacement of the minor fissure. Increasing opacity of the lower lobe projects over the lower thoracic spine and obscures the adjacent hemidiaphragm. (**Right**) Composite image with PA (left) and lateral (right) chest radiographs shows right lower lobe atelectasis with displaced major ➜ and minor fissures ➜.*

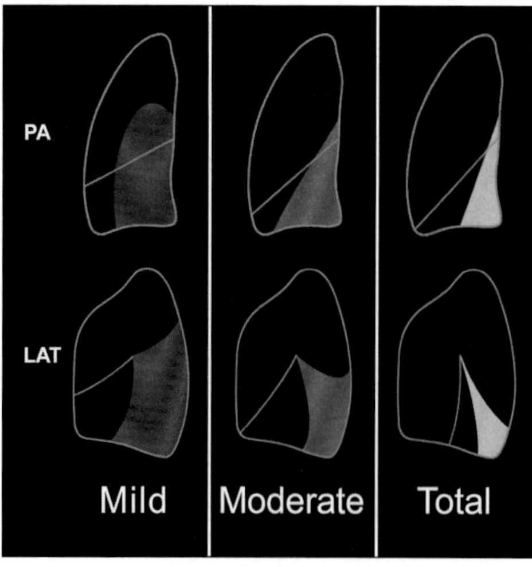

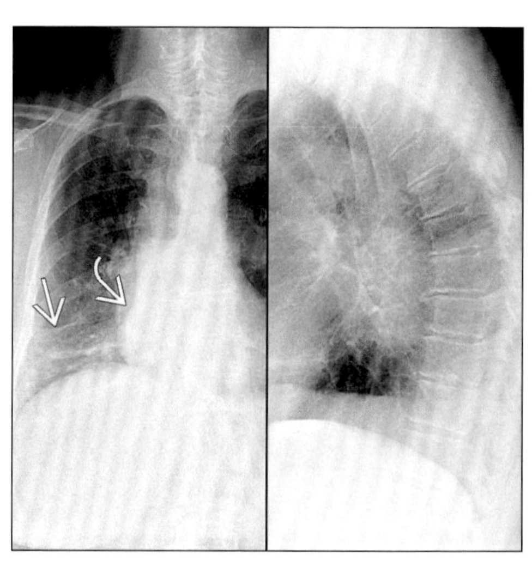

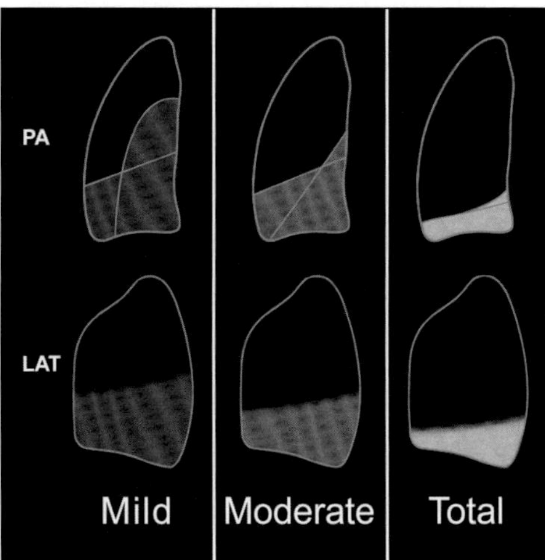

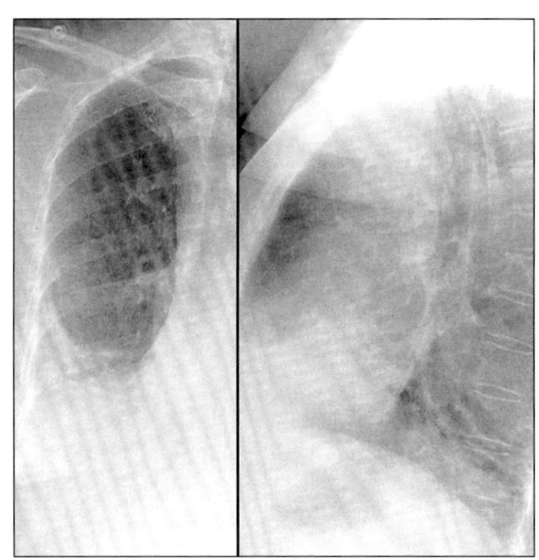

*(**Left**) Graphic shows findings of progressive combined middle and right lower lobe atelectasis, usually caused by obstruction at the bronchus intermedius. A band of increased opacity extends across the entire lung base on both PA and lateral views. (**Right**) Composite image with PA (left) and lateral (right) chest radiographs shows opacity across the right lung base on both views and inferior displacement of the right hilum caused by a carcinoid tumor in the bronchus intermedius.*

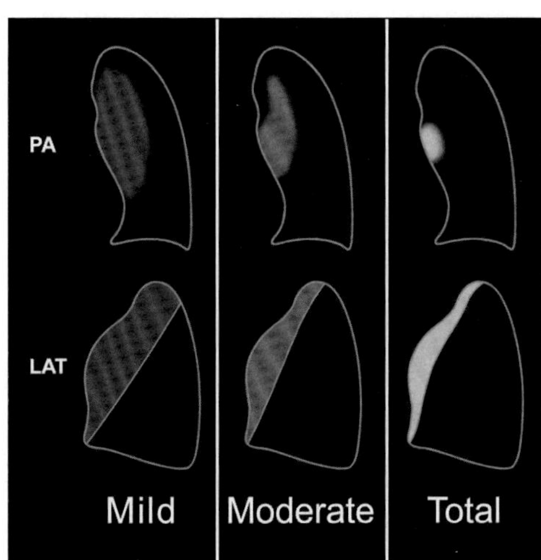

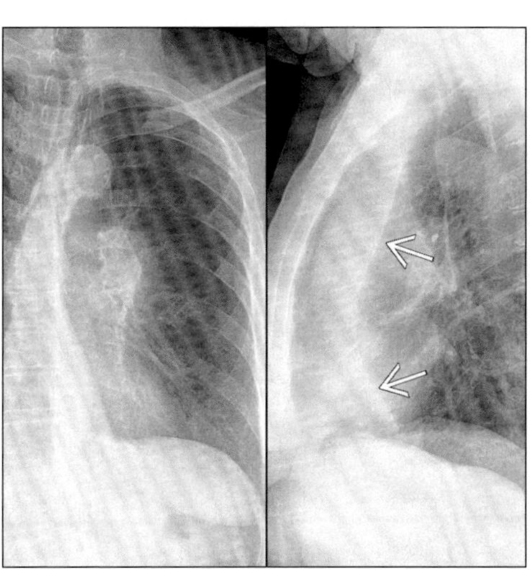

*(**Left**) Graphic shows findings of progressive left upper lobe atelectasis with increasing opacity in the perihilar and retrosternal regions and characteristic anterior displacement of the major fissure on the lateral view. (**Right**) Composite image with PA (left) and lateral (right) chest radiographs shows left upper lobe atelectasis. The displaced major fissure forms a sharp interface ➔ along the posterior edge of the opaque atelectatic left upper lobe. Bronchoscopy revealed lung cancer.*

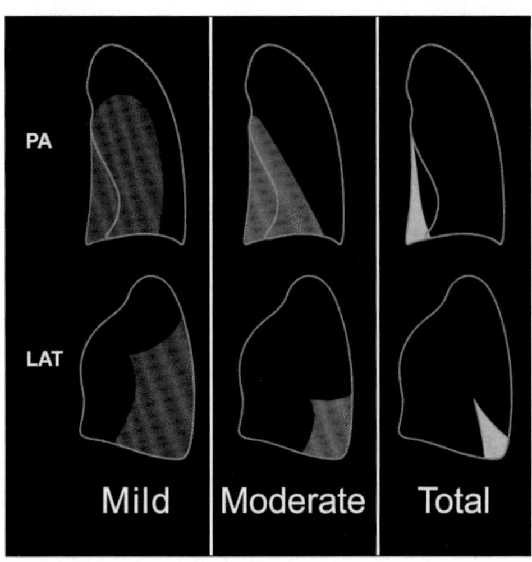

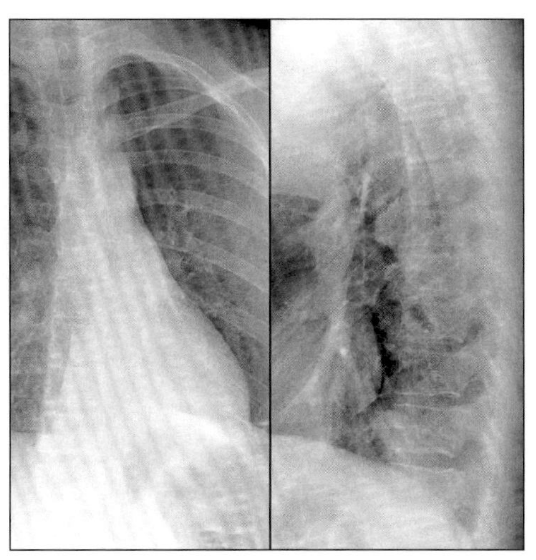

*(**Left**) Graphic shows findings of progressive left lower lobe atelectasis with medial displacement of the major fissure on the PA view, forming a triangular opacity. On the lateral view, increasing opacity of the lower lobe projects over the lower thoracic spine. (**Right**) Composite image with PA (left) and lateral (right) chest radiographs shows these findings. Note subtle increased opacity over the lower thoracic spine that obscures the adjacent elevated left hemidiaphragm.*

RIGHT UPPER LOBE ATELECTASIS

Key Facts

Imaging

- Frontal chest radiograph
  - Right upper lung zone opacity
  - Obscuration of right superior mediastinum
  - Superior displacement of right minor fissure with clockwise rotation laterally
  - Superior displacement of right hilum
  - Rightward shift of trachea
  - Juxtaphrenic peak of right hemidiaphragm
- Lateral chest radiograph
  - Opacity in right upper lung zone
  - Superior displacement of minor fissure
  - Anterior displacement of major fissure
- **S-sign of Golden**
  - Inferior concavity of lateral minor fissure
  - Inferior bulge of medial minor fissure by central hilar mass
  - Right hilar enlargement
- CT
  - Opaque, atelectatic, triangular right upper lobe
  - Anterior & medial rotation of minor fissure

Top Differential Diagnoses

- Pneumonia
- Lung cancer
- Lobectomy

Pathology

- Endobronchial obstruction
  - Malignant > benign tumors
  - Mucous plugging
- Extrinsic bronchial compression

Clinical Issues

- Symptoms depend on severity of atelectasis & rapidity of development
- Shortness of breath, dyspnea, & chest pain

*(**Left**) PA chest radiograph demonstrates right upper lobe atelectasis with elevation of the minor fissure ➡, rightward shift of the trachea ⇨, and elevation of an enlarged right hilum ➡. This constellation of findings is called the S-sign of Golden and is characteristic of right upper lobe atelectasis caused by a central mass. (**Right**) Lateral chest radiograph of the same patient shows increased opacity due to right upper lobe atelectasis with anterior displacement of the major fissure ➡.*

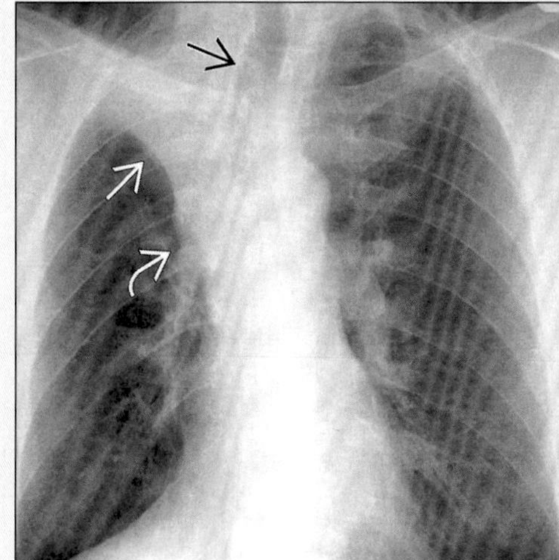

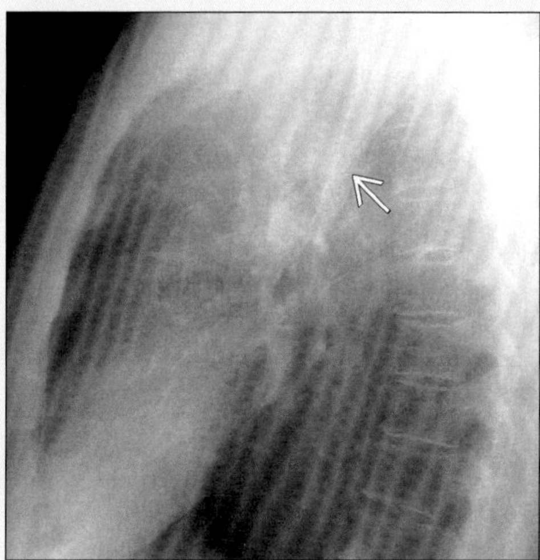

*(**Left**) Axial NECT of the same patient shows an opaque atelectatic right upper lobe, which assumes a triangular shape and exhibits no internal air bronchograms, suggesting a central obstructing lesion. Note the anterior and medial rotation of the minor fissure ➡. (**Right**) Axial NECT of the same patient shows the atelectatic right upper lobe with narrowing and obliteration of the right upper lobe bronchus ➡. Surgery revealed squamous cell lung cancer and mediastinal lymphadenopathy.*

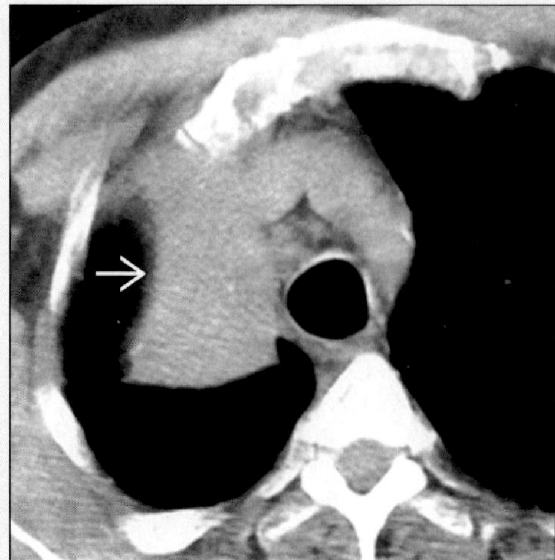

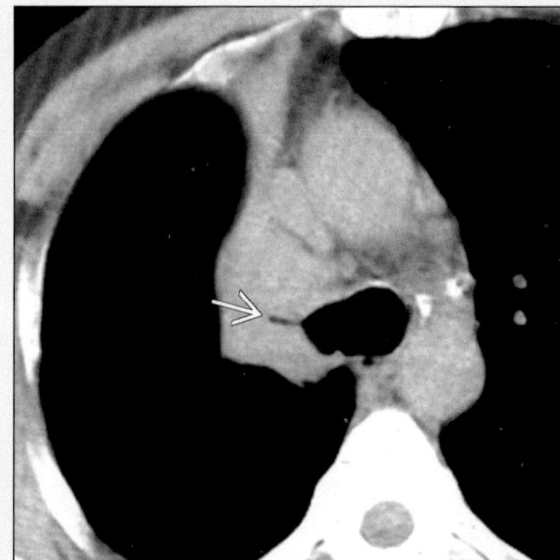

MIDDLE LOBE ATELECTASIS

Key Facts

Imaging

- Frontal chest radiograph
  - Opacity in right mid-lung zone that obscures right heart border
  - Nonvisualization of minor fissure secondary to inferior displacement
- Lateral chest radiograph
  - Thin band-like opacity with apex located at right hilum
  - Inferior displacement of minor fissure
  - Anterior displacement of right major fissure
- CT
  - Opacification of triangular-shaped right middle lobe
  - Right upper lobe located anterior & lateral to atelectatic right middle lobe
  - Right lower lobe located posterior & lateral (sometimes medial) to atelectatic right middle lobe

Top Differential Diagnoses

- Pneumonia
- Lobectomy
- Lung cancer

Pathology

- Endobronchial obstruction
  - Malignant > benign tumors
  - Mucus plugging
- Right middle lobe syndrome
  - Recurrent or chronic middle lobe atelectasis
  - Tumors, inflammatory states, infection

Clinical Issues

- Symptoms depend on severity of atelectasis & rapidity of development
- Shortness of breath, dyspnea, & chest pain most common

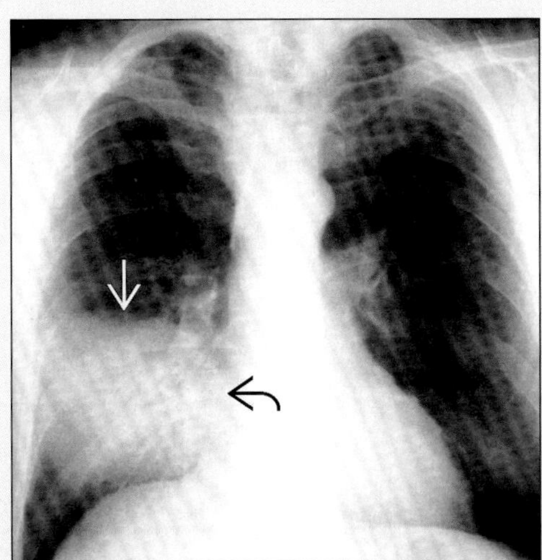

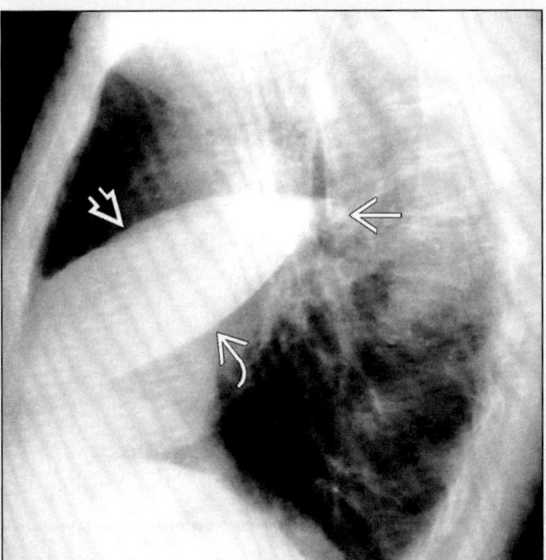

(Left) *PA chest radiograph of a patient with middle lobe atelectasis demonstrates opacity ➡ in the right mid-lung zone that obscures the right heart border ⇨.* ***(Right)*** *Lateral chest radiograph of the same patient shows a band-like opacity in the anatomic location of the middle lobe, the apex of which is located at the right hilum ➡. Note the inferior displacement of the minor fissure ➡ and the anterior displacement of the right major fissure ➡.*

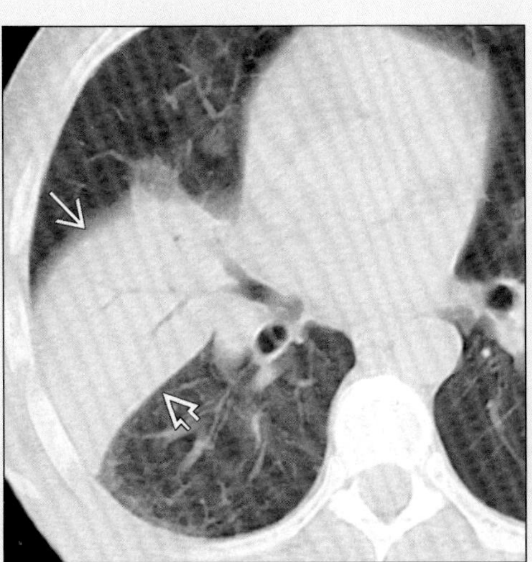

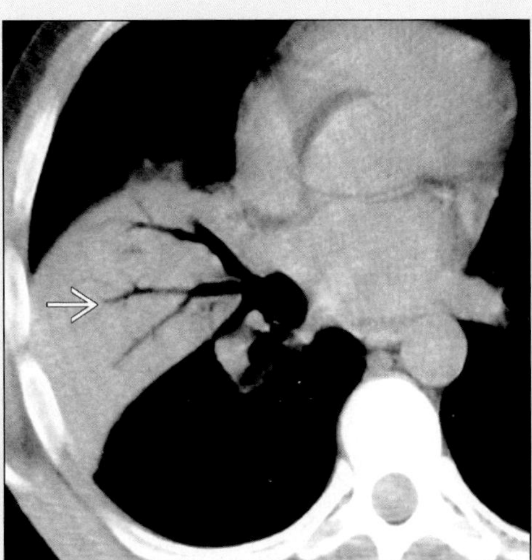

(Left) *Axial NECT of the same patient shows opacification of the right middle lobe, which is bordered by the minor fissure anteriorly ➡ and the major fissure posteriorly ➡.* ***(Right)*** *Axial NECT of the same patient demonstrates middle lobe atelectasis and intrinsic air bronchograms ➡. The most common cause of lobar atelectasis is endobronchial obstruction, usually from endoluminal lesion or mucus plugging. Middle lobe syndrome is chronic middle lobe atelectasis from a variety of etiologies.*

RIGHT LOWER LOBE ATELECTASIS

Key Facts

Imaging

- Frontal chest radiograph
  - Triangular-shaped opacity in right lower lung zone
  - Triangle apex: Right hilum
  - Triangle base: Right hemidiaphragm
  - Obscuration of right hemidiaphragm
  - Displacement of right major fissure toward mediastinum
  - Inferior displacement of right hilum
- Lateral chest radiograph
  - Opacity projecting over lower thoracic spine
  - Displacement of right major fissure posteriorly & inferiorly
  - Major fissure may not be visualized depending on extent of atelectasis
  - Posterior displacement of right hilum
- CT
  - Opacification of collapsed right lower lobe
  - Right lower lobe contacts right hemidiaphragm & paravertebral region
  - Displacement of right major fissure posteriorly & medially

Top Differential Diagnoses

- Pneumonia
- Lobectomy
- Lung cancer

Pathology

- Endobronchial obstruction
  - Malignant > benign tumors
  - Mucus plugging
- Extrinsic bronchial compression

Clinical Issues

- Symptoms depend on severity of atelectasis & rapidity of development

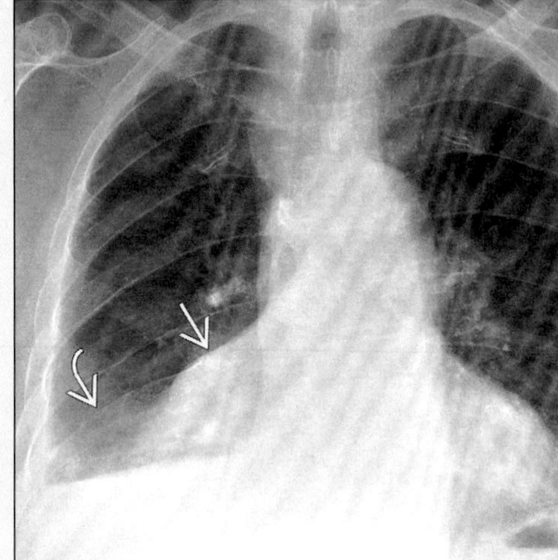

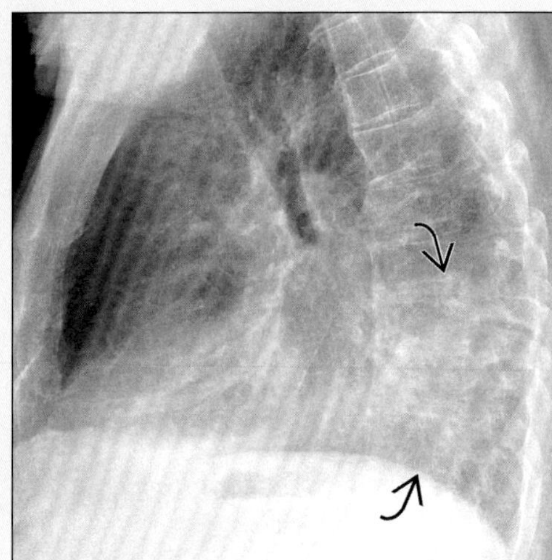

(Left) *PA chest radiograph shows right lower lobe atelectasis manifesting with increased opacity in the right lower lung zone that partly obscures the right hemidiaphragm. The major fissure forms a sharp interface along the edge of the collapsing right lower lobe ➡. The minor fissure is displaced inferomedially ➡.* ***(Right)*** *Lateral chest radiograph of the same patient shows opacity projecting posteriorly over the lower thoracic spine ➡ and obscuration of the right hemidiaphragm.*

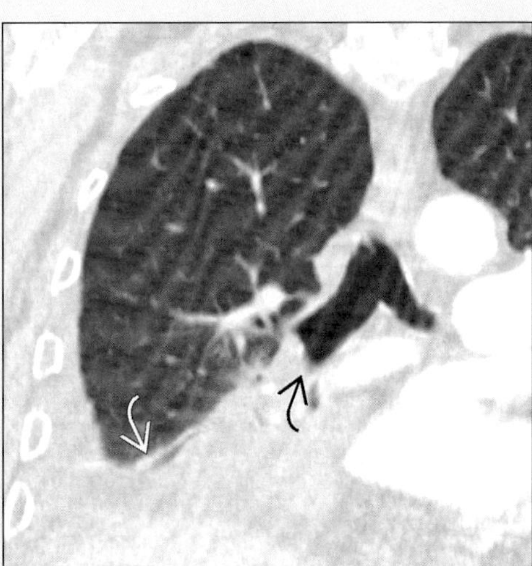

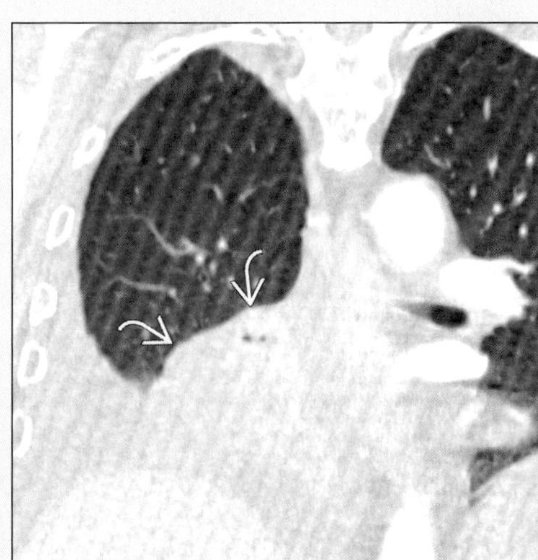

(Left) *Coronal CECT shows right lower lobe atelectasis manifesting as a triangular opacity with its apex at the hilum and its base along the right hemidiaphragm. A central lung cancer obstructs the right lower lobe bronchus ➡. Note inferomedial displacement of the minor fissure ➡.* ***(Right)*** *Coronal CECT of the same patient shows the displaced major fissure forming a sharp interface along the edge of the triangular-shaped atelectatic right lower lobe ➡.*

LEFT UPPER LOBE ATELECTASIS

Key Facts

Imaging

- Frontal chest radiograph
  - Opacity in left upper lung zone
  - "**Silhouette" sign**: Obscuration of left heart border & superior mediastinum
  - "**Luftsichel" sign**: Crescentic lucency caused by interposition of aerated superior segment of left lower lobe between collapsed left upper lobe & mediastinum
- Lateral chest radiograph
  - Anterior displacement of left major fissure
  - Left major fissure parallels chest wall
  - Opaque atelectatic lung anterior to left major fissure
  - Anterior displacement of left hilum
- CT
  - Opaque atelectatic left upper lobe
  - Displacement of left major fissure anteriorly & medially
  - "**Luftsichel" sign**

Top Differential Diagnoses

- Pneumonia
- Lobectomy
- Lung cancer

Pathology

- Endobronchial obstruction
  - Malignant > benign tumors
  - Mucus plugging
- Extrinsic bronchial compression

Clinical Issues

- Symptoms depend on severity of atelectasis & rapidity of development
- Shortness of breath, dyspnea, & chest pain

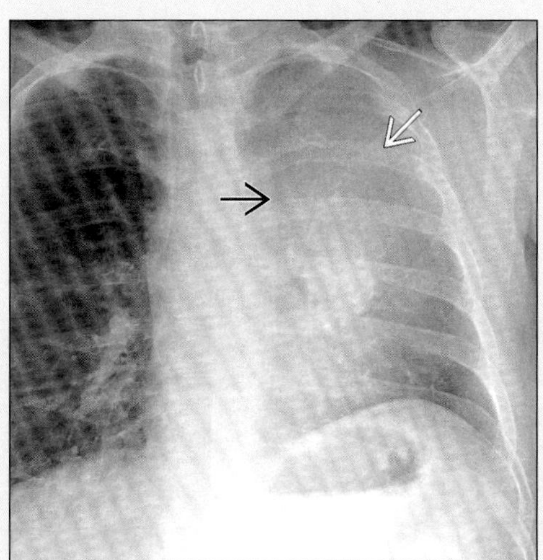

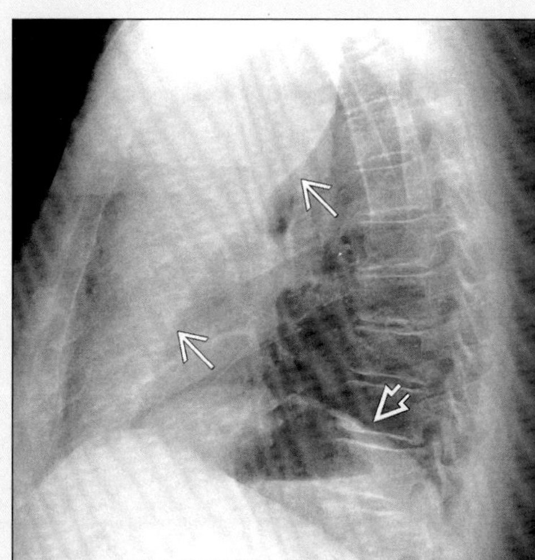

(Left) *PA chest radiograph shows left upper lung opacity ➡ that obscures the left superior mediastinum. Interposition of the aerated superior segment of the left lower lobe between the opacity and the mediastinum forms a vertical band of lucency ➡, the "luftsichel" sign.* ***(Right)*** *Lateral chest radiograph of the same patient shows anterior displacement of the major fissure ➡ with anterior opacity representing the atelectatic left upper lobe and associated elevation of the left hemidiaphragm ➡.*

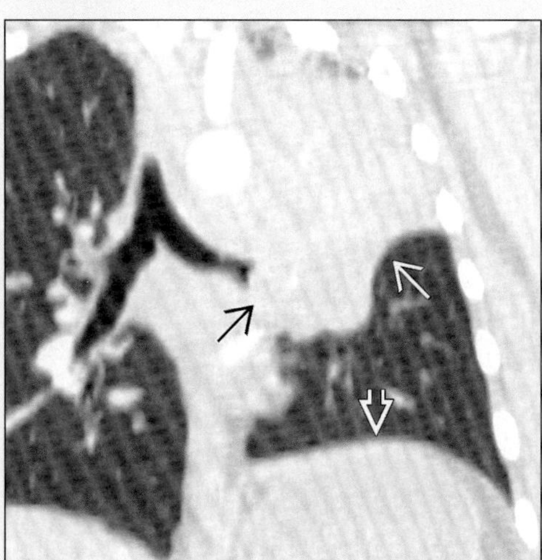

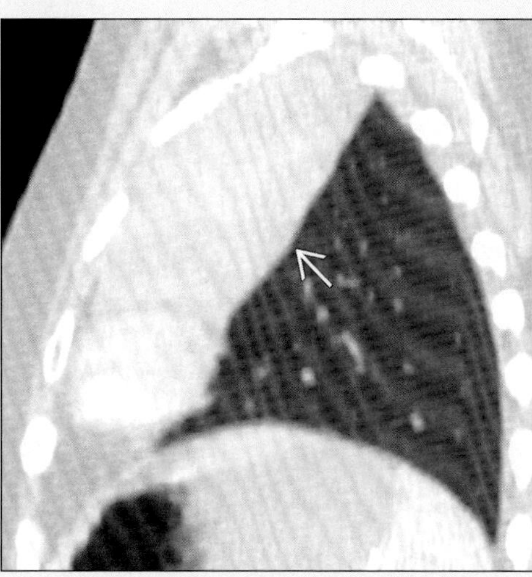

(Left) *Coronal CECT shows opacification of the atelectatic left upper lobe, displacement of the major fissure ➡, and elevation of the left hemidiaphragm ➡. Absence of air bronchograms within the atelectatic lobe suggests complete endobronchial obstruction, here produced by a central lung cancer ➡.* ***(Right)*** *Sagittal CECT of the same patient shows anterior displacement of the major fissure ➡ and opacification of the atelectatic left upper lobe, findings typically apparent on lateral chest radiography.*

LEFT LOWER LOBE ATELECTASIS

Key Facts

Imaging

- Frontal chest radiograph
  - Triangular left lower lung zone opacity: Apex of triangle is left hilum; base of triangle is left hemidiaphragm
  - Obscuration of left hemidiaphragm
  - Displacement of major fissure toward mediastinum
  - Inferior displacement of left hilum
- Lateral chest radiograph
  - Opacity projecting over lower thoracic spine
  - Posterior inferior displacement of major fissure
  - Major fissure may not be visualized depending on extent of atelectasis
  - Posterior displacement of left hilum
  - Obscuration of posterior left hemidiaphragm
- CT
  - Opaque atelectatic left lower lobe
  - Atelectatic left lower lobe contacts left hemidiaphragm & paravertebral region
  - Major fissure is displaced posteriorly & medially

Top Differential Diagnoses

- Pneumonia
- Lobectomy
- Lung cancer

Pathology

- Endobronchial obstruction
  - Malignant > benign tumors
  - Mucus plugging
- Extrinsic bronchial compression

Clinical Issues

- Symptoms depend on severity of atelectasis & rapidity of development
- Shortness of breath, dyspnea, & chest pain

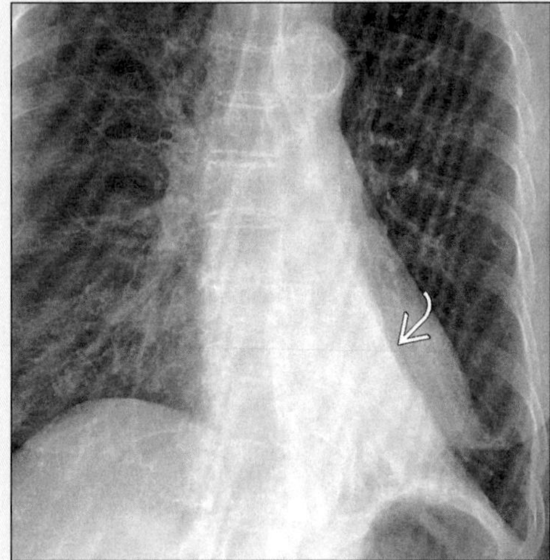

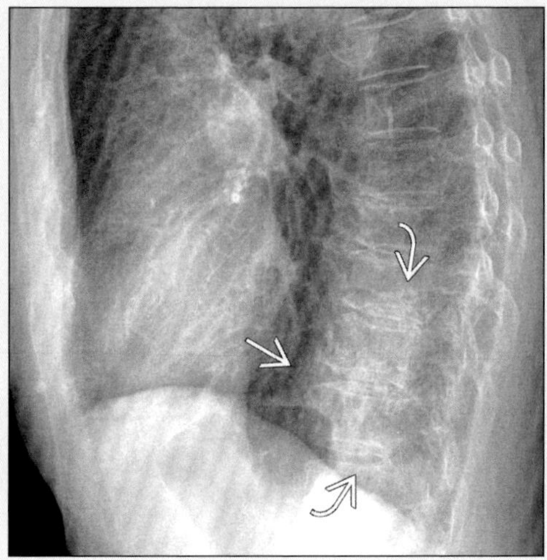

(Left) *PA chest radiograph shows left lower lobe atelectasis forming a triangular retrocardiac opacity that obscures the descending aorta and the left hemidiaphragm. The major fissure is displaced inferomedially, forming a sharp interface along the edge of the atelectatic lobe ➲.* ***(Right)*** *Lateral chest radiograph of the same patient shows opacity projecting over the lower thoracic spine ➲, posterior and inferior displacement of the major fissure ➔, and obscuration of the posterior left hemidiaphragm.*

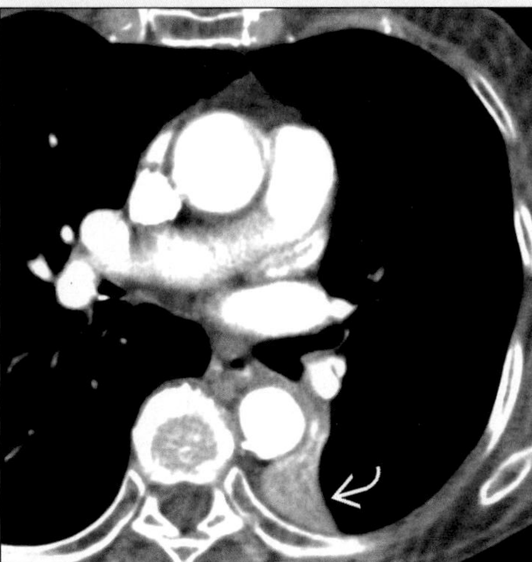

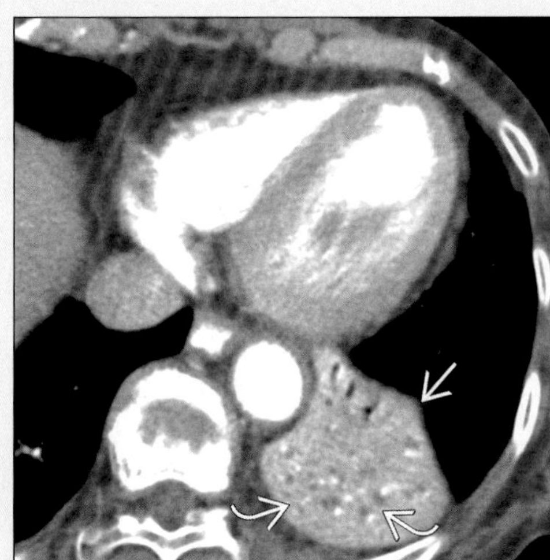

(Left) *Axial CECT of the same patient shows left lower lobe atelectasis forming a triangular opacity along the left aortic margin and paravertebral region with posteromedial displacement of the left major fissure ➲ and enhancing vessels within the atelectatic lung.* ***(Right)*** *Axial CECT of the same patient shows crowding of bronchi and vessels ➲, indicative of volume loss. The displaced left major fissure forms a sharp interface along the margin of the atelectatic left lower lobe ➔.*

Key Facts

Terminology
- Loss of alveolar air within entire lung

Imaging
- Radiography
  - Complete opacification of affected lung
  - Elevation of ipsilateral hemidiaphragm
  - Shift of mediastinum toward affected lung
  - Compensatory overinflation of contralateral lung
- CT
  - Evaluation of atelectatic lung
  - Identification of bronchovascular crowding
  - Evaluation of underlying etiology for complete atelectasis: Central tumor, mucus plug, extrinsic compression
  - Evaluation of pleural space for pleural effusion or pneumothorax

Top Differential Diagnoses
- Pneumonia
- Pleural effusion
- Pneumothorax

Pathology
- Endobronchial obstruction
  - Malignant > benign tumors
  - Mucus plugging
- Extrinsic bronchial compression
- Intubation of contralateral main bronchus
- Relaxation or passive atelectasis: Pneumothorax, pleural effusion

Clinical Issues
- Symptoms depend on severity & rapidity of atelectasis
- Shortness of breath, dyspnea, & chest pain

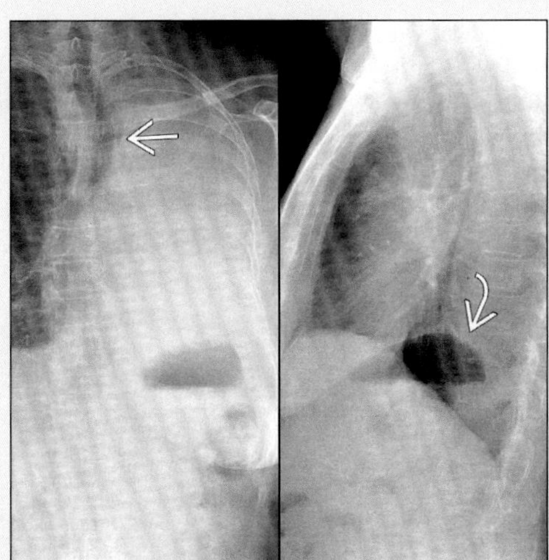

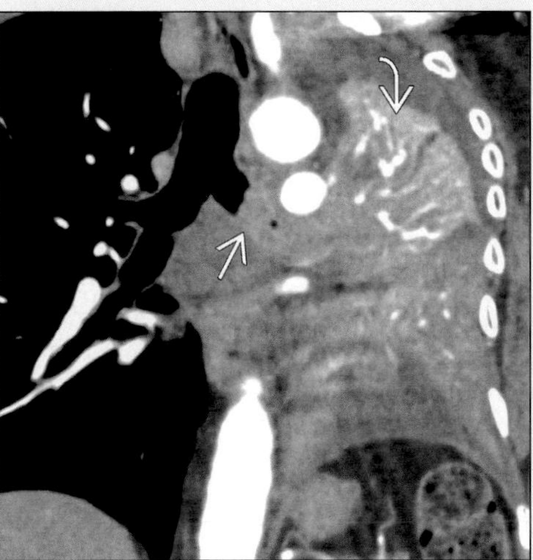

(Left) *Composite image with PA (left) and lateral (right) chest radiographs shows complete left lung atelectasis with elevation of the ipsilateral hemidiaphragm ➡ and shift of the trachea ➡ and other mediastinal structures toward the affected lung.* ***(Right)*** *Coronal CECT of the same patient shows a central endoluminal lung cancer obstructing the left main bronchus ➡ and confirms elevation of the left hemidiaphragm. Note crowding of bronchovascular structures in the affected lung ➡.*

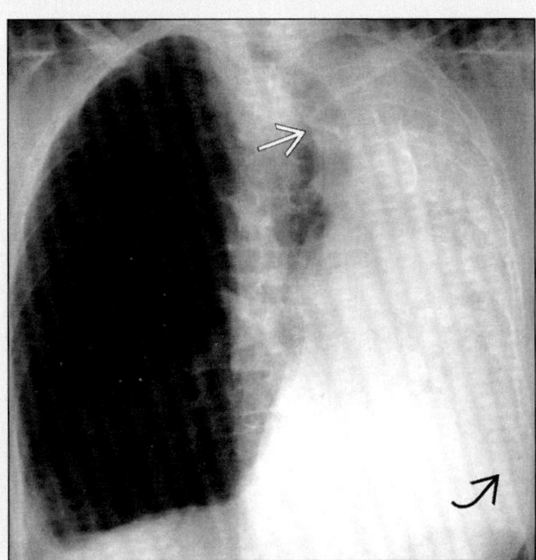

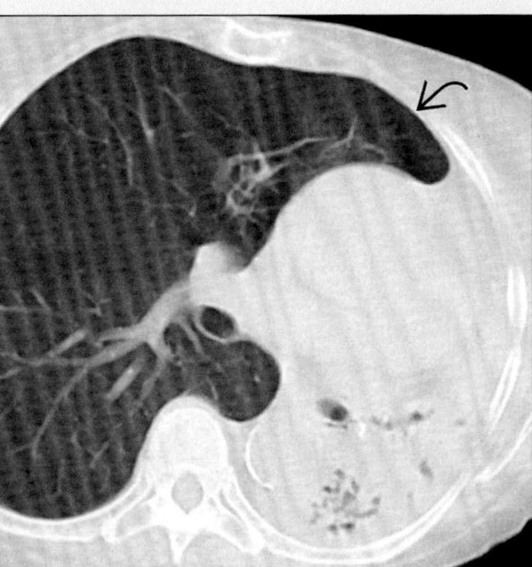

(Left) *PA chest radiograph shows left lung atelectasis caused by a mucus plug with opacification of the affected hemithorax, elevation of the ipsilateral hemidiaphragm ➡, and shift of the trachea ➡ and other mediastinal structures toward the affected lung.* ***(Right)*** *Axial NECT of the same patient shows shift of the mediastinal structures toward the affected lung and hyperinflation of the right lung across the midline into the left hemithorax ➡. The findings resolved following bronchoscopy.*

SUBSEGMENTAL ATELECTASIS

Key Facts

Terminology

- Atelectasis involving airways smaller than a bronchopulmonary segment

Imaging

- Linear band of atelectasis that crosses segmental boundaries
  - May be horizontally or obliquely oriented
  - Abuts pleura, perpendicular to pleural surface
  - Most common in mid & lower lung zones
- "**Nordenstrom**" **sign**: Lingular subsegmental atelectasis in patients with left lower lobe atelectasis
- CT may show extent of disease & underlying cause

Top Differential Diagnoses

- Fissures & pulmonary ligaments
- Fibrotic bands
- Interlobular septal thickening

Pathology

- Hypoventilation or decreased diaphragmatic excursion
  - General anesthesia, mechanical ventilation
  - Surgery, trauma
  - Eventration & phrenic nerve paralysis
- Endobronchial obstruction
  - Mucus plugging, asthma
  - Atypical pneumonia
  - Aspirated foreign bodies

Clinical Issues

- Usually asymptomatic
  - Most commonly incidental discovery on radiography or CT
- May signify greater degree of peripheral atelectasis than radiologically evident

*(**Left**) PA chest radiograph shows bands of subsegmental atelectasis extending from and perpendicular to the mediastinal pleural surface. The patient had general anesthesia 1 day prior to the date of this radiograph. The bands of atelectasis resolved completely on a radiograph obtained 1 week later. (**Right**) Axial CECT shows bibasilar subsegmental atelectasis, manifesting as areas of ground-glass opacity. Oblique bands of atelectasis on CECT may appear as ground-glass opacity on axial imaging.*

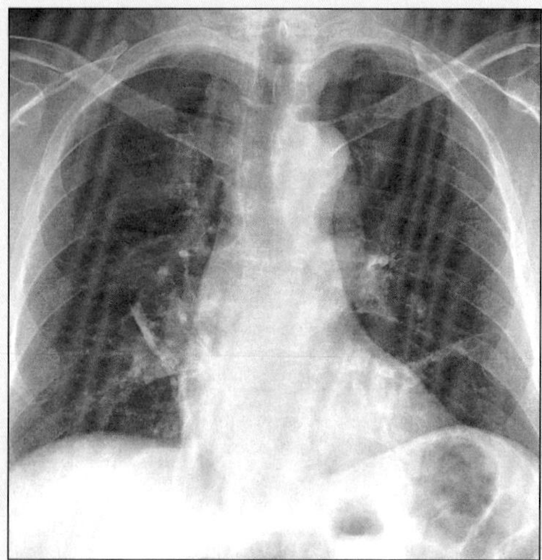

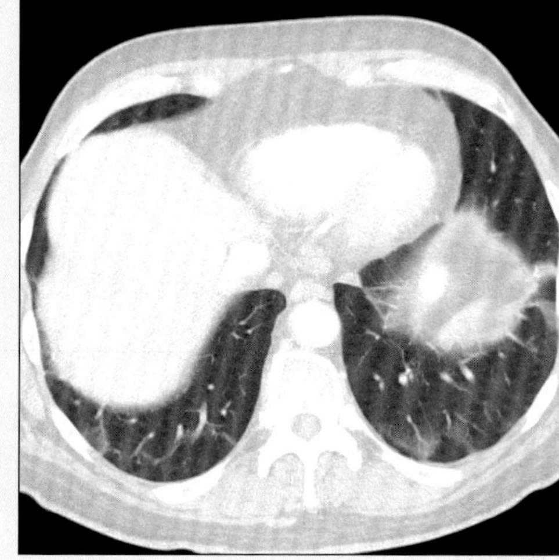

*(**Left**) Coronal CECT of a patient with abdominal ascites shows elevation of both hemidiaphragms and adjacent linear and band-like areas of subsegmental atelectasis in both lower lungs ➡. (**Right**) Sagittal CECT of the same patient shows linear and band-like areas of subsegmental atelectasis ➡ adjacent to the elevated left hemidiaphragm. Note underlying abdominal ascites ➡. CT may show associated abdominal or subphrenic disease in patients with basilar subsegmental atelectasis.*

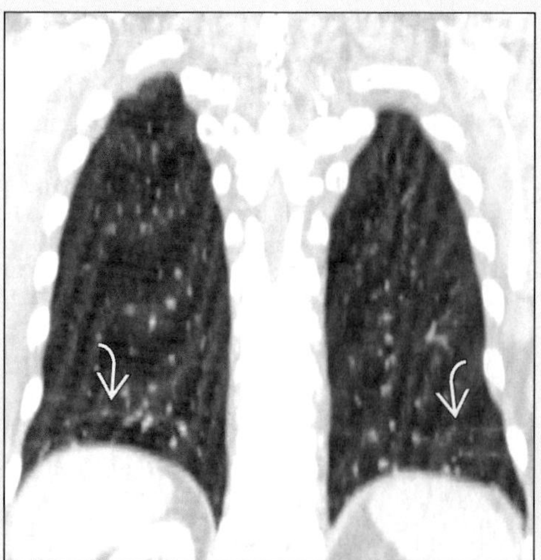

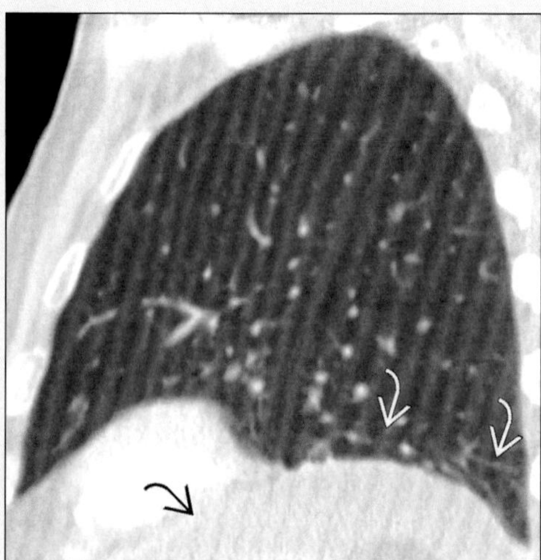

Key Facts

Terminology

- Synonym: Passive atelectasis

Imaging

- Best diagnostic clue
  - Patchy opacity adjacent to space-occupying process that is cause of atelectasis
- Chest radiographs
  - Patchy or dense pulmonary opacity usually in lower lung zones
  - Commonly seen alongside space-occupying lesions: Pleural effusions & intrathoracic masses
  - May not be apparent in presence of pneumothorax
- CT
  - Patchy or dense opacity, usually in lower lobes
  - Enhances with contrast administration
  - Crowding of bronchovascular structures
  - Visualization of underlying cause of atelectasis

Top Differential Diagnoses

- Aspiration
- Pneumonia

Pathology

- Any abnormality that limits elasticity of lung
  - Pleural effusion
  - Pneumothorax
  - Intrathoracic mass

Clinical Issues

- Symptoms usually due to underlying etiology of atelectasis
- Shortness of breath, dyspnea, chest pain most common

Diagnostic Checklist

- Underlying pulmonary infection may be difficult to exclude in cases of relaxation atelectasis

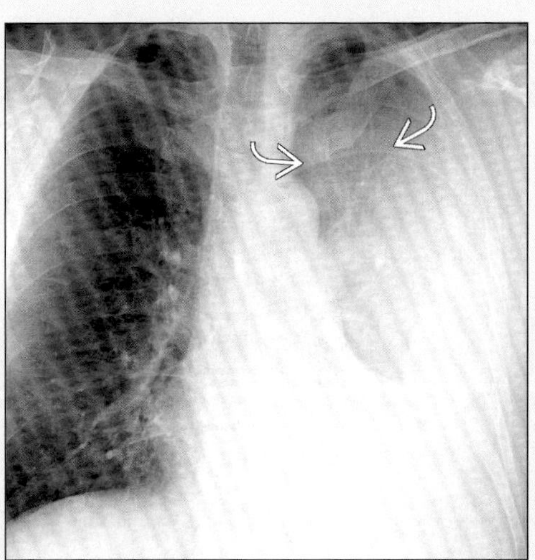

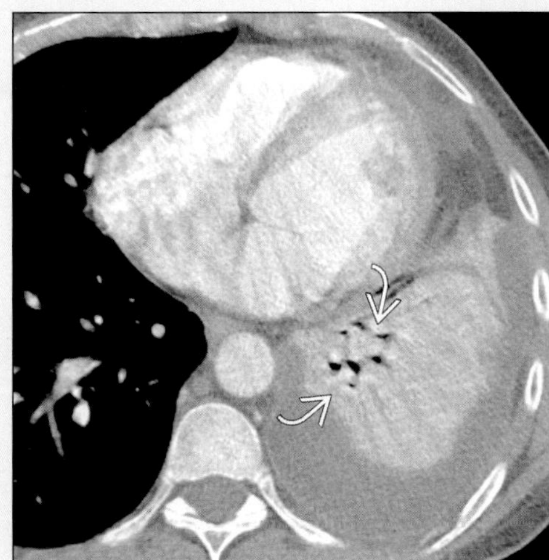

(Left) *PA chest radiograph demonstrates a large left pleural effusion that causes relaxation/compressive atelectasis in the left lung. Note crowding of bronchovascular structures in the left upper lobe ➔.* ***(Right)*** *Axial CECT of the same patient shows a large left pleural effusion and relaxation atelectasis in the left lower lobe. Note crowding of bronchovascular structures in the left lower lobe ➔, a direct imaging sign of volume loss.*

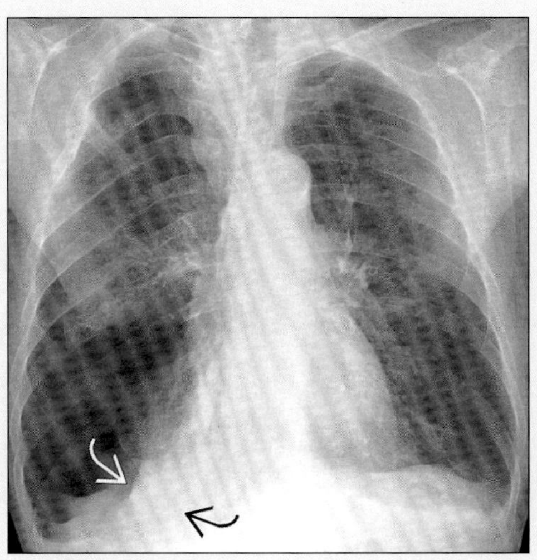

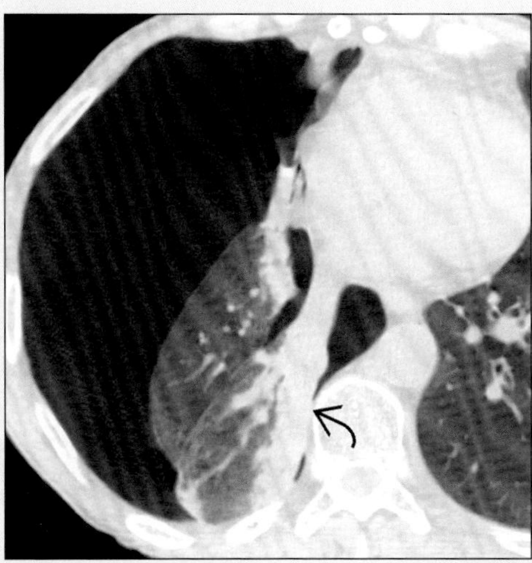

(Left) *PA chest radiograph shows a large right pneumothorax that exerts mass effect on and compresses the right lower lobe. Note inferomedial displacement of the major fissure ➔ and crowding of bronchovascular structures ➔, both primary imaging signs of atelectasis.* ***(Right)*** *Axial NECT of the same patient shows a right pneumothorax and relaxation atelectasis of the right lung manifesting as crowding of bronchovascular structures and a band-like opacity ➔.*

ROUNDED ATELECTASIS

Key Facts

Terminology

- Rounded volume loss of portion of lung

Imaging

- Radiography
  - Subpleural mass-like opacity
  - Distortion of vessels & bronchi in involved lobe
  - Calcified plaques in asbestos-related pleural disease
  - Blunt or obliterated costophrenic angles
- CT
  - Wedge-shaped or rounded peripheral opacity
  - Adjacent focal or diffuse pleural thickening
  - "**Comet tail**" **sign**: Distortion, displacement, & convergence of vessels into lesion
  - Volume loss in affected lobe
  - Hyperlucency of surrounding nonatelectatic lobe
  - Air bronchogram in hilar aspect of peripheral opacity
- Best diagnostic clue: Mass-like opacity with comet tail sign & adjacent calcified pleural plaques or pleural thickening

Top Differential Diagnoses

- Lung cancer
- Localized fibrous tumor of the pleura
- Pulmonary infarction

Pathology

- Asbestos exposure
- Pleural effusions (including prior thoracotomy)
- Pulmonary infection

Clinical Issues

- Typically asymptomatic
  - Incidentally discovered on chest radiographs or CT
- Chest pain or shortness of breath may be present

*(**Left**) Lateral chest radiograph of a patient with rounded atelectasis demonstrates an opacity ➡ projecting over the lower thoracic spine in the posterior aspect of the thorax. (**Right**) Axial NECT of the same patient shows a rounded peripheral mass-like opacity ➡ in the posterior subpleural right lower lobe. Note surrounding lung hyperlucency and thickening of the adjacent pleura ⇨. Rounded atelectasis is often incidentally discovered on chest CT.*

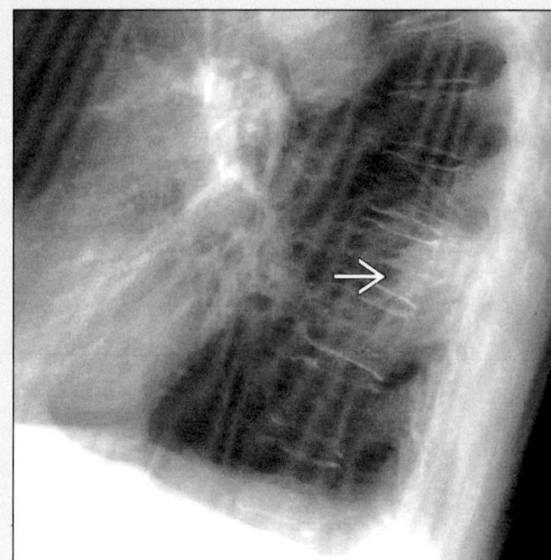

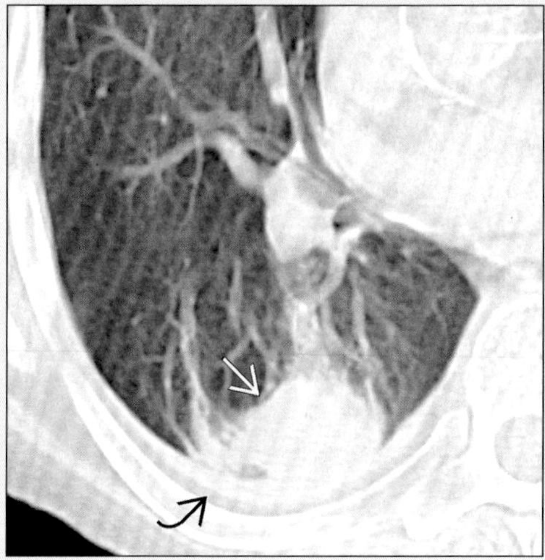

*(**Left**) Axial NECT of a patient with rounded atelectasis shows a rounded opacity in the posterior subpleural right lower lobe. Distortion, displacement, and convergence of vessels ➡ into the lesion represent the "comet tail" sign of rounded atelectasis. (**Right**) Axial NECT of the same patient demonstrates thickening of the adjacent pleura ➡. The most common causes of rounded atelectasis include asbestos exposure, pleural effusion (including that related to prior surgery), and infection.*

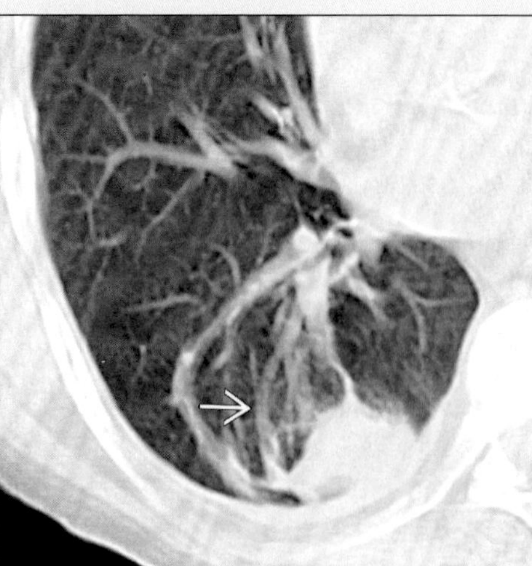

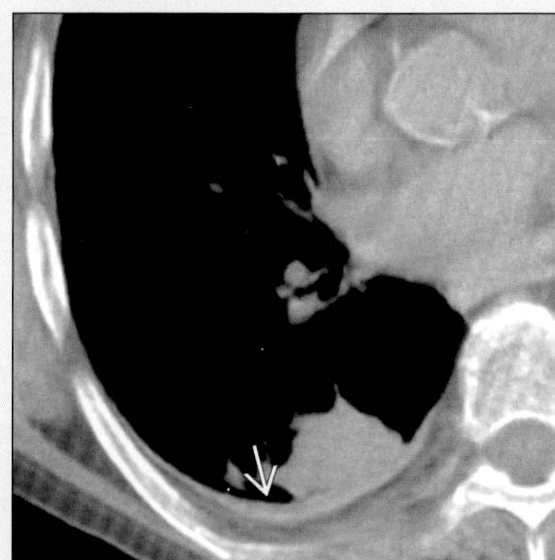

Key Facts

Terminology

- Reduction in alveolar volume in setting of pulmonary fibrosis
- Localized & diffuse forms

Imaging

- Localized
  - Typically seen in 1 or more lobes
  - Opacity of affected lung
  - Reduced lung volumes
  - Scarring
  - Bronchiectasis
  - Hyperinflation of unaffected lung
- Diffuse
  - Opacity of affected lung
  - Reduced lung volumes
  - Reticular opacities
- Findings usually evident on chest radiographs
- CT useful in evaluating underlying etiology

Top Differential Diagnoses

- Pneumonia
- Sublobar resection

Pathology

- Localized
  - Chronic tuberculosis: Typically in upper lobes
  - Necrotizing pneumonia
  - Radiation fibrosis: Limited to radiation port
- Diffuse
  - Interstitial fibrosis

Clinical Issues

- Clinical symptoms related to underlying etiology of cicatricial atelectasis
- Most common symptoms
  - Shortness of breath, dyspnea
  - Cough

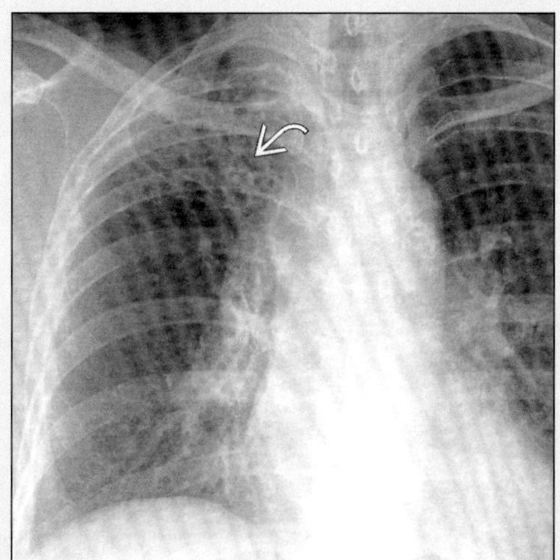

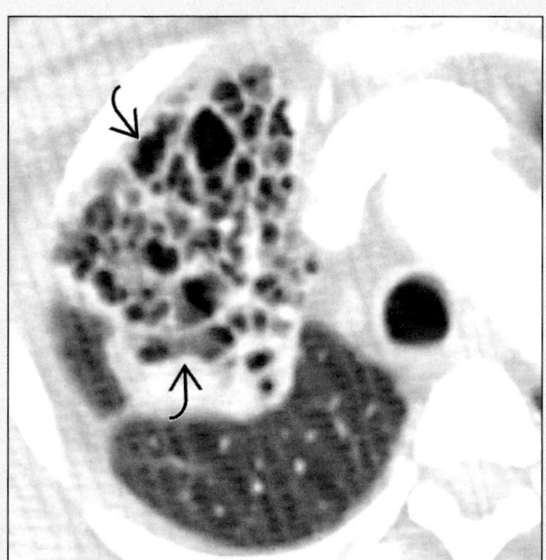

(Left) *PA chest radiograph of a patient with healed tuberculosis demonstrates heterogeneous opacity in the right upper lobe with intrinsic bronchiectasis ➔, right hilar retraction, and volume loss.* ***(Right)*** *Axial CECT of the same patient shows right upper lobe volume loss with focal dense fibrosis and scarring and marked intrinsic bronchiectasis ➔. These findings represent localized cicatricial atelectasis. Note mild displacement of the superior mediastinum toward the atelectasis.*

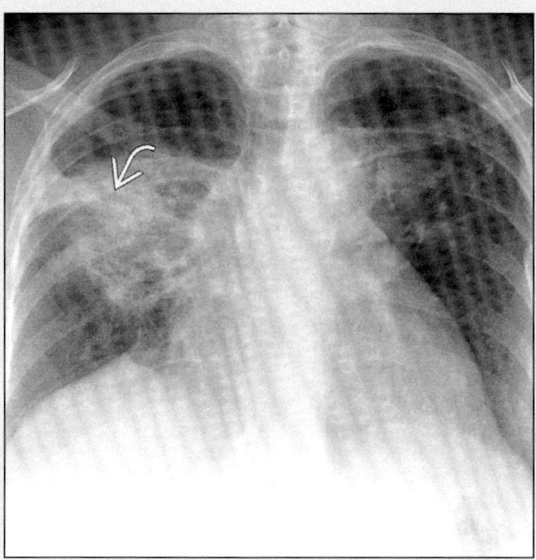

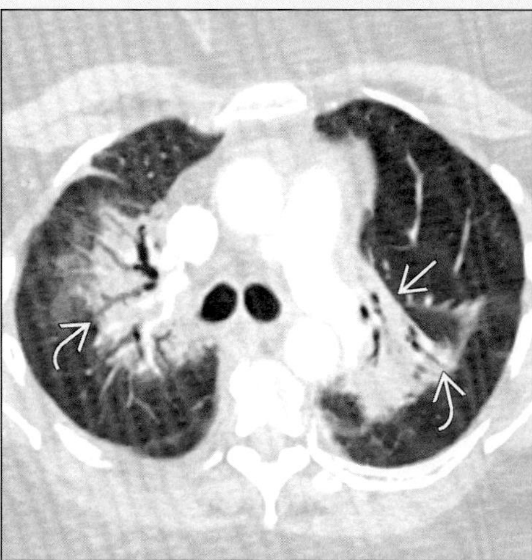

(Left) *PA chest radiograph of a patient 2 years following radiation therapy shows dense bilateral paramediastinal opacities with architectural distortion, bronchiectasis ➔, and volume loss.* ***(Right)*** *Axial CECT of the same patient shows dense perihilar opacities with intrinsic bronchiectasis ➔ and architectural distortion. The straight interface along the margin of the left consolidation ➔ is characteristic of radiation fibrosis and represents the boundary of a treatment port.*

SECTION 2
Developmental Abnormalities

Introduction and Overview

Airways

Lung

Pulmonary Circulation

Systemic Circulation

Cardiac, Pericardial, and Valvular Defects

Chest Wall & Diaphragm

Introduction

Developmental abnormalities of the thorax characteristically manifest in neonates, infants, and young children. With the increasing utilization of obstetrical ultrasound, many developmental conditions are diagnosed antenatally and healthcare providers are thus prepared to manage their manifestations and complications at the time of birth. In some cases, the diagnosis is initially made in the neonatal period. Infants with respiratory distress are usually imaged with portable chest radiography to exclude common neonatal diseases such as surfactant deficiency syndrome, meconium aspiration, and retained fetal fluid. Occasionally, infants with respiratory distress have an undiagnosed developmental abnormality. The radiologist must be familiar with the imaging features of the more common anomalies in order to suggest the most likely diagnosis and expedite treatment.

Many developmental chest lesions are not diagnosed antenatally or during infancy or childhood. Affected adult patients are often asymptomatic or only minimally symptomatic and may be diagnosed because of an incidental abnormality detected on chest imaging obtained for other reasons. Recognition and careful analysis of such lesions should enable the radiologist to formulate a differential diagnosis and suggest further imaging and management. Focal lung and mediastinal abnormalities in adults often raise the possibility of primary or metastatic lung cancer, but cross-sectional imaging studies may help distinguish neoplasms from developmental lesions.

Spectrum of Developmental Thoracic Abnormalities

Developmental abnormalities may affect any of the anatomic compartments of the chest, including the airways, lung, mediastinum, heart, systemic and pulmonary vasculature, diaphragm, and the chest wall. Generally speaking, developmental lesions that manifest in adults tend to originate later in embryologic development, although there are exceptions to this rule.

Tracheobronchial Tree

The normal development of the tracheobronchial tree is intimately related to the development of the primitive foregut. The trachea and bronchi originate as a ventral foregut bud (lung bud) that undergoes sequential branching to form the intrapulmonary airways. Invagination of the developing airways into the surrounding primitive mesenchyma induces development of the lung parenchyma. Vascularization of the lung brings airways in contact with the pulmonary capillary bed and establishes the alveolar capillary membrane, which allows gas exchange and respiration. Congenital lobar overinflation (CLO) and congenital pulmonary airway malformation (CPAM) are airway abnormalities that affect neonates and infants. Both lesions may produce mass effect within the lung, but CPAM is more likely to produce pulmonary hypoplasia and may result in neonatal pneumothorax and/or pneumomediastinum. CLO may produce progressive respiratory distress that may require emergent neonatal surgery.

On the other hand, some congenital tracheobronchial anomalies are completely asymptomatic. The most common relate to anomalous bronchial branching, a frequent incidental finding on thoracic CT studies of adults evaluated for other reasons. Even though the "best known" anomalous bronchial branching pattern is the tracheal bronchus, anomalous displaced pre-eparterial segmental bronchi are actually more common. Although these lesions typically have no clinical significance, their recognition allows the radiologist to contribute to the planning of bronchoscopic procedures in selected cases.

Lung

Lung development occurs in synchrony with tracheobronchial development. Thus, it is difficult to separate airway anomalies such as CPAM from pulmonary anomalies. CPAM is considered an anomaly of the airways, but its imaging manifestations characteristically involve the lung parenchyma, with findings ranging from microscopic to small or large "lung" cysts. Congenital bronchial atresia is characterized by abrupt focal interruption of the lumen of a segmental airway with resultant formation of a distal mucocele. However, identification of abnormal hyperlucency of the surrounding lung is critical to suggesting the diagnosis. A confident prospective diagnosis of such lesions is of utmost importance since surgical management is rarely indicated.

One of the most debated and poorly understood developmental lung anomalies is pulmonary sequestration. Sequestered lung does not normally communicate with the tracheobronchial tree and is supplied by the systemic circulation. Pulmonary sequestration may be extralobar or intralobar. Extralobar sequestration (ELS) is clearly a congenital lesion thought to arise from an anomalous primitive foregut bud that induces parenchymal development forming extrapulmonary lung tissue. There is controversy regarding the etiology of intralobar sequestration (ILS). As the name implies, ILS occurs within the confines of an otherwise normal pulmonary lobe. Unlike ELS, ILS affects males and females equally, does not have a strong association with other congenital anomalies, and is often diagnosed in adulthood. Because affected patients often present with signs and symptoms of infection (which may be recurrent), and because the affected lung often exhibits chronic inflammation, it has been postulated that this lesion may result from postobstructive pulmonary infection with loss of normal blood supply and parasitization of adjacent systemic vessels. Systemic feeders typically course through the pulmonary ligament, giving rise to the usual posteromedial lower lobe location of ILS. Whatever its etiology, the diagnosis of ILS requires a high index of suspicion, and radiologists must thoroughly evaluate recurrent and chronic lower lobe abnormalities for identification of a systemic blood supply to establish the diagnosis.

Pulmonary Circulation

Partial anomalous pulmonary venous return (PAPVR) is often diagnosed in asymptomatic adult patients. Given the variable degree of enhancement of the pulmonary veins during CT angiography, PAPVR may be overlooked in patients presenting with chest pain and dyspnea who are referred for evaluation of possible pulmonary thromboembolic disease. However, it is important to correctly diagnose this lesion since the patient's symptoms may be related to an accompanying left-to-right shunt or an occult sinus venosus atrial septal defect (ASD).

Arteriovenous malformations (AVM) produce a direct communication between a pulmonary artery and a pulmonary vein without an intervening capillary bed. As a result, affected patients are at risk for systemic embolic events and may present with stroke and peripheral infarcts and abscesses. Evaluation of the pulmonary parenchyma with maximum-intensity projection (MIP) images may be particularly helpful in identifying small AVMs. Radiologists also contribute to the treatment of these lesions by performing selective catheter embolization to obliterate the shunt.

Systemic Circulation

Developmental anomalies of the systemic arterial circulation are common and easily recognized, and cross-sectional imaging features are diagnostic. Thus, aberrant right subclavian and left vertebral arteries are readily identified and characterized as normal variants. Interestingly, the radiographic diagnosis of aortic arch anomalies (right aortic arch, double aortic arch, coarctation) may prove challenging, and such lesions may be mistaken for a mediastinal mass on radiography. It is important to remember that arterial vascular anomalies often manifest as mediastinal contour abnormalities and that approximately 10% of such contour abnormalities are vascular. Cross-sectional imaging should be performed to exclude a potential vascular lesion prior to any invasive or interventional procedure.

Developmental anomalies also affect the systemic veins. Accessory azygos fissure is a common anomaly considered a normal variant with no clinical significance. Persistent left superior vena cava (PLSVC) may exhibit subtle radiographic findings characterized by lateralization of the aortopulmonary reflection. It is rarely diagnosed prospectively on radiography, but is often identified after placement of central vascular lines and pacemakers that follow a characteristic craniocaudad left paramediastinal course into the coronary sinus and right atrium. Many PLSVC are found incidentally on chest CT.

Heart and Valves

The majority of significant congenital lesions of the heart manifest in the neonatal period. However, some congenital heart lesions escape early detection and manifest in adulthood. Atrial septal defect is the most common shunt lesion to be initially diagnosed in an adult. Many patients are asymptomatic early in life and become increasingly symptomatic with advancing age due to the effects of a chronic left-to-right intracardiac shunt that may be complicated by pulmonary arterial hypertension. Radiologists performing non-gated CT angiography should pay special attention to cardiac anatomy since these lesions are occasionally evident.

Pulmonic stenosis is a congenital valvular lesion often detected in asymptomatic adults who are diagnosed incidentally because of a mediastinal contour abnormality produced by an enlarged pulmonary trunk and left pulmonary artery. Bicuspid aortic valve may manifest with valvular calcifications indicative of aortic stenosis associated with left ventricular hypertrophy and dilatation of the ascending aorta. Both lesions can be diagnosed by echocardiography.

Diaphragm

Congenital diaphragmatic hernia (CDH) is the most severe congenital anomaly of the diaphragm and results from partial agenesis of one or both hemidiaphragms with intrauterine herniation of abdominal viscera, stomach, and bowel into the thorax. The lesion may be diagnosed antenatally and typically affects neonates and infants. Prognosis is related to the presence or absence of associated congenital anomalies, the size of the diaphragmatic defect, and the extent of herniation. As early lung development is greatly influenced by the available thoracic volume, large CDH may produce severe pulmonary hypoplasia that may be incompatible with life. CDH is not to be confused with Bochdalek hernia, in which fat and sometimes abdominal organs herniate through a patulous Bochdalek foramen (a normal remnant of the pleuroperitoneal canal). This lesion typically affects asymptomatic adults, may mimic an intrathoracic mass, and is readily diagnosed on cross-sectional imaging. Morgagni hernias also affect adults and manifest as cardiophrenic angle lesions that may contain variable amounts of peritoneal fat and bowel. Patients are often asymptomatic, although symptoms related to vascular engorgement have been described.

Chest Wall

Many congenital chest wall anomalies manifest in adults who are asymptomatic or minimally symptomatic, including scoliosis, Poland syndrome, and pectus deformities that may come to medical attention because of an observable thoracic deformity. Some affected patients are symptomatic and others are referred for cosmetic surgery. Pectus excavatum deformity is a depression of the distal sternum that produces mass effect on the heart and cardiac rotation. The anatomic effects result in obscuration of the right cardiac border on frontal chest radiography. In the absence of lateral chest radiography, the patient may be misdiagnosed with middle lobe atelectasis or pneumonia. Fortunately, the diagnosis is readily made on the lateral chest radiograph. Radiologists must be familiar with the indications for surgical management of these conditions and with the postsurgical imaging findings. For example, the Nuss procedure is a minimally invasive corrective surgery for pectus excavatum and has shown favorable results. A metallic bar is placed behind the sternum through small lateral chest wall incisions and is manipulated to effectively "lift" the depressed sternum, thus correcting pectus excavatum deformity.

Summary

Congenital anomalies of the thorax have protean manifestations and affect virtually all the organs and anatomic locations in the chest. While many lesions are diagnosed antenatally and in the neonate and infant, some escape early detection and manifest in adults. Familiarity with the characteristic imaging features of such lesions allows the radiologist to suggest the diagnosis prospectively and to guide further imaging and management. As lesions located in the lung and mediastinum may mimic common neoplastic conditions such as lung cancer and lymphoma, careful and thorough imaging assessment is required prior to performing any invasive diagnostic procedures.

*(**Left**) AP chest radiograph of a newborn with respiratory distress shows a heterogeneous right lung lesion with small intrinsic lucencies suggestive of congenital pulmonary airway malformation (CPAM) and pneumomediastinum. (**Right**) Coronal CECT of a patient with chest pain shows an accessory azygos fissure ➔ and a displaced pre-eparterial right upper lobe apical segmental bronchus ➔. Variant bronchial branching is frequently found incidentally on chest CT.*

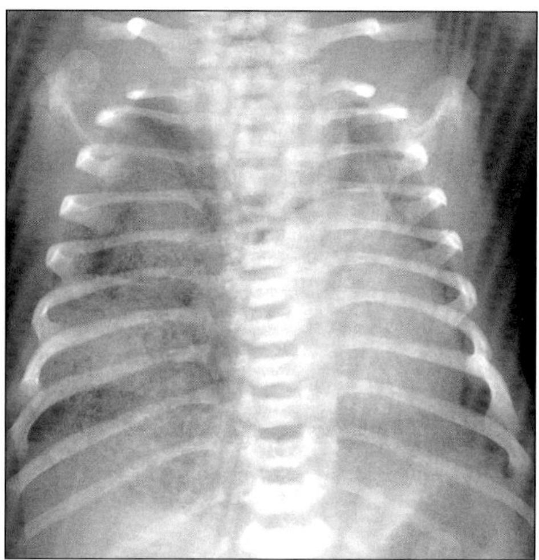

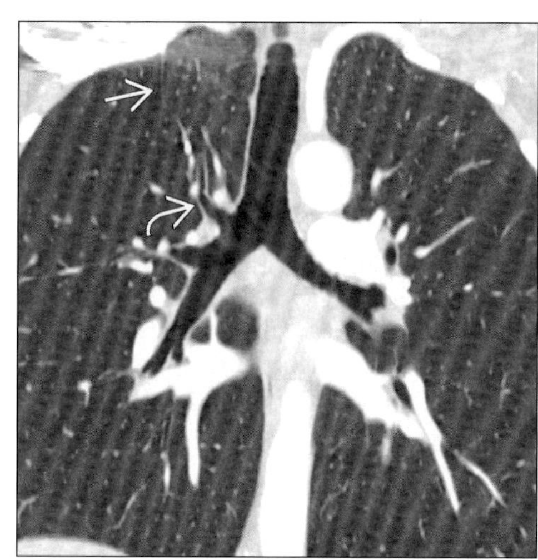

*(**Left**) Coronal CECT (lung window) of a 43-year-old man who presented with seizures shows areas of left upper and left lower lobe hyperlucency with a tubular opacity ➔ coursing into the left lower lobe. (**Right**) Coronal CECT (soft tissue window) of the same patient shows that the tubular structure exhibits low attenuation and no contrast enhancement ➔. The findings are diagnostic of bronchial atresia. As the lesion is not infected or symptomatic, treatment is not required.*

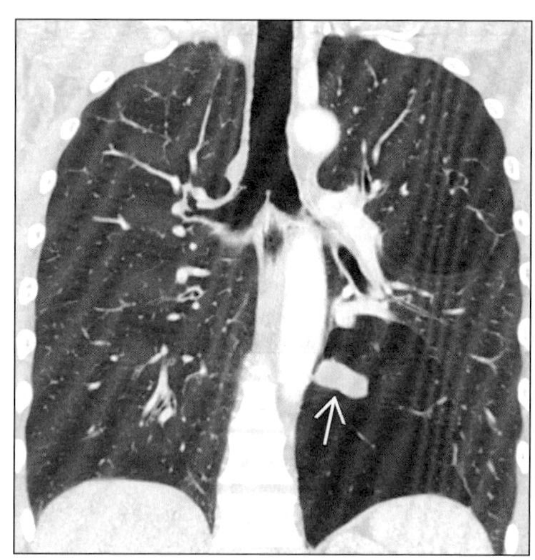

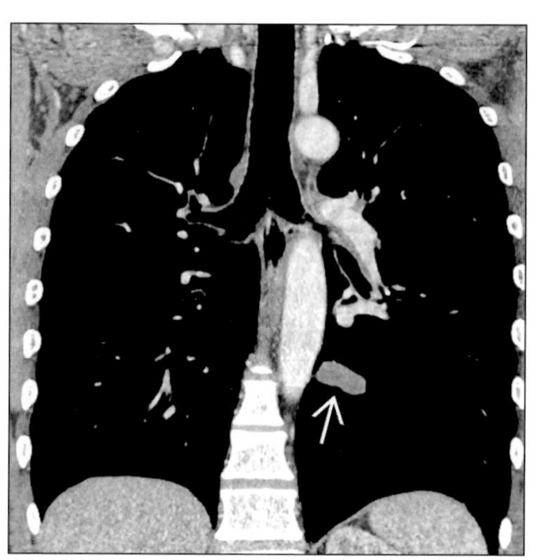

*(**Left**) Composite image with CECT in lung (left) and soft tissue (right) window shows heterogeneous left lower lobe attenuation with systemic vascular supply ➔, diagnostic of intralobar sequestration. (**Right**) Coronal oblique CTA (MIP image) shows left upper lobe partial anomalous pulmonary venous return ➔. This congenital vascular anomaly is associated with sinus venosus atrial septal defect (ASD), here treated with an ASD closure device ➔.*

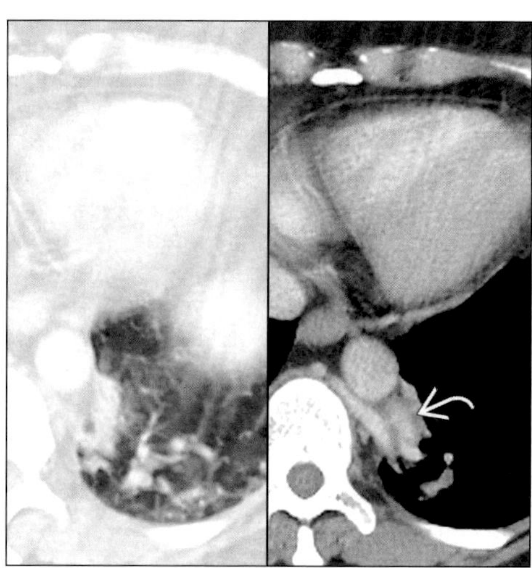

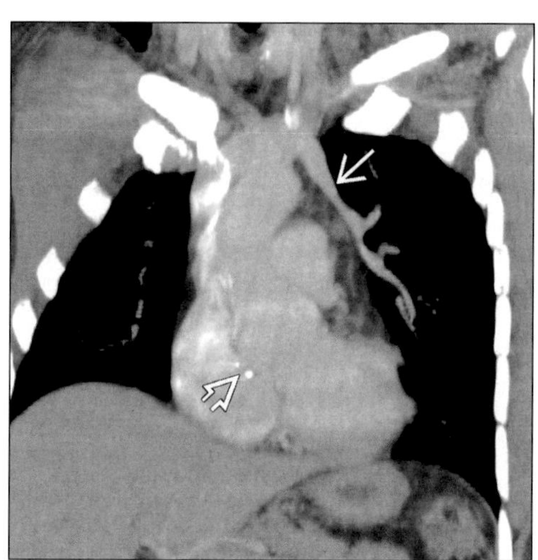

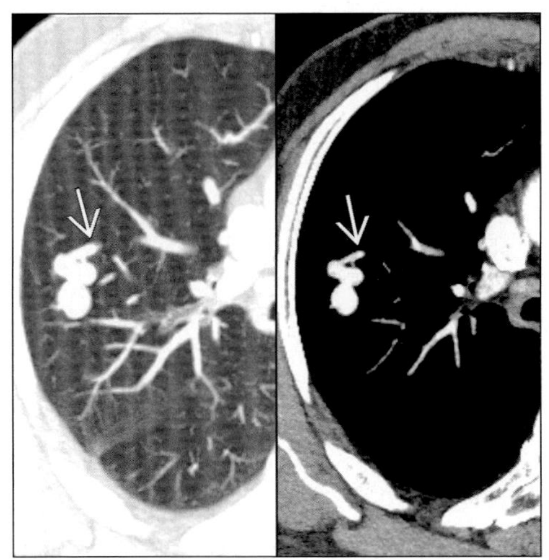

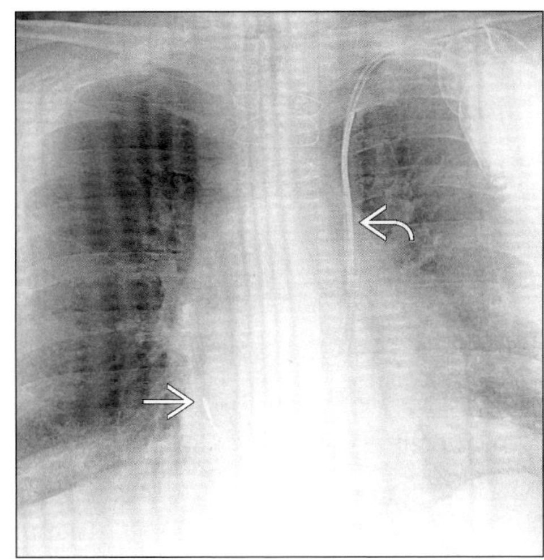

(Left) *Composite image with axial CECT in lung (left) and soft tissue (right) window shows a polylobular right upper lobe nodule that exhibits a feeding vessel ➔ and enhances intensely, consistent with arteriovenous malformation. Embolotherapy is indicated to prevent systemic embolization.* ***(Right)*** *AP chest radiograph of a patient with chest pain shows left pectoral dual chamber pacer leads coursing into the right atrium ➔ via a persistent left superior vena cava ↩.*

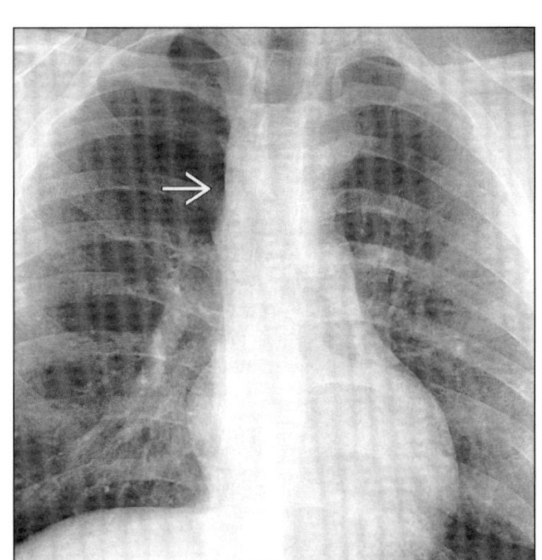

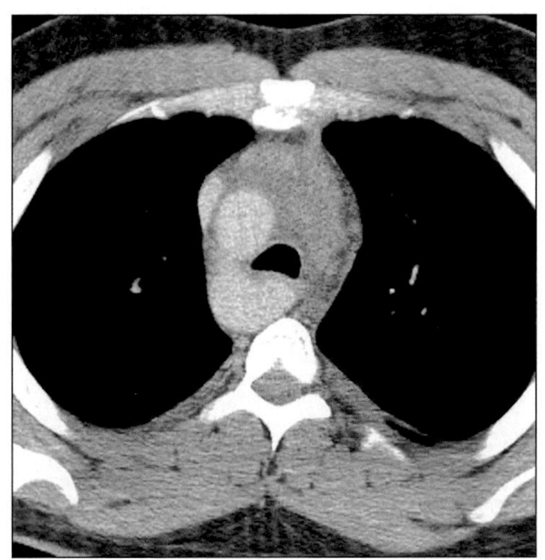

(Left) *PA chest radiograph of a patient who presented with left brachiocephalic vein thrombosis shows an abnormal mediastinal contour representing a right-sided aortic arch ➔. The vascular anomaly was not recognized and a mediastinal mass was suspected.* ***(Right)*** *Axial CECT of the same patient shows a right aortic arch and thymic engorgement related to thymic vein occlusion from venous thrombosis. Based on the initial diagnosis, exploratory surgery was performed and revealed engorged thymic tissue.*

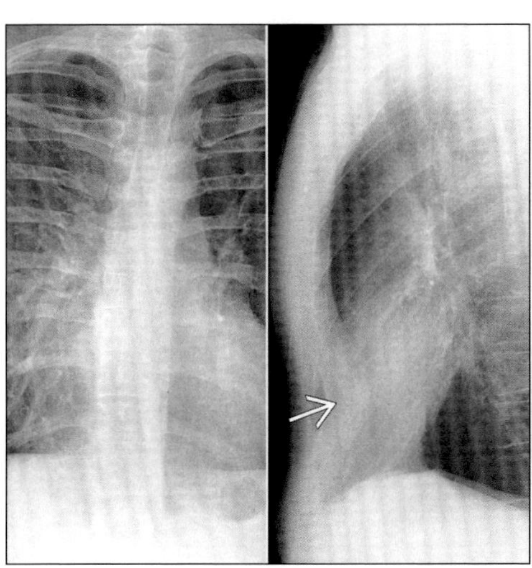

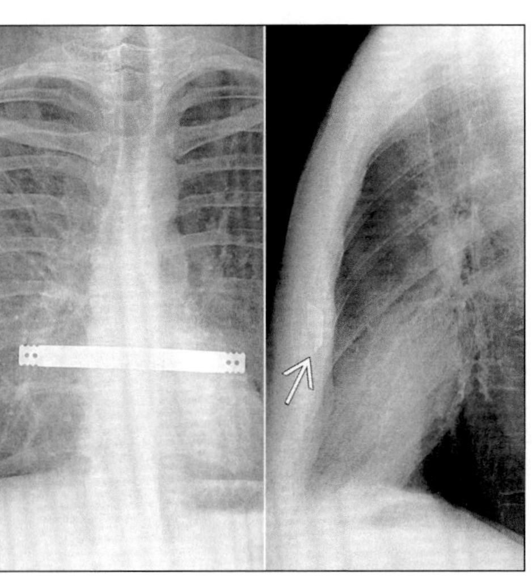

(Left) *Composite image with PA (left) and lateral (right) chest radiographs shows obscuration of the right cardiac border by pectus excavatum deformity ➔.* ***(Right)*** *Composite image with PA (left) and lateral (right) chest radiographs of the same patient status post Nuss procedure shows elevation of the sternum and correction of the sternal deformity by the Nuss bar ➔. Pectus excavatum deformity may mimic pulmonary disease. The diagnosis is readily made on lateral radiography.*

TRACHEAL BRONCHUS AND OTHER ANOMALOUS BRONCHI

Key Facts

Terminology

- Different congenital variations in number, length, diameter, & position of bronchi

Imaging

- Anomalies arising from normal higher order bronchial divisions
  - Accessory superior segmental bronchi
  - Axillary bronchi
- Anomalies arising from sites typically lacking branches
  - Tracheal bronchus
  - Spectrum of "tracheal bronchus"
  - Bridging bronchus
  - Accessory cardiac bronchus
- Anomalies associated with abnormalities of situs
  - Bronchial isomerism: Bilateral left-sided or right-sided airway anatomy

Top Differential Diagnoses

- Endobronchial obstruction
  - Children: Foreign bodies
  - Adults: Lung cancer
- Aspiration
- Intralobar pulmonary sequestration
- Congenital pulmonary airway malformation

Clinical Issues

- Usually asymptomatic
- Tracheal bronchus, accessory cardiac bronchus
  - Recurrent infection, atelectasis, or bronchiectasis

Diagnostic Checklist

- Anomalous bronchial abnormalities should be suspected in recurrent pneumonia &/or atelectasis
- Some congenital airway anomalies are found incidentally on conventional radiography or CT of asymptomatic adults

__(Left)__ Axial NECT minimum-intensity projection (MinIP) image shows an anomalous tracheal bronchus ➡ arising from the right lateral tracheal wall. In this case, note the presence of adjacent small air bubbles ➡ distal to the bronchus. Tracheal bronchus almost exclusively arises on the right side. __(Right)__ Virtual bronchoscopy shows the orifice ➡ of the tracheal bronchus located proximal to the carina ➡. Virtual bronchoscopy is useful in the evaluation of central bronchial anomalies.

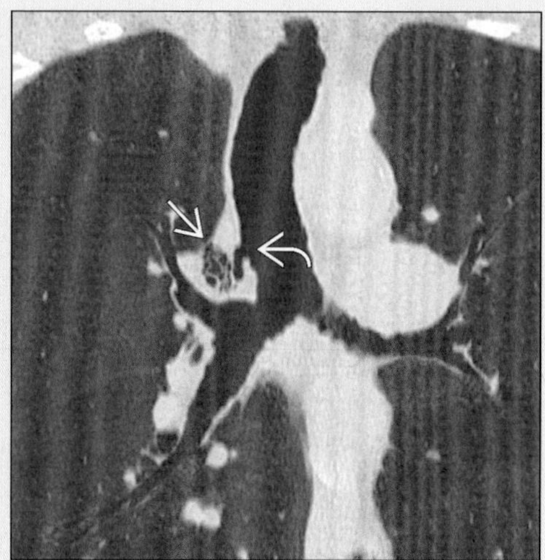

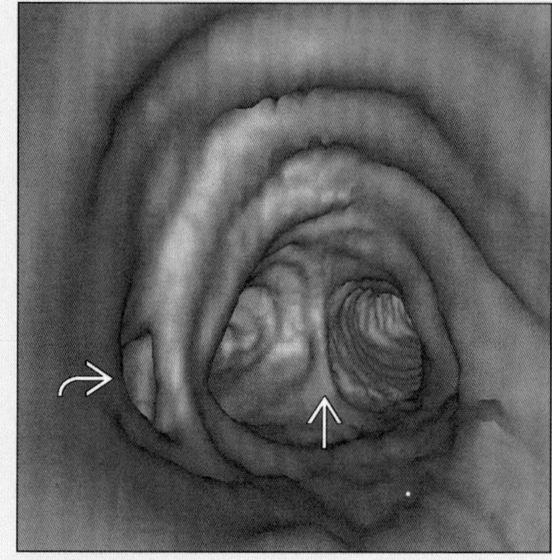

__(Left)__ Composite image with axial (left) and coronal (right) NECT shows a displaced right apical segmental tracheal bronchus ➡ arising from the right lateral tracheal wall. The right upper lobe bronchus ➡ lacked an apical segmental branch. __(Right)__ Composite image with coronal CECT shows a supernumerary tracheal bronchus ➡ arising from the right lateral tracheal wall and coursing under the azygos arch ➡ and cephalad toward the right apex and a normal right upper lobe apical segmental bronchus ➡.

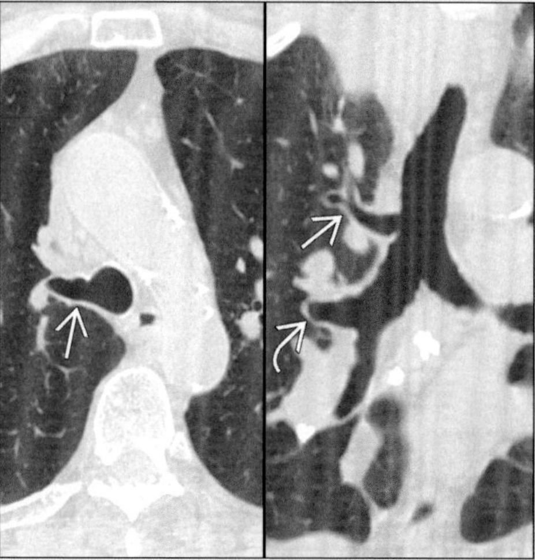

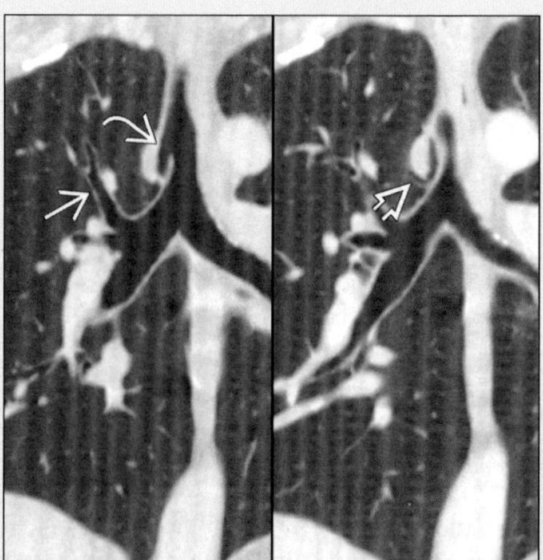

TRACHEAL BRONCHUS AND OTHER ANOMALOUS BRONCHI

TERMINOLOGY

Synonyms

- **Congenital anomalies of bronchi**

Definitions

- **Tracheocele**: Tracheal diverticulum
- **Tracheal bronchus**: "Pig" bronchus, bronchus suis

IMAGING

General Features

- Best diagnostic clue
  - Different congenital variations in number, length, diameter, & position of bronchi
- Other general features
  - Anomalies arising from normal higher order bronchial divisions
    - Accessory superior segmental bronchi
    - Axillary bronchi
  - Anomalies arising from sites typically lacking branches
    - Tracheal bronchus
    - Bridging bronchus
    - Accessory cardiac bronchus
  - Anomalies associated with abnormalities of situs
    - Bronchial isomerism: Bilateral left-sided or right-sided airway anatomy
  - Congenital bronchial atresia
  - Agenesis-hypoplasia complex

CT Findings

- **Accessory superior segmental bronchi**
  - 2 closely aligned bronchi both supplying superior segment of right lower lobe (RLL)
- **Axillary bronchus**
  - Supernumerary segmental bronchus supplying lateral aspect of right upper lobe (RUL)
  - One of the most frequently encountered bronchial abnormalities (5-16%)
- **Tracheal bronchus**
  - Various types
    - Supernumerary (23%): Coexists with normal branching upper lobe bronchus
    - Displaced (77%): In addition to aberrant bronchus, a branch of upper lobe bronchus is lacking
  - Distinct from tracheocele
  - Most cases located on right
  - Tracheal origin of right upper lobe bronchus ("pig" bronchus)
  - Arises from right lateral tracheal wall
  - Usually within 2 cm of carina, may be up to 6 cm from carina
  - Variable length, sometimes blind-ending pouch
  - Left tracheal bronchus: Early origin of apicoposterior left upper lobe (LUL) bronchus from terminal portion of left main bronchus
- **Spectrum of "tracheal bronchus"** (upper lobe)
  - **Normal bronchi**
    - **Eparterial**: Normal right upper lobe bronchus, arises above right pulmonary artery
    - **Hyparterial**: Normal left upper lobe bronchus, arises below left pulmonary artery
  - **Anomalous bronchi**
    - **Supernumerary**: Coexistent with normal branching bronchi
    - **Displaced**: Missing branch of upper lobe bronchus
    - Nomenclature for right anomalous bronchi
      - **Pre-eparterial**: Anomalous bronchus arising proximal to right upper lobe bronchus
      - **Posteparterial**: Arises distal to right upper lobe bronchus
    - Nomenclature for left anomalous bronchi
      - **Eparterial**: (Left "tracheal") arises from left mainstem bronchus proximal to left pulmonary artery
      - **Prehyparterial**: Arises proximal to left upper lobe bronchus
      - **Posthyparterial**: Arises distal to left upper lobe bronchus
    - Displaced pre-eparterial apical segmental bronchus is most common variant
- **Bridging bronchus**
  - Ectopic bronchus arising from left mainstem bronchus
  - Crosses through mediastinum to supply RLL
  - Bronchus intermedius originates from left mainstem bronchus
- **Accessory cardiac bronchus**
  - Distinct airway originating from medial wall of mainstem bronchus or bronchus intermedius
  - Up to 0.5% of population
  - Cephalic to middle lobe bronchus origin
  - Located in azygo-esophageal recess
  - Demarcated from RLL by anomalous fissure
  - Potential reservoir for retained secretions
    - Recurrent episodes of aspiration
    - Hemoptysis
- Bronchial isomerism
  - Pattern of bronchial branching & pulmonary lobe formation identical in both lungs
    - Bilateral left-sided airway anatomy
    - Bilateral right-sided airway anatomy
  - Equal number of bronchi within each lung
- Agenesis-hypoplasia complex
  - Agenesis: Total absence of bronchus & lung
  - Aplasia: Total absence of lung with rudimentary main bronchus
  - Hypoplasia: Hypoplastic bronchi & associated variable amount of lung tissue

Imaging Recommendations

- Best imaging tool
  - MDCT; consider multiplanar reformations
- Protocol advice
  - MDCT has helped improve understanding of complex tracheobronchial abnormalities

DIFFERENTIAL DIAGNOSIS

Endobronchial Obstruction

- Children: Foreign bodies
- Adults: Lung cancer
  - 10% of nonresolving pneumonias due to underlying carcinoma
- May exhibit volume loss in addition to chronic consolidation
- CT useful to exclude airway obstruction

TRACHEAL BRONCHUS AND OTHER ANOMALOUS BRONCHI

Aspiration

- Predisposing conditions: Alcoholism, neuromuscular disorders, structural abnormalities of esophagus, reflux disease
- Recurrent opacities in dependent locations
- May be unilateral
- Esophagram useful to determine esophageal motility & evaluate for reflux

Intralobar Pulmonary Sequestration

- Abnormal pulmonary tissue that does not communicate with tracheobronchial tree via normal bronchial connection
- Anomalous systemic vascularization
- Recurrent pulmonary infections usually in lower lobe

Congenital Pulmonary Airway Malformation

- Usually manifest in neonatal period
- Hamartomatous pulmonary lesion
- Recurrent episodes of pneumonia

PATHOLOGY

General Features

- Etiology
  - Congenital
  - Pathogenesis
    - Controversial
    - Various developmental theories
      - Reduction
      - Migration
      - Selection
    - Tracheal bronchus: Occurs 29-30 days after onset of differentiation of lobar bronchi
    - Accessory cardiac bronchus: Always a supernumerary bronchus
- Associated abnormalities
  - Congenital diaphragmatic hernia (CDH) sometimes associated with airway anomalies, such as congenital stenosis, abnormal bronchial branching, & pulmonary hypoplasia
  - Variable bronchial branching associated with isolated lobar agenesis, aplasia, or hypoplasia (hypogenetic lung syndrome)
  - Isomerism with bilateral left-sided airway anatomy: Associated with venolobar syndrome, absence of inferior vena cava with azygous continuation, polysplenia
    - Absence of inferior vena cava (IVC) normally visible on lateral chest radiography
    - Azygous continuation normally visible on frontal chest radiography
  - Isomerism with bilateral right-sided airway anatomy: Associated with asplenia & severe congenital heart disease
  - Agenesis-hypoplasia complex: May be associated with partial anomalous venous return (congenital pulmonary venolobar syndrome) & pectus excavatum

CLINICAL ISSUES

Presentation

- Most common signs/symptoms
  - Usually asymptomatic
  - Tracheal bronchus, accessory cardiac bronchus
    - Often asymptomatic incidental finding
    - Recurrent infections
    - Atelectasis, bronchiectasis
- Other signs/symptoms
  - Intubated patients with tracheal bronchus may have recurrent or chronic partial atelectasis of upper lobe

Demographics

- Age
  - Any age
- Epidemiology
  - Prevalence
    - Proximal or distal segmental or subsegmental bronchial displacement in 10% of individuals
    - Right tracheal bronchus: 0.1-2%
    - Left tracheal bronchus: 0.3-1%
    - Accessory cardiac bronchus: 0.09-0.5%

Natural History & Prognosis

- Prognosis: Very good

Treatment

- Usually no treatment
- Treat complications
  - Antibiotics for infections
  - Surgery in complicated cases

DIAGNOSTIC CHECKLIST

Consider

- Anomalous bronchial abnormalities should be suspected in recurrent pneumonia &/or atelectasis
- Some congenital airway anomalies are found incidentally on conventional radiography or CT of asymptomatic adults
- Knowledge of bronchial abnormalities is necessary for fiberoptic bronchoscopy, endobronchial treatment, & transplantation

Image Interpretation Pearls

- MDCT is modality of choice to evaluate anomalous bronchi, particularly those affecting central airways
- Some bronchial anomalies are associated with specific clinical & imaging features

SELECTED REFERENCES

1. Kang EY: Large airway diseases. J Thorac Imaging. 26(4):249-62, 2011
2. Desir A et al: Congenital abnormalities of intrathoracic airways. Radiol Clin North Am. 47(2):203-25, 2009
3. Kumagae Y et al: An adult case of bilateral true tracheal bronchi associated with hemoptysis. J Thorac Imaging. 21(4):293-5, 2006
4. Ghaye B et al: Congenital bronchial abnormalities revisited. Radiographics. 21(1):105-19, 2001
5. Ghaye B et al: Accessory cardiac bronchus: 3D CT demonstration in nine cases. Eur Radiol. 9(1):45-8, 1999

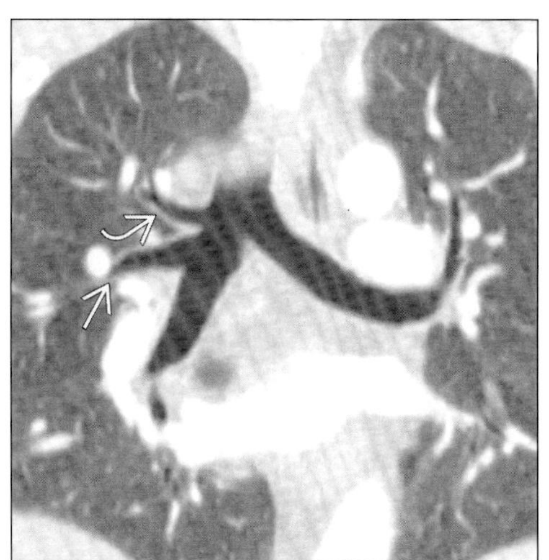

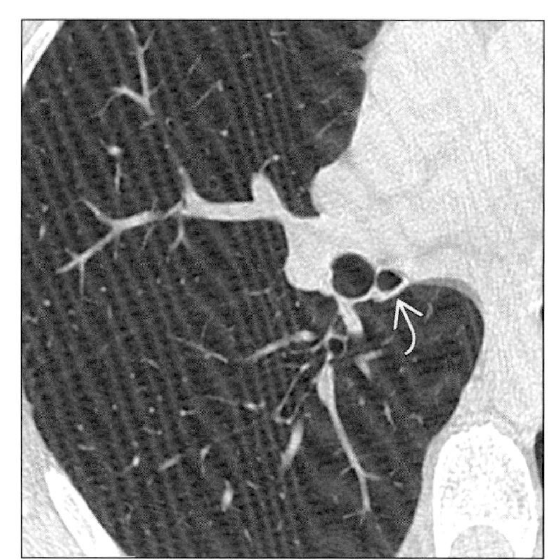

(Left) *Coronal CECT shows a displaced right upper lobe apical segmental pre-eparterial bronchus ➔ arising from the right mainstem bronchus. The right upper lobe bronchus ➔ lacked a right apical segmental branch. This is one of the most frequently seen anomalous bronchi.* ***(Right)*** *Axial NECT shows an accessory cardiac bronchus ➔ arising from the medial wall of the bronchus intermedius. Accessory cardiac bronchus may be associated with aspiration pneumonitis or hemoptysis.*

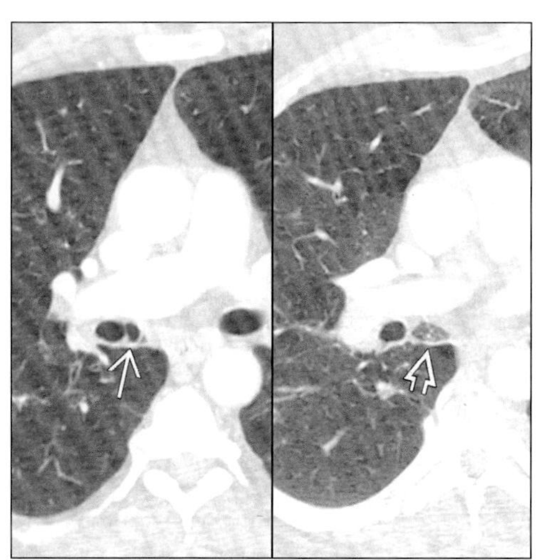

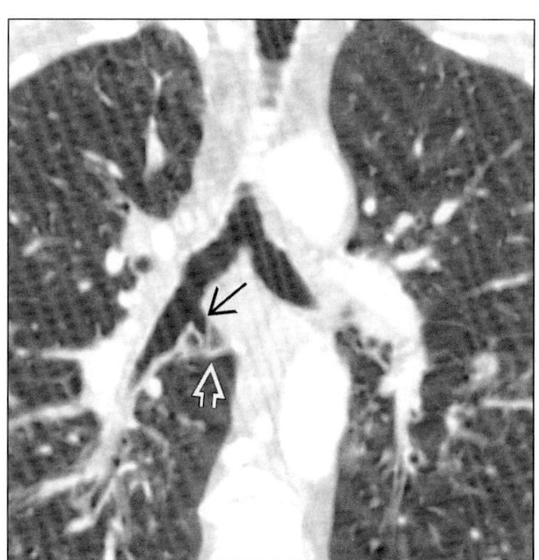

(Left) *Composite image with axial CECT shows an accessory cardiac bronchus ➔ arising from the medial wall of the bronchus intermedius and coursing caudally toward a rudimentary lung lobule ➔.* ***(Right)*** *Coronal CECT of the same patient shows the accessory cardiac bronchus ➔ arising from the medial wall of the bronchus intermedius and coursing caudally toward a rudimentary lung lobule ➔.*

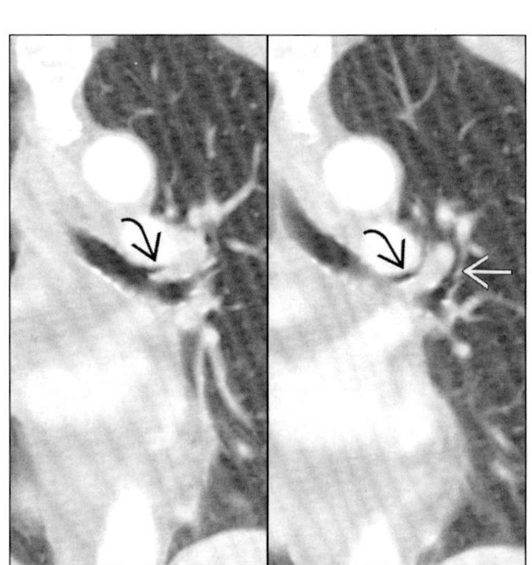

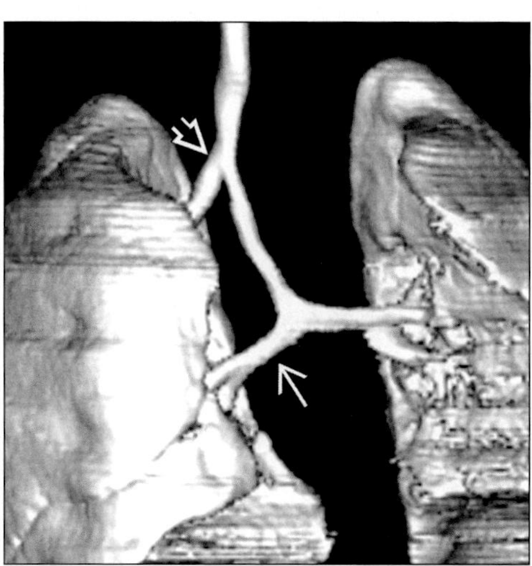

(Left) *Composite image with coronal CECT shows an anomalous supernumerary left upper lobe apicoposterior segmental prehyparterial bronchus ➔ arising proximal to the normal left upper lobe bronchus ➔ and coursing cephalad toward the lung apex.* ***(Right)*** *Volumetric 3D reformation shows a bridging bronchus. The right mainstem bronchus ➔ supplies the RUL. The bronchus intermedius arises from the distal aspect of the left main bronchus ➔. (Courtesy J. Kim, MD.)*

PARATRACHEAL AIR CYST

Key Facts

Terminology

- Mucosal herniation through tracheal wall
- Synonyms
  - Tracheal diverticulum
  - Tracheocele
  - Lymphoepithelial cyst

Imaging

- Radiography
  - Not visible
- CT
  - Small rounded air-filled cyst
  - Right posterior paratracheal region at thoracic inlet
  - Near right posterolateral tracheal wall at thoracic inlet (> 95%)
  - No calcification, air-fluid level or lung markings
  - Visible tracheal communication in only 35%

Top Differential Diagnoses

- Pneumomediastinum
- Paraseptal emphysema
- Apical lung hernia
- Zenker diverticulum

Pathology

- Cyst lined with normal ciliated columnar epithelium & communicates with trachea

Clinical Issues

- Usually asymptomatic
- Rarely chronic cough & dyspnea
- Common incidental finding on CT

Diagnostic Checklist

- Paratracheal air cyst should not be mistaken for pneumomediastinum or pneumothorax

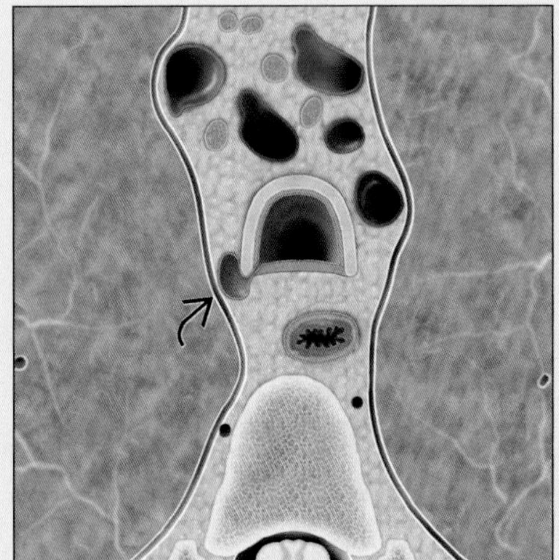

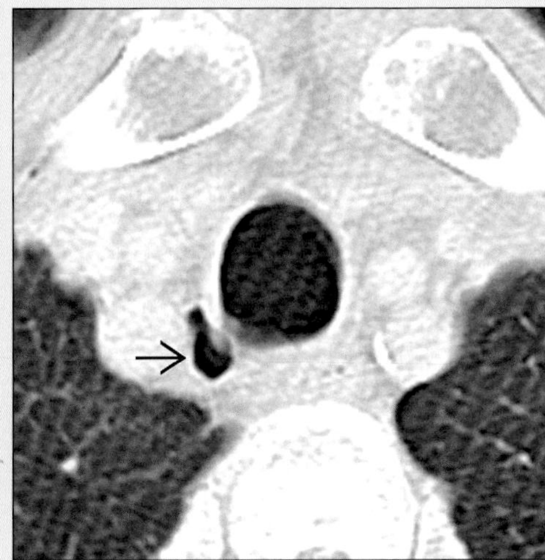

*(**Left**) Graphic shows a right paratracheal air cyst ⮫ with a narrow tracheal communication. Paratracheal cysts are most common on the right at the thoracic inlet, but can occur anywhere along the trachea. (**Right**) Axial NECT of a 48-year-old woman undergoing pulmonary nodule follow-up shows a 12 mm cyst adjacent to the right posterolateral tracheal wall ➔. The tracheal connection is not usually seen. This is an incidental finding, and follow-up or treatment are not required.*

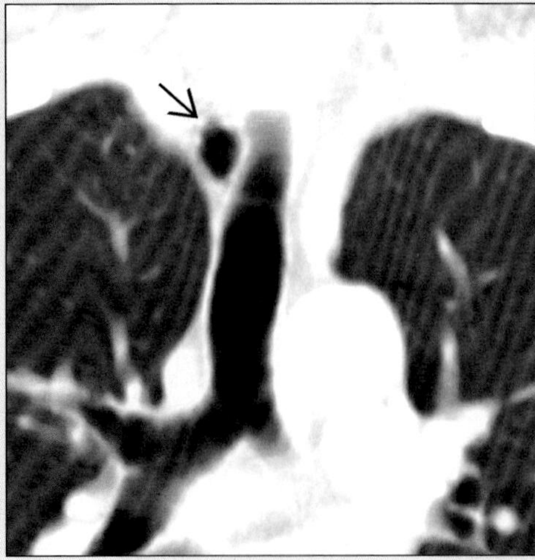

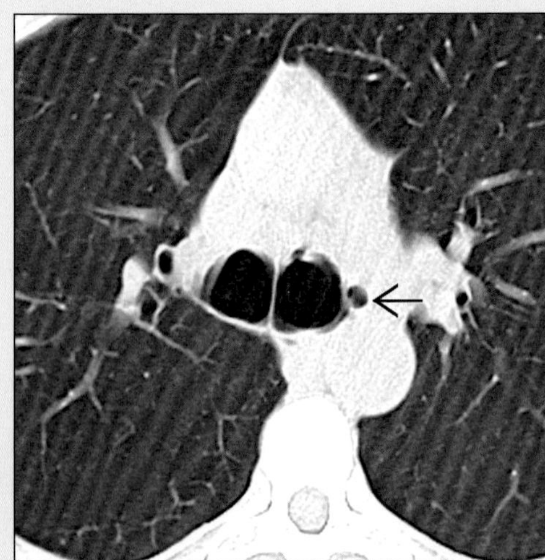

*(**Left**) Coronal CECT of a 28-year-old man obtained following trauma shows a 15 mm air-filled cyst ➔ adjacent to the right posterolateral tracheal wall. Given the typical location and absence of other gas collections, the misdiagnosis of pneumomediastinum was avoided. (**Right**) Axial HRCT of a 48-year-old man with chronic cough shows a 5 mm cyst lateral to the wall of the left mainstem bronchus, just below the carina ➔. Cysts can occur anywhere along the trachea or central airways.*

PARATRACHEAL AIR CYST

TERMINOLOGY

Synonyms

- Tracheal diverticulum
- Tracheocele
- Lymphoepithelial cyst

Definitions

- Mucosal herniation through tracheal wall

IMAGING

General Features

- Best diagnostic clue
  - Small rounded air-filled cyst posterior to trachea
- Location
  - Near right posterolateral tracheal wall at thoracic inlet (> 95%)
- Size
  - Usually < 2 cm in diameter
  - Variable
    - Enlarge on expiration
    - Shrink on inspiration
- Morphology
  - No calcification, air-fluid level or lung markings
  - Wall thickening uncommon (33%)
  - Usually single, but rarely multiple

Imaging Recommendations

- Best imaging tool
  - CT is modality of choice for assessment of airways
- Protocol advice
  - Multiplanar reconstruction to find tracheal communication

Radiographic Findings

- Radiography
  - Not visible

CT Findings

- NECT
  - **Air-filled cyst usually adjacent to right posterolateral tracheal wall**
  - **Visible tracheal communication in only 35%**

Ultrasonographic Findings

- Grayscale ultrasound
  - May be mistaken for calcified parathyroid mass due to location & echogenicity of air

DIFFERENTIAL DIAGNOSIS

Pneumomediastinum

- Often multifocal & usually more extensive

Paraseptal Emphysema

- Usually several subpleural cysts aligned in rows

Apical Lung Hernia

- Larger and contains lung markings

Zenker Diverticulum

- Usually located more cephalad & often contains fluid

PATHOLOGY

General Features

- Etiology
  - Congenital
    - Supernumerary lung buds contain all layers of tracheal wall including smooth muscle & cartilage, often filled with mucus
  - Acquired
    - Theory: Chronic increased intraluminal pressure from coughing
    - Association with emphysema is questionable

Gross Pathologic & Surgical Features

- Cyst communicates with trachea, channel measures 1.5-2 mm in length, 1 mm in diameter
- Location at transition point between intrathoracic & extrathoracic trachea

Microscopic Features

- Cyst lined with normal ciliated columnar epithelium

CLINICAL ISSUES

Presentation

- Most common signs/symptoms
  - Usually asymptomatic
  - Chronic cough & dyspnea
- Other signs/symptoms
  - May be large enough for endotracheal tube insertion

Demographics

- Age
  - Seen in all ages
- Epidemiology
  - Common incidental finding on CT, reported in up to 3.7% of cases

Treatment

- No treatment if asymptomatic
- Surgical resection if symptomatic

DIAGNOSTIC CHECKLIST

Image Interpretation Pearls

- Vast majority of paratracheal cysts are incidental findings
- Should not be mistaken for pneumomediastinum or pneumothorax

SELECTED REFERENCES

1. Oshiro Y et al: Subcarinal air cysts: multidetector computed tomographic findings. J Comput Assist Tomogr. 34(3):402-5, 2010
2. Buterbaugh JE et al: Paratracheal air cysts: a common finding on routine CT examinations of the cervical spine and neck that may mimic pneumomediastinum in patients with traumatic injuries. AJNR Am J Neuroradiol. 29(6):1218-21, 2008
3. Goo JM et al: Right paratracheal air cysts in the thoracic inlet: clinical and radiologic significance. AJR Am J Roentgenol. 173(1):65-70, 1999

BRONCHIAL ATRESIA

Key Facts

Terminology

- Bronchial atresia (BA)
- Congenital focal atresia of subsegmental, segmental, or lobar bronchus

Imaging

- Radiography
  - Well-defined rounded, ovoid, tubular, or branching mucocele
  - Surrounded by hyperlucent lung parenchyma
  - Expiratory air-trapping in affected lung
- CT
  - Rounded, tubular, or branching mucocele
  - Nonenhancing, low-attenuation mucocele
  - Surrounding wedge-shaped hyperlucent lung
  - Exclusion of central obstructing neoplasm
- V/Q scintigraphy: Hypoperfusion & absent or delayed ventilation of affected pulmonary segment

Top Differential Diagnoses

- Other causes of mucoid impaction
- Arteriovenous malformation
- Intralobar sequestration

Clinical Issues

- Symptoms/signs
  - Asymptomatic adult (60%)
  - Cough, recurrent infection, dyspnea, chest pain
- Imaging diagnosis after exclusion of central obstructing lesion

Diagnostic Checklist

- Consider bronchial atresia in asymptomatic patient with focal pulmonary hyperlucency surrounding nodular or tubular opacity
- Prospective imaging diagnosis allows conservative management of asymptomatic patients

*(**Left**) PA chest radiograph of an asymptomatic patient with bronchial atresia shows left upper lung zone hyperlucency and hyperexpansion surrounding a tubular branching opacity →, representing a mucocele. The radiographic findings are diagnostic. (**Right**) Composite image with ventilation (top) and perfusion (bottom) scintigraphy of the same patient shows matching left upper lobe ventilation → and perfusion ⇨ defects. Delayed imaging may demonstrate delayed ventilation of the affected lung.*

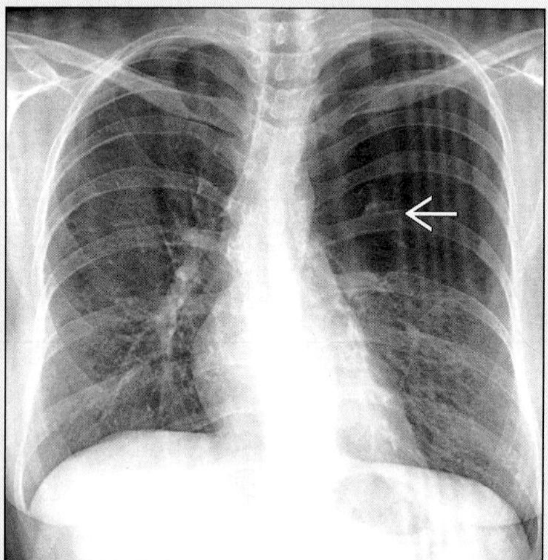

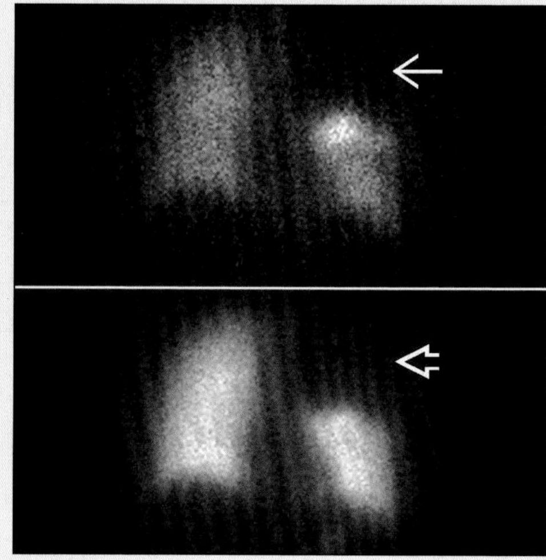

*(**Left**) PA chest radiograph of a patient with bronchial atresia shows a right lower lobe branching opacity consistent with mucoid impaction →. (**Right**) Composite image with axial CECT of the same patient in lung (left) and soft tissue (right) window shows a low-attenuation right lower lobe branching mucocele ⇨ surrounded by hyperlucent lung parenchyma →. After exclusion of a central obstructing neoplasm, the imaging findings are diagnostic of bronchial atresia.*

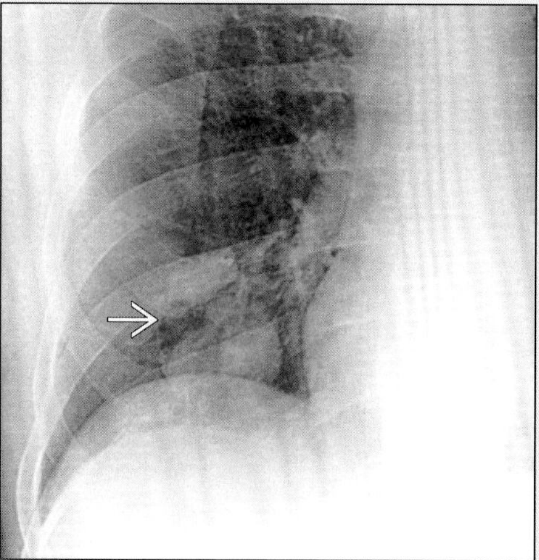

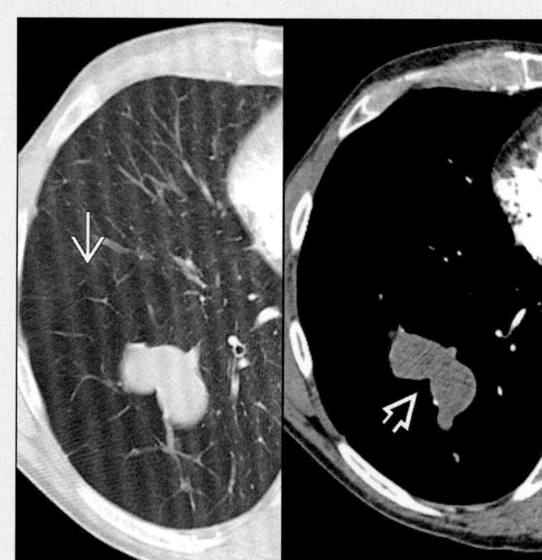

BRONCHIAL ATRESIA

TERMINOLOGY

Abbreviations

- **Bronchial atresia (BA)**

Synonyms

- **Congenital bronchial atresia (CBA)**

Definitions

- Congenital focal atresia of subsegmental, segmental, or lobar bronchus
  - Normal distal bronchial tree
- Mucocele: Mucoid impaction distal to bronchial atresia
  - Synonym: Bronchocele

IMAGING

General Features

- Best diagnostic clue
  - Rounded, tubular, or branching opacity with surrounding pulmonary hyperlucency
- Location
  - In decreasing order
    - Left upper lobe
      - Apicoposterior segment most commonly affected
    - Right upper lobe
    - Left lower lobe
    - Middle lobe
    - Right lower lobe
  - Typically segmental
    - Rarely lobar or subsegmental
- Size
  - Variable
- Morphology
  - Mucocele
    - Rounded, ovoid
    - Tubular
    - May exhibit branching morphology

Radiographic Findings

- Radiography
  - **Mucocele surrounded by hyperlucent lung parenchyma**
  - Visualization & characterization of **mucocele**
    - Well-defined round, ovoid, tubular, or branching morphology
    - Central location
    - Longitudinal axis of mucocele oriented toward ipsilateral hilum
    - Air-fluid levels within mucocele consistent with superimposed infection
  - **Hyperlucent lung parenchyma**
    - Surrounds mucocele
    - Decreased markings & vascularity
  - **Expiratory air-trapping of hyperlucent lung**

CT Findings

- NECT
  - Identification & characterization of **mucocele**
    - Well-defined borders
    - Spherical, ovoid
    - Tubular
    - Branching
    - Longitudinal axis of mucocele oriented toward ipsilateral hilum
    - Low attenuation: -5 to 25 HU
  - Evaluation of bronchial tree to determine relationship of normal bronchi to mucocele
  - **Assessment of hyperlucent lung parenchyma**
    - Wedge-shaped hyperlucent lung
      - Hyperlucent lung surrounds mucocele
    - Hyperlucency related to collateral ventilation, air-trapping, & hypoperfusion
  - Finding of mucocele & peripheral hyperinflation seen in up to 83% of BA cases
- CECT
  - **Mucocele**
    - **Low attenuation**
    - **Absence of contrast enhancement**
      - Distinction from vascular lesion such as arteriovenous malformation
  - Exclusion of central obstructing neoplasm

Nuclear Medicine Findings

- V/Q scan
  - Hypoperfusion of affected pulmonary segment
  - Absent or delayed ventilation of affected segment
  - Affected segment may exhibit delayed washout secondary to air-trapping

MR Findings

- Identification & assessment of mucocele
  - High signal intensity mucocele on T1WI & T2WI
- Fetal MR imaging
  - Focal lung mass
  - Homogeneous high signal intensity on T2WI

Ultrasonographic Findings

- Prenatal diagnosis
  - Echogenic fluid-filled lung distal to atresia

Imaging Recommendations

- Best imaging tool
  - Diagnosis may be suspected on radiography
  - CT is imaging modality of choice to assess suspected bronchial atresia
    - Exclusion of centrally obstructing neoplasm
- Protocol advice
  - Multiplanar reformatted images for evaluation of bronchial anatomy & extent of involvement
  - Expiratory radiography or CT for documentation of air-trapping distal to mucocele

DIFFERENTIAL DIAGNOSIS

Other Causes of Mucoid Impaction

- Allergic bronchopulmonary aspergillosis
  - History of asthma
  - Upper lobe bronchiectasis with mucus plugging
- Endobronchial neoplasm
  - May be associated with distal mucus plugging
  - CECT for differentiation of central neoplasm from peripheral mucus plug
- Bronchiectasis
  - May exhibit mucus plugging, particularly with superimposed infection
  - Typically multifocal

Arteriovenous Malformation

- Direct communication between feeding pulmonary artery & draining pulmonary vein

BRONCHIAL ATRESIA

- Contrast enhancement
- No bronchial obstruction, hyperlucency, or hyperinflation

Intralobar Sequestration

- Heterogeneous attenuation
- May exhibit areas of hyperlucency
- Anomalous feeding artery typically arising from descending aorta
- Characteristic lower lobe location

Intrapulmonary Bronchogenic Cyst

- Lower lobes
- Medial 1/3 of lung
- May be fluid-filled, air-filled, or both (air-fluid level)

Congenital Lobar Overinflation

- Neonates & infants with respiratory distress
- Typically lobar, not segmental
- Left upper lobe most commonly affected
- Progressive lobar hyperinflation with mass effect

PATHOLOGY

General Features

- Etiology
  - 2 theories of pathogenesis
    - Disconnection of bronchial cells from bronchial bud
      - Postulated to occur at 4th to 6th weeks of gestation
      - Disconnected cells undergo normal division resulting in normal distal bronchial branching
    - In utero vascular insult
      - Focal ischemia after 16th week of gestation
      - Focal bronchial injury results in atresia with normal development of distal bronchi
      - Obstruction to proximal drainage with mucocele formation
      - Distal hyperinflation
- Associated abnormalities
  - Pediatric patients
    - Bronchogenic cyst
    - Congenital pulmonary adenomatoid malformation
    - Sequestration
    - Reports of systemic arterial supply

Gross Pathologic & Surgical Features

- Focal short-segment bronchial atresia
  - No connection between bronchus distal to atresia & proximal feeding bronchus
- Mucocele distal to atresia
- Overexpanded lung distal to atresia
  - Likely due to chronic collateral ventilation
    - Pores of Kohn
    - Canals of Lambert

Microscopic Features

- Alveolar overexpansion
- Signs of infection/inflammation in complicated BA
- Airways plugged with mucus
- No evidence of lung destruction

CLINICAL ISSUES

Presentation

- Most common signs/symptoms
  - Asymptomatic adult (60%)
    - Incidental imaging finding
  - Cough, recurrent pulmonary infection
  - Dyspnea
  - Chest pain
- Other signs/symptoms
  - Wheezing
  - Hemoptysis
  - Decreased breath sounds over affected lung

Demographics

- Age
  - Wide age range
  - Mean age at diagnosis: 17 years
- Gender
  - M:F = 2:1

Natural History & Prognosis

- Excellent

Diagnosis

- **Imaging diagnosis after exclusion of central obstructing lesion**
- Bronchoscopy may be normal or may reveal blind-ending bronchus

Treatment

- None for asymptomatic patients
- Surgical resection for intractable or recurrent superimposed infection

DIAGNOSTIC CHECKLIST

Consider

- Bronchial atresia in asymptomatic patient with focal pulmonary hyperlucency surrounding nodular or tubular opacity

Image Interpretation Pearls

- Prospective imaging diagnosis allows conservative management of asymptomatic patients

SELECTED REFERENCES

1. Biyyam DR et al: Congenital lung abnormalities: embryologic features, prenatal diagnosis, and postnatal radiologic-pathologic correlation. Radiographics. 30(6):1721-38, 2010
2. Desir A et al: Congenital abnormalities of intrathoracic airways. Radiol Clin North Am. 47(2):203-25, 2009
3. Gipson MG et al: Bronchial atresia. Radiographics. 29(5):1531-5, 2009
4. Martinez S et al: Mucoid impactions: finger-in-glove sign and other CT and radiographic features. Radiographics. 28(5):1369-82, 2008

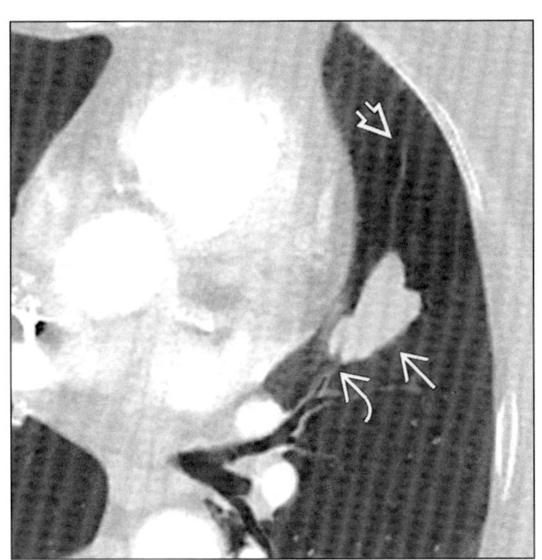

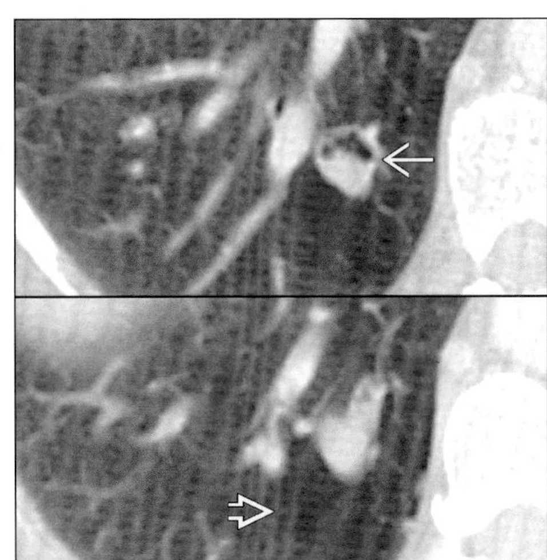

(Left) *Axial CECT minimum-intensity projection (MinIP) image of a patient with bronchial atresia shows a lingular branching mucocele* ➔ *with surrounding hyperlucency* ➔ *and allows identification of the proximal aspect of the affected bronchus* ➔. ***(Right)*** *Composite image with axial CECT of a patient with persistent fever shows a right lower lobe branching opacity with an intrinsic air-fluid level* ➔ *and surrounding hyperlucency* ➔. *The findings are consistent with BA with infected mucocele.*

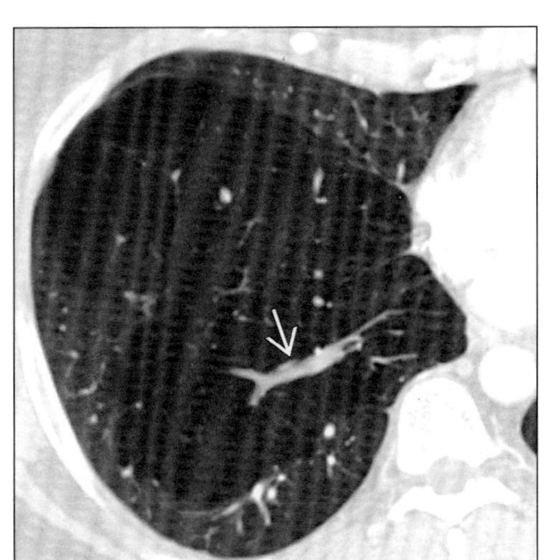

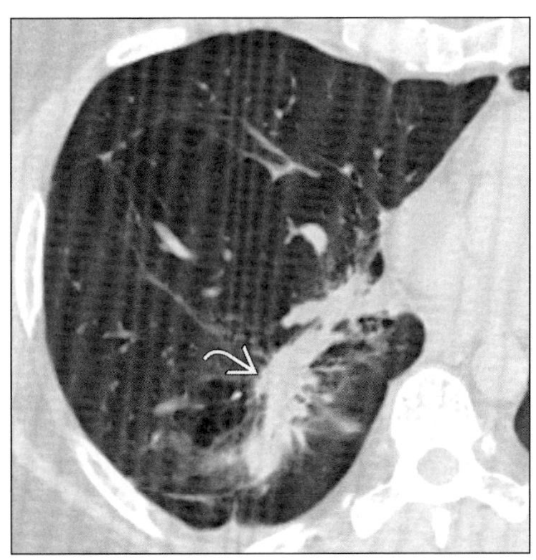

(Left) *Axial CECT shows extensive right lower lobe hyperlucency and 1 of several extensions of a branching mucocele* ➔. *The patient was prospectively diagnosed with bronchial atresia.* ***(Right)*** *Axial CECT of the same patient obtained at a later date because of cough and fever shows a new irregular consolidation* ➔ *in the affected right lower lobe consistent with pneumonia. Patients who fail to respond to antibiotic treatment may require surgical excision of the affected lung.*

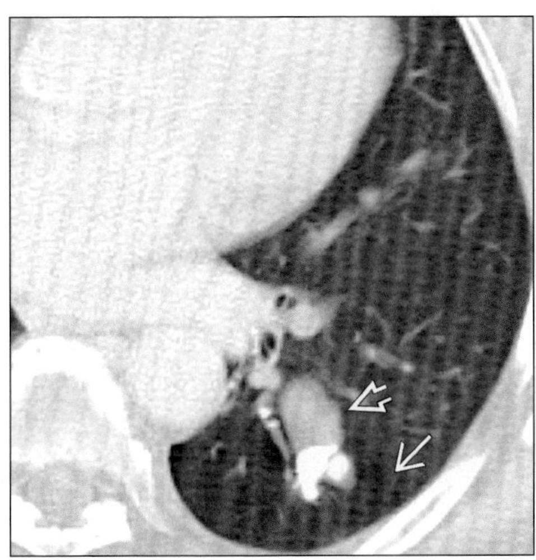

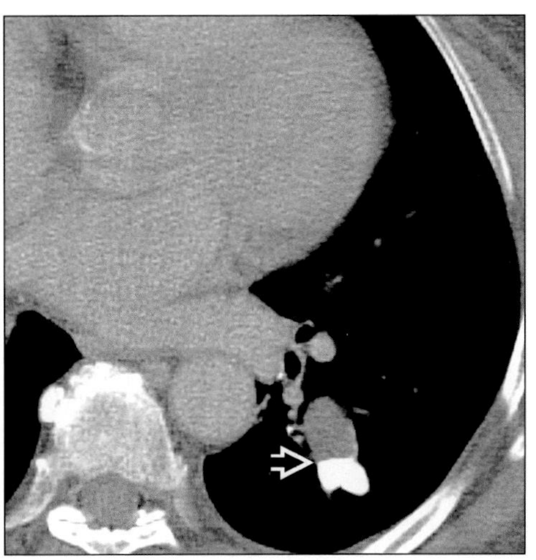

(Left) *Axial NECT (lung window) of an asymptomatic patient with a left lower lobe segmental bronchial atresia shows a branching opacity* ➔ *with dependent high attenuation surrounded by mild peripheral hyperlucency* ➔. ***(Right)*** *Axial NECT (soft tissue window) of the same patient shows the branching morphology of the mucocele. In this case, the mucocele exhibits internal layering milk of calcium* ➔. *Although this is an atypical manifestation of BA, the other morphologic features are diagnostic.*

TRACHEOBRONCHOMEGALY

Key Facts

Terminology

- Synonym: Mounier-Kuhn syndrome
- Dilatation of trachea & central bronchi that impairs ability to clear mucus

Imaging

- Radiography
  - Marked dilatation of trachea & central bronchi
  - Tracheal collapse with expiration
  - Central bronchiectasis
- CT
  - Large tracheal/bronchial diameters on inspiration
  - Corrugated effect due to redundant mucosa prolapsing between tracheal rings
  - Central bronchiectasis, 1st to 4th order bronchi
  - Tracheobronchial diverticula
  - Tracheobronchial collapse with expiration

Top Differential Diagnoses

- Ehlers-Danlos syndrome
- Cutis laxa (generalized elastolysis)
- Upper lobe or diffuse pulmonary fibrosis
- Immune deficiency states & recurrent childhood infections

Pathology

- Atrophy or absence of elastic fibers & thinning of smooth muscle layer in trachea & main bronchi

Clinical Issues

- Symptoms of recurrent infection & bronchiectasis
- Prognosis: Variable from minimal disease to respiratory failure and death

Diagnostic Checklist

- Evaluate tracheal caliber in patients with bronchiectasis &/or recurrent pneumonia

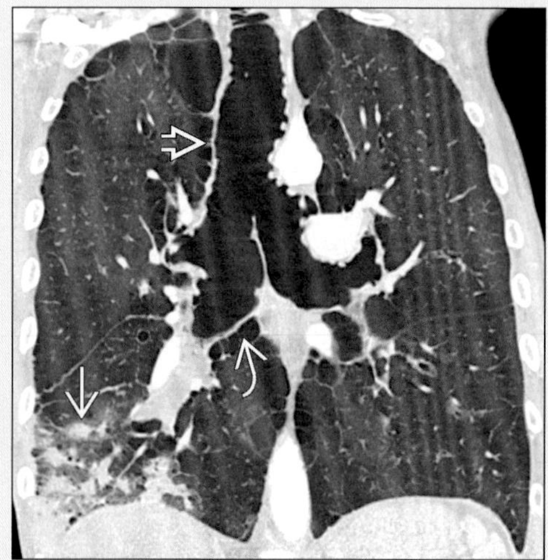

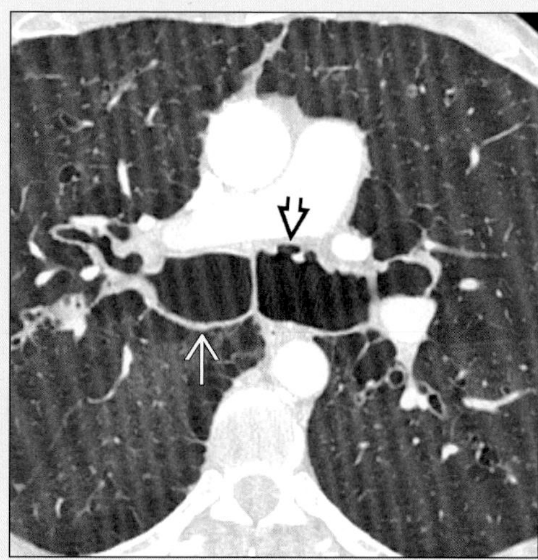

(Left) *Coronal CECT of a patient with tracheobronchomegaly shows marked dilatation of the trachea ➡ and mainstem bronchi ➡. The large airways have a corrugated appearance. Right lower lobe pneumonia ➡ and paraseptal emphysema are also present.* ***(Right)*** *Axial CECT of the same patient shows enlarged mainstem bronchi ➡ and bronchial diverticula ➡. The corrugated appearance of the airways results from redundant mucosa interdigitating between cartilaginous rings.*

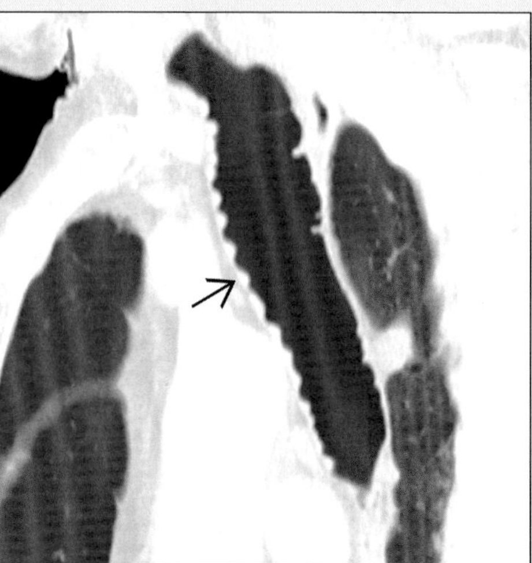

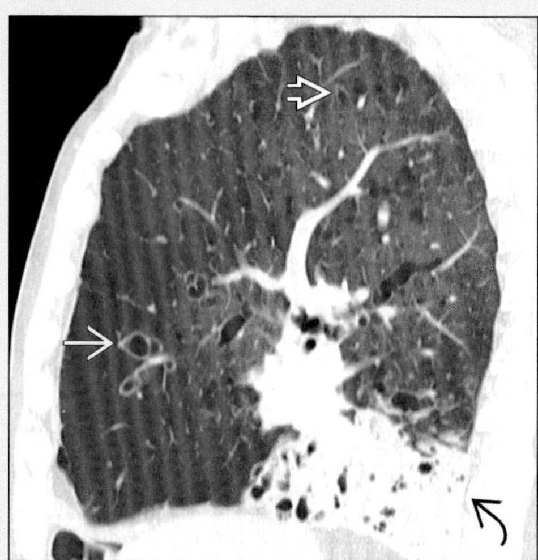

(Left) *Sagittal NECT of a patient with tracheobronchomegaly shows a markedly enlarged and corrugated trachea ➡.* ***(Right)*** *Sagittal NECT of the same patient shows centrilobular emphysema ➡, bronchiectasis ➡, segmental air-trapping, and lower lobe consolidation ➡. Patients with tracheobronchomegaly are predisposed to recurrent infection due to poor secretory clearance, which may result in bronchiectasis, air-trapping, and pulmonary fibrosis.*

TRACHEOBRONCHOMEGALY

TERMINOLOGY

Synonyms

- Mounier-Kuhn syndrome

Definitions

- Rare disorder characterized by dilatation of trachea & central bronchi that impairs ability to clear mucus from lungs

IMAGING

General Features

- Best diagnostic clue
  - Tracheal diameter > 27 mm in men & > 23 mm in women
  - Recurrent pulmonary infections; bronchiectasis

Radiographic Findings

- **Marked dilatation of trachea & central bronchi**
- Normal tracheal diameters
  - Men: Coronal 13-25; sagittal 13-27 mm
  - Women: Coronal 10-21; sagittal 10-23 mm
  - Mainstem bronchi, normal (right-left): Men 21mm, 18.4 mm; women 19.8 mm, 17.4 mm
- Central bronchiectasis, 1st to 4th order bronchi
- Hyperinflation & emphysema
- Secondary pulmonary fibrosis from recurrent infections (less common)

CT Findings

- NECT
  - **Abnormally large tracheal & bronchial diameters on inspiration**
  - **Airways dilated on inspiration, collapsed on expiration**
  - Corrugated effect due to redundant mucosa prolapsing between tracheal rings
  - **Tracheobronchial diverticula**
  - **Normal diameter of subglottic trachea**
  - **Tracheobronchial collapse with expiration**
  - Bronchiectasis, pulmonary fibrosis, hyperinflation

Imaging Recommendations

- Best imaging tool
  - CT is optimal imaging modality for identification & assessment of airway abnormalities

DIFFERENTIAL DIAGNOSIS

Tracheobronchomegaly

- Ehlers-Danlos syndrome
  - Inherited connective tissue disorder
  - Pulmonary artery stenoses, bronchiectasis, thin-walled cavitary lesions, cysts
- Cutis laxa (generalized elastolysis)
  - Hereditary connective tissue disorder
  - Premature aging, loose skin, & subcutaneous tissue
  - Tracheobronchomegaly, panacinar emphysema, bronchiectasis, aortic aneurysms
- Upper lobe or diffuse pulmonary fibrosis
- Immune deficiency states & recurrent childhood infections

PATHOLOGY

General Features

- Etiology
  - Many cases familial, autosomal recessive
- Atrophy or absence of elastic fibers & thinning of tracheal & mainstem bronchial smooth muscle layer

Gross Pathologic & Surgical Features

- Enlarged trachea with thinning of tracheal wall; may contain diverticula
- Both cartilage & membranous portions of trachea affected

CLINICAL ISSUES

Presentation

- Most common signs/symptoms
  - Related to recurrent infection & bronchiectasis
- Symptoms may date back to childhood with ineffective cough
- Loud, productive cough, hoarseness, dyspnea, recurrent pneumonia
- Recurrent infection may lead to bronchiectasis & pulmonary fibrosis
- Obstructive airway disease from collapse of trachea & bronchi (tracheobronchomalacia)
- Pulmonary function tests: Increased dead space, total lung capacity, residual volume, & airflow obstruction

Demographics

- Age
  - Usually diagnosed at 30-50 years of age
- Gender
  - M:F = 19:1
- Ethnicity
  - Predisposition in black patients
- Epidemiology
  - Most cases are sporadic
  - Rare, seen in approximately 1% of bronchograms

Natural History & Prognosis

- Prognosis: Variable from minimal disease to respiratory failure & death

Treatment

- Physiotherapy
- Reduction of infection risk, pneumococcal immunization
- Smoking cessation

DIAGNOSTIC CHECKLIST

Consider

- Expiratory CT to evaluate for tracheomalacia

Image Interpretation Pearls

- Evaluate tracheal caliber in patients with bronchiectasis &/or recurrent pneumonia

SELECTED REFERENCES

1. Javidan-Nejad C et al: Bronchiectasis. Radiol Clin North Am. 47(2):289-306, 2009

CONGENITAL LOBAR OVERINFLATION

Key Facts

Terminology

- Congenital lobar overinflation (CLO)
- Congenital lobar emphysema (CLE)

Imaging

- Radiography
  - Hyperlucent pulmonary lobe
  - Progressive lobar enlargement
  - Ipsilateral rib space widening
  - Initially opaque due to retained fetal lung fluid
- CT
  - Hyperlucent, hyperexpanded lobe with paucity of vascular markings
  - Mass effect on ipsilateral lobes, mediastinum, & hemidiaphragm
  - Demonstration of extrinsic obstructing lesion: Vascular anomaly, congenital cyst

Top Differential Diagnoses

- Congenital pulmonary airway malformation
- Bronchial atresia

Pathology

- 1-way valve obstruction: Air enters distal airways → does not exit → progressive lobar expansion
- Loss of lobar shape, sponge-like appearance on cut section

Clinical Issues

- Symptoms/signs
  - Neonatal respiratory distress, may be progressive
  - Occasionally diagnosed in older children with minimal symptoms
- Treatment
  - Lobectomy
  - Supportive care & observation

__(Left)__ AP chest radiograph of a neonate with respiratory distress shows characteristic findings of CLO, including left upper lobe hyperinflation, mass effect on the lingula ➡ and mediastinum, and contralateral displacement of the anterior junction line ↪. __(Right)__ Axial NECT of the same patient shows a hyperexpanded hyperlucent left upper lobe producing mass effect on the mediastinum and increased attenuation of the normal compressed right lung. CLO most commonly affects the left upper lobe.

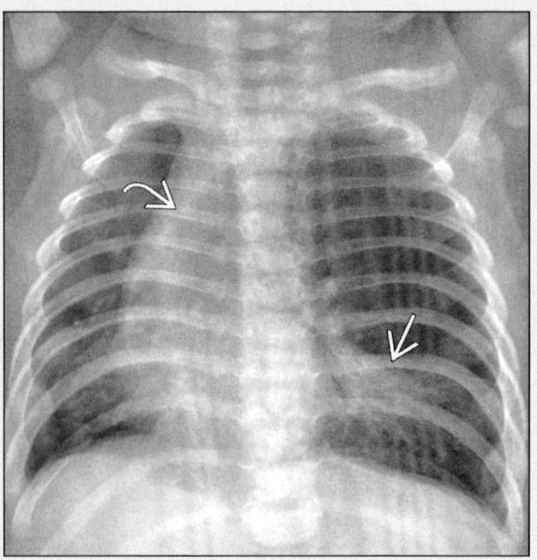

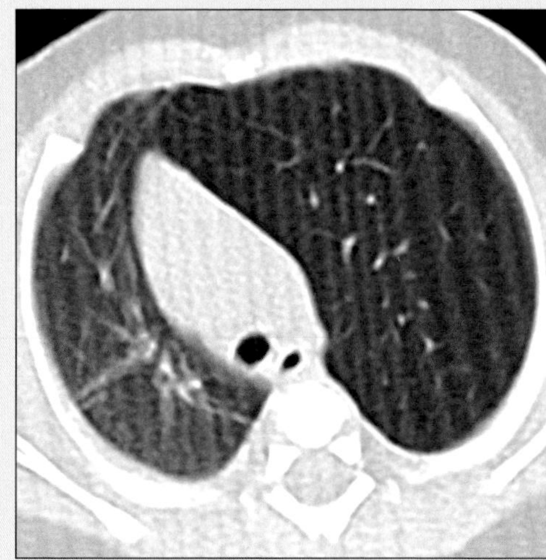

__(Left)__ NECT of a neonate with CLO and respiratory distress shows a hyperinflated hyperlucent right upper lobe with paucity of vascular markings, mass effect on the mediastinum, and contralateral displacement of the anterior junction line ➡. Note normal attenuation of the uninvolved left lung ↪. __(Right)__ 3D surface-rendered NECT of a patient with right upper lobe CLO shows hyperinflation of the right upper lobe ➡ and increased attenuation ⇨ of the normal but compressed adjacent and contralateral lungs.

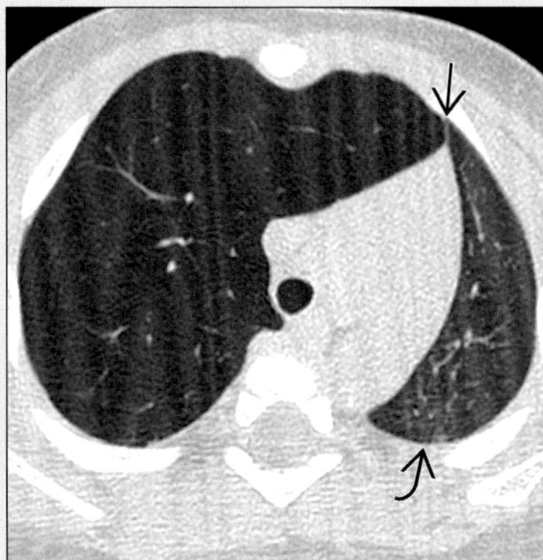

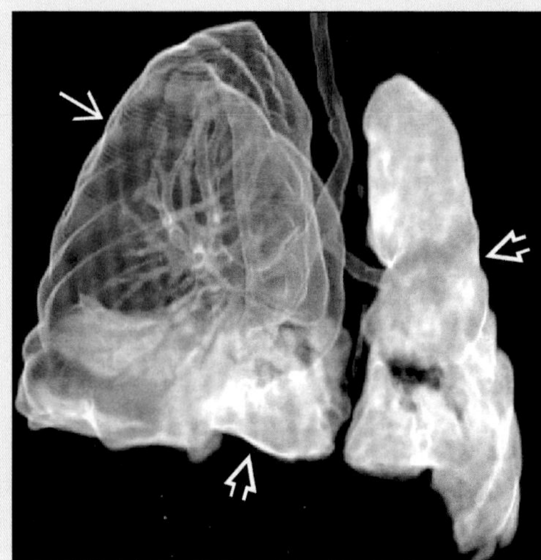

CONGENITAL LOBAR OVERINFLATION

TERMINOLOGY

Abbreviations

- Congenital lobar overinflation (CLO)

Synonyms

- Congenital lobar emphysema (CLE)
- Infantile lobar emphysema (ILE)

Definitions

- Progressive overdistention of a pulmonary lobe due to 1-way valve airway obstruction

IMAGING

General Features

- Best diagnostic clue
  - Progressively hyperlucent & hyperexpanded lobe
- Location
  - Left upper lobe: 42%
  - Middle lobe: 35%
  - Right upper lobe: 21%
  - Either lower lobe: < 1%

Radiographic Findings

- Hyperlucent pulmonary lobe
  - Paucity of vascular markings
- Progressive lobar enlargement
  - Mass effect on ipsilateral lobes
  - Contralateral mediastinal deviation
  - Depression of ipsilateral hemidiaphragm
  - Ipsilateral rib space widening
- Initially opaque due to retained fetal lung fluid
  - Fluid clearance via pulmonary lymphatics
  - Lymphatics may be visible as "reticular" opacities

CT Findings

- NECT
  - Hyperlucent, hyperexpanded lobe with paucity of vascular markings
  - Mass effect on ipsilateral lobes, mediastinum, & hemidiaphragm
  - Demonstration of extrinsic obstructing lesion: Vascular anomaly, congenital cyst

Ultrasonographic Findings

- Prenatal ultrasound: Homogeneous hyperechoic mass, mass effect

MR Findings

- Fetal MR: High signal expanded lobe with mass effect

Imaging Recommendations

- Best imaging tool
  - Diagnosis typically made on chest radiography
  - CT: Confirmation & exclusion of extrinsic lesion

DIFFERENTIAL DIAGNOSIS

Congenital Pulmonary Airway Malformation

- Multifocal air-containing cysts of varying sizes
- May be initially opaque, may develop air-fluid levels

Bronchial Atresia

- Central tubular, rounded, or branching mucocele
- Surrounding hyperlucent lung parenchyma

Pneumothorax

- Hyperlucent hemithorax, visible pleural line

Congenital Diaphragmatic Hernia

- Initially opaque from fluid-filled bowel loops
- Visualization of air within bowel loops

PATHOLOGY

General Features

- Etiology
  - Cause found in approximately 50% of cases
  - 1-way valve bronchial obstruction: Air enters distal airways → does not exit → progressive lobar expansion
    - Abnormal bronchial cartilage
    - Abnormal mucosal folds
    - Mucoid impaction
    - Extrinsic compression: Congenital cyst, anomalous vasculature
- Associated abnormalities
  - Association with congenital heart disease (up to 15%)
    - PDA, ASD, VSD, TAPVR, tetralogy of Fallot

Gross Pathologic & Surgical Features

- Loss of lobar shape
- Sponge-like appearance on cut section
- Resected lobe does not deflate

Microscopic Features

- Dilated alveoli
- Alveolar walls are thinned but intact

CLINICAL ISSUES

Presentation

- Most common signs/symptoms
  - Neonatal respiratory distress
  - May be progressive

Demographics

- Age
  - Most symptomatic in neonatal period & infancy
    - 50% in first 4 weeks; 75% in first 6 months
  - Occasionally diagnosed in late childhood
- Gender
  - M:F = 1.8:1

Treatment

- Lobectomy: Symptomatic patients, life-threatening progressive hyperinflation
- Supportive care & observation: Mildly symptomatic, asymptomatic

SELECTED REFERENCES

1. Dillman JR et al: Expanding upon the unilateral hyperlucent hemithorax in children. Radiographics. 31(3):723-41, 2011
2. Biyyam DR et al: Congenital lung abnormalities: embryologic features, prenatal diagnosis, and postnatal radiologic-pathologic correlation. Radiographics. 30(6):1721-38, 2010

CONGENITAL PULMONARY AIRWAY MALFORMATION

Key Facts

Terminology

- Congenital pulmonary airway malformation (CPAM)
- Abnormal mass of pulmonary tissue with varying degrees of cystic change

Imaging

- Radiography
  - Unilateral hyperlucent lung lesion
  - Multiple thin-walled cysts
  - Single dominant cyst surrounded by smaller cysts
  - Homogeneous opacity: Cystic CPAM with retained fetal fluid, solid CPAM
- CT
  - Multilocular cystic lesion within pulmonary lobe
  - Variable cyst size, thin or thick cyst walls
  - Cysts may contain air, fluid, &/or air-fluid levels
- Antenatal diagnosis
  - Prenatal ultrasound
  - Prenatal MR
- Radiologic classification
  - Large cyst CPAM
  - Small cyst CPAM
  - Microcystic CPAM (solid appearing)

Top Differential Diagnoses

- Congenital lobar overinflation
- Pulmonary sequestration
  - Intralobar & extralobar sequestration

Clinical Issues

- Symptoms/signs
  - Acute progressive neonatal respiratory distress
  - Incidental diagnosis on prenatal ultrasound

Diagnostic Checklist

- Consider CPAM in patient with cystic lung lesion found in perinatal period

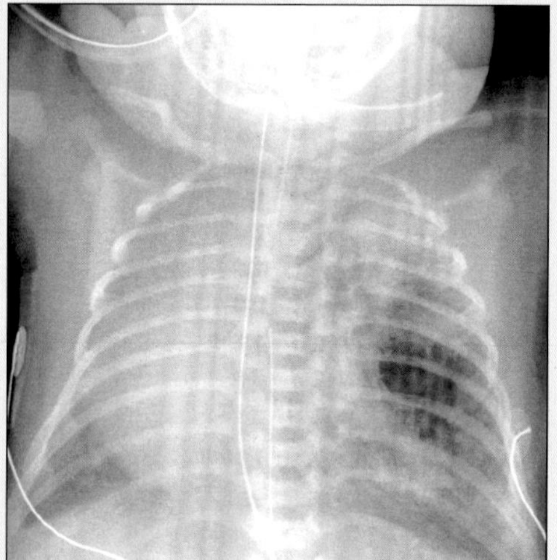

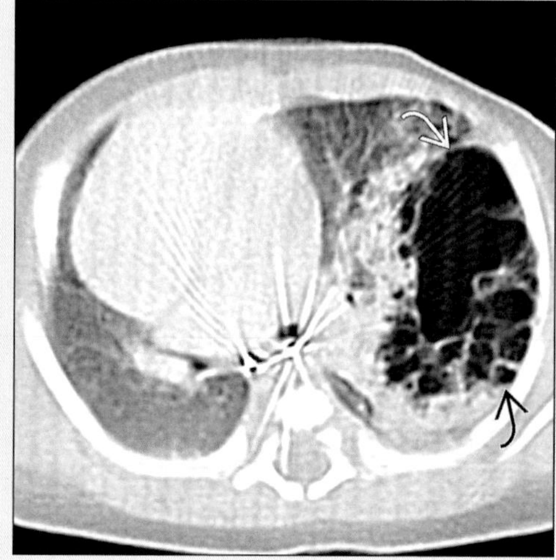

(Left) *AP chest radiograph of a neonate with respiratory distress shows a large air-filled left lung lesion with mediastinal shift to the right and mass effect on the esophageal enteric tube.* ***(Right)*** *Axial CECT of the same patient shows a predominantly air-filled multilocular cystic lesion in the left lung. A dominant cyst ➙ is surrounded by smaller cysts ➙ and there are air-fluid levels in the dependent aspect of the lesion. The morphologic features of the lesion are consistent with large cyst CPAM.*

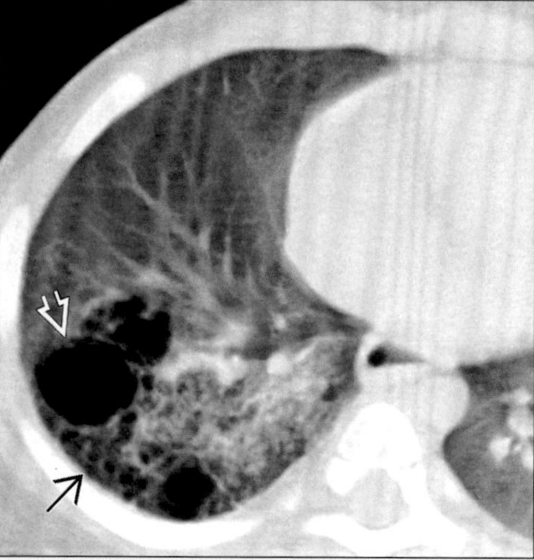

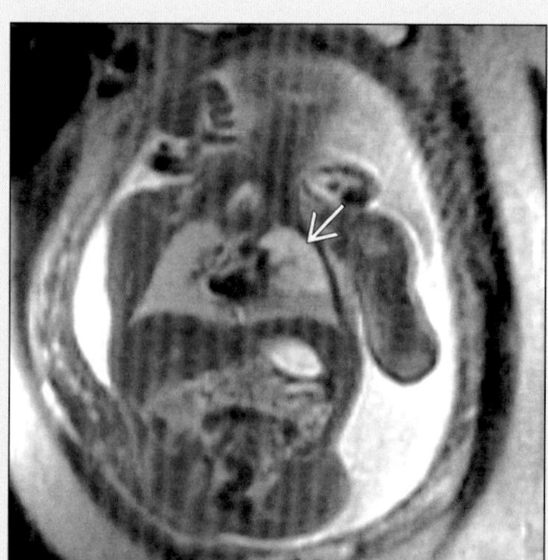

(Left) *Axial NECT of an infant with small cyst CPAM shows a right lower lobe heterogeneous lesion consisting of larger cysts ➙ (surrounded by numerous small cysts ➙) and scattered areas of interspersed normal-appearing lung parenchyma.* ***(Right)*** *Coronal T2WI MR through the fetal thorax shows a high signal intensity lesion ➙ in the left upper lobe, consistent with a large cyst CPAM with thin internal septa. There is no evidence of mass effect, pleural effusion, or fetal hydrops.*

CONGENITAL PULMONARY AIRWAY MALFORMATION

TERMINOLOGY

Definitions

- Congenital pulmonary airway malformation (CPAM)
  - Spectrum of lesions affecting various portions of tracheobronchial tree & distal airways
- Abnormal mass of pulmonary tissue with varying degrees of cystic change
- Communicates with tracheobronchial tree; normal blood supply & venous drainage

IMAGING

General Features

- Best diagnostic clue
  - Multilocular cystic pulmonary lesion in fetus, neonate, or infant
    - Rarely diagnosed beyond infancy since chronic inflammation may preclude confident histologic diagnosis
- Location
  - Usually affects single lung lobe
- Size
  - Variable: Large lesions associated with pulmonary hypoplasia, fetal hydrops, & fetal demise
- Morphology
  - Cystic CPAM is most common; multilocular cysts with thick or thin walls

Radiographic Findings

- Unilateral hyperlucent lung lesion
  - Thin-walled cysts may not be visible
  - May produce mass effect, atelectasis
- Multiple thin- or thick-walled cysts
  - Air-filled, fluid-filled, or air-fluid levels
- Single dominant cyst surrounded by smaller cysts
- Heterogeneous airspace disease with intrinsic small cysts
- Homogeneous opacity: Cystic CPAM with retained fetal fluid, microcystic CPAM

CT Findings

- Multilocular cystic lesion within pulmonary lobe
- Thin or thick cyst walls
- Variable cyst size
  - Dominant cyst surrounded by small cysts
  - Uniform cyst size in small cyst CPAM
    - Interspersed normal lung
- Cysts may contain air, fluid, &/or air-fluid levels
  - May be initially fluid-filled; retained fetal fluid
- Solid lesion within pulmonary lobe
  - May replace lobe or lung & produce mass effect

Ultrasonographic Findings

- Prenatal ultrasound
  - Cystic mass in fetal thorax
  - Solid mass in fetal thorax
  - Assessment of mediastinal shift, polyhydramnios, fetal hydrops

MR Findings

- Prenatal diagnosis of fetal anomalies
  - Evaluation of lesion & adjacent structures
  - Evaluation of associated abnormalities

DIFFERENTIAL DIAGNOSIS

Congenital Lobar Overinflation

- Increasing size of pulmonary lobe after birth
- Hyperlucent enlarged lobe without cystic change

Pulmonary Sequestration

- Intralobar sequestration
  - Multilocular cysts surrounded by consolidated or normal lung
  - Systemic blood supply; pulmonary venous drainage
- Extralobar sequestration
  - Solid mass; small fluid-filled cysts may represent intrinsic focal small cyst CPAM
  - Systemic blood supply; systemic venous drainage

Bronchogenic Cyst

- Congenital mediastinal lesion; rarely intrapulmonary
- Unilocular air- or fluid-filled cyst in central lung

PATHOLOGY

General Features

- Approximately 25% of congenital lung lesions
- Epidemiology: Typically diagnosed in perinatal period

Staging, Grading, & Classification

- Radiologic classification
  - Large cyst CPAM
    - Most common lesion
  - Small cyst CPAM
  - Microcystic CPAM (solid appearing)

Microscopic Features

- Classification of CPAM: Types 0 through 4
  - Based on major lesion components reflecting area or stage of development of tracheobronchial tree

CLINICAL ISSUES

Presentation

- Most common signs/symptoms
  - Acute progressive neonatal respiratory distress
  - Incidental diagnosis on prenatal ultrasound

Demographics

- Age: Neonates, mature & premature

Natural History & Prognosis

- Good prognosis for large cyst CPAM

Treatment

- Surgical excision

DIAGNOSTIC CHECKLIST

Consider

- CPAM in patients with cystic lung lesions found in perinatal period

SELECTED REFERENCES

1. Biyyam DR et al: Congenital lung abnormalities: embryologic features, prenatal diagnosis, and postnatal radiologic-pathologic correlation. Radiographics. 30(6):1721-38, 2010

EXTRALOBAR SEQUESTRATION

Key Facts

Terminology

- Extralobar sequestration (ELS)
- Sequestered lung
  - No communication with tracheobronchial tree
  - Systemic blood supply
  - Thoracic ELS invested by pleura

Imaging

- Radiography
  - Basilar homogeneous mass, well-defined borders
  - Adjacent to posterior medial hemidiaphragm
  - Large lesions may produce opaque hemithorax
- CT
  - Homogeneous or heterogeneous soft tissue mass
  - May exhibit cystic changes from intrinsic pulmonary airway malformation
  - Visualization of systemic vascular supply

Top Differential Diagnoses

- Congenital pulmonary airway malformation
- Neuroblastoma

Pathology

- Well-defined supernumerary lung tissue with systemic blood supply
- Associated congenital anomalies (65%)

Clinical Issues

- Neonates, infants; M:F = 4:1
- Symptoms/signs: Respiratory distress, feeding difficulties
- Surgical excision

Diagnostic Checklist

- Consider ELS in neonates with intrathoracic soft tissue mass & evaluate for systemic blood supply

*(**Left**) AP chest radiograph of a newborn with a left basilar cystic lesion diagnosed on prenatal ultrasound shows a homogeneous spherical lobular mass ➔ in the left inferior hemithorax. (**Right**) Composite image with axial (top) and coronal (bottom) T2WI MR of the same patient shows a multilocular cystic lesion with thin low signal intensity tissue septa. Although a systemic feeding vessel was not identified, ELS with intrinsic pulmonary airway malformation type 2 was diagnosed at surgery.*

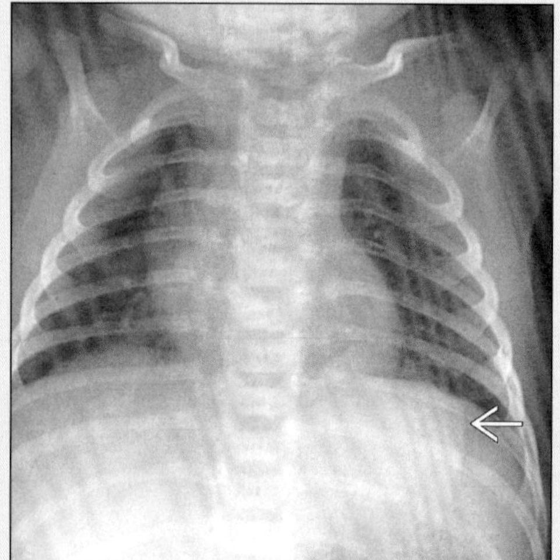

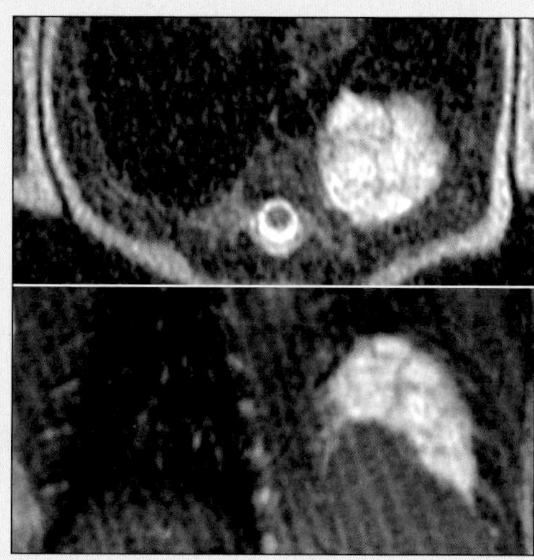

*(**Left**) Coronal CECT of an infant with ELS shows a well-defined triangular mass in the left inferior hemithorax supplied by an anomalous vessel ➔ arising from the descending aorta. (Courtesy D. Frush, MD.) (**Right**) Graphic illustrates the morphologic features of extralobar sequestration characterized by supernumerary lung tissue invested in pleura and located in the left inferior hemithorax. There is no communication with the tracheobronchial tree and the lesion is supplied by the systemic circulation.*

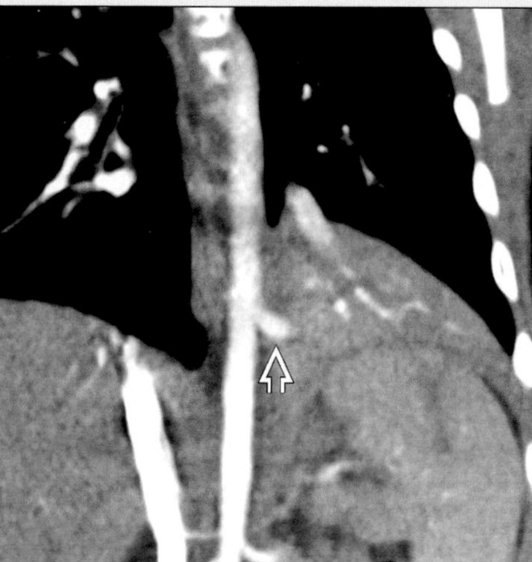

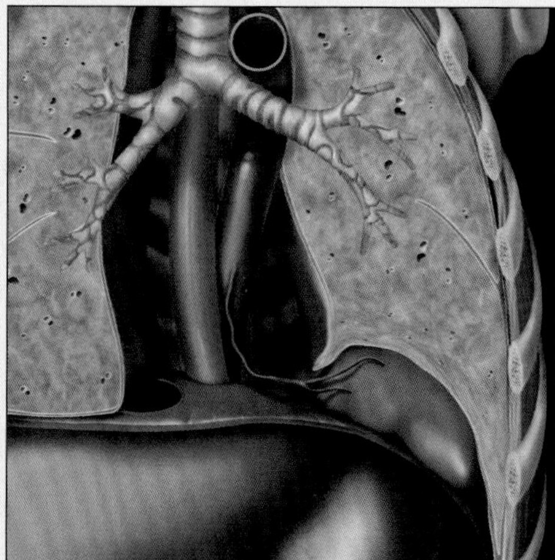

EXTRALOBAR SEQUESTRATION

TERMINOLOGY

Abbreviations

- **Extralobar sequestration (ELS)**

Definitions

- Sequestered lung
  - No normal communication to tracheobronchial tree
  - Systemic blood supply
- Extralobar sequestration
  - Supernumerary lung tissue covered by pleura, separate from adjacent lung

IMAGING

General Features

- Best diagnostic clue
  - Left lower thoracic soft tissue mass with systemic blood supply in neonate
- Location
  - Basilar thorax adjacent to hemidiaphragm
- Size
  - Wide range: May occupy entire hemithorax
- Morphology
  - Ovoid, spherical, or pyramidal

Radiographic Findings

- Basilar triangular opacity, well-defined borders
- Adjacent to posterior medial hemidiaphragm
- Large lesions may produce opaque hemithorax

CT Findings

- CECT
  - Homogeneous or heterogeneous soft tissue mass with well-defined borders
    - May exhibit fluid-filled cysts with associated pulmonary airway malformation
  - Visualization of systemic vascular supply
    - Single or multiple feeding vessels

MR Findings

- Homogeneous or heterogeneous lesion
- Visualization of cystic spaces
- Identification of systemic blood supply

Angiographic Findings

- Rarely performed
- Identification of arterial blood supply
  - Thoracic or abdominal aorta (80%)
  - Other (15%): Splenic, gastric, subclavian, intercostals
  - Multiple arteries (20%)

Prenatal Ultrasound

- Homogeneous, echogenic mass with well-defined borders
  - Mass effect on mediastinum in large lesions
- Identification of intralesional cysts
- Identification of systemic blood supply

Imaging Recommendations

- Best imaging tool
  - Prenatal ultrasound for early diagnosis
  - Multidetector CT angiography for surgical planning & identification of vascular supply

DIFFERENTIAL DIAGNOSIS

Congenital Pulmonary Airway Malformation (CPAM)

- Congenital lung lesion of neonates & infants
- Microcystic CPAM (solid-appearing) may mimic ELS
  - Normal blood supply & venous drainage

Neuroblastoma

- Malignant neoplasm of sympathetic ganglia
- May be congenital
- Elongate paravertebral soft tissue mass

PATHOLOGY

General Features

- Associated abnormalities
  - Associated congenital anomalies (65%)
    - Bronchogenic cyst
    - Congenital diaphragmatic hernia

Gross Pathologic & Surgical Features

- Ovoid, spherical, or pyramidal soft tissue mass
- Pleural investment in thoracic lesions
- Characteristic systemic blood supply & systemic venous drainage
- May exhibit internal cystic changes

Microscopic Features

- Resembles normal lung with bronchial, bronchiolar, & alveolar dilatation
- Intrinsic pulmonary airway malformation type 2 in 50%

CLINICAL ISSUES

Presentation

- Most common signs/symptoms
  - Respiratory distress, feeding difficulties

Demographics

- Age
  - Neonates, infants
- Gender
  - M:F = 4:1

Natural History & Prognosis

- Excellent prognosis after excision in absence of congenital anomalies or pulmonary hypoplasia

Treatment

- Surgical excision

DIAGNOSTIC CHECKLIST

Consider

- ELS in neonates with intrathoracic soft tissue mass & evaluate for systemic blood supply

SELECTED REFERENCES

1. Biyyam DR et al: Congenital lung abnormalities: embryologic features, prenatal diagnosis, and postnatal radiologic-pathologic correlation. Radiographics. 30(6):1721-38, 2010

INTRALOBAR SEQUESTRATION

Key Facts

Terminology
- Intralobar sequestration (ILS)
- Sequestration: No normal communication with tracheobronchial tree, systemic blood supply
- ILS: Shares visceral pleura of affected lobe

Imaging
- Radiography
  - Lower lobe lung mass or consolidation
  - Well-defined, lobular, irregular, or ill-defined margins
  - Homogeneous or heterogeneous
- CT
  - Lesion identification & characterization
  - Basilar consolidation or mass
  - Solid &/or cystic components
  - May contain fluid, air, air-fluid levels
- Identification of systemic blood supply

Top Differential Diagnoses
- Pneumonia
- Lung abscess
- Lung cancer
- Extralobar sequestration

Pathology
- Systemic arterial supply, pulmonary venous drainage
- Chronic inflammation, cysts, & extensive fibrosis

Clinical Issues
- Signs & symptoms of pulmonary infection
  - Fever, productive cough, chest pain
- Treatment: Lobectomy

Diagnostic Checklist
- Consider ILS in patient with persistent lower lobe abnormality & history of recurrent infection

*(**Left**) PA chest radiograph of a 42-year-old woman with ILS who presented with recurrent pulmonary infection shows a left lower lobe retrocardiac opacity ➡ with irregular borders. The lesion did not resolve with antibiotic treatment. (**Right**) Axial CECT of the same patient shows a triangular left lower lobe soft tissue mass ➡ with surrounding architectural distortion. The lesion exhibited heterogeneous attenuation at this level on soft tissue window images (not shown).*

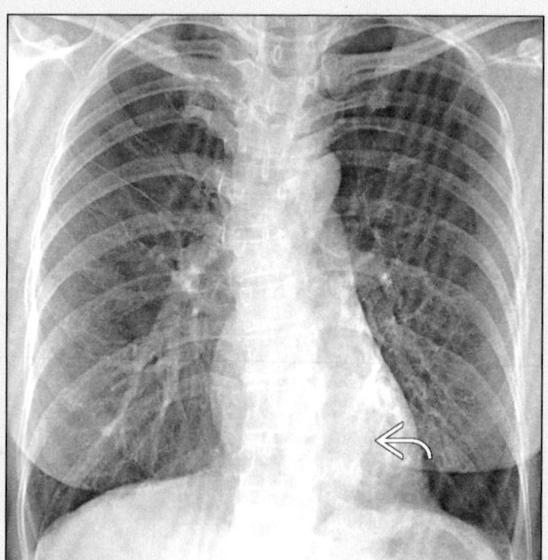

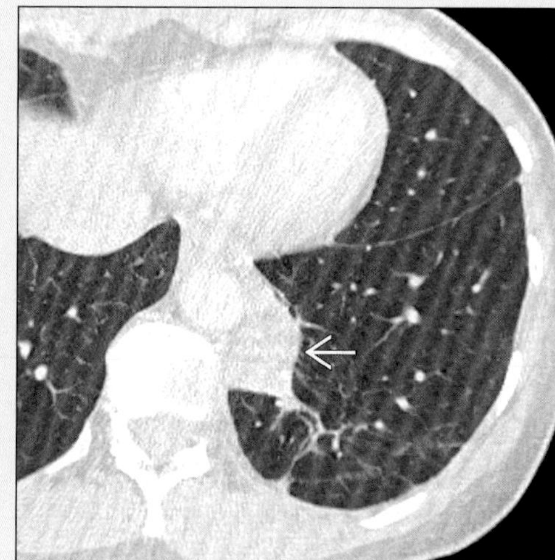

*(**Left**) Axial CECT of the same patient shows the systemic aortic branch ➡ that supplied the ILS. Such vessels characteristically course within the pulmonary ligament. (**Right**) Graphic shows the morphologic features of intralobar sequestration. ILS is typically a heterogeneous lower lobe lesion with irregular borders that often contains solid and cystic components. The latter may contain air, fluid, &/or air-fluid levels. An anomalous systemic aortic branch ➡ courses in the pulmonary ligament to supply the lesion.*

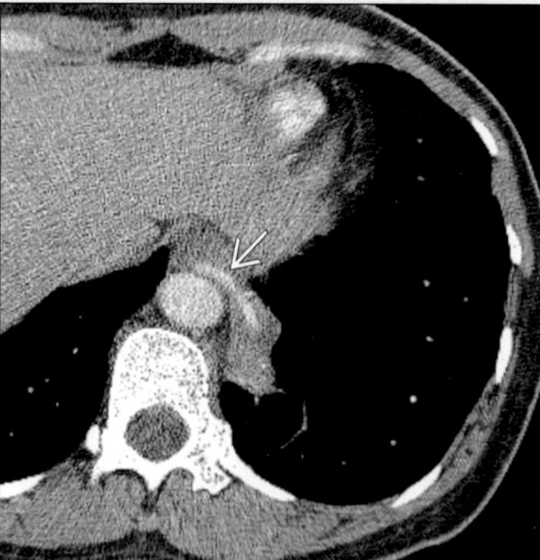

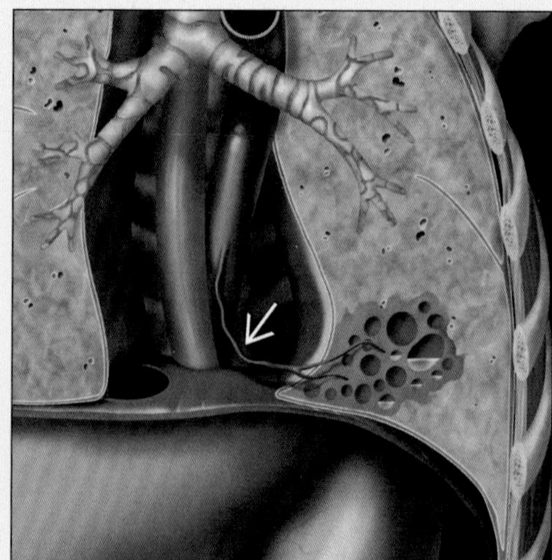

TERMINOLOGY

Abbreviations

- **Intralobar sequestration (ILS)**

Definitions

- From Latin "sequestrare" (to be separated)
- Intralobar sequestration (~ 75%)
  - Shares visceral pleura of affected lobe
- Pulmonary sequestration
  - No normal communication with tracheobronchial tree
  - Systemic blood supply
- Extralobar sequestration (~ 25%)
  - Supernumerary lung tissue
  - Separate pleural investment
- Bronchopulmonary foregut malformation
  - Pulmonary sequestration (ELS or ILS) with foregut communication (esophagus, stomach) (rare)

IMAGING

General Features

- Best diagnostic clue
  - Chronic basilar mass, consolidation, or cystic lesion in patient with recurrent infection
- Location
  - Lower lobes, slightly more common on left (55-64%)
    - Posterior basal segments > medial basal segments
- Size
  - Variable
- Morphology
  - Irregular borders
  - Often heterogeneous with solid &/or cystic components

Radiographic Findings

- **Lower lobe lung mass or consolidation**
- Well-defined, lobular, irregular, or ill-defined margins
- Homogeneous lesion
  - May mimic mass or consolidation
- Heterogeneous lesion
  - May exhibit cystic spaces with air/air-fluid levels
  - Predominantly cystic lesions may occur
- Large lesions may produce mass effect on adjacent lung & mediastinum

CT Findings

- Lesion identification & characterization
- **Basilar consolidation or mass**
- Irregular borders with adjacent nonsequestered lung
  - May exhibit well-defined lobular borders
  - May mimic neoplasm
- Surrounding lung may appear hyperlucent or emphysematous
  - May mimic air-trapping
- CECT
  - Heterogeneous attenuation accentuated by contrast enhancement of solid areas
    - Intrinsic air, fluid, & soft tissue components
    - Single or multiple intralesional cystic changes
      - May contain air, fluid, &/or air-fluid levels
    - Solid lesions may mimic consolidation
      - May exhibit intralesional branching vessels
  - Identification of systemic blood supply
    - ~ 80% of cases on CECT or CT angiography
    - Systemic artery arising from distal thoracic or upper abdominal aorta
      - Anomalous artery typically 6-7 mm in diameter
    - Multiple systemic arteries in up to 20% of cases
    - Feeding artery often courses within pulmonary ligament
    - Nonvisualization of systemic artery does not exclude diagnosis

MR Findings

- MR not routinely performed
- Lesion characterization
  - Variable signal intensity of cystic components
    - Typically high signal intensity on T2WI
- MRA
  - Identification of systemic feeding vessel(s)

Angiographic Findings

- Angiography rarely performed
- Identification of feeding vessel(s)
  - Thoracic aorta (75%)
  - Abdominal aorta (20%)
  - Intercostal artery (5%)
  - Multiple arteries (16%)
- May allow identification of venous drainage
  - 95% have pulmonary venous drainage
  - 5% systemic venous drainage, usually via azygos, hemiazygos, superior vena cava, or intercostal routes

Imaging Recommendations

- Best imaging tool
  - CTA is imaging modality of choice for characterization of ILS & identification of systemic blood supply
- Protocol advice
  - Multiplanar reformatted images & maximum-intensity projection (MIP) images for optimal identification & characterization of vascular supply & venous drainage

DIFFERENTIAL DIAGNOSIS

Pneumonia

- Consolidation, mass-like consolidation
- No systemic blood supply
- Complete resolution with antibiotics

Lung Abscess

- Mass/mass-like consolidation
- Intrinsic cavitation
- No systemic blood supply
- Slow response to antibiotic treatment
- May rarely require external drainage

Lung Cancer

- Preferential upper lobe involvement
- Mass/mass-like consolidation
- May exhibit cavitation
- Locally invasive
- No systemic blood supply

Postobstructive Pneumonia

- Endoluminal tumor/obstructing lesion
  - Volume loss
  - Peripheral consolidation

INTRALOBAR SEQUESTRATION

- No systemic blood supply

Extralobar Sequestration

- Supernumerary lung tissue
- Well-defined pyramidal basilar soft tissue mass
  - May exhibit intrinsic fluid-filled cysts
- 90% in left inferior hemithorax
  - Other locations: Within diaphragm, abdomen, mediastinum
- Systemic arterial supply
- Systemic venous drainage

PATHOLOGY

General Features

- Etiology
  - Controversy regarding etiology
  - Postulated acquired etiology
    - Most lesions originally described in adults
    - Rare association with other congenital anomalies
    - Normal pulmonary venous drainage
    - Postulated chronic lower lobe pneumonia with loss of pulmonary artery supply/airway communication & acquisition of systemic blood supply from parasitized pulmonary ligament arteries
  - Postulated congenital etiology
    - Increasing reports of ILS in neonates & infants with increased utilization of prenatal ultrasound
    - Reports of coexistent ILS & ELS in same infant

Gross Pathologic & Surgical Features

- 98% of cases in lower lobes
  - Left slightly more common than right
- Intralobar location
  - No normal communication with tracheobronchial tree
- Thick, fibrous visceral pleura over lesion
- Cut section
  - Solid &/or cystic components
    - Dense fibrotic consolidated lung
    - Cysts contain blood, pus, or gelatinous material
    - Cystic spaces resemble ectatic bronchi
- ILS surrounded by nonsequestered lung
- Systemic arterial supply
- Pulmonary venous drainage

Microscopic Features

- Chronic inflammation, vascular sclerosis, cystic changes, & extensive fibrosis
- Atherosclerosis of anomalous feeding arteries

CLINICAL ISSUES

Presentation

- Most common signs/symptoms
  - Signs & symptoms of pulmonary infection
  - Fever
  - Productive cough
  - Chest pain, may be pleuritic
- Other signs/symptoms
  - Hemoptysis
  - 15-20% asymptomatic: Incidental imaging abnormality

Demographics

- Age
  - Any age
    - Infancy
    - Late childhood
    - Young adulthood
    - Adulthood
  - 50% > 20 years of age
- Gender
  - M = F

Natural History & Prognosis

- Excellent prognosis following surgical excision

Treatment

- Lobectomy
  - Symptomatic lesions, recurrent infection
  - Preoperative imaging for identification of systemic feeding vessels

DIAGNOSTIC CHECKLIST

Consider

- ILS in patient with recurrent or persistent lower lobe pulmonary abnormality & history of recurrent infection

SELECTED REFERENCES

1. Wei Y et al: Pulmonary sequestration: a retrospective analysis of 2625 cases in China. Eur J Cardiothorac Surg. 40(1):e39-42, 2011
2. Biyyam DR et al: Congenital lung abnormalities: embryologic features, prenatal diagnosis, and postnatal radiologic-pathologic correlation. Radiographics. 30(6):1721-38, 2010
3. Lee EY et al: Multidetector CT evaluation of congenital lung anomalies. Radiology. 247(3):632-48, 2008
4. Newman B: Congenital bronchopulmonary foregut malformations: concepts and controversies. Pediatr Radiol. 36(8):773-91, 2006
5. Corbett HJ et al: Pulmonary sequestration. Paediatr Respir Rev. 5(1):59-68, 2004
6. Zylak CJ et al: Developmental lung anomalies in the adult: radiologic-pathologic correlation. Radiographics. 22 Spec No:S25-43, 2002
7. Bratu I et al: The multiple facets of pulmonary sequestration. J Pediatr Surg. 36(5):784-90, 2001
8. Do KH et al: Systemic arterial supply to the lungs in adults: spiral CT findings. Radiographics. 21(2):387-402, 2001
9. Saygi A: Intralobar pulmonary sequestration. Chest. 119(3):990-2, 2001
10. Frazier AA et al: Intralobar sequestration: radiologic-pathologic correlation. Radiographics. 17(3):725-45, 1997

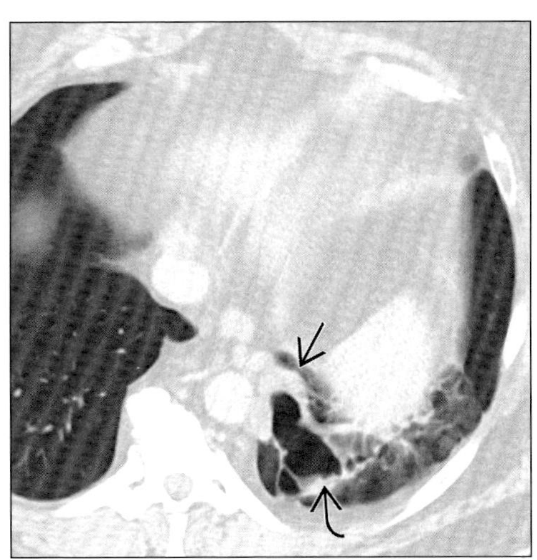

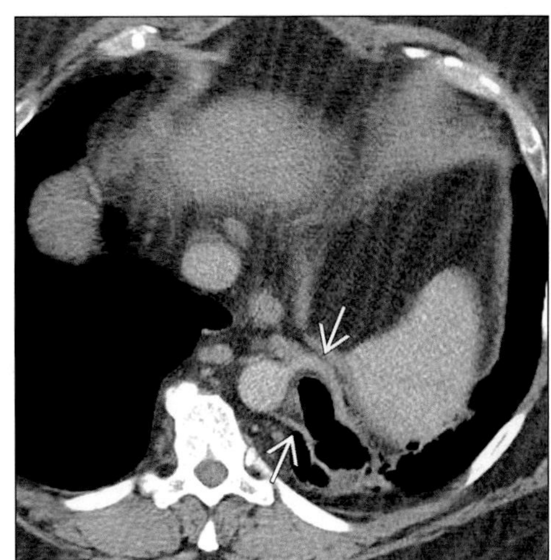

(Left) *Axial CECT (lung window) of a 67-year-old man with a chronic radiographic abnormality shows a left lower lobe heterogeneous lesion with a dominant cystic component ⇾ and surrounding bronchiectasis and ground-glass opacity. A tubular structure ⇾ courses into the lesion.* ***(Right)*** *Axial CECT (soft tissue window) of the same patient shows 2 arteries ➡ that arise from the distal descending thoracic aorta to supply the lesion. Up to 20% of ILS have more than 1 feeding artery.*

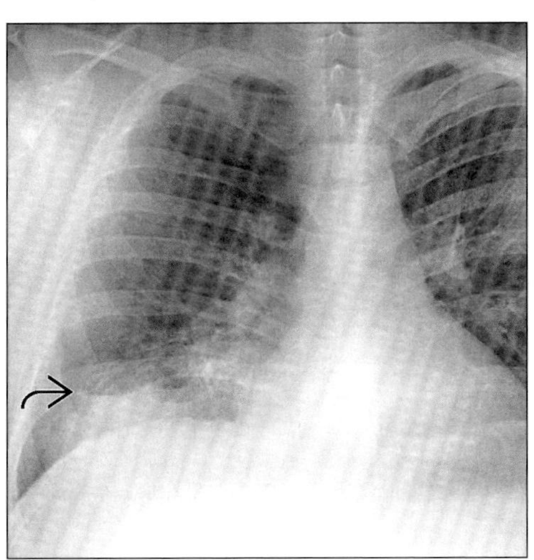

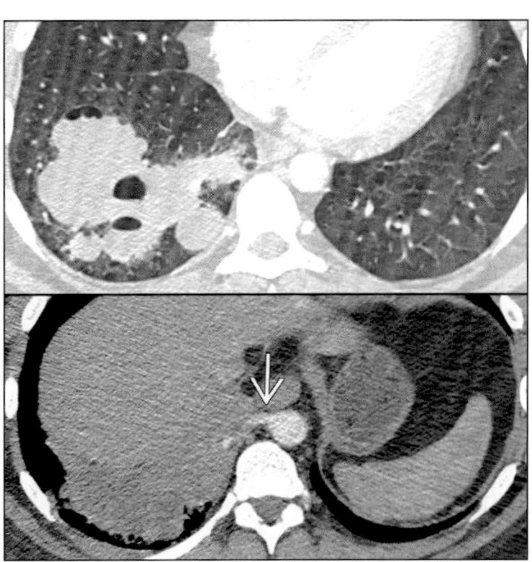

(Left) *PA chest radiograph of a patient with recurrent pulmonary infection demonstrates a complex right lower lobe mass-like consolidation with cystic/cavitary components and intrinsic air-fluid levels ⇾.* ***(Right)*** *Composite image with axial NECT in lung (top) and soft tissue (bottom) window demonstrates a polylobular right lower lobe lesion with intrinsic fluid, soft tissue, and air-fluid levels. The lesion is supplied by an anomalous systemic artery ➡ arising from the descending aorta.*

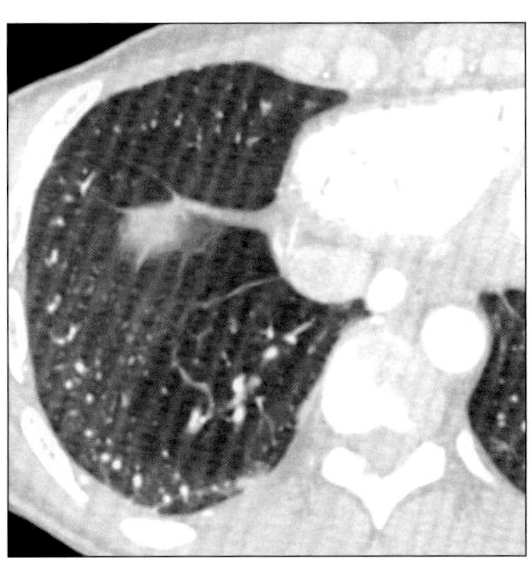

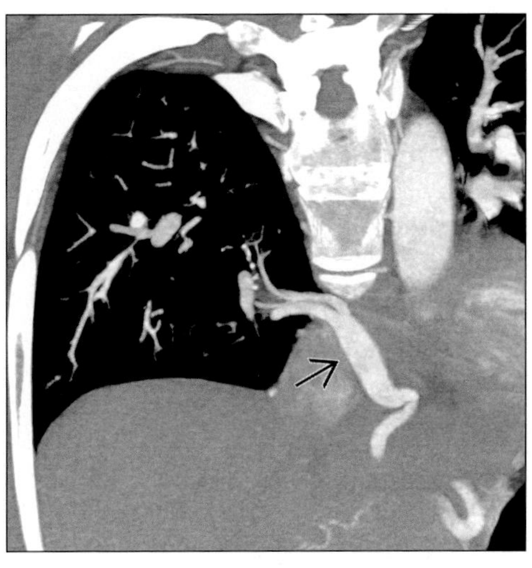

(Left) *Axial NECT of a 28-year-old woman with ILS shows a hyperlucent right lower lobe posterior basal segment with intrinsic dilated vascular structures. A large anomalous vessel was identified in the adjacent mediastinum.* ***(Right)*** *Coronal oblique CECT of the same patient shows the large systemic artery ⇾ that supplied the ILS and originated from the celiac axis. Intralobar sequestration may exhibit soft tissue attenuation, cystic changes, &/or hyperlucent lung.*

DIFFUSE PULMONARY LYMPHANGIOMATOSIS

Key Facts

Terminology

- Diffuse pulmonary lymphangiomatosis (DPL)
- Congenital disorder: Increased number & complexity of lymphatic channels
- Involves lymphatics in interlobular septa, pleura, & peribronchovascular regions

Imaging

- Radiography
  - Diffuse bilateral reticular opacities
  - Unilateral or bilateral pleural effusion
  - Cardiomegaly from pericardial effusion
- CT
  - Smooth interlobular septal thickening
  - Patchy ground-glass opacities
  - Pleural effusion; pleural thickening
  - Mediastinal soft tissue infiltration
  - Pericardial effusion

Top Differential Diagnoses

- Pulmonary lymphangiectasis
- Pulmonary edema
- Lymphangitic carcinomatosis
- Erdheim-Chester disease

Clinical Issues

- Symptoms/signs
  - Dyspnea, wheezing
  - Pleural effusion, chylothorax
- Children & young adults
- Progressive, often fatal disease

Diagnostic Checklist

- Consider DPL in children or adults with unexplained diffuse interlobular septal thickening & chylous pleural effusions

*(**Left**) Axial CECT of a patient with diffuse pulmonary lymphangiomatosis shows typical CT features including smooth thickening of interlobular septa ➡ and centrilobular nodules ⇨. The latter likely result from thickened peribronchovascular lymphatics. (**Right**) Axial CECT of the same patient shows soft tissue infiltration ➡ of the mediastinum due to proliferation of abnormal lymphatic tissue. Mediastinal soft tissue infiltration is a common finding in diffuse pulmonary lymphangiomatosis.*

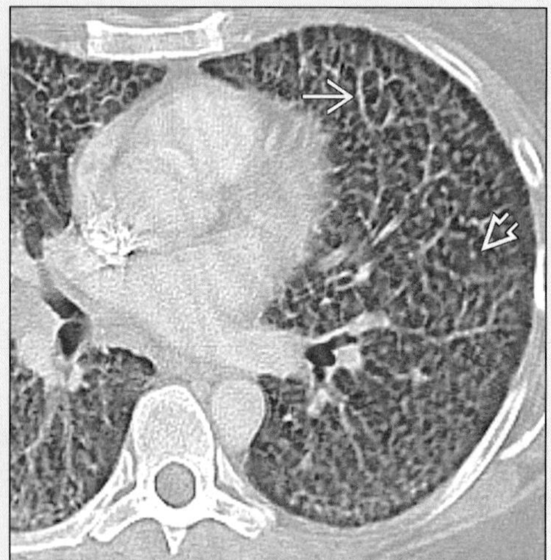

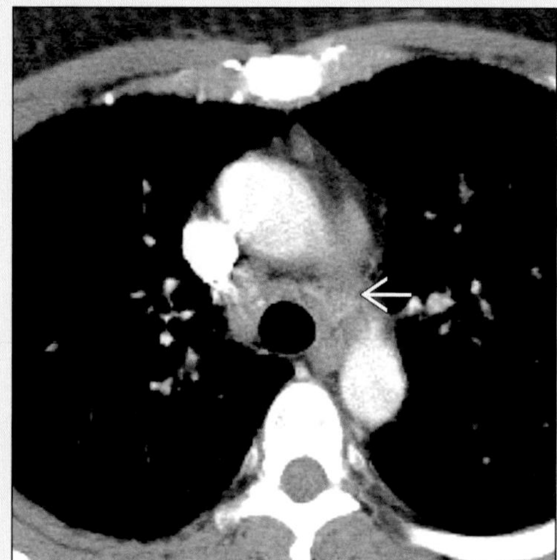

*(**Left**) Axial CECT of a patient with dyspnea shows diffuse bilateral smooth interlobular septal thickening ⇨ due to diffuse pulmonary lymphangiomatosis. Scattered ground-glass opacities ➡ are present, which are typically related to edema or hemorrhage. (**Right**) Coronal CECT of the same patient shows diffuse, bilateral, smooth, interlobular septal thickening ⇨. Thickening of the peribronchovascular interstitium ➡ is likely related to proliferation of lymphatic tissue.*

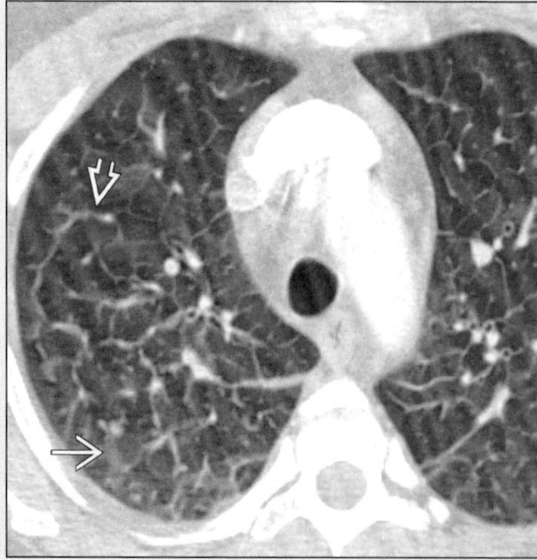

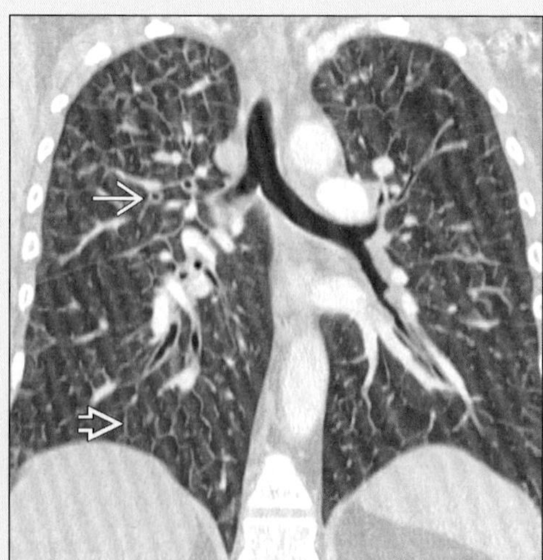

DIFFUSE PULMONARY LYMPHANGIOMATOSIS

TERMINOLOGY

Abbreviations

- **Diffuse pulmonary lymphangiomatosis (DPL)**

Synonyms

- **Diffuse pulmonary angiomatosis**; uncertain nature of vascular abnormalities

Definitions

- Congenital disorder: Increased number & complexity of anastomosing lymphatic channels
- Involves lymphatics in interlobular septa, pleura, & peribronchovascular regions

IMAGING

General Features

- Best diagnostic clue
  - Diffuse thickening of interlobular septa & bronchovascular structures with infiltration of mediastinal fat

Radiographic Findings

- Diffuse bilateral reticular opacities
- Unilateral or bilateral pleural effusion; chylothorax
- Cardiomegaly from pericardial effusion

CT Findings

- Smooth interlobular septal thickening
- Thickening of peribronchovascular interstitium
- Patchy ground-glass opacities
- Pleural effusion; pleural thickening
- Mediastinal soft tissue infiltration
- Pericardial effusion

Imaging Recommendations

- Best imaging tool
  - CT & HRCT optimally demonstrate peribronchovascular/septal thickening & mediastinal fat infiltration

DIFFERENTIAL DIAGNOSIS

Pulmonary Lymphangiectasis

- Dilated pulmonary lymphatics, no increase in number
- Neonates with respiratory distress
- Interlobular septal thickening, chylous pleural effusion

Pulmonary Edema

- Cardiogenic & noncardiogenic
- Smooth septal & peribronchovascular thickening
- Patchy ground-glass opacities, pleural effusion

Lymphangitic Carcinomatosis

- Advanced malignancy; typically adenocarcinoma
- Smooth or nodular asymmetric septal thickening
- Pleural effusion, lymphadenopathy

Erdheim-Chester Disease

- Perilymphatic cellular infiltration
- Smooth interlobular septal & pleural thickening
- Symmetric osteosclerosis

PATHOLOGY

General Features

- Etiology
  - Unknown
- Associated abnormalities
  - Chylothorax
  - Chylopericardium
  - Chylous ascites
  - Reports of protein-wasting enteropathy & lymphopenia

Gross Pathologic & Surgical Features

- Thick interlobular septa, peribronchovascular interstitium, & pleura

Microscopic Features

- Increased diameter, number, & complexity of lymphatic channels in pulmonary interstitium
- Reports of involvement of other organs (any tissue in which lymphatics are normally found)

CLINICAL ISSUES

Presentation

- Most common signs/symptoms
  - Dyspnea, wheezing, hemoptysis, chyloptysis, bronchial casts
- Other signs/symptoms
  - Restrictive & obstructive pulmonary function abnormalities
  - Pleural effusion, chylothorax

Demographics

- Age
  - Children & young adults
- Gender
  - No gender predilection

Natural History & Prognosis

- Progressive, often fatal disease

Treatment

- Dietary treatment
- Surgical treatment of pleural effusions
- Thoracic duct ligation
- Radiation therapy with variable success

DIAGNOSTIC CHECKLIST

Consider

- DPL in children or adults with unexplained diffuse interlobular septal thickening & chylous pleural effusions

SELECTED REFERENCES

1. Raman SP et al: Imaging of thoracic lymphatic diseases. AJR Am J Roentgenol. 193(6):1504-13, 2009
2. El Hajj L et al: Diagnostic value of bronchoscopy, CT and transbronchial biopsies in diffuse pulmonary lymphangiomatosis: case report and review of the literature. Clin Radiol. 60(8):921-5, 2005

APICAL LUNG HERNIA

Key Facts

Terminology

- Protrusion of lung apex into neck through defect in Sibson fascia, which covers lung apex

Imaging

- Radiography
  - Apical lucency extending into base of neck
  - Lateral deviation of trachea
- CT
  - Continuity of apical lucency with rest of lung
  - Lung constriction at hernia aperture
  - Obtain images at maximal inspiration to improve detection

Top Differential Diagnoses

- Paratracheal air cyst
- Esophageal diverticula
- Laryngocele

Pathology

- Weakening or tearing of Sibson fascia anteromedially, between anterior scalene & sternocleidomastoid muscles
- Etiology
  - Usually congenital in infants & children
  - Usually acquired in adults

Clinical Issues

- Signs/symptoms
  - Soft, bulging mass in supraclavicular region
  - Cough
- Male > female
- Treatment
  - None required
  - Usually reduces easily
  - Surgery if incarcerated, symptomatic, or for cosmetic reasons

(Left) Graphic shows the anatomy of apical lung hernia. The herniation of the lung apex ➩ occurs through a defect in Sibson fascia ➡, allowing extension of the lung apex into the neck. *(Right)* Axial CECT shows extension of the right lung apex into the lower neck, consistent with a small right apical lung hernia ➙.

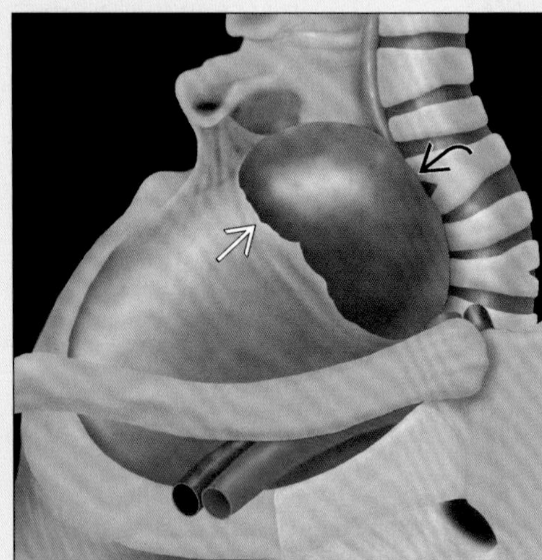

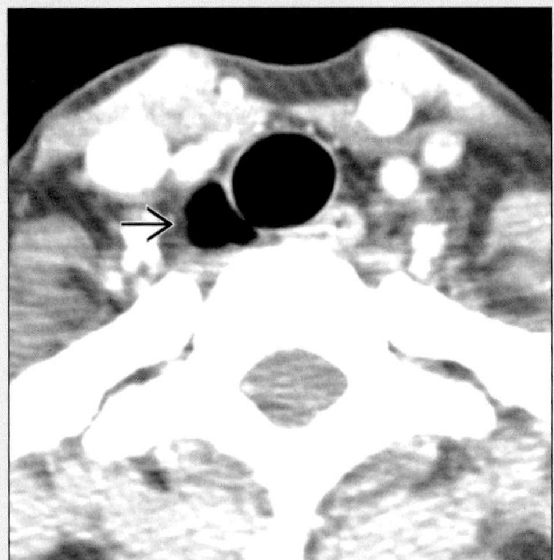

(Left) PA chest radiograph shows air lucency in the right neck with mild deviation of the trachea to the left, consistent with an apical lung hernia ➡. *(Right)* PA chest radiograph magnification view shows a right apical lung hernia extending into the right neck ➙.

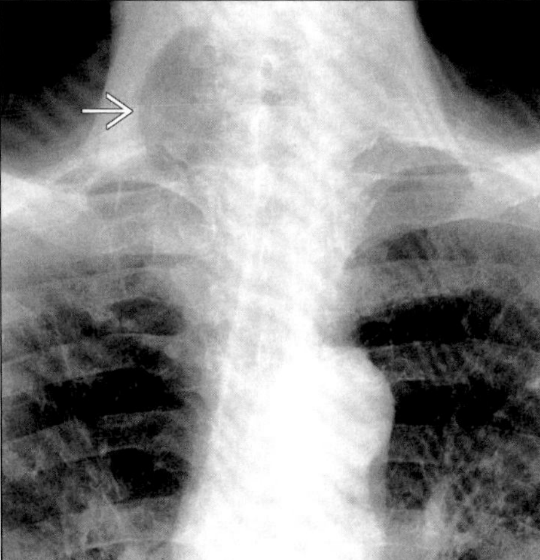

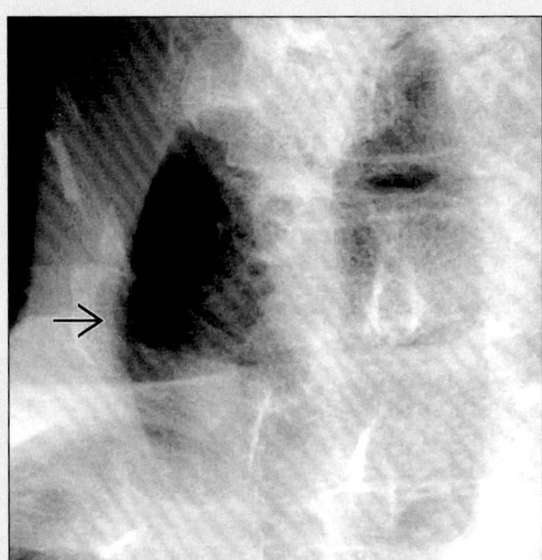

APICAL LUNG HERNIA

TERMINOLOGY

Synonyms

- Cervical lung hernia

Definitions

- Protrusion of lung apex into neck through defect in Sibson fascia, which covers lung apex

IMAGING

General Features

- Location
  - Typically unilateral, but can be bilateral
  - Right > left
- Size
  - Can enlarge to 10 cm

Imaging Recommendations

- Best imaging tool
  - Fluoroscopy
    - Reducibility of hernia can be assessed dynamically
    - Hernia worsens with Valsalva maneuver, cough, maximum inspiration
- Protocol advice
  - Coronal & sagittal CT reformations improve delineation of anatomy of apical hernia

Radiographic Findings

- Apical lucency extending into base of neck
- Lateral deviation of trachea
- Best seen with maximal inspiration or Valsalva

CT Findings

- Shows continuity of apical lucency with rest of lung
- Constriction of lung at hernia aperture
- Deviation of trachea
- False-negative CT can occur given intermittent nature of some apical hernias
  - Obtain images at maximal inspiration to improve detection

DIFFERENTIAL DIAGNOSIS

Paratracheal Air Cyst

- Mucosal herniation through tracheal wall

Esophageal Diverticula

- Do not usually cause lateral tracheal deviation
- Unlike apical hernia, may have air-fluid level
- Contrast esophagram helpful

Lateral Pharyngeal Diverticulum

- Mucosal herniation through thyrohyoid membrane

Laryngocele

- Dilated appendix of laryngeal ventricle

PATHOLOGY

General Features

- Etiology
  - Usually congenital in infants & children
    - 60% of congenital lung hernias are apical
    - Associated with hernia in other locations (umbilical, inguinal)
  - Usually acquired in adults
    - Penetrating trauma
    - Surgery
    - Chest wall neoplasm, infection
    - Increased intrathoracic pressure
      - Wind instrumentalists
      - Emphysema, chronic cough
      - Weight lifters
      - Repeated, prolonged Valsalva maneuver

Gross Pathologic & Surgical Features

- Weakening or tearing of Sibson fascia, which covers lung apex
  - Usually anteromedially, between anterior scalene & sternocleidomastoid muscles
  - Defect usually large, so hernia easily reducible

CLINICAL ISSUES

Presentation

- Most common signs/symptoms
  - Asymptomatic
- Other signs/symptoms
  - Soft, bulging mass in supraclavicular region
  - Cough
  - Dyspnea
  - Dysphagia
  - Hoarseness

Demographics

- Age
  - Patients may present in childhood or adulthood
- Gender
  - Male > female
- Epidemiology
  - Very rare condition
  - Apical lung hernia accounts for ~ 33% of lung hernias
    - ~ 65% lung hernias are "thoracic"; around lateral margin of thorax, through ribs
    - Diaphragmatic lung hernia rarest

Natural History & Prognosis

- Congenital apical hernias tend to resolve spontaneously
- Incarceration rare
- ↑ risk of pneumothorax with placement of central venous catheter or tracheostomy

Treatment

- None required; usually reduces easily
- Surgery may be appropriate for incarcerated or symptomatic hernias or for cosmetic reasons

SELECTED REFERENCES

1. McAdams HP et al: Apical lung hernia: radiologic findings in six cases. AJR Am J Roentgenol. 167(4):927-30, 1996
2. Moncada R et al: Congenital and acquired lung hernias. J Thorac Imaging. 11(1):75-82, 1996
3. Bhalla M et al: Lung hernia: radiographic features. AJR Am J Roentgenol. 154(1):51-3, 1990

PROXIMAL INTERRUPTION OF THE PULMONARY ARTERY

Key Facts

Terminology

- Proximal interruption of pulmonary artery (PIPA)
- Failed development of proximal pulmonary artery

Imaging

- Radiography
  - Small ipsilateral lung & hilum
  - Aortic arch contralateral to interrupted pulmonary artery
- CT
  - Absence of pulmonary artery
  - Visualization of ipsilateral collateral systemic & bronchial arteries
  - Contralateral aortic arch
  - Normal bronchial branching pattern
  - Bronchiectasis from recurrent infections
  - Mosaic attenuation from variable perfusion

Top Differential Diagnoses

- Swyer-James-McLeod syndrome
- Mediastinal fibrosis
- Scimitar syndrome

Pathology

- Left PIPA: Higher incidence of congenital cardiovascular anomalies

Clinical Issues

- Symptoms/signs
  - May be asymptomatic
  - Recurrent pulmonary infection, dyspnea, hemoptysis
  - Pulmonary hypertension
- Prognosis: Determined by associated cardiac anomalies & pulmonary artery hypertension

*(**Left**) PA chest radiograph of a patient with PIPA shows a small right hilum ⇒ and a small right lung with compensatory hyperinflation of the left lung. As in this case, the aortic arch ➡ is typically contralateral to the interrupted pulmonary artery. (**Right**) Axial CECT of the same patient shows interruption of the right pulmonary artery at its expected origin ⇧. Serrated right-sided pleural thickening ↶ is produced by systemic collateral vessels supplying the lung.*

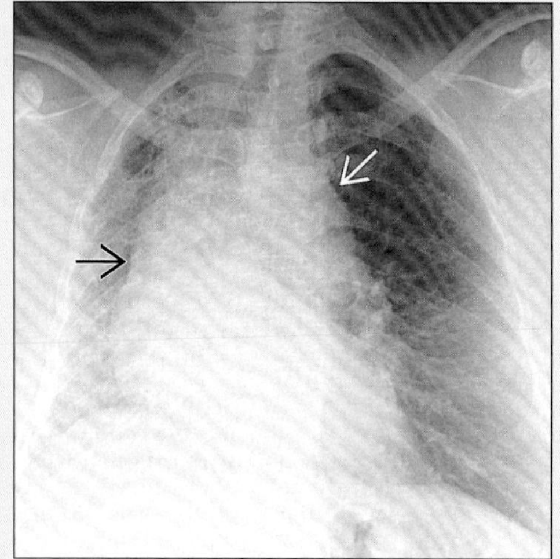

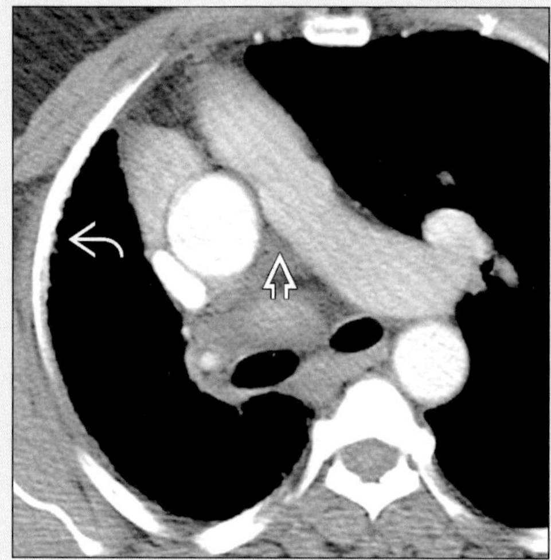

*(**Left**) Axial CECT of the same patient shows a small hypoplastic right lung with cystic changes and subtle peripheral reticular opacities ⇒ related to systemic collateral vessels supplying the lung. Bronchiectasis ➡ is a frequent finding related to chronic pulmonary infections. (**Right**) Axial CECT of the same patient shows bilateral areas of mosaic attenuation. Ipsilateral low attenuation ⇨ is likely due to hypoperfusion. Contralateral areas of low attenuation ➡ may be due to surrounding overperfusion.*

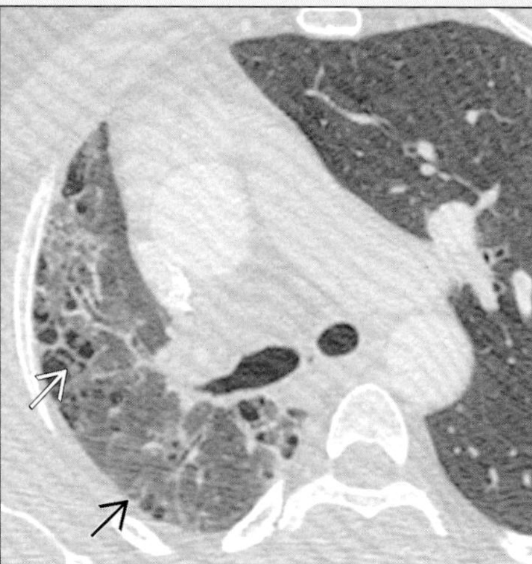

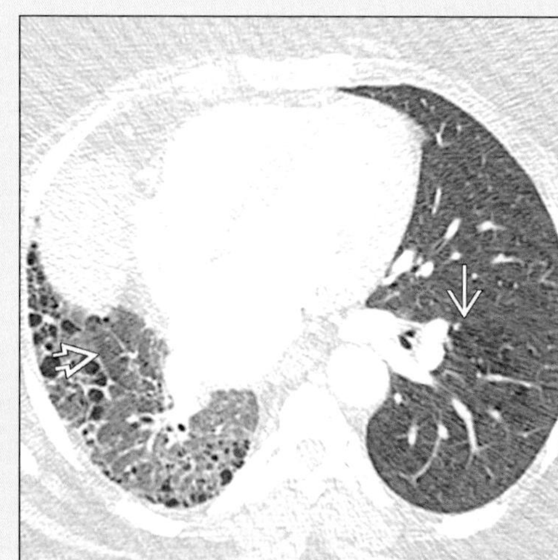

PROXIMAL INTERRUPTION OF THE PULMONARY ARTERY

TERMINOLOGY

Abbreviations

- **Proximal interruption of pulmonary artery (PIPA)**

Synonyms

- Unilateral absence of pulmonary artery
- "Interruption" preferred over "absence"
  - Intrapulmonary portion of pulmonary artery is intact

Definitions

- Failed development of proximal pulmonary artery

IMAGING

General Features

- Best diagnostic clue
  - Small hilum with small ipsilateral lung
  - Contralateral aortic arch
- Location
  - Right > left

Radiographic Findings

- Radiography
  - Affected hemithorax
    - **Volume loss with ipsilateral mediastinal shift & ipsilateral hemidiaphragm elevation**
    - **Small or indistinct hilum**
    - Fine linear peripheral opacities
      - Systemic collateral vessels supplying hypoplastic lung
    - Rib notching (intercostal collaterals)
  - Unaffected hemithorax
    - Compensatory lung hyperinflation
    - Enlarged hilum from increased blood flow
  - Aortic arch typically on opposite side of interrupted pulmonary artery
  - Cardiomegaly due to associated cardiac anomalies & pulmonary hypertension

CT Findings

- CECT
  - **Proximal pulmonary artery may be completely absent or terminate within 1 cm of origin**
  - Normal bronchial branching pattern
  - Bronchiectasis from recurrent infections
  - Mosaic attenuation
    - Affected lung likely from hypoxic vasoconstriction
    - Unaffected lung likely from overperfusion
    - No expiratory air-trapping
  - **Signs of collateral circulation**
    - Enlarged vessels
      - Bronchial arteries
      - Internal mammary arteries
      - Intercostal arteries
    - Serrated pleural thickening
    - Subpleural parenchymal bands

Angiographic Findings

- Documentation of systemic collateral vessels

Nuclear Medicine Findings

- V/Q scan
  - No perfusion of affected side
  - Normal ventilation of affected side

Imaging Recommendations

- Best imaging tool
  - CECT is optimal modality for evaluation of pulmonary arteries

DIFFERENTIAL DIAGNOSIS

Swyer-James-McLeod Syndrome

- Obliterative bronchiolitis in infant or child
- Unilateral hyperlucent lung with small ipsilateral pulmonary artery
- Expiratory air-trapping

Mediastinal Fibrosis

- Hilar or mediastinal (often calcified) soft tissue with narrowing of adjacent airways & vessels
- Focal & diffuse types

Scimitar Syndrome

- Right lung hypoplasia
- Anomalous return of right basilar pulmonary (scimitar) vein resembling Turkish sword

PATHOLOGY

General Features

- Etiology
  - Involution of proximal 6th primitive arch
    - Intrapulmonary vessels remain intact
- Associated abnormalities
  - Left interruption has higher incidence of congenital cardiovascular anomalies
    - Most commonly tetralogy of Fallot

CLINICAL ISSUES

Presentation

- Most common signs/symptoms
  - May be asymptomatic
  - Recurrent pulmonary infections, dyspnea, hemoptysis
- Other signs/symptoms
  - Pulmonary hypertension
  - High altitude pulmonary edema

Natural History & Prognosis

- Determined by associated cardiac anomalies or pulmonary artery hypertension

Treatment

- Revascularization of interrupted artery in infancy may prevent some degree of lung hypoplasia
- Hemoptysis: Angiographic embolization of systemic collaterals

SELECTED REFERENCES

1. Dillman JR et al: Expanding upon the unilateral hyperlucent hemithorax in children. Radiographics. 31(3):723-41, 2011
2. Castañer E et al: Congenital and acquired pulmonary artery anomalies in the adult: radiologic overview. Radiographics. 26(2):349-71, 2006

PROXIMAL INTERRUPTION OF THE PULMONARY ARTERY

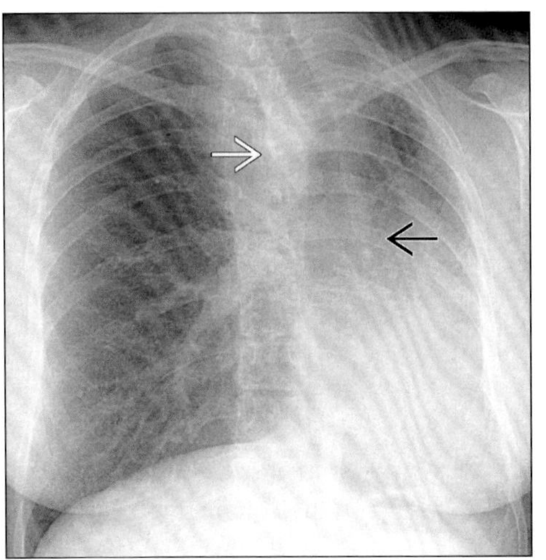

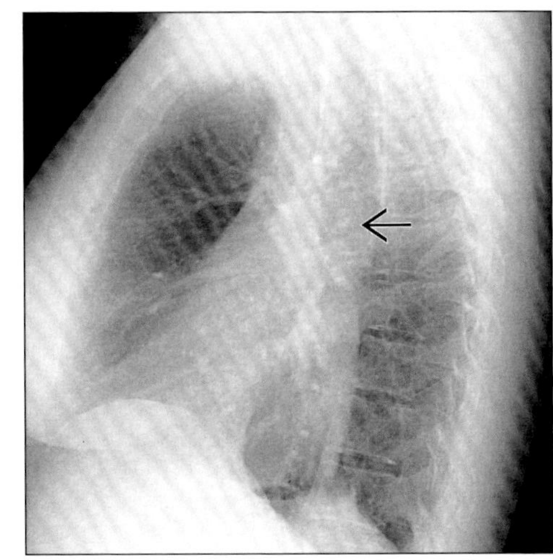

(Left) *PA chest radiograph of an asymptomatic patient with proximal interruption of the left pulmonary artery shows a small left lung, a small left hilum →, a right aortic arch ➡, and shift of the mediastinal structures to the left.* ***(Right)*** *Lateral chest radiograph of the same patient demonstrates absence of the left pulmonary artery →. The mediastinum is shifted posteriorly due to left lung hypoplasia and compensatory anterior herniation of the hyperinflated right lung.*

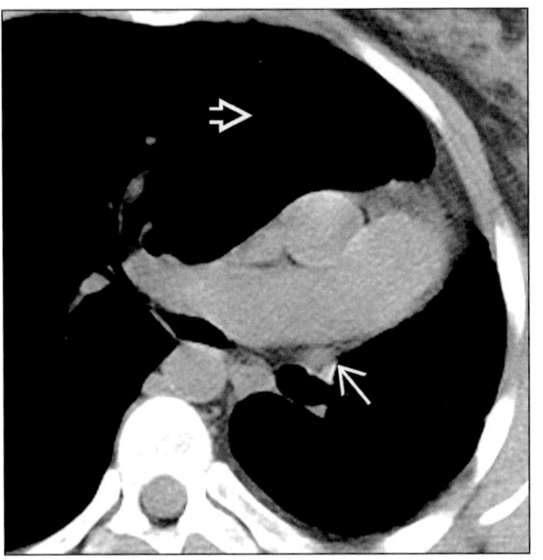

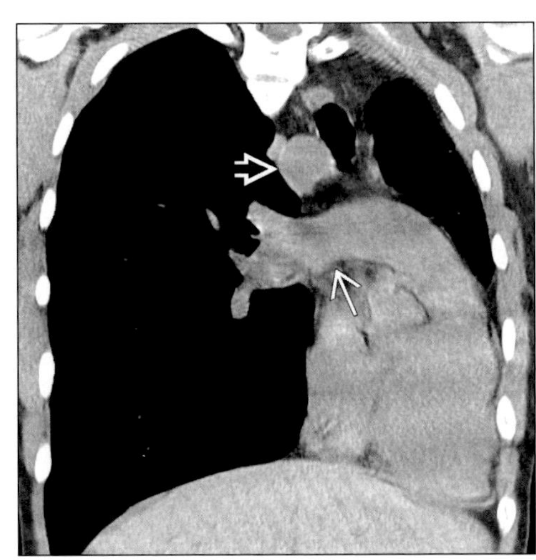

(Left) *Axial NECT of the same patient shows marked mediastinal shift to the left due to left lung hypoplasia. The left pulmonary artery is interrupted ➡ and the right lung herniates across the midline ➡ due to compensatory hyperinflation.* ***(Right)*** *Coronal NECT of the same patient shows that the right pulmonary artery ➡ is larger than the aortic arch ➡. This suggests pulmonary arterial hypertension, which is often found in patients with PIPA.*

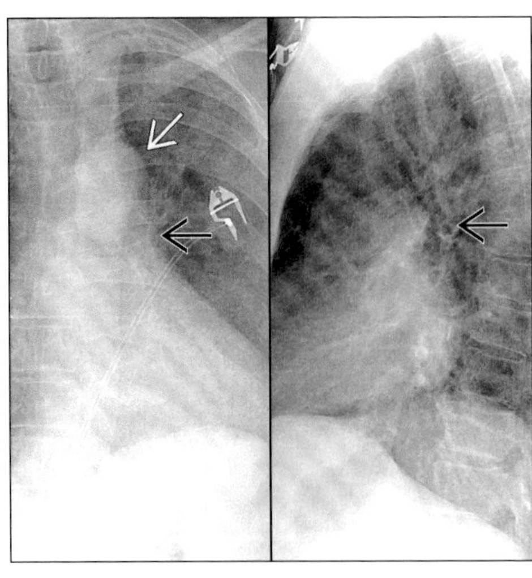

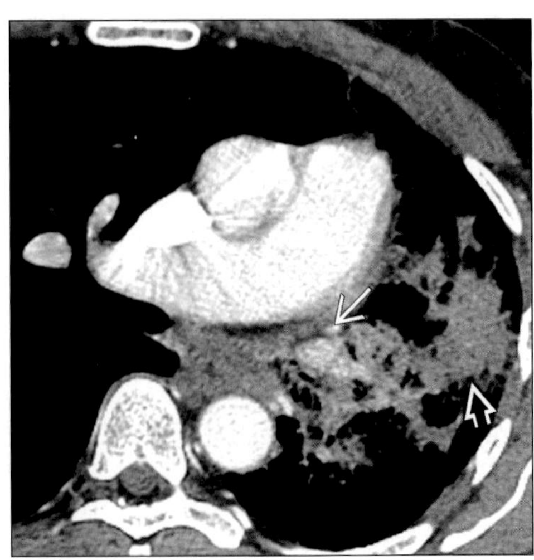

(Left) *Composite image with PA (left) and lateral (right) chest radiographs of a patient with proximal interruption of the left pulmonary artery shows absence of the left pulmonary artery →. This case illustrates an uncommon variant in that the aortic arch ➡ is ipsilateral to the interrupted artery.* ***(Right)*** *Axial CECT of the same patient obtained for evaluation of pneumonia shows interruption of the left pulmonary artery ➡ and left lung consolidation ➡. Infection commonly affects the hypoplastic lung.*

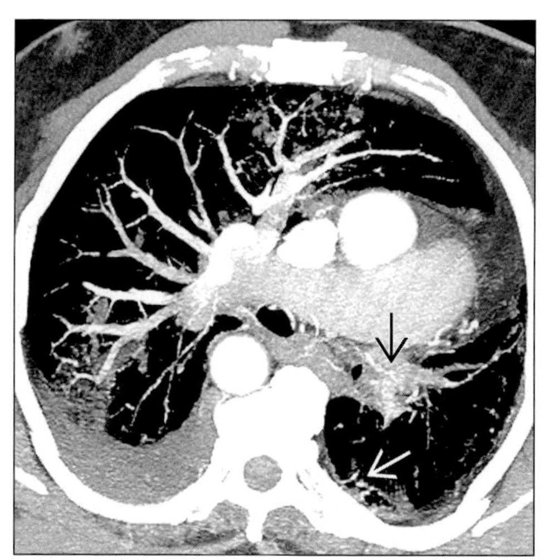

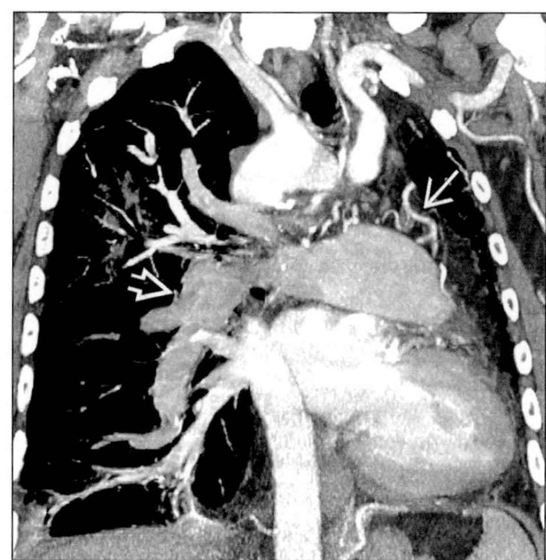

(Left) *Axial CECT maximum-intensity projection (MIP) image shows asymmetric blood supply to the lungs. The left lung is supplied by bronchial* → *and intercostal* ➡ *collateral vessels.* ***(Right)*** *Coronal CECT MIP image of the same patient shows enlarged bronchial arteries* ➡ *supplying the hypoplastic left lung due to proximal interruption of the left pulmonary artery. There is dilatation of the right pulmonary artery* ⇨*. Patients with PIPA may develop pulmonary hypertension.*

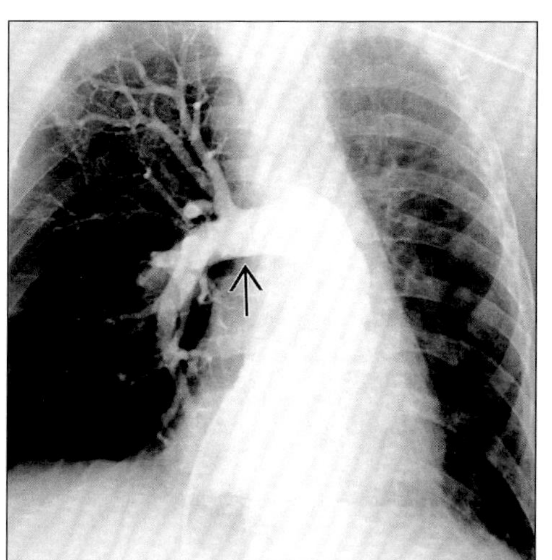

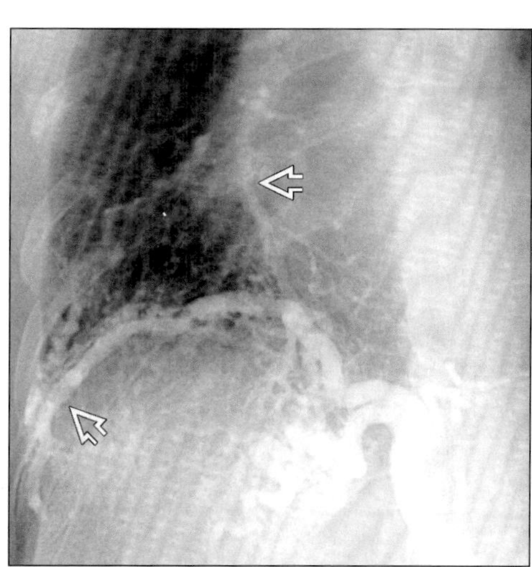

(Left) *Frontal pulmonary artery angiography of a patient with proximal interruption of the left pulmonary artery shows an enlarged right pulmonary artery* → *and nonvisualization of the left pulmonary artery.* ***(Right)*** *Frontal angiography of a patient with hemoptysis and interrupted right pulmonary artery shows multiple enlarged systemic collateral arteries* ⇨ *supplying the right lung. Angiography and embolization may be required to treat recurrent or severe hemoptysis.*

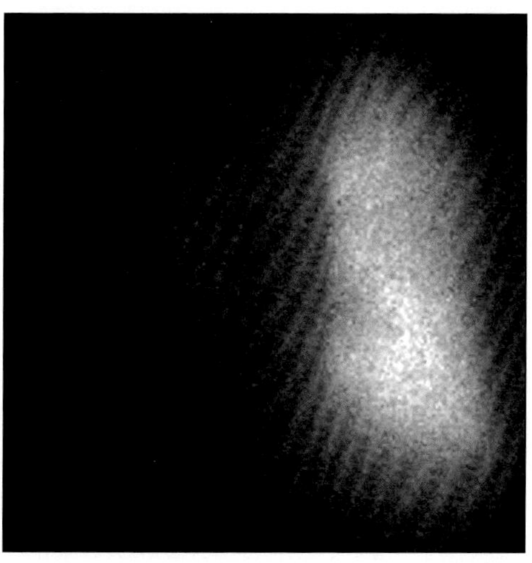

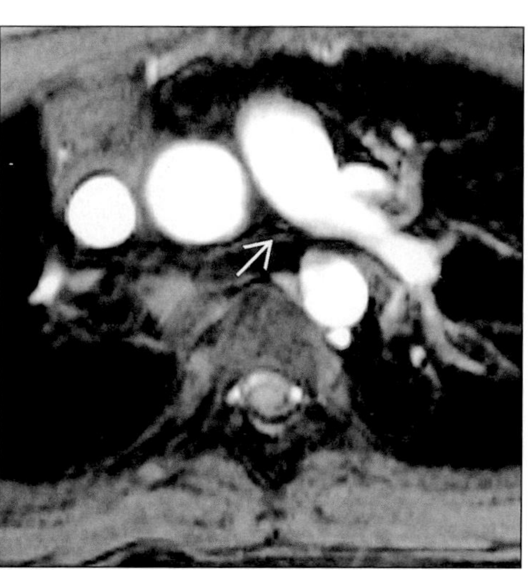

(Left) *Anterior projection from a perfusion scintigram shows absence of perfusion to the right lung secondary to proximal interruption of the right pulmonary artery.* ***(Right)*** *Axial T2WI MR shows a normal pulmonary trunk, a normal left pulmonary artery, and proximal interruption of the right pulmonary artery* ➡*. MR imaging may be obtained in patients with PIPA to evaluate associated congenital cardiac abnormalities.*

ABERRANT LEFT PULMONARY ARTERY

Key Facts

Terminology
- Abbreviations
  - Aberrant left pulmonary artery (ALPA)
  - Pulmonary artery sling (PAS)
- Definition
  - ALPA arises from posterior right pulmonary artery and courses between trachea and esophagus

Imaging
- Radiography
  - Mass effect on right lower trachea
  - Hyperinflation/atelectasis of right lung
  - Ovoid opacity (ALPA) between trachea and esophagus on lateral chest radiograph
- CT/MR
  - Left pulmonary artery origin from posterior aspect of distal right pulmonary artery
  - ALPA course between trachea and esophagus

Top Differential Diagnoses
- Vascular ring
- Mediastinal mass
- Congenital interruption of pulmonary artery
- Paraesophageal varices

Clinical Issues
- Signs/symptoms
  - Stridor, wheezing
  - Recurrent pneumonia
- Associated conditions
  - Complete tracheal rings, tracheomalacia
- Demographics
  - 2/3 of affected patients present on 1st day of life
  - Isolated ALPA reported in asymptomatic adults
- Treatment
  - Surgical ligation & reanastomosis of ALPA
  - Tracheoplasty for associated tracheal anomalies

*(**Left**) NECT shows that the right pulmonary artery (R) arises from the main pulmonary artery (M) while the ALPA (L) arises from the posterior aspect of the right pulmonary artery and courses between a moderately narrowed trachea ➔ and the esophagus ➲. (**Right**) CECT shows the ALPA (L) arising from the posterior aspect of the right pulmonary artery (R) and coursing between the carina ➔ and the esophagus ➲. The sling-like morphology of the ALPA accounts for the term "pulmonary artery sling."*

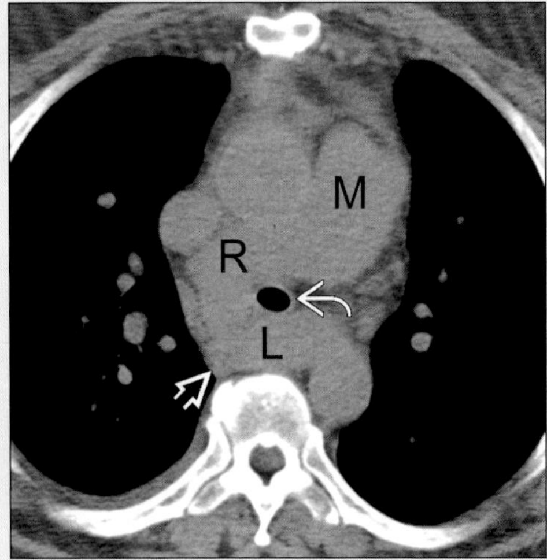

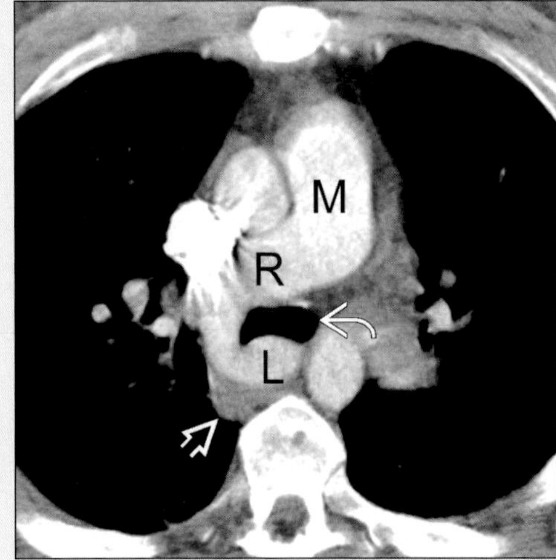

*(**Left**) Axial CECT of the same patient shows the ALPA (L) located between the carina ➔ and the esophagus ➲. (**Right**) Axial CECT of the same patient shows the ALPA (L) coursing toward the left hilum (*) between the proximal mainstem bronchi anteriorly and the esophagus ➲, which is located posteriorly and deviated to the right. The ALPA produces mass effect on the central airways and may result in tracheomalacia &/or postobstructive effects of the right tracheobronchial tree and right lung.*

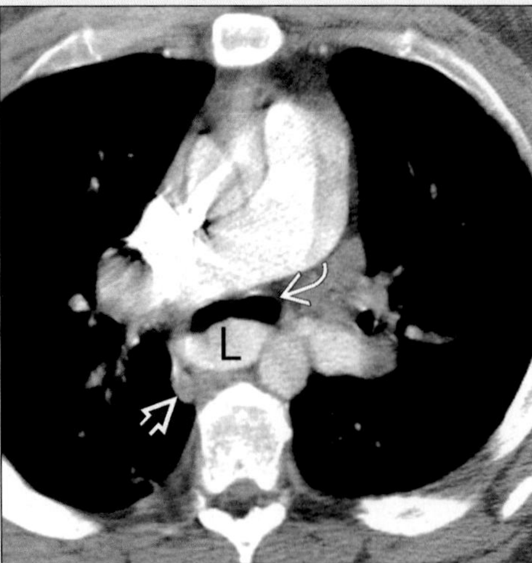

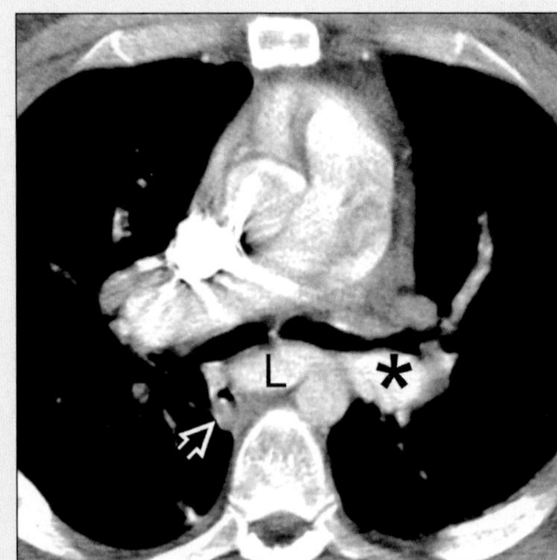

ABERRANT LEFT PULMONARY ARTERY

TERMINOLOGY

Abbreviations

- **Aberrant left pulmonary artery (ALPA)**

Synonyms

- **Anomalous pulmonary artery**
- **Pulmonary artery sling (PAS)**

Definitions

- ALPA arises from posterior right pulmonary artery & courses between trachea & esophagus toward left hilum

IMAGING

General Features

- Best diagnostic clue
  - **Left pulmonary artery between trachea & esophagus**
- Location
  - Middle-posterior mediastinum
- Size
  - ALPA may be smaller than normal left pulmonary artery

Radiographic Findings

- Right-sided mass effect on lower trachea
- Leftward deviation of lower trachea
- Hyperinflation or atelectasis of right lung or middle and right lower lobes
  - Vascular compression of trachea & right bronchi
- **Ovoid opacity (ALPA) between trachea & esophagus on lateral chest radiography**

Fluoroscopic Findings

- Upper GI
  - **Anterior impression on mid esophagus**
  - **Rightward deviation of esophagus**

CT Findings

- CECT
  - **ALPA**
    - **Left pulmonary artery origin from posterior aspect of distal right pulmonary artery**
    - **Courses between trachea & esophagus**
    - Courses toward left lung
    - Normal pulmonary artery branching
    - No normal vascular connection between pulmonary trunk & left lung
  - Associated findings
    - Hyperinflation or atelectasis of right lung or middle & right lower lobes
    - Complete tracheal rings
    - Tracheomalacia
    - Tracheal bronchus
    - Congenital heart disease in children

MR Findings

- T1WI
  - ALPA origin from distal right pulmonary artery
  - ALPA course between trachea & esophagus

Imaging Recommendations

- Best imaging tool
  - Cross-sectional imaging with CT or MR for assessment of vascular anatomy
- Protocol advice
  - CT pulmonary angiography
  - MR with black blood or bright blood sequences

DIFFERENTIAL DIAGNOSIS

Vascular Ring

- Posterior to esophagus

Mediastinal Mass

- Rarely localized to tracheoesophageal groove

Congenital Interruption of Pulmonary Artery

- Small hemithorax & small ipsilateral hilum

Paraesophageal Varices

- May course between trachea & esophagus

PATHOLOGY

General Features

- Etiology
  - Embryonic regression of left pulmonary artery
  - ALPA develops from right pulmonary artery
- Associated abnormalities
  - Assorted congenital heart lesions in 15% of cases

CLINICAL ISSUES

Presentation

- Most common signs/symptoms
  - Respiratory symptoms in infancy
    - **Stridor** most common; occasional apnea
    - **Wheezing**
    - **Recurrent pneumonia**
- Other signs/symptoms
  - Dysphagia; failure to thrive

Demographics

- Age
  - 2/3 of affected patients present on 1st day of life
  - Isolated ALPA reported in asymptomatic adults
- Gender
  - No gender predilection

Treatment

- Surgical ligation of ALPA with reanastomosis to normal location
- Tracheoplasty for associated tracheal anomalies

DIAGNOSTIC CHECKLIST

Consider

- ALPA in asymptomatic adult with ovoid opacity between trachea & esophagus on lateral radiography

Image Interpretation Pearls

- Anterior impression on esophagus on esophagram
- ALPA course between trachea & esophagus on CT

SELECTED REFERENCES

1. Fiore AC et al: Surgical treatment of pulmonary artery sling and tracheal stenosis. Ann Thorac Surg. 79(1):38-46; discussion 38-46, 2005

PULMONARY ARTERIOVENOUS MALFORMATION

Key Facts

Terminology

- Pulmonary arteriovenous malformation (PAVM)
- Communication between pulmonary arteries & pulmonary veins, right-to-left shunt

Imaging

- Radiography
  - Nodule with feeding artery(ies) & draining vein(s)
- CT/MR
  - Sharply defined round or oval nodule with feeding artery/arteries & draining vein(s)
  - Simple: 1 or more feeding arteries from same segmental artery
  - Complex (10%): Multiple feeding arteries from different segmental arteries
- Contrast echocardiography: Evaluation of cardiac & intrapulmonary shunts
- Nuclear medicine (Tc-99m labeled macroaggregates)
  - Estimation of size of right-to-left shunt

Top Differential Diagnoses

- Metastases
- Septic emboli
- Solitary pulmonary nodule
- Pulmonary artery pseudoaneurysm

Pathology

- Multiple AVMs highly associated with HHT

Clinical Issues

- Asymptomatic: Single PAVM < 2 cm in diameter
- Symptomatic: 40-60 years of age
  - Hemorrhage
  - Paradoxic embolism to central nervous system

Diagnostic Checklist

- Consider PAVM in lung nodule with associated tubular opacities representing feeding artery & draining vein

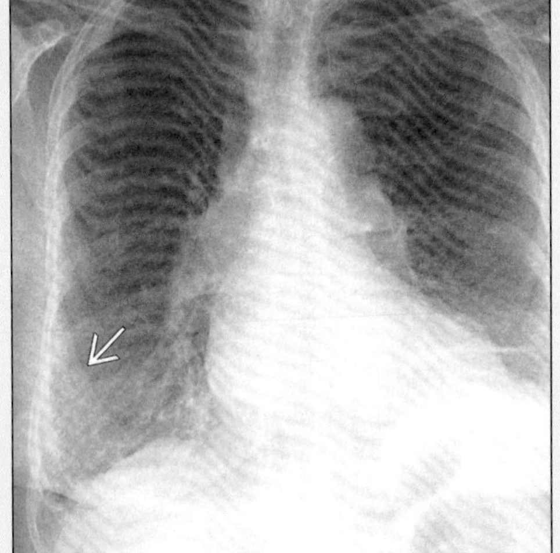

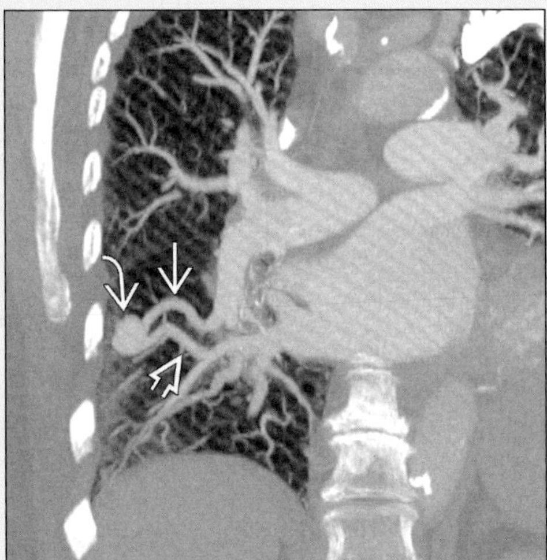

(Left) *PA chest radiograph of a young woman shows an ill-defined "rounded" opacity in the right lung base ➡. Chest radiography is of limited value in the detection of small PAVMs.* ***(Right)*** *Coronal CTA (MIP image) of the same patient shows a right lower lobe PAVM ➡. A single afferent arterial pedicle arises from a branch of the right lower lobe pulmonary artery ➡ to supply the PAVM. The draining vein ➡ drains into the left atrium. A complex PAVM is supplied by more than 1 pulmonary artery.*

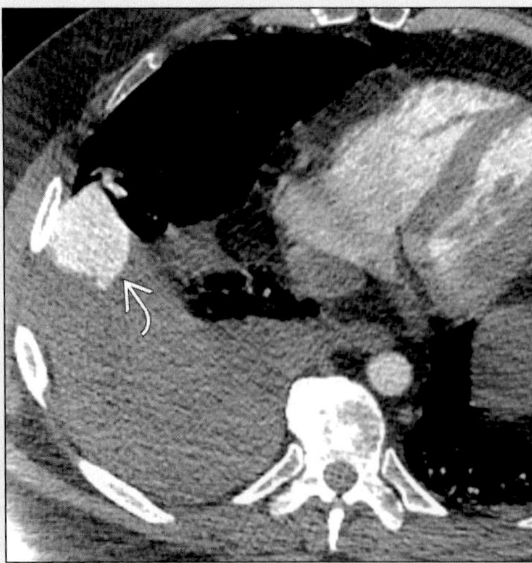

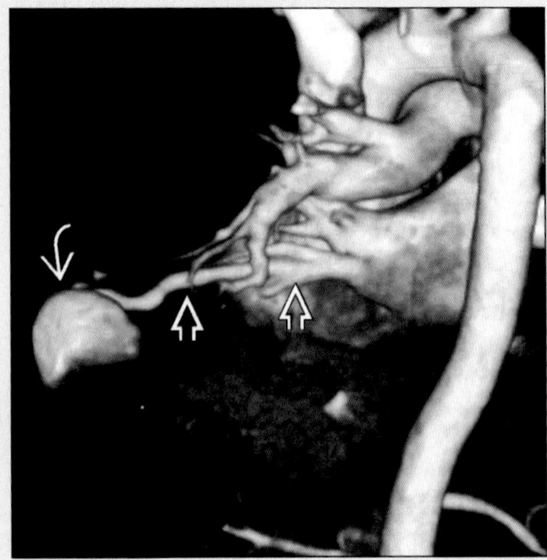

(Left) *Axial CECT of a patient with a ruptured PAVM shows a moderate hemothorax and enhancement of the aneurysmal sac ➡ in the right lower lobe. PAVM rupture is a life-threatening complication. Expeditious diagnosis is lifesaving.* ***(Right)*** *CTA volume-rendered image of the same patient shows the aneurysmal sac ➡ of the PAVM and the draining vein ➡. Three-dimensional reformatted images may be useful for providing information regarding the angioarchitecture of the PAVM.*

PULMONARY ARTERIOVENOUS MALFORMATION

TERMINOLOGY

Abbreviations

- **Pulmonary arteriovenous malformation (PAVM)**

Definitions

- Abnormal direct communication between pulmonary arteries & pulmonary veins, direct right-to-left shunt
  - **Congenital**: Hereditary hemorrhagic telangiectasia (HHT) or Osler-Weber-Rendu syndrome
  - **Acquired**: Hepatopulmonary syndrome, systemic diseases, venous anomalies, after palliation of complex cyanotic congenital heart disease

IMAGING

General Features

- Best diagnostic clue
  - Nodule(s) with feeding artery(ies) & draining vein(s)
- Location
  - Peripheral lower lobes (50-70%): Medial 1/3 of lung
- Size
  - Variable: 1-5 cm in diameter

Radiographic Findings

- Radiography
  - Sensitivity for PAVMs: 50-70%
  - Round, oval, or lobulated well-defined nodule with feeding artery(ies) & draining vein(s)
  - Consolidation-like lesions in diffuse PAVM

CT Findings

- Sharply defined round or oval nodule with **feeding artery/arteries & draining vein(s)**
  - **Simple**: 1 or more feeding arteries from same segmental artery
  - **Complex** (10%): Multiple feeding arteries from different segmental arteries
    - Diffuse PAVM (5% of complex PAVMs): Innumerable feeders, frequently lobar

MR Findings

- MRA: Similar to CT for detection

Echocardiographic Findings

- Contrast echocardiography: Evaluation of cardiac & intrapulmonary shunts

Nuclear Medicine Findings

- Tc-99m MAA: Right-to-left shunt size estimate

Imaging Recommendations

- Best imaging tool
  - MDCT with MIP images
- Protocol advice
  - Screen for PAVMs with CT every 3-5 years
    - Unenhanced CT low dose (30 mAs)
    - Review with thin-slab MIP (5 mm)
  - Pulmonary angiography for treatment, not for diagnosis

DIFFERENTIAL DIAGNOSIS

Metastases

- History of malignancy, usually multiple

Septic Emboli

- Rapid growth, cavitation frequent
- Blood or central line culture

Solitary Pulmonary Nodule

- Most commonly lung cancer, granuloma, hamartoma

Pulmonary Artery Pseudoaneurysm

- Complication related to pulmonary artery catheter, trauma, & bacterial endocarditis

PATHOLOGY

General Features

- Genetics
  - HHT: Autosomal dominant disorder
    - Mutations in *ENG* & *ALK1* on chromosome 9 (75%)

Gross Pathologic & Surgical Features

- Draining veins usually larger than feeding arteries

CLINICAL ISSUES

Presentation

- Most common signs/symptoms
  - **Asymptomatic**: Single PAVM < 2 cm in diameter
  - **Symptomatic**: 40-60 years of age
    - **Hemorrhage**: Hemoptysis (10%), epistaxis from nasal telangiectasia in 90% of HHT
    - **CNS complications** (40%): Paradoxical embolism & cerebral abscess
- Other signs/symptoms
  - Desaturation, exercise intolerance, cyanosis, & clubbing with large PAVMs

Demographics

- Age
  - 10% of cases identified in infancy or childhood
- Gender
  - M:F = 1:2

Diagnosis

- Blood test for identification of mutation (80% of patients)
- Genetic screening
- Screening of at risk patients with contrast echocardiography

Natural History & Prognosis

- Growth postulated in puberty & pregnancy

Treatment

- Coil embolotherapy
  - Recanalization in up to 20%
  - Long-term imaging follow-up post therapy

DIAGNOSTIC CHECKLIST

Consider

- Consider PAVM in lung nodule with associated tubular opacities representing feeding artery & draining vein

SELECTED REFERENCES

1. Trerotola SO et al: PAVM embolization: an update. AJR Am J Roentgenol. 195(4):837-45, 2010

PARTIAL ANOMALOUS PULMONARY VENOUS RETURN

Key Facts

Terminology

- Partial anomalous pulmonary venous return (PAPVR)
- Congenital pulmonary venous anomaly involving drainage of 1-3 pulmonary veins into systemic venous circulation or right atrium; left-to-right shunt

Imaging

- Distribution in adults
  - Left upper lobe (47%), right upper lobe (38%)
- Radiography
  - Left upper lobe PAPVR: Lateralization of aortopulmonary reflection
- CT
  - Left upper lobe PAPVR drains to left brachiocephalic via vertical vein
  - Right upper lobe PAPVR drains to SVC
- MR
  - Allows shunt quantification (QP/QS)

Top Differential Diagnoses

- Persistent left superior vena cava
  - May simulate vertical vein
  - Often associated with dilated coronary sinus
- Lateralization of aortopulmonary reflection
  - Mediastinal lipomatosis
  - Mediastinal lymphadenopathy
  - Lung cancer

Clinical Issues

- Often asymptomatic with only 1 anomalous vein
- Symptoms as shunt ↑: Dyspnea, palpitations, chest pain, tachycardia, edema, systolic murmur
- Surgical correction may be indicated for symptomatic PAPVR &/or QP/QS > 2:1, vascular rings, coexistent congenital heart disease
- Outcome depends on associated conditions (e.g., sinus venosus atrial septal defect)

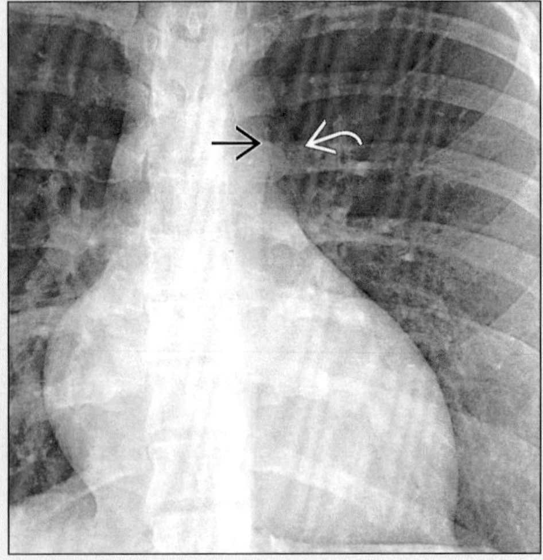

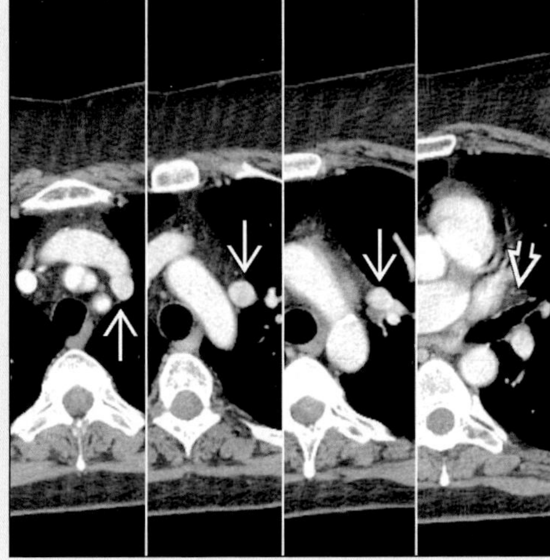

(Left) *PA chest radiograph of a patient with left upper lobe PAPVR shows soft tissue ➔ lateral to the aortic arch → and lateralization of the AP reflection. In normal circumstances, no soft tissue should be seen lateral to the aortic arch.* ***(Right)*** *Composite axial CECT of the same patient shows the vertical vein ➔ coursing lateral to the aortic arch. Note absence of the left superior pulmonary vein from its normal location, anterior to the left mainstem bronchus ➔.*

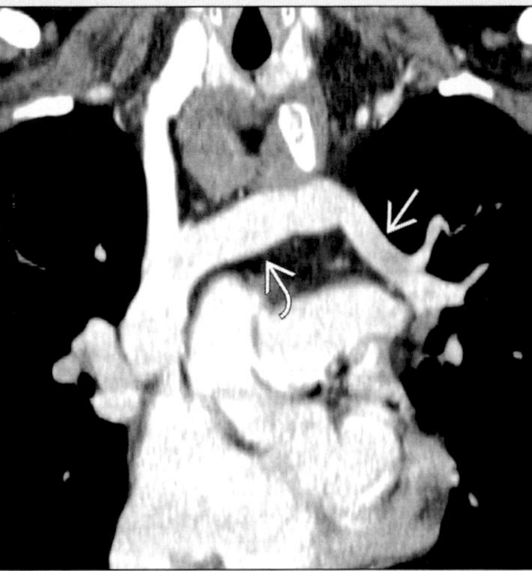

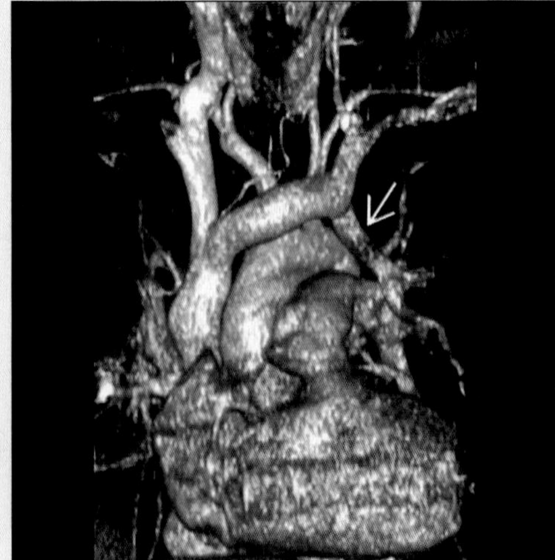

(Left) *Curved coronal CECT reformation of the same patient shows the vertical vein ➔ arising from segmental left upper lobe veins and draining into the ipsilateral left brachiocephalic vein ➔.* ***(Right)*** *Coronal CECT 3D SSD reformation of the same patient shows the left upper lobe PAPVR ➔. This lesion is the most common form of PAPVR in the left hemithorax. When isolated, the left-to-right shunt is small and, consequently, hardly ever symptomatic.*

PARTIAL ANOMALOUS PULMONARY VENOUS RETURN

TERMINOLOGY

Abbreviations

- Partial anomalous pulmonary venous return (PAPVR)

Definitions

- Congenital pulmonary venous anomaly involving drainage of 1-3 pulmonary veins into systemic venous circulation or right atrium; left-to-right shunt

IMAGING

General Features

- Best diagnostic clue
  - Direct drainage of a pulmonary vein into systemic circulation (e.g., superior vena cava, inferior vena cava, right atrium, left brachiocephalic vein)
- Location
  - Distribution in adults
    - Left upper lobe, most common (47%)
    - Right upper lobe (38%)
    - Right lower lobe (13%)
    - Left lower lobe (2%)

Radiographic Findings

- Radiography
  - **Frequently normal**
  - **Left upper lobe PAPVR**: Vertical vein may cause **lateralization of aortopulmonary interface**
  - If significant shunt
    - Cardiomegaly; right heart enlargement
    - Pulmonary artery enlargement
    - Increased number & size of sharply defined pulmonary vessels (shunt vascularity)

CT Findings

- CECT
  - **Left upper lobe PAPVR**
    - Drains to left brachiocephalic vein via vertical vein; may occasionally drain into coronary sinus, hemiazygos vein, subclavian, or subdiaphragmatic vein
    - Absence of left superior pulmonary vein from normal location (i.e., anterior to left mainstem bronchus)
  - **Right upper lobe PAPVR**
    - Most cases also involve right middle lobe pulmonary vein
    - Drains into superior vena cava; occasionally drains into azygos vein, right atrium, IVC, hepatic vein, or portal vein
    - Often associated with sinus venosus atrial septal defect (ASD) & rarely with ostium primum ASD
  - **Right lower lobe PAPVR**
    - Scimitar syndrome: Right PAPVR draining left lower lobe & occasionally right middle or upper lobes into inferior vena cava
    - May drain directly into right atrium (rare) when associated with sinus venosus ASD
  - **Bilateral upper lobe PAPVR** is uncommon (4% of all cases)
  - If significant left-to-right shunt
    - Right heart enlargement
    - Pulmonary artery > 3 cm (pulmonary hypertension)
  - Ancillary findings
    - Persistent left SVC
    - Azygos continuation of inferior vena cava

MR Findings

- MR equivalent to CT for morphologic characterization of PAPVR
- MR superior to CT for identification of ASD
- Allows shunt quantification (QP/QS)
  - Significant left-to-right shunt may occur when 2 or more anomalous pulmonary veins exist or with coexistent sinus venosus ASD

Echocardiographic Findings

- Echocardiography findings frequently diagnostic
- Consider cardiac MR or CT for equivocal cases

Imaging Recommendations

- Best imaging tool
  - CT & MR are equivalent modalities for detection of PAPVR if echocardiography is equivocal

DIFFERENTIAL DIAGNOSIS

Persistent Left Superior Vena Cava

- May mimic vertical vein
- Typically associated with dilated coronary sinus
- Left superior pulmonary vein identified anterior to left mainstem bronchus

PATHOLOGY

Staging, Grading, & Classification

- Partial anomalous pulmonary venous **connection**: Anomalous vein connection with systemic vein
- Partial anomalous pulmonary venous **drainage**: Anomalous vein delivers oxygenated blood to right atrium because of presence of a sinus venosus ASD

CLINICAL ISSUES

Presentation

- Most common signs/symptoms
  - Frequently asymptomatic with only 1 anomalous pulmonary vein
  - Symptoms occur as shunt ↑: Dyspnea, palpitations, chest pain, tachycardia, edema, systolic murmur

Natural History & Prognosis

- Outcome depends on associated conditions (e.g., sinus venosus ASD)

Treatment

- Surgical correction may be indicated for symptomatic PAPVR &/or QP/QS > 2:1, vascular rings, coexistent congenital heart disease

SELECTED REFERENCES

1. Ho ML et al: MDCT of partial anomalous pulmonary venous return (PAPVR) in adults. J Thorac Imaging. 24(2):89-95, 2009
2. Haramati LB et al: Computed tomography of partial anomalous pulmonary venous connection in adults. J Comput Assist Tomogr. 27(5):743-9, 2003

*(**Left**) PA chest radiograph of a patient with left upper lobe PAPVR shows obscuration of the aortic arch due to the presence of the adjacent vertical vein. (**Right**) Coronal CTA MIP image of the same patient shows a left upper lobe PAPVR draining into a vertical vein. This anomaly should be distinguished from persistent left SVC (PLSVC). In the latter, the left superior pulmonary vein courses anterior to the left mainstem bronchus, and the coronary sinus is often dilated.*

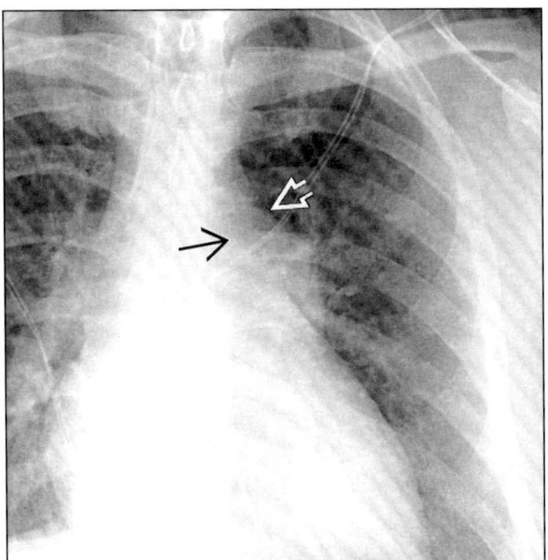

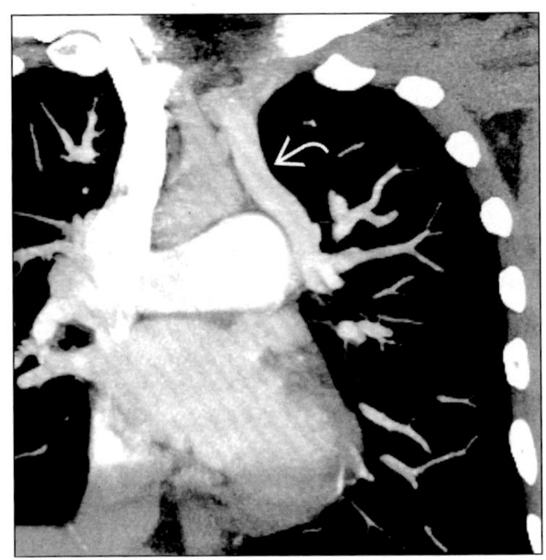

*(**Left**) Axial CTA of a patient with right upper lobe PAPVR and sinus venosus ASD shows anomalous drainage of the right upper lobe pulmonary vein into the SVC. (**Right**) Axial CTA of the same patient demonstrates a sinus venosus ASD. Note also that the right middle lobe pulmonary vein drains directly to the left atrium, contributing to the left-to-right shunt. The association with sinus venosus ASD is typically seen in right upper lobe PAPVR, which constitutes approximately 40% of all cases.*

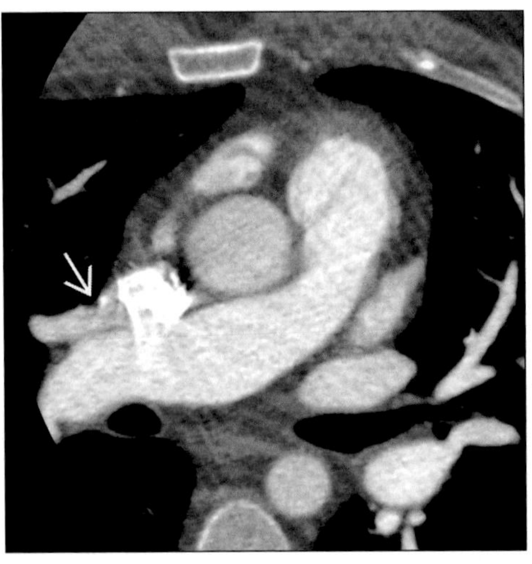

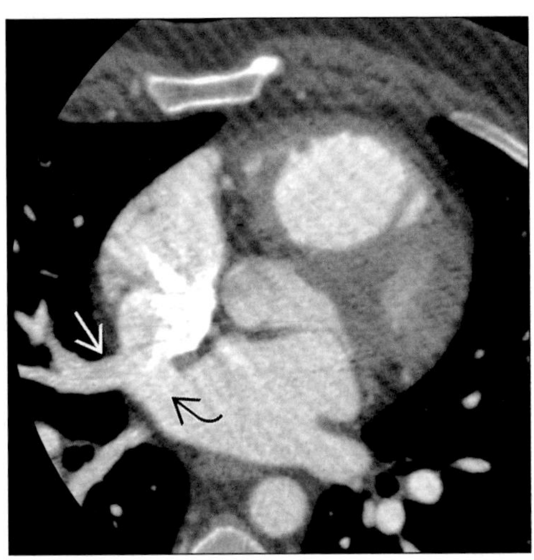

*(**Left**) Axial CTA of the same patient demonstrates enlargement of the right heart with inversion of the interventricular septum, consistent with increased right heart pressures secondary to a significant left-to-right shunt. (**Right**) Axial CTA shows a sinus venosus ASD and a right lower lobe pulmonary vein draining into the left atrium and contributing to the left-to-right shunt produced by the sinus venosus ASD. (Courtesy S. Abbara, MD.)*

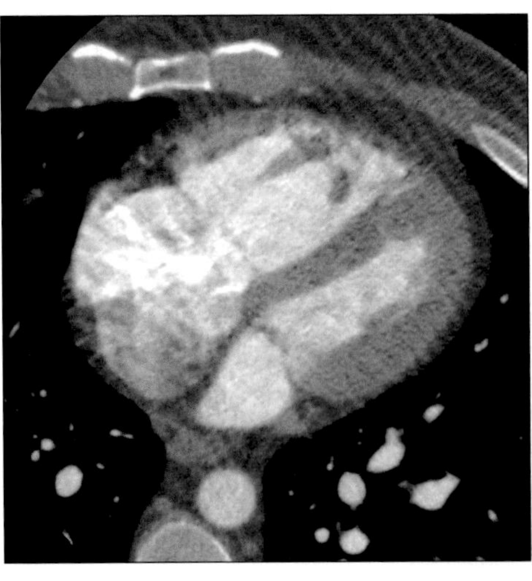

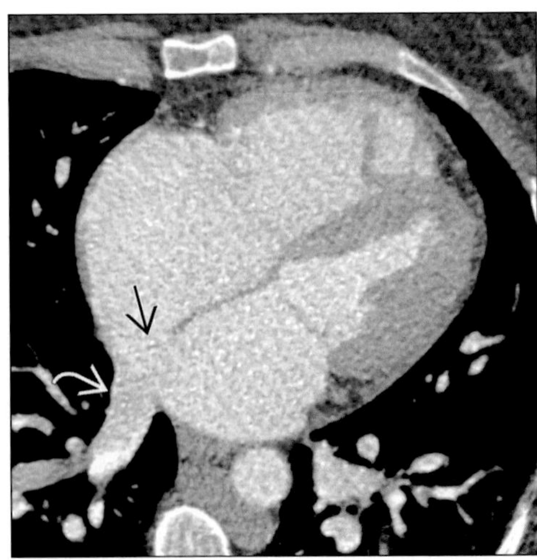

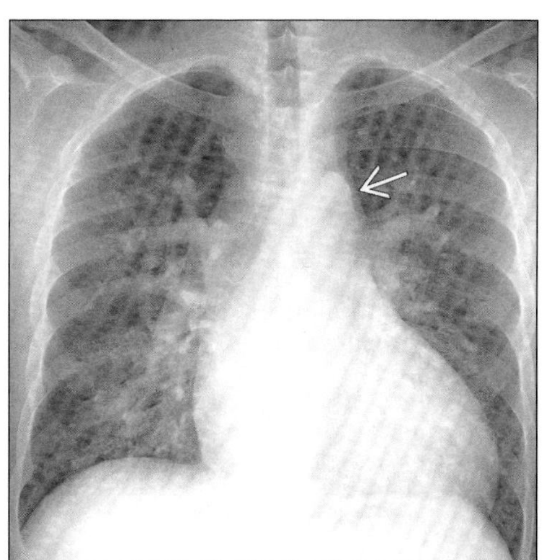

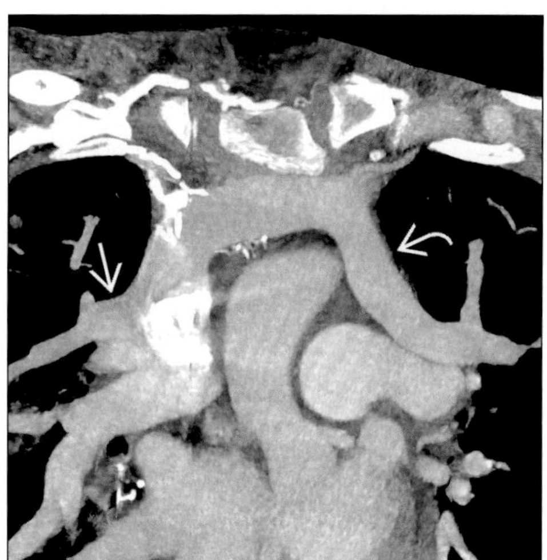

(Left) *PA chest radiograph of a patient with bilateral upper lobe PAPVR but no sinus venosus ASD shows cardiomegaly and markedly increased pulmonary vascularity (shunt vascularity). There is an abnormal sot tissue interface lateral to the aortic arch* ➡. ***(Right)*** *Curved coronal CTA MIP image of the same patient shows left upper lobe* ➡ *and right upper lobe* ➡ *pulmonary veins draining to the left brachiocephalic vein and the superior vena cava, respectively.*

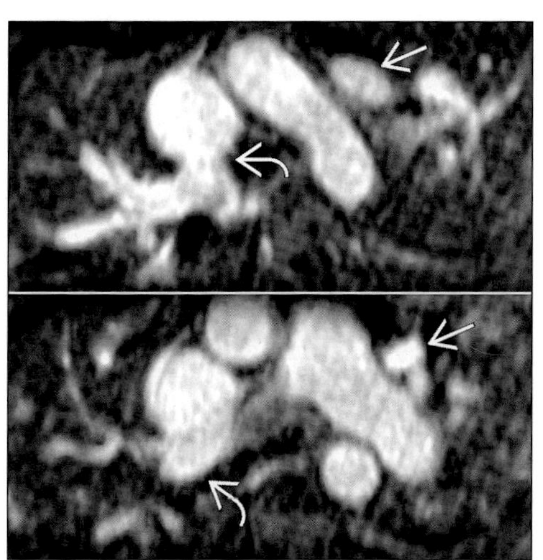

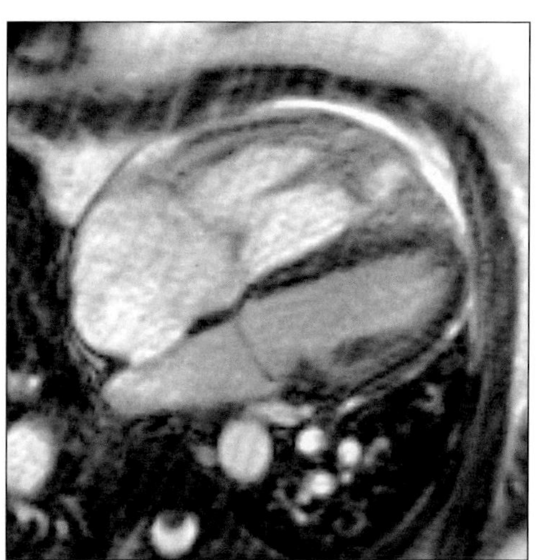

(Left) *Composite image with axial MRA shows bilateral upper lobe PAPVR without associated sinus venosus ASD. Note the vertical vein on the left* ➡ *and direct drainage of the right upper lobe pulmonary vein* ➡ *into the SVC.* ***(Right)*** *Four chamber view of SSFP cine MR of the same patient shows dilatation of the right heart with flattening of the interventricular septum in keeping with a significant left-to-right shunt. Cardiac MR allows quantification of the shunt with velocity encoded imaging.*

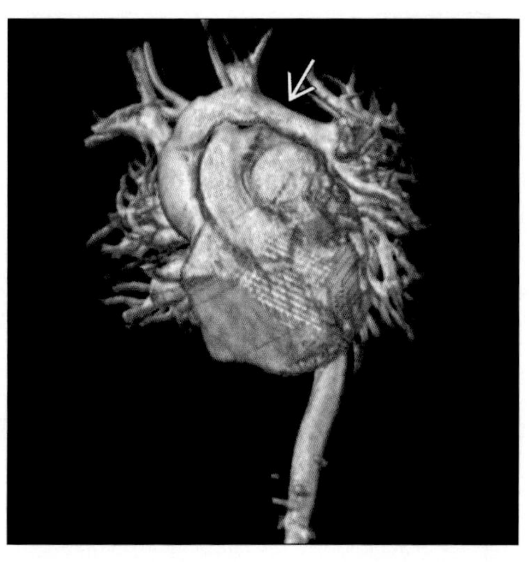

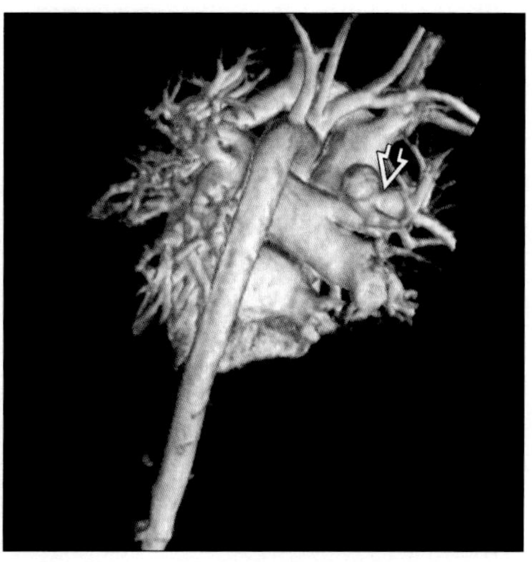

(Left) *Coronal anterior 3D reconstruction of an MRA of the same patient demonstrates the vertical vein* ➡ *receiving all left upper lobe pulmonary vein branches.* ***(Right)*** *Coronal posterior 3D reconstruction of an MRA of the same patient shows the right upper lobe pulmonary vein* ➡ *draining into the SVC. While PAPVR is often asymptomatic, symptoms may arise in direct proportion to the amount of blood being shunted as in this patient with bilateral PAPVR.*

Key Facts

Terminology
- Synonyms: Hypogenetic lung syndrome, pulmonary venolobar syndrome
- Partial or total anomalous pulmonary venous return of right lung to vena cava above or below diaphragm

Imaging
- Radiography
  - Curved tubular opacity (scimitar vein) descending toward midline, paralleling right heart border
  - Small right hilum
  - Small right hemithorax, hyperlucent lung
- CT
  - Visualization of course & drainage of anomalous pulmonary vein
  - Drainage to infradiaphragmatic IVC
- MR: Equivalent to CT for scimitar vein characterization, allows shunt quantification

Top Differential Diagnoses
- Unilateral absence of the pulmonary artery
- Pulmonary sequestration
- Meandering pulmonary vein

Pathology
- Congenital, sporadic

Clinical Issues
- Infantile form: Associated cardiovascular anomalies
- Pediatric/adult form: May be asymptomatic
- Surgical treatment: Symptomatic patients, significant shunts, associated anomalies

Diagnostic Checklist
- Triad of respiratory distress, right lung hypoplasia, & heart dextroposition should suggest scimitar syndrome

(Left) PA chest radiograph of a patient with scimitar syndrome shows a small right lung with mild dextroposition of the heart related to pulmonary hypoplasia. The anomalous pulmonary vein or scimitar vein ➡ is identified in the medial right lower lung coursing medially to the mediastinum. This appearance is nearly always diagnostic. (Right) Lateral chest radiograph of the same patient shows a band-like opacity ➡ paralleling the anterior chest wall resulting from rotation of the mediastinum to the right.

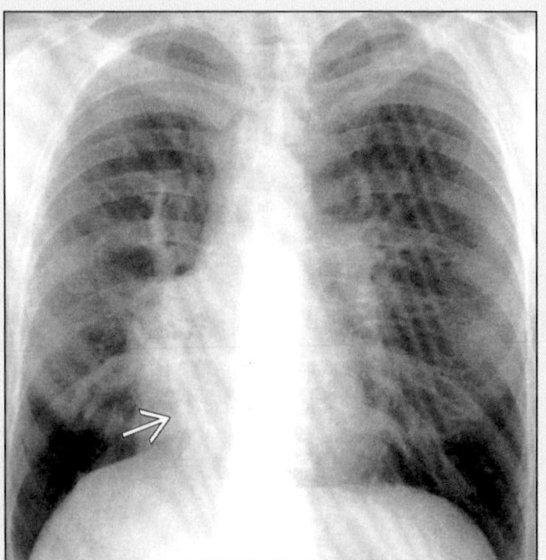

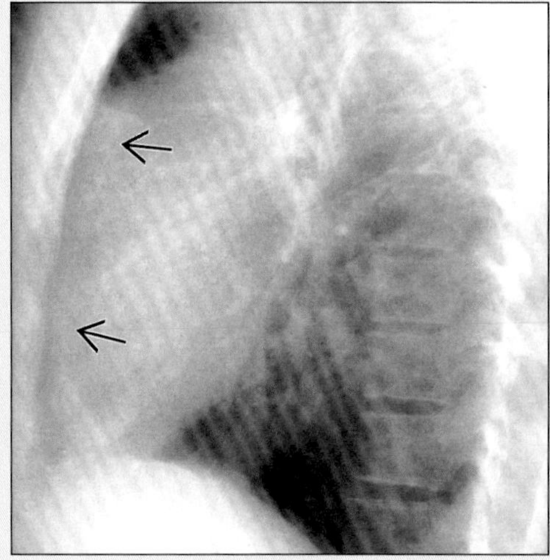

(Left) AP chest angiography of the same patient shows contrast enhancement of the anomalous pulmonary vein ➡. In this case, the entire lung is drained through the PAPVR constituting a significant left-to-right shunt. Today, angiography is hardly ever necessary to establish the diagnosis. (Right) Coronal CTA (MIP image) of a patient with scimitar syndrome shows the anomalous pulmonary vein ➡ coursing inferomedially and across the diaphragm to drain into the inferior vena cava.

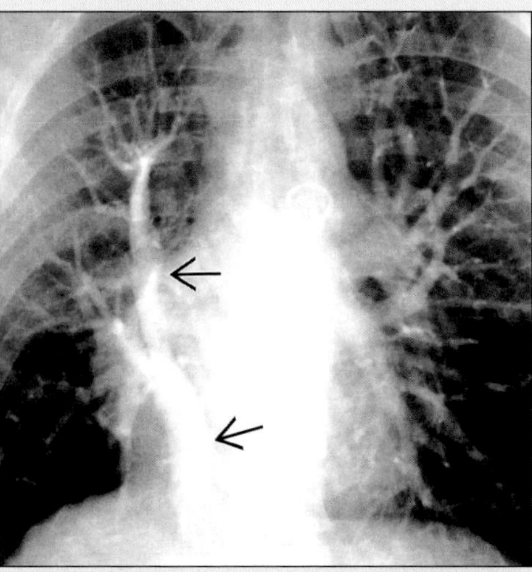

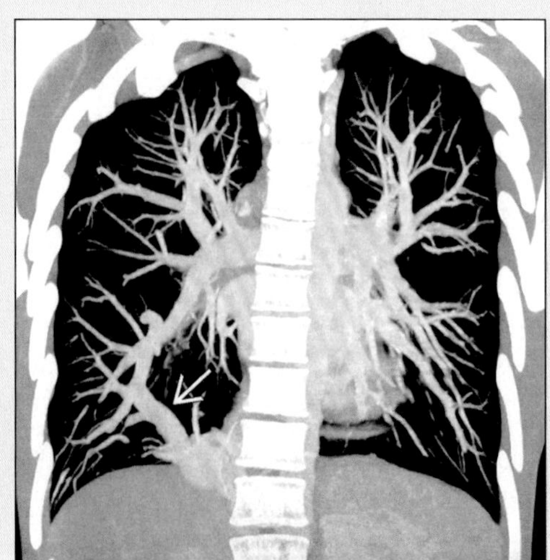

SCIMITAR SYNDROME

TERMINOLOGY

Synonyms

- **Hypogenetic lung syndrome**
- **Pulmonary venolobar syndrome**

Definitions

- **Partial or total anomalous pulmonary venous return of right lung to inferior vena cava just above or below diaphragm**
- Infantile & pediatric/adult variants
- Associated abnormalities in descending frequency
  - Abnormal right lung lobation & right lung hypoplasia (~ 100%)
  - Dextroposition of heart; right pulmonary artery hypoplasia (60%)
  - Systemic arterialization of right lower lung (60%)
  - Secundum atrial septal defect (ASD) (40% overall, 80-90% in infantile variant)
  - Right diaphragmatic hernia (15%)
  - Infantile form: Ventricular septal defect, patent ductus, hypoplastic aortic arch, coarctation, tetralogy of Fallot, anomalous origin of left coronary artery, truncus arteriosus

IMAGING

General Features

- Best diagnostic clue
  - Curved vertical vein paralleling right heart border directed toward midline
  - Shaped like Turkish sword (or scimitar)
- Location
  - Majority are right sided
  - Left-sided scimitar (extremely rare); drains into IVC
- Size
  - Variable

Radiographic Findings

- Radiography
  - **Partial anomalous pulmonary venous return** (PAPVR), 75%
    - Gently curved tubular opacity (**scimitar vein**) descending from right mid-lung toward midline, paralleling right heart border
    - Vein broadens as it courses inferiorly toward diaphragm
    - **Scimitar vein only seen in 50% of patients overall**, 70% of pediatric/adult, & 10% of infantile
      - Less conspicuous small, multiple, or obscured veins in the rest
  - **Cardiovascular findings**
    - Small right hilum
    - Shift of cardiomediastinal silhouette to right (dextroposition)
    - Rotation of cardiomediastinal silhouette to right; retrosternal band-like interface on lateral chest radiograph
  - **Pulmonary findings**
    - No lung abnormalities (10%)
    - Small right hemithorax (hypoplasia), lung may be hyperlucent
    - Reticular opacities may be seen with recurrent infection & bronchiectasis
  - Other: Elevated hemidiaphragm

CT Findings

- CECT
  - PAPVR
    - **Visualization of course & drainage of anomalous pulmonary vein**
    - **Drainage to infradiaphragmatic IVC (more common)**
  - Cardiovascular findings
    - Pulmonary artery may be normal, hypoplastic, or absent
    - Dilated right heart in left-to-right shunts
    - Enlarged pulmonary trunk (pulmonary hypertension)
    - Systemic arterialization of lung from descending aorta or upper abdominal aorta
  - Pulmonary findings
    - **Right hypoplastic lung**
    - Mosaic perfusion of hypoplastic lung
    - Bronchiectasis from recurrent infection
    - Absent minor fissure & left bronchial isomerism
    - Horseshoe lung: Lung bridge fusing lungs across posterior mediastinum; association with lethal cardiac anomalies

MR Findings

- **Equivalent to CT for characterization of scimitar vein**
- Superior to CT for assessment of congenital heart disease & aortic hypoplasia
- Allows shunt quantification, QP/QS with velocity encoding sequences
- Disadvantages: Less useful for assessment of lung or bronchial anatomy

Echocardiographic Findings

- 1st approach to diagnosis & postsurgical follow-up
- Evaluation of shunts & estimation of pulmonary artery pressure

Angiographic Findings

- Gold standard for diagnosis, pressure measurements, & determination of size of left-to-right shunt

Imaging Recommendations

- Best imaging tool
  - CT & MR for assessment of morphologic features including lung abnormalities
- Protocol advice
  - MR must include angiography with gadolinium & velocity-encoding imaging for shunt quantification
  - CTA allows comprehensive morphologic characterization

DIFFERENTIAL DIAGNOSIS

Unilateral Absence of Pulmonary Artery

- Also associated with pulmonary hypoplasia
- No vertical (scimitar) vein
- Normal bronchial branching

Pulmonary Sequestration

- Systemic supply to sequestered lung, usually from descending or abdominal aorta
- No vertical (scimitar) vein
- Normal venous drainage in intralobar sequestration

SCIMITAR SYNDROME

Meandering Pulmonary Vein

- Anatomic variant
- Pulmonary vein "meanders" in lung but drains normally into left atrium

PATHOLOGY

General Features

- Etiology
  - Congenital
- Genetics
  - Sporadic (most)
  - Autosomal dominant (some cases)
- Associated abnormalities
  - **Cardiovascular anomalies in infantile form**
    - Atrial septal defect (80%)
    - Patent ductus arteriosus (75%)
    - Ventricular septal defect (30%)
    - Pulmonic stenosis (20%)
    - Aortic coarctation
    - Subaortic stenosis
    - Aortic arch hypoplasia
    - Tetralogy of Fallot
    - Persistent left superior vena cava
  - **Cardiovascular anomalies in pediatric/adult form**
    - Atrial septal defect, ostium secundum (20%)
    - Patent ductus arteriosus
    - Other: Persistent left SVC, coronary artery fistula, azygos continuation of inferior vena cava, cor triatrium
  - Airway anomalies: Bronchiectasis, left bronchial isomerism, hypoplasia/anomalies of segmentation of right bronchial tree
  - Vertebral anomalies: Hemivertebra, scoliosis
  - Other: Bronchogenic cyst, accessory diaphragm, diaphragmatic hernia, horseshoe lung

Gross Pathologic & Surgical Features

- Typically single scimitar vein, occasionally multiple
- Scimitar vein drains right lung
  - Entire lung (2/3 of all cases)
  - Right lower lobe (1/3 of cases)
- Course of scimitar vein: Anterior to right hilum
- Scimitar drainage
  - Infradiaphragmatic IVC (most common)
  - Less common: Hepatic veins, portal vein, azygos vein, coronary sinus, right atrium
- Lung morphology
  - Lobar agenesis to focal hypoplasia: Equal incidence of uni-, bi-, & trilobar right lung
- Pulmonary arterial supply
  - Absent, hypoplastic, or normal right pulmonary artery
  - Systemic supply from thoracic or abdominal aorta to right lower lobe

CLINICAL ISSUES

Presentation

- Most common signs/symptoms
  - Infantile form
    - Severe tachypnea, cyanosis, & congestive heart failure from left-to-right shunt, resulting in failure to thrive
    - Diagnosed within 1st months of age
  - Pediatric/adult form
    - Absent or mild symptoms
      - Frequently asymptomatic
      - Recurrent pneumonia, mild dyspnea, or increased fatigue
    - Hemoptysis may occur with left-to-right shunt due to bronchial wall varices
    - Diagnosed within first 3 decades
- Other signs/symptoms
  - Infantile form
    - Average QP/QS is > 3.0
  - Pediatric/adult form
    - Mild deficits in vital capacity and FEV1 (~ 80% of predicted)
    - Average QP/QS is 2.0

Demographics

- Age
  - Bimodal: Infantile & pediatric/adult forms
- Gender
  - M:F = 1:2
- Epidemiology
  - 1-3 cases per 100,000 births

Natural History & Prognosis

- Infantile form: Significant mortality, poor prognosis without treatment
- Pediatric/adult form: Milder form, good prognosis

Treatment

- In absence of pulmonary hypertension, medical treatment during infancy allows growth before surgical repair
- Indications for surgical treatment
  - Coexistent ASD, pulmonary hypertension, stenosis of scimitar vein
  - Symptomatic patients & asymptomatic patients with QP:QS shunt > 1.5:1

DIAGNOSTIC CHECKLIST

Image Interpretation Pearls

- Triad of respiratory distress, right lung hypoplasia, & heart dextroposition should suggest scimitar syndrome
- Scimitar vein may be subtle, identification requires careful evaluation of small hyperlucent right hemithorax

SELECTED REFERENCES

1. Korkmaz AA et al: Scimitar syndrome: a complex form of anomalous pulmonary venous return. J Card Surg. 26(5):529-34, 2011
2. Midyat L et al: Eponym. Scimitar syndrome. Eur J Pediatr. 169(10):1171-7, 2010

SCIMITAR SYNDROME

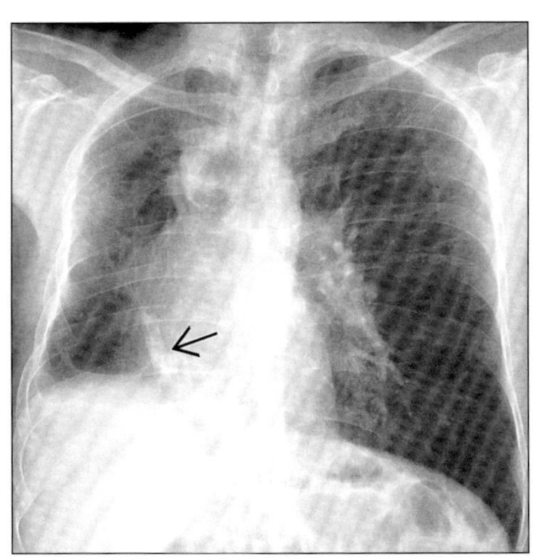

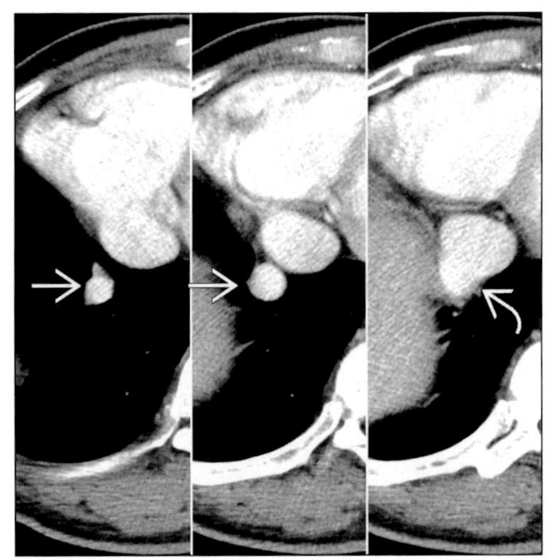

(Left) *PA chest radiograph of a patient with scimitar syndrome shows a small hypoplastic right lung, dextroposition of the heart, and a scimitar vein → paralleling the right cardiac border. The scimitar vein constitutes a form of partial anomalous venous return.* ***(Right)*** *Axial CTA of the same patient demonstrates the scimitar vein → and its drainage ↪ into the inferior vena cava. Less commonly, a scimitar vein may drain into the hepatic, portal, or azygos veins.*

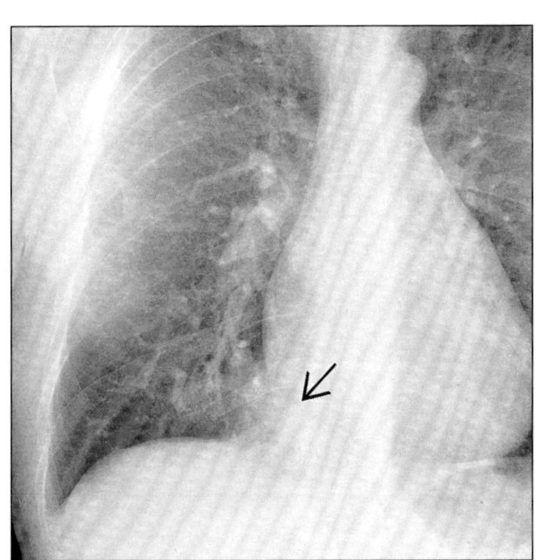

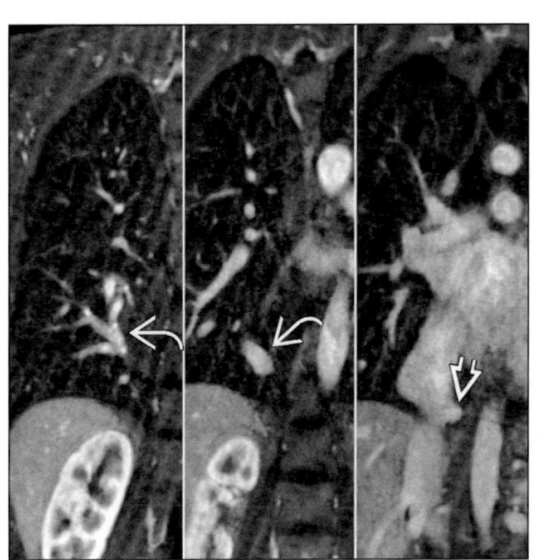

(Left) *PA chest radiograph of an adult patient with scimitar syndrome shows a scimitar vein → but no evidence of right pulmonary hypoplasia.* ***(Right)*** *Coronal MRA of the same patient shows the anomalous pulmonary vein ↪ draining the right lower lobe and anastomosing with the infradiaphragmatic inferior vena cava ⇨. While frequently associated with pulmonary hypoplasia, milder forms of scimitar syndrome occur without associated right pulmonary hypoplasia.*

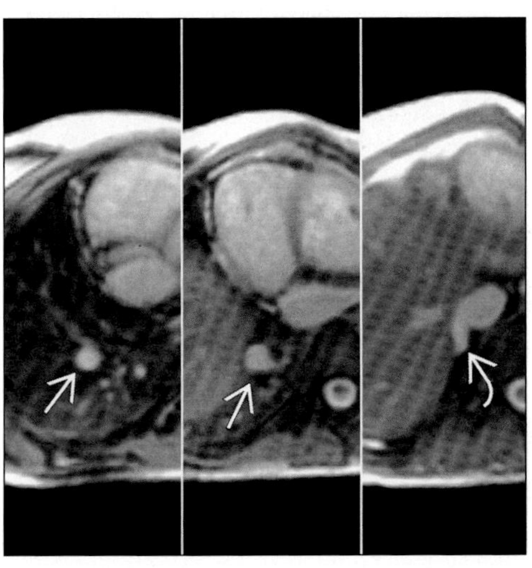

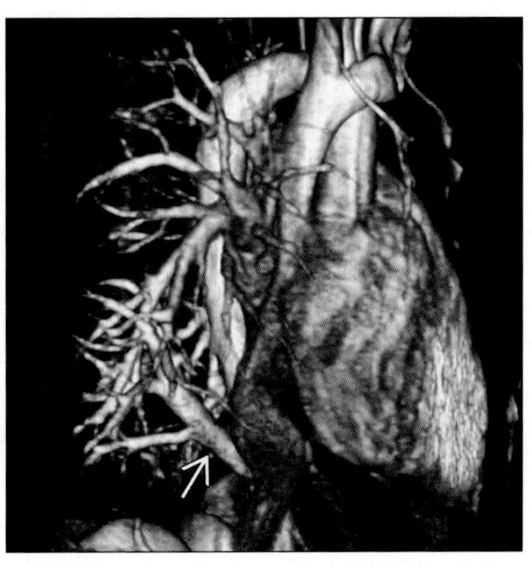

(Left) *Axial SSFP (bright blood) MR of a patient with scimitar syndrome shows the scimitar vein → draining into the infradiaphragmatic IVC ↪.* ***(Right)*** *Coronal MRA 3D reconstruction of the same patient shows the right lower lobe scimitar vein → as it courses inferomedially to drain into the inferior aspect of the IVC. Angiographic techniques are superb in depicting morphologic features of scimitar syndrome.*

PULMONARY VARIX

Key Facts

Terminology

- Synonyms
  - Pulmonary venous aneurysm
- Definition: Nonobstructive dilatation of 1 or more pulmonary veins at insertion into left atrium
  - May be an isolated radiologic finding

Imaging

- Radiography
  - Left atrial enlargement (LAE)
  - Soft tissue opacity adjacent to LAE in expected location of pulmonary vein
- CT
  - Enlarged confluence of pulmonary vein(s)
  - Maximum enhancement during pulmonary venous phase
  - May be dilated 2-3x normal venous diameter
  - No soft tissue mass

Top Differential Diagnoses

- Unilateral common pulmonary vein
- Arteriovenous malformation
- Pericardial recess
- Lung cancer
- Intralobar sequestration

Clinical Issues

- Symptoms/signs
  - Most patients are asymptomatic; associated with mitral valve disease & pulmonary venous hypertension
  - Incidental imaging finding
- Treatment
  - Not clinically significant
  - Typically no therapy or follow-up needed
  - Surgical repair if progressive increase in size

*(**Left**) PA chest radiograph of a 65-year-old man with known coronary artery disease and ischemic cardiomyopathy shows postsurgical changes of CABG, a left pectoral dual chamber biventricular implanted cardiac defibrillator (ICD), cardiomegaly, pulmonary hypertension, and mild interstitial edema. (**Right**) Lateral chest radiograph of the same patient demonstrates a dense retrocardiac opacity ➔, likely related to the left atrial enlargement and confluence of the inferior pulmonary veins.*

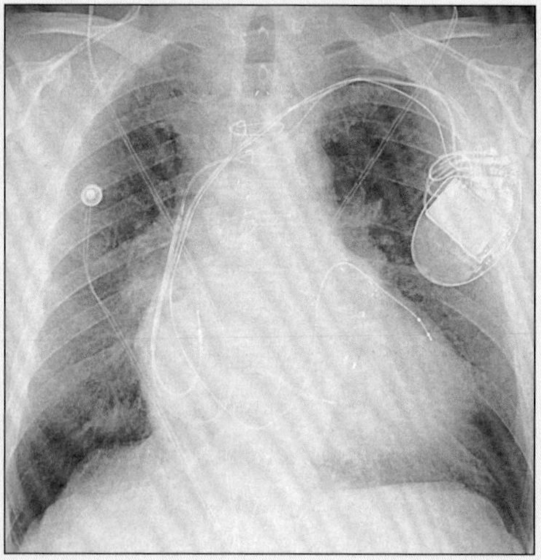

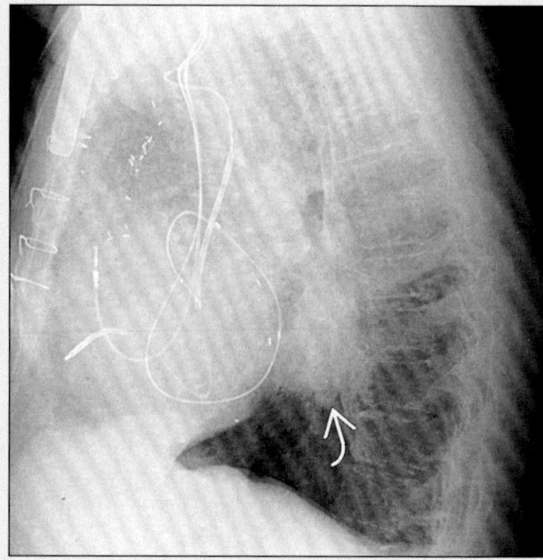

*(**Left**) Axial CECT of the same patient shows left atrial enlargement and a large varix ➔ of the right inferior pulmonary vein. (**Right**) Coronal CECT maximum-intensity projection (MIP) image of the same patient shows the right inferior pulmonary vein varix ➔ and associated left atrial enlargement.*

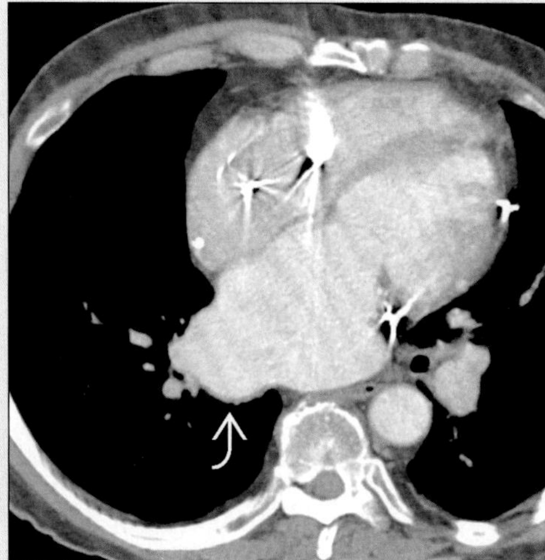

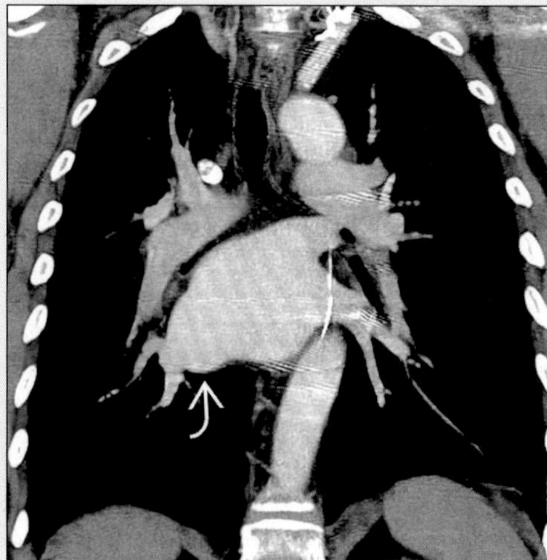

PULMONARY VARIX

TERMINOLOGY

Synonyms

- Pulmonary venous aneurysm

Definitions

- Nonobstructive dilatation of 1 or more pulmonary veins at insertion into left atrium (LA)
- May be isolated radiologic finding
- Typically associated with acquired heart disease (e.g., mitral stenosis ± regurgitation)
- No enlarged feeding artery or soft tissue mass
- May be mistaken for mediastinal or hilar mass

IMAGING

General Features

- Best diagnostic clue
  - Left atrial enlargement (LAE) & enlarged confluence of pulmonary vein(s)
- Location
  - Typically affects an inferior pulmonary vein
- Size
  - May be dilated 2-3x normal venous diameter
- Morphology
  - Fusiform dilatation of 1 of major central pulmonary veins
    - At insertion into left atrium

Radiographic Findings

- Radiography
  - Soft tissue opacity adjacent to LAE in expected location of pulmonary vein

CT Findings

- CECT
  - Maximum enhancement during pulmonary venous phase
  - No soft tissue mass

Imaging Recommendations

- Best imaging tool
  - Contrast-enhanced CT is imaging modality of choice
- Protocol advice
  - Administer contrast to evaluate right & left cardiac chambers

DIFFERENTIAL DIAGNOSIS

Unilateral Common Pulmonary Vein

- Superior & inferior pulmonary veins share common insertion into LA; a normal variant

Arteriovenous Malformation

- Feeding artery & large draining pulmonary vein

Pericardial Recess

- Water attenuation collection around inferior pulmonary vein
  - No encasement or soft tissue component

Lung Cancer

- May arise adjacent to &/or invade a pulmonary vein

Intralobar Sequestration

- Draining vein empties into pulmonary vein
- Systemic feeding artery

Cor Triatriatum

- LA divided into 2 chambers by fibromuscular band
  - Pulmonary veins drain into upper portion
  - Associated congenital heart disease

PATHOLOGY

Staging, Grading, & Classification

- Histologically benign

Gross Pathologic & Surgical Features

- Dilated pulmonary vein at insertion of LA

CLINICAL ISSUES

Presentation

- Most common signs/symptoms
  - Most patients are asymptomatic
  - Incidental imaging finding
- Other signs/symptoms
  - Associated with acquired heart disease
    - Mitral valve disease, typically stenosis
    - Pulmonary venous hypertension
  - Rarely congenital

Natural History & Prognosis

- Not clinically significant
- Not to be confused with mediastinal or hilar mass
- Rupture is rare
- Size may decrease following treatment of pulmonary venous hypertension

Treatment

- Typically no treatment required
- Surgical repair if progressive increase in size

DIAGNOSTIC CHECKLIST

Image Interpretation Pearls

- Enlarged pulmonary vein with acquired heart disease
- May decrease with Valsalva & enlarge with Müller maneuvers

Reporting Tips

- Finding of no clinical significance in most cases

SELECTED REFERENCES

1. Sirivella S et al: Pulmonary venous aneurysm presenting as a mediastinal mass in ischemic cardiomyopathy. Ann Thorac Surg. 68(1):241-3, 1999
2. Bhaktaram VJ et al: Large pulmonary vein varix diagnosed by transesophageal echocardiography: an unusual site for thrombus in atrial fibrillation. J Am Soc Echocardiogr. 11(2):213-5, 1998
3. Twersky J et al: Further observations on pulmonary venous varix. AJR Am J Roentgenol. 127(3):435-40, 1976

Key Facts

Terminology

- Accessory fissure surrounding portion of right upper lobe (RUL)

Imaging

- Radiography
  - Azygos fissure: Thin curvilinear opacity convex toward chest wall extending from right tracheobronchial angle to right lung apex
  - Azygos vein: Ovoid, tear-shaped opacity in inferior aspect of accessory fissure
  - Trigone: Triangular opacity that marks superior aspect of azygos fissure
- CT findings
  - Arcuate linear opacity extending from posterolateral aspect of upper thoracic spine to superior vena cava (SVC)
  - Traverses lung before entering SVC

Top Differential Diagnoses

- Enlarged paratracheal lymph nodes
- Tortuous supraaortic vessels
- Right upper lobe atelectasis

Pathology

- Failure of normal azygos vein migration over right lung apex

Clinical Issues

- Azygos fissure: Seen in 1% of individuals

Diagnostic Checklist

- Enlarged azygos vein should prompt
  - Exclusion of elevated central venous pressure
  - Vena cava obstruction
  - Heterotaxy syndrome
- Dense lung medial to fissure does not signify underlying disease

*(**Left**) PA chest radiograph (coned down to the right upper lobe) shows an accessory azygos fissure manifesting as a thin curvilinear opacity ➡, extending obliquely across the right apex and terminating in a teardrop-shaped opacity ➡ caused by the azygos arch. Note the triangular-shaped "trigone" ➡ at the cranial aspect of the fissure. (**Right**) Coronal CECT shows the "trigone" ➡, the azygos fissure ➡, and a partially calcified azygos arch ➡.*

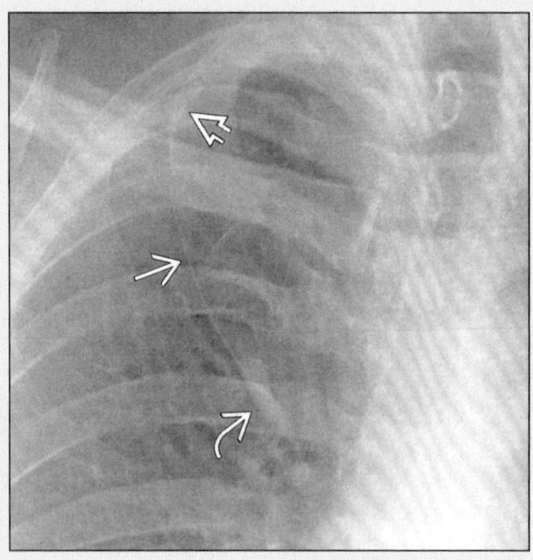

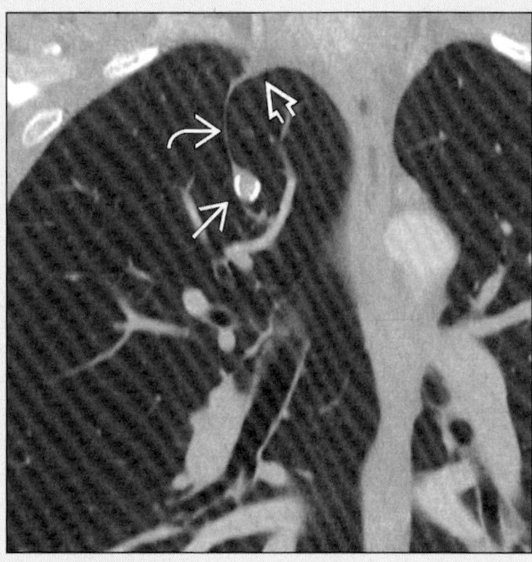

*(**Left**) Composite image with axial CECT in lung (left) and soft tissue window (right) shows the azygos arch coursing within the inferior aspect of the accessory azygos fissure and draining into the superior vena cava. (**Right**) Coronal CECT of a patient with a right pneumothorax shows air surrounding the 2 parietal pleura components ➡ of the accessory azygos fissure and the azygos arch ➡ at the inferior aspect of the fissure. The visceral pleura components have "fallen away" from the fissure.*

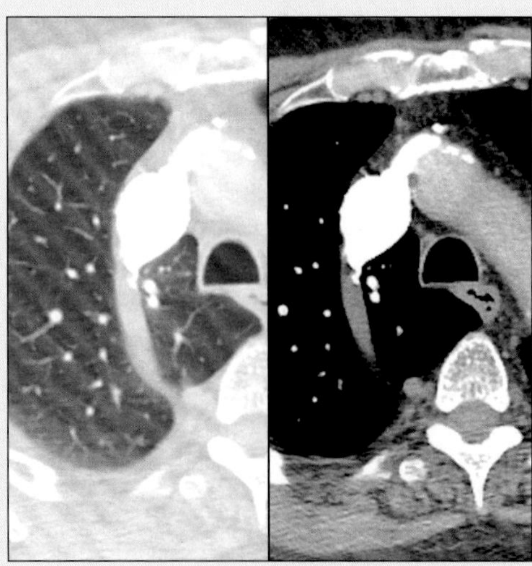

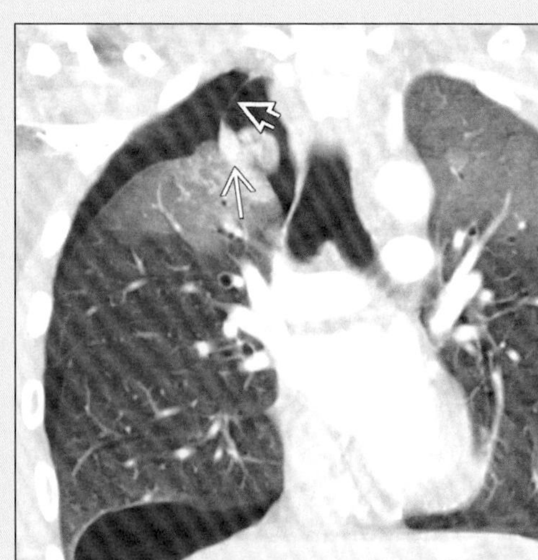

ACCESSORY AZYGOS FISSURE

TERMINOLOGY

Synonyms

- Azygos fissure

Definitions

- Accessory fissure surrounding portion of right upper lobe (RUL); lobe is supplied by branches of apical segmental bronchus
- Variable size
- **Anomalous intrapulmonary course of azygos vein creating an accessory fissure**
  - **4 layers of pleura** invaginating into lung apex
  - **Trigone**
    - Most cranial part of fissure (triangular shape)
    - Determines size of lung medial to fissure
  - Contains azygos vein within its lower margin

IMAGING

Imaging Recommendations

- Azygos vein: Oval opacity normally occupying right tracheobronchial angle

Radiographic Findings

- **Azygos fissure**: Thin curvilinear opacity convex toward chest wall extending from right tracheobronchial angle to right lung apex
- **Azygos vein**: Ovoid, tear-shaped opacity in inferior aspect of accessory fissure
- **Trigone**: Triangular opacity that marks superior aspect of azygos fissure
- Lung limited by fissure is normally aerated
- Increased density of lung medial to fissure may be seen
  - Overlapping tortuous supraaortic vessels
  - Increased thickness of upper mediastinal soft tissues
  - Young infants: Thymus

CT Findings

- Arcuate linear opacity extending from posterolateral aspect of upper thoracic spine to superior vena cava (SVC)
- Traverses lung before entering SVC
- Useful for excluding pulmonary pathology medial to accessory fissure
- Azygos vein calcification
- **Migration of azygos vein to mediastinum**
  - Associated with pneumothorax
  - Disappearance of fissure

DIFFERENTIAL DIAGNOSIS

Enlarged Paratracheal Lymph Nodes

- Widening of right paratracheal stripe

Tortuous Supraaortic Vessels

- Wide mediastinum without tracheal displacement

Right Upper Lobe Atelectasis

- Elevated minor fissure
- Secondary signs of volume loss: Tracheal shift, elevated right hilum, elevated right hemidiaphragm (often with juxtaphrenic peak)

PATHOLOGY

General Features

- Etiology
  - Failure of normal azygos vein migration over right lung apex
- Associated abnormalities
  - Dense lung medial to azygos fissure
    - Potential diagnostic pitfall
    - May simulate pathology
  - Azygos vein dilatation
    - Elevated central venous pressure: Cardiac decompensation, tricuspid stenosis, acute pericardial tamponade, constrictive pericarditis
    - Intrahepatic & extrahepatic portal vein obstruction
    - Anomalous pulmonary venous drainage
    - Polysplenia syndrome
      - Polysplenia, azygos continuation of IVC, left superior vena cava, left thoracic isomerism, abdominal heterotaxy, short pancreas
    - Acquired occlusion of SVC or inferior vena cava (IVC)
  - Azygos vein calcification
  - Azygos vein migration to normal position in mediastinum
    - Pneumothorax
    - Shorter fissures
  - Vanishing azygos fissure
    - Apical pulmonary fibrosis may retract fissure upward (short fissure)

CLINICAL ISSUES

Presentation

- Most common signs/symptoms
  - None; usually incidental radiographic finding

Demographics

- Epidemiology
  - Azygos fissure: Seen in 1% of individuals

DIAGNOSTIC CHECKLIST

Image Interpretation Pearls

- Dense lung medial to fissure does not signify underlying disease
- Enlarged azygos vein should prompt exclusion of elevated central venous pressure
  - Obstruction of vena cava
  - Heterotaxy (polysplenia syndrome & azygos continuation)
    - Lateral chest radiograph: Absence of retrocardiac IVC interface

SELECTED REFERENCES

1. Villanueva A et al: Migrating azygos vein and vanishing azygos lobe: MDCT findings. AJR Am J Roentgenol. 194(3):599-603, 2010
2. Maldjian PD et al: The empty azygos fissure: sign of an escaped azygos vein. J Thorac Imaging. 23(1):54-6, 2008
3. Shin MS et al: Clinical significance of azygos vein enlargement: radiographic recognition and etiologic analysis. Clin Imaging. 23(4):236-40, 1999

Key Facts

Terminology

- IVC interrupted above renal veins, hepatic veins drain into right atrium, azygos vein carries venous return from lower extremities

Imaging

- Radiography
  - Focal enlargement of azygos arch in right tracheobronchial angle
  - Dilated if > 10 mm diameter in erect position
  - Bilateral left lungs & bronchi with heterotaxy
- CT
  - Absent suprarenal & intrahepatic portions of IVC
  - Hepatic veins enter directly into right atrium
  - Dilated azygos courses upward & drains to SVC
  - Dilated hemiazygos in hemiazygos continuation
  - Polysplenia heterotaxy syndrome

Top Differential Diagnoses

- Azygos enlargement from SVC obstruction
- Azygos enlargement from pulmonary artery hypertension
- Azygos enlargement from high volume states
- Enlargement of azygos-region lymph node
- Intrahepatic IVC occlusion by tumor/thrombus

Clinical Issues

- Often asymptomatic
- Symptoms related to congenital heart disease
- Prognosis related to associated anomalies
- If inadvertently ligated at surgery, may be lethal

Diagnostic Checklist

- Difficulties may arise during catheter-based intervention through IVC, such as right heart catheterization

__(Left)__ Graphic shows characteristic features of azygos continuation. The inferior vena cava is absent, the hepatic veins drain directly into the right atrium, and the azygos vein ➡ is enlarged and provides the main venous drainage below the diaphragm. Identification of azygos continuation is vital in surgical planning to avoid inadvertent surgical ligation of the azygos vein. __(Right)__ PA chest radiograph shows enlargement of the azygos arch ➡ in this patient with azygos continuation of the IVC.

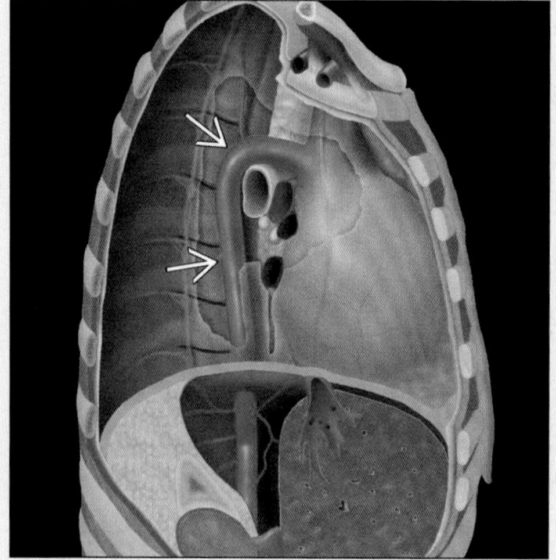

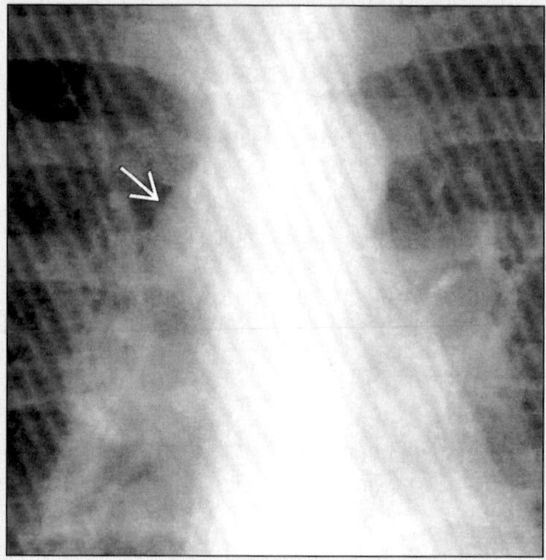

__(Left)__ Axial CECT of a patient with azygos continuation of the inferior vena cava shows an enlarged azygos arch ➡. __(Right)__ Axial CECT of the abdomen of the same patient shows the enlarged azygous vein ⇨ and heterotaxy with a midline liver, a right-sided stomach ➡, and polysplenia ➡. Azygos continuation of the inferior vena cava is associated with heterotaxy syndrome.

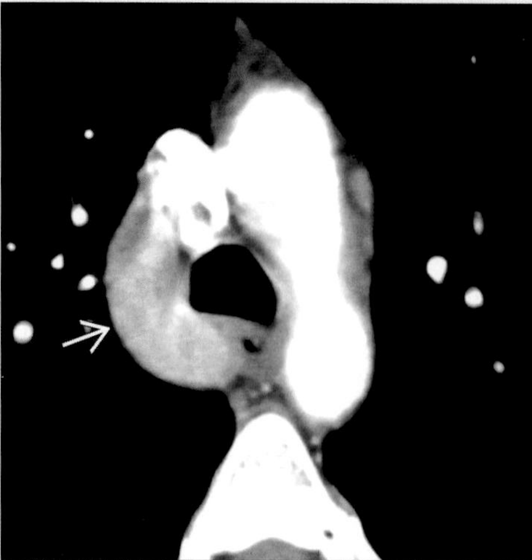

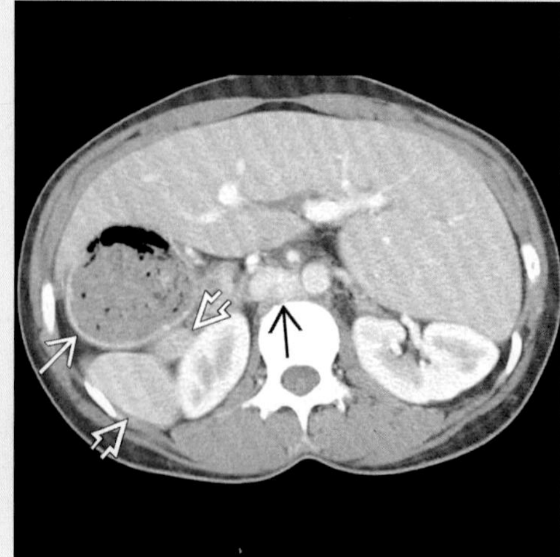

AZYGOS AND HEMIAZYGOS CONTINUATION OF THE IVC

TERMINOLOGY

Synonyms

- **Azygos continuation of inferior vena cava (IVC)**
- **Interruption of IVC**
- Absence of hepatic segment of IVC with azygos continuation

Definitions

- IVC interrupted above renal veins
- Hepatic veins drain directly into right atrium
- Large azygos vein carries venous return from lower extremities
  - Occasionally, a large hemiazygos vein carries venous return
- Caused by persistence of embryonic right supracardinal vein & failure of development of suprarenal part of subcardinal vein
- Associated with congenital heart disease & situs abnormalities, especially polysplenia (heterotaxy syndrome)

IMAGING

General Features

- Best diagnostic clue
  - Absence of intrahepatic segment of IVC with dilated azygos or hemiazygos vein on contrast-enhanced CT
- Size
  - Azygos arch located in right tracheobronchial angle
    - Dilatation: > 10 mm short-axis diameter in erect position
    - Dilatation: > 15 mm short-axis diameter in supine position

Radiographic Findings

- Posteroanterior (PA)
  - **Focal enlargement of azygos arch in right tracheobronchial angle**
    - Round or oval shape
    - Considered dilated when > 10 mm diameter in erect position
    - Considered dilated when > 15 mm diameter in supine position
  - **Visualization of azygos vein interface**
  - Visualization of aortic nipple may occur with hemiazygos continuation
  - **Bilateral left lungs & bronchi if associated with polysplenia**
  - Transverse or transposed liver if associated with polysplenia
- Lateral
  - Thickening of retroesophageal stripe
  - Absence of retrocardiac IVC interface (sometimes)
  - Suprahepatic portions of IVC may be present

CT Findings

- CECT
  - Absent suprarenal & intrahepatic portion of IVC
  - Hepatic veins enter directly into right atrium
  - **Large posterior, paraspinal vessel corresponding to azygos (right) or hemiazygos (left) continuation**
  - Dilated azygos courses upward & drains into SVC
    - Look for dilated azygos arch
  - Dilated hemiazygos courses upward
    - Typically drains into a left SVC with a dilated coronary sinus
    - May cross midline and join azygos vein
    - Rarely drains to accessory hemiazygos, left superior intercostal, & left brachiocephalic veins
    - Look for dilated left-sided venous arch lateral to aorta in typical drainage
  - **Polysplenia findings (heterotaxy)**
    - Multiple spleens
    - Situs ambiguus
    - Bilateral bilobed (left-sided morphology) lungs
    - Bilateral hyparterial (left-sided morphology) bronchi
    - Congenital heart disease (especially atrial septal defect, ventricular septal defect)
    - Midline or transposed abdominal viscera, intestinal malrotation, preduodenal portal vein, truncated pancreas

MR Findings

- T1WI
  - Absent suprarenal & intrahepatic portion of IVC
  - Hepatic veins enter directly into right atrium
  - Large posterior, paraspinal vessel corresponding to azygos (right) or hemiazygos (left) continuation
  - Dilated azygos courses upward & drains to SVC
    - Look for dilated azygos arch
  - Dilated hemiazygos courses upward along left side of spine
    - Typically drains to left SVC with dilated coronary sinus
    - May cross midline & join azygos
    - Rarely drains to accessory hemiazygos vein, left superior intercostal vein, & left brachiocephalic vein
    - Look for dilated left-sided venous arch lateral to aorta in typical drainage
  - Polysplenia findings identical to CT findings
    - Multiple spleens
    - Situs ambiguus
- MRA
  - Azygos continuation, interrupted IVC observed on venous phase

Imaging Recommendations

- Best imaging tool
  - Contrast-enhanced CT is imaging study of choice to evaluate azygos continuation

DIFFERENTIAL DIAGNOSIS

Enlargement of Azygos Arch & Vein Due to Superior Vena Cava (SVC) Obstruction

- Distal occlusion of SVC by mass or thrombosis
- Azygos serves as collateral pathway
- Normal IVC

Enlargement of Azygos Arch Due to Pulmonary Artery Hypertension

- Dilated right heart chambers & SVC
- Enlarged central pulmonary arteries
- Normal IVC

AZYGOS AND HEMIAZYGOS CONTINUATION OF THE IVC

Enlargement of Azygos Arch Due to High Volume States

- Enlarged heart & increased pulmonary vessels
- Normal or dilated IVC
- Seen with pregnancy, sickle cell disease, renal disease

Enlargement of Azygos-region Lymph Node

- Azygos arch & vein normal & separate from node
- Normal IVC

Occlusion of Intrahepatic IVC Due to Tumor or Thrombosis

- Liver mass, especially hepatocellular carcinoma, which grows intravascularly
- Infrahepatic IVC normal

Double Aortic Arch

- Azygos arch & vein normal
- IVC normal

PATHOLOGY

General Features

- Etiology
  - Persistence of embryonic right supracardinal vein
  - Failure of development of suprarenal part of subcardinal vein
- Genetics
  - Sporadic
- Associated abnormalities
  - **Polysplenia**
    - Bilateral hyparterial bronchi & bilobed lungs
    - Midline liver
    - Multiple spleens
    - Congenital heart disease: Atrial & ventricular septal defects
  - Rare in asplenia

Gross Pathologic & Surgical Features

- Complicates surgical planning for
  - Esophagectomy
  - Liver transplantation
  - IVC filter placement
  - Abdominal aortic aneurysm repair

CLINICAL ISSUES

Presentation

- Most common signs/symptoms
  - Often asymptomatic
- Other signs/symptoms
  - Symptoms related to congenital heart disease
  - May be associated with sick sinus syndrome

Demographics

- Age
  - Variable, often discovered incidentally
  - Early in life if associated with severe congenital heart disease
- Gender
  - No predilection
- Epidemiology
  - Prevalence < 0.6%
  - 0.2-4.3% of cardiac catheterizations for congenital heart disease

Natural History & Prognosis

- Related to associated anomalies, particularly congenital heart disease
- If inadvertently ligated at surgery, may be lethal

Treatment

- Related to associated anomalies, particularly congenital heart disease
- May complicate surgical procedures such as liver transplantation

DIAGNOSTIC CHECKLIST

Consider

- Difficulties may arise during catheter-based intervention through IVC such as right heart catheterization

Image Interpretation Pearls

- Lateral chest radiograph may not show absence of retrocardiac IVC interface due to drainage of hepatic veins in that location

SELECTED REFERENCES

1. Yildirim A et al: An unusual case of heterotaxy and polysplenia syndrome associated with hemiazygous continuation of the left-sided vena cava inferior, dilated azygous vein and large venous ectasia. Congenit Heart Dis. 6(3):262-5, 2011
2. Mamidipally S et al: Azygous continuation of inferior vena cava. J Am Coll Cardiol. 56(21):e41, 2010
3. Demos TC et al: Venous anomalies of the thorax. AJR Am J Roentgenol. 182(5):1139-50, 2004
4. Yilmaz E et al: Interruption of the inferior vena cava with azygos/hemiazygos continuation accompanied by distinct renal vein anomalies: MRA and CT assessment. Abdom Imaging. 28(3):392-4, 2003
5. Bass JE et al: Spectrum of congenital anomalies of the inferior vena cava: cross-sectional imaging findings. Radiographics. 20(3):639-52, 2000
6. Gayer G et al: Polysplenia syndrome detected in adulthood: report of eight cases and review of the literature. Abdom Imaging. 24(2):178-84, 1999

AZYGOS AND HEMIAZYGOS CONTINUATION OF THE IVC

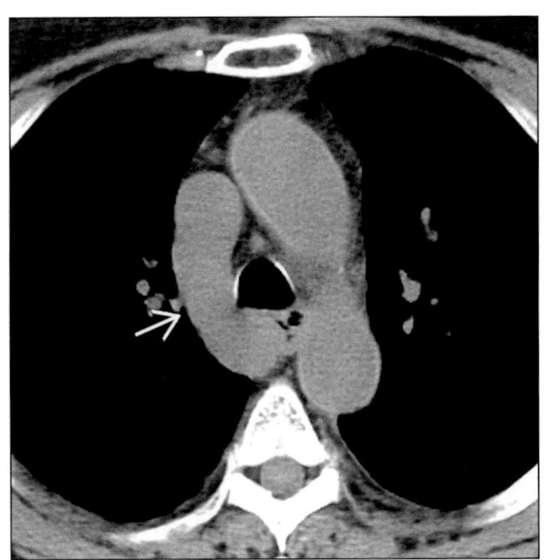

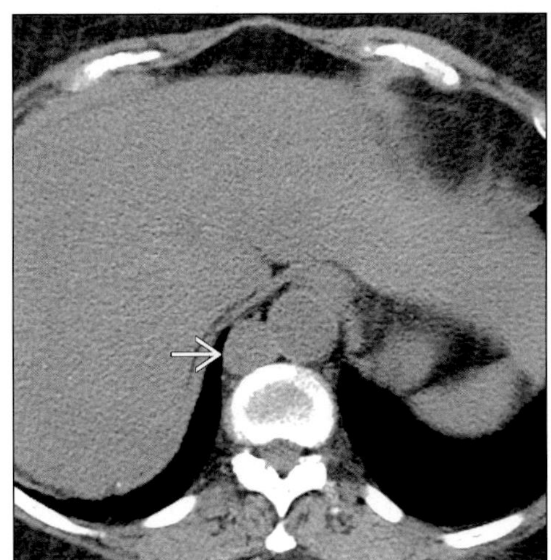

(Left) *Axial NECT shows an enlarged azygos vein* ➔ *in this case of azygos continuation of the IVC. Acquired obstruction of the IVC could also result in dilatation of the azygos vein and should be excluded.* ***(Right)*** *Axial NECT of the same patient shows the typical appearance of the enlarged azygos vein* ➔ *coursing alongside the descending aorta. Azygos continuation of the IVC is typically easily recognized on CT studies even in the absence of intravenous contrast.*

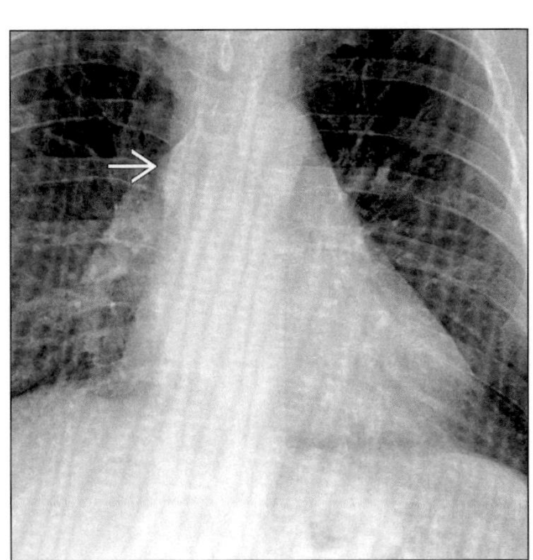

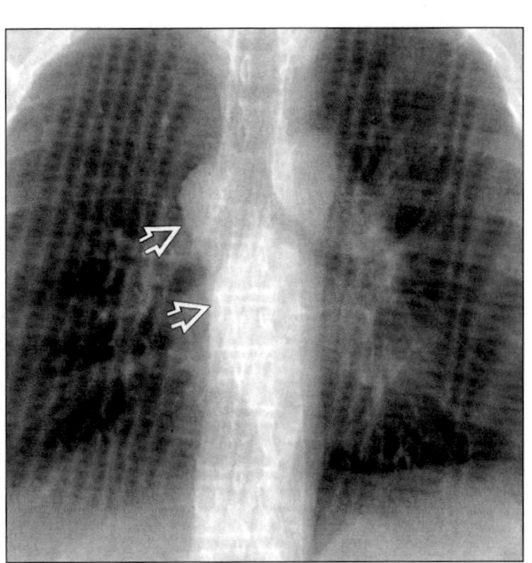

(Left) *PA chest radiograph of a patient with azygos continuation shows an enlarged azygos vein* ➔ *and nonvisualization of the superior aspect of the azygoesophageal recess.* ***(Right)*** *Coronal NECT thick MPR average shows the dilated azygos vein* ⇨ *as it courses obliquely across the superior aspect of the azygoesophageal recess, explaining the obliteration of the superior aspect of the recess on frontal chest radiography.*

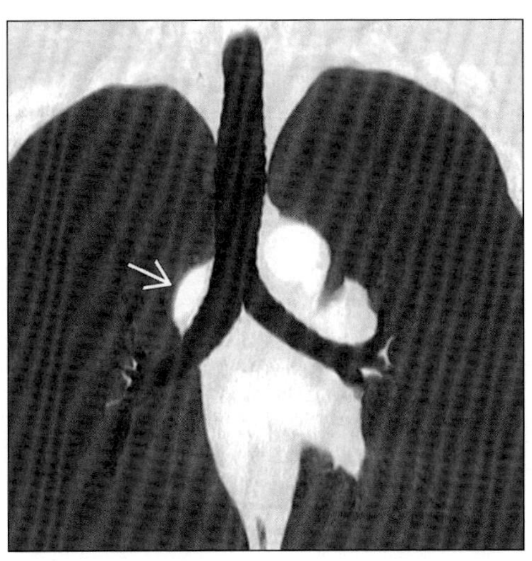

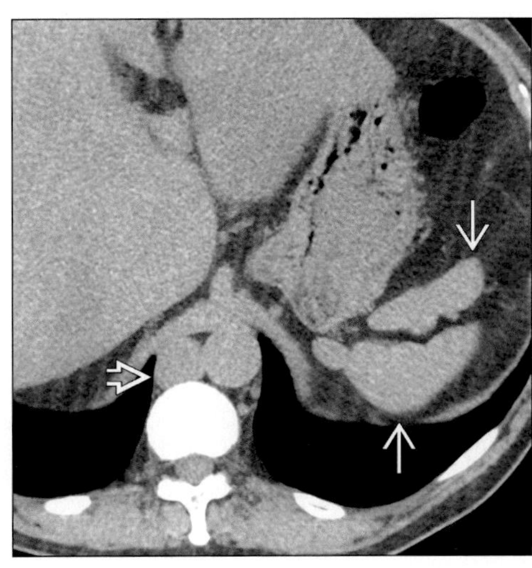

(Left) *Coronal MinIP reformation shows bilateral left-sided bronchi and an enlarged azygos arch* ➔ *in this patient with azygos continuation of the IVC. The lungs were bilobed (not shown). Airway anatomy is shown in high detail using thick MinIP reformatted images.* ***(Right)*** *Axial NECT of the same patient shows the dilated azygos vein* ⇨ *coursing alongside the descending aorta and multiple left-sided spleens related to polysplenia* ➔.

PERSISTENT LEFT SUPERIOR VENA CAVA

Key Facts

Terminology

- Persistent left superior vena cava (PLSVC)
- Left-sided superior vena cava arising from confluence of ipsilateral subclavian & internal jugular veins
- Typically drains to coronary sinus & occasionally to left atrium ± unroofed coronary sinus (i.e., coronary sinus atrial septal defect)

Imaging

- Radiography
  - Lateralization of aortopulmonary reflection
  - Left vertical course of catheters & pacer leads
- CT/MR
  - Vertical vessel in left superior mediastinum
  - Originates from confluence of left internal jugular & subclavian veins
  - Typically drains into dilated coronary sinus
  - Right SVC may be normal, small, or absent

Top Differential Diagnoses

- Left upper lobe partial anomalous pulmonary venous return (PLSVC)
  - Anomalous left upper lobe veins join vertical vein
  - Vertical vein courses in prevascular space of left mediastinum lateral to aortic arch
  - No enlargement of coronary sinus

Clinical Issues

- Usually asymptomatic
- Cyanosis: PLSVC draining to left atrium &/or ASD
- Most common congenital thoracic venous anomaly
  - 0.3-0.5% of general population
- Treatment: None if isolated; surgical correction if significant shunt

Diagnostic Checklist

- Suggest PLSVC in patient with left-sided vertical course of central catheter/lead lateral to aortic arch

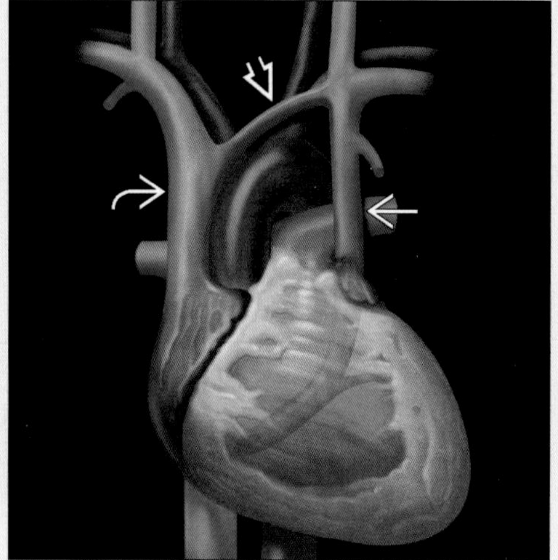

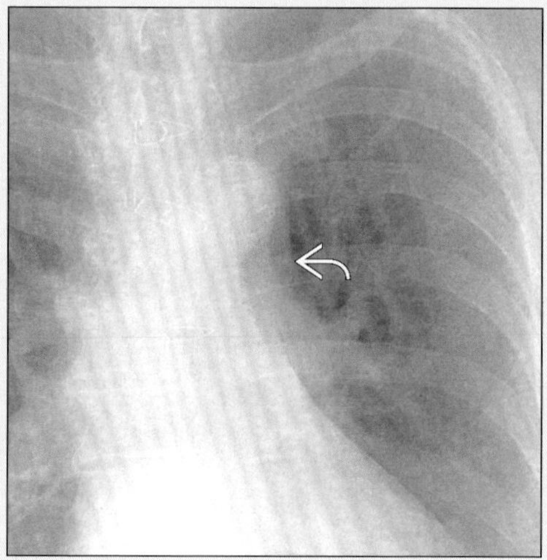

(Left) *Graphic shows the typical appearance of PLSVC ➡ coursing vertically and medially into the coronary sinus with an associated right SVC ➡ and a bridging vein ➡.* ***(Right)*** *PA chest radiograph of an asymptomatic patient with PLSVC shows lateralization of the aortopulmonary reflection ➡. Normally, no soft tissue should be seen lateral to the aortic arch. However, this is a nonspecific finding that can also be seen in partial anomalous venous return, lymphadenopathy, and mediastinal lipomatosis.*

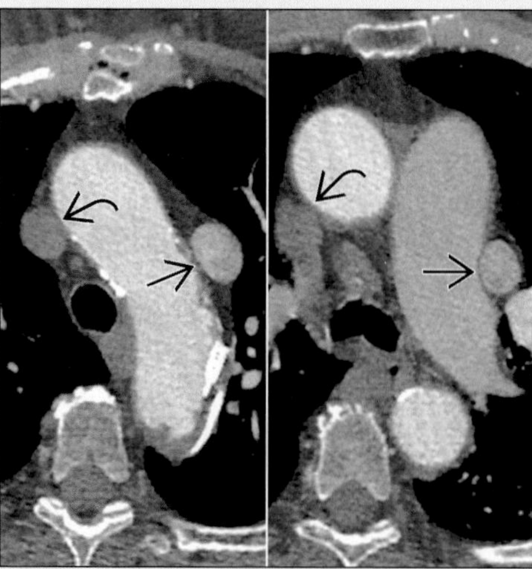

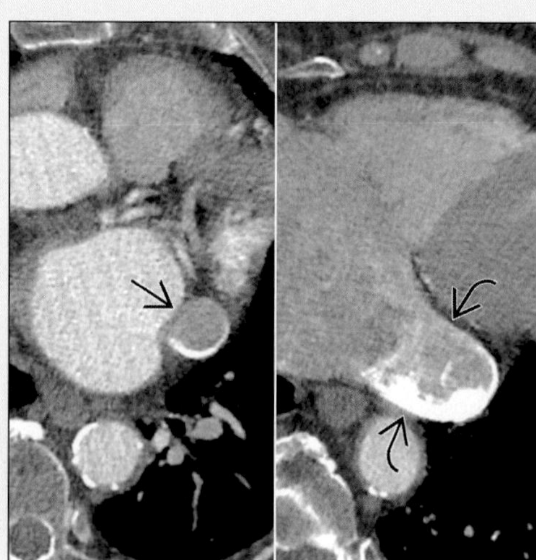

(Left) *Composite image with axial CTA shows a PLSVC ➡ coursing along the left mediastinal border. There is also a right-sided superior vena cava ➡. Often no communication (i.e., bridging vein) is identified between the 2 vena cavas.* ***(Right)*** *Axial CTA of the same patient shows the PLSVC ➡ coursing along the left mediastinal border between the left atrial appendage and the superior pulmonary vein. The coronary sinus ➡ is often dilated in cases of PLSVC.*

PERSISTENT LEFT SUPERIOR VENA CAVA

TERMINOLOGY

Abbreviations

- **Persistent left superior vena cava (PLSVC)**

Definitions

- Left-sided superior vena cava arising from confluence of ipsilateral subclavian & internal jugular veins
- Typically drains to coronary sinus & occasionally to left atrium ± unroofed coronary sinus (i.e., coronary sinus atrial septal defect)

IMAGING

General Features

- Best diagnostic clue
  - Vertical vessel lateral to aortic arch associated with coronary sinus dilatation
- Size
  - Variable

Radiographic Findings

- Radiography
  - **May be normal**
  - **Lateralization of aortopulmonary reflection**
    - Normally there should be no soft tissue lateral to aortic arch
    - May also occur in left upper lobe partial anomalous pulmonary venous return (PAPVR); radiographically indistinguishable entities
  - Left-sided central catheter or pacemaker/defibrillator lead coursing lateral to aortic arch

CT Findings

- CECT
  - **PLSVC: Vertical vessel coursing along left superior mediastinum**
    - Originates from confluence of left internal jugular & subclavian veins
    - Receives drainage from left superior intercostal vein
    - Courses inferiorly in prevascular space
      - Lateral to aortic arch & pulmonary trunk
      - Anterior to left mainstem bronchus
      - May be difficult to identify as it courses posterior to left atrium
  - **Drainage**
    - **Most into coronary sinus; frequently dilated**
    - **May drain into left atrium**
      - Always constitutes a right-to-left shunt of variable size
      - May be associated with unroofed coronary sinus; constitutes coronary sinus atrial septal defect (ASD), a left-to-right shunt
  - Right SVC may be normal, small, or absent
  - Left brachiocephalic (bridging vein) frequently absent (65%)
  - May receive drainage from left hemiazygous system, particularly with hemiazygous continuation

MR Findings

- Equivalent to CT for morphologic assessment
  - Same findings as in CT
- Allows shunt quantification in cases of drainage to left atrium &/or coronary sinus ASD
  - Velocity encoding sequences
- Superior to CT for assessment of associated congenital heart disease

Angiographic Findings

- DSA
  - Injection through left-sided catheter shows vessel coursing inferiorly into coronary sinus & right atrium

Imaging Recommendations

- Best imaging tool
  - CT & MR are equivalent for morphologic assessment
- Protocol advice
  - Injection in left arm for optimal vessel opacification

Echocardiographic Findings

- Dilated coronary sinus
- Confirmed by use of saline contrast (bubble study)
- Criteria
  - Dilated coronary sinus on 2-dimensional echocardiography without evidence of elevated right-sided filling pressures
  - Enhancement of dilated coronary sinus before right atrium after saline contrast infusion into left arm vein
  - Normal contrast transit with opacification of right atrium before coronary sinus when saline contrast injected into right arm vein

DIFFERENTIAL DIAGNOSIS

Dilated Coronary Sinus

- Other etiologies
  - Elevated right atrial pressure (most common)
  - Coronary arteriovenous fistula
  - Partial anomalous pulmonary venous return
  - Coronary sinus ASD (unroofed coronary sinus)

Left Upper Lobe Partial Anomalous Pulmonary Venous Return (PAPVR)

- Anomalous left upper lobe veins join vertical vein
- Vertical vein courses in prevascular space of left mediastinum lateral to aortic arch
- Absence of left superior pulmonary vein from normal location anterior to left main bronchus
- No enlargement of coronary sinus
- Normal to enlarged left brachiocephalic vein & right SVC
- Cephalic (not caudal) direction of blood flow on MRV

Lateralization of Aortopulmonary Interface

- Other etiologies
  - Mediastinal lipomatosis (most common)
  - Left upper lobe PAPVR (i.e., vertical vein)
  - Lymphadenopathy
  - Neoplasm (e.g., lung cancer)

Enlarged Left Superior Intercostal Vein

- Courses along lateral margin of aorta
- Typically smaller than left SVC
- Provides anastomotic connection between left brachiocephalic vein & accessory hemiazygous vein

Lymph Node

- Not tubular on contiguous images

PERSISTENT LEFT SUPERIOR VENA CAVA

PATHOLOGY

General Features

- Etiology
  - Persistence of left superior cardinal vein
- Genetics
  - No known genetic predisposition
  - Higher prevalence in patients with congenital heart disease
- Associated abnormalities
  - **Congenital heart disease**
    - Present in 40% of all cases of PLSVC
    - More common with absent right SVC
      - ASD
      - Bicuspid aortic valve
      - Aortic coarctation
      - Coronary sinus ostial atresia
      - Cor triatriatum
  - PLSVC occurs in 30-50% of patients with heterotaxy syndrome

Staging, Grading, & Classification

- **Unroofed coronary sinus ASD classification**
  - Type I: Completely unroofed with PLSVC
  - Type II: Completely unroofed without PLSVC
  - Type III: Partially unroofed mid portion
  - Type IV: Partially unroofed terminal portion

Gross Pathologic & Surgical Features

- Subtypes
  - Right & left SVC
    - Most common
    - Bridging vein may or may not be present (absent in 65%)
  - PLSVC & absent right SVC
    - Related to regression of caudal right superior cardinal vein
- Termination
  - Right atrium (80-90%)
  - Left atrium (~ 10%)

CLINICAL ISSUES

Presentation

- Most common signs/symptoms
  - Usually asymptomatic
- Other signs/symptoms
  - Cyanosis may occur with PLSVC draining to left atrium &/or ASD
  - Risk of paradoxical embolism or cerebral abscess when associated with ASD, unroofed coronary sinus, or direct communication of vein to left atrium
  - Rarely, cardiac arrhythmias due to atrioventricular nodal stretching in setting of catheter placement
  - Rarely, left ventricular outflow obstruction due to incomplete occlusion of mitral valve
  - Congenital heart disease
    - May exhibit symptoms related to ASD or heterotaxy syndrome
  - Challenging placement of Swan Ganz catheter; imaging guidance is recommended
  - Challenging placement of pacemakers & implantable cardioverter defibrillators
    - Complications: Arrhythmia, cardiogenic shock, cardiac tamponade, coronary sinus thrombosis
  - PLSVC is a relative contraindication for administration of retrograde cardioplegia

Demographics

- Age
  - Usually incidental finding at any age
  - Patients with complex associated congenital anomalies may present early in life
- Gender
  - No predilection
- Epidemiology
  - Most common congenital thoracic venous anomaly
  - Left superior vena cava occurs in 0.3-0.5% of general population
  - Prevalence: 3-10% in children with congenital heart disease
    - In congenital heart disease, PLSVC often drains directly into left atrium
    - Drainage into top of left atrium usually between left atrial appendage & pulmonary veins
    - Coronary sinus often absent or unroofed, producing intraatrial communication

Natural History & Prognosis

- Related to associated congenital anomalies

Treatment

- None if isolated; surgical correction if significant shunt

DIAGNOSTIC CHECKLIST

Consider

- Injection in left arm for optimal opacification of PLSVC
- Evaluation for associated congenital anomalies in patients with PLSVC

Image Interpretation Pearls

- Suggest diagnosis in patient with left-sided vertical course of central catheter or pacemaker lead lateral to aortic arch

SELECTED REFERENCES

1. Thangaroopan M et al: Images in cardiovascular medicine. Rare case of an unroofed coronary sinus: diagnosis by multidetector computed tomography. Circulation. 119(16):e518-20, 2009
2. Kong PK et al: Unroofed coronary sinus and persistent left superior vena cava. Eur J Echocardiogr. 8(5):398-401, 2007
3. Piacentini G et al: Persistent left superior vena cava into unroofed coronary sinus. Lancet. 368(9551):1963-4, 2006
4. Sueyoshi E et al: Persistent left superior vena cava into left atrium. Lancet. 368(9543):1270, 2006
5. Gonzalez-Juanatey C et al: Persistent left superior vena cava draining into the coronary sinus: report of 10 cases and literature review. Clin Cardiol. 27(9):515-8, 2004
6. Tak T et al: Persistent left superior vena cava: incidence, significance and clinical correlates. Int J Cardiol. 82(1):91-3, 2002

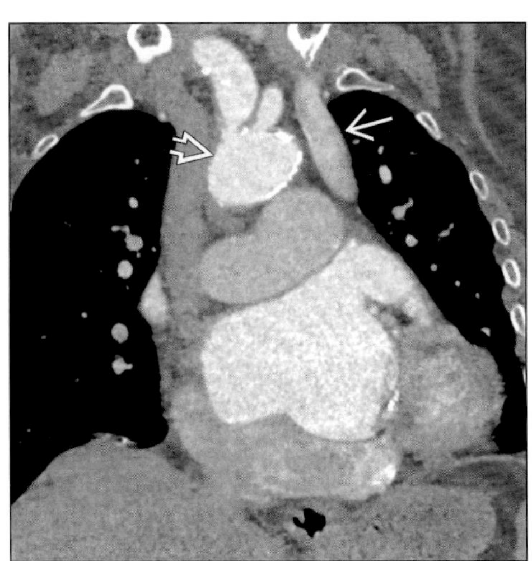

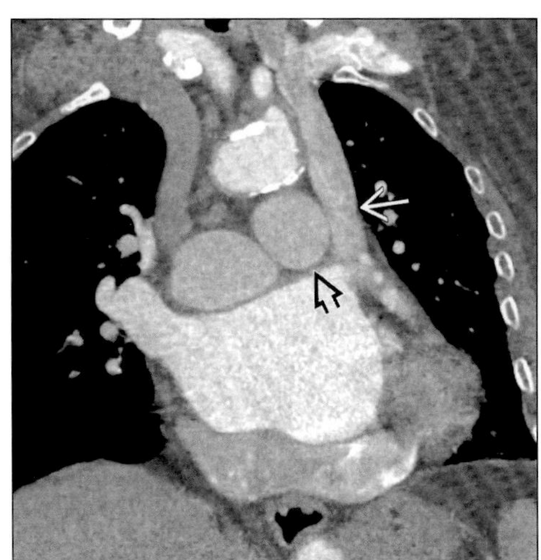

(Left) *Coronal CTA of the same patient shows the relationship of the PLSVC ➔ to the aortic arch ⇨, which explains the radiographic finding of lateralization of the aortopulmonary reflection.* ***(Right)*** *Coronal CTA of the same patient shows the relationship of the PLSVC ➔ to the left pulmonary artery ⇨. Normally, no soft tissue should be identified lateral to the aortic arch or the pulmonary artery.*

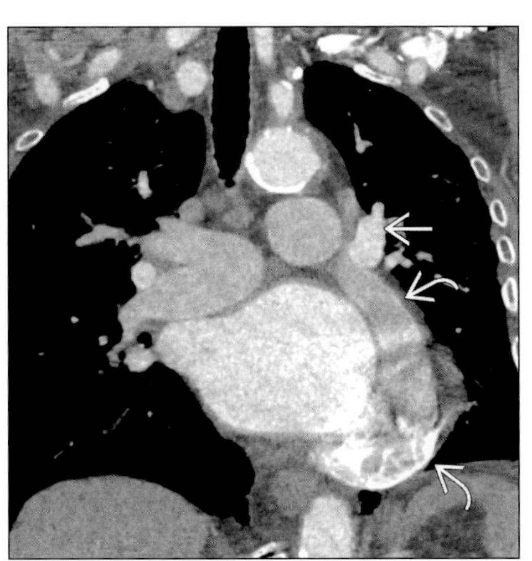

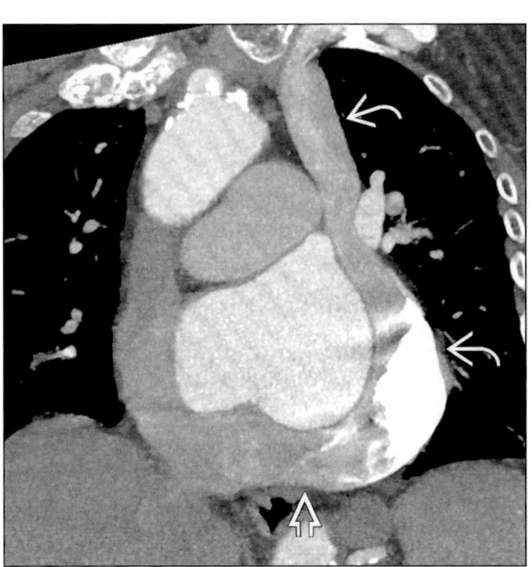

(Left) *Coronal CTA of the same patient shows the PLSVC ↷ coursing inferiorly toward the coronary sinus in close relationship with the left atrium. The PLSVC is often located between the left atrial appendage and the left superior pulmonary vein ➔.* ***(Right)*** *Curved coronal CTA of the same patient shows the entire course of the PLSVC ↷. The dilated coronary sinus ⇨ is a characteristic finding that helps differentiate PLSVC from left upper lobe partial anomalous pulmonary venous return.*

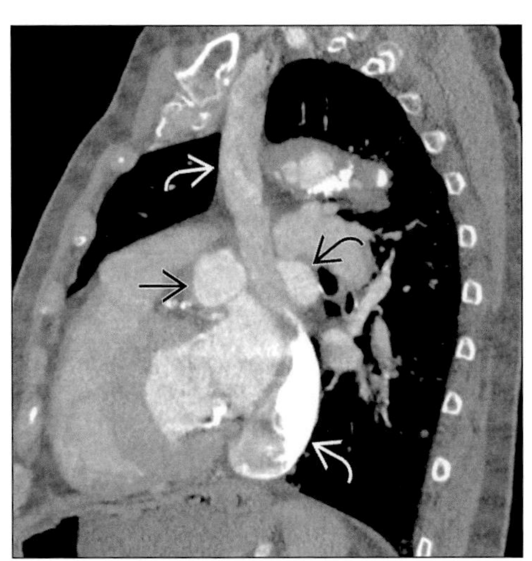

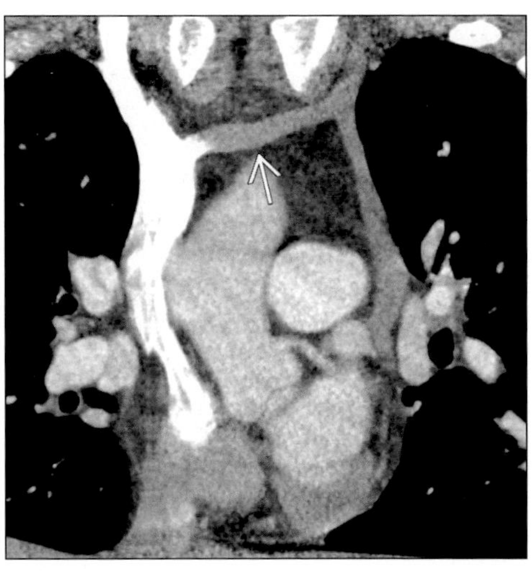

(Left) *Sagittal CTA of the same patient shows the course of the PLSVC ↷. The atrial appendage ➔ is anterior to the PLSVC, and the left superior pulmonary vein ↷ is posterior to the PLSVC.* ***(Right)*** *Curved coronal CTA of a patient with a PLSVC shows a bridging vein ➔ that connects the PLSVC to the right SVC. A bridging vein between the left and right superior vena cavas is absent in approximately 65% of all patients with PLSVC.*

*(**Left**) Axial MRA of a patient with PLSVC draining into the left atrium shows the PLSVC ➚ lateral to the aortic arch. (**Right**) Axial MRA of the same patient shows the PLSVC ➚ lateral to the pulmonary trunk. While MR is equivalent to CT for the assessment PLSVC, it is superior in the assessment of associated congenital heart disease and allows measurement of the size of vascular shunts.*

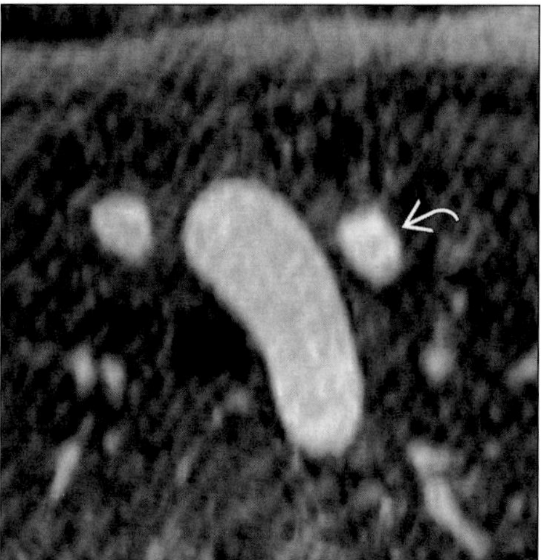

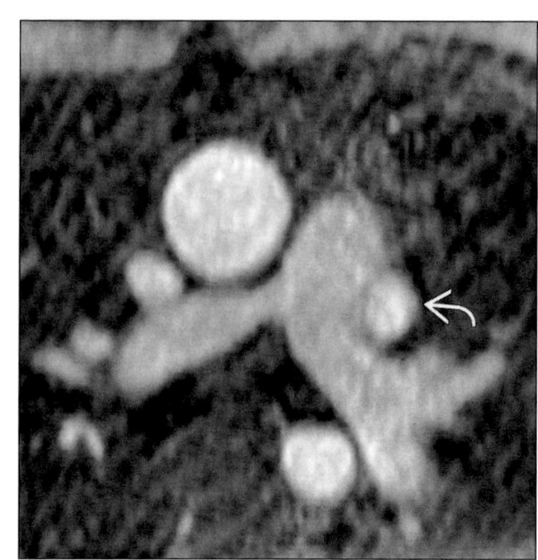

*(**Left**) Axial MRA of the same patient shows the PLSVC ➚ draining into the left atrium ➡. (**Right**) Coronal MRA MIP image of the same patient shows the complete course of the PLSVC ➚ and its drainage ➡ into the left atrium. If isolated, this abnormality results in a mild right-to-left shunt, and affected patients are frequently asymptomatic. However, a concomitant coronary sinus atrial septal defect should be excluded as this is a common associated condition.*

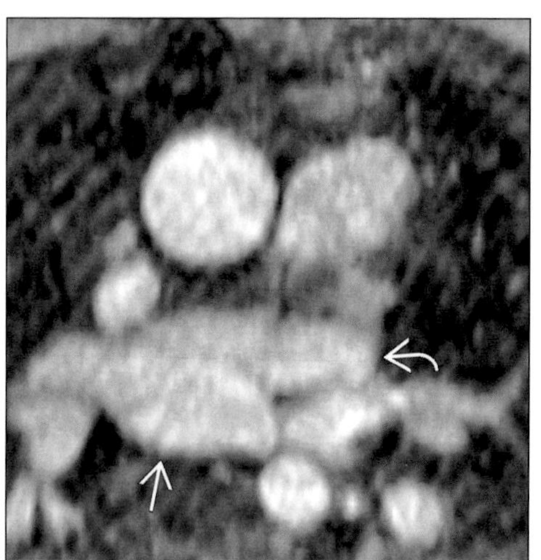

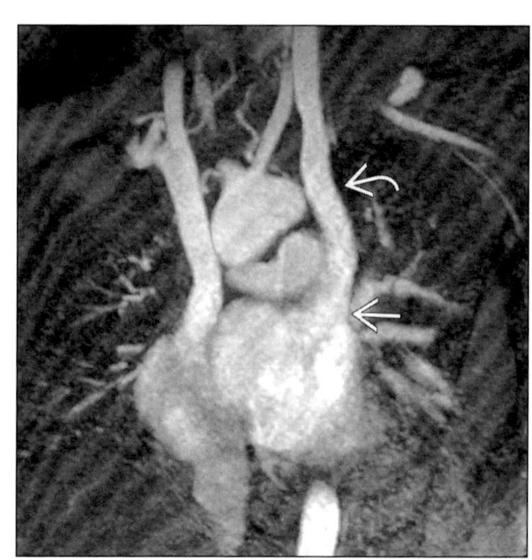

*(**Left**) 3D reformatted oblique sagittal image from a chest MRA of the same patient demonstrates the PLSVC ➡ draining into the left atrium. (**Right**) Curved coronal CTA of a patient with PLSVC draining into the left atrium shows the entire course of the PLSVC ➚. While uncommon, this abnormality is frequently asymptomatic and is characteristically associated with unroofing of the coronary sinus, which results in a right-to-left shunt.*

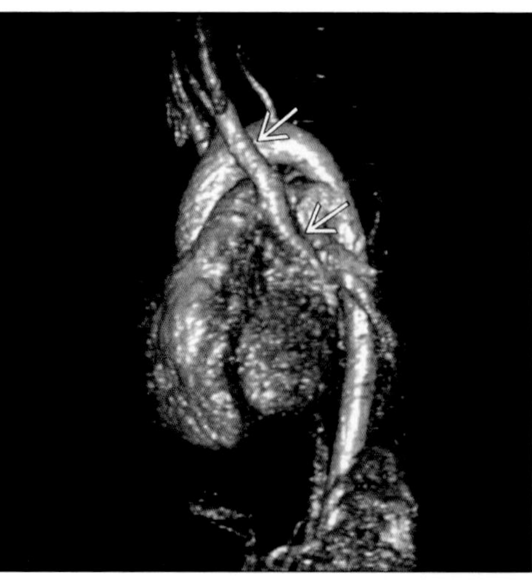

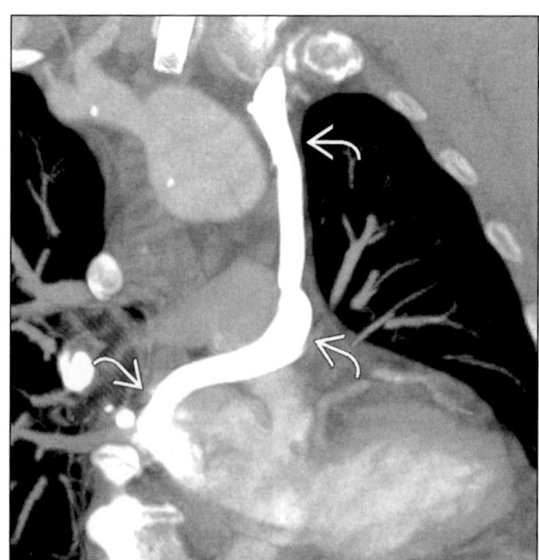

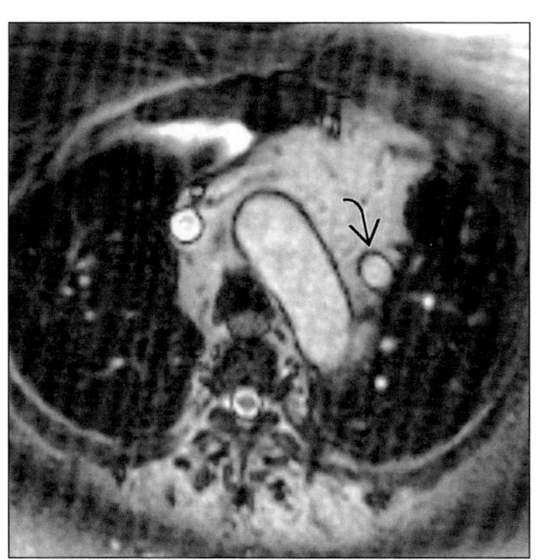

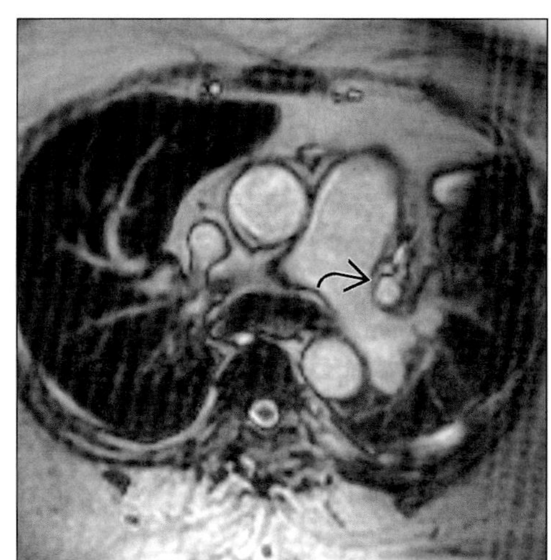

(Left) *Axial SSFP MR of a patient with PLSVC draining into the left atrium and a coronary sinus atrial septal defect (i.e., unroofed coronary sinus) shows the PLSVC coursing along the prevascular space, lateral to the aortic arch.* ***(Right)*** *Axial SSFP MR of the same patient shows the PLSVC descending along the left lateral portion of the mediastinum, lateral to the pulmonary trunk. At this level, the findings are identical to those seen in PLSVC without coronary sinus ASD.*

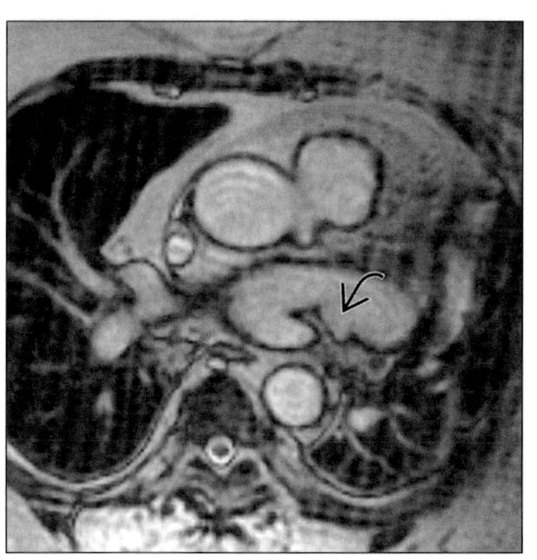

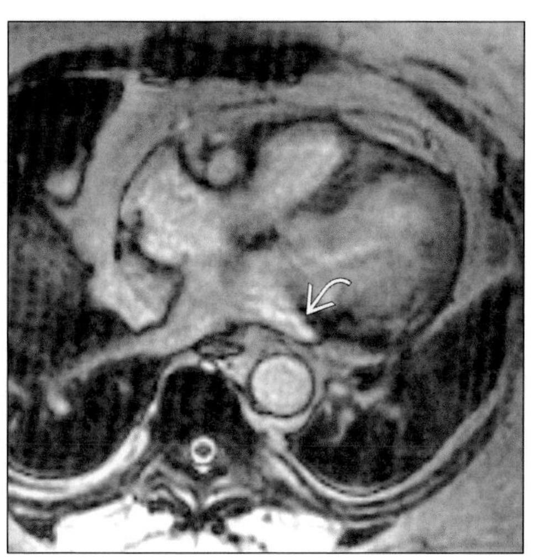

(Left) *Axial SSFP MR of the same patient shows the PLSVC draining directly into the left atrium.* ***(Right)*** *Axial SSFP MR of the same patient shows a coronary sinus of normal size. Note that in this sequence it is uncertain whether the coronary sinus is unroofed. Multiplanar imaging through the coronary sinus is recommended to demonstrate the unroofing. Velocity encoded sequences may be necessary to establish the presence of a right-to-left shunt.*

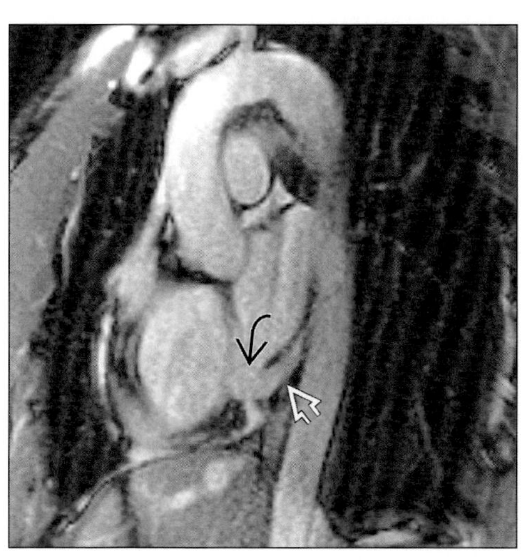

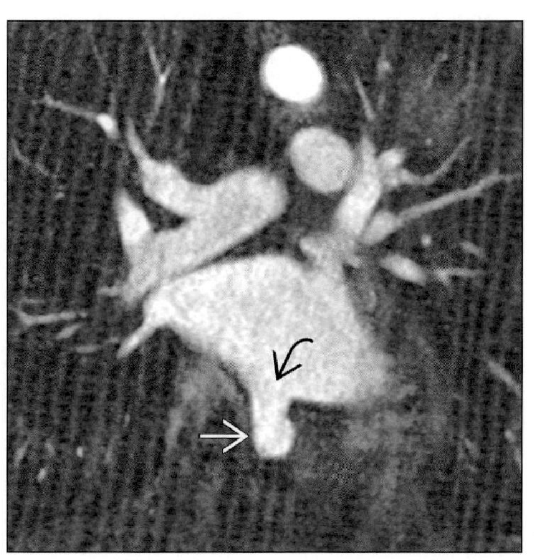

(Left) *Oblique sagittal SSFP MR of the same patient shows a coronary sinus of normal size as well as the unroofing of the distal portion of the coronary sinus constituting a right-to-left shunt.* ***(Right)*** *Oblique coronal MRA of the same patient shows a short-axis view of the coronary sinus with unroofing and communication with the left atrium. MR is superior to CT in confirming and quantifying the amount of right-to-left shunt in these cases.*

ABERRANT SUBCLAVIAN ARTERY

Key Facts

Imaging

- Radiography
  - Frontal chest radiograph: Oblique edge extending to right, arising from aortic arch (60%), often seen through trachea
  - Ill-defined mass in right medial clavicular area
  - Lateral chest radiograph: Mass posterior to trachea in Raider triangle
- Esophagram: Oblique posterior impression on esophagram directed superiorly toward right shoulder
- CT
  - Aberrant subclavian artery: Last branch of 4-branch vessel aortic arch
  - Courses posterior to trachea & esophagus
  - Extends superiorly from left to right
  - Diverticulum of Kommerell: Dilatation of origin of aberrant subclavian artery

Top Differential Diagnoses

- Right aortic arch
- Double aortic arch
- Foregut cyst
- Esophagus: Tumor, achalasia, foreign body
- Substernal thyroid

Clinical Issues

- Most common congenital anomaly of aortic arch
- Symptoms/signs: Most asymptomatic, dysphagia (lusoria) due to esophageal compression
- Treatment
  - None unless symptomatic
  - Major symptoms may require surgery

Diagnostic Checklist

- All mediastinal masses should be considered vascular until proven otherwise

__(Left)__ Graphic shows a left aortic arch and an aberrant right subclavian artery ➔ that crosses to the right side, posterior to the trachea and esophagus. Aberrant right subclavian arteries are almost always retroesophageal in location. __(Right)__ Coronal gadolinium-enhanced MRA shows an aberrant right subclavian artery ➔ arising from the proximal aspect of the descending aorta and crossing the midline to supply the right upper extremity.

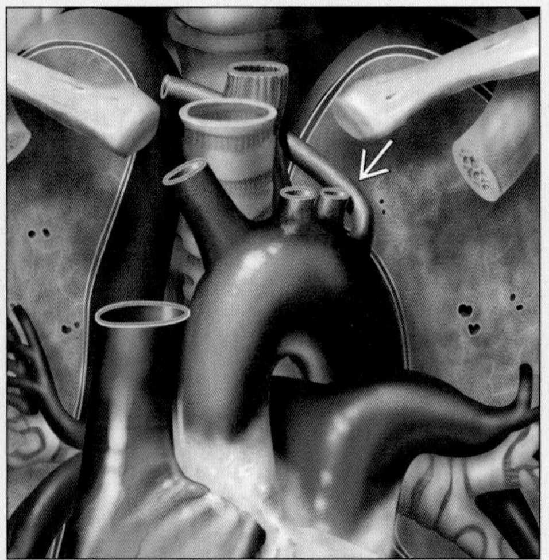

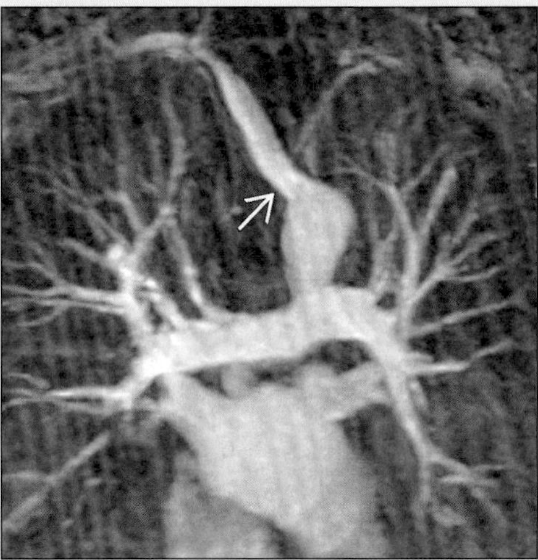

__(Left)__ Oblique image from esophagram shows an extrinsic posterior indentation ➔ on the esophagus, highly suggestive of an aberrant right subclavian artery. __(Right)__ Axial CECT demonstrates an aberrant right subclavian artery ➔ that originates from the distal aortic arch. Although the origin of the aberrant vessel is normal in this case, it is often enlarged (diverticulum of Kommerell). Local vascular dilation may cause mass effect on the esophagus and dysphagia (dysphagia lusoria).

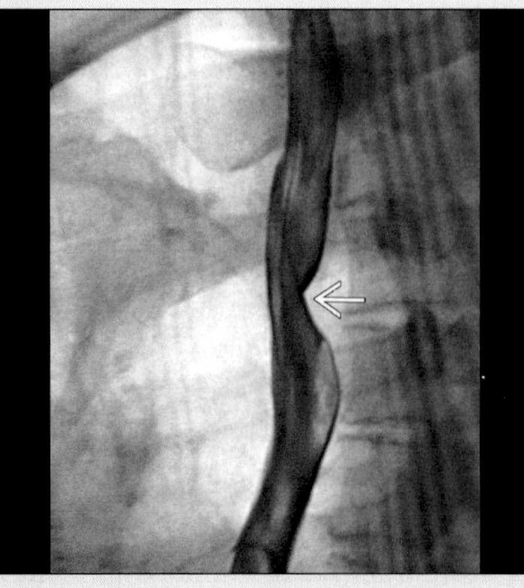

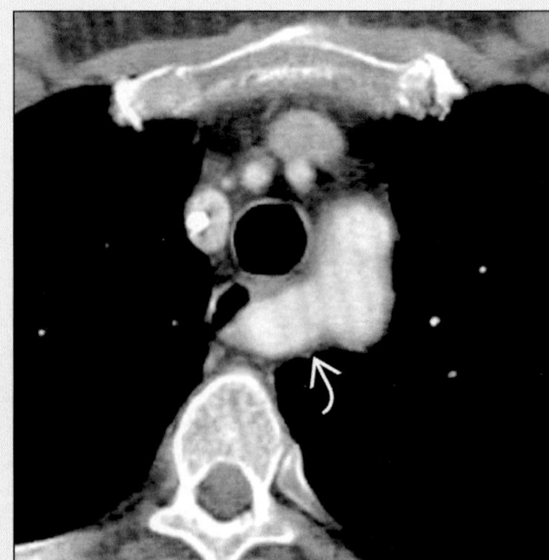

ABERRANT SUBCLAVIAN ARTERY

TERMINOLOGY

Synonyms

- **Aberrant right subclavian artery (ARSA)**

IMAGING

General Features

- Best diagnostic clue
  - Tubular enhancing structure posterior to esophagus
- Location
  - Retroesophageal & anterior to spine

Radiographic Findings

- Radiography
  - Frontal radiograph
    - Oblique edge extending to right, arising from aortic arch (60%), often seen through trachea
    - Ill-defined mass in right medial clavicular area
  - Lateral radiograph: Mass posterior to trachea in Raider triangle
    - **Raider triangle**: Clear space posterior to trachea, anterior to vertebral bodies, superior to aorta
    - Obscuration of aortic arch (60%)
    - Indentation on posterior tracheal wall (50%)
  - Chest radiography often normal

Fluoroscopic Findings

- Esophagram
  - Oblique posterior impression on esophagram directed superiorly toward right shoulder

CT Findings

- **ARSA is last branch of 4-branch vessel aortic arch**
  - Courses posterior to trachea & esophagus
    - Extends superiorly from left to right
    - Esophageal compression frequently evident
  - No brachiocephalic artery
  - **Diverticulum of Kommerell**
    - Dilatation of origin of aberrant subclavian artery
    - Visible as tapering tubular structure arising from posterior aortic arch
    - May contain thrombus or calcification

Imaging Recommendations

- Best imaging tool
  - Contrast-enhanced CT is optimal imaging modality for visualization & characterization of ARSA

DIFFERENTIAL DIAGNOSIS

Mass in Retrotracheal Triangle

- Vascular
  - Right aortic arch
  - Double aortic arch
- Foregut cyst
- Esophagus
  - Tumor
  - Achalasia
  - Foreign body
- Substernal thyroid

PATHOLOGY

General Features

- Etiology
  - Involution of embryonic right 4th aortic arch between left carotid & left subclavian artery
- Associated abnormalities
  - Congenital heart disease
  - Down syndrome
  - Anomalous recurrent laryngeal nerve (nonrecurrent laryngeal nerve)
  - Thoracic duct may terminate on right

Gross Pathologic & Surgical Features

- Aberrant right subclavian artery course on pathology series
  - Retroesophageal (50%)
  - Retrotracheal, between trachea & esophagus (12%)
  - Pre-tracheal (< 2%)
- Diverticulum of Kommerell (60%)
- Aberrant left subclavian artery
  - Right aortic arch
  - Last branch off aorta, no increased incidence of congenital heart disease
  - 1st branch off aorta (mirror image branching), high incidence of congenital heart disease
    - Most commonly tetralogy of Fallot, ventricular septal defect, truncus arteriosus

CLINICAL ISSUES

Presentation

- Most common signs/symptoms
  - Most patients asymptomatic
- Other signs/symptoms
  - Dysphagia (lusoria) due to esophageal compression
  - Dyspnea, cough from tracheal compression

Demographics

- Epidemiology
  - Frequency approximately 0.5% (1 in 200)
  - Most common congenital anomaly of aortic arch (ignoring bovine arch variant)

Treatment

- None unless symptomatic
- Mild symptoms: Dietary modification
- Major symptoms may require surgery

DIAGNOSTIC CHECKLIST

Consider

- Other aortic arch abnormalities: Right aortic arch, double aortic arch
- All mediastinal masses should be considered vascular until proven otherwise
- Important anomaly for ENT surgeon who must be aware of nonrecurrent laryngeal nerve

SELECTED REFERENCES

1. Donnelly LF et al: Aberrant subclavian arteries: cross-sectional imaging findings in infants and children referred for evaluation of extrinsic airway compression. AJR Am J Roentgenol. 178(5):1269-74, 2002

RIGHT AORTIC ARCH

Key Facts

Terminology

- Congenital anomaly in which aortic arch courses to right of trachea
  - Different types based on branching patterns
  - Right aortic arch (RAA) with aberrant left subclavian artery (ALSA)
  - Right aortic arch with mirror image branching

Imaging

- Radiography
  - Round, mass-like opacity in right paratracheal region
  - Indentation of right lateral margin of trachea
  - Normal left aortic arch absent
  - ± small, round opacity in expected left arch location due to diverticulum of Kommerell
  - ± retroesophageal opacity due to ALSA + diverticulum of Kommerell
  - Right descending aorta in most cases
- CT
  - Aortic arch courses to right of trachea
  - RAA with ALSA: Left carotid, right carotid, right subclavian, followed by retroesophageal ALSA
  - RAA with mirror image branching: Left innominate, right carotid, right subclavian arteries

Top Differential Diagnoses

- Mediastinal mass
- Double aortic arch

Pathology

- 98% of RAA with mirror image branching associated with congenital heart disease

Clinical Issues

- Usually asymptomatic
- Dysphagia due to esophageal compression by ALSA or complete vascular ring

*(**Left**) PA chest radiograph shows a right paratracheal opacity that indents the right lateral margin of the trachea. A normal left aortic arch is absent. The descending aorta ➡ is to the right of the midline. (**Right**) Lateral chest radiograph shows a retroesophageal opacity ➡ with anterior deviation of the trachea. These findings are characteristic of right aortic arch with aberrant left subclavian artery (ALSA).*

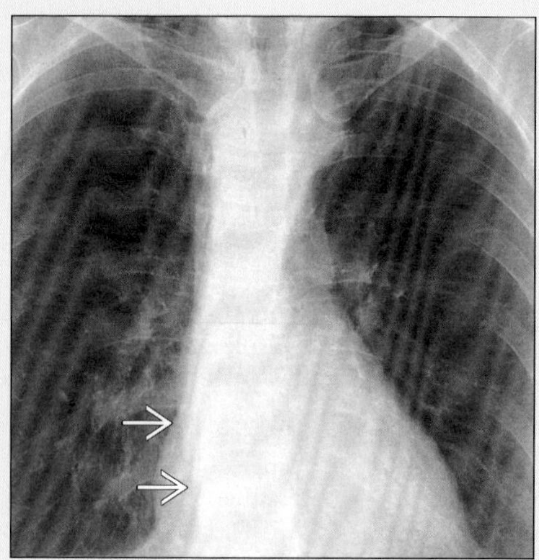

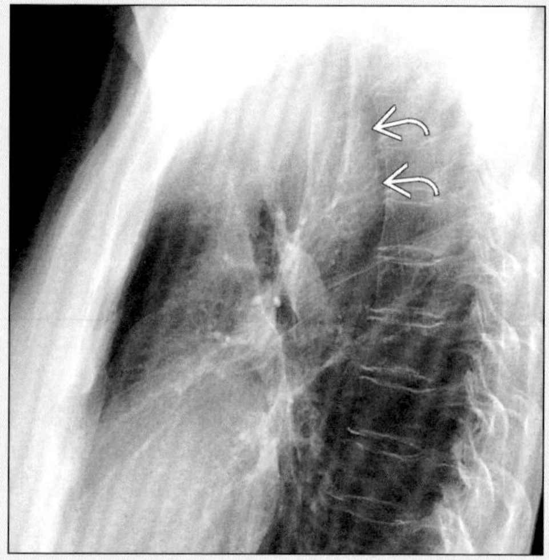

*(**Left**) Frontal 3D reformatted image of the same patient confirms a right aortic arch with an aberrant left subclavian artery ➡ arising from a diverticulum of Kommerell ➡ that accounts for the left paratracheal opacity seen on radiography. The aorta ➡ descends to the right of midline. (**Right**) Axial CECT shows an aberrant left subclavian artery ➡ coursing posterior to the esophagus ➡, which accounts for the retroesophageal opacity seen on lateral chest radiography.*

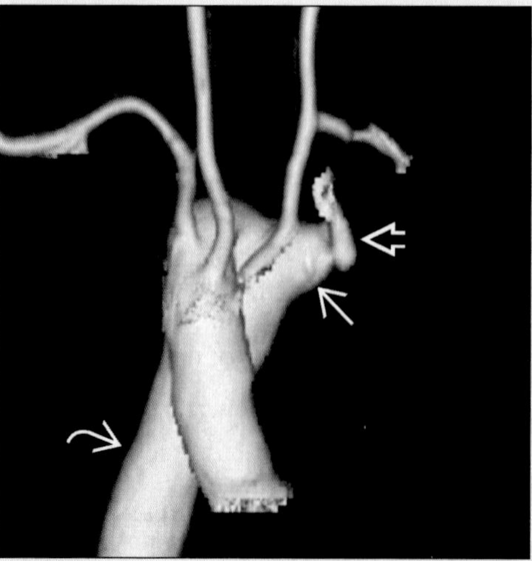

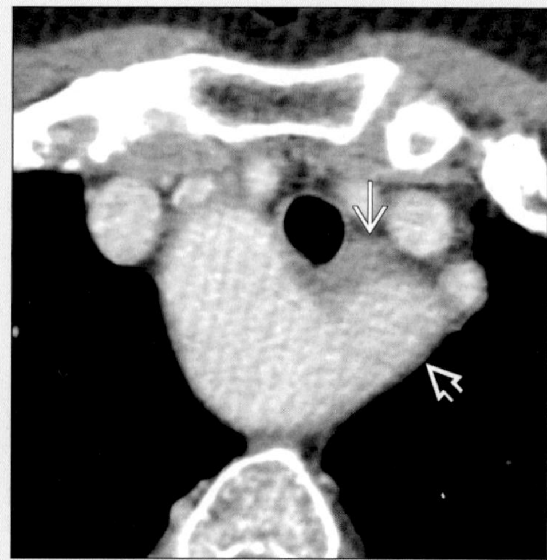

RIGHT AORTIC ARCH

TERMINOLOGY

Abbreviations

- **Right aortic arch (RAA)**

Synonyms

- Right arch

Definitions

- Congenital anomaly in which aortic arch courses to right of trachea; different types based on branching patterns
  - RAA with aberrant left subclavian artery (ALSA)
    - 4 great vessel branches in following order: Left carotid, right carotid, right subclavian, aberrant left subclavian arteries
    - ALSA has retroesophageal course
    - ± diverticulum of Kommerell at origin of ALSA
  - RAA with mirror image branching
    - Left innominate artery followed by right carotid & right subclavian arteries
  - RAA with isolation of left subclavian artery
    - Left carotid artery followed by right carotid & right subclavian arteries
    - Left subclavian artery, not connected to aorta, is connected to pulmonary artery by left ductus arteriosus
  - RAA with left descending aorta
    - a.k.a. circumflex aorta or retroesophageal aortic segment
    - Transverse arch courses posterior to esophagus then continues as left descending aorta
    - May be variant of double arch with atretic left arch
  - RAA with aberrant brachiocephalic
    - Right carotid artery followed by right subclavian artery & left innominate artery
    - Left innominate artery has a retroesophageal course

IMAGING

General Features

- Best diagnostic clue
  - Right paratracheal rounded opacity on radiography with leftward tracheal deviation
- Location
  - Right paratracheal region
- Size
  - Usually 2.5-4 cm
- Morphology
  - Soft tissue density often convex in right paratracheal region enhances on CT

Radiographic Findings

- Radiography
  - Round mass-like opacity in right paratracheal region
  - Indentation of right lateral margin of trachea
  - Leftward tracheal deviation
  - Normal left aortic arch absent
    - Normal indentation of left tracheal margin absent
  - ± small round opacity in expected left arch location due to diverticulum of Kommerell
  - ± absent normal descending aortic interface
    - Descending aorta to right of midline in most cases
  - Retroesophageal opacity
    - Diverticulum of Kommerell + aberrant left subclavian artery
    - Displaced proximal descending aorta

CT Findings

- CTA
  - RAA with ALSA
    - Arch passes to right of trachea
    - 4 branches: Left carotid, right carotid, right subclavian, retroesophageal aberrant left subclavian arteries
    - Dilated origin of ALSA (diverticulum of Kommerell) may cause esophageal compression
    - Coronal reconstructions show aortic arch rightward of trachea
    - Sagittal reconstructions show retroesophageal left subclavian artery
  - Right aortic arch with mirror image branching
    - Arch passes to right of trachea
    - 3 branch vessels: Left innominate, right carotid, right subclavian arteries
    - No retroesophageal vessel
    - No tracheal or esophageal compression typically

MR Findings

- MR findings similar to CT findings
- Advantages over CT
  - No ionizing radiation
  - Allows better evaluation of cardiac morphology & function in case of associated congenital heart disease
  - Can be performed without intravenous contrast
- Disadvantages compared to CT
  - Long scanning time
    - Sedation needed in pediatric population
  - Esophagus & trachea compression not as well evaluated

Imaging Recommendations

- Best imaging tool
  - Multidetector CT angiography
- Protocol advice
  - Contrast enhancement
  - Thin sections to allow multiplanar reformation
    - 3D volume rendering (VR) & 2D maximum-intensity projection (MIP) helpful for structural overview
  - Expiratory CT helpful to identify tracheomalacia in patients with stridor

Angiographic Findings

- Similar to CTA findings
- Not usually necessary given advances in CTA & MRA

Fluoroscopic Findings

- Esophagram
  - Obtained to evaluate dysphagia
  - Right esophageal indentation
  - Posterior indentation of esophagus if ALSA present
  - Impression on left side of esophagus by diverticulum of Kommerell can simulate double aortic arch

DIFFERENTIAL DIAGNOSIS

Mediastinal Mass

- Consider vascular origin of mediastinal "mass" if
  - Adjacent to known vascular structures

- Mural calcification
- Oval or round shape with smooth contour
- Poor visualization in orthogonal view

Double Aortic Arch

- Right arch typically higher & larger than left arch
- Difficult to distinguish if left arch is atretic

PATHOLOGY

General Features

- Genetics
  - 4% of patients with aortic arch anomalies have 12q11.2 deletion
- Associated abnormalities
  - RAA with mirror image branching
    - 98% with associated congenital heart disease
      - 90% with tetralogy of Fallot (TOF); 25% of TOF have RAA
      - 2.5% with truncus arteriosus (TA); 25-50% of TA have RAA
      - 1.5% with transposition of great vessels (TGV); 10% of TGV have RAA
      - Also associated with tricuspid atresia, atrial & ventricular septal defect
  - RAA with ALSA
    - Rarely associated with other congenital cardiovascular anomalies
      - Tetralogy of Fallot, atrial septal defect, coarctation
    - Esophageal compression in elderly with ectasia, tortuosity, or aneurysm of ALSA
    - Rarely forms a complete vascular ring when ligamentum arteriosum is left sided
      - Tracheal compression + stridor
  - RAA with isolation of left subclavian artery
    - Congenital subclavian steal syndrome, vertebrobasilar insufficiency
    - Rarely associated with congenital heart disease
      - Tetralogy of Fallot
  - RAA with aberrant left brachiocephalic artery
    - Can be associated with complete vascular ring when ligamentum arteriosum is left sided
- RAA with ALSA
  - Interruption of dorsal segment of left arch between left common carotid & left subclavian arteries
  - Regression of right ductus arteriosus
  - ± diverticulum of Kommerell, a remnant of left dorsal aortic root
- RAA with mirror image branching
  - Interruption of dorsal segment of left arch between left subclavian artery & descending aorta
  - Regression of right ductus arteriosis
- RAA with isolation of left subclavian artery
  - Interruption of left arch at 2 levels
    - Between left common carotid & left subclavian arteries
    - Distal to attachment of distal ductus
- RAA with aberrant left brachiocephalic artery
  - Interruption of left arch before left common carotid artery

CLINICAL ISSUES

Presentation

- Most common signs/symptoms
  - Usually asymptomatic
- Other signs/symptoms
  - Dysphagia lusoria due to esophageal compression by ALSA
  - Difficulty feeding &/or stridor in infant due to vascular ring
  - Heart failure related to associated congenital heart disease

Demographics

- Age
  - RAA with mirror image branching usually detected in neonate or childhood
  - RAA with ALSA often incidentally detected on imaging studies in adults
    - Patients with RAA with ALSA & complete vascular ring tend to present early
- Epidemiology
  - Uncommon (~ 0.05-0.1% of population)
  - RAA with aberrant left subclavian artery is most common subtype

Natural History & Prognosis

- Dysphagia may worsen with time due to tightening of vascular ring or atherosclerosis/ectasia of retroesophageal vessel & compression of esophagus
- Overall prognosis depends on associated congenital heart disease, if present

Treatment

- None unless symptomatic
- Surgery for relief of dysphagia or stridor
- Surgery for aneurysmal dilatation of diverticulum of Kommerell

DIAGNOSTIC CHECKLIST

Image Interpretation Pearls

- Look for evidence of associated congenital heart disease, particularly in RAA with mirror image branching

SELECTED REFERENCES

1. Hellinger JC et al: Congenital thoracic vascular anomalies: evaluation with state-of-the-art MR imaging and MDCT. Radiol Clin North Am. 49(5):969-96, 2011
2. Kanne JP et al: Right aortic arch and its variants. J Cardiovasc Comput Tomogr. 4(5):293-300, 2010
3. Türkvatan A et al: Congenital anomalies of the aortic arch: evaluation with the use of multidetector computed tomography. Korean J Radiol. 10(2):176-84, 2009
4. Felson B et al: The two types of right aortic arch. Radiology. 81:745-59, 1963

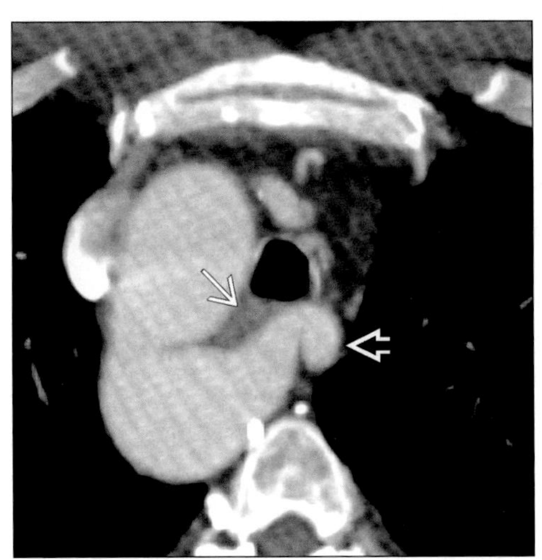

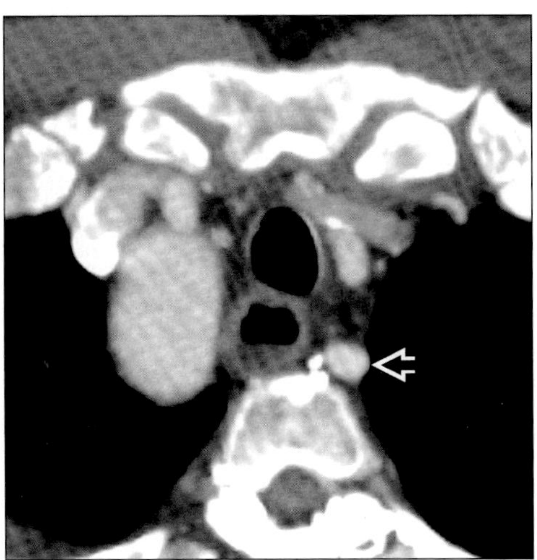

(Left) *Axial CECT of a patient with right aortic arch shows an aberrant left subclavian artery ⇨ arising from a diverticulum of Kommerell. The esophagus → is compressed at this level.* ***(Right)*** *Axial CECT of the same patient shows dilatation of the proximal esophagus with an internal air-fluid level due to extrinsic compression by the diverticulum of Kommerell. Note the left subclavian artery ⇨ coursing to the left of the esophagus.*

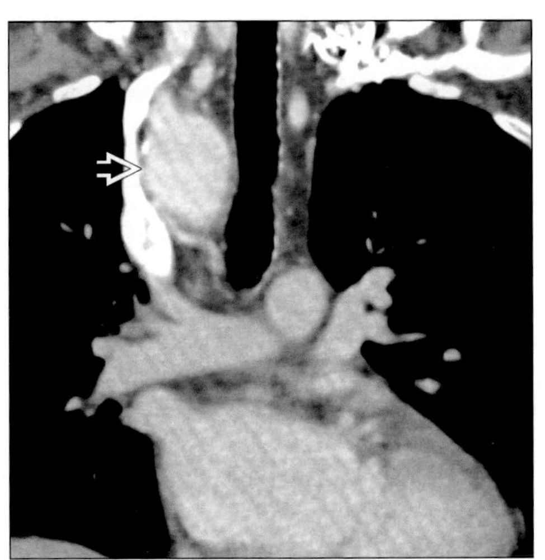

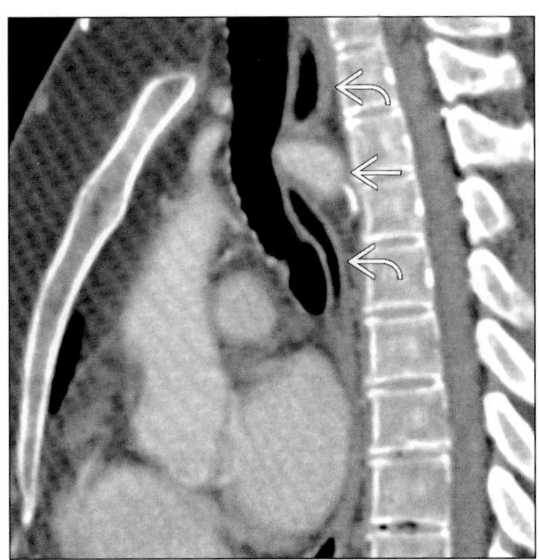

(Left) *Coronal CECT shows a right aortic arch ⇨ in the right paratracheal region that produces mild indentation of the right lateral wall of trachea.* ***(Right)*** *Sagittal CECT of the same patient shows a diverticulum of Kommerell → coursing posterior to and compressing the esophagus ↗ and indenting the posterior wall of the trachea.*

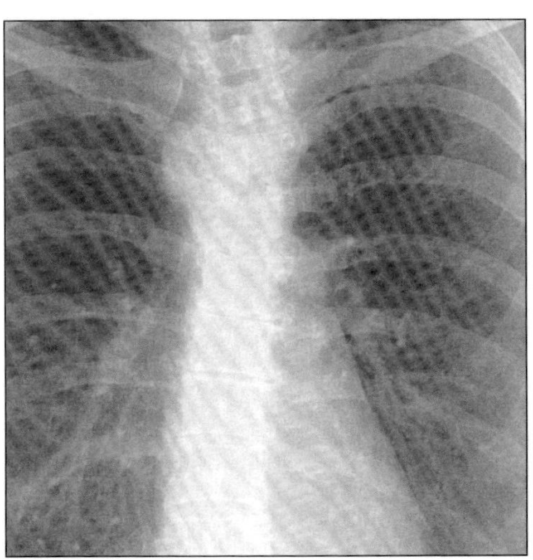

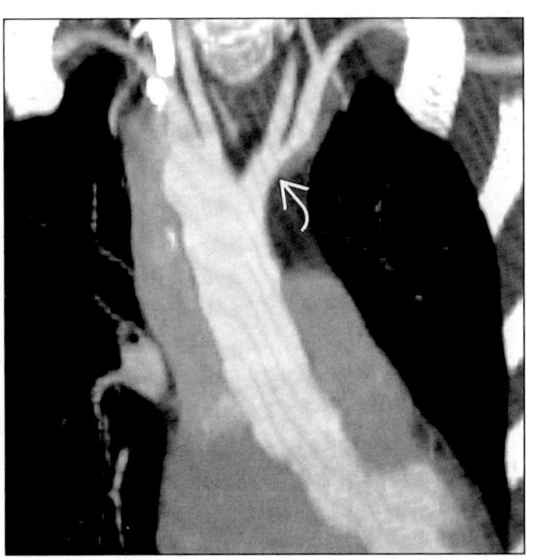

(Left) *PA chest radiograph shows a rounded right paratracheal opacity indenting the right margin of the trachea. No normal left aortic arch or paraaortic interface are seen. These findings should prompt consideration of a right aortic arch.* ***(Right)*** *Coronal CECT MIP image confirms a right aortic arch with mirror image branching. The left innominate artery ↗ arises as the 1st branch of the arch. This patient does not have associated congenital heart disease.*

DOUBLE AORTIC ARCH

Key Facts

Terminology

- Congenital aortic arch anomaly
- Most common symptomatic vascular ring (55%)

Imaging

- Radiography
  - Bilateral tracheal indentations
  - Right arch indentation typically higher & more pronounced than left
  - Lateral chest radiograph: Anterior & posterior tracheal compression at level of arch
- CT/MR
  - "4 artery" sign: Symmetric takeoff of 4 aortic branches on axial image at thoracic inlet
  - 2 arches encircle trachea & esophagus
  - Right aortic arch typically larger & more superior
  - Severe tracheal compression at level of double arch
  - Descending thoracic aorta is typically on the left

Top Differential Diagnoses

- Right arch with aberrant left subclavian artery (LSA) & other arch abnormalities
- Aberrant left pulmonary artery
- Innominate artery compression syndrome
- Nonvascular masses

Clinical Issues

- Symptoms/signs
  - Typically manifests early in life, soon after birth
  - Inspiratory stridor, worsens with feeding
  - May be minimally symptomatic incidental finding
- Treatment: Thoracotomy with division of smaller of 2 arches

Diagnostic Checklist

- "4 artery" sign on axial image at thoracic inlet should suggest double aortic arch

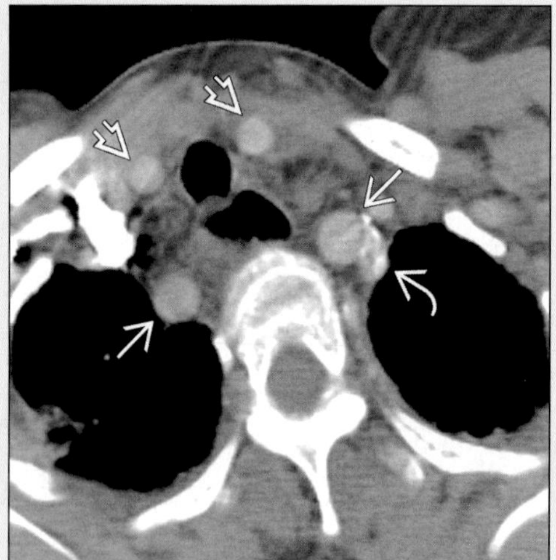

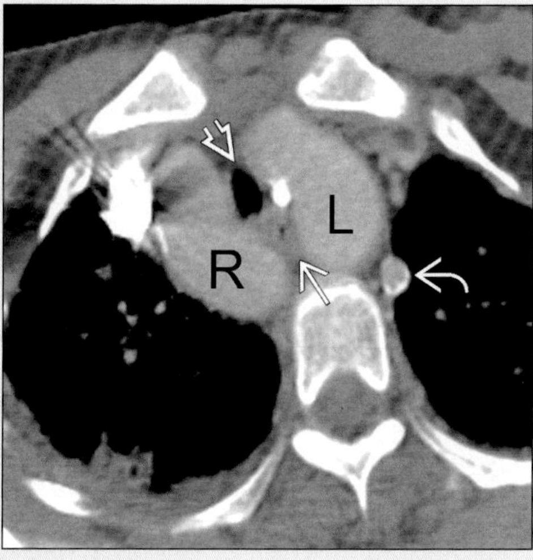

*(**Left**) Axial CECT of an adult with double aortic arch who had repair of congenital heart disease shows that the common carotid ➔ and subclavian arteries ➔ arise from their respective arches ("4 artery" sign). A Blalock-Taussig (BT) conduit from the left subclavian artery to pulmonary artery is present ➔. (**Right**) Axial CECT of the same patient shows that the right (R) and left (L) arches have equal size and encircle and narrow the trachea ➔ and esophagus ➔. The BT conduit ➔ courses caudally.*

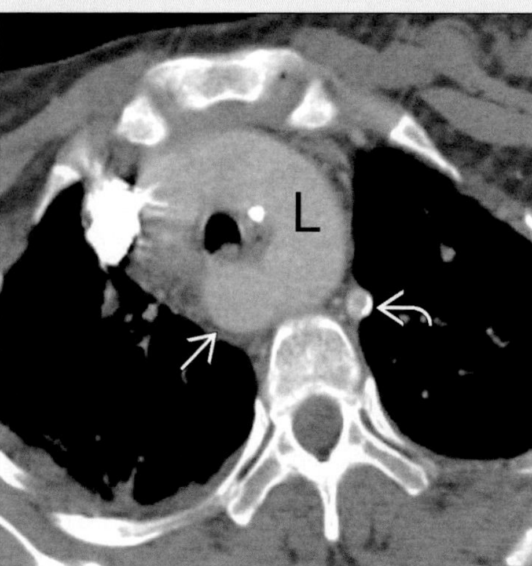

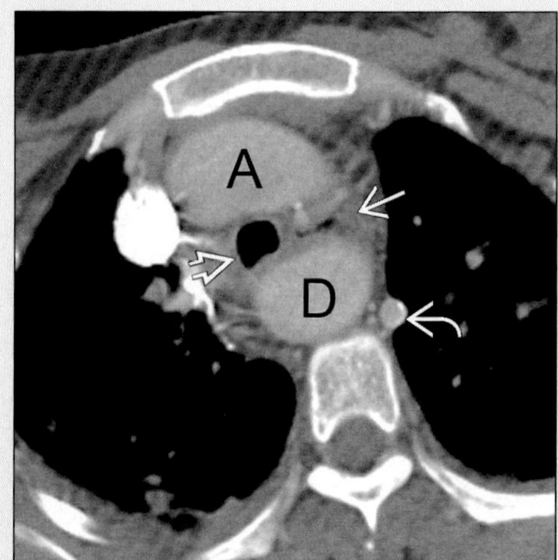

*(**Left**) Axial CECT of the same patient shows the more inferior left (L) arch joining with the right arch posteriorly ➔ to form the descending aorta. The BT conduit ➔ courses caudally. (**Right**) Axial CECT of the same patient shows the ascending aorta (A), which divides superiorly into right and left aortic arches. The descending aorta (D) courses inferiorly in the midline. The trachea ➔ and esophagus ➔ are encircled and compressed. The BT conduit ➔ courses caudally to the left pulmonary artery.*

DOUBLE AORTIC ARCH

TERMINOLOGY

Definitions

- **Congenital aortic arch anomaly**
  - Persistent right & left 4th embryonic aortic arches
  - Complete vascular ring encases trachea & esophagus
- **Most common symptomatic vascular ring (55%)**
- Typically occurs with other congenital abnormalities
- May be isolated anomaly, especially in adults

IMAGING

General Features

- Best diagnostic clue
  - Right & left aortic arches compressing trachea
- Location
  - Ascending aorta divides into right & left arches
  - Right aortic arch typically larger & more superior
  - Each arch gives rise to respective carotid & subclavian arteries
    - Symmetric "**4 artery**" sign
    - No brachiocephalic artery is present
  - Arches rejoin posterior to esophagus
    - Right arch courses behind esophagus to join left
  - Descending thoracic aorta is typically on left
- Part of left arch may be atretic, but patent portions remain connected by fibrous band

Radiographic Findings

- Radiography
  - **Soft tissue on both sides of mid trachea**
  - **Bilateral tracheal indentations, mid-tracheal stenosis**
    - Trachea may be deviated by dominant arch
    - Trachea may be in abnormal midline position
  - **Right arch indentation typically higher & more pronounced than left**
  - **Lateral chest radiograph: Anterior & posterior tracheal compression at level of aortic arch**
  - Symmetric lung aeration, no unilateral air trapping

Fluoroscopic Findings

- Frontal view: Bilateral indentations on contrast-filled esophagus, often at different levels
- Lateral view: Oblique or nearly horizontal posterior indentation

CT Findings

- CTA
  - "**4 artery**" sign: Symmetric takeoff of 4 aortic branches on axial image at thoracic inlet
    - **2 anterior carotid & 2 posterior subclavian arteries**
  - 2 arches encircle trachea & esophagus
  - Smaller of 2 arches may be partially atretic
  - Severe tracheal compression at level of double arch

MR Findings

- Axial & coronal images are most helpful
- Findings comparable with those of CTA

Echocardiographic Findings

- Echocardiogram
  - Suprasternal notch view shows 2 aortic arches, each with separate carotid & subclavian arteries
  - Often insufficient for preoperative diagnosis

Angiographic Findings

- Conventional angiography
  - Rarely required with use of CT & MR

Imaging Recommendations

- Best imaging tool
  - Radiography remains primary diagnostic test
    - Absence of tracheal compression excludes vascular ring
  - Esophagram rarely obviates need for CT or MR
    - However, many asymptomatic arch anomalies are initially diagnosed by esophagram
  - CT or MR confirm diagnosis & depict anatomic variations
- Protocol advice
  - Axial & coronal reformations
  - Multidetector CTA faster to perform than MR, typically with no need for sedation & intubation
  - CT shows airway compromise better than MR

DIFFERENTIAL DIAGNOSIS

Right Arch with Aberrant Left Subclavian Artery (LSA) & Other Arch Abnormalities

- Differentiation with cross-sectional imaging

Aberrant Left Pulmonary Artery

- Compression on anterior aspect of esophagus & posterior aspect of trachea on radiography
- Often associated with tracheomalacia & congenital heart disease

Innominate Artery Compression Syndrome

- Anterior tracheal compression
- No esophageal compression

Nonvascular Masses

- Neoplasm or foregut cyst may compress trachea

PATHOLOGY

General Features

- Genetics
  - No specific genetic defect identified
- Associated abnormalities
  - Typically isolated lesion
  - 20% have congenital heart disease (CHD)
    - Tetralogy of Fallot
    - Ventricular septal defect
    - Coarctation
    - Patent ductus arteriosus
    - Transposition of great arteries
    - Truncus arteriosus
- Pathophysiology
  - Severe airway & esophageal compression
  - Tracheomalacia is common
- No hemodynamic sequelae, unless associated CHD

Gross Pathologic & Surgical Features

- **Complete vascular ring encircles trachea & esophagus**
  - Dominant right arch, left descending aorta: 75%
  - Dominant left arch, right descending aorta: 20%
  - Arches equal in size: 5%
- Smaller of 2 arches may be partially atretic

DOUBLE AORTIC ARCH

CLINICAL ISSUES

Presentation

- Most common signs/symptoms
  - Inspiratory stridor
  - Stridor worsens with feeding
  - May be minimally symptomatic, incidental finding on imaging
- Other signs/symptoms
  - Apneic attacks
  - Noisy breathing
  - "Seal bark" cough

Demographics

- Age
  - Patients typically present early in life, soon after birth

Treatment

- Thoracotomy with division of smaller of 2 arches, atretic segments & ligamentum arteriosum
  - Rare complication: Aortoesophageal fistula
    - Associated with prolonged esophageal tube placement
- < 30% have persistent symptoms postoperatively
  - Tracheobronchomalacia ± extrinsic compression
    - Midline/circumflex descending aorta
    - Previously ligated arch
- 11% of patients require 2nd surgery to repair airway
  - Aortopexy or other vascular suspension procedures
  - Tracheal ring resection & airway reconstruction

DIAGNOSTIC CHECKLIST

Consider

- Look for signs of atretic arch segment that does not opacify on CTA or MRA & does not show flow void on MR

Image Interpretation Pearls

- "4 artery" sign on axial image at thoracic inlet should suggest double aortic arch

SELECTED REFERENCES

1. Cerillo AG et al: Sixteen-row multislice computed tomography in infants with double aortic arch. Int J Cardiol. 99(2):191-4, 2005
2. Chan MS et al: Angiography and dynamic airway evaluation with MDCT in the diagnosis of double aortic arch associated with tracheomalacia. AJR Am J Roentgenol. 185(5):1248-51, 2005
3. Greil GF et al: Diagnosis of vascular rings and slings using an interleaved 3D double-slab FISP MR angiography technique. Pediatr Radiol. 2005
4. Schlesinger AE et al: Incomplete double aortic arch with atresia of the distal left arch: distinctive imaging appearance. AJR Am J Roentgenol. 184(5):1634-9, 2005
5. Backer CL et al: Pediatric Cardiac Surgery. 3rd ed. Philadelphia: Mosby. 234-50, 2003
6. Subramanyan R et al: Vascular rings: an important cause of persistent respiratory symptoms in infants and children. Indian Pediatr. 40(10):951-7, 2003
7. Yilmaz M et al: Vascular anomalies causing tracheoesophageal compression: a 20-year experience in diagnosis and management. Heart Surg Forum. 6(3):149-52, 2003
8. Fleck RJ et al: Imaging findings in pediatric patients with persistent airway symptoms after surgery for double aortic arch. AJR Am J Roentgenol. 178(5):1275-9, 2002
9. Park SC et al: Pediatric Cardiology. Vol 2. 2nd ed. London: Churchill Livingstone. 1559-75, 2002
10. Skinner LJ et al: Complete vascular ring detected by barium esophagography. Ear Nose Throat J. 81(8):554-5, 2002
11. Brockes C et al: Double aortic arch: diagnosis missed for 29 years. Vasa. 29(1):77-9, 2000
12. Gustafson LM et al: Spiral CT versus MRI in neonatal airway evaluation. Int J Pediatr Otorhinolaryngol. 52(2):197-201, 2000
13. McMahon CJ et al: Double aortic arch in D-transposition of the great arteries: confirmation of dominant arch by magnetic resonance imaging. Tex Heart Inst J. 27(4):398-400, 2000
14. Krinsky GA et al: Thoracic aorta: comparison of single-dose breath-hold and double-dose non-breath-hold gadolinium-enhanced three-dimensional MR angiography. AJR Am J Roentgenol. 173(1):145-50, 1999
15. Beghetti M et al: Double aortic arch. J Pediatr. 133(6):799, 1998
16. Donnelly LF et al: The spectrum of extrinsic lower airway compression in children: MR imaging. AJR Am J Roentgenol. 168(1):59-62, 1997
17. Fattori R et al: Intramural posttraumatic hematoma of the ascending aorta in a patient with a double aortic arch. Eur Radiol. 7(1):51-3, 1997
18. Hopkins KL et al: Pediatric great vessel anomalies: initial clinical experience with spiral CT angiography. Radiology. 200(3):811-5, 1996
19. Murdison KA: Ultrasonic Imaging of Vascular Rings and Other Anomalies Causing Tracheobronchial Compression. Echocardiography. 13(3):337-356, 1996
20. Othersen HB Jr et al: Aortoesophageal fistula and double aortic arch: two important points in management. J Pediatr Surg. 31(4):594-5, 1996
21. Ito K et al: A case of the incomplete double aortic arch diagnosed in adulthood by MR imaging. Radiat Med. 13(5):263-7, 1995
22. Katz M et al: Spiral CT and 3D image reconstruction of vascular rings and associated tracheobronchial anomalies. J Comput Assist Tomogr. 19(4):564-8, 1995
23. Simoneaux SF et al: MR imaging of the pediatric airway. Radiographics. 15(2):287-98; discussion 298-9, 1995
24. Tuma S et al: Double aortic arch in d-transposition of the great arteries complicated by tracheobronchomalacia. Cardiovasc Intervent Radiol. 18(2):115-7, 1995
25. van Son JA et al: Demonstration of vascular ring anatomy with ultrafast computed tomography. Thorac Cardiovasc Surg. 43(2):120-1, 1995
26. van Son JA et al: Imaging strategies for vascular rings. Ann Thorac Surg. 57(3):604-10, 1994
27. Kramer LA et al: Rare case of double aortic arch with hypoplastic right dorsal segment and associated tetralogy of Fallot: MR findings. Magn Reson Imaging. 11(8):1217-21, 1993

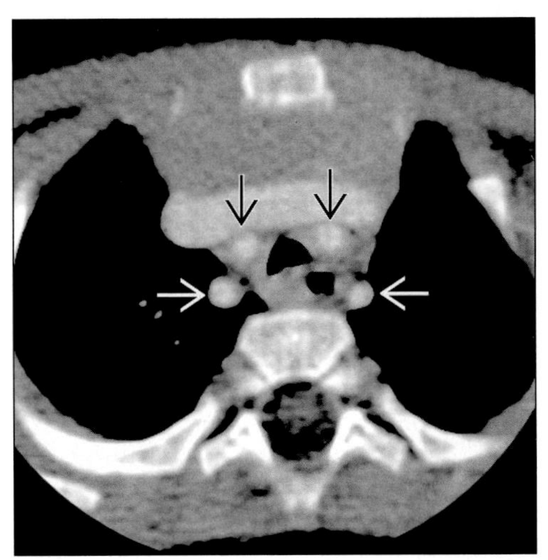

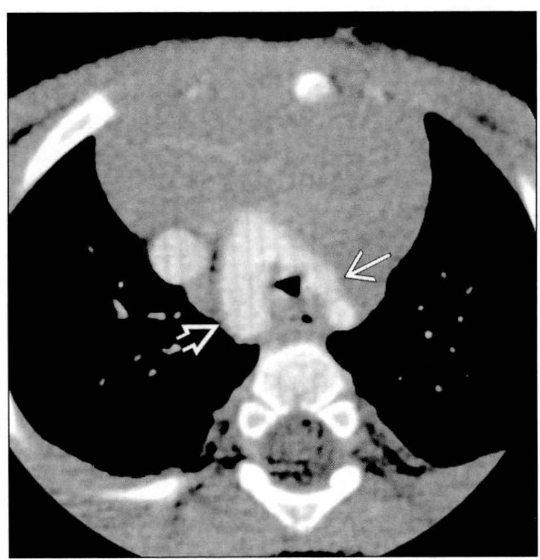

(Left) *Axial CTA of an infant with stridor secondary to an isolated double aortic arch shows that the common carotid ➙ and subclavian arteries ➙ symmetrically arise from their respective arches ("4 artery" sign) and encircle the trachea and esophagus.* ***(Right)*** *Axial CTA of the same infant shows a dominant right arch ➙ and a smaller left arch ➙. The arches encircle the trachea and esophagus. Severe tracheal narrowing resulted in stridor. Residual thymic tissue is normal for age.*

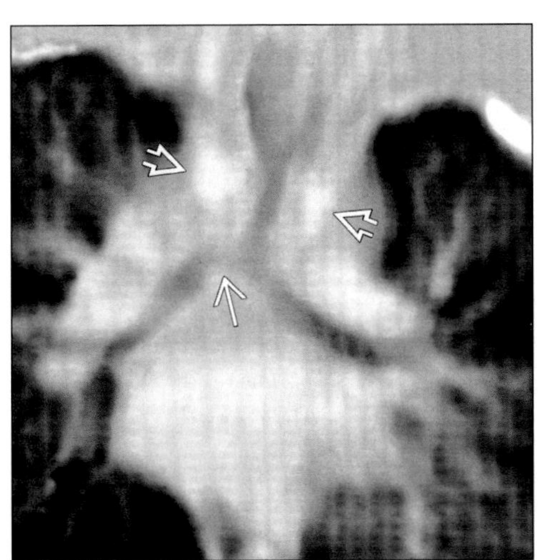

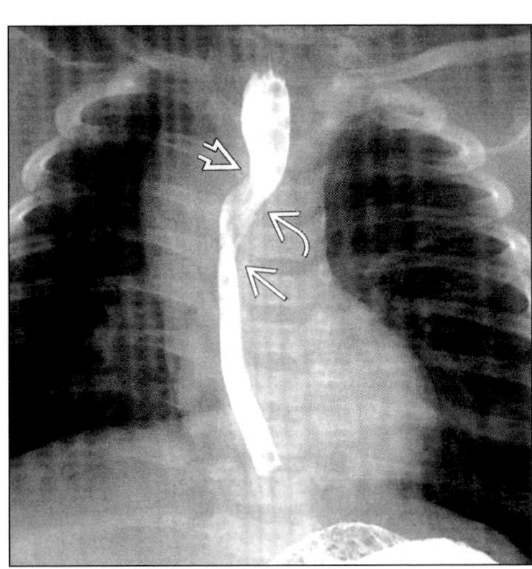

(Left) *Coronal CTA of the central airways of the same infant shows that the trachea is moderately compressed between the arches ➙. Moderate stenosis of the right mainstem bronchus ➙ is not related to the vascular ring and likely represents bronchomalacia.* ***(Right)*** *AP esophagram of the same infant shows typical indentations from the higher dominant right arch ➙, the lower left arch ➙, and the left-sided proximal descending aorta ➙. Affected infants may present with difficulty feeding.*

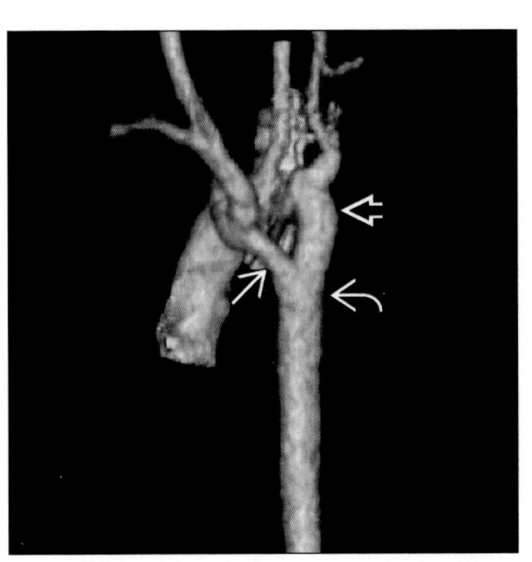

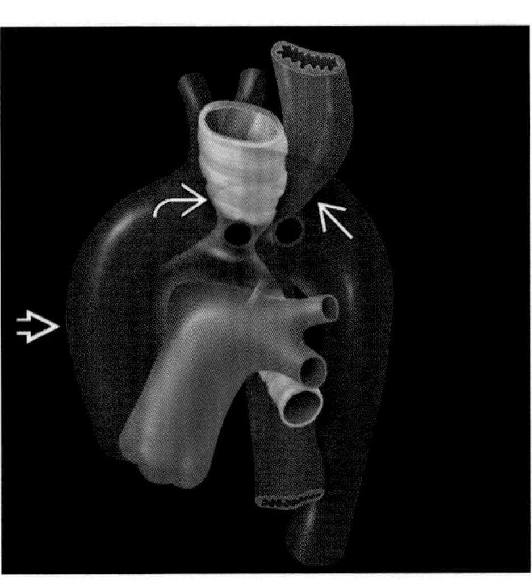

(Left) *Coronal 3D reformatted image (posterior view) of the same infant shows the right arch ➙ superior to the smaller left arch ➙. The arches join posteriorly to form the descending aorta ➙. A double aortic arch may be an isolated anomaly.* ***(Right)*** *Graphic shows the morphology of double aortic arch with arches arising from the ascending aorta ➙ to form a complete vascular ring that encircles and compresses the trachea ➙ and the esophagus ➙. The right arch is typically larger and more superior.*

AORTIC COARCTATION

Key Facts

Terminology

- Congenital narrowing of aorta, most commonly occurring just distal to left subclavian artery origin

Imaging

- Chest radiograph: Inferior rib notching, "figure 3" sign
- Esophagram: "Reverse figure 3" sign
- CTA: Focal shelf-like narrowing of posterior/lateral aorta just distal to left subclavian origin
- MR
  - Contrast-enhanced 3D MRA for vessel morphology & depiction of enlarged collateral arteries
  - Velocity encoded cine (VENC) used to estimate pressure gradients & flow volumes
- Angiography
  - Morphology of coarctation & collateral vessels
  - Measurement of pressure gradients

Top Differential Diagnoses

- Pseudocoarctation
- Takayasu arteritis

Pathology

- Associations
  - Bicuspid aortic valve, ventricular septal defect (VSD), patent ductus arteriosus (PDA)
  - Turner syndrome

Clinical Issues

- Surgical correction used for infants
- Balloon angioplasty used for children and adults
- Stent placement typically for recoarctation

Diagnostic Checklist

- Search for subtle signs of coarctation in any young patient with hypertension

*(**Left**) PA chest radiograph shows inferior rib notching, a classic radiographic sign of aortic coarctation produced by collateral vasculature. (Courtesy L. Heyneman, MD.) (**Right**) Composite PA chest radiographs of patients with coarctation show the "figure 3" sign (left) produced by a proximal convexity ➪ from a tortuous left subclavian artery, an indentation → representing the coarctation, a distal convexity ↪ from a dilated post-stenotic aorta, and obscuration of the aortic arch (right).*

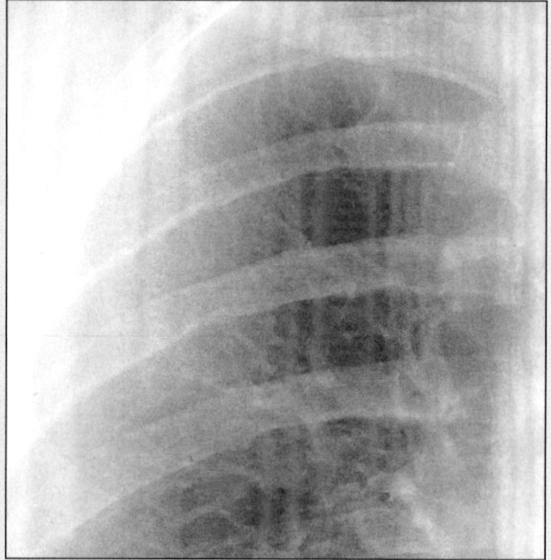

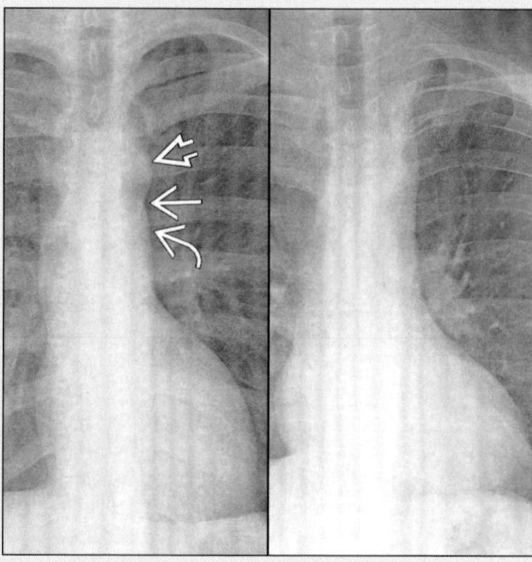

*(**Left**) Composite image with axial CTA at the prestenotic level (left) and the coarctation (right) shows characteristic features, including focal narrowing at the coarctation ➪ and dilated internal mammary → and intercostal ↪ arteries that serve as collaterals. (**Right**) Oblique CTA MIP reformation of the same patient better delineates the coarctation →, the poststenotic dilatation ↪, tortuous and dilated internal mammary artery ➪, and intercostal collaterals.*

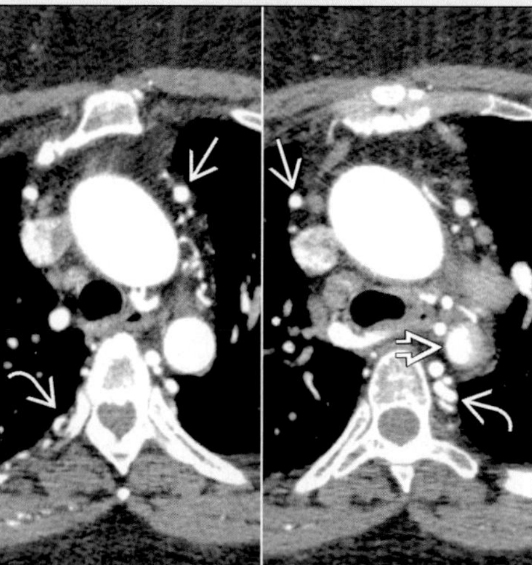

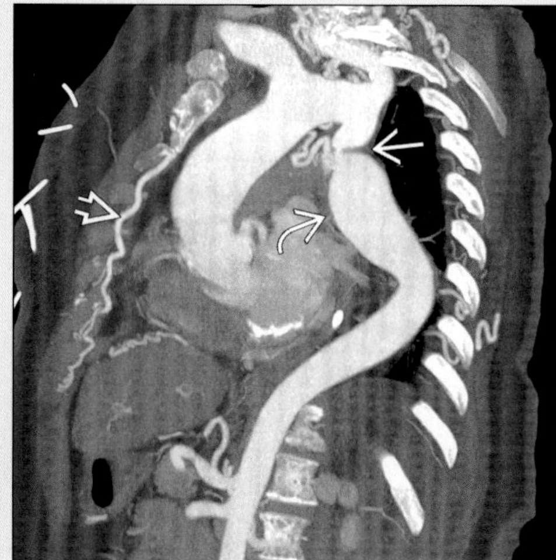

AORTIC COARCTATION

TERMINOLOGY

Definitions

- Congenital narrowing of aorta, most commonly occurring just distal to left subclavian artery origin

IMAGING

General Features

- Best diagnostic clue
  - Inferior rib notching on radiography
- Location
  - May occur anywhere in aorta or at multiple sites
  - Preductal, ductal, & postductal

Radiographic Findings

- Radiography
  - **Inferior rib notching (Roesler sign)**
    - Related to enlargement of intercostal arteries serving as collaterals
    - Rare before 5 years of age
    - Affects ribs 3 through 8; 1st & 2nd ribs not affected as they arise from costocervical trunk & do not anastomose with distal aorta
    - May regress post repair
  - **"Figure 3" sign in up to 50% of cases**
    - Dilated left subclavian artery produces proximal convexity
    - Indentation at coarctation
    - Poststenotic descending aorta produces distal convexity
  - **Ill-defined or obscured aortic arch**
- Esophagram
  - "Reverse figure 3" sign
    - Compression on esophagus from dilated left subclavian artery & poststenotic dilatation of descending aorta

CT Findings

- CTA
  - Multiplanar reformations (sagittal oblique plane) & 3D volume-rendered images
  - **Defines location & severity of stenosis**
  - Focal shelf-like narrowing of posterior/lateral aorta just distal to left subclavian origin
  - Demonstration of enlarged collateral arteries

MR Findings

- Contrast-enhanced MRA
  - Vessel morphology & demonstration of enlarged collateral arteries
  - Detection of bicuspid aortic valve
- Velocity encoded cine (VENC)
  - Used to estimate pressure gradients & flow volumes
- Cardiac MR
  - Diagnosis of associated cardiac anomalies
  - Assessment of bicuspid aortic valve with quantification of stenosis &/or aortic regurgitation

Angiographic Findings

- Vessel morphology & direct measurement of pressure gradient
  - < 20 mmHg: Mild coarctation
  - > 20 mmHg: Suggests need for intervention

Imaging Recommendations

- Best imaging tool
  - Echocardiography in infancy
  - MR in older child or adult
  - Angiography for pressure gradients

DIFFERENTIAL DIAGNOSIS

Pseudocoarctation

- Older adult with elongation & kinking of aorta related to atherosclerosis
- No hemodynamically significant stenosis, no collateral vessels

Takayasu Arteritis

- Inflammatory narrowing of unknown etiology
- Narrowing &/or occlusion of aorta & branch vessels, rarely isolated to aortic isthmus

Interrupted Aortic Arch

- Complete absence of continuity between 2 segments of aorta
- Nearly always manifests in neonates

Traumatic Pseudoaneurysm

- History of trauma, healed rib & other skeletal fractures
- Narrowing of descending thoracic aorta may coexist with pseudoaneurysm

Inferior Rib Notching Differential

- Neurofibromatosis
- Venous collaterals (SVC obstruction)
- Decreased pulmonary blood flow (tetralogy of Fallot, pulmonary atresia)
- Blalock-Taussig shunt (1st & 2nd ribs)

PATHOLOGY

General Features

- Etiology
  - Muscular theory
    - Migration of tissue from ductus arteriosus into aortic wall & subsequent contraction
  - Hemodynamic theory
    - Decreased aortic blood flow during fetal development may not allow proper aortic growth
    - Increased incidence of coarctation in disorders where left ventricular outflow tract obstruction reduces aortic blood flow; conversely, decreased incidence of coarctation in disorders where decreased ductal flow is present (e.g., tetralogy of Fallot)
- Associated abnormalities
  - **Bicuspid aortic valve (reported in 50-85%)**
  - Ventricular septal defect (VSD)
  - Patent ductus arteriosus (PDA)
  - Cerebral aneurysms

Staging, Grading, & Classification

- No agreed upon classification; previously used classifications, including infantile & adult type, are discouraged due to overlapping manifestations
- **Simple coarctation**
  - Occurs in isolation

AORTIC COARCTATION

- Often localized just beyond left subclavian artery origin (postductal)
- **Complex coarctation**
  - Occurs in presence of other intracardiac anomalies; thus, tends to manifest in infancy
  - Often preductal

Gross Pathologic & Surgical Features

- Obstructing membrane or ridge of tissue near aortic isthmus
- May develop cystic medial necrosis adjacent to coarctation site; predisposes to aneurysm or dissection

CLINICAL ISSUES

Presentation

- Most common signs/symptoms
  - **Neonates**
    - Asymptomatic if coarctation not severe or patent PDA
    - If severe coarctation or closed ductus arteriosus, may have heart failure
    - Decreased femoral pulses, associated murmurs
  - **Children & adults**
    - Usually asymptomatic unless severe hypertension
    - May have claudication & chest pain with exercise
    - Differential hypertension between upper & lower extremities, diminished femoral pulses
    - Murmur associated with bicuspid aortic valve

Demographics

- Age
  - Related to degree of narrowing & presence of associated abnormalities
- Gender
  - M:F = 2:1
- Epidemiology
  - Incidence: 2-6 per 10,000 births
  - Comprises 5-8% of cases of congenital heart disease

Natural History & Prognosis

- Without repair
  - Average age of death: 35-42 years
  - 75% mortality by age 46
  - Due to aortic dissection or rupture, heart failure, myocardial infarct, & cerebral hemorrhage
- With repair
  - Approximately 90% survival at 20 years; decreased survival with increased age at repair
  - Recoarctation (2-14%)
  - Postoperative aneurysms (increased risk after patch aortoplasty)
  - Long-term survival decreased due to hypertension, coronary artery disease, dissection
- Pregnancy-related issues
  - Untreated coarctation: Increased risk of dissection & intracranial hemorrhage
  - Treated coarctation: Increased rate of miscarriage & preeclampsia

Treatment

- Indications for treatment
  - Infant with severe stenosis & heart failure
  - Longstanding hypertension
  - Hemodynamically significant stenosis (gradient > 20 mmHg)
  - Extensive collateral flow
  - Female patient contemplating pregnancy
- Surgical correction: First-line treatment for infants
  - Resection with end-to-end anastomosis
    - Higher risk of spinal artery injury & restenosis
  - Left subclavian flap aortoplasty
    - Sacrifice left subclavian artery & vertebral artery (to avoid subclavian steal)
  - Bypass graft
    - Used if area of narrowing is too long for end-to-end repair
  - Prosthetic patch or interposition graft
    - Rarely used due to long-term risk of infection or aneurysm with prosthetic material
  - Acute complications
    - Surgical mortality rare
    - Paradoxic hypertension, recoarctation, hypertension, paraplegia due to spinal artery damage, recurrent laryngeal or phrenic nerve injury, subclavian steal
  - Late complications
    - Aortic aneurysm, recurrent coarctation, hypertension
- Balloon angioplasty
  - First-line treatment for older children & adults for native coarctation or recoarctation
  - Not recommended for infants due to ↑ rate of recurrence
  - Acute complications rare
    - Dissection, stroke
  - Late complications
    - Recoarctation, aneurysm, endocarditis, hypertension
- Stent placement
  - Generally reserved for recoarctation
  - Complications
    - Acute rupture, dissection, stent fracture or migration
    - Aneurysm in up to 11%

DIAGNOSTIC CHECKLIST

Consider

- Search for subtle signs of coarctation in any young patient with hypertension

Image Interpretation Pearls

- Enlarged collaterals imply significant stenosis

SELECTED REFERENCES

1. Gaca AM et al: Repair of congenital heart disease: a primer--Part 2. Radiology. 248(1):44-60, 2008
2. Hom JJ et al: Velocity-encoded cine MR imaging in aortic coarctation: functional assessment of hemodynamic events. Radiographics. 28(2):407-16, 2008
3. Konen E et al: Coarctation of the aorta before and after correction: the role of cardiovascular MRI. AJR Am J Roentgenol. 182(5):1333-9, 2004
4. Sloan RD et al: Coarctation of the aorta; the roentgenologic aspects of one hundred and twenty-five surgically confirmed cases. Radiology. 61(5):701-21, 1953

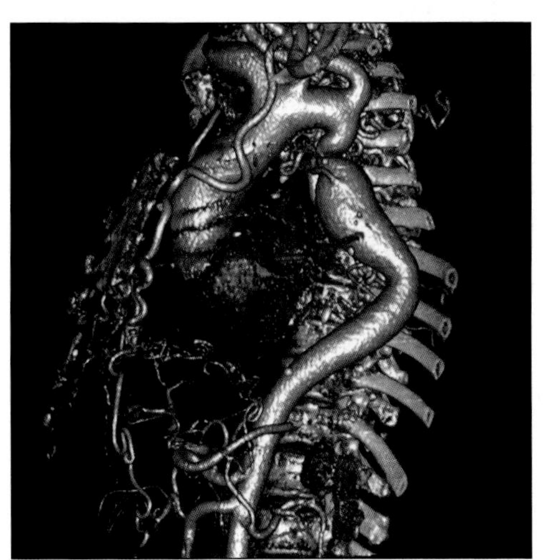

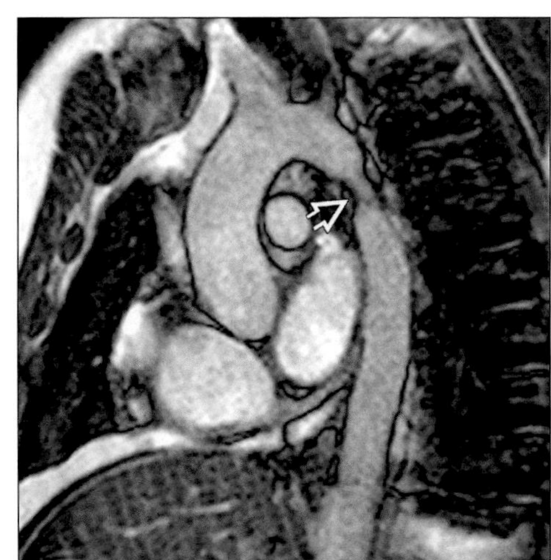

(Left) *Volume-rendered 3D CTA of a patient with aortic coarctation shows the use of this technique for morphologic assessment of coarctation and for providing an overall view of chest wall collaterals. 3D reformations are useful to help clinicians and surgeons better understand the tridimensional configuration of the lesion.* **(Right)** *Sagittal oblique MR SSFP cine (bright blood) sequence shows the aortic morphology and the area of stenosis ➔. Spin dephasing jets can be seen in regions of stenosis.*

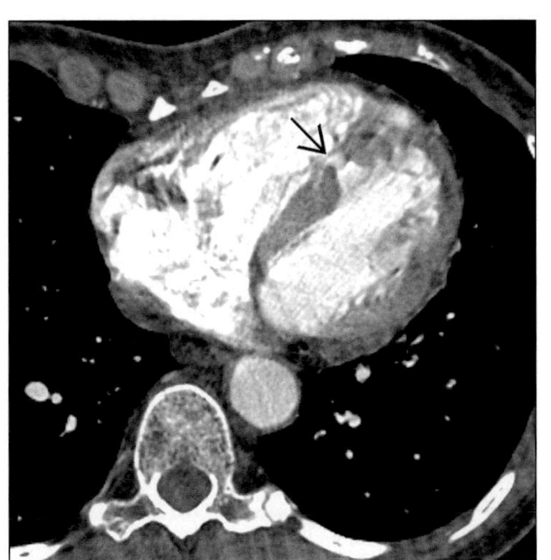

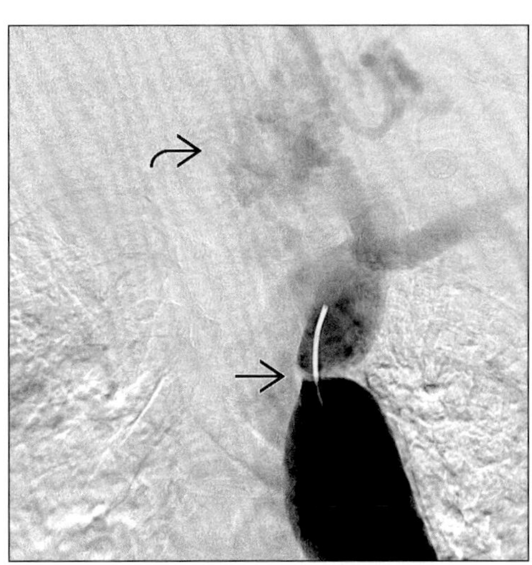

(Left) *Axial CECT of a patient with coarctation shows a ventricular septal defect (VSD) ➔, a known associated finding.* **(Right)** *DSA of a patient undergoing cerebral angiography for subarachnoid hemorrhage shows the catheter tip proximal to a severe coarctation ➔. Because of their association with intracranial aneurysms, coarctations may be incidentally discovered during conventional angiography. Note dilated thyrocervical and costocervical trunk branches ➔.*

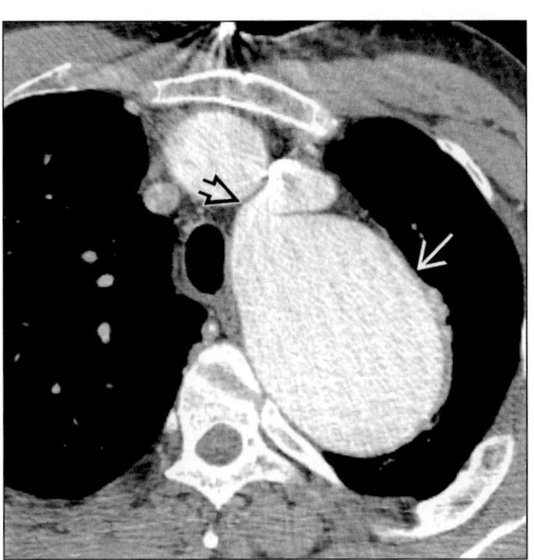

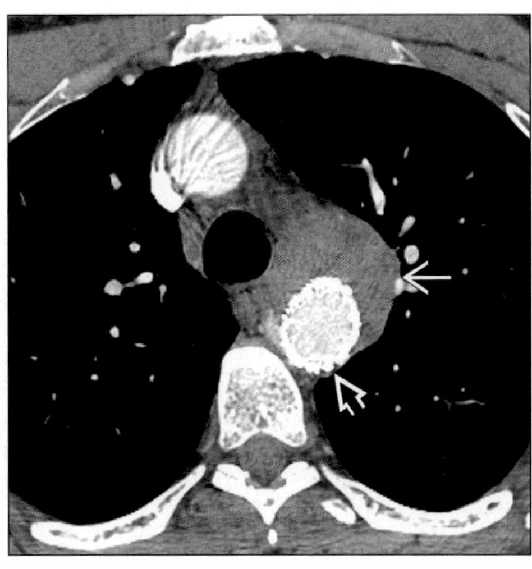

(Left) *Axial CTA of a patient who underwent surgical repair of aortic coarctation demonstrates a postoperative recoarctation ➔ and a poststenotic aneurysm ➔.* **(Right)** *Axial CECT of a patient who underwent surgical repair of a coarctation shows a postoperative pseudoaneurysm ➔. Such pseudoaneurysms can subsequently be excluded with a stent graft ➔, as in this case.*

ATRIAL SEPTAL DEFECT

Key Facts

Terminology
- Atrial septal defect (ASD)

Imaging
- Radiography
  - Cardiac silhouette usually normal
  - Shunt vascularity
  - Pulmonary edema & pleural effusions
  - Pulmonary artery hypertension
- Cardiac gated CTA
  - Direct visualization of ASD
  - Determination of direction & extent of shunt
  - Associated abnormalities
- MR
  - Evaluation of shunt volume & direction
  - Evaluation of valvular function
  - Assessment of pressure gradients across valves

Top Differential Diagnoses
- Ventricular septal defect
- Patent ductus arteriosus
- Pulmonary artery hypertension

Clinical Issues
- Usually asymptomatic in early life
- Becomes symptomatic with advancing age
- 90% of patients symptomatic by 40 years
  - Exertional dyspnea, fatigue, palpitations, & congestive heart failure
- Surgical repair
  - Open repair with extracorporeal support most common
  - Minimally invasive approaches
- Percutaneous transcatheter therapy
  - Small ostium secundum defects most amenable
  - Fewer complications vs. surgical repair

*(**Left**) AP chest radiograph of a patient with an atrial septal defect (ASD) shows shunt vascularity ➔, especially within the upper lung zones. (**Right**) Axial cardiac gated CTA demonstrates a small defect ➔ within the interatrial septum, consistent with an ASD. Cardiac gated CTA not only enables direct visualization of an ASD, but may also provide information regarding the direction and extent of intracardiac shunting.*

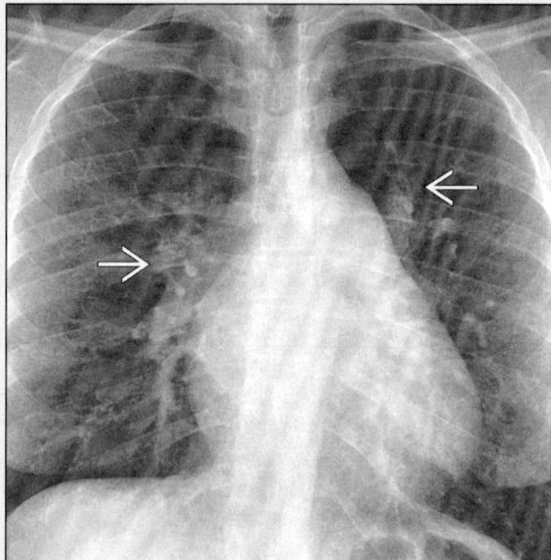

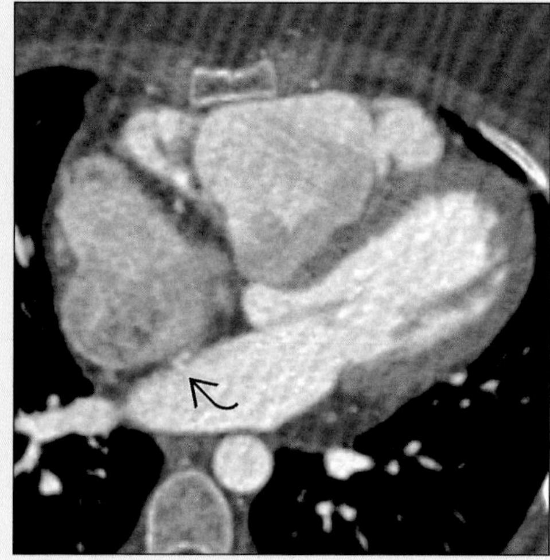

*(**Left**) Axial CECT shows a sinus venosus ASD ➔. Sinus venosus defects are the least common type of ASD, accounting for approximately 5-10% of ASDs. (**Right**) Axial cine MR of a different patient demonstrates a sinus venosus defect ➔. ASDs account for approximately 10% of all congenital cardiac anomalies, but they are the most common congenital cardiac anomalies in adults.*

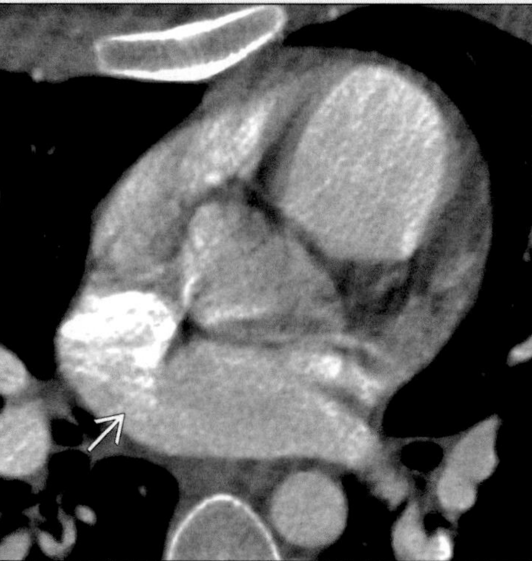

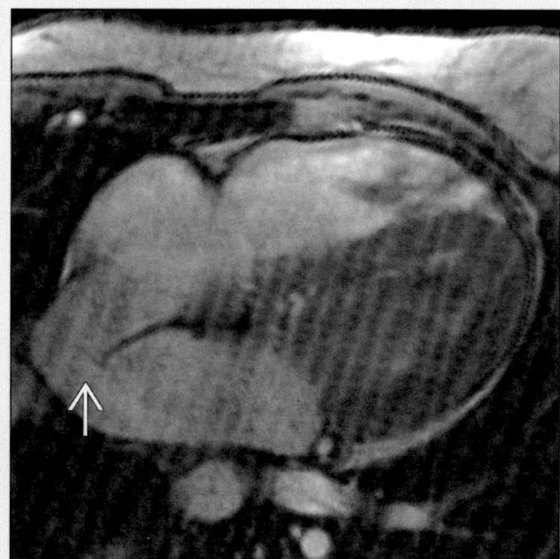

ATRIAL SEPTAL DEFECT

TERMINOLOGY

Abbreviations

- **Atrial septal defect (ASD)**

IMAGING

General Features

- Best diagnostic clue
  - Normal cardiac silhouette & shunt vascularity on chest radiography
- Location
  - Ostium secundum (75%)
    - Mid interatrial septum
    - Oval defect bordered by fossa ovalis
  - Ostium primum (15-20%)
    - Anterior/inferior interatrial septum
    - Located adjacent to atrioventricular (AV) valves
  - Sinus venosus (5-10%)
    - Superior interatrial septum near superior vena cava
    - Posterior to fossa ovalis

Radiographic Findings

- Radiography
  - Cardiac silhouette usually normal
    - Left atrium typically normal in size
      - Differentiates ASD from ventricular septal defect (VSD) & patent ductus arteriosus (PDA)
    - May be enlarged in severe mitral regurgitation
    - Enlargement of right atrium & ventricle may be seen in pulmonary artery hypertension
  - **Shunt vascularity**
  - Pulmonary edema & pleural effusions
  - Pulmonary artery hypertension
    - Enlarged pulmonary trunk & pulmonary arteries
    - Pruning of peripheral pulmonary artery branches
    - Enlargement of right atrium & ventricle

CT Findings

- Cardiac gated CTA
  - Direct visualization of ASD
  - Determination of direction & extent of shunt
  - Associated abnormalities
    - Partial anomalous pulmonary venous return
      - Pulmonary vein draining into SVC
      - Usually involves right upper lobe
      - Strongest association with sinus venosus ASD

MR Findings

- Phase contrast & cine MR
  - Assessment of shunt volume & direction
  - Assessment of valvular function
  - Determination of pressure gradients across valves

Echocardiographic Findings

- Echocardiogram
  - Direct visualization of ASD
    - 2-dimensional (2D) imaging subcostal approach
  - Mitral valve prolapse may be visualized
  - Anterior systolic motion of interventricular septum
  - Gooseneck deformity of ostium primum defect
    - Subxiphoid long-axis view of left ventricular outflow tract (LVOT)
  - Enlargement of pulmonary trunk & right ventricle in pulmonary artery hypertension
- Color Doppler
  - Direct visualization of ASD

Angiographic Findings

- Cardiac catheterization
  - Performed when echocardiography is inconclusive or to evaluate associated abnormalities
  - Extension of catheter across defect
- Left ventricular angiography
  - Evaluation of mitral valve prolapse & extent of mitral regurgitation
  - Gooseneck deformity in ostium primum defect
    - Best seen on right anterior oblique (RAO) view

Imaging Recommendations

- Best imaging tool
  - Cardiac gated CTA or MR to visualize defect

DIFFERENTIAL DIAGNOSIS

Ventricular Septal Defect (VSD)

- Left-to-right intracardiac shunt
- Enlarged cardiac silhouette: LA & LV
- Shunt vascularity
- Pulmonary edema
- Pulmonary artery hypertension
  - Enlarged pulmonary trunk & pulmonary arteries
  - Pruning of peripheral pulmonary artery branches
  - Enlargement of right ventricle

Patent Ductus Arteriosus (PDA)

- Persistent connection between descending thoracic aorta & proximal left pulmonary artery
- Left-to-right intracardiac shunt
- Enlarged cardiac silhouette: LA & LV
- Enlarged aortic arch: Distinguishes PDA from VSD
- Shunt vascularity
- Pulmonary edema
- Pulmonary artery hypertension
  - Enlarged pulmonary trunk & pulmonary arteries
  - Pruning of peripheral pulmonary artery branches
  - Enlargement of right ventricle

Pulmonary Artery Hypertension (PAH)

- Enlarged pulmonary trunk & central pulmonary arteries
- CTA: Enlargement of pulmonary trunk > 30 mm
- HRCT
  - Pre-capillary etiologies: Emphysema, fibrosis, honeycomb lung
  - Post-capillary etiologies: Centrilobular ground-glass nodules, pulmonary edema, pleural effusions
  - Chronic PAH: Patchy, ground-glass opacities
- Pre-capillary etiologies: Chronic pulmonary emboli, congenital left-to-right shunts, lung disease, idiopathic PAH
- Post-capillary etiologies: Left heart failure & mitral stenosis

PATHOLOGY

General Features

- Etiology
  - Congenital cardiac anomaly characterized by defects within interatrial septum

ATRIAL SEPTAL DEFECT

- Ostium secundum
  - Incomplete adhesion of septum secundum to flap valve of foramen ovale
- Ostium primum
  - Incomplete fusion of septum primum with endocardial cushion
- Sinus venosus
  - Abnormal fusion of sinus venosus & right atrium
- Genetics
  - Ellis van Creveld
    - Skeletal dysplasia with a common atrium
    - Autosomal recessive pattern of inheritance
  - Holt-Oram syndrome
    - ASD & upper extremity anomalies
    - Autosomal dominant pattern of inheritance
  - Trisomy 21
    - Associated with ostium primum defects
  - Other syndromes
    - Familial ASD associated with progressive atrioventricular block
      - Autosomal dominant pattern of inheritance
- Associated abnormalities
  - Mitral valve abnormalities
    - Double-orifice mitral valve
      - 2% of ostium primum defects
  - Partial anomalous pulmonary venous return
    - Strongest association with sinus venosus ASD

CLINICAL ISSUES

Presentation

- Most common signs/symptoms
  - Usually asymptomatic in early life
    - Some patients may be symptomatic
      - Exertional dyspnea
      - Fatigue
      - Recurrent respiratory infections
      - Congestive heart failure
  - Typically become symptomatic with advancing age
    - 90% of patients with ASD symptomatic by age 40
    - Exertional dyspnea
    - Fatigue
    - Palpitations
    - Congestive heart failure
  - Pulmonary artery hypertension
    - Dyspnea on exertion, fatigue, syncope, & chest pain
  - Eisenmenger syndrome
    - Symptoms related to polycythemia
    - Headache, fatigue, & marked dyspnea

Demographics

- Gender
  - F:M = 2:1
- Epidemiology
  - 10% of all congenital cardiac anomalies
  - Most common congenital cardiac anomaly in adults

Natural History & Prognosis

- 20% close spontaneously during 1st year of life
- Spontaneous closure in adulthood is unlikely
- 1% become symptomatic during 1st year of life
  - 0.1% mortality
- Defects may result in pulmonary artery hypertension
  - May be reversible if treated early
  - Development of Eisenmenger syndrome
    - Reversal of left-to-right shunt
- 25% lifetime mortality if unrepaired

Treatment

- Medical therapy
  - Limited to atrial arrhythmias & volume overload
- Surgical repair
  - Indications
    - Right ventricular overload
    - Pulmonary flow:systemic flow > 1.5
  - Contraindications
    - Pulmonary flow:systemic flow < 0.7
    - Severe pulmonary artery hypertension
  - Open repair with extracorporeal support most common
    - Direct closure & patch repair
  - Minimally invasive approaches
    - Types: Limited thoracotomy, hemisternotomy, & submammary
    - No difference in morbidity & mortality
- Percutaneous transcatheter therapy
  - Use of atrial septal occluder device
  - Small ostium secundum defects most amenable
  - Success rates approach 96%
  - Fewer complications & decreased hospitalization time vs. surgical repair

DIAGNOSTIC CHECKLIST

Consider

- Atrial septal defect in setting of normal cardiac silhouette & shunt vascularity on chest radiography

SELECTED REFERENCES

1. Kafka H et al: Cardiac MRI and pulmonary MR angiography of sinus venosus defect and partial anomalous pulmonary venous connection in cause of right undiagnosed ventricular enlargement. AJR Am J Roentgenol. 192(1):259-66, 2009
2. Lee T et al: MDCT evaluation after closure of atrial septal defect with an Amplatzer septal occluder. AJR Am J Roentgenol. 188(5):W431-9, 2007
3. Piaw CS et al: Use of non-invasive phase contrast magnetic resonance imaging for estimation of atrial septal defect size and morphology: a comparison with transesophageal echo. Cardiovasc Intervent Radiol. 29(2):230-4, 2006
4. Webb G et al: Atrial septal defects in the adult: recent progress and overview. Circulation. 114(15):1645-53, 2006

ATRIAL SEPTAL DEFECT

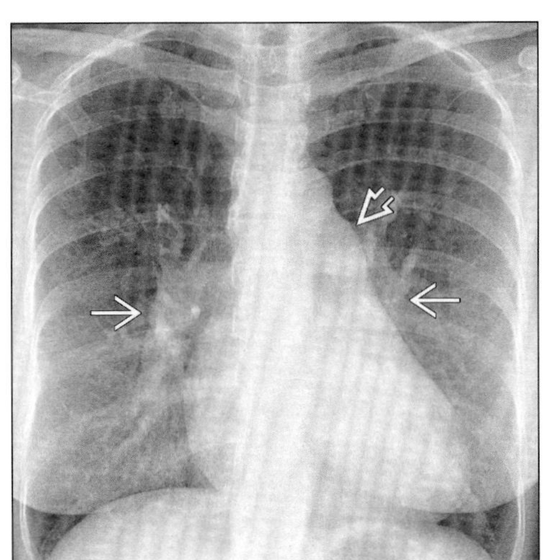

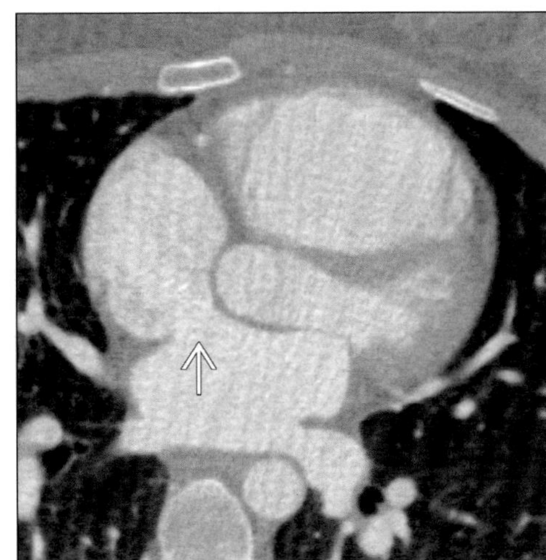

(Left) *AP chest radiograph demonstrates increased size and number of pulmonary vessels, enlargement of the left and right pulmonary arteries →, and enlargement of the pulmonary trunk →. These findings are consistent with shunt vascularity and pulmonary artery hypertension in this patient with an ASD.* ***(Right)*** *Axial cardiac gated CTA shows an ostium secundum defect →, which is the most common type of ASD.*

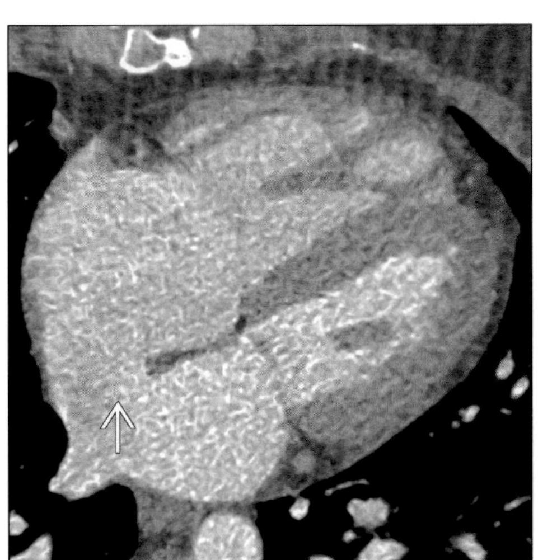

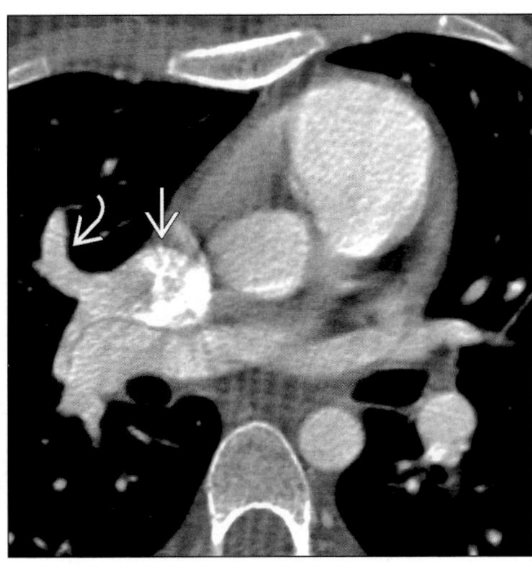

(Left) *Axial cardiac gated CTA shows a sinus venosus ASD →. Note the enlargement of the right atrium and right ventricle.* ***(Right)*** *Axial CECT of a different patient with a sinus venosus ASD demonstrates partial anomalous pulmonary venous return, with the right upper lobe pulmonary vein → draining directly into the superior vena cava →. Partial anomalous pulmonary venous return is strongly associated with sinus venosus defects.*

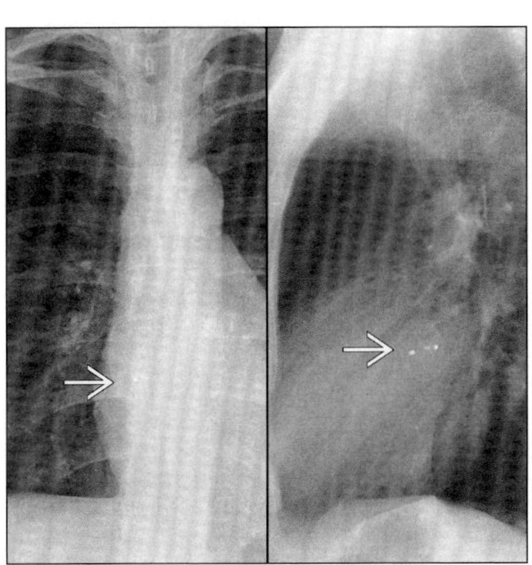

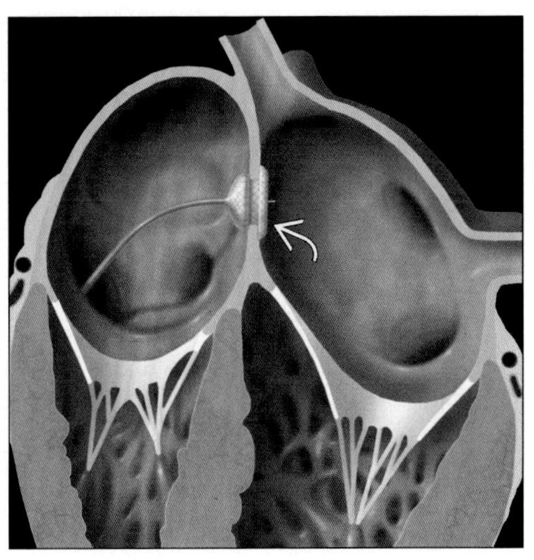

(Left) *PA chest radiograph of a patient following percutaneous closure of an ASD demonstrates an atrial septal occluder → projecting over the expected position of the interatrial septum.* ***(Right)*** *Graphic shows placement of an atrial septal occluder introduced into the right atrium via inferior vena cava approach. The device is placed and expanded within the ASD → so that its double-disc morphology secures it within the defect, resulting in closure.*

VENTRICULAR SEPTAL DEFECT

Key Facts

Terminology

- Ventricular septal defect (VSD)

Imaging

- Chest radiographs may be normal with small defects
- Cardiac enlargement with larger defects
  - Left atrial enlargement: Distinguishes VSD & PDA from ASD
- Aortic arch normal in size: Distinguishes VSD from PDA
- Enlarged pulmonary vasculature
- Findings of pulmonary artery hypertension
- Direct visualization of VSD on CT & MR
- MR: Ventricular volume, mass, function
  - Shunt volume & direction
  - Valvular function
  - Pressure gradients across valves

Top Differential Diagnoses

- Atrial septal defect (ASD)
- Patent ductus arteriosus (PDA)
- Pulmonary artery hypertension (PAH)

Pathology

- Most commonly congenital in etiology

Clinical Issues

- Patients with small defects may be asymptomatic
- Small VSDs typically close spontaneously
- Large VSDs require surgical correction
- Defects may result in PAH & Eisenmenger syndrome
- Treatment
  - Medical management of congestive heart failure & Eisenmenger syndrome
  - Surgical management: Closure & percutaneous device occlusion

*(**Left**) PA chest radiograph of a patient with a ventricular septal defect (VSD) shows marked enlargement of the pulmonary trunk ➔ and left ➔ and right ➔ pulmonary arteries. These findings are consistent with pulmonary artery hypertension secondary to the left-to-right intracardiac shunt. (**Right**) Lateral chest radiograph of the same patient demonstrates enlargement of the left atrium ➔, which extends posteriorly and exerts mass effect on the anterior aspect of the trachea.*

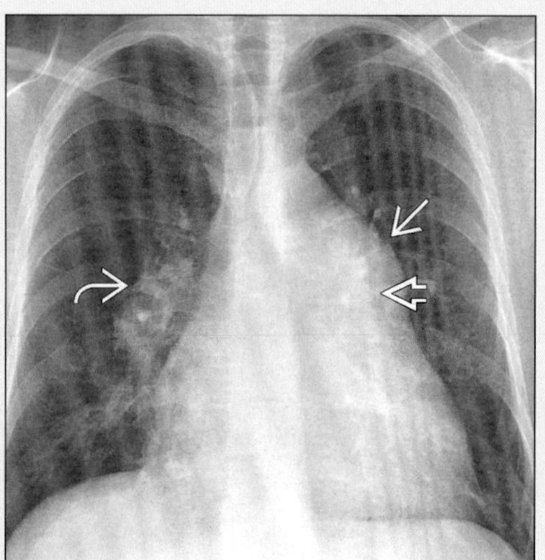

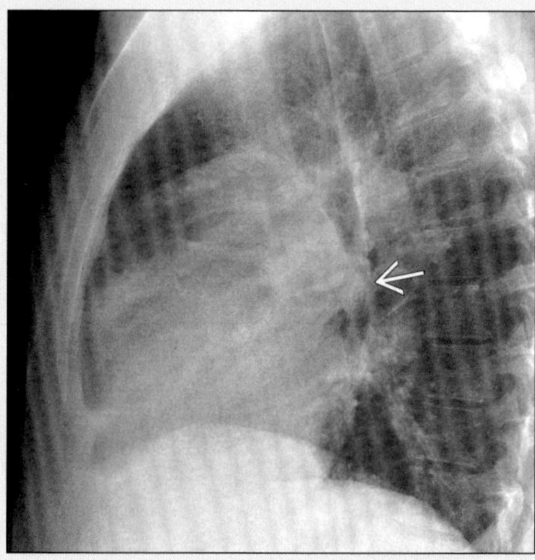

*(**Left**) Axial cardiac gated CTA demonstrates a defect ➔ within the high aspect of the interventricular septum, allowing communication between the left and right ventricles. (**Right**) Axial GRE MR image of the same patient shows the defect ➔, which is consistent with a perimembranous type of ventricular septal defect. Perimembranous VSDs are the most common types of defect, accounting for approximately 75% of VSDs.*

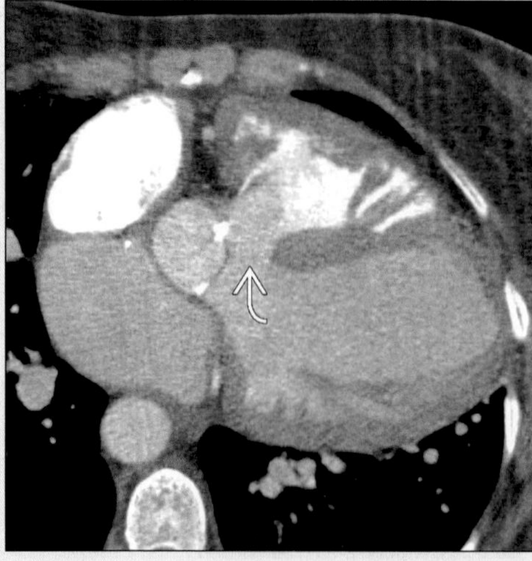

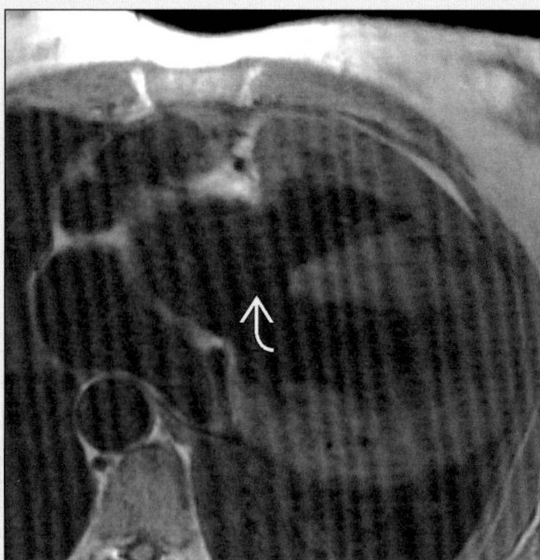

VENTRICULAR SEPTAL DEFECT

TERMINOLOGY

Abbreviations

- **Ventricular septal defect (VSD)**

IMAGING

General Features

- Best diagnostic clue
  - **Enlargement of left atrium & ventricle & enlarged pulmonary vasculature on chest radiography**
- Location
  - Perimembranous (75%)
  - Inlet (8-10%)
  - Muscular or trabecular (5-10%)
  - Outlet or supracristal (5%)
- Morphology
  - Multiple defects may occur
    - More common in muscular or trabecular septum

Radiographic Findings

- Radiography
  - **Chest radiographs may be normal in patients with small defects**
  - **Medium-sized defects**
    - Mild enlargement of cardiac silhouette
    - Enlarged pulmonary vasculature
  - **Large defects**
    - Enlargement of cardiac silhouette
      - Left ventricle
      - Left atrial enlargement: Distinguishes VSD & patent ductus arteriosus (PDA) from atrial septal defect (ASD)
    - Aortic arch normal in size: Distinguishes VSD from PDA
    - Enlarged pulmonary vasculature
    - Pulmonary edema & pleural effusions may be present
    - Pulmonary artery hypertension (PAH)
      - Enlarged pulmonary trunk & central pulmonary arteries
      - Pruning of peripheral pulmonary artery branches
      - Enlargement of right ventricle

CT Findings

- Cardiac gated CTA
  - **Direct visualization of VSD**
  - Determination of direction & extent of shunting

MR Findings

- Phase contrast & cine MR
  - Ventricular volume, mass, function
  - Shunt volume & direction
  - Valvular function
  - Pressure gradients across valves

Echocardiographic Findings

- Echocardiogram
  - Most VSDs identified & characterized by echocardiography
  - Direct visualization of defects
- Color Doppler
  - Helpful in detecting small defects
  - Direction & velocity of shunting

Angiographic Findings

- Small defects
  - Normal right heart pressures
  - Normal pulmonary vascular resistance
- Large defects
  - Pulmonary flow > systemic flow
  - Pulmonary & systemic systolic pressures equivalent
- **Eisenmenger syndrome**
  - Elevated systolic & diastolic pulmonary artery pressures
  - Desaturation of blood in left ventricle
  - Minimal left-to-right shunting

Imaging Recommendations

- Best imaging tool
  - Cardiac gated CTA or MR to visualize defect

DIFFERENTIAL DIAGNOSIS

Atrial Septal Defect

- Left-to-right intracardiac shunt
- Left atrium typically normal in size: Distinguishes ASD from VSD
- Enlarged pulmonary vasculature
- Pulmonary edema
- Pulmonary artery hypertension
  - Enlarged pulmonary trunk & central pulmonary arteries
  - Pruning of peripheral pulmonary artery branches
  - Enlargement of right ventricle

Patent Ductus Arteriosus

- Persistent connection between descending thoracic aorta & proximal left pulmonary artery
- Left-to-right intracardiac shunt
- Enlargement of cardiac silhouette
  - Left atrium & left ventricle
- Enlargement of aortic arch: Distinguishes PDA from VSD
- Enlarged pulmonary vasculature
- Pulmonary edema
- Pulmonary artery hypertension
  - Enlarged pulmonary trunk & central pulmonary arteries
  - Pruning of peripheral pulmonary artery branches
  - Enlargement of right ventricle

Pulmonary Artery Hypertension

- Enlarged pulmonary trunk & central pulmonary arteries
- CTA: Enlargement of pulmonary trunk > 30 mm
- HRCT
  - Pre-capillary etiologies: Emphysema, fibrosis, honeycomb lung
  - Post-capillary etiologies: Centrilobular ground-glass nodules, pulmonary edema, pleural effusions
  - Chronic PAH: Patchy ground-glass opacity
- Pre-capillary etiologies: Chronic pulmonary emboli, congenital left-to-right shunts, lung disease, idiopathic PAH
- Post-capillary etiologies: Left heart failure & mitral stenosis

VENTRICULAR SEPTAL DEFECT

PATHOLOGY

General Features

- Etiology
  - **Congenital**
    - Most common etiology
    - 4 types described by location along interventricular septum
  - **Traumatic**
    - Blunt or penetrating chest trauma
  - **Postmyocardial infarction**
- Associated abnormalities
  - Tetralogy of Fallot, truncus arteriosus, & double outlet right ventricle
  - Coarctation & tricuspid atresia less common

Staging, Grading, & Classification

- Interventricular septum divided into 2 parts
  - Membranous part
    - Divided into atrioventricular & interventricular parts by apical attachment of septal leaflet of tricuspid valve
  - Muscular part
    - Divided into inlet, trabecular, & outlet components

CLINICAL ISSUES

Presentation

- Most common signs/symptoms
  - **Patients with small defects may be asymptomatic**
    - "Maladie de Roger"
      - Small, asymptomatic VSD
  - Development of symptoms depends on several factors
    - Size & location
    - Pulmonary arterial pressure
    - Left ventricular outflow resistance
  - Most common symptoms
    - Shortness of breath
    - Tachypnea
    - Failure to thrive
    - Tachycardia
  - Pulmonary artery hypertension
    - Dyspnea on exertion
    - Fatigue
    - Syncope
    - Chest pain
  - Eisenmenger syndrome
    - Symptoms related to polycythemia
    - Headache, fatigue, & marked dyspnea
  - Physical examination
    - Holo- or pansystolic murmur
- Other signs/symptoms
  - Recurrent respiratory infections

Demographics

- Gender
  - M:F = 1:1
- Epidemiology
  - VSD accounts for 20% of all congenital cardiac anomalies
  - Incidence: 2-6 of every 1,000 live births

Natural History & Prognosis

- Defects that spontaneously close or decrease in size early in life usually require no treatment
- Small VSDs typically close spontaneously
  - Inlet VSDs rarely close spontaneously
- Large VSDs require surgical correction
- Defects may result in pulmonary artery hypertension
  - May be reversible if treated early
  - Development of Eisenmenger syndrome
    - Reversal of left-to-right shunt

Treatment

- Medical management
  - Treatment of congestive heart failure
    - Diuretics
    - Afterload reduction
  - Treatment of Eisenmenger syndrome
    - Partial exchange transfusion
  - Endocarditis prophylaxis
  - Treatment of recurrent respiratory infections
- Surgical management
  - Pulmonary artery banding
    - Dilatable banding of the pulmonary trunk ± branch vessels
    - May enable postponement of surgery
    - Constriction of VSD may be seen
  - Surgical closure
    - Indications
      - Symptomatic patients
      - Large defects
      - Elevated pulmonary vascular resistance
  - Minimally invasive surgical closure
    - Typically for perimembranous VSD
  - Percutaneous transcatheter device occlusion
    - Use of septal occluder device
    - Typically for perimembranous VSD
    - Complications
      - Complete heart block
      - Aortic regurgitation
      - Tricuspid regurgitation

DIAGNOSTIC CHECKLIST

Consider

- Ventricular septal defect in patient with left atrial & ventricular enlargement & prominent pulmonary vasculature on chest radiography

SELECTED REFERENCES

1. Mongeon FP et al: Indications and outcomes of surgical closure of ventricular septal defect in adults. JACC Cardiovasc Interv. 3(3):290-7, 2010
2. Rajiah P et al: Computed tomography of septal defects. J Cardiovasc Comput Tomogr. 4(4):231-45, 2010
3. Spanos GP et al: Time-resolved contrast-enhanced MRI in ventricular septal defect evaluation. Clin Radiol. 63(6):724-6, 2008
4. Goo HW et al: CT of congenital heart disease: normal anatomy and typical pathologic conditions. Radiographics. 23 Spec No:S147-65, 2003
5. Wang ZJ et al: Cardiovascular shunts: MR imaging evaluation. Radiographics. 23 Spec No:S181-94, 2003

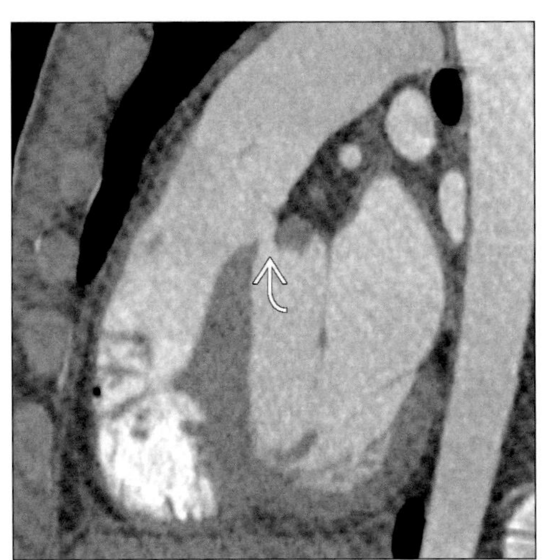

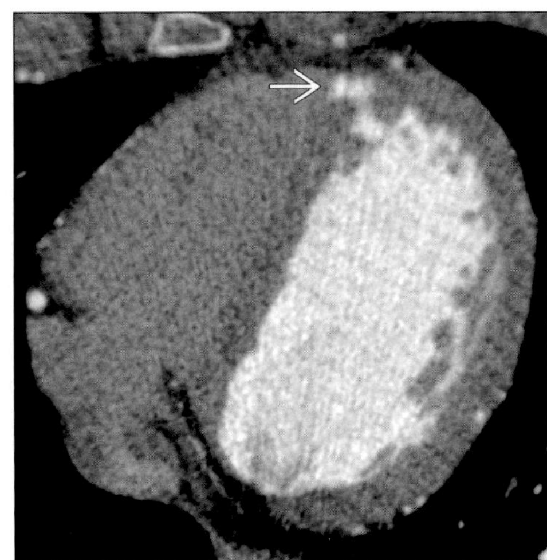

(Left) *Sagittal reformatted image from a cardiac gated CTA shows a supracristal ventricular septal defect ➲. VSDs account for approximately 20% of congenital cardiac anomalies.* ***(Right)*** *Axial image from a cardiac gated CTA demonstrates an irregular defect ➡ within the anterior interventricular septum connecting the left and right ventricles. Cardiac gated CTA can directly identify VSDs, as well as provide information regarding direction and extent of intracardiac shunting.*

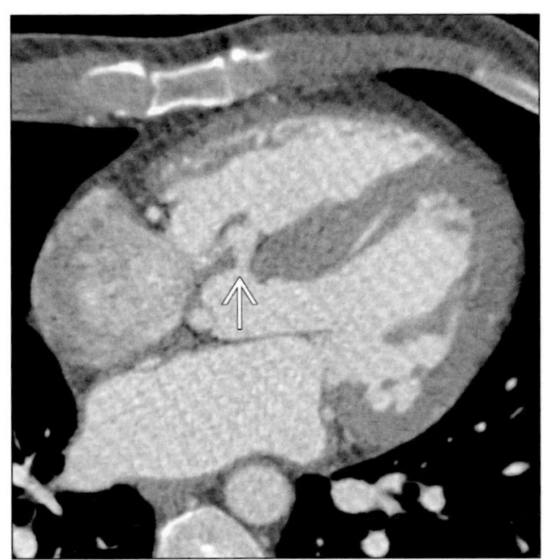

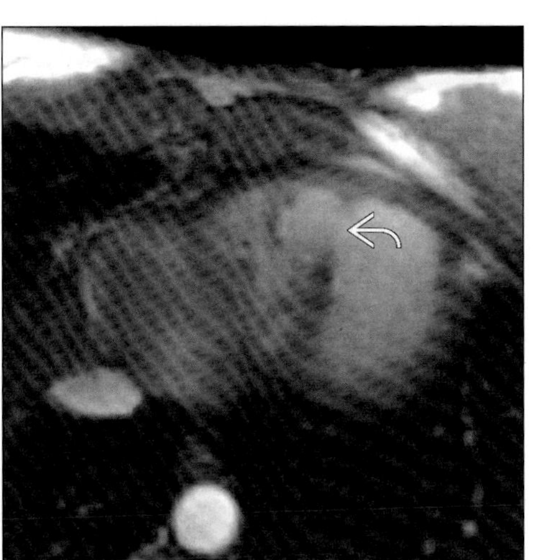

(Left) *Axial image from a cardiac gated CTA demonstrates a perimembranous ventricular septal defect ➡.* ***(Right)*** *Axial image from a cine MR shows a defect ➲ in the anterior interventricular septum near the cardiac apex, which allows communication between the left and right ventricles. In addition to identifying the defect, MR provides functional information such as shunt volume and direction, as well as information regarding ventricular and valvular function.*

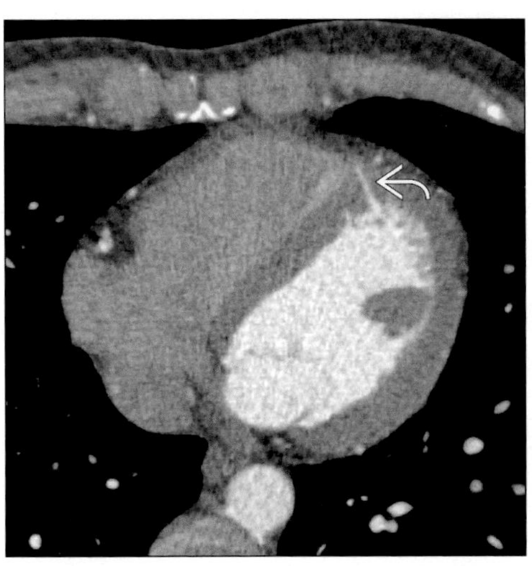

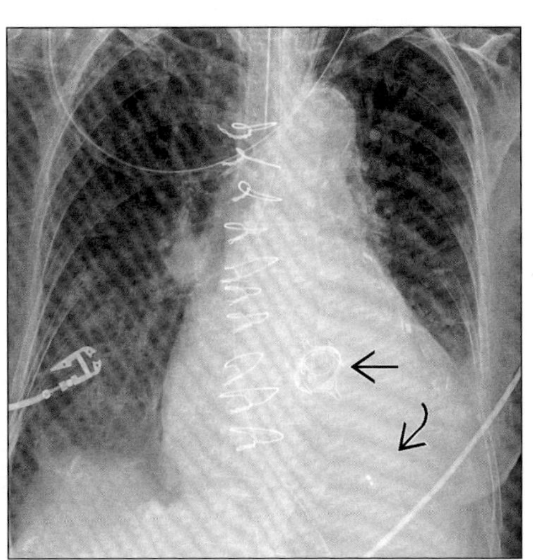

(Left) *Axial image from a cardiac gated CTA demonstrates a linear defect ➲ within the anterior interventricular septum extending between the left and right ventricles.* ***(Right)*** *Portable chest radiograph obtained following percutaneous device closure of a VSD shows an occluder device ➲ in the expected position of the interventricular septum. Note is made of sternotomy wires in this patient with a previous aortic valve replacement ➡.*

BICUSPID AORTIC VALVE

Key Facts

Terminology

- Bicuspid aortic valve (BAV)
- BAV has only 2 leaflets

Imaging

- Radiography: Ascending aortic aneurysm: Contour abnormality of right cardiomediastinal silhouette
- CT/MR
  - Direct visualization of aortic valve, cardiac gating may be necessary

Top Differential Diagnoses

- Aortic stenosis in tricuspid aortic valve
  - 3 leaflets & triangular systolic aperture
- Marfan syndrome
  - Effacement of sinotubular junction
- Aortic aneurysm
  - More common in aortic arch & descending aorta

Pathology

- Type 1 (~ 80%): Fusion of right & left coronary cusps (anterior-posterior BAV)
- Type 2 (~ 20%): Fusion of right & noncoronary cusps (right-left BAV)

Clinical Issues

- Type 1 BAV
  - Normal aortic shape & ↑ aortic root dimensions
  - Associated with aortic coarctation & less aortic valve pathology
  - M:F = 2.7:1
- Type 2 BAV
  - More rapid progression of valvular disfunction, ascending aortic dilatation, larger arch diameters
  - ↑ prevalence of myxomatous mitral valve disease
  - M:F = 1.3:1
- Aortic reconstruction when diameter > 4.5 cm

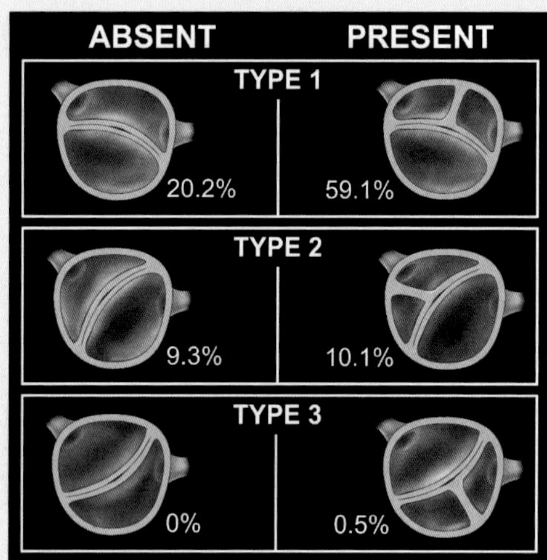

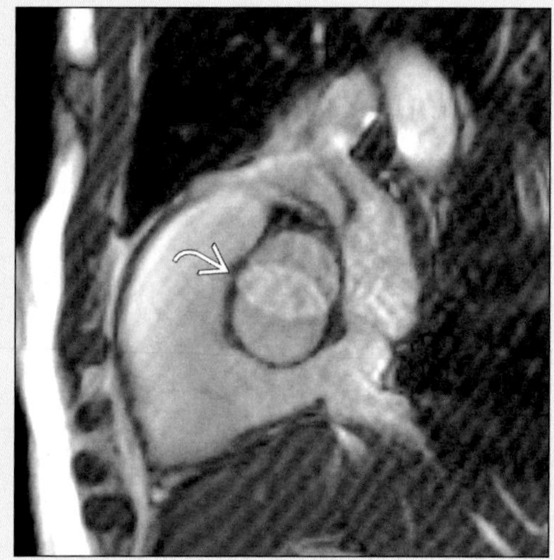

(Left) *Graphic shows the morphologic features of the different types of bicuspid aortic valve. Approximately 80% are type 1 and 20% are type 2. Type 3 is very uncommon.* ***(Right)*** *Short axis SSFP cardiac MR of a patient with type 1 BAV without raphe shows a "fish-mouth" aperture ➔ of the aortic valve during systole. In this case, no significant stenosis is appreciated, and both coronaries arose from the anterior coronary sinus that resulted from fusion of the right and left coronary sinuses.*

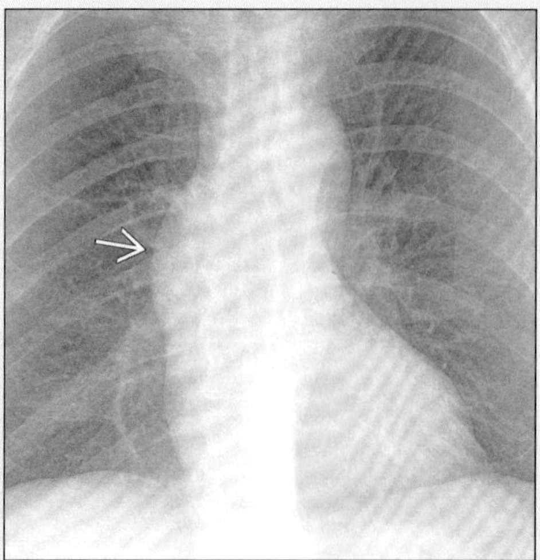

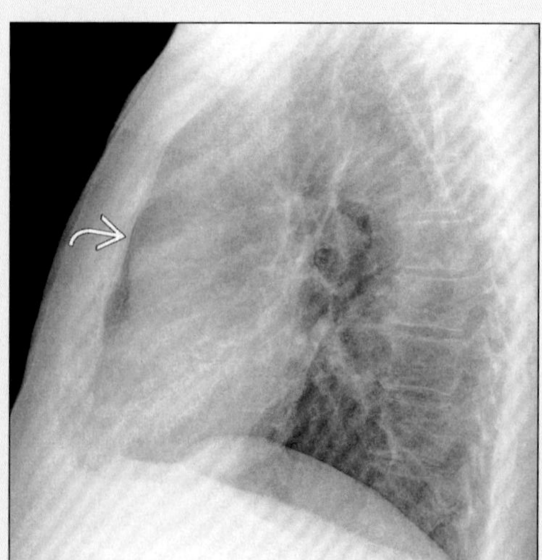

(Left) *PA chest radiograph of a patient with BAV and an aneurysm of the ascending aorta shows the characteristic contour abnormality of the superior right cardiomediastinal border ➔ representing the dilated aorta. This finding can also be seen in other other etiologies of ascending aortic aneurysm such as Marfan syndrome and atherosclerosis.* ***(Right)*** *Lateral chest radiograph of the same patient demonstrates filling of the retrosternal space ➔ related to a dilated ascending aorta.*

BICUSPID AORTIC VALVE

TERMINOLOGY

Abbreviations

- **Bicuspid aortic valve (BAV)**

Definitions

- Normal aortic valve has 3 leaflets
- **BAV has only 2 leaflets**

IMAGING

General Features

- Best diagnostic clue
  - Ascending aortic aneurysm on chest radiograph in young patient without Marfan syndrome

Radiographic Findings

- Indirect findings
  - **Visualization of calcified raphe** is diagnostic but difficult to ascertain
  - **Ascending aortic aneurysm**: Contour abnormality of right cardiomediastinal silhouette

CT Findings

- CTA
  - **Calcifications** confined to raphe & base of cusps (commissures)
  - Often accurately differentiates between bicuspid & tricuspid aortic valves
  - Bicuspid aortic valve best assessed with cardiac gating & multiplanar reformations
  - BAV without raphe identified on diastolic short axis reformations
  - BAV with raphe better identified on systolic short axis (i.e., "fish-mouth" appearance)
    - **Normal tricuspid valve has triangular aperture**
  - Planimetry during mid systole (maximum aperture) allows for grading of aortic stenosis
- Cardiac gated CTA
  - Helpful for assessment of preoperative coronary artery morphology

MR Findings

- Cardiac gated MR is as accurate as echocardiography & CTA for morphologic diagnosis (including planimetry)
- Allows calculation of additional functional parameters in aortic stenosis
  - e.g., peak velocity
- Determination & quantification of aortic regurgitation
- Promising 4-dimensional MR evaluation can assess flow patterns

Echocardiographic Findings

- Specificity 96%, sensitivity 78%, & accuracy 93%
- 2 cusps & 2 commissures on short axis
- Cusp redundancy & eccentric valve closure
- Single coaptation line between cusps during diastole
- BAV may be obscured by severe fibrosis or calcification; false-negative results may be produced by prominent raphe

Imaging Recommendations

- Best imaging tool
  - Echocardiography
- **American College of Cardiology (ACC)/ American Heart Association (AHA) follow-up recommendations**
  - Consider echocardiographic follow-up
    - If sinuses of Valsalva, sinotubular junction, & ascending aorta are not well visualized, consider CT or MR
  - **Follow-up intervals**
    - Every year for severe stenosis or severe regurgitation
    - Every 1 or 2 years for moderate aortic stenosis or moderate aortic regurgitation
    - Every 3-5 years for mild aortic stenosis or mild aortic regurgitation
    - Every year if aortic root > 4 cm

DIFFERENTIAL DIAGNOSIS

Aortic Stenosis in Tricuspid Aortic Valve

- 3 leaflets & triangular systolic aperture
- May be difficult to differentiate in heavily calcified & stenotic aortic valves
- Calcification typically extends to commissure

Marfan Syndrome

- Dilatation of ascending aorta with tricuspid aortic valve
- Effacement of sinotubular junction

Aortic Aneurysm

- More common in aortic arch & descending thoracic aorta
- Often associated with extensive atherosclerotic plaques

PATHOLOGY

General Features

- Etiology
  - Etiologies of aneurysm formation
    - Hemodynamic hypothesis
      - Orientation of systolic jet in BAV may lead to differential distribution of wall stress & eventual remodeling of vessel wall
      - Abnormal systolic helical flow
      - Type 2 BAV more prone to significant aortic stenosis
    - Congenital hypothesis
      - Intrinsic congenital disorder of vascular connective tissue
- Genetics
  - Exact genetic cause & inheritance pattern remain unknown
  - Familial or hereditary form of BAV described in 10-30% of individuals
  - Mutation in *NOTCH1* causes cardiac abnormalities including BAV with severe calcifications
  - Disruption of expression of fibroblast growth factor 8 in pharyngeal arch ectoderm & endoderm leads to BAV & other vascular abnormalities
- Associated abnormalities
  - **Aortic coarctation**
    - BAV present in 20-85% of all cases of coarctation
  - Hypoplastic left heart syndrome
  - Interrupted aortic arch: BAV present in 27%

BICUSPID AORTIC VALVE

Staging, Grading, & Classification

- **BAV leaflet morphology**
  - Type 1 (~ 80%): Fusion of right and left coronary cusps (anterior-posterior BAV)
    - Without raphe (20.2%)
    - With raphe (59.1%)
  - Type 2 (~ 20%): Fusion of right and noncoronary cusps (right-left BAV)
    - Without raphe (9.3%)
    - With raphe (10.1%)
  - Type 3: Fusion of noncoronary & left coronary cusp
    - Without raphe (0.5%)
- **Morphology of aortic root**
  - Normal (type N)
    - Definition: Diameter sinuses of Valsalva > diameter sinotubular junction; diameter sinuses of Valsalva ≥ diameter mid ascending aorta
    - More common in type 1 BAV
  - Ascending aortic dilatation (type A)
    - Definition: Diameter sinuses of Valsalva > diameter sinotubular junction; diameter sinuses of Valsalva < diameter mid ascending aorta
    - More common in type 2 BAV
  - Effacement of sinotubular junction (type E)
    - Definition: Diameter sinuses of Valsalva ≤ diameter sinotubular junction
    - Infrequent in patients with dilated ascending aorta in BAV
    - Common in patients with dilated ascending aorta in Marfan syndrome

Gross Pathologic & Surgical Features

- Calcification increases with age & is largely confined to raphe
- Left coronary artery dominance more common in BAV
- Short left main coronary artery
- Asymmetric leaflet size more prone to develop rapid calcification
- Unicuspid or quadricuspid aortic valves are rare

Microscopic Features

- Congenital bicuspid aortic valve shows valve tissue in raphe
- Aortic stenosis in tricuspid aortic valve (functionally bicuspid)
  - Shows evidence of prior valvulitis

CLINICAL ISSUES

Presentation

- Most common signs/symptoms
  - Asymptomatic until aortic stenosis develops (2nd decade)
    - Aortic ejection click ± ejection systolic murmur
  - Aortic stenosis or regurgitation
    - Incidence of aortic stenosis: 15-71%
    - Incidence of aortic regurgitation: 1.3-3%
    - Angina, syncope, & heart failure: Peak incidence in 5th to 6th decades
    - Survival after development of symptoms < 5 years
      - ↑ incidence of sudden death (15-20%)
  - Aortic dissection (9x risk): Chest pain
    - Incidence: 5%
  - Aortic aneurysm
    - ↑ risk of dissection & rupture
    - Often asymptomatic; chest pain in setting of rupture
  - Infective endocarditis
    - Incidence 9.5-40%
  - Sudden death
- Clinical profile
  - **Type 1 BAV**
    - Normal aortic shape & ↑ aortic root dimensions
    - Associated with aortic coarctation & less aortic valve pathology
  - **Type 2 BAV**
    - Associated with more rapid progression of valve disfunction (i.e., aortic stenosis & regurgitation), ascending aortic dilatation, larger arch diameters
    - ↑ prevalence of myxomatous mitral valve disease
  - **Type 3 BAV**
    - Uncommon

Demographics

- Age
  - Symptoms & complications of bicuspid aortic valve stenosis increase with age
- Gender
  - Type 1 BAV
    - M:F = 2.7:1
  - Type 2 BAV
    - M:F = 1.3:1
- Epidemiology
  - Most common congenital heart disease (0.5-2% of general population)
  - Most common reason for aortic valve replacement
  - 50% of all adults with aortic stenosis have BAV

Treatment

- Close follow-up; ascending aortic reconstruction when diameter > 4.5 cm

DIAGNOSTIC CHECKLIST

Consider

- Ascending aortic aneurysms in young patients are common in Marfan syndrome & BAV
- Chest radiography is often insensitive for detection of ascending aortic aneurysm
- Echocardiography: Standard initial evaluation with high sensitivity & specificity
- CT and MR
  - Helpful to assess for complications
  - Consider cardiac gating if actual assessment of aortic valve required

SELECTED REFERENCES

1. Tanaka R et al: Diagnostic value of cardiac CT in the evaluation of bicuspid aortic stenosis: comparison with echocardiography and operative findings. AJR Am J Roentgenol. 195(4):895-9, 2010
2. Schaefer BM et al: The bicuspid aortic valve: an integrated phenotypic classification of leaflet morphology and aortic root shape. Heart. 94(12):1634-8, 2008

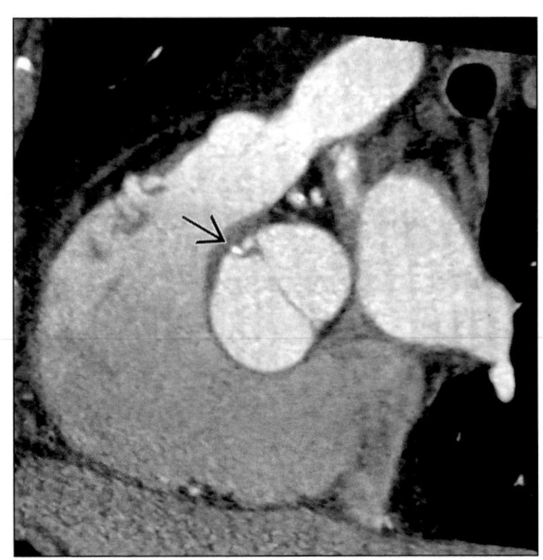

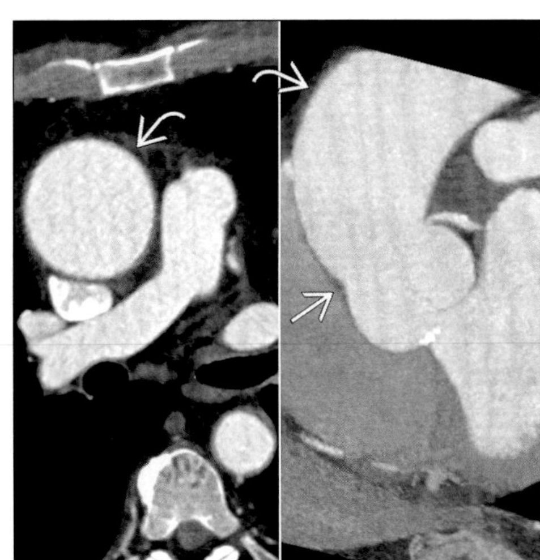

(Left) *Short axis cardiac CTA during diastole shows a type 1 BAV without raphe. Early calcification along the commissures → eventually results in aortic stenosis.* ***(Right)*** *Composite image with axial (left) and oblique (right) sagittal cardiac CTA of the same patient shows ascending aorta dilatation → and preservation of the sinotubular junction → (type A morphology). Patients with type 1 BAV tend toward a preserved ascending aortic shape (type N morphology) with larger sinuses of Valsalva.*

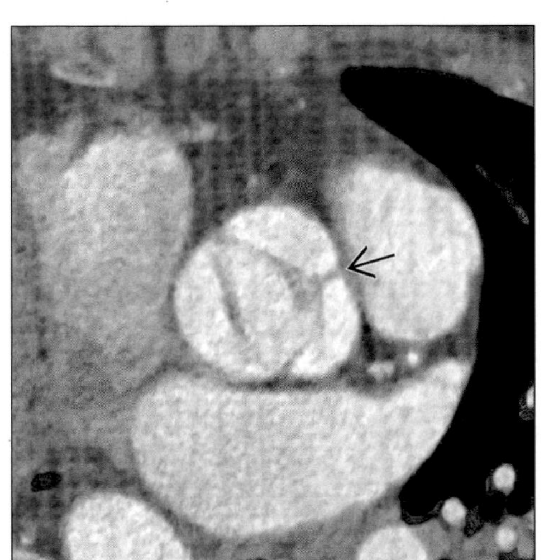

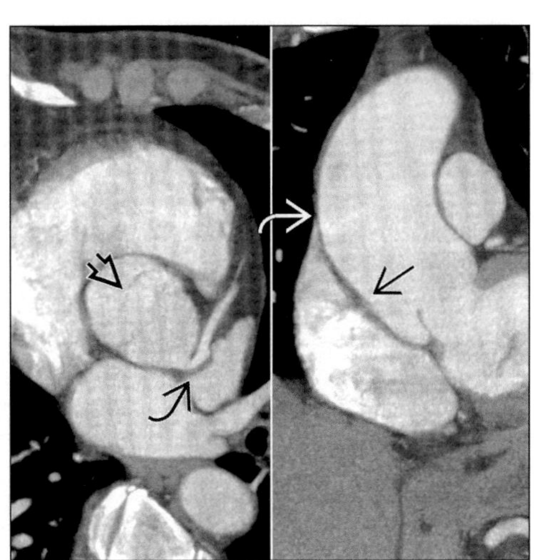

(Left) *Short axis MIP reformation of a cardiac CTA of a patient with type 1 BAV with raphe during mid-diastole shows normal aperture of the aortic valve and a raphe →.* ***(Right)*** *Composite image with short (left) and long (right) axis reformations from a cardiac CTA of a patient with type 2 BAV without raphe → shows the left coronary artery → arising from the left coronary sinus and dilatation of the ascending aorta → with effacement of the sinotubular junction → (aortic type E morphology).*

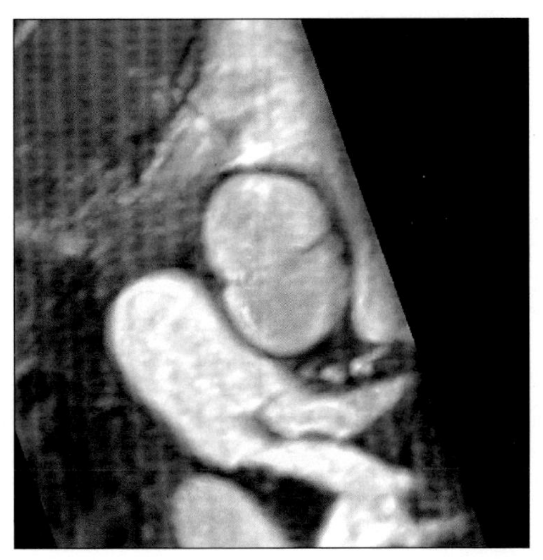

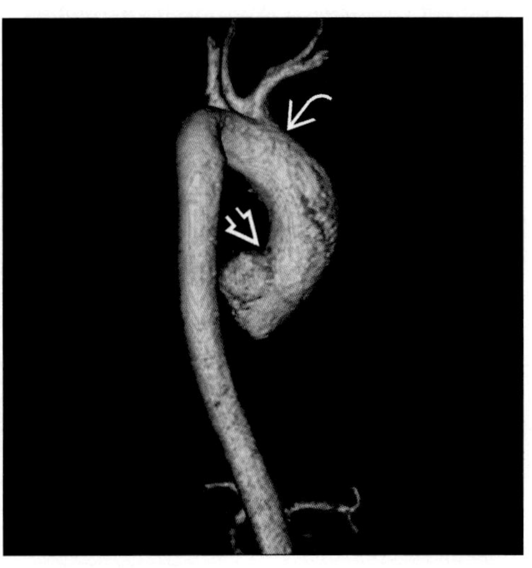

(Left) *Short axis MRA after intravenous gadolinium injection shows a BAV type 2 without a raphe and dilatation of the coronary sinuses.* ***(Right)*** *Posterior 3D reformation from MRA after gadolinium of the same patient shows dilatation of the ascending aorta and the aortic arch → with preservation of the sinotubular junction → (aortic type A morphology). Type 2 BAV exhibits a female predominance, larger aortic arch dimensions, and myxomatous mitral valve disease.*

PULMONIC STENOSIS

Key Facts

Terminology

- Pulmonic stenosis (PS)
- Lesion resulting in obstruction of right ventricular outflow tract (RVOT)

Imaging

- Radiography: Enlargement of pulmonary trunk & left pulmonary artery
- CT
  - Poststenotic dilation of pulmonary trunk & left pulmonary artery
  - Thickened, immobile valve leaflets
  - Small valvular annulus
  - Pericardial calcification involving aorta & pulmonary trunk may rarely produce acquired PS
- MR: Determination of presence & extent of PS
  - Doming or windsock appearance of pulmonic valve
  - Narrowing of valve orifice

Top Differential Diagnoses

- Pulmonary artery hypertension
- Idiopathic dilatation of pulmonary trunk
- Proximal interruption of pulmonary artery

Pathology

- Majority of cases are congenital in etiology
- Acquired: Rheumatic heart disease, carcinoid syndrome, & infective endocarditis
- Severity of PS determined by pressure gradient across pulmonic valve or pulmonic valve area

Clinical Issues

- Treatment
  - Trivial & mild PS: Observation & endocarditis prophylaxis prior to surgical procedures
  - Moderate & severe PS: Balloon valvuloplasty or surgical valvotomy

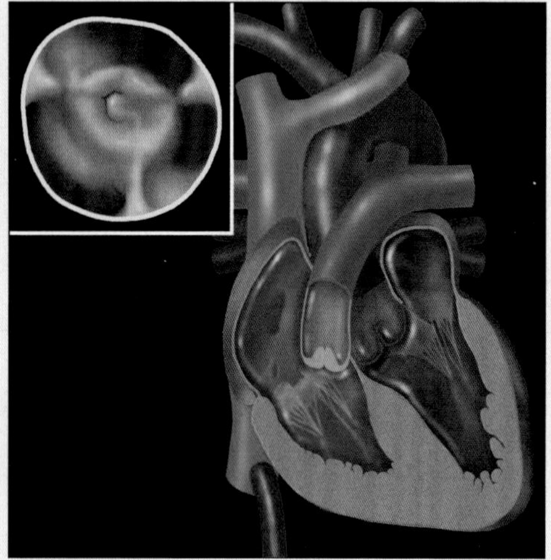

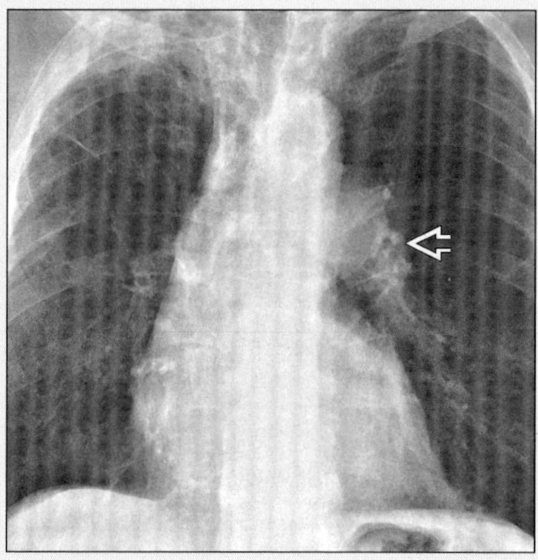

(Left) *Graphic shows morphologic features of pulmonic stenosis (PS) characterized by diffuse thickening of the pulmonic valve leaflets and resultant marked narrowing of the valve orifice (insert).* ***(Right)*** *PA chest radiograph of a patient with congenital pulmonic stenosis shows enlargement of the pulmonary trunk and the left pulmonary artery ⇨. Pulmonary artery enlargement is the most common radiographic manifestation of pulmonic stenosis.*

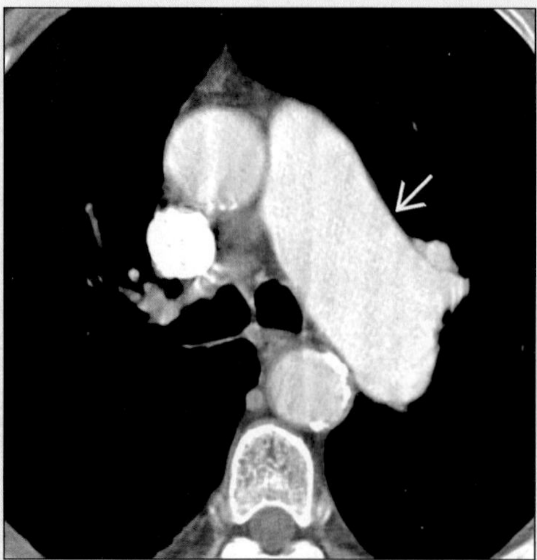

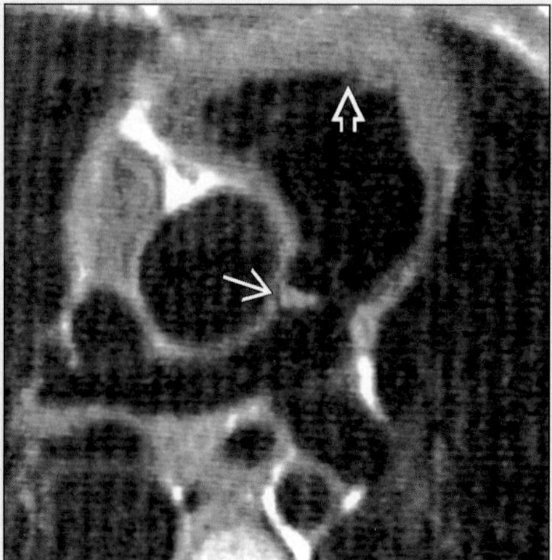

(Left) *Axial CECT of a patient with pulmonic stenosis shows enlargement of the left pulmonary artery ➔, representing poststenotic dilatation.* ***(Right)*** *Oblique axial "black blood" FSE STIR MR through the pulmonary trunk demonstrates thickening of a leaflet of the pulmonic valve ➔ and right ventricular hypertrophy ⇨ secondary to pulmonic stenosis.*

PULMONIC STENOSIS

TERMINOLOGY

Abbreviations

- **Pulmonic stenosis (PS)**

Definitions

- Lesion resulting in obstruction of right ventricular outflow tract (RVOT) & poststenotic dilatation of pulmonary trunk & left pulmonary artery

IMAGING

General Features

- Best diagnostic clue
  - **Enlargement of pulmonary trunk & left pulmonary artery**
- Location
  - Valvular (90%)
  - Subvalvular
  - Supravalvular

Radiographic Findings

- Radiography
  - Most common abnormality is **enlargement of pulmonary trunk**
    - Convexity along left mediastinal border inferior to aortic arch
  - Enlargement of left pulmonary artery may be present
  - Right ventricular enlargement

CT Findings

- CECT
  - **Poststenotic dilatation of pulmonary trunk & left pulmonary artery**
  - **Right ventricular enlargement**
  - Focal pericardial calcification involving aorta & pulmonary trunk reported as unusual cause of acquired PS
- Cardiac gated CTA
  - **Thickened, immobile valve leaflets**
  - Small valvular annulus
  - Hypoplasia of supravalvular pulmonary trunk may be present

MR Findings

- MRA
  - Enlargement of pulmonary trunk & left pulmonary artery
- MR cine
  - Evaluation of pulmonic valve morphology
    - Thickening ± fusion of valve leaflets
    - Narrowing of valve orifice
    - Doming or windsock appearance of pulmonic valve
- Phase contrast imaging
  - Determination of presence & extent of pulmonic stenosis
  - Determination of volume flow rates across pulmonic valve

Echocardiographic Findings

- Echocardiogram
  - **Thickening of valve leaflets**
  - Restricted systolic motion & reduced mobility of valve leaflets
  - Doming or windsock appearance of pulmonic valve
  - Poststenotic dilatation of pulmonary artery
- Color Doppler
  - Systolic high-velocity flow jet in pulmonary outflow tract

Angiographic Findings

- Conventional
  - Not indicated in mild or moderate PS
  - Patients with severe PS usually undergo cardiac catheterization for confirmatory pressure assessment
    - Concomitant balloon valvuloplasty may be performed
  - Useful in evaluating morphology of pulmonary outflow tract, pulmonary arteries, & right ventricle

DIFFERENTIAL DIAGNOSIS

Pulmonary Artery Hypertension (PAH)

- Enlarged pulmonary trunk & central pulmonary arteries
- CTA: Enlargement of pulmonary trunk > 30 mm
- HRCT
  - Pre-capillary etiologies: Emphysema, fibrosis, honeycomb lung
  - Post-capillary etiologies: Centrilobular ground-glass nodules, pulmonary edema, pleural effusions
  - Chronic PAH: Patchy ground-glass opacities
- Pre-capillary etiologies: Chronic pulmonary emboli, congenital left-to-right shunts, idiopathic PAH
- Post-capillary etiologies: Left heart failure & mitral stenosis

Idiopathic Dilation of Pulmonary Trunk

- Congenital dilatation of pulmonary trunk ± involvement of left & right pulmonary arteries
- Pulmonary & cardiac causes of pulmonary artery enlargement must be excluded
- Normal pressures in pulmonary artery & right ventricle
- Enlarged pulmonary artery may appear as rounded opacity along left mediastinal border
  - May mimic mediastinal mass

Proximal Interruption of Pulmonary Artery

- Failed development of proximal pulmonary artery
- Small ipsilateral lung & hilum on chest radiography
- Absence of pulmonary artery on CT
- Visualization of ipsilateral collateral systemic & bronchial arteries
- Mosaic attenuation may be seen on HRCT

Aberrant Left Pulmonary Artery

- a.k.a. pulmonary artery sling
- Congenital anomaly in which left pulmonary artery arises from right pulmonary artery
- Forms "sling" around trachea as it passes between trachea & esophagus
- May be associated with abnormalities of tracheobronchial tree & cardiovascular system
- May appear as a nodular opacity projecting between trachea anteriorly and esophagus posteriorly on lateral chest radiographs
- CT & MR useful for definitive diagnosis

PULMONIC STENOSIS

PATHOLOGY

General Features

- Etiology
  - Congenital
    - Most common etiology of PS
    - Isolated in 80% of cases
    - Additional forms of congenital heart disease present in 20% of cases
  - Acquired
    - Rheumatic heart disease
      - Associated with mitral & aortic valvular disease
    - Carcinoid syndrome
      - Associated with tricuspid valvular disease
    - Infective endocarditis
- Genetics
  - Generally considered to be multifactorial in origin
  - Familial forms have been described
  - May be associated with genetic disorders
    - Valvular PS
      - Noonan syndrome
    - Supravalvular PS
      - Congenital rubella syndrome
      - Williams syndrome
- Associated abnormalities
  - Atrial septal defect (ASD)
  - Ventricular septal defect (VSD)
  - Patent foramen ovale (PFO)
  - Tetralogy of Fallot

Staging, Grading, & Classification

- **Severity classification by pressure gradient across pulmonic valve**
  - Trivial stenosis (gradient < 25 mmHg)
  - Mild stenosis (gradient 25-50 mmHg)
  - Moderate stenosis (gradient 50-80 mmHg)
  - Severe stenosis (gradient > 80 mmHg)
- **Severity classification by pulmonic valve area**
  - Normal: 2.5-4.0 cm^2
  - Mild PS: < 1 cm^2
  - Severe PS: < 0.5 cm^2

Gross Pathologic & Surgical Features

- Thickening of valve leaflets
  - Calcification may be present
- Partial fusion of commissures
- Valve is typically dome-shaped or conical in configuration
- Narrowing of central orifice

Microscopic Features

- Thickening of valve leaflets
- Dysplastic valves may be composed of myxomatous tissue
  - Present in 10-15% of patients with valvular PS

CLINICAL ISSUES

Presentation

- Most common signs/symptoms
  - Presentation depends on severity of symptoms
    - Mild PS: Typically asymptomatic
    - Moderate or severe PS
      - Signs & symptoms of systemic venous congestion
      - Mimics congestive heart failure
- Other signs/symptoms
  - Cyanosis in setting of concomitant PFO or ASD

Demographics

- Age
  - Age of presentation depends on severity of obstruction
- Gender
  - M:F = 1:1
- Epidemiology
  - Represents 10% of all congenital cardiac defects
  - 8-12% of all congenital cardiac defects in children
    - Isolated PS with intact ventricular septum is 2nd most common defect

Natural History & Prognosis

- Severity of stenosis determines morbidity & mortality
  - Mild to moderate PS is usually well tolerated
  - Severe PS
    - Decreased cardiac output, right ventricular hypertrophy, congestive heart failure, & cyanosis may develop

Treatment

- Trivial & mild PS: Observation & endocarditis prophylaxis prior to surgical procedures
- Moderate & severe PS: Balloon valvuloplasty or surgical valvotomy
  - Mild pulmonic regurgitation & right ventricular dilatation may develop following valvuloplasty

DIAGNOSTIC CHECKLIST

Consider

- Pulmonic stenosis in patients with pulmonary trunk & left pulmonary artery enlargement

SELECTED REFERENCES

1. Harrild DM et al: Long-term pulmonary regurgitation following balloon valvuloplasty for pulmonary stenosis risk factors and relationship to exercise capacity and ventricular volume and function. J Am Coll Cardiol. 2010 Mar 9;55(10):1041-7. Erratum in: J Am Coll Cardiol. 55(16):1767, 2010
2. Ryan R et al: Cardiac valve disease: spectrum of findings on cardiac 64-MDCT. AJR Am J Roentgenol. 190(5):W294-303, 2008
3. Castañer E et al: Congenital and acquired pulmonary artery anomalies in the adult: radiologic overview. Radiographics. 26(2):349-71, 2006
4. Hwang YJ et al: Severe pulmonary artery stenosis by a calcified pericardial ring. Eur J Cardiothorac Surg. 29(4):619-21, 2006
5. Gielen H et al: Natural history of congenital pulmonary valvar stenosis: an echo and Doppler cardiographic study. Cardiol Young. 9(2):129-35, 1999
6. Gikonyo BM et al: Anatomic features of congenital pulmonary valvar stenosis. Pediatr Cardiol. 8(2):109-16, 1987

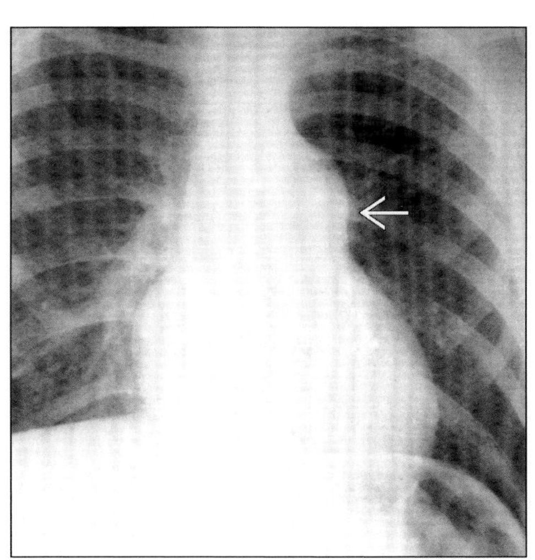

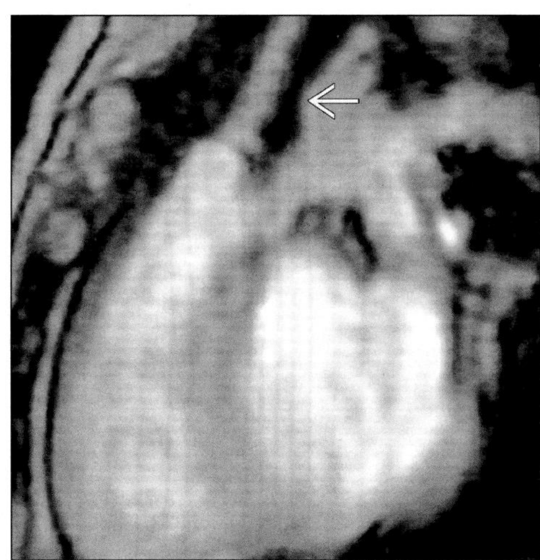

(Left) *PA chest radiograph of a patient with PS shows enlargement of the pulmonary trunk ➡, consistent with poststenotic dilatation characteristically seen in patients with pulmonic stenosis.* ***(Right)*** *Sagittal right ventricular outflow tract (RVOT) magnitude image shows linear hypointensity ➡ arising from the pulmonic valve, consistent with severe PS. Severity of PS may be classified according to the pressure gradient across the pulmonic valve or the pulmonic valve area.*

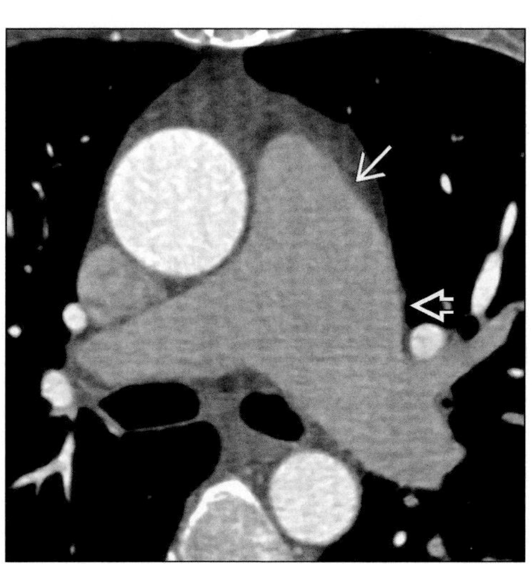

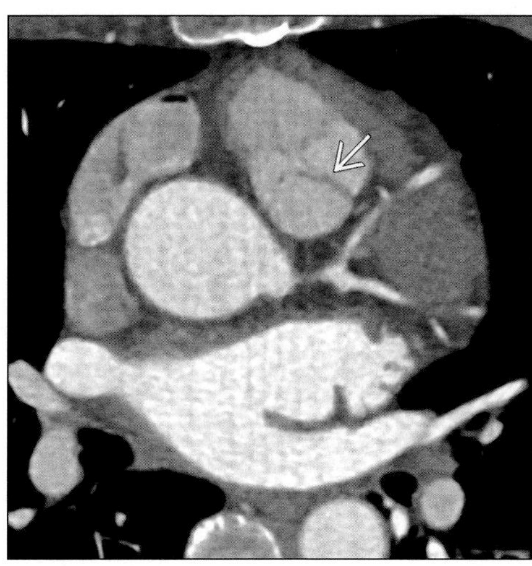

(Left) *Axial CTA of a patient with pulmonic stenosis shows enlargement of the pulmonary trunk ➡ and the left pulmonary artery ➡. Although PS is most commonly congenital in etiology, acquired etiologies include rheumatic heart disease, carcinoid, and endocarditis.* ***(Right)*** *Axial CTA of the same patient demonstrates thickening of a leaflet of the pulmonic valve ➡. CT may demonstrate thickened and immobile pulmonic valve leaflets in patients with PS. Calcification may also be present.*

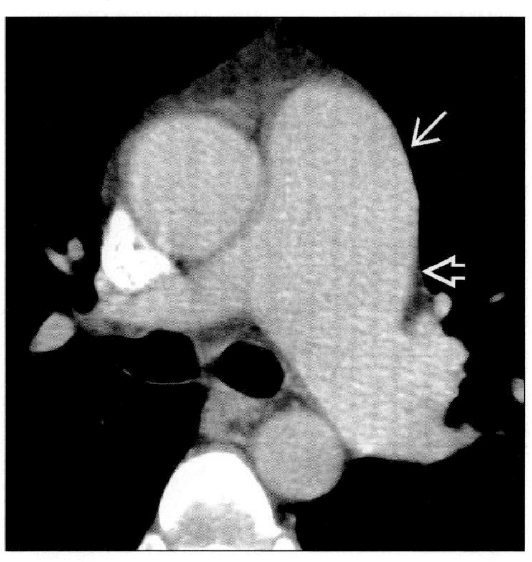

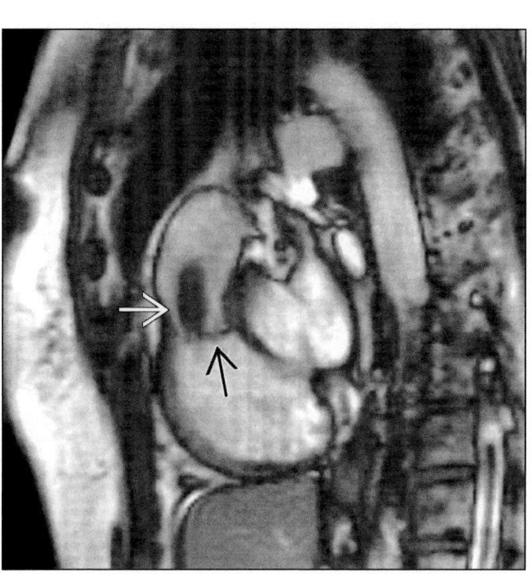

(Left) *Axial CECT of a patient with congenital PS demonstrates enlargement of the pulmonary trunk ➡ and the left pulmonary artery ➡.* ***(Right)*** *Oblique sagittal RVOT SSFP cardiac MR shows a focal region of signal dephasing ➡ arising from the pulmonic valve, consistent with severe PS. Thickening of the pulmonic valve leaflets ➡ is also noted. Patients with moderate and severe PS are typically treated with balloon valvuloplasty or surgical valvulotomy.*

Key Facts

Terminology

- Synonym: Situs ambiguous
- Definition: Abnormal arrangement of thoraco-abdominal organs across left-right axis

Imaging

- Best clue: Cardiac apex usually ipsilateral to stomach bubble; if not, suspect heterotaxy syndrome
- 2 classic forms
  - Asplenia: Bilateral right-sidedness
  - Polysplenia: Bilateral left-sidedness
- Chest radiograph useful as preliminary survey: Assessment of central tracheobronchial tree
- CT for characterization of visceral situs abnormalities
- Echocardiography and MR to evaluate cardiac chamber anomalies
- Upper GI in infants with heterotaxy to exclude intestinal malrotation

Top Differential Diagnoses

- Situs inversus
- Scimitar syndrome
- Mislabeled images

Clinical Issues

- Long-term prognosis usually determined by severity of cardiovascular anomalies

Diagnostic Checklist

- Classification schemes
  - Van Praagh segmental method
  - "Heterotaxy syndrome" followed by description of specific anatomy in parentheses
- Consider heterotaxy syndrome with polysplenia in asymptomatic or minimally symptomatic patient with radiographic findings of bilateral hyparterial bronchi & azygos continuation of IVC

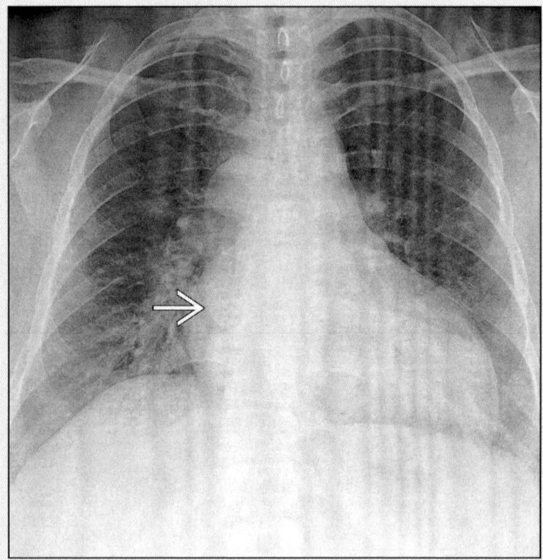

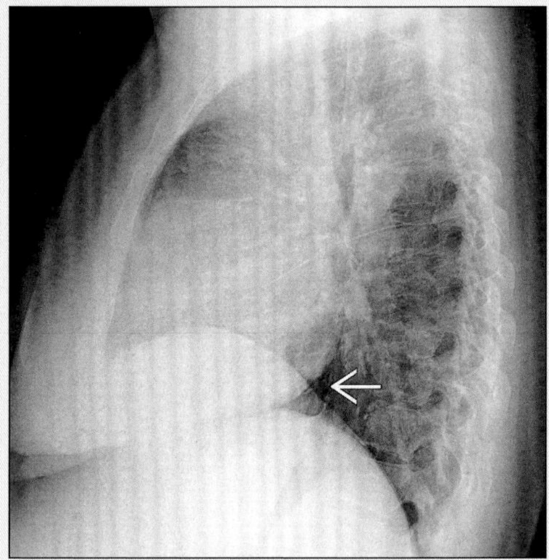

(Left) *PA chest radiograph of a patient with heterotaxy syndrome demonstrates an abnormal right mediastinal interface ➔ due to azygos continuation of the IVC and bilateral hyparterial bronchi, consistent with left isomerism.* ***(Right)*** *Lateral chest radiograph of the same patient shows absence of the normal IVC interface ➔. This is a common finding in situs ambiguous, typically associated with left isomerism. The minor fissure is also absent, consistent with bilateral bilobed lungs.*

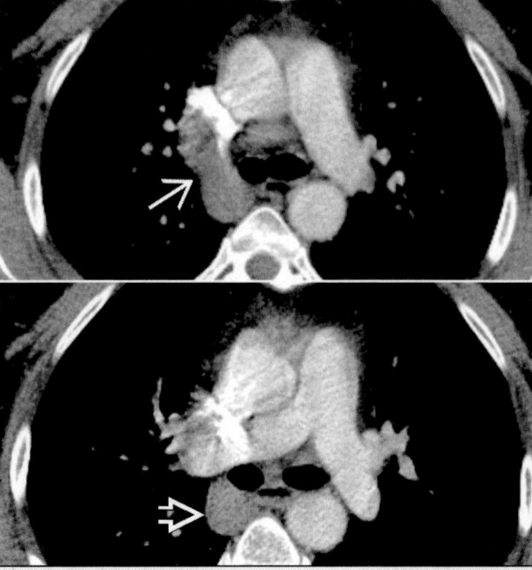

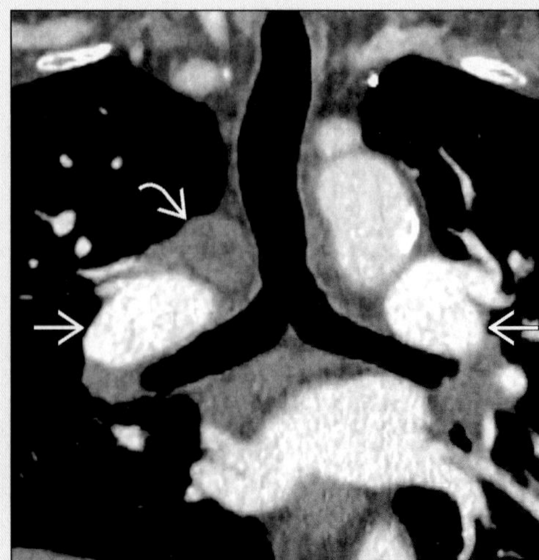

(Left) *Composite image with axial CECT shows an enlarged azygos arch ➔ (top) and azygos continuation of the IVC ➔ (bottom). Azygos continuation of the IVC is a common finding in heterotaxy syndrome.* ***(Right)*** *Coronal CECT of the same patient shows bilateral hyparterial bronchi with the first bronchial branches arising below the respective pulmonary arteries ➔, consistent with left isomerism. The azygos arch ➔ is enlarged, consistent with azygos continuation of the IVC.*

HETEROTAXY

TERMINOLOGY

Synonyms

- Situs ambiguous

Definitions

- **Situs**
  - Position of cardiac atria & viscera relative to midline
  - Independent of cardiac apex position
- **Situs solitus**
  - Normal position of cardiac atria & viscera
- **Situs inversus**
  - Mirror image of normal position
- **Situs ambiguous (heterotaxy)**
  - Abnormal arrangement of thoraco-abdominal organs across left-right axis
- **Isomerism**
  - Equal parts (bilateral left- or right-sidedness)
- **Cardiac position**
  - Refers to global location of heart in chest
  - Left (levoposition), midline (mesoposition), right (dextroposition)
- Levocardia & dextrocardia refer only to location of cardiac apex
  - Levoversion: Situs inversus with levocardia
  - Dextroversion: Situs solitus with dextrocardia

IMAGING

General Features

- Best diagnostic clue
  - Suspect heterotaxy if cardiac apex is contralateral to gastric bubble

Radiographic Findings

- **Tracheobronchial morphology (hyparterial or eparterial bronchi): A reliable predictor of ipsilateral atrial morphology**
- Cardiac apex may be ipsilateral or contralateral to gastric bubble
  - Levocardia or dextrocardia
- Dilated azygos vein from azygos continuation of IVC
- Lateral chest radiograph may or may not show absence of IVC interface

CT Findings

- **Situs solitus**
  - Right sided: Systemic atrium, trilobed lung, eparterial bronchus, liver
  - Left sided: Pulmonary atrium, bilobed lung, hyparterial bronchus, aorta, cardiac apex, single spleen, gastric bubble
- **Situs inversus**
  - Left sided: Systemic atrium, trilobed lung, eparterial bronchus, liver
  - Right sided: Pulmonary atrium, bilobed lung, hyparterial bronchus, aorta, cardiac apex, single spleen, stomach
- **Situs ambiguous (heterotaxy)**
  - 2 classic forms: Asplenia & polysplenia; inconsistent features
  - **Right isomerism (asplenia)**
    - Bilateral minor fissures
    - Bilateral trilobed lungs
    - Bilateral eparterial bronchi: 1st bronchial branch above ipsilateral pulmonary artery
  - **Left isomerism (polysplenia)**
    - No minor fissures
    - Bilateral bilobed lungs
    - Bilateral hyparterial bronchi: 1st bronchial branch below ipsilateral pulmonary artery
    - Interrupted IVC with azygos/hemiazygos continuation
  - Midline transverse liver & discordant location of stomach & cardiac apex

MR Findings

- Excellent modality to evaluate patients with heterotaxy, no ionizing radiation
- **Direct evaluation of atrial morphology (situs)**
  - Right atrium
    - Contains coronary sinus ostium
    - Connects to suprahepatic portion of inferior vena cava (IVC)
    - Atrial appendage: Pyramidal shape with broad base
    - Contains crista terminalis & coarse pectinate muscles
  - Left atrium
    - Receives blood from pulmonary veins
    - Atrial appendage: Narrow base & tubular shape

Fluoroscopic Findings

- Upper GI
  - Malrotation
    - Frequent finding in heterotaxy
    - Displacement of duodenal/jejunal junction below level of duodenal bulb

Echocardiographic Findings

- Diagnosis & characterization of cardiovascular anomalies

Imaging Recommendations

- Best imaging tool
  - Chest radiography useful as preliminary survey
  - CT for characterization of visceral situs abnormalities
  - Echocardiography & MR for evaluation of cardiovascular anomalies
  - Upper GI in infant with heterotaxy to exclude intestinal malrotation

DIFFERENTIAL DIAGNOSIS

Situs Inversus

- Complete reversal of thoraco-abdominal organs
- Congenital heart disease in 3-5%
- Kartagener syndrome (20%)
  - Structural abnormality of cilia
  - Bronchiectasis
  - Chronic sinusitis
  - Situs inversus

Scimitar Syndrome

- Hypoplasia of right lung
- Heart displaced into right hemithorax, not true dextrocardia
- Scimitar-shaped vein in right inferior hemithorax
  - Partial anomalous pulmonary venous return

HETEROTAXY

Mislabeled Images

- Most common cause of misinterpretation
- Confirm accuracy of image labeling with technicians prior to diagnosis of situs abnormalities

PATHOLOGY

General Features

- Genetics
  - Most occur sporadically
  - Evidence of both autosomal & X-linked inheritance, likely multifactorial
- Associated abnormalities
  - **Situs ambiguous**
    - Classic asplenia & polysplenia categories misleading
    - Extensive overlap of abnormalities
    - **Asplenia**
      - Associated with more severe (cyanotic) congenital heart disease: AV canal, TGA, TAPVR, single ventricle, double outlet right ventricle
      - Right aortic arch, dextrocardia
      - Midline liver & gallbladder
      - Gastrointestinal malrotation
    - **Polysplenia**
      - Less severe congenital heart disease: Left-to-right shunts (ASD, VSD), PAPVR, TGA, double outlet RV
      - Interruption IVC with azygos/hemiazygos continuation
      - Biliary atresia
      - Midline liver & gallbladder
      - Gastrointestinal malrotation
      - Truncated pancreas

Staging, Grading, & Classification

- **Segmental approach to congenital heart disease**
  - 3-step approach
    - 1. Determination of viscero-atrial situs: S (solitus), I (inversus), A (ambiguous)
    - 2. Determination of ventricular loop orientation: D (dextro; normal), L (levo; reversed)
    - 3. Determination of great vessel orientation: S (situs), I (inverted), D-TGA, L-TGA
  - Segmental analysis coded with 3 letters, that address each of the 3 steps (e.g., normal would be S, D, S)
  - Atrioventricular & ventriculoarterial connections, & other malformations also reported
- **Alternative scheme**: "Heterotaxy syndrome" followed by description of specific anatomy in parentheses
  - Heterotaxy syndrome (bilateral trilobed lungs, dextrocardia, asplenia)

CLINICAL ISSUES

Presentation

- Most common signs/symptoms
  - Ranges from severe cardiac anomalies in infants to asymptomatic adults
  - Midgut volvulus due to malrotation in heterotaxy
- Other signs/symptoms
  - Asplenia: Howell-Jolly bodies on blood smear

Demographics

- Age
  - Asplenia likely to manifest in infancy due to severe congenital heart disease
  - Polysplenia may be incidental finding in adult
- Epidemiology
  - Situs ambiguous: 1 per 10,000 live births
  - Situs inversus: 0.01%

Natural History & Prognosis

- Asplenia: Immunosuppressed for encapsulated bacteria
- Long-term prognosis usually determined by cardiac defects
- Incidence of congenital heart disease
  - Situs solitus: < 1%
  - Situs solitus + dextrocardia (dextroversion): 95%
  - Situs inversus: 3-5%
  - Situs inversus + levocardia (levoversion): 99%
  - Polysplenia: 90%
  - Asplenia: 99%

Treatment

- Surgical repair of cardiac anomalies
- Prophylactic Ladd procedure to prevent midgut volvulus
- Prophylactic antibiotics for asplenia
- Pneumococcal vaccination for asplenia

DIAGNOSTIC CHECKLIST

Consider

- Heterotaxy syndrome with polysplenia in asymptomatic or minimally symptomatic patient with radiographic findings of bilateral hyparterial bronchi & azygos continuation of IVC

Image Interpretation Pearls

- Discordance between cardiac apex & abdominal situs suggests congenital heart disease
- Visceroatrial concordance rule
  - Liver should be ipsilateral to right atrium
  - Stomach should be ipsilateral to left atrium, but not to degree seen with liver and right atrium

Reporting Tips

- Classic classification schemes of asplenia & polysplenia discouraged due to extensive overlap
- Alternative schemes
  - "Heterotaxy syndrome" followed by description of specific anatomy in parentheses
    - Heterotaxy syndrome (bilateral trilobed lungs, dextrocardia, asplenia)
  - Van Praagh segmental method

SELECTED REFERENCES

1. Lapierre C et al: Segmental approach to imaging of congenital heart disease. Radiographics. 30(2):397-411, 2010
2. Maldjian PD et al: Approach to dextrocardia in adults: review. AJR Am J Roentgenol. 188(6 Suppl):S39-49; quiz S35-8, 2007
3. Applegate KE et al: Situs revisited: imaging of the heterotaxy syndrome. Radiographics. 19(4):837-52; discussion 53-4, 1999

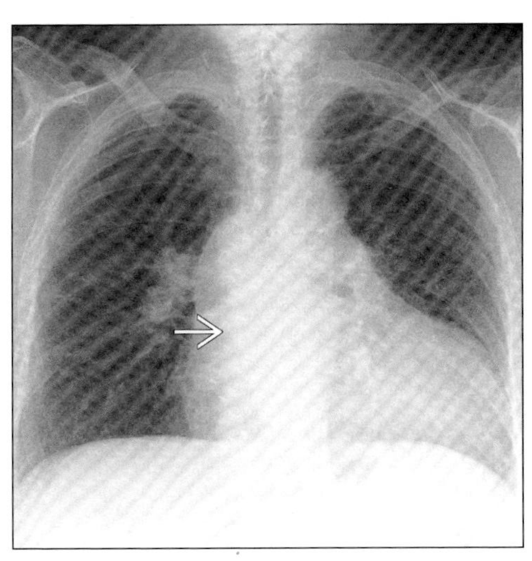

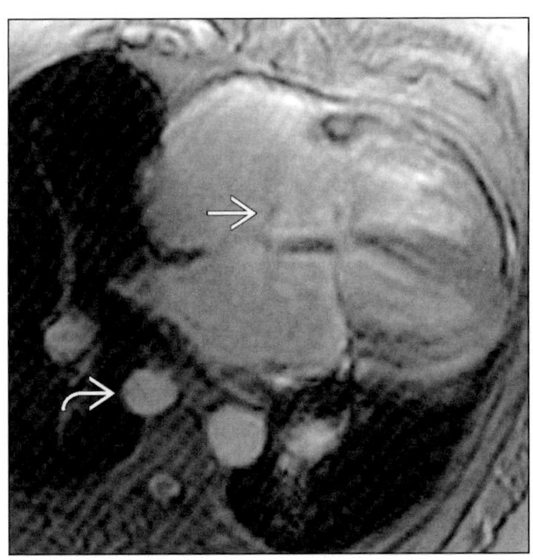

(Left) *PA chest radiograph shows bilateral hyparterial bronchi and azygos continuation → of the IVC. This patient also has cardiomegaly and pulmonary artery enlargement.* ***(Right)*** *Horizontal long axis (4 chamber) FIESTA (bright blood) MR of the same patient shows azygos continuation → of the IVC and biatrial enlargement. A spin dephasing jet → is present in the right atrium due to a small ASD. Patients with heterotaxy have an increased incidence of congenital heart disease.*

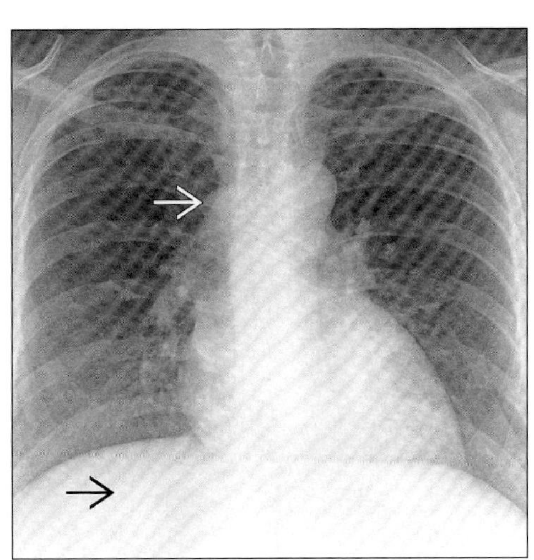

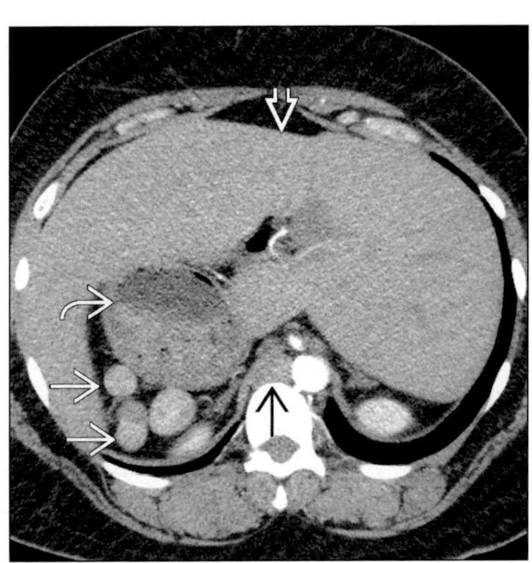

(Left) *PA chest radiograph of a patient with situs ambiguous demonstrates discordance of the cardiac apex and the gastric bubble →, highly indicative of heterotaxy syndrome. Note enlarged azygos arch → from azygos continuation of the IVC.* ***(Right)*** *Axial CECT of the same patient shows a midline liver → with the major hepatic lobe on the left, a right-sided gastric bubble →, multiple right-sided spleens →, and azygos continuation → of the IVC.*

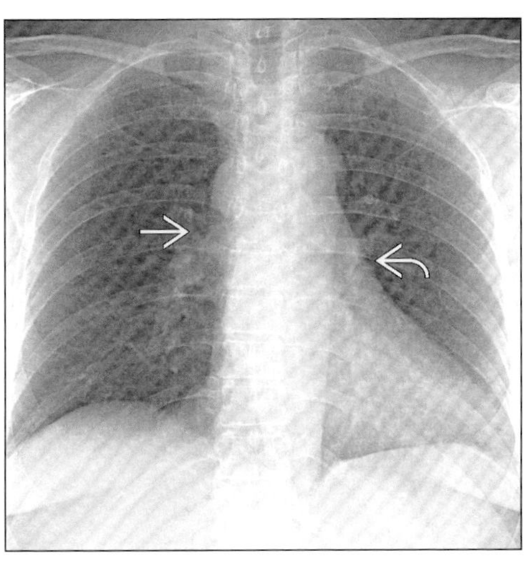

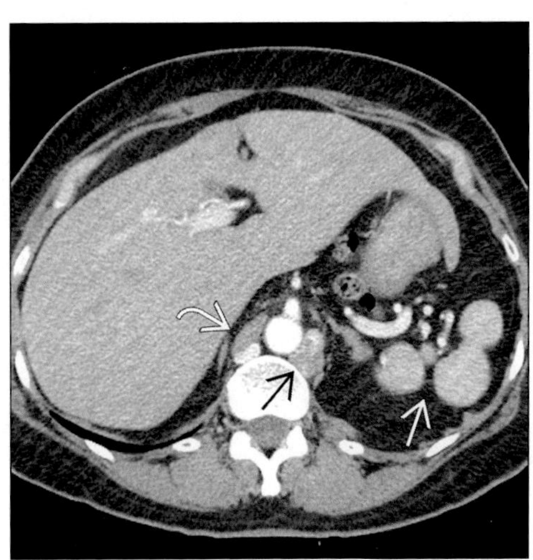

(Left) *PA chest radiograph shows a right eparterial bronchus → and a left hyparterial bronchus →, suggesting normal situs. Note enlargement of the azygos arch and mild cardiomegaly.* ***(Right)*** *Axial CECT of the same patient shows heterotaxy syndrome with polysplenia →, transverse liver, and azygos → and hemiazygos → continuation of the IVC secondary to IVC interruption. The thoracic findings of heterotaxy are inconsistent in this patient.*

ABSENCE OF THE PERICARDIUM

Key Facts

Terminology
- Congenital absence of pericardium; may be partial or complete

Imaging
- Radiography
  - Lung interposition between pulmonary trunk & aortic arch
  - Lung interposition between left hemidiaphragm & base of heart
  - Conspicuous left atrial appendage
  - Leftward shift of cardiac silhouette
- CT: Leftward shift & rotation of heart
  - Absence of visible pericardium in affected region
- MR: Absence of hypointense pericardial line
  - Excessive mobility of myocardium
  - Large difference in heart volume between end-systole & end-diastole in affected patients

Top Differential Diagnoses
- Pericardial cyst
- Pericardial effusion
- Loculated pleural effusion
- Left ventricular aneurysm

Pathology
- Interruption of vascular supply to developing pericardium during embryogenesis

Clinical Issues
- Most complete defects are clinically insignificant
- Subtype of partial absence ("foramen-type" defects) may be lethal
- Treatment
  - Surgical closure of pericardial defect
  - Enlargement of pericardial defect to prevent strangulation of heart

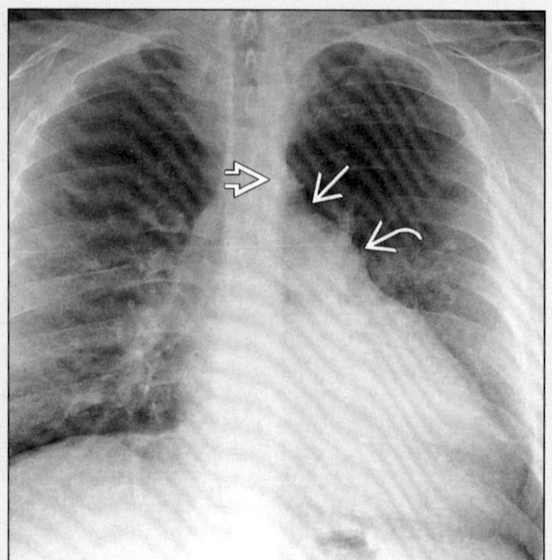

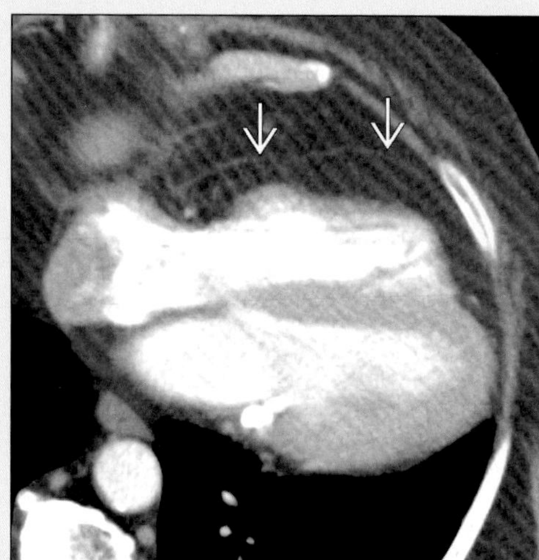

(Left) *AP chest radiograph demonstrates partial absence of the pericardium manifesting as lung interposition ➔ between the pulmonary trunk ➔ and the aortic arch ➔ and leftward shift of the heart.* ***(Right)*** *Axial CECT shows complete shift of the heart into the left hemithorax. Normal pericardium ➔ is present anterior to the right ventricle, but there is no visible pericardium posterior to the left ventricle. Partial absence of the pericardium is most common along the lateral left ventricular wall.*

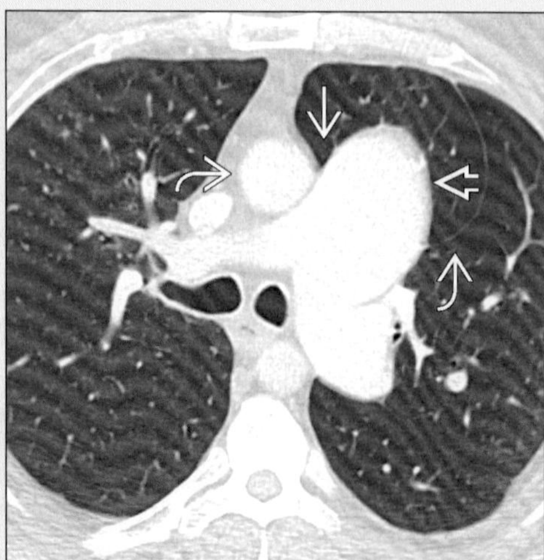

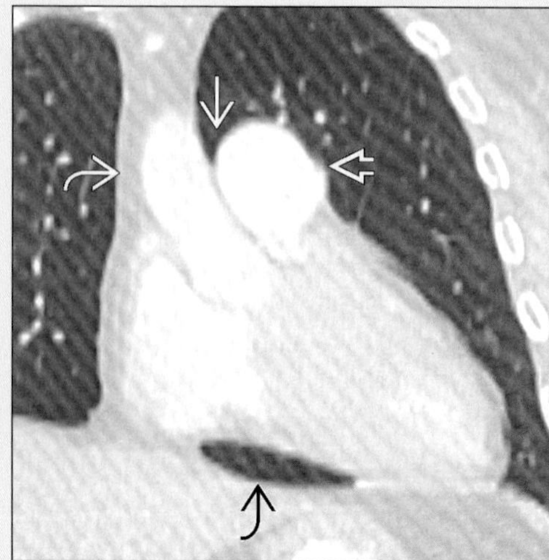

(Left) *Axial CECT of a patient with partial absence of the pericardium shows interposition of lung ➔ between the pulmonary trunk ➔, which is enlarged, and the ascending thoracic aorta ➔. A left minor fissure is incidentally identified.* ***(Right)*** *Coronal CECT of the same patient shows lung interposition ➔ between the pulmonary trunk ➔ and the ascending thoracic aorta ➔. There is also interposition of lung ➔ between the left hemidiaphragm and the base of the heart.*

ABSENCE OF THE PERICARDIUM

TERMINOLOGY

Definitions

- Congenital absence of pericardium; may be partial or complete

IMAGING

General Features

- Location
  - Partial defects usually occur along lateral left ventricular wall

Radiographic Findings

- Radiography
  - **Lung interposition between pulmonary trunk & aortic arch**
  - Lung interposition between left hemidiaphragm & base of heart
  - **Leftward shift of cardiac silhouette** ("Snoopy's nose")
    - Classically described in complete absence of pericardium
      - May not be seen in younger patients with complete absence
      - May also be seen in partial absence of left pericardium
  - **Conspicuous left atrial appendage** ("Snoopy's ear")
    - Common in partial absence of left pericardium

CT Findings

- NECT
  - **Lung interposition between pulmonary trunk & ascending aorta**
  - Leftward shift & rotation of heart
  - Absence of visible pericardium in affected region

MR Findings

- Absence of hypointense pericardial line
- Excessive myocardium mobility
- Large difference in heart volume between end-systole & end-diastole in affected patients

Echocardiographic Findings

- Echocardiogram
  - Enlargement of left atrial appendage
  - Hypermobility of heart
  - Abnormal ventricular septal motion
  - Swinging heart motion

Imaging Recommendations

- Best imaging tool
  - CT & MR findings are diagnostic

DIFFERENTIAL DIAGNOSIS

Pericardial Cyst

- Cardiophrenic angle mass abutting heart
- Imperceptible wall
- Water attenuation on CT
- Fluid signal intensity on MR

Pericardial Effusion

- Globular symmetric enlargement of cardiopericardial silhouette on frontal chest radiography: "Water bottle" sign
- > 2 mm water density stripe between retrosternal & subepicardial fat on lateral chest radiography
  - "Fat pad" sign or "Oreo cookie" sign

Loculated Pleural Effusion

- Usually can be separated from uninvolved pericardium
- Typically water attenuation on CT

Left Ventricular Aneurysm

- Rare complication of myocardial infarction
- Calcification may be present

PATHOLOGY

General Features

- Etiology
  - Interruption of vascular supply to developing pericardium during embryogenesis
- Associated abnormalities
  - Atrial septal defect, patent ductus arteriosus, mitral valve stenosis, & tetralogy of Fallot

CLINICAL ISSUES

Presentation

- Most common signs/symptoms
  - Complete absence: Usually asymptomatic
  - Partial absence: Nonexertional paroxysmal chest pain, tachycardia, & palpitations

Demographics

- Epidemiology
  - Prevalence: 0.002-0.004%

Natural History & Prognosis

- Most complete defects are clinically insignificant
- Subtype of partial absence may be lethal
  - "Foramen-type" defects may result in herniation of left atrial appendage or left ventricle that results in strangulation of myocardium

Treatment

- Surgical
  - Closure of pericardial defect
  - Enlargement of pericardial defect to prevent strangulation of heart

DIAGNOSTIC CHECKLIST

Consider

- Absence of pericardium when there is lung interposition between pulmonary trunk & aortic arch, particularly if associated with left shift of the heart

SELECTED REFERENCES

1. Psychidis-Papakyritsis P et al: Functional MRI of congenital absence of the pericardium. AJR Am J Roentgenol. 189(6):W312-4, 2007

POLAND SYNDROME

Key Facts

Terminology

- Definition
  - Pectoral aplasia-syndactyly syndrome
  - Congenital unilateral partial or total absence of pectoralis major muscle

Imaging

- Radiography
  - Unilateral hyperlucency
  - Absence of normal axillary fold on affected side
- CT/MR
  - Absence or hypoplasia of pectoral girdle musculature
- Associated abnormalities
  - Hypoplasia of affected hand
  - Hypoplastic middle phalanx
  - Rib deformities

Top Differential Diagnoses

- Radiographic artifact
- Swyer-James-McLeod
- Radical mastectomy/prosthesis
- Chest wall soft tissue mass

Clinical Issues

- Asymptomatic cosmetic deformity
- Increased incidence of leukemia, non-Hodgkin lymphoma, lung cancer, breast cancer

Diagnostic Checklist

- Consider conditions involving lung parenchyma, airway, pulmonary vasculature, pleural space, chest wall, & technical factors in patients with unilateral hyperlucent hemithorax
- Evaluate patients with Poland syndrome for occult lung cancer (increased incidence)

(Left) Axial CECT of a patient with Poland syndrome demonstrates absence of the major and minor left pectoral muscles ➔. CT is helpful in demonstrating other associated abnormalities of the pectoralis minor, serratus anterior, and latissimus dorsi. ***(Right)*** *Coronal CECT of the same patient demonstrates asymmetric absence of the left pectoralis major muscle ➔. Cross-sectional imaging plays a fundamental role in the detection and characterization of this and other chest wall disorders.*

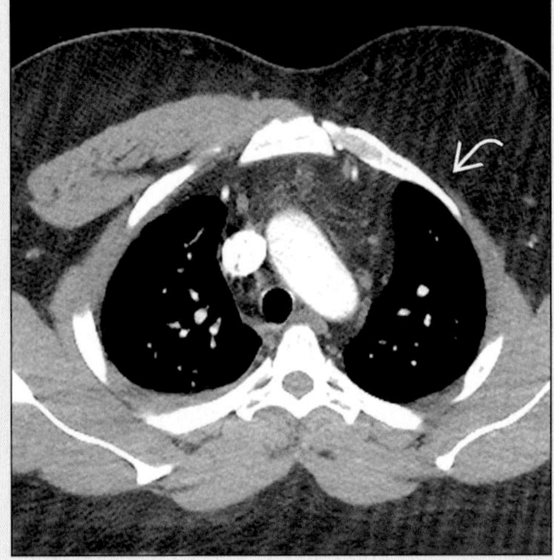

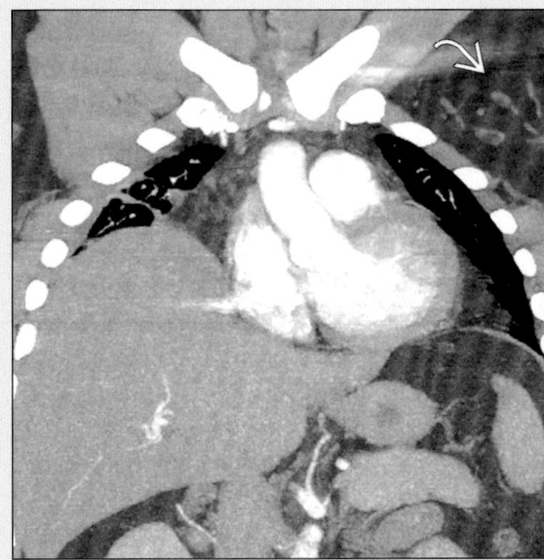

(Left) Axial NECT of a patient who presented with pneumonia ➔ shows complete absence of the right pectoralis muscle ➔. CT and MR are the most sensitive techniques for detecting and evaluating chest wall soft tissue abnormalities. ***(Right)*** *PA chest radiograph of a patient with Poland syndrome shows radiolucency of the right hemithorax. In an asymptomatic patient, these findings are strongly suggestive of congenital absence of the pectoralis muscle, which may be partial or total.*

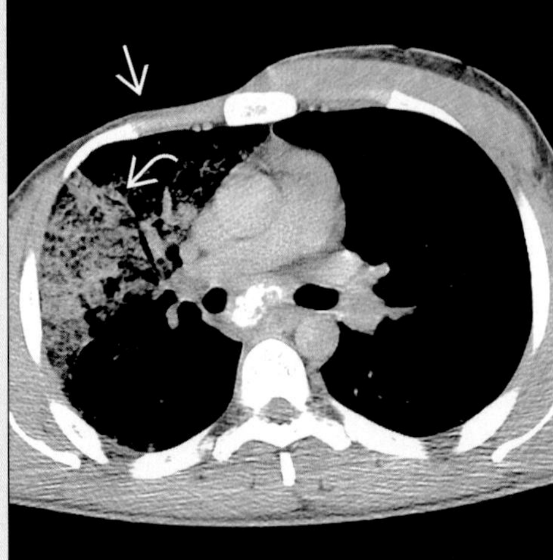

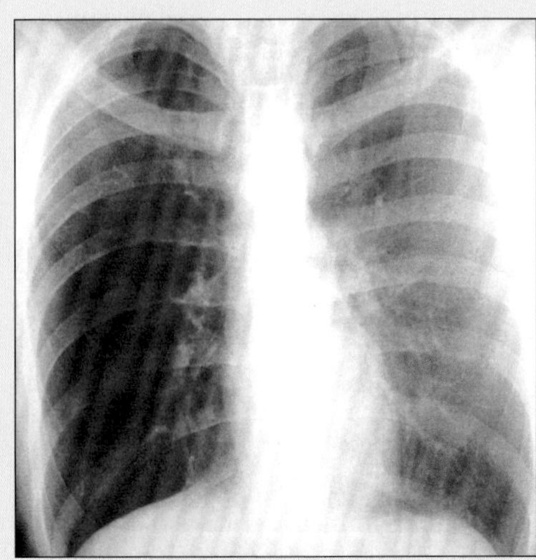

POLAND SYNDROME

TERMINOLOGY

Synonyms

- Pectoral aplasia-syndactyly syndrome

Definitions

- Congenital unilateral partial or total absence of pectoralis major muscle
  - Rarely bilateral

IMAGING

General Features

- Best diagnostic clue
  - Clinical suspicion: Syndactylism with deformity of pectoral muscle

Radiographic Findings

- Unilateral hyperlucency
- Absence of normal axillary fold on affected side
- Rib deformities
- Affected hand with hypoplastic middle phalanx

CT Findings

- Absence or hypoplasia of pectoral girdle musculature
- Hypoplastic ipsilateral breast

Imaging Recommendations

- Best imaging tool
  - Chest radiography usually sufficient to document thoracic abnormalities
  - CT & MR: More sensitive in detecting soft tissue abnormalities

DIFFERENTIAL DIAGNOSIS

Technical Factors and Artifacts

- Malaligned grid
- Abnormal image density extending outside thorax

Swyer-James-McLeod

- Unilateral hyperlucent lung
- Small pulmonary vasculature in affected lung
- Expiratory air-trapping on affected side
- Mosaic attenuation at HRCT

Radical Mastectomy/Prosthesis

- Absent or altered breast shadow
- Surgical clips in axilla (often)
- History of breast cancer

Chest Wall Soft Tissue Mass

- Increased, often asymmetric density of affected side

PATHOLOGY

General Features

- Genetics
  - Autosomal recessive condition
- Associated abnormalities
  - Skeletal dysostoses affecting hand
    - Brachymesophalangy with
      - Syndactyly
      - Biphalangy
      - Ectrodactyly
  - Pectus excavatum
  - Anomalies of ipsilateral upper limb
  - **Other anomalies**
    - Absence of pectoralis minor
    - Hypoplasia of latissimus dorsi & serratus anterior muscles
    - Hypoplasia or aplasia of nipple & breast
    - Lung herniation
    - Hypoplasia of hemithorax or ribs

CLINICAL ISSUES

Presentation

- Most common signs/symptoms
  - Asymptomatic cosmetic deformity
- Other signs/symptoms
  - Increased incidence of leukemia, non-Hodgkin lymphoma, lung cancer, breast cancer

Demographics

- Gender
  - M > F
- Epidemiology
  - True incidence/prevalence difficult to predict
    - Variable between groups (male vs. female)
    - Prevalence: Ranges from 1/7,000 to 1/100,000 live births

Treatment

- Muscle flaps and breast implants: To correct muscle deficiency & breast hypoplasia
- Chest wall reconstruction if thoracic skeleton involved
  - Homologous preservation of costal cartilage: Improves chest wall stability
  - Bone grafts or prosthetic mesh: Reconstruction of aplastic ribs

DIAGNOSTIC CHECKLIST

Consider

- Unilateral hyperlucent hemithorax
  - Conditions involving pulmonary parenchyma, airway, pulmonary vasculature, pleural space, chest wall
  - In adult woman, hyperlucent hemithorax mimics mastectomy
  - Technical factors & artifacts

Image Interpretation Pearls

- Evaluate patients with Poland syndrome for occult lung cancer (increased incidence)
- Chest radiography, CT, & MR depict (when present) absent or hypoplastic ipsilateral ribs & scoliosis

SELECTED REFERENCES

1. Dillman JR et al: Expanding upon the unilateral hyperlucent hemithorax in children. Radiographics. 31(3):723-41, 2011
2. Jeung MY et al: Imaging of chest wall disorders. Radiographics. 19(3):617-37, 1999
3. Wright AR et al: MR and CT in the assessment of Poland syndrome. J Comput Assist Tomogr. 16(3):442-7, 1992
4. Pearl M et al: Poland's syndrome. Radiology. 101(3):619-23, 1971

PECTUS DEFORMITY

Key Facts

Terminology
- Pectus excavatum: Sternum depressed; anterior ribs protrude anterior to sternum
- Pectus carinatum: Anterior protrusion of sternum; congenital or acquired

Imaging
- Right heart border frequently obliterated because depressed sternum replaces aerated lung at the right heart border
- Heart displaced to left & rotated (mitral configuration), may cause spurious cardiomegaly
- Degree of depression best evaluated on lateral chest radiography

Top Differential Diagnoses
- Right middle lobe atelectasis
- Right middle lobe pneumonia
- Cardiophrenic angle mass

Pathology
- Pectus excavatum: Mitral valve prolapse (20-60%)
- Pectus carinatum: Cyanotic congenital heart disease

Clinical Issues
- Pectus excavatum and carinatum: Usually asymptomatic
- Pectus excavatum: 1 in 300-400 births; most common chest wall abnormality (90%)
- Scoliosis in 21% of patients with pectus excavatum & in 11% of patients with pectus carinatum
- M:F = 4:1

Diagnostic Checklist
- Consider pectus excavatum in asymptomatic patients with obscuration of right heart border on PA chest radiography

*(**Left**) PA chest radiograph of an asymptomatic 23-year-old woman shows leftward displacement of the heart and obscuration of the right heart border ➔. The findings may mimic middle lobe atelectasis or pneumonia. (**Right**) Lateral chest radiograph of a 75-year-old man shows anterior sternal protrusion (pectus carinatum) ➔ associated with severe hypertrophic chondrosternal junctions ➔. Sagittal and coronal CT reformations are useful for evaluation of abnormalities of the sternum and costal cartilages.*

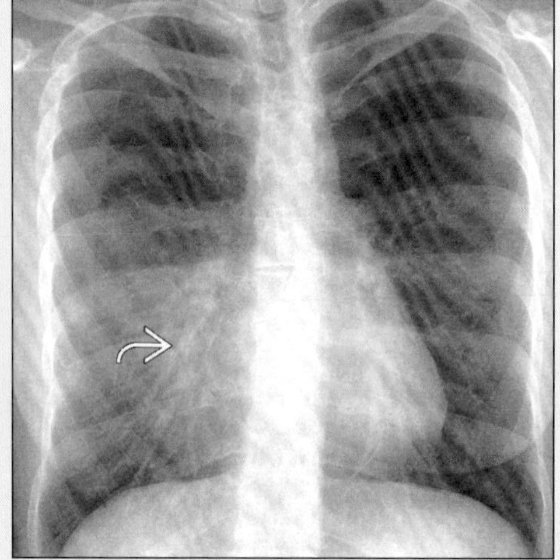

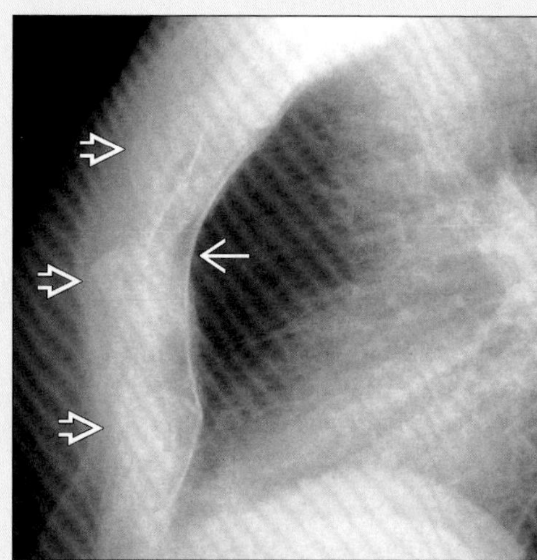

*(**Left**) Sagittal NECT of an asymptomatic patient with pectus excavatum ➔ shows surgical placement of a subcutaneous silicone implant ➔. In patients with no physiologic compromise, this treatment avoids a major reconstruction surgery of the chest wall with its attendant risks and complications. (**Right**) 3D reformation of the thoracic cage shows slight outward convexity of the upper sternal body ➔ (pectus carinatum) and depression of the xiphoid appendix ➔.*

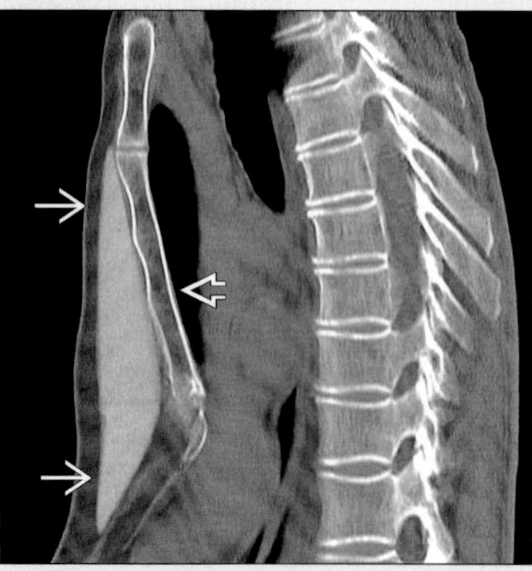

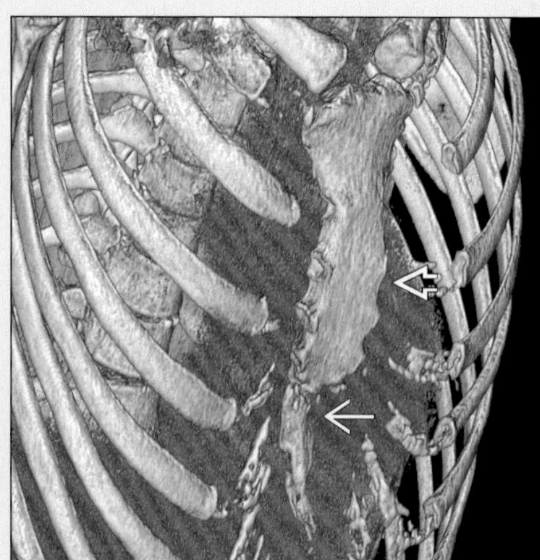

PECTUS DEFORMITY

TERMINOLOGY

Synonyms

- Pectus excavatum: Funnel chest
- Pectus carinatum: Chicken breast or pouter pigeon breast

Definitions

- Pectus excavatum: Sternum depressed; anterior ribs protrude anterior to sternum
- Pectus carinatum: Anterior protrusion of sternum; congenital or acquired

IMAGING

Radiographic Findings

- Radiography
  - **Pectus excavatum**
    - Right heart border frequently obscured because depressed sternum replaces aerated lung at the right heart border
    - Heart displaced to left & rotated (mitral configuration), may cause spurious cardiomegaly
    - Degree of depression best evaluated on lateral chest radiograph
  - **Pectus carinatum:** 3 different types
    - Chondrogladiolar protrusion (chicken breast): Anterior displacement of sternum & symmetric concavity of costal cartilages (most common)
    - Lateral depression of ribs on 1 or both sides of sternum (frequently associated with Poland syndrome)
    - Chondromanubrial prominence (pouter pigeon breast): Upper prominence with protrusion of manubrium & depression of sternal body (least common)

CT Findings

- Severity of defect can be quantified by CT or MR (Haller index)
  - "Pectus index" = transverse diameter/AP diameter
  - "Pectus index" > 3.25 requires surgical correction

DIFFERENTIAL DIAGNOSIS

Right Middle Lobe Atelectasis

- Obscuration of right heart border without cardiac displacement to left
- Other signs of atelectasis

Right Middle Lobe Pneumonia

- Consolidation on lateral chest radiograph

Cardiophrenic Angle Mass

- Smooth, sharply marginated mass (usually homogeneous)

PATHOLOGY

General Features

- Etiology
  - Pathogenesis unclear
    - Overgrowth of costal cartilage
    - Abnormalities of diaphragm
    - Elevated intrauterine pressure
- Genetics
  - Pectus excavatum: Familial history (40%)
  - Pectus carinatum: Familial history (26%)
- Associated abnormalities
  - Musculoskeletal abnormalities: Marfan syndrome, Noonan syndrome, osteogenesis imperfecta
  - Scoliosis (15-20%)
  - Pectus excavatum: Mitral valve prolapse (20-60%)
  - Pectus carinatum: Cyanotic congenital heart disease

CLINICAL ISSUES

Presentation

- Most common signs/symptoms
  - Pectus excavatum & carinatum: Usually asymptomatic
- Other signs/symptoms
  - Pectus excavatum & carinatum: Nonspecific chest or back pain
  - Pectus excavatum: Exercise-induced decrease in respiratory reserve or pain along costal cartilages
  - Pectus excavatum: Occasionally, cardiac symptoms/signs (pulmonic murmur, mitral valve prolapse, Wolff-Parkinson-White syndrome)

Demographics

- Gender
  - M:F = 4:1
  - Family history in 20-40% of cases
- Epidemiology
  - Pectus excavatum: 1 in 300-400 births; most common chest wall abnormality (90%)
  - Pectus carinatum: Less frequent by ratio of approximately 1:5; 5-7% of chest wall deformities

Natural History & Prognosis

- Scoliosis in 21% of patients with pectus excavatum and in 11% of patients with pectus carinatum

Treatment

- Surgical correction
  - Pectus index > 3.25
  - Respiratory or cardiovascular insufficiency
  - Psychosocial factors & cosmesis

DIAGNOSTIC CHECKLIST

Consider

- Pectus excavatum in asymptomatic patients with obscuration of right heart border on PA radiography

Image Interpretation Pearls

- Degree of sternal depression best evaluated on lateral chest radiography

SELECTED REFERENCES

1. Haje SA et al: Pectus deformities: tomographic analysis and clinical correlation. Skeletal Radiol. 39(8):773-82, 2010
2. Rattan AS et al: Pectus excavatum imaging: enough but not too much. Pediatr Radiol. 40(2):168-72, 2010
3. Restrepo CS et al: Imaging appearances of the sternum and sternoclavicular joints. Radiographics. 29(3):839-59, 2009

KYPHOSCOLIOSIS

Key Facts

Terminology
- Complex 3-dimensional rotational curvature of spine

Imaging
- Scoliosis: > 10° lateral deviation of spine from central axis
- Cobb angle: Scoliotic curve's angle
- Idiopathic kyphoscoliosis
  - Usually convex to right; most cases, no kyphosis (hypokyphosis)
- Neurofibromatosis type 1
  - Sharply angled at thoracolumbar junction
  - Lateral thoracic meningocele
  - Neurofibromas that may extend into spinal canal
- Pott disease
  - Erosive scalloping of anterolateral surface of vertebral bodies
  - Collapse of intervertebral disc space
  - Angular kyphotic deformity & gibbus formation
- Ankylosing spondylitis
  - Kyphosis, squared vertebral bodies
  - Vertebral syndesmophytes, usually T9 to T12
- Mitral valve prolapse
  - Idiopathic scoliosis (25%)
  - Straight back syndrome (33%)

Top Differential Diagnoses
- Neurofibromatosis type 1
- Infectious spondylitis
- Neuromuscular etiology

Clinical Issues
- Restrictive lung disease
- Pulmonary artery hypertension; cor pulmonale
- Respiratory failure
- Treatment of scoliosis
  - Observation, orthosis, and surgical correction & stabilization

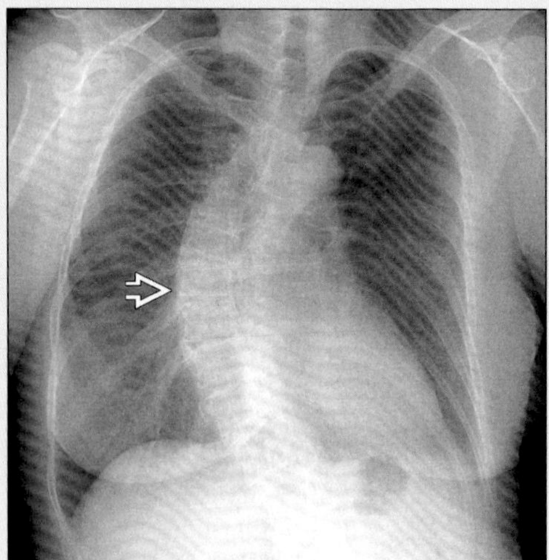
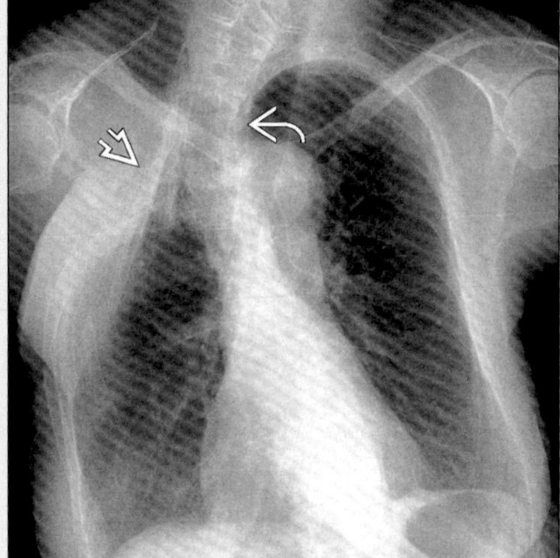

(Left) *PA chest radiograph of a 51-year-old woman shows typical features of idiopathic scoliosis manifesting as a right convex scoliosis ➡. The lateral chest radiograph (not shown) demonstrated hypokyphosis.* ***(Right)*** *PA chest radiograph of a 73-year-old woman status post thoracoplasty ➡ for tuberculosis shows a right convex scoliosis ➡ at the cervicothoracic spine that developed as a result of the chest wall surgery.*

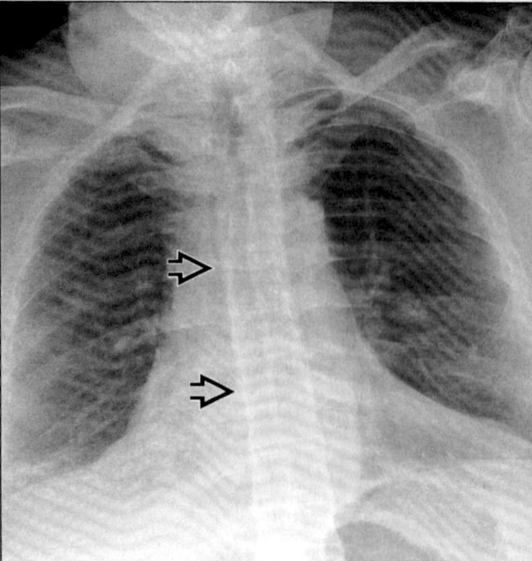
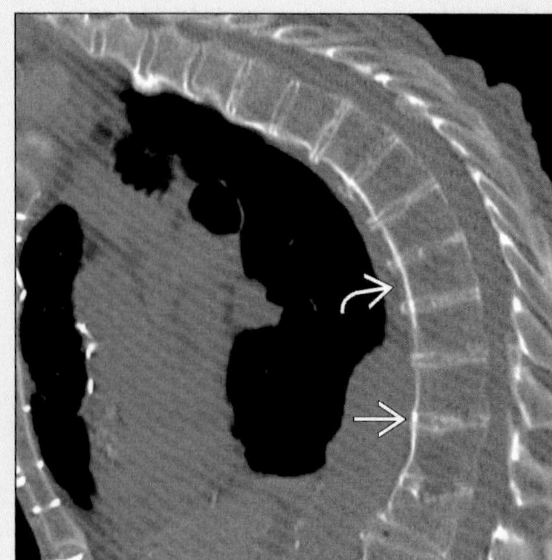

(Left) *AP chest radiograph of a 63-year-old man with ankylosing spondylitis shows the typical bamboo spine ➡ deformity resulting from spinal ankylosis.* ***(Right)*** *Sagittal NECT of a patient with ankylosing spondylitis shows typical findings of kyphosis, squared vertebrae ➡, syndesmophytes ➡, and spinal ankylosis.*

KYPHOSCOLIOSIS

TERMINOLOGY

Synonyms

- Scoliosis
- Kyphosis
- Gibbus deformity

Definitions

- Complex 3-dimensional rotational curvature of spine

IMAGING

General Features

- Best diagnostic clue
  - Abnormal spinal curvature on anteroposterior & lateral radiographs
- Location
  - Cervical, thoracic, lumbar, sacral spine
- Size
  - Partial or entire spine involvement
- Morphology
  - Scoliosis: > 10° lateral deviation of spine from central axis
  - **Cobb angle**: Scoliotic curve's angle
    - Calculated by selecting upper & lower end vertebrae in a curve
    - Erecting perpendiculars to their transverse axes
    - At their point of intersection, angle is measured

Radiographic Findings

- Idiopathic kyphoscoliosis
  - Usually convex to right
  - Most cases, no kyphosis (hypokyphosis)
  - Chest radiograph is difficult to interpret in severe cases because of rotation of thorax & heart
- Neurofibromatosis type 1, (NF1, von Recklinghausen disease)
  - Short segment angular scoliosis
    - Kyphosis more pronounced than scoliosis
    - Involves 5 vertebrae or fewer in primary curve
    - NF1: Sharply angled at thoracolumbar junction
  - Intervertebral foramina enlargement
    - NF1: Lateral thoracic meningocele, neurofibromas that may extend into spinal canal
  - Lateral thoracic meningocele
    - Herniation of meninges through intervertebral foramen
    - Kyphoscoliosis with meningocele on convex side
    - Round, well-defined, paravertebral mass
    - Right > left
    - Rib erosion & erosion of adjacent neural foramen
    - 10% multiple meningoceles
  - Scalloping of vertebral body
    - Anterior, posterior, lateral
  - Wedge-shaped vertebra
  - Hypoplastic or pressure remodeled pedicles
  - Transverse process spindling
  - Spondylolisthesis, spinal clefts, osteolysis
  - Unstable spine, leading to subluxation or dislocation
  - Spinal fusion, complicated by pseudoarthrosis, curve progression
  - Inferior rib notching; twisted, ribbon-like upper ribs
  - Pectus excavatum
- Infectious spondylitis: Kyphosis, paraspinal mass, bone destruction, disc space loss
- Pott disease
  - L1 vertebra corpus is most common site; 3 or more contiguous vertebrae
  - Erosive scalloping of anterolateral surfaces of vertebral bodies (gouge defect)
  - Collapse of intervertebral disc space
  - Progressive vertebral collapse with anterior wedging
  - Angular kyphotic deformity & gibbus formation
  - Paravertebral "cold" abscesses that may calcify
- Congenital: Hemivertebra, fused ribs may lead to scoliosis
- Senile osteoporotic kyphosis: Compression fractures of multiple vertebra & cortical thinning
- Ankylosing spondylitis
  - Kyphosis, squared vertebral bodies
  - Vertebral syndesmophytes, usually T9 to T12
  - Interspinous ossification
  - Ossification of costotransverse joints
  - Manubriosternal joint erosion or fusion

CT Findings

- CECT
  - Lateral thoracic meningocele
    - Well-circumscribed, low-attenuation paravertebral masses
    - Peripheral rim enhancement may occur
    - CT myelography: Filling with intrathecally injected contrast
  - Neurofibromas
    - May show very low attenuation (10-20 HU)

MR Findings

- Neurofibromatosis type 1
  - Dural dysplasia: Lateral meningoceles, dural ectasia
    - Shows cerebrospinal fluid content of meningoceles
  - Neurofibromas
    - T1WI: Low to intermediate signal intensity; T1 C+ (enhance after contrast)
    - T2WI: Often heterogeneous, high signal intensity regions, myxoid tissue or cystic degeneration; central low signal intensity, collagen & fibrous tissue

Echocardiographic Findings

- Echocardiogram
  - Mitral valve prolapse in idiopathic scoliosis (25%) & straight back syndrome (33%)

Imaging Recommendations

- Best imaging tool
  - Radiography: Serial studies to assess for progression
    - Assessment of skeletal maturity
  - Complex cases: MR or CT with multiplanar reconstructions
- Protocol advice
  - Upright standing anteroposterior & lateral radiographs, entire spine
    - Sitting radiographs for patients who cannot stand
    - Supine radiographs for patients who cannot sit
  - Close surveillance during greatest growth (puberty & early adolescence)
  - Radiation dose approximately 140 μSv
- MR to detect peri/intraspinal abnormalities

KYPHOSCOLIOSIS

DIFFERENTIAL DIAGNOSIS

Neurofibromatosis Type 1

- Stigmata of neurofibromatosis

Infectious Spondylitis

- Disc space involvement, vertebral destruction, sepsis

Neuromuscular Etiology

- Upper motor neuron lesions: Cerebral palsy, syringomyelia, spinal cord trauma
- Lower motor neuron lesions: Poliomyelitis, spinal muscular atrophy
- Myopathic conditions: Arthrogryposis, muscular dystrophy, & other myopathies

Congenital

- Hemivertebra, fused ribs, spina bifida, Klippel-Feil syndrome
- VATER complex (**v**ertebral, **a**norectal, **t**racheal, **e**sophageal, **r**enal)

Post Thoracoplasty

- Chest wall deformity, surgical history

Complications after Radiation Treatment for Childhood Malignancy

- Hypoplasia ipsilateral pedicles in radiation port

PATHOLOGY

General Features

- Etiology
  - Majority are idiopathic
- Genetics
  - Variety of diseases associated with scoliosis: Friedrich ataxia, Morquio syndrome, Ehlers-Danlos, Marfan syndrome, muscular dystrophy
  - Neurofibromatosis type 1, autosomal dominant
- Associated abnormalities
  - Scoliosis associated with pectus excavatum or carinatum deformities

Gross Pathologic & Surgical Features

- Pathophysiology: Not well understood

CLINICAL ISSUES

Presentation

- Most common signs/symptoms
  - Most patients are symptom free; many discovered at school screening
  - Indications for CT or MR imaging
    - Abnormal neurological examination
    - Painful scoliosis; neck pain & headache, especially with exertion
    - Clinical signs of dysraphism; weakness, pes cavus, ataxia
  - Neuromuscular disease: Poor cough reflex
    - Susceptibility for pneumonia
- Cardiac symptoms
  - Pulmonic murmur, mitral valve prolapse, syncope, Wolff-Parkinson-White syndrome
  - Ankylosing spondylitis
    - Aortic valve stenosis
  - Neurofibromatosis type 1
    - Hypertension, aortic coarctation, coronary artery disease
    - Pulmonic valve stenosis, atrial septal defect, ventricular septal defect, idiopathic hypertrophic subaortic stenosis
- Respiratory symptoms
  - Kyphoscoliosis
    - Decreased compliance of lung & chest wall
    - Restrictive lung disease
    - Hypoventilation, hypoxic vasoconstriction, hypercapnia
    - Pulmonary artery hypertension; cor pulmonale
    - Respiratory failure
  - Neurofibromatosis type 1
    - Interstitial lung disease, basilar predominance
    - Pulmonary artery hypertension, peripheral vessel pruning
    - Upper lobe bullae & honeycomb lung
    - Spontaneous pneumothorax/hemothorax
  - Ankylosing spondylitis
    - Upper lobe fibrosis, mycetomas

Demographics

- Age
  - Age at presentation
    - Congenital
    - Infantile (< 3 years)
    - Juvenile (3–10 years)
    - Adolescent (> 10 years)
- Gender
  - Idiopathic scoliosis: M:F = 1:4
- Epidemiology
  - Idiopathic scoliosis
    - Prevalence 1-3% for curves > 10°
    - 80% of severe cases are idiopathic
  - Neurofibromatosis type 1 (50% of patients with kyphosis)
  - Neuromuscular diseases
    - 90% of males with Duchenne muscular dystrophy
    - 60% of patients with myelodysplasia
    - 20% of children with cerebral palsy

Natural History & Prognosis

- Most severe in nonambulatory patients; progression in neuromuscular disorders
- Juvenile idiopathic scoliosis: Nearly 90% of curves progress, almost 70% require surgery
- Longstanding severe kyphoscoliosis
  - Pulmonary artery hypertension
  - Respiratory failure associated with Cobb angle > 100°

Treatment

- Scoliosis: Observation, orthosis, surgical correction & stabilization

SELECTED REFERENCES

1. Grissom LE et al: Thoracic deformities and the growing lung. Semin Roentgenol. 33(2):199-208, 1998
2. Barnes PD et al: Atypical idiopathic scoliosis: MR imaging evaluation. Radiology. 186(1):247-53, 1993

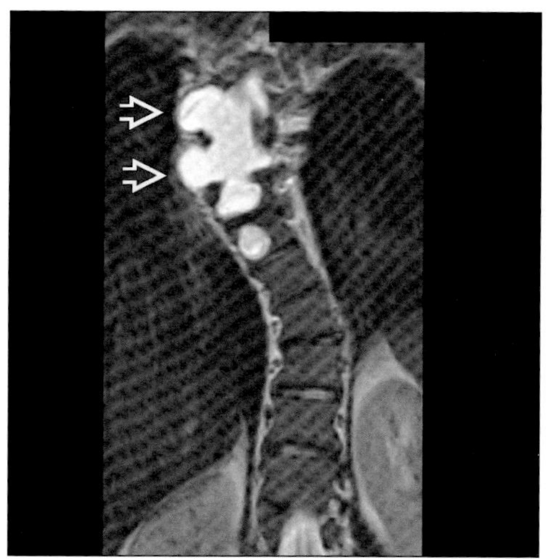

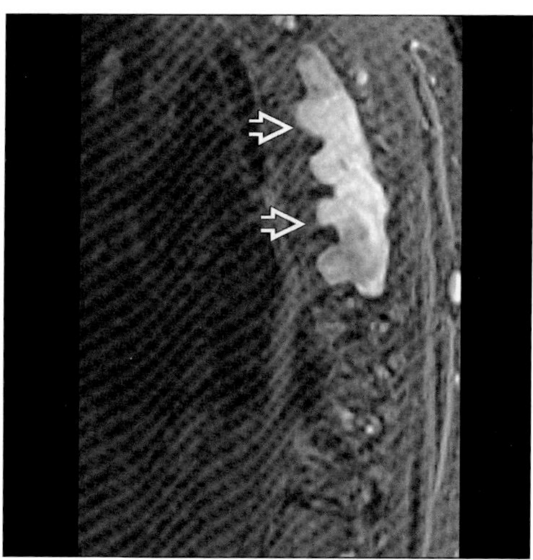

(Left) Coronal T2WI MR of a 20-year-old patient with neurofibromatosis type 1 shows dextroscoliosis extending from T3 to T7 with right-sided lateral thoracic meningoceles ➔. Meningoceles in this condition typically occur at the convex side of the scoliotic curve. ***(Right)*** Sagittal STIR MR of the same patient shows dural ectasia with posterior scalloping ➔ of the T3 through T7 vertebral bodies, typical imaging features of patients with neurofibromatosis type 1.

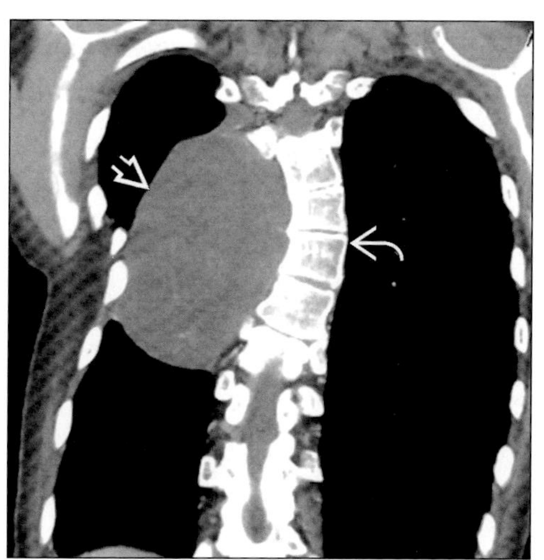

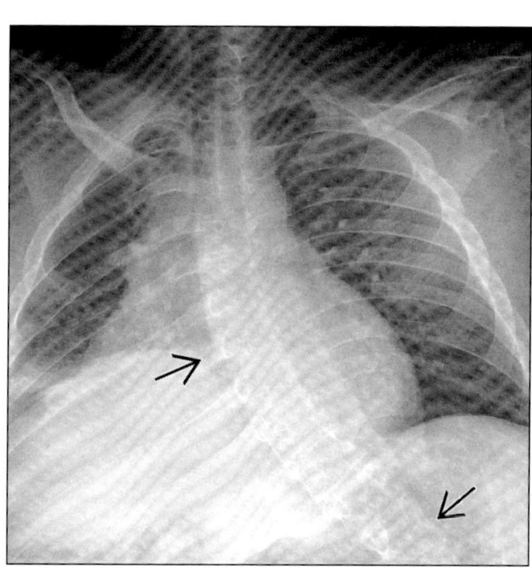

(Left) Coronal CECT of a 30-year-old patient with neurofibromatosis shows a large paravertebral mass ➔ that was shown to represent a neurofibroma. The lesion extended into the T7 neural foramen (not shown). Neurofibromas typically occur at the concave side of the scoliosis ➔. ***(Right)*** PA chest radiograph of a 23-year-old man with Duchenne muscular dystrophy shows an S-shaped scoliosis ➔ of the thoracic and lumbar spine, the result of muscular wasting.

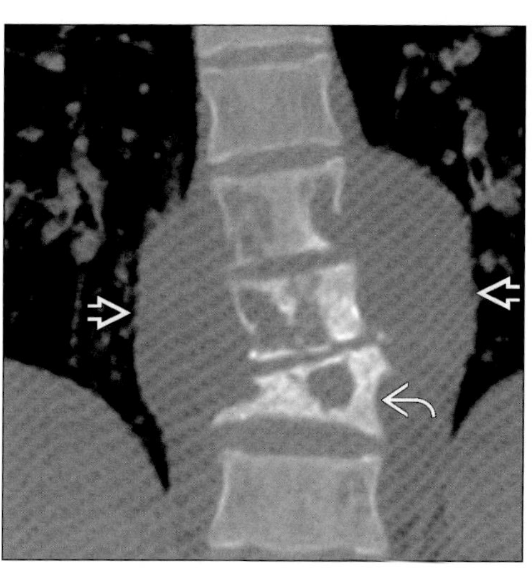

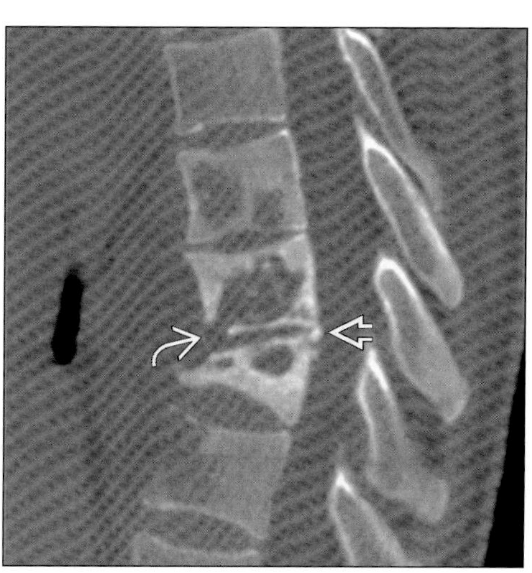

(Left) Coronal NECT of a 29-year-old woman with HIV infection and Pott disease shows bilateral large paravertebral soft tissue masses ➔, lytic and sclerotic lesions at T8-T10, and compression of T10 ➔. ***(Right)*** Sagittal NECT of the same patient shows disc space narrowing and gibbus deformity at the T9-T10 level ➔ and erosion of the anterior inferior endplate of T9 ➔, consistent with osteomyelitis and discitis. Percutaneous biopsy cultures grew M. tuberculosis.

MORGAGNI HERNIA

Key Facts

Terminology

- Anterior diaphragmatic hernia
- Protrusion of abdominal cavity contents through retrosternal defect in diaphragm

Imaging

- Radiography
  - 90% are located on right side
  - Well-circumscribed mass with smooth borders, possibly containing bowel gas
- CT with multiplanar reformats is best imaging tool
  - Anterolateral diaphragmatic defect with hernia sac containing omental fat ± bowel
  - Assessment of complications (incarceration, strangulation)
- MR
  - Allows direct multiplanar imaging
  - Better resolution of diaphragm muscle & defect

Top Differential Diagnoses

- Mediastinal fat pad
- Cardiophrenic mass

Pathology

- Congenital defect secondary to maldevelopment of septum transversum (precursor of diaphragm)
- Most defects small, containing only omental fat
- Covered by peritoneal sac

Clinical Issues

- Potential for incarceration or strangulation if hernia contains bowel

Diagnostic Checklist

- Consider Morgagni hernia in patient with pericardiophrenic mass containing bowel on radiography or mesenteric vessels on CT/MR

*(**Left**) PA chest radiograph of an asymptomatic patient with a Morgagni hernia shows a right cardiophrenic opacity obscuring the right heart border. Note lucency within the mass indicating bowel ⇒. 90% of Morgagni hernias are on the right side. (**Right**) Oblique coronal NECT of the same patient shows an anterior/retrosternal diaphragmatic defect through which bowel ➡ and mesenteric vessels ➦ course. Mesenteric vessels within the hernia sac are an important diagnostic clue.*

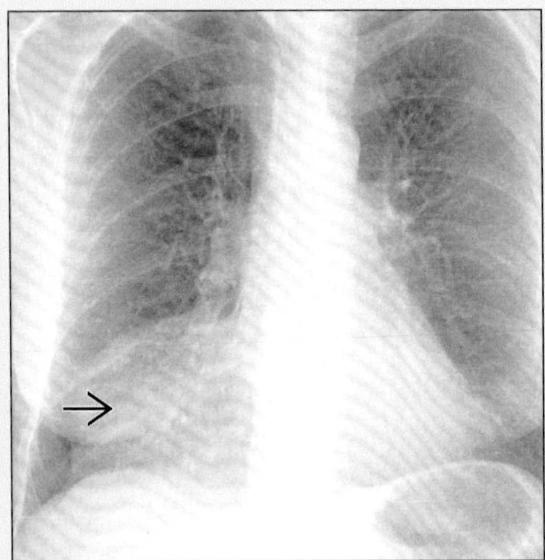

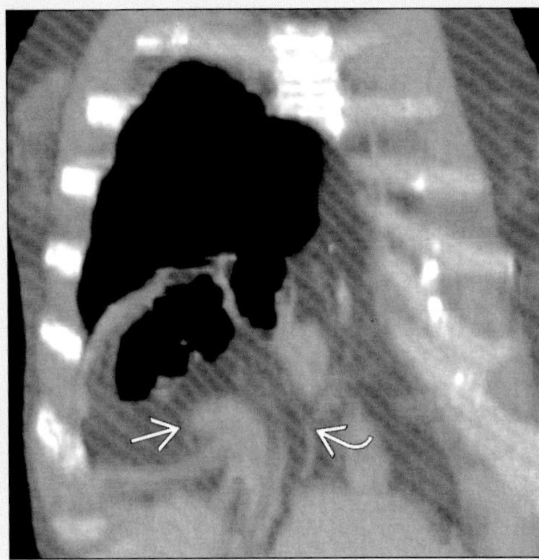

*(**Left**) Axial CECT of a patient with a Morgagni hernia shows a large anterior diaphragmatic defect that contains liver ➡ and stomach ➦. Mesenteric fat and transverse colon are the most common hernia sac contents, followed by liver and stomach. (**Right**) Axial CT image of a patient with abdominal pain and Morgagni hernia shows free air ➦ and herniated bowel within the hernia sac. Gastric volvulus, gastric outlet obstruction, and bowel strangulation are rare complications of Morgagni hernias.*

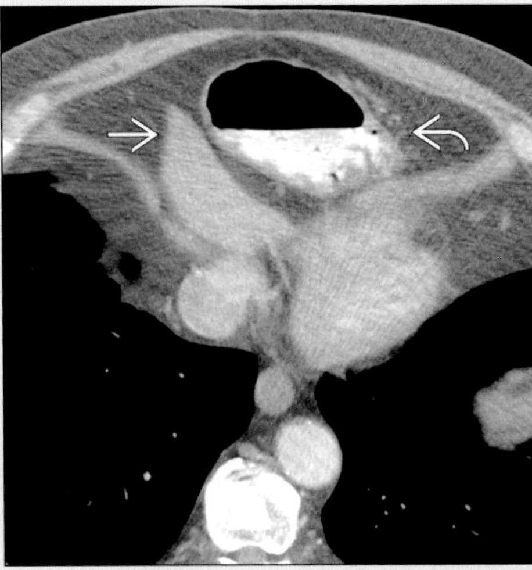

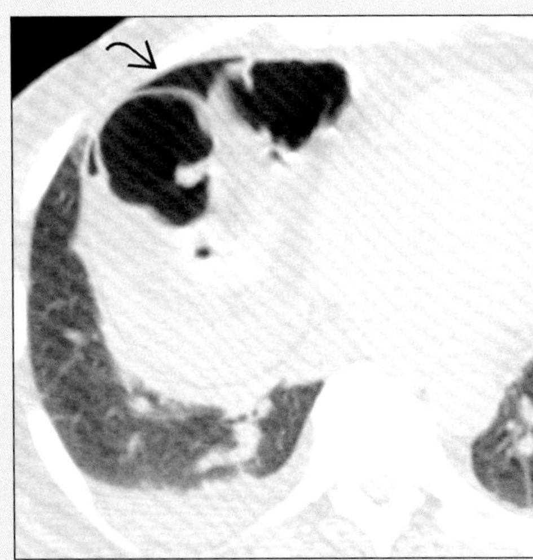

MORGAGNI HERNIA

TERMINOLOGY

Synonyms

- Anterior diaphragmatic hernia

Definitions

- Protrusion of abdominal cavity contents through retrosternal defect in diaphragm

IMAGING

General Features

- Best diagnostic clue
  - Retrosternal diaphragmatic defect with hernia sac containing omental fat ± bowel
- Location
  - Retrosternal diaphragm
  - **90% located on right side**
- Size
  - Variable; most cases are small
- Morphology
  - Disruption in anteromedial part of diaphragm

Radiographic Findings

- Radiography
  - Soft tissue, fat, or air density along heart border
    - Smooth margin; obscuration of heart border
    - Right cardiophrenic angle; anterior to heart

Fluoroscopic Findings

- Upper GI contrast studies may show or confirm bowel within hernia sac
- Hernias that only contain mesenteric fat or solid organs are not excluded

CT Findings

- Defect in retrosternal part of diaphragm
- Hernia sac with air, fat, &/or soft tissue
  - Most cases contain only omental fat
  - Other contents
    - Transverse colon > liver > small bowel > stomach
- Coronal & sagittal reformats may better delineate diaphragmatic defect
  - Visualization of abdominal vessels, fat, & organs leading into hernia
- With pericardial defect, hernia sac may protrude into pericardial cavity
  - Rarely, heart may protrude through defect down into abdominal cavity
- CECT helpful for assessment of complications (incarceration, strangulation)

MR Findings

- Allows direct multiplanar imaging
- Single-shot, fast spin-echo with respiratory triggering used to eliminate motion artifact
- Better resolution of diaphragm muscle & defect
- Signal characteristics depend on content of hernia sac
  - Hyperintense on T1WI & T2WI due to fat content

Imaging Recommendations

- Best imaging tool
  - CT with multiplanar reformats or MR

DIFFERENTIAL DIAGNOSIS

Mediastinal Fat Pad

- Intact diaphragm
- Homogeneous fat density; no bowel content

Cardiophrenic Mass

- Pericardial cyst, mediastinal lipoma/liposarcoma
- Intact diaphragm

PATHOLOGY

General Features

- Etiology
  - Congenital defect secondary to maldevelopment of septum transversum (precursor of diaphragm)
  - Can be traumatic (rarely)
- Associated abnormalities
  - Pericardial defect

Gross Pathologic & Surgical Features

- Covered by peritoneal sac
- Usually small, containing only omental fat

CLINICAL ISSUES

Presentation

- Most common signs/symptoms
  - Usually asymptomatic in adults; epigastric or retrosternal discomfort, bloating
- Other signs/symptoms
  - Incarceration, strangulation with infarction of herniated fat or bowel

Demographics

- Age
  - Most cases are diagnosed in adults
  - > 50% of congenital forms diagnosed after 5 years of age
- Epidemiology
  - Rare (2-4% of all diaphragmatic hernias)

Natural History & Prognosis

- Less herniated bowel than in congenital diaphragmatic hernia
- In congenital forms with herniated bowel, malrotation of bowel is common
- Potential for strangulation if containing bowel

Treatment

- Surgical repair if hernia contains bowel (risk of strangulation): Laparoscopic or open approach

DIAGNOSTIC CHECKLIST

Consider

- Morgagni hernia in patient with pericardiophrenic mass containing bowel on radiography or mesenteric vessels on CT/MR

SELECTED REFERENCES

1. Sandstrom CK et al: Diaphragmatic hernias: a spectrum of radiographic appearances. Curr Probl Diagn Radiol. 40(3):95-115, 2011

BOCHDALEK HERNIA

Key Facts

Terminology

- Protrusion of abdominal contents through normal remnant of pleuroperitoneal canal
  - Distinguished from Bochdalek-type congenital diaphragmatic hernia, a maldevelopment of posterior diaphragm

Imaging

- Radiography
  - Posterior basilar mass obscuring hemidiaphragm
- CT
  - Posterior diaphragmatic defect with herniated retroperitoneal fat, kidney, &/or spleen
  - Coronal & sagittal reformations helpful to optimally delineate defect
  - Helpful for assessment of complications (incarceration, strangulation)
- Best imaging tools: Multiplanar CT or MR

Top Differential Diagnoses

- Diaphragmatic eventration
- Paravertebral mass
- Congenital diaphragmatic hernia
- Diaphragmatic rupture

Pathology

- Herniation through normal remnant of pleuroperitoneal canal

Clinical Issues

- Usually of no clinical significance in adults
  - Associated with chronic obstructive lung disease

Diagnostic Checklist

- Consider Bochdalek hernia in patient with asymptomatic posterior basilar opacity obscuring hemidiaphragm on radiography

(Left) PA chest radiograph of an asymptomatic patient with a left Bochdalek hernia shows a vague opacity ➔ at the left inferior hemithorax. (Right) Lateral chest radiograph of the same patient shows a mass-like lesion ➔ at the posterior left costophrenic angle. The lesion obscures the posterior aspect of the left hemidiaphragm and exhibits a sharply marginated superior border.

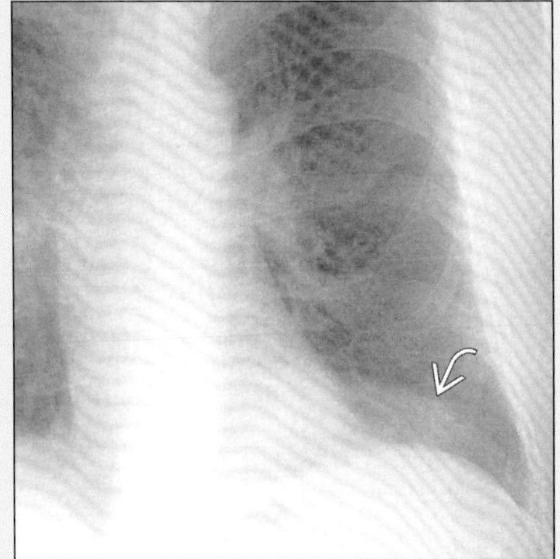

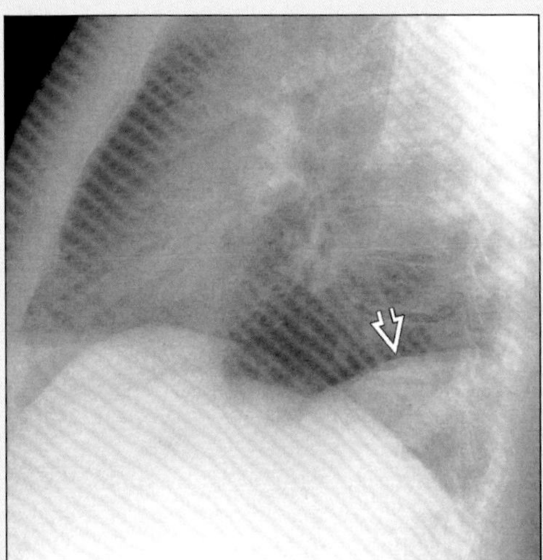

(Left) Axial NECT of the same patient shows a left Bochdalek hernia manifesting as a focal left posterior diaphragmatic defect ➔ through which retroperitoneal fat and vessels course. The superior pole of the left kidney ➔ has also herniated through this defect. The spleen may rarely herniate through a Bochdalek hernia. (Right) Coronal CECT of a patient with a right Bochdalek hernia shows a right-sided diaphragmatic defect with herniation of the liver and right kidney into the right hemithorax.

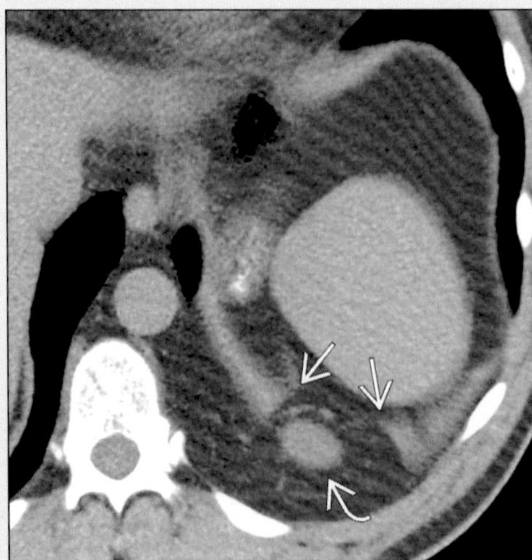

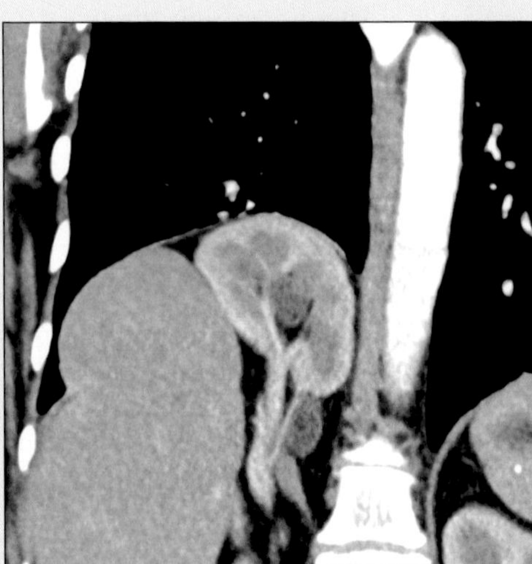

BOCHDALEK HERNIA

TERMINOLOGY

Synonyms

- Posterior diaphragmatic hernia

Definitions

- Protrusion of abdominal contents through normal remnant of pleuroperitoneal canal
  - Distinguished from Bochdalek-type congenital diaphragmatic hernia, a maldevelopment of posterior diaphragm

IMAGING

General Features

- Location
  - Posterolateral diaphragm
  - **Incidentally discovered, Bochdalek hernias in adults are more frequent on the right**
  - 14% are bilateral
- Size
  - Variable; usually small in adults
- Morphology
  - **Usually contains retroperitoneal fat**
  - May contain kidney, bowel, stomach, spleen, or liver

Radiographic Findings

- Posterior mass obscuring portion of hemidiaphragm
- Well-defined margins

CT Findings

- Posterior diaphragmatic defect
- Visualization of herniated retroperitoneal fat, kidney, &/or spleen
- Coronal & sagittal reformations optimally delineate defect
- CECT helpful for assessment of complications (incarceration, strangulation)

MR Findings

- MR allows direct multiplanar imaging
- Single-shot, fast spin-echo with respiratory triggering may eliminate motion artifact
- Better resolution of diaphragm muscle & defect

Imaging Recommendations

- Best imaging tool
  - **Multiplanar CT or MR** for optimal evaluation of diaphragmatic integrity & herniated contents

DIFFERENTIAL DIAGNOSIS

Diaphragmatic Eventration

- Thin but intact hemidiaphragm
- Most common on left

Paravertebral Mass

- Neurogenic neoplasm, vascular aneurysm, lymphadenopathy

Congenital Diaphragmatic Hernia

- Diaphragmatic malformation
- Bochdalek-type occurs at posterolateral diaphragm, more common on left
- Most common congenital diaphragmatic hernia
- Usually manifests in neonates & infants

Diaphragmatic Rupture

- Traumatic diaphragmatic laceration
- Affects right & left hemidiaphragms equally

PATHOLOGY

General Features

- Etiology
  - Herniation through normal remnant of pleuroperitoneal canal
    - Normal morphologic communication between thorax & abdomen during early fetal life
- Associated abnormalities
  - Chronic obstructive lung disease

Gross Pathologic & Surgical Features

- No hernia sac
  - Peritoneal membrane seen in only 10%

CLINICAL ISSUES

Presentation

- Most common signs/symptoms
  - Almost always asymptomatic in adults, usually diagnosed incidentally
  - Chest pain & bowel symptoms have been reported

Demographics

- Epidemiology
  - Prevalence of 6% in adults
    - More common & larger in elderly patients
    - Reported prevalence of up to 20% at age 70 years

Natural History & Prognosis

- Usually of no clinical significance in adults
  - More common in elderly patients & those with chronic lung disease

DIAGNOSTIC CHECKLIST

Consider

- Bochdalek hernia in patient with asymptomatic posterior basilar opacity obscuring hemidiaphragm on radiography

Image Interpretation Pearls

- Identification of diaphragmatic defect & herniated retroperitoneal fat are diagnostic
  - Retroperitoneal vessels may help identify fat as retroperitoneal

SELECTED REFERENCES

1. Sandstrom CK et al: Diaphragmatic hernias: a spectrum of radiographic appearances. Curr Probl Diagn Radiol. 40(3):95-115, 2011
2. Kinoshita F et al: Late-presenting posterior transdiaphragmatic (Bochdalek) hernia in adults: prevalence and MDCT characteristics. J Thorac Imaging. 24(1):17-22, 2009

CONGENITAL DIAPHRAGMATIC HERNIA

Key Facts

Terminology
- Congenital diaphragmatic hernia (CDH)
- Intrathoracic herniation of abdominal contents via diaphragmatic defect

Imaging
- Radiography
  - Variable appearance based on hernia contents & whether herniated bowel contains air
  - Opaque hemithorax
  - Unilateral, intrathoracic, air-filled bowel
  - Mass effect on lung & mediastinum
  - Abnormal position of support apparatus
  - Decreased/absent abdominal bowel gas
- Prenatal ultrasound
  - Intrathoracic mass of mixed echogenicity
  - Displacement of cardiac structures
  - Stomach bubble at level of heart

Top Differential Diagnoses
- Congenital pulmonary airway malformation
- Congenital lobar overinflation

Pathology
- Mass effect on lung by herniated abdominal contents may lead to pulmonary hypoplasia
- Congenital heart disease is most common associated abnormality

Clinical Issues
- Symptoms/signs
  - Severe neonatal respiratory distress
  - Patients with small CDH may present later in life
- Prognosis related to degree of lung hypoplasia

Diagnostic Checklist
- Consider CDH in neonate with respiratory distress & opaque hemithorax or intrathoracic bowel loops

*(**Left**) Graphic shows posterior left hemidiaphragm defect and herniation of stomach & small bowel into left hemithorax, producing rightward mediastinal shift and mass effect on the ipsilateral and contralateral lungs. (**Right**) AP chest radiograph of a neonate with respiratory distress and CDH shows air-filled bowel loops in the left hemithorax with mass effect on the lung and mediastinum. Note mass effect on the umbilical artery catheter ⇨ and the umbilical vein catheter tip in the left portal vein ➡.*

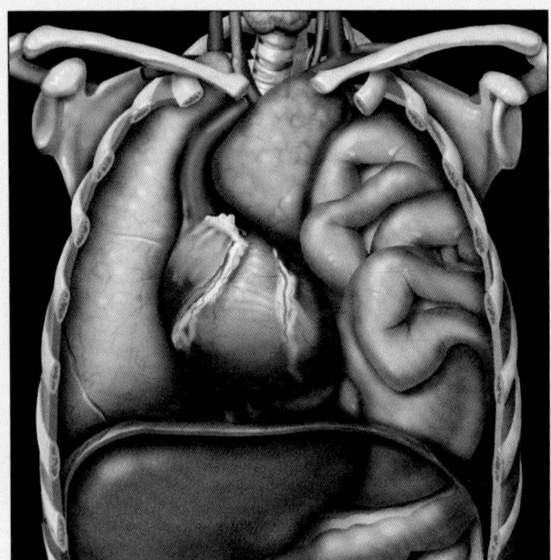

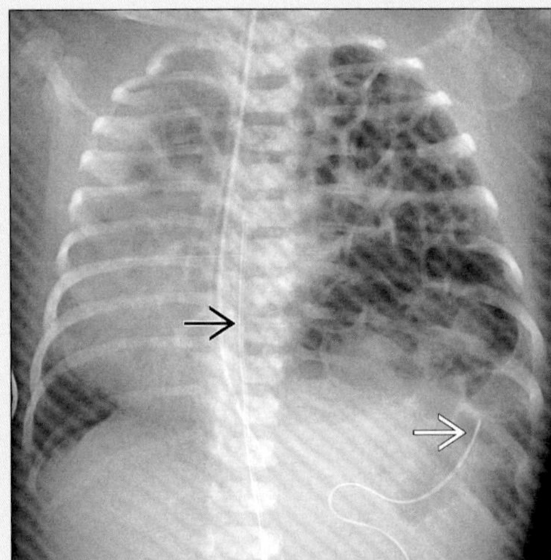

*(**Left**) AP chest radiograph of an infant with respiratory distress and CDH shows opacification of the left hemithorax due to herniation of multiple nonaerated bowel loops with contralateral shift of the mediastinum and the esophageal enteric tube ⇨. (**Right**) AP chest radiograph of a neonate with a large CDH shows coiling of the enteric tube ⇨ in the herniated intrathoracic stomach. The umbilical artery catheter ➡ is markedly displaced to the right due to mass effect from the CDH.*

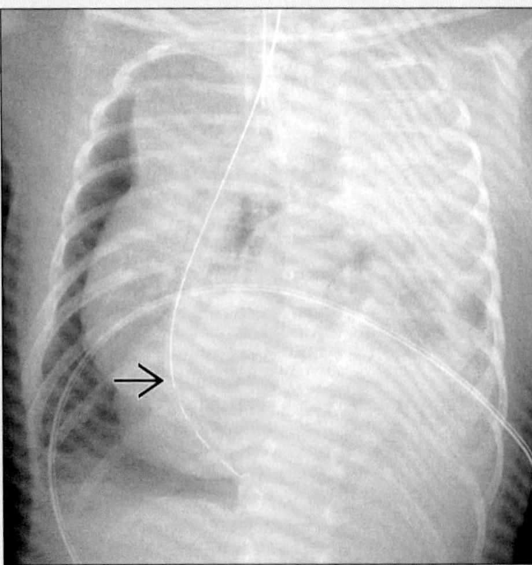

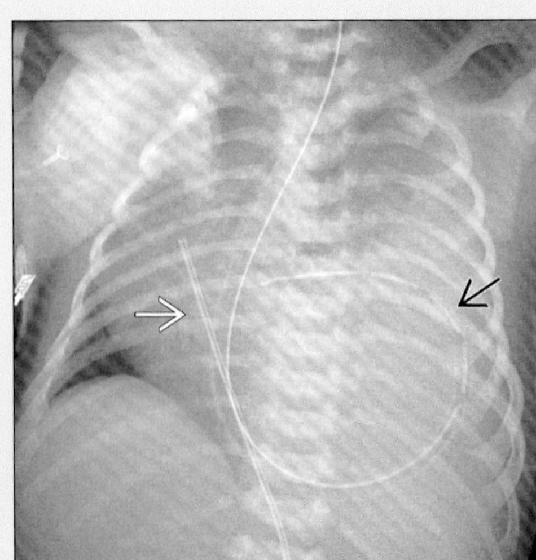

CONGENITAL DIAPHRAGMATIC HERNIA

TERMINOLOGY

Abbreviations

- **Congenital diaphragmatic hernia (CDH)**

Definitions

- Intrathoracic herniation of abdominal contents via diaphragmatic defect
  - **Bochdalek type**: Posterolateral hernia (most common type of CDH)
  - **Morgagni type**: Anterior (retrosternal); much less common in neonates

IMAGING

General Features

- Best diagnostic clue
  - Intrathoracic air-filled bowel loops
- Location
  - Left > right
    - Left-to-right ratio = 5:1
  - Bochdalek type: Posterolateral, 80% left sided

Radiographic Findings

- Variable appearance based on hernia contents & whether herniated bowel contains air
  - **Opaque hemithorax**
    - Early finding prior to air entering stomach & bowel
  - **Intrathoracic, air-filled bowel loops**
  - **Right-sided hernia may contain liver rather than bowel**
- **Mass effect**
  - Mediastinal shift away from hernia
- **Low volumes of ipsilateral &/or contralateral lung (pulmonary hypoplasia)**
- **Decreased/absent bowel gas in abdomen**
- **Abnormal position of support apparatus**
  - Enteric tube with tip at GE junction or coiled above diaphragm in herniated stomach
  - Deviation of umbilical venous catheter toward side of hernia

Ultrasonographic Findings

- Grayscale ultrasound
  - Prenatal ultrasound
    - Intrathoracic mass of mixed echogenicity
    - Displacement of cardiac structures
    - Stomach bubble at level of heart

MR Findings

- Fetal MR
  - **Assessment of liver herniation & other anomalies**

Imaging Recommendations

- Best imaging tool
  - Prenatal ultrasound, postnatal chest radiography

DIFFERENTIAL DIAGNOSIS

Congenital Pulmonary Airway Malformation

- Multicystic, air-containing lung lesion
- CPAM more likely to exhibit air-fluid levels than CDH

Congenital Lobar Overinflation

- Hyperlucent lobe rather than air-filled bowel
- Often involves upper lobe

PATHOLOGY

General Features

- Etiology
  - Not completely understood
    - Postulated failure of pleuroperitoneal fold closure during 4th-10th week of gestation
  - Mass effect on lung by herniated abdominal contents prevents normal development
    - Pulmonary hypoplasia
- Associated abnormalities
  - Associated congenital anomalies in 25-50% of cases of CDH
  - Congenital heart disease is most common associated abnormality
    - VSD, ASD, PFO, tetralogy of Fallot, hypoplastic left heart
  - Gastrointestinal, genitourinary, central nervous system, & musculoskeletal anomalies

CLINICAL ISSUES

Presentation

- Most common signs/symptoms
  - **Severe neonatal respiratory distress**
  - Patients with small CDH may present later in life or may be diagnosed incidentally

Demographics

- Epidemiology
  - Incidence: 1 in 2,500-5,000 live births

Natural History & Prognosis

- Widely variable survival rates, some as high as 88%
  - Do not account for frequent in utero demise
- Prognosis related to degree of lung hypoplasia & associated anomalies
- Prenatal US/MR indicators of poor prognosis
  - Bilateral CDH
  - Herniation of liver & stomach
  - Polyhydramnios & fetal hydrops
  - Pulmonary hypoplasia

Treatment

- "Gentle ventilation" for pulmonary hypoplasia & respiratory failure
- Severe respiratory failure may require extracorporeal membrane oxygenation (ECMO)
- Surgical repair of diaphragmatic defect

DIAGNOSTIC CHECKLIST

Consider

- CDH in neonate with respiratory distress & opaque hemithorax or intrathoracic bowel loops

SELECTED REFERENCES

1. Kline-Fath BM: Congenital diaphramatic hernia. Pediatr Radiol. Epub ahead of print, 2011

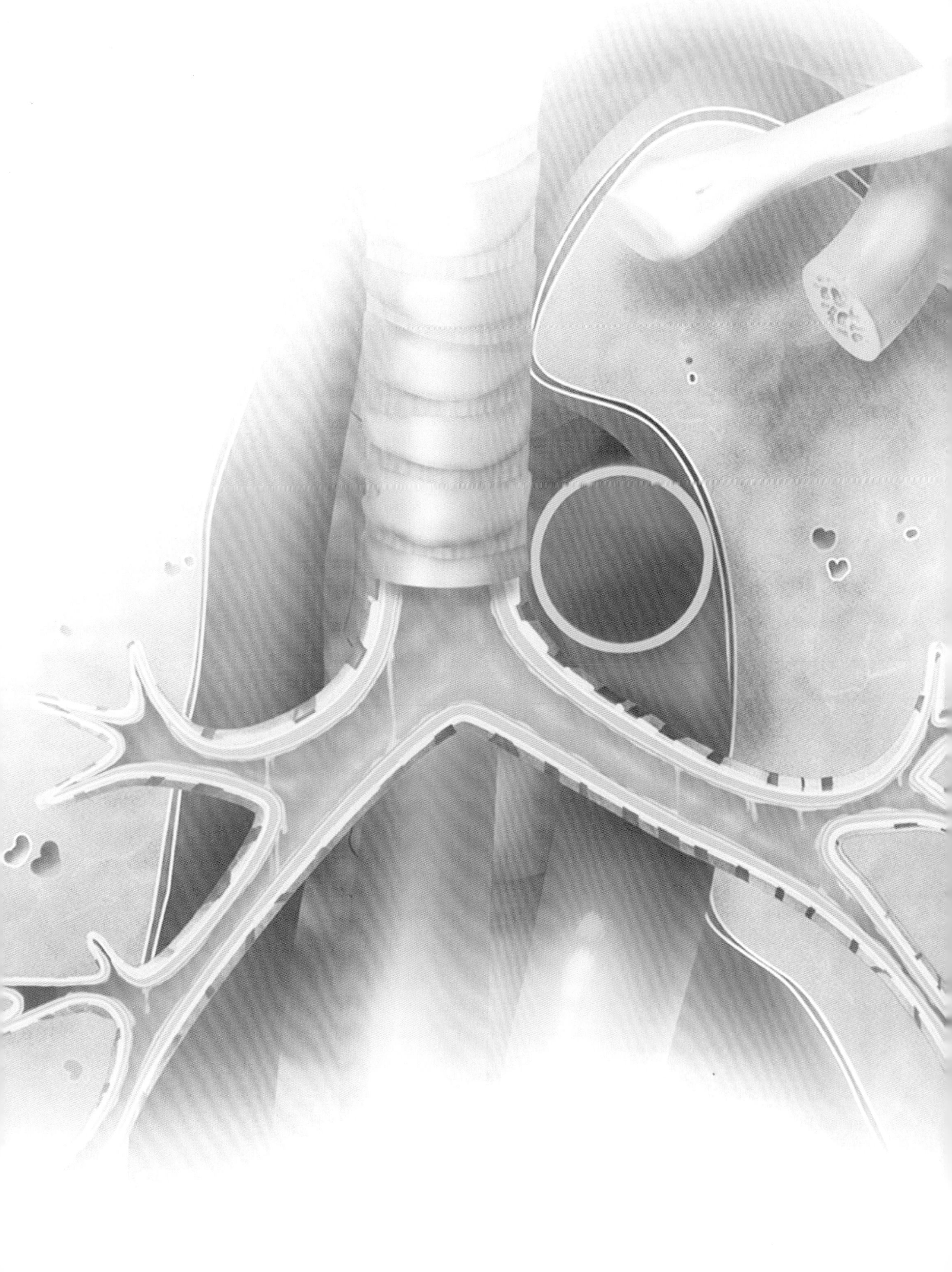

SECTION 3
Airway Diseases

Introduction and Overview

Benign Neoplasms

Malignant Neoplasms

Airway Narrowing and Wall Thickening

Bronchial Dilatation and Impaction

Emphysema and Small Airway Diseases

Introduction

In recent years there have been major advances in the imaging evaluation of airways diseases. The advent of multidetector computed tomography (CT) and increased experience with image post-processing techniques have enabled advanced methods of airways imaging, including virtual bronchoscopic techniques and dynamic CT imaging. Volume and surface rendered displays provide three-dimensional views of the external airway walls and the airway lumina. Imaging of the trachea and central bronchi performed during forced expiration allows assessment of tracheobronchomalacia. In addition, inspiratory and expiratory high-resolution computed tomography (HRCT) of the chest offers a noninvasive method for assessing the small airways.

Anatomic Considerations

The airways are tubular structures that conduct air through their lumina and represent twenty-four generations of dichotomous branching. They can be divided into large airways (trachea, bronchi) and small airways (bronchioles, terminal bronchioles, respiratory bronchioles, and alveolar ducts). The airways are important components in the functional organization of the lung into three zones with overlapping characteristics: 1) conductive zone (air conduction only) consisting of the trachea, bronchi, and membranous bronchioles, 2) transitional zone (conductive and respiratory) comprised of respiratory bronchioles and alveolar ducts, and 3) respiratory zone (respiratory only) consisting of the alveoli and alveolar sacs.

A variety of diseases may involve the airways, including congenital, neoplastic, infectious, and inflammatory processes. For practical purposes, airway diseases can be categorized based on whether they involve the large or the small airways. Large airway diseases include congenital abnormalities, airway neoplasms, and morphologic alterations that may produce airway narrowing, dilatation, and/or airway wall thickening. Small airway diseases include chronic progressive disorders, cellular infiltrations, and fibrotic processes. Emphysema is characterized by destruction of structures within the secondary pulmonary lobule. Cellular and constrictive bronchiolitis are small airway diseases characterized by peribronchiolar cellular infiltration and concentric fibrosis, respectively.

Airway Neoplasms

Lung cancer is generally regarded as a neoplasm of the lung. However, both squamous cell carcinoma and small cell carcinoma are central neoplasms and often manifest with an irregular endoluminal airway lesion or extrinsic encasement of the central airways, respectively. Other malignant airway neoplasms are uncommon or rare and include **bronchial carcinoid**, **adenoid cystic carcinoma**, and **mucoepidermoid carcinoma**. **Metastatic disease** may also involve the airway and may be the first manifestation of occult malignancy, particularly in cases of metastatic renal cell carcinoma, in which airway metastases may antedate the diagnosis of the primary malignancy. Such neoplasms characteristically manifest as sharply marginated or irregular polylobular endoluminal lesions within the airways. As a result, these tumors may come to clinical attention because of postobstructive effects such as atelectasis or pneumonia. Endoluminal airway neoplasms may transgress the airway wall to invade adjacent structures, including the lung and mediastinum. Alternatively, these neoplasms may circumferentially encase the airway, producing focal or diffuse airway stenosis. Generally speaking, patients with central neoplasms that produce airway obstruction are likely to present with symptoms, including cough, wheezing, and hemoptysis. However, it is also recognized that central tracheal tumors may compromise up to 75% of the tracheal lumen before producing symptoms.

Although airway neoplasms may be suspected because of radiographic abnormalities, CT is the imaging modality of choice for their initial assessment and staging. Such tumors are typically accessible to bronchoscopic visualization and biopsy. Thus, a description of the size and location of the lesion with specific mention of the airway branches involved and any variations in airway anatomy is very helpful to the pulmonologist performing bronchoscopic evaluation of such lesions. Cross-sectional imaging allows evaluation of surrounding structures and may demonstrate local invasion and/or lymphadenopathy. Multiplanar reformatted images and volume-rendered techniques may provide valuable information for surgical planning, including the length of airway involvement.

Morphologic Alterations of the Airway Lumen

Airway Narrowing

Saber-sheath trachea is a morphologic abnormality associated with chronic obstructive pulmonary disease (COPD) and characterized by a decrease in the coronal tracheal diameter and an increase in the sagittal tracheal diameter. The morphologic features of saber-sheath trachea may be accentuated with imaging during forced expiration where the lateral tracheal walls may show more pronounced medial displacement. Although the intrathoracic trachea may appear severely narrowed on frontal radiography, this abnormality rarely requires stenting or surgical intervention.

Tracheal stenosis is usually an acquired lesion that occurs as a complication of endobronchial intubation. Stenosis may be focal or diffuse, and symptomatic patients may require dilatation, stent placement, or surgical correction. Congenital tracheal stenosis related to complete cartilaginous tracheal rings is rare, may be associated with other congenital anomalies, and is typically seen in neonates and infants.

Tracheal narrowing may be strictly functional, as in cases of **tracheomalacia** or **tracheobronchomalacia** where weakness of tracheal and bronchial cartilages results in expiratory airway collapse. Prior to the era of multidetector CT, radiologists contributed little to the diagnosis of this condition. Tracheobronchomalacia is typically recognized by pulmonologists who may observe expiratory airway collapse during bronchoscopy. Today, radiologists can also participate in the assessment of abnormal tracheal collapsibility with the use of dynamic CT of the central airways and expiratory imaging. However, it should be noted that broad ranges of expiratory large airway collapse have been observed in normal subjects.

Tracheal narrowing may also result from inflammatory diseases, including **Wegener granulomatosis**, **amyloidosis**, and **relapsing polychondritis**. These diseases may produce focal or diffuse tracheal wall thickening and may also involve the central bronchi. Thus, radiologists must thoroughly assess the large airways in patients with these diseases in order to exclude significant stenoses that may require treatment.

While findings of airway narrowing are characteristically described in the trachea, the bronchi may also be affected. A well-recognized form of bronchial stenosis is **middle lobe syndrome** in which chronic middle lobe atelectasis results from a variety of etiologies, including neoplasms, nonneoplastic endoluminal lesions (e.g., broncholiths), and chronic infectious and noninfectious inflammatory conditions.

Patients with symptomatic airway stenosis may be treated with airway dilatation, airway stents, or surgical excision of the stenotic segment, each with varying results. Radiologists should familiarize themselves with the different treatment methods, particularly the appearance of appropriately positioned airway stents and potential complications related to their use.

Airway Dilatation

Bronchiectasis refers to irreversible bronchial dilatation. It may be categorized and graded as cylindrical, varicose, or cystic (in increasing order of severity). Bronchiectasis may be identified on radiography, but is best visualized and assessed on chest CT. Normal bronchial diameter generally equals the diameter of its adjacent paired pulmonary artery branch. Bronchial diameters larger than those of adjacent pulmonary arteries are consistent with bronchiectasis. Airway dilatation may result from infectious or inflammatory processes and may be seen in association with the retractile effects of fibrosis (i.e., traction bronchiectasis). Congenital abnormalities (e.g., cystic fibrosis, primary ciliary dyskinesia, immunodeficiency, etc.) may result in severe symptomatic, diffuse bronchiectasis. The radiologist should provide a comprehensive differential diagnosis in such cases in order to guide the clinical assessment, definitive diagnosis, and appropriate treatment of affected patients.

Small Airways Disease

Emphysema

In spite of the decline in tobacco use in the United States of America, COPD remains the fourth leading cause of chronic morbidity and mortality. In fact, emphysema is so prevalent that most radiologists are routinely exposed to the imaging findings of this disease since it is frequently found incidentally on chest CT obtained for a wide variety of other clinical indications. Advances in multidetector CT technology make it possible to rapidly obtain diagnostic images of the lung in less than ten seconds, even in patients with severe dyspnea. CT allows the identification and characterization of emphysema as centrilobular, paraseptal, or panlobular types. In addition, noninvasive quantification of emphysema can be performed using visual quantification of disease severity as well as computer assisted quantification. Regardless of the method used, identification of emphysema usually confirms a history of cigarette smoking. Also, given the increased risk of lung cancer in this patient population, any focal lung abnormalities should be viewed with suspicion.

Cellular Bronchiolitis

Cellular bronchiolitis manifests on CT as centrilobular opacities situated in the bronchovascular core of the secondary pulmonary lobule 5-10 mm from the pleural surfaces and interlobular septa. Cellular bronchiolitis may be focal, multifocal, or diffuse. Although bronchiolitis may be identified on chest radiography, it is typically detected on conventional and thin-section chest CT. It manifests with centrilobular nodules of soft tissue or ground-glass attenuation that may be associated with tree-in-bud opacities, which are branching opacities that resemble the morphology of a budding tree. The linear component of these opacities corresponds to the dilated centrilobular bronchiole impacted with mucus, fluid, or pus, while the nodular component corresponds to peribronchiolar inflammation.

Cellular bronchiolitis is frequently secondary to pulmonary **infection** by bacteria, mycobacteria, fungi, or viruses. Although the presence of associated tree-in-bud opacities is highly suggestive of infection, it can also be seen in cases of aspiration bronchiolitis. Other common etiologies of cellular bronchiolitis include **respiratory bronchiolitis (RB)**, **respiratory bronchiolitis-associated interstitial lung disease (RB-ILD)**, and **hypersensitivity pneumonitis**. RB and RB-ILD are smoking-related diseases characterized by upper lobe predominant, poorly defined centrilobular nodules that are often seen in association with centrilobular emphysema. Hypersensitivity pneumonitis is an allergic lung disease characterized by alveolitis and inflammatory granulomatous bronchiolitis in response to a variety of inhaled substances. Other causes of cellular bronchiolitis include **follicular bronchiolitis** and **diffuse panbronchiolitis**. Correlation with clinical presentation and history is helpful in determining the etiology of cellular bronchiolitis.

Constrictive Bronchiolitis

Constrictive bronchiolitis is characterized by mosaic lung attenuation, manifesting with geographic areas of alternating decreased and increased lung attenuation. These characteristically appear accentuated on expiratory HRCT (air-trapping) and may be associated with bronchial dilatation and bronchial wall thickening. Among other etiologies, constrictive bronchiolitis may be a manifestation of infectious, connective tissue, or inhalational lung diseases, or as a complication of transplantation.

Summary

Airways disease has protean imaging manifestations. Imaging diagnosis requires a systematic assessment of the large and small airways and careful characterization of the specific airway abnormalities seen on imaging. CT and HRCT are valuable tools in the imaging assessment of affected patients.

Selected References

1. Kang EY: Large airway diseases. J Thorac Imaging. 26(4):249-62, 2011
2. Abbott GF et al: Imaging of small airways disease. J Thorac Imaging. 24(4):285-98, 2009

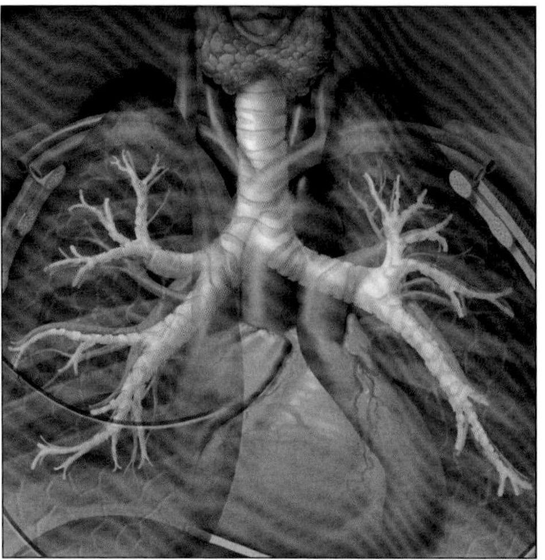

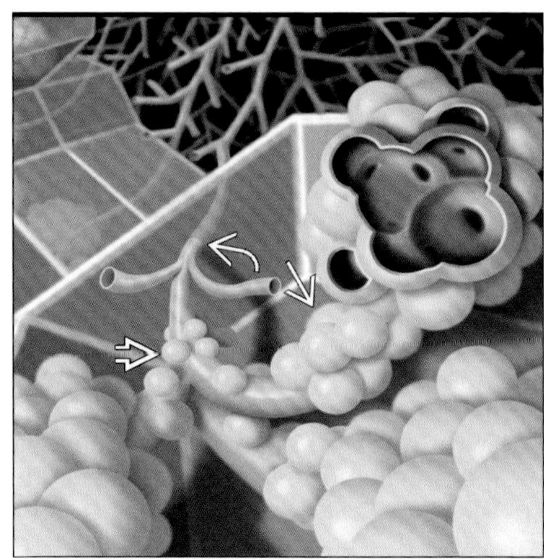

(Left) Graphic shows the anatomy of the large airways. The trachea bifurcates into right and left mainstem bronchi, which in turn branch into lobar, segmental, and subsegmental bronchi that continue to branch and taper as they course toward the lung periphery. The trachea, bronchi, and bronchioles are conducting airways. ***(Right)*** Graphic shows the small airways of the secondary pulmonary lobule: Terminal ➚ and respiratory ➩ bronchioles and alveolar ducts ➔ leading to alveolar sacs and alveoli.

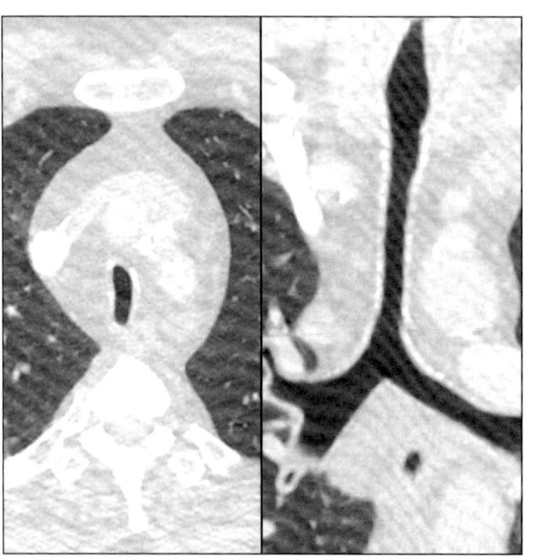

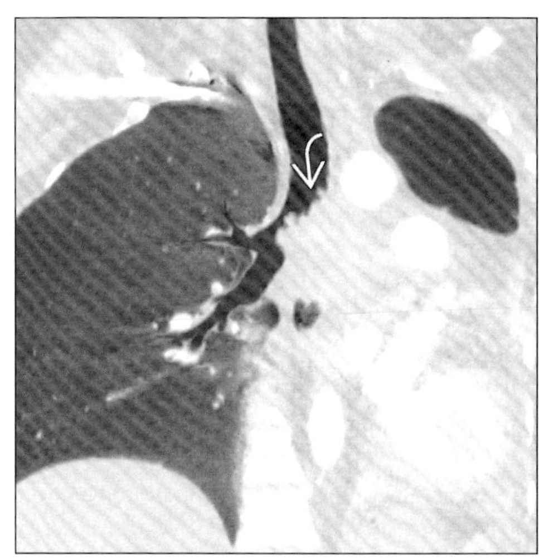

(Left) Composite image with axial (left) and coronal (right) NECT of a patient with COPD shows coronal narrowing of the lumen of the intrathoracic trachea with normal caliber of the extrathoracic trachea and the central bronchi characteristic of saber-sheath trachea. Saber-sheath trachea is a common cause of tracheal narrowing. ***(Right)*** Coronal CECT MinIP image of a patient with adenoid cystic carcinoma shows a polylobular mass ➚ in the tracheal lumen with resultant severe left lung atelectasis.

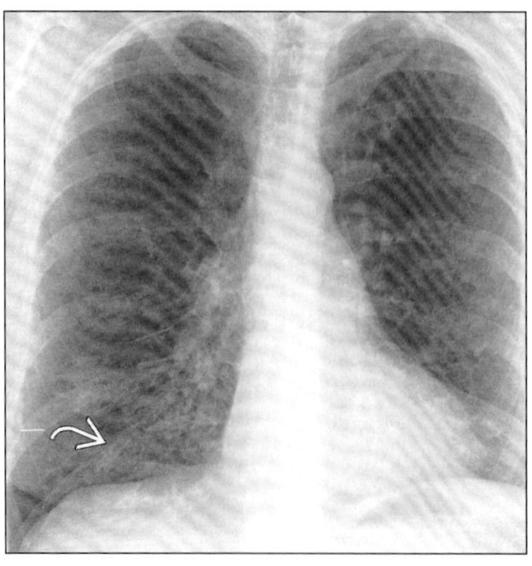

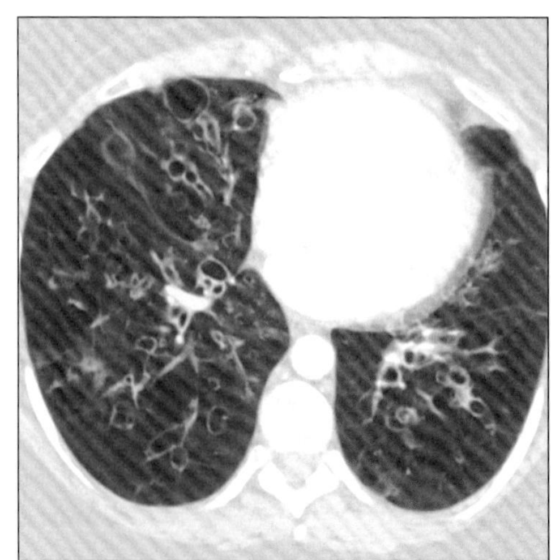

(Left) PA chest radiograph of a young woman with recurrent respiratory infections since childhood shows characteristic radiographic features of bronchiectasis manifesting with tram-track opacities ➚ representing the thickened walls of dilated bronchi. ***(Right)*** Axial NECT of the same patient shows severe bilateral bronchiectasis with bronchial wall thickening, mucus plugs, and mosaic attenuation of the lung parenchyma. The patient was evaluated and diagnosed with IgA deficiency.

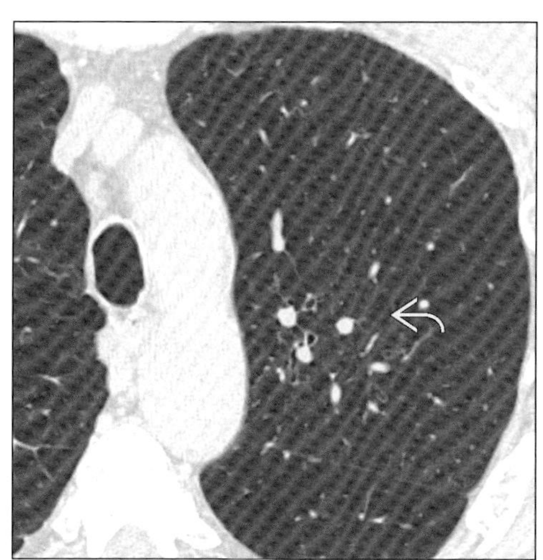

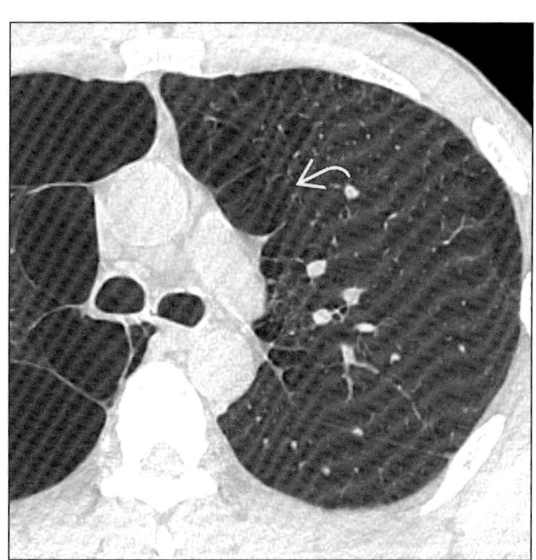

*(**Left**) Axial NECT shows centrilobular emphysema manifesting with multifocal centrilobular foci of low attenuation with imperceptible walls with characteristic central "dot-like" structures ➔ representing lobular arteries. Centrilobular emphysema is a common incidental finding on chest CT. (**Right**) Axial NECT shows paraseptal emphysema manifesting as small subpleural "cystic" spaces ➔ of varying sizes separated by intact interlobular septa.*

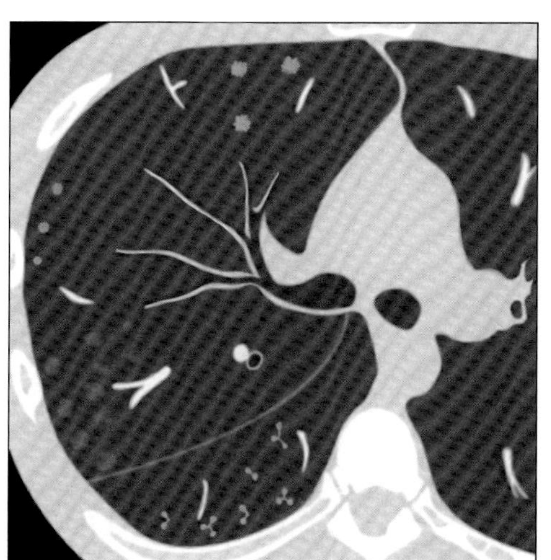

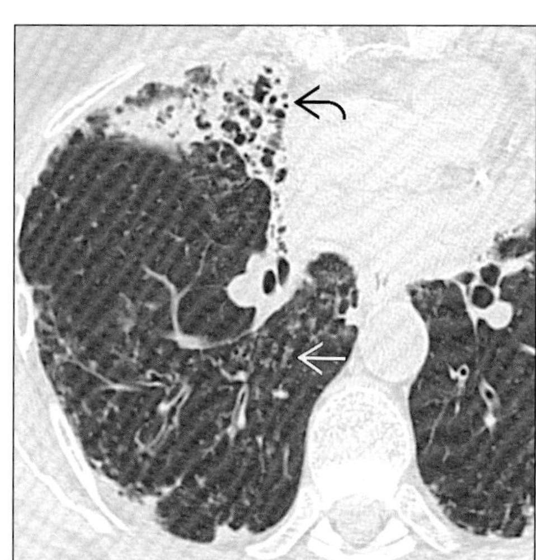

*(**Left**) Graphic shows the CT manifestations of cellular bronchiolitis characterized by centrilobular soft tissue and ground-glass nodular opacities as well as branching and tree-in-bud opacities that occur 5-10 mm from the adjacent pleura. (**Right**) Axial NECT of a patient with nontuberculous mycobacterial infection shows multifocal centrilobular nodules and tree-in-bud opacities ➔ associated with bronchial wall thickening and characteristic middle lobe volume loss and bronchiectasis ➔.*

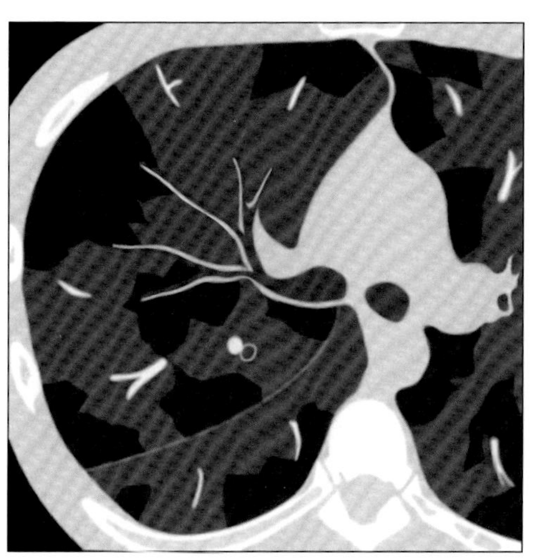

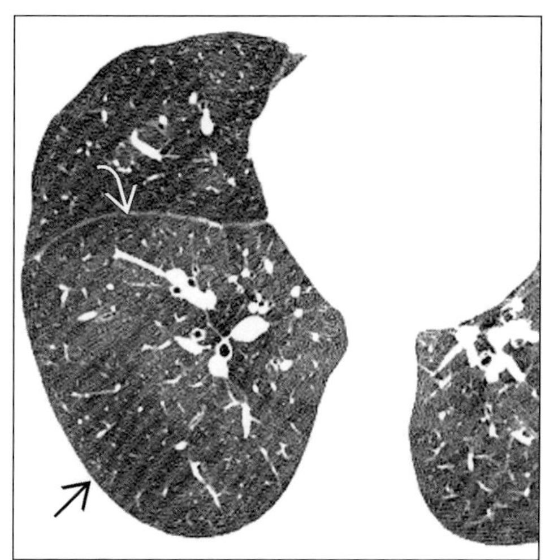

*(**Left**) Graphic shows the typical features of mosaic attenuation characterized by abnormal geographic areas of sharply defined low attenuation adjacent to areas of higher attenuation. (**Right**) Axial NECT of a patient with constrictive bronchiolitis secondary to graft-vs.-host disease shows mosaic lung attenuation with areas of abnormal hyperlucent lung ➔ adjacent to areas of normal higher attenuation parenchyma ➔.*

TRACHEOBRONCHIAL HAMARTOMA

Key Facts

Terminology

- Benign neoplasm comprised of mesenchymal tissues of varying proportions

Imaging

- Radiography
  - May be normal
  - Endoluminal nodule in central airway
  - Postobstructive findings: Atelectasis, consolidation, bronchiectasis
- CT
  - Focal endoluminal lesion in central airway
  - Internal fat &/or calcification suggest diagnosis
  - Fat in endoluminal nodule only seen in airway hamartoma or lipoma
  - Postobstructive findings: Atelectasis, consolidation, bronchiectasis

Top Differential Diagnoses

- Squamous cell carcinoma
- Metastasis
- Lipoma
- Chondroma

Pathology

- Multiple tissue elements: Cartilage, fat, bone
- 1.4-20% of all pulmonary hamartomas

Clinical Issues

- Asthma-like symptoms
- Treatment: Bronchoscopic resection if small; surgical resection may be required in larger lesions

Diagnostic Checklist

- Consider airway hamartoma in patient with endoluminal nodule with fat &/or calcification

*(**Left**) Axial CECT of a patient with an endobronchial hamartoma shows an endoluminal tumor in the distal left mainstem bronchus ⇨ that exhibits central calcification. (**Right**) Axial NECT shows a lobular soft tissue nodule ➡ with intrinsic calcification and fat, consistent with a hamartoma. The nodule originated from a subsegmental right upper lobe bronchus. Visualization of fat within the lesion is virtually diagnostic. Lipoma also exhibits fat attenuation, but is typically completely endoluminal.*

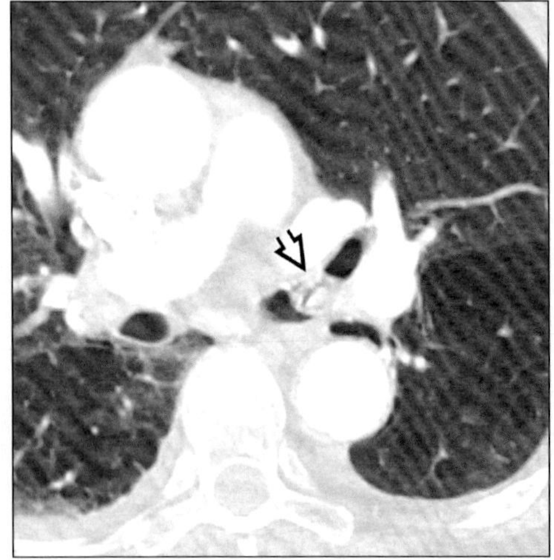

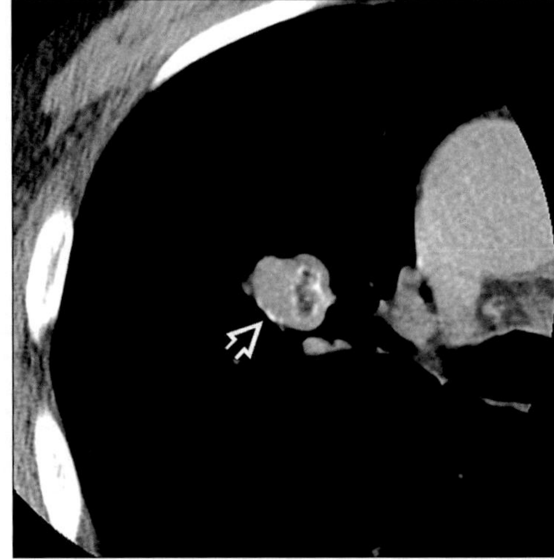

*(**Left**) Axial NECT shows a bronchial hamartoma ⇨ obstructing the right mainstem bronchus with postobstructive bronchiectasis and mucoid impaction ➡. Other scattered pulmonary nodules ➡ are consistent with pulmonary hamartomas in this patient with Cowden syndrome. (**Right**) Axial CECT shows an endobronchial nodule in a left lower lobe bronchus ➡ proven to represent a small bronchial hamartoma at surgery. Unfortunately, the imaging appearance of many hamartomas is nonspecific.*

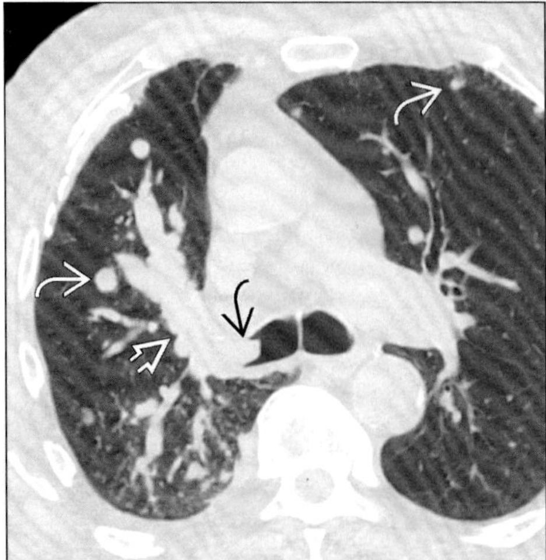

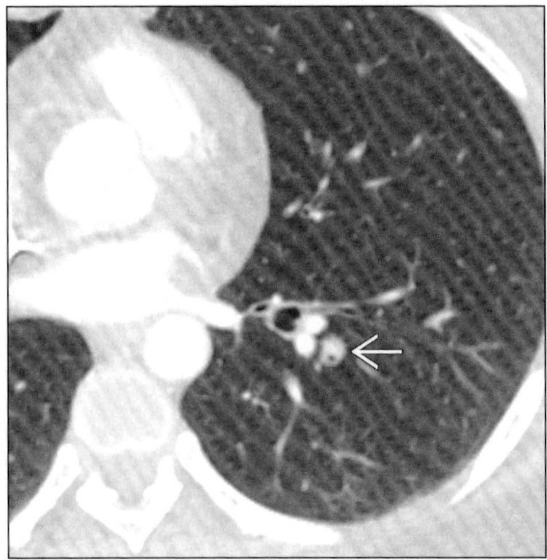

TRACHEOBRONCHIAL HAMARTOMA

TERMINOLOGY

Synonyms

- Endobronchial hamartoma
- Mesenchymoma
- Chondroid mesenchymoma

Definitions

- Benign neoplasm comprised of mesenchymal tissues of varying proportions

IMAGING

General Features

- Best diagnostic clue
  - Indolent or slowly growing endobronchial lesion with internal fat &/or calcification
- Location
  - Central bronchus, trachea
- Size
  - Usually < 2 cm; larger lesions may completely obstruct airway
- Morphology
  - Smooth or lobular, sharply marginated

Radiographic Findings

- Radiography
  - May be normal
  - Endoluminal nodule in central airway
  - Postobstructive effects
    - Atelectasis, often lobar
    - Consolidation
    - Distal bronchiectasis in longstanding obstruction

CT Findings

- NECT
  - Focal endoluminal lesion in central airway
  - Internal fat &/or calcification suggest diagnosis
    - Fat in endoluminal nodule only seen in airway hamartoma or lipoma
  - Postobstructive effects
    - Atelectasis, often lobar
    - Consolidation, bronchiolitis, ground-glass opacity
    - Distal bronchiectasis in longstanding obstruction
    - Chronic obstruction may result in distal lung destruction

MR Findings

- Identification of intralesional fat
  - T1 & T2 hyperintense

Imaging Recommendations

- Best imaging tool
  - CT is imaging study of choice for assessment of endoluminal lesions

DIFFERENTIAL DIAGNOSIS

Squamous Cell Carcinoma

- Middle-aged/elderly man with smoking history
- Endoluminal lesion with extraluminal extension & circumferential involvement
- 10% multifocal
- Lymphadenopathy

Metastasis

- Endoluminal lesion of variable size
- Hematogenous spread: Breast, colon, & renal cancer, melanoma
- Direct invasion from lung cancer

Lipoma

- Fatty endoluminal tumor

Chondroma

- Endoluminal lesion with calcification
- Calcification may also occur in malignant lesions

PATHOLOGY

General Features

- Etiology
  - Benign neoplasm

Gross Pathologic & Surgical Features

- Inflamed tumor surface mimics squamous cell carcinoma

Microscopic Features

- Multiple tissue elements
  - Cartilage (most profuse), fat, bone
- Bronchoscopic biopsy often misleading
  - Squamous metaplasia of tumor surface

CLINICAL ISSUES

Presentation

- Most common signs/symptoms
  - **Asthma-like symptoms**
  - Cough, dyspnea, stridor, pneumonia

Demographics

- Age
  - 40-60 years of age
- Epidemiology
  - Rare benign airway neoplasm
  - 1.4-20% of all pulmonary hamartomas

Natural History & Prognosis

- Morbidity related to chronic postobstructive effects

Treatment

- Bronchoscopic resection if small
- Surgical resection may be required for large lesions
  - Lobectomy in end-stage postobstructive lung disease

DIAGNOSTIC CHECKLIST

Consider

- Airway hamartoma in patient with endoluminal nodule with intrinsic fat &/or calcification

SELECTED REFERENCES

1. Tsitouridis I et al: Endobronchial lipomatous hamartoma with mediastinal extension. J Thorac Imaging. 25(1):W6-9, 2010
2. Cosío BG et al: Endobronchial hamartoma. Chest. 122(1):202-5, 2002

TRACHEOBRONCHIAL PAPILLOMATOSIS

Key Facts

Terminology
- Airway nodules due to human papilloma virus (HPV) infection
- Invasive papillomatosis: Spread to lungs

Imaging
- Thickening or nodularity of airway walls
- Multiple pulmonary nodules/masses
  - Larger nodules more likely to cavitate
  - Seeding of posterior lungs
- Growth rate
  - Most nodules grow slowly
  - Rapid growth suspicious for squamous cell carcinoma
- Complications
  - Squamous cell carcinoma, secondary infection, & airway obstruction with atelectasis &/or postobstructive pneumonia

Top Differential Diagnoses
- Tracheobronchopathia osteochondroplastica
- Wegener granulomatosis
- Tracheobronchial amyloidosis
- Relapsing polychondritis

Pathology
- Infection with HPV; types 6 & 11 most common
- Larynx most commonly affected
- Diagnosis made by laryngoscopy & biopsy

Clinical Issues
- Asymptomatic in mild cases
- May be mistaken for asthma when symptomatic
- Treatment
  - Self-limited disease usually requires no treatment
  - Surgical & medical therapies for lesions causing airway obstruction

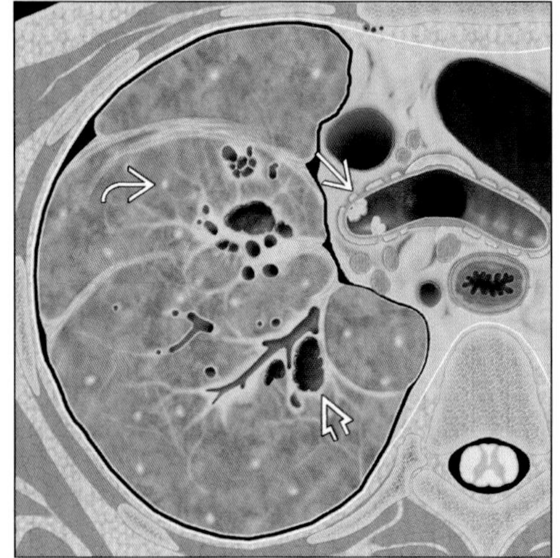

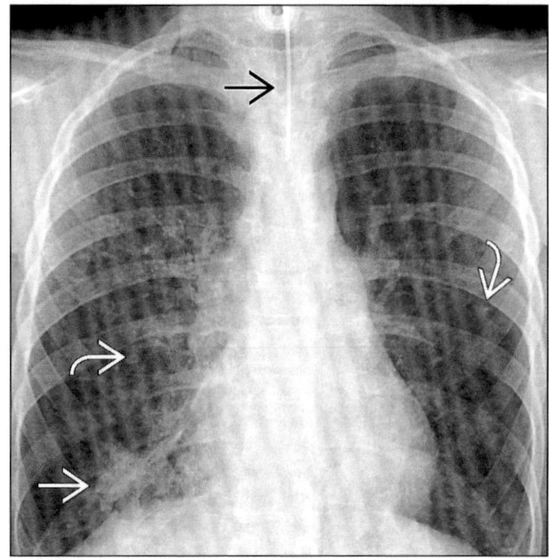

***(Left)** Axial graphic shows the morphologic features of tracheobronchial papillomatosis that produce the characteristic imaging findings of central airway nodules ➔, peribronchovascular nodules, cavitary lesions ➔, and scattered parenchymal nodules ➔. **(Right)** AP chest radiograph of a patient with papillomatosis shows endotracheal intubation ➔, multiple small bilateral lung nodules ➔ (some with cavitation), and larger nodular lesions (such as those within the right lower lung zone ➔).*

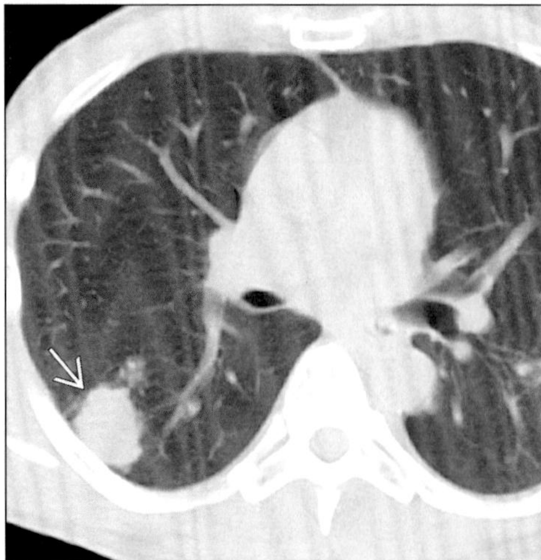

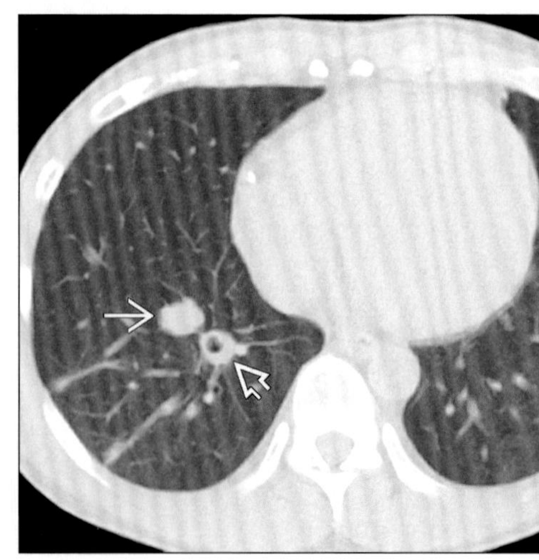

***(Left)** Axial NECT of the same patient shows a squamous cell carcinoma in the superior segment of the right lower lobe ➔. The incidence of squamous cell carcinoma in patients with tracheobronchial papillomatosis is approximately 2% and should be suspected when pulmonary nodules grow rapidly. **(Right)** Axial NECT of the same patient shows solid ➔ and cavitary ➔ nodules within the right lower lobe. The presence of lung nodules in tracheobronchial papillomatosis indicates invasive papillomatosis.*

TRACHEOBRONCHIAL PAPILLOMATOSIS

TERMINOLOGY

Synonyms

- **Recurrent respiratory papillomatosis (RRP)**

Definitions

- Airway nodules due to human papilloma virus (HPV) infection
  - Upper > lower airways
- Invasive papillomatosis
  - Spread to lungs

IMAGING

General Features

- Best diagnostic clue
  - Thickening or nodularity of airways
  - Multiple solid & cavitary pulmonary nodules &/or masses
- Location
  - Larynx is most commonly affected site
    - Variable involvement of lower airways
      - 5-29% of cases
  - Invasive papillomatosis
    - Perihilar & central location in coronal plane
    - Posterior distribution in axial plane
- Size
  - Invasive papillomatosis
    - Variable in size
    - Most nodules 1-3 cm in diameter
- Morphology
  - Invasive papillomatosis
    - Smaller nodules usually solid
    - Larger nodules more likely to cavitate

Radiographic Findings

- Radiography
  - Airways
    - Thickening or nodularity of airway walls
      - May not be visible on chest radiography
  - Multiple pulmonary nodules &/or masses
    - May exhibit cavitation

CT Findings

- NECT
  - Airways
    - **Thickening or nodularity of airway walls**
      - Upper > lower airways
      - No calcification
    - Solitary papillomas
      - Less common than multiple papillomas
      - Typically located in lobar or segmental bronchi
    - Bronchiectasis
      - Recurrent infection & airway obstruction
  - **Multiple pulmonary nodules**
    - Larger nodules more likely to cavitate
    - Walls may be thin or thick & irregular
    - Posterior lung involvement may be related to gravity
      - Represents dependent seeding of lung
    - Nodules may communicate with adjacent airways
    - Nodule growth manifestations
      - Ground-glass opacity
      - Consolidation
    - Growth rate
      - Most pulmonary nodules demonstrate slow growth
      - Rapid growth suspicious for squamous cell carcinoma
      - Growth rate may increase during pregnancy
  - Complications
    - Squamous cell carcinoma
    - Secondary infection
      - Air-fluid levels
    - Atelectasis ± postobstructive pneumonia
      - Usually secondary to intraluminal papillomas

Imaging Recommendations

- Best imaging tool
  - CT is optimal imaging modality to visualize airway nodules & evaluate lungs for invasive papillomatosis & development of squamous cell carcinoma

DIFFERENTIAL DIAGNOSIS

Tracheobronchopathia Osteochondroplastica

- Multiple small airway nodules; ± calcification
- Involvement of anterolateral tracheal & proximal bronchial walls
- Sparing of posterior membranous airway wall
- Asymmetric airway stenosis

Wegener Granulomatosis

- Multiple cavitary pulmonary nodules or masses
- Subglottic stenosis
- Thickening of airway walls

Tracheobronchial Amyloidosis

- Calcified or noncalcified submucosal nodules with narrowing of tracheal lumen
- Posterior membrane not spared

Relapsing Polychondritis

- Noncalcified diffuse thickening & narrowing of trachea & mainstem bronchi
- Anterior & lateral tracheal walls; tracheal cartilage

Sarcoidosis

- Airway distortion/stenosis
  - May lead to atelectasis
- Nodular thickening of airway wall
- Mosaic attenuation, expiratory air-trapping

Squamous Cell Carcinoma

- Most common lung cancer to cavitate
  - Present in 15% of cases
- Strongly associated with cigarette smoking
- Increased risk with invasive papillomatosis

Pulmonary Metastases

- Well-formed pulmonary nodules or masses
- Squamous cell carcinomas & sarcomas may cavitate
- Trachea normal

Septic Emboli

- Poorly defined pulmonary nodules or masses
- Varying degrees of cavitation

TRACHEOBRONCHIAL PAPILLOMATOSIS

PATHOLOGY

General Features

- Etiology
  - HPV infection of respiratory tract
    - Peripartum sexual transmission of HPV
      - Risk factors: Firstborn child, vaginal delivery, & mother < 20 years of age
    - Types 6 & 11 are most common
    - Any portion of respiratory tract may be affected
      - 95% of cases involve larynx
      - Solitary papillomas more common in middle-aged male smokers
    - Airway dissemination (invasive papillomatosis)
      - < 1% seed lung
      - Surgical manipulation of laryngeal papillomas increases risk of dissemination
      - Lung seeding usually apparent in children or young adults
- HPV infection
  - Cutaneous & genital warts
  - Tropism for keratinizing epithelium
  - Cervical cancer

Gross Pathologic & Surgical Features

- Sessile or papillary lesions with vascular core covered by squamous epithelium
- Airway papillomas may be exophytic or endophytic
- Cauliflower-like shape

Microscopic Features

- Laryngeal & pulmonary lesions composed of squamous cells
- Cavities lined with squamous epithelium
  - Squamous epithelium may spread from airspace to airspace across pores of Kohn

CLINICAL ISSUES

Presentation

- Most common signs/symptoms
  - Asymptomatic in mild cases
  - Hoarseness most common symptom due to laryngeal involvement
  - Wheezing & stridor may be mistaken for asthma
  - Presence of other symptoms depends on size, number, & location of papillomas
    - Dyspnea, hemoptysis, & obstructive pneumonia
- Pulmonary function tests
  - Upper airway obstructive pattern
- Laryngoscopy
  - Visualization of nodules
  - Biopsy necessary for typing of HPV

Demographics

- Age
  - Adults: 2 cases per 100,000 population
  - Bimodal age distribution
    - Children: 18 months to 3 years of age
    - Adults: 4th decade
- Gender
  - Children: M = F
  - Adults: M > F

Natural History & Prognosis

- Usually self-limited disease in young patients
- Pulmonary nodules typically grow very slowly
  - Rapid growth suspicious for squamous cell carcinoma
- Invasive papillomatosis
  - Death due to respiratory failure
  - Mortality as high as 50%
  - 2% incidence of squamous cell carcinoma
    - Usually occurs > 15 years after development of papillomatosis
    - Carcinomas often multicentric

Treatment

- Self-limited disease usually requires no treatment
- Surgical & medical therapies for lesions causing airway obstruction
  - Laser ablation of airway lesions
    - Numerous procedures usually necessary
    - Technically difficult with involvement of lower airways
    - Viral respiratory precautions important for health care providers
      - Aerosolization of virus
  - Tracheostomy
    - Treatment of airway obstruction
    - More commonly required in younger patients
  - Antiviral agents may slow growth
  - Interferon may slow growth
    - Systemic or direct intralesional injection
- Smoking cessation
  - Decreases risk of squamous cell carcinoma
  - Tobacco carcinogen synergistic with papillomas

DIAGNOSTIC CHECKLIST

Consider

- Tracheobronchial papillomatosis in patients with multiple airway nodules

Image Interpretation Pearls

- Evaluation of lungs for evidence of invasive papillomatosis & lesions suspicious for squamous cell carcinoma

SELECTED REFERENCES

1. Colt HG et al: Multimodality bronchoscopic imaging of recurrent respiratory papillomatosis. Laryngoscope. 120(3):468-72, 2010
2. Thorne MC et al: Transoral trans-stomal microdebrider excision of tracheal papillomatosis. Laryngoscope. 119(5):964-6, 2009
3. Prince JS et al: Nonneoplastic lesions of the tracheobronchial wall: radiologic findings with bronchoscopic correlation. Radiographics. 22 Spec No(S215-30, 2002
4. Armstrong LR et al: Initial results from the national registry for juvenile-onset recurrent respiratory papillomatosis. RRP Task Force. Arch Otolaryngol Head Neck Surg. 125(7):743-8, 1999
5. Guillou L et al: Squamous cell carcinoma of the lung in a nonsmoking, nonirradiated patient with juvenile laryngotracheal papillomatosis. Evidence of human papillomavirus-11 DNA in both carcinoma and papillomas. Am J Surg Pathol. 15(9):891-8, 1991

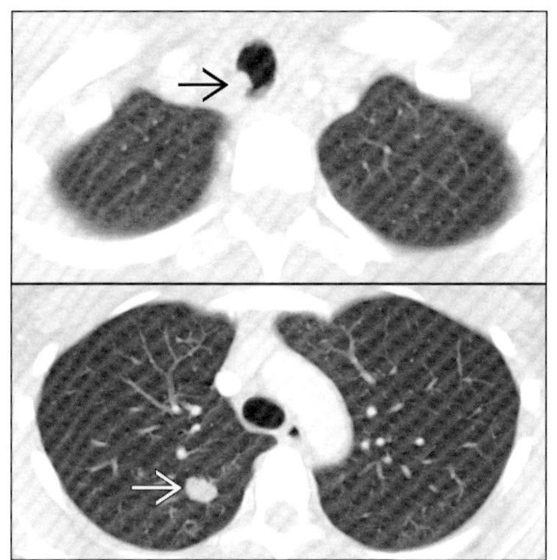

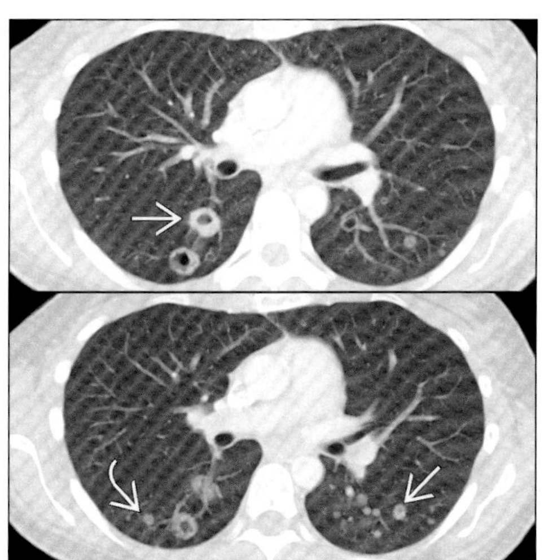

*(**Left**) Composite image with axial NECT of a patient with tracheobronchial papillomatosis shows lobular endoluminal tracheal nodules ➔ and a parenchymal nodule ➔ in the right upper lobe. (**Right**) Composite image with axial NECT of the same patient obtained caudad to the carina shows multiple solid ➔ and cavitary ➔ pulmonary nodules bilaterally. The constellation of findings is characteristic of invasive tracheobronchial papillomatosis.*

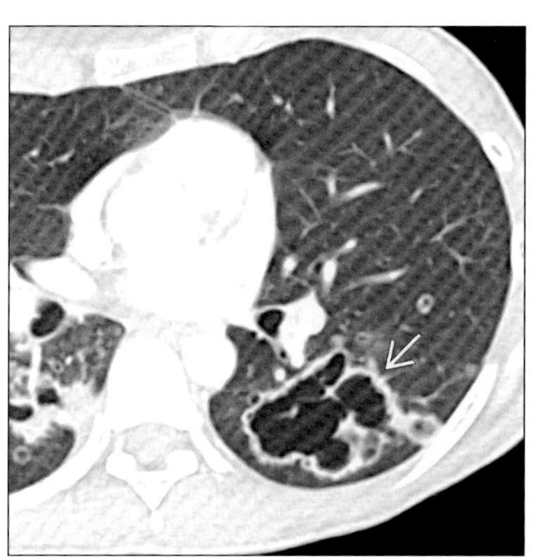

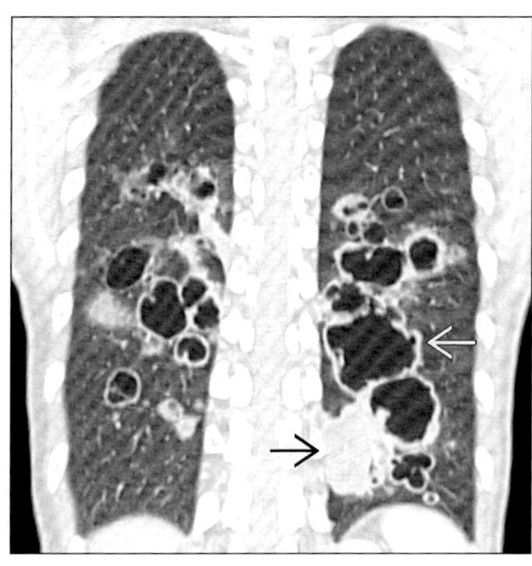

*(**Left**) Axial CECT demonstrates multiple bilateral cavitary nodules and a cavitary mass of irregular borders ➔ that exhibit a predilection for the posterior aspects of the lower lobes. Invasive papillomatosis preferentially affects the posterior lungs due to dependent seeding through the airways. (**Right**) Coronal NECT of the same patient shows multiple solid ➔ and cavitary ➔ nodules and masses bilaterally. Larger nodules are more likely to exhibit cavitation.*

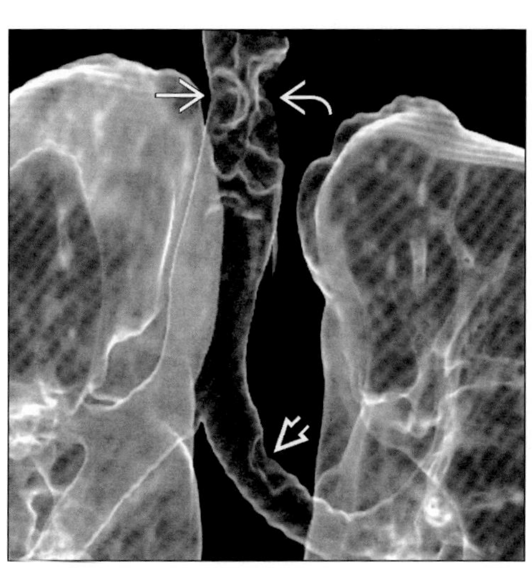

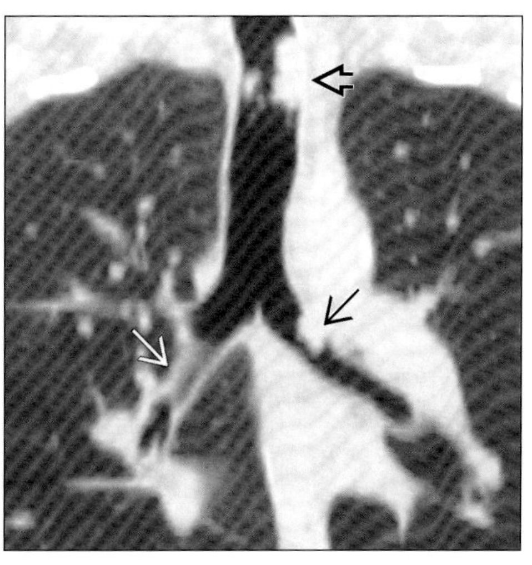

*(**Left**) Coronal 3D reformation of a patient with tracheobronchial papillomatosis shows irregular nodular lesions of the tracheal wall ➔ and multiple nodules within the trachea ➔ and left mainstem bronchus ➔. (**Right**) Coronal NECT of the same patient demonstrates nodules of various sizes in the proximal trachea ➔ and in the left mainstem bronchus ➔. Note bronchial wall thickening of the right mainstem bronchus ➔. The tracheal lesion exhibits a characteristic cauliflower-like morphology.*

SQUAMOUS CELL CARCINOMA, AIRWAYS

Key Facts

Terminology

- Squamous cell carcinoma (SCC)
- Malignant tumor of trachea

Imaging

- Distal 1/3 of trachea
- Radiography
  - Trachea classic "blind spot" for radiologists
  - Often subtle; detection requires careful inspection on PA & lateral radiography
  - Focal endoluminal tracheal nodule or mass
- CT
  - Nonspecific findings; difficult differentiation from other malignant tracheal tumors
  - Nodular or lobular tracheal nodule or mass
  - Extraluminal extension & circumferential involvement suggestive of malignancy
  - Local lymphadenopathy that may be necrotic

Top Differential Diagnoses

- Adenoid cystic carcinoma
- Benign neoplasms
- Metastases (rare)

Clinical Issues

- Nonspecific symptoms; may mimic asthma
- Dyspnea, cough, hemoptysis, wheezing, stridor
- Age: 6th to 7th decades
- Men affected up to 4x as often as women
- Association with cigarette smoking
- Prognosis worse than that of adenoid cystic carcinoma

Diagnostic Checklist

- Consider SCC in middle-aged or elderly men with smoking history & tracheal tumor

*(**Left**) PA chest radiograph (coned down to the trachea) shows an eccentric nodular endoluminal left tracheal lesion ➔. The trachea and central bronchi are traditional "blind spots" for radiologists and must be carefully assessed to detect endoluminal lesions. (**Right**) Axial NECT of the same patient shows an infiltrative squamous cell carcinoma narrowing the tracheal lumen with extraluminal extension of the lesion ➔, highly suggestive of malignancy. Specific pathological diagnosis requires tissue sampling.*

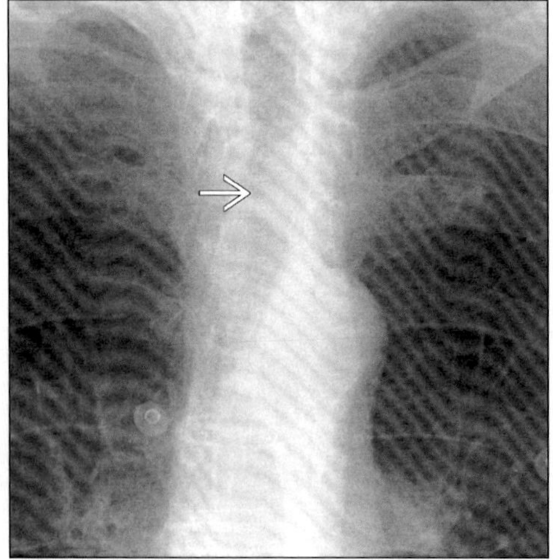

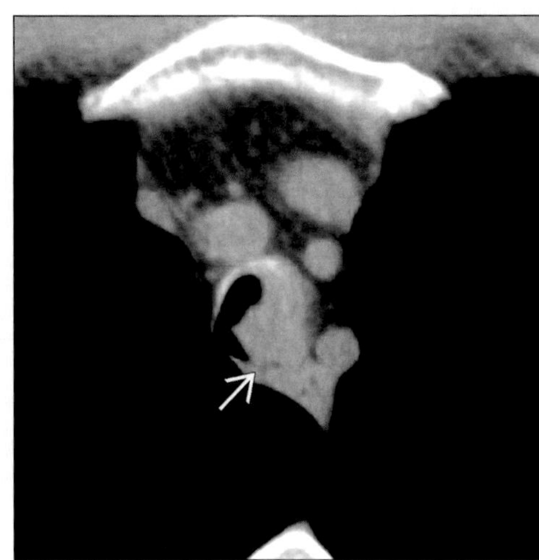

*(**Left**) Axial CECT of SCC shows a large enhancing mass ➔ with endoluminal involvement of the trachea, moderate airway narrowing, and extension into the right paratracheal region. (**Right**) Axial CECT shows a large lobular mass invading the superior mediastinum and markedly narrowing the tracheal lumen, consistent with squamous cell carcinoma. Severe narrowing of the large airways prior to clinical presentation is not uncommon, as in this case.*

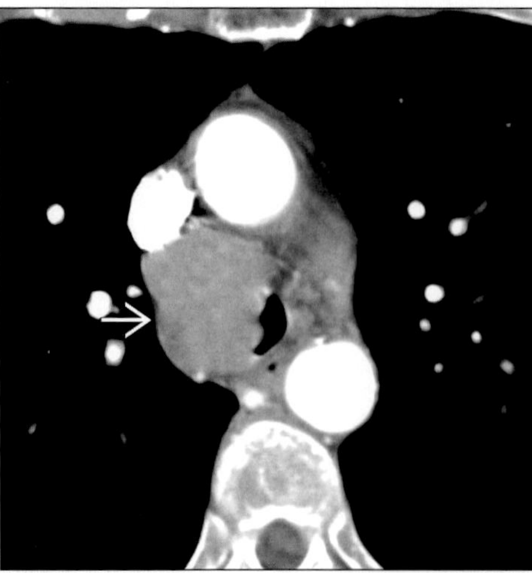

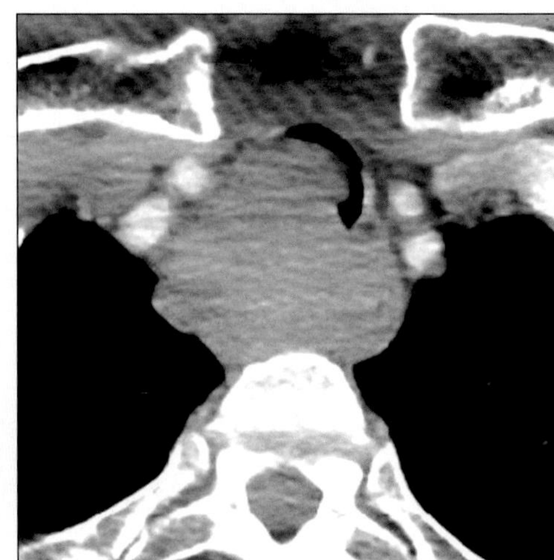

SQUAMOUS CELL CARCINOMA, AIRWAYS

TERMINOLOGY

Abbreviations

- **Squamous cell carcinoma (SCC)**

Definitions

- Malignant tumor of trachea, which arises from surface epithelium

IMAGING

General Features

- Best diagnostic clue
  - Nodular or irregularly marginated mass or nodule within tracheal lumen; frequent infiltration/invasion of adjacent mediastinal structures
- Location
  - **Distal 1/3 of trachea**
- Size
  - Usually < 2.5 cm in maximum diameter at presentation

Radiographic Findings

- Radiography
  - Trachea is classic "blind spot" for radiologists
  - Often subtle; detection requires careful tracheal inspection on PA & lateral radiography
  - **Focal endoluminal tracheal nodule or mass**
  - Asymmetric thickening of tracheal wall or focal thickening of paratracheal or retrotracheal stripes

CT Findings

- NECT
  - Nonspecific findings; difficult differentiation from other malignant tracheal tumors
  - Nodular or lobular tracheal nodule or mass
  - Extraluminal extension & circumferential involvement suggestive of malignancy
  - **May be multifocal (10%)**
  - Local lymphadenopathy, which may be necrotic

Imaging Recommendations

- Best imaging tool
  - CT is optimal imaging modality for evaluation of tracheal neoplasms
- Protocol advice
  - Multiplanar reformatted images to show length of involvement may be helpful for surgical planning

DIFFERENTIAL DIAGNOSIS

Adenoid Cystic Carcinoma

- M = F (as opposed to SCC)
- May affect long segments of trachea
- Growth along submucosa & perineural structures

Benign Neoplasms

- Hamartoma & lipoma: Internal macroscopic fat is diagnostic of these benign tumors
- Chondroma: Internal calcification
  - Calcification not indicative of benignity

Metastases (Rare)

- Direct invasion of trachea from bronchogenic or esophageal cancer
- Hematogenous metastases from any primary malignancy, but most commonly
  - Breast cancer
  - Colon cancer
  - Melanoma
  - Renal cell carcinoma

CLINICAL ISSUES

Presentation

- Most common signs/symptoms
  - Nonspecific symptoms; may mimic asthma
  - Dyspnea, cough, hemoptysis, wheezing, stridor
  - Upper airway obstructive symptoms usually do not develop until > 50% tracheal narrowing

Demographics

- Age
  - 6th to 7th decades of life
- Gender
  - Men affected up to 4x as often as women
- Epidemiology
  - Rare tumor of respiratory tract, but most common tracheal malignancy in adults
  - **Association with cigarette smoking**

Natural History & Prognosis

- **Prognosis worse than that of adenoid cystic carcinoma**
- 1/3 have pulmonary or mediastinal lymph node metastases at diagnosis
- 5-year survival rate: 39-73%
- 10-year survival rate: 18-53%

Treatment

- Surgery only curative option
- Radiotherapy in cases in which surgery not feasible or as adjuvant or palliative measure
- Tracheal stents as palliative measure
- Chemotherapy has no established role currently

DIAGNOSTIC CHECKLIST

Consider

- SCC in middle-aged or elderly men with smoking history & tracheal tumor
- Tracheal tumor in adult with new onset asthma

Image Interpretation Pearls

- Multifocal primary tracheal tumors not uncommon in SCC

SELECTED REFERENCES

1. Kang EY: Large airway diseases. J Thorac Imaging. 26(4):249-62, 2011
2. Javidan-Nejad C: MDCT of trachea and main bronchi. Radiol Clin North Am. 48(1):157-76, 2010
3. Lee KS et al: Update on multidetector computed tomography imaging of the airways. J Thorac Imaging. 25(2):112-24, 2010
4. Ferretti GR et al: Imaging of tumors of the trachea and central bronchi. Radiol Clin North Am. 47(2):227-41, 2009
5. Boiselle PM: Imaging of the large airways. Clin Chest Med. 29(1):181-93, vii, 2008

ADENOID CYSTIC CARCINOMA

Key Facts

Terminology
- Adenoid cystic carcinoma (ACC)
- Rare primary malignant tracheal neoplasm arising from bronchial glands

Imaging
- Radiography
  - Trachea is common "blind spot" for radiologists
  - Tracheal lesions often subtle on radiography
  - Focal tracheal nodule or mass
  - Abrupt nodular thickening of paratracheal or retrotracheal stripes
- CT
  - Polypoid tracheal nodule or mass; may also involve central bronchi
  - May exhibit circumferential airway involvement
  - Often affects long segments of trachea
  - Metastatic mediastinal lymphadenopathy

Top Differential Diagnoses
- Squamous cell carcinoma
- Benign neoplasms
- Metastases

Pathology
- Perineural extension classic

Clinical Issues
- Symptoms/signs: Often misdiagnosed as asthma
  - Dyspnea, cough, stridor, wheezing, hemoptysis
- Treatment
  - Surgical resection with end-to-end anastomosis of trachea ± adjuvant radiotherapy

Diagnostic Checklist
- Consider ACC in differential diagnosis of tracheal tumors, especially if long segment involvement

*(**Left**) Axial CECT of a patient with ACC shows marked circumferential tracheal wall thickening ➔ with extensive narrowing of the airway lumen, consistent with malignancy. (**Right**) Coronal CECT of the same patient shows extensive longitudinal tracheal involvement ➔ extending into the right mainstem bronchus. Adenoid cystic carcinoma commonly affects long segments of the trachea. Even in cases of apparent focal tracheal involvement, long segmental tracheal extension may be present.*

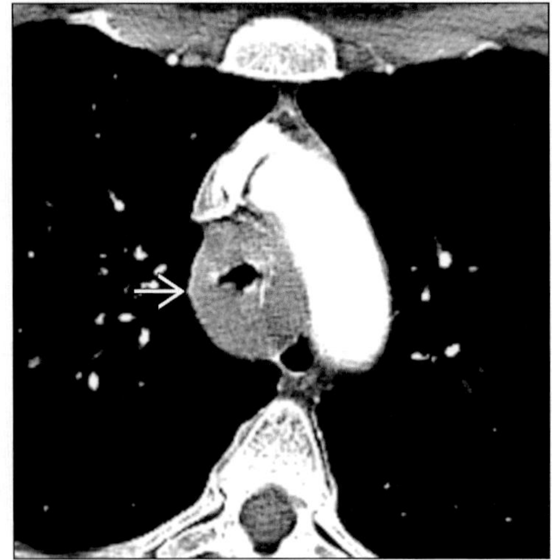

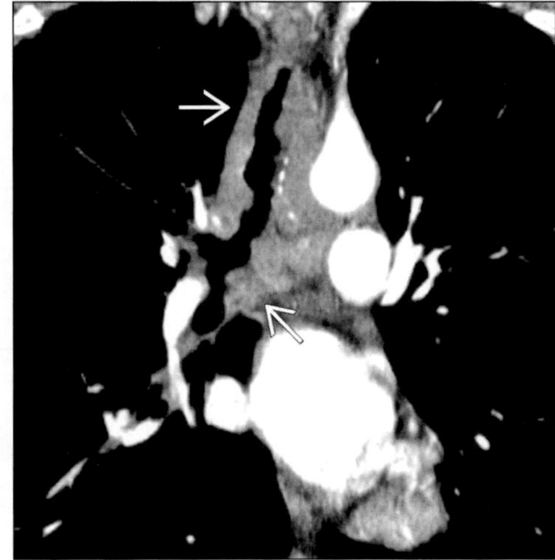

*(**Left**) Lateral chest radiograph of a patient with ACC demonstrates a focal endoluminal tracheal nodule ➔ arising from the anterior tracheal wall. CT is the optimal modality for imaging assessment of these lesions. However, definitive diagnosis always relies on tissue sampling. (**Right**) Axial CECT of a patient with ACC shows characteristic nodular tracheal wall thickening ➔, typical of adenoid cystic carcinoma. Asymmetric nodular tracheal wall thickening is highly suggestive of malignancy.*

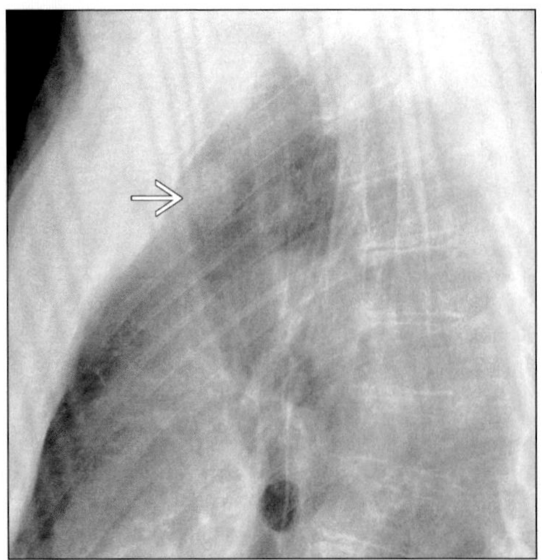

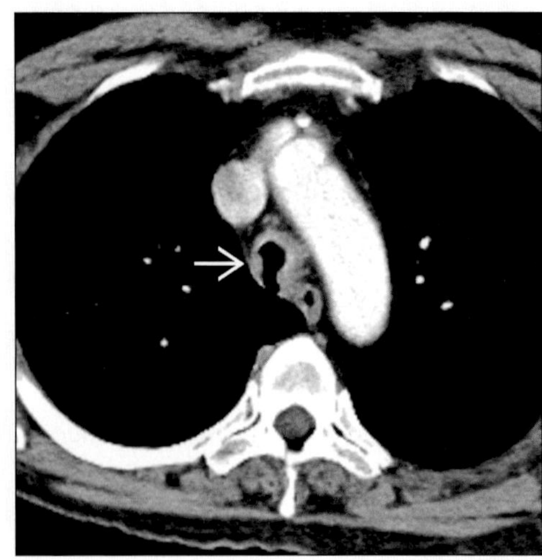

ADENOID CYSTIC CARCINOMA

TERMINOLOGY

Abbreviations

- **Adenoid cystic carcinoma** (ACC)

Definitions

- Rare primary malignant tracheal neoplasm arising from bronchial glands

IMAGING

General Features

- Best diagnostic clue
  - Tracheal endoluminal nodule or mass; may involve long segment of trachea
  - Signs of malignant tracheal tumor
    - Tracheal lesion > 2 cm
    - Irregular or lobular borders
    - Adjacent tracheal wall thickening
    - Extraluminal extension, local invasion
- Morphology
  - Irregular margins; often infiltrates adjacent mediastinal structures

Radiographic Findings

- Radiography
  - Trachea is common "blind spot" for radiologists
  - Tracheal lesions often subtle on radiography; detection requires careful assessment of airway on both PA & lateral radiographs
  - Focal tracheal nodule or mass
  - Abrupt nodular thickening of paratracheal or retrotracheal stripes (> 4 mm)
  - Mediastinal lymphadenopathy
    - Evaluate paratracheal regions, AP window, AP stripe, intermediate stem line

CT Findings

- NECT
  - **Polypoid or broad-based nodule or mass**
  - Endoluminal tracheal involvement, may also involve central bronchi
  - May exhibit circumferential airway involvement
  - Often affects long segments of trachea
  - Metastatic mediastinal lymphadenopathy
  - Microscopic invasion along tracheal submucosa & into mediastinum, often occult on imaging

Imaging Recommendations

- Best imaging tool
  - CT is imaging modality of choice for assessment of tracheal neoplasms
- Protocol advice
  - Multiplanar reformatted images to show length of involvement may be useful in surgical planning

DIFFERENTIAL DIAGNOSIS

Squamous Cell Carcinoma

- Men much more often affected than women
- History of cigarette smoking
- May be ulcerative or necrotic
- May be multifocal

Benign Neoplasms

- Hamartoma & lipoma: Internal macroscopic fat is diagnostic
- Chondroma: Internal calcification
- Papilloma or papillomatosis

Metastases

- Direct tracheal invasion by bronchogenic or esophageal cancers
- Hematogenous metastases from any primary, but most commonly
  - Breast cancer
  - Colon cancer
  - Melanoma
  - Renal cell carcinoma

PATHOLOGY

General Features

- Perineural extension classic
- Infiltrative cribriform pattern of uniform tumor cells arranged in cords & nests
- High nuclear:cytoplasmic ratio

CLINICAL ISSUES

Presentation

- Most common signs/symptoms
  - Indolent symptoms
  - Often misdiagnosed as asthma
  - Nonspecific respiratory symptoms: Dyspnea, cough, stridor, wheezing, hemoptysis
- Clinical profile
  - M = F
  - Average age: 45-60 years

Natural History & Prognosis

- **5-year survival: 65-100%**
- 10-year survival: 50-60%
- Up to 50% of patients with ACC have hematogenous metastases, most commonly pulmonary (indolent growth)
- At risk for tracheoesophageal fistula, especially in setting of previous radiation treatment

Treatment

- Surgical resection with end-to-end tracheal anastomosis ± adjuvant radiotherapy
- Palliative radiotherapy in nonsurgical cases
- Chemotherapy not generally indicated

DIAGNOSTIC CHECKLIST

Consider

- ACC in differential diagnosis of solid tracheal tumors, especially if long segment involvement

SELECTED REFERENCES

1. Dean CW et al: AIRP best cases in radiologic-pathologic correlation: adenoid cystic carcinoma of the trachea. Radiographics. 31(5):1443-7, 2011
2. McCarthy MJ et al: Tumors of the trachea. J Thorac Imaging. 10(3):180-98, 1995

MUCOEPIDERMOID CARCINOMA

Key Facts

Terminology
- Mucoepidermoid carcinoma (MEC)
- Primary bronchial gland neoplasm arising in lung & tracheobronchial tree
  - 0.1-0.2% of all primary pulmonary malignant neoplasms

Imaging
- Radiography
  - Endoluminal lesion may be subtle
  - Visualization of postobstructive pneumonia/ atelectasis
- CT
  - Well-circumscribed endobronchial lesion
  - Central airway: ~ 45% (main bronchus > trachea)
  - Distal obstructive pneumonia or atelectasis
  - Punctate calcification: ~ 50%
  - Mild heterogeneous contrast enhancement

Top Differential Diagnoses
- Non-small cell lung cancer
- Squamous cell carcinoma of airways
- Carcinoid
- Adenoid cystic carcinoma
- Airways metastasis

Pathology
- Indistinguishable from primary salivary gland MEC

Clinical Issues
- Cough, hemoptysis, wheeze, stridor, pneumonia
- ~ 50% of patients younger than 30 years
- Surgical resection; prognosis usually good

Diagnostic Checklist
- Primary lung carcinoma is far more common than MEC & should be considered in differential diagnosis

(Left) PA chest radiograph of a young woman with minimal symptoms shows a right lower lobe nodule ➔ with well-defined margins. There is no associated atelectasis or obstructive sequela. ***(Right)*** *Axial NECT of the same patient shows a homogeneous, well-defined, large soft tissue nodule ➔ in the right lower lobe. The differential diagnosis is broad and includes lung cancer, less common neoplasms (such as carcinoid and mucoepidermoid carcinoma), and inflammatory and infectious lesions.*

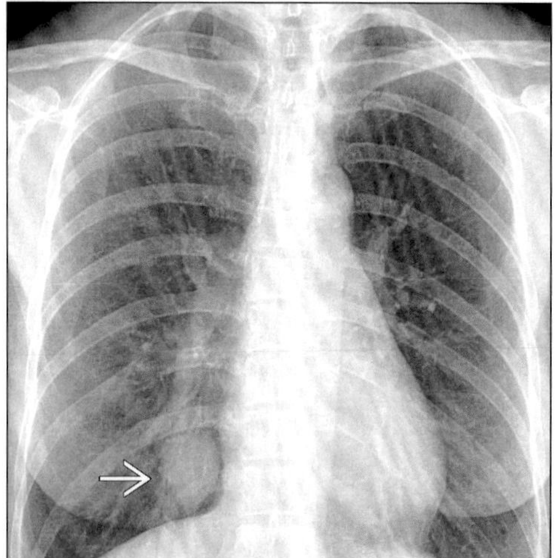

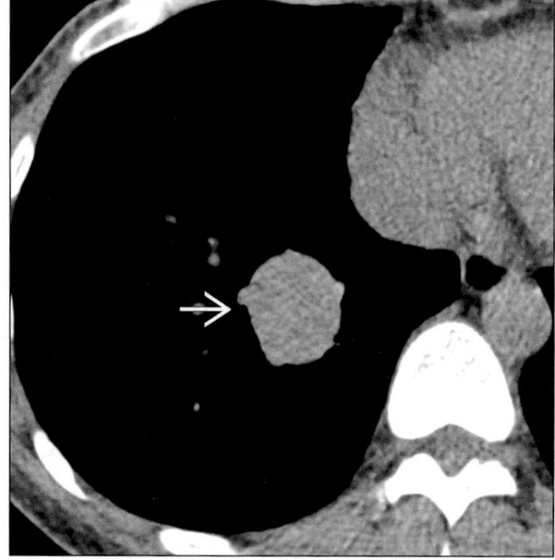

(Left) *Axial NECT of patient with MEC who presented with cough and hemoptysis shows hyperlucency and hyperexpansion of the left upper lobe secondary to a central polylobular soft tissue mass ➔ within the left mainstem bronchus with extension into the left upper and left lower lobe bronchi.* ***(Right)*** *Axial CECT of a patient with MEC who presented with hemoptysis and left upper lobe atelectasis shows a low-attenuation lesion ➔ obstructing the left upper lobe bronchus with resultant left upper lobe atelectasis.*

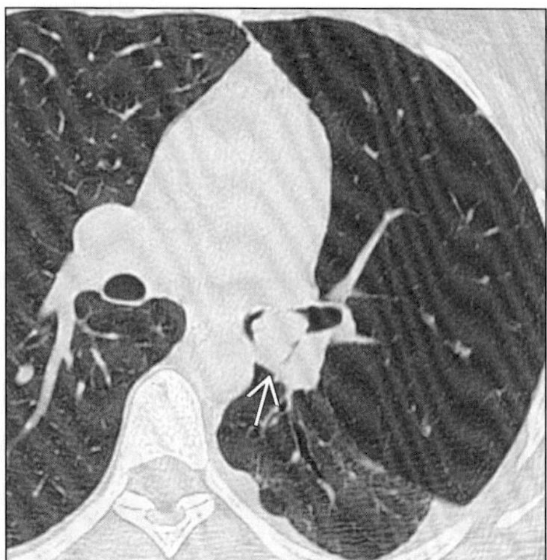

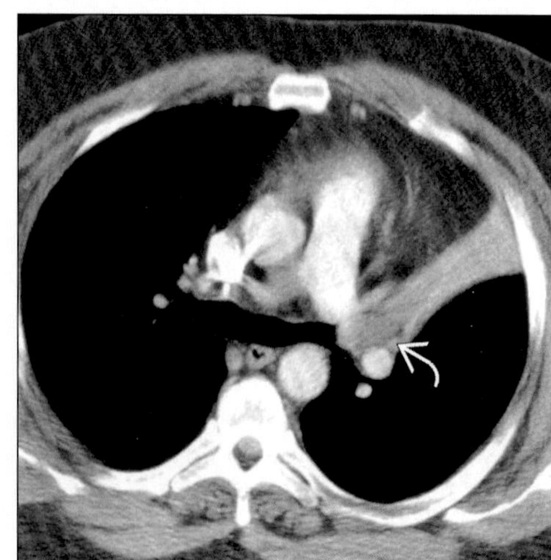

MUCOEPIDERMOID CARCINOMA

TERMINOLOGY

Abbreviations

- **Mucoepidermoid carcinoma** (MEC)

Definitions

- Primary bronchial gland neoplasm arising in lung & tracheobronchial tree
  - 0.1-0.2% of all primary pulmonary malignant neoplasms

IMAGING

General Features

- Best diagnostic clue
  - Endoluminal smooth or lobulated mass in segmental bronchus
- Location
  - Central airway: ~ 45% (mainstem bronchus > trachea)
  - Peripheral lung: ~ 55% (segmental bronchus most common)
- Size
  - 1-2 cm
- Morphology
  - Smooth or lobular endoluminal nodule

Radiographic Findings

- Endoluminal lesion may be subtle
- Visualization of postobstructive pneumonia/atelectasis

CT Findings

- CECT
  - **Well-circumscribed endobronchial lesion**
    - Ovoid or lobulated margins
    - May conform to branching airway morphology
  - Distal obstructive pneumonia or atelectasis
  - Punctate calcification: ~ 50%
  - Mild heterogeneous contrast enhancement

Imaging Recommendations

- Best imaging tool
  - CT more sensitive than radiography
  - CT is imaging modality of choice for assessment of airway neoplasms

DIFFERENTIAL DIAGNOSIS

Non-Small Cell Lung Cancer

- May extend into airway from adjacent lung
- Associated with cigarette smoking
- Patients typically older than those with MEC

Squamous Cell Carcinoma of Airways

- Most common primary malignant airway neoplasm
- Frequent extraluminal extension
- Irregular margins
- Associated with cigarette smoking

Carcinoid

- Far more common than MEC
- More common in lobar bronchi
- Marked contrast enhancement

Adenoid Cystic Carcinoma

- More common in trachea, especially near carina
  - Irregular margins
  - Extraluminal extension

Airways Metastasis

- Known primary neoplasm elsewhere
  - Non-small cell lung cancer, melanoma, renal cell carcinoma, colon cancer, & breast cancer are common primary malignancies
  - Pulmonary, pleural, & lymph node metastases far more common than with MEC

PATHOLOGY

Staging, Grading, & Classification

- Higher grade tumors (grades 2 & 3) propensity for transmural invasion

Microscopic Features

- Indistinguishable from primary salivary gland MEC
  - Presence of mucous cells mixed with epidermoid, clear, & "intermediate"-type cells

CLINICAL ISSUES

Presentation

- Most common signs/symptoms
  - Cough, hemoptysis, wheezing, stridor, pneumonia

Demographics

- Age
  - ~ 50% of patients younger than 30 years
- Gender
  - M = F
- Epidemiology
  - No significant association with cigarette smoking

Natural History & Prognosis

- Prognosis usually good
  - Survival with MEC better than with adenoid cystic carcinoma & non-small cell lung carcinoma
  - Complete resection usually curative
- Metastases in ~ 10%

Treatment

- Surgical resection
- Adjuvant external beam radiation therapy in select few patients

DIAGNOSTIC CHECKLIST

Consider

- Primary lung carcinoma is far more common than MEC & should be considered in differential diagnosis of peripheral & central neoplasms

Image Interpretation Pearls

- Endoluminal location in segmental airway suggestive

SELECTED REFERENCES

1. Ishizumi T et al: Mucoepidermoid carcinoma of the lung: high-resolution CT and histopathologic findings in five cases. Lung Cancer. 60(1):125-31, 2008

METASTASIS, AIRWAYS

Key Facts

Terminology
- Hematogenous spread of neoplasm to airway

Imaging
- Radiography
  - Atelectasis: Lung, lobar, segmental
  - Obstructive pneumonitis
  - Endotracheal or endobronchial lesion rarely apparent
- CT
  - Endoluminal soft tissue nodule or mass
  - Obstructive pneumonitis
  - Consolidation in distribution of affected airway
  - Fluid-filled bronchi distal to obstruction
  - Atelectasis distal to obstructing lesion
  - Atelectasis with associated shift of pulmonary fissures

Top Differential Diagnoses
- Non-small cell lung cancer
- Carcinoid
- Tracheal neoplasms
- Hamartoma

Pathology
- Renal cell & colon carcinoma most common

Clinical Issues
- Symptoms/signs: Cough, hemoptysis, wheezing, pneumonia, atelectasis
- Prognosis usually poor because of disseminated neoplasm elsewhere

Diagnostic Checklist
- Consider airway metastasis in patient with malignancy & endobronchial lesion with obstructive pneumonia or atelectasis

__(Left)__ PA chest radiograph of a patient with metastatic melanoma shows right middle lobe consolidation ➔. Endobronchial metastases are usually occult on radiography, but their effects (e.g., atelectasis, pneumonia) may be evident. CT is the imaging study of choice for assessment of suspected endobronchial metastases. __(Right)__ Axial NECT of the same patient shows a mass lesion ➔ filling and obstructing the lumen of the bronchus intermedius. Biopsy confirmed metastatic melanoma.

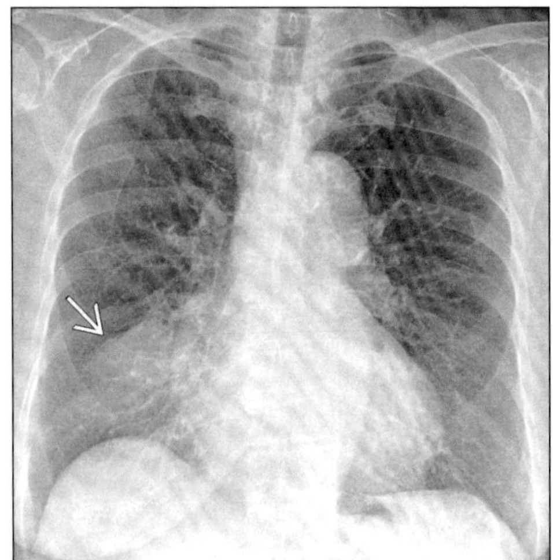

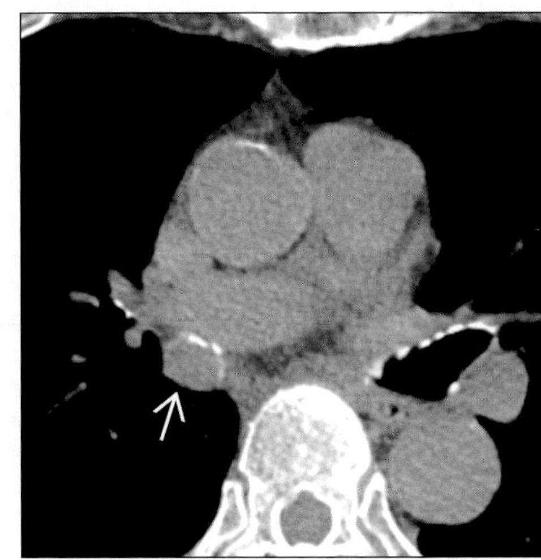

__(Left)__ Axial CECT of a patient with metastatic renal cell carcinoma shows an ovoid, enhancing soft tissue lesion ➔ at the orifice of the left upper lobe bronchus with resultant left upper lobe atelectasis ➔ and leftward mediastinal shift. __(Right)__ Coronal oblique CECT of a patient with metastatic breast cancer shows a mass ➔ that completely occludes the left main bronchus. The presence of metastases elsewhere typically obviates the need for biopsy of a new endobronchial lesion in such patients.

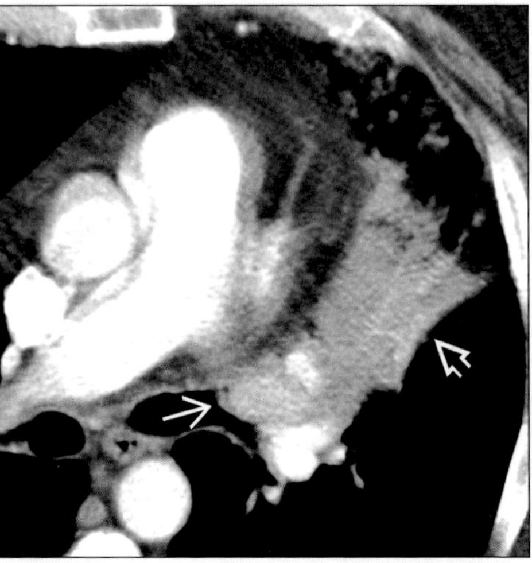

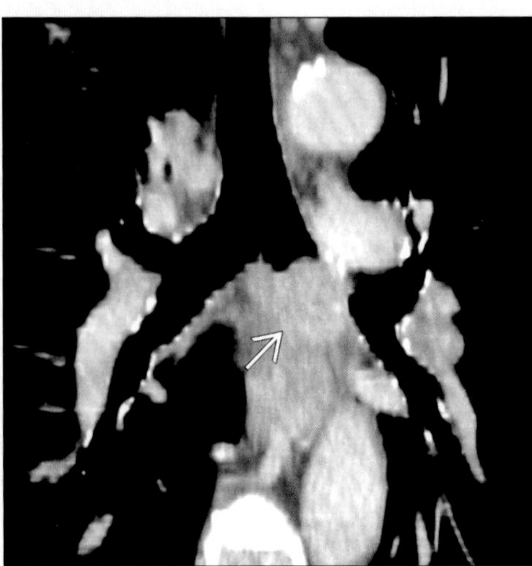

METASTASIS, AIRWAYS

TERMINOLOGY

Synonyms

- **Endobronchial metastasis**
- **Endotracheal metastasis**

Definitions

- Hematogenous spread of neoplasm to airway

IMAGING

General Features

- Best diagnostic clue
  - Endobronchial or endotracheal nodule or mass on CT
- Location
  - Trachea & larger bronchi
- Size
  - Range from small mural nodule to large obstructing mass
- Morphology
  - Smooth or polypoid endoluminal lesion

Radiographic Findings

- **Atelectasis**
  - Lung, lobar, segmental
- Endotracheal or endobronchial lesion rarely apparent

CT Findings

- **Endoluminal soft tissue nodule or mass**, may obstruct airway
- **Obstructive pneumonitis**
  - Consolidation in distribution of affected airway
  - Fluid-filled bronchi distal to obstruction
- **Atelectasis distal to obstructing lesion**
  - Shift of pulmonary fissures

Imaging Recommendations

- Best imaging tool
  - CT: Superior to radiography
    - Optimal imaging modality for evaluation of airway neoplasia
- Protocol advice
  - Use of intravenous contrast may be helpful for delineating obstructing mass & distinguishing it from adjacent atelectasis/pneumonitis
  - Volumetric thin-section imaging useful for detecting small lesions
    - Multiplanar reformations may help delineate tumor extent

DIFFERENTIAL DIAGNOSIS

Non-Small Cell Lung Cancer

- No known primary malignancy
- Usually occurs in current or former cigarette smokers

Carcinoid

- Often hypervascular
- No known primary malignancy

Tracheal Neoplasms

- No known primary malignancy
- Primary tracheal neoplasms more common than metastases
- Squamous cell carcinoma & adenoid cystic carcinoma most common primary neoplasms

Hamartoma

- No known primary malignancy
- Usually heterogeneous with dystrophic calcification
- Presence of macroscopic fat usually diagnostic

PATHOLOGY

General Features

- Renal cell & colon carcinoma most common
- Numerous other extrathoracic solid tumors also reported

CLINICAL ISSUES

Presentation

- Most common signs/symptoms
  - Cough
  - Hemoptysis
    - Especially with hypervascular tumors, such as renal cell carcinoma & melanoma
  - Wheezing
  - Pneumonia
  - Atelectasis
- Other signs/symptoms
  - Rarely, patients may expectorate tissue fragments

Demographics

- Epidemiology
  - ~ 2% of patients die from solid malignancies

Natural History & Prognosis

- Prognosis usually poor because of disseminated neoplasm elsewhere
- Chronic obstruction can lead to pneumonia & sepsis

Treatment

- Dependent on site & status of primary neoplasm
  - Chemotherapy & palliative radiation therapy
  - Endobronchial cryoablation or laser therapy for palliation
  - Surgery can be considered if no active malignancy elsewhere

DIAGNOSTIC CHECKLIST

Consider

- Primary airway neoplasm in differential diagnosis of endoluminal obstructing airway lesions

Image Interpretation Pearls

- Endobronchial lesion with obstructive pneumonia or atelectasis in patient with known malignancy

SELECTED REFERENCES

1. Plavsic BM et al: Melanoma metastatic to the bronchus: radiologic features in two patients. J Thorac Imaging. 9(2):67-70, 1994
2. Heitmiller RF et al: Endobronchial metastasis. J Thorac Cardiovasc Surg. 106(3):537-42, 1993

SABER-SHEATH TRACHEA

Key Facts

Terminology

- Abnormal configuration of intrathoracic trachea in which coronal dimension is ≤ 2/3 of sagittal dimension

Imaging

- Best diagnostic clue: Side-to-side narrowing of intrathoracic trachea
- Frontal chest radiograph: Narrowing of coronal diameter of intrathoracic trachea
- Lateral chest radiograph: Widening of sagittal diameter of intrathoracic trachea
- Frontal tracheal diameter (FTD)/lateral tracheal diameter (LTD) < 2/3
  - Specificity: 95%; sensitivity: < 10%
- CT: Side-to-side narrowing of intrathoracic trachea
  - Inward bowing of lateral tracheal walls during expiration or Valsalva maneuver

Top Differential Diagnoses

- Tracheal stenosis
- Tracheobronchomalacia
- Tracheobronchomegaly
- Diffuse tracheal narrowing

Pathology

- Most commonly associated with emphysema, COPD

Clinical Issues

- Prognosis depends on severity of narrowing and tracheomalacia
- Treatment directed at emphysema
- Tracheal stenting & surgery uncommon

Diagnostic Checklist

- Consider saber-sheath trachea in smokers with characteristic tracheal deformity on imaging

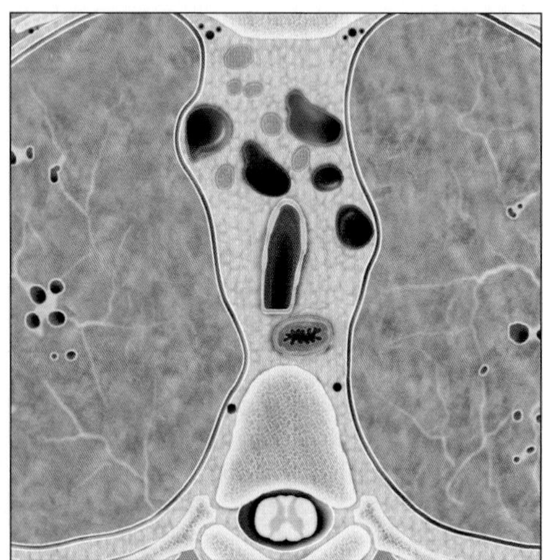

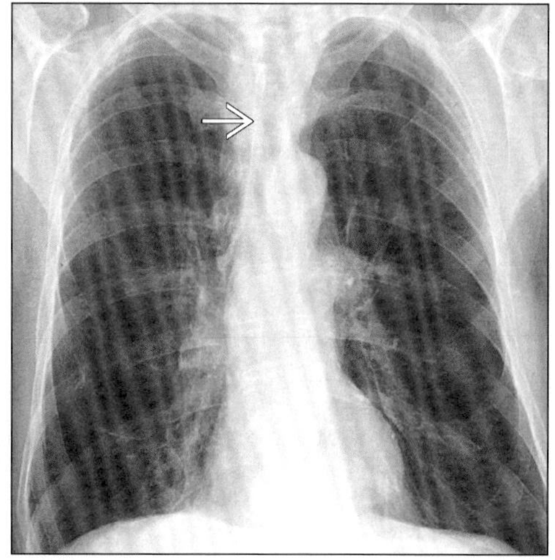

(Left) *Graphic shows an abnormal configuration of the intrathoracic trachea, with narrowing of its coronal diameter and widening of its sagittal diameter. The shape and configuration are characteristic findings of saber-sheath trachea.* ***(Right)*** *PA chest radiograph demonstrates side-to-side narrowing of the intrathoracic trachea ➔. Note hyperexpansion and hyperlucency of the lungs in this patient with emphysema and clinical features of chronic obstructive pulmonary disease (COPD).*

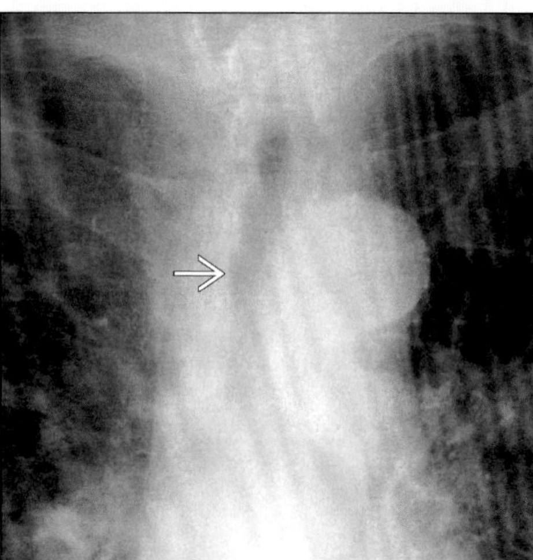

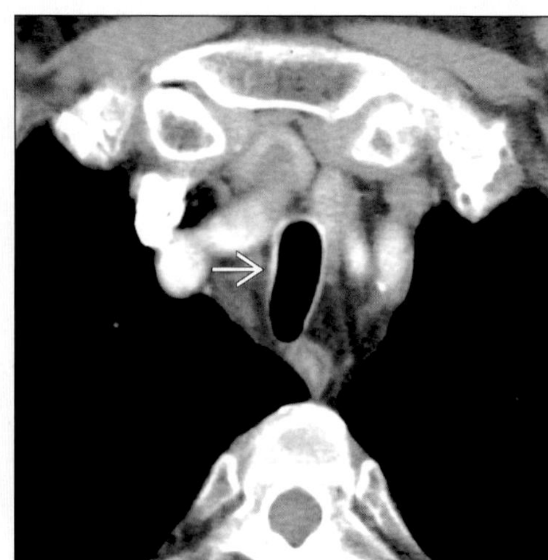

(Left) *Coned-down PA chest radiograph demonstrates narrowing of the coronal diameter of the intrathoracic trachea ➔ resulting in a characteristic "saber-sheath" configuration.* ***(Right)*** *Axial CECT of the same patient shows side-to-side narrowing of the intrathoracic trachea ➔. Inward bowing of the lateral tracheal walls may be seen during expiration or with the Valsalva maneuver in patients with saber-sheath trachea.*

SABER-SHEATH TRACHEA

TERMINOLOGY

Definitions

- Abnormal configuration of intrathoracic trachea in which coronal dimension is ≤ 2/3 of sagittal dimension

IMAGING

General Features

- Best diagnostic clue
  - Side-to-side narrowing of intrathoracic trachea that occurs abruptly at thoracic inlet
- Location
  - Intrathoracic trachea
    - Early: Trachea at thoracic inlet
    - Late: Entire intrathoracic trachea
  - Mainstem bronchi & extrathoracic trachea are normal
- Size
  - Normal tracheal dimensions
    - Sagittal diameter: 13-27 mm in men & 10-23 mm in women
    - Coronal diameter: 13-25 mm in men & 10-21 mm in women
  - **Saber-sheath trachea**
    - Coronal & sagittal diameters < 13 mm in men & < 10 mm in women
    - Frontal tracheal diameter (FTD)/lateral tracheal diameter (LTD) < 2/3

Radiographic Findings

- Frontal chest radiograph: Narrowing of coronal diameter of intrathoracic trachea
- Lateral chest radiograph: Widening of sagittal diameter of intrathoracic trachea
- FTD/LTD < 2/3
  - Specificity for emphysema: 95%
  - Sensitivity for emphysema: < 10%

CT Findings

- Side-to-side narrowing of intrathoracic trachea
- Inward bowing of lateral tracheal walls during expiration or Valsalva maneuver

Imaging Recommendations

- Best imaging tool
  - CT with multiplanar reformatted images
- Protocol advice
  - CT during forced expiration or Valsalva maneuver

DIFFERENTIAL DIAGNOSIS

Tracheal Stenosis

- Segmental narrowing of intrathoracic trachea on expiratory CT

Tracheobronchomalacia

- Weakness of central airway walls
- At least 70% tracheal collapse on expiratory CT

Tracheobronchomegaly

- a.k.a. Mounier-Kuhn syndrome
- Marked dilation of trachea & mainstem bronchi

Diffuse Tracheal Narrowing

- Infection: Bacterial, fungal, & viral organisms
- Tracheobronchopathia osteochondroplastica
  - Osteocartilaginous lesions in anterior & lateral tracheal walls; posterior wall spared
- Wegener granulomatosis
  - Involves upper & lower respiratory tracts
- Amyloidosis
  - Submucosal nodules or masses involving any portion of tracheal wall
- Relapsing polychondritis
  - Rare autoimmune connective tissue disorder
  - Inflammation & destruction of cartilaginous tissue
- Sarcoidosis
  - Intraluminal granulomatous lesions
  - Extrinsic compression from nodes or fibrosis

PATHOLOGY

General Features

- Etiology
  - Restricted dimensions of paratracheal mediastinum due to retained air in upper lobes
  - Calcification of cartilaginous rings secondary to injury from chronic coughing
- Associated abnormalities
  - Most commonly associated with emphysema
  - Tracheobronchopathia osteochondroplastica less commonly

Gross Pathologic & Surgical Features

- Deformity of tracheal cartilage results in narrowing
- Calcification of cartilaginous rings

CLINICAL ISSUES

Presentation

- Most common signs/symptoms
  - Dyspnea, shortness of breath, & chronic cough

Demographics

- Age
  - Older patients (> 50 years) with emphysema

Natural History & Prognosis

- Depends on severity of narrowing & tracheomalacia

Treatment

- Directed at emphysema
- Tracheal stenting & surgery uncommon

DIAGNOSTIC CHECKLIST

Consider

- Saber-sheath trachea in smokers with characteristic tracheal deformity on imaging

SELECTED REFERENCES

1. Stark P et al: Imaging of the trachea and upper airways in patients with chronic obstructive airway disease. Radiol Clin North Am. 36(1):91-105, 1998
2. Trigaux JP et al: CT of saber-sheath trachea. Correlation with clinical, chest radiographic and functional findings. Acta Radiol. 35(3):247-50, 1994

TRACHEAL STENOSIS

Key Facts

Terminology
- Focal or diffuse tracheal narrowing

Imaging
- Radiography
  - Focal or diffuse narrowing of tracheal air column
- CT
  - Stenosis involving tracheal cartilage & membranous posterior wall
  - Expiratory imaging may show associated malacia
  - Evaluation for extrinsic compression
  - Multiplanar reformations, volume rendering, & virtual bronchoscopy possible
- MR
  - Particularly useful in pediatric patients
  - Identification & characterization of adjacent soft tissue masses & vasculature

Top Differential Diagnoses
- Idiopathic tracheal stenosis
- Tracheal neoplasms
- Iatrogenic tracheal stenosis
- Saber-sheath trachea
- Infectious/inflammatory tracheal stenosis

Clinical Issues
- May mimic chronic obstructive physiology

Diagnostic Checklist
- Look for associated soft tissue component & associated lymphadenopathy
- Include larynx in evaluation for subglottic stenosis
- Classification systems typically rely on location, severity, & transition of stenosis

*(**Left**) PA chest radiograph of a 51-year-old man with post-intubation tracheal stenosis shows focal, short segment stenosis of the upper tracheal air column ➔. (**Right**) Composite image with coronal NECT (left) and coronal volume-rendered CT reformation (right) of the same patient shows focal tracheal stenosis with characteristic hourglass shape. Location, severity, and transition margins of tracheal stenosis are important descriptors for classification and clinical management.*

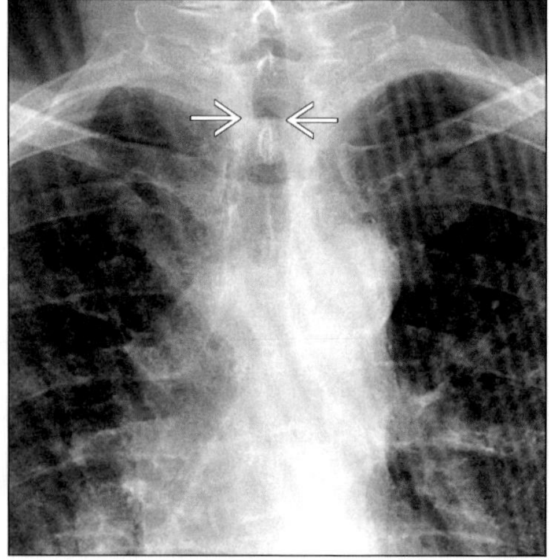

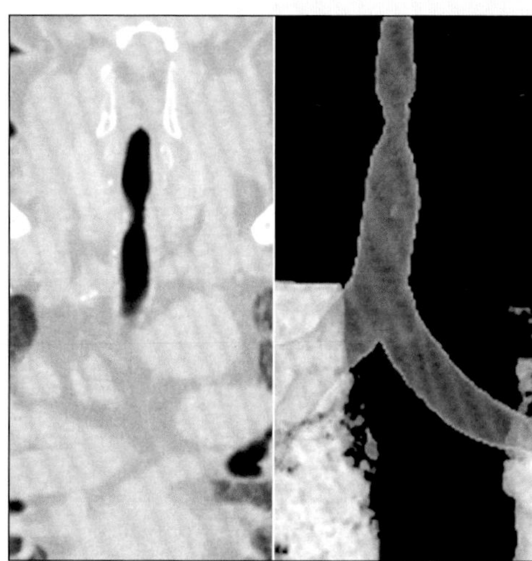

*(**Left**) Composite image with PA chest radiograph (left) and axial CECT (right) of a 67-year-old man with relapsing polychondritis shows diffuse, severe tracheal narrowing. Expiratory phase imaging may be important to evaluate for associated tracheomalacia. (**Right**) Coronal volume-rendered CT reformation of a patient with pulmonary sling shows distal tracheal narrowing and a tracheal bronchus ➔. CECT may be helpful in identifying vascular compression or evaluating the vascular anatomy in preparation for surgery.*

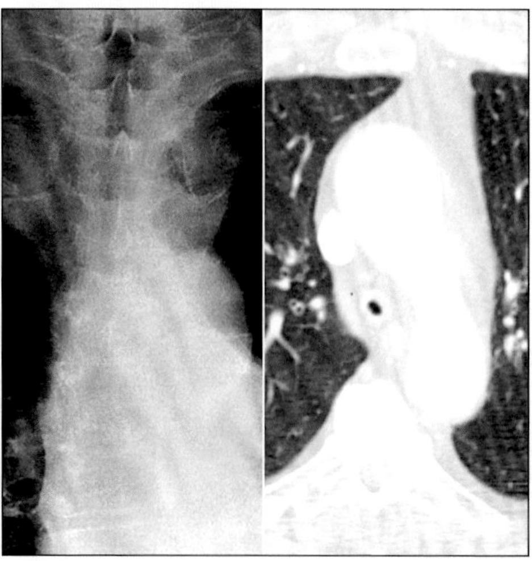

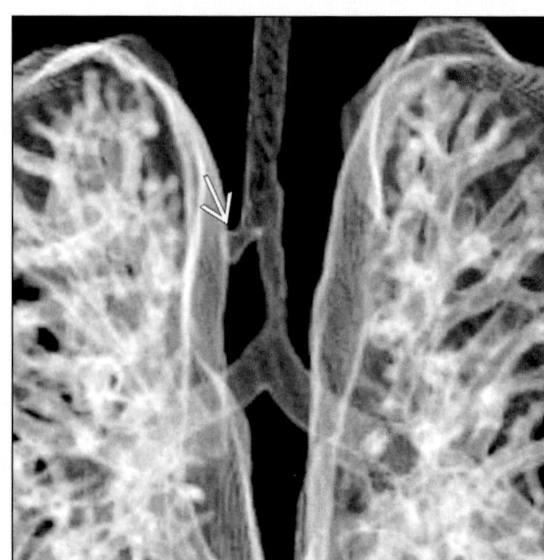

TRACHEAL STENOSIS

TERMINOLOGY

Definitions

- Focal or diffuse tracheal narrowing

IMAGING

General Features

- Best diagnostic clue
  - Tracheal narrowing relative to proximal/distal segment
- Location
  - Upper, mid, &/or lower 1/3 of trachea
- Morphology
  - Post-intubation stenosis hourglass-shaped

Radiographic Findings

- Focal or diffuse narrowing of tracheal air column
- Tracheal cartilage rings may be visible if calcified

CT Findings

- Stenosis involving tracheal cartilage & membranous posterior wall
- Evaluation for extrinsic compression
- Multiplanar reformations, volume rendering, & virtual bronchoscopy

MR Findings

- Particularly useful in pediatric patients
- Identification & characterization of adjacent soft tissue masses & vasculature

Imaging Recommendations

- Best imaging tool
  - CT with multiplanar reformations provides fine anatomic detail & allows evaluation of extent of stenosis
- Protocol advice
  - Expiratory imaging may show associated malacia
  - Inclusion of larynx to evaluate for subglottic narrowing
  - CECT may help identify vascular compression

DIFFERENTIAL DIAGNOSIS

Tracheal Neoplasms

- Benign: Tracheobronchial papillomatosis, carcinoid
- Malignant: Squamous cell carcinoma, adenoid cystic carcinoma, mucoepidermoid carcinoma
- Secondary involvement from lung, esophageal, thyroid cancers
- Typically eccentric, ± lymphadenopathy

Idiopathic Tracheal Stenosis

- Smooth, tapered narrowing, 2-4 cm long
- Typically subglottic

Iatrogenic Tracheal Stenosis

- Post-intubation or tracheostomy
- Typically short segment, proximal, concentric
- Edema & granulation tissue cause acute stenosis
- Fibrosis & tracheal deformity in chronic stenosis
- Typically affects middle-aged females

Congenital Tracheal Stenosis

- Vascular abnormalities cause characteristic patterns of tracheal narrowing
- Associated with ring-shaped tracheal cartilages

Tracheobronchomalacia

- Expiratory tracheal collapse
- Diffuse or focal

Saber-Sheath Trachea

- Most common in males with COPD
- Coronal diameter narrowing starts at thoracic inlet

Infectious/Inflammatory Tracheal Stenosis

- Viral, fungal, bacterial etiologies
  - Tuberculous tracheal stenosis
    - Granulomatous involvement of tracheal wall
    - Extrinsic compression from lymphadenopathy
- Pulmonary Wegener granulomatosis, ulcerative colitis, sarcoidosis, amyloidosis
- Tracheobronchopathia osteochondroplastica, relapsing polychondritis

PATHOLOGY

Staging, Grading, & Classification

- Trachea divided into upper, mid, & lower 1/3
- Degree of cross-sectional narrowing reported
  - ≤ 25%, 26-50%, 51-75%, 75-90%, > 90%
- Transition (abrupt or tapered) clinically relevant

Gross Pathologic & Surgical Features

- Tracheal cartilage &/or membranous portion involved
- Hyperplastic & fibrostenotic stages in tuberculosis

CLINICAL ISSUES

Presentation

- Most common signs/symptoms
  - Progressive dyspnea, cough
  - Wheezing, stridor, hoarseness
- Other signs/symptoms
  - May mimic chronic obstructive physiology

Treatment

- Dilatation ± stenting for unresectable disease
- Resection & end-to-end anastomosis in surgical cases
- Endobronchial brachytherapy

DIAGNOSTIC CHECKLIST

Image Interpretation Pearls

- Look for associated soft tissue component & associated lymphadenopathy
- Include larynx in evaluation for subglottic stenosis

Reporting Tips

- Classification systems typically rely on location, severity, & transition of stenosis

SELECTED REFERENCES

1. Grenier PA et al: Nonneoplastic tracheal and bronchial stenoses. Thorac Surg Clin. 20(1):47-64, 2010

TRACHEOBRONCHOMALACIA

Key Facts

Terminology
- Increased compliance & excessive collapsibility of trachea or bronchi

Imaging
- Fluoroscopy
  - Diagnosis based upon > 50% decrease in airway lumen during expiration or coughing
- CT
  - Paired inspiratory-dynamic expiratory CT
  - Malacia defined as > 70% decrease in cross-sectional area with expiration
  - Most common finding during dynamic expiration: Tracheal collapse with crescentic bowing of posterior membranous trachea ("frown" sign)
  - Coughing is most sensitive method for eliciting tracheal collapse

Top Differential Diagnoses
- Chronic obstructive pulmonary disease
- Tracheal stenosis
- Relapsing polychondritis
- Longstanding extrinsic compression
- Radiation

Pathology
- Weakening of cartilage &/or hypotonia of posterior membranous trachea with degeneration & atrophy of longitudinal elastic fibers

Clinical Issues
- Intractable cough, dyspnea, wheezing, recurrent respiratory infections
- Underdiagnosed condition
- Acquired form relatively common in adults, incidence increases with advancing age

__(Left)__ Axial NECT during full inspiration shows normal tracheal diameter. The posterior wall of the trachea (composed mainly of the trachealis muscle) bows outward ⇒, which indicates that this is an inspiratory image. __(Right)__ At full expiration there is severe narrowing of the trachea ➡ in a "frown" sign (crescentic narrowing of tracheal lumen that resembles a frown) configuration, which is highly suggestive of tracheomalacia. Inspiratory CT is insensitive for the detection of tracheomalacia.

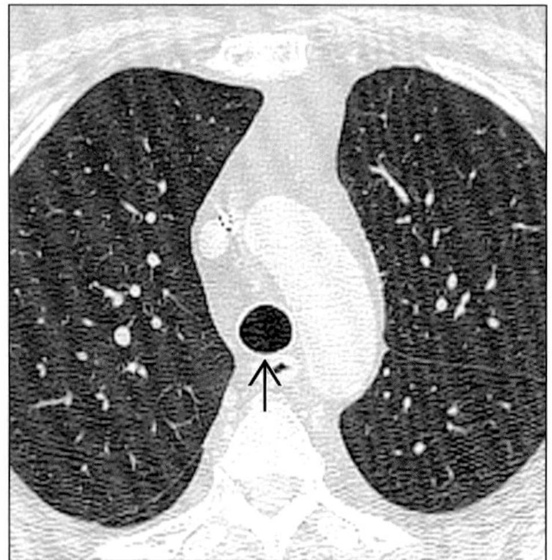

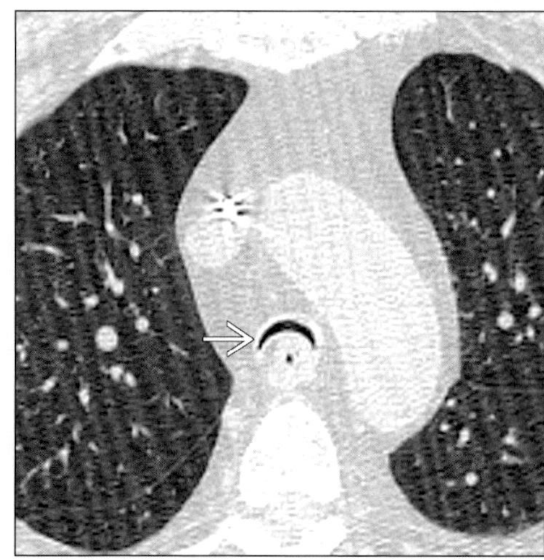

__(Left)__ Axial NECT during expiration shows a normal extrathoracic trachea. __(Right)__ Axial NECT of the same patient obtained during expiration shows marked expiratory tracheal narrowing ➡, which is highly suggestive of tracheomalacia. The extrathoracic trachea is not affected by pressure changes from respiration.

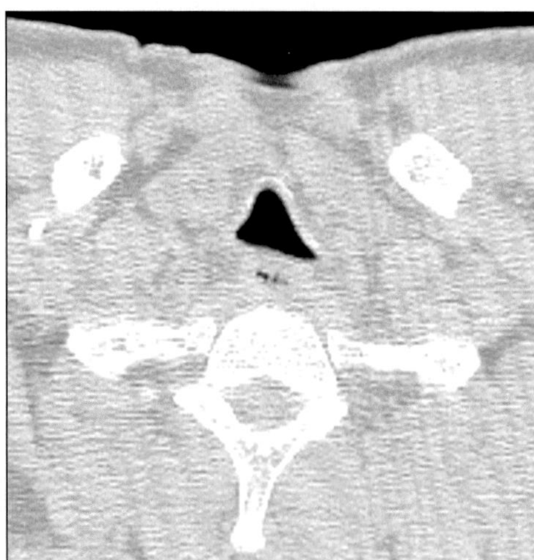

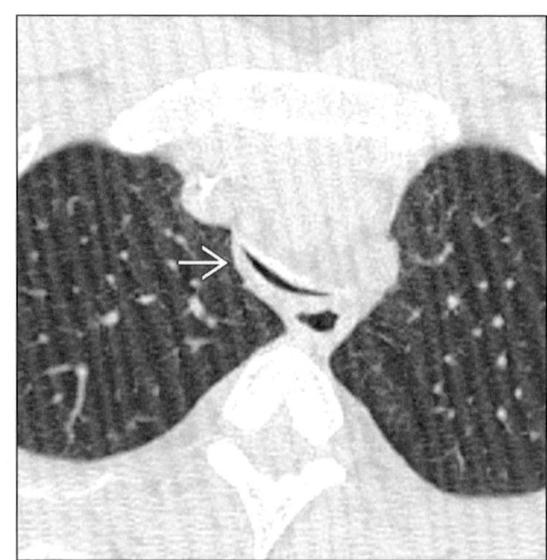

TRACHEOBRONCHOMALACIA

TERMINOLOGY

Synonyms

- **Tracheomalacia, bronchomalacia**

Definitions

- Increased compliance & excessive collapsibility of trachea or bronchi

IMAGING

General Features

- Best diagnostic clue
  - **"Frown" sign during expiration (crescentic narrowing of tracheal lumen that resembles frown)**
- Location
  - Diffuse
    - May involve entire trachea &/or bronchi
  - Focal
    - May be seen following intubation, in conjunction with focal stenosis, or at site of longstanding compression
- Size
  - At end-inspiration, tracheal lumen may be normal in size, widened in coronal (lunate trachea) or sagittal (saber sheath trachea) diameter, or focally narrowed (malacia may accompany focal stenosis)
  - **> 70% reduction in airway lumen at expiration is diagnostic**
- Morphology
  - Intrathoracic trachea: Collapse with expiration due to positive extratracheal pressures
  - Extrathoracic trachea: Collapse with inspiration due to negative intratracheal pressures

Radiographic Findings

- Radiography
  - Usually escapes detection on routine, end-inspiratory radiography

Fluoroscopic Findings

- Chest fluoroscopy
  - Cine fluoroscopy historically used to evaluate tracheal wall mobility between inspiration & forced expiration or during coughing
  - Diagnosis based upon > 50% decrease in airway lumen during expiration or coughing
  - Limitations: Subjective interpretation; operator-dependent; inability to simultaneously evaluate anteroposterior & lateral tracheal walls; limited visualization of tracheal anatomy & adjacent mediastinal structures

CT Findings

- NECT
  - Paired inspiratory-dynamic expiratory CT
    - Inspiratory CT provides comprehensive assessment of airway anatomy
    - Dynamic expiratory CT provides assessment of central airway collapse during 1 helical acquisition
    - **Malacia defined as > 70% decrease in cross-sectional area with expiration**
    - Most common finding during dynamic expiration: **Tracheal collapse with crescentic bowing of posterior membranous trachea ("frown" sign)**
    - Multiplanar & 3D reformations not required for diagnosis, but help display extent of disease
  - Cine CT during coughing
    - Coughing most sensitive method for eliciting tracheal collapse
    - Can be performed with electron beam CT or multidetector row CT
    - Requires multiple acquisitions to cover entire central airways

MR Findings

- 50-100 msec imaging time allows cine evaluation of tracheal collapse during coughing
- Only limited data in the literature using this technique

Imaging Recommendations

- Best imaging tool
  - Paired inspiratory-dynamic expiratory helical CT imaging
- Protocol advice
  - Helical CT with 2.5 or 3.0 mm collimation
    - 50% overlapping reconstruction intervals for multiplanar reformations & 3D reconstructions
  - Perform at suspended inspiration & during dynamic, forced exhalation
    - Forced exhalation elicits greater collapse than end-expiration
  - Dynamic expiratory portion of scan can be performed with low-dose (40 mAs) technique to reduce radiation exposure

DIFFERENTIAL DIAGNOSIS

Chronic Obstructive Pulmonary Disease (COPD)

- Emphysema
- Saber-sheath trachea

Tracheal Stenosis

- Post-intubation tracheal stenosis

Relapsing Polychondritis

- Look for wall thickening ± calcification that spares posterior membranous wall

Longstanding Extrinsic Compression

- Mass adjacent to trachea
  - Thyroid
  - Ectatic/anomalous vasculature

Radiation

- Geographically marginated fibrosis in paramediastinal region with traction bronchiectasis

Mounier-Kuhn Syndrome

- Tracheobronchomegaly

PATHOLOGY

General Features

- Etiology
  - **Primary tracheomalacia: Congenital weakness**
    - Abnormal cartilaginous matrix (chondromalacia, mucopolysaccharidoses, such as Hurler syndrome)

- Inadequate maturity of cartilage (e.g., premature infants)
- Congenital tracheoesophageal fistula
- Mounier-Kuhn syndrome (congenital tracheobronchomegaly)
- **Secondary (acquired) tracheobronchomalacia**
  - Chronic obstructive pulmonary disease
  - Prior intubation (endotracheal tube or tracheostomy tube)
  - Prior surgery (e.g., lung resection, lung transplantation)
  - Radiation therapy
  - Longstanding extrinsic compression (e.g., thyroid mass, vascular ring, aneurysm)
  - Chronic inflammation (e.g., relapsing polychondritis)
  - Tracheoesophageal fistula
  - Idiopathic
- Associated abnormalities
  - Congenital form often associated with cardiovascular abnormalities, bronchopulmonary dysplasia, & gastroesophageal reflux
- Weakening of cartilage &/or hypotonia of posterior membranous trachea with degeneration & atrophy of longitudinal elastic fibers

CLINICAL ISSUES

Presentation

- Most common signs/symptoms
  - Intractable cough, dyspnea, wheezing, recurrent respiratory infections
  - Congenital form usually manifests in first weeks to months of life with expiratory stridor, cough, & difficulty feeding
- Underdiagnosed condition
- **Patients often misdiagnosed as having asthma**
  - If imaging requisition states asthma, always look for tracheal stenosis, tracheal mass, or malacia
- Rarely, hypoventilation, hypoxemia, hypercarbia, pulmonary artery hypertension, cor pulmonale
- Inspiratory wheeze if lesion extrathoracic; expiratory wheeze if lesion intrathoracic
- Post-intubation: Symptoms may appear several weeks to years after intubation
- Bronchoscopic findings in tracheomalacia
  - > 50% narrowing of lumen in AP diameter (normal: < 40%)
  - In children, expiratory-inspiratory cross-sectional area ratio < 0.35 (normal: 0.82)

Demographics

- Age
  - Neonates to elderly
- Gender
  - Acquired form has male predominance
- Epidemiology
  - Congenital form more common in premature infants
  - Acquired form relatively common in adults, incidence increases with advancing age
  - 5-23% of patients undergoing bronchoscopy for respiratory symptoms
  - 5-10% of patients referred to pulmonologists for chronic cough
  - 10% of patients referred for CTA for suspected pulmonary embolism
  - Up to 20% of autopsies

Natural History & Prognosis

- Acquired form usually progressive over time without therapy
- Congenital form sometimes self-limited (especially in premature infants with malacia due to immature cartilage)

Treatment

- Conservative therapy for mildly symptomatic patients
- Nasal continuous positive airway pressure can help to relieve nocturnal symptoms
- Silicone stents for severely symptomatic patients who are poor surgical candidates
- Surgical repair with tracheoplasty procedure for severely symptomatic patients with diffuse malacia
  - Goals are to remodel trachea & increase its rigidity by placing Marlex graft along posterior wall
- Surgical repair with aortopexy procedure when due to longstanding extrinsic compression by vascular lesion
  - Mechanical fixation of trachea releases compression & widens anteroposterior dimension of trachea

DIAGNOSTIC CHECKLIST

Image Interpretation Pearls

- Recognize characteristics of expiratory CT scan to ensure that expiratory component of scan is diagnostic
  - Increased lung attenuation
  - Decreased anteroposterior dimension of thorax
  - Posterior wall of trachea should be flat or bowed forward
- Malacia defined on basis of percentage change in tracheal lumen between inspiration & expiration
  - If either component of the scan is not performed during appropriate phase of respiration, diagnostic errors may occur
  - Coaching patient with careful breathing instructions necessary to ensure diagnostic study

SELECTED REFERENCES

1. Ridge CA et al: Tracheobronchomalacia: Current Concepts and Controversies. J Thorac Imaging. 26(4):278-289, 2011
2. Javidan-Nejad C: MDCT of trachea and main bronchi. Radiol Clin North Am. 48(1):157-76, 2010
3. Lee KS et al: Update on multidetector computed tomography imaging of the airways. J Thorac Imaging. 25(2):112-24, 2010
4. Sverzellati N et al: Airway malacia in chronic obstructive pulmonary disease: prevalence, morphology and relationship with emphysema, bronchiectasis and bronchial wall thickening. Eur Radiol. 19(7):1669-78, 2009
5. Boiselle PM et al: Tracheal morphology in patients with tracheomalacia: prevalence of inspiratory lunate and expiratory "frown" shapes. J Thorac Imaging. 21(3):190-6, 2006

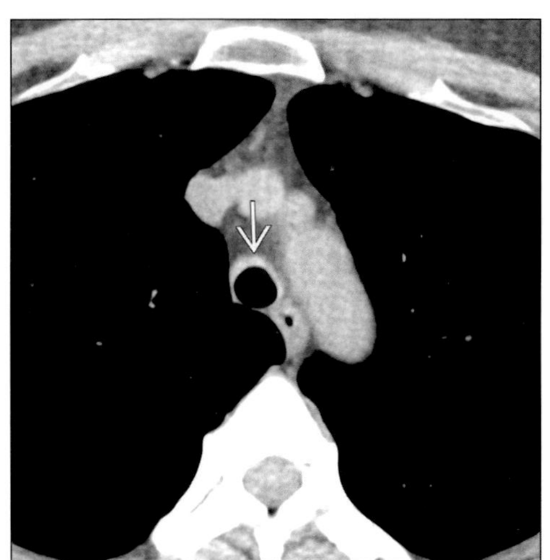

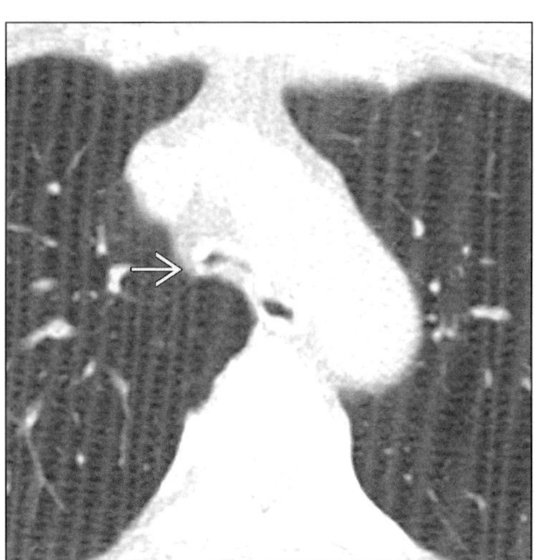

(Left) *Axial NECT shows thickening ➔ of the anterior wall of the trachea in this patient with relapsing polychondritis. As is typical in cases of relapsing polychondritis, the posterior wall of the trachea is spared because there is no cartilage in this portion of the airway.* ***(Right)*** *Axial NECT of the same patient obtained during expiration shows marked collapse of the trachea ➔, highly suggestive of tracheomalacia. Relapsing polychondritis is a well-described cause of tracheobronchomalacia.*

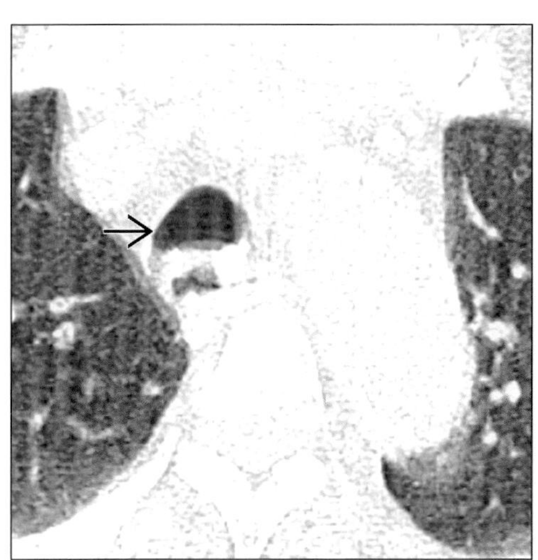

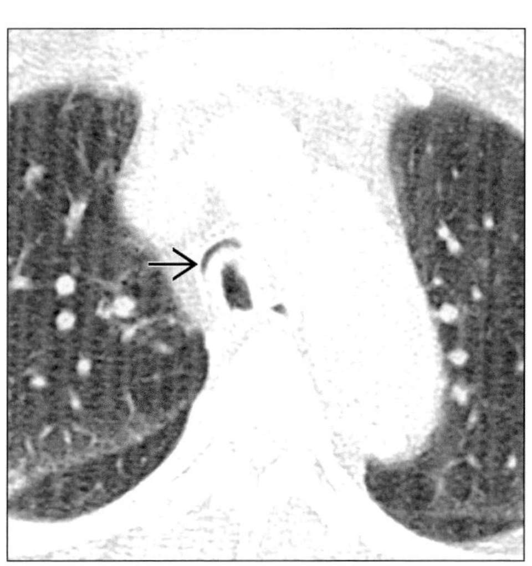

(Left) *Axial NECT during end-expiration shows normal caliber of the trachea ➔.* ***(Right)*** *Axial NECT of the same patient obtained during dynamic expiration shows severe collapse of the trachea with anterior bowing of the posterior wall ➔, highly consistent with tracheomalacia. Dynamic expiratory CT is more sensitive than end-expiratory CT in the detection of tracheobronchomalacia.*

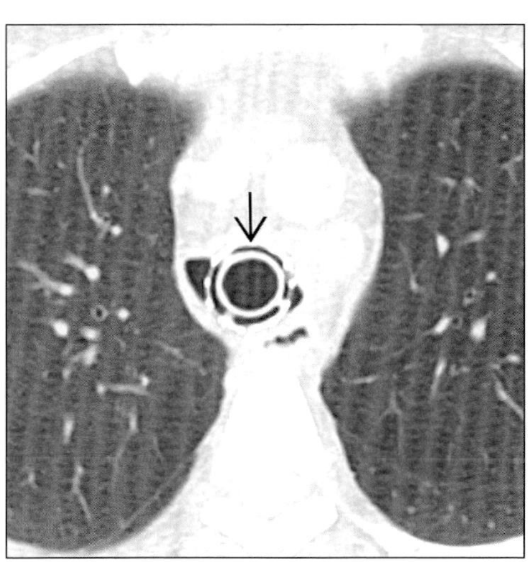

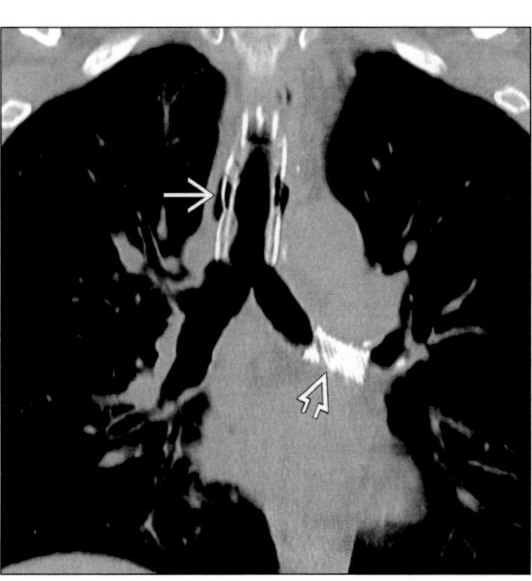

(Left) *Axial NECT of a patient with a history of tracheobronchomalacia shows a stent ➔ placed for treatment of a lunate-shaped trachea.* ***(Right)*** *Coronal NECT of the same patient shows stents ➔ in the trachea and left mainstem bronchus ➔ for treatment of tracheobronchomalacia. Stents are most useful for symptomatic improvement of patients with tracheobronchomalacia when surgery is contraindicated or refused by the patient.*

MIDDLE LOBE SYNDROME

Key Facts

Terminology
- Chronic or recurrent nonobstructive middle lobe atelectasis

Imaging
- Radiography
  - Focal opacity obscuring right heart border
  - Wedge-shaped opacity on lateral radiography, sharply marginated by major & minor fissures
  - ± air bronchograms
- CT
  - Atelectatic middle lobe
  - Bronchiectasis
  - Patent middle lobe bronchus; no endobronchial lesion
  - Pleural thickening
  - ± surrounding calcified lymph nodes or lung nodules related to prior granulomatous infection

Top Differential Diagnoses
- Bacterial pneumonia
- Nontuberculous mycobacterial infection
- Endobronchial tumor

Pathology
- Chronic inflammation with lung destruction & fibrosis
- ± bronchial compression by adjacent enlarged lymph nodes

Clinical Issues
- Symptoms: Cough, hemoptysis, recurrent pneumonia
- Treatment: Bronchoscopic intervention, lobectomy

Diagnostic Checklist
- Consider CT for evaluation of patients with chronic middle lobe atelectasis to exclude endoluminal tumor

*(**Left**) PA chest radiograph of a woman with cough and hemoptysis shows airspace opacity obscuring the right heart border with inferior displacement of the minor fissure ➡, consistent with middle lobe atelectasis. (**Right**) Lateral chest radiograph of the same patient shows a middle lobe opacity sharply marginated by an inferiorly displaced minor fissure ➡ and an anteriorly displaced major fissure ➡. The findings are consistent with middle lobe volume loss.*

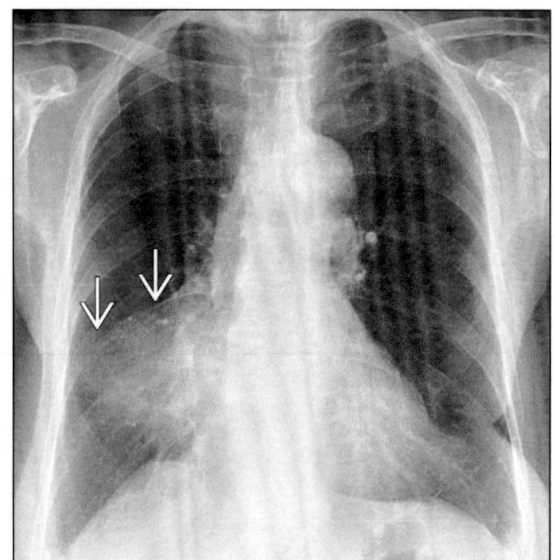

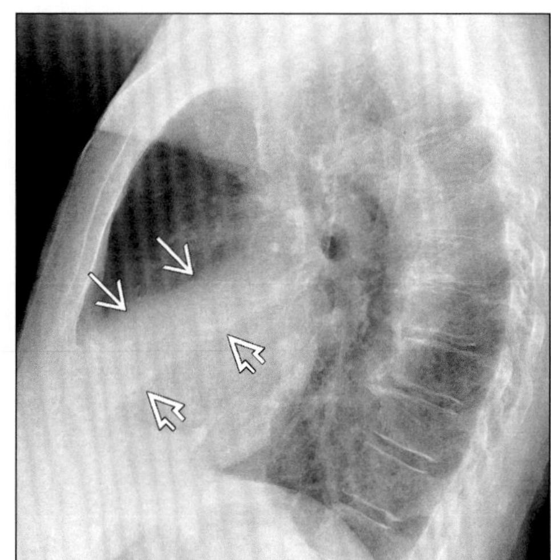

*(**Left**) Axial CECT of the same patient confirms middle lobe atelectasis with internal fluid attenuation branching opacities, consistent with mucus plugging ➡. Lobectomy specimen showed chronic inflammation, bronchiectasis, and fibrosis, consistent with middle lobe syndrome. (**Right**) Axial CECT of a patient with recurrent pneumonia shows an atelectatic middle lobe with patent bronchiectatic airways, consistent with middle lobe syndrome. No endobronchial lesion was found on CT or bronchoscopy.*

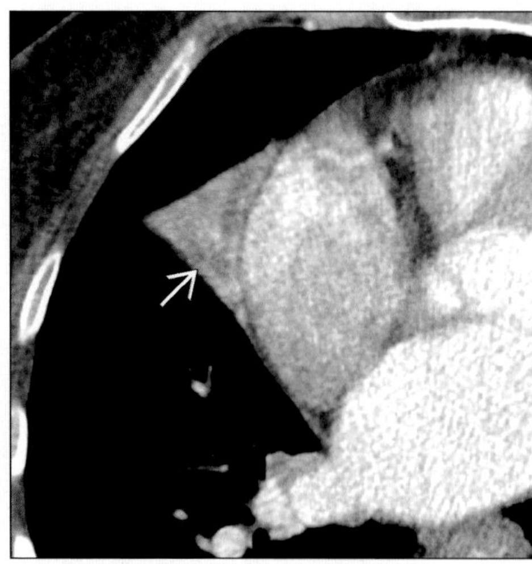

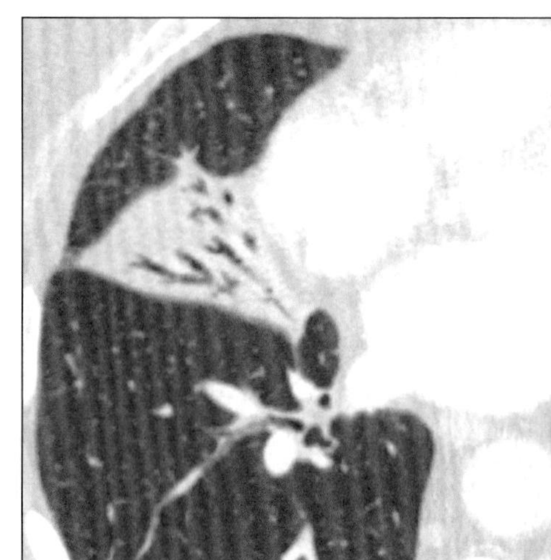

MIDDLE LOBE SYNDROME

TERMINOLOGY

Synonyms

- **Right middle lobe syndrome**

Definitions

- Chronic or recurrent nonobstructive middle lobe atelectasis

IMAGING

General Features

- Best diagnostic clue
  - Chronic middle lobe atelectasis or opacification
- Location
  - Middle lobe most commonly affected, followed by lingula

Radiographic Findings

- Radiography
  - **Focal opacity obscuring right heart border**
  - Wedge-shaped opacity on lateral chest radiograph, sharply marginated by major & minor fissures
  - ± air bronchograms

CT Findings

- **Atelectatic middle lobe**
  - Triangular opacity bound by major fissure posteriorly & minor fissure anteriorly
- **Bronchiectasis**
  - Hypodense branching opacities: Mucus plugs or air within bronchiectatic airways
- Patent middle lobe bronchus; no endobronchial lesion
- Pleural thickening
- ± surrounding calcified lymph nodes or lung nodules related to prior granulomatous infection

Imaging Recommendations

- Best imaging tool
  - CT is optimal imaging modality to evaluate bronchiectasis & endobronchial obstruction

DIFFERENTIAL DIAGNOSIS

Bacterial Pneumonia

- Acute illness, should resolve in 4-6 weeks

Nontuberculous Mycobacterial Infection

- Typically elderly women
- Bronchiectasis of middle lobe, lingula, or both
- Scattered nodules & tree-in-bud opacities
- May be a cause of middle lobe syndrome

Endobronchial Tumor

- Can cause middle lobe atelectasis & postobstructive pneumonia
- Bronchoscopy for evaluation of endobronchial tumor

Cystic Fibrosis

- Chronic mucus plugging may produce chronic middle lobe or lingular atelectasis
- Bronchiectasis & bronchial wall thickening, usually involves other lobes

Pectus Excavatum Deformity

- Vague middle lobe opacity on frontal radiography
- Lateral radiograph shows characteristic depression of sternum & no middle lobe airspace disease

PATHOLOGY

General Features

- Etiology
  - Chronic inflammatory process with lung destruction & fibrosis
  - Complete fissures prevent collateral ventilation with impaired clearing of secretions
  - ± bronchial compression by adjacent enlarged lymph nodes
  - Reported association with
    - Tuberculosis & atypical mycobacterial infection
    - Fungal infection
    - Sarcoidosis
    - Cystic fibrosis
    - Asthma; allergic bronchopulmonary aspergillosis

Gross Pathologic & Surgical Features

- Combination of bronchiectasis, bronchitis, bronchiolitis, & organizing pneumonia

CLINICAL ISSUES

Presentation

- Most common signs/symptoms
  - Chronic cough, hemoptysis
  - Recurrent pulmonary infection
- Other signs/symptoms
  - Dyspnea, chest pain, wheezing

Demographics

- Age
  - Any age
- Gender
  - F > M

Diagnosis

- CT for evaluation of bronchi to exclude endobronchial tumor
- Bronchoscopy to evaluate bronchial stenosis & exclude endobronchial tumor

Treatment

- Long-term antibiotics
- Balloon dilatation, stent placement, or laser therapy for focal stenosis
- Surgical lobectomy for recurrent pneumonia & failed medical management

DIAGNOSTIC CHECKLIST

Consider

- CT for evaluation of patients with chronic middle lobe atelectasis to exclude endoluminal tumor

SELECTED REFERENCES

1. Gudmundsson G et al: Middle lobe syndrome. Am Fam Physician. 53(8):2547-50, 1996

AIRWAY WEGENER GRANULOMATOSIS

Key Facts

Terminology
- Wegener granulomatosis (WG)
- Granulomatous polyangiitis, granulomatosis with polyangiitis (newly accepted name for WG)
- Multisystem necrotizing granulomatous small to medium vessel vasculitis

Imaging
- Radiography
  - Subglottic stenosis often visible, but overlooked
  - Segmental or lobar atelectasis from peripheral airway stenosis
- CT: Optimal modality for evaluation of airways
  - Trachea & bronchi concentrically thickened
  - Smooth or irregular wall thickening, may be circumferential
  - Focal or long segment stenosis
  - Focal involvement common in subglottic area

Top Differential Diagnoses
- Tuberculosis infection
- Tracheobronchial amyloidosis
- Relapsing polychondritis
- Inflammatory bowel disease

Pathology
- Necrotizing vasculitis of small to medium vessels, necrotizing granulomatosis, & hemorrhage

Clinical Issues
- Symptoms/signs
  - Voice changes & stridor
  - Sinusitis, rhinitis, & otitis media

Diagnostic Checklist
- WG should be strongly considered in patients with airway wall thickening/stenosis with associated lung nodules & glomerulonephritis

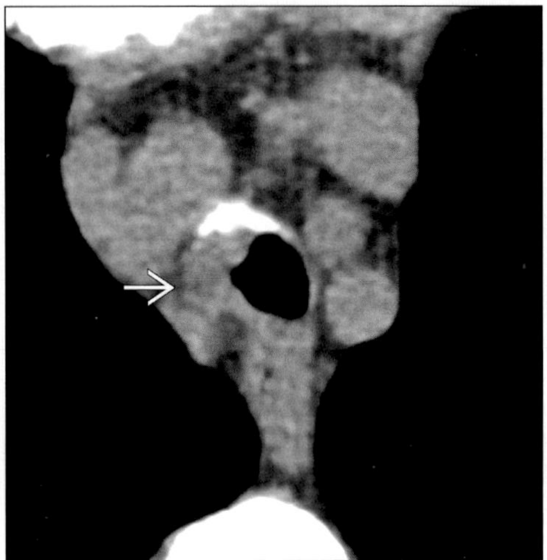
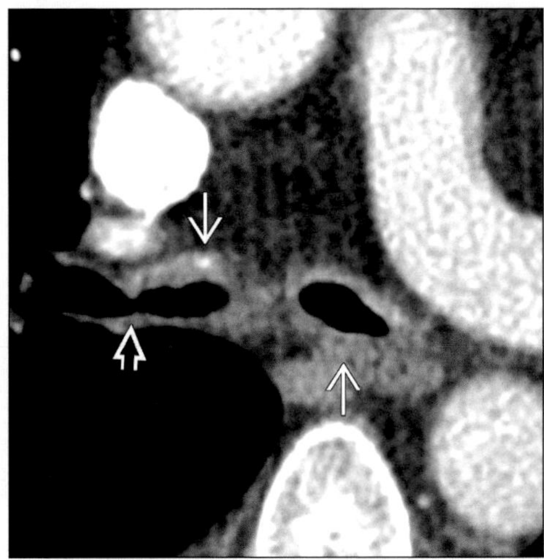

(Left) *Axial NECT shows irregular tracheal wall thickening ➔ with luminal distortion and narrowing. Airway involvement in WG can be focal, as in this patient, or can be more diffuse.* ***(Right)*** *Axial CECT shows circumferential thickening of the walls of the mainstem bronchi ➔, resulting in mild luminal stenosis. Note the more severe focal stenosis ➔ at the origin of the right upper lobe bronchus. Involvement of the posterior membrane helps distinguish WG from relapsing polychondritis.*

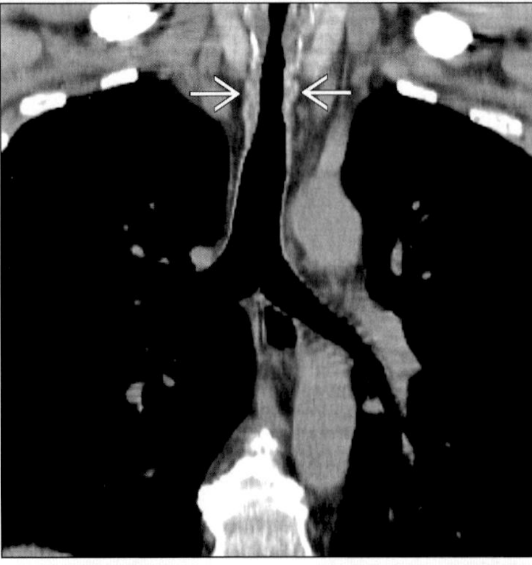
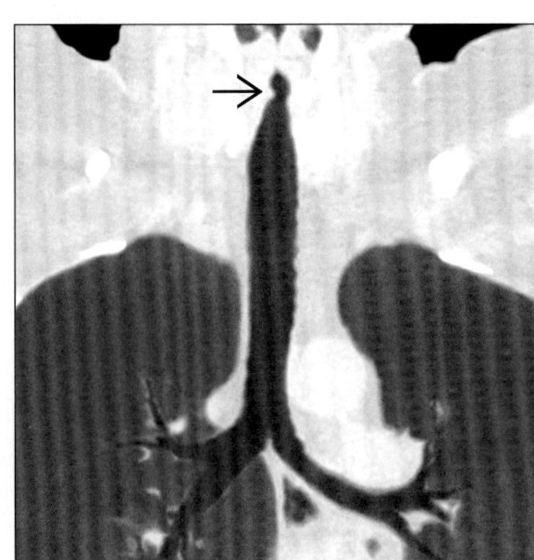

(Left) *Coronal NECT of a patient with WG and airway involvement shows long segment tracheal wall thickening ➔, resulting in mild luminal narrowing.* ***(Right)*** *Coronal CECT minimum-intensity projection (MinIP) image shows focal severe stenosis ➔ of the subglottic trachea. The subglottic trachea is the most common site of lower airway involvement in WG. While usually a later manifestation of the disease, some patients with WG will present with subglottic stenosis as the only manifestation of WG.*

AIRWAY WEGENER GRANULOMATOSIS

TERMINOLOGY

Abbreviations

- **Wegener granulomatosis (WG)**

Synonyms

- Granulomatous polyangiitis, **granulomatosis with polyangiitis** (newly accepted name for WG)

Definitions

- Multisystemic necrotizing granulomatous vasculitis of small to medium vessels without associated infection

IMAGING

General Features

- Best diagnostic clue
  - Large airway narrowing
- Location
  - **Focal airway involvement most common in subglottic area** (20%)
- Morphology
  - Smooth or irregular airway wall thickening
  - May be circumferential, involving posterior membrane

Radiographic Findings

- Peripheral airway stenosis can result in segmental or lobar atelectasis
- Subglottic stenosis often visible, but overlooked on chest radiography

CT Findings

- Trachea & bronchi concentrically thickened, either focal or long segments

Imaging Recommendations

- Best imaging tool
  - CT is optimal imaging modality for evaluation of possible airway involvement
- Protocol advice
  - Thin section unenhanced chest CT for optimal airway imaging
    - Multiplanar reformations particularly useful for evaluating airways
    - Including glottis is helpful because of frequent subglottic involvement

DIFFERENTIAL DIAGNOSIS

Tuberculosis Infection

- Radiographic findings can be indistinguishable
- Diagnosis based on culture or special stains

Tracheobronchial Amyloidosis

- Airway involvement usually diffuse
- Stippled calcifications may be present

Relapsing Polychondritis

- Spares posterior membrane of trachea & central bronchi
- Involvement of extrathoracic cartilage

Inflammatory Bowel Disease

- Airway involvement typically late manifestation
- Biopsy required for diagnosis

CLINICAL ISSUES

Presentation

- Most common signs/symptoms
  - Sinusitis, rhinitis, & otitis media
- Other signs/symptoms
  - Voice changes & stridor
  - Cough, fever, night sweats, dyspnea, wheezing, hemoptysis, & chest pain
- Frequency of systemic involvement during disease course
  - Upper airways (92%), lower airways (85%), kidney (80%), joints (67%), eye (52%), skin (46%), nerve (20%)
- Circulating antineutrophil cytoplasmic antibodies (c-ANCA)
  - In patients with WG, c-ANCA is usually directed against proteinase-3 (PR3), an antigen found in neutrophils
    - 96% sensitive for generalized disease & 83% sensitive for limited disease
  - Positive c-ANCA supports diagnosis, but is neither necessary nor sufficient

Demographics

- Age
  - Any age; mean age at diagnosis 40-55 years
- Gender
  - M = F
  - Airway involvement much more common in women
- Ethnicity
  - 80-97% Caucasian, 2-8% African-American
- Epidemiology
  - Prevalence: 3/100,000 persons in USA

Natural History & Prognosis

- Renal failure: Most common cause of death
- Subglottic stenosis occurs later in course of disease

Treatment

- Systemic involvement
  - Corticosteroids & cyclophosphamide
  - Rituximab
- Less extensive involvement or cyclophosphamide toxicity
  - Corticosteroids and cytotoxic agents
- Tracheobronchial disease may require tracheostomy or stent placement

DIAGNOSTIC CHECKLIST

Image Interpretation Pearls

- WG should be strongly considered in patients with airway wall thickening/stenosis with associated lung nodules & glomerulonephritis

SELECTED REFERENCES

1. Ananthakrishnan L et al: Wegener's granulomatosis in the chest: high-resolution CT findings. AJR Am J Roentgenol. 192(3):676-82, 2009
2. Daum TE et al: Tracheobronchial involvement in Wegener's granulomatosis. Am J Respir Crit Care Med. 151(2 Pt 1):522-6, 1995

TRACHEOBRONCHIAL AMYLOIDOSIS

Key Facts

Terminology
- Focal or diffuse submucosal deposition of amyloid in tracheobronchial tree
  - Characterized by amyloid light chain (AL) protein

Imaging
- Nodular soft tissue thickening of airway wall
  - Multifocal submucosal plaques (most common)
  - May involve posterior tracheal wall
  - Focal airway nodules
  - May exhibit foci of calcification
- May affect larynx, trachea, & central to segmental bronchi
- Obstructive effects
  - Bronchiectasis
  - Atelectasis
  - Consolidation
  - Hyperinflation

Top Differential Diagnoses
- Acquired tracheal stenosis
- Tracheobronchopathia osteochondroplastica
- Wegener granulomatosis
- Relapsing polychondritis
- Tracheal neoplasms

Pathology
- Abnormal protein deposition in submucosal aspects of airway walls

Clinical Issues
- Symptoms/signs (gradual onset over several years)
  - Chronic cough, dyspnea, wheezing, hemoptysis
- Wide age range: 16-85 years (mean: 53 years)
- 5-year survival rates range from 30-50%
- Treatment: Bronchoscopic/surgical resection, radiation therapy for progressive disease

__(Left)__ PA chest radiograph (coned down to the trachea) shows smooth bilateral paratracheal stripe thickening ➔, suggestive of tracheal wall thickening. __(Right)__ Coronal CECT shows diffuse tracheobronchial wall thickening ➔ with foci of significant luminal narrowing ➔ and scattered amorphous calcification ➔ in areas of airway wall thickening. Diffuse, undulating circumferential airway wall thickening with or without calcification is typical of tracheobronchial amyloidosis.

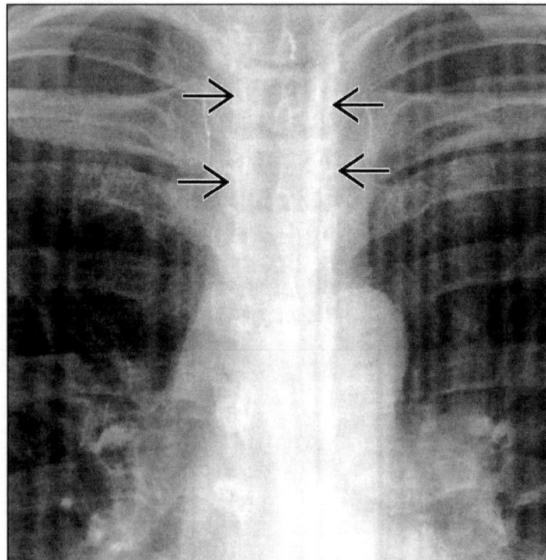

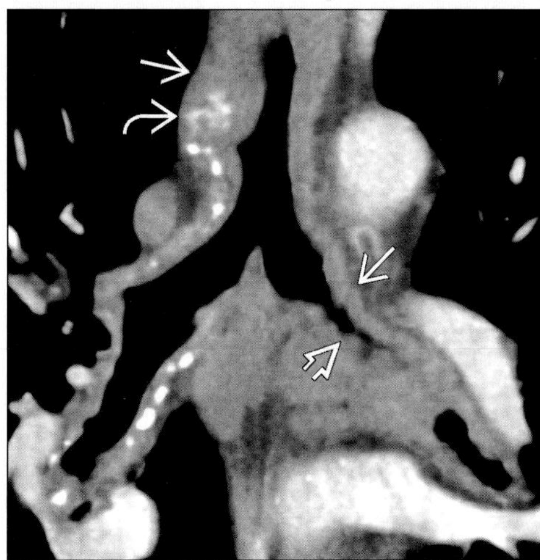

__(Left)__ Axial CECT shows smooth, circumferential wall thickening ➔ involving the right upper lobe and mainstem bronchi with smooth luminal narrowing. Calcification may or may not be present with amyloidosis. Involvement of the posterior airway wall helps distinguish amyloidosis from relapsing polychondritis. __(Right)__ Axial CECT shows soft tissue thickening in and around the right upper lobe bronchial wall with faint calcification and obstruction of the anterior segmental bronchus ➔.

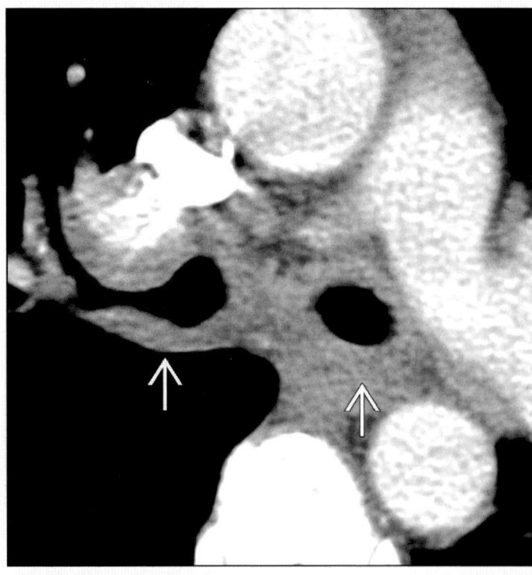

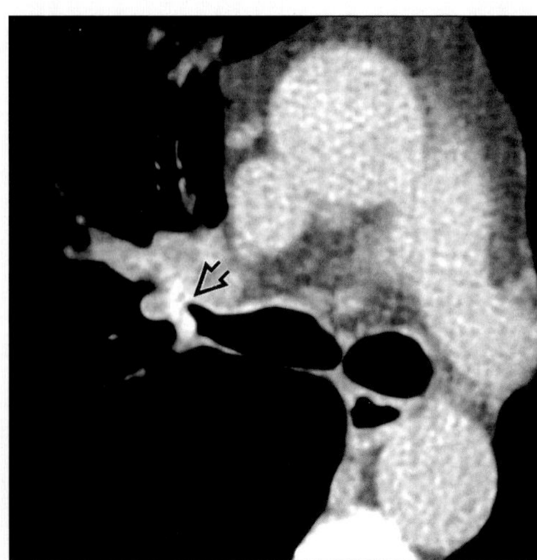

TRACHEOBRONCHIAL AMYLOIDOSIS

TERMINOLOGY

Synonyms

- Airway amyloidosis

Definitions

- Focal or diffuse submucosal deposition of amyloid in tracheobronchial tree
  - Characterized by amyloid light chain (AL) protein

IMAGING

General Features

- Best diagnostic clue
  - Focal or diffuse nodular soft tissue thickening of airway walls ± calcification

Radiographic Findings

- **Chest radiography is often normal**
- Atelectasis or consolidation from airway obstruction

CT Findings

- **Nodular soft tissue thickening of airway wall**
  - Multifocal submucosal plaques (most common)
    - Eccentric or circumferential
    - May involve posterior tracheal wall
  - **Focal airway nodules**
  - **May exhibit foci of calcification**
  - May produce **luminal narrowing & obstruction**
- May affect larynx, trachea, & central to segmental bronchi
  - Associated postobstructive effects
    - Atelectasis
    - Consolidation
    - Bronchiectasis
    - Hyperinflation

Imaging Recommendations

- Best imaging tool
  - Volumetric thin-section CT
    - Identification of submucosal airway abnormalities
    - Determination of extent of airway involvement
    - Evaluation of secondary effects of airway obstruction

DIFFERENTIAL DIAGNOSIS

Acquired Tracheal Stenosis

- History of prolonged intubation
- Focal, circumferential, or eccentric soft tissue thickening of airway wall
- Located at tracheal stoma or level of tube balloon cuff

Tracheobronchopathia Osteochondroplastica

- Nodular osseous &/or chondroid lesions in tracheobronchial walls
  - Typically calcified
  - Spares posterior tracheal wall

Wegener Granulomatosis

- Typical subglottic involvement with abnormal soft tissue thickening of tracheal wall & resultant luminal stenosis
- Posterior tracheobronchial walls may be involved
- May affect distal tracheobronchial tree

Relapsing Polychondritis

- Soft tissue thickening of airway wall
  - Spares posterior tracheal wall
  - May exhibit calcification; typically limited to airway cartilages

Tracheal Neoplasms

- Typically focal airway soft tissue nodule
- May exhibit local invasion or mediastinal lymphadenopathy

PATHOLOGY

General Features

- Etiology
  - Unknown
- Extracellular deposition of abnormal eosinophilic proteins

Gross Pathologic & Surgical Features

- Thick irregular airway wall with waxy or firm deposits

Microscopic Features

- Abnormal protein deposition in submucosal aspects of airway walls
- Stains with **Congo red**
  - Characteristic **apple-green birefringence on polarized microscopy**

CLINICAL ISSUES

Presentation

- Most common signs/symptoms
  - Symptoms (gradual onset over several years)
    - Chronic cough
    - Dyspnea
    - Wheezing
    - Hemoptysis

Demographics

- Age
  - Wide range: 16-85 years (mean: 53 years)
- Gender
  - M:F = 2:1

Natural History & Prognosis

- 5-year survival rates range from 30-50%

Treatment

- Bronchoscopic resection of obstructing airway lesions
- Surgical resection; usually for extensive involvement
- Medical therapy; limited success
- Radiation therapy for progressive disease

SELECTED REFERENCES

1. Chung JH et al: CT of diffuse tracheal diseases. AJR Am J Roentgenol. 196(3):W240-6, 2011
2. Aylwin AC et al: Imaging appearance of thoracic amyloidosis. J Thorac Imaging. 20(1):41-6, 2005
3. Dahl KA et al: Tracheobronchial amyloidosis: a surgical disease with long-term consequences. J Thorac Cardiovasc Surg. 128(5):789-92, 2004

TRACHEOBRONCHOPATHIA OSTEOCHONDROPLASTICA

Key Facts

Terminology

- Tracheobronchopathia osteochondroplastica (TO)
- Rare idiopathic benign condition characterized by multiple submucosal osteocartilaginous nodules in central airway walls (trachea & proximal bronchi)

Imaging

- Radiography
  - Chest radiograph may be normal in mild disease
  - Nodular irregularity of tracheal wall
  - Asymmetric tracheal stenosis
  - Central bronchial narrowing/obstruction
- CT
  - Multiple small mural nodules; ± calcification
  - Involvement of anterolateral tracheal & proximal bronchial walls
  - Sparing of posterior membranous tracheal wall
  - Postobstructive atelectasis/consolidation

Top Differential Diagnoses

- Tracheobronchial amyloidosis
- Tracheolaryngeal papillomatosis
- Wegener granulomatosis
- Relapsing polychondritis

Pathology

- Multifocal submucosal tracheal & bronchial nodules; intact mucosa
- Hyalinized fibrocollagenous tissue with fibrosis, calcification, necrosis

Clinical Issues

- Usually asymptomatic
- Dyspnea, cough, wheezing, hemoptysis, recurrent pneumonia
- Treatment: Endoscopic therapy or surgery for obstructing lesions

__(Left)__ PA chest radiograph (coned-down to the trachea) of a patient with tracheobronchopathia osteochondroplastica shows irregular, nodular thickening ➔ of the tracheal wall and focal narrowing of the tracheal lumen. __(Right)__ Axial NECT of the same patient demonstrates calcified plaque-like nodules ↪ of the anterolateral tracheal walls that protrude into the airway lumen and spare the posterior membranous tracheal wall. Mural tracheal nodules in patients with TO may produce asymmetric tracheal stenosis.

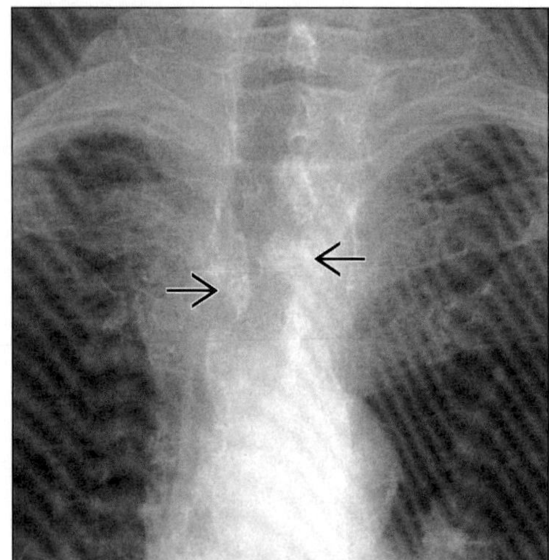

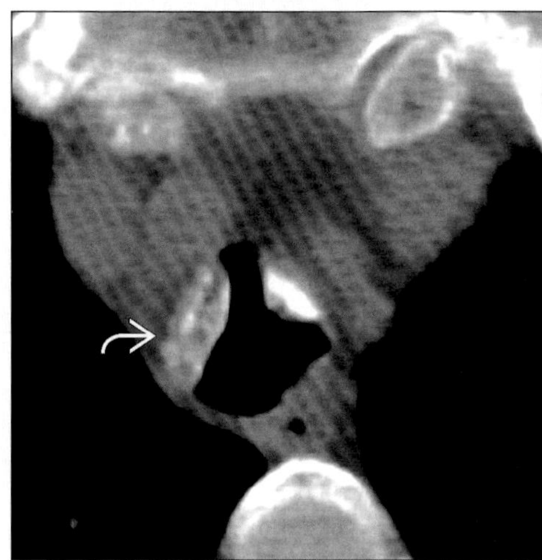

__(Left)__ Axial NECT of a patient with TO shows nodular mural calcification ↪ along the lateral tracheal walls and resultant saber-sheath configuration of the trachea. __(Right)__ Axial CECT of a patient with TO shows calcified mural nodules ➔ involving the anterior and lateral aspects of the bilateral mainstem bronchi. Such nodules can grow to produce obstruction of the airway lumen and postobstructive effects including atelectasis and postobstructive pneumonia.

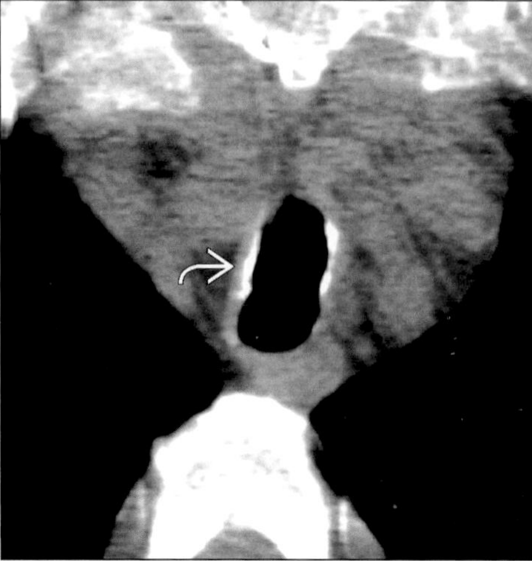

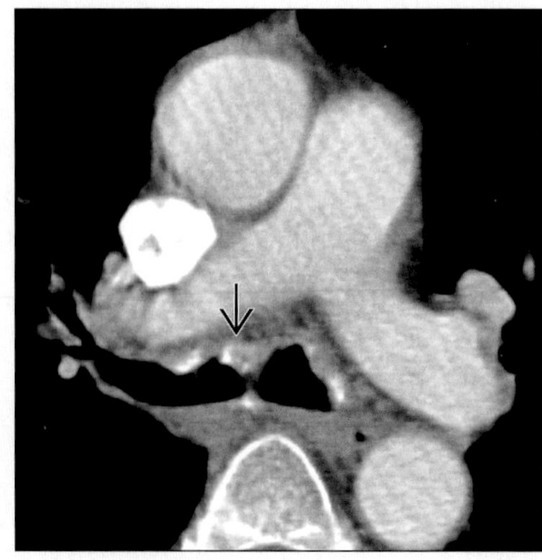

TRACHEOBRONCHOPATHIA OSTEOCHONDROPLASTICA

TERMINOLOGY

Abbreviations

- **Tracheobronchopathia osteochondroplastica (TO)**

Synonyms

- Tracheopathia osteoplastica
- Tracheopathia osteochondroplastica

Definitions

- Rare idiopathic benign condition characterized by multiple submucosal osteocartilaginous nodules in central airway walls (trachea & proximal bronchi)

IMAGING

General Features

- Best diagnostic clue
  - Nodular tracheal wall
- Location
  - Anterolateral tracheal walls
    - Predilection for distal 2/3 of trachea
    - Sparing of posterior membranous tracheal wall
  - Central bronchial walls
- Size
  - Small uniform nodules; 1-3 mm
- Morphology
  - Typically round; may appear plaque-like or polypoid, may coalesce

Radiographic Findings

- Radiography
  - Chest radiograph may be **normal** in mild disease
  - **Nodular irregularity of tracheal wall**
  - Asymmetric tracheal stenosis
  - Central bronchial narrowing/obstruction
    - Lobar collapse
    - Consolidation related to postobstructive pneumonia

CT Findings

- Direct visualization of tracheal wall abnormalities
- **Multiple small mural nodules**; protrude into airway lumen
  - Calcified or noncalcified
- Involvement of **anterolateral tracheal & proximal bronchial walls**
- **Sparing of posterior membranous tracheal wall** (where there is no cartilage)
- Variable degree of airway stenosis
- Saber-sheath appearance of trachea in some patients
- Direct visualization & assessment of postobstructive effects
  - Atelectasis
  - Postobstructive pneumonia

Imaging Recommendations

- Best imaging tool
  - CT is imaging modality of choice for visualization & characterization of TO
- Protocol advice
  - Intravenous contrast administration is not required

DIFFERENTIAL DIAGNOSIS

Tracheobronchial Amyloidosis

- Calcified or noncalcified submucosal tracheal nodules with narrowing of tracheal lumen
- Posterior membrane is not spared, unlike in TO

Tracheolaryngeal Papillomatosis

- Noncalcified mucosal nodules; also affect larynx
- Childhood or young adulthood presentation
- Distal dissemination may lead to cavitary pulmonary nodules

Wegener Granulomatosis

- Noncalcified, diffuse, nodular or smooth circumferential tracheal wall thickening
- Association with multiple pulmonary nodules, masses, or consolidations with frequent cavitation

Relapsing Polychondritis

- Thickening of tracheal & mainstem bronchial cartilages
- Anterolateral tracheal walls; membranous trachea spared

PATHOLOGY

Gross Pathologic & Surgical Features

- Multifocal submucosal tracheal & bronchial nodules; intact mucosa

Microscopic Features

- Hyalinized fibrocollagenous tissue with fibrosis, calcification, necrosis
- Cartilaginous, osseous, & hematopoietic tissue

CLINICAL ISSUES

Presentation

- Most common signs/symptoms
  - **Usually asymptomatic**
  - Dyspnea, cough, wheezing, hemoptysis, recurrent pneumonia
  - May be discovered during difficult intubation or bronchoscopy

Demographics

- Age
  - Usually > 50 years of age
- Gender
  - Male > female
- Epidemiology
  - 0.5% prevalence at autopsy

Natural History & Prognosis

- Slow progression
- Usually incidental diagnosis at autopsy

Treatment

- Endoscopic therapy or surgery for obstructing lesions

SELECTED REFERENCES

1. Restrepo S et al: Tracheobronchopathia osteochondroplastica: helical CT findings in 4 cases. J Thorac Imaging. 19(2):112-6, 2004

RELAPSING POLYCHONDRITIS

Key Facts

Terminology

- Relapsing polychondritis (RPC)
- Rare autoimmune disorder resulting in cartilage inflammation & destruction

Imaging

- Tracheobronchial tree
  - Focal or diffuse involvement
  - Airway wall thickening
  - Posterior tracheobronchial membrane spared
- Early
  - Increased attenuation of airway wall
- Late
  - Airway wall stenosis & calcification
  - Stenosis typically smooth, ranges from 1 cm to entire tracheal length
- Trachea & main bronchi may show dynamic collapse from malacia on expiratory CT

Top Differential Diagnoses

- Wegener granulomatosis
- Post-intubation stenosis
- Amyloidosis

Pathology

- Other autoimmune disorders

Clinical Issues

- Prolonged remitting disease, diagnosis usually delayed 3 years
- Airway involvement more common in women (3:1)
- Respiratory complications account for 30% of deaths
  - 75% 5-year survival

Diagnostic Checklist

- Anterolateral central airway wall thickening with posterior sparing highly suggestive of RPC

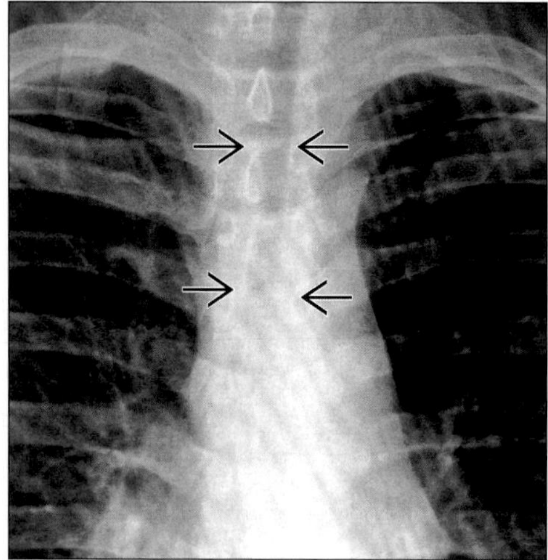

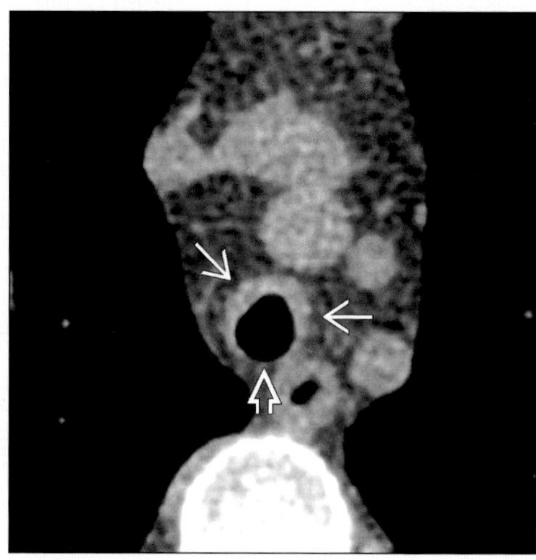

(Left) *PA chest radiograph of a patient with relapsing polychondritis shows diffuse, smooth tracheal wall thickening ⇒ and narrowing of the tracheal lumen. CT is superior in showing the extent and morphology of tracheal disease.* ***(Right)*** *Axial NECT of the same patient shows diffuse tracheal narrowing with smooth thickening ➡ of the anterior and lateral aspects of the tracheal wall. Note the conspicuous sparing of the posterior tracheal membrane ➡, characteristic of relapsing polychondritis.*

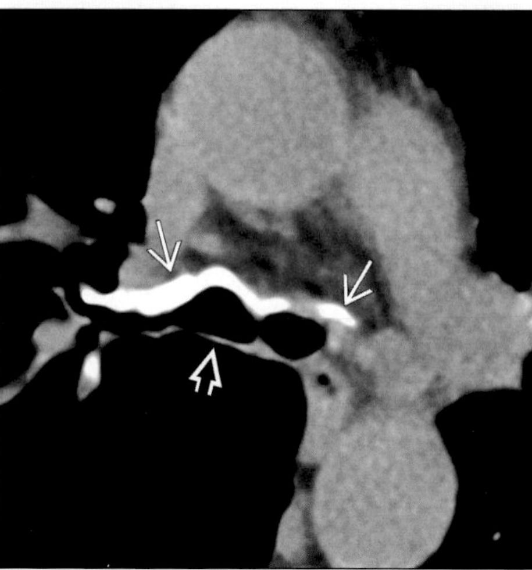

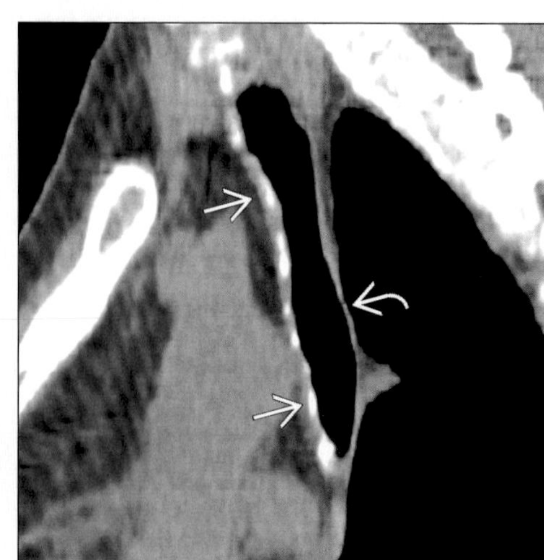

(Left) *Axial NECT of a patient with relapsing polychondritis shows thickening and calcification ➡ of the anterior walls of the mainstem bronchi with characteristic posterior membrane sparing ➡.* ***(Right)*** *Sagittal NECT of the same patient shows the craniocaudad extent of anterior tracheal wall thickening and calcification ➡ and characteristic sparing of the posterior tracheal membrane ➡. Tracheobronchopathia osteochondroplastica also spares the posterior tracheobronchial membrane.*

RELAPSING POLYCHONDRITIS

TERMINOLOGY

Abbreviations

- **Relapsing polychondritis (RPC)**

Definitions

- Rare autoimmune disorder resulting in cartilage inflammation & destruction
  - Ear, nose, laryngotracheobronchial tree

IMAGING

General Features

- Best diagnostic clue
  - ↑ thickness & attenuation of cartilaginous tracheal/bronchial wall, spared posterior trachea & bronchi
- Size
  - Stenosis usually focal & short segment
- Morphology
  - Diffuse thickening of tracheal wall, sparing posterior tracheal membrane

CT Findings

- NECT
  - Tracheobronchial tree
    - Focal or diffuse involvement
      - Posterior tracheobronchial membrane spared
    - Early
      - Airway wall thickening
      - Increased airway wall attenuation
    - Late
      - Airway wall stenosis & calcification
      - Stenosis typically smooth, ranges from 1 cm to entire tracheal length
- CECT
  - Aorta
    - Ascending aortic aneurysm
    - Aortic wall thickening
- Expiratory CT
  - Trachea & main bronchi may show dynamic collapse from malacia

Imaging Recommendations

- Best imaging tool
  - Volumetric HRCT

DIFFERENTIAL DIAGNOSIS

Wegener Granulomatosis

- Subglottic or diffuse tracheal involvement
- Nodular or smooth tracheal wall thickening
- Posterior tracheobronchial membrane often affected
- Often associated with multiple thick-walled pulmonary cavities

Post-intubation Stenosis

- History of endotracheal intubation or tracheostomy
- Smooth subglottic narrowing
- Airway wall not calcified

Amyloidosis

- Diffuse thickening & nodularity of tracheal wall, usually circumferential
- Nodules often calcify

PATHOLOGY

General Features

- Etiology
  - Autoimmune disorder: Anticartilage antibodies
- Associated abnormalities
  - Other autoimmune disorders

CLINICAL ISSUES

Presentation

- Most common signs/symptoms
  - Prolonged remitting disease, diagnosis usually delayed 3 years
    - Swelling & redness of ears (90%)
    - Arthralgias & arthritis (80%) especially costochondral joints, usually spares forefeet
    - Nasal chondritis (50%) may result in saddle nose deformity
    - Hearing loss (50%), often sudden
    - Cardiovascular disease (25%): Aortic or mitral valvular regurgitation, aortic aneurysm, pericarditis
  - Respiratory tract (50%)
    - Initial presentation in 20%
    - Dyspnea, cough hoarseness, stridor, wheezing
    - Respiratory tract may be involved without other sites
  - Glomerulonephritis (20%) may result from circulating immune complexes

Demographics

- Age
  - Any age; average at diagnosis is 50 years
- Gender
  - Equal
    - Airway involvement more common in women (3:1)
- Epidemiology
  - 3.5 cases per million

Natural History & Prognosis

- Respiratory complications account for 30% of deaths
- 75% 5-year survival

Treatment

- Corticosteroid bolus with tapered long-term maintenance
- Tracheostomy & airway stents for stenosed airways

DIAGNOSTIC CHECKLIST

Image Interpretation Pearls

- Anterolateral central airway wall thickening with posterior sparing highly suggestive of RPC

SELECTED REFERENCES

1. Rafeq S et al: Pulmonary manifestations of relapsing polychondritis. Clin Chest Med. 31(3):513-8, 2010
2. Prince JS et al: Nonneoplastic lesions of the tracheobronchial wall: radiologic findings with bronchoscopic correlation. Radiographics. 2002 Oct;22 Spec No:S215-30. Review. Erratum in: Radiographics. 23(1):191, 2003

RHINOSCLEROMA

Key Facts

Terminology

- Scleroma, *Klebsiella rhinoscleromatis*
- Progressive upper respiratory tract granulomatous infection by *Klebsiella rhinoscleromatis*

Imaging

- Nasal polyps & enlarged turbinates
- Paranasal sinuses characteristically spared unless nasal disease obstructs ostiomeatal units
- Thickening of nasopharyngeal soft tissues
  - Fascial planes preserved
- Laryngeal involvement in 15-80% of patients
- Tracheobronchial involvement far less common
  - Subglottic tracheal narrowing
  - Crypt-like spaces nearly diagnostic
  - Nodularity of tracheal mucosa
  - Concentric tracheobronchial narrowing
  - Calcification not common

Top Differential Diagnoses

- Laryngotracheal papillomatosis
- Relapsing polychondritis
- Wegener granulomatosis
- Post-intubation stricture

Pathology

- Mikulicz cells: Large vacuolated macrophages containing bacilli

Clinical Issues

- Symptoms/signs
  - Nasal obstruction, stridor, epistaxis, rhinorrhea
- Endemic in Central America, Africa, India
  - Females more commonly affected
  - 10-30 years of age
- Treatment: Long-term antibiotics for months or years; surgery may be required for obstructive lesions

*(**Left**) Axial CECT shows circumferential subglottic narrowing and mucosal thickening ➔ containing crypt-like airspaces ➲, which are highly suggestive of rhinoscleroma since they are not typical of other causes of subglottic tracheal narrowing. (**Right**) Axial CECT shows subglottic tracheal mucosal thickening and nodularity ➔ typical of rhinoscleroma. Other diseases, such as tuberculosis, Wegener granulomatosis, and inflammatory bowel disease can also exhibit this appearance.*

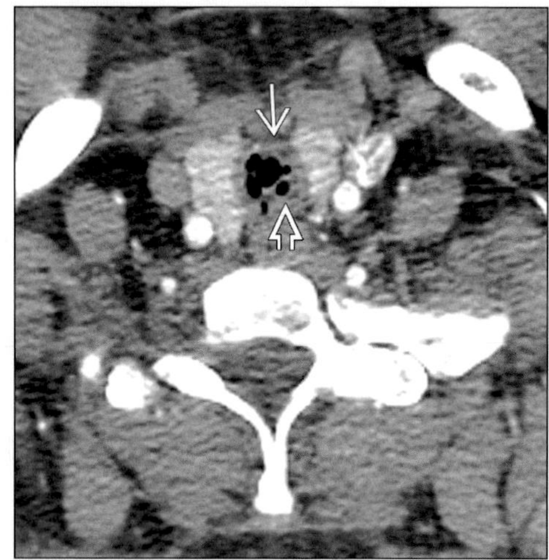

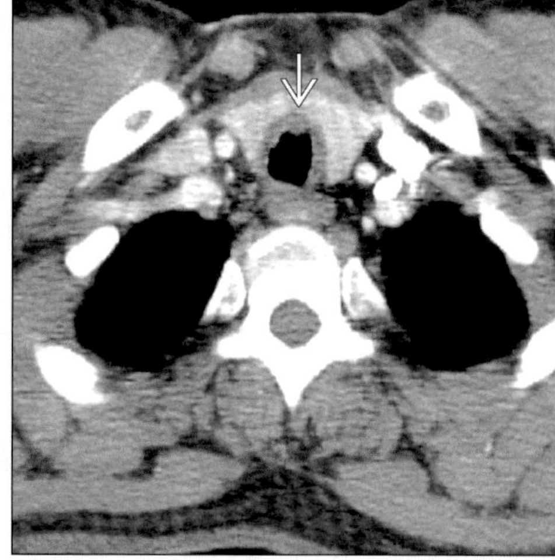

*(**Left**) Axial CECT shows diffuse and smooth circumferential thickening ➲ of the mid trachea. This smooth appearance is similar to that of relapsing polychondritis (RPC). However, in contrast to rhinoscleroma, RPC spares the posterior tracheal membrane. (**Right**) Axial CECT of the same patient 6 months following antibiotic treatment shows marked reduction in tracheal wall thickening ➔. Some patients may make a full recovery with prolonged antibiotic therapy; however, relapses are not uncommon.*

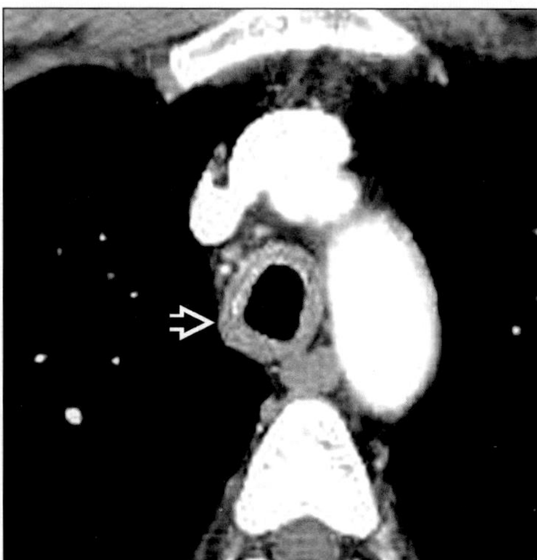

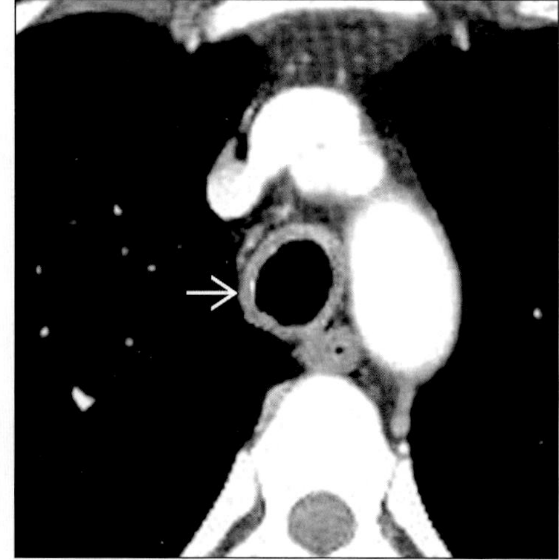

RHINOSCLEROMA

TERMINOLOGY

Synonyms

- Scleroma, *Klebsiella rhinoscleromatis*

Definitions

- Progressive upper respiratory tract granulomatous infection by *Klebsiella rhinoscleromatis*

IMAGING

General Features

- Best diagnostic clue
  - Irregular subglottic mucosal thickening with crypt-like spaces
- Location
  - Nasal vault, nasopharynx, subglottic trachea

CT Findings

- Nasal polyps & enlarged turbinates
- Paranasal sinuses characteristically spared unless nasal disease obstructs ostiomeatal units
- Thickening of nasopharyngeal soft tissues
  - Fascial planes preserved
- Laryngeal involvement in 15-80% of patients
- Tracheobronchial involvement far less common
  - Subglottic tracheal narrowing
    - Crypt-like spaces nearly diagnostic
  - Nodularity of tracheal mucosa
  - Concentric tracheobronchial narrowing
  - Calcification not common

Imaging Recommendations

- Best imaging tool
  - CT or MR to fully evaluate upper respiratory tract

DIFFERENTIAL DIAGNOSIS

Laryngotracheal Papillomatosis

- Discrete laryngeal & tracheal polypoid masses
- May spread to lung, forming solid & cavitary nodules

Relapsing Polychondritis

- Cartilage thickening: Ear, nose, tracheal rings
- Posterior tracheal membrane spared

Wegener Granulomatosis

- Smooth subglottic narrowing
- Lung nodules, cavities, consolidations, & ground-glass opacities
- Renal disease
- c-ANCA positivity

Post-Intubation Stricture

- History of prolonged or traumatic intubation
- Smooth tracheal narrowing
- Hourglass configuration on coronal oblique reformation

PATHOLOGY

General Features

- Etiology
  - Direct inhalation of contaminated droplets
  - Impaired cellular immunity with impaired T-cell function & decreased macrophage activation

Staging, Grading, & Classification

- Stage I: Catarrhal
  - Purulent rhinitis for weeks or months
- Stage II: Atrophic
  - Mucosal changes & crust formation
- Stage III: Granulomatous
  - Nasal polyps & nodular thickening of affected epithelium
- Stage IV: Sclerosis
  - Fibrosis & scarring of affected structures

Gross Pathologic & Surgical Features

- Nasal cavity: 95%
- Nasopharynx: 50%
- Larynx & trachea: 15-40%

Microscopic Features

- Mikulicz cells: Large vacuolated macrophages containing bacilli

CLINICAL ISSUES

Presentation

- Most common signs/symptoms
  - Nasal obstruction
  - Stridor
  - Epistaxis & rhinorrhea
- Other signs/symptoms
  - Cultures positive in only 50%

Demographics

- Age
  - 10-30 years of age
- Gender
  - Females more commonly affected
- Epidemiology
  - Endemic in Central America, Africa, India

Natural History & Prognosis

- Chronic debilitating progressive disease
- May relapse with discontinuation of therapy

Treatment

- Long-term antibiotic therapy for months or years
- Surgery may be required for obstructive lesions

SELECTED REFERENCES

1. Zhong Q et al: Rhinoscleroma: a retrospective study of pathologic and clinical features. J Otolaryngol Head Neck Surg. 40(2):167-74, 2011
2. Ingegnoli A et al: Uncommon causes of tracheobronchial stenosis and wall thickening: MDCT imaging. Radiol Med. 112(8):1132-41, 2007
3. Prince JS et al: Nonneoplastic lesions of the tracheobronchial wall: radiologic findings with bronchoscopic correlation. Radiographics. 2002 Oct;22 Spec No:S215-30. Review. Erratum in: Radiographics. 23(1):191, 2003

CHRONIC BRONCHITIS

Key Facts

Terminology
- Chronic bronchitis (CB)
- Productive cough on most days for ≥ 3 months in each of 2 consecutive years without other causes

Imaging
- Radiography
  - Normal chest radiograph in most
  - Bronchial wall thickening: Tram-tracking, peribronchial cuffing, increased interstitial markings
  - Hyperinflation
- CT
  - Bronchial wall thickening
  - Mosaic attenuation, air-trapping
  - Mucus in tracheobronchial tree
  - Cor pulmonale: Enlarged central pulmonary arteries & right heart chambers

Top Differential Diagnoses
- Centrilobular emphysema
- Asthma
- Acute bronchitis

Pathology
- Mucous gland hypertrophy & hyperplasia

Clinical Issues
- Etiologies: Smoking, occupational exposure, air pollution
- Symptoms: Productive cough, dyspnea, wheezing
- 4% of U.S. adults > 18 years have diagnosis of CB
- Treatment: Bronchodilators, steroids

Diagnostic Checklist
- Clinical criteria must be fulfilled for diagnosis; therefore, imaging findings are only supportive

*(**Left**) Graphic shows generalized thickening of the trachea and the central bronchi. The central airway walls are coated with a thick layer of mucus. The inset depicts a thickened bronchiole in cross section with thick endoluminal mucus. (**Right**) PA chest radiograph of a heavy smoker shows "tram-tracking" ➡ and peribronchial cuffing ↪ of central airways, consistent with the thickened airway walls characteristic of chronic bronchitis.*

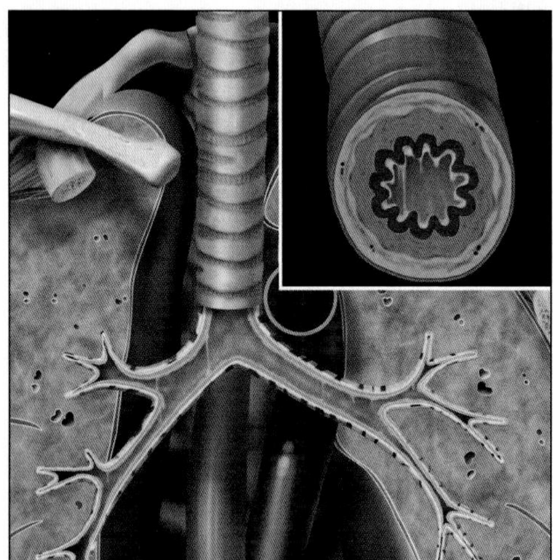

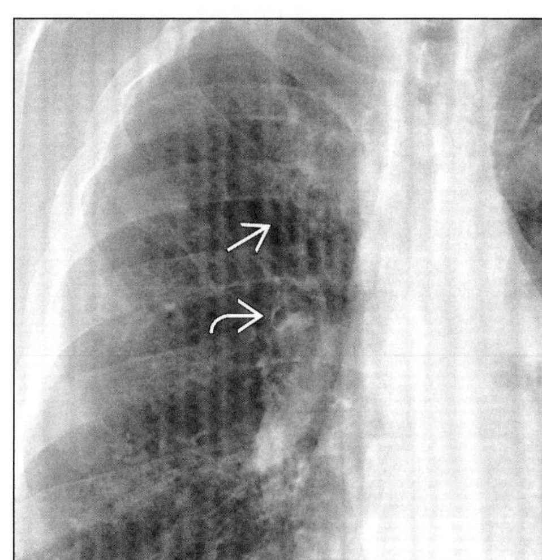

*(**Left**) Coronal CECT of a smoker with productive cough shows diffuse mild to moderate bronchial wall thickening ➡ and an incidentally discovered ground-glass nodule in the left upper lobe ↪. Patients with chronic bronchitis due to smoking are also at risk for lung cancer. (**Right**) Axial CECT of a smoker with a clinical diagnosis of COPD shows severe bilateral centrilobular emphysema and diffuse central bronchial wall thickening ➡. Emphysema and chronic bronchitis often coexist.*

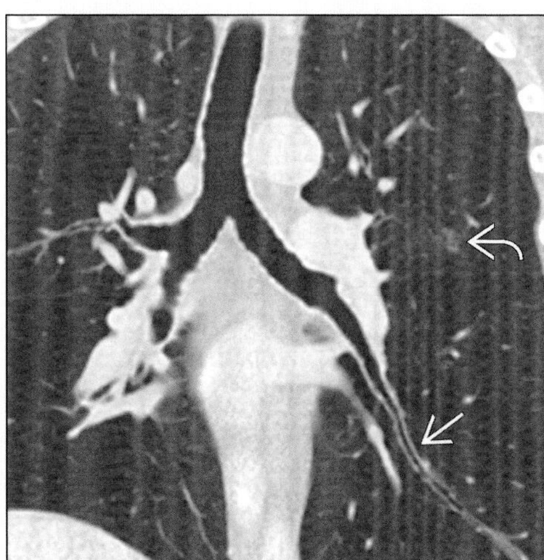

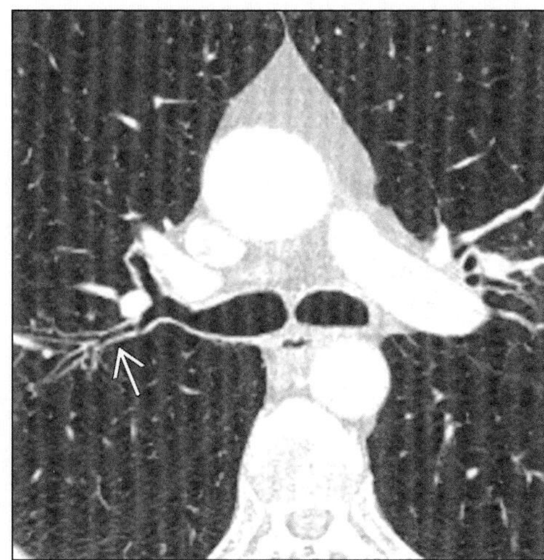

CHRONIC BRONCHITIS

TERMINOLOGY

Abbreviations

- **Chronic bronchitis (CB)**

Definitions

- CB defined clinically, not anatomically
  - Productive cough on most days for ≥ 3 months in each of 2 consecutive years without other causes
- Chronic obstructive pulmonary disease (COPD) encompasses patients with CB, emphysema, & combination of both

IMAGING

Radiographic Findings

- Radiography
  - Many, if not most, patients with isolated CB have normal chest radiographs
  - **Bronchial wall thickening**
    - **Tram-tracking**, tramline opacities
      - Longitudinally oriented bronchi with thickened walls
    - **Peribronchial cuffing**, ring shadows
      - Thickened bronchi seen on end, adjacent to pulmonary arteries
    - Increased interstitial lung markings; "dirty lungs"
      - Increased linear opacities in central lungs
  - **Hyperinflation**; may be related to coexisting emphysema
  - Cor pulmonale
    - Enlarged right ventricle, dilated central pulmonary arteries, & peripheral arterial pruning

CT Findings

- Bronchial wall thickening
  - Bronchi in patients with CB shown to have significantly higher thickness:diameter ratio
  - Multivariate analysis has shown correlation between bronchial measurements & indices of bronchial obstruction
- Mucus in tracheobronchial tree
- Mosaic attenuation, air-trapping on expiratory images
- Cor pulmonale
  - Enlarged central pulmonary arteries
  - Enlarged right heart chambers

DIFFERENTIAL DIAGNOSIS

Centrilobular Emphysema

- Commonly coexists with CB
- Also found in smokers
- Hyperinflated lungs on radiography
  - Relative upper lung lucency characteristic of emphysema not seen in isolated CB
- Reliably diagnosed on HRCT

Asthma

- May coexist with CB
- May exhibit bronchial wall thickening & hyperinflation
- Airflow obstruction reversible with bronchodilator treatment

Acute Bronchitis

- Often superimposed on CB
- Acute onset, often after viral upper respiratory infection

PATHOLOGY

General Features

- Etiology
  - Cigarette smoking
  - Occupational exposure: Mining, textile industry
  - Air pollution
  - Genetics

Gross Pathologic & Surgical Features

- Inflamed, erythematous bronchial mucosa with increased mucus on bronchial surfaces

Microscopic Features

- Mucous gland hypertrophy & hyperplasia
- Goblet cell hyperplasia

CLINICAL ISSUES

Presentation

- Most common signs/symptoms
  - Productive cough
- Other signs/symptoms
  - Dyspnea, wheezing, chest tightness, hemoptysis
  - Cor pulmonale: Peripheral edema
  - "Blue bloater"
    - Cyanosis related to hypoxemia
    - Peripheral edema from right heart failure
- Pulmonary function tests often normal in pure CB

Demographics

- Gender
  - Male > female
- Epidemiology
  - 4% of U.S. adults > 18 years have diagnosis of CB
  - CB frequency proportional to cigarette smoking

Natural History & Prognosis

- Acute exacerbation due to lower respiratory tract infection

Treatment

- Smoking cessation
- Bronchodilators, steroids
- Pulmonary rehabilitation
- Supplemental oxygen
- Immunizations against influenza & pneumococcus

DIAGNOSTIC CHECKLIST

Consider

- Clinical criteria must be fulfilled for diagnosis; therefore, imaging findings are only supportive

SELECTED REFERENCES

1. Orlandi I et al: Chronic obstructive pulmonary disease: thin-section CT measurement of airway wall thickness and lung attenuation. Radiology. 234(2):604-10, 2005

BRONCHIECTASIS

Key Facts

Terminology
- Irreversible dilatation of bronchus or bronchi, often with bronchial wall thickening

Imaging
- Bronchial wall thickening
- Dilated bronchi with bronchoarterial ratio > 1
- Signet ring sign
- "V" or "Y" opacities or "finger in glove" sign
- When diffuse, distribution may be characteristic
- **Cylindrical bronchiectasis**: Tram-tracking, nontapering, uniform diameter
- **Varicose bronchiectasis**: "String of pearls," alternating dilatation & narrowing
- **Cystic bronchiectasis**: "Cluster of grapes," marked dilatation, rounded
- Bronchial wall thickening & decreased attenuation on expiratory CT scans correlate with obstruction

Top Differential Diagnoses
- Cystic fibrosis
- Allergic bronchopulmonary aspergillosis
- Primary ciliary dyskinesia
- Bronchial atresia

Clinical Issues
- Cough, sputum production, & hemoptysis

Diagnostic Checklist
- Consider bronchiectasis in cases of tubular or cystic lesions, particularly when associated with bronchial wall thickening
- In young patient with diffuse bronchiectasis, confirm cystic fibrosis by identifying pancreatic atrophy
- Look for bronchial artery enlargement in affected patient with hemoptysis &/or preoperatively
- Consider expiratory imaging to identify obstructive physiology

__(Left)__ PA chest radiograph of a 22-year-old man with cystic fibrosis shows diffuse upper lobe predominant bronchiectasis with associated architectural distortion, fibrosis, and volume loss. __(Right)__ Axial CECT of a patient with cystic fibrosis shows bilateral bronchiectasis most pronounced in the left upper lobe with an associated cystic space ⮫ containing a mycetoma, a known complication of cystic fibrosis. Bronchiectasis is present on CT in all patients with advanced cystic fibrosis.

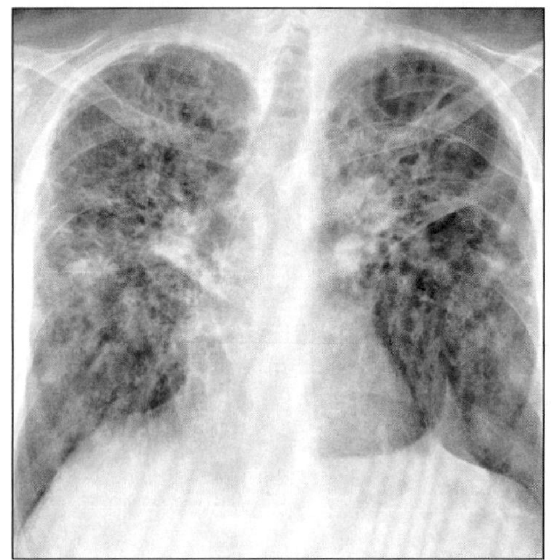

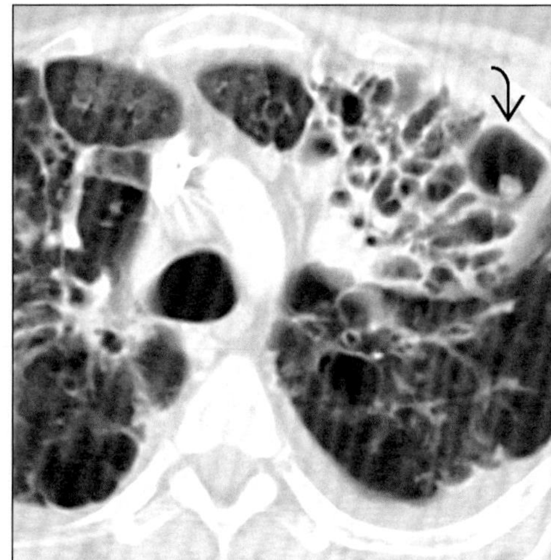

__(Left)__ Axial NECT of a 39-year-old man with focal left lower lobe cystic bronchiectasis shows dilated airways that appear ballooned and lack a normal branching pattern. Bronchi affected by cystic bronchiectasis can exceed 2 cm in diameter. __(Right)__ Axial NECT of a patient with varicose bronchiectasis shows dilated, irregular, beaded bronchi ➔. Increased bronchoarterial ratio, lack of normal bronchial tapering, and visible airways in the peripheral 1 cm of the lung are specific for bronchiectasis.

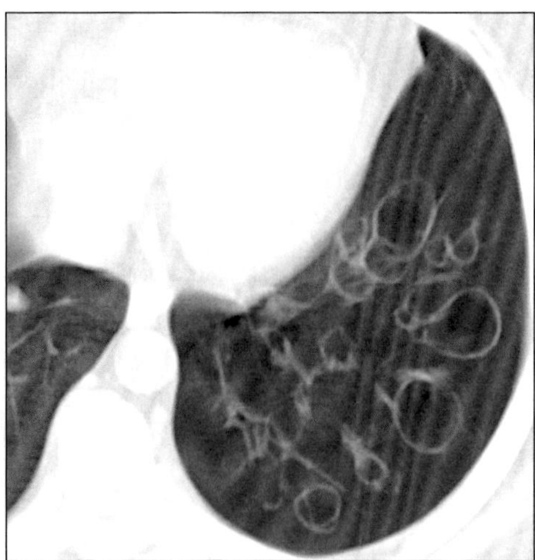

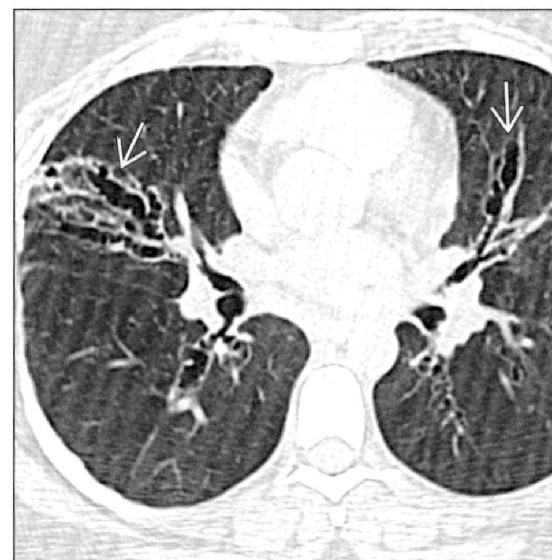

BRONCHIECTASIS

TERMINOLOGY

Definitions

- Irreversible dilatation of bronchus or bronchi, often with bronchial wall thickening

IMAGING

General Features

- Best diagnostic clue
  - Dilated bronchi with thickened walls
- Location
  - May be focal or diffuse
  - Focal bronchiectasis often post-infectious or from airway obstruction
  - When diffuse, distribution may be characteristic
    - **Upper lobe predominance**
      - Cystic fibrosis: Central & peripheral
      - Allergic bronchopulmonary aspergillosis (ABPA): Often bilateral, asymmetric, central
      - Tuberculosis: Often unilateral or asymmetric
    - **Middle lobe & lingular predominance**
      - Nontuberculous mycobacterial infection
    - **Lower lobe predominance**
      - Viral infection
      - Chronic aspiration
      - Primary ciliary dyskinesia
      - Immunodeficiency
- Size
  - Bronchi affected by cystic bronchiectasis can be up to 2 cm in diameter
- Morphology
  - **Cylindrical bronchiectasis**: Tram-tracking, nontapering, uniform diameter
  - **Varicose bronchiectasis**: "String of pearls," alternating dilatation & narrowing
  - **Cystic bronchiectasis**: "Cluster of grapes," marked dilatation, rounded

Radiographic Findings

- Bronchial dilatation
- Bronchi
  - Bronchial wall thickening
  - Tram-tracking
    - Parallel lines of thickened bronchial walls
  - Ring shadows
    - Thickened bronchi seen on end
  - "V" or "Y" opacities, band shadows, or "finger in glove" sign
    - Fluid or mucus-filled bronchi may branch
- Lung
  - Volume loss
    - Subsegmental to lobar
    - Scarring or endobronchial obstruction
    - Compensatory hyperinflation of uninvolved lung
  - Cystic changes: May contain fluid/air-fluid level
  - Bullae

CT Findings

- HRCT
  - **Dilated bronchi with bronchoarterial ratio** > 1
  - Bronchial wall thickening
  - **Signet ring sign**
    - Dilated bronchus > adjacent pulmonary artery
  - "V" or "Y" opacities or "finger in glove" sign
    - Mucus or secretions in bronchioles or bronchi
  - Bronchi not tapering appropriately &/or seen ≤ 1 cm of costal or paravertebral pleura
  - **Bronchial artery enlargement**
  - Air-trapping, mosaic attenuation
- Bronchial wall thickening & decreased attenuation on expiratory CT scans correlate with obstruction
  - Correlations suggest that obliterative bronchiolitis is cause for airway obstruction in bronchiectasis
- HRCT of idiopathic bronchiectasis shows interlobular septal thickening in 60%
  - Possibly from impaired lymphatic drainage
- Traction bronchiectasis, distortion, & honeycombing in pulmonary fibrosis

Imaging Recommendations

- Best imaging tool
  - HRCT for diagnosis & characterization of severity & extent of bronchiectasis
- Protocol advice
  - Expiratory imaging may confirm areas of obstructive physiology

DIFFERENTIAL DIAGNOSIS

Cystic Fibrosis (CF)

- Autosomal recessive disorder of chloride transport causing thick mucus, recurrent infection
- Diffuse cylindrical to cystic bronchiectasis, bronchial wall thickening
- Upper lobe predominant, right upper lobe often worse
- Onset in childhood, female predominant, higher incidence in Caucasians

Allergic Bronchopulmonary Aspergillosis

- Hypersensitivity reaction to *Aspergillus fumigatus*
- Cystic or varicose bronchiectasis
- Upper lobe & central predominant
- High-attenuation mucoid impaction

Primary Ciliary Dyskinesia

- Abnormal ciliary ultrastructure, poor mucus clearing
- Cylindrical, varicose, & cystic bronchiectasis
- Predominant in lingula, middle & lower lobes
- 50% have triad of abnormal situs, bronchiectasis, sinusitis (**Kartagener syndrome**)

Bronchial Atresia

- Dilated, mucus-filled bronchi distal to atretic airway segment
- Associated with marked hyperlucency & hypoperfusion of involved segment

Pneumonia

- Airway dilation sometimes associated with pneumonia
- Short-interval re-imaging after resolution of pneumonia to confirm that bronchi have returned to normal

Cystic Lung Disease

- May mimic cystic bronchiectasis
- Langerhans cell histiocytosis
  - Irregular cysts of Langerhans cell histiocytosis may simulate bronchiectasis
- Lymphangioleiomyomatosis

BRONCHIECTASIS

- Uniform distribution of cysts in young women
- Bullae in emphysema
- Laryngotracheal papillomatosis
  - Airway nodules; solid & cystic lung nodules

Asthma

- Bronchiectasis & asthma can coexist
- Tram-tracking, mucus plugs, & hyperinflation in both

PATHOLOGY

General Features

- Etiology
  - Idiopathic in up to 40% of cases
  - **Congenital**
    - Cystic fibrosis
    - Primary ciliary dyskinesia
    - Mounier-Kuhn syndrome
    - Williams-Campbell syndrome
    - Immunodeficiency (e.g., HIV)
    - Bronchial atresia
  - **Infectious**
    - Allergic bronchopulmonary aspergillosis
    - Chronic mycobacterial infection
    - Post-infectious from fungal, bacterial, or viral pathogens
  - **Acquired**
    - Chronic aspiration
    - Toxic inhalation
    - Obstruction
      - Tumor, foreign body, lymphadenopathy
  - **Inflammatory**
    - Rheumatoid arthritis
    - Sarcoidosis
    - Post-transplant chronic rejection
  - Pulmonary fibrosis
    - Traction bronchiectasis, architectural distortion
- Genetics
  - Dependent on etiology
- Associated abnormalities
  - Pneumonia, pneumothorax, & empyema
  - Cor pulmonale, hypertrophic osteoarthropathy
  - Brain abscess & amyloidosis: Rare
- Defect of mucous clearance
- Traction bronchiectasis occurs in pulmonary fibrosis

Gross Pathologic & Surgical Features

- Bronchial wall dilatation, thickening, & chronic inflammation with granulation tissue & fibrosis
- Bronchial wall weakness, recurrent infections, parenchymal volume loss, & distortion
- Bronchial artery enlargement
- Lymph node enlargement

Microscopic Features

- Edema, inflammation, ulceration, organizing pneumonia, & fibrosis

CLINICAL ISSUES

Presentation

- Most common signs/symptoms
  - Cough, sputum production, & hemoptysis
- Other signs/symptoms
  - Digital clubbing, dyspnea, crackles, & wheezing
- Mild bronchiectasis can be asymptomatic
- ↓ FEV1, ↓ FEV1/forced vital capacity ratio

Demographics

- Age
  - Prevalence of acquired disease increases with age
  - Ranges from 4.2/100,000 for patients 18-34 years to 271.8/100,000 for ≥ 75 years
- Gender
  - Prevalence among women higher at all ages
  - Bronchiectasis often more severe in women
  - Nontuberculous mycobacterial infection more common in elderly women
- Epidemiology
  - ~ 30,000 patients with CF in US
  - > 110,000 patients (exclusive of CF) receiving treatment for bronchiectasis in U.S.
  - Prevalence lower with antibiotics & immunization

Natural History & Prognosis

- Depends on severity & underlying cause

Treatment

- Smoking cessation, vaccination
- Postural drainage
- Antibiotic treatment for superimposed infection
- **Bronchial artery embolization for severe hemoptysis**
- Surgery for localized disease unresponsive to medical therapy
- Lung transplant for selected cases

DIAGNOSTIC CHECKLIST

Consider

- Bronchiectasis in cases of tubular or cystic lesions, particularly when associated with bronchial wall thickening
- Expiratory imaging to identify obstructive physiology

Image Interpretation Pearls

- In young patient with diffuse bronchiectasis, confirm cystic fibrosis by identifying pancreatic atrophy
- Look for bronchial artery enlargement in affected patient with hemoptysis &/or preoperatively

SELECTED REFERENCES

1. Devaraj A et al: Pulmonary hypertension in patients with bronchiectasis: prognostic significance of CT signs. AJR Am J Roentgenol. 196(6):1300-4, 2011
2. Loeve M et al: Bronchiectasis and pulmonary exacerbations in children and young adults with cystic fibrosis. Chest. 140(1):178-85, 2011
3. Cantin L et al: Bronchiectasis. AJR Am J Roentgenol. 193(3):W158-71, 2009

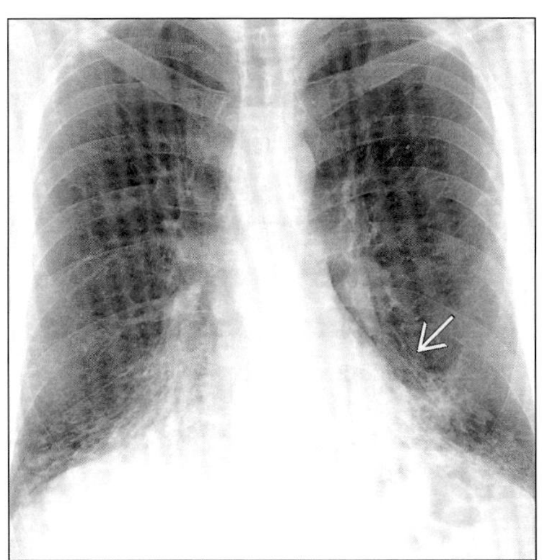

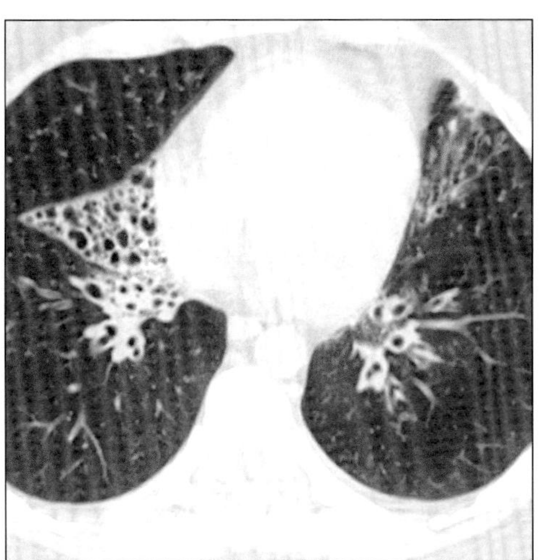

(Left) PA chest radiograph of a 38-year-old man with chronic nontuberculous mycobacterial infection shows tubular lucencies ➡ and scarring in the middle lobe and lingula. *(Right)* Axial NECT of the same patient shows bronchiectasis, bronchial wall thickening, and scarring in the lingula and middle and lower lobes. This distribution is characteristic of nontuberculous mycobacterial infection. Scattered tree-in-bud opacities are also present.

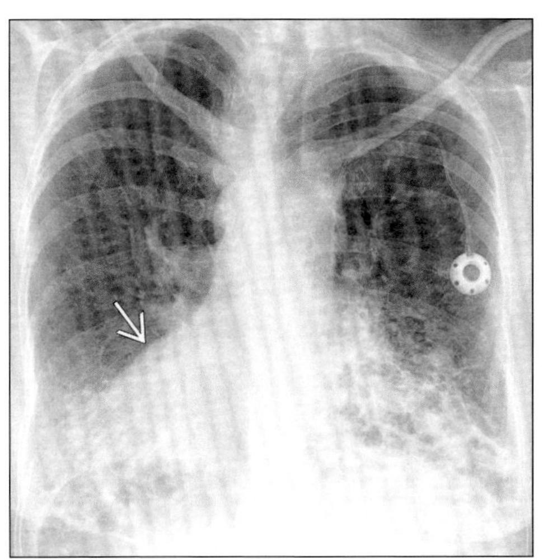

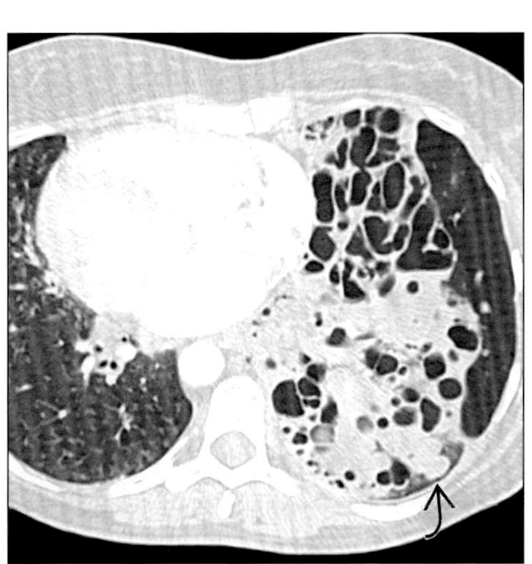

(Left) PA chest radiograph of a patient with Kartagener syndrome shows bilateral lower lobe tubular lucencies and patchy opacities. Note the situs abnormalities, including dextrocardia ➡ and the right-sided aortic arch. *(Right)* Axial CECT of the same patient shows bronchiectasis primarily involving the left lower lobe with extensive mucus plugging ➦. Note dextrocardia and a right-sided aortic arch. The triad of abnormal situs, bronchiectasis, and sinusitis defines Kartagener syndrome.

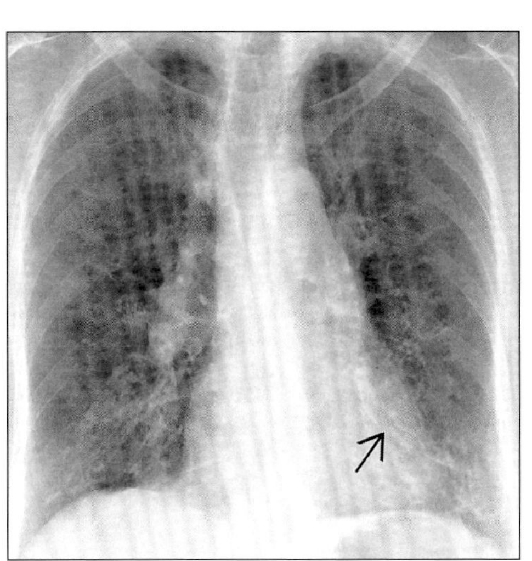

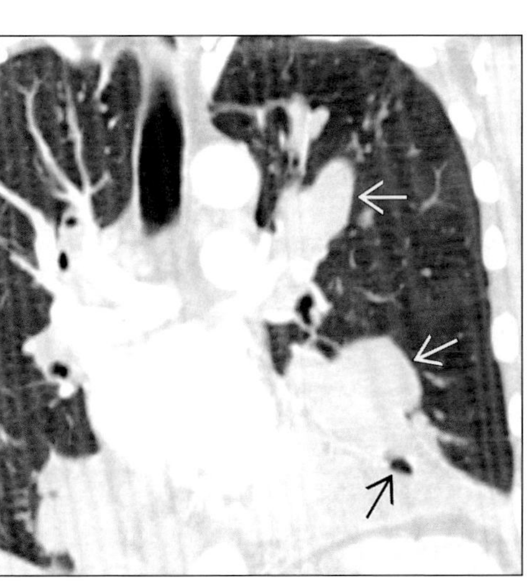

(Left) PA chest radiograph of a patient with tracheobronchomegaly shows dilation of the trachea and bronchi bilaterally. Lower lobe predominant bronchiectasis is evidenced by tubular lucencies and tram-tracking ➔. *(Right)* Coronal CECT of a patient with allergic bronchopulmonary aspergillosis shows dilated proximal airways with extensive mucus plugging ➡, which is the CT correlate of the "finger in glove" sign. Distal bronchiectasis is also present ➔.

CYSTIC FIBROSIS

Key Facts

Terminology
- Cystic fibrosis (CF)

Imaging
- Radiography
  - Bronchial wall thickening; peribronchial cuffing
  - Upper lobe predominant bronchiectasis
  - Mucoid impaction: "Finger in glove," nodular opacities
  - Hyperinflation
- CT
  - Bronchiectasis
  - Bronchial wall thickening
  - Mucoid impaction; "tree-in-bud" opacities
  - Consolidation, atelectasis
  - Mosaic attenuation; air-trapping
  - Enlarged central pulmonary arteries
  - Hilar & mediastinal lymphadenopathy

Top Differential Diagnoses
- Allergic bronchopulmonary aspergillosis
- Primary ciliary dyskinesia
- Post-infectious bronchiectasis

Pathology
- Chronic inflammation, airway wall fibrosis

Clinical Issues
- Childhood onset, recurrent respiratory infection
- Complications
  - Pulmonary arterial hypertension
  - Massive hemoptysis: Bronchial artery hypertrophy
- Treatment: Bronchodilators, antibiotics, transplant

Diagnostic Checklist
- Consider CF in any young adult with unexplained bronchiectasis

*(**Left**) PA chest radiograph of a 26-year-old woman with cystic fibrosis shows upper lobe predominant bronchial wall thickening, bronchiectasis, hyperinflation, and bilateral hilar enlargement. (**Right**) Lateral chest radiograph of the same patient shows hyperinflation with increased anteroposterior diameter of the chest and enlargement of the retrosternal clear space. "Tram-tracking" due to bronchiectasis is best seen in the retrocardiac region.*

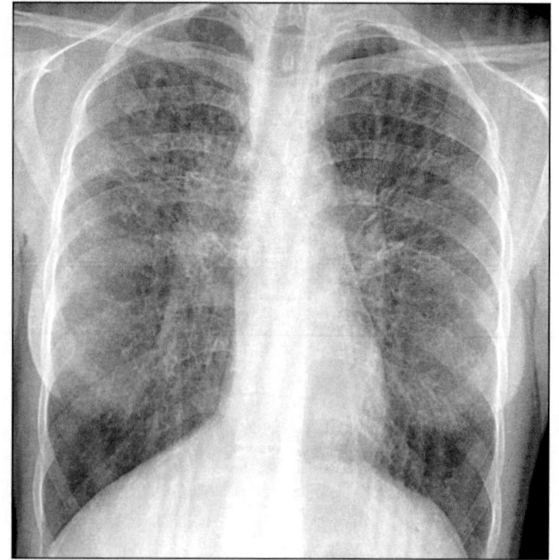

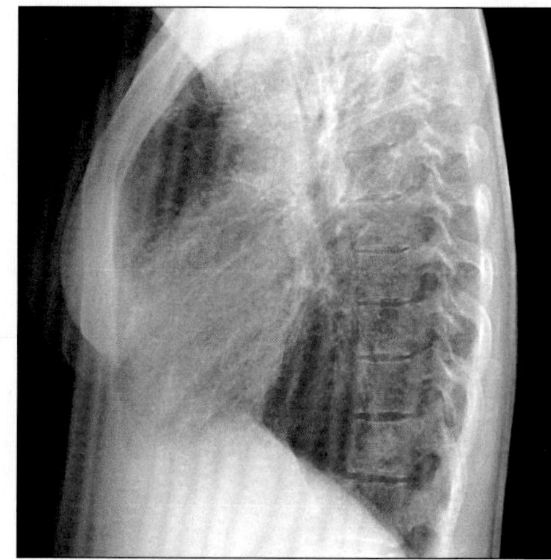

*(**Left**) Axial CECT of the same patient shows bilateral upper lobe varicose and cystic bronchiectasis and marked bronchial wall thickening. An endobronchial tubular opacity ➡ is consistent with mucus plugging. Note associated reactive mediastinal lymphadenopathy ➡. (**Right**) Axial CECT of the same patient shows less severe lower lung zone involvement with cylindrical bronchiectasis ➡ and scattered tree-in-bud opacities ➡ due to small airway mucus plugging and peribronchiolar inflammation.*

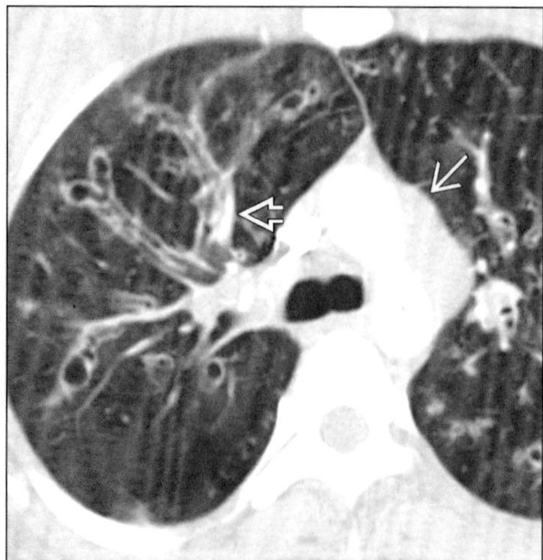

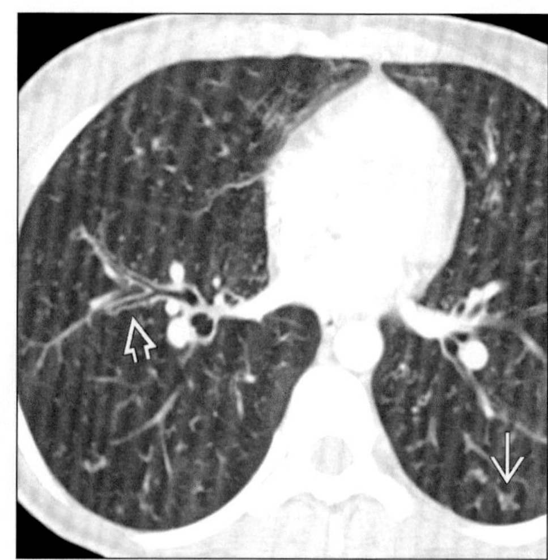

CYSTIC FIBROSIS

TERMINOLOGY

Abbreviations

- **Cystic fibrosis** (CF)

Synonyms

- Fibrocystic disease
- Mucoviscidosis

Definitions

- Autosomal recessive hereditary disorder; abnormality in gene regulating chloride transport → thick viscous secretions affecting primarily lung & pancreas
- Thick mucus → reduced mucociliary clearance → airway obstruction → recurrent infections → airway destruction

IMAGING

General Features

- Best diagnostic clue
  - Upper lobe predominant diffuse bronchiectasis & bronchial wall thickening with mucous plugging
- Location
  - Upper lobe predominance, often worse in right upper lobe

Radiographic Findings

- Radiography
  - Normal or minimal linear opacities in patients with early or mild disease
  - **Airways**
    - **Bronchial wall thickening**: Peribronchial cuffing
    - **Bronchiectasis**: Cylindrical most common, evolves into varicose & cystic forms
      - Tram-tracking
      - Cystic lucency
      - Upper lobe predominance, right > left
    - **Mucoid impaction**
      - "Finger in glove"
      - Nodular opacities
  - **Lung**
    - **Atelectasis**; ranges from subsegmental to cicatricial lobar atelectasis
      - Mostly in upper lobes
    - **Consolidation**
    - Hyperinflation due to air-trapping
      - Increased AP diameter
      - Flattened diaphragm
    - Subpleural bullae
  - Pleura
    - Pleural effusions uncommon
    - Spontaneous pneumothorax
  - Hilum
    - Reactive lymphadenopathy from chronic inflammation
    - Enlarged central pulmonary arteries from pulmonary artery hypertension

CT Findings

- CT more sensitive than radiography & pulmonary function measurements in detecting early disease
- CT of patients with normal radiographs may show
  - Mosaic attenuation secondary to small-airway abnormalities
  - Expiratory air-trapping
    - Imaging in lateral decubitus position in infants & toddlers unable to cooperate with expiratory scans
  - Mucus plugging within peripheral small bronchioles may produce V- or Y-shaped "tree-in-bud" opacities, or centrilobular nodules
- **Bronchiectasis**: Cylindrical, varicose, cystic
  - More severe in upper lobes
  - Air-fluid levels in cystic bronchiectasis correlate with acute exacerbation
- **Bronchial wall thickening**
- Focal atelectasis or consolidation
- Subpleural bullae or cystic change
- Hilar & mediastinal lymphadenopathy
- Enlargement of pulmonary trunk
- Quantitation CT measurements: Reproducible, objective
  - Regional air-trapping
    - More sensitive in detecting disease & treatment change than pulmonary function measurements
  - Airway wall thickness & airway lumen diameter
- Fat replacement of pancreas

MR Findings

- More sensitive than radiography for detecting hilar lymphadenopathy
  - Differentiation of hilar lymph nodes from pulmonary artery enlargement
- Hyperintensity on T2WI & contrast enhancement of bronchial wall may be related to inflammatory activity
- Mucus plugging: High signal within bronchial lumen on T2WI
- Hyperpolarized ^{3}He-enhanced MR
  - Sensitive for detection of ventilatory defects
  - Correlates with pulmonary function tests
  - Can detect treatment-related changes
- Contrast-enhanced MR used to evaluate abnormality in pulmonary perfusion

Angiographic Findings

- Dilated, hypertrophied bronchial arteries
- Bronchial artery embolization effective for control of bleeding/hemoptysis

Imaging Recommendations

- Best imaging tool
  - Cystic Fibrosis Foundation recommends chest radiographs
    - Every 2-4 years for clinically stable patients
    - Every year for those with deteriorating pulmonary function or frequent infections
  - HRCT: Best imaging modality for detection of early disease, complications, & progression
  - Efforts must be made to reduce radiation dose important for patients followed with serial CT
    - Low-dose CT
    - Shielding
  - MR being investigated for evaluation of disease progression
    - Lack of ionizing radiation desirable for repeated scanning
    - Provides functional information

CYSTIC FIBROSIS

DIFFERENTIAL DIAGNOSIS

Allergic Bronchopulmonary Aspergillosis

- Upper lobe predominant central bronchiectasis
- History of asthma, often eosinophilia
- Hyperdense impacted mucus

Primary Ciliary Dyskinesia

- No upper lobe predominance
- Dextrocardia or situs inversus
- Sinusitis

Postinfectious Bronchiectasis

- Usually unilateral, lobar or sublobar
- Often affects lower lobes

Endobronchial Obstruction

- Generally localized, lobar or sublobar, may exhibit associated volume loss or hyperinflation
- Etiology
  - Foreign body
  - Carcinoid tumor
  - Bronchial atresia

Radiation-induced Lung Disease

- Cicatricial scarring & bronchiectasis conforming to radiation port
- History of intrathoracic malignancy

Tuberculosis

- Can produce upper lobe volume loss & bronchiectasis
- May exhibit calcifications in lung granulomas & hilar/mediastinal lymph nodes

PATHOLOGY

General Features

- Etiology
  - Abnormal chloride ion transport leads to
    - Thick mucus
    - Mucus not expectorated, becomes secondarily infected
    - Repeated infections eventually destroy airways
    - Airways colonized with *Pseudomonas aeruginosa*, *Burkholderia cepacia*, *Stenotrophomonas maltophilia*, & atypical mycobacteria
  - Increased lower lobe respiratory excursion aids removal of secretions, thus upper lobe airways predominately affected
- Genetics
  - Autosomal recessive
  - Various mutations of a gene on chromosome 7 that codes for cystic fibrosis transmembrane conductance regulator (CFTR)
    - *ΔF508*, a deletion (Δ) of 3 nucleotides resulting in a loss of amino acid phenylalanine (F) at the 508th position on the protein, accounts for ~ 90% of CF cases in USA
- Associated abnormalities
  - Exocrine pancreatic insufficiency
  - Pansinusitis
    - Almost all will have underdeveloped & opacified paranasal sinuses on imaging
  - Infertility

Microscopic Features

- Chronic inflammation, fibrosis of airway wall
- Purulent material in airway lumen

CLINICAL ISSUES

Presentation

- Most common signs/symptoms
  - Onset in childhood
    - Meconium ileus at birth
    - Failure to thrive
    - Recurrent respiratory infection: *P. aeruginosa*, *S. aureus*, *H. influenzae*
  - Cough
  - Wheezing
  - Dyspnea
- Other signs/symptoms
  - Hemoptysis, sometimes massive
  - Pneumothorax

Demographics

- Age
  - Most diagnosed by age 5
  - Occasional mild cases not diagnosed until adulthood
- Ethnicity
  - More common in Caucasians, rare in African-Americans or Asians
- Epidemiology
  - 3,200 cases each year in U.S.; 30,000 cases total in USA

Natural History & Prognosis

- More patients surviving into 40s, 50s, & older
- Death due to pulmonary arterial hypertension & cor pulmonale or hemoptysis

Treatment

- Bronchodilators
- Promotion of airway secretion clearance
  - Inhaled DNase I
  - Inhaled hypertonic saline
  - Chest physiotherapy
- Lung transplant
  - Bilateral transplant to prevent infection of transplanted lung by native lung

DIAGNOSTIC CHECKLIST

Consider

- CF in any young adult with unexplained bronchiectasis

SELECTED REFERENCES

1. Daines C et al: The importance of imaging in cystic fibrosis. Am J Respir Crit Care Med. 184(7):751-2, 2011
2. Eichinger M et al: Computed tomography and magnetic resonance imaging in cystic fibrosis lung disease. J Magn Reson Imaging. 32(6):1370-8, 2010
3. Robinson TE: Imaging of the chest in cystic fibrosis. Clin Chest Med. 28(2):405-21, 2007
4. Berrocal T et al: Pancreatic cystosis in children and young adults with cystic fibrosis: sonographic, CT, and MRI findings. AJR Am J Roentgenol. 184(4):1305-9, 2005

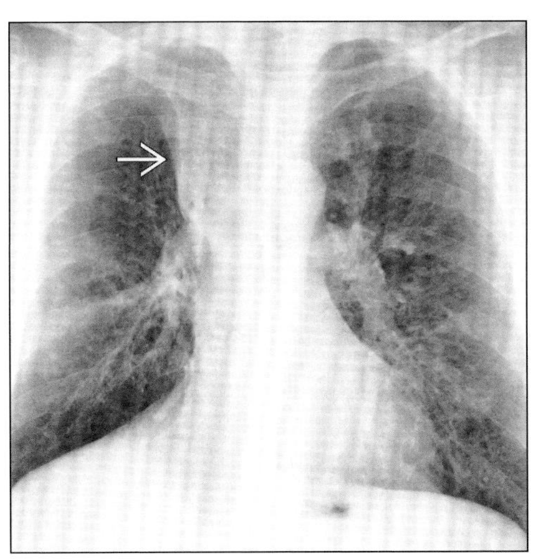

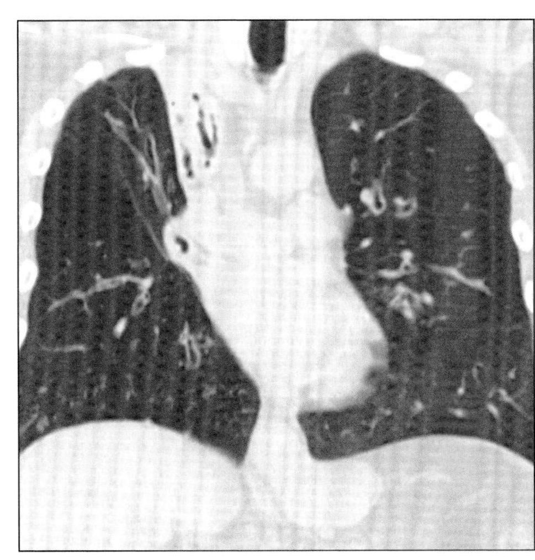

(Left) PA chest radiograph of a patient with cystic fibrosis shows chronic right upper lobe atelectasis ➡, bilateral bronchiectasis, and bronchial wall thickening. **(Right)** Coronal NECT of the same patient confirms right upper lobe atelectasis with intrinsic patent bronchiectatic airways. Cicatricial atelectasis of the upper lobes, commonly seen in cystic fibrosis, may be related to recurrent pulmonary infection.

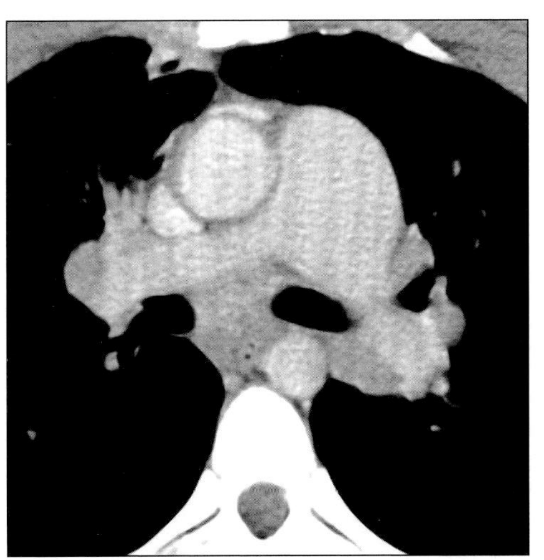

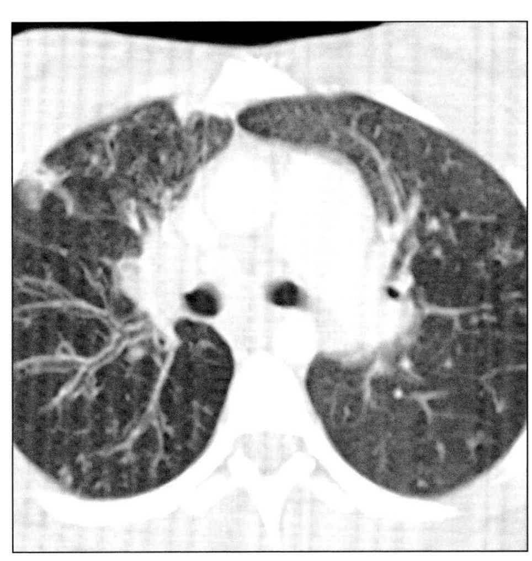

(Left) Axial NECT of a patient with CF shows dilatation of the pulmonary trunk, consistent with pulmonary arterial hypertension and bilateral hilar lymphadenopathy. Both pulmonary hypertension and hilar lymphadenopathy may produce hilar enlargement, which is frequently seen on chest radiographs of patients with CF. **(Right)** Axial CECT of the same patient shows bronchiectasis, bronchial wall thickening, and nodular consolidations. Note mosaic attenuation secondary to air-trapping.

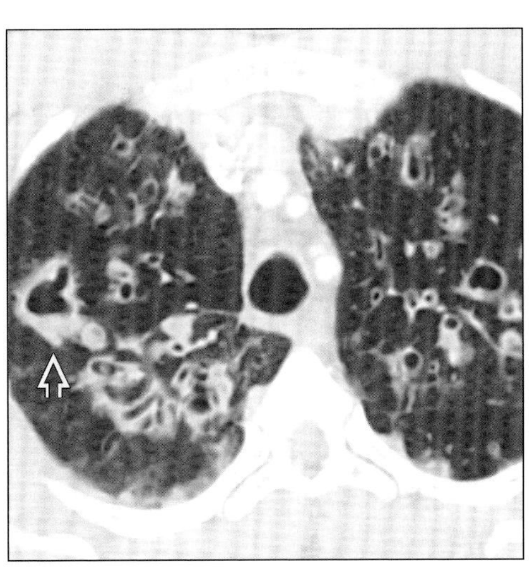

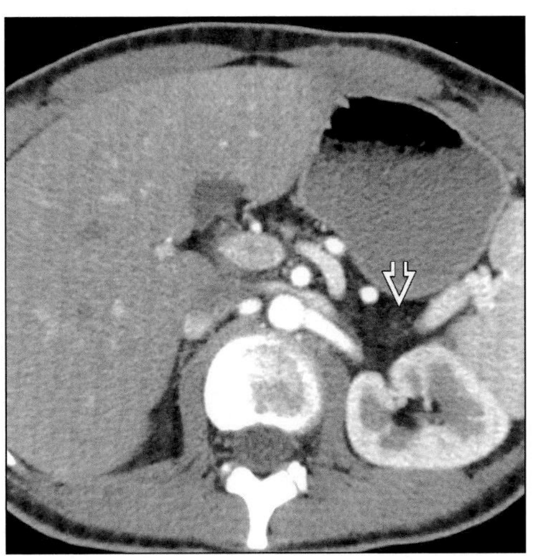

(Left) Axial CECT of a patient with cystic fibrosis shows cystic bronchiectasis with an air-fluid level in a right upper lobe thick-walled dilated bronchus ➡, a CT finding associated with acute exacerbation of CF. **(Right)** Axial CECT of a patient with CF shows the characteristic finding of fatty replacement of the pancreas ➡.

ALLERGIC BRONCHOPULMONARY ASPERGILLOSIS

Key Facts

Terminology
- Allergic bronchopulmonary aspergillosis (ABPA)
- Hypersensitivity reaction to *Aspergillus fumigatus*
- Often associated with asthma & cystic fibrosis

Imaging
- Radiography
  - Fleeting areas of consolidation
  - "Tram-track" parallel lines indicating thick-walled central bronchiectatic airways
  - Pulmonary nodules
- HRCT
  - Central multifocal bronchiectasis with mucoid impactions
  - Atelectasis related to bronchial obstruction
  - Centrilobular nodules that may be branching
  - Areas of consolidation & ground-glass opacities
  - Mosaic perfusion or air-trapping

Top Differential Diagnoses
- Lung cancer with central obstruction
- Other forms of bronchiectasis
- Bronchial atresia
- Primary ciliary dyskinesia

Pathology
- Type I hypersensitivity reaction with IgE & IgG release

Clinical Issues
- Diagnosis based on combination of clinical, laboratory, and imaging criteria
- Oral corticosteroids treatment of choice

Diagnostic Checklist
- Consider ABPA in patients with asthma or cystic fibrosis with new consolidations or mucoid impactions

*(**Left**) PA chest radiograph of a 36-year-old steroid-dependent asthmatic with increasing cough and dyspnea shows middle lobe consolidation and central bronchiectasis ➔. Note left upper lobe mucoid impaction ➔. (**Right**) Axial CECT of the same patient shows dense middle lobe consolidation and bilateral varicose bronchiectasis ➔ with mild surrounding ground-glass opacity. An elevated serum IgE and positive skin reaction to Aspergillus antigen confirmed the diagnosis.*

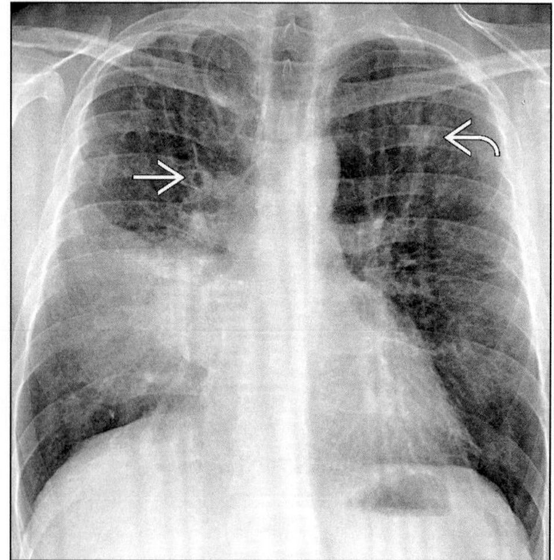

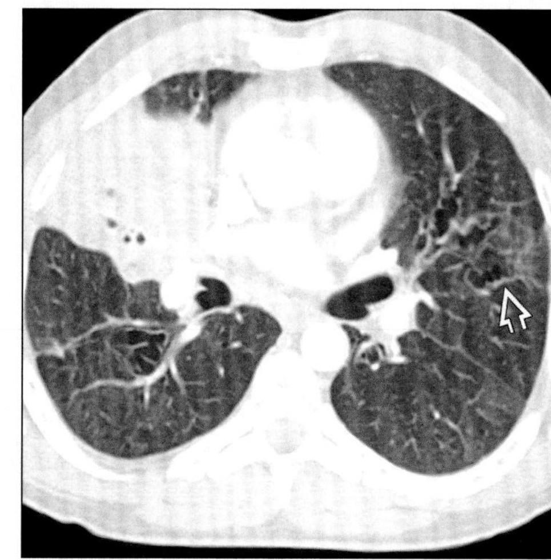

*(**Left**) Axial CECT of a 55-year-old asthmatic woman who presented with fever, dyspnea, and weight loss shows markedly dilated central bronchi filled with high-attenuation mucus ➔. (**Right**) Sagittal CECT of the same patient shows markedly dilated and mucus-filled central airways ➔ with a "finger in glove" appearance, characteristic for ABPA. Note hyperlucent areas ➔, likely due to air-trapping from small airways disease in this patient with asthma.*

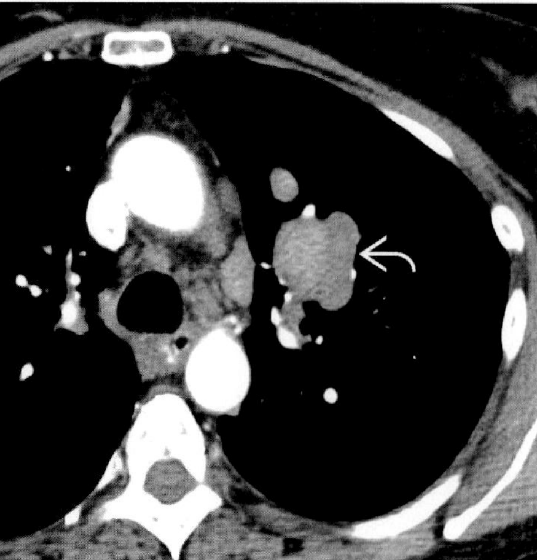

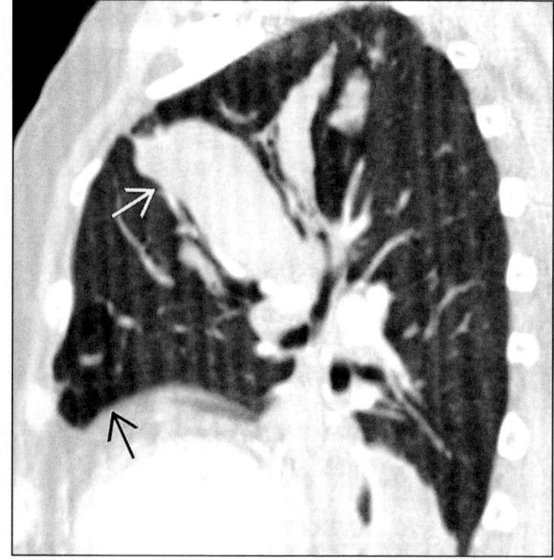

ALLERGIC BRONCHOPULMONARY ASPERGILLOSIS

TERMINOLOGY

Abbreviations

- **Allergic bronchopulmonary aspergillosis (ABPA)**

Synonyms

- Allergic bronchopulmonary mycosis

Definitions

- Hypersensitivity reaction to *Aspergillus fumigatus*
  - Colonization of tracheobronchial tree
- Often occurs in conjunction with asthma & cystic fibrosis
- Allergic fungal sinusitis may occur alone or with ABPA
- May be associated with chronic eosinophilic pneumonia or cryptogenic organizing pneumonia (COP)

IMAGING

General Features

- Best diagnostic clue
  - Central bronchiectasis with mucoid impactions
- Location
  - Predominantly upper lobes

Radiographic Findings

- Radiography
  - **Mucoid impaction**
    - Tubular, "**finger in glove**" opacities in bronchial distribution
    - Y-shaped opacities
    - May result in lobar collapse
  - Fleeting areas of consolidation
  - "**Tram-track**" parallel lines indicating thick-walled central bronchiectatic airways
  - Pleural effusions
  - Pulmonary nodules, may exhibit branching morphology

CT Findings

- HRCT
  - **Bronchiectasis**
    - Often involving multiple lobes bilaterally
    - Cystic or saccular bronchiectasis ± air-fluid levels
    - Varicose bronchiectasis has bulbous appearance with dilated bronchi & interspersed sites of constriction
  - Mucus-filled dilated bronchi
    - High-attenuation mucus
  - Lobulated masses
  - Centrilobular nodules
  - Areas of consolidation, ground-glass opacity (GGO)
  - Atelectasis related to bronchial obstruction
  - Mosaic perfusion or air-trapping
  - Combination of above findings highly suggestive of ABPA

Imaging Recommendations

- Best imaging tool
  - HRCT is modality of choice for evaluation of airways diseases

DIFFERENTIAL DIAGNOSIS

Lung Cancer with Central Obstruction

- Mucoid impaction may exhibit mass-like appearance & is sometimes resected as undiagnosed lung mass
- Carcinoid may manifest as central endobronchial lesion with distal mucoid impaction
- Differentiating features
  - Endobronchial lesion
  - Associated lymphadenopathy

Bronchial Atresia

- Likely sequela of vascular insult to lung during early fetal development
- Branching, tubular mass, representing mucoid impaction
- Segmental bronchus does not communicate with central airway
- Difficult to distinguish from ABPA
  - Hyperinflation of lung with decreased vascular markings
  - No history of allergies or cystic fibrosis

Primary Ciliary Dyskinesia

- Manifested by dyskinetic cilia with poor mucociliary clearing, recurrent infection, & bronchiectasis
- Hearing loss, male infertility
- Bronchiectasis in setting of dyskinetic cilia
- Dextrocardia in patients with Kartagener syndrome

Airway Obstruction from Foreign Body

- Radiopaque foreign body
- Air-trapping on expiratory radiography
- History of aspiration

Bronchocentric Granulomatosis

- Rare hypersensitivity lung disease, may be caused by *Aspergillus* species
- May be seen with ABPA or as response to infection with mycobacteria, other fungi, or *Echinococcus*
- Distal airway lumen replacement by necrotizing granulomas
- Radiographically same as ABPA
- May exhibit focal mass or lobar consolidation with atelectasis

Tuberculosis

- Associated cavitary changes; lobar consolidation; more predominant centrilobular nodularity/septal thickening; lymphadenopathy
- Cutaneous reactivity with tuberculin skin test

Distinct from Other Pulmonary Aspergillosis Syndromes

- Semi-invasive aspergillosis (chronic necrotizing pneumonia)
  - Subacute process in patients with some degree of immunosuppression (COPD, alcoholism, diabetes mellitus, steroids)
- Aspergilloma (fungus ball; mycetoma)
  - Develops in preexisting lung cavity
- Invasive aspergillosis
  - Occurs in severely immunosuppressed patients
  - Halo sign: Nodules surrounded by ground-glass opacity halo

ALLERGIC BRONCHOPULMONARY ASPERGILLOSIS

PATHOLOGY

General Features

- Etiology
  - Aspergillus fumigatus
    - Ubiquitous soil fungi
  - Type I hypersensitivity reaction with IgE & IgG release
- Genetics
  - Higher frequencies of specific *HLA-DR2* & *HLA-DR5* genotypes found in association with ABPA

Staging, Grading, & Classification

- May be progressive
  - Not all patients progress
- 5 stages
  - Stage I: Acute disease
  - Stage II: Remission
  - Stage III: Exacerbation or recurrence
  - Stage IV: Corticosteroid-dependent asthma
  - Stage V: End-stage fibrosis

Microscopic Features

- Septate hyphae branching at 45° angles
- Plugs of inspissated mucus containing *Aspergillus* & eosinophils
  - Fungi do not invade mucosa

CLINICAL ISSUES

Presentation

- Most common signs/symptoms
  - Cough
  - Wheezing
  - Low-grade fever
  - Malaise
  - Sputum with thick mucous plugs (contain hyphae)
- Other signs/symptoms
  - No single test is diagnostic
- Diagnosis usually determined based upon combination of clinical, laboratory, & imaging criteria; occasionally requires pathologic diagnosis
- **Major criteria**
  - Asthma
  - Immediate skin reactivity with *Aspergillus* antigen reaction manifested by wheal & flare
  - Serum precipitating antibodies to *Aspergillus fumigatus*
  - Increased total serum IgE concentration (> 1,000 ng/mL)
  - Peripheral blood eosinophilia
  - Elevated serum IgE &/or IgG antibodies to *Aspergillus fumigatus*
  - Central bronchiectasis on HRCT
  - Airspace disease on radiography
- **Minor criteria**
  - Sputum *Aspergillus fumigatus*
  - Expectoration of brown mucous plugs
  - Late skin reactivity with *Aspergillus* antigen reaction manifested by wheal & flare
- Pulmonary function tests: Airflow obstruction, air-trapping, reduced FEV1
  - Patients with fibrosis may exhibit mixed obstruction & restriction

Demographics

- Age
  - Occurs at all ages, most commonly 3rd to 4th decade
- Epidemiology
  - Occurs in approximately 1-15% patients with cystic fibrosis
  - Occurs in 2-32% patients with asthma
  - Most common cause of eosinophilic lung disease

Natural History & Prognosis

- Recurrent ABPA may result in widespread bronchiectasis & fibrosis
- 35% of exacerbations are asymptomatic but may result in lung damage

Treatment

- Oral corticosteroids treatment of choice
  - Inhaled steroids alleviate asthma symptoms, not effective treating or preventing ABPA
  - Response monitored by serum IgE concentration
- Addition of oral itraconazole may allow steroid tapering & faster response
- Voriconazole & nebulized amphotericin B have been used successfully
- Omalizumab (monoclonal antibody to IgE): Has been used with mixed results to treat ABPA in children with cystic fibrosis
- Allergic fungal sinusitis may require endoscopic sinus surgery to improve drainage

DIAGNOSTIC CHECKLIST

Consider

- ABPA in patients with asthma or cystic fibrosis with new consolidations or mucoid impactions

SELECTED REFERENCES

1. Agarwal R: Allergic bronchopulmonary aspergillosis: Lessons for the busy radiologist. World J Radiol. 3(7):178-81, 2011
2. Agarwal R: Allergic bronchopulmonary aspergillosis. Chest. 135(3):805-26, 2009
3. Segal BH: Aspergillosis. N Engl J Med. 360(18):1870-84, 2009
4. Greene R: The radiological spectrum of pulmonary aspergillosis. Med Mycol. 43 Suppl 1:S147-54, 2005
5. Franquet T et al: Aspergillus infection of the airways: computed tomography and pathologic findings. J Comput Assist Tomogr. 28(1):10-6, 2004
6. Stevens DA et al: Allergic bronchopulmonary aspergillosis in cystic fibrosis--state of the art: Cystic Fibrosis Foundation Consensus Conference. Clin Infect Dis. 2003 Oct 1;37 Suppl 3:S225-64. Review. Erratum in: Clin Infect Dis. 38(1):158, 2004
7. Buckingham SJ et al: Aspergillus in the lung: diverse and coincident forms. Eur Radiol. 13(8):1786-800, 2003
8. Gotway MB et al: The radiologic spectrum of pulmonary Aspergillus infections. J Comput Assist Tomogr. 26(2):159-73, 2002
9. Franquet T et al: Spectrum of pulmonary aspergillosis: histologic, clinical, and radiologic findings. Radiographics. 21(4):825-37, 2001

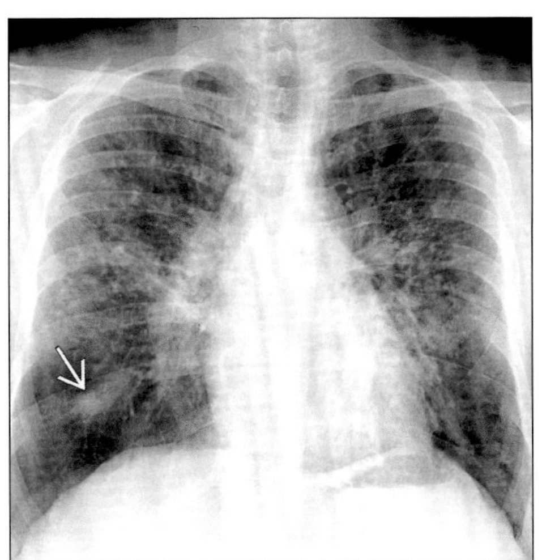

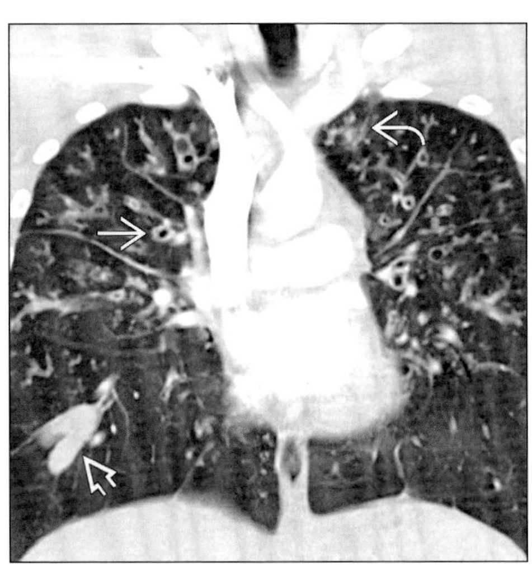

(Left) *PA chest radiograph of a 33-year-old man with cystic fibrosis, ABPA, and new hemoptysis shows extensive bronchiectasis and a dilated branching tubular opacity ➔ in the right lung base that was new when compared to prior studies (not shown).* ***(Right)*** *Coronal CECT of the same patient shows extensive cylindrical bronchiectasis ➔, scattered centrilobular tree-in-bud nodules ➔, and areas of mucoid impaction ➔. ABPA is commonly seen in patients with cystic fibrosis.*

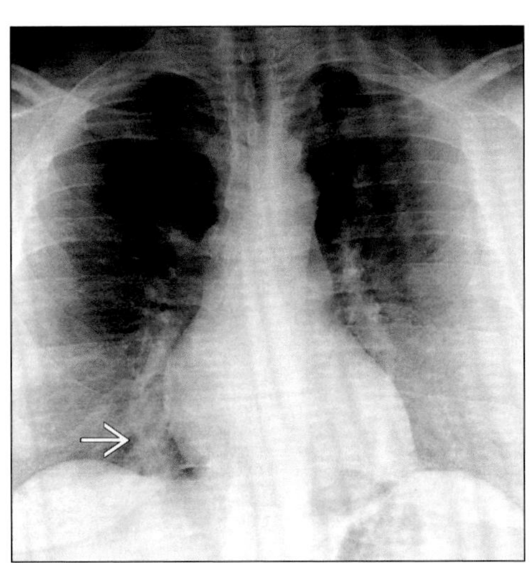

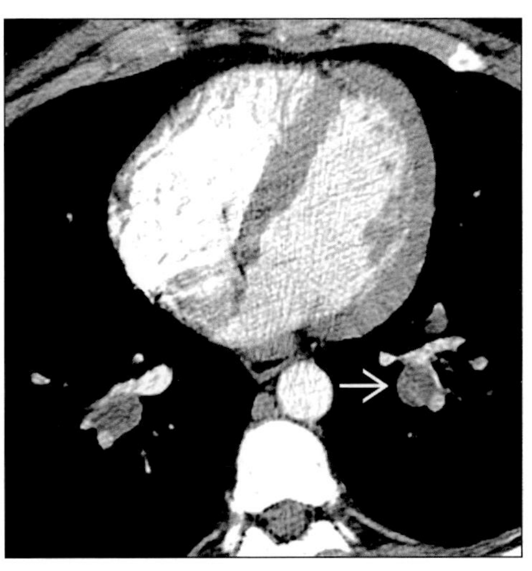

(Left) *PA chest radiograph of a 22-year-old man with dyspnea and cough shows bilateral tubular branching opacities ➔. These are more numerous and larger than would be expected for normal pulmonary vessels.* ***(Right)*** *Axial CTA of the same patient shows bilateral lower lobe high-density mucoid impactions ➔ within bronchiectatic airways. While ABPA is commonly seen in patients with longstanding asthma, occasionally the diseases are diagnosed concurrently.*

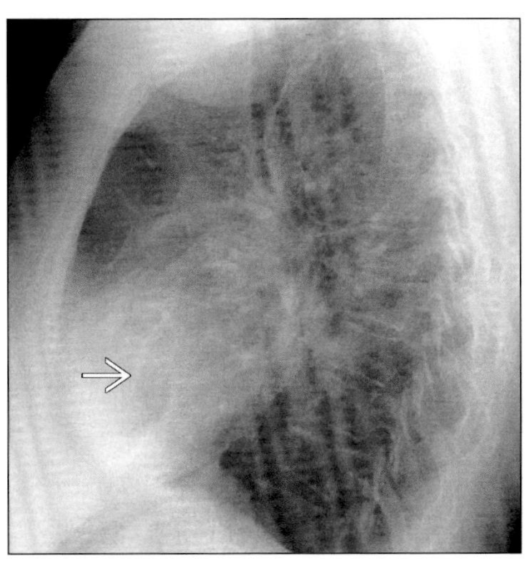

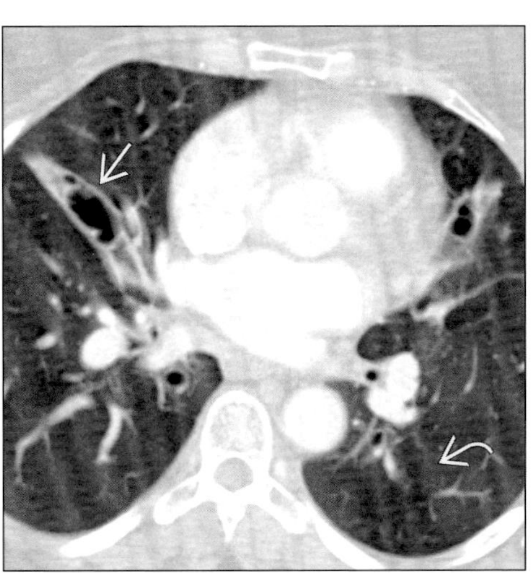

(Left) *Lateral chest radiograph of a 40-year-old asthmatic patient with increasing dyspnea shows extensive severe bronchiectasis ➔ overlying the cardiac silhouette.* ***(Right)*** *Axial CECT of the same patient shows cylindrical and cystic bronchiectasis ➔ predominantly affecting the middle lobe and lingula. There is volume loss related to chronic collapse of the middle lobe. Note bilateral areas of lower lobe mosaic attenuation related to the sequela of asthma ➔.*

PRIMARY CILIARY DYSKINESIA

Key Facts

Terminology

- Primary ciliary dyskinesia (PCD)
- Abnormal ciliary ultrastructure with resultant mucociliary dysfunction & sinopulmonary disease
  - Kartagener syndrome: 50% of PCD

Imaging

- Radiography
  - Hyperinflation
  - Bronchial wall thickening & bronchiectasis
  - Atelectasis, consolidation
- CT
  - Bronchial wall thickening
  - Bronchiectasis with predilection for lingula, middle & lower lobes
  - Mucus plugs within dilated airways
  - Centrilobular nodules & tree-in-bud opacities
  - Mosaic attenuation, air trapping on expiratory CT

Top Differential Diagnoses

- Cystic fibrosis
- Allergic bronchopulmonary aspergillosis (ABPA)
- Immune deficiency disorders

Pathology

- Cilia: Absence of dynein arms, central microtubule pairs, inner sheath, radial spokes, or nexin links

Clinical Issues

- Symptoms/signs
  - Productive cough, wheezing, coarse crackles, exertional dyspnea
  - Recurrent pulmonary infection
  - Infertility in males, lowered fertility in females
- Diagnosis: Nasal brush biopsy
- Good prognosis, particularly with early diagnosis & aggressive treatment

*(**Left**) PA chest radiograph of a 41-year-old man with cough and wheezing demonstrates dextrocardia ➔, a right-sided aortic arch, and a left-sided gastric bubble →, indicating situs ambiguous. Note the bilateral basilar bronchiolitis is most pronounced in the right lower lobe. (**Right**) Axial NECT of the same patient shows bilateral bronchiectasis, bronchial wall thickening ➔, bronchiolitis, and tree-in-bud opacities ➔. The left lung is trilobed, and the right lung is bilobed consistent with situs abnormality.*

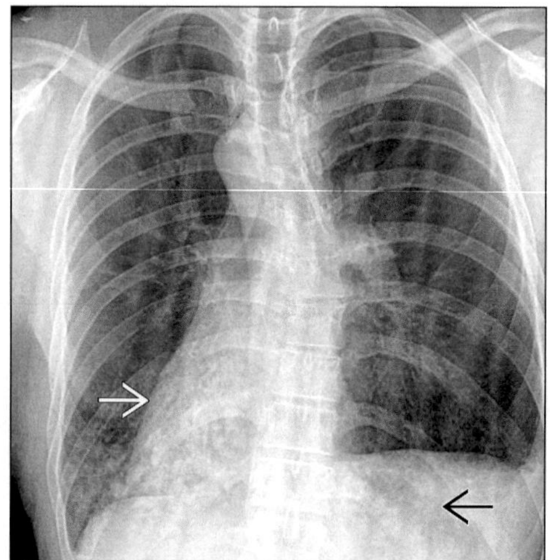

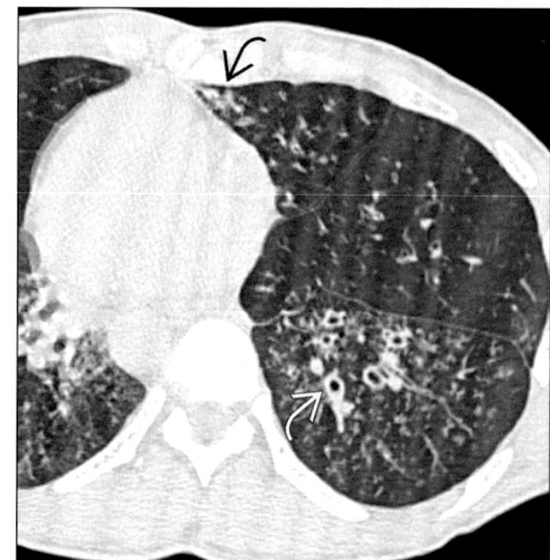

*(**Left**) Axial NECT of the same patient shows opacification of the bilateral maxillary sinuses ➔. Other images (not shown) demonstrated bilateral pansinusitis. (**Right**) Axial CECT of the same patient shows a left-sided stomach ➔, polysplenia ➔, and a midline liver ➔. The location of the thoracic and abdominal organs is consistent with situs ambiguous. The sinopulmonary features are the result of chronic infections due to abnormal ciliary function from primary ciliary dyskinesia.*

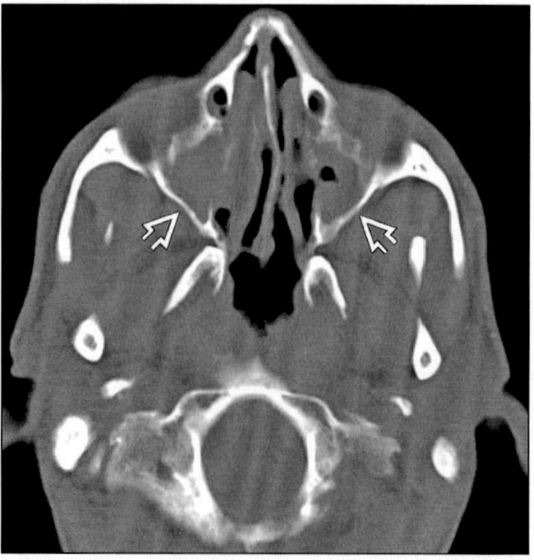

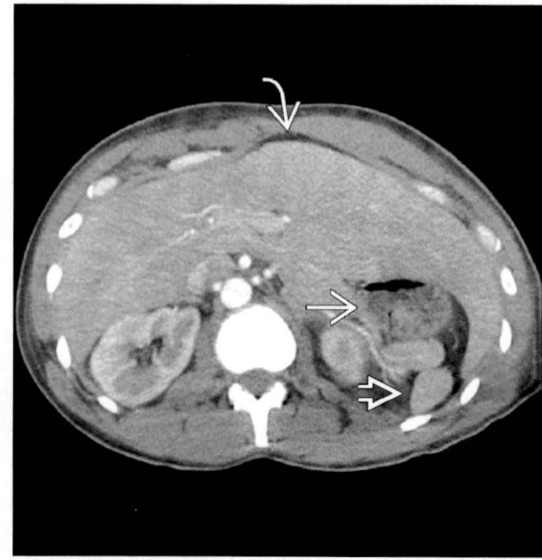

PRIMARY CILIARY DYSKINESIA

TERMINOLOGY

Abbreviations

- **Primary ciliary dyskinesia (PCD)**

Synonyms

- Dyskinetic cilia syndrome, immotile cilia syndrome

Definitions

- **PCD**
  - Includes all genetic disorders that cause ciliary defects & impaired mucociliary clearance
  - Ciliary motion is usually present but abnormal
  - Abnormal ciliary ultrastructure with resultant mucociliary dysfunction & sinopulmonary disease
  - Abnormalities of situs in 50% of cases (including situs inversus & situs ambiguous)
- **Kartagener syndrome**: 50% of PCD
  - Triad of situs inversus, sinusitis or nasal polyposis, & bronchiectasis
  - Subset of PCD
  - Kartagener-Afzelius syndrome: Kartagener described sinusitis, bronchiectasis, & situs inversus; Afzelius described associated infertility

IMAGING

General Features

- Best diagnostic clue
  - Triad of abnormal situs, bronchiectasis, & sinusitis
- Location
  - Bronchiectasis with predilection for middle & lower lobes
- Size
  - Bronchial dilatation ranges from mild to severe
- Morphology
  - Bronchial dilatation, bronchial wall thickening, & surrounding airspace disease

Radiographic Findings

- Hyperinflation
- **Bronchial wall thickening**
- **Bronchiectasis of variable severity**
- Atelectasis
- **Consolidation**, may be recurrent
- **Dextrocardia & abnormalities of situs**
- Findings of prior pulmonary resection

CT Findings

- **Bronchial wall thickening**
- **Bronchiectasis with predilection for lingula, middle & lower lobes**
  - Variable severity: Cylindrical, varicose, & cystic
  - **Signet-ring sign**: Bronchial diameter > adjacent pulmonary artery
    - CT section perpendicular to bronchial long axis
    - "Ring" is dilated bronchus
    - "Stone" is adjacent pulmonary artery
- **Mucus plugs within dilated airways**
- Centrilobular nodules & tree-in-bud opacities
- Peribronchial airspace disease
  - Ground-glass opacity
  - Consolidation
- Mosaic attenuation, air trapping on expiratory CT
- Atelectasis, often segmental
- Findings of prior pulmonary resection
- Associated conditions
  - **Abnormalities of situs**
    - Situs inversus
    - Situs ambiguous
  - Congenital heart disease
  - Sinusitis

Imaging Recommendations

- Best imaging tool
  - HRCT is imaging study of choice for diagnosis & assessment of bronchiectasis
  - Chest radiographic abnormalities may suggest diagnosis in cases of Kartagener syndrome
- Protocol advice
  - Full inspiration HRCT at 10 mm intervals or volumetrically through chest

DIFFERENTIAL DIAGNOSIS

Cystic Fibrosis

- Autosomal recessive condition; abnormal exocrine gland secretions
- Caucasian patients; typically diagnosed in childhood
- Recurrent infections, wheezing, dyspnea
- Upper lobe predominant severe bronchiectasis, mucus plugging, bronchial wall thickening, mosaic attenuation

Allergic Bronchopulmonary Aspergillosis (ABPA)

- Patients with asthma or cystic fibrosis
- Reactivity to *Aspergillus*
- Worsening of asthma, cough, wheezing
- Upper lobe predominant central bronchiectasis
  - Mucoid impaction; may exhibit high attenuation

Postinfectious Bronchiectasis

- Recurrent pulmonary infection
  - Bacteria, mycobacteria, viruses
- Pulmonary infection may result in abnormal ciliary function & poor clearance of airway mucus
  - Subsequent bacterial colonization & host effects may lead to irreversible airway damage

Immune Deficiency Disorders

- HIV/AIDS, common variable immunodeficiency
- Recurrent pulmonary infection resulting in bronchiectasis

Young Syndrome

- Abnormal viscosity of airway mucus
- Bronchiectasis, rhinosinusitis, infertility
  - Infertility secondary to functional obstruction of genital tract & abnormal sperm transport

PATHOLOGY

General Features

- Etiology
  - Compromised mucociliary clearance secondary to structural and functional ciliary abnormalities
    - Leads to vicious cycle of pulmonary infection → airway destruction → pulmonary infection
    - Airway abnormalities predispose to recurrent pulmonary infection

PRIMARY CILIARY DYSKINESIA

- Genetics
  - Autosomal recessive; genetic heterogeneity with other genetic patterns described
- Associated abnormalities
  - Situs abnormalities
  - Congenital heart disease
  - Infertility
- Abnormal ciliary ultrastructure with abnormal ciliary beat frequency
- Abnormal ciliary orientation
  - May have normal ultrastructure & beat frequency
    - Transient abnormalities of ciliary orientation may occur with airway infection & inflammation

Gross Pathologic & Surgical Features

- Diffuse bronchiectasis
- Pulmonary infection
- Dextrocardia, abnormal situs

Microscopic Features

- Bronchial inflammation, squamous metaplasia, ulceration
- Bronchial wall fibrosis & destruction
- Acute & chronic pneumonia, organizing pneumonia
- Electron microscopy: Ultrastructural ciliary defect
  - Absence of dynein arms, central microtubule pairs, inner sheath, radial spokes, or nexin links
  - Most commonly: Absence of dynein arms

CLINICAL ISSUES

Presentation

- Most common signs/symptoms
  - Neonates: Respiratory distress, rhinitis, pneumonia
  - Infants & children: Cough, asthma, rhinorrhea, nose blowing, otitis, recurrent pneumonia
  - Older patients: Recurrent sinus, ear, & pulmonary infection & male infertility
  - Chronic rhinosinusitis, nasal polyposis, chronic secretory otitis media with hearing impairment
    - History of sinus surgery, adenotonsillectomy, nasal polypectomy
  - Recurrent pulmonary infection
    - *Haemophilus influenzae* most commonly cultured pathogen
    - *Neisseria meningitidis* and *Streptococcus pneumoniae* cause most infections
  - Productive cough, wheezing, coarse crackles, exertional dyspnea
  - Infertility in males, lowered fertility in females
  - Pulmonary function
    - Mild to severe obstructive abnormalities
    - Mixed obstructive & restrictive abnormalities
- Other signs/symptoms
  - Situs abnormalities in patients with Kartagener syndrome
    - 23% of patients with situs inversus have PCD
  - Rarely: Esophageal atresia, complex congenital heart disease, biliary atresia, hydrocephalus
    - Usually associated with situs abnormalities

Demographics

- Age
  - Typically diagnosed in childhood or adolescence
    - Median age at diagnosis is 4 years
- Gender
  - No predilection
- Epidemiology
  - Incidence estimated at 1:12,000-20,000 births
  - True incidence unknown

Diagnosis

- Nasal brush biopsy
  - Functional studies: Direct measurement of ciliary beat frequency
  - Ultrastructural studies: Evaluation of ciliary orientation & ciliary ultrastructure on electron microscopy

Screening

- Measurement of nasal nitric oxide (NO)
  - Low levels of exhaled NO in patients with PCD

Natural History & Prognosis

- Affected patients may present as newborns
- Diagnosis in late childhood and adolescence; nonresponsive cough, wheezing, or recurrent infection
- Good prognosis, particularly with early diagnosis & aggressive treatment

Treatment

- Aggressive airway clearance with rigorous lung physiotherapy
- Prophylactic & organism-specific antibiotics against common pulmonary pathogens to prevent bronchiectasis
- Immunization for common pathogens
- Advanced disease
  - Surgical intervention for severe bronchiectasis
  - Lung transplantation for end-stage lung disease

DIAGNOSTIC CHECKLIST

Consider

- PCD in young patients with chronic bronchial infection since infancy & patients with abnormal situs & bronchiectasis

Image Interpretation Pearls

- Basilar bronchiectasis in young patient ± situs abnormality

SELECTED REFERENCES

1. Jain K et al: Primary ciliary dyskinesia in the paediatric population: range and severity of radiological findings in a cohort of patients receiving tertiary care. Clin Radiol. 62(10):986-93, 2007
2. Kennedy MP et al: High-resolution CT of patients with primary ciliary dyskinesia. AJR Am J Roentgenol. 188(5):1232-8, 2007
3. Kennedy MP et al: Primary ciliary dyskinesia and upper airway diseases. Curr Allergy Asthma Rep. 6(6):513-7, 2006
4. Berdon WE et al: Situs inversus, bronchiectasis, and sinusitis and its relation to immotile cilia: history of the diseases and their discoverers-Manes Kartagener and Bjorn Afzelius. Pediatr Radiol. 34(1):38-42, 2004

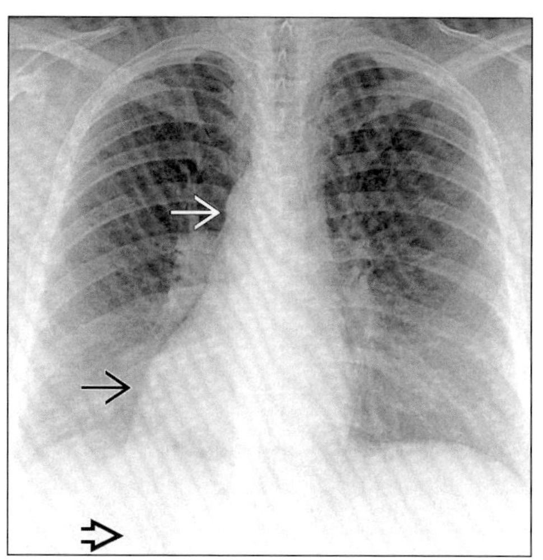

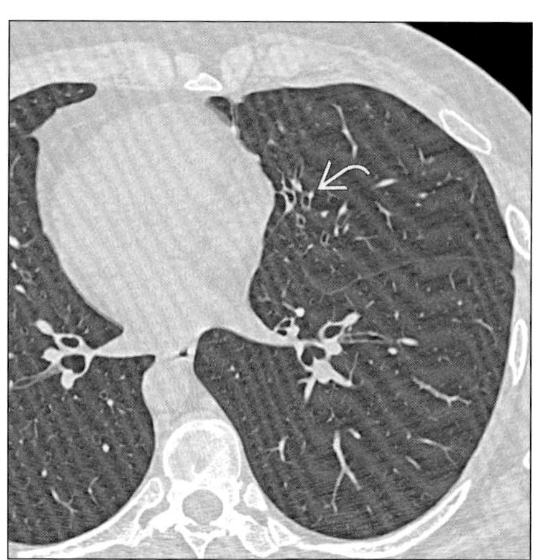

(Left) *PA chest radiograph of a 38-year-old man shows dextrocardia, a right-sided aortic arch, and a right-sided stomach, indicating situs inversus totalis.* ***(Right)*** *Axial CECT of the same patient shows mild left middle lobe bronchiectasis without surrounding bronchiolitis. Prophylactic antibiotic treatment and aggressive lung physiotherapy can prevent bronchiectasis in patients with primary ciliary dyskinesia.*

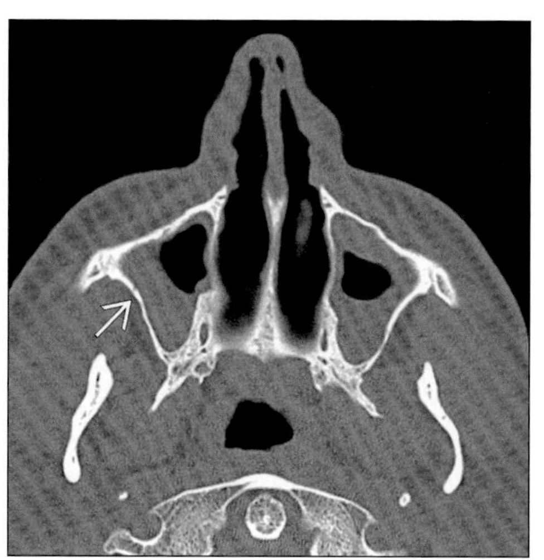

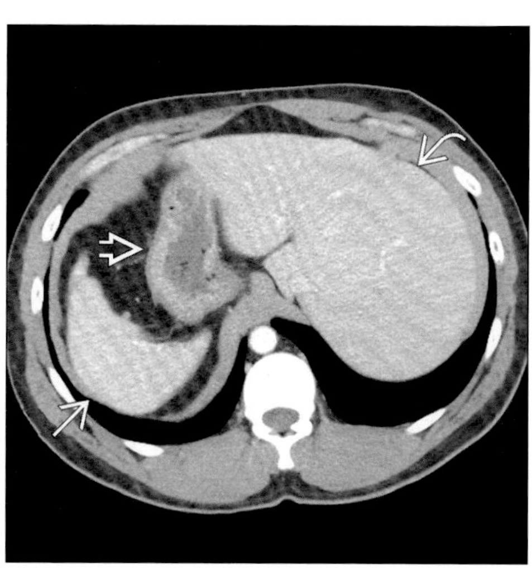

(Left) *Axial NECT of the same patient shows bilateral maxillary sinusitis with bilateral mucosal thickening and an air-fluid level in the left maxillary sinus.* ***(Right)*** *Axial CECT of the same patient shows a left-sided liver, a right-sided stomach, and a single right-sided spleen. The findings of situs inversus totalis, bronchiectasis, and sinusitis are consistent with Kartagener syndrome. Bronchiectasis and sinusitis are related to chronic infections from ciliary dysmotility.*

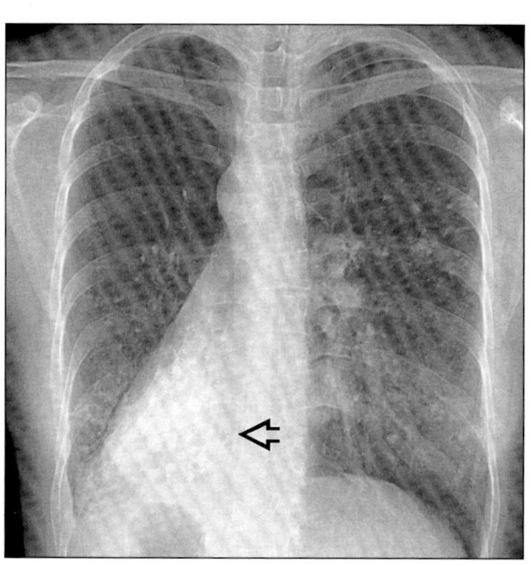

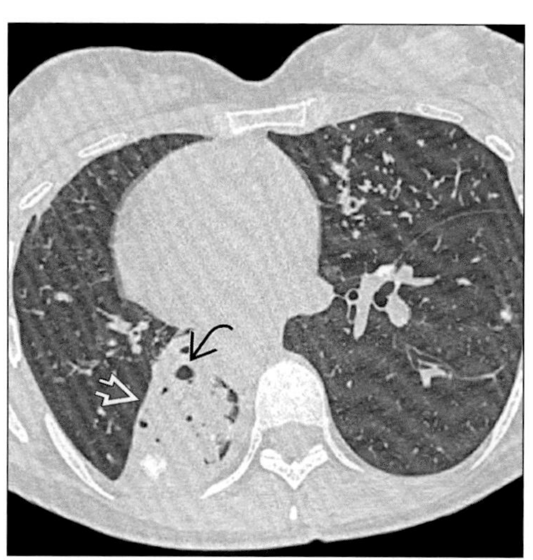

(Left) *PA chest radiograph of a young woman with Kartagener syndrome shows situs inversus totalis. Note the retrocardiac opacity, representing right lower lobe consolidation.* ***(Right)*** *Axial HRCT of the same patient obtained 6 months later shows persistent right lower lobe consolidation with volume loss, bronchiectasis and cavitation, left middle lobe bronchiectasis, mucus plugging, and bronchiolitis. These findings are related to chronic infection secondary to ciliary dysmotility.*

WILLIAMS-CAMPBELL SYNDROME

Key Facts

Terminology

- Congenital form of bronchiectasis related to cartilage deficiency in subsegmental bronchi

Imaging

- Radiography
  - Bronchiectasis of 4th through 6th order bronchi
  - Bronchial wall thickening
  - Cystic spaces
- HRCT
  - Varicoid & cystic bronchiectasis
  - 4th to 6th order bronchi involved
  - Other central airways normal
  - Bronchial wall thickening, mucus plugs, fluid
  - Expiratory imaging for detection of bronchomalacia & distal air-trapping
- Absent normal cartilaginous ring impressions on virtual bronchoscopy

Top Differential Diagnoses

- Cystic fibrosis, lung disease
- Allergic bronchopulmonary aspergillosis
- Bronchiectasis
- Primary ciliary dyskinesia

Pathology

- Absence of cartilage in medium to small airways
- Cystic bronchiectasis

Clinical Issues

- Recurrent pulmonary infection, usually in infancy & childhood
- Cough, dyspnea, wheezing

Diagnostic Checklist

- Cystic bronchiectasis of 4th to 6th order bronchi should suggest Williams-Campbell syndrome

__(Left)__ PA chest radiograph shows coarse perihilar tubular opacities ➦ (consistent with bronchiectasis) and left lower lobe airspace disease ➔ with ipsilateral mediastinal shift (consistent with volume loss). __(Right)__ Lateral chest radiograph of the same patient shows a dense posterior basal opacity ➔. Bronchiectatic airways are not readily apparent. The radiographic findings of Williams-Campbell syndrome are nonspecific and can be masked by superimposed pneumonia, atelectasis, or scar.

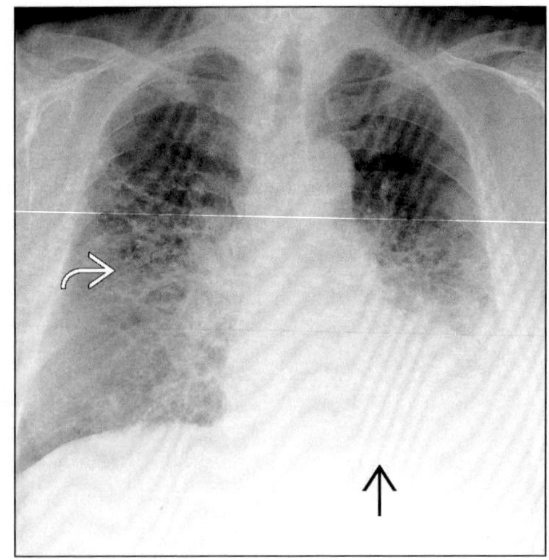

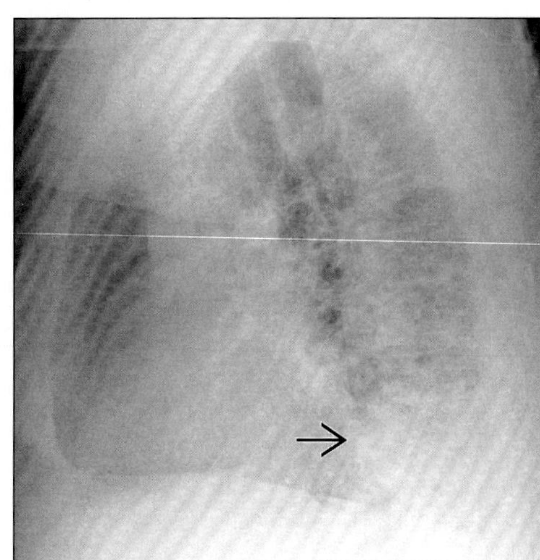

__(Left)__ Axial NECT of the same patient shows cystic bronchiectasis ➔ with fluid pooling dependently in some bronchiectatic airways. Note leftward mediastinal shift ➦ secondary to left lung volume loss. __(Right)__ Axial NECT of the same patient shows extensive cystic bronchiectasis ➔ in the lower lobes and left lung volume loss. Note the normal more proximal airways ➦. The 4th through 6th order bronchi are affected in Williams-Campbell syndrome.

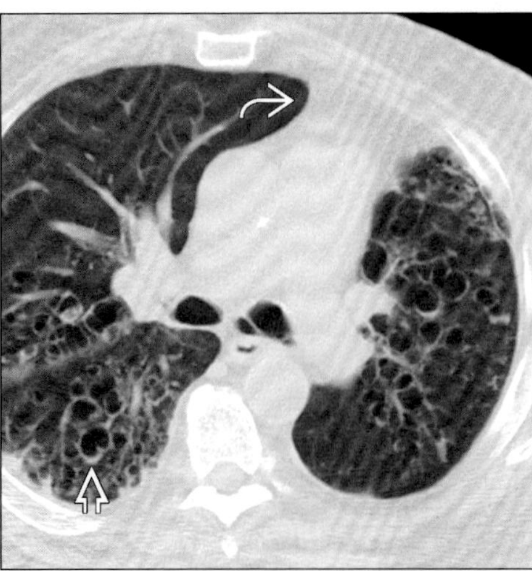

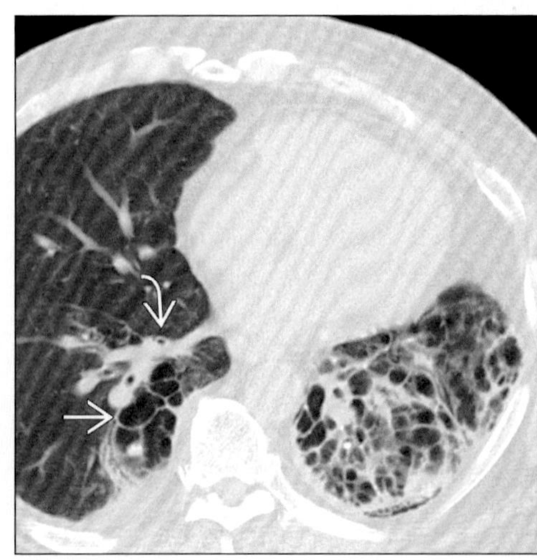

WILLIAMS-CAMPBELL SYNDROME

TERMINOLOGY

Definitions

- Congenital form of bronchiectasis related to deficiency of cartilage in subsegmental bronchi

IMAGING

General Features

- Best diagnostic clue
  - Bronchiectasis of 4th through 6th order bronchi
- Location
  - Central lungs
- Size
  - Segmental airways
- Morphology
  - Varicoid & cystic bronchiectasis

Radiographic Findings

- Radiography
  - Bronchial wall thickening
  - Bronchiectasis & cystic spaces

CT Findings

- HRCT
  - Varicoid & cystic bronchiectasis
    - 4th to 6th order bronchi involved
    - Other central airways normal
    - Bronchial wall thickening, mucus plugs, fluid
    - Ballooning on inspiration
  - Expiratory imaging
    - Bronchomalacia (bronchial collapse)
    - Distal air-trapping
  - CT virtual bronchoscopy
    - Absent normal cartilaginous ring impressions

Imaging Recommendations

- Best imaging tool
  - HRCT is imaging modality of choice to evaluate airways disease
- Protocol advice
  - Expiratory imaging useful for detecting bronchomalacia & air-trapping

DIFFERENTIAL DIAGNOSIS

Cystic Fibrosis

- Mid & upper lung predominant bronchiectasis
- More proximal & distal airways usually involved
- Fatty or cystic replacement of pancreas
- Positive sweat chloride test

Cystic Lung Disease

- Cysts evident on volumetric HRCT or coronal reformations
- Airways usually normal

Allergic Bronchopulmonary Aspergillosis

- Occurs primarily in asthmatics
- Central varicoid bronchiectasis with high-attenuation mucoid impaction, a characteristic finding
- Tree-in-bud opacities & air-trapping may be present distally

Bronchiectasis

- Focal or diffuse
- Classic distribution (4th to 6th order) of bronchiectasis usually diagnostic of Williams-Campbell syndrome

Primary Ciliary Dyskinesia

- Bronchiectasis usually basal predominant
- Associations
  - Situs inversus
  - Chronic sinusitis
  - Male infertility

PATHOLOGY

General Features

- Etiology
  - Believed to be result of airway wall cartilage deficiency

Gross Pathologic & Surgical Features

- Absence of cartilage in medium to small airways
- Cystic bronchiectasis

CLINICAL ISSUES

Presentation

- Most common signs/symptoms
  - Recurrent pulmonary infection
    - Usually in infancy or early childhood
    - Uncommon presentation in adulthood
- Other signs/symptoms
  - Cough
  - Dyspnea
  - Wheezing

Demographics

- Age
  - Most present in infancy because of recurrent infection
- Epidemiology
  - Familial clustering often apparent

Natural History & Prognosis

- Recurrent infection common
  - Bronchiectasis may worsen

Treatment

- Directed & prophylactic anti-infectives for pulmonary infections

DIAGNOSTIC CHECKLIST

Consider

- Other causes of severe bronchiectasis

Image Interpretation Pearls

- Cystic bronchiectasis limited to 4th to 6th order bronchi should suggest Williams-Campbell syndrome

SELECTED REFERENCES

1. Di Scioscio V et al: The role of spiral multidetector dynamic CT in the study of Williams-Campbell syndrome. Acta Radiol. 47(8):798-800, 2006

BRONCHOLITHIASIS

Key Facts

Terminology

- Calcified or ossified endobronchial material, usually due to erosion from adjacent lymph nodes

Imaging

- Radiography
  - Airway obstruction: Atelectasis, mucoid impaction, bronchiectasis, air-trapping
  - Mediastinal or hilar lymph node calcification
  - Actual broncholith rarely appreciated
- CT
  - Endobronchial or peribronchial calcified lymph node
  - Usually solitary, rarely multiple
  - Middle lobe & upper lobe anterior segmental bronchi most commonly involved
  - Extraluminal air nearly diagnostic of endobronchial erosion

Top Differential Diagnoses

- Carcinoid
- Airway hamartoma
- Airway amyloidosis

Pathology

- Etiology
  - Erosion by & extrusion of calcified lymph nodes
  - Aspiration of radiopaque material or in situ foreign body calcification

Clinical Issues

- Symptoms: Cough, hemoptysis, recurrent pneumonia
- Treatment
  - Bronchoscopic removal of loose broncholith
  - Surgical lobectomy or segmentectomy often required

*(**Left**) PA chest radiograph of a 60-year-old man with persistent cough shows focal middle lobe opacity and volume loss with inferior displacement of the minor fissure ➡. Note adjacent calcified granuloma ➡. (**Right**) Axial CECT of the same patient shows a broncholith obstructing the lateral segmental middle lobe bronchus with associated partial atelectasis and postobstructive consolidation. The patient underwent middle lobectomy. The middle lobe bronchi are common locations for broncholithiasis.*

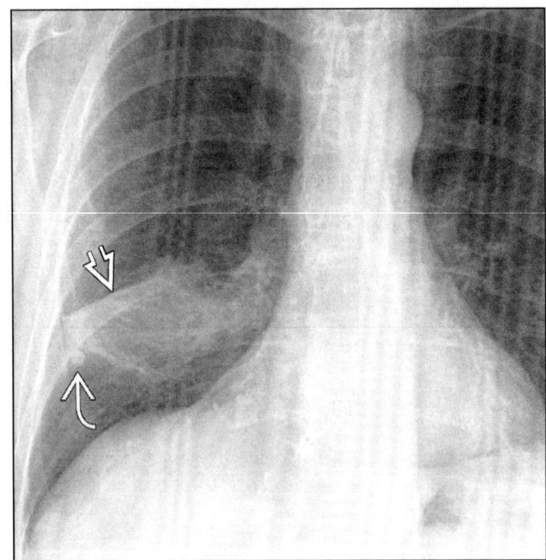

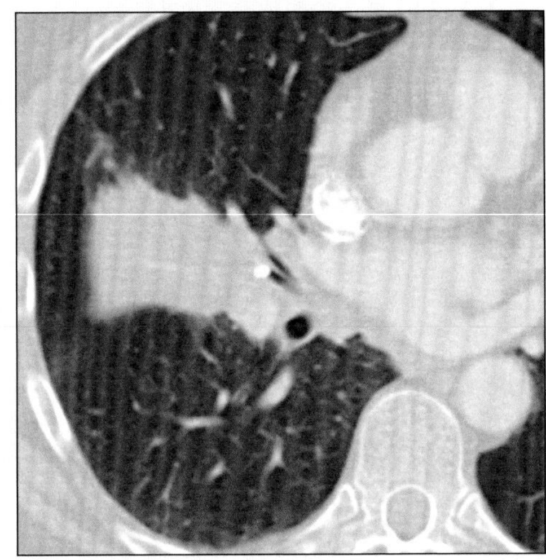

*(**Left**) PA chest radiograph of a 40-year-old woman with recurrent pneumonia shows calcified right paratracheal and hilar lymph nodes ➡ and a subtle linear opacity in the right lung base ➡. (**Right**) Axial CECT of the same patient shows a calcified nodule ➡ occluding the anterior basal segmental bronchus of the right lower lobe; this is consistent with broncholithiasis, which was confirmed at bronchoscopy. The broncholith appeared mobile during bronchoalveolar lavage and was successfully extracted bronchoscopically.*

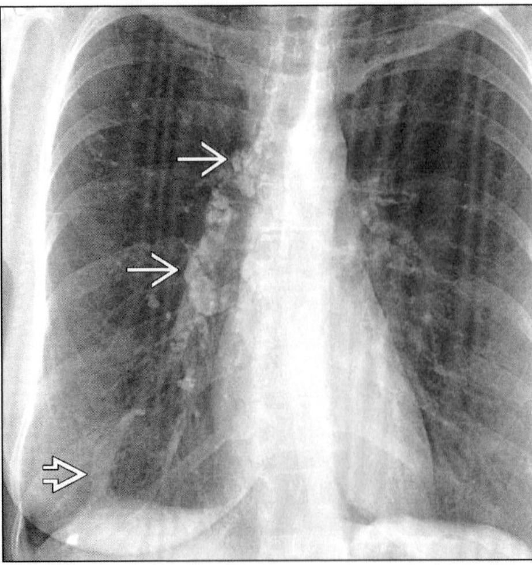

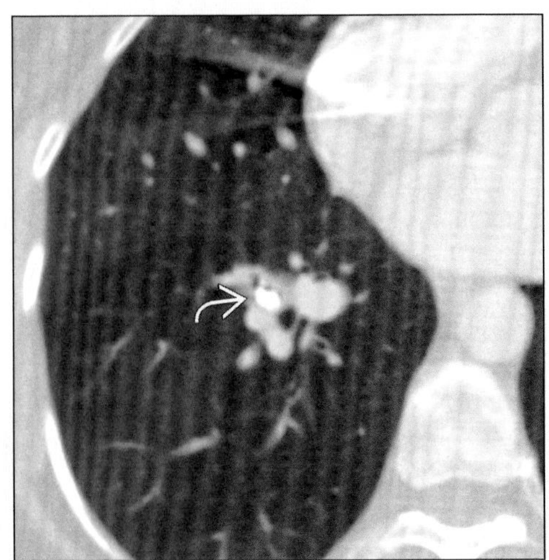

BRONCHOLITHIASIS

TERMINOLOGY

Definitions

- Calcified or ossified material within bronchial lumen, usually due to erosion from adjacent lymph nodes

IMAGING

General Features

- Best diagnostic clue
  - Endobronchial or peribronchial calcified nodule with signs of bronchial obstruction
- Location
  - Most common: Middle lobe & upper lobe anterior segmental bronchi
  - Right > left (2:1)
  - Anywhere from trachea to subsegmental airways, most common in lobar to segmental airways
- Size
  - 2-15 mm
- Morphology
  - Irregular shape, angular margins
  - Majority of lesion calcified; minimal soft tissue component

Radiographic Findings

- Airway obstruction
  - Atelectasis
  - Mucoid impaction
    - "Finger in glove" opacities
  - Bronchiectasis
  - Expiratory air-trapping
- Calcified mediastinal or hilar lymph nodes
- Actual broncholiths not usually appreciated

CT Findings

- Endobronchial or peribronchial calcified nodule/ lymph node
  - Distortion & narrowing of adjacent airway (50%)
  - Complete airway obstruction (50%)
  - Extraluminal air nearly diagnostic of endobronchial erosion
  - Usually solitary, rarely multiple
  - Does not enhance with intravenous contrast
- Signs of bronchial obstruction
  - Atelectasis (66%)
  - Postobstructive pneumonia (33%)
  - Bronchiectasis (33%)
  - Air-trapping (5%)
  - Mucoid impaction

Imaging Recommendations

- Best imaging tool
  - CT for localization of calcified lymph nodes & evaluation of adjacent airways

DIFFERENTIAL DIAGNOSIS

Carcinoid

- 39% of central carcinoids exhibit calcification or ossification
- May enhance with intravenous contrast

Airway Hamartoma

- May exhibit internal calcification & fat attenuation

Tracheobronchopathia Osteochondroplastica

- Idiopathic condition characterized by submucosal osteocartilaginous growths along cartilaginous rings
  - Anterior & lateral tracheal margins
    - May circumferentially involve lobar & segmental airways
  - Calcified nodules usually numerous & diffuse

Airway Amyloidosis

- Airway narrowed by submucosal amyloid deposits
- Calcification usually amorphous or stippled
- Usually diffuse & multifocal rather than solitary

PATHOLOGY

General Features

- Etiology
  - Erosion by & extrusion of calcified lymph nodes
    - Longstanding foci of necrotizing granulomatous lymphadenitis
      - *Mycobacterium tuberculosis* worldwide
      - *Histoplasma capsulatum, Coccidioides immitis* in endemic regions
    - Silicosis: Few reported cases
  - Aspiration of radiopaque material or in situ foreign body calcification
  - Erosion by & extrusion of calcified bronchial cartilage

Microscopic Features

- Laminated necrotic material with dystrophic calcification
- Organisms responsible for granulomatous lymphadenitis may be identified with special stains
- Inflammation, ulceration of adjacent bronchial wall

CLINICAL ISSUES

Presentation

- Most common signs/symptoms
  - Nonproductive cough
  - Hemoptysis
  - Recurrent pneumonia
- Other signs/symptoms
  - **Lithoptysis**: Expectoration of calcified material

Treatment

- Bronchoscopy for loose broncholith
  - Hemorrhage may result if broncholith is attached to bronchial wall due to proximity of pulmonary artery branches to airways
- Surgical lobectomy or segmentectomy for failed bronchoscopic removal

SELECTED REFERENCES

1. Seo JB et al: Broncholithiasis: review of the causes with radiologic-pathologic correlation. Radiographics. 22 Spec No:S199-213, 2002
2. Conces DJ Jr et al: Broncholithiasis: CT features in 15 patients. AJR Am J Roentgenol. 157(2):249-53, 1991

CENTRILOBULAR EMPHYSEMA

Key Facts

Terminology

- Centrilobular emphysema (CLE)
- Synonyms
  - Centriacinar emphysema
  - Proximal acinar emphysema
- Enlargement & destruction of respiratory bronchioles near center of secondary pulmonary lobule

Imaging

- Radiography
  - Mild disease: Radiography may be normal
  - Advanced disease: Heterogeneous lung density, vascular distortion/disruption
  - Hyperinflated & hyperlucent lungs
- CT/HRCT
  - Centrilobular low attenuation, no discernible wall
  - May visualize central lobular artery surrounded by destroyed lung

Top Differential Diagnoses

- Panlobular emphysema
- Paraseptal emphysema
- Cystic lung disease
- Constrictive bronchiolitis
- Asthma

Pathology

- Precursor may be respiratory bronchiolitis

Clinical Issues

- Symptoms: Dyspnea, shortness of breath
- Strongly associated with cigarette smoking
- Treatment
  - Smoking cessation
  - Lung volume reduction/endobronchial valves
  - Lung transplantation

__(Left)__ PA chest radiograph of a female smoker with severe centrilobular emphysema shows marked hyperinflation and upper lung zone hyperlucency with relative paucity of vascular markings. __(Right)__ Lateral chest radiograph of the same patient shows flattening of the diaphragm, an increased AP diameter of the chest, and enlargement of the retrosternal space. Chest CT (not shown) confirmed the presence of severe centrilobular emphysema.

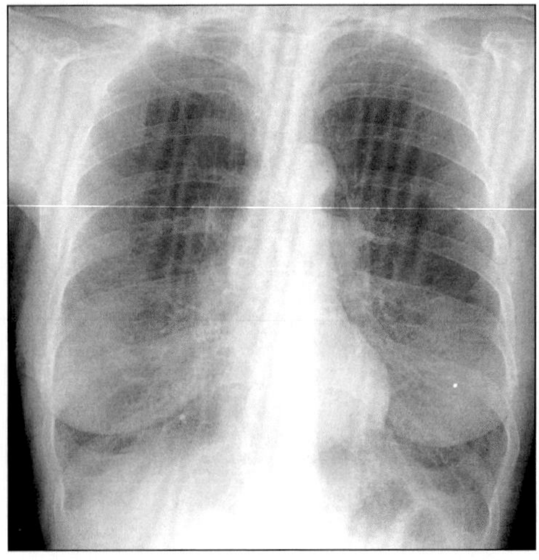

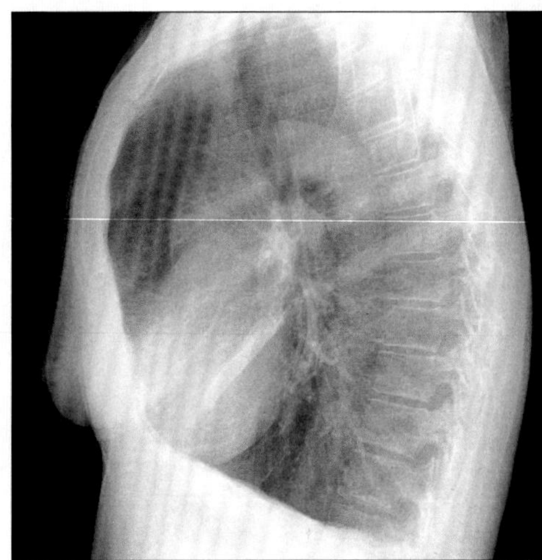

__(Left)__ Graphic depicts the morphologic appearance of centrilobular emphysema characterized by parenchymal destruction at the center of the secondary pulmonary lobules surrounding the central lobular arteries ➔. __(Right)__ Coronal CECT of a 60-year-old female smoker who presented with increasing dyspnea on exertion shows upper lung zone predominant centrilobular emphysema and bullae. Centrilobular emphysema exhibits a predilection for the upper lung zones.

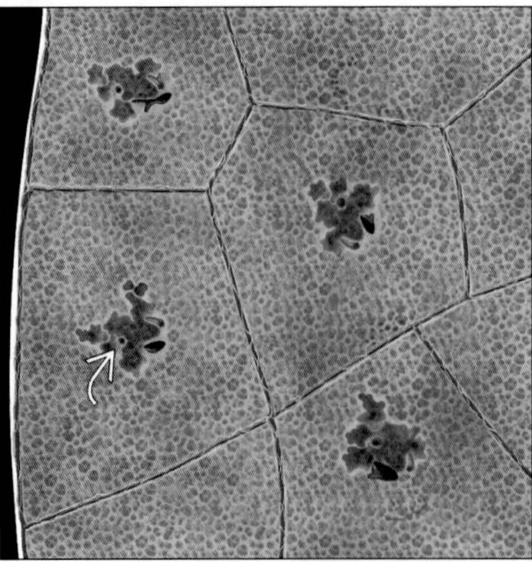

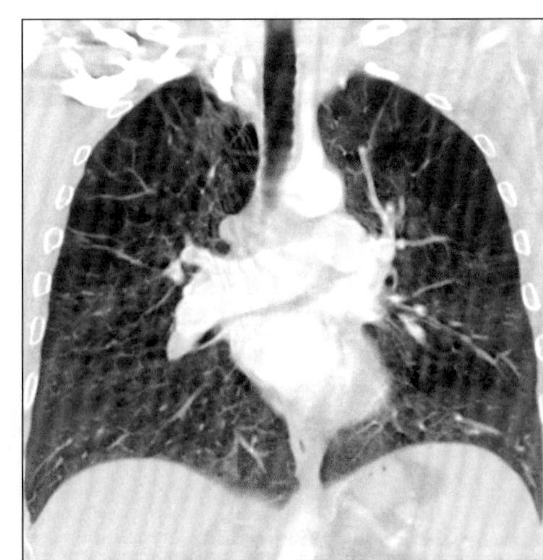

CENTRILOBULAR EMPHYSEMA

TERMINOLOGY

Abbreviations

- **Centrilobular emphysema** (CLE)

Synonyms

- Centriacinar emphysema
- Proximal acinar emphysema

Definitions

- Enlargement & destruction of respiratory bronchioles located near center of secondary pulmonary lobule

IMAGING

General Features

- Best diagnostic clue
  - Well-defined round lucencies in centrilobular portion of secondary pulmonary lobule on HRCT
  - Anatomical borders of secondary pulmonary lobule are preserved
- Location
  - **Upper lung zone predominant**
    - Lung apices
    - Lower lobe superior segments
- Size
  - Mild disease: 1-2 mm centrilobular "holes"
  - Advanced disease: May occupy entire secondary pulmonary lobule & mimic panlobular emphysema
    - Also referred to as centrilobular emphysema with panlobular features
- Morphology
  - Destruction of lung parenchyma near lobular arteriole & bronchiole
  - Well-defined margins between normal & emphysematous lungs result in heterogeneous attenuation

Radiographic Findings

- Radiography
  - Mild disease: Very insensitive, radiography may be completely normal
    - Normal lung is 90% air, making radiographic detection of slight increases in air nearly impossible
    - Consequence: Weak correlation between functional indices & radiographic findings
  - Advanced disease: May be visible on radiograph
    - Heterogeneous lung density
    - Vascular distortion & disruption
    - Increased branching angle of remaining vessels
- **Hyperinflation**
  - Flat hemidiaphragms
  - Increased AP diameter of thorax
  - Enlarged retrosternal space
  - Small narrow heart
- Secondary manifestations
  - **Pulmonary arterial hypertension**
    - Enlarged central pulmonary arteries
    - Peripheral arterial pruning

CT Findings

- HRCT
  - More sensitive than chest radiography
  - Detection of clinically & functionally "silent" CLE
  - Low-attenuation areas located in center of secondary pulmonary lobule
    - No discernible wall
    - Surrounded by normal lung
    - May visualize central lobular artery surrounded by destroyed lung
    - Borders of secondary pulmonary lobule are preserved
  - Objectively measured by assuming that lung with threshold HU < -950 is emphysema

Imaging Recommendations

- Best imaging tool
  - HRCT is imaging modality of choice for assessment & characterization of emphysema
- Protocol advice
  - Acquire scans at end inspiration only
  - Expiratory scans are of little value in CLE
  - Careful evaluation of lung apices & superior segments of lower lobes
  - Minimum-intensity projection (MinIP) images increase sensitivity for detecting mild disease
  - CT quantification analysis more accurate at grading extent of disease compared to subjective visual grading

MR Findings

- Hyperpolarized 3He at both 1.5 & 3.0 Tesla
  - Shows significantly increased ADC values for emphysematous lungs
- Used rarely in clinical practice; ongoing research

DIFFERENTIAL DIAGNOSIS

Panlobular Emphysema

- Pattern of destruction more homogeneous than CLE
- Uniform distribution, no upper lobe predominance
- Uniform destruction of secondary pulmonary lobule

Paraseptal Emphysema

- Single tier of subpleural cystic spaces of varying sizes
- Often seen in association with CLE

Cystic Lung Disease

- Cysts with definable walls (e.g., lymphangioleiomyomatosis)
- Nonvisualization of central lobular artery

Constrictive Bronchiolitis

- No parenchymal destruction, mosaic attenuation
- Air-trapping on expiratory CT

Langerhans Cell Histiocytosis

- Smoking-related disease
- Nodules that may cavitate & evolve into cysts with irregular nodular walls
- Upper/mid lung zone distribution
- Longstanding disease may mimic advanced centrilobular emphysema

Asthma

- No parenchymal destruction
- Hyperinflation may be reversible

CENTRILOBULAR EMPHYSEMA

PATHOLOGY

General Features

- Etiology
  - CLE strongly associated with cigarette smoking
    - Severity related to magnitude of exposure
  - CLE also occurs after inhalation of industrial dusts (silica)
- Genetics
  - Potential genetic predisposition to CLE
    - Could explain varying extent of CLE in individuals with comparable smoking habits
- Associated abnormalities
  - Respiratory bronchiolitis
  - Chronic bronchitis
  - Hyperinflation
  - Secondary pulmonary hypertension
- Pathologic functional correlation
  - Patients may have anatomic emphysema without alteration of pulmonary function
  - 30% of normal lung must be destroyed before pulmonary function deteriorates
  - Pulmonary function usually determined by structural integrity of lower lung zones
  - Pulmonary function tests are global summation of airways & lung, but HRCT provides regional information

Staging, Grading, & Classification

- HRCT allows objective quantification of emphysema

Gross Pathologic & Surgical Features

- Centrilobular location
  - Dilatation of 2nd-order respiratory bronchioles
  - Primarily involves upper lung zones
  - Precursor may be respiratory bronchiolitis

Microscopic Features

- Enlargement & destruction of alveolar walls
- Emphysematous spaces become confluent within acinus

CLINICAL ISSUES

Presentation

- Most common signs/symptoms
  - Mild disease
    - Often asymptomatic
    - May be incidental finding on HRCT
  - Moderate/advanced disease
    - Dyspnea, shortness of breath
    - Increased total & residual lung volumes
    - Residual volume > 120% predicted
    - FEV1 < 80% predicted
    - Diffusion capacity decreased < 80% predicted
    - CLE most common form of emphysema associated with symptomatic or fatal COPD
- Other signs/symptoms
  - Pulmonary hypertension

Demographics

- Age
  - Incidence peak between 45-75 years
- Gender
  - Slight male predominance (due to smoking habits)
- Epidemiology
  - Very common disease in industrialized world
  - Geographic variations according to regional smoking habits

Natural History & Prognosis

- With smoking cessation: Stabilization or slow progression
- Without smoking cessation: Accelerated progression to clinically symptomatic form that requires treatment

Treatment

- Smoking cessation
  - Pulmonary function will continue to decline
- Bronchodilators
- Lung volume reduction surgery
  - Candidates with heterogeneous emphysema (usually upper lobe predominant)
- Endobronchial valve placement in patients with advanced emphysema shown to modestly improve pulmonary function, exercise tolerance, & symptoms
  - 1-way valves which allow air to exit but not enter treated bronchus
  - Placed bronchoscopically
  - Complications include hemoptysis, pneumonia, and COPD exacerbation
- Lung transplantation: Unfortunately too few organs for those in need

DIAGNOSTIC CHECKLIST

Consider

- CLE is very common "incidental" CT finding in smokers

Image Interpretation Pearls

- Focal areas of low attenuation with imperceptible walls
- Predominates in upper lung zones
- Best seen on HRCT

SELECTED REFERENCES

1. Gietema HA et al: Quantifying the extent of emphysema: factors associated with radiologists' estimations and quantitative indices of emphysema severity using the ECLIPSE cohort. Acad Radiol. 18(6):661-71, 2011
2. Mets OM et al: Identification of chronic obstructive pulmonary disease in lung cancer screening computed tomographic scans. JAMA. 306(16):1775-81, 2011
3. Gietema HA et al: Distribution of emphysema in heavy smokers: impact on pulmonary function. Respir Med. 104(1):76-82, 2010
4. Sciurba FC et al: A randomized study of endobronchial valves for advanced emphysema. N Engl J Med. 363(13):1233-44, 2010
5. Akira M et al: Quantitative CT in chronic obstructive pulmonary disease: inspiratory and expiratory assessment. AJR Am J Roentgenol. 192(1):267-72, 2009
6. Litmanovich D et al: CT of pulmonary emphysema--current status, challenges, and future directions. Eur Radiol. 19(3):537-51, 2009
7. Parraga G et al: Hyperpolarized 3He ventilation defects and apparent diffusion coefficients in chronic obstructive pulmonary disease: preliminary results at 3.0 Tesla. Invest Radiol. 42(6):384-91, 2007

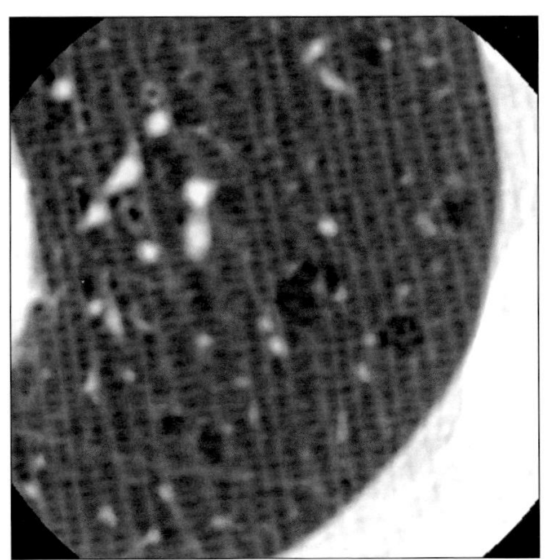

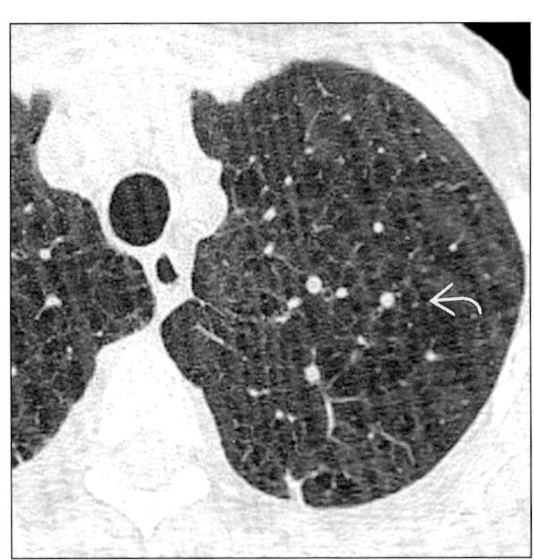

(Left) *Axial NECT of a 40-year-old smoker shows CLE manifesting with scattered small foci of low attenuation with imperceptible walls located in a centrilobular distribution. CLE is commonly found incidentally in smokers undergoing chest CT.* ***(Right)*** *Axial HRCT of a heavy smoker with oxygen-dependent COPD shows moderate CLE predominantly involving the upper lung zones and manifesting with low-attenuation foci, some with a visible central "dot" ➔ representing the central lobular artery.*

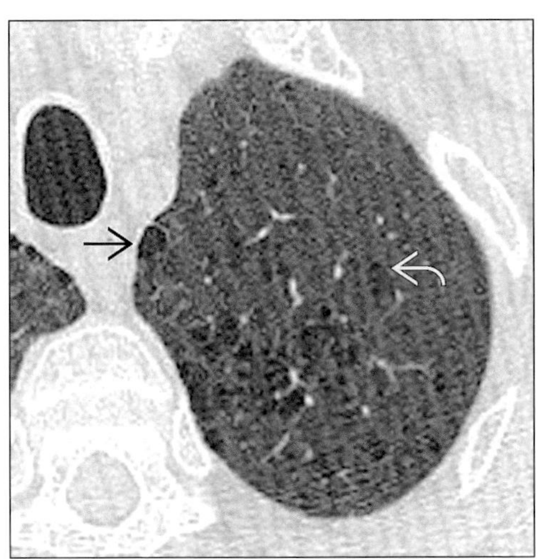

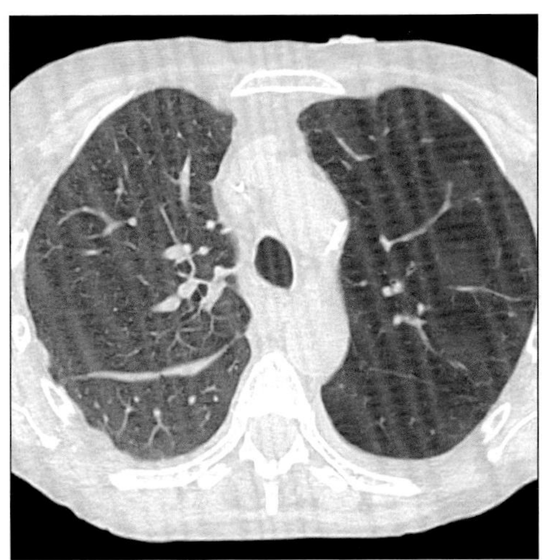

(Left) *Axial HRCT of a 49-year-old smoker with dyspnea and airway obstruction on pulmonary function tests shows centrilobular ➔ and paraseptal ➔ emphysema, both often seen concurrently in smokers.* ***(Right)*** *Axial NECT of a 50-year-old woman following right lung transplantation for treatment of CLE shows a normal transplanted right lung and severe centrilobular emphysema in the native left lung. There is a limited supply of organs available for this treatment option.*

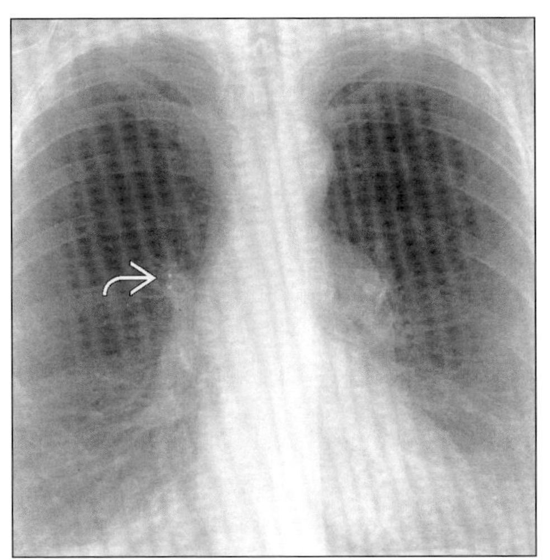

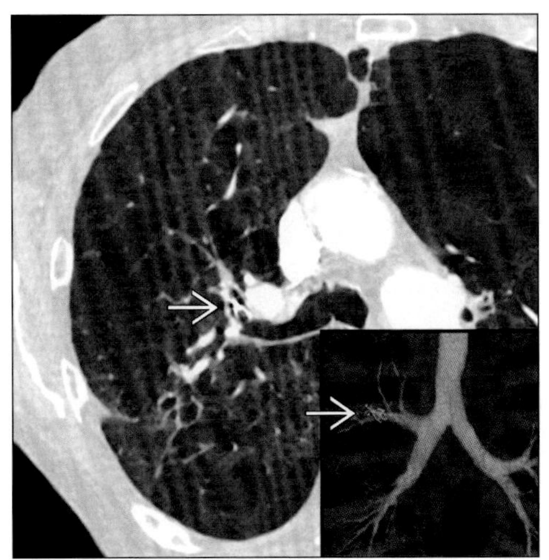

(Left) *PA chest radiograph shows upper lung zone hyperlucency and metallic bronchial valves ➔ in the upper lobe bronchi used to treat severe CLE.* ***(Right)*** *Axial CECT and coronal volume-rendered image (see insert) of a patient with severe centrilobular emphysema shows an endobronchial valve in the anterior segmental right upper lobe bronchus ➔. Endobronchial valves look like IVC filters and have been used clinically to treat postoperative air leaks and in trials to treat severe COPD.*

PARASEPTAL EMPHYSEMA

Key Facts

Terminology

- Paraseptal emphysema (PSE)
- Synonym: Distal acinar emphysema
- Permanently enlarged distal acinus with destruction of alveolar ducts & sacs

Imaging

- Radiography
  - Mild paraseptal emphysema difficult to detect
  - Radiography may be normal
  - Peripheral lung lucencies with thin walls
- CT/HRCT
  - Subpleural & peribronchovascular single tier of cystic spaces
  - Separated by intact interlobular septa
  - Minimum-intensity projection (MinIP) images may improve detection
- HRCT is imaging modality of choice

Top Differential Diagnoses

- Cystic lung disease
- Centrilobular emphysema
- Panlobular emphysema
- Honeycomb lung (pulmonary fibrosis)

Pathology

- ↑ incidence: Smokers, IV drug users, HIV(+) patients

Clinical Issues

- Often incidentally detected
- Treatment
  - Smoking cessation
  - Pleurodesis for recurrent pneumothorax

Diagnostic Checklist

- Consider paraseptal emphysema as a cause of spontaneous pneumothorax

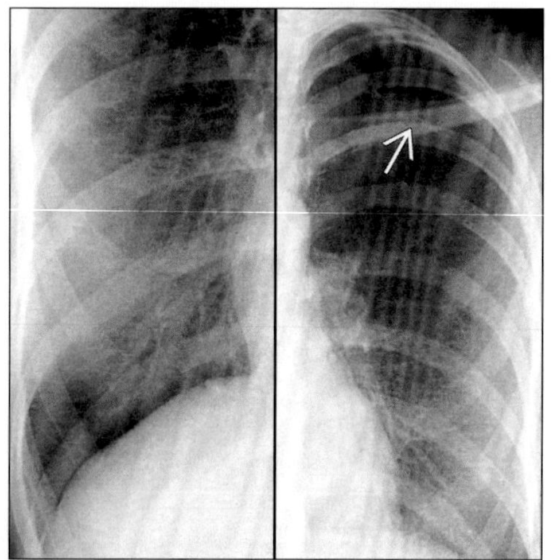

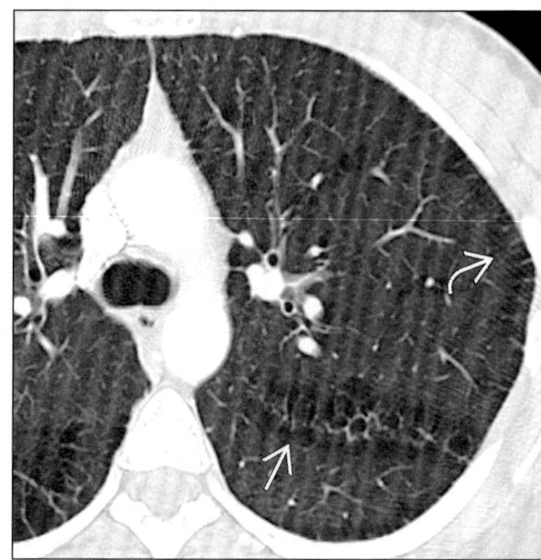

(Left) *Composite image with coned-down PA chest radiographs of a young woman who presented with chest pain shows a small left apical spontaneous pneumothorax ➔. In this case, severe PSE produces diffuse bilateral fine reticular markings.* ***(Right)*** *Axial CECT of the same patient shows numerous small lucencies distributed throughout the peripheral ➔ and perifissural ➔ subpleural spaces. Unlike honeycombing with multi-tiered cysts, PSE manifests with a single tier of cysts with intact interlobular septa.*

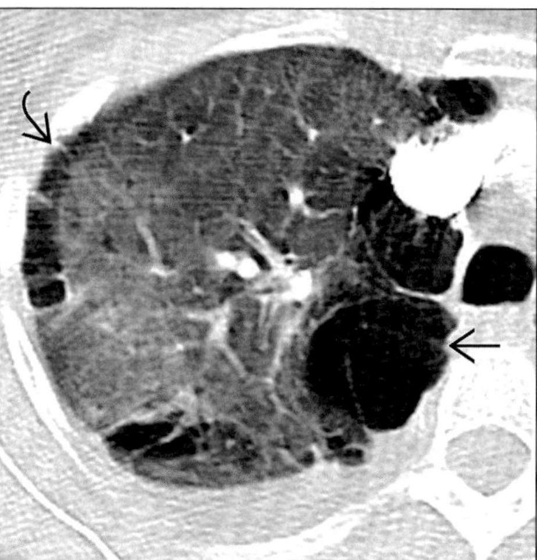

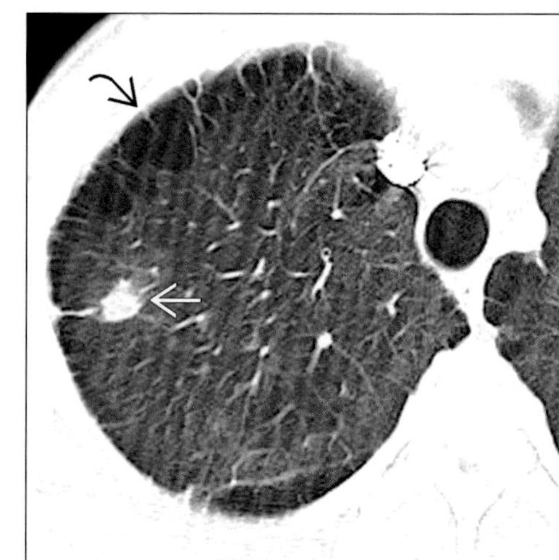

(Left) *Axial CECT of a 44-year-old woman with increasing dyspnea shows paraseptal emphysema ➔ and apical bullae ➔. Two months later, the patient presented with a spontaneous pneumothorax.* ***(Right)*** *Axial CECT of a 32-year-old woman with acute chest pain following cocaine use shows paraseptal emphysema ➔ and a spiculated right upper lobe nodule ➔. Biopsy confirmed the diagnosis of adenocarcinoma. Despite her young age, a 30 pack-year smoking history was documented.*

PARASEPTAL EMPHYSEMA

TERMINOLOGY

Abbreviations

- **Paraseptal emphysema (PSE)**

Synonyms

- **Distal acinar emphysema**

Definitions

- Permanently enlarged distal acinus
- Destruction of alveolar ducts & sacs
- Bullae
  - Circumscribed, well demarcated
  - Thin-walled dilated airspace measuring > 1 cm

IMAGING

General Features

- Best diagnostic clue
  - Small subpleural lucencies arranged as single tier of "cystic" spaces
- Location
  - Upper lung zone predominant

Radiographic Findings

- Radiography
  - Mild paraseptal emphysema difficult to detect
    - Radiography may be normal
  - **Peripheral lung lucencies with thin walls**

CT Findings

- HRCT
  - **Subpleural & peribronchovascular arcades of cystic spaces**
  - **Cystic spaces separated by intact interlobular septa**
  - Minimum-intensity projection (MinIP) images may improve detection
  - Quantitative data may be obtained from CT densitometry software

Imaging Recommendations

- Best imaging tool
  - HRCT is imaging modality of choice for assessment & characterization of emphysema

DIFFERENTIAL DIAGNOSIS

Cystic Lung Disease

- Cysts with thin walls
- Not confined to subpleural location

Centrilobular Emphysema

- Frequently associated with paraseptal emphysema
- Foci of low attenuation with imperceptible walls
- Most common type of emphysema
- Affects cigarette smokers

Panlobular Emphysema

- Diffuse regions of low attenuation with a paucity of vascular structures
- Lower zone predominant hyperlucency

Honeycomb Lung (Pulmonary Fibrosis)

- Multiple tiers of subpleural cystic spaces with thicker walls
- Predilection for lower lung zones

PATHOLOGY

General Features

- Etiology
  - Association with tall & thin body habitus: Postulated gravitational forces with increased negative pressure at lung apices as cause
  - Higher incidence in smokers, IV drug users, HIV-positive patients
  - Associated with Marfan & Ehlers-Danlos syndromes

Microscopic Features

- Dilated alveoli adjacent to pleural surfaces & interlobular septa

CLINICAL ISSUES

Presentation

- Most common signs/symptoms
  - Asymptomatic
- Other signs/symptoms
  - Acute dyspnea & chest pain with spontaneous pneumothorax

Demographics

- Age
  - 4th decade
- Gender
  - Female > male

Natural History & Prognosis

- Progression with advancing age
- Progression with cumulative smoking pack-years

Treatment

- Smoking cessation
- Pleurodesis for recurrent pneumothorax

DIAGNOSTIC CHECKLIST

Consider

- Paraseptal emphysema as a potential cause of spontaneous pneumothorax

Image Interpretation Pearls

- Characteristic subpleural location allows differentiation from lymphangioleiomyomatosis & Langerhans cell histiocytosis, which affect a similar population that may present with spontaneous pneumothorax

SELECTED REFERENCES

1. Litmanovich D et al: CT of pulmonary emphysema--current status, challenges, and future directions. Eur Radiol. 19(3):537-51, 2009
2. Satoh K et al: CT assessment of subtypes of pulmonary emphysema in smokers. Chest. 120(3):725-9, 2001

PANLOBULAR EMPHYSEMA

Key Facts

Terminology
- Panlobular emphysema (PLE)

Imaging
- Radiography
  - Very insensitive
  - May be normal
  - Hyperinflation, flat diaphragm, increased retrosternal space
- HRCT
  - Diffuse areas of low attenuation with a paucity of vessels
  - Difficult distinction between normal & affected lung

Top Differential Diagnoses
- Centrilobular emphysema (advanced)
- Paraseptal emphysema
- Asthma

Pathology
- Alpha-1-antitrypsin deficiency (α1AD)
- Destruction of entire acinus

Clinical Issues
- Mild disease
  - Often asymptomatic
  - May be incidental finding on HRCT
- Advanced disease
  - Dyspnea
- > 3 million people worldwide with severe α1AD
- Treatment
  - Bronchodilators & prevention of infection
  - May require surgery or transplant

Diagnostic Checklist
- Consider PLE in patients with diffuse homogeneous decreased lung attenuation on CT/HRCT

*(**Left**) PA chest radiograph of a 45-year-old man who presented with dyspnea shows hyperinflation and asymmetric paucity of basilar markings, most pronounced in the left lung base. (**Right**) Axial HRCT of the same patient shows diffuse low attenuation (most pronounced in the lower lobes), which is consistent with PLE. The patient was subsequently diagnosed with α1AD. The lung destruction is diffuse without discrete cystic spaces as seen in other types of emphysema.*

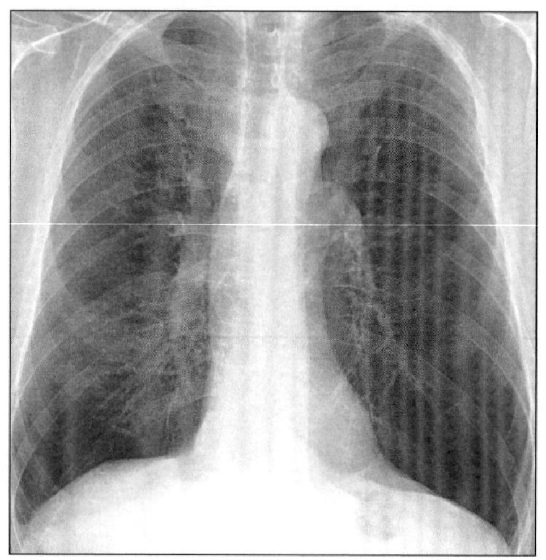

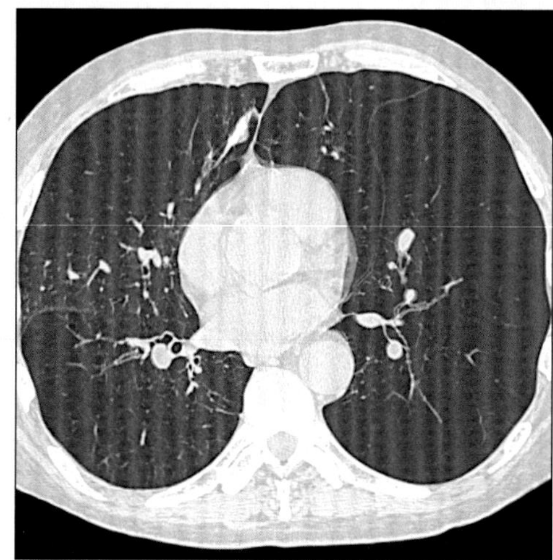

*(**Left**) PA chest radiograph of a 23-year-old woman who presented to the emergency department with progressive dyspnea shows hyperinflation and hyperlucency with a paucity of vascular markings predominantly affecting the upper lung zones. (**Right**) Axial CECT of the same patient shows diffuse low attenuation bilaterally with associated paucity of vascular structures and scattered areas of normal lung ⇨. Given these imaging findings, the patient was tested for and diagnosed with α1AD.*

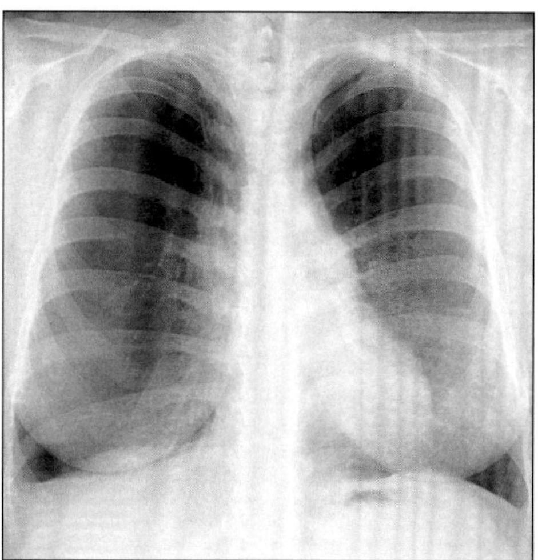

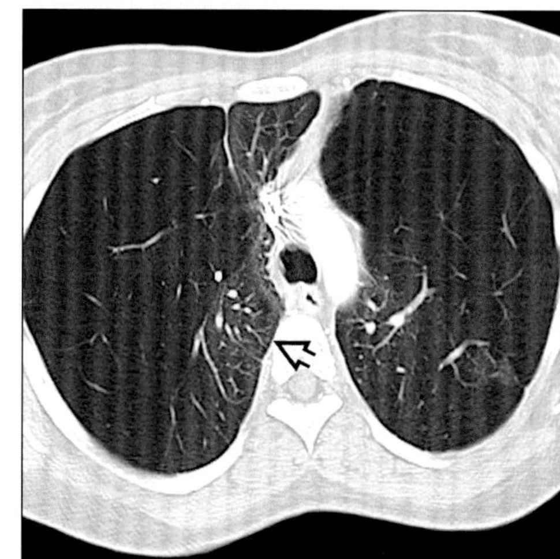

PANLOBULAR EMPHYSEMA

TERMINOLOGY

Abbreviations

- Panlobular emphysema (PLE)

Synonyms

- Panacinar emphysema

Definitions

- Enlargement & destruction of entire secondary pulmonary lobule

IMAGING

General Features

- Best diagnostic clue
  - Ill-defined areas of low attenuation & a paucity of vessels
  - Difficult to distinguish between normal lung & PLE
- Location
  - Homogeneously distributed in lungs with lower lobe predominance

Radiographic Findings

- Radiography
  - Mild disease: Very insensitive, may be normal
  - **Advanced disease: Vascular distortion & disruption, a paucity of vascular markings**
  - Hyperinflation
    - Flat hemidiaphragms
    - Increased AP diameter of thorax
    - Increased retrosternal/retrocardiac spaces

CT Findings

- HRCT
  - **Diffuse regions of low attenuation** with a paucity of vessels in affected areas
  - Difficult to distinguish between normal lung & PLE
  - Bronchiectasis

Imaging Recommendations

- Best imaging tool
  - HRCT for optimal visualization & assessment of PLE

DIFFERENTIAL DIAGNOSIS

Centrilobular Emphysema

- More common in upper lung zones
- Centrilobular lung destruction
- Distinction between normal & emphysematous lung more apparent

Paraseptal Emphysema

- Single tier of subpleural cystic spaces
- Bullae often present

Cystic Lung Disease

- Cysts with definable walls

Asthma

- Mosaic attenuation & air-trapping
- No parenchymal destruction

PATHOLOGY

General Features

- Etiology
  - Alpha-1-antitrypsin deficiency (α1AD)
    - Protease inhibitor for elastase enzyme
    - Encoded by the gene *PI (GSTP1), MIM (MTSS1)* + 107400, > 100 alleles identified
  - Incidental PLE: 5-10% of random autopsies
  - Associated centrilobular emphysema in smokers
  - Congenital bronchial atresia (around mucocele)
  - Intravenous drug use (chronic effect)
- Associated abnormalities
  - Chronic bronchitis
  - Recurrent infection
  - Secondary pulmonary hypertension

Microscopic Features

- Destruction of entire acinus; very few, if any, alveolar septa seen

CLINICAL ISSUES

Presentation

- Most common signs/symptoms
  - Mild disease: Often asymptomatic, may be incidental finding on HRCT
  - Advanced disease: Dyspnea
    - Abnormal pulmonary function
      - Increased total & residual lung volumes
      - FEV1 < 80% predicted
      - Diffusion capacity < 80% predicted

Demographics

- Age
  - α1AD typically diagnosed in 3rd to 4th decade
- Gender
  - Slight male predominance
- Epidemiology
  - > 3 million people worldwide have severe α1AD
  - Under-recognized disease

Natural History & Prognosis

- Rapidly progresses if untreated

Treatment

- Bronchodilators & prevention of infection
- Lung volume reduction: Surgery or endobronchial valves
- Lung transplantation may be required

DIAGNOSTIC CHECKLIST

Consider

- PLE in patients with diffuse homogeneous decreased lung attenuation on CT/HRCT

SELECTED REFERENCES

1. Litmanovich D et al: CT of pulmonary emphysema--current status, challenges, and future directions. Eur Radiol. 19(3):537-51, 2009

INFECTIOUS BRONCHIOLITIS

Key Facts

Terminology

- Inflammation of bronchioles secondary to infectious organisms

Imaging

- Best diagnostic clue: Centrilobular nodules & tree-in-bud opacities on HRCT
- Chest radiography
  - Nodular or reticulonodular opacities
  - Airway wall thickening & peribronchial consolidation
  - Hyperinflation
- CT/HRCT
  - Centrilobular nodules & tree-in-bud opacities
  - Mosaic attenuation secondary to air-trapping
  - Ground-glass opacity, cavitary lesions, bronchiectasis, & consolidation

Top Differential Diagnoses

- Hypersensitivity pneumonitis
- Aspiration bronchiolitis
- Respiratory bronchiolitis & respiratory bronchiolitis-associated interstitial lung disease
- Follicular bronchiolitis

Pathology

- Etiologies
  - Children: Viral & bacterial organisms
  - Immunocompromised: Fungal organisms

Clinical Issues

- Treatment: Antimicrobial therapy

Diagnostic Checklist

- Infectious bronchiolitis in patients with appropriate clinical symptoms & centrilobular nodules & tree-in-bud opacities on CT/HRCT

*(**Left**) Graphic shows CT/HRCT findings of infectious bronchiolitis with centrilobular nodules ➦ and tree-in-bud opacities ➞. Centrilobular distribution is characterized by nodules that appear evenly spaced and do not contact the pleural surfaces, including the interlobar fissures. (**Right**) Axial CECT MIP image of a patient with infectious bronchiolitis demonstrates clustered centrilobular nodules and tree-in-bud opacities in the right lung.*

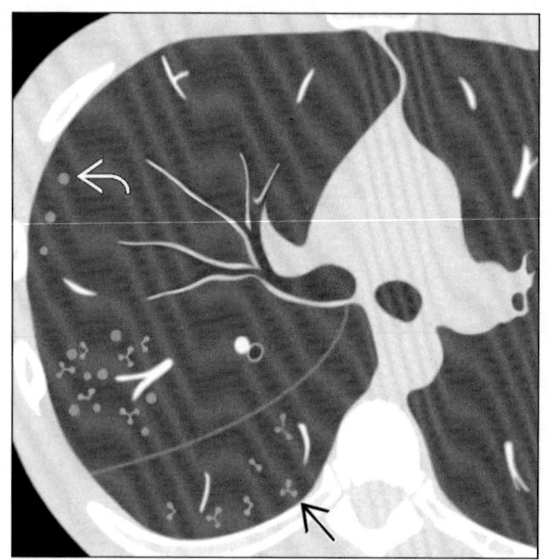

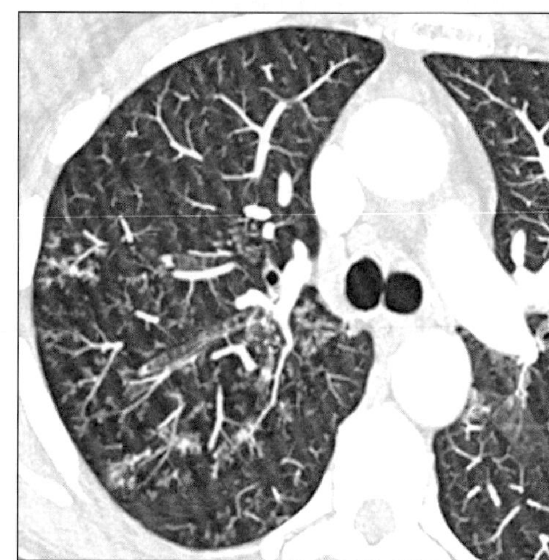

*(**Left**) Coronal NECT MIP image of a patient with viral bronchiolitis demonstrates centrilobular nodules and tree-in-bud opacities throughout both lungs. (**Right**) Axial CECT of a patient with active Mycobacterium tuberculosis pulmonary infection shows centrilobular nodules in the left upper and lower lobes, in association with a thick-walled cavitary lesion ➦ in the left lower lobe. The diagnosis was established by identification and culture of acid-fast bacilli in the patient's sputum.*

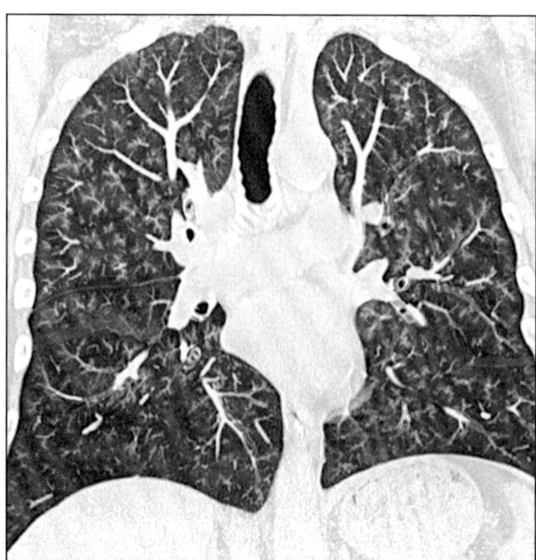

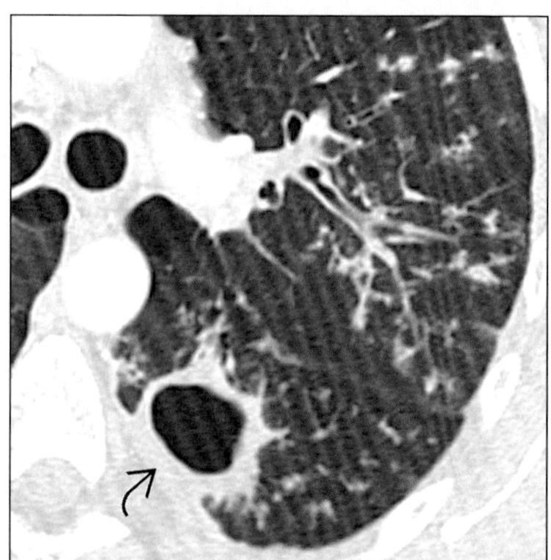

INFECTIOUS BRONCHIOLITIS

TERMINOLOGY

Definitions

- Inflammation of bronchioles secondary to infectious organisms

IMAGING

General Features

- Best diagnostic clue
  - Centrilobular nodules & tree-in-bud opacities on HRCT
- Location
  - Terminal & respiratory bronchioles
  - Alveolar ducts & spaces less commonly involved

Radiographic Findings

- Radiography
  - Bilateral parenchymal opacities
    - Nodular or reticulonodular
  - Airway wall thickening & peribronchial consolidation
    - Common in children
  - Hyperinflation
    - Partial small airway obstruction
  - Patchy consolidation
    - Bronchopneumonia
    - More common with bacterial organisms

CT Findings

- HRCT
  - Abnormalities common, but nonspecific
    - **Centrilobular nodules & tree-in-bud opacities**
  - Centrilobular nodules & ground-glass opacity
    - Bronchiolar mural inflammation
    - *Mycoplasma pneumoniae*
  - **Tree-in-bud opacities**
    - Highly suggestive of infectious bronchiolitis
  - **Mosaic attenuation**
    - Represents air-trapping
  - **Cavitary lesions**
    - *Mycobacterium tuberculosis*
    - Atypical mycobacteria
    - Fungal organisms
  - **Bronchiectasis**
    - Atypical mycobacteria
      - Right middle lobe & lingula in elderly women = "**Lady Windermere syndrome**"
  - Consolidation
    - Bronchopneumonia
    - More common with bacterial organisms

Imaging Recommendations

- Best imaging tool
  - HRCT for optimal visualization & characterization of bronchiolitis

DIFFERENTIAL DIAGNOSIS

Hypersensitivity Pneumonitis

- Inhalational allergic lung disease
- Acute: Pulmonary edema & airspace consolidation
- Subacute: Bilateral ground-glass opacity & centrilobular nodules
- Air-trapping on expiratory CT

Aspiration Pneumonia and Pneumonitis

- Chronic peribronchiolar inflammation
- Diffuse small nodular opacities & hyperinflation on chest radiographs
- Centrilobular nodules & tree-in-bud opacities
  - Lobular consolidation
  - Distribution reflects body position at time of aspiration

Respiratory Bronchiolitis (RB) & RB-associated Interstitial Lung Disease (RB-ILD)

- Bronchiolitis found in smokers
- Submucosal inflammation & fibrosis of respiratory bronchioles
- RB
  - Poorly defined centrilobular nodules on HRCT
  - Patchy ground-glass opacity often present
  - Most commonly involves upper lobes
- RB-ILD
  - Patchy ground glass opacity
  - Air-trapping

Follicular Bronchiolitis

- Characterized by peribronchial & peribronchiolar lymphoid follicles
- Common associations
  - Congenital or acquired immunodeficiency syndromes
    - HIV & acquired immunoglobulin deficiencies
  - Collagen vascular disease
    - Rheumatoid arthritis & Sjögren syndrome
  - Systemic hypersensitivity reactions
  - Infection
  - Lymphoproliferative disorders
  - Diffuse panbronchiolitis
- Bilateral reticular or reticulonodular opacities on chest radiography
- Poorly defined centrilobular nodules on HRCT
  - Less common findings
    - Peribronchial & subpleural nodules
    - Patchy ground-glass opacity
    - Bronchial wall thickening

Diffuse Panbronchiolitis

- Progressive form of bronchiolitis
- Patients may present with sinusitis
- Respiratory tract often colonized by *P. aeruginosa*
- Nonspecific imaging features overlap with other causes of small airways disease
  - Centrilobular nodules & tree-in-bud opacities
  - Bronchiolectasis, bronchiectasis, mosaic attenuation

Constrictive Bronchiolitis

- Bronchiolar inflammation → luminal obstruction
- Mosaic attenuation
  - Alternating areas of decreased & increased lung attenuation
  - Decreased lung attenuation: Decreased vessel caliber from hypoxic vasoconstriction
  - Increased (normal) lung attenuation: Increased vessel caliber & blood flow
  - Air-trapping on expiratory CT
  - Associated findings
    - Bronchial dilation, bronchiectasis, & bronchial wall thickening
    - Scattered centrilobular nodules

INFECTIOUS BRONCHIOLITIS

- Causes include infection, inhalational injury, collagen vascular disease, drugs & toxins, graft-vs.-host disease, chronic rejection of lung transplant

PATHOLOGY

General Features

- Etiology
  - Children
    - Viral
      - Respiratory syncytial virus
      - Adenovirus
      - Parainfluenza and influenza
      - Human metapneumovirus
    - Bacterial
      - *Mycoplasma pneumoniae*
  - Immunocompromised
    - Fungal
      - *Aspergillus*
    - Viral
      - Cytomegalovirus
  - Other bacterial causes
    - *Chlamydia*
    - Mycobacteria
      - *Mycobacterium tuberculosis*
      - Atypical mycobacteria: *M. avium-intracellulare* complex (MAC), *M. kansasii*, *M. fortuitum*, and *M. chelonei*
    - *Staphylococcus aureus*
    - *Legionella pneumophila*
    - *Haemophilus influenzae*
    - *Pseudomonas aeruginosa*
- Associated abnormalities
  - Etiologies of immunocompromised status
    - Immunosuppressive medication following solid organ or hematopoietic stem cell transplantation
    - Malignancy
    - Immunodeficiency syndromes

Microscopic Features

- Acute bronchiolar injury
  - Epithelial necrosis
  - Bronchiolar wall inflammation
    - Lymphoplasmacytic & bronchiolar wall infiltrates
    - Edema & fibrosis may be seen
  - Neutrophil-rich intraluminal exudates
  - Injury to respiratory mucosa
    - Destruction of cilia & ciliated cells
- Specific findings related to causative organism
  - Aspergillus
    - Fungal hyphae
  - *Mycobacterium tuberculosis*
    - Presence of acid-fast bacilli

CLINICAL ISSUES

Presentation

- Most common signs/symptoms
  - Clinical presentation in children usually more severe than in adults
    - Symptoms of upper respiratory tract infection
    - Dyspnea, tachypnea, & fever typically develop 2-3 days later

Demographics

- Age
  - Children more commonly affected than adults

Natural History & Prognosis

- Most with acute bronchiolitis develop no sequelae
  - Some may develop constrictive bronchiolitis
- Children with RSV bronchiolitis have increased morbidity as compared with non-RSV bronchiolitis
  - Longer hospitalization
  - Admission to intensive care unit
  - Requirement of supplemental oxygen & mechanical ventilation
- Lower incidence of adult hospitalization
- Restrictive & obstructive defects have been described
- Occasionally fatal

Treatment

- Therapy directed at specific organism (if known)
- Bronchodilators
- Corticosteroids
  - Documented efficacy against *Mycoplasma pneumoniae*
  - Suppress exuberant cell-mediated immune response

DIAGNOSTIC CHECKLIST

Consider

- Infectious bronchiolitis in patients with appropriate symptoms & centrilobular nodules & tree-in-bud opacities on CT/HRCT

SELECTED REFERENCES

1. García CG et al: Risk factors in children hospitalized with RSV bronchiolitis versus non-RSV bronchiolitis. Pediatrics. 126(6):e1453-60, 2010
2. Abbott GF et al: Imaging of small airways disease. J Thorac Imaging. 24(4):285-98, 2009
3. Visscher DW et al: Bronchiolitis: the pathologist's perspective. Proc Am Thorac Soc. 3(1):41-7, 2006
4. Pipavath SJ et al: Radiologic and pathologic features of bronchiolitis. AJR Am J Roentgenol. 185(2):354-63, 2005
5. Rossi SE et al: Tree-in-bud pattern at thin-section CT of the lungs: radiologic-pathologic overview. Radiographics. 25(3):789-801, 2005
6. Franquet T et al: Infectious pulmonary nodules in immunocompromised patients: usefulness of computed tomography in predicting their etiology. J Comput Assist Tomogr. 27(4):461-8, 2003
7. Chan ED et al: Mycoplasma pneumoniae-associated bronchiolitis causing severe restrictive lung disease in adults: report of three cases and literature review. Chest. 115(4):1188-94, 1999
8. Hartman TE et al: CT of bronchial and bronchiolar diseases. Radiographics. 14(5):991-1003, 1994

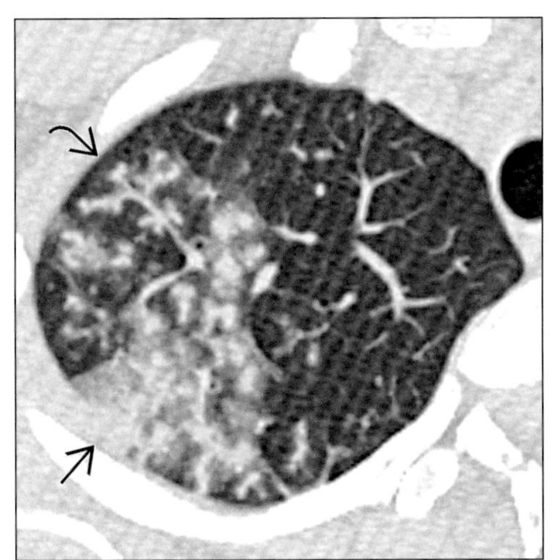

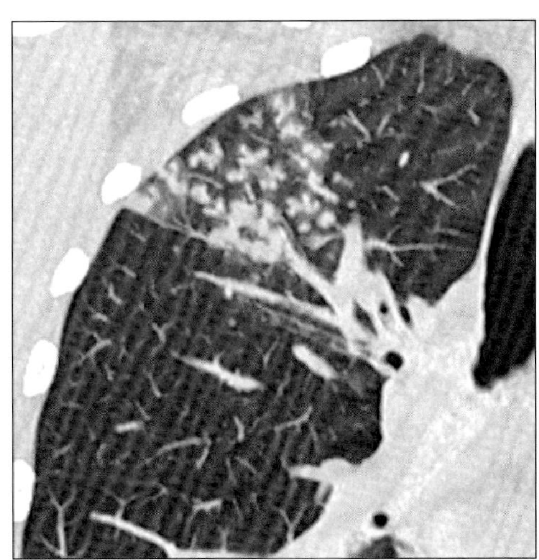

(Left) *Axial NECT (MIP image) of a patient with tuberculosis demonstrates numerous centrilobular nodules and tree-in-bud opacities ➩ in the right lung apex, some of which are surrounded by patchy ground-glass opacity and consolidation ➙.* ***(Right)*** *Coronal NECT (MIP image) of the same patient demonstrates numerous clustered centrilobular tree-in-bud opacities in the right lung apex. Maximum-intensity projection (MIP) images enable improved detection of pulmonary nodules.*

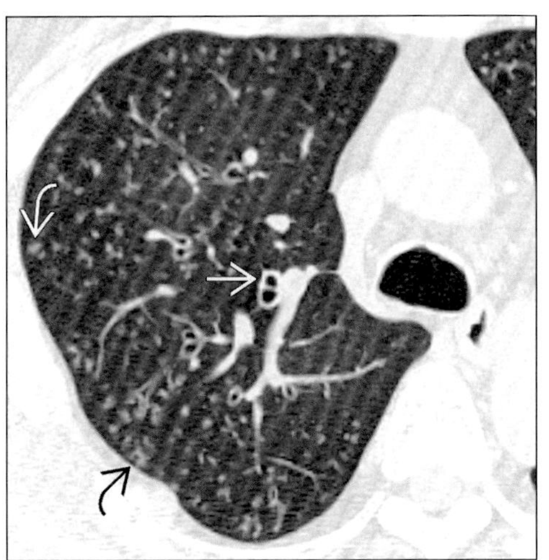

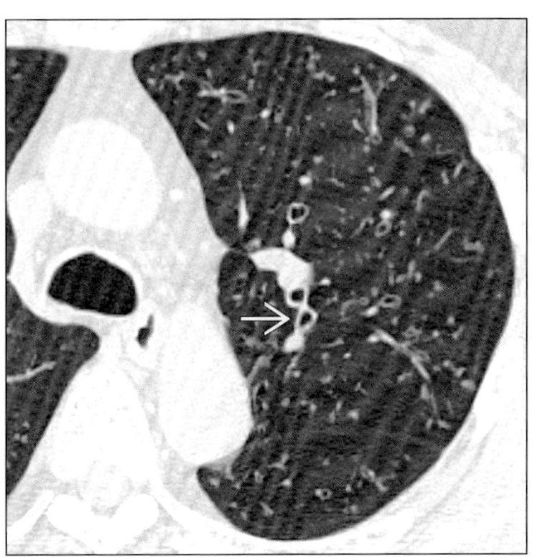

(Left) *Axial NECT of a patient with bacterial infectious bronchiolitis shows centrilobular nodules ➡, tree-in-bud opacities ➩, and mild bronchial wall thickening ➡. Centrilobular nodules appear evenly spaced and do not make contact with the pleura.* ***(Right)*** *Axial NECT of the same patient shows centrilobular nodules and bronchial wall thickening ➡. Infectious bronchiolitis may be caused by bacterial (including mycobacterial), viral, and fungal etiologies.*

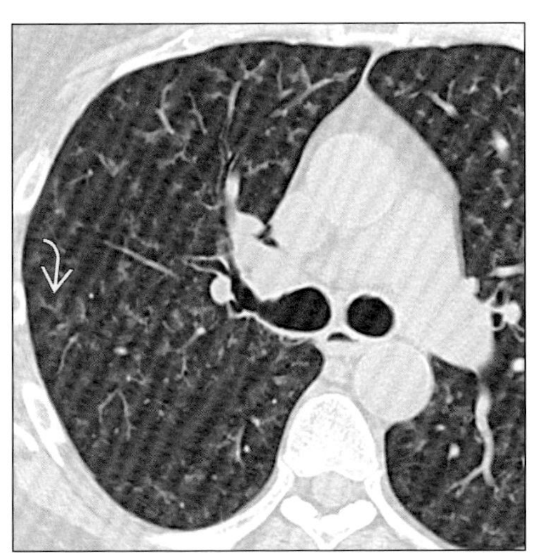

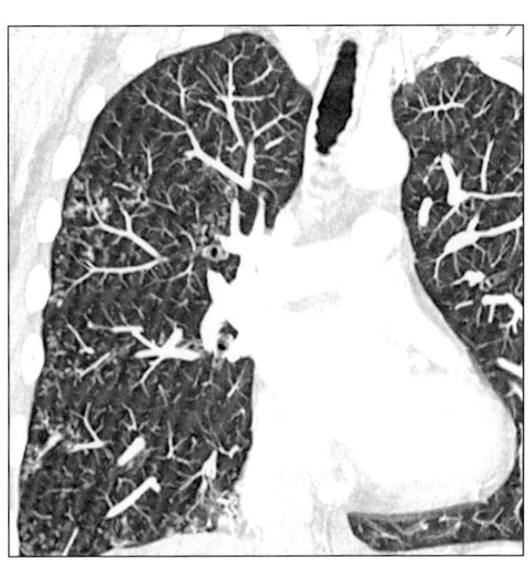

(Left) *Axial NECT of a patient with viral infectious bronchiolitis demonstrates centrilobular nodules and tree-in-bud opacities ➡ that also extend along bronchovascular bundles. Viral organisms are the most common cause of infectious bronchiolitis.* ***(Right)*** *Coronal reformatted CECT (MIP image) shows centrilobular tree-in-bud opacities in the peripheral aspect of the right lung. Tree-in-bud opacities are the most common imaging manifestations of infectious bronchiolitis.*

CONSTRICTIVE BRONCHIOLITIS

Key Facts

Terminology

- Constrictive bronchiolitis (CB)

Imaging

- Best diagnostic clue: Mosaic attenuation & expiratory air-trapping on HRCT
- Radiography
  - Normal chest radiographs
  - Hyperinflation, peripheral attenuation of vascular structures, multiple small nodules, air-trapping on expiratory radiography
- HRCT: Mosaic attenuation with alternating areas of decreased & increased lung attenuation
  - Inspiratory CT may be normal
  - Air-trapping on expiratory CT
  - Bronchial dilation, bronchiectasis, & bronchial wall thickening
  - Scattered centrilobular nodules

Top Differential Diagnoses

- Panlobular emphysema
- Pulmonary artery hypertension
- Asthma

Pathology

- Etiologies
  - Postinfectious
  - Lung and heart-lung transplantation
  - Hematopoietic stem cell transplantation
  - Connective tissue disease

Clinical Issues

- Chronic & slowly progressive course

Diagnostic Checklist

- Consider constrictive bronchiolitis in patients with HRCT findings of mosaic attenuation & air-trapping in appropriate clinical setting

*(**Left**) Graphic illustrates CT findings of CB with alternating areas of increased ⇗ and decreased ⇒ lung attenuation with borders that conform to the contours of underlying secondary pulmonary lobules. (**Right**) Axial inspiratory NECT of a patient status post lung transplantation for cystic fibrosis shows mosaic attenuation, which is an imaging manifestation of constrictive bronchiolitis. The most common symptoms at the time of clinical presentation are dyspnea and chronic cough.*

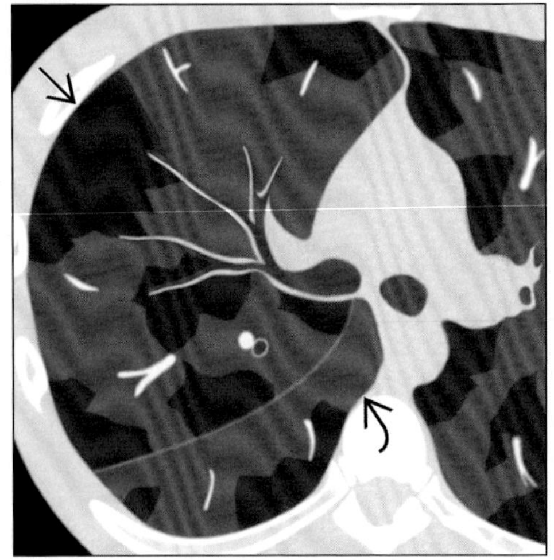

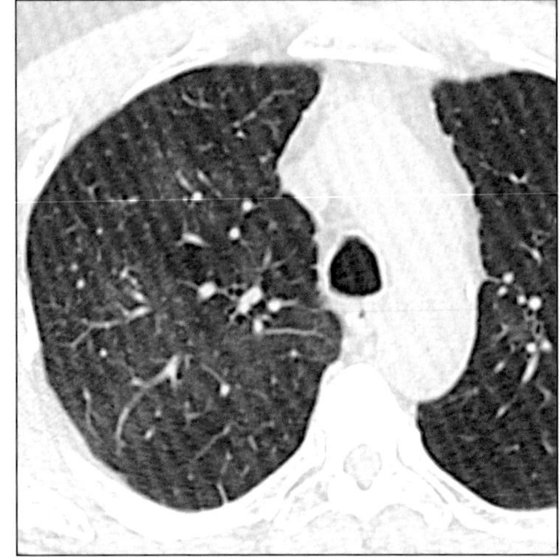

*(**Left**) Axial NECT of a patient with postinfectious constrictive bronchiolitis (CB) shows areas of decreased attenuation ⇒ in the right lung with associated decrease in the caliber and number of vessels. Other etiologies of CB include transplantation, collagen vascular disorders, inhalational lung injury, and ingested toxins. (**Right**) Axial expiratory HRCT of a patient with rheumatoid arthritis shows mosaic attenuation within the left lung. Scattered centrilobular nodules ➡ are also present.*

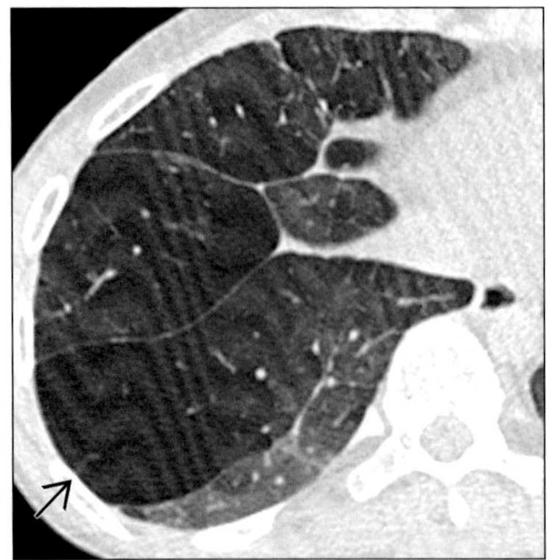

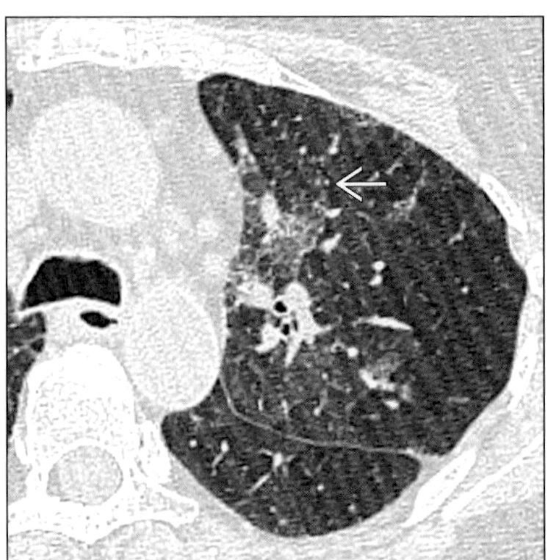

CONSTRICTIVE BRONCHIOLITIS

TERMINOLOGY

Definitions

- **Bronchiolitis**: Spectrum of inflammatory & fibrotic processes affecting small airways
  - Multiple classification schemes
    - Clinical features, setting, etiologies
    - Histology & HRCT findings
- **Bronchiolitis obliterans**
  - **Constrictive bronchiolitis (CB)**
    - Peribronchiolar fibrosis with resultant bronchiolar narrowing or obstruction
    - Collagen deposition extrinsic to airway lumen
    - Irreversible process
  - Cryptogenic organizing pneumonia (COP)
    - Previously known as bronchiolitis obliterans organizing pneumonia (BOOP)
    - Cellular bronchiolitis with fibroblastic proliferation
    - Typically responds to treatment
- **Obliterative bronchiolitis**: Clinical syndrome of airflow obstruction, may be associated with CT or HRCT findings of small airways disease
- **Swyer-James-MacLeod syndrome**: Unilateral or focal postinfectious constrictive bronchiolitis
- **Bronchiolitis obliterans syndrome (BOS)**: Clinical syndrome of chronic rejection following lung transplantation

IMAGING

General Features

- Best diagnostic clue
  - Mosaic attenuation & expiratory air-trapping on HRCT

Radiographic Findings

- Radiography
  - Chest radiographs are usually normal
  - Nonspecific findings
    - Hyperinflation
    - Peripheral attenuation of vascular structures
    - Multiple small nodules
  - Swyer-James-MacLeod syndrome
    - Unilateral hyperlucent lung
    - Decreased pulmonary vascularity
    - Normal or decreased volume of affected lung
    - Small ipsilateral hilum
    - Air-trapping on expiratory radiography

CT Findings

- HRCT
  - **Mosaic attenuation**: Alternating areas of decreased & increased lung attenuation
    - Decreased lung attenuation
      - Decreased vessel caliber from hypoxic vasoconstriction
      - No decrease in lung cross-sectional area
    - Increased (normal) lung attenuation
      - Increased vessel caliber & blood flow
  - **Air-trapping on expiratory CT**
    - May be lobular, segmental, or lobar
      - Large confluent areas of decreased attenuation may be present
    - Not diagnostic of CB in absence of functional abnormalities
    - Mild expiratory air trapping may be seen in normal patients
    - Inspiratory CT in CB may be completely normal
  - Associated findings
    - Bronchial dilation, bronchiectasis, bronchial wall thickening
    - Scattered centrilobular nodules
    - Pulmonary nodules
      - Consider diffuse idiopathic neuroendocrine cell hyperplasia
  - **Swyer-James-MacLeod syndrome**
    - Focal lung hyperlucency & decreased vascularity
    - Normal or decreased volume of affected lung
    - Air-trapping in affected lung on expiratory CT
    - Areas of air-trapping and hyperlucency typically found in other lobes & contralateral lung

MR Findings

- Hyperpolarized 3-helium MR imaging
  - Delineates extent of air-trapping
  - Earlier detection of disease than with spirometry or HRCT

Imaging Recommendations

- Best imaging tool
  - Expiratory HRCT for detection & characterization of air-trapping

DIFFERENTIAL DIAGNOSIS

Panlobular Emphysema

- Parenchymal destruction & vascular distortion
- Decreased lung attenuation
- Decreased vessel caliber
- Diffuse or lower lung zone predominance

Pulmonary Artery Hypertension

- Mosaic lung attenuation
  - Decreased vessel caliber in areas of low attenuation
  - Increased vessel caliber in areas of high attenuation
- Air-trapping may occur
- Enlarged pulmonary trunk & pulmonary arteries

Asthma

- Reversible reactive small airway obstruction
- Common disease
  - 5% of adults, 10% of children
- Mosaic attenuation less frequent than in CB
- Severe asthma may be indistinguishable from CB
- Bronchial wall thickening, bronchial dilation, & mucus plugging may be present in severe cases

PATHOLOGY

General Features

- Etiology
  - **Postinfectious**
    - Childhood infection
      - Viral: Adenovirus type 7 most common; also RSV, measles, parainfluenza, influenza
      - Bacterial: *Mycoplasma pneumoniae*
    - Swyer-James-MacLeod syndrome
      - Subset of affected patients
      - Typically unilateral involvement following childhood viral bronchiolitis

CONSTRICTIVE BRONCHIOLITIS

    - Cystic fibrosis
      - Sequela of recurrent episodes of pulmonary infection
  - **Lung & heart-lung transplantation**
    - Chronic rejection or graft-vs.-host disease
      - Prevalence of 50% in survivors 5 years post transplantation
    - Severe infection, particularly Cytomegalovirus pneumonia
  - **Hematopoietic stem cell transplantation**
    - Manifestation of graft-vs.-host disease
    - Classically described in allogeneic transplants
      - Less common in autologous transplants
  - **Connective tissue diseases**
    - Rheumatoid arthritis
      - Middle-aged women with longstanding disease
      - May or may not be associated with penicillamine therapy
    - Systemic lupus erythematosus
    - Scleroderma
    - Sjögren syndrome
  - **Inhalational lung diseases**
    - Nitrous gases: NO, NO_2, N_2O_2
    - Sulfur dioxide: SO_2
    - Ammonia, chlorine, phosgene
    - Occupational exposure to diacetyl
  - **Diffuse idiopathic pulmonary neuroendocrine cell hyperplasia (DIPNECH)**
    - Proliferation of pulmonary neuroendocrine cells
    - Tumorlets manifesting as pulmonary nodules
    - Nodular proliferations > 5 mm: Carcinoid tumors
    - Women > 40 years of age
  - **Idiopathic**
    - Older women
    - Variable history of cigarette smoking
  - Miscellaneous conditions
    - Ingestion of uncooked *Sauropus androgynous*
    - Inflammatory bowel disease
    - Paraneoplastic pemphigus
    - Gold & penicillamine therapy

Microscopic Features

- Narrowing of membranous & respiratory bronchioles
  - Concentric involvement
  - Inflammation & fibrosis of submucosal & peribronchiolar tissues
  - No polyps or granulation tissue
- Lung or heart-lung transplantation
  - Chronic rejection
    - Submucosal & intraepithelial lymphocytic & histiocytic infiltrates

CLINICAL ISSUES

Presentation

- Most common signs/symptoms
  - Dyspnea & chronic cough
- Other signs/symptoms
  - Symptoms of lower respiratory tract infection
    - Mid-inspiratory squeaks, wheezes, & crackles on auscultation
  - Swyer-James-MacLeod syndrome
    - Patients may be asymptomatic
    - Cough, recurrent infection, or hemoptysis
  - Inhalational lung disease
    - Mild symptoms
    - May progress to pulmonary edema & acute respiratory distress syndrome
    - Patients who recover may initially become asymptomatic
      - Subsequently develop progressive cough, dyspnea, and hypoxemia

Natural History & Prognosis

- Chronic & slowly progressive course is most common
- Rapidly progressive course has been described
  - More common in idiopathic CB
  - Eventual respiratory failure
- Pulmonary function tests
  - Mixed restrictive & obstructive abnormalities
- Lung transplantation
  - Median time between transplantation & CB: 16-20 months
  - Leading cause of death after 1st year post transplantation
  - Survival after constrictive bronchiolitis: 30-40%
- Graft-vs.-host disease
  - Mortality: 12% at 5 years; 18% at 10 years

Treatment

- Limited success of treatment regimens
- Treatment of concomitant infection
- Macrolide antibiotics for chronic inflammatory lung diseases
- Corticosteroids & augmentation of immunosuppression in transplant recipients
- Extracorporeal photopheresis
  - Prophylaxis & treatment of acute rejection in heart transplantation
  - Preliminary results in lung transplantation encouraging
    - Significant reduction in rate of decline of lung function & improved forced expiratory volume in 1 second (FEV_1)

DIAGNOSTIC CHECKLIST

Consider

- CB in patients with HRCT findings of mosaic attenuation & air-trapping in appropriate clinical setting

SELECTED REFERENCES

1. Epler GR: Diagnosis and treatment of constrictive bronchiolitis. F1000 Med Rep. 2, 2010
2. Abbott GF et al: Imaging of small airways disease. J Thorac Imaging. 24(4):285-98, 2009
3. Lynch DA: Imaging of small airways disease and chronic obstructive pulmonary disease. Clin Chest Med. 29(1):165-79, vii, 2008
4. Cordier JF: Challenges in pulmonary fibrosis. 2: Bronchiolocentric fibrosis. Thorax. 62(7):638-49, 2007

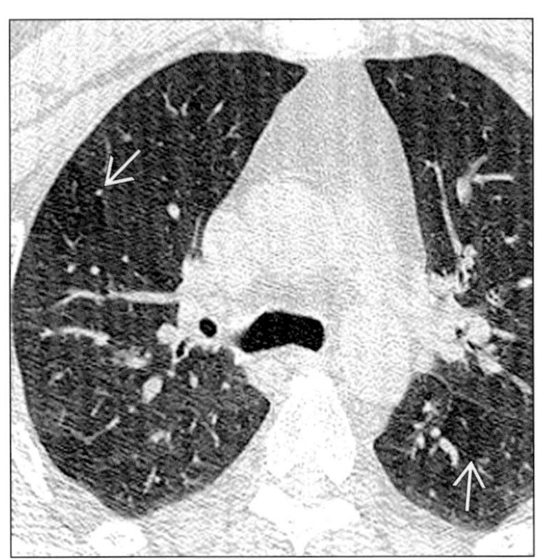

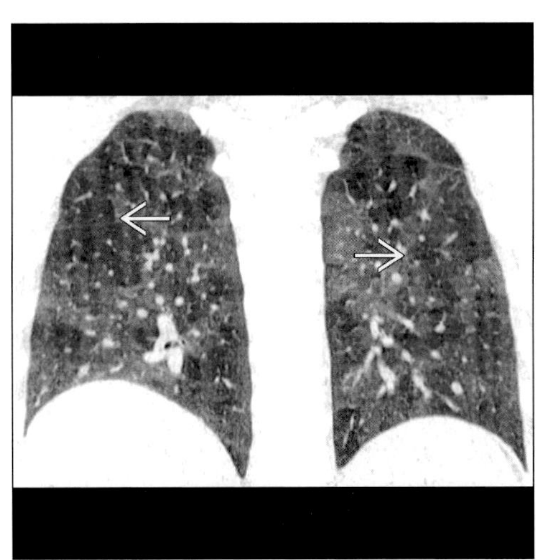

(Left) *Axial expiratory HRCT of a patient who survived severe smoke inhalation in a house fire demonstrates multiple areas of bilateral air-trapping ➔. Air-trapping is not diagnostic of constrictive bronchiolitis, and small degrees of lobular air-trapping may be seen in normal patients.* ***(Right)*** *Coronal HRCT of the same patient demonstrates mosaic attenuation throughout both lungs and multifocal areas of bilateral air-trapping ➔.*

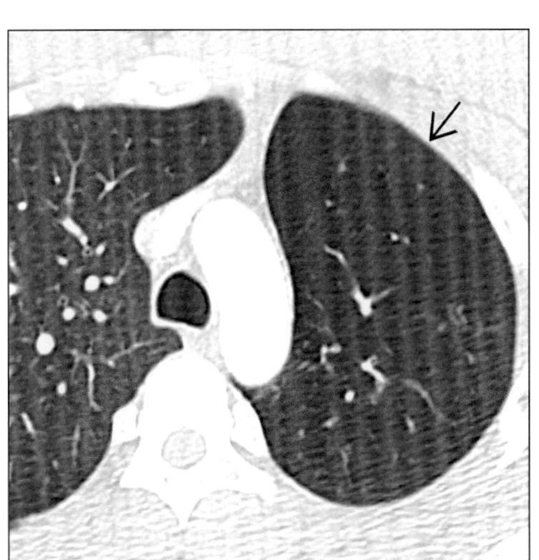

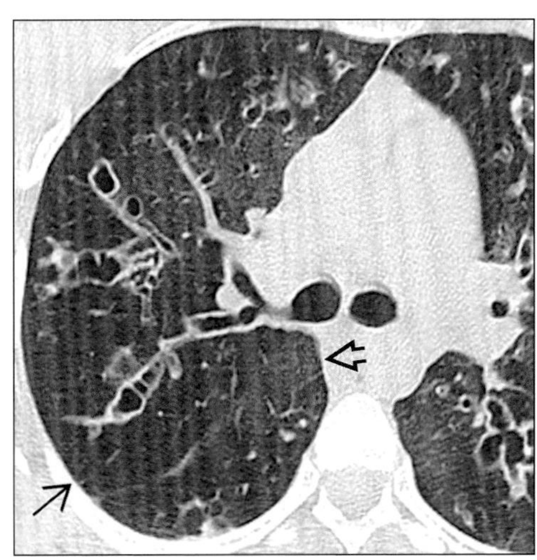

(Left) *Axial CECT of a patient with Swyer-James-McLeod syndrome demonstrates decreased lung attenuation ➔ throughout the left lung. The vessels within the regions of hypoattenuation are markedly diminished in size and number.* ***(Right)*** *Axial NECT of a patient with cystic fibrosis demonstrates alternating areas of decreased ➔ and increased ⇨ lung attenuation, indicative of mosaic attenuation. The small vessel caliber within areas of hypoattenuation represents hypoxic vasoconstriction.*

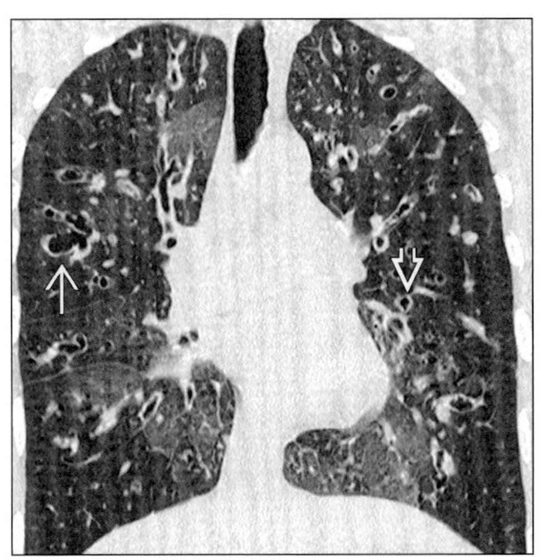

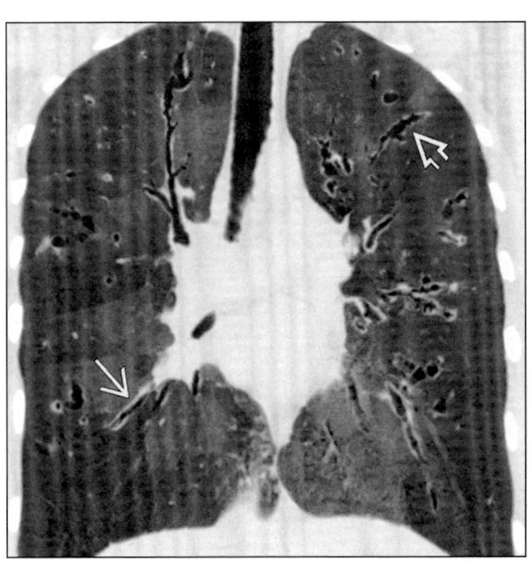

(Left) *Coronal NECT of a patient with cystic fibrosis and constrictive bronchiolitis shows multifocal mosaic attenuation with alternating areas of increased and decreased lung attenuation associated with bronchial wall thickening ⇨, bronchiectasis ➔, and mucus plugging.* ***(Right)*** *Coronal NET MinIP image of the same patient highlights the finding of bilateral mosaic attenuation associated with bronchial wall thickening ➔ and bronchiectasis ⇨.*

SWYER-JAMES-MCLEOD

Key Facts

Terminology

- Swyer-James-McLeod syndrome (SJMS)
- Unilateral hyperlucent lung syndrome
- First described in 1953 as unilateral hyperlucent, hypovascular lung with small ipsilateral hilum

Imaging

- Radiography
  - Unilateral hyperlucent lung with a paucity of peripheral vessels
  - Normal or slightly decreased volume & small ipsilateral hilum
- CT
  - Heterogeneous geographic low-attenuation hypovascular regions, often multifocal & bilateral
  - Bronchiectasis, bronchial wall thickening, & scarring are common
  - Expiratory air-trapping

Top Differential Diagnoses

- Congenital lobar overinflation
- Bronchial atresia
- Centrilobular emphysema
- Allergic bronchopulmonary aspergillosis
- Scimitar syndrome
- Congenital interruption of pulmonary artery

Pathology

- Postinfectious bronchiolitis occurring in childhood

Clinical Issues

- Asymptomatic adult
- Productive cough, dyspnea, wheezing, hemoptysis

Diagnostic Checklist

- Consider SJMS in patients with incidentally found unilateral hyperlucent, hypovascular lung

*(**Left**) PA chest radiograph of a 40-year-old man with dyspnea shows hyperlucency and hypovascularity of the right upper lung. (**Right**) Coronal NECT of the same patient shows right upper lung zone mosaic attenuation due to air-trapping, paucity of pulmonary vessels, and cylindrical ➔ and cystic bronchiectasis ➔. These findings are also present to a lesser extent in the bilateral lower lobes. The patient had a history of childhood "pneumonia." Imaging findings of SJMS may be subtle.*

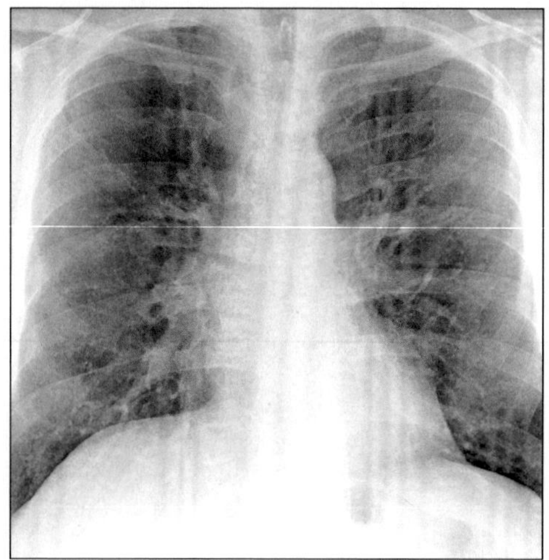

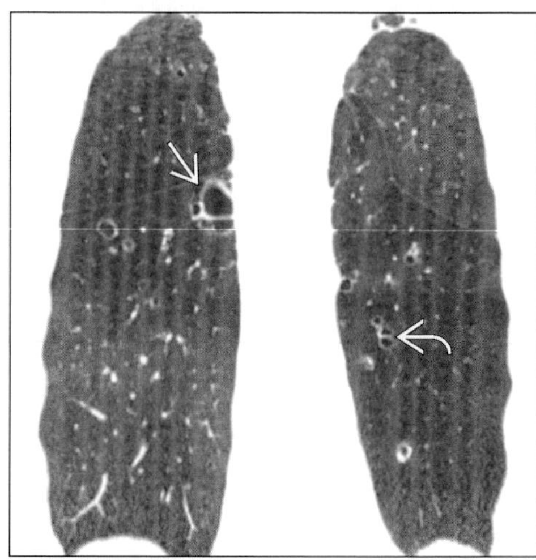

*(**Left**) PA chest radiograph of an asymptomatic 48-year-old man obtained for preoperative evaluation shows a hyperlucent and hypovascular left lower lobe. (**Right**) Axial NECT of the same patient shows marked hypovascularity and low attenuation throughout the left lower lobe. Expiratory images confirmed air-trapping. There were no centrally dilated or impacted bronchi. The history of a viral illness during childhood confirmed the diagnosis of Swyer-James-McLeod syndrome.*

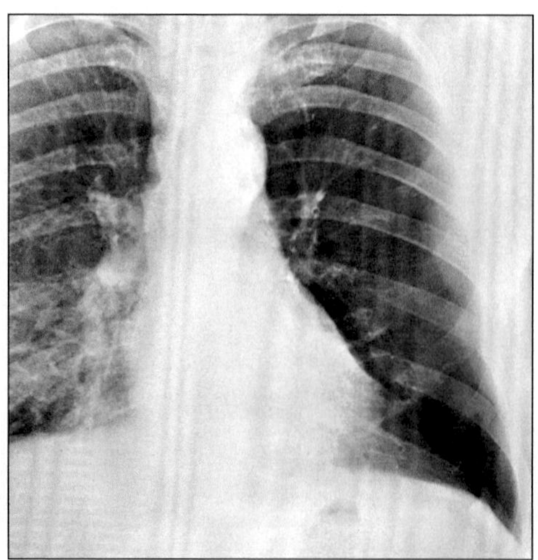

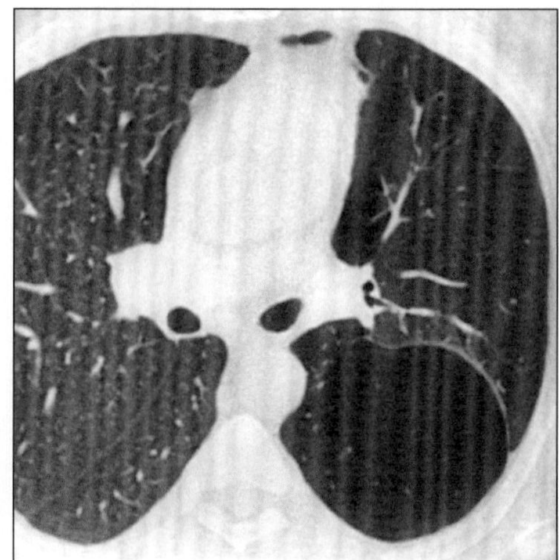

SWYER-JAMES-MCLEOD

TERMINOLOGY

Abbreviations

- **Swyer-James-McLeod syndrome (SJMS)**

Synonyms

- Unilateral hyperlucent lung syndrome

Definitions

- First described in 1953 as unilateral hyperlucent, hypovascular lung with small ipsilateral hilum

IMAGING

General Features

- Best diagnostic clue
  - Hyperlucent lung with slightly decreased volume & small ipsilateral hilum
- Location
  - Unilateral or bilateral
- Size
  - Range from subsegmental to lobar

Radiographic Findings

- **Unilateral hyperlucent lung with a paucity of peripheral vessels**
- Normal or slightly decreased volume with small ipsilateral hilum

CT Findings

- HRCT
  - **Heterogeneous geographic low-attenuation hypovascular regions**, often multifocal & bilateral
  - **Bronchiectasis, bronchial wall thickening, & scarring** are common
  - **Expiratory air-trapping**
- CTA
  - Small caliber vessels supplying affected regions

Imaging Recommendations

- Best imaging tool
  - Inspiratory & expiratory HRCT to document constrictive bronchiolitis

DIFFERENTIAL DIAGNOSIS

Congenital Lobar Overinflation

- Hyperinflated lobe results in contralateral mediastinal shift
- Typically diagnosed in infants with respiratory distress

Bronchial Atresia

- Mucus-filled bronchocele with surrounding hyperlucent & hypovascular lung
- Expiratory air-trapping

Centrilobular Emphysema

- Upper lobe predominant centrilobular low attenuation
- Increased lung volumes
- No expiratory air-trapping

Allergic Bronchopulmonary Aspergillosis

- Central bronchiectasis ± mucoid impaction
- Increased lung volumes

Scimitar Syndrome

- Hypoplastic right lung drained by anomalous vein usually adjacent to right heart border extending below diaphragm

Congenital Interruption of Pulmonary Artery

- Synonym: Proximal interruption of pulmonary artery
- Small hemithorax, small hilum
- Aortic arch on opposite side
- No expiratory air-trapping

PATHOLOGY

General Features

- Etiology
  - Postinfectious bronchiolitis occurring in childhood, usually < 8 years of age
    - *Paramyxovirus* (*Morbillivirus*), *Bordetella pertussis*, *Mycobacterium tuberculosis*, *Mycoplasma pneumoniae*, influenza A, respiratory syncytial virus, several adenoviruses
- Associated abnormalities
  - Small ipsilateral pulmonary arteries

Microscopic Features

- Constrictive bronchiolitis, bronchiectasis, & areas of parenchymal destruction

CLINICAL ISSUES

Presentation

- Most common signs/symptoms
  - Asymptomatic adult
- Other signs/symptoms
  - Productive cough, dyspnea, wheezing, hemoptysis

Natural History & Prognosis

- Recurrent infections may result in bronchiectasis & hemoptysis

Treatment

- Treatment of symptoms
- Pulmonary resection reserved for severe cases

DIAGNOSTIC CHECKLIST

Consider

- SJMS in patients with incidentally found unilateral hyperlucent, hypovascular lung

Image Interpretation Pearls

- Expiratory HRCT optimally demonstrates air-trapping

SELECTED REFERENCES

1. Dillman JR et al: Expanding upon the unilateral hyperlucent hemithorax in children. Radiographics. 31(3):723-41, 2011
2. Ghossain MA et al: Swyer-James syndrome documented by spiral CT angiography and high resolution inspiratory and expiratory CT: an accurate single modality exploration. J Comput Assist Tomogr. 21(4):616-8, 1997

ASTHMA

Key Facts

Terminology
- Typically reversible airway obstruction, chronic airway inflammation, & nonspecific airway hyperreactivity

Imaging
- Radiography
  - Bronchial wall thickening
  - Hyperinflation: Transient or fixed
  - Atelectasis, pneumothorax, pneumonia
- CT
  - Bronchiectasis
  - Assessment of extent & severity of airway wall thickness/luminal narrowing
  - Bronchiolitis
  - Identification of associated conditions
- Imaging of patients with asthma only when complications are suspected

Top Differential Diagnoses
- Vocal cord paralysis
- Tracheal or carinal obstruction
- Constrictive bronchiolitis
- Infiltrative lung disease

Pathology
- Chronic inflammation of mid & small-sized bronchi
- Bronchiolar findings: Constrictive bronchiolitis

Clinical Issues
- Symptoms/signs
  - Cough, shortness of breath, wheezing, & chest discomfort
- Affects 7% of USA population
  - Children & adults
- Treatment: Combination of anti-inflammatory drugs & bronchodilators

*(**Left**) PA chest radiograph of a patient with longstanding asthma shows hyperinflation and nonspecific bilateral reticular opacities. (**Right**) Lateral chest radiograph of the same patient shows flattening of the diaphragm and enlargement of the retrosternal clear space, consistent with marked hyperinflation. There is also diffuse peribronchial cuffing. While nonspecific, hyperinflation and peribronchial cuffing are common findings in patients with asthma.*

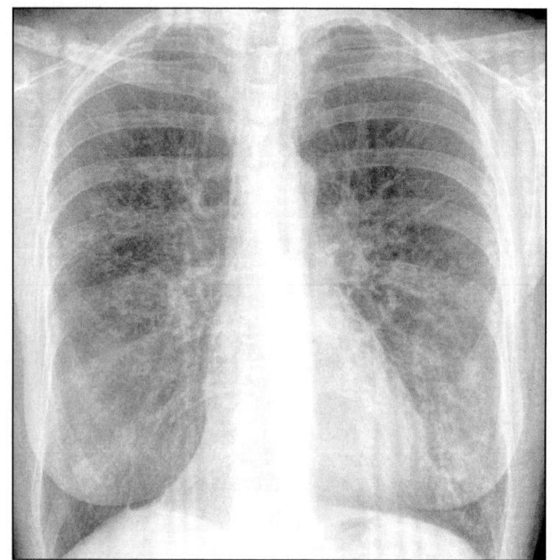

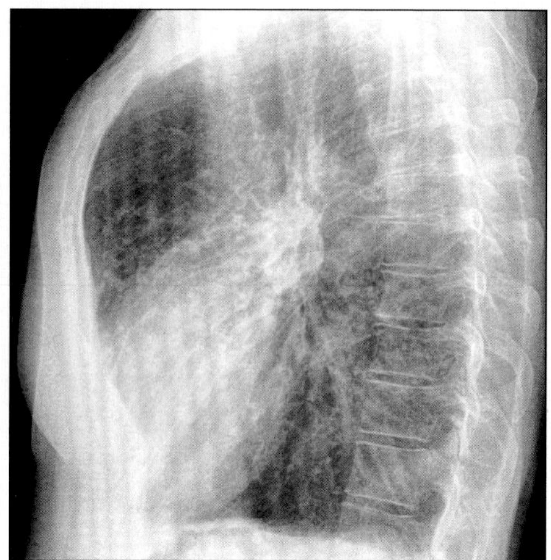

*(**Left**) Axial NECT of the same patient demonstrates extensive bronchiectasis, bronchial wall thickening ➔, and branching opacities representing mucoid impactions ➔. (**Right**) Coronal NECT MIP image of the same patient shows bilateral dilated bronchi with mucoid impactions ➔ and tree-in-bud opacities ➔ from bronchiolar mucoid impactions. Cylindrical bronchiectasis is more commonly seen in asthma, whereas cystic or varicoid bronchiectasis tends to occur in ABPA. (Courtesy S. Rossi, MD.)*

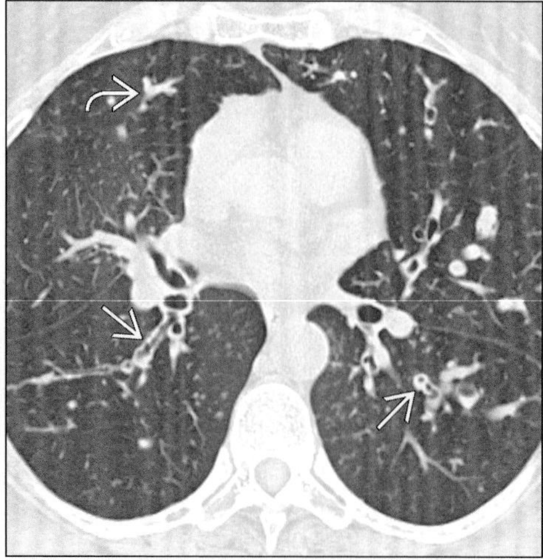

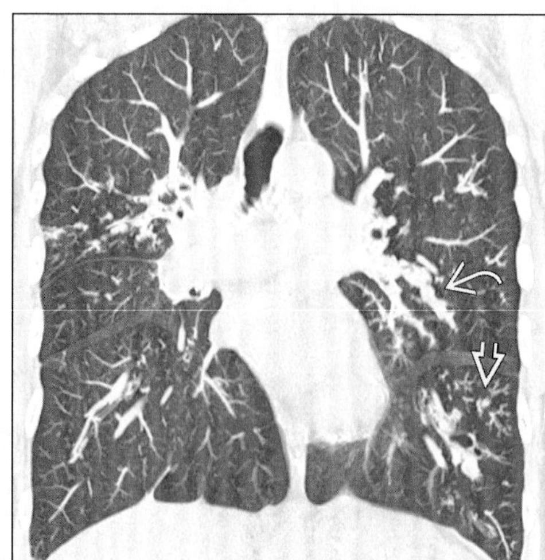

ASTHMA

TERMINOLOGY

Definitions

- Typically reversible airway obstruction, chronic airway inflammation, & nonspecific airway hyperreactivity

IMAGING

Radiographic Findings

- **Bronchial wall thickening** or **peribronchial cuffing** (most common)
- **Hyperinflation**: Transient or fixed
- **Complications**
  - **Atelectasis**
    - Often related to mucoid impaction
    - Right middle lobe commonly affected
  - **Pneumothorax & pneumomediastinum**
  - Pneumopericardium, pneumoretroperitoneum
  - Rarely pneumorrhachis & subdural air
  - **Pneumonia**

CT Findings

- Assessment of extent & severity of airway wall thickness/luminal narrowing
  - ↑ thickness correlates with severity of disease
- **Bronchiectasis**
  - Signet ring sign, absence of bronchial tapering
  - Mucoid impactions
  - Cylindrical bronchiectasis more likely in asthma without allergic bronchopulmonary aspergillosis (ABPA)
  - Central cystic or varicoid bronchiectasis, mucoid impaction, & centrilobular nodules more likely in ABPA
- **Bronchiolitis**
  - Mosaic attenuation during inspiration
  - Expiratory air-trapping
    - More likely to be associated with history of asthma-related hospitalization, ICU admissions, &/or mechanical ventilation
  - Small centrilobular nodules

Imaging Recommendations

- Best imaging tool
  - Consider imaging only when complications are suspected
- Protocol advice
  - Indications for chest radiography in patients with asthma
    - Chronic obstructive pulmonary disease
    - Fever or temperature > 37.8° C
    - History of intravenous drug abuse
    - Seizures
    - Immunosuppression
    - Clinical suspicion of pneumothorax

DIFFERENTIAL DIAGNOSIS

Vocal Cord Paralysis

- Severe symptoms, inspiratory or expiratory stridor, episodic hoarseness
- No bronchial wall thickening
- Laryngoscopic diagnosis

Tracheal or Carinal Obstruction

- Etiologies: Benign/malignant neoplasm, post-intubation tracheal stenosis, vascular rings, foreign body, sarcoidosis, Wegener granulomatosis, amyloidosis, relapsing polychondritis, tracheobronchopathia osteochondroplastica
- Imaging studies for visualization & assessment of obstructing lesion

Constrictive Bronchiolitis

- Etiology: Idiopathic, post-infectious, autoimmune disease, asthma
- Often refractory to bronchodilators
- May be radiologically indistinguishable from asthma

PATHOLOGY

General Features

- Etiology
  - Common asthma triggers: Animals (pet hair or dander), dust, weather changes, air or food chemicals, exercise, mold, pollen, respiratory infections (e.g., common cold), emotional stress, tobacco smoke, medications (e.g., aspirin)
- Associated abnormalities
  - Allergic bronchopulmonary aspergillosis
  - Bronchocentric granulomatosis
  - Chronic eosinophilic pneumonia
  - Churg-Strauss syndrome

Microscopic Features

- Chronic inflammation of mid & small-sized bronchi
- Bronchiolar findings
  - Constrictive bronchiolitis

CLINICAL ISSUES

Presentation

- Most common signs/symptoms
  - Cough, shortness of breath, wheezing, & chest discomfort

Demographics

- Age
  - Adults & children
- Epidemiology
  - Affects 7% of USA population

Treatment

- Complex; combination of anti-inflammatory drugs (e.g., corticosteroids, cromolyn) & bronchodilators

DIAGNOSTIC CHECKLIST

Consider

- "All that wheezes is not asthma" when interpreting imaging studies of affected patients

SELECTED REFERENCES

1. Woods AQ et al: Asthma: an imaging update. Radiol Clin North Am. 47(2):317-29, 2009
2. Silva CI et al: Asthma and associated conditions: high-resolution CT and pathologic findings. AJR Am J Roentgenol. 183(3):817-24, 2004

ASTHMA

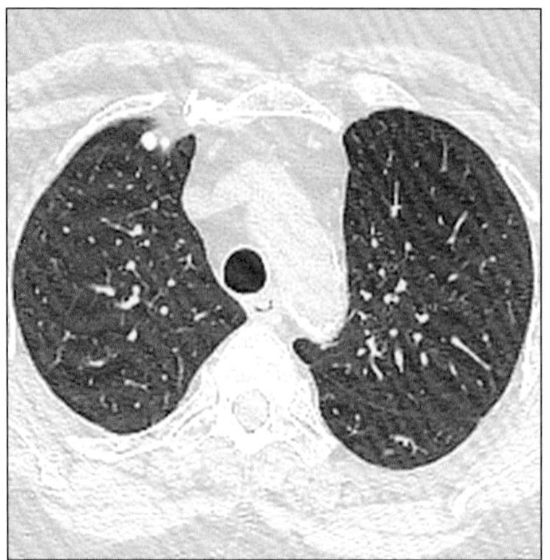

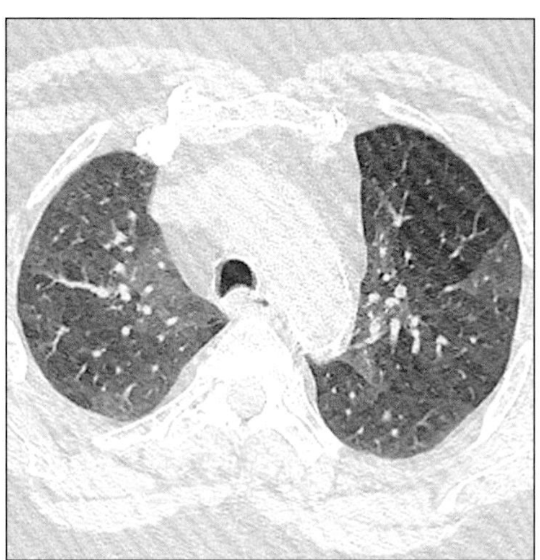

(Left) *Axial inspiratory HRCT of a patient with asthma shows a very subtle pattern of mosaic attenuation bilaterally.* ***(Right)*** *Axial expiratory HRCT of the same patient shows scattered areas of subsegmental air-trapping bilaterally, consistent with small airways disease. This finding often correlates with severity of asthma and is associated with a history of asthma-related hospitalization, ICU admissions, &/or mechanical ventilation.*

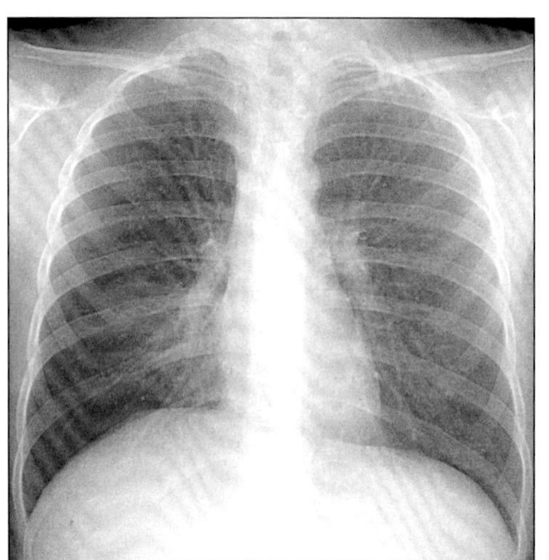

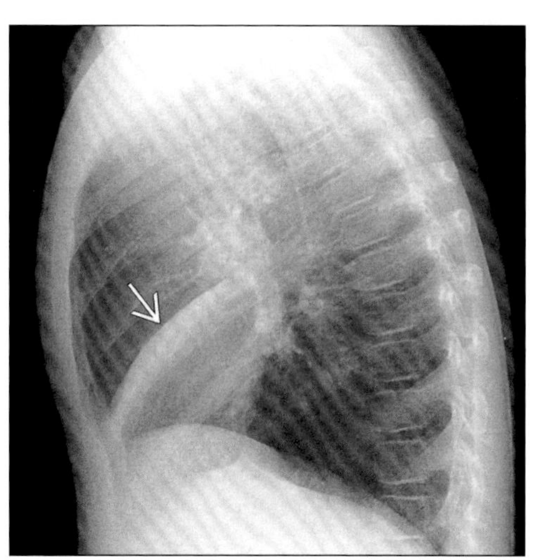

(Left) *PA chest radiograph of a young patient with asthma shows mild elevation of the right hemidiaphragm and obscuration of the right cardiac border secondary to atelectasis of the middle lobe.* ***(Right)*** *Lateral chest radiograph of the same patient shows a band-like opacity ➔ caudal to the inferiorly displaced horizontal fissure that confirms middle lobe atelectasis. Atelectasis is one of the most common abnormalities found on chest radiographs of patients with asthma.*

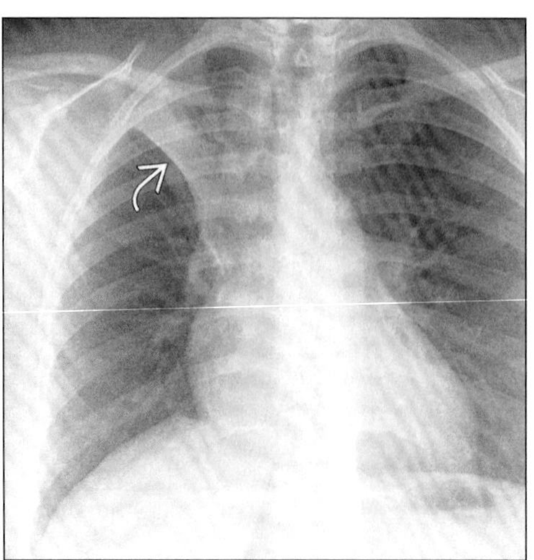

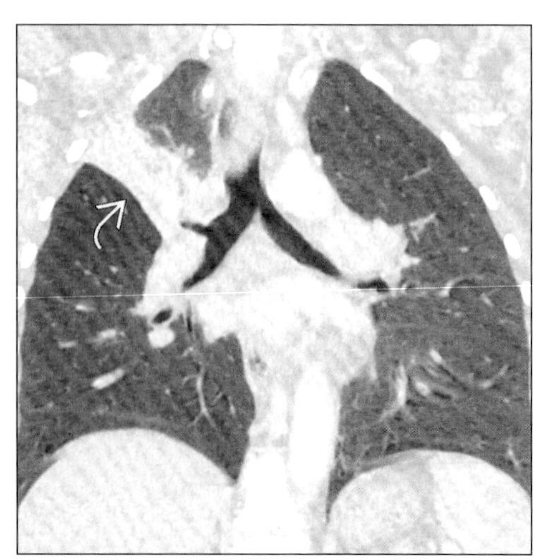

(Left) *PA chest radiograph of a patient with asthma shows a right upper lobe opacity with elevation of the minor fissure ↗, consistent with right upper lobe atelectasis.* ***(Right)*** *Coronal CECT of the same patient shows sublobar right upper lobe atelectasis ↗. Atelectasis in asthma is typically associated with mucous plugs and does not necessarily imply acute illness, infection, or worsening asthma.*

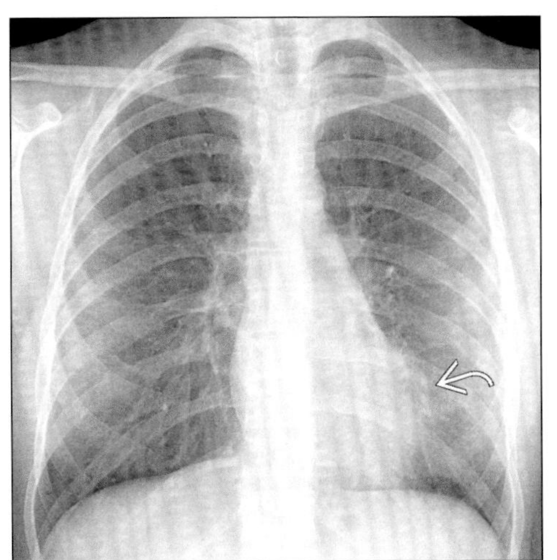

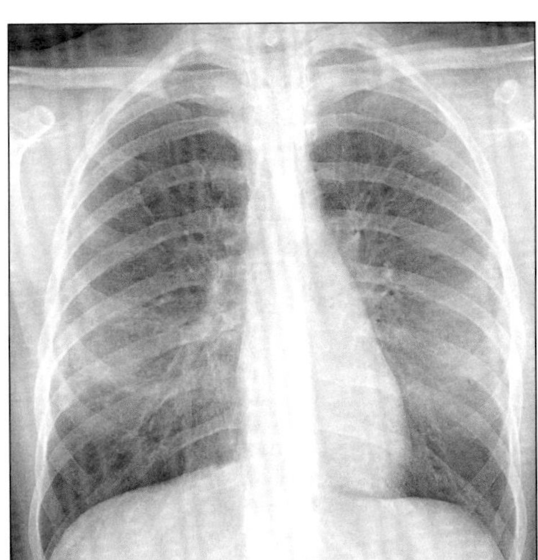

*(**Left**) PA chest radiograph of a patient with asthma who presented with dyspnea, fever, and leukocytosis shows obscuration of the left heart border ➦, consistent with lingular pneumonia given the history. (**Right**) PA chest radiograph of the same patient shows post-treatment resolution of the lingular consolidation. Pneumonia is a common complication of asthma and an indication for imaging asthmatic patients. Since asthma is so prevalent, efforts should be made to image affected patients as little as possible.*

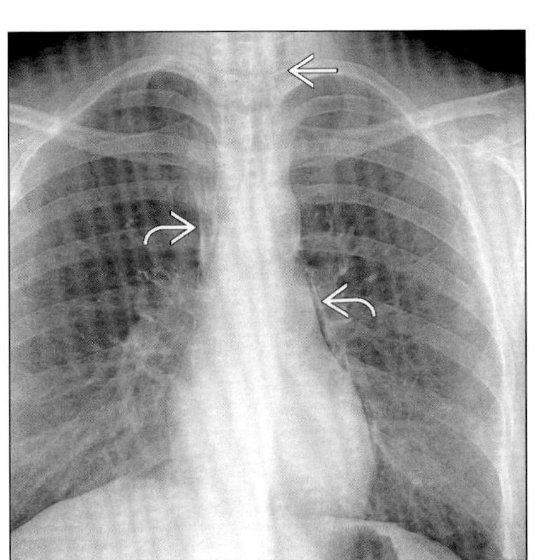

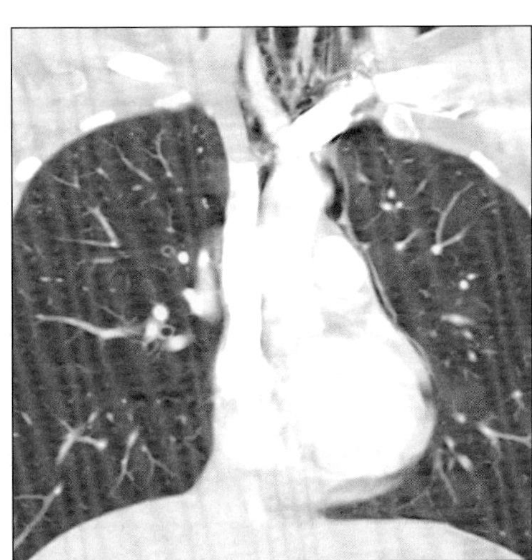

*(**Left**) PA chest radiograph of a patient with asthma who presented with acute dyspnea and chest pain shows extensive pneumomediastinum ➦ and subcutaneous air in the neck ➔. (**Right**) Coronal CECT of the same patient shows pneumomediastinum and subcutaneous air in the neck. Pneumomediastinum as a complication of asthma is more common in children and more frequent than pneumothorax. Rarely, pneumomediastinum may be associated with air within the spinal canal.*

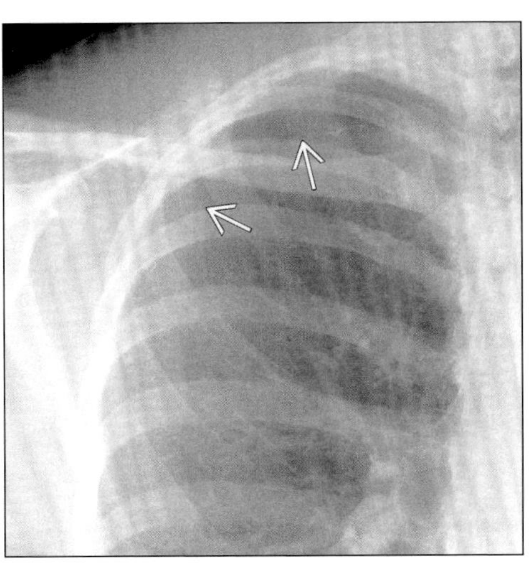

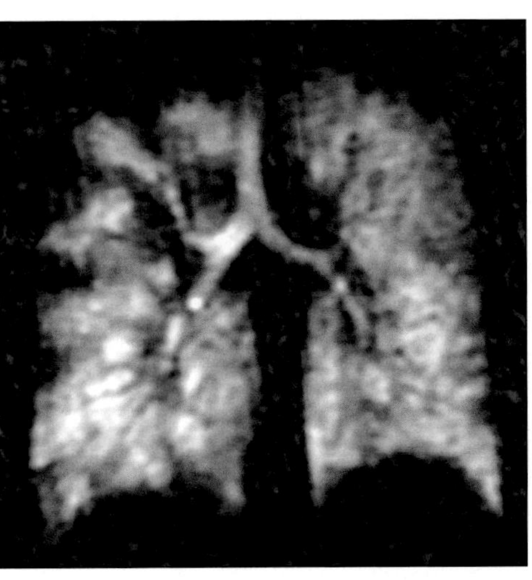

*(**Left**) PA chest radiograph of a patient with asthma shows a pneumothorax manifesting with a visible visceral pleural line at the right apex ➔. (**Right**) Coronal MR with hyperpolarized ^{129}Xe of an asthmatic patient shows heterogeneous distribution of ^{129}Xe due to extensive ventilation defects. ^{3}He and ^{129}Xe have been used successfully in research studies designed to assess ventilatory abnormalities and are promising techniques for future clinical practice. (Courtesy H. P. McAdams, MD.)*

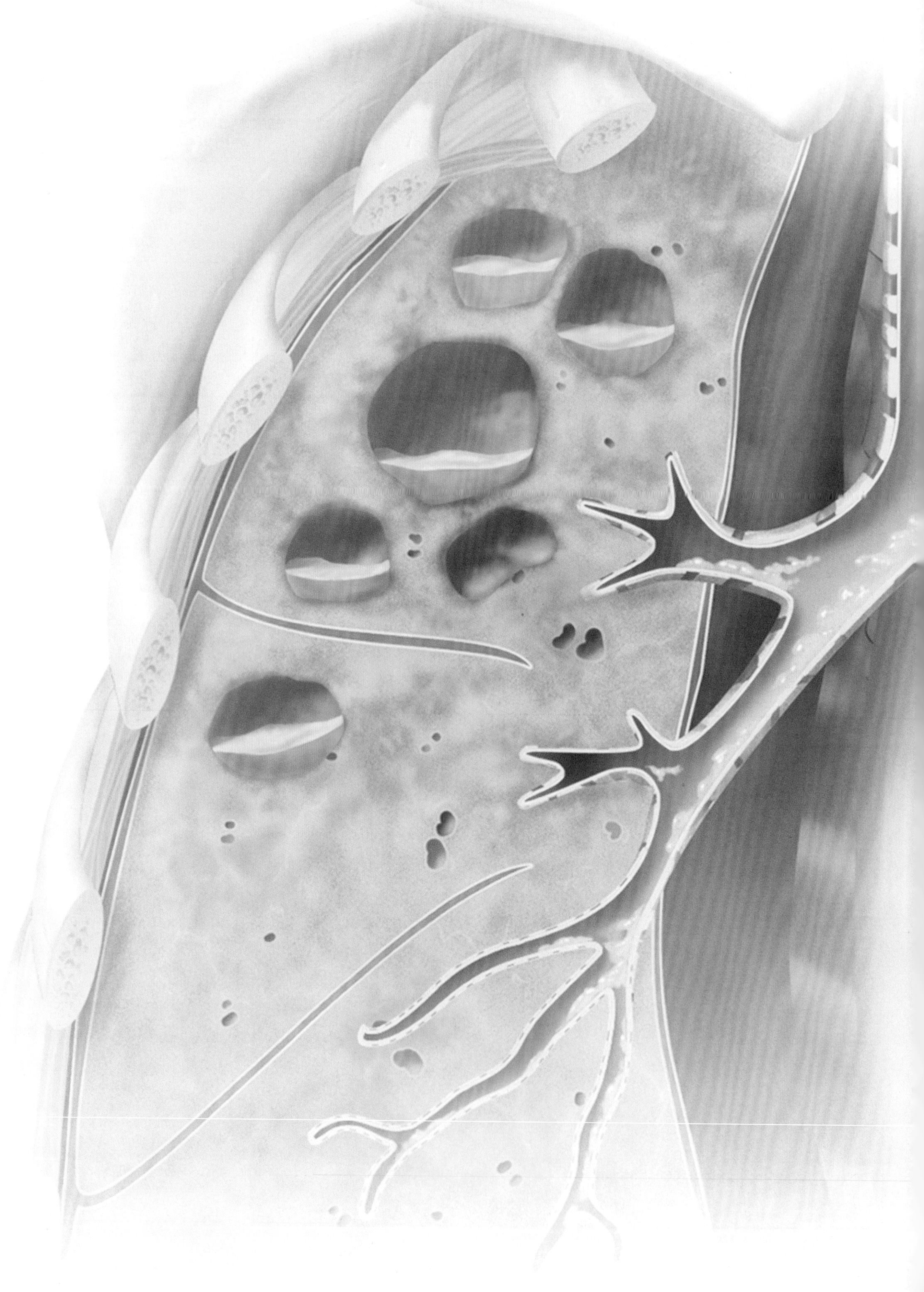

SECTION 4
Infections

Introduction and Overview

General

Bacteria

Mycobacteria and Mycoplasma

Viruses

Fungi

Parasites

APPROACH TO INFECTIONS

Introduction

Imaging of pulmonary infection is challenging due to the numerous infectious organisms that may affect the lung and the protean radiologic abnormalities these may produce. The radiologist may be the first healthcare provider to raise the possibility of pulmonary infection based on the identification of an imaging abnormality. Furthermore, imaging studies are often performed before microbiologic and immunologic testing results become available. In some cases, the radiologist may be able to suggest an unsuspected pulmonary infection and/or a specific pulmonary pathogen. For example, identification of cavitary disease in the upper lobe should suggest the possibility of tuberculosis. In such a case, the radiologist must promptly alert the referring physician and/or other members of the clinical team. Sputum analysis can then be expeditiously performed and respiratory isolation procedures instituted to prevent spread of infection to individuals who may come in contact with the patient. At times, the imaging data is so compelling that empiric treatment is instituted while awaiting definitive microbiologic proof of tuberculosis. Thus, radiologists may play a critical role in the identification, assessment, and management of patients with pulmonary infection. Although imaging features may not provide information about a specific pathogen, communication with other members of the healthcare team may lead to the formulation of a focused differential diagnosis or the identification of a likely causative microorganism, which may have a positive impact on early treatment and likelihood of recovery.

There are various algorithms for approaching the patient with suspected pulmonary infection. Some of these may be favored by the radiologist and/ or the clinicians based on past experience. Several patient factors may also influence the approach to the diagnosis of infection, including age, immune status, and underlying conditions. Although an exhaustive discussion of diagnostic algorithms is beyond the scope of this work, some essential considerations are discussed below. It should be noted that, in some cases of suspected infection, patients respond to conventional antimicrobial treatment before a specific infectious etiology can be identified. However, every effort should be made to objectively identify the pulmonary infection that best fits the clinical scenario using scientific data and evidence-based medicine. This allows the institution of appropriate treatment and surveillance regimens.

While findings are often nonspecific, chest radiography remains a reasonable first step in the identification of a suspected pulmonary infection, particularly in the immunocompetent patient. CT and more invasive procedures are characteristically reserved for complicated cases. Nevertheless, immunocompromised patients may benefit from an early thin-section CT evaluation if they have signs and symptoms of infection and normal chest radiographs.

Immune Status

Diagnostic algorithms used in patients with pulmonary infections must take into account various aspects of the patient's history and demographic characteristics. In all cases, host immunity is an important consideration and is used to stratify a population of potentially infected patients into two groups: patients with normal immunity and immunocompromised patients. Knowledge of the patient's immune status allows healthcare providers to significantly narrow the differential diagnosis. For example, a patient with acquired immunodeficiency syndrome (AIDS) who presents with symptoms may be suffering from one or more infectious, inflammatory, or neoplastic processes. However, when such a patient exhibits diffuse bilateral hazy pulmonary opacities on chest radiography and bilateral ground-glass opacities on chest CT, the most likely diagnosis is infection with *Pneumocystis jiroveci*, also known as *Pneumocystis* pneumonia (PCP).

The radiologist must be familiar with the various types of immunosuppression which may affect surface barriers (skin, mucosa), humoral immunity, and cell-mediated immunity. Pulmonary pathogens will vary with the type of immune suppression affecting a given patient. For example, patients with AIDS are unlikely to develop PCP when CD4 levels are > 500 cells/mm³. However, in patients with CD4 levels < 500 cells/mm³, the rate of PCP infection increases significantly. On the other hand, patients with other forms of immunosuppression, such as steroid therapy, neutropenia, and diabetes, are at risk of developing specific pulmonary infections related to the nature of their immune compromise.

Unfortunately, the radiologist does not always have access to information regarding the patient's immune status, either because the clinical history is initially unavailable or because the patient is not known to be immunosuppressed. Certain imaging findings may suggest specific disease processes, and the radiologist may be able to suggest further testing to exclude immunosuppressive states. For example, if symptomatic patients exhibit characteristic imaging features of PCP, the radiologist may raise the possibility of HIV/AIDS and suggest specific testing to determine HIV status. In these instances, the radiologist may make a significant contribution to a timely diagnosis and appropriate management.

Assessment of pulmonary infection in patients who have undergone allogeneic hematopoietic cell transplantation warrants additional discussion. In these cases, pulmonary infection must be considered on the basis of the time elapsed since transplantation. Specific bacteria (e.g., *S. aureus, S. viridans)*, fungi (e.g., *Candida, Aspergillus*), and viruses (e.g., reactivation of HSV, respiratory syncytial virus [RSV], and influenza) commonly infect patients in the pre-engraftment period (i.e., < three weeks) following transplantation. In the immediate post-engraftment period (i.e., three weeks to three months), other bacterial (e.g., *Listeria monocytogenes, Legionella pneumophila)*, fungal (invasive aspergillosis, PCP), and viral (e.g., CMV, HHV-6, -7, & -8, EBV, and adenovirus) infections are most common. Finally, in the late post-engraftment period (i.e., > three months) still other bacterial (e.g., *S. pneumoniae, H. influenzae, N. meningitidis)* and viral (e.g., VZV reactivation and EBV and associated lymphoproliferative disorders) infections should be suspected and specifically excluded. Analysis of imaging findings after consideration of the time elapsed after transplantation may allow the radiologist to suggest a focused and appropriate differential diagnosis.

Community-acquired vs. Hospital-acquired Infection

There are well-recognized differences between infections acquired in the community and nosocomial infections that affect hospitalized patients. Overall, community-acquired pneumonia often manifests on chest radiography as lobar (lobar pneumonia) or multifocal consolidation (e.g., bronchopneumonia). Common causative microorganisms include *Pneumococcus pneumoniae, Haemophilus influenzae, Staphylococcus aureus, Mycoplasma pneumoniae, Chlamydia pneumoniae, Legionella pneumophila,* and viral agents such as influenza and RSV. *P. pneumoniae* is the most common cause of lobar pneumonia, but a bronchopneumonia pattern of pulmonary involvement is more characteristic of *S. aureus* or *H. influenzae.*

Nosocomial (hospital-acquired) pneumonia should be considered if the patient acquires the pulmonary infection at least 48 hours after admission to the hospital. Most common pathogens include gram-negative bacilli (e.g., *P. aeruginosa* and *Enterobacter* spp.) and *S. aureus*. These infections manifest on chest radiography as new or progressive consolidations in a patient with clinical signs and symptoms of infection.

Clinical Manifestations

The clinical presentation of an infected patient may vary with the offending organism. Patients with bacterial pneumonia typically present with acute onset of chest pain, fever, productive cough, and neutrophilia. Patients with viral and mycoplasmal pneumonias may exhibit mild fever, productive cough, and mildly elevated white blood cell count. Febrile neutropenia following bone marrow transplant should suggest angioinvasive fungal infection.

Knowledge of preexisting conditions may help suggest specific infections. For example, *Pseudomonas* pneumonia is common in patients with cystic fibrosis, anaerobic pneumonia and abscess should be considered in the setting of aspiration (alcoholism, postanesthesia, deglutition anomalies), and *Haemophilus* infection is typical of patients with COPD.

Age, Gender, and Race

Age, gender, and race play an important role in the evaluation of pulmonary infection. For example, bronchiectatic atypical mycobacterial infection manifesting with bronchiectasis, centrilobular nodules, and mosaic attenuation is characteristically seen in elderly white women. On the other hand, classic atypical mycobacterial infection manifesting with upper lobe cavitary disease is frequently seen in men with underlying pulmonary conditions such as COPD or pulmonary fibrosis. Finally, infections in infants are commonly viral, and infections in young children are often related to *Mycoplasma*.

Link between Infection and Neoplasia

It is very important to recognize that certain infections may be associated with malignancy. This association is predominantly described in patients with viral infections. For example, Kaposi sarcoma (KS), primary effusion lymphoma, and multicentric Castleman disease are related to KS-associated herpesvirus or human herpes virus (HHV) type 8. Hodgkin lymphoma, non-Hodgkin lymphoma, post-transplantation lymphoproliferative disorder, and AIDS-associated lymphoma are associated with Epstein-Barr virus (EBV). Squamous cell papilloma of the upper respiratory tract, recurrent respiratory papillomatosis, and esophageal squamous cell cancers are associated with human papilloma virus (HPV); malignant mesothelioma is associated with simian virus 40 (SV-40).

Parasitic Infection

Parasitic infections are commonly overlooked in the formulation of a differential diagnosis. Indeed, the overwhelming majority of pulmonary infections are bacterial, fungal, and viral. Most parasitic infections in North America are diagnosed in immigrants from areas in which these infections are endemic. However, *Strongyloides stercoralis* is an important pathogen that affects patients on chronic immunosuppression therapy (e.g., corticosteroids). Infected patients may develop a fulminant pulmonary infection that can progress to respiratory failure and result in the patient's death. Because imaging findings of pulmonary strongyloidiasis are nonspecific, a high degree of suspicion is required to suggest the diagnosis prospectively.

When to Intervene

To identify the causative microorganism, radiologists may be asked to perform image-guided biopsy of pulmonary lesions in patients with presumed infection. Whether percutaneous biopsy is the appropriate method of obtaining microbiologic confirmation in patients with suspected infection remains open to debate. In some patients, biopsy specimens allow the identification of a specific pathogen, but a causative organism cannot be found in 33-45%. It is not clear whether these procedures result in a significant reduction in morbidity or mortality that would outweigh the related risks. In most cases, the patient is treated empirically and percutaneous biopsy is only considered in patients who fail to respond to therapy and in patients with nosocomial superinfection, immunosuppression, or suspected tuberculosis not confirmed on sputum or gastric lavage analysis.

Nonetheless, radiologists who perform percutaneous tissue sampling for diagnosis of suspected infection must obtain tissue samples under aseptic technique to avoid false-positive results due to contaminants. In addition, it is advisable to obtain samples for culture, including anaerobic cultures that require the use of special sealed containers. All specimens must also be submitted for histologic analysis given that infections may mimic malignancy &/or inflammatory conditions and vice versa.

Selected References

1. Franquet T: Imaging of pulmonary viral pneumonia. Radiology. 260(1):18-39, 2011
2. Ferguson PE et al: Parainfluenza virus type 3 pneumonia in bone marrow transplant recipients: multiple small nodules in high-resolution lung computed tomography scans provide a radiological clue to diagnosis. Clin Infect Dis. Epub ahead of print, 2009
3. Masterton RG et al: Guidelines for the management of hospital-acquired pneumonia in the UK: report of the working party on hospital-acquired pneumonia of the British Society for Antimicrobial Chemotherapy. J Antimicrob Chemother. 62(1):5-34, 2008

*(**Left**) PA chest radiograph of a patient with HIV infection and P. pneumoniae pneumonia shows a well-defined area of sublobar right upper lobe consolidation ➡. (**Right**) Axial NECT of the same patient shows dense right upper lobe consolidation with an intrinsic air bronchogram ⇨. The patient had a CD4 count > 500 cells/mm³. Correlation with CD4 levels is always suggested in patients with HIV infection as it helps formulate a focused and more appropriate differential diagnosis.*

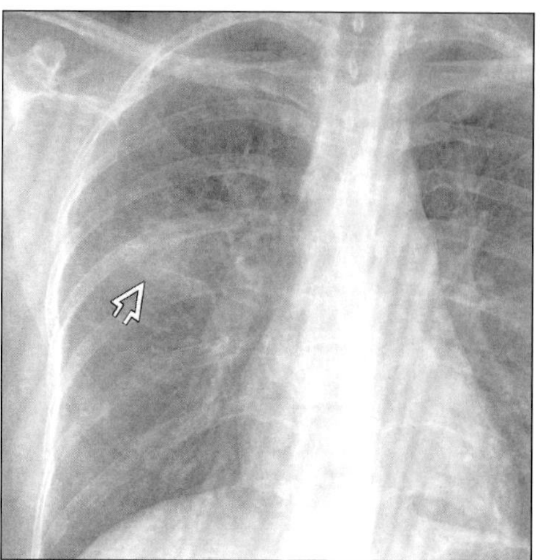

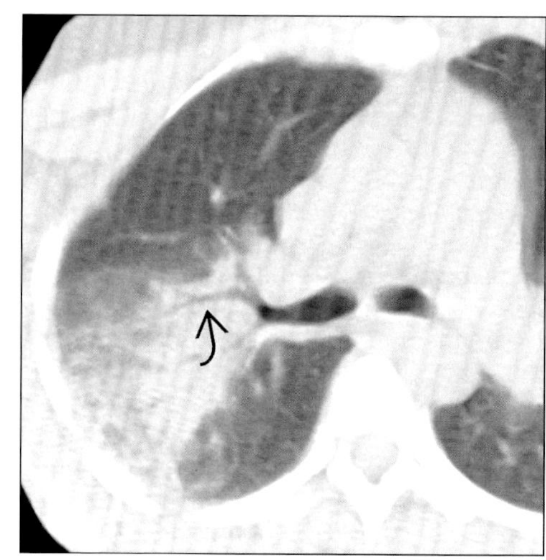

*(**Left**) PA chest radiograph of a patient with Mycoplasma pneumoniae pneumonia and upper respiratory symptoms shows scattered multifocal heterogeneous airspace disease. (**Right**) Axial CECT of the same patient better characterizes the extent of pulmonary consolidation and shows associated ground-glass opacities. Mycoplasma pneumonia is a common cause of community-acquired pneumonia in children and a common cause of discordance between radiologic findings and severity of clinical illness.*

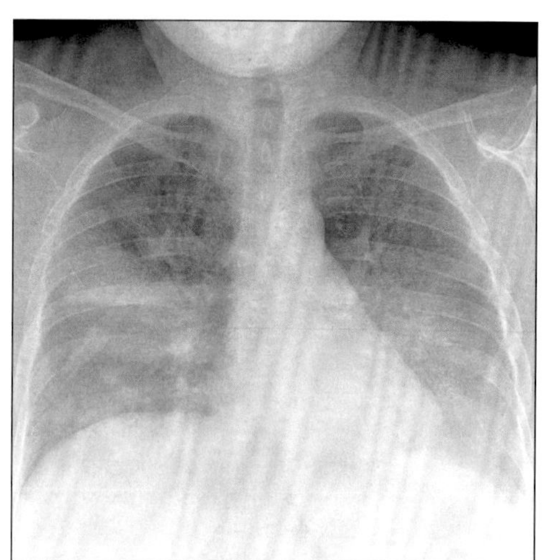

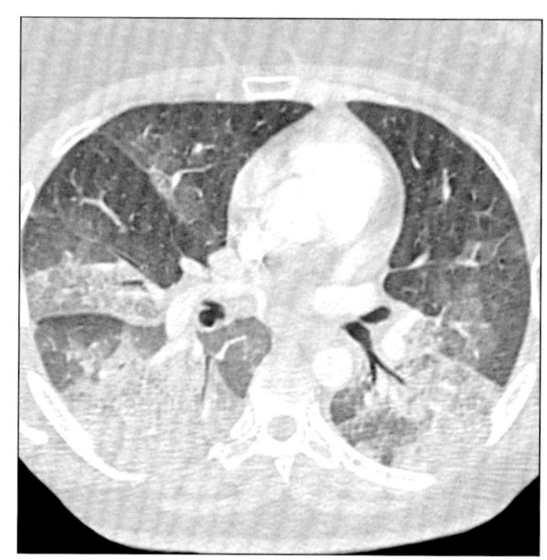

*(**Left**) PA chest radiograph of a neutropenic patient with angioinvasive aspergillosis secondary to A. flavum after bone marrow transplant shows a right lower lobe cavitary nodule ➡. (**Right**) Axial NECT of the same patient confirms a right lower lobe cavitary nodule ➡ with nodular cavity walls. A. flavum is the 2nd most common pathogen to cause angioinvasive aspergillosis after A. fumigatus and is considered 100x more virulent in terms of the inoculum required for infection.*

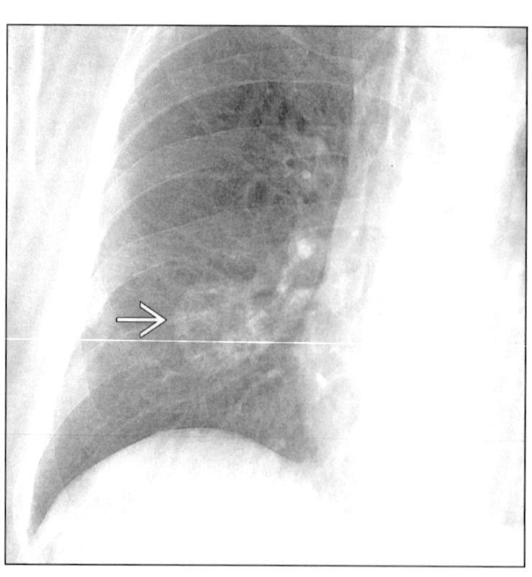

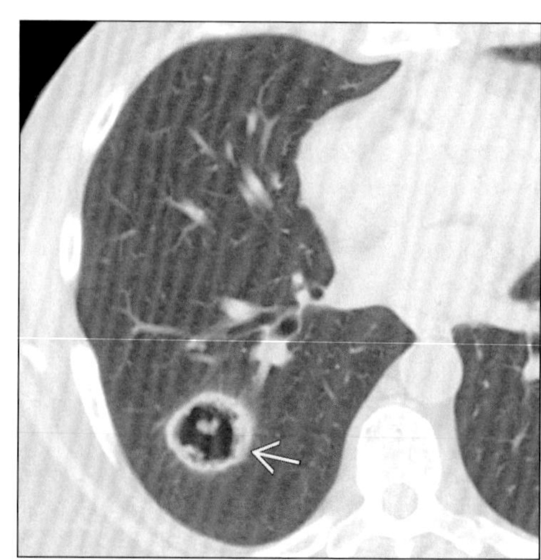

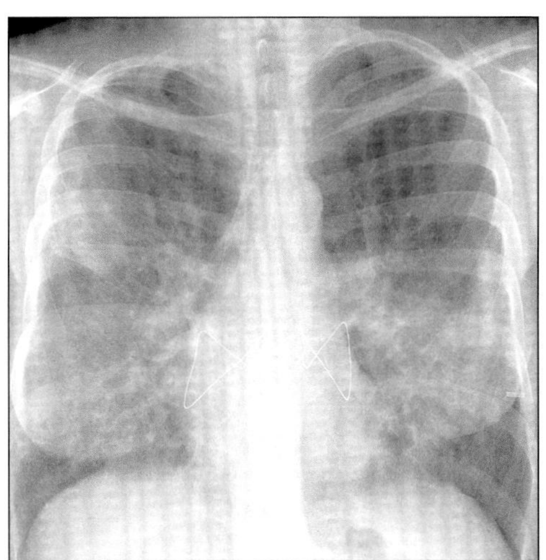

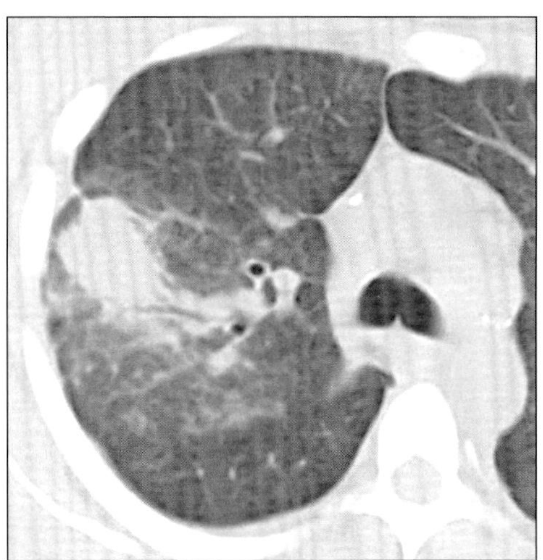

(Left) *PA chest radiograph of a patient with CMV pneumonia status post bilateral orthotopic lung transplantation shows scattered bilateral heterogeneous opacities.* ***(Right)*** *Axial NECT of the same patient shows a mass-like right upper lobe consolidation with a surrounding ground-glass opacity halo. CMV pneumonia commonly affects immunosuppressed patients who have AIDS and patients post bone marrow or solid-organ transplant &/or chemotherapy.*

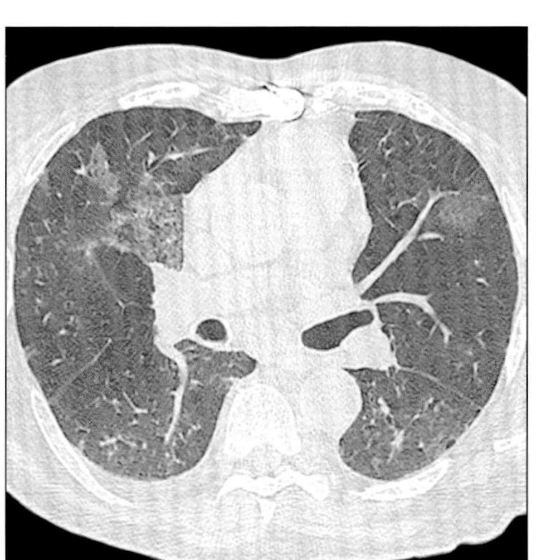

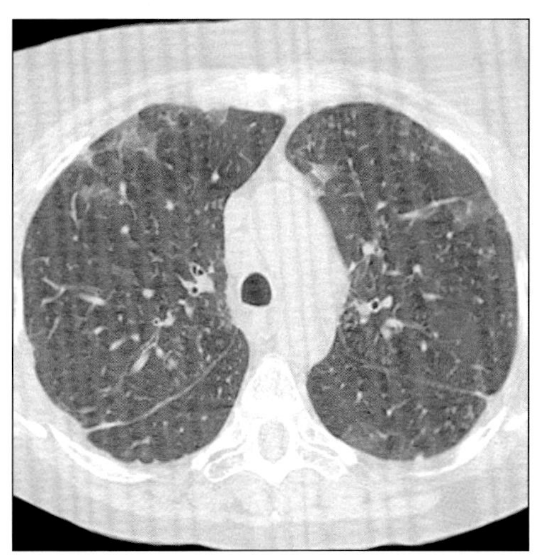

(Left) *Axial HRCT of a patient with fever secondary to parainfluenza 3 pneumonia after bone marrow transplant shows scattered bilateral ground-glass opacities. Influenza, RSV, rhinovirus, and parainfluenza are the most common pathogens in this patient population.* ***(Right)*** *Axial NECT of a patient with IgG deficiency and Haemophilus influenzae infection shows scattered bilateral peripheral ground-glass opacities, a common but nonspecific imaging finding in patients with pulmonary infection.*

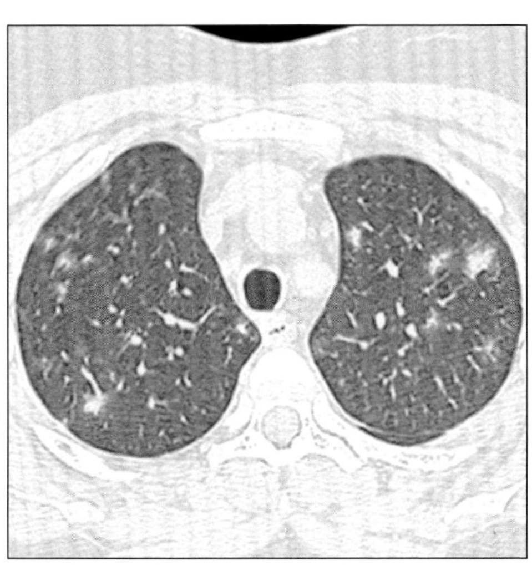

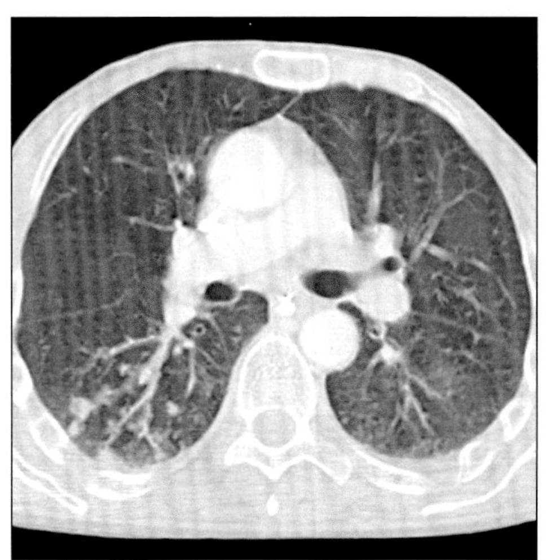

(Left) *Axial HRCT of a patient with varicella-zoster virus (VZV) pneumonia shows bilateral lung nodules with surrounding ground-glass halos. VZV pneumonia is common among patients with lymphoma and immunosuppression.* ***(Right)*** *Axial NECT of a patient on chronic corticosteroids who presented with respiratory failure due to Strongyloides stercoralis found on bronchoalveolar lavage shows subtle diffuse miliary nodules with clustered larger nodules in the right lower lobe.*

BRONCHOPNEUMONIA

Key Facts

Terminology

- Lobular pneumonia
- Multifocal inflammatory exudate centered on large inflamed airways

Imaging

- Radiography
  - Multifocal lobular or confluent consolidations
  - Aspiration pneumonia (dependent lungs)
  - Air bronchograms usually absent
  - Cavitation (abscess)
  - Pneumatoceles (*S. aureus* or *P. jiroveci*)
- CT
  - Centrilobular nodules & tree-in-bud opacities
  - Patchy airspace nodules (4-10 mm in diameter)
  - Lobular, subsegmental, segmental consolidations
  - Identification of necrosis/cavitation

Top Differential Diagnoses

- Aspiration
- Alveolar hemorrhage
- Organizing pneumonia

Pathology

- Aspiration of secretions from colonized trachea
- *S. aureus, E. coli, P. aeruginosa, H. influenza*, anaerobes

Clinical Issues

- Symptoms/signs
  - Acute onset of fever, chills, cough, sputum
  - Elevated white blood cell count with left-shift
- Any age, but elderly at increased risk
- 5th leading cause of death
- Treatment: Antibiotics & empyema drainage
- Nonsmokers & outpatients: Resolution in 2-3 weeks

*(**Left**) PA chest radiograph shows patchy bilateral areas of consolidation with ill-defined nodular opacities in the right upper lobe. Lobular consolidations and ill-defined nodules suggest bronchopneumonia. (**Right**) Coronal NECT shows multifocal bilateral basilar predominant areas of lobular consolidation ⇒ and diffuse bilateral ill-defined centrilobular nodules and branching tree-in-bud opacities ➡, which is consistent with endobronchial dissemination of pulmonary infection.*

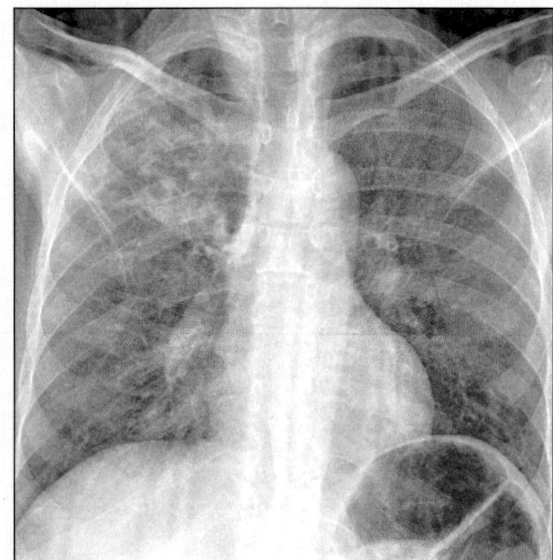

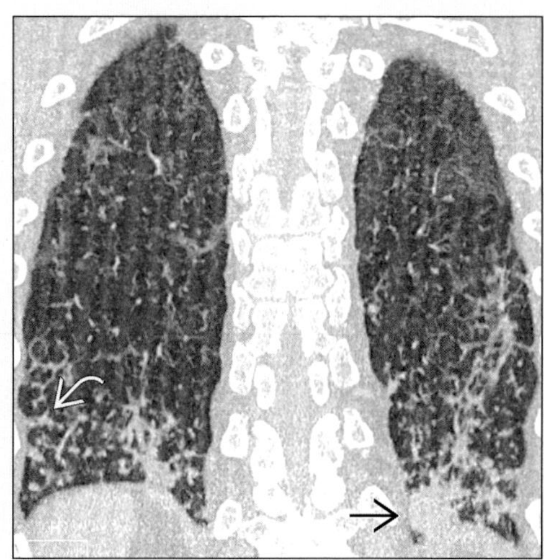

*(**Left**) Axial CECT shows multifocal bilateral areas of lobular consolidation ➡ associated with faint surrounding ground-glass opacities and ground-glass attenuation in the superior segment of the left lower lobe ➡. These findings in a patient with fever are highly suggestive of bronchopneumonia. (**Right**) PA chest radiograph shows bilateral lower lobe consolidations ➡ affecting the basal segments. The gravity-dependent distribution of airspace disease suggests aspiration pneumonia.*

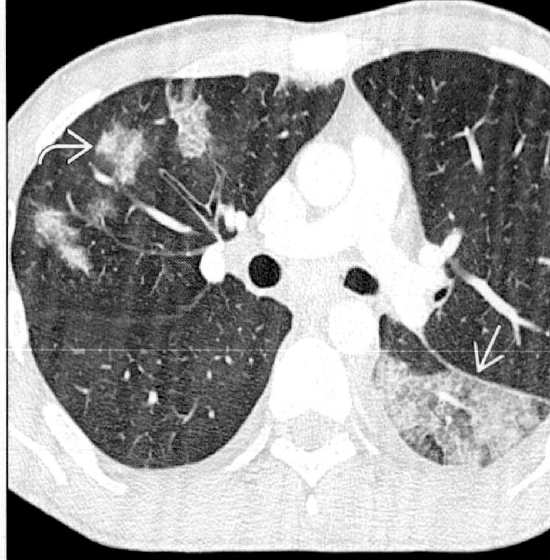

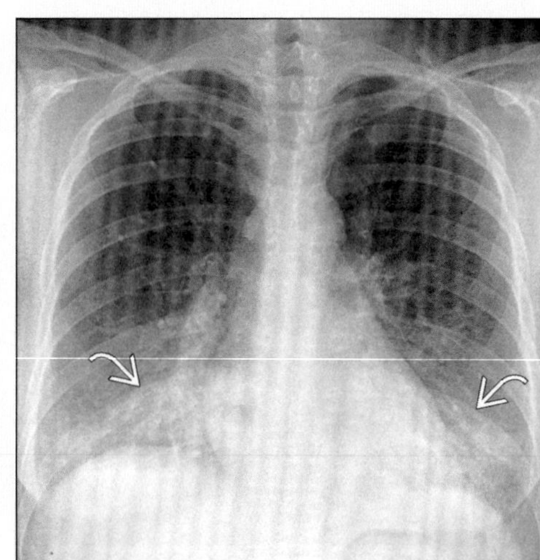

BRONCHOPNEUMONIA

TERMINOLOGY

Synonyms

- **Lobular pneumonia**

Definitions

- Multifocal inflammatory exudate centered on large inflamed airways

IMAGING

General Features

- Best diagnostic clue
  - Acute multifocal (patchy) lobular or confluent areas of consolidation in febrile patient
- Location
  - Aspiration pneumonia: Dependent portions of lungs
    - Usually multilobar & bilateral
    - Upper lobe posterior segments (supine position)
    - Lower lobe basal segments (upright position)

Radiographic Findings

- Radiography
  - Multifocal lobular or confluent areas of consolidation
    - Air bronchograms usually absent on radiography
  - Lobular, subsegmental, or segmental distribution
  - Pneumatoceles (*S. aureus* or *P. jiroveci*)
  - Cavitation (abscess)
    - More common in upper lobes: *S. aureus*, anaerobes, gram-negative bacteria

CT Findings

- NECT
  - Centrilobular nodules & branching opacities (tree-in-bud)
  - Patchy airspace nodules (4-10 mm in diameter)
  - Lobular, subsegmental, or segmental areas of consolidation
  - Necrosis/cavitation
- CECT
  - Necrosis: Low-attenuation areas ± cavitation & rim enhancement (within consolidation or as isolated finding)

Imaging Recommendations

- Best imaging tool
  - Chest radiograph: Useful for detection of disease & documentation of response to therapy
- Protocol advice
  - CT
    - Useful in clinically suspected infection with normal chest radiograph
    - Sensitive & specific for detection of underlying structural abnormalities & complications

DIFFERENTIAL DIAGNOSIS

Aspiration

- Unilateral/bilateral consolidation with gravitational distribution
- Predisposing conditions: Esophageal motility disorder, alcoholism

Alveolar Hemorrhage

- Bilateral centrilobular, geographic, or diffuse airspace disease
- Anemia, hemoptysis

Organizing Pneumonia

- Subpleural & peribronchovascular consolidations
- Patients often treated for pneumonia for variable length of time

PATHOLOGY

General Features

- Etiology
  - Commonly caused by aspiration of secretions from colonized trachea
    - *S. aureus*, *E. coli*, *P. aeruginosa*, *H. influenza*, and anaerobes

Gross Pathologic & Surgical Features

- **Exudate centered on terminal bronchioles** (centrilobular)
- Respects septal boundaries
- Patchy distribution: Adjacent lobules may be normal

Microscopic Features

- Bronchial inflammation with epithelial ulcerations & fibrinopurulent exudate
- Spread to contiguous pulmonary lobules

CLINICAL ISSUES

Presentation

- Most common signs/symptoms
  - Acute onset fever, chills, cough, sputum production
  - Elevated white blood cell count with left-shift
  - Identification of etiology in < 50%
- Clinical profile
  - Associated with hospital-acquired pneumonia
    - *S. aureus*, *P. aeruginosa*, *E. coli*, anaerobes, gram-negative organisms
    - *Pseudomonas aeruginosa*: Most common & lethal form of hospital-acquired pneumonia
  - **Associated conditions**
    - **COPD**: *P. aeruginosa*, *H. influenza*, *M. catarrhalis*
    - **Cystic fibrosis**: *P. aeruginosa*

Demographics

- Age
  - Any age, elderly at increased risk

Natural History & Prognosis

- **5th leading cause of death**
- Prognosis depends on virulence of organism, antibiotic susceptibility, & host response
- Resolution
  - Nonsmokers & outpatients: Within 2-3 weeks

Treatment

- Appropriate antibiotics & empyema drainage

SELECTED REFERENCES

1. Reynolds JH et al: Pneumonia in the immunocompetent patient. Br J Radiol. 83(996):998-1009, 2010

COMMUNITY-ACQUIRED PNEUMONIA

Key Facts

Terminology

- Pneumonia developing in patient who has not been hospitalized or in long-term care facility for at least 14 days before onset of symptoms

Imaging

- Chest radiography for detection of abnormality, assessment of extent of disease, detection of complications, & evaluation of treatment response
  - Limited value in predicting causative organism
  - Immunocompromised, especially if neutropenic, may have normal radiographs
- CT is problem-solving tool for nondiagnostic chest radiographs, used in cases of unresolved pneumonia or suspected complications
- Complications
  - Cavitation, abscess formation
  - Empyema

Top Differential Diagnoses

- Cardiogenic pulmonary edema
- Hemorrhage
- Aspiration

Pathology

- Common pathogens: *Streptococcus pneumoniae* (50%), viral pneumonia (20%), *Haemophilus influenzae* (20%), *Chlamydia pneumoniae* (15%), *Mycoplasma pneumoniae* (5%), *Moraxella catarrhalis*

Clinical Issues

- Symptoms/signs: Fever, chills, cough, sputum

Diagnostic Checklist

- Careful imaging assessment of patients with CAP for early detection of complications, such as abscess & empyema

*(**Left**) PA chest radiograph of a patient with pneumococcal pneumonia shows focal consolidation ➔ in the periphery of the right lower lung zone. S. pneumoniae is the most common cause of community-acquired pneumonia and typically manifests as a lobar consolidation. (**Right**) PA chest radiograph of a patient with pneumococcal pneumonia shows a patchy left upper lobe consolidation with air bronchograms ➔ and central bronchial wall thickening ➔.*

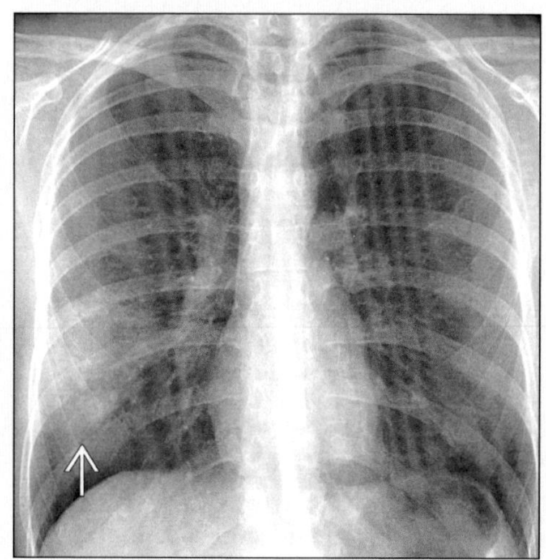

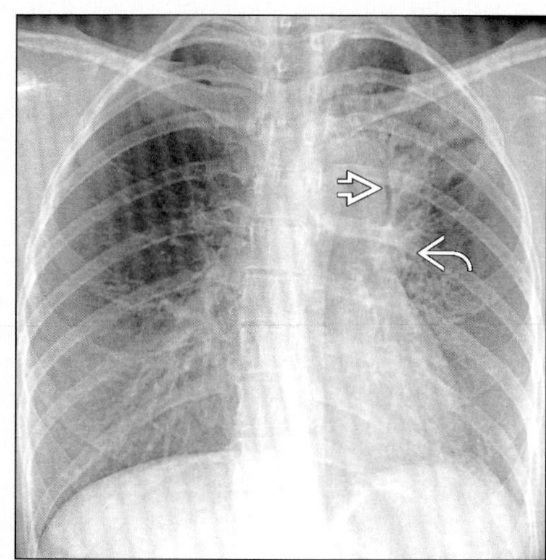

*(**Left**) PA chest radiograph of a patient with bacterial community-acquired pneumonia shows a diffuse lingular consolidation ➔. Extension of pulmonary infection into adjacent lung lobes depends on whether the interlobar fissure is complete and may follow collateral pathways such as airflow via pores of Kohn and canals of Lambert. (**Right**) Axial HRCT of a patient with community-acquired adenovirus pneumonia shows tiny miliary nodules and mild mosaic attenuation of the lung parenchyma.*

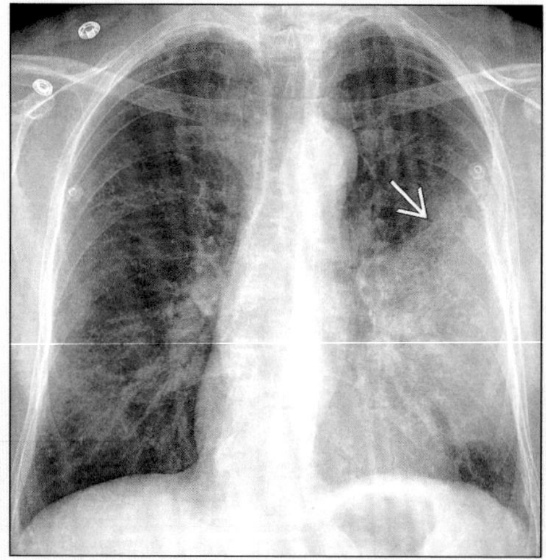

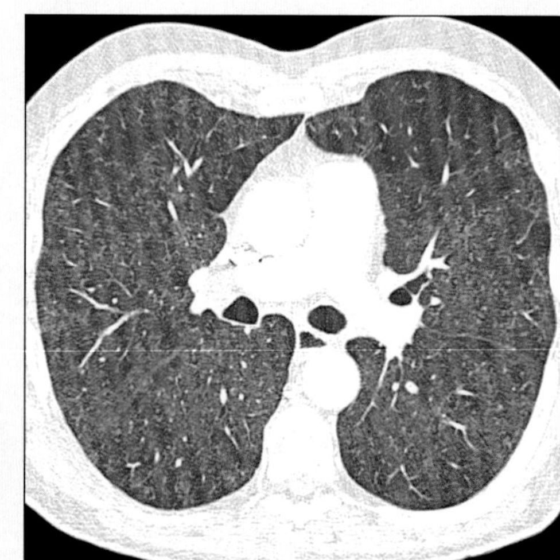

COMMUNITY-ACQUIRED PNEUMONIA

TERMINOLOGY

Abbreviations

- **Community-acquired pneumonia (CAP)**

Definitions

- Pneumonia developing in patient who has not been hospitalized or in long-term care facility for at least 14 days before onset of symptoms

IMAGING

General Features

- Best diagnostic clue
  - Focal parenchymal abnormality in patient with fever
- Location
  - Single lobe or multiple lobes
- Size
  - Range from small opacity to lobar or multilobar consolidation
- Morphology
  - Range from ground-glass opacity to frank consolidation

Radiographic Findings

- High sensitivity
  - Immunocompromised, especially if neutropenic, may have normal radiographs
- Typical distribution: Unilateral or bilateral segmental consolidation
- Significant interobserver variability in pattern recognition
  - May exhibit nearly any pattern, from ground-glass opacity to frank consolidation
  - Pattern not diagnostic of organism
    - Single organism may cause multiple patterns
  - Poor agreement for disease pattern, presence of air bronchogram, bronchial wall thickening
  - Good to excellent agreement for pleural effusion & extent of radiographic abnormalities
- Lobar vs. bronchopneumonia
  - Pathologic designation difficult to reliably identify radiographically
- Unusual patterns
  - Hyperinflation common with viral pneumonia (due to obstruction of distal airways)
  - Lobar enlargement with bulging fissures: *Klebsiella* pneumonia
  - Round pneumonia is common pattern of CAP in children
  - Pneumatoceles
    - Develop later in course of pneumonia (classically *S. aureus*), may persist for months, resolve spontaneously
  - Hilar lymphadenopathy
    - Rare, limits differential to tuberculosis, mycoplasma, fungi, mononucleosis, measles, plague, tularemia, anthrax, pertussis
- Complications
  - Cavitation
    - Suggests bacterial disease (*S. aureus*, gram-negative bacteria, anaerobes)
    - Can occur in pulmonary blastomycosis
  - Empyema
    - Pleural effusion in 20-60%, reactive parapneumonic effusion
    - Up to 5% progress to empyema
    - Suspect if effusion enlarges or becomes loculated
- Resolution
  - Delayed with advancing age & involvement of multiple lobes
    - Faster resolution in nonsmokers & outpatients
  - Expected timetable
    - 50% resolve in 2 weeks; 66% in 4 weeks; 75% in 6 weeks
- Mortality associated with 2 radiographic abnormalities
  - Bilateral pleural effusions
  - Multilobar disease

CT Findings

- Ground-glass opacity
- Consolidation
- Nodules
  - Diffuse or patchy tree-in-bud opacities highly suggestive of infectious bronchiolitis (especially *Mycoplasma* & viruses)
- More sensitive and specific for detection of complications
  - Abscess vs. empyema
    - Abscess: Thick, irregular wall; round shape; small area of contact with chest wall
    - Empyema: Thin, uniform wall; lenticular shape; broad area of contact with chest wall; pleural thickening & enhancement; edema in adjacent extrapleural fat
- In patients with recurrent pneumonia, consider
  - Lung cancer, bronchiectasis, COPD

Imaging Recommendations

- Best imaging tool
  - Chest radiography for detection of abnormality, assessment of extent of disease, detection of complications, & evaluation of treatment response
  - Limited value in predicting causative organism
- Protocol advice
  - CT is problem-solving tool for nondiagnostic chest radiographs, used in cases of unresolved pneumonia or suspected complications

DIFFERENTIAL DIAGNOSIS

Cardiogenic Pulmonary Edema

- Cardiomegaly & pulmonary venous hypertension
- Edema will shift with patient position
- Focal right upper lobe edema may occur with mitral regurgitation

Pulmonary Hemorrhage

- Patients usually anemic & often have hemoptysis
- Multifocal bilateral ground-glass opacities

Aspiration

- May have predisposing condition, such as esophageal motility disorder
- Gravity-dependent location of airspace disease

Cryptogenic Organizing Pneumonia

- Patients often treated for pneumonia for variable length of time
- Patchy chronic or migratory bibasilar consolidation

Chronic Eosinophilic Pneumonia
- Typically chronic peripheral upper lobe consolidation
- Does not respond to antibiotics
- Most patients have asthma

Hypersensitivity Pneumonitis
- Often mistaken for pneumonia
- History of antigen exposure
- Chest radiograph often normal
- CT: Diffuse ground-glass opacities, poorly defined centrilobular nodules, & geographic lobular hyperinflation

Pulmonary Infarction
- Infarcts exhibit "melting snowball" sign with resolution
- Pneumonia, in contrast, "fades" away like ghost

Atelectasis
- Fissural displacement or indirect signs of volume loss

PATHOLOGY

General Features
- Etiology
  - Most common pathogens: *Streptococcus pneumoniae* (50%), viral pneumonia (20%), *Haemophilus influenzae* (20%), *Chlamydia pneumoniae* (15%), *Mycoplasma pneumoniae* (5%), *Moraxella catarrhalis*
- Offending organism cultured in < 50%
- Portal of entry: Inhalation or aspiration of oral secretions

Staging, Grading, & Classification
- Pneumonia Outcomes Research Team (PORT) Severity Index useful in determining inpatient vs. outpatient treatment

Gross Pathologic & Surgical Features
- Lobar vs. bronchopneumonia
  - Lobar
    - Alveolar flooding with inflammatory exudate, especially neutrophils
    - Rapidly spreads throughout lobe, only stopped by intact fissures
    - Usually peripheral in lung
  - Bronchopneumonia
    - Exudate centered on terminal bronchioles (centrilobular)
    - Respects septal boundaries
    - Patchy: Adjacent secondary pulmonary lobules may be normal, patchwork quilt pattern

Microscopic Features
- Nonspecific acute &/or chronic inflammatory cells
- Organism identified with special stains (such as Gram or acid fast)

CLINICAL ISSUES

Presentation
- Most common signs/symptoms
  - No individual or combinations of signs & symptoms on history or physical examination can reliably confirm or refute presence of pneumonia
  - Classic findings: Fever, chills, cough, sputum
  - Empyema: Patient may be surprisingly free of toxic symptoms
  - Pulmonary cavity in patient with poor dentition = lung abscess

Demographics
- Age
  - Any age
- Epidemiology
  - 8-15 per 1,000 persons per year

Natural History & Prognosis
- Depends on virulence of organism, antibiotic susceptibility, host immune factors
- Pneumonia 6th most common cause of death

Treatment
- Appropriate antibiotics
- Drain empyemas, not abscesses

DIAGNOSTIC CHECKLIST

Image Interpretation Pearls
- Absence of parenchymal abnormality excludes pneumonia (except in immunocompromised)

Reporting Tips
- Diagnosis of CAP is based on culture
- Careful imaging assessment of patients with CAP for early detection of complications, such as abscess & empyema

SELECTED REFERENCES

1. Mandell LA et al: Infectious Diseases Society of America/ American Thoracic Society consensus guidelines on the management of community-acquired pneumonia in adults. Clin Infect Dis. 44 Suppl 2:S27-72, 2007
2. Sharma S et al: Radiological imaging in pneumonia: recent innovations. Curr Opin Pulm Med. 13(3):159-69, 2007
3. Lutfiyya MN et al: Diagnosis and treatment of community-acquired pneumonia. Am Fam Physician. 73(3):442-50, 2006
4. Apisarnthanarak A et al: Etiology of community-acquired pneumonia. Clin Chest Med. 26(1):47-55, 2005
5. Tarver RD et al: Radiology of community-acquired pneumonia. Radiol Clin North Am. 43(3):497-512, viii, 2005
6. Herold CJ et al: Community-acquired and nosocomial pneumonia. Eur Radiol. 14 Suppl 3:E2-20, 2004
7. Reittner P et al: Pneumonia: high-resolution CT findings in 114 patients. Eur Radiol. 13(3):515-21, 2003

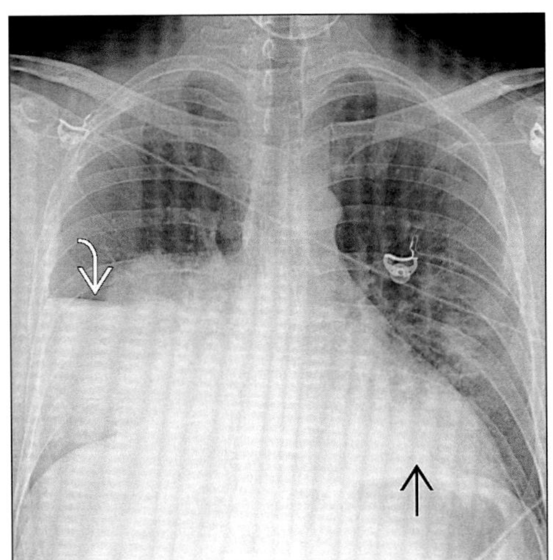

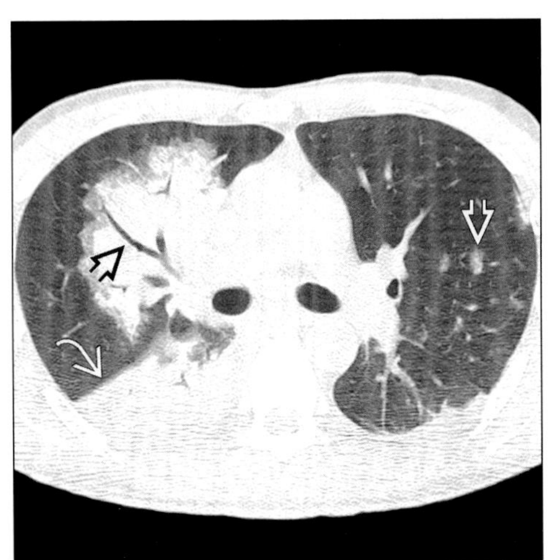

(Left) *AP chest radiograph of a patient with community-acquired pneumococcal pneumonia shows bilateral multilobar consolidations* →*. Note sharp demarcation of the minor fissure* → *by adjacent middle lobe consolidation.* **(Right)** *Axial HRCT of the same patient shows dense right upper and lower lobe consolidations with adjacent ground-glass opacity and air bronchograms* → *and small foci of nodular ground-glass opacity* → *on the left. Note sharp demarcation of the right major fissure* →*.*

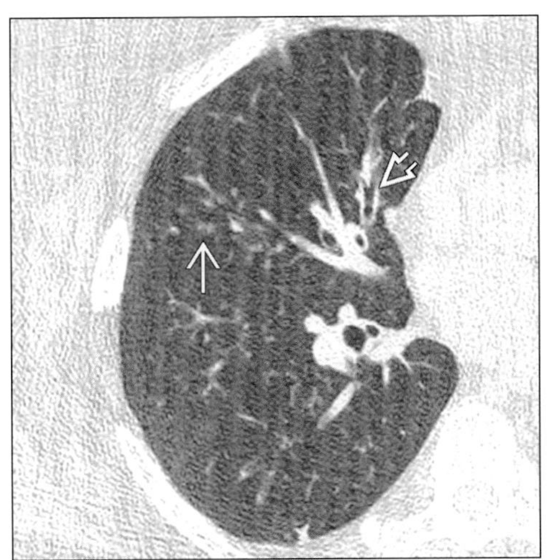

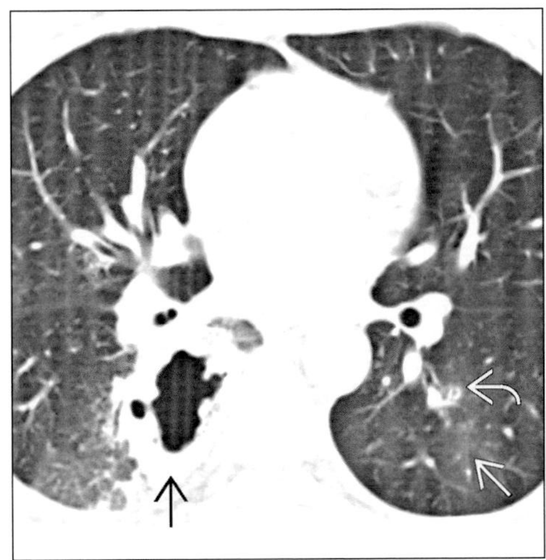

(Left) *Axial HRCT of a patient with community-acquired pulmonary infection shows clusters of small centrilobular nodules* → *and mild bronchial wall thickening* →*. Mycoplasma, Chlamydia, and viruses are common causes of this pattern.* **(Right)** *Axial CECT of a patient with lung abscess shows a cavitary right lower lobe lesion* →*, bilateral lower lobe patchy ground-glass opacities* →*, and a small poorly defined left lower lobe nodule* →*.*

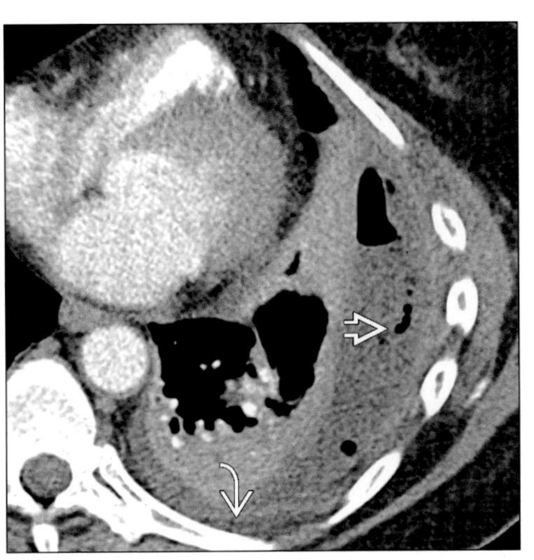

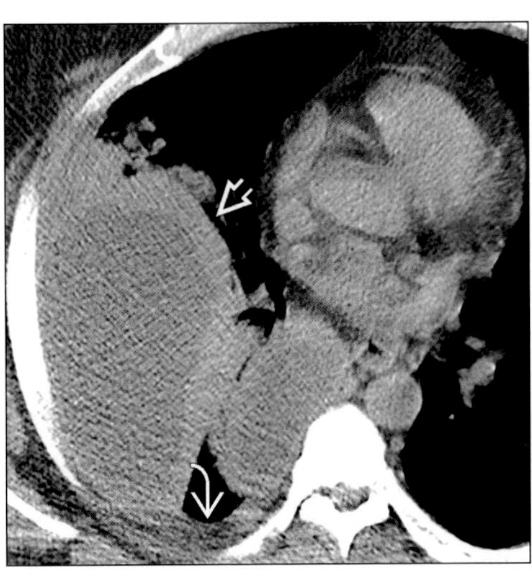

(Left) *Axial CECT of a patient with empyema resulting from CAP shows a complex left pleural collection containing several loculations of gas* → *and edema of the extrapleural fat* →*.* **(Right)** *Axial NECT of a patient with CAP-related empyema shows a complex, multiloculated right pleural fluid collection compressing adjacent collapsed lung* →*. Note that the extrapleural fat* → *is hazy as compared to the deep chest wall fat. This finding is highly suggestive of empyema.*

HEALTHCARE-ASSOCIATED PNEUMONIA

Key Facts

Terminology
- Healthcare-associated pneumonia (HCAP)
- Pneumonia developing in patients receiving outpatient healthcare services

Imaging
- Radiography
  - Patchy unilateral or bilateral consolidation (bronchopneumonia)
  - Confluent consolidation
  - Abscesses (usually solitary)
  - Pleural effusion & empyema
- CT
  - Centrilobular nodules
  - Lobular, subsegmental, or segmental consolidations
  - Abscess formation (15-30%)
  - Pleural effusion (30-50%); 1/2 are empyemas

Top Differential Diagnoses
- Tuberculosis
- Aspiration
- Pulmonary vasculitis

Pathology
- Methicillin-resistant *S. aureus* (MRSA), *P. aeruginosa*, *Acinetobacter* species, gram-negatives

Clinical Issues
- Symptoms/signs
  - Mild respiratory symptoms
  - Frequent extrapulmonary manifestations
- Treatment
  - Multidrug broad-spectrum antibiotic therapy

Diagnostic Checklist
- Absence of parenchymal abnormality excludes pneumonia (except in immunocompromised)

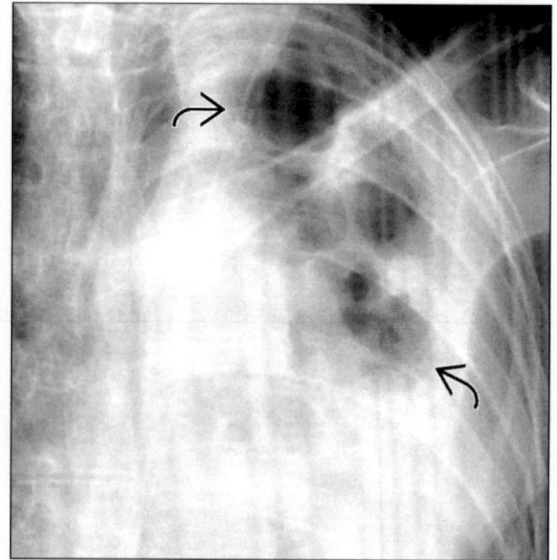
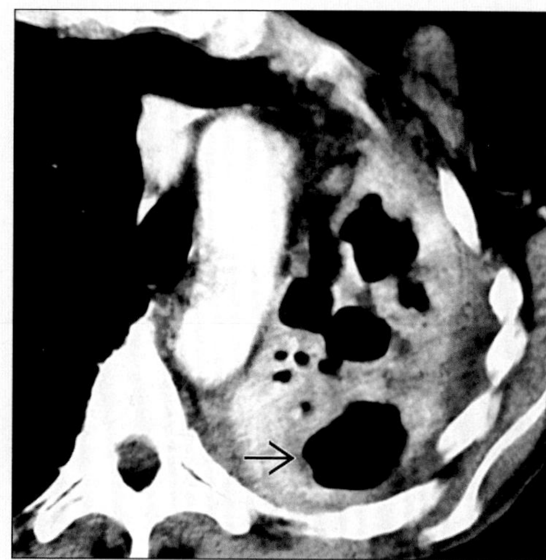

***(Left)** PA chest radiograph of a 68-year-old nursing home resident who developed methicillin-resistant Staphylococcus aureus (MRSA) pulmonary infection shows diffuse dense left lung consolidation with multiple areas of cavitation ⮫. **(Right)** Axial CECT of the same patient shows multiple left upper lobe abscesses ⇥, some with intrinsic air-fluid levels surrounded by dense pulmonary consolidation. Healthcare-associated pneumonias typically require therapy for multidrug-resistant pathogens.*

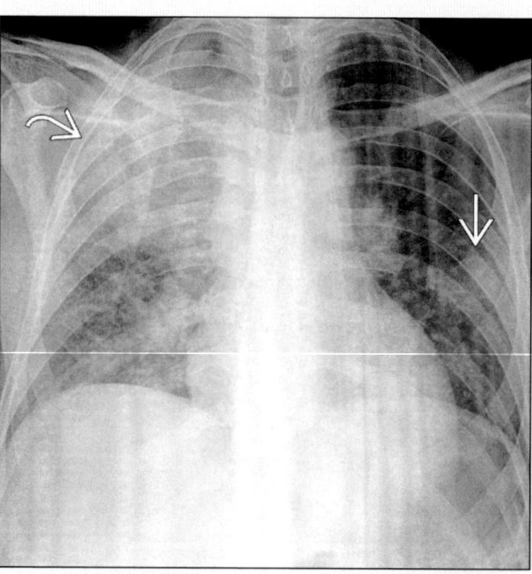
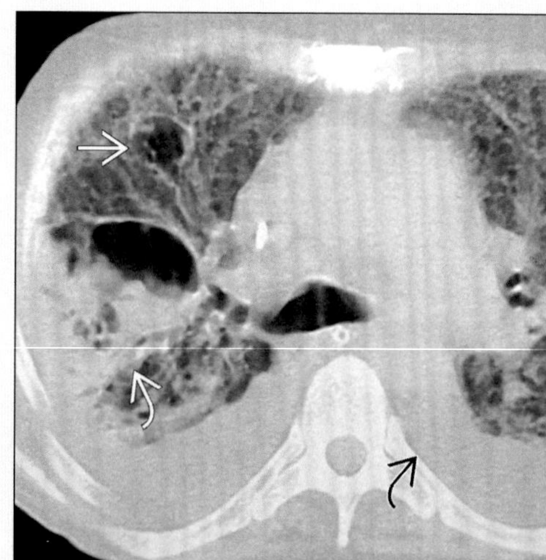

***(Left)** AP chest radiograph of a patient with HCAP shows dense right upper lobe consolidation ⮫ and bilateral multifocal heterogeneous consolidations ⮕. Bronchopneumonia is the most common imaging manifestation of HCAP. **(Right)** Axial NECT of a patient with emphysema and HCAP shows a right upper lobe consolidation ⮫, pneumatoceles ⮕, bilateral ground-glass opacities, and bilateral pleural effusions ⮫. HCAP may manifest with multifocal lung involvement & carries a high mortality rate.*

HEALTHCARE-ASSOCIATED PNEUMONIA

TERMINOLOGY

Abbreviations

- Healthcare-associated pneumonia (HCAP)

Synonyms

- Nursing home-acquired pneumonia

Definitions

- Pneumonia developing in patients receiving outpatient healthcare services
  - **HCAP criteria** (risk factors)
    - Hospitalization > 2 days in preceding 90 days
    - Resident of nursing home or long-term care facility
    - Recipient of recent intravenous antibiotic therapy, chemotherapy, or wound care within past 30 days
    - Long-term dialysis
    - Exposure to family members with multiple drug-resistant pathogens

IMAGING

General Features

- Best diagnostic clue
  - Consolidation in patient with fever

Radiographic Findings

- Patchy unilateral or bilateral consolidation (bronchopneumonia)
- Confluent consolidation
- Abscesses (usually solitary)
- Pleural effusion & empyema

CT Findings

- Centrilobular nodules
- Lobular, subsegmental, or segmental consolidations
  - Unilateral or bilateral
- Abscess formation (15-30%)
- Pneumatoceles
- Pleural effusion (30-50%); 1/2 are empyemas

Imaging Recommendations

- Best imaging tool
  - Chest radiography for disease detection, assessment of disease extent, detection of complications, evaluation of response to treatment
  - Limited value in predicting causative organism
- Protocol advice
  - Main role of CT: Nondiagnostic chest radiographs, unresolved pneumonia, suspected complication

DIFFERENTIAL DIAGNOSIS

Tuberculosis

- Apical heterogeneous consolidation with cavitation
- Associated centrilobular nodules & tree-in-bud opacities

Aspiration

- Focal or multifocal consolidation with gravity-dependent distribution

Pulmonary Vasculitis

- Multifocal nodules, masses, consolidations
- Frequent cavitation

PATHOLOGY

General Features

- Etiology
  - Methicillin-resistant *S. aureus* (MRSA), *P. aeruginosa*, *Acinetobacter* species, multidrug-resistant gram-negatives

CLINICAL ISSUES

Presentation

- Most common signs/symptoms
  - Mild respiratory symptoms
  - Frequent extrapulmonary manifestations
    - Advanced age, neurological disorders, multiple chronic comorbidities

Demographics

- Epidemiology
  - More comorbid illness than patients with CAP
    - Immunosuppression, diabetes, chronic renal disease, heart disease, stroke

Natural History & Prognosis

- More severe clinical course than community-acquired pneumonia (CAP)
- Increased risk for multidrug-resistant organisms
- Clinically & etiologically similar to hospital-acquired pneumonia (HAP)
  - Mortality rate close to that of HAP

Treatment

- Multidrug broad-spectrum empirical antibiotic therapy

DIAGNOSTIC CHECKLIST

Consider

- **Extensive microbiological testing to overcome high prevalence of multidrug-resistant infection**
  - Urinary antigens for *Legionella* & *S. pneumoniae*
  - Blood cultures
  - Gram stain of low respiratory tract secretions
    - Sputum, tracheobronchial aspirate, fibrobronchial aspirate, protected specimen brush, bronchoalveolar lavage fluid
  - Cultures for aerobic, anaerobic, mycobacterial, & fungal pathogens
- **PCR-based techniques in respiratory samples**

Image Interpretation Pearls

- Absence of parenchymal abnormality excludes pneumonia (except in immunocompromised)

SELECTED REFERENCES

1. Tablan OC et al: Guidelines for preventing health-care--associated pneumonia, 2003: recommendations of CDC and the Healthcare Infection Control Practices Advisory Committee. MMWR Recomm Rep. 53(RR-3):1-36, 2004

NOSOCOMIAL PNEUMONIA

Key Facts

Terminology
- Hospital-acquired pneumonia (HAP)
- Pneumonia that occurs > 48 hours after hospital admission or within 48 hours of hospital discharge

Imaging
- Radiography
  - Segmental & subsegmental consolidation
  - Lobe enlargement, bulging fissures: *K. pneumonia*
  - Pneumatoceles: *S. aureus*
  - Cavitation: *S. aureus*, gram-negatives, anaerobes
  - Pleural effusion/empyema
- CT findings
  - Centrilobular nodules, acinar/ground-glass opacities
  - Segmental & subsegmental consolidation
  - Enhancing consolidation with low-density areas & cavity formation

Top Differential Diagnoses
- Cardiogenic pulmonary edema
- Acute respiratory distress syndrome (ARDS)
- Cryptogenic organizing pneumonia
- Drug-induced lung disease

Clinical Issues
- Symptoms/signs
  - Fever, leukocytosis or leukopenia
  - Cough, purulent sputum
- Most common in elderly patients
- Factors increasing risk of HAP: Old age (> 80 years), severe comorbidities, immunosuppression
- Treatment: Appropriate antibiotics

Diagnostic Checklist
- Combination of clinical history, physical exam, serologic tests, & diagnostic imaging

(Left) AP chest radiograph of a patient with HAP shows extensive right upper lobe consolidation with cavitation ➦ and bulging major fissure ➡. Klebsiella pneumonia has a peculiar tendency to produce a large volume of consolidation, resulting in the typical "bulging fissure" sign. ***(Right)*** Axial NECT of a patient with HAP shows bilateral lower lobe subsegmental consolidations ➡ with cavitation ➡ and right lower lobe ground-glass opacity ➦. Anaerobes and S. aureus frequently produce cavitation.

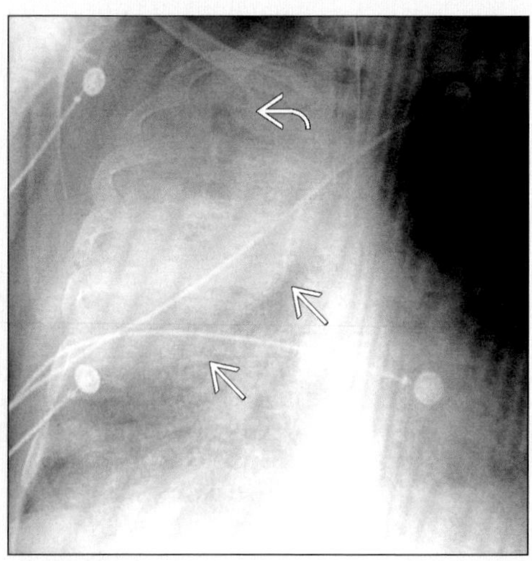

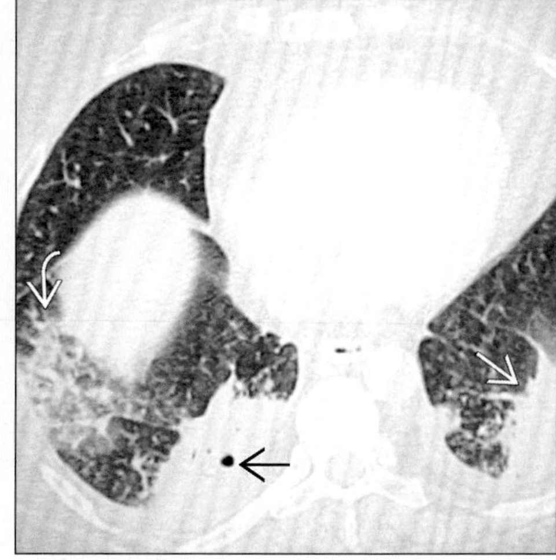

(Left) Axial CECT of a patient with Pseudomonas bronchopneumonia shows dense right upper lobe consolidation with multiple variably sized lucencies ➦, representing areas of necrosis and early cavitation. Subsegmental consolidations were also present in the left lung (not shown). ***(Right)*** Coronal CECT shows patchy bilateral ill-defined acinar nodules ➡ and an associated significant right pleural effusion ➡. These findings may progress to multifocal, often bilateral, consolidations.

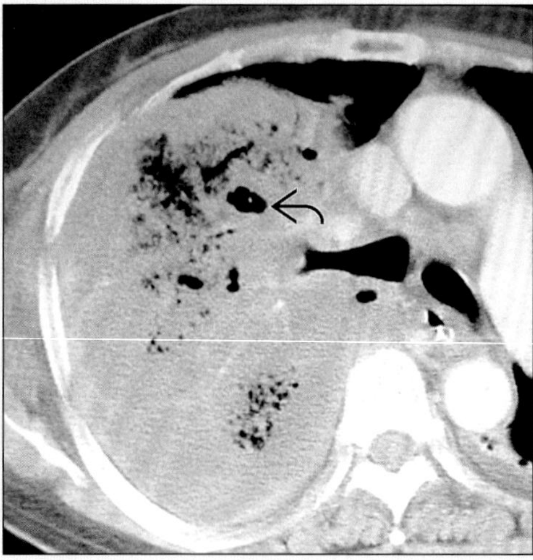

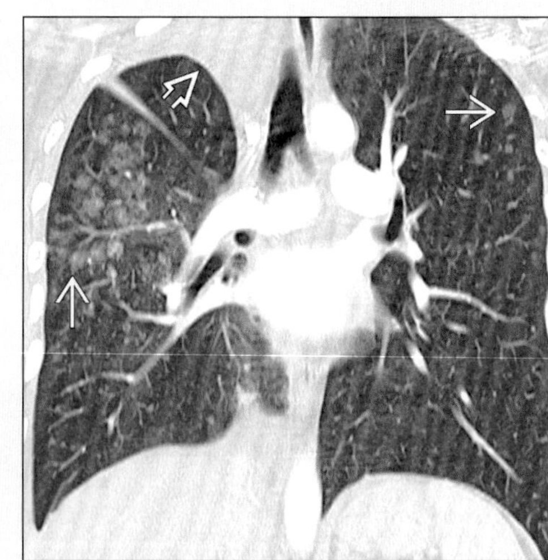

NOSOCOMIAL PNEUMONIA

TERMINOLOGY

Synonyms

- Hospital-acquired pneumonia (HAP)

Definitions

- **American Thoracic Society**: Pneumonia that occurs > 48 hours after hospital admission or within 48 hours of discharge from hospital

IMAGING

General Features

- Best diagnostic clue
  - Focal/multifocal consolidation in patient with fever

Radiographic Findings

- Segmental & subsegmental consolidation (unilateral or bilateral)
- Lobar enlargement with bulging fissures: *K. pneumonia*
- Pneumatoceles: *S. aureus*
- Cavitation: *S. aureus*, gram-negative bacteria, anaerobes
- Pleural effusion/empyema

CT Findings

- Centrilobular nodules, acinar & ground-glass opacities
- Segmental & subsegmental consolidation (multilobar; unilateral or bilateral)
- Enhancing consolidation with low-density areas & cavity formation
- Empyema ("split pleura" sign)

Imaging Recommendations

- Best imaging tool
  - Chest radiography: Detection of abnormality, assessment of extent of disease, identification of complications, evaluation of treatment response
  - Limited value in predicting causative organism
- Protocol advice
  - CT (complementary study): Nondiagnostic radiographs, unresolved pneumonia, complications

DIFFERENTIAL DIAGNOSIS

Cardiogenic Pulmonary Edema

- Bilateral & symmetric (perihilar) airspace disease

Acute Respiratory Distress Syndrome (ARDS)

- Progressive respiratory failure associated with diffuse airspace disease

Cryptogenic Organizing Pneumonia

- Changing multifocal peripheral consolidations

Drug-induced Lung Disease

- History of drug use: Pharmaceutic & illicit
  - Focal or multifocal consolidation
  - Multifocal or diffuse ground-glass opacities

PATHOLOGY

General Features

- Etiology
  - Microaspiration of oral & pharyngeal contents
  - **Gram-negative bacteria** (*P. aeruginosa*, *Enterobacter*, *Acinetobacter*, enteric gram-negative rods) in 55-85% of cases, **gram-positive cocci** (*S. aureus*) in 20-30% of cases, and **polymicrobial** in 40-60% of cases
  - **Viruses**: Herpes simplex virus (HSV) and Cytomegalovirus (CMV) in nonimmunosuppressed ICU patients
  - **Emerging resistant bacterial pathogens**: Methicillin-resistant *S. aureus*, vancomycin-resistant *Enterococcus sp.*, *C. difficile*, multidrug-resistant gram-negative bacteria
  - **Etiologic diagnosis**: 40-50% of cases

Gross Pathologic & Surgical Features

- Lobar vs. bronchopneumonia
- Necrotizing or nonnecrotizing

Microscopic Features

- Nonspecific acute &/or chronic inflammatory cells
- Organism identified with special stains (such as Gram or acid-fast)

CLINICAL ISSUES

Presentation

- Most common signs/symptoms
  - Fever, leukocytosis, or leukopenia
  - Cough, purulent sputum

Demographics

- Age
  - Most common in elderly patients
- Epidemiology
  - Nosocomial pneumonia is 2nd most frequent nosocomial infection
    - 0.5-2.0% of hospitalized patients

Natural History & Prognosis

- Factors increasing risk of HAP: Old age (> 80 years), severe comorbidities, immunosuppression

Treatment

- Appropriate antibiotics
  - 20-50% of patients do not respond adequately to empirical antibiotic treatment
- Drainage of empyemas, not abscesses

DIAGNOSTIC CHECKLIST

Consider

- Combination of clinical history, physical exam, serologic tests, & diagnostic imaging

Image Interpretation Pearls

- Radiologic resolution may lag behind clinical improvement

SELECTED REFERENCES

1. Niederman MS: Hospital-acquired pneumonia, health care-associated pneumonia, ventilator-associated pneumonia, and ventilator-associated tracheobronchitis: definitions and challenges in trial design. Clin Infect Dis. 51 Suppl 1:S12-7, 2010

LUNG ABSCESS

Key Facts

Terminology
- Lung necrosis secondary to microbial infection

Imaging
- Radiography
  - Spherical thick-walled cavity surrounded by consolidation
  - Equal length air-fluid levels on frontal & lateral
  - Usually related to aspiration: Gravitationally dependent lung
  - Pleural effusion common
- CT
  - Abscess: Thick, irregular wall, spherical, narrow contact with chest wall, and bronchovascular markings extend to abscess
  - Empyema: Thin, uniform wall, lenticular shape, broad contact with chest wall, split pleura sign, and adjacent compressed lung

Top Differential Diagnoses
- Tuberculosis
- Lung cancer
- Wegener granulomatosis

Pathology
- Aspiration: Mixed aerobic & anaerobic polymicrobial bacterial infection originating in gingiva

Clinical Issues
- Cough, foul-smelling sputum, periodontal disease
- Usually responds to antibiotics in contrast to abscesses elsewhere that usually require drainage
- < 10% require surgery

Diagnostic Checklist
- Consider CT to assess complications, such as empyema & bronchopleural fistula

__(Left)__ PA chest radiograph of a 51-year-old man with poor dentition shows a mass-like opacity ➔ with central lucency consistent with cavitation overlying the right hilum. The lesion exhibits the hilum overlay sign, which indicates that it is not in the hilum. __(Right)__ Lateral chest radiograph of the same patient shows the mass-like opacity ➔ in the superior segment of the right lower lobe. Although tuberculosis should be considered based on location, lung abscess must also be considered.

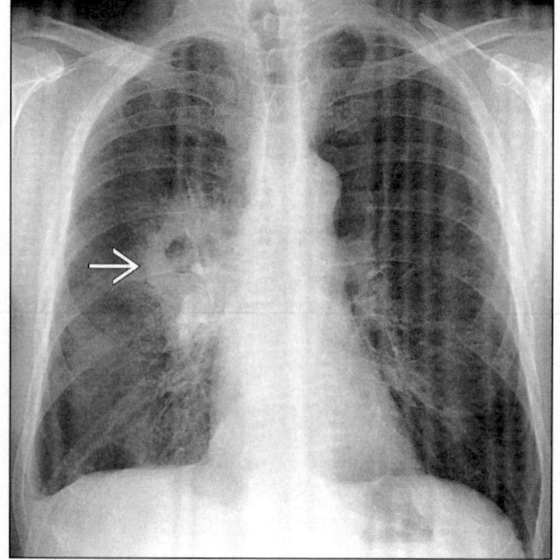

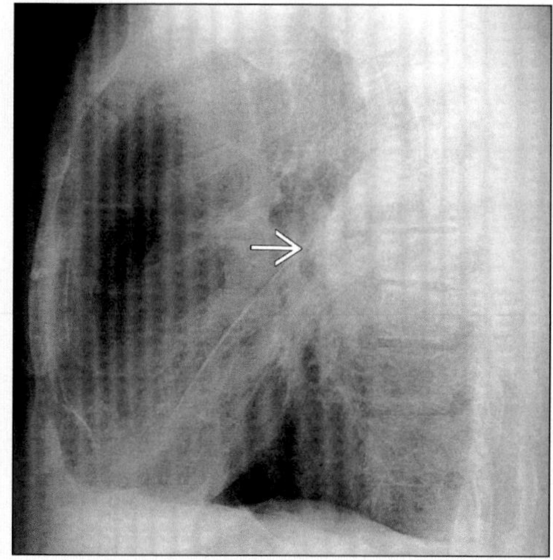

__(Left)__ Coronal CECT of the same patient shows a spherical lesion of lobular borders with cavitation and a thick, nodular cavity wall surrounded by a ground-glass opacity halo ➔. __(Right)__ Axial CECT of the same patient shows the cavitary lesion in the superior segment of the right lower lobe ➔ abutting the paravertebral region with associated mildly enlarged reactive right hilar lymph nodes ➔. The location in the dependent aspect of the right lower lobe suggests aspiration in the supine position.

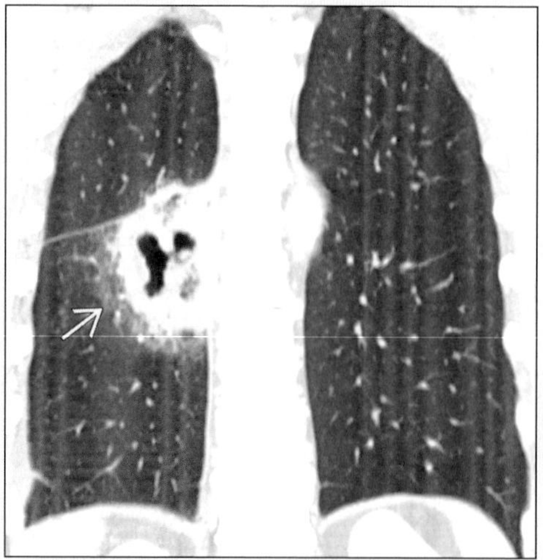

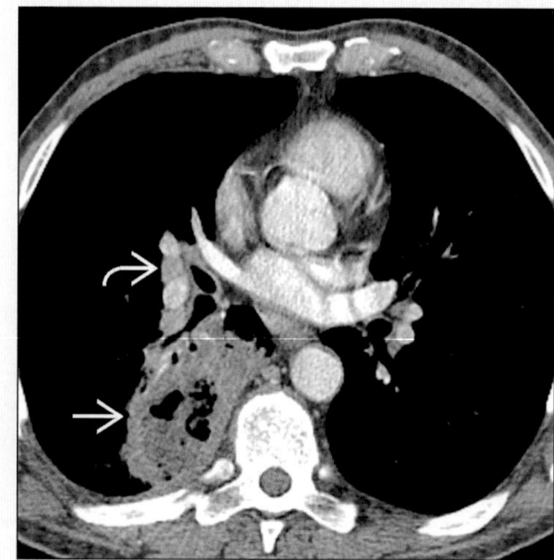

LUNG ABSCESS

TERMINOLOGY

Synonyms

- Necrotizing pneumonia, pulmonary gangrene

Definitions

- Lung necrosis secondary to microbial infection
- Cavity: Air-containing lesion with relatively thick wall (> 4 mm) ± surrounding consolidation or mass

IMAGING

General Features

- Best diagnostic clue
  - Irregular thick-walled lung cavity, often containing air, air-fluid level
- Location
  - Gravitationally dependent segments in aspiration
- Morphology
  - Spherical thick-walled cavity with relatively smooth inner margin

Radiographic Findings

- Evolution of consolidation from pneumonia to abscess cavity over 7-14 days
- **Pulmonary cavity**
  - Often solitary
  - Wall thickness: < 4 mm (5%); 5-15 mm (80%); > 15 mm (15%)
  - Air-fluid level in 75%
  - Often surrounded by consolidation (50%)
- Location usually relates to aspiration in gravitationally dependent locations
  - Supine position: Upper lobe posterior segments, lower lobe superior segments
  - Decubitus position: Upper lobe posterior segments, lower lobe lateral basilar segments
  - Upright position: Lower lobe basilar segments, middle lobe
- Lower lobe abscesses usually larger than upper lobe abscesses
- Pleural effusions common (50%), may evolve into empyema
- Multiple abscesses
  - Bronchogenic spread from initial abscess
    - Daughter abscesses usually smaller than parent
    - Located in areas gravitationally dependent from parent abscess
  - **Lemierre syndrome**
    - Sore throat with internal jugular vein thrombosis
    - Usually secondary to *Fusobacterium*
- **Distinction of lung abscess from empyema**
  - Cavity: Spherical shape, equal length of air-fluid levels on orthogonal radiographs, acute angles with chest wall
  - Empyema: Lenticular shape, unequal length of air-fluid levels on orthogonal radiographs, obtuse angles with chest wall
  - 33% of lung abscesses accompanied by empyema
- Slow resolution with treatment, often months
  - Larger the abscess, longer the time to resolution

CT Findings

- Optimal visualization & assessment of lung abscess
- Abscess may be fluid-filled
- Air-fluid level or central air collection indicates bronchial communication
- Cavity wall thickness: Variable, 4 mm to < 15 mm; thick wall more common
  - Luminal interior wall usually smooth (90%), shaggy (10%)
- Surrounding airspace or ground-glass opacity may show air bronchograms or tiny air bubbles
- Abscess vs. empyema
  - Abscess: Thick, irregular wall, spherical, narrow contact with chest wall, bronchovascular markings extend toward abscess
  - Empyema: Thin, uniform wall, lenticular shape, broad contact with chest wall, split pleura sign, adjacent compressed lung
- Reactive hilar & mediastinal lymphadenopathy common, usually < 2.5 cm short axis diameter
- Bronchopleural fistula: Development of hydropneumothorax, empyema
- Air crescent: Suggests invasive aspergillosis or mycetoma in preexisting cavity

Imaging Recommendations

- Best imaging tool
  - CT for distinction of lung abscess from empyema, exclusion of lung cancer
- Protocol advice
  - Antibiotics should be continued until chest radiograph shows resolution or stability

DIFFERENTIAL DIAGNOSIS

Pneumatoceles

- Difficult to distinguish from abscess, especially in staphylococcal pneumonia

Tuberculosis

- Upper lobe consolidation with cavitation
- May be bilateral

Infected Bulla

- Emphysema & history of smoking
- Thin-walled bulla with air-fluid level
- Considered pneumonia variant, responds to antibiotics

Lung Cancer

- Lung cavity in edentulous patient more likely from cancer than abscess
- Thickest portion of cavity wall > 15 mm suggests tumor
- Nodular cavity wall
- Less likely to exhibit surrounding consolidation

Septic Emboli

- Endocarditis, extrathoracic site of infection, indwelling catheter, or IV drug abuse
- Often multiple consolidations, rapidly evolve into cavities (24 hours)

Wegener Granulomatosis

- History of sinus & renal disease
- Nodules or masses ± cavitation, air-fluid levels rare
- Subglottic stenosis may be associated

Necrobiotic Nodules

- History of rheumatoid arthritis &/or dust inhalation
- Few, small, & subpleural cavitary nodules

LUNG ABSCESS

Intralobar Sequestration

- Recurrent pneumonia in same site, especially basilar segments of lower lobes
- May exhibit intrinsic air, air-fluid levels, fluid
- Supplied by systemic artery(ies)

PATHOLOGY

General Features

- Etiology
  - Aspiration: Mixed aerobic & anaerobic polymicrobial bacterial infection originating from gingiva
  - Abscess-forming organisms
    - Anaerobes: *Peptostreptococcus*, *Bacteroides*, *Fusobacterium*, microaerophilic streptococci
    - Aerobes: *Staphylococcus aureus*, *Streptococcus pyogenes*, *Klebsiella pneumoniae*, *Haemophilus influenzae*, *Actinomyces*, *Nocardia*, *Mycobacterium* species
    - Parasites: *Paragonimus*, *Entamoeba*
    - Fungi: *Aspergillus*, *Cryptococcus*, *Histoplasma*, *Blastomyces*, *Coccidioides immitis*
- Associated abnormalities
  - May progress to empyema & bronchopleural fistula

Gross Pathologic & Surgical Features

- Parenchymal destruction: Heals with scarring, bronchiectasis, cyst formation
- Uncommon complication: Pulmonary gangrene with necrotic lung fragments in abscess cavity (pulmonary sequestrum)

Microscopic Features

- 1/2 of cases due to anaerobic organisms; must be cultured with anaerobic techniques
  - Any antibiotic administration makes retrieval of anaerobes nearly impossible
- Gram stain of sputum classically polymicrobial with many neutrophils
- TB or *Nocardia* detected with acid-fast stain; fungi detected with silver stain

CLINICAL ISSUES

Presentation

- Most common signs/symptoms
  - Often subacute illness of weeks to months
  - Fever
  - Leukocytosis in 90% of patients
  - Cough, foul-smelling sputum
  - Periodontal disease
  - Hemoptysis may occur, may be fatal

Demographics

- Age
  - Any age, but more common in elderly
- Gender
  - M:F = 4:1
- Epidemiology
  - High risk: Poor dentition, seizure disorder, alcoholism
  - Predisposition in patients with immune deficiency, bronchiectasis, malignancy, emphysema, steroid treatment
  - May develop in patients with inappropriate/ inadequate antibiotic treatment of pneumonia
  - 70-80% are smokers; 12% have associated lung cancer; infected lung cancer, rare

Diagnosis

- Image-guided aspiration
  - No bronchoscopy in acute phase for abscesses > 4 cm because of potential spillover of contents to normal lung

Natural History & Prognosis

- Good prognosis with early diagnosis & treatment
  - 33% mortality if untreated
- Aspiration leads to pneumonia, pneumonia progresses to lung abscess in 7-14 days
  - Resolution slower than noncavitary pneumonia
  - Heals with scarring, bronchiectasis, cystic change
  - Mortality higher in elderly debilitated immunocompromised patients with large abscesses

Treatment

- Usually responds to antibiotics (clindamycin 4-6 weeks of therapy) in contrast to abscesses elsewhere that usually require drainage
- Bronchoscopy to assess for endobronchial lesion or foreign body if medical treatment has failed
- < 10% require surgery
- Percutaneous drainage (controversial)
  - Reserved for nonresolving abscess or empyema that abuts chest wall (10-20%)

DIAGNOSTIC CHECKLIST

Consider

- Lung cancer in edentulous patient (most abscesses arise from periodontal bacteria)
- CT to evaluate for complications, such as empyema and bronchopleural fistula

SELECTED REFERENCES

1. Bartlett JG: The role of anaerobic bacteria in lung abscess. Clin Infect Dis. 40(7):923-5, 2005
2. Lai C et al: Images in clinical medicine. Lemierre's Syndrome. N Engl J Med. 350(16):e14, 2004
3. Ryu JH et al: Cystic and cavitary lung diseases: focal and diffuse. Mayo Clin Proc. 78(6):744-52, 2003
4. Mueller PR et al: Complications of lung abscess aspiration and drainage. AJR Am J Roentgenol. 178(5):1083-6, 2002
5. Franquet T et al: Aspiration diseases: findings, pitfalls, and differential diagnosis. Radiographics. 20(3):673-85, 2000
6. Shaham D et al: Lemierre's syndrome presenting as multiple lung abscesses. Clin Imaging. 24(4):197-9, 2000
7. Marom EM et al: The many faces of pulmonary aspiration. AJR Am J Roentgenol. 172(1):121-8, 1999
8. Woodring JH et al: Solitary cavities of the lung: diagnostic implications of cavity wall thickness. AJR Am J Roentgenol. 135(6):1269-71, 1980

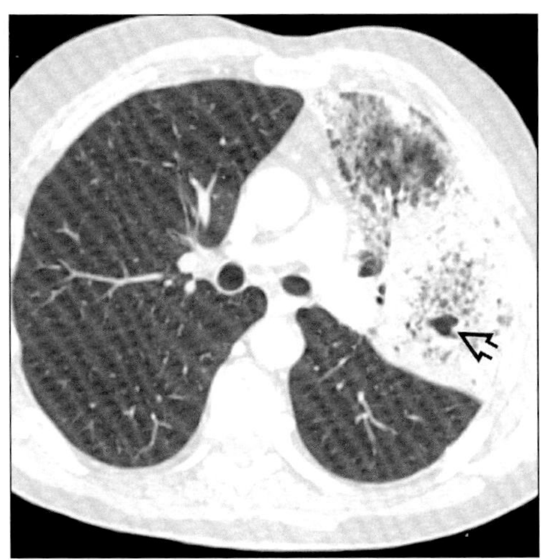

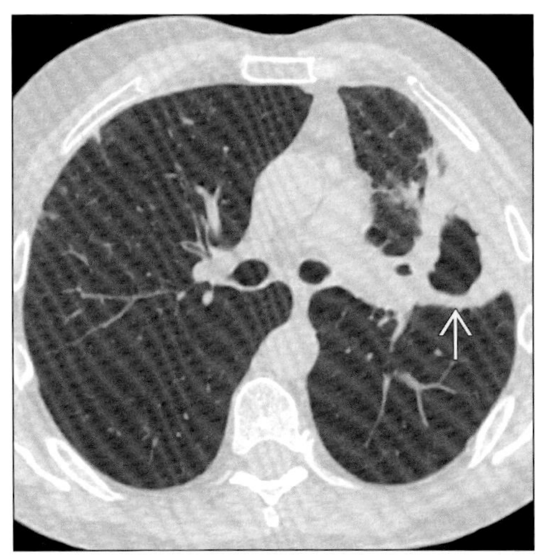

*(**Left**) Axial CECT of a 61-year-old alcoholic man with productive cough and dyspnea shows a heterogeneous left upper lobe consolidation with central lucencies ⊳, consistent with cavitation and suggestive of necrotizing pneumonia. Blood cultures revealed Streptococcus pneumoniae. (**Right**) Axial NECT of the same patient obtained 2 months later shows improving but persistent left upper lobe cavitary disease with a thick, nodular abscess wall →.*

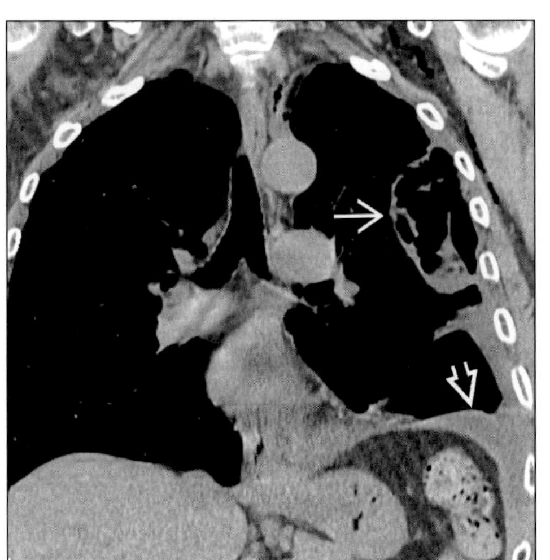

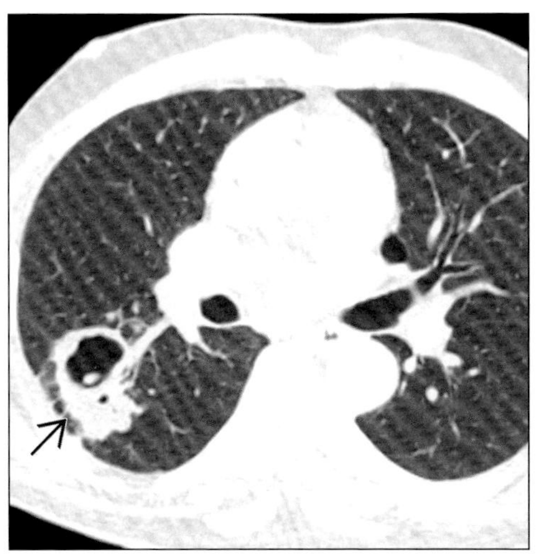

*(**Left**) Coronal NECT of a patient with hemoptysis shows a complex left upper lobe abscess → secondary to methicillin-sensitive Staphylococcus aureus infection. The left pleural effusion ⊳ represented an empyema, which required decortication. (**Right**) Axial NECT of a 62-year-old man with fever and cough shows a right lung cavitary lesion → with a thick, nodular wall and intraluminal debris. Culture of bronchoalveolar lavage specimens showed coccidioidomycosis.*

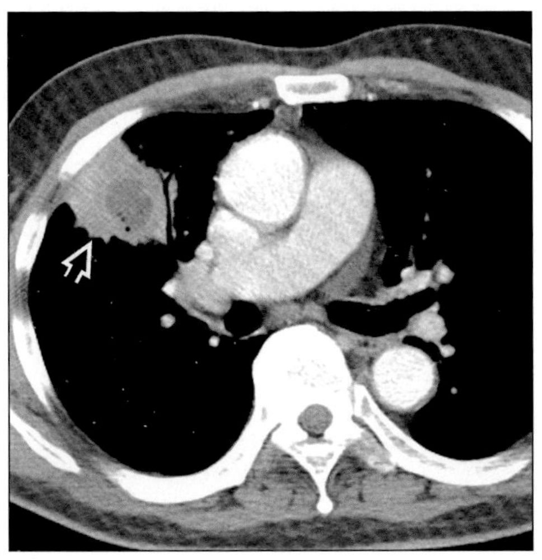

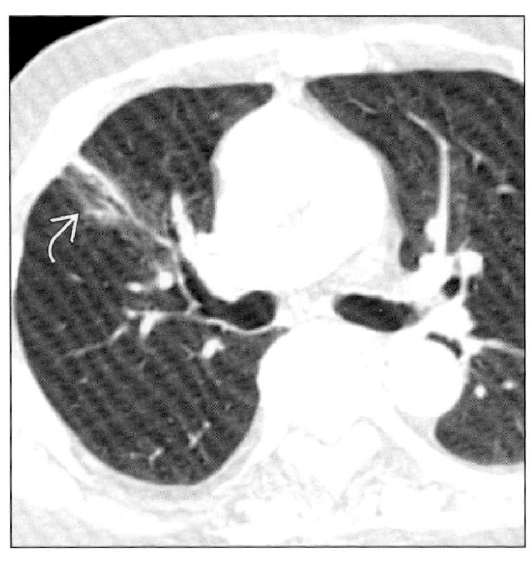

*(**Left**) Axial CECT of an 84-year-old man shows a large right upper lobe mass-like opacity ⊳ with spherical central low attenuation. The lesion was thought to represent a lung abscess rather than a pulmonary neoplasm. (**Right**) Axial NECT of the same patient obtained 2 months later after antibiotic treatment shows marked interval improvement with resolution of the mass-like lesion and a residual linear scar ↗ at the site of the previously noted lung abscess.*

SEPTIC EMBOLI

Key Facts

Terminology

- Infected embolic material seeding lung from extrapulmonary source; often foreign body or infective endocarditis

Imaging

- Radiography
  - Peripheral, poorly marginated, 1-3 cm, nodular or wedge-shaped opacities
  - Rapid cavitation, often within 24 hours
  - Pleural effusions, may be loculated
- CT
  - Multifocal peripheral & basilar lung nodules
  - Cavities in various stages of evolution (thick- to thin-walled)
  - Subpleural wedge-shaped consolidations due to hemorrhage or infarction
  - Empyema

Top Differential Diagnoses

- Pulmonary emboli
- Pneumonia
- Pulmonary metastases

Pathology

- *Staphylococcus aureus* is most common organism related to foreign bodies & IV drug use
- Etiology: Infective endocarditis, Lemierre syndrome, infected venous catheters, or pacemaker wires
- Risk factors: IV drug use, indwelling catheters

Clinical Issues

- Symptoms/signs: Fever, dyspnea, chest pain

Diagnostic Checklist

- Consider septic emboli in IV drug user or patient with indwelling catheter with multiple lung nodules

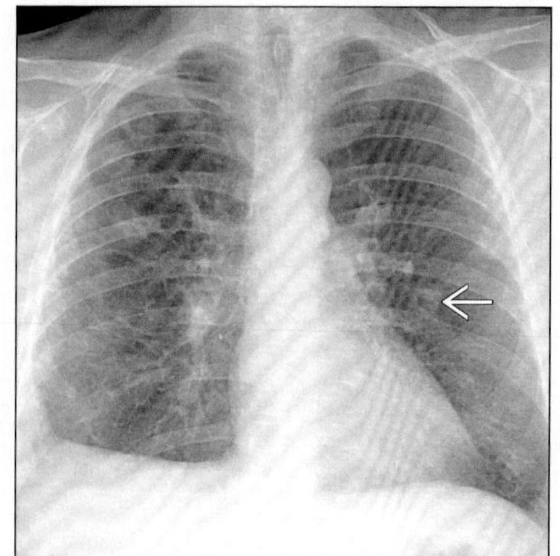

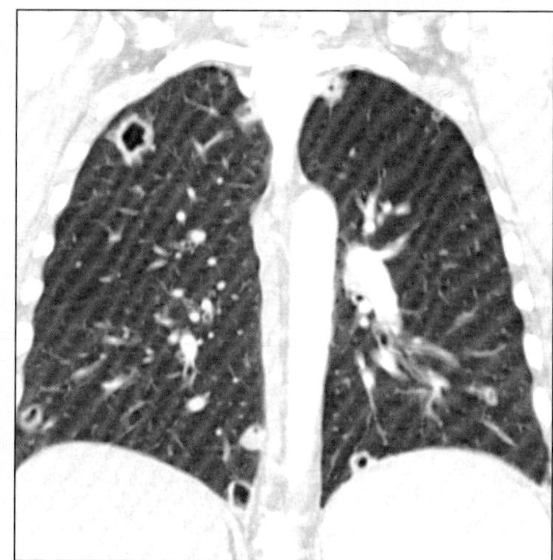

(Left) *PA chest radiograph of an intravenous drug user who presented with dyspnea and fever shows multiple bilateral pulmonary nodules, some of which demonstrate central cavitation ➔.* ***(Right)*** *Coronal CECT of the same patient confirms bilateral cavitary lung nodules, which exhibit a peripheral distribution consistent with septic emboli. Echocardiogram demonstrated a tricuspid valve vegetation, and blood culture was positive for MRSA.*

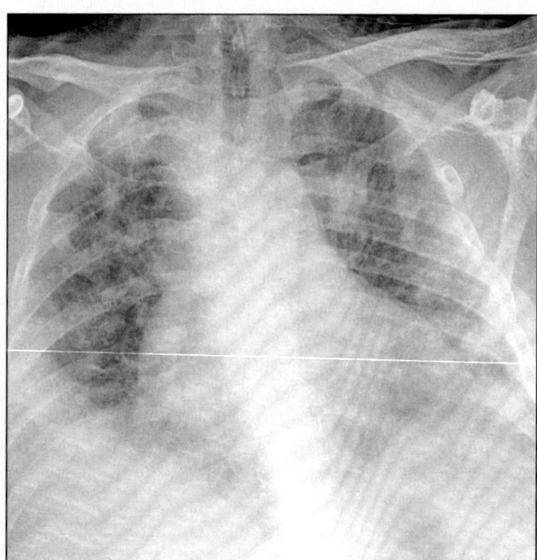

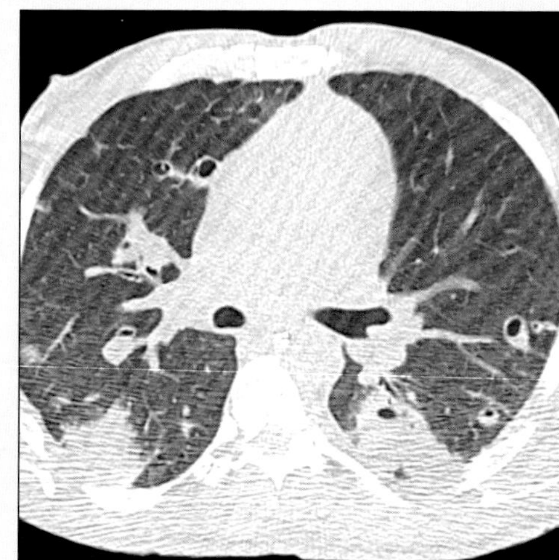

(Left) *AP chest radiograph of an intravenous drug user with septic emboli shows bilateral nodules of varying sizes and ill-defined borders.* ***(Right)*** *Axial NECT of the same patient shows bilateral cavitary nodules and bilateral lower lobe subpleural wedge-shaped opacities. Septic emboli can occlude small pulmonary arterioles leading to pulmonary infarcts. Septic emboli should be the leading consideration in intravenous drug users with multiple cavitary lung nodules.*

SEPTIC EMBOLI

TERMINOLOGY

Definitions

- Infected embolic material seeding lung from extrapulmonary source; often foreign body or infective endocarditis

IMAGING

General Features

- Best diagnostic clue
  - Multiple nodules or patchy areas of consolidation with rapid cavitation
- Location
  - Peripheral & basilar predominance
- Size
  - Usually small (< 3 cm in diameter)

Radiographic Findings

- Radiography
  - Peripheral, poorly marginated, 1-3 cm, nodular or wedge-shaped opacities
    - May change in number or appearance (size or degree of cavitation) from day to day
  - Target sign: Thin-walled cyst with central density
  - Usually basilar (due to gravity & blood flow)
  - Evolve rapidly, cavitation common within 24 hours (50%)
    - Cavity wall often thick
    - Lack air-fluid level
    - Cavities typically in various stages of evolution
  - Complications
    - Loculated pleural effusion
    - Pneumothorax (rare)

CT Findings

- **Multiple discrete nodules**
  - Average number: 15
  - Size: 0.5-3.5 cm; larger nodules rare
  - Peripheral & bilateral
  - **Cavitation**
    - Cavities in various stages of evolution (thick- to thin-walled)
  - Air bronchograms
    - More common in gram-positive septic emboli
  - **Ground-glass halo**
    - More common in gram-negative septic emboli
- Subpleural wedge-shaped consolidation
  - Occlusion of pulmonary arteries by septic emboli → hemorrhage or infarction
  - Cavitation slightly more common in nodules than in wedge-shaped consolidations
- **Feeding vessel sign**: Vessel leading directly to nodule or wedge-shaped opacity
  - Found in 60-70% of patients with nodules, less common with wedge-shaped opacities
  - Multiplanar reformatted images often show that vessel actually courses around nodules
  - "Feeding vessel" sometimes represents draining vein
- Mediastinal lymphadenopathy (CT only) in 20%
- No intravascular clots
- Pleural effusion, may be loculated in 80%
  - Often evolves into empyema

Echocardiographic Findings

- Detection of valve vegetations/endocarditis as source of septic emboli

Imaging Recommendations

- Best imaging tool
  - CT for characterization of nodules initially detected on radiographs & detection of complications
  - Chest radiographs usually sufficient for monitoring response to therapy

DIFFERENTIAL DIAGNOSIS

Pulmonary Emboli

- Infarct: Increased opacities from hemorrhage
  - Hampton sign: Subpleural wedge-shaped opacities
  - Pulmonary infarct may cavitate (rare)
    - Cavity usually single & large (> 4 cm)
  - Infarct evolves from ill-defined consolidation to well-defined opacity
- CTA shows filling defect(s) in pulmonary arterial system

Pneumonia

- Bacterial, fungal, mycobacterial
  - Solitary or multiple nodules & consolidation
    - Not necessarily peripheral in location
    - *M. tuberculosis* & classic atypical mycobacterial infection with upper lobe predominance
  - Cavitation or pneumatoceles common with *Staphylococcus*, gram-negative organisms (such as *Klebsiella*), fungal & mycobacterial infection
  - Invasive aspergillosis
    - Ground-glass halo
    - Air crescent sign

Pulmonary Metastases

- Multiple variably sized pulmonary nodules
  - Tend to be peripheral, 80% within 2 cm of pleural surface
  - Usually sharply marginated in contrast to septic emboli
  - May also exhibit "feeding vessel" sign
  - Indistinct margins or ground-glass halo in hemorrhagic metastases: Renal cell carcinoma, choriocarcinoma, melanoma
  - Cavitation common in metastases from squamous cell carcinoma or sarcoma
    - Less common: Primary GI tract adenocarcinomas
- Do not rapidly evolve

Pneumatoceles

- Transient, usually follow known insult (trauma, infection, hydrocarbon ingestion)
- May also evolve rapidly
- Typically thin-walled without air-fluid level

Wegener Granulomatosis

- Nodules with varying degrees of cavitation
  - Do not rapidly evolve
- May exhibit subglottic airway stenosis

Laryngeal Papillomatosis

- Multiple solid & cystic nodules: Grow extremely slowly
- Perihilar & central in location
- Laryngeal infection with human papilloma virus

SEPTIC EMBOLI

PATHOLOGY

General Features

- Etiology
  - **Organisms**
    - *Staphylococcus aureus* most common organism related to foreign bodies & IV drug abuse
    - Burn patients: *Pseudomonas aeruginosa* most common
    - Other organisms include streptococci, fungi, gram-negative rods (*Serratia*)
    - Fungi: ICU patients on broad-spectrum antibiotics as well as IV drug users
  - **Infective endocarditis**
    - Tricuspid valve most commonly affected, aortic valve may also be involved
    - Secondary to nonbacterial thrombotic endocarditis, with injury to endothelial surface of heart
    - Transient bacteremia leads to seeding of lesions with adherent bacteria
    - Subsequent development of infective endocarditis
  - **Lemierre syndrome**
    - Uncommon but potentially life-threatening complication of acute pharyngotonsillitis
    - Jugular vein septic thrombophlebitis from adjacent peritonsillar abscess leads to septic emboli
    - Anaerobic infection from gram-negative bacilli (*Fusobacterium* most common)
    - Immunocompetent host
  - Infected venous catheter or pacemaker wires
  - Pelvic thrombophlebitis
  - Osteomyelitis

Gross Pathologic & Surgical Features

- Necrotic infected lung
  - Usually sharply demarcated from adjacent normal lung

Microscopic Features

- Acute inflammatory cells and necrosis are not specific and can be seen in infections, neoplasms, etc.
- May see colonies of organisms

CLINICAL ISSUES

Presentation

- Most common signs/symptoms
  - Fever
  - Dyspnea
  - Chest pain
  - Hemoptysis
- Other signs/symptoms
  - Endocarditis
    - **Osler nodes**: Tender subcutaneous nodules usually found on distal pads of digits
    - **Janeway lesions**: Nontender maculae on palms & soles
    - **Roth spots**: Retinal hemorrhages with small, clear centers
    - Petechiae, splinter hemorrhages (dark red linear lesions in nailbed)
  - **Lemierre syndrome**
    - Sore throat
    - Neck pain, swelling
    - Cervical lymphadenopathy
    - "Cord" sign (palpable thrombosed jugular vein)

Demographics

- Epidemiology
  - Risk factors
    - Indwelling venous catheters
    - Intravenous drug abuse
    - Immunologic deficiencies, particularly lymphoma, organ transplants
    - Periodontal disease
    - Burns

Natural History & Prognosis

- Radiographic abnormalities may precede positive blood cultures
- Mean duration of symptoms before diagnosis: 18 days

Treatment

- Therapy with broad spectrum antibiotics
  - In cases of infective endocarditis: 6-8 weeks
- Drainage of associated empyema
- Surgery
  - Remove source of infection; drain abscess
  - Replace heart valves

DIAGNOSTIC CHECKLIST

Consider

- Septic emboli in intravenous drug user or patient with long-term indwelling catheters with multiple pulmonary nodules

SELECTED REFERENCES

1. Kwon WJ et al: Computed tomographic features of pulmonary septic emboli: comparison of causative microorganisms. J Comput Assist Tomogr. 31(3):390-4, 2007
2. Dodd JD et al: High-resolution MDCT of pulmonary septic embolism: evaluation of the feeding vessel sign. AJR Am J Roentgenol. 187(3):623-9, 2006
3. Cook RJ et al: Septic pulmonary embolism: presenting features and clinical course of 14 patients. Chest. 128(1):162-6, 2005
4. Goldenberg NA et al: Lemierre's and Lemierre's-like syndromes in children: survival and thromboembolic outcomes. Pediatrics. 116(4):e543-8, 2005
5. Gormus N et al: Lemierre's syndrome associated with septic pulmonary embolism: a case report. Ann Vasc Surg. 18(2):243-5, 2004
6. Han D et al: Thrombotic and nonthrombotic pulmonary arterial embolism: spectrum of imaging findings. Radiographics. 23(6):1521-39, 2003

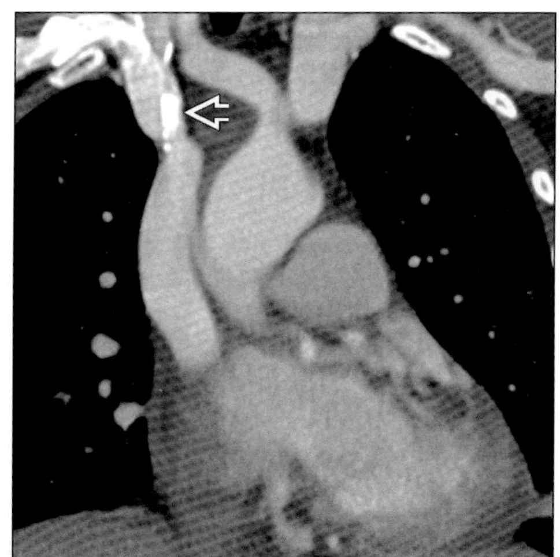

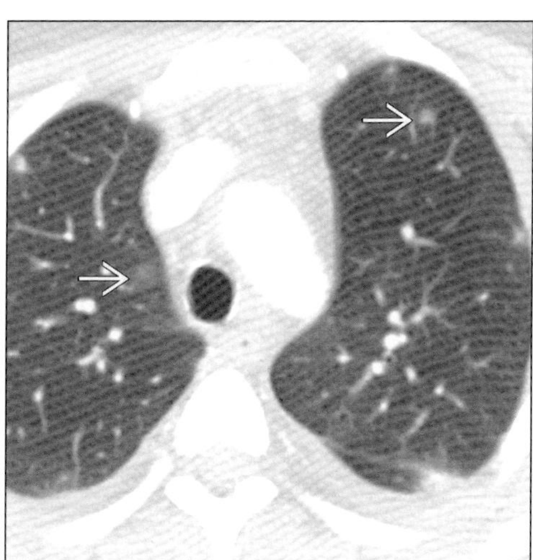

(Left) *Coronal CECT of a patient who presented with fever shows a retained catheter fragment ⇨ in the right brachiocephalic vein.* ***(Right)*** *Axial CECT of the same patient shows multiple bilateral small peripheral pulmonary nodules ⇨, consistent with pulmonary emboli. Blood culture was positive for S. aureus. An infected central line is a common cause of pulmonary septic emboli.*

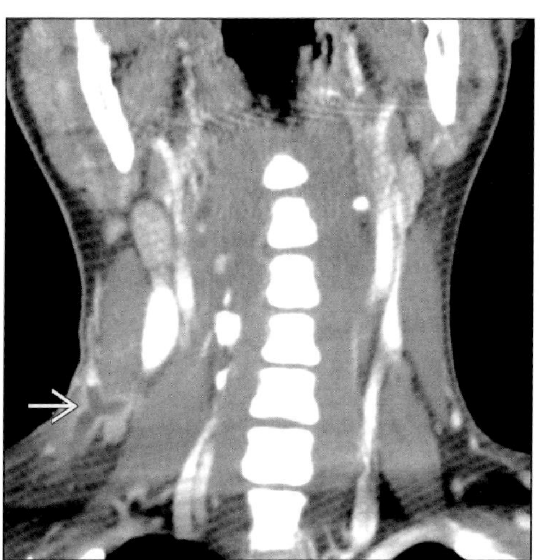

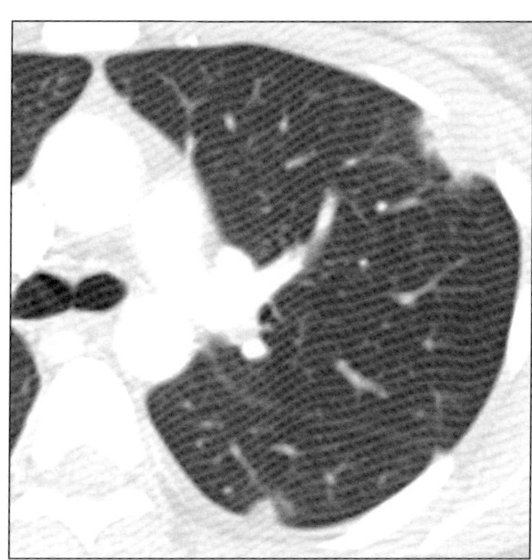

(Left) *Coronal CECT of a patient who presented with sore throat, neck pain, and dyspnea shows thrombosis of right external jugular vein ⇨ with enhancement of the vascular walls, consistent with thrombophlebitis.* ***(Right)*** *Axial CECT of the same patient shows multiple subpleural nodules (2 of which are shown here), consistent with septic emboli. Blood culture grew Fusobacterium necrophorum. These findings are consistent with Lemierre syndrome, an uncommon cause of septic emboli.*

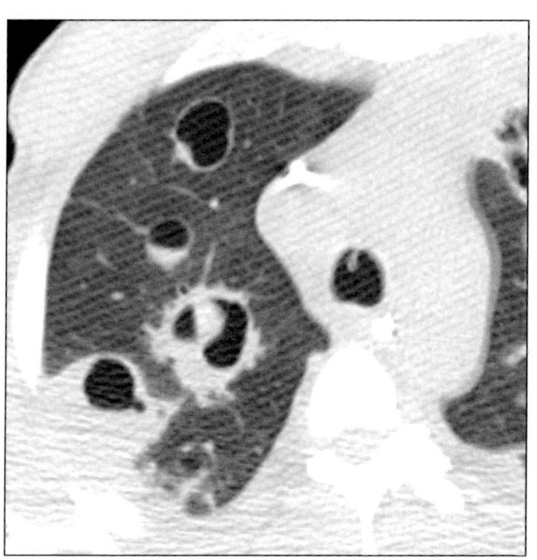

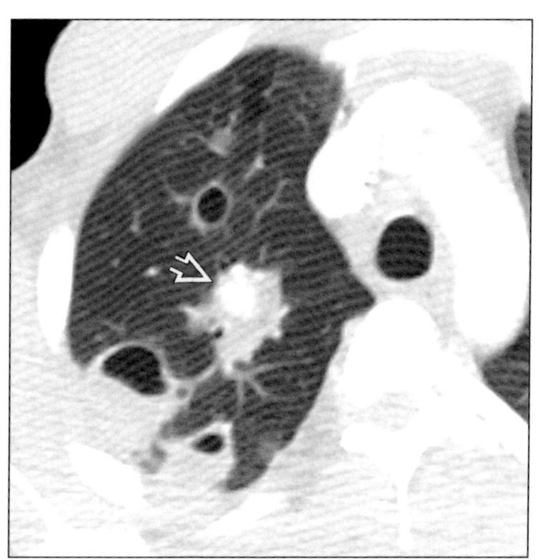

(Left) *Axial NECT of an intravenous drug user with tricuspid endocarditis and MRSA bacteremia shows multiple cavitary lesions of varying sizes and variable wall thicknesses, consistent with septic emboli.* ***(Right)*** *Axial CECT of the same patient obtained 2 weeks later shows focal dilatation of a pulmonary artery branch ⇨, consistent with pulmonary artery pseudoaneurysm (a rare complication of septic emboli).*

PNEUMOCOCCAL PNEUMONIA

Key Facts

Terminology

- Lung infection caused by *Streptococcus pneumoniae*

Imaging

- Radiography
  - Lobar consolidation with air bronchograms, may be multifocal & bilateral
  - Mass-like consolidation ("round pneumonia")
  - Pleural effusion in up to 50% of cases
- CT
  - Consolidation frequently more extensive than expected based on radiography
  - Ground-glass opacities surround consolidation
  - Bronchopneumonia with reticular &/or nodular opacities
  - Diffuse bronchial wall thickening ± interlobular septal thickening
  - Cavitation & abscess formation are rare

Top Differential Diagnoses

- Other bacterial pneumonias
- Viral pneumonia
- Aspiration pneumonia and pneumonitis
- Pulmonary hemorrhage
- Lung cancer

Pathology

- Highly variable yield (40-80%) of Gram stain & culture on sputum samples

Clinical Issues

- *S. pneumoniae* is most common type of bacterial pneumonia, accounting for ~ 65% of cases

Diagnostic Checklist

- Consider pneumonococcal pneumonia in patient with fever, chills, productive cough, & pleuritic chest pain

*(**Left**) PA chest radiograph of a 43-year-old otherwise healthy man with acute onset of fever, chills, cough, and pleuritic chest pain shows a large, dense right upper lobe consolidation. The patient was treated for community-acquired pneumonia. (**Right**) Coronal NECT of the same patient obtained 7 days later shows new right upper lobe cavitation and new middle lobe consolidation. Streptococcus pneumoniae was recovered from the sputum. The patient had not been compliant with his outpatient antibiotics.*

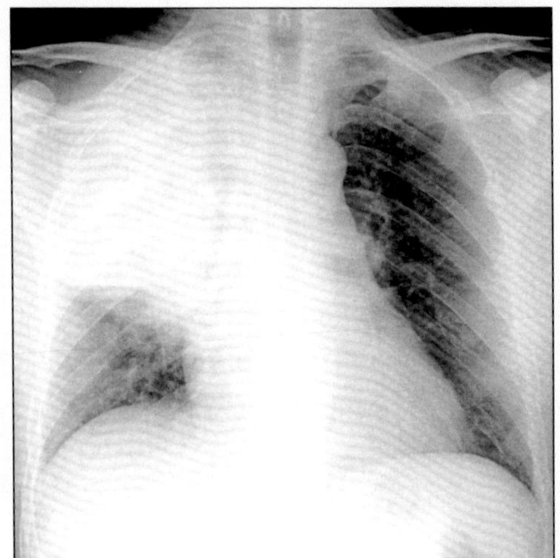

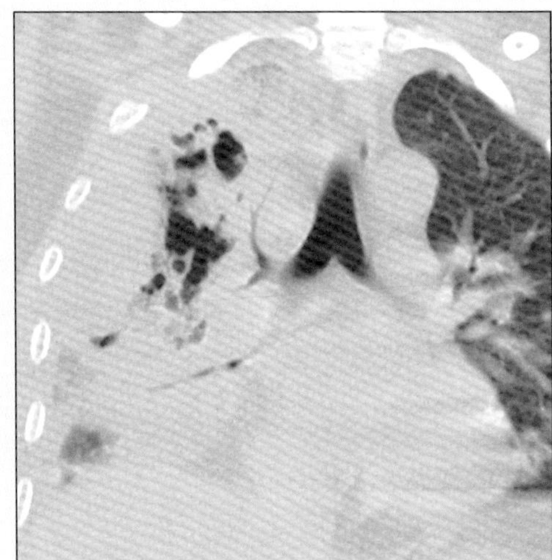

*(**Left**) Axial CECT of a 48-year-old man with dyspnea, cough, pleuritic chest pain, and a normal chest radiograph shows a 3.5 cm mass in the superior segment of the right lower lobe ➔. (**Right**) Axial NECT of the same patient obtained 4 weeks following antibiotic therapy shows complete resolution of the mass. While round pneumonias are frequently seen in children, they do occur in adults, and short interval follow-up is suggested in such cases to exclude the possibility of malignancy.*

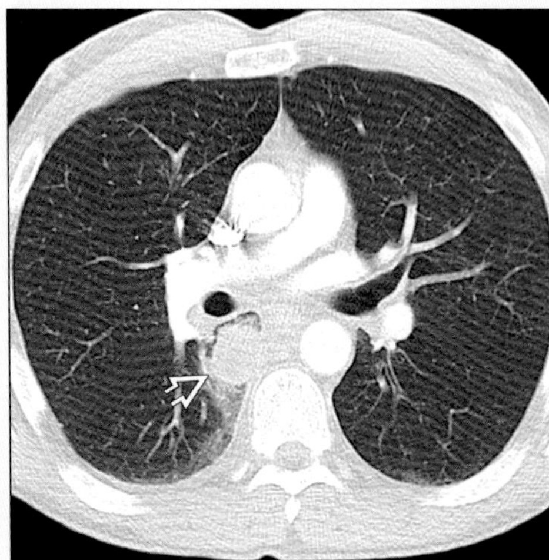

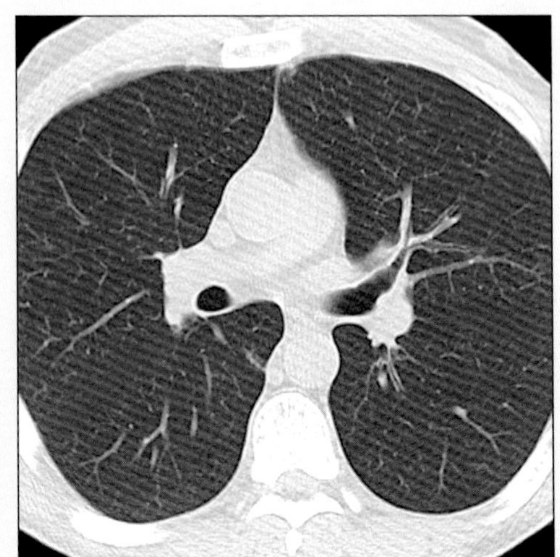

PNEUMOCOCCAL PNEUMONIA

TERMINOLOGY

Definitions

- Lung infection caused by *Streptococcus pneumoniae*

IMAGING

General Features

- Best diagnostic clue
  - Consolidation with air bronchograms, may be lobar or bilateral & multifocal
- Location
  - Tends to be peripheral & spread via pores of Kohn
- Size
  - Range from small centrilobular nodules to lobar consolidations
- Morphology
  - Dense consolidation (most common)

Radiographic Findings

- Radiography
  - **Lobar consolidation with air bronchograms**
    - May be multifocal & bilateral
  - Patchy airspace disease
  - Round, mass-like consolidation ("round pneumonia")
    - More common in pediatric population
  - **Bronchopneumonia** with reticular &/or nodular opacities
  - Pleural effusion in up to 50% of cases
  - Cavitation is rare

CT Findings

- **Consolidation** frequently more extensive than expected based on radiography
  - **Lobar consolidation most common**
  - Peribronchial consolidation also common in some series
- Ground-glass opacities frequently surround consolidation
- Cavitation & abscess formation are rare
  - When present consider co-infection with anaerobic organisms or *S. aureus*
- **Pleural effusion in up to 50% of cases**
- **Lymphadenopathy in up to 50% of cases**
- CECT
  - Pleural effusion with pleural thickening & enhancement (**"split pleura" sign)** suggests empyema
- HRCT
  - **Centrilobular nodules, branching & tree-in-bud opacities**
  - Diffuse bronchial wall thickening ± interlobular septal thickening

Ultrasonographic Findings

- Pleural effusions may be free or loculated
- Commonly used for guidance during thoracentesis & pleural drain placement

Imaging Recommendations

- Best imaging tool
  - Chest radiograph remains modality of choice for initial diagnosis & monitoring response to therapy
  - CT for assessment of complications: Cavitation, empyema, lymphadenopathy
- Protocol advice
  - Contrast-enhanced CT helpful in evaluation of pleura & mediastinum

DIFFERENTIAL DIAGNOSIS

Other Bacterial Pneumonia

- Gram-positive organisms, such as *Staphylococcus aureus*
  - Cavitation/abscess formation more common
- Gram-negative organisms, such as *Pseudomonas, Klebsiella, Enterobacter, Serratia*
- No single imaging finding is diagnostic of particular organism

Viral Pneumonia

- Similar imaging findings
- Perihilar linear opacities, bronchial wall thickening, atelectasis, & air-trapping most common findings

Aspiration Pneumonia and Pneumonitis

- Can be bland with rapidly clearing perihilar opacities or polymicrobial pneumonia resulting in lung abscess
- Typically located in dependent portions of lung

Pulmonary Hemorrhage

- Alveolar hemorrhage syndromes
  - Diffuse or patchy bilateral ground-glass opacities
- Trauma: Pulmonary laceration may mimic abscess

Pneumocystis jiroveci Pneumonia

- Immunocompromised host
- Ground-glass opacities & cysts are more common

Lung Cancer

- Postobstructive pneumonia commonly initial presentation in patients subsequently diagnosed with lung cancer
  - Rationale for performing follow-up radiography in adult patients diagnosed with pneumonia
- Malignancy with highest mortality rate in both men & women

Alveolar Edema

- History usually suggestive of heart failure
- May mimic multifocal pneumonia with diffuse bilateral airspace disease
- Bilateral pleural effusions

PATHOLOGY

General Features

- Etiology
  - *Pneumococci* colonize nasopharynx via aerosol inhalation
    - 40-50% of adults are asymptomatic carriers
    - Invasive infection when immune system is overwhelmed by amount inhaled; bacteria invade type II pneumocytes, multiply in alveoli spreading via pores of Kohn

Microscopic Features

- Highly variable yield (40-80%) of Gram stain & culture on sputum samples
- Pneumococcal urinary antigen: Sensitivity (70-90%), specificity (80-100%)

◦ Utilization: Failed outpatient antibiotic treatment, intensive care admission, asplenic patient, pleural effusion, alcohol abuse, leukopenic patient

CLINICAL ISSUES

Presentation

- Most common signs/symptoms
  - Acute onset fever, chills, productive cough, pleuritic chest pain
  - Occasionally sputum is blood-tinged or rust-colored
  - Hypoxia & cyanosis in severe cases
  - Dullness to percussion, egophony, & whispered pectoriloquy in areas of consolidation
- Other signs/symptoms
  - Increased incidence
    - Chronic diseases of heart, lungs, kidneys
    - Immunocompromised host
    - Advanced age
    - Cirrhosis
    - Splenectomy
      - All patients should receive pneumococcal vaccine
    - Malignancy, especially hematopoietic
    - Dementia
    - Smoking & exposure to second-hand smoke
    - Influenza infection
  - Complications
    - Empyema
    - Acute respiratory distress syndrome (ARDS)
    - Meningitis
    - Sepsis
- Clinical profile
  - Colonization: 20% of population, higher percentage of patients with chronic lung disease
  - Significant portion of sputum-negative cases of community-acquired pneumonia
    - Sputum culture negative in 50% with (+) blood culture for pneumococcal bacteremia
    - Majority of these cases respond to penicillin
  - Accounts for 2/3 of bacteremic pneumonias

Demographics

- Age
  - Elderly patients often exhibit fewer signs & symptoms
    - May present with mental status change
- Epidemiology
  - *S. pneumoniae* is most common type of bacterial pneumonia, accounting for ~ 65% of cases
    - Isolated in only 5-18% of patients
  - Most common type of pneumonia requiring hospitalization in all age groups
  - Most common type of pneumonia resulting in death
    - Up to 25% mortality in certain populations

Natural History & Prognosis

- Ranges from mild illness with rapid response to antibiotics to progressive disease with sepsis & death
  - Seeding of other organs in ~ 1% of bacteremic patients
- Consolidation usually takes several weeks to clear following treatment

Treatment

- Polyvalent polysaccharide vaccination recommended for high-risk patients
- Macrolide or doxycycline used commonly in outpatient setting
- β-lactam + aminoglycoside + azithromycin or fluoroquinolone among others used for hospitalized patients with suspected pneumonia
- Improved outcomes with adherence to Infectious Disease Society of America/American Thoracic Society guidelines
- Multi-drug-resistant strains are becoming more common
- Tube thoracostomy for empyema; surgical debridement may be required

DIAGNOSTIC CHECKLIST

Consider

- Pneumonococcal pneumonia in patient with fever, chills, productive cough, & pleuritic chest pain

Image Interpretation Pearls

- Lobar consolidation with air bronchograms is classic finding
- No single imaging finding can differentiate bacterial from nonbacterial pneumonia

Reporting Tips

- If initial radiograph is negative & clinical history is convincing for pneumonia, suggest follow-up chest radiograph in 24-48 hours
- Chest CT may also be performed to document radiographically occult pulmonary infection

SELECTED REFERENCES

1. Pande A et al: The incidence of necrotizing changes in adults with pneumococcal pneumonia. Clin Infect Dis. 54(1):10-6, 2012
2. Marrie TJ et al: Pneumococcal pneumonia in adults. UpToDate.com. Accessed December 6, 2011
3. Watkins RR et al: Diagnosis and management of community-acquired pneumonia in adults. Am Fam Physician. 83(11):1299-306, 2011
4. Yagihashi K et al: Correlations between computed tomography findings and clinical manifestations of Streptococcus pneumoniae pneumonia. Jpn J Radiol. 29(6):423-8, 2011
5. Metersky ML et al: Determining the optimal pneumococcal vaccination strategy for adults: is there a role for the pneumococcal conjugate vaccine? Chest. 138(3):486-90, 2010
6. Mandell LA et al: Infectious Diseases Society of America/ American Thoracic Society consensus guidelines on the management of community-acquired pneumonia in adults. Clin Infect Dis. 44 Suppl 2:S27-72, 2007

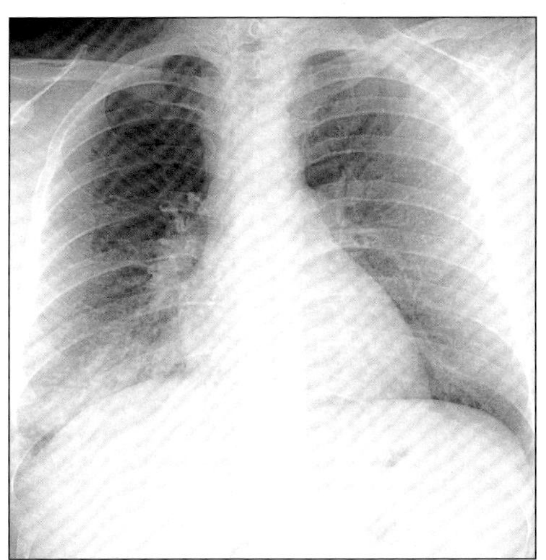

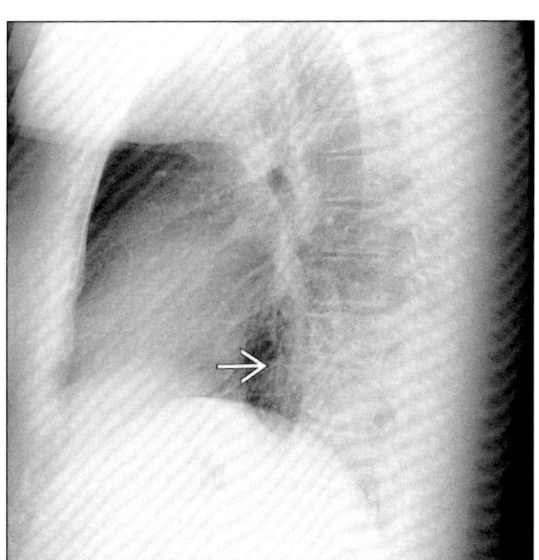

(Left) *PA chest radiograph of an 18-year-old man with fever, cough, and chest pain shows focal dense right lower lobe consolidation.* ***(Right)*** *Lateral chest radiograph of the same patient shows focal dense consolidation ➔ projecting over the lower thoracic spine and obscuring the adjacent posterior right hemidiaphragm. Increasing opacity over the distal thoracic spine is consistent with the spine sign.*

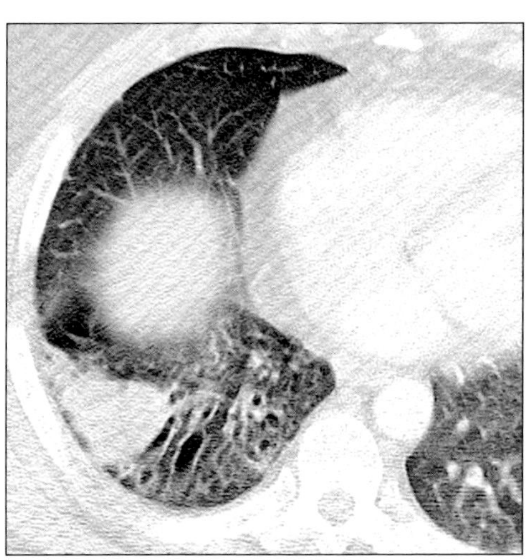

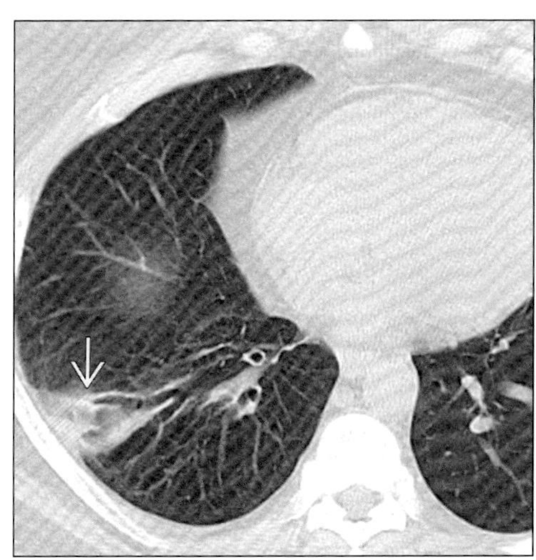

(Left) *Axial NECT of a 43-year-old HIV(+) man who presented with cough and pleuritic chest pain shows a mass-like right lower lobe consolidation. Adjacent right lower lobe cylindrical bronchiectasis is likely the sequela of prior infection. Bronchoscopy was performed, and Streptococcus pneumoniae was cultured.* ***(Right)*** *Axial NECT of the same patient obtained 2 months later shows near complete resolution of the consolidation with a small residual scar ➔.*

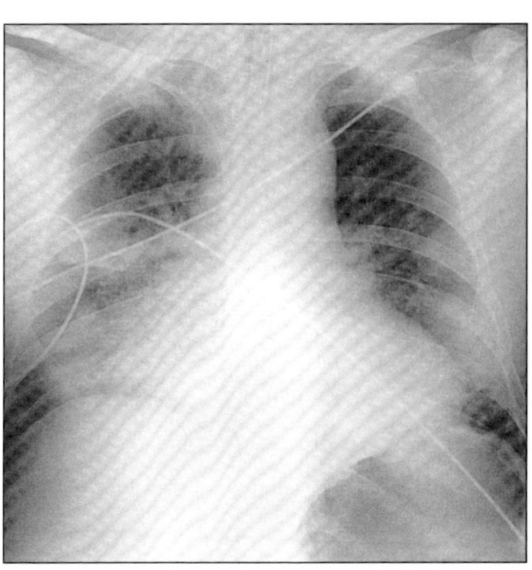

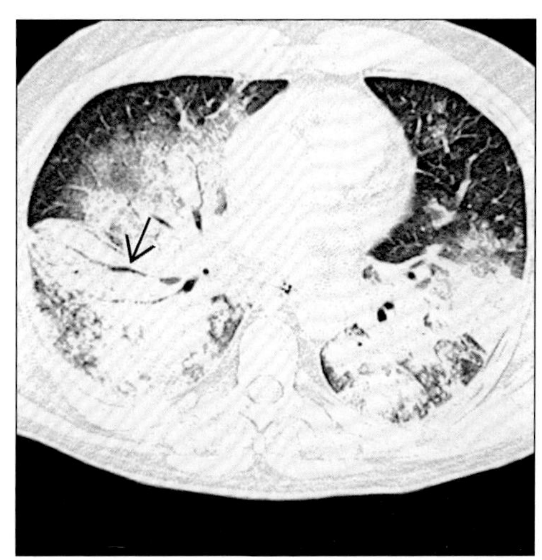

(Left) *AP chest radiograph shows dense bilateral heterogeneous lung consolidations from streptococcal pneumonia. The patient was critically ill, requiring admission to the intensive care unit and intubation.* ***(Right)*** *Axial NECT of the same patient confirms dense bilateral consolidations that obscure bronchial and vascular margins. Note the air bronchograms ➔ produced by aerated airways outlined by dense adjacent pulmonary consolidation.*

STAPHYLOCOCCAL PNEUMONIA

Key Facts

Terminology
- Lung infection caused by gram-positive organism *Staphylococcus*, usually *S. aureus*

Imaging
- Radiography
  - Patchy or lobar consolidation, marked by widespread, rapid, severe lung destruction & abscess formation
  - Cavitation in up to 30%
  - Rapid progression of disease on serial radiography
  - Pleural effusions, may be loculated
- CT
  - Consolidation, ranging from patchy nonsegmental to bilateral multilobar
  - Detection of cavitation & abscess
  - Small centrilobular lung nodules to large masses
  - Pleural effusion common

Top Differential Diagnoses
- Other bacterial pneumonias
- Viral pneumonia
- Aspiration pneumonia & pneumonitis
- Alveolar hemorrhage
- *Pneumocystis jiroveci* pneumonia

Pathology
- Gram-positive cocci in clusters

Clinical Issues
- Children & elderly more susceptible
- Mortality varies widely depending upon strain of organism, expression of virulence, & host factors

Diagnostic Checklist
- Consider staphylococcal pneumonia in patient with fever, cough, & multifocal consolidation

*(**Left**) PA chest radiograph of a 48-year-old man with fever, cough, and chest pain shows multifocal bilateral areas of dense consolidation and blunting of the right costophrenic angle secondary to pleural effusion. (**Right**) Coronal CECT of the same patient obtained on the same day shows bilateral mass-like consolidations, bilateral nodular opacities, and small bilateral pleural effusions. Sputum samples were positive for Staphylococcus aureus.*

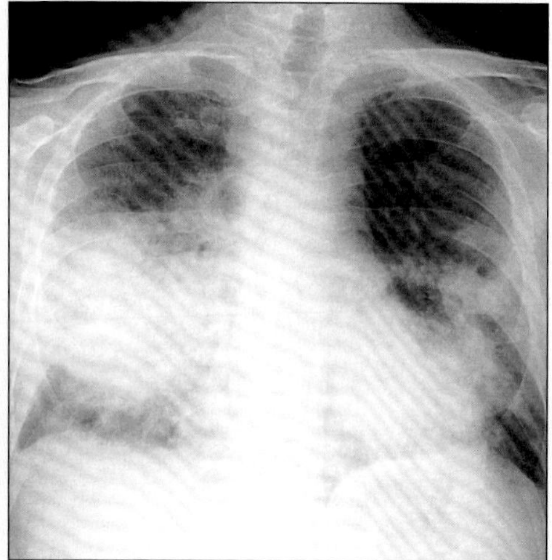

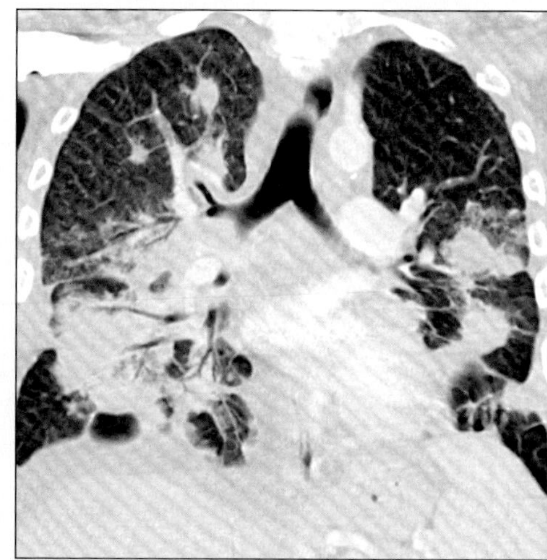

*(**Left**) Axial CECT of a 39-year-old man with fever and dyspnea shows a large left-sided pleural effusion with associated pleural enhancement ➔ (the "split pleura" sign) in this patient with a Staphylococcus aureus empyema. Empyema is a common complication of S. aureus infection. (**Right**) PA chest radiograph of the same patient was obtained after placement of a pigtail pleural drainage catheter. Although early drainage has been associated with better outcomes, some patients will require surgical drainage.*

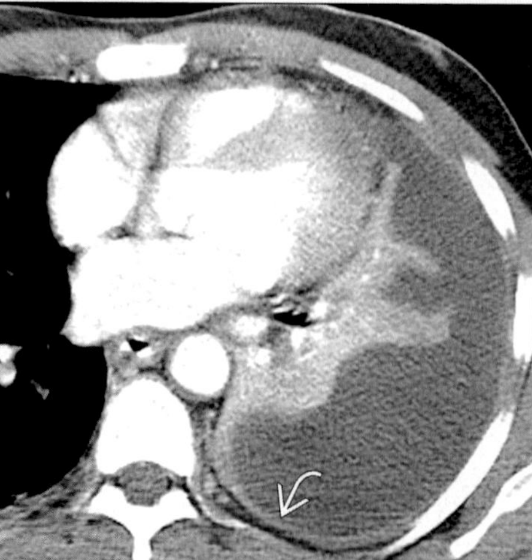

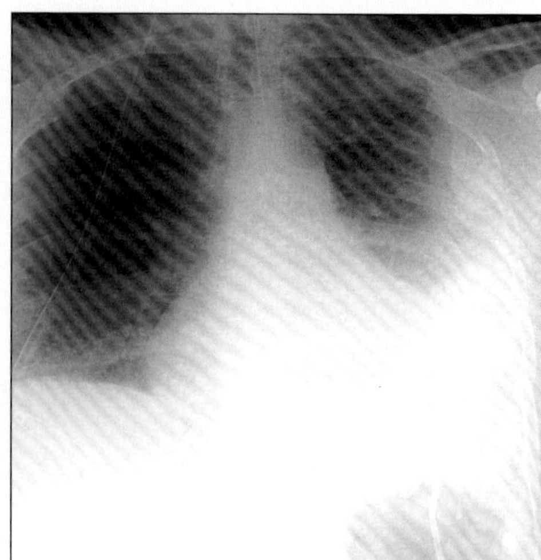

STAPHYLOCOCCAL PNEUMONIA

TERMINOLOGY

Abbreviations

- Methicillin-resistant *Staphylococcus aureus* (MRSA)

Synonyms

- *Staphylococcus aureus* pneumonia

Definitions

- Lung infection caused by gram-positive organism *Staphylococcus*, usually *S. aureus*

IMAGING

General Features

- Best diagnostic clue
  - Patchy or lobar consolidation, marked by widespread, rapid, severe lung destruction with abscess formation
  - Parapneumonic pleural effusions very common (up to 2/3 of patients)
  - Pathogen not reliably predicted based on imaging features alone
- Location
  - Frequently multifocal & bilateral
- Size
  - Range from small patchy air space opacities to lobar pneumonia to diffuse alveolar damage & acute respiratory distress syndrome (ARDS)
- Morphology
  - Dense consolidation (most common)

Radiographic Findings

- Radiography
  - Consolidation, ranging from patchy nonsegmental to bilateral multilobar
  - Cavitation in up to 30%
  - Rapid progression of disease on serial radiography
  - Pleural effusions, may be loculated
    - Consider empyema with loculation &/or air, air-fluid level
  - Pneumothorax (rare)

CT Findings

- NECT
  - Consolidations often more extensive than expected based on radiography
  - More sensitive than radiography in detection of cavitation & abscess formation
    - Abscesses may heal with pneumatocele formation
    - Resolution in weeks to months but may persist for years
  - Small centrilobular lung nodules to large parenchymal masses
  - Septal thickening occasionally seen
  - Pleural effusion (common)
  - Pneumothorax (rare)
- CECT
  - Pleural enhancement "**split pleura**" **sign** around loculated pleural fluid suggests empyema

Ultrasonographic Findings

- Pleural effusion may be simple or multilocular
- Commonly used for image guidance during thoracentesis & pleural drain placement

Imaging Recommendations

- Best imaging tool
  - Chest radiography: Initial detection of disease & evaluation of severity/extent
  - CT: Detection of lung abscess & empyema
- Protocol advice
  - Contrast administration helpful in diagnosing empyema

DIFFERENTIAL DIAGNOSIS

Other Bacterial Pneumonias

- Gram-positive organisms: *Streptococcus pneumoniae* & *S. pyogenes*
- Gram-negative organisms: *Pseudomonas, Klebsiella, Enterobacter, Serratia*
- Parenchymal consolidation, may be multifocal
- No single imaging finding is diagnostic of particular pathogen

Viral Pneumonia

- Centrilobular nodules, tree-in-bud opacities
- Perihilar linear opacities, bronchial wall thickening, atelectasis, & air-trapping most commonly seen

Aspiration Pneumonia & Pneumonitis

- May produce rapidly clearing perihilar opacities vs. polymicrobial pneumonia progressing to lung abscess
- Typically located in dependent portions of lung

Hemorrhage

- History of trauma, anemia, or hemoptysis
- Diffuse airspace opacities with spontaneous hemorrhage
- Pulmonary laceration may mimic cavitation

Pneumocystis jiroveci Pneumonia

- Immunocompromised patients
- Ground-glass opacities & cysts

Lung Cancer

- Postobstructive pneumonia may be initial abnormality in patients subsequently diagnosed with lung cancer
- Radiographic follow-up to resolution in adult patients with consolidation

Alveolar Edema

- Imaging can be similar, clinical history usually suggests heart failure
- Interstitial and alveolar opacities
- Pleural effusions typically bilateral

Anthrax

- Encapsulated gram-positive rod
- Farmers & butchers at highest risk
- Lymphadenopathy and pleural effusions are common

PATHOLOGY

General Features

- Etiology
  - Hospital- or community-acquired pneumonia
  - Hospital-acquired pneumonias are often polymicrobial
- Genetics

- Gene responsible for methicillin resistance located on staphylococcal cassette chromosome
  - 5 types described (I-V), differing in size & genetics
  - Community-acquired MRSA typically type IV
    - Does not carry multiple drug-resistance genes
    - Susceptible to other β-lactams & erythromycin
- *Staphylococcus aureus* strains carrying gene for Panton-Valentine leukocidin (PVL) cause rapidly progressive, hemorrhagic, necrotizing pneumonia
  - Typically immunocompetent children & young adults
  - Associated with skin & soft tissue infections
  - Mortality up to 56%

- Associated abnormalities
  - Community-acquired MRSA pneumonia associated with outbreaks of influenzavirus
    - 17 affected patients reported to CDC during 2003 influenza season: 5 deaths
    - 10 patients reported to CDC during 2006 influenza season: 6 deaths

Microscopic Features

- Gram-positive cocci in clusters
- *S. aureus* commonly colonizes nasal passages

CLINICAL ISSUES

Presentation

- Most common signs/symptoms
  - Acute onset chest pain
  - Dyspnea
  - Productive cough ± blood-tinged sputum
  - Fever, leukocytosis
  - Massive hemoptysis
- Other signs/symptoms
  - Viral prodrome during influenza season
  - Hematogenous spread may result in septic emboli
    - Endocarditis
    - Infected indwelling catheter
    - Thrombophlebitis
    - Cellulitis

Demographics

- Age
  - Children & elderly more susceptible
- Gender
  - Women may have higher rate of colonization by *S. aureus*
- Epidemiology
  - Most common hospital-acquired pneumonia
  - Vast majority of MRSA are hospital-acquired
    - Increased prevalence worldwide since 1960s
  - Common cause of death during outbreaks of influenza
    - Community-acquired disease in these instances
    - Increased morbidity & mortality in elderly
  - Higher incidence in patients with chronic medical diseases
    - Chronic obstructive pulmonary disease
    - Cystic fibrosis
    - Immunosuppression

Natural History & Prognosis

- Mortality varies widely depending upon strain of organism, expression of virulence, & host factors
- Imaging follow-up depends upon underlying comorbidities & complications

Treatment

- Community-acquired pneumonia
  - β-lactams
  - Macrolides
  - Fluoroquinolones
- Methicillin-resistant *Staphylococcus aureus* (MRSA) pneumonia
  - Clindamycin & linezolid both inhibit protein synthesis, thus reducing PVL & exotoxin production
- Aggressive pleural drainage improves outcomes
  - Video-assisted thoracic surgery may be required

DIAGNOSTIC CHECKLIST

Consider

- Staphylococcal pneumonia in patient with fever, cough, & multifocal consolidation

Image Interpretation Pearls

- Unable to predict MRSA based on imaging findings

Reporting Tips

- Presence of pleural effusion on radiography should suggest possibility of empyema, which may require aggressive drainage

SELECTED REFERENCES

1. Lobo LJ et al: Expanded clinical presentation of community-acquired methicillin-resistant Staphylococcus aureus pneumonia. Chest. 138(1):130-6, 2010
2. Hayden GE et al: Chest radiograph vs. computed tomography scan in the evaluation for pneumonia. J Emerg Med. 36(3):266-70, 2009
3. Nguyen ET et al: Community-acquired methicillin-resistant Staphylococcus aureus pneumonia: radiographic and computed tomography findings. J Thorac Imaging. 23(1):13-9, 2008
4. Centers for Disease Control and Prevention (CDC): Severe methicillin-resistant Staphylococcus aureus community-acquired pneumonia associated with influenza--Louisiana and Georgia, December 2006-January 2007. MMWR Morb Mortal Wkly Rep. 56(14):325-9, 2007
5. Hageman JC et al: Severe community-acquired pneumonia due to Staphylococcus aureus, 2003-04 influenza season. Emerg Infect Dis. 12(6):894-9, 2006
6. Hodina M et al: Imaging of cavitary necrosis in complicated childhood pneumonia. Eur Radiol. 12(2):391-6, 2002
7. Macfarlane J et al: Radiographic features of staphylococcal pneumonia in adults and children. Thorax. 51(5):539-40, 1996

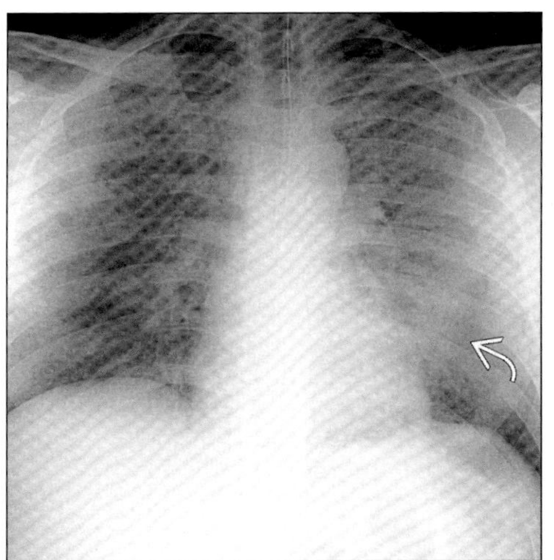

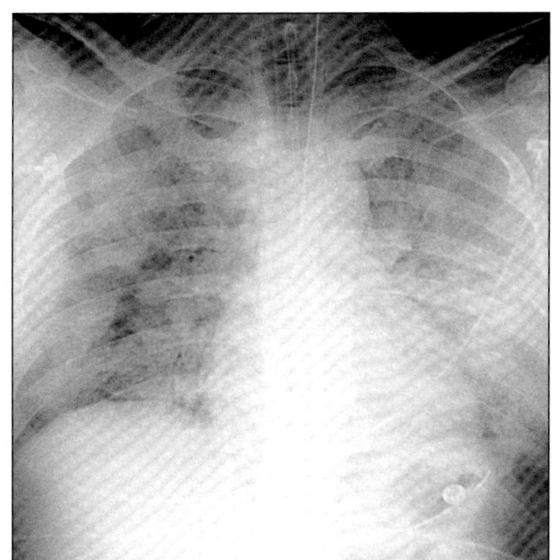

(Left) *PA chest radiograph of a 39-year-old woman who developed fever on postoperative day 1 following abdominal surgery shows a patchy left infrahilar airspace opacity ➚.* ***(Right)*** *AP chest radiograph of the same patient obtained 18 hours later shows diffuse bilateral airspace disease and areas of consolidation. The patient required mechanical ventilation and was scheduled for a CT pulmonary angiogram because of suspicion of pulmonary embolism.*

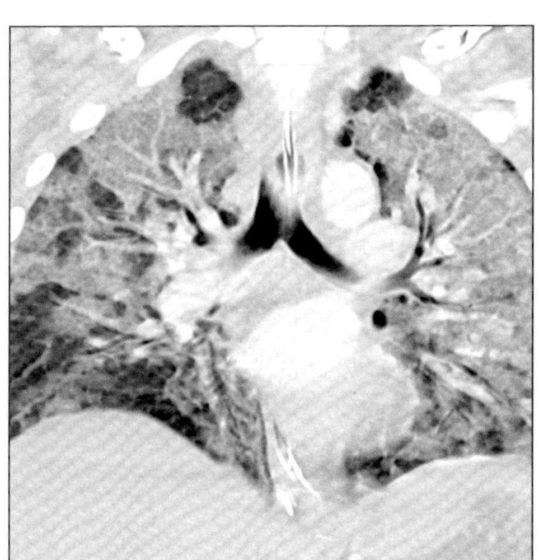

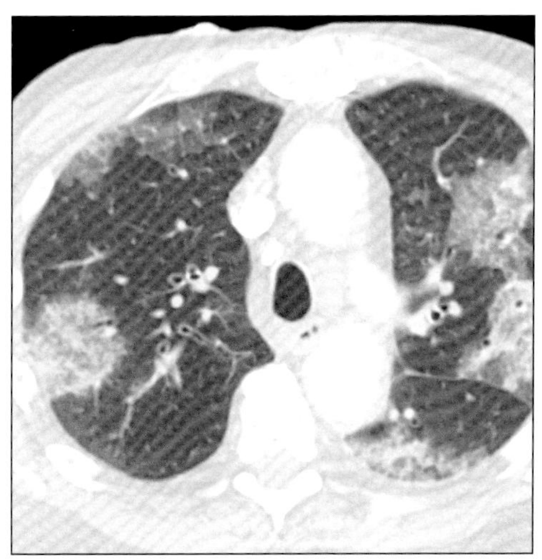

(Left) *Coronal CTPA of the same patient shows diffuse bilateral ground-glass opacities. No pulmonary embolism was identified. The imaging features are consistent with ARDS. S. aureus was isolated from bronchoscopic washings.* ***(Right)*** *Axial CECT of a 34-year-old man with endocarditis shows multiple peripheral nodular areas of ground-glass opacity and consolidation. The sputum was positive for MRSA.*

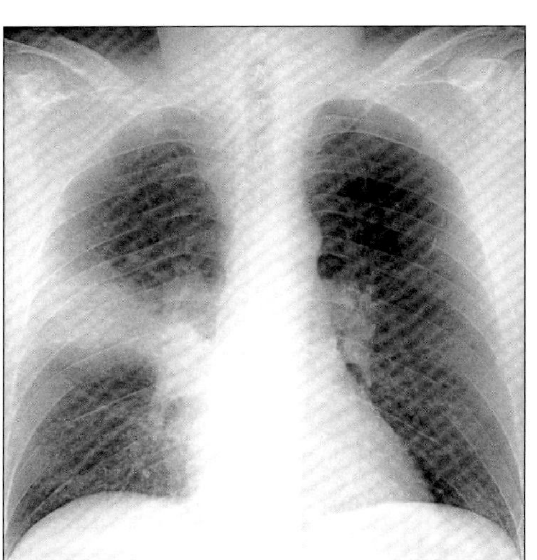

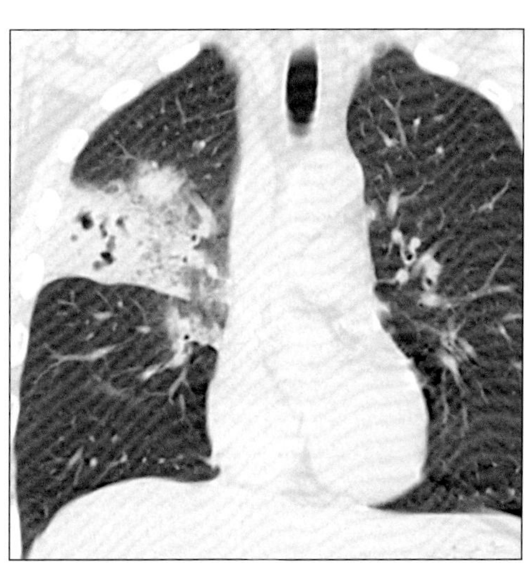

(Left) *PA chest radiograph of a 42-year-old man with fever and cough shows a focal right upper lobe consolidation. The patient was treated as an outpatient for community-acquired pneumonia.* ***(Right)*** *Coronal NECT of the same patient obtained 2 days later because of progressive dyspnea and productive cough shows cavitation within the right upper lobe consolidation. Cavitation is commonly associated with staphylococcal pneumonia.*

KLEBSIELLA PNEUMONIA

Key Facts

Terminology

- Friedländer pneumonia
- *Klebsiella pneumoniae*, gram-negative bacteria

Imaging

- Radiography
  - Lobar consolidation
  - Bulging interlobar fissures
  - Cavitation in 30-50% of cases
- CT
  - Ground-glass opacity
  - Consolidation with lobar expansion
  - Small air cavities within consolidation
  - Pulmonary abscess
  - Pulmonary gangrene
  - Empyema
  - Chronic infection: Upper lobe consolidation, cavitation

Top Differential Diagnoses

- Bacterial pneumonia
- Tuberculosis

Clinical Issues

- Symptoms/signs
  - High fever, cough
  - Currant-jelly sputum
- Risk factors
  - Alcohol abuse, cigarette smoking
  - Diabetes
- Treatment
  - Antibiotics
  - Surgical resection of pulmonary gangrene

Diagnostic Checklist

- Consider *Klebsiella* pneumonia in alcoholic with rapidly progressing community-acquired pneumonia

__(Left)__ PA chest radiograph of a patient with Klebsiella pneumonia shows lobar consolidation and mild convex contour of the minor fissure. __(Right)__ Lateral chest radiograph of the same patient shows dense middle lobe consolidation and mild bulging of the surrounding interlobar fissures. Sputum culture was positive for Klebsiella. A bulging fissure is a characteristic radiographic feature of Klebsiella pneumonia caused by the large volume of inflammatory exudate.

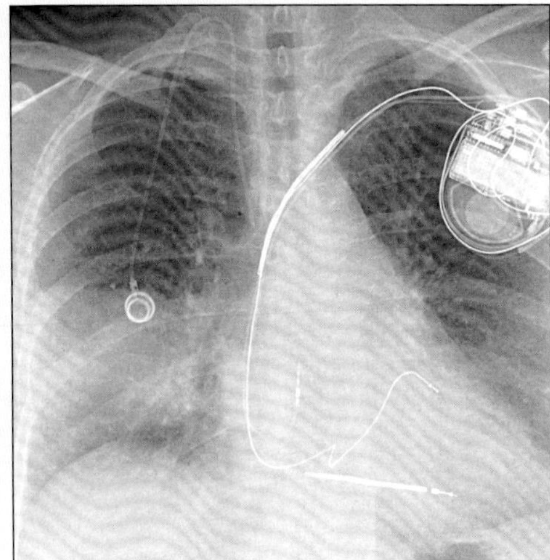

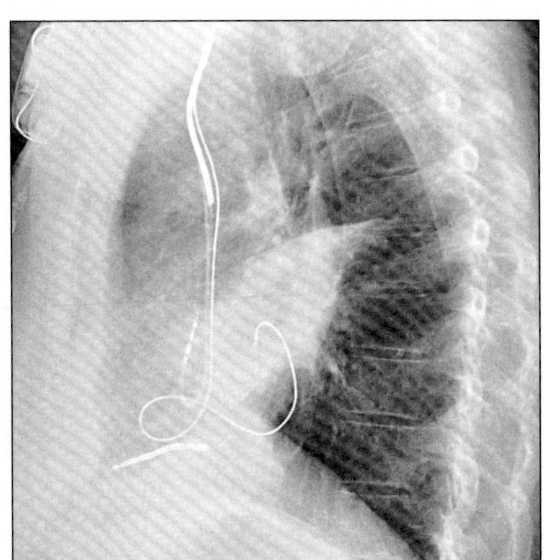

__(Left)__ PA chest radiograph of a patient with metastatic prostate cancer, failure to thrive, and fever shows a thick-walled cavitary lesion ➔ in the right upper lobe and a loculated left pleural effusion. __(Right)__ Coronal CECT of the same patient confirms a right upper lobe cavity with thick nodular walls, a loculated left pleural effusion, and left upper lobe patchy opacities. Sputum culture was positive for Klebsiella. Cavitation and pleural effusions are not infrequently seen in Klebsiella pneumonia.

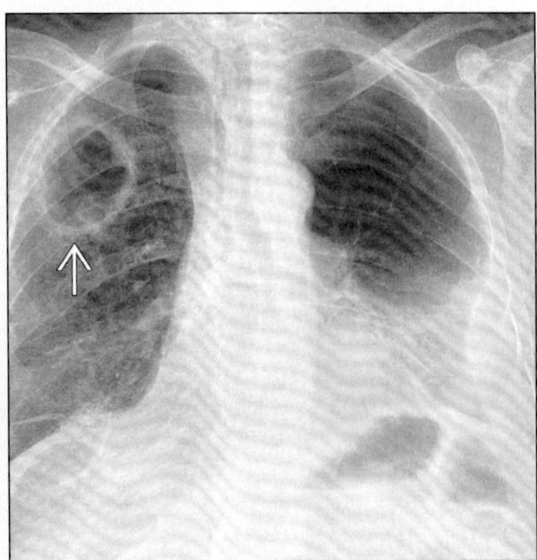

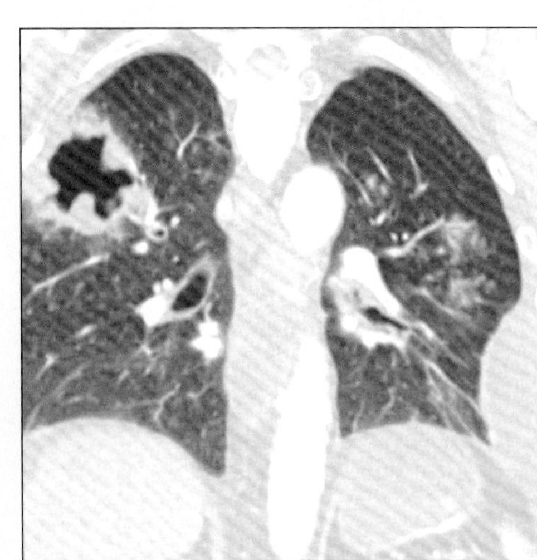

KLEBSIELLA PNEUMONIA

TERMINOLOGY

Synonyms

- **Friedländer pneumonia**

Definitions

- *Klebsiella pneumoniae,* gram-negative bacteria
- Accounts for 0.5-5% of community-acquired pneumonia & 15% of nosocomial pneumonias

IMAGING

Radiographic Findings

- **Consolidation**
  - Lobar distribution
  - Bulging interlobar fissures (30%)
    - Voluminous inflammatory exudate
    - Positive predictive value (67%)
  - Sharp margins of advancing border
  - Most common in right upper lobe
- **Cavitation (30-50%)**
  - Frequently multiple
  - May be chronic, simulating tuberculosis
- **Pleural effusion**

CT Findings

- **Ground-glass opacity**
- **Consolidation**
  - Initially nonsegmental but quickly becomes lobar
    - More common in community-acquired pneumonia
  - May be multilobar & bilateral
    - More common in nosocomial pneumonia
  - Expansion of consolidated lobes
  - Enhancing consolidation with low-density areas (necrosis)
  - Small air cavities within consolidation suggest necrosis; may result in bronchopleural fistula
- **Lung abscesses (cavitary lesions)**: 16-50%
  - Occur early, within days
- **Pulmonary gangrene** from pulmonary vessel thrombosis
  - Massive necrosis & sloughed lung
  - Large cavity with air-crescent & intracavitary mass
- Interlobular septal thickening
- Bronchial wall thickening
- Pleural effusion, empyema
- Lymphadenopathy not common
- Fibrosis or bronchiectasis
- Chronic *Klebsiella* pneumonia: Symptoms > 1 month
  - Abscess &/or consolidation almost exclusively in upper lobe
  - Empyema

Imaging Recommendations

- Best imaging tool
  - Chest radiography for initial detection of pneumonia
  - CT helps in detection of complications in patients without appropriate response to treatment

DIFFERENTIAL DIAGNOSIS

Bacterial Pneumonia

- Anaerobic bacterial pneumonia also considered in alcoholics with cavitary lesions
  - Some patients have concomitant anaerobic & *Klebsiella* infection
- Pneumococcal, *Haemophilus,* & anaerobic bacteria are more frequent causes of community-acquired pneumonia than *Klebsiella*

Tuberculosis

- Chronic *Klebsiella* pneumonia with upper lobe cavitary consolidation may mimic TB

Pulmonary Gangrene

- Also reported with *S. pneumoniae,* anaerobes, *M. tuberculosis, Aspergillus,* & mucormycosis

PATHOLOGY

Microscopic Features

- Gram-negative bacilli, surrounded by clear capsule

CLINICAL ISSUES

Presentation

- Most common signs/symptoms
  - High fever, cough
  - Thick & gelatinous, currant-jelly sputum
- Other signs/symptoms
  - Dyspnea, pleuritic chest pain, leukopenia

Demographics

- Gender
  - M > F
- Epidemiology
  - Risk factors
    - Alcohol abuse, cigarette smoking
    - Diabetes, chronic bronchopulmonary disease
    - Malnutrition, chronic debilitating disease
  - Additional pathogens frequently coexist
    - 37% have methicillin-resistant *S. aureus* (MRSA)
    - 23% have *P. aeruginosa* (PA)

Natural History & Prognosis

- Nosocomial infection with mortality rate of 32%
- Mortality in alcoholics reported to be 50-60%

Treatment

- Antibiotics, based on susceptibility
- Surgical resection for pulmonary gangrene

DIAGNOSTIC CHECKLIST

Consider

- *Klebsiella* pneumonia in alcoholic with rapidly progressing severe community-acquired pneumonia

SELECTED REFERENCES

1. Okada F et al: Acute Klebsiella pneumoniae pneumonia alone and with concurrent infection: comparison of clinical and thin-section CT findings. Br J Radiol. 83(994):854-60, 2010

METHICILLIN-RESISTANT *STAPHYLOCOCCUS AUREUS* PNEUMONIA

Key Facts

Terminology
- Methicillin-resistant *Staphylococcus aureus* (MRSA)
- Important cause of severe nosocomial & community-acquired necrotizing pneumonia & septic emboli

Imaging
- Radiography
  - Multifocal patchy or nodular consolidations
  - Cavitary lesions
  - Pleural effusions
- CT
  - Multifocal consolidations, ground-glass opacities
  - Internal necrosis; small cavities within consolidation
  - Cavitary nodules, abscess formation
  - Centrilobular nodules
  - Empyema with pleural thickening & enhancement
  - Septic emboli: Multiple nodules ± cavitations

Pathology
- Gram-positive cocci in clusters

Clinical Issues
- Symptoms/signs
  - Fever, cough, chest pain
- 20-40% of hospital-acquired pneumonia
  - Risk factors: Elderly, ventilatory support, indwelling lines
- 9% of community-acquired pneumonia
  - Young, previously healthy, may follow influenza
- Treatment: Vancomycin, linezolid
- High mortality of up to 56%

Diagnostic Checklist
- Consider MRSA pneumonia in patients with bilateral patchy or nodular multifocal consolidations with internal cavitation

__(Left)__ AP chest radiograph of a 75-year-old man hospitalized for treatment of smoke inhalation injury and tracheostomy tube placement shows bilateral patchy opacities that developed 17 days after admission. __(Right)__ Coronal NECT of the same patient shows bilateral patchy consolidations, ground-glass opacities, and lower lobe tree-in-bud opacities. Sputum culture confirmed MRSA pneumonia. Hospital-acquired MRSA pneumonia is particularly common in elderly patients on ventilatory support.

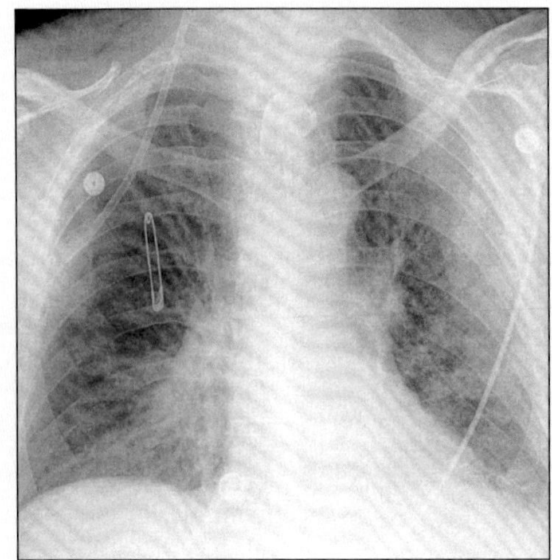

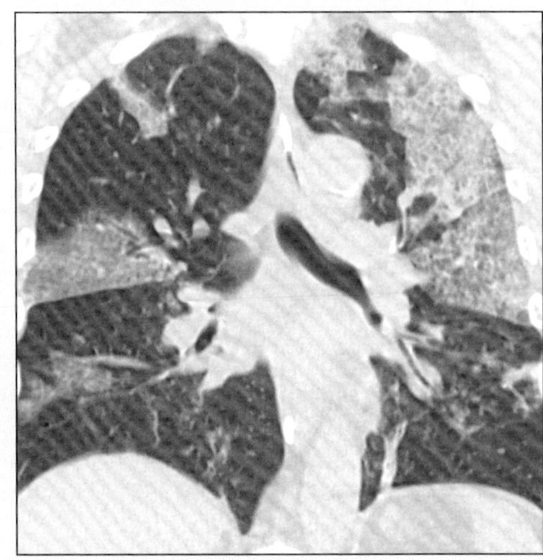

__(Left)__ Axial NECT of a young man who presented with high fever and respiratory distress shows patchy opacities in the right lower and left upper lobes and dense right upper lobe consolidation with small internal low-attenuation foci from early cavitation ⇨. Sputum culture was positive for MRSA. __(Right)__ Axial CECT of a 42-year-old woman with fever and cough shows right upper lobe cavitary nodules ➡. Bronchoalveolar lavage was positive for MRSA. Community-acquired MRSA pneumonia tends to affect younger patients.

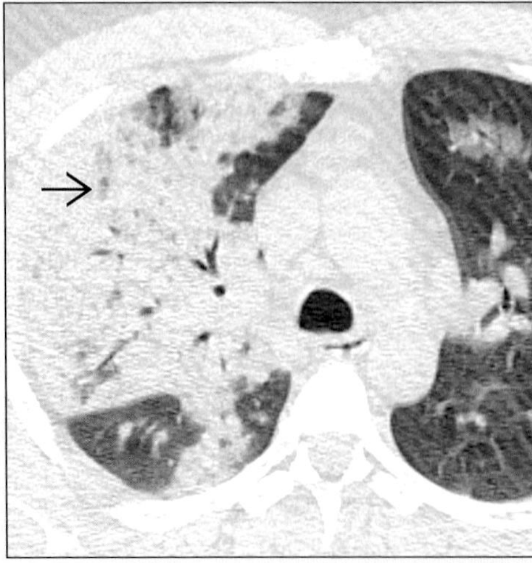

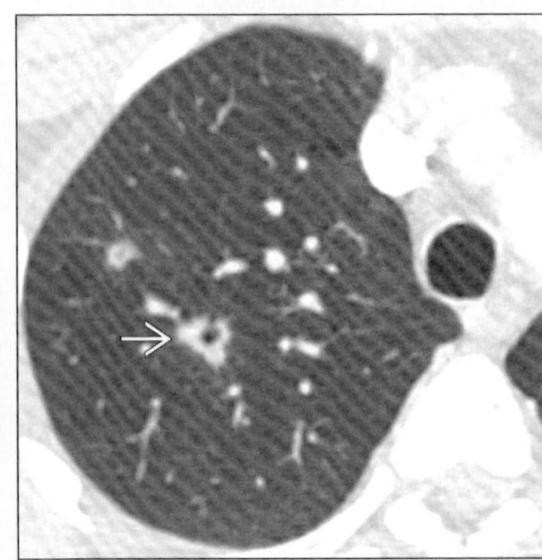

METHICILLIN-RESISTANT *STAPHYLOCOCCUS AUREUS* PNEUMONIA

TERMINOLOGY

Abbreviations

- Methicillin-resistant *Staphylococcus aureus* (MRSA)

Definitions

- MRSA emerged in 1960, within short time of introduction of methicillin
- Important cause of severe nosocomial & community-acquired necrotizing pneumonia & septic emboli

IMAGING

Radiographic Findings

- Multifocal patchy or nodular consolidations
  - Often bilateral
- Cavitary lesions
- Pleural effusions

CT Findings

- Multifocal consolidations, ground-glass opacities
  - Patchy or segmental
  - Often bilateral
  - Peripheral predominance
  - Necrosis with small internal cavitations
- Septal thickening
- Bronchial wall thickening
- Centrilobular nodules
- Cavitary nodules, abscess formation
- Pleural effusions
- Empyema in 20% of patients
  - **"Split pleura" sign**; smoothly thickened & enhancing parietal & visceral pleural surfaces
- Pneumatoceles, pneumothorax
- Mediastinal/hilar lymphadenopathy uncommon
- Hematogenous spread (septic emboli)
  - Multiple nodules ± cavitations

DIFFERENTIAL DIAGNOSIS

Methicillin-susceptible Staphylococcus aureus (MSSA) Pneumonia

- Higher frequency of cardiovascular disease, malignancy, & diabetes in patients with MRSA compared to those with MSSA
- Difficult to distinguish by imaging
  - Higher frequency of centrilobular nodules with tree-in-bud opacities in MSSA than in MRSA
  - Pleural effusions more frequent with MRSA than with MSSA

Other Bronchopneumonia

- Such as *P. aeruginosa*, *M catarrhalis*, or *H. influenza*

PATHOLOGY

General Features

- Genetics
  - CA-MRSA strains frequently carry Panton-Valentine leukocidin (*PVL*) genes

Microscopic Features

- Gram-positive cocci in clusters

CLINICAL ISSUES

Presentation

- Most common signs/symptoms
  - Fever
  - Productive cough
    - Purulent secretions in intubated patients
  - Chest pain
- Other signs/symptoms
  - Flu-like prodrome in community-acquired MRSA pneumonia
  - Hemoptysis

Demographics

- Epidemiology
  - MRSA colonizes nasal passages of up to 50% of population
  - MRSA causes skin & soft tissue infection, osteomyelitis, bacteremia, endocarditis, & pneumonia
  - 20-40% of hospital-acquired pneumonia
  - 9% of community-acquired pneumonia
  - Pulmonary infection also from hematogenous spread of endocarditis, thrombophlebitis, infected indwelling catheters, intravenous drug use
- Hospital-acquired MRSA pneumonia
  - Elderly
  - Ventilatory support
  - Indwelling tubes & lines
  - Chronic obstructive pulmonary disease (COPD)
- Community-acquired MRSA pneumonia
  - Young, < 35 years old
  - Previously healthy
  - Sometimes follows influenza

Natural History & Prognosis

- Higher mortality than MSSA
- Hospital-acquired MRSA pneumonia, mortality of 28-56%
- Community-acquired MRSA pneumonia
  - Rapid progression of symptoms requiring hospitalization
  - Mortality: 20-50%

Treatment

- Antibiotics: Vancomycin, linezolid

SELECTED REFERENCES

1. Morikawa K et al: Methicillin-resistant Staphylococcus aureus and methicillin-susceptible S. aureus pneumonia: comparison of clinical and thin-section CT findings. Br J Radiol. Epub ahead of print, 2011
2. Dean N: Methicillin-resistant Staphylococcus aureus in community-acquired and health care-associated pneumonia: incidence, diagnosis, and treatment options. Hosp Pract (Minneap). 38(1):7-15, 2010
3. Nguyen ET et al: Community-acquired methicillin-resistant Staphylococcus aureus pneumonia: radiographic and computed tomography findings. J Thorac Imaging. 23(1):13-9, 2008

LEGIONELLA PNEUMONIA

Key Facts

Terminology

- Legionnaires disease
- Pneumonia caused by infection with any *Legionella* species, most commonly *Legionella pneumophila*

Imaging

- Radiography
  - Rapidly progressive, asymmetric consolidation
  - Expands to occupy majority of lobe
  - Progresses to involve additional lobes or contralateral lung (3-4 days)
  - Pleural effusion in up to 2/3 of patients
- CT
  - Lobar or multilobar consolidation
  - Ground-glass opacity adjacent to consolidation
  - Perihilar > peripheral distribution
  - Pleural effusion (~ 1/3 of patients)
  - Mild mediastinal & hilar lymphadenopathy

Top Differential Diagnoses

- Pneumococcal pneumonia
- *Mycoplasma* pneumonia
- Viral pneumonia
- *Klebsiella* pneumonia
- *Staphylococcus* pneumonia

Pathology

- Inhaled aerosolized contaminated water droplets

Clinical Issues

- Most patients have preexisting disease
- Most common in adults > 50 years
- M:F = 2-3:1
- Prognosis varies with underlying conditions
  - Patients with impaired T-cell-mediated immunity have greatest mortality risk
- Treatment: Doxycycline, fluoroquinolones

*(**Left**) AP chest radiograph of a patient with Legionella pneumonia shows dense peripheral consolidation → in the left lung. Mechanical ventilation ⇨ was required. (**Right**) Axial NECT of a patient with Legionella pneumonia who presented with fever, chills, and cough shows a left lower lobe mass-like consolidation with surrounding ground-glass opacity. There was subsequent disease progression with eventual involvement of the right lung (not shown). Legionella pneumonia commonly exhibits progression on imaging.*

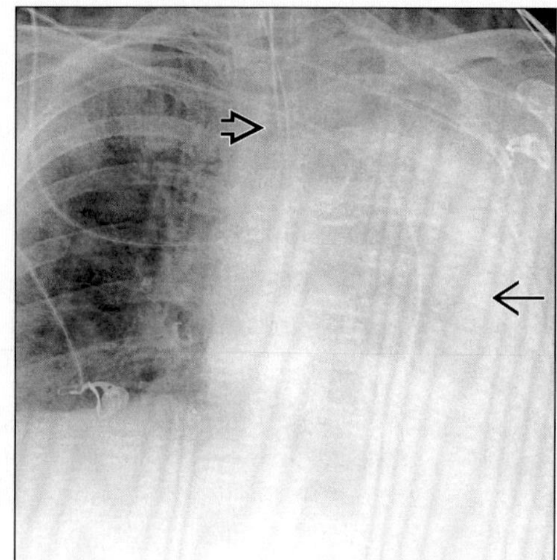

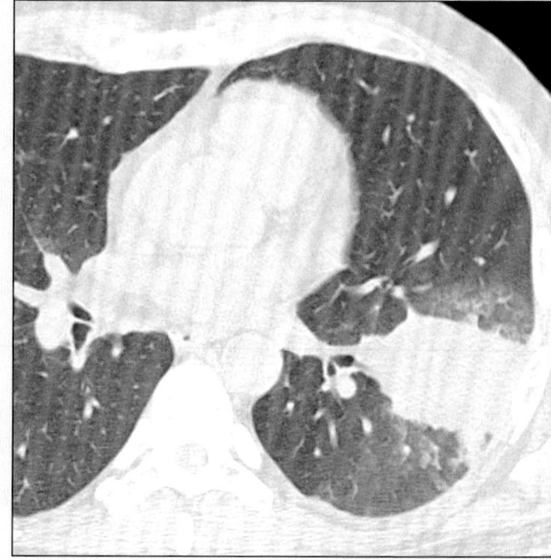

*(**Left**) AP chest radiograph shows large bilateral consolidations → in this patient with Legionella pneumophila-induced pneumonia. Radiographically apparent pleural effusions and hilar lymph node enlargement are uncommon in these patients but may be observed on CT. (**Right**) PA chest radiograph of a kidney-pancreas transplant recipient with non-pneumophila Legionella pneumonia shows bilateral, asymmetric peripheral mass-like pulmonary consolidations →.*

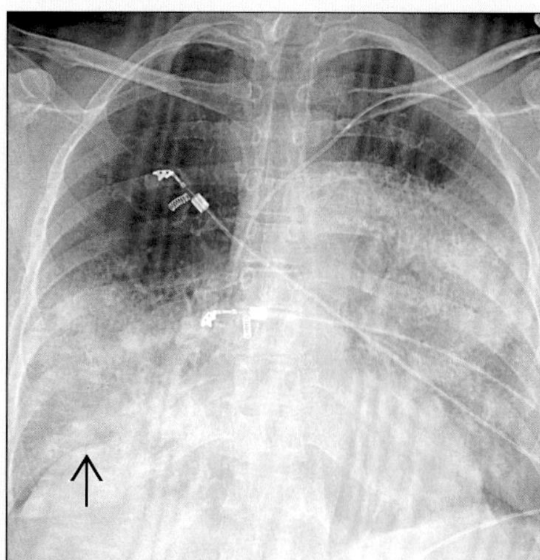

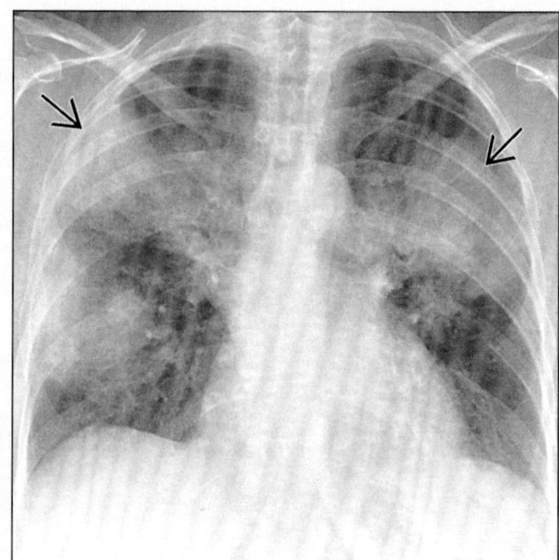

LEGIONELLA PNEUMONIA

TERMINOLOGY

Synonyms

- **Legionnaires disease**

Definitions

- Pneumonia caused by infection with any *Legionella* species, most commonly *Legionella pneumophila*

IMAGING

General Features

- Best diagnostic clue
  - Rapidly progressive, asymmetric consolidation
- Size
  - Initially lobar, then multilobar
- Morphology
  - Consolidation

Radiographic Findings

- **Rapidly progressive, asymmetric lung consolidation**
  - Initially lobar, expanding to occupy majority of lobe
  - Progresses to involve additional lobes or contralateral lung (3-4 days)
- Less common manifestations
  - Spherical consolidation
  - Solitary or multiple mass, nodule- or mass-like consolidations
  - Cavitation & lymphadenopathy unusual except in immunocompromised patients
- **Pleural effusion** in up to 2/3 of patients

CT Findings

- NECT
  - Lobar or multilobar consolidation most common
    - Perihilar distribution more common than peripheral distribution
    - Ground-glass opacity, often adjacent to consolidation
  - Pleural effusion (~ 1/3 of patients), may be small
  - Mild mediastinal & hilar lymphadenopathy

Imaging Recommendations

- Best imaging tool
  - Chest radiography usually sufficient to diagnose pneumonia

DIFFERENTIAL DIAGNOSIS

Pneumococcal Pneumonia

- Consolidation usually limited to 1 lobe
  - Almost always abuts visceral pleural surface
  - Air bronchograms usually present
  - Usually does not progress with appropriate therapy
  - Typically lacks extrapulmonary features, such as headache, diarrhea, & relative bradycardia

Mycoplasma Pneumonia

- Bronchopneumonia or bronchiolitis pattern more common
- Patients usually younger
- More insidious onset of symptoms

Viral Pneumonia

- Bronchopneumonia or bronchiolitis pattern more common
  - Adenovirus infection may manifest as lobar pneumonia
- Cough, typically nonproductive

Klebsiella Pneumonia

- Usually nosocomial infection
- Radiographic abnormalities may mimic *Legionella* pneumonia
- Typically lacks extrapulmonary features, such as headache, diarrhea, & relative bradycardia

Staphylococcus Pneumonia

- Often nosocomial infection, especially in ICU
- Bronchopneumonia pattern most common
  - Air bronchograms uncommon
- Abscesses in 15-30%

PATHOLOGY

General Features

- Etiology
  - Inhaled or aspirated aerosolized droplets of contaminated water

CLINICAL ISSUES

Presentation

- Most common signs/symptoms
  - Fever, chills, cough (initially dry), dyspnea
  - Pleuritic chest pain in ~ 30%
- Other signs/symptoms
  - Headache, confusion, lethargy
  - Relative bradycardia
  - Loose stools or watery diarrhea
  - Microscopic hematuria, acute renal insufficiency

Demographics

- Age
  - May affect any age group
    - Most common in adults > 50 years
- Gender
  - M:F = 2-3:1
- Epidemiology
  - Seasonal peak in late summer & early autumn
  - Sporadic cases associated with exposure to colonized water (construction, travel)
  - Nosocomial outbreaks related to exposure to contaminated water sources (air conditioners, showers)

Natural History & Prognosis

- Prognosis varies with underlying conditions
  - Patients with impaired T-cell-mediated immunity have greatest mortality risk

SELECTED REFERENCES

1. Cunha BA: Legionnaires' disease: clinical differentiation from typical and other atypical pneumonias. Infect Dis Clin North Am. 24(1):73-105, 2010

NOCARDIOSIS

Key Facts

Terminology
- Infection by organisms in *N. asteroides* complex

Imaging
- Radiography
  - Consolidation, nodules/masses ± cavitation
  - Upper lobe fibrocavitary disease
  - Reticulonodular interstitial opacities
  - Pleural effusion, unilateral or bilateral
- CT
  - Homogeneous consolidation (65%)
  - Cavitation (40%)
  - Nodules (60%) &/or masses (20%)
  - Pleural effusion (30%)
  - Lymphadenopathy (15%)
- May involve extrapulmonary structures
- Best clue: Necrotizing pneumonia in immunocompromised patient

Top Differential Diagnoses
- Other infections that traverse tissue planes
- Lung cancer

Pathology
- Gram-positive bacilli, weakly acid-fast

Clinical Issues
- Symptoms/signs: Fever, chills, fatigue, dyspnea, productive cough, hemoptysis, sweats, weight loss
- Immunocompromised in 50% of infections
- Underlying lung disease
- Dissemination in 50% of pulmonary infections
- Treatment: Sulfa-containing antibiotic (3-6 months)

Diagnostic Checklist
- Consider brain imaging in patients with nocardiosis to exclude metastatic infection

__(Left)__ Axial NECT of a 32-year-old patient with Fanconi anemia and Nocardia pneumonia shows a right lower lobe consolidation ↪. The diagnosis was established via bronchoalveolar lavage. __(Right)__ Axial CECT of a 66-year-old man post bilateral lung transplantation for emphysema shows middle → and lower lobe pneumonia, right pleural effusion, and chest wall abscesses ↪. Thoracentesis revealed nocardiosis. This infection may traverse anatomic boundaries, resulting in chest wall involvement.

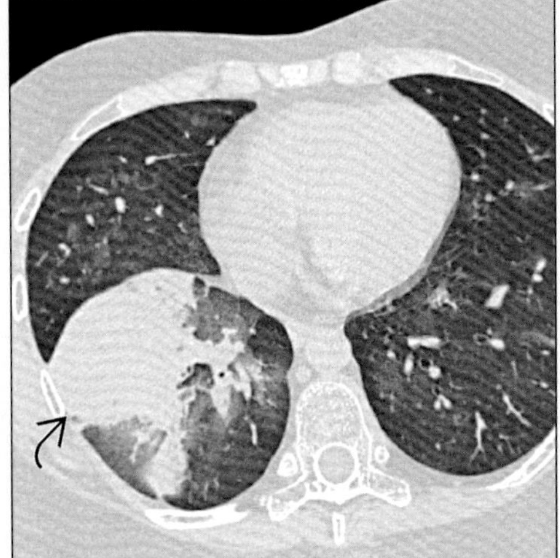

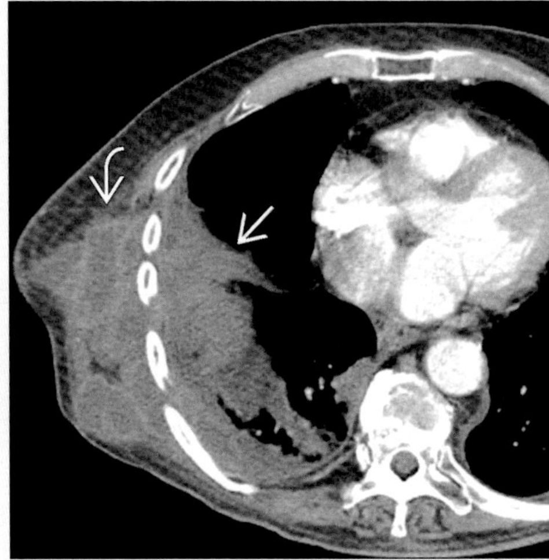

__(Left)__ Axial NECT of a 72-year-old woman with a history of immunosuppression shows a large right lower lobe cavitary mass →, patchy left lower lobe airspace opacities ↪, and trace bilateral pleural effusions. Blood cultures recovered Nocardia. __(Right)__ Axial NECT of a 74-year-old woman with Nocardia pneumonia shows multiple indistinct left upper and lower lobe pulmonary nodules →, a right lower lobe consolidation, and bilateral pleural effusions. Nocardiosis may manifest with cavitation &/or multifocal nodules.

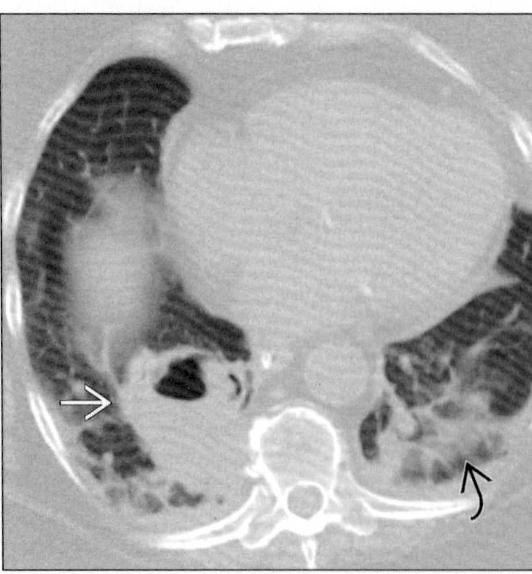

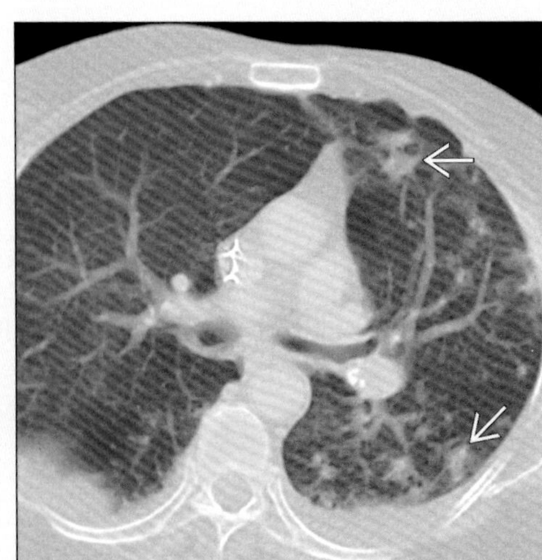

NOCARDIOSIS

TERMINOLOGY

Synonyms

- *Nocardia asteroides* complex: *Nocardia nova, Nocardia farcinica, Nocardia transvalensis*

Definitions

- Infection by organisms in *N. asteroides* complex

IMAGING

General Features

- Best diagnostic clue
  - Necrotizing or cavitary pneumonia in immunocompromised patient
- Location
  - Typically unilateral disease
- Morphology
  - May traverse tissue planes

Radiographic Findings

- Radiography
  - Consolidation, nodules/masses ± cavitation
  - Upper lobe fibrocavitary disease
  - Reticulonodular interstitial opacities
  - Pleural effusion, ~ 1/3 of cases, unilateral or bilateral

CT Findings

- NECT
  - **Homogeneous consolidation (65%)**
    - Lobar or diffuse, indistinct margins, frequently abuts pleura
    - Bronchopneumonia (10%)
  - **Cavitation (40%)**
    - Abscess, single/multiple thick-walled cavities
  - **Nodules (60%)** &/or masses (20%)
    - Solitary or multiple
    - Well-defined or irregular borders
    - Indolent, slowly enlarging pulmonary nodule
    - Associated reticular or fine nodular opacities
  - Bronchiectasis (10%)
  - Pleural effusion (30%)
  - Lymphadenopathy (15%)
- CECT
  - Chronic infection may involve adjacent pleura, chest wall, pericardium, mediastinum, superior vena cava
    - Pleural effusion/empyema (80%)
  - AIDS: Irregular spiculated nodules & cavitary masses

Imaging Recommendations

- Best imaging tool
  - CECT optimally demonstrates extension of disease to chest wall & mediastinum

DIFFERENTIAL DIAGNOSIS

Other Infections that Traverse Tissue Planes

- Tuberculosis, actinomycosis, invasive aspergillosis, mucormycosis

Lung Cancer

- Pulmonary mass; may invade adjacent pleura, chest wall, mediastinum

PATHOLOGY

Microscopic Features

- Gram-positive, branching, beaded bacilli, weakly acid-fast, ubiquitous, soil-borne
- Slow growth: 3-5 weeks to grow in culture
- Polymerase chain reaction, rapid & reliable diagnosis

CLINICAL ISSUES

Presentation

- Most common signs/symptoms
  - Fever, chills, fatigue, dyspnea, productive cough, hemoptysis, sweats, weight loss, anorexia
- Other signs/symptoms
  - AIDS, CD4 count < 50 cells/mL, not on *Pneumocystis* prophylaxis

Demographics

- Gender
  - More common in males
- Epidemiology
  - In USA, 1,000 cases/year
  - Immunocompromised in 50% of infections
    - Transplant recipients: Kidney, lung, heart, liver, bone marrow
    - Malignancy on antineoplastic therapy; leukemia, lymphoma, colon cancer
    - AIDS
    - Intravenous drug use
    - Prolonged corticosteroid or other immunosuppressive treatment, such as Infliximab
    - Sternal wound infection, indwelling catheter/line infection
  - Underlying lung disease: Silicosis, pulmonary fibrosis, emphysema, alveolar proteinosis

Natural History & Prognosis

- Bacteremia with dissemination in 50% of pulmonary infections
  - Brain abscess, most common site (up to 33%)
  - Retina, joints, soft tissues (psoas), liver, adrenal, skin
- Mortality with CNS involvement (up to 90%)

Treatment

- Sulfa-containing antibiotic (3-6 months)
- Surgery or drainage for extensive lung destruction & empyema

DIAGNOSTIC CHECKLIST

Consider

- Brain imaging in all patients with nocardiosis to exclude metastatic infection
- In severely immunocompromised, brain abscess may be asymptomatic for up to 3 years

SELECTED REFERENCES

1. Blackmon KN et al: Pulmonary nocardiosis: computed tomography features at diagnosis. J Thorac Imaging. 26(3):224-9, 2011
2. Oszoyoglu AA et al: Pulmonary nocardiosis after lung transplantation: CT findings in 7 patients and review of the literature. J Thorac Imaging. 22(2):143-8, 2007

ACTINOMYCOSIS

Key Facts

Terminology

- Granulomatous infection caused by *Actinomyces* species

Imaging

- Radiography
  - Unilateral, peripheral, patchy consolidation
  - Cavitary mass
  - Pleural effusion, chest wall involvement
- CT
  - Focal/patchy consolidation, central low attenuation
  - Peripheral rim enhancement
  - Bronchiectatic: Bronchiectasis, bronchial wall thickening, peribronchial consolidation
  - Pleural effusion
  - Chest wall involvement: Soft tissue/skeletal abnormalities

Top Differential Diagnoses

- Bronchopneumonia
- Fungal infection
- Aspiration pneumonia
- Tuberculosis (empyema necessitatis)
- Lung cancer

Pathology

- Microabscess or necrotic material
- *Actinomyces* colonies or sulfur granules

Clinical Issues

- Symptoms/signs: Cough, fever, chest pain
- Treatment: Antibiotics, surgical resection

Diagnostic Checklist

- Consider actinomycosis in patients with alcoholism & poor oral hygiene with chronic consolidation

*(**Left**) Axial CECT of a patient with actinomycosis shows a left lower lobe consolidation with multifocal low-attenuation areas, intrinsic ring-like enhancement ➡ surrounding a low-attenuation area with small air bubbles, and pleural effusion with associated enhancing thickened parietal pleura ⮚. (**Right**) Axial NECT of a patient with actinomycosis shows a middle lobe consolidation involving the adjacent pleura ➡ and chest wall ↪. A locally invasive neoplasm must also be considered.*

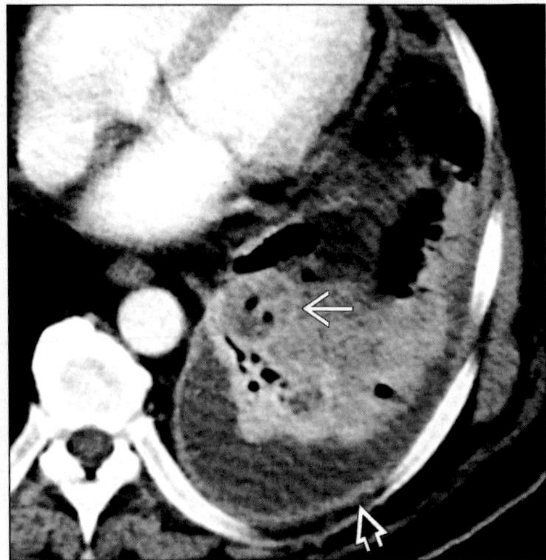

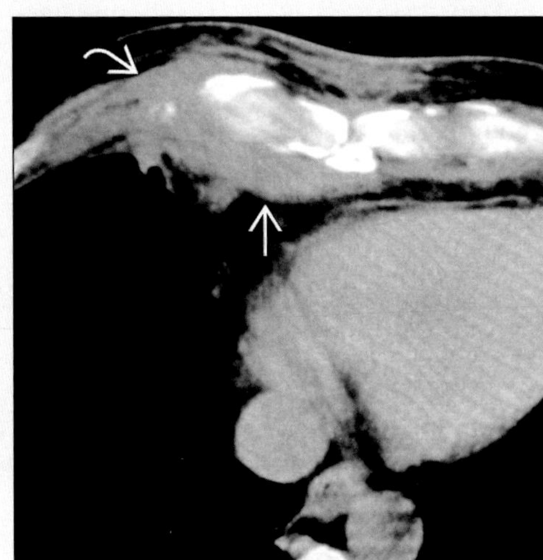

*(**Left**) Axial NECT of a patient with actinomycosis shows abnormal soft tissue obstructing the middle lobe bronchus ➡, subsegmental consolidation with cavitation ⮚, and irregular bronchial dilatation ↪. Endobronchial actinomycosis may mimic lung cancer. (**Right**) Axial CECT of a patient with actinomycosis shows bilateral pulmonary masses with central low attenuation from necrosis. Note peripheral rim enhancement ↪ of the left upper lobe lesion. Malignancy and vasculitis should also be considered.*

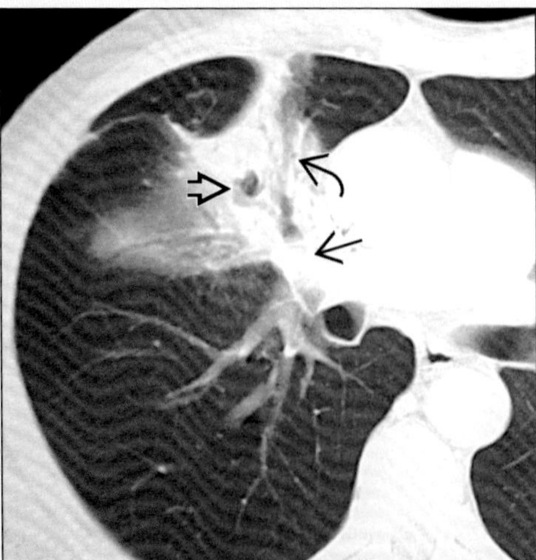

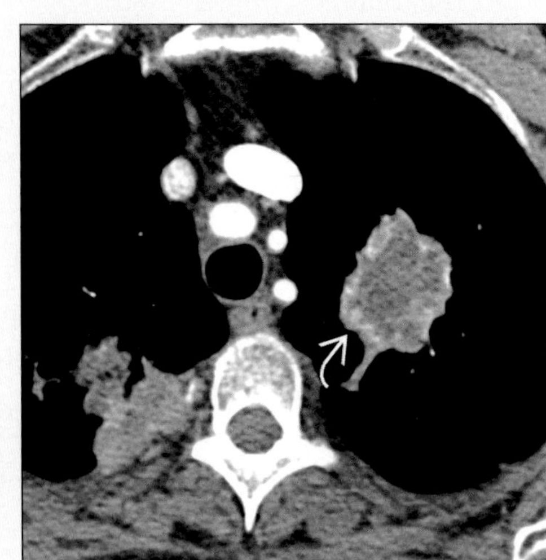

ACTINOMYCOSIS

TERMINOLOGY

Definitions

- Granulomatous infection caused by *Actinomyces* species, most commonly *A. israelii,* gram-positive anaerobic saprophytic organism
  - **Parenchymal actinomycosis**: Aspiration of endogenous oropharyngeal organisms into lungs
  - **Bronchiectatic form**: Colonization of devitalized tissue & bronchiectasis
  - **Endobronchial actinomycosis associated with broncholithiasis or foreign body**: Colonization of preexisting endobronchial broncholith/foreign body

IMAGING

Radiographic Findings

- Parenchymal actinomycosis
  - Unilateral, peripheral, patchy consolidations
  - Cavitary mass
  - Pleural effusion, chest wall involvement

CT Findings

- Parenchymal actinomycosis
  - Focal/patchy consolidation with central low attenuation
    - CECT: Rim enhancement around central low attenuation
  - Pleural effusion
  - Chest wall involvement: Soft tissue/skeletal abnormalities
- Bronchiectatic form
  - Localized bronchiectasis, irregular bronchial wall thickening, irregular peribronchial consolidation ± abscess formation
- Endobronchial actinomycosis associated with broncholithiasis or foreign body
  - Radiopaque endobronchial nodule/calcification with distal obstructive pneumonia
- Hilar or mediastinal lymphadenopathy

Imaging Recommendations

- Best imaging tool
  - CT: More sensitive for disease characterization & extent of involvement

DIFFERENTIAL DIAGNOSIS

Bronchopneumonia

- Focal or multifocal areas of consolidation

Fungal Infection

- Actinomycotic intracavitary lung colonization by fungus forming fungus ball
  - Radiologic features (air crescent sign) similar to fungus ball typically caused by *Aspergillus* species

Aspiration Pneumonia

- Gravity-dependent focal or multifocal consolidation

Tuberculosis (Empyema Necessitatis)

- Empyema may communicate with chest wall (empyema necessitatis)

Lung Cancer

- May mimic cancer as it does not respect anatomic borders

PATHOLOGY

General Features

- Etiology
  - Gram-positive anaerobic saprophytic organism in oral cavity (poor oral hygiene)

Gross Pathologic & Surgical Features

- Chronic inflammation with varying degrees of fibrosis
  - Microabscess or necrotic material

Microscopic Features

- Difficulty in isolating *Actinomyces*: Normal inhabitant of oropharynx
- *Actinomyces* colonies or sulfur granules

CLINICAL ISSUES

Presentation

- Most common signs/symptoms
  - Nonproductive cough, low-grade fever
- Other signs/symptoms
  - Pleuritic chest pain (chest wall involvement)

Demographics

- Majority of patients are alcoholic men

Natural History & Prognosis

- Prognosis generally good with appropriate antibiotic therapy

Treatment

- Antibiotic therapy: Intravenous or oral amoxicillin-clavulanate
- Surgical resection: Patients unresponsive to antibiotic therapy

DIAGNOSTIC CHECKLIST

Consider

- Actinomycosis in patients with alcoholism & poor oral hygiene with chronic consolidation

Image Interpretation Pearls

- Chronic segmental airspace consolidation with frequent cavity formation and chest wall involvement

Reporting Tips

- Malignancy should be excluded

SELECTED REFERENCES

1. Song JU et al: Treatment of thoracic actinomycosis: A retrospective analysis of 40 patients. Ann Thorac Med. 5(2):80-5, 2010
2. Kim TS et al: Thoracic actinomycosis: CT features with histopathologic correlation. AJR Am J Roentgenol. 186(1):225-31, 2006

TUBERCULOSIS

Key Facts

Terminology
- Tuberculosis (TB)
- Airborne communicable infection by *M. tuberculosis*

Imaging
- Primary pattern
  - Consolidation
  - Lymphadenopathy
  - Pleural effusion, self-limited
- Post-primary pattern
  - Upper lobe heterogeneous consolidation ± cavitation
  - Centrilobular nodules, tree-in-bud opacities, acinar/ lobular consolidations
  - Tuberculomas
- Complications
  - Miliary TB
  - Tuberculous empyema

Top Differential Diagnoses
- Sarcoidosis
- Chronic fungal infection
- Lung cancer

Clinical Issues
- Symptoms/signs
  - Self-limited mildly symptomatic respiratory infection, may be undiagnosed
  - Cough, pleuritic chest pain
  - Hemoptysis
- Treatment
  - Antituberculous drugs over prolonged time
  - Vascular embolization for hemoptysis

Diagnostic Checklist
- Consider active tuberculosis infection in patients with apical consolidation ± cavitation

*(**Left**) PA chest radiograph of a 22-year-old Somalian man with cough and fever shows a left upper lobe consolidation with cavitation and an intracavitary air-fluid level ➔. Based on risk factors and imaging findings, the patient was placed on respiratory isolation. Sputum was positive for acid-fast bacilli, and M. tuberculosis was cultured. (**Right**) PA chest radiograph of a young woman with tuberculosis shows left upper lobe nodular opacities and patchy airspace disease. Antituberculous drug therapy was initiated.*

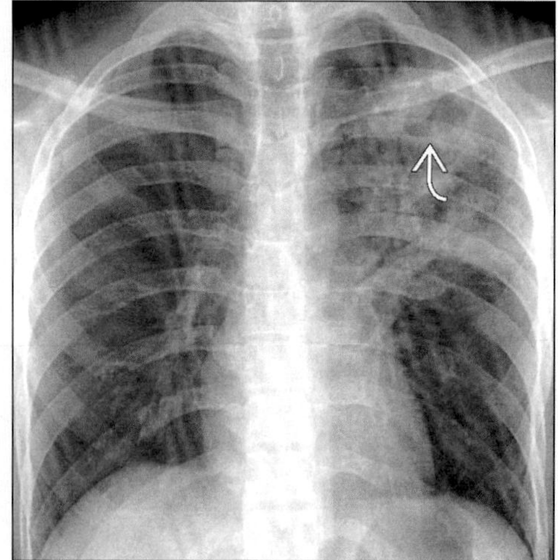

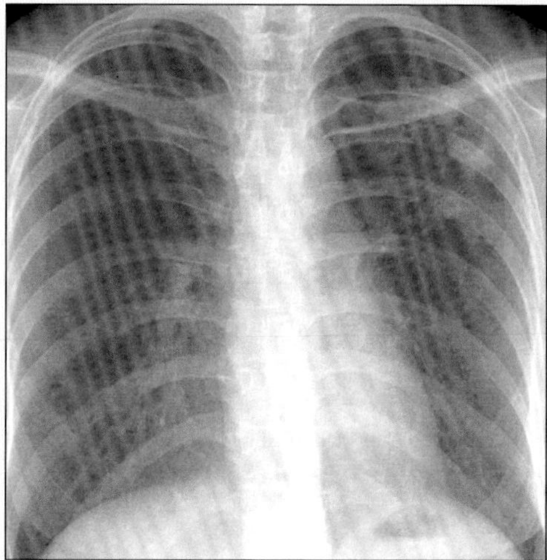

*(**Left**) PA chest radiograph of the same patient obtained 2 years later shows progression of left upper lobe nodular lesions and cavitation. The patient was noncompliant on antituberculous drug treatment. Inappropriately or incompletely treated patients may develop drug-resistant tuberculosis. (**Right**) Axial CECT of the same patient obtained after reinstitution of antituberculous drug therapy shows improving but persistent left apical nodules. In spite of improvement, activity of disease cannot be excluded.*

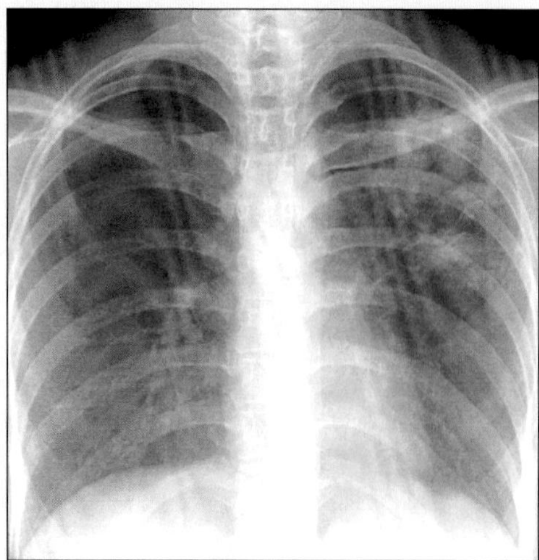

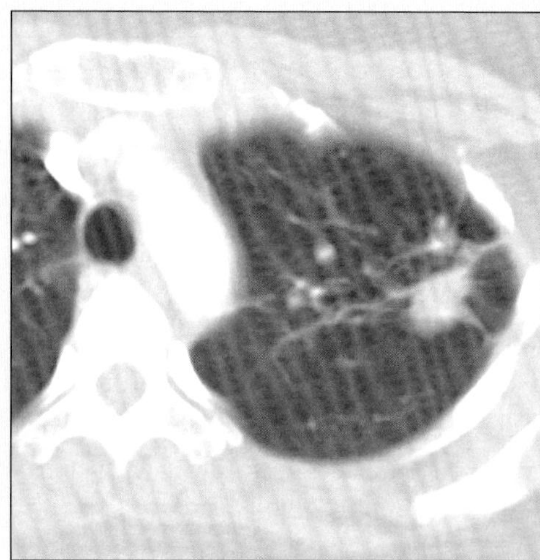

TUBERCULOSIS

TERMINOLOGY

Abbreviations

- **Tuberculosis (TB)**

Definitions

- Airborne communicable infection by inhaled bacteria
  - *Mycobacterium tuberculosis*
- Imaging patterns of TB
  - Primary pattern: Immunocompromised host
  - Post-primary pattern: Immunocompetent host

IMAGING

General Features

- Best diagnostic clue
  - Apical consolidation ± cavitation
- Location
  - Upper lobe apical/posterior segments
  - Lower lobe superior segments

Radiographic Findings

- **Primary pattern**
  - **Unilateral consolidation**
    - Middle/lower lobes, predilection for right lung
    - Segmental, lobar, multifocal
  - Unilateral **lymphadenopathy**, typically in children
    - Right hilar & paratracheal
    - Ipsilateral to lung consolidation
  - **Pleural effusion**
    - Unilateral, ipsilateral to pulmonary disease
    - Usually self-limited, resolves in several weeks
- Progressive primary pattern
  - Cavitary consolidation
  - Bronchogenic dissemination (acinar nodules)
- **Post-primary pattern**
  - Upper lobe apical/posterior segments & lower lobe superior segments, multiple segments involved
  - Poorly defined airspace disease
  - **Heterogeneous consolidation ± cavitation**
  - Pleural effusion: Small, loculated, ± calcification

CT Findings

- **Primary pattern**
  - **Consolidation**
    - Segmental, lobar, multifocal
    - Linear, nodular, mass-like components
  - **Lymphadenopathy**
    - Central low attenuation
    - Peripheral enhancing rim
- Progressive primary TB
  - Consolidation ± cavitation
  - Acute bronchogenic dissemination
- **Post-primary pattern**
  - Upper lobe predominant involvement
  - **Heterogeneous consolidation**
    - Segmental, lobar, multifocal
  - **Cavitation (45%)**
    - Thin, thick, nodular, or irregular walls
    - May exhibit air-fluid levels
    - Surrounding consolidation
  - **Bronchiolitis: Endobronchial dissemination**
    - Tree-in-bud opacities
    - Centrilobular nodules (2-4 mm)
    - Acinar nodules & lobular consolidations
  - **Airway involvement**
    - Bronchial stenosis, bronchial wall thickening
    - Associated volume loss, hyperinflation, postobstructive pneumonia
  - **Nodules (tuberculomas)**
    - Dominant lesion with satellite nodules
    - Calcification
  - Pleural effusion
    - Unilateral, small, loculated
    - Smooth pleural thickening, calcification
  - Lymphadenopathy (5%)

Complications

- **Miliary TB**
  - Radiography may be normal in early disease
  - Profuse, bilateral, well-defined nodules (2-3 mm)
  - Random distribution (hematogenous dissemination)
- **Tuberculous empyema**
  - Large to moderate loculated pleural effusion
  - Pleural calcification, enlargement of adjacent ribs
  - Enhancing thick pleura ± calcification
  - Bronchopleural fistula
    - Air-fluid levels within pleural space
  - Empyema necessitatis
    - Communication with adjacent chest wall
    - Chest wall soft tissue mass ± calcification
- **Cavitary TB**
  - **Mycetoma**
    - Soft tissue mass in dependent aspect of cavity, air crescent sign
    - May completely fill cavity or adhere to walls
    - Adjacent pleural thickening
  - **Hemoptysis**
    - Hypertrophied bronchial arteries related to cavities
    - Pulmonary artery pseudoaneurysm (Rasmussen aneurysm)
- **Acute respiratory distress syndrome (ARDS)**
  - Extensive pulmonary involvement
  - Miliary TB, diffuse endobronchial dissemination, extensive consolidation

Immunocompromised Patients

- HIV infection is potent risk factor for progression from latent TB to active TB disease
- Early HIV infection with near normal immunity
  - Post-primary pattern of TB
- **Severe immunosuppression**
  - Normal chest radiographs in 20%
  - Primary pattern of TB
    - Mediastinal & hilar lymphadenopathy in 75%
  - **Miliary TB**
  - Extrapulmonary involvement
- Highly active antiretroviral therapy (HAART)
  - Immune reconstitution inflammatory syndrome
    - Restoration of cellular inflammatory response
    - Progression of lymphadenopathy, lung disease, & pleural effusion
    - Absence of progression of mycobacterial infection

Sequelae of TB

- Pulmonary nodules (tuberculomas)
  - May exhibit calcification
- Calcified hilar/mediastinal lymph nodes
- Architectural distortion
  - Upper lobe volume loss, bronchiectasis, emphysema

TUBERCULOSIS

Imaging Recommendations

- Best imaging tool
  - Chest radiography: Detection of disease & monitoring response to therapy; **not sensitive for detection of active disease**
  - CT: Detection of **cavities & endobronchial dissemination, indicative of active TB disease**; evaluation of complications

DIFFERENTIAL DIAGNOSIS

Sarcoidosis

- End-stage disease
- Upper lobe volume loss, architectural distortion, cystic spaces

Chronic Fungal Infection

- Histoplasmosis, coccidioidomycosis
- Upper lobe fibrocavitary disease, volume loss, architectural distortion

Lung Cancer

- Predilection for upper lobes
- Irregular mass, may exhibit cavitation

PATHOLOGY

Staging, Grading, & Classification

- **TB infection**
  - **Latent TB infection**: Positive tuberculin skin test; no clinical, radiologic, or bacteriologic evidence of disease
  - **Active TB infection**: Clinical, radiologic, or bacteriologic evidence of active disease

Gross Pathologic & Surgical Features

- **Ghon focus**: Lung nodule
- **Ranke complex**: Lung nodule + ipsilateral, often calcified lymph nodes
- **Caseous necrosis**: Central necrosis with dry, cheesy appearance

Microscopic Features

- *M. tuberculosis*: Aerobic, nonmotile bacillus
  - Stains red with Ziehl-Neelsen stain
  - Acid-fast: Resists discoloration with acid alcohol
- Granulomatous infection/inflammation
  - Macrophage aggregates transform into epithelioid cells, epithelioid cells fuse to form multinucleated Langhans giant cells
  - Central necrosis, satellite granulomas

CLINICAL ISSUES

Presentation

- Most common signs/symptoms
  - Self-limited, mildly symptomatic respiratory infection, may be undiagnosed
  - Cough, pleuritic chest pain
  - Hemoptysis
  - Insidious onset & fever of unknown origin in elderly
  - Pneumonia, unresponsive to standard antibiotics
- Other signs/symptoms
  - Malaise, fever, night sweats, weight loss
  - Severe symptomatic systemic infection vs. insidious nonspecific symptoms in disseminated disease
  - Dyspnea & respiratory failure from diffuse lung involvement

Demographics

- Epidemiology
  - Leading cause of death from infection worldwide
  - U.S. 2010: 11,182 cases, 3.6 cases/100,000 persons
  - Increased susceptibility in patients with impaired cellular immunity
    - HIV infection, elderly, prisoners, congregate settings, indigent/homeless

Diagnosis

- Microscopic analysis & culture of body fluids or tissue specimens
- Isolation & culture of *M. tuberculosis*

Natural History & Prognosis

- Inhaled bacteria deposited in mid/lower lung
- Organisms ingested by macrophages & monocytes
- Lymphatic dissemination to regional lymph nodes
- Hematogenous dissemination
- Development of cell-mediated immunity & delayed hypersensitivity halts & controls organism growth
  - Positive tuberculin skin test
  - 5% risk of developing active TB within first 2 years & 10% lifetime risk of developing active TB
  - HIV-infected individuals: Up to 50% risk of active TB in first 2 years

Treatment

- Multiple antituberculous drugs administered over prolonged time
- Treatment regimens vary with drug susceptibility of organisms, imaging findings, & clinical factors
- Hemoptysis: Bronchial artery embolization or surgery
- Symptomatic TB empyema: Drainage

Prevention

- Respiratory isolation
- Identification & treatment of latent TB infection
  - Positive tuberculin skin test
  - Positive whole-blood δ-interferon release assay
  - Radiographic screening

DIAGNOSTIC CHECKLIST

Consider

- Tuberculosis in patients with apical consolidation ± cavitation

Reporting Tips

- Cavitation, bronchiolitis, & progressive consolidation consistent with active disease
- Stability over ≥ 6 months reported as stable, rather than inactive, disease

SELECTED REFERENCES

1. Jeong YJ et al: Pulmonary tuberculosis: up-to-date imaging and management. AJR Am J Roentgenol. 191(3):834-44, 2008

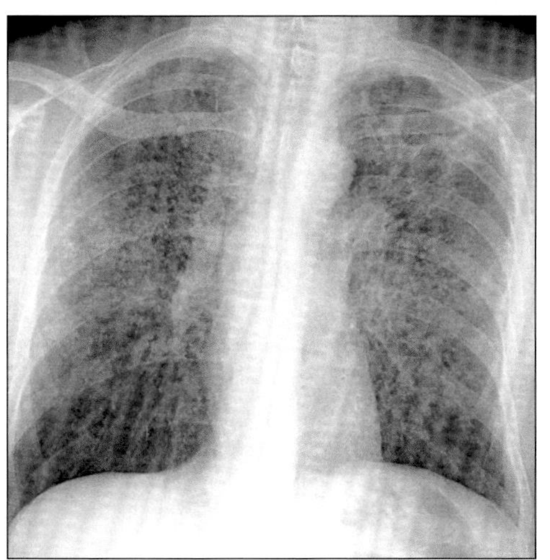

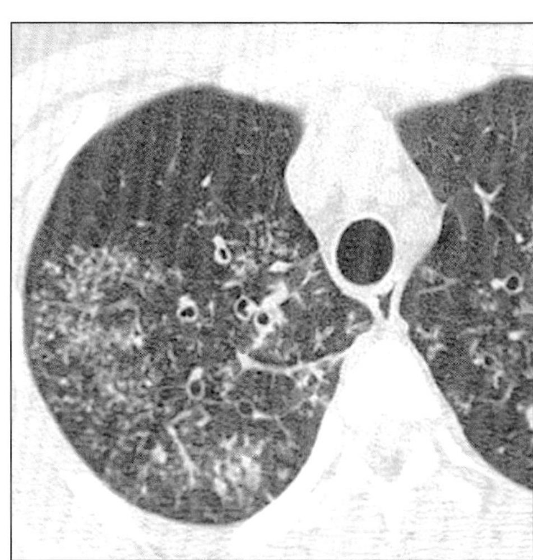

(Left) *PA chest radiograph of a 49-year-old man with active TB shows left upper lobe cavities and profuse bilateral micronodules secondary to endobronchial dissemination of pulmonary infection. Such patients are infectious and should be placed on respiratory isolation until therapy is instituted and sputum Gram stain becomes negative.* ***(Right)*** *Axial NECT of a 22-year-old indigent woman with active TB shows profuse right upper lobe centrilobular and tree-in-bud opacities and upper lobe bronchiectasis.*

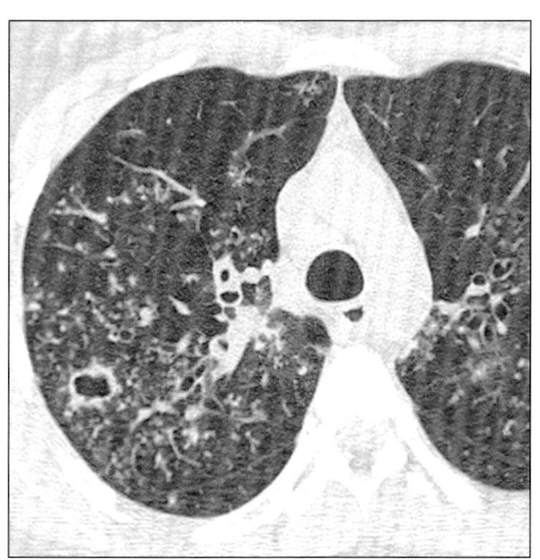

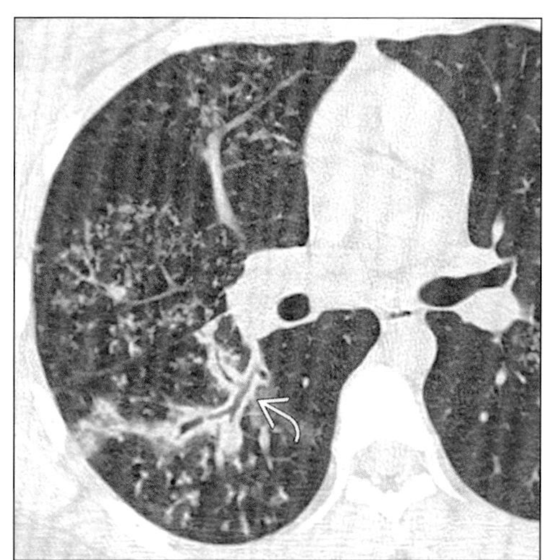

(Left) *Axial NECT of the same patient shows a right upper lobe cavity with nodular walls and surrounding bronchiolitis and tree-in-bud opacities. Although bacterial, viral, and fungal infections may produce bronchiolitis, documentation of associated cavitation is highly suggestive of TB.* ***(Right)*** *Axial NECT of the same patient shows marked right lower lobe bronchial wall thickening ➔ and bronchiolitis. Cavitation, bronchiolitis, and bronchial wall thickening on CT are consistent with active TB disease.*

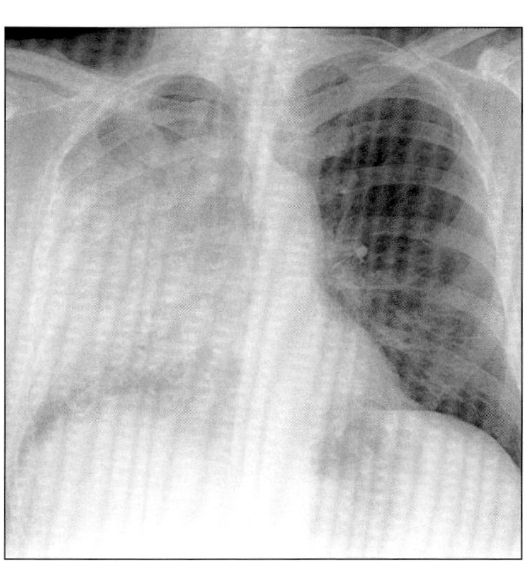

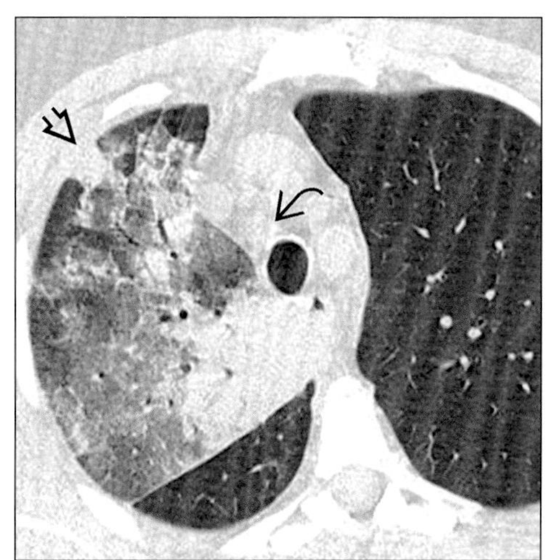

(Left) *PA chest radiograph of a febrile heroin addict shows right upper lobe consolidation with air bronchograms. The patient did not respond to antimicrobial therapy, and active TB was diagnosed on bronchoscopy.* ***(Right)*** *Axial NECT of the same patient shows a heterogeneous right upper lobe consolidation with lobular ⇨ and ground-glass opacities, as well as mediastinal lymph node enlargement ➔. The primary pattern of TB is associated with immunocompromise and does not necessarily imply initial infection.*

*(**Left**) PA chest radiograph of a Cambodian man with fever and chest pain shows a left upper lobe consolidation and left hilar and mediastinal lymphadenopathy. Consolidation associated with lymphadenopathy should suggest atypical infection, including TB. (**Right**) Composite image with axial CECT of the same patient shows left upper lobe consolidation ➔ and left hilar and mediastinal enlarged lymph nodes with central low attenuation and peripheral rim enhancement ➔, consistent with necrosis.*

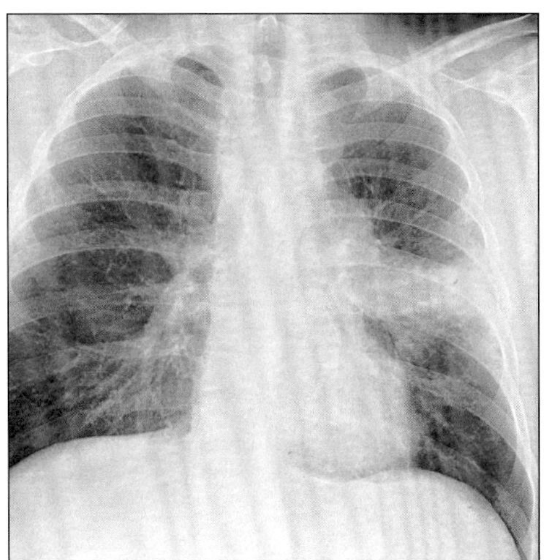

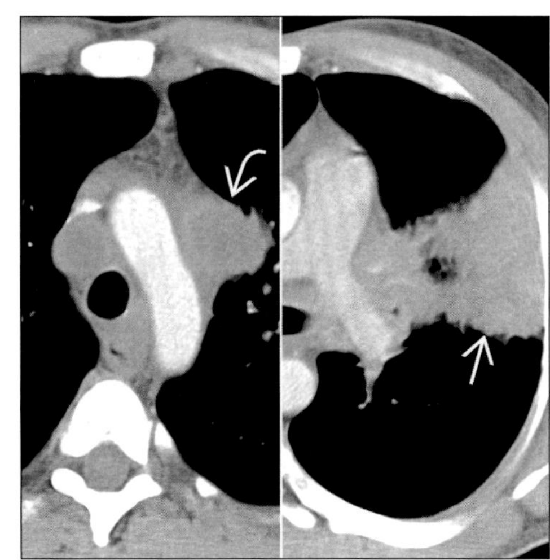

*(**Left**) Axial CECT of a 51-year-old woman status post renal transplant complicated by miliary TB shows left superior mediastinal lymphadenopathy with central low attenuation and peripheral enhancement ➔. (**Right**) Axial CECT of the same patient shows multifocal 2-3 mm randomly distributed well-defined miliary nodules that were not visible on radiography. Miliary TB typically affects immunocompromised patients and may be associated with extrapulmonary TB.*

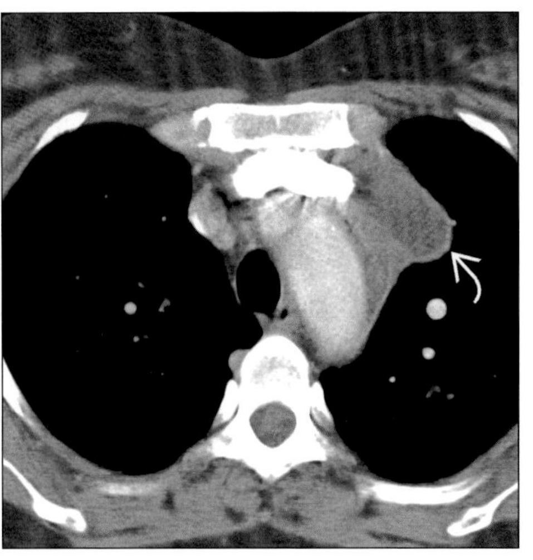

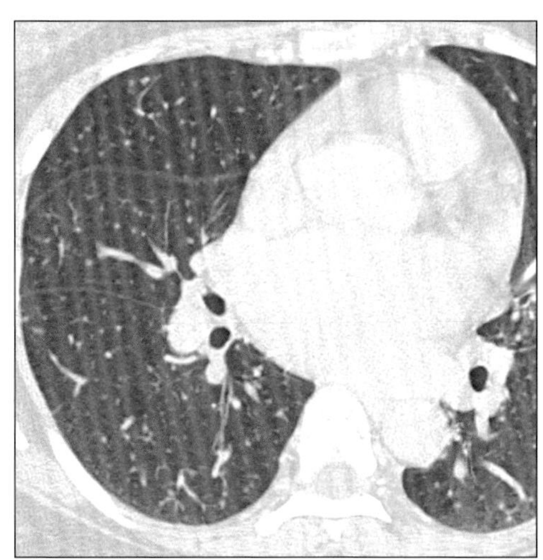

*(**Left**) PA chest radiograph of a young man with tuberculous empyema who presented with fever and left chest pain shows a loculated left pleural effusion or pleural thickening and asymmetric thickening of the adjacent left chest wall soft tissues. (**Right**) Axial CECT of the same patient shows a loculated left basilar pleural effusion with intrinsic calcification ➔ and thickening and enhancement of the pleural surfaces ➔. Note left paravertebral abscess ➔ with destruction of an adjacent rib.*

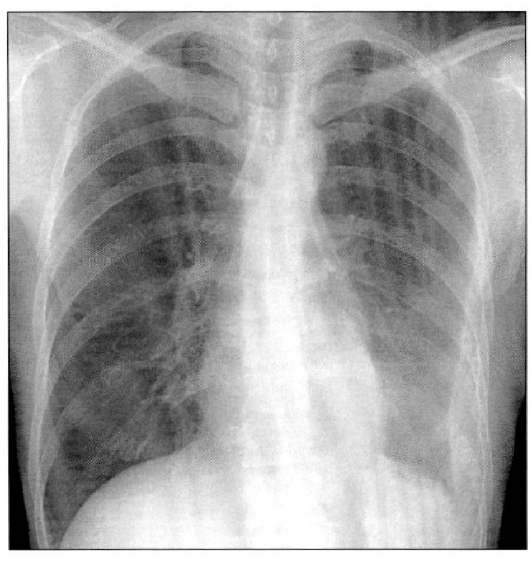

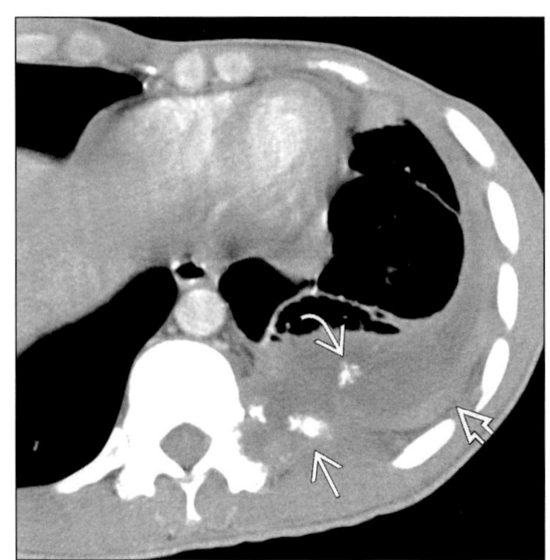

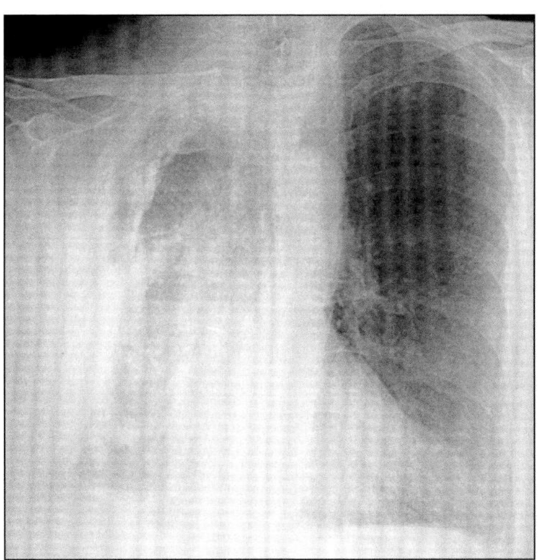

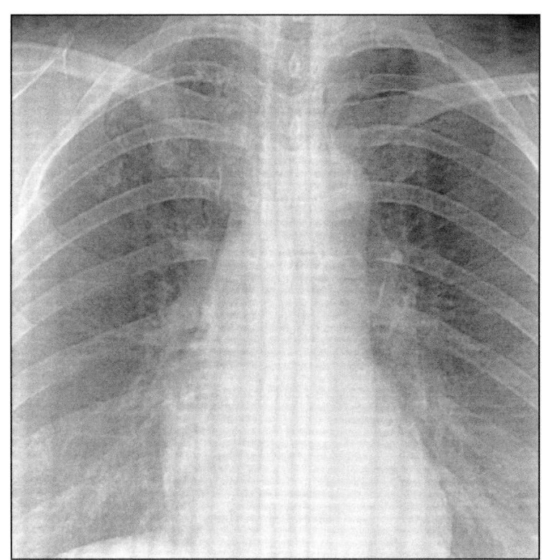

(Left) *PA chest radiograph of an asymptomatic man with prior tuberculous empyema complicated by fibrothorax shows asymmetric right lung volume loss and dense right pleural calcification. The abnormalities had been stable for years, sputum analysis was negative, and the patient had presumed inactive disease.* ***(Right)*** *PA chest radiograph of an asymptomatic 42-year-old woman with known prior tuberculosis shows stable multifocal right apical calcified lung nodules, consistent with healed tuberculomas.*

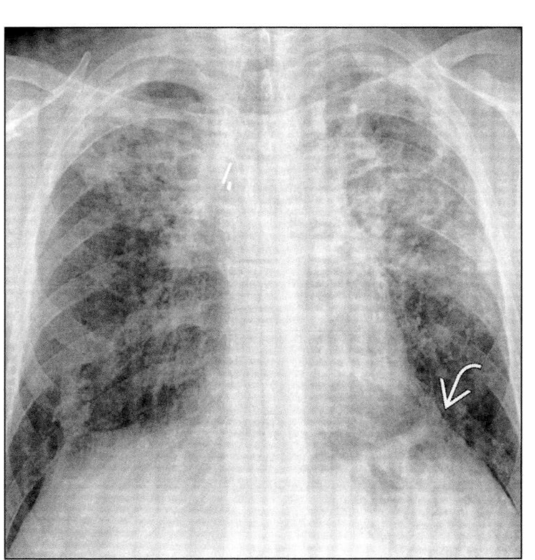

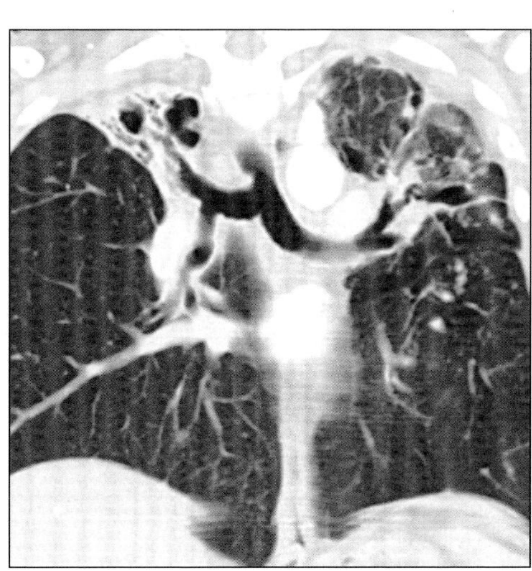

(Left) *PA chest radiograph of a 41-year-old man with active tuberculosis shows bilateral upper lobe heterogeneous consolidations, pulmonary cavities, and surrounding bronchiolitis, consistent with active disease. Note upper lobe volume loss and bilateral juxtaphrenic peaks* ➔. ***(Right)*** *Coronal CECT of a patient with sputum-negative healed tuberculosis shows bilateral upper lobe volume loss with intrinsic bronchiectasis and architectural distortion representing the sequela of prior TB.*

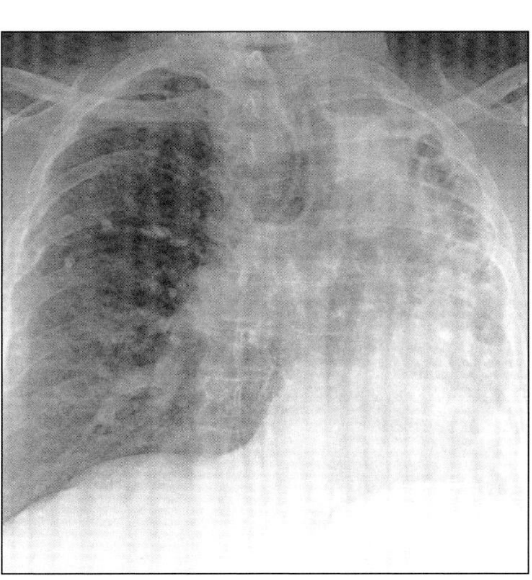

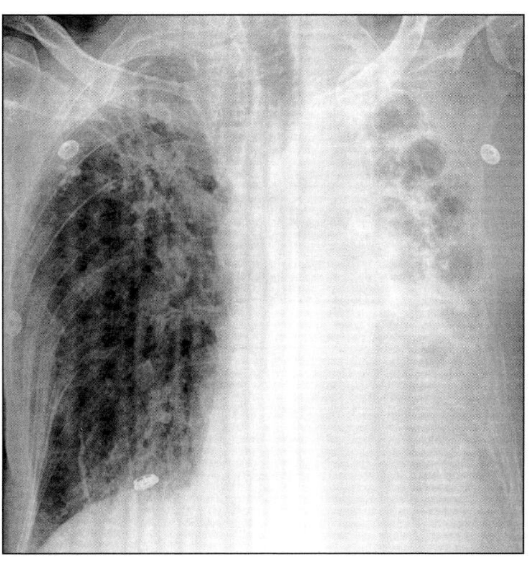

(Left) *PA chest radiograph of a sputum-negative patient with prior tuberculosis shows marked left lung volume loss with intrinsic rounded lucencies related to bronchiectasis and left tracheal and mediastinal shift. Note right lung hyperinflation and calcified tuberculomas.* ***(Right)*** *PA chest radiograph of a patient with prior plombage treatment of tuberculosis shows a virtually opaque left hemithorax with intrinsic air-containing lucite balls and right upper lobe architectural distortion and volume loss.*

NONTUBERCULOUS MYCOBACTERIAL INFECTION

Key Facts

Terminology
- Nontuberculous mycobacterial infection (NTMBI)
- *Mycobacterium avium-intracellulare complex* (MAC)
- NTMBI, most commonly caused by MAC

Imaging
- Cavitary form (classic)
  - Upper lobe thin-walled cavities, indistinguishable from TB
- Bronchiectatic form (nonclassic)
  - Middle lobe & lingular bronchiectasis, centrilobular micronodules, tree-in-bud opacities
- Nodular lesions of variable size: Miliary to 30 mm
- Immunocompromised/AIDS
  - Hilar/mediastinal lymphadenopathy, pleural effusions
- Hypersensitivity pneumonitis: Hot tub lung
  - Ill-defined centrilobular nodules, air-trapping

Top Differential Diagnoses
- Tuberculosis
- Other infections
- Lung cancer

Clinical Issues
- Cavitary form: Elderly men
  - Underlying lung disease, emphysema, pulmonary fibrosis
- Bronchiectatic form: Elderly white women
  - Lady Windermere syndrome
- Treatment
  - Multiple antimycobacterial drugs for 12-36 months; curative in up to 80%
  - AIDS, with antiretroviral treatment: 5-year survival (50%)
  - Hypersensitivity: Cessation of hot tub use, steroids, ± antimycobacterial drugs

*(**Left**) PA chest radiograph of a 35-year-old woman on azathioprine for systemic lupus erythematosus shows bilateral fibrocavitary pneumonias with volume loss and upper lobe predominance. Cultures of bronchoalveolar lavage specimens showed M. avium-intracellulare. (**Right**) Axial NECT of a patient with chronic bronchiectatic MAC infection shows bronchiectasis, tree-in-bud opacities, and hyperlucent hypoperfused lung indicating air-trapping due to small airways disease.*

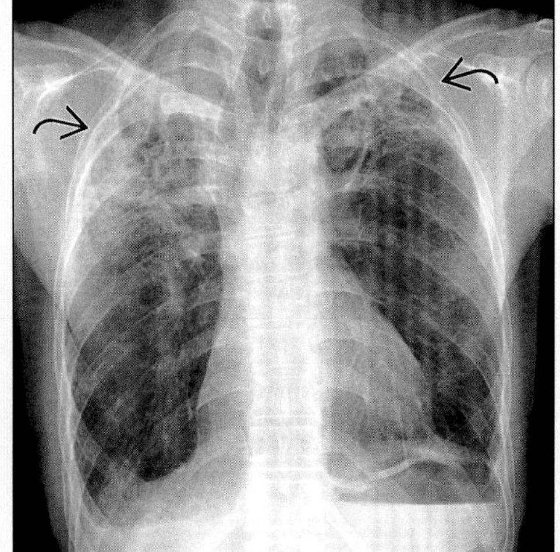

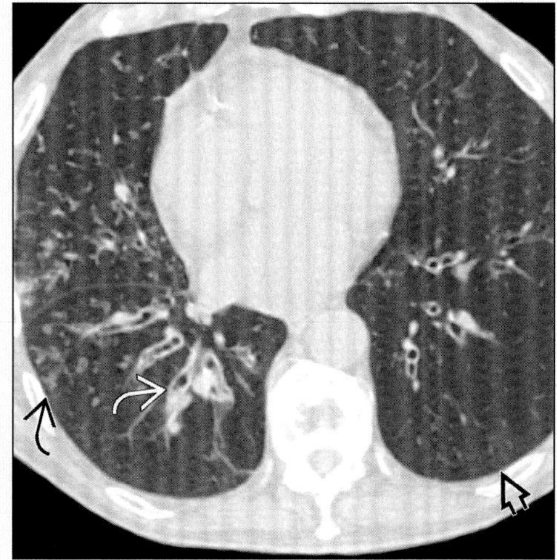

*(**Left**) Composite image with axial NECT of an asymptomatic 60-year-old man shows a right upper lobe nodule, which exhibits a tiny focus of nonspecific calcification. Fine needle aspiration biopsy specimens grew M. xenopi. (**Right**) Axial CECT of a patient with chronic lymphocytic leukemia shows diffuse bilateral miliary lung nodules secondary to disseminated M. avium-intracellulare infection. The appearance suggests hematogenous spread of infection to the lungs.*

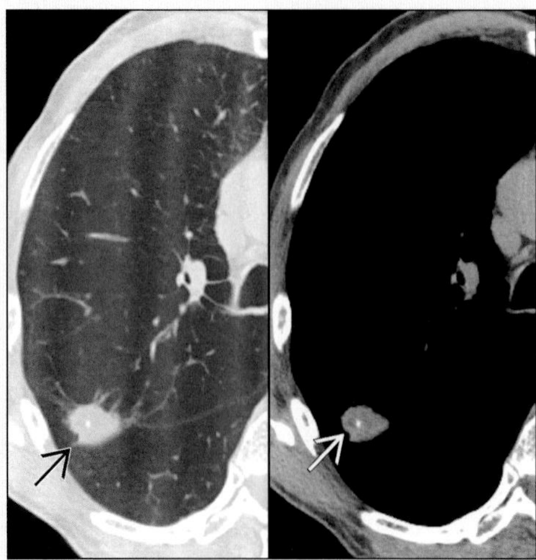

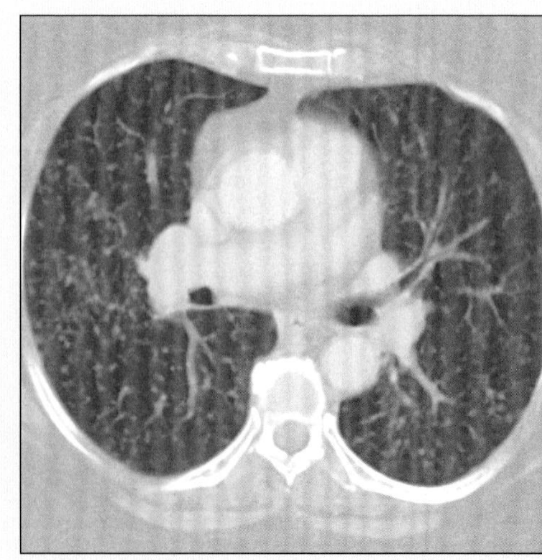

NONTUBERCULOUS MYCOBACTERIAL INFECTION

TERMINOLOGY

Abbreviations

- **Nontuberculous mycobacteria (NTM)**
- **Nontuberculous mycobacterial infection (NTMBI)**
- *Mycobacterium avium-intracellulare complex* (MAC)

Definitions

- NTMBI, most commonly caused by MAC
  - NTMBI also caused by *M. kansasii, M. xenopi, M. fortuitum, M. chelonae, M. abscessus*
- 5 types of disease
  - Cavitary form (classic)
  - Bronchiectatic form (nonclassic)
  - Solitary or multiple pulmonary nodules
  - Pneumonia in immunosuppressed host
  - Hot tub lung: Hypersensitivity pneumonitis to NTM

IMAGING

General Features

- Best diagnostic clue
  - Slowly progressive bronchiectasis, bronchiolectasis, nodules
- Location
  - Middle lobe & lingular involvement

Radiographic Findings

- Radiography
  - **Cavitary form (classic)**
    - **Upper lobe cavitary disease** (indistinguishable from tuberculosis)
      - Thin- or thick-walled cavities, usually < 3 cm
      - Upper lobe apical posterior segments, lower lobe superior segments
    - Unilateral or bilateral
    - Adjacent pleural thickening
    - Endobronchial spread of disease: Small nodules
    - Linear, nodular, or mass-like opacities
    - Volume loss & architectural distortion
  - **Bronchiectatic form (nonclassic)**
    - **Bronchiectasis & bronchial wall thickening**
    - **Scattered ill-defined reticular/nodular opacities**
    - **Middle lobe & lingula involvement**
    - Hyperinflation
  - **Nodule(s)**
    - Single or multiple, may be clustered
  - **Immunosuppressed host, AIDS**
    - Normal radiograph with positive sputum cultures (common)
    - Small scattered alveolar & nodular opacities, miliary nodules, mass-like lesions
    - Cavitation in non-AIDS immunosuppressed
    - Hilar/mediastinal lymphadenopathy & pleural effusions common; may be isolated findings
  - **Hypersensitivity pneumonitis** (hot tub lung)
    - Interstitial/nodular opacities, consolidation
    - Normal radiograph (22%)

CT Findings

- **Cavitary form (classic)**
  - Upper lobe predominance
  - **Thin-walled cavities**; thick-walled cavities less common
  - Apical pleural thickening
  - Airspace disease, consolidation, masses, nodules
  - **Bronchogenic spread**: 5-15 mm peripheral centrilobular nodules & tree-in-bud opacities
  - Bronchial wall thickening
  - Lymphadenopathy, miliary disease, & pleural effusion are uncommon
- **Bronchiectatic form (nonclassic)**
  - **Bronchiectasis mainly in middle lobe & lingula**
  - Bilateral multifocal **bronchiolitis**
    - Tree-in-bud opacities, centrilobular nodules, bronchial wall thickening, mucus plugging
  - Well-defined small peribronchial nodules
  - Consolidation, ground-glass opacities
  - Mosaic attenuation from small airways disease
  - Scarring, volume loss, architectural distortion
- **Nodule(s) of variable size**
  - **Often < 10 mm**
  - Larger nodules, mass-like lesions: 10-30 mm
  - Miliary, small or medium size
- **Immunosuppressed host, AIDS**
  - Normal or subtle pulmonary findings of scattered centrilobular nodules
  - Airspace opacification, mass-like opacities, nodules, miliary disease
  - Cavitation in immunosuppressed non-AIDS
  - Patients with AIDS: Hilar/mediastinal lymphadenopathy, central low attenuation
  - Pleural effusions
- Hypersensitivity pneumonitis
  - Diffuse centrilobular micronodules
  - Ground-glass opacities
  - Expiratory air-trapping

Imaging Recommendations

- Best imaging tool
  - CT: Superior for demonstration & assessment of cavities, nodules, bronchiolitis, bronchiectasis, lymphadenopathy
    - MAC-related airway involvement: Sensitivity (80%), specificity (87%), accuracy (86%)
- Protocol advice
  - Inspiratory & expiratory thin-section CT for assessment of small airways disease
    - Identification of mosaic attenuation &/or air-trapping

DIFFERENTIAL DIAGNOSIS

Tuberculosis

- Imaging appearance identical to classic form
- Unlike NTMBI, human-to-human transmission

Other Infections

- Cryptococcosis, sporotrichosis, nocardiosis, abscess
- Similar radiologic appearance
- Clinical presentation may suggest pathogenic etiology
  - Renal transplant recipient: *Cryptococcus, Nocardia*
  - Rose gardener: Sporotrichosis
  - Aspiration: Aerobic & anaerobic abscess

Lung Cancer

- Nodule, mass, consolidation, lymphadenopathy
- Biopsy for diagnosis

NONTUBERCULOUS MYCOBACTERIAL INFECTION

Progressive Massive Fibrosis

- History of coal or silica dust exposure
- Background of small, sometimes calcified nodules
- Lymphadenopathy with eggshell calcifications
- Masses are pancake-shaped, may cavitate

PATHOLOGY

General Features

- Etiology
  - Water is likely source of human infection
    - Inhalation, ingestion, or direct inoculation
  - Hot tub lung: Hypersensitivity reaction to NTM
- Associated abnormalities
  - Lung disease: Emphysema, chronic bronchitis, bronchiectasis, cystic fibrosis
  - Cardiac disease: Mitral valve prolapse
  - Skeletal anomalies: Pectus excavatum, mild scoliosis, straight back
  - Immunosuppressed patients
    - AIDS, rheumatoid arthritis, diabetes mellitus, alcoholism
    - Lung cancer, nonpulmonary malignancies

Gross Pathologic & Surgical Features

- MAC
  - Nonphotochromogen colonies, type III, beige or white
  - Does not change color on exposure to light
  - Low-grade pathogen, 2-4 weeks to grow in culture
- Consolidation, cavities, bronchiectasis, bronchostenosis, bronchopleural fistula, architectural distortion

Microscopic Features

- Peribronchial & peribronchiolar granulomas
- Bronchiolectasis, centrilobular bronchiolar granulomas or necrotic debris

CLINICAL ISSUES

Presentation

- Most common signs/symptoms
  - Chronic, minimally productive cough, sputum production
  - Malaise, fever, weight loss, hemoptysis
  - AIDS: Fever, sweats, weight loss, fatigue, diarrhea, shortness of breath
  - Purified protein derivative (PPD) skin test may be positive
- Other signs/symptoms
  - Cavitary form
    - Elderly white men
    - Underlying lung disease, emphysema, pulmonary fibrosis
  - Bronchiectatic form
    - Infection ± preexisting lung disease
    - Lady Windermere syndrome
      - Middle lobe & lingular volume loss & bronchiectasis
      - Almost exclusively in elderly white women
      - Nonsmokers
      - Immunocompetent
      - Chronic pulmonary MAC infection
      - No underlying lung disease other than nodular bronchiectatic disease
  - Immunosuppressed, AIDS
    - Infection with CD4(+) lymphocyte count of < 50 cells per μL
    - Disseminated disease (uncommon, 2%)
  - Hot tub lung
    - Hypersensitivity pneumonitis
    - Hot tub use, aerosolized water in showers

Demographics

- Age
  - Many infected patients are > 50 years
- Gender
  - Classic infection: Primarily men
  - Bronchiectatic form: Primarily women
- Ethnicity
  - More common in whites, excluding patients with AIDS
- Epidemiology
  - Ubiquitous throughout environment
  - Water, soil, milk, fish, birds, animals
  - Common infection in southeast United States
  - No human-to-human transmission

Diagnosis

- Diagnosis by isolation from 2 separate sputum samples, transbronchial or open lung biopsy specimens
- AIDS patients: Positive sputum or bronchoalveolar lavage fluid cultures diagnostic of infection

Natural History & Prognosis

- Slowly progressive radiographic abnormalities
  - Localized disease may involve other lobes & contralateral lung
  - Progressive fibrosis with volume loss & traction bronchiectasis
- Mycetomas may form in residual cavities
- Bronchopleural fistula
- Death from respiratory failure (uncommon)
- AIDS, with antiretroviral treatment: 5-year survival (50%)

Treatment

- Multiple antimycobacterial drugs for 12-36 months
  - Curative in up to 80%
- Surgery for localized disease, followed by antimycobacterial drugs
- Hypersensitivity pneumonitis: Cessation of hot tub use, steroids, ± antimycobacterial drugs

SELECTED REFERENCES

1. Martinez S et al: The many faces of pulmonary nontuberculous mycobacterial infection. AJR Am J Roentgenol. 189(1):177-86, 2007
2. Hanak V et al: Hot tub lung: presenting features and clinical course of 21 patients. Respir Med. 100(4):610-5, 2006
3. Jeong YJ et al: Nontuberculous mycobacterial pulmonary infection in immunocompetent patients: comparison of thin-section CT and histopathologic findings. Radiology. 231(3):880-6, 2004

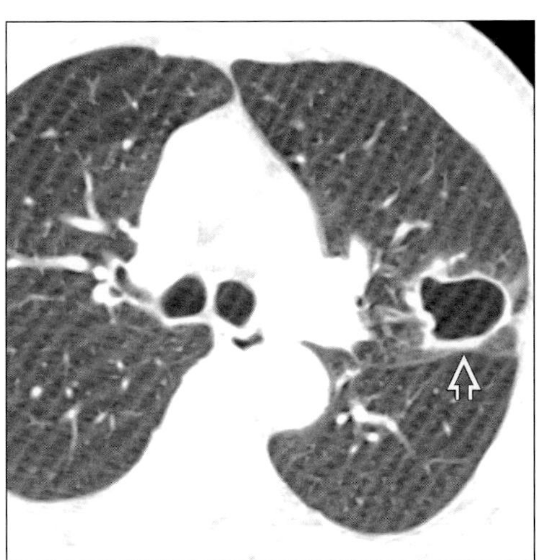

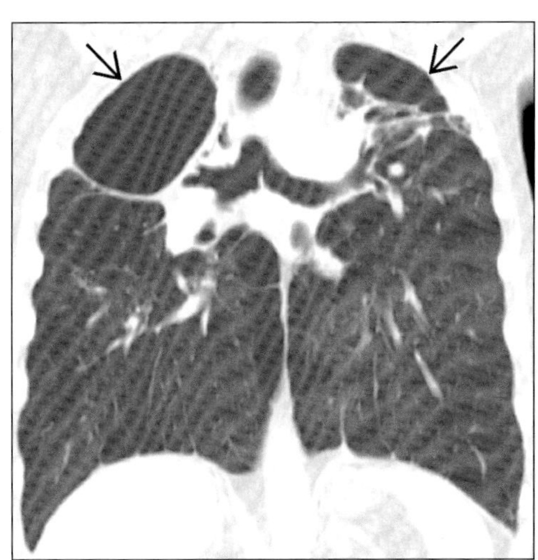

(Left) *Axial NECT of a patient who presented with cough shows a solitary left upper lobe cavity with variable wall thickness ➡. Culture of bronchoscopy specimens confirmed M. avium-intracellulare infection.* **(Right)** *Coronal NECT of a patient with chronic emphysema shows bilateral upper lobe cavitary disease → with severe upper lobe volume loss, hilar retraction, and architectural distortion. Repeated cultures were positive for M. chelonae.*

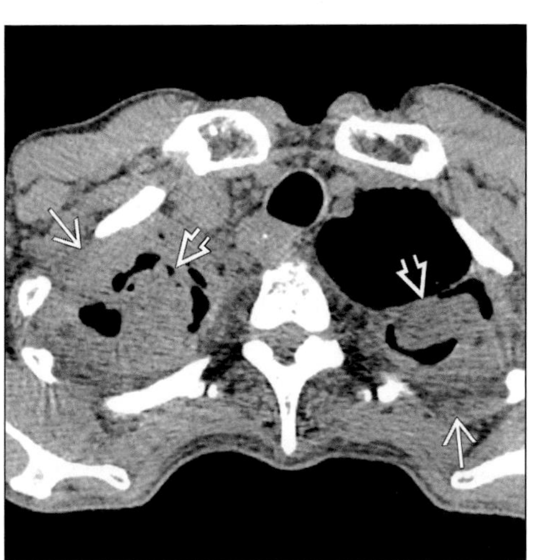

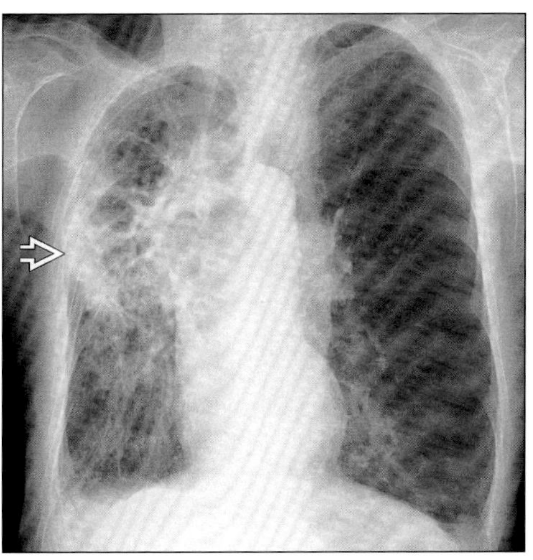

(Left) *Axial NECT of a 62-year-old man with chronic M. kansasii pulmonary infection shows large mycetomas ➡ manifesting as soft tissue masses within biapical lung cavities. Note thick cavity wall, adjacent pleural thickening, and extrapleural fat edema ➡ (the result of active infection).* **(Right)** *PA chest radiograph of a 60-year-old man with emphysema shows a small right lung and severe ipsilateral fibrocavitary lung disease ➡ due to chronic MAC infection, indistinguishable from tuberculosis.*

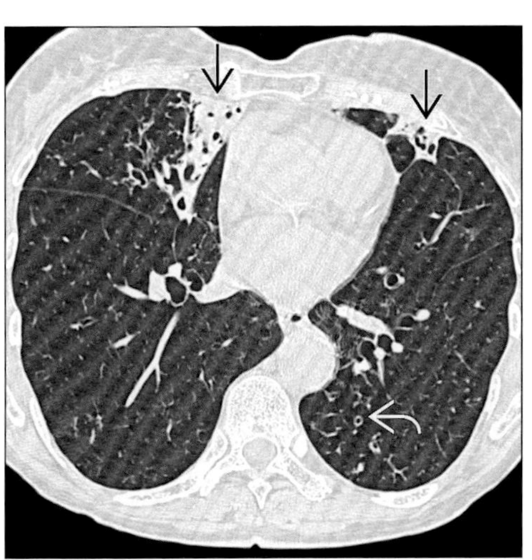

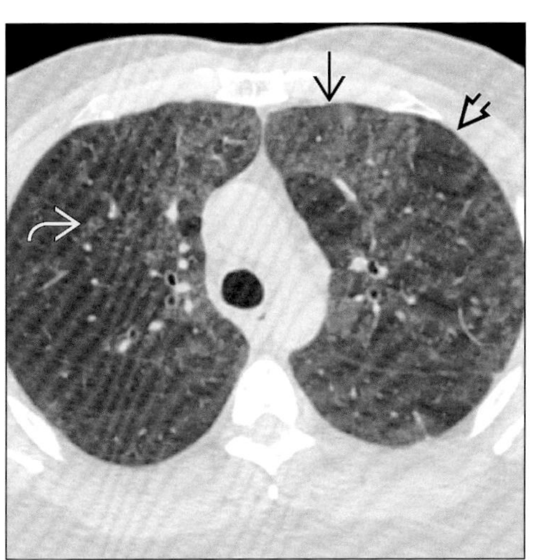

(Left) *Axial HRCT of a 75-year-old woman with the bronchiectatic form of NTMBI shows middle lobe and lingular volume loss, bronchiectasis, and bronchial wall thickening →, with milder bronchiectasis in the left lower lobe ➡.* **(Right)** *Axial NECT of a patient with hot tub lung from hypersensitivity to M. avium-intracellulare shows mosaic attenuation with geographic regions of ground-glass opacity → and ground-glass nodules ➡. Hyperlucent lung ➡ and air-trapping indicate small airways disease.*

MYCOPLASMA PNEUMONIA

Key Facts

Terminology

- Pneumonia caused by *Mycoplasma pneumoniae*
  - Most common atypical community-acquired pneumonia of children & young adults

Imaging

- Radiography
  - Unilateral or bilateral patchy consolidation
  - Nodular or reticular opacities, resembling interstitial process
  - Pleural effusion (small)
- CT
  - Patchy consolidation
  - Ground-glass opacities
  - Centrilobular nodules
  - Bronchial wall thickening
  - Tree-in-bud opacities
  - Regional lymphadenopathy

Top Differential Diagnoses

- Community-acquired pneumonia
- Cryptogenic organizing pneumonia

Pathology

- Small bacterium in class of Mollicutes
- Lacks peptidoglycan cell wall: Resistance to penicillins & other β-lactam antibiotics

Clinical Issues

- Signs and symptoms
  - Fever, malaise
  - Cough with minimal sputum
  - Bullous myringitis
- Spread through respiratory droplets
- Treatment
  - Macrolides, quinolones
  - Supportive measures

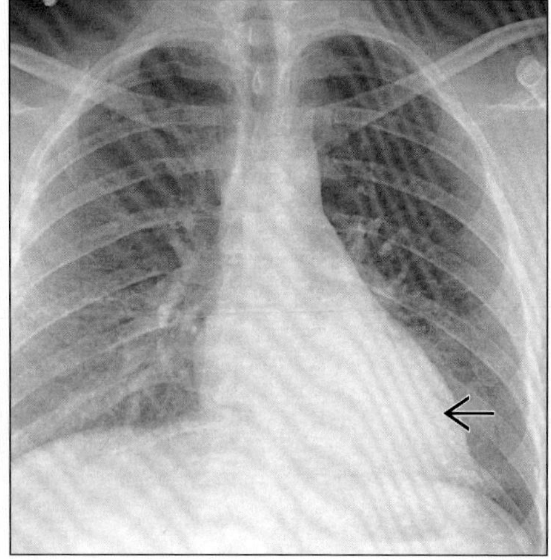

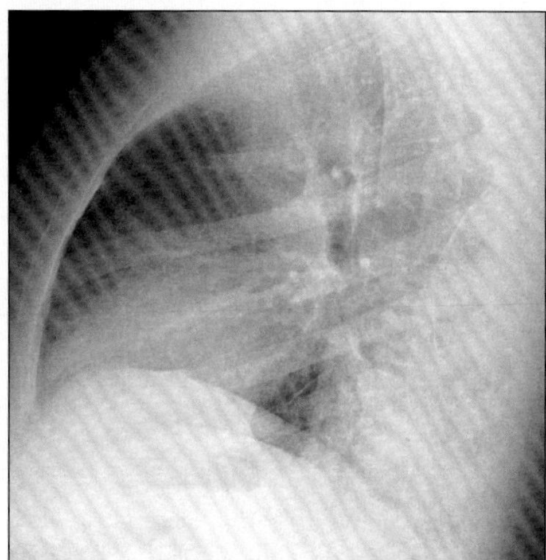

(Left) *PA chest radiograph of a 19-year-old patient who presented with fever, cough, and headache shows a retrocardiac consolidation* → *that obscures the left paraaortic interface, consistent with left lower lobe pneumonia.* ***(Right)*** *Lateral chest radiograph of the same patient confirms a left lower lobe consolidation. Sputum Mycoplasma pneumoniae PCR was positive. Mycoplasma is a common cause of community-acquired pneumonia in young adults.*

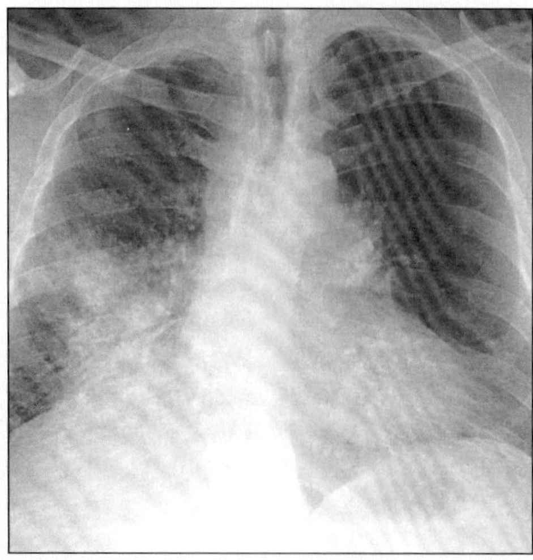

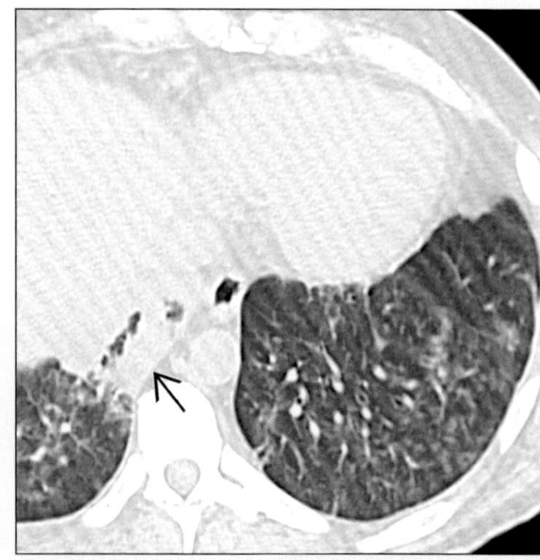

(Left) *PA chest radiograph of a patient who presented with fever and cough shows patchy consolidations in the right mid and lower lung zones and reticulonodular opacities in the left lower lung.* ***(Right)*** *Axial NECT of the same patient shows a right lower lobe confluent consolidation* → *and extensive bilateral lower lobe centrilobular nodules and tree-in-bud opacities. The sputum M. pneumoniae PCR test was positive. Mycoplasma pneumonia has a predilection for involving the lower lobes.*

MYCOPLASMA PNEUMONIA

TERMINOLOGY

Definitions

- Pneumonia caused by *Mycoplasma pneumoniae*
- Most common atypical community-acquired pneumonia of children & young adults

IMAGING

General Features

- Location
  - Lower lobe predominance

Radiographic Findings

- Unilateral or bilateral patchy consolidation
- Nodular or reticular opacities, resembling interstitial process
- Pleural effusion (small)

CT Findings

- **Patchy consolidation**
- **Ground-glass opacities**
  - Multifocal
  - Centrilobular or peribronchovascular distribution
- **Centrilobular nodules**
- Bronchial wall thickening
- Tree-in-bud opacities
- Regional lymphadenopathy
- Complications
  - Pericarditis
    - Pericardial effusion
    - Pericardial thickening
  - Swyer-James-McLeod syndrome
    - Typically as sequela of childhood infection
    - Mosaic attenuation, air-trapping
    - Bronchiectasis

Imaging Recommendations

- Best imaging tool
  - Chest radiography is usually sufficient for detection of pneumonia and monitoring response to treatment

DIFFERENTIAL DIAGNOSIS

Community-acquired Pneumonia

- Lobular distribution of ground-glass opacities; centrilobular nodules more common in *M. pneumoniae* than in other bacterial pneumonias
- Mycoplasma pneumonia has more gradual onset of symptoms

Idiopathic Pulmonary Hemorrhage

- Clinical history of hemoptysis, bleeding diathesis, or coagulopathy
- Diffuse bilateral airspace disease

Cryptogenic Organizing Pneumonia

- Clinical & imaging findings may be similar to those of *Mycoplasma* pneumonia
- Infection must be excluded as cause

PATHOLOGY

Gross Pathologic & Surgical Features

- Edema & inflammatory cellular infiltrate in alveolar septa & peribronchovascular interstitium
- Extension into adjacent parenchyma leads to peribronchiolar inflammation & consolidation

Microscopic Features

- Small bacterium in class of Mollicutes
  - Lacks peptidoglycan cell wall
    - Resistance to penicillins & other β-lactam antibiotics
  - Smallest free-living organisms

CLINICAL ISSUES

Presentation

- Most common signs/symptoms
  - Fever, malaise
  - Cough with minimal sputum
  - Headache
  - Sore throat
- Other signs/symptoms
  - Erythematous tympanic membranes or bullous myringitis
  - Myalgia or arthralgia
  - Stevens-Johnson syndrome
    - Skin rash
    - Stomatitis
    - Ophthalmia
  - Exacerbation of asthma symptoms

Demographics

- Age
  - Children & young adults
- Epidemiology
  - Outbreaks can occur in schools, homeless shelters, or military recruits
  - Causes up to 15-50% of pneumonia in school-age children & young adults
  - Most frequently during fall & winter

Natural History & Prognosis

- Spread through respiratory droplets
- 10-20 day incubation period

Treatment

- Antibiotics
  - Macrolides
  - Quinolones
- Supportive measures
  - Nonsteroidal anti-inflammatory drugs (NSAID), acetaminophen

SELECTED REFERENCES

1. Reynolds JH et al: Pneumonia in the immunocompetent patient. Br J Radiol. 83(996):998-1009, 2010
2. Lee I et al: Mycoplasma pneumoniae pneumonia: CT features in 16 patients. Eur Radiol. 16(3):719-25, 2006

INFLUENZA PNEUMONIA

Key Facts

Terminology
- Lower respiratory tract viral infection
- Influenza A: Avian flu H5N1
- Swine flu: H1N1

Imaging
- Radiography
  - Interstitial opacities
  - Nodular opacities
  - Extensive airspace disease from hemorrhagic edema
  - Acute pneumonia with rapid progression to ARDS
- CT
  - Mosaic attenuation
  - Ground-glass opacity & consolidation
  - Nodules: Centrilobular, 1-10 mm
  - Tree-in-bud opacities
- HRCT: Expiratory air-trapping

Top Differential Diagnoses
- Mycoplasma pneumonia

Pathology
- Airway epithelial necrosis, submucosal chronic inflammation
- Nucleic acid amplification tests, improved virus detection

Clinical Issues
- Symptoms/signs
  - Often confined to upper respiratory tract
  - Dry cough, rhinorrhea, sore throat
- Most viral pneumonias in immunocompetent adults
- Seasonal upper respiratory tract infections

Diagnostic Checklist
- Imaging features cannot enable prediction of etiologic agent

__(Left)__ AP chest radiograph of a 61-year-old man with chronic lymphocytic leukemia who presented with cough and dyspnea shows bilateral asymmetric patchy airspace and interstitial opacities more pronounced in the right lung. __(Right)__ Axial CECT of the same patient shows tree-in-bud opacities ➘, centrilobular nodules, and a right lower lobe consolidation ⇨ associated with small bilateral pleural effusions. The patient succumbed 1 week later to ARDS, a complication of influenza A pneumonia.

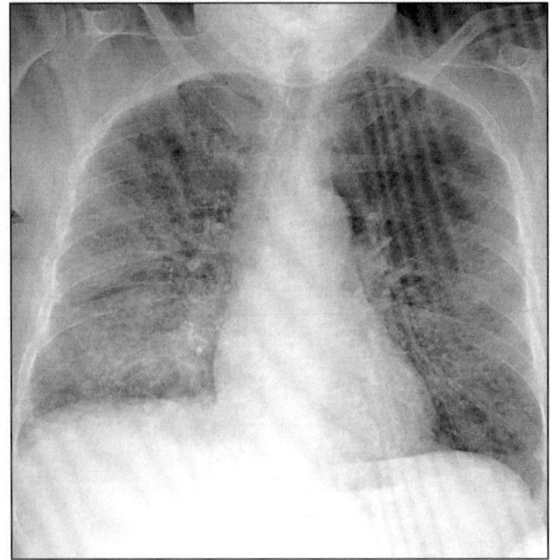

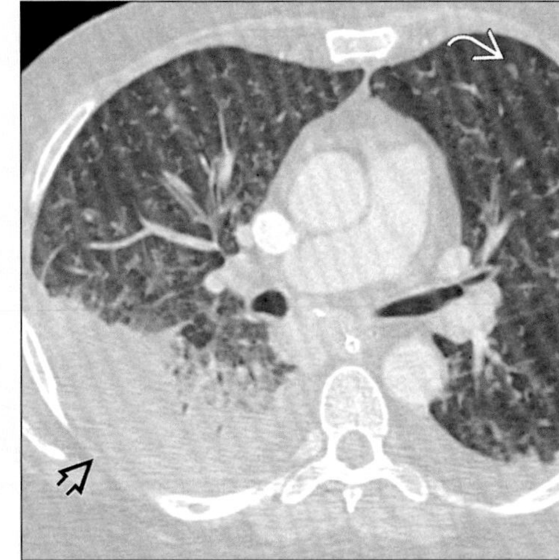

__(Left)__ Axial CECT of a 71-year-old man who presented with dyspnea shows right lower lobe ground-glass opacities and consolidation ➔ without evidence of pleural effusion. Similar opacities were present in the left lower lobe (not shown). The patient was diagnosed with H1N1 influenza infection. __(Right)__ Axial CECT of a 75-year-old woman diagnosed with influenza A pneumonia shows geographic regions of patchy ground-glass opacity ➘, which are nonspecific findings of multifocal pneumonia.

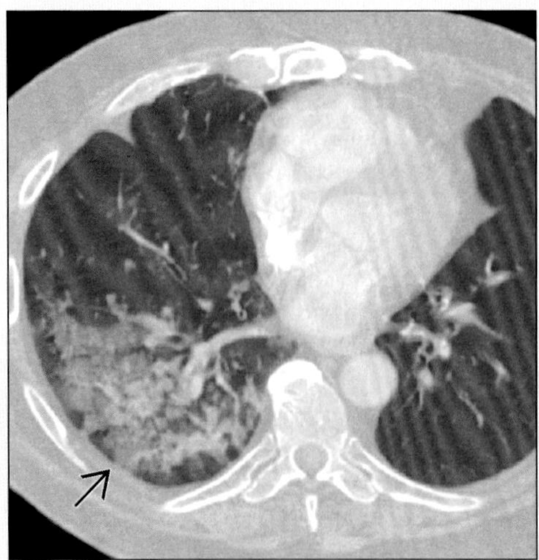

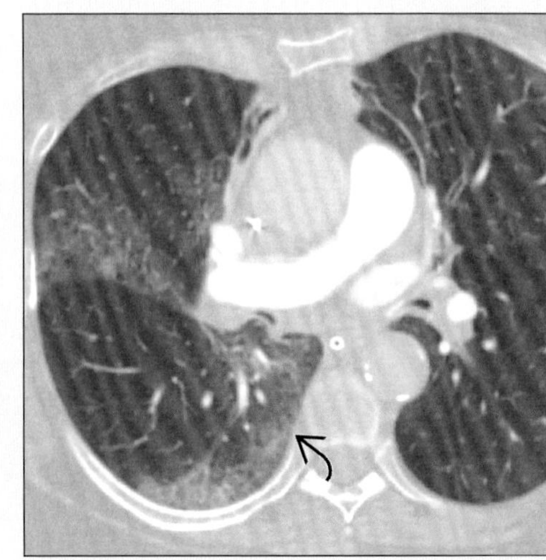

INFLUENZA PNEUMONIA

TERMINOLOGY

Synonyms

- Influenza A: Avian flu H5N1, swine flu H1N1

Definitions

- Lower respiratory tract viral infection

IMAGING

General Features

- Location
  - Unilateral or bilateral
- Size
  - Patchy areas of consolidation
- Morphology
  - Lobar consolidation uncommon

Radiographic Findings

- Radiography
  - Interstitial opacities
  - Nodular opacities, "patchwork quilt" pattern of bronchopneumonia
    - 1-2 cm patchy areas of consolidation
  - Extensive airspace disease due to hemorrhagic edema
  - Cavity formation suggests superinfection with *Staphylococcus* organisms
  - Small pleural effusions (rare); usually represent superimposed bacterial infection
  - Acute pneumonia with rapid progression to ARDS

CT Findings

- NECT
  - Mosaic attenuation: Patchy heterogeneous lung attenuation
    - Lucent lung due to small airways disease with air-trapping & hypoperfusion
    - Opacified lung due to redistribution of flow & pneumonia
  - Lobular ground-glass opacity & consolidation: Patchy, poorly defined bronchopneumonia or focal well-defined lobar pneumonia
  - Nodules & tree-in-bud opacities: 1-10 mm, centrilobular, dense or ground-glass nodules
  - H5N1 infection
    - Focal, multifocal, or diffuse ground-glass opacities or consolidation
    - Pseudocavitation, cavitation, pneumatoceles, pleural effusion, lymphadenopathy
  - H1N1 infection
    - Ground-glass opacities & consolidations
    - Predominant peribronchovascular & subpleural distribution
- HRCT
  - Hypoperfused lung shows expiratory air-trapping

Imaging Recommendations

- Best imaging tool
  - Radiography: Detection of disease, assessment of extent of involvement, monitoring response to treatment, for intervention guidance

DIFFERENTIAL DIAGNOSIS

Mycoplasma Pneumonia

- Segmental peribronchial patchy opacities, similar to viral pneumonias; less symptomatic than expected for extent of radiographic disease
- Seasonal: Spring & fall

PATHOLOGY

General Features

- Diffuse epithelial infection

Microscopic Features

- Airway epithelial necrosis, submucosal chronic inflammation
- Necrotizing bronchitis &/or bronchiolitis
- Diffuse alveolar damage, hemorrhage

Laboratory Identification

- Single-stranded RNA viruses, Orthomyxoviridae family
- Viral culture results in 3-14 days
- Nucleic acid amplification tests, improved ability to detect viruses; H5N1, H1N1, reverse transcriptase PCR

CLINICAL ISSUES

Presentation

- Most common signs/symptoms
  - Often confined to upper respiratory tract with dry cough, rhinorrhea, sore throat
  - **Influenza syndrome**: Abrupt fever, headache, myalgias, malaise

Demographics

- Age
  - Infants to elderly
- Epidemiology
  - Severe pneumonia
    - Infants with influenza A infection
    - Immunocompromised, including solid organ transplant recipients

Natural History & Prognosis

- Influenza accounts for most viral pneumonias in immunocompetent adults
- Seasonal upper respiratory tract infections, periodic & unpredictable pandemics
- Lower respiratory tract infections in 10% of cases
- H5N1 avian flu, 60% mortality

DIAGNOSTIC CHECKLIST

Image Interpretation Pearls

- Imaging features cannot enable prediction of etiologic agent

SELECTED REFERENCES

1. Franquet T: Imaging of pulmonary viral pneumonia. Radiology. 260(1):18-39, 2011
2. Shiley KT et al: Chest CT features of community-acquired respiratory viral infections in adult inpatients with lower respiratory tract infections. J Thorac Imaging. 25(1):68-75, 2010

CYTOMEGALOVIRUS PNEUMONIA

Key Facts

Terminology

- Cytomegalovirus (CMV)
- CMV pneumonia is serious cause of mortality & morbidity in immunocompromised adults
- Severe viral community-acquired pneumonia in immunocompetent adults

Imaging

- Radiography
  - Bilateral patchy or diffuse opacities
  - Small or large lung nodules
  - Pulmonary consolidation
  - Pleural effusion
- CT
  - Pulmonary consolidation
  - Patchy or diffuse ground-glass opacities
  - Small nodules in random distribution
  - Tree-in-bud opacities

Top Differential Diagnoses

- *Pneumocystis jiroveci* pneumonia
- Drug reaction
- Viral pneumonia
- Lung transplant rejection

Clinical Issues

- Symptoms/signs
  - Fever, dyspnea
- Treatment
  - Ganciclovir, valganciclovir, foscarnet
  - Correction of underlying immunosuppression
- Mortality > 50% in immunocompromised host
- Good prognosis in immunocompetent host

Diagnostic Checklist

- Consider CMV pneumonia in immunocompromised patients with diffuse pulmonary abnormalities

__(Left)__ AP chest radiograph of a patient with acute myeloid leukemia and neutropenic fever shows bilateral symmetrical reticulonodular opacities, later confirmed to represent CMV pneumonia. __(Right)__ Axial CECT of the same patient shows bilateral patchy ground-glass and nodular ➚ opacities and small bilateral pleural effusions. CMV pneumonia usually affects immunocompromised patients, but may also cause a severe community-acquired pneumonia in immunocompetent adults.

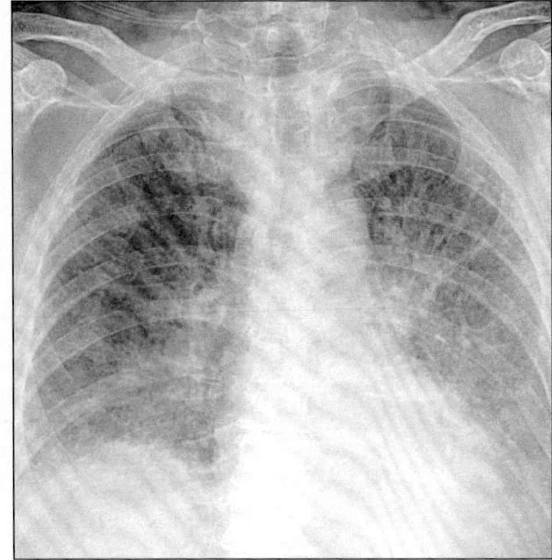

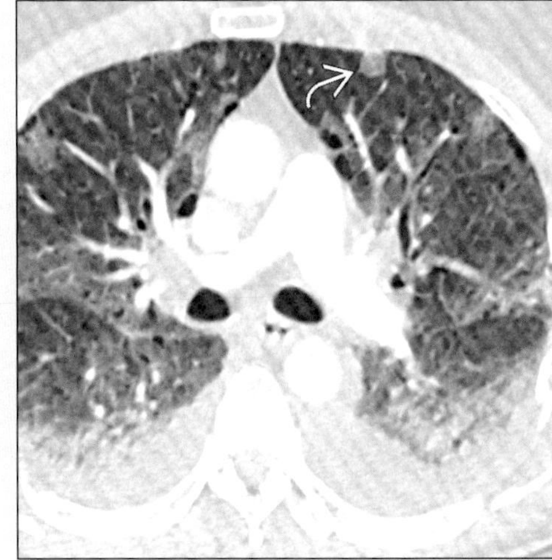

__(Left)__ PA chest radiograph of a patient who presented with dyspnea 3 months after a hematopoietic stem cell transplantation shows bilateral diffuse hazy opacities. __(Right)__ Axial NECT of same patient shows bilateral symmetrical diffuse ground-glass opacities. CMV pneumonia was confirmed by bronchoalveolar lavage. Hematopoietic stem cell transplant recipients are particularly susceptible to CMV infection 30-100 days post transplant. Ground-glass opacities are a common manifestation of CMV pneumonia.

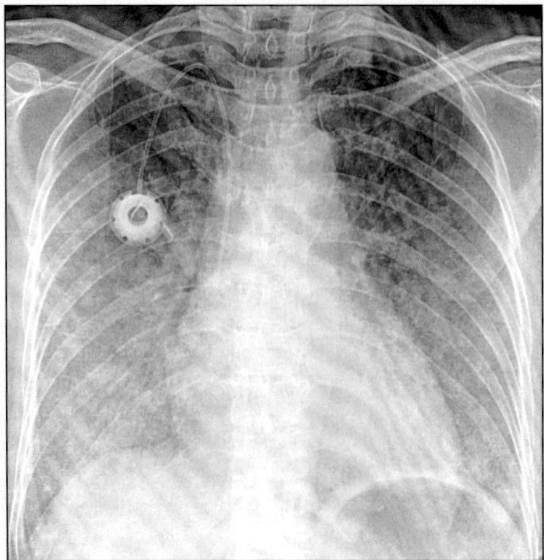

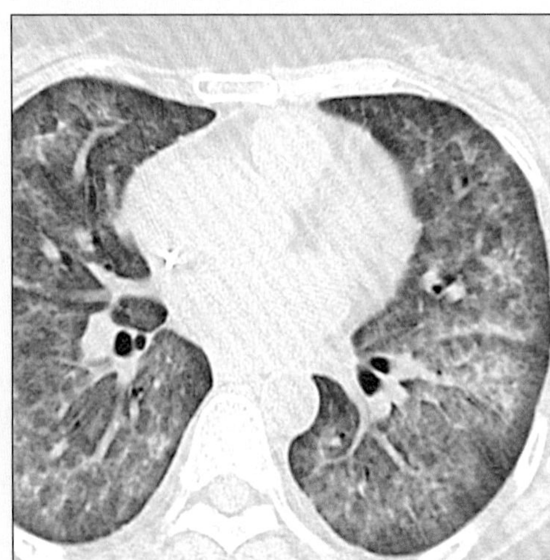

CYTOMEGALOVIRUS PNEUMONIA

TERMINOLOGY

Abbreviations

- Cytomegalovirus (CMV)

Synonyms

- Formerly known as human herpesvirus 5 (HHV-5)

Definitions

- **Cytomegalovirus**
  - Member of herpesvirus family
  - Variety of disease manifestations
- CMV pneumonia is serious cause of mortality & morbidity in immunocompromised adults
  - Patients with AIDS
  - Allogeneic stem cell transplant recipients
  - Solid organ transplant recipients
- CMV pneumonia
  - Severe viral community-acquired pneumonia in immunocompetent adults

IMAGING

General Features

- Location
  - Diffuse or lower lung zone predominance

Radiographic Findings

- Bilateral patchy or diffuse opacities
  - Ground-glass &/or reticular patterns
- Small or large lung nodules
- Bronchial wall thickening
- Pulmonary consolidation
  - Segmental or lobar
- Pleural effusion

CT Findings

- Pulmonary consolidation
  - May be mass-like
- Ground-glass opacities
  - Patchy
  - Diffuse
- Nodules < 10 mm
  - Random or subpleural distribution
  - ± ground-glass opacity halo
  - Bilateral, symmetric, diffuse distribution
- Tree-in-bud opacities
- Interlobular septal thickening
- Bronchial wall thickening
- Traction bronchiectasis
- Pleural effusion

Imaging Recommendations

- Best imaging tool
  - Chest radiograph is typically used for initial evaluation
  - CT is indicated if radiograph is negative, particularly in evaluation of immunocompromised patients
    - Guides bronchoscopic or surgical biopsy

DIFFERENTIAL DIAGNOSIS

Pneumocystis jiroveci Pneumonia (PCP)

- CMV present in lungs of approximately 75% of patients with HIV & PCP
- Presence of CMV in patients with HIV infection & PCP does not indicate causal role of CMV in patient pneumonia
- If PCP is treated, respiratory symptoms usually resolve without anti-CMV therapy
- CMV more likely if nodules or masses present on CT

Drug Reaction

- May exhibit diffuse or patchy ground-glass opacities

Decompensation of Preexisting Interstitial Lung Disease (ILD)

- New opacities in patients with ILD on immunosuppressive therapy
  - Exacerbation of ILD
  - Pulmonary infection

Viral Pneumonia

- Influenza, adenovirus, & CMV may exhibit similar clinical & imaging findings
- CMV, unlike influenza, is not seasonal

Lung Transplant Rejection

- CMV & lung transplant rejection have similar clinical presentation
  - Low-grade fever
  - Dyspnea
  - Cough
- Time course of symptoms is helpful
  - Acute rejection more likely < 2 weeks after transplantation
  - CMV pneumonia usually occurs in first 3 months after discontinuation of CMV prophylaxis

PATHOLOGY

Microscopic Features

- Interstitial mononuclear infiltrate with foci of necrosis
- Enlarged infected cells with intranuclear & cytoplasmic inclusion bodies
- ± associated organizing pneumonia or diffuse alveolar damage

CLINICAL ISSUES

Presentation

- Most common signs/symptoms
  - Fever
  - Dyspnea
- Other signs/symptoms
  - Elevated lactate dehydrogenase (LDH) level
  - Leukopenia
  - Atypical lymphocytes
  - Thrombocytopenia
  - Hypoxemia

Demographics

- Epidemiology
  - 50-100% of adults have serum anti-CMV antibodies, suggesting exposure
  - Virus remains latent within leukocytes in seropositive asymptomatic individuals
- CMV pneumonia in immunocompromised hosts
  - **Recipients of solid organ transplant**

CYTOMEGALOVIRUS PNEUMONIA

    - CMV from seropositive donors or de novo infection more serious than reactivation of latent infection
      - CMV status match between donor & recipient to avoid combination of seronegative recipient & seropositive donor
    - Associated with acute rejection in lung, renal, & liver transplant
    - Lung transplant
      - 1-12 months post lung transplant, peak at 1-3 months
      - 2nd most common infection in lung transplant recipients, after bacterial pneumonia
      - Associated with acute & chronic rejection
  - **Recipients of allogeneic stem cell transplant**
    - Immunosuppression + graft-vs.-host disease
    - Usually reactivation of latent CMV
    - Occurs 30-100 days after transplantation
  - **AIDS**
    - CMV: Most common viral pulmonary pathogen
      - Can also cause retinitis, acalculous cholecystitis, esophagitis, colitis, encephalitis
    - Infection by sexual partners or reactivation of latent infection
    - CMV pneumonitis usually when CD4 < 100 cells/ mm^3
    - Incidence reduced by effective antiretroviral medications (HAART)
  - **Systemic lupus erythematosus (SLE)**
    - CMV has immunomodulatory effects & may cause SLE flare
    - SLE flare with mildly elevated serum transaminases & pneumonitis, likely caused by CMV
  - Other causes of immunosuppression
    - Steroid therapy for connective disease or inflammatory bowel disease
    - Chemotherapy
- CMV pneumonia in immunocompetent hosts
  - Uncommon cause of severe community-acquired viral pneumonia

Natural History & Prognosis

- Routes of transmission
  - Transplacental
  - Cervical or vaginal secretions at birth
  - Breast milk
  - Saliva
  - Respiratory secretions
  - Venereal transmission
  - Iatrogenic
    - Organ transplants
    - Transfusion of blood products
- Accounts for 4% of deaths in 1st year after lung transplant
- Suppresses T-cell-mediated immunity
  - Associated with *Pneumocystis*, *Aspergillus*, & *Cryptococcus* infections
- Good prognosis in immunocompetent host
- Mortality > 50% in immunocompromised patient despite therapy

Treatment

- Ganciclovir (intravenous) or valganciclovir (oral)
  - Also used as prophylaxis
- Foscarnet
  - Used in patients who cannot tolerate ganciclovir
  - Used to treat ganciclovir-resistant CMV infection
- Anti-CMV immunoglobulin
  - Prophylaxis when seronegative host receives solid organ or stem cell transplant from seropositive donor
- Correction of underlying immunosuppression
  - Decrease in dose of immunosuppressant in transplant patients

DIAGNOSTIC CHECKLIST

Consider

- CMV pneumonia in immunocompromised patients with diffuse pulmonary abnormalities, particularly transplant recipients

SELECTED REFERENCES

1. Cunha BA: Cytomegalovirus pneumonia: community-acquired pneumonia in immunocompetent hosts. Infect Dis Clin North Am. 24(1):147-58, 2010
2. Ison MG et al: Cytomegalovirus pneumonia in transplant recipients. Clin Chest Med. 26(4):691-705, viii, 2005
3. Chan KM et al: Infectious pulmonary complications in lung transplant recipients. Semin Respir Infect. 17(4):291-302, 2002
4. Kang EY et al: Cytomegalovirus pneumonia in transplant patients: CT findings. J Comput Assist Tomogr. 20(2):295-9, 1996
5. McGuinness G et al: Cytomegalovirus pneumonitis: spectrum of parenchymal CT findings with pathologic correlation in 21 AIDS patients. Radiology. 192(2):451-9, 1994

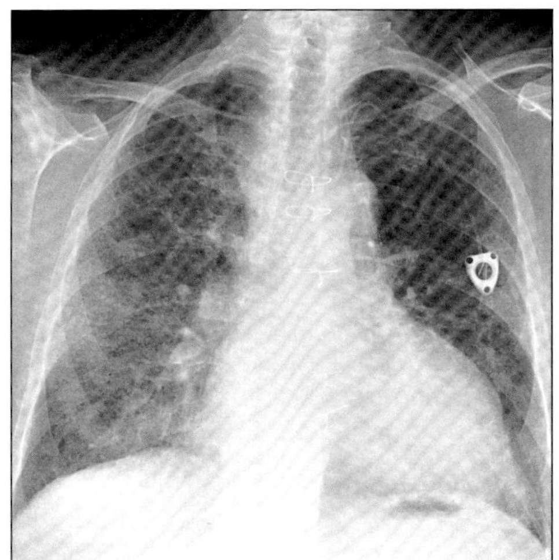

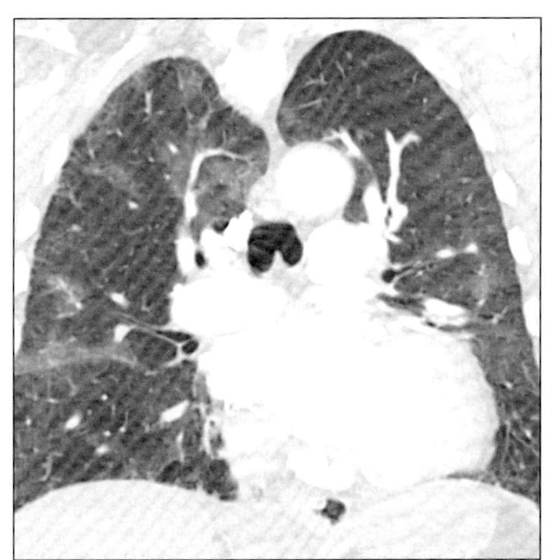

(Left) *PA chest radiograph of a patient undergoing chemotherapy for pancreatic cancer shows bilateral patchy airspace opacities.* ***(Right)*** *Coronal CECT of the same patient shows bilateral patchy ground-glass opacities with a peribronchovascular and subpleural distribution. CMV infection was confirmed by bronchoalveolar lavage. Bronchoalveolar lavage is important in the diagnostic work-up of immunocompromised patients with nonspecific CT findings, such as ground-glass opacity.*

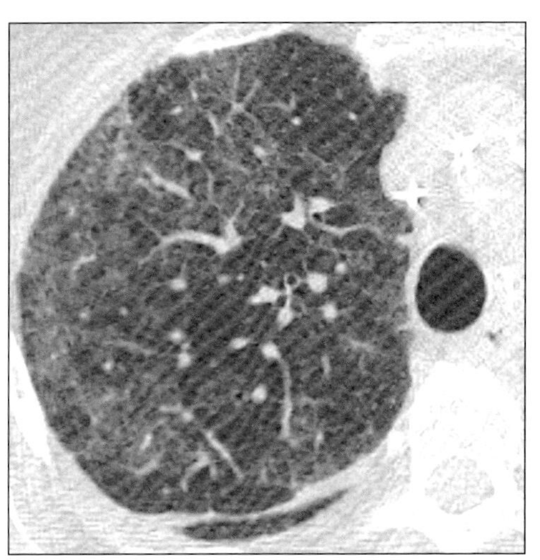

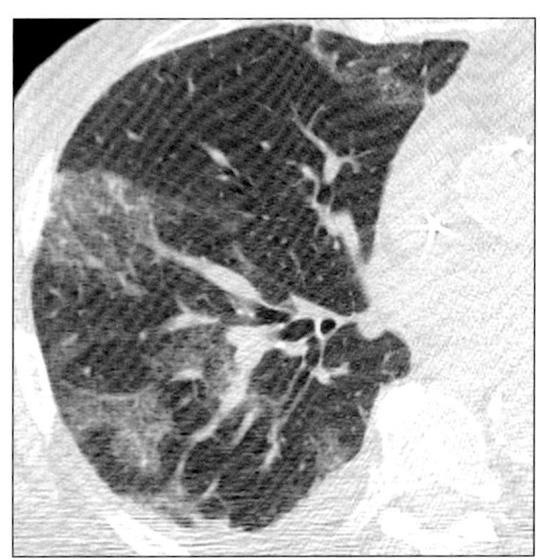

(Left) *Axial NECT of a patient with acute myeloid leukemia, respiratory distress, and confirmed CMV pneumonia shows patchy ground-glass and reticular opacities and thickening of the superior aspect of the major fissure.* ***(Right)*** *Axial NECT of the same patient shows patchy ground-glass and reticular opacities involving the right lower lobe. Differential considerations include other viral pneumonias, Pneumocystis jiroveci pneumonia, drug reaction, and pulmonary hemorrhage.*

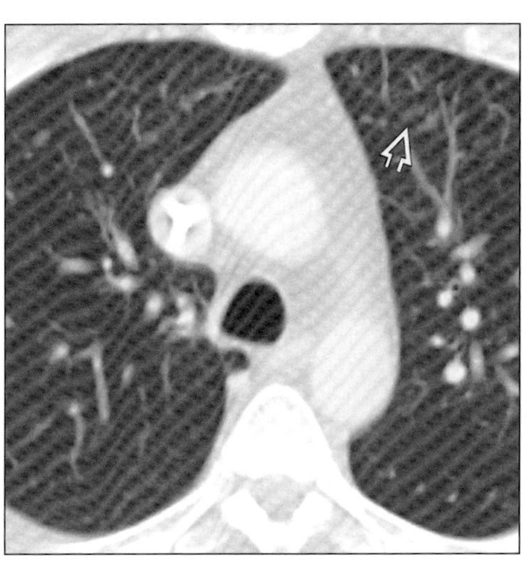

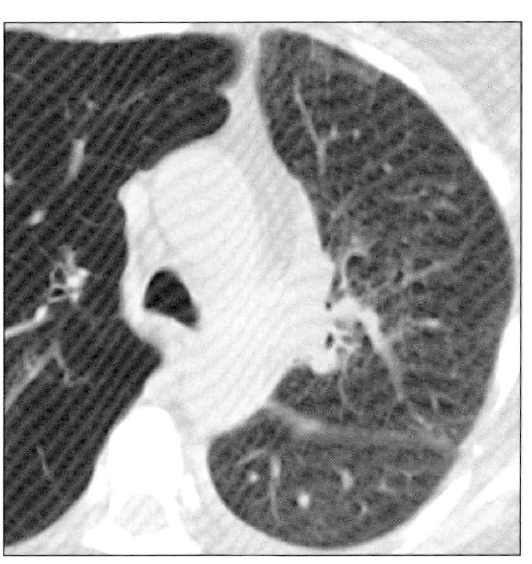

(Left) *Axial NECT of a patient with AIDS, 34 days post stem cell transplantation for non-Hodgkin lymphoma, shows subtle bilateral tree-in-bud opacities ➡. CMV pneumonia was confirmed by bronchoalveolar lavage.* ***(Right)*** *Axial NECT of a left lung transplant recipient who presented with dyspnea shows mild patchy ground-glass opacities in the transplanted lung. CT findings of CMV pneumonia can be quite subtle, and the radiologist must have a high index of suspicion in the appropriate clinical setting.*

SEVERE ACUTE RESPIRATORY SYNDROME

Key Facts

Terminology
- Severe acute respiratory syndrome (SARS)
- Outbreak of atypical pneumonia caused by newly discovered SARS-associated coronavirus (SARS-CoV)

Imaging
- Radiography
  - Normal at presentation (20%)
  - Focal opacity: Peripheral middle & lower lung zones (40%)
  - Multifocal opacities (consolidations)
  - Diffuse consolidation
- CT
  - Ground-glass opacities ± consolidation
  - Focal/multifocal consolidations
  - Intralobular lines & septal thickening
  - Follow-up CT: Bronchial dilatation or bronchiectasis with architectural distortion

Top Differential Diagnoses
- Pulmonary edema
- Organizing pneumonia
- Acute hypersensitivity pneumonitis

Pathology
- Diffuse alveolar damage (DAD)

Clinical Issues
- Symptoms/signs: Fever, dyspnea, hypoxia
- CDC diagnostic criteria

Diagnostic Checklist
- Imaging abnormalities of SARS are nonspecific
- Consider SARS in patient with abnormal chest radiograph or CT in appropriate clinical scenario using CDC diagnostic criteria
- Positive RT-PCR for SARS-CoV

__(Left)__ AP chest radiograph of a patient with SARS shows diffuse bilateral multifocal ground-glass opacities ➔ with a peripheral distribution. Focal lower lung zone peripheral opacities are the most common abnormalities seen on initial chest radiographs of patients with SARS (40%), although chest radiographs are normal in 20% of symptomatic patients. __(Right)__ Axial NECT of a patient with SARS shows a focal middle lobe consolidation with air bronchograms and an ipsilateral small right pleural effusion.

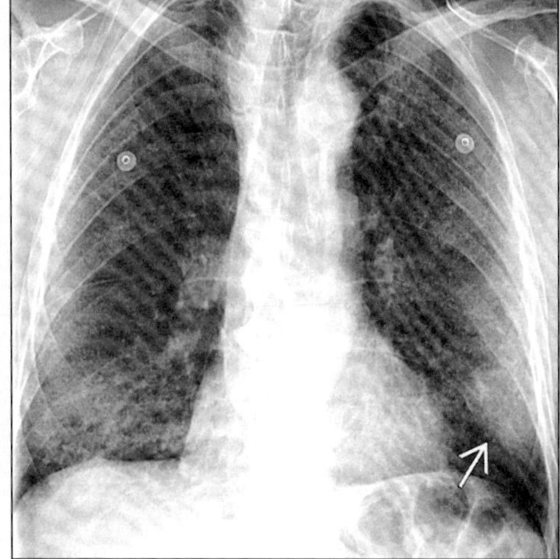

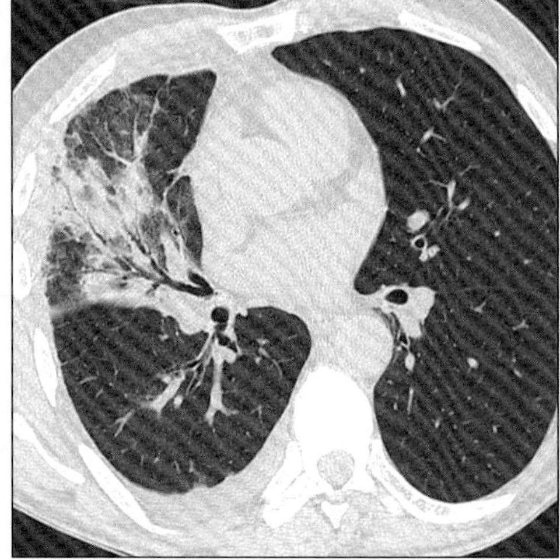

__(Left)__ PA chest radiograph of a symptomatic 28-year-old man with SARS shows bilateral lower lung zone airspace disease, more extensive in the left lower lobe ➔. Such multifocal consolidations represent the 2nd most common radiographic abnormality found on initial chest radiographs of patients with SARS and are seen in 27% of cases. __(Right)__ Coronal NECT of a symptomatic 71-year-old man with SARS shows multifocal centrilobular ground-glass opacities predominantly affecting the left lower lobe.

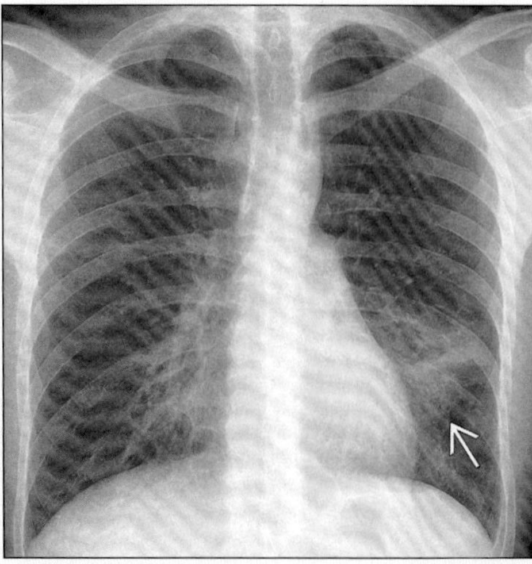

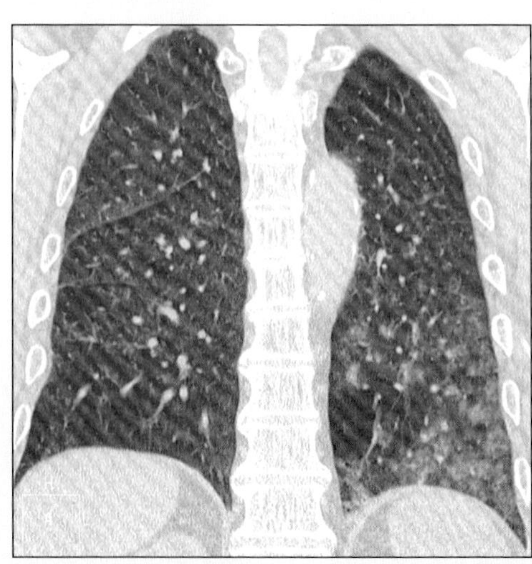

SEVERE ACUTE RESPIRATORY SYNDROME

TERMINOLOGY

Synonyms

- **Severe acute respiratory syndrome (SARS)**

Definitions

- Outbreak of atypical pneumonia caused by newly discovered SARS-associated coronavirus (SARS-CoV)

IMAGING

General Features

- Location
  - Lower lobes preferentially affected
  - Bilateral involvement in advanced cases

Radiographic Findings

- Radiography
  - **Normal** at presentation (20%)
  - **Focal opacity**: Predominantly in periphery & mid/ lower lung zones (40%)
    - May progress to extensive consolidation
    - Resolution to normal appearance: Mean interval of 16 days
  - **Multifocal opacities (consolidations)**: Predominantly peripheral & confined to mid/lower lung zones (27%)
  - **Diffuse consolidation** (14%)

CT Findings

- NECT
  - Ground-glass opacities ± consolidation
  - Focal/multifocal areas of consolidation
  - Intralobular lines & interlobular septal thickening
  - "Crazy-paving" pattern
  - Follow-up CT
    - Bronchial dilatation or bronchiectasis with architectural distortion

DIFFERENTIAL DIAGNOSIS

Pulmonary Edema

- Usually bilateral & symmetric (perihilar) opacities

Organizing Pneumonia

- Changing multifocal peripheral consolidations

Acute Hypersensitivity Pneumonitis

- Abrupt onset of symptoms within a few hours after heavy antigen exposure
  - Mimics acute pulmonary edema

PATHOLOGY

General Features

- Etiology
  - SARS-associated coronavirus (SARS-CoV)
  - Isolated from respiratory secretions, stool, & blood specimens (living patients); from lungs & other organs (postmortem specimens)

Gross Pathologic & Surgical Features

- Predominant pulmonary pathology: Diffuse alveolar damage (DAD)
  - First 7-10 days
    - **Acute exudative DAD**: Extensive edema, hyaline membrane formation, alveolar collapse, desquamation of alveolar epithelial cells, fibrous tissue in alveolar spaces
  - After ~ 10-14 days
    - **Fibrotic/organizing phase**: Interstitial/airspace fibrosis & pneumocyte hyperplasia

CLINICAL ISSUES

Presentation

- Most common signs/symptoms
  - Fever, dyspnea, hypoxia
- Other signs/symptoms
  - **CDC diagnostic criteria**
    - Fever (temperature ≥ 38°C)
    - 1 or more clinical findings of lower respiratory tract illness (e.g., cough, shortness of breath, difficulty breathing, hypoxia, radiographic findings of either pneumonia or ARDS)
    - Travel within 10 days of onset of symptoms to area with documented or suspected community transmission of SARS
    - Close contact with person with respiratory illness who traveled to SARS area, or person known to be suspected SARS case, within 10 days of onset of symptoms
    - Absence of alternative diagnosis

Natural History & Prognosis

- Atypical pneumonia among previously healthy adults; emerged from Guangdong province, China
- From November (2002) to August (2003): 8,422 probable cases of SARS & 916 deaths; mortality 11%
- 1/5 of patients required admission to ICU & majority required mechanical ventilation
- Follow-up in survivors
  - Air-trapping in 50-60% of asymptomatic subjects with normal pulmonary function tests (significance unclear)
  - Long-term follow-up required in patients who recover from SARS

DIAGNOSTIC CHECKLIST

Consider

- SARS in patient with abnormal chest radiograph or CT in appropriate clinical scenario using CDC diagnostic criteria
- Positive RT-PCR for SARS-CoV

Image Interpretation Pearls

- Imaging abnormalities of SARS are nonspecific

SELECTED REFERENCES

1. Antonio GE et al: Radiographic-clinical correlation in severe acute respiratory syndrome: study of 1373 patients in Hong Kong. Radiology. 237(3):1081-90, 2005
2. Paul NS et al: Radiologic pattern of disease in patients with severe acute respiratory syndrome: the Toronto experience. Radiographics. 24(2):553-63, 2004

HISTOPLASMOSIS

Key Facts

Terminology

- Infection with *Histoplasma capsulatum*

Imaging

- Histoplasmoma: Lung nodule ± calcification
- Acute histoplasmosis: Solitary or multiple lower lobe airspace disease ± lymphadenopathy
- Disseminated histoplasmosis: Miliary or diffuse airspace disease; cavitation
- Hilar/mediastinal lymphadenopathy
- Broncholith: Calcified node eroding into bronchus
- Fibrosing mediastinitis: Soft tissue infiltration of mediastinum with encasement & stenosis of airways, veins, arteries, esophagus
- Middle lobe syndrome: Bronchial obstruction by lymphadenopathy with chronic lobar collapse
- Chronic histoplasmosis: Progressive upper lobe volume loss, fibrosis, bullae

Top Differential Diagnoses

- Tuberculosis
- Lung cancer
- Other fungal infection

Pathology

- Inhalation of airborne spores

Clinical Issues

- Symptoms/signs
  - Immunocompetent: Asymptomatic
  - Immunosuppressed: Symptomatic
- Diagnosis: Smears & culture of bronchoscopic specimens, lymph nodes, bone marrow, radioimmunoassay of antigen in urine or serum
- Treatment
  - Immunocompetent: Resolves without treatment
  - Immunosuppressed or large inoculum: Antifungals

(Left) PA chest radiograph of a patient with a history of massive inhalational histoplasmosis shows profuse tiny calcified lung nodules ➔ that represent the residua of remote granulomatous fungal infection. ***(Right)*** *Axial NECT of a patient with acute histoplasmosis shows a left lower lobe mass-like consolidation with a surrounding ground-glass opacity halo ➔. Such mass-like lesions may mimic primary lung cancer.*

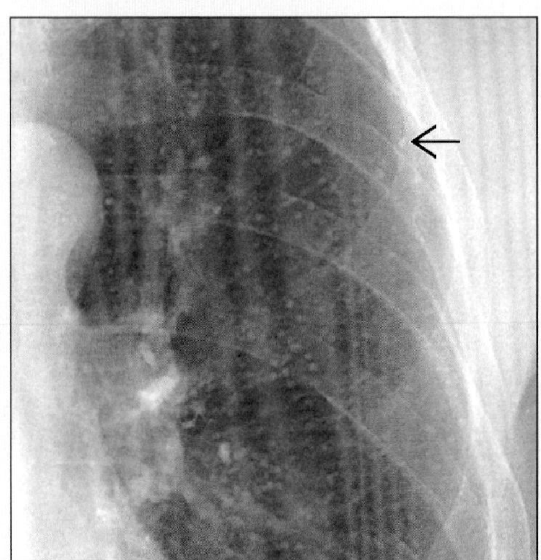

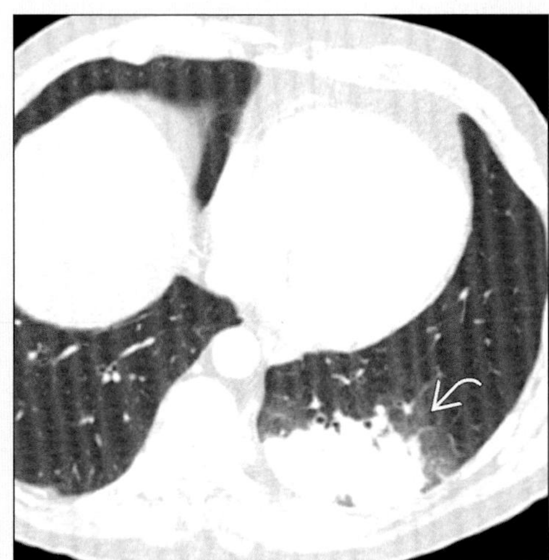

(Left) *Composite image with axial CECT in lung (left) and soft tissue (right) window shows a small right lower lobe nodule ➔ representing focal Histoplasma pneumonitis with associated ipsilateral right hilar lymphadenopathy ➔. The appearance is typical for acute histoplasmosis.* ***(Right)*** *Coronal NECT of a patient with chronic active histoplasmosis shows bilateral upper lobe volume loss, architectural distortion, and thick-walled cavitary lesions ➔. These abnormalities may mimic those produced by tuberculosis.*

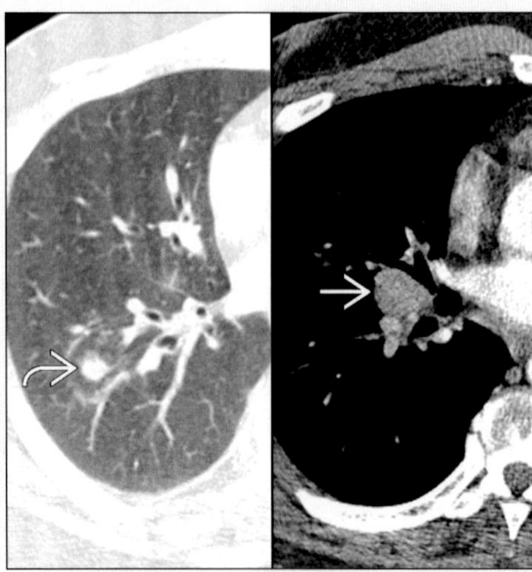

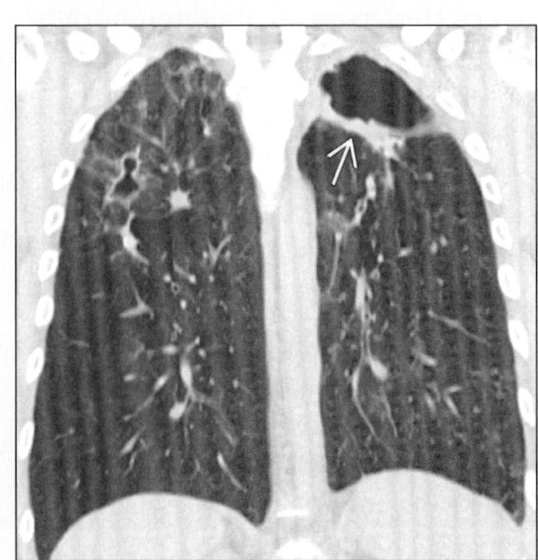

HISTOPLASMOSIS

TERMINOLOGY

Definitions

- Infection with *Histoplasma capsulatum*
- Disease manifestations
  - **Histoplasmoma**
  - **Acute, massive inhalational histoplasmosis**
  - **Acute disseminated histoplasmosis**
  - **Chronic pulmonary or mediastinal histoplasmosis**
  - **Fibrosing mediastinitis**

IMAGING

General Features

- Best diagnostic clue
  - Lung nodule with central, laminated, or diffuse calcification is virtually diagnostic of histoplasmoma
- Location
  - Lung, mediastinum most commonly affected
- Size
  - In endemic areas, > 90% of lung nodules < 2 cm are granulomas
- Morphology
  - Variable

Radiographic Findings

- **Acute histoplasmosis**
  - Airspace disease in any lobe, solitary or multiple; usually lower lungs
  - Ipsilateral hilar/mediastinal lymphadenopathy (common)
  - Pleural or pericardial effusion & cavitation (uncommon)
- **Massive inhalational histoplasmosis**
  - Multilobar pneumonitis, hilar lymphadenopathy
  - Complete resolution or evolution to tiny calcified or noncalcified lung nodules
- **Disseminated histoplasmosis**
  - Miliary or diffuse airspace disease ± cavitation
  - Chest radiograph may be normal
- **Hilar/mediastinal lymphadenopathy ± calcification**
- **Right middle lobe syndrome**: Chronic middle lobe collapse due to bronchial compression
- **Mediastinal involvement**
  - **Mediastinal granuloma**
    - Partially calcified mediastinal mass, especially in superior mediastinum, unilateral or bilateral
  - **Fibrosing mediastinitis**
    - Encasement/stenosis of airways, systemic veins, pulmonary arteries, esophagus
- **Broncholithiasis**: Calcified lymph node that has eroded into bronchus
  - Postobstructive pneumonia, interstitial opacities, atelectasis, oligemia, pleural effusion
- **Chronic histoplasmosis**
  - Progressive upper lobe patchy opacities, volume loss, fibrosis, bullae, honeycombing (20%)
  - Emphysema, unilateral or bilateral
  - Opacities outline emphysematous spaces; simulate cavities with thin or thick walls
  - Mycetomas may develop in upper lobe emphysematous spaces
  - Apical pleural thickening; no pleural effusion or lymphadenopathy

Fluoroscopic Findings

- **Barium swallow** to evaluate esophageal stenosis, fistula, diverticula, downhill varices

CT Findings

- NECT
  - Thin-section CT to characterize lung nodules
    - **Histoplasmoma**: Well-defined nodule, usually < 2 cm (range: 0.5-3 cm)
      - Single or multiple
      - May enlarge slowly (2 mm/year)
      - Visualization of satellite nodules surrounding dominant pulmonary nodule
      - Smooth or lobular nodule margins, sometimes irregular
      - Calcification (50%): Central, laminated, diffuse
      - Ipsilateral hilar/mediastinal lymph nodes with mulberry-like calcification (common); mimics tuberculous Ranke complex
      - Nodule cavitation uncommon
  - Thin-section CT & multiplanar reformations to show endobronchial location of broncholith
  - Calcified hepatic & splenic granulomas
- CECT
  - **Lymph nodes with central low attenuation** from caseous necrosis
  - **Mediastinal granuloma**
    - Enlarged mediastinal coalescent lymph nodes, may impinge on adjacent mediastinal structures
    - Does not progress to fibrosing mediastinitis
  - **Fibrosing mediastinitis**
    - Soft tissue infiltration of mediastinal fat with encasement, narrowing, & obliteration of airways, veins, arteries, esophagus
    - Superior vena cava (SVC) syndrome: Narrowed or obstructed veins & collateral venous pathways
  - **Right middle lobe syndrome**: Lymphadenopathy compressing & obstructing bronchus with chronic lobar collapse
    - Exclusion of endoluminal obstructing neoplasm
- HRCT
  - Disseminated disease: Miliary nodules, 1-3 mm diameter, random distribution

MR Findings

- Decreased signal in lymph nodes may represent calcification

Imaging Recommendations

- Best imaging tool
  - Radiography usually sufficient to demonstrate manifestations of thoracic histoplasmosis
- Protocol advice
  - NECT, 1-3 mm thick sections to identify & assess calcification in pulmonary nodules
  - CECT for assessment of mediastinal fibrosis

DIFFERENTIAL DIAGNOSIS

Consolidation with Lymphadenopathy

- Tuberculosis
- Infectious mononucleosis

HISTOPLASMOSIS

- Bacterial pneumonia in children
- Other fungal infection

Fibrosing Mediastinitis

- Tuberculosis
- Drug reaction (methysergide)
- Radiation-induced lung disease

Solitary Pulmonary Nodule

- Malignant
  - Lung cancer
  - Carcinoid
  - Solitary metastasis
- Benign
  - Fungal: Blastomycosis, coccidioidomycosis
  - Hamartoma
  - Intrapulmonary lymph node

PATHOLOGY

General Features

- Etiology
  - Septate mycelium in soil; temperate zones
  - Inhalation of airborne spores from soil infected by bird excreta & feathers, infected bats
  - Yeast form in human tissues

Gross Pathologic & Surgical Features

- Benign extrapulmonary spread in most infections, liver/spleen exhibit calcified granulomas

Microscopic Features

- Yeast forms in tissues; granulomas with caseous necrosis; fibrous capsule, calcification
- Progressive disseminated disease: Bone marrow involvement
- Usually not isolated from mediastinal fibrosis, pleural or pericardial effusions

CLINICAL ISSUES

Presentation

- Most common signs/symptoms
  - Malaise, fever, headache, muscle pain, nonproductive cough, wheezing, dysphagia, oropharyngeal ulcers, hemoptysis, chest pain
  - Lymphadenopathy, hepatosplenomegaly, erythema nodosum, erythema multiforme, pericarditis
  - **Acute respiratory distress syndrome**: Immunosuppression or large inoculum
  - **Progressive disseminated disease**: Abnormal T-cell immunity, AIDS, chemotherapy, steroids, organ transplants, lymphoma
    - May result in adrenal insufficiency
  - Symptoms influenced by patient's immune status
    - **Immunocompetent**: Asymptomatic or minimal symptoms; self-limited disease
    - **Immunosuppressed, patients with emphysema**: Symptomatic

Demographics

- Age
  - Any age
  - Clinical symptoms more common in infants & elderly patients
- Gender
  - Disseminated disease, M:F = 4:1
- Epidemiology
  - Central & eastern United States (Ohio, Mississippi river valleys); central & South America; Africa
  - > 80% in endemic areas infected

Diagnosis

- Smears & culture of bronchoscopic specimens, lymph nodes, bone marrow
- Antigen radioimmunoassay, urine or serum

Natural History & Prognosis

- Pulmonary & lymph node abnormalities may resolve completely
- Late sequelae
  - Histoplasmoma
    - Calcified granulomas in healed disease; 3 months to years for foci to calcify
  - Chronic hilar & mediastinal lymphadenopathy
  - Calcific or constrictive pericarditis: Residua from histoplasma pericarditis
  - Broncholithiasis: Calcified lymph nodes eroding into airways, mainstem, lobar, segmental bronchi
    - Airway obstruction: Atelectasis, postobstructive pneumonia, mucoid impaction, bronchiectasis, expiratory air-trapping
- Death from respiratory failure (rare); cor pulmonale with fibrosing mediastinitis

Treatment

- Immunocompetent: Usually resolves without treatment (99%)
- Immunosuppressed or large inoculum exposure: Ketoconazole, itraconazole therapy; amphotericin B for overwhelming infection
- Mediastinal granuloma: Surgery usually not indicated
- Fibrosing mediastinitis: Does not respond to drug treatment; surgery often dangerous & unsuccessful
  - Vascular & airway stents for treatment of stenoses

DIAGNOSTIC CHECKLIST

Consider

- Histoplasmosis in patients from endemic areas with pulmonary &/or mediastinal abnormalities

SELECTED REFERENCES

1. Marom EM et al: Imaging studies for diagnosing invasive fungal pneumonia in immunocompromised patients. Curr Opin Infect Dis. 24(4):309-14, 2011
2. Franquet T et al: Imaging of opportunistic fungal infections in immunocompromised patient. Eur J Radiol. 51(2):130-8, 2004
3. Seo JB et al: Broncholithiasis: review of the causes with radiologic-pathologic correlation. Radiographics. 22 Spec No:S199-213, 2002
4. Gurney JW et al: Pulmonary histoplasmosis. Radiology. 199(2):297-306, 1996

HISTOPLASMOSIS

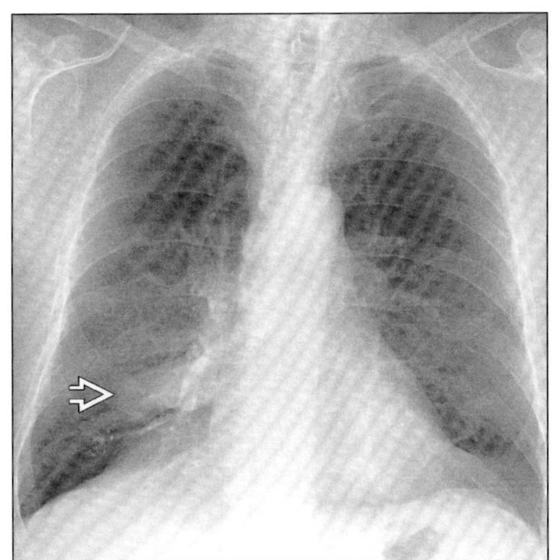

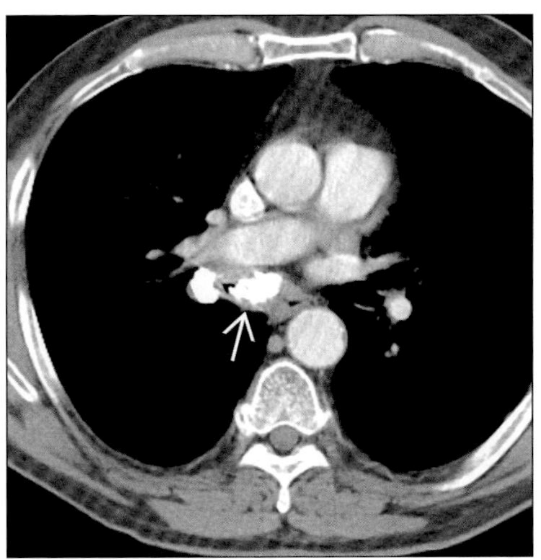

(Left) *PA chest radiograph of a patient with remote granulomatous infection related to histoplasmosis shows middle lobe atelectasis ➔ that was stable from prior studies (not shown).* ***(Right)*** *Axial CECT of the same patient shows a large calcified mediastinal lymph node ➔ that has eroded into the bronchus intermedius. The middle lobe bronchus was occluded by adjacent lymphadenopathy (not shown). The findings were secondary to broncholithiasis and resultant right middle lobe syndrome.*

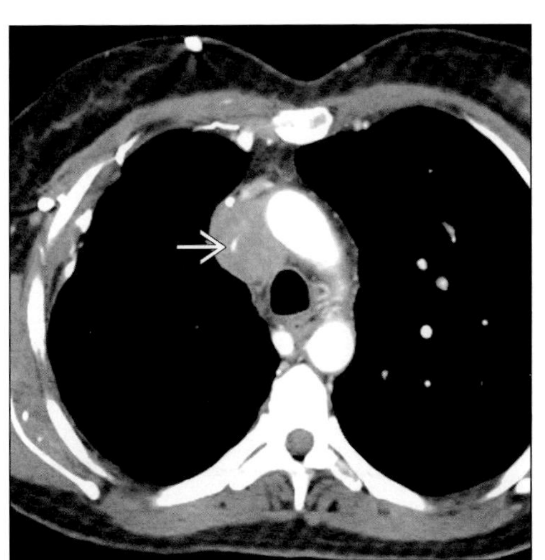

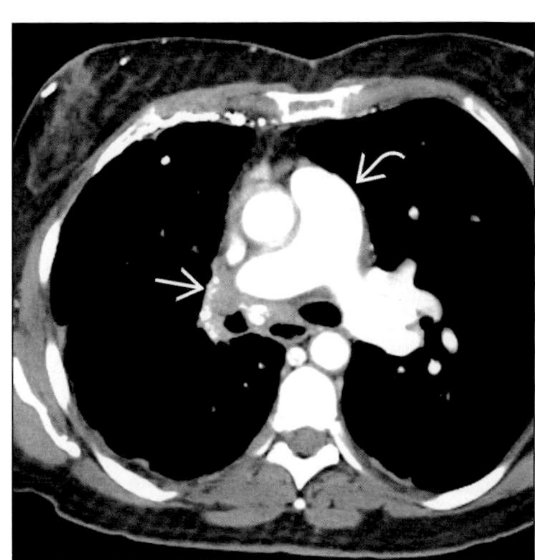

(Left) *Axial CECT of a patient with fibrosing mediastinitis shows right paratracheal bulky lymphadenopathy, which produces superior vena cava ➔ stenosis and impending occlusion.* ***(Right)*** *Axial CECT of the same patient shows right hilar partially calcified soft tissue ➔ producing obstruction of the distal right pulmonary artery. Enlargement of the pulmonary trunk ➔ is consistent with pulmonary artery hypertension. Note chest wall and mediastinal vascular collaterals.*

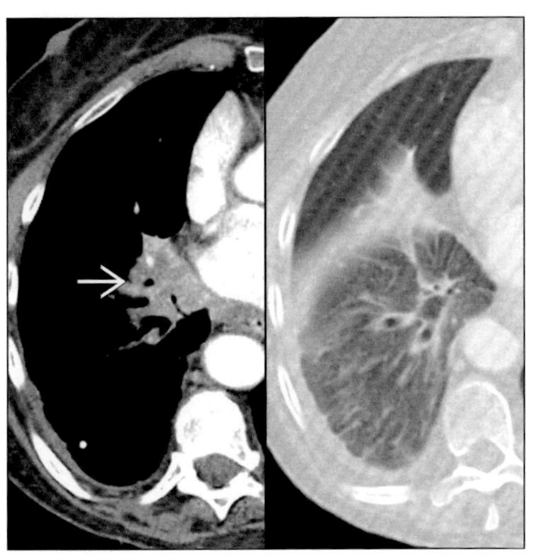

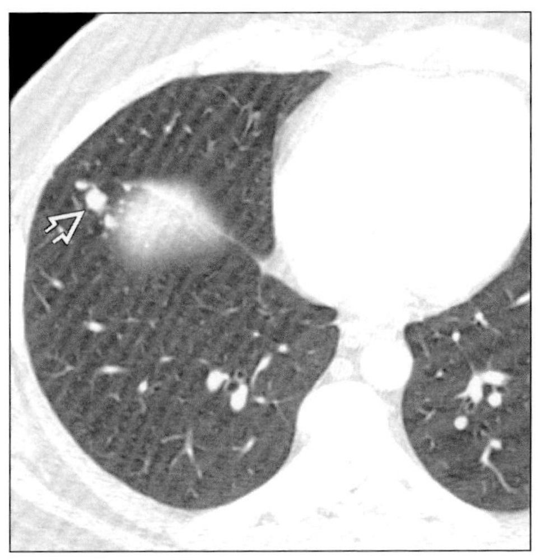

(Left) *Composite image with axial CECT in soft tissue (left) and lung (right) windows of a patient with fibrosing mediastinitis shows a heterogeneous soft tissue mass ➔ occluding the right inferior pulmonary vein with resultant right lower lobe volume loss and hazy opacity secondary to lobar edema from obstructed venous and lymphatic outflow.* ***(Right)*** *Axial NECT of a patient with histoplasmosis shows clustered Histoplasma granulomas manifesting with a dominant nodule ➔ and adjacent satellite nodules.*

COCCIDIOIDOMYCOSIS

Key Facts

Terminology

- Fungal infection with *Coccidioides immitis*
- Inhalation of fungal arthrospores

Imaging

- Radiography
  - Solitary or multifocal segmental or lobar consolidation
  - Solitary or multiple lung nodules, may cavitate with thick or thin ("grape-skin") walls
  - Hilar lymphadenopathy in 20%
  - Pleural effusion in 20%
  - Mediastinal lymphadenopathy typical of disseminated disease
- CT
  - Evaluation of airspace disease, nodules, cavities
  - Thoracic lymphadenopathy
  - Evaluation of immunocompromised patients

Top Differential Diagnoses

- Bacterial pneumonia
- Fungal pneumonia
- Mycobacterial pneumonia
- Lung cancer

Clinical Issues

- Endemic to arid regions of western hemisphere
- Signs/symptoms: Asymptomatic, mild flu-like symptoms, severe infection in immunocompromised
- Most infections resolve
- Chronic lung disease 5%; disseminated disease < 1%
- Exogenous reinfection may occur in endemic areas
- Reactivation of latent disease in immune impaired

Diagnostic Checklist

- Consider coccidioidomycosis in nonresolving consolidations in patients from endemic areas

*(**Left**) PA chest radiograph of a patient with cough, fever, and a history of recent travel to Arizona shows a left lower lobe consolidation that did not respond to antibiotics. Serologic and skin tests were positive for coccidioidomycosis. This infection may mimic community-acquired pneumonia. (**Right**) PA chest radiograph of the same patient obtained 4 months later shows resolution of the consolidation with a residual thin-walled "grape-skin" cavity ➡. Coccidioidomycosis may take months to resolve.*

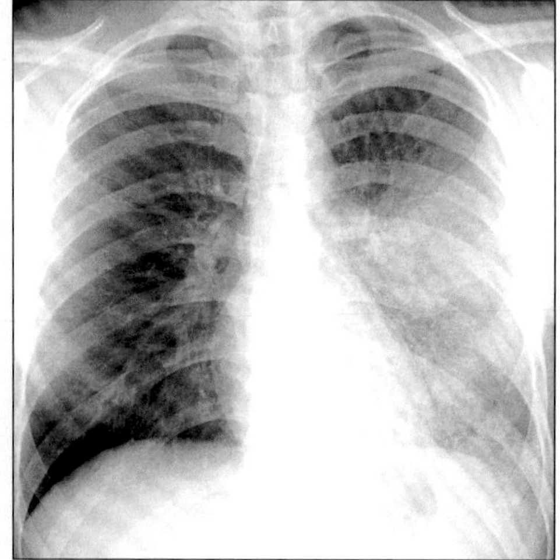

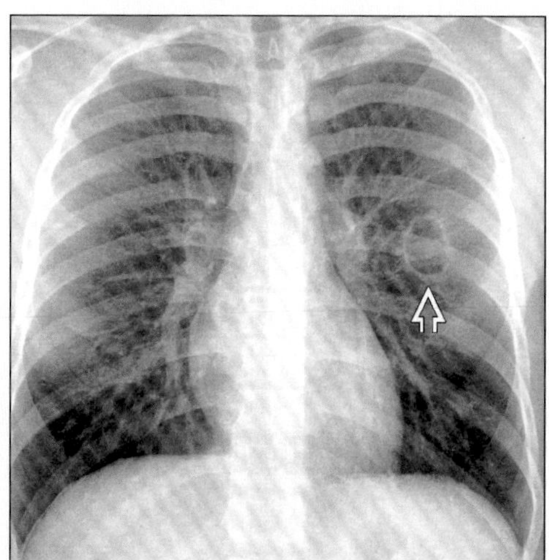

*(**Left**) Axial NECT of a 45-year-old man status post heart transplantation shows a left upper lobe consolidation ➡, left hilar lymphadenopathy ➡, and multiple small nodules →. Coccidioides spherules were recovered from the sputum. The patient was originally from Arizona and likely developed reactivation disease secondary to immunocompromise. (**Right**) Axial CECT of a patient with coccidioidomycosis shows a right upper lobe cavitary consolidation ➡ and mediastinal → and hilar ➡ lymphadenopathy.*

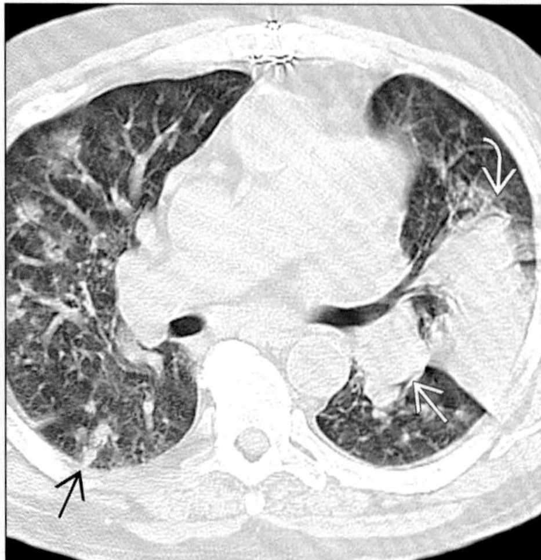

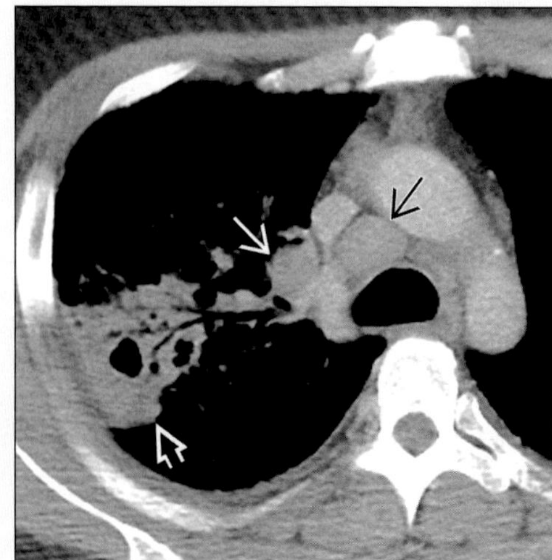

COCCIDIOIDOMYCOSIS

TERMINOLOGY

Synonyms

- **Valley fever**

Definitions

- Fungal infection with *Coccidioides immitis*
- Inhalation of fungal arthrospores

IMAGING

General Features

- Best diagnostic clue
  - Cavitary segmental or lobar consolidation in patient from endemic area
- Location
  - Primary form limited to lungs, thoracic lymph nodes
  - Disseminated form spreads to nearly any tissue
- Size
  - Range from lung nodule to disseminated disease
- Morphology
  - Foci of consolidation may evolve into nodule(s) or thin-walled ("grape-skin") cysts

Radiographic Findings

- Solitary or multifocal segmental or lobar consolidation
- Solitary or multiple lung nodules
  - Nodules may cavitate with thick or thin ("grape-skin") walls
- Hilar lymphadenopathy in 20%
- Pleural effusion in 20%
- Mediastinal lymphadenopathy typical of disseminated disease

CT Findings

- Evaluation of focal airspace disease, lung nodules, cavitary lesions
- Evaluation of hilar & mediastinal lymphadenopathy
- Evaluation of immunocompromised patients

Imaging Recommendations

- Best imaging tool
  - Chest radiographs for disease detection & follow-up
- Protocol advice
  - Consider chest CT for assessment of lung & mediastinal involvement, particularly in immunocompromised patient

DIFFERENTIAL DIAGNOSIS

Bacterial Pneumonia

- Patients typically symptomatic with fever & cough
- Parenchymal consolidation

Fungal Pneumonia

- Nodules, consolidation, cavitation, lymphadenopathy

Mycobacterial Pneumonia

- Cavitary consolidation, chronic fibrocavitary disease
- Miliary nodules with disseminated disease

Lung Cancer

- Persistent cavity or granuloma may mimic lung cancer

PATHOLOGY

General Features

- Etiology
  - Inhalation of arthroconidia of *Coccidioides immitis*

Microscopic Features

- Endemic dimorphic fungus: Virulent, resistant to drying
  - Soil: Mycelium, produces 2-5 μm arthrospores
  - Host (humans & animals): Arthrospore inhalation

CLINICAL ISSUES

Presentation

- Most common signs/symptoms
  - **Asymptomatic acute infection**
  - **Mild flu-like symptoms** in some patients
  - Immune compromised at risk for severe infection
- Other signs/symptoms
  - **Valley fever**: Syndrome of fever, rash, arthralgias
    - Erythema nodosum & erythema multiforme
- Clinical profile
  - Large mature spherules with endospores found in sputum, gastric contents, pus, skin lesions
  - Serologic & skin testing become positive within 3 weeks after exposure
  - Anergic patients: Complement factor titer > 1:16 is pathognomonic

Demographics

- Age
  - Incidence increases with increasing age
- Gender
  - More common in males
- Ethnicity
  - African-Americans & Hispanics: High risk
- Epidemiology
  - Endemic to arid regions of western hemisphere
    - U.S.: California, Arizona, New Mexico, & Texas
  - Persons with high dust exposure at risk
  - 100,000 new cases/year in U.S.

Natural History & Prognosis

- Incubation period of 1-4 weeks
- Most infections resolve
- Chronic lung disease 5%; disseminated disease < 1%
- Exogenous reinfection may occur in endemic areas
- Reactivation of latent disease in immune impaired

Treatment

- **Amphotericin B** is drug of choice
- Treatment of severe disease & patients with risk factors

DIAGNOSTIC CHECKLIST

Consider

- Coccidioidomycosis in nonresolving consolidations in patients from endemic areas

SELECTED REFERENCES

1. Galgiani JN et al: Coccidioidomycosis. Clin Infect Dis. 41(9):1217-23, 2005

BLASTOMYCOSIS

Key Facts

Terminology
- Synonym: North American blastomycosis
- Fungal infection with *Blastomyces dermatitidis*
- Dimorphic fungus: Disease caused by inhalation of airborne spores

Imaging
- Radiography
  - Acute patchy consolidation, may be mass-like
  - Lung nodules of variable size, may be miliary
  - Most common in upper lungs
  - Cavitation in 15-35%
  - Pleural thickening common, pleural effusion 20%
  - Lymph node enlargement in 10%
- CT
  - Characterization of airspace disease
  - Evaluation of mass-like consolidations, cavitation, complications

Top Differential Diagnoses
- Lung cancer
- Bacterial pneumonia
- Mycobacterial or fungal infection
- Rounded atelectasis

Pathology
- Inhalation of conidia of *Blastomyces dermatitidis*
- Endemic to southeastern USA, Great Lakes region

Clinical Issues
- Asymptomatic or flu-like illness
- Skin lesions common, draining sinus tract
- Young to middle-aged outdoorsmen

Diagnostic Checklist
- Consider culture of lung biopsy specimens for *Blastomyces* in endemic areas

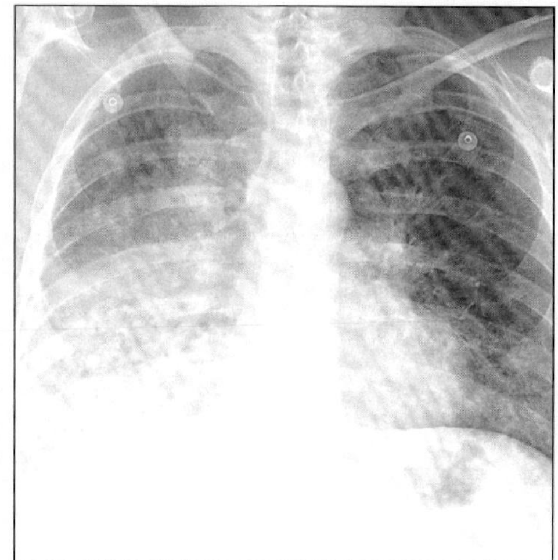
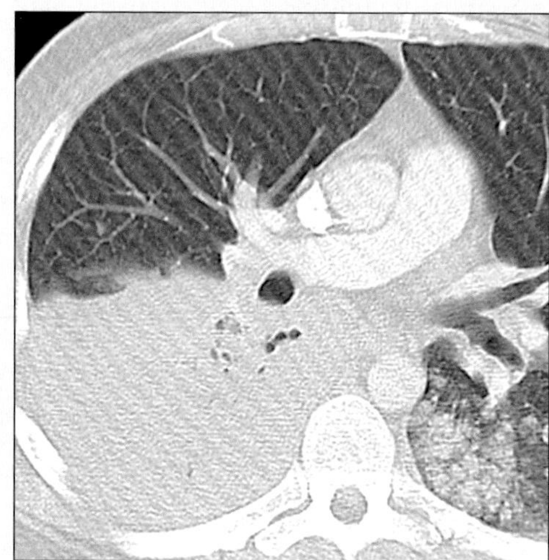

(Left) *PA chest radiograph of a 38-year-old man with blastomycosis who presented with fever shows extensive right lung consolidation and multifocal small lung nodules.* ***(Right)*** *Axial CECT of the same patient shows extensive right lower lobe consolidation and centrilobular left lower lobe nodules and patchy lobular consolidations. The imaging findings are nonspecific and mimic those of bacterial pneumonia. The diagnosis of blastomycosis was established on bronchial washings.*

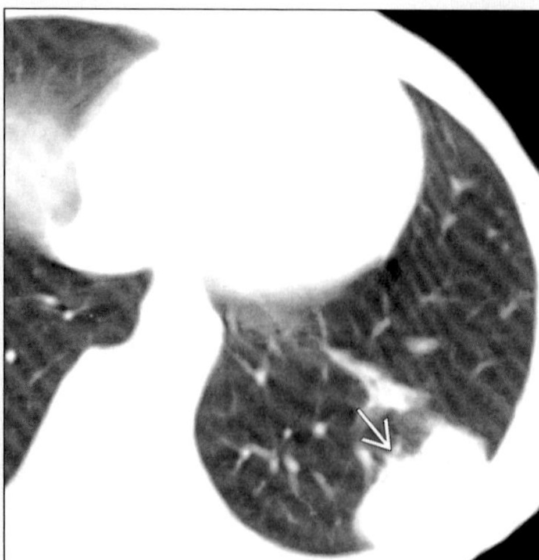
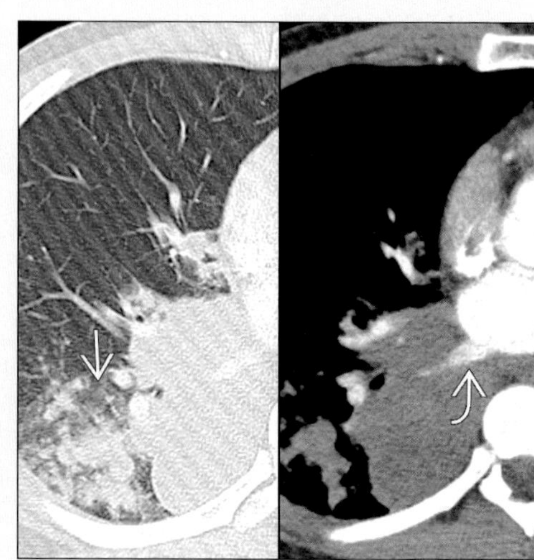

(Left) *Axial NECT of a 43-year-old man with blastomycosis who presented with fever and weight loss shows a peripheral left lower lobe lobular mass ➔.* ***(Right)*** *Composite image with axial CECT in lung (left) and soft tissue (right) window of a 39-year-old man who presented with cough and fever shows patchy right lower lobe consolidation ➔ and centrilobular nodules adjacent to a lobular soft tissue mass that encases the right inferior pulmonary vein ➔ and the adjacent left atrium. Blastomycosis may mimic lung cancer.*

BLASTOMYCOSIS

TERMINOLOGY

Synonyms

- **North American blastomycosis**
- Chicago disease
- Gilchrist disease

Definitions

- Fungal infection with *Blastomyces dermatitidis*
  - Dimorphic fungus: Disease caused by inhalation of airborne spores
  - Found in dead, decaying, or moist material
  - Pulmonary & disseminated forms

IMAGING

General Features

- Best diagnostic clue
  - Consolidation or mass in outdoorsmen from endemic area
- Location
  - Upper lungs more commonly involved
- Size
  - Range from tiny nodules to lobar consolidation
- Morphology
  - Consolidation or lung nodule(s)
  - Cavitation & lymph node enlargement uncommon

Radiographic Findings

- Acute patchy consolidation
  - Nonsegmental, segmental, &/or lobar
  - Mass-like consolidation
    - Lung nodules of variable size, may be miliary
- Most common in upper lungs
- Cavitation (15-35%)
- Pleural thickening common, pleural effusion (20%)
- Lymph node enlargement (10%)
- **Chronic blastomycosis**: Upper lung fibrocavitary disease

CT Findings

- Characterization of airspace disease
- Evaluation of mass-like consolidations, cavitation, complications
- Identification of lymph node involvement

Imaging Recommendations

- Best imaging tool
  - Radiography usually suffices for detection & follow-up

DIFFERENTIAL DIAGNOSIS

Lung Cancer

- Indeterminate nodule or mass ± pleural thickening
- Fungal osteomyelitis may mimic metastasis

Pneumonia

- Bacterial: Patchy, segmental, or lobar consolidation
- Mycobacterial or fungal: Consolidation, nodules, cavitation, lymphadenopathy, miliary nodules

Rounded Atelectasis

- Mass-like appearance & pleural thickening

PATHOLOGY

General Features

- Etiology
  - Inhalation of conidia of *Blastomyces dermatitidis*
  - Exposure typically occurs in heavily wooded areas
- Associated abnormalities
  - Ulcerative skin, bone, & genitourinary infections

Microscopic Features

- Bronchopneumonia evolves into noncaseating granulomas with central microabscesses
- Pyogranulomas
- Thermally dimorphic fungus
  - Source (soil): Mycelial form (room temperature)
  - Host (humans & animals): Inhalation of spores
    - Forms 8-15 μm round budding yeast (37°C)
- Characteristic yeast form found in sputum, pus, tissue

CLINICAL ISSUES

Presentation

- Most common signs/symptoms
  - Asymptomatic or flu-like illness
  - Skin lesions common, draining sinus tract
- Other signs/symptoms
  - Dissemination to skin, bone, genitourinary system
    - Hematogenous spread from lung infection
    - Osteomyelitis of vertebral body, pelvis, sacrum
- Clinical profile
  - Young to middle-aged outdoorsmen
  - Incubation period of ~ 6 weeks after exposure
  - Severity varies with inoculum size & immune status
  - Immune-impaired host at increased risk

Demographics

- Age
  - Most patients are adults, uncommon in children
- Gender
  - Strong male predominance
- Epidemiology
  - Endemic to southeastern USA, Great Lakes region, Central & South America, Africa

Natural History & Prognosis

- Mortality for untreated blastomycosis nearly 60%
- May develop progressive or disseminated disease

Diagnosis

- No reliable skin or serologic tests

Treatment

- Most symptomatic patients should be treated
- Itraconazole: Usual drug of choice

DIAGNOSTIC CHECKLIST

Consider

- Culture of lung biopsy specimens for *Blastomyces* in endemic areas

SELECTED REFERENCES

1. Wheat LJ et al: State-of-the-art review of pulmonary fungal infections. Semin Respir Infect. 17(2):158-81, 2002

CRYPTOCOCCOSIS

Key Facts

Terminology

- Infection of respiratory system by *Cryptococcus neoformans*

Imaging

- Radiography
  - Multiple pulmonary nodules
  - Less commonly pulmonary masses
  - Patchy airspace consolidation
  - Lesions may exhibit cavitation
- CT
  - Pulmonary nodules or masses
  - Cavitation, more common in immunocompromised patients
  - Ground-glass opacity, CT halo sign
  - Mediastinal lymphadenopathy
  - Air-fluid levels in abscesses
  - Pleural effusions

Top Differential Diagnoses

- Squamous cell carcinoma
- Pulmonary metastases
- Septic emboli
- Wegener granulomatosis

Clinical Issues

- Symptoms/signs
  - Cough, fever, chest pain, dyspnea, headache
- Serum cryptococcal antigen (sCRAG) used for diagnosis & monitoring
- Immunocompromised patients with more aggressive disease may have higher sCRAG titers
- Treatment: Oral & intravenous antifungals

Diagnostic Checklist

- Consider cryptococcosis in immunocompromised patients with 1 or more lung nodules or masses

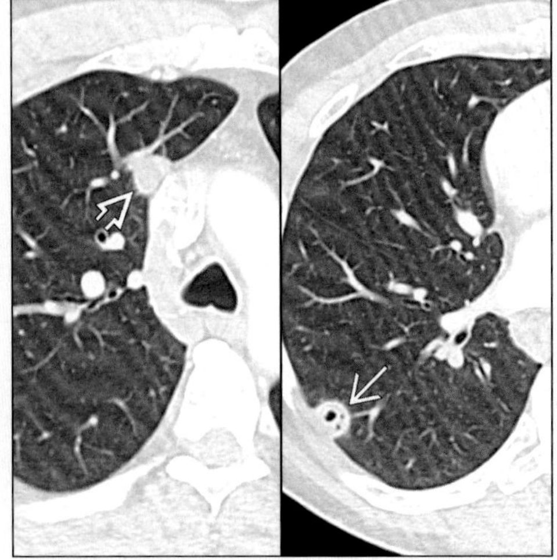

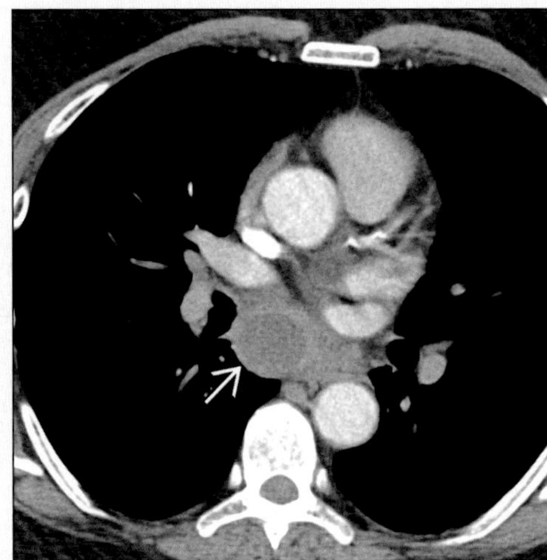

(Left) *Composite image with axial CECT of a patient with AIDS complicated by pulmonary cryptococcosis demonstrates solid ➢ and cavitary ➡ pulmonary nodules in the right lung. The most common manifestation of pulmonary cryptococcosis is multiple pulmonary nodules. Cavitation is more common in larger nodules and in immunocompromised patients.* ***(Right)*** *Axial CECT of the same patient shows an enlarged subcarinal lymph node ➡ that exhibits peripheral enhancement and central hypoattenuation.*

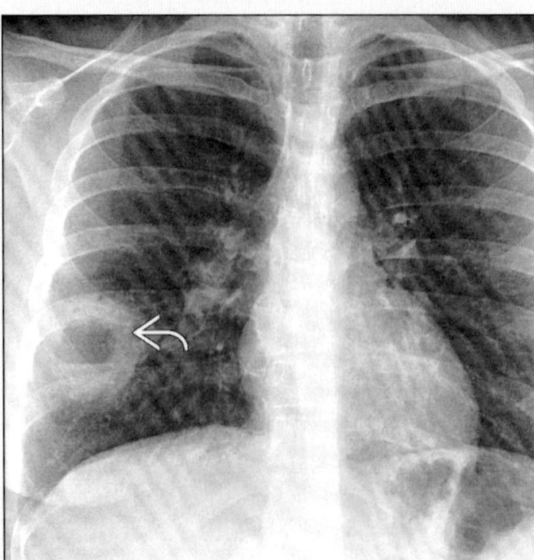

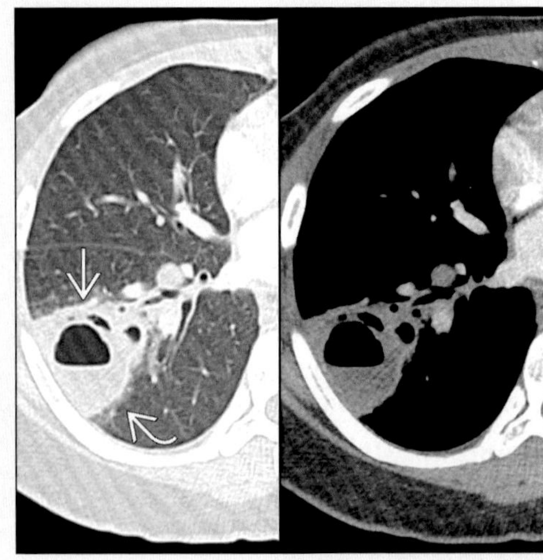

(Left) *PA chest radiograph of an immunocompromised patient with pulmonary cryptococcosis shows a cavitary mass ➡ in the right lower lung zone with an intrinsic air-fluid level.* ***(Right)*** *Composite image with axial CECT of the same patient on lung (left) and soft tissue (right) window demonstrates the cavitary right lower lobe mass ➡ with an internal air-fluid level consistent with abscess formation. Patchy ground-glass opacity ➡ is present in the adjacent lung parenchyma.*

CRYPTOCOCCOSIS

TERMINOLOGY

Definitions

- Infection of respiratory system by *Cryptococcus neoformans*

IMAGING

General Features

- Best diagnostic clue
  - Multiple pulmonary nodules that may cavitate
- Location
  - Peripheral > central lung
- Size
  - Most 7-20 mm
    - May exceed 30 mm
- Morphology
  - Poorly circumscribed margins
  - Clustered nodules most common
  - Solitary & scattered nodules less common

Radiographic Findings

- Pulmonary nodule(s) or mass(es)
- Patchy airspace consolidation
- Lesions may exhibit cavitation

CT Findings

- Pulmonary nodules
- Pulmonary masses less common
- Cavitation
  - More common in immunocompromised patients
  - Air-fluid levels in abscesses
- Patchy airspace consolidation
- Ground-glass opacity
  - CT halo sign
- Mediastinal lymphadenopathy
  - May exhibit central low attenuation
- Pleural effusions

Nuclear Medicine Findings

- PET/CT
  - FDG uptake variable
    - FDG-avid nodules or masses may mimic lung cancer & metastatic disease

Imaging Recommendations

- Best imaging tool
  - CT for assessment of lung nodules, masses, consolidations

DIFFERENTIAL DIAGNOSIS

Squamous Cell Carcinoma

- Most common lung cancer to cavitate
  - Cavitation in 15% of cases
- Strongly associated with cigarette smoking

Pulmonary Metastases

- Well-defined pulmonary nodules or masses
- Hemorrhagic metastases may exhibit irregular margins & surrounding ground-glass opacity
  - Renal cell cancer, melanoma, & choriocarcinoma
- Squamous cell carcinomas & sarcomas may cavitate

Septic Emboli

- Poorly defined pulmonary nodules or masses
- Varying degrees of cavitation

Wegener Granulomatosis

- Multiple cavitary pulmonary nodules or masses
- Consolidation & ground-glass opacity less common

PATHOLOGY

General Features

- Etiology
  - *Cryptococcus neoformans*
    - Fungus typically affects respiratory system
    - Immunocompromised > immunocompetent

Microscopic Features

- Macrophages & proteinaceous fluid within airspaces
  - Correspond to ground-glass opacity surrounding pulmonary lesions

CLINICAL ISSUES

Presentation

- Most common signs/symptoms
  - Cough & fever
- Other signs/symptoms
  - Chest pain, shortness of breath, headache
- Clinical profile
  - Serum cryptococcal antigen (sCRAG) used for diagnosis & monitoring
    - Immunocompromised patients with more aggressive disease may have higher sCRAG titers

Natural History & Prognosis

- Immunocompromised patients
  - Radiographic abnormalities may improve, stabilize, or progress over time
    - Imaging abnormalities improve more slowly
  - sCRAG titers decrease more slowly or fluctuate
- Immunocompetent patients
  - Radiographs improve & sCRAG titers decrease more rapidly over time in most

Treatment

- Antifungals
  - Oral: Fluconazole
  - Intravenous: Amphotericin B

DIAGNOSTIC CHECKLIST

Consider

- Cryptococcosis in immunocompromised patients with 1 or more lung nodule(s) or mass(es)

SELECTED REFERENCES

1. Song KD et al: Pulmonary cryptococcosis: imaging findings in 23 non-AIDS patients. Korean J Radiol. 11(4):407-16, 2010
2. Chang WC et al: Pulmonary cryptococcosis: comparison of clinical and radiographic characteristics in immunocompetent and immunocompromised patients. Chest. 129(2):333-40, 2006

ASPERGILLOSIS

Key Facts

Terminology
- Aspergillosis: Fungal infection caused by organisms of genus *Aspergillus*
- Most mycetomas are aspergillomas: Terms often used interchangeably

Imaging
- Aspergilloma
  - Nodule/mass within preexisting cavity
- Invasive aspergillosis
  - Radiography: Rapidly progressing lung nodules or consolidations, air crescent sign
  - CT: Halo sign suggests diagnosis in febrile neutropenic patient
- Semi-invasive aspergillosis
  - Radiography: Apical slow-growing nodule or consolidation
  - CT: Nodule, mass, or consolidation

Top Differential Diagnoses
- Other infection: Fungal, mycobacterial, bacterial
- Pulmonary emboli
- Wegener granulomatosis

Pathology
- Most *Aspergillus* infections caused by *A. fumigatus*

Clinical Issues
- Aspergilloma: Immunocompetent
- Invasive aspergillosis: Severely immunocompromised
- Voriconazole is treatment of choice
- Bronchial artery embolization or surgery may be needed in patients with hemoptysis

Diagnostic Checklist
- Consider invasive aspergillosis in febrile neutropenic patients with pulmonary abnormalities

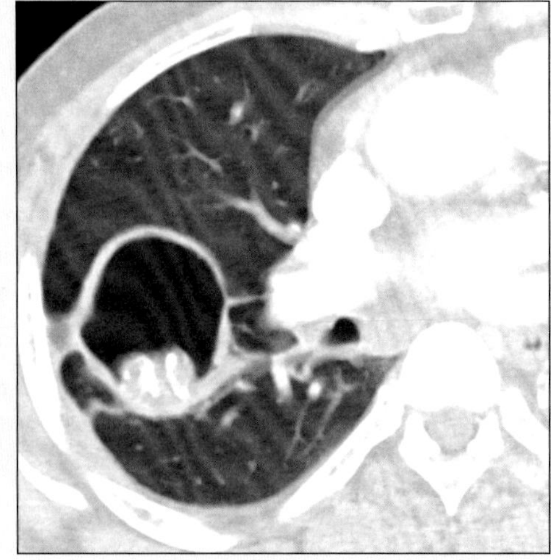
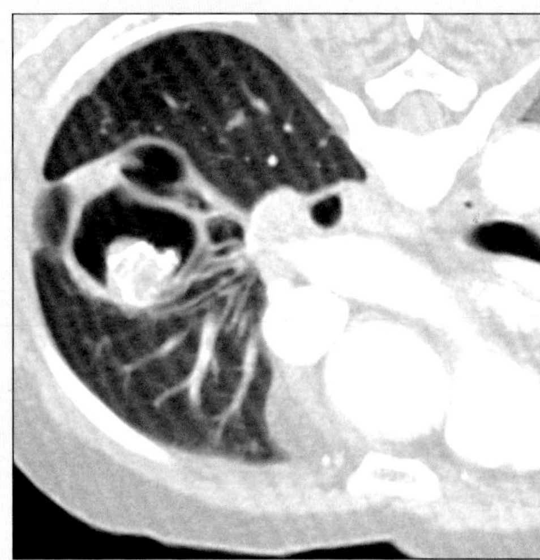

(Left) *Axial CECT of a 40-year-old man with a chronic right upper lobe cavity from prior tuberculosis shows an aspergilloma manifesting as an intracavitary, partially calcified nodule in the dependent aspect of the cavity. (Courtesy S. Digumarthy, MD.)* ***(Right)*** *Axial prone CECT of the same patient shows the aspergilloma in the dependent aspect of the cavity. Repeat low-dose CT in the prone position may help demonstrate intracavitary mobility of a suspected aspergilloma. (Courtesy S. Digumarthy, MD.)*

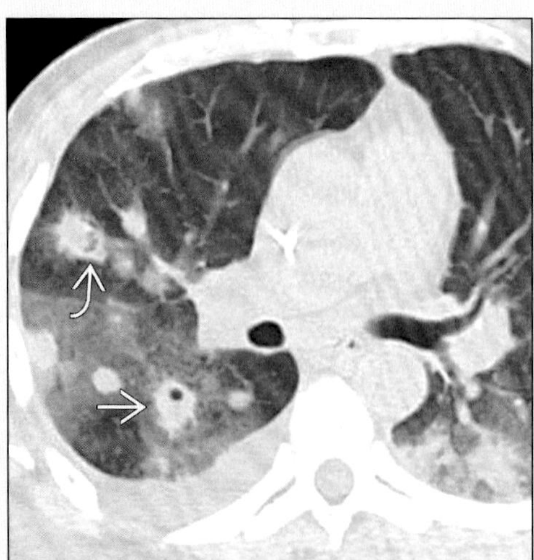
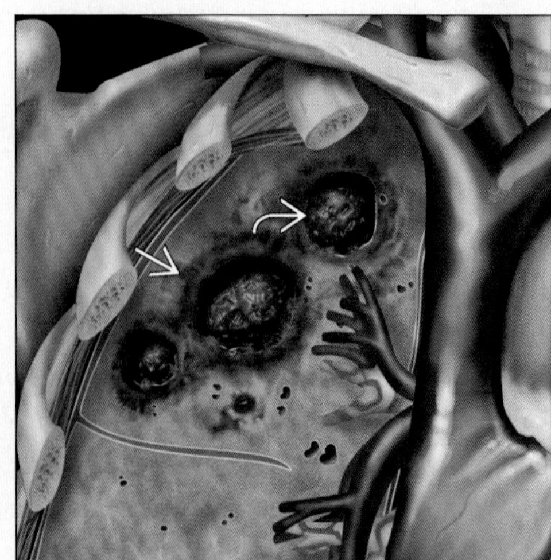

(Left) *Axial NECT of a patient with acute myelogenous leukemia and invasive aspergillosis shows multiple lung nodules, some with cavitation ➔ with surrounding ground-glass opacity. An air crescent ➔ outlines necrotic lung in one of the nodules, characteristic of angioinvasive fungal infection.* ***(Right)*** *Graphic illustrates typical features of invasive aspergillosis, characterized by multifocal cavitary lesions containing devitalized lung ➔ surrounded by air crescents and peripheral halos of hemorrhage ➔.*

ASPERGILLOSIS

TERMINOLOGY

Synonyms

- **Mycetoma, aspergilloma**
- Most mycetomas are aspergillomas: Terms often used interchangeably

Definitions

- **Aspergillosis**: Fungal infection caused by organisms of genus *Aspergillus* (> 100 species)
- **Aspergilloma**: Fungus ball developing in preexisting cavity
- **Semi-invasive aspergillosis**: Chronic necrotizing pulmonary aspergillosis
  - Subacute disease in immunosuppressed patient
- **Invasive aspergillosis**: Rapidly progressive angioinvasive fungal infection affecting severely immunocompromised patients

IMAGING

General Features

- Best diagnostic clue
  - **Aspergilloma**: Dependent spherical or ovoid nodule developing in preexisting cavity or cystic space
  - **Invasive aspergillosis**: CT halo sign
    - Nodule, mass, consolidation surrounded by ground-glass opacity related to hemorrhage
- Location
  - **Aspergillomas**: Preexisting cavities, most frequent in upper lobes
- Size
  - Range from miliary nodules to widespread bilateral consolidations

Radiographic Findings

- **Aspergilloma**
  - Intracavitary, dependent, spherical or ovoid nodule with surrounding gas
  - May not be visible on radiography
- **Invasive aspergillosis**
  - Chest radiograph may initially be normal
  - Rapidly progressing lung nodules or consolidations
  - **Air crescent sign**
    - Crescent-shaped gas collection within lung nodule, mass, or consolidation
    - Consistent with development of invasive aspergillosis in setting of immune compromise
    - Indicates recovery of white blood cell function & is associated with favorable outcome
  - May progress to extensive cavitation & necrosis
  - May invade pleura causing pleural effusion, empyema, or pneumothorax
- **Semi-invasive aspergillosis**
  - Varied appearance: Slow-growing nodule or focus of apical lung consolidation
  - May exhibit coexistent aspergilloma
  - Associated with preexisting lung disease

CT Findings

- **Aspergilloma**
  - Fungus ball or sponge-like heterogeneous mass
  - May fill entire cavity or move within cavity; typically gravity dependent within cavity
  - May exhibit air crescent sign
- **Invasive aspergillosis**
  - Lobar or peribronchial consolidation, centrilobular nodules, ground-glass opacity
  - Peripheral wedge-shaped consolidation mimicking pulmonary infarct
  - **CT halo sign**
    - Represents surrounding parenchymal hemorrhage
    - Highly suggestive of invasive aspergillosis in appropriate clinical setting
      - May be seen with other angioinvasive fungal infections
    - Warrants initiation of antifungal therapy before confirmation by other tests
    - Correlate of air crescent sign, suggests invasive aspergillosis
      - Air crescent sign has limited utility
      - Seen in less than 1/2 of affected patients, often appears late or after initiation of therapy
  - Invasive tracheobronchial aspergillosis
    - Tracheal & central bronchial ulcerations
    - May be associated with atelectasis & consolidation
    - May be seen in lung transplant recipients
- **Semi-invasive aspergillosis**
  - Nodule, mass, or consolidation
  - Cavitary disease

Imaging Recommendations

- Best imaging tool
  - Chest CT for assessment of lung abnormalities & features of angioinvasive fungal disease
- Protocol advice
  - Decubitus radiography may demonstrate intracavitary mobility of aspergilloma
  - Supine & prone CT may likewise demonstrate intracavitary mobility of aspergilloma

DIFFERENTIAL DIAGNOSIS

Other Fungal Infection

- Mucormycosis & candidiasis
- May produce angioinvasive disease

Mycobacterial Infection

- May exhibit consolidation, halo sign, & cavitation
- Cavitary tuberculosis may mimic mycetoma

Bacterial Pneumonia

- Lung abscess may cavitate & mimic angioinvasive aspergillosis

Pulmonary Emboli

- Wedge-like consolidations or nodular opacities from pulmonary infarcts
- Bland or septic pulmonary emboli

Wegener Granulomatosis

- Multifocal nodules, masses, consolidations
- May exhibit cavitation & halo sign

Non-Small Cell Lung Cancer

- Cavitary lung cancer may simulate mycetoma
- Tumor may cause angioinvasion & lung infarction

ASPERGILLOSIS

PATHOLOGY

General Features

- Etiology
  - Most *Aspergillus* infections caused by *A. fumigatus*

Gross Pathologic & Surgical Features

- Invasive aspergillosis: Hyphae invade pulmonary arteries
  - Occlusion, hemorrhage, & infarction
- Necrotic lung within cavitary invasive aspergillosis mimics aspergilloma

Microscopic Features

- *Aspergillus* is dimorphic fungus: Conidial & hyphal forms with 45° angle branching
- Inhaled conidia transform into hyphal forms
- Aspergilloma: Mass containing hyphae, fibrin, & mucus

CLINICAL ISSUES

Presentation

- Most common signs/symptoms
  - Cough, fever, chills, dyspnea, & chest pain
- Other signs/symptoms
  - Weight loss & hemoptysis
- Clinical profile
  - Aspergilloma
    - No serious immunologic abnormality
    - Preexisting lung cavity or cystic space
  - Invasive aspergillosis
    - Severely immunocompromised, characteristically with neutropenia
    - No preexisting lung abnormality
  - Semi-invasive aspergillosis
    - Mildly immunocompromised
    - Preexisting lung disease

Demographics

- Age
  - Older, debilitated patients are more susceptible, but any age group can be affected
  - Most patients with semi-invasive aspergillosis are middle-aged
- Epidemiology
  - **Aspergillomas occur in preexisting cavities**
    - Mycobacterial infection
    - Fungal disease
    - Sarcoidosis
  - **Invasive aspergillosis occurs in immunocompromised patients**
    - Bone marrow, lung, & liver transplants (up to 25%)
    - Acute leukemia (up to 20%)
    - Chemotherapy-induced immune deficiency (up to 20%)
    - Increasing incidence in patients with steroid-dependent COPD
  - **Semi-invasive aspergillosis occurs in mildly immunocompromised patients**
    - Steroid use, malignancy, diabetes mellitus, alcoholism, sarcoidosis
  - No increased risk for aspergillosis in patients with AIDS without additional predisposing factors
    - Neutropenia & steroid use raise risk

Diagnostic Options

- Sputum culture, bronchoalveolar lavage, transthoracic biopsy, & open lung biopsy
- Serum *Aspergillus* precipitin test
- Elevated serum galactomannan levels
  - *Aspergillus* cell wall component

Natural History & Prognosis

- Aspergilloma may remain stable for years
  - Prognosis is generally good
  - Hemoptysis in 40%; may be life threatening
- Invasive aspergillosis progresses over days to weeks
  - Poor prognosis, high mortality
- Semi-invasive aspergillosis progresses over weeks to years
  - Prognosis is often good, but some report up to 40% mortality

Treatment

- Aspergilloma
  - Oral itraconazole & intracavitary amphotericin B have shown mixed success
- Invasive & semi-invasive aspergillosis
  - Voriconazole is treatment of choice
  - Amphotericin B, posaconazole, caspofungin also effective
- Hemoptysis may require bronchial artery embolization or surgical resection

DIAGNOSTIC CHECKLIST

Consider

- Invasive aspergillosis in febrile neutropenic patients with pulmonary abnormalities

Image Interpretation Pearls

- Aspergillomas develop in preexisting cavities
  - Sentinel sign for aspergilloma: Development of pleural thickening adjacent to cavity
  - Cavities should be examined for mycetoma & observed closely on serial exams
- Invasive aspergillosis develops in previously normal lungs of patients with neutropenia
  - Development of low-density rim around invasive aspergillosis
    - May indicate improvement of neutropenia
    - Presages development of air crescent

SELECTED REFERENCES

1. Kousha M et al: Pulmonary aspergillosis: a clinical review. Eur Respir Rev. 20(121):156-74, 2011
2. Segal BH: Aspergillosis. N Engl J Med. 360(18):1870-84, 2009
3. Pinto PS: The CT halo sign. Radiology. 230(1):109-10, 2004
4. Abramson S: The air crescent sign. Radiology. 218(1):230-2, 2001
5. Franquet T et al: Spectrum of pulmonary aspergillosis: histologic, clinical, and radiologic findings. Radiographics. 21(4):825-37, 2001
6. Gefter WB: The spectrum of pulmonary aspergillosis. J Thorac Imaging. 7(4):56-74, 1992

ASPERGILLOSIS

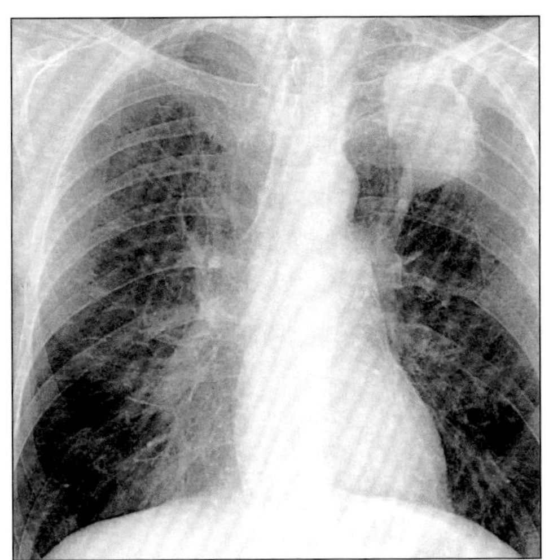

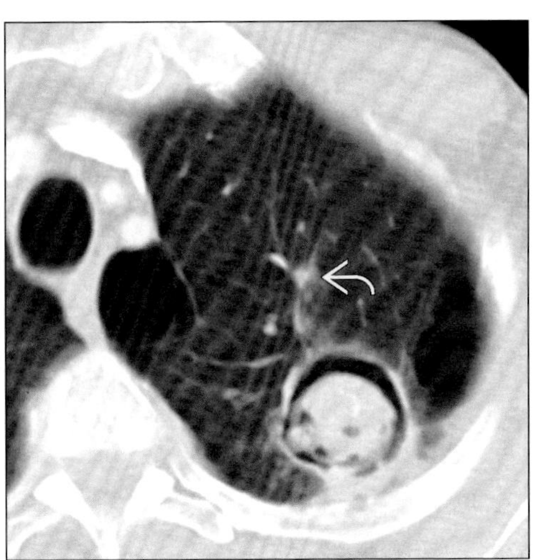

(Left) *PA chest radiograph of a 50-year-old man with HIV infection and new massive hemoptysis shows a right upper lobe mass with irregular borders and intrinsic lucency, suggestive of an air crescent sign.* ***(Right)*** *Axial CECT of the same patient shows a cavitary thick-walled lesion containing central heterogeneous soft tissue. Note surrounding ground-glass opacity related to hemorrhage and adjacent small lung nodules ➥. Invasive aspergillosis was diagnosed after surgical excision.*

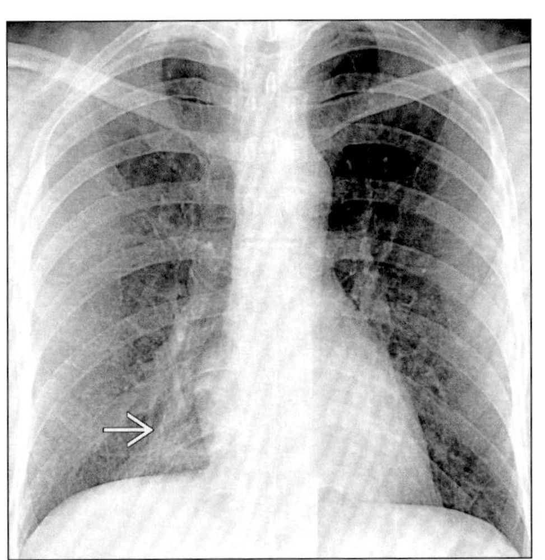

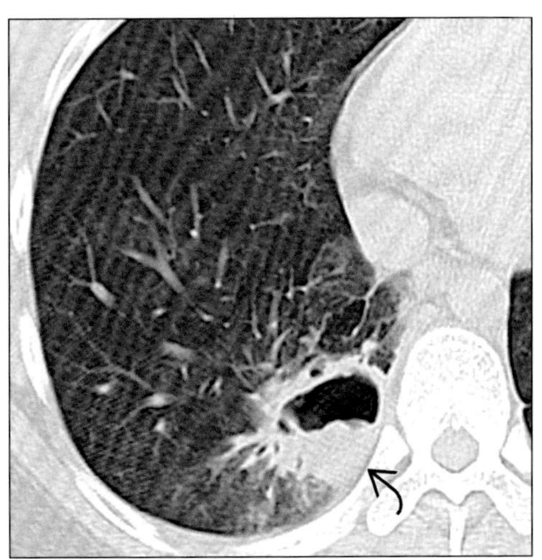

(Left) *PA chest radiograph of a 23-year-old man who presented with massive hemoptysis shows a cavitary lesion ➡ in the right lower lobe.* ***(Right)*** *Axial NECT of the same patient shows a cavitary right lower lobe lesion with thick walls, dependent internal soft tissue ↷, and surrounding ground-glass opacity related to hemorrhage. The patient was scheduled for urgent angiography and potential bronchial artery embolization to treat massive hemoptysis.*

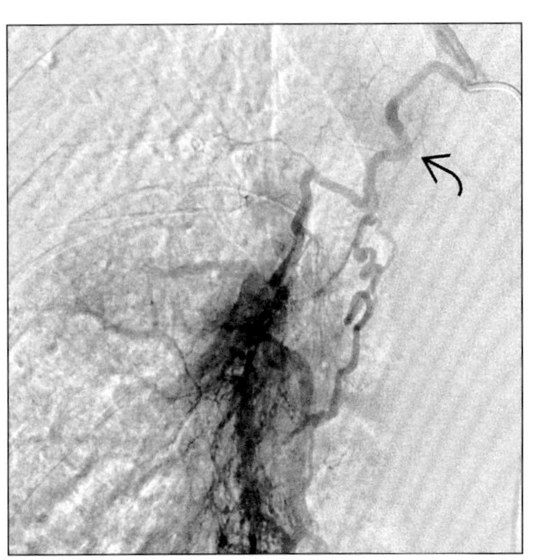

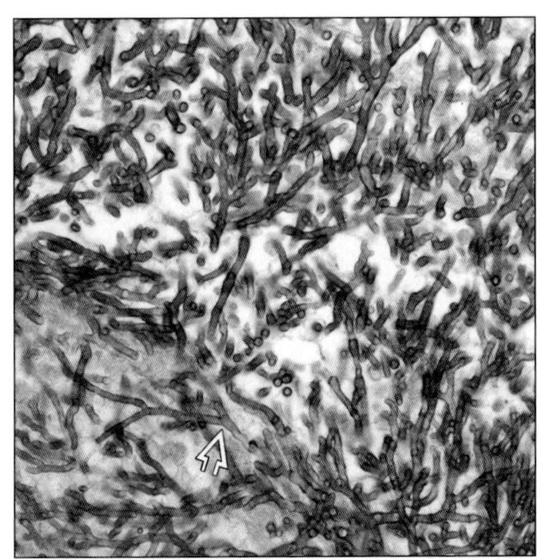

(Left) *AP DSA image of the same patient obtained during bronchial artery embolization demonstrates markedly hypertrophied bronchial arteries ↷ and a blush of contrast in the region of the cavitary lesion. Embolization was only temporarily successful, and resection was ultimately required. Pathology revealed an intralobar sequestration with an aspergilloma.* ***(Right)*** *High-power photomicrograph (H&E stain) shows fungal hyphae branching at 45° angles ⇨, typical of Aspergillus species.*

*(**Left**) PA chest radiograph of a 72-year-old man with acute lymphocytic leukemia and neutropenic fever shows numerous bilateral ill-defined nodules ➔. (**Right**) Axial NECT of the same patient shows multiple part-solid nodules characterized by central soft tissue attenuation and peripheral ground-glass opacity halos ➔. While CT-guided biopsy confirmed invasive aspergillosis in this case, treatment can often be instituted based on presentation and characteristic imaging findings.*

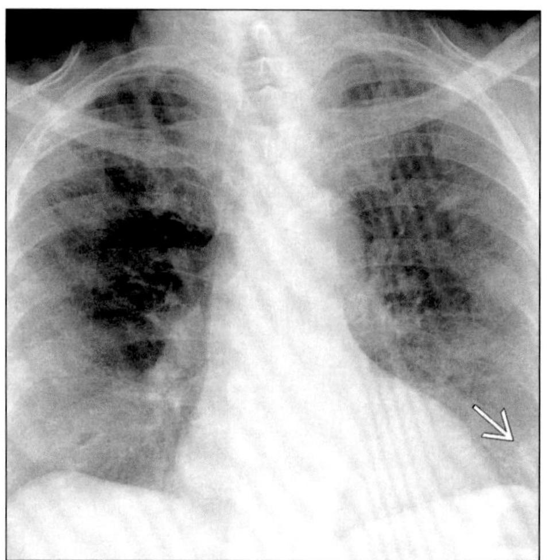

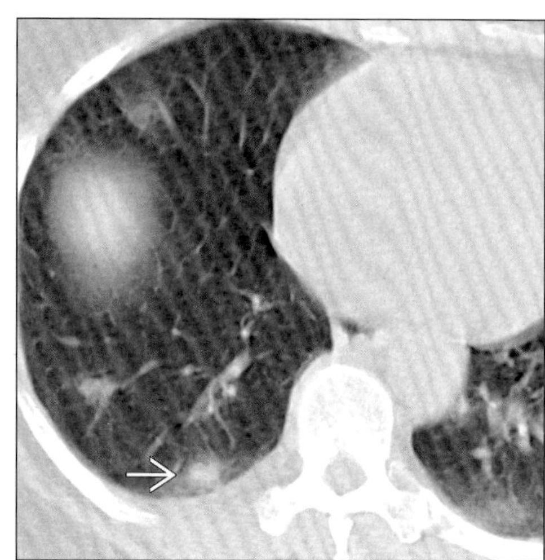

*(**Left**) Coronal NECT of a 26-year-old man with acute myelogenous leukemia and neutropenic fever shows multiple bilateral lung nodules ➔, some with ground-glass opacity halos. The serum galactomannan level was elevated, and the patient received 2 months of voriconazole treatment for the presumed diagnosis of invasive aspergillosis. (**Right**) Axial NECT of the same patient following treatment shows resolution of all lesions except for a small right upper lobe cavitary nodule.*

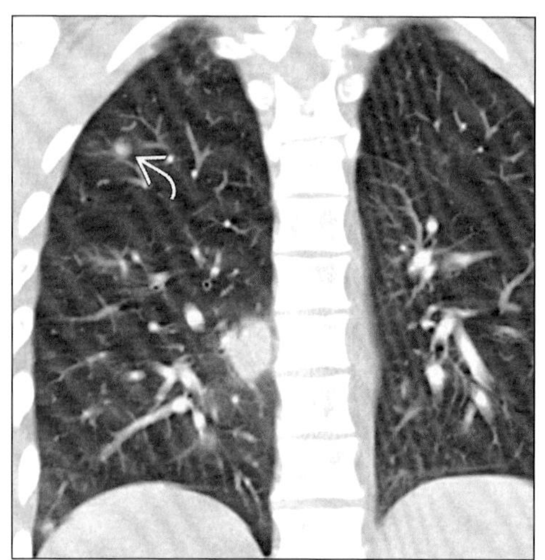

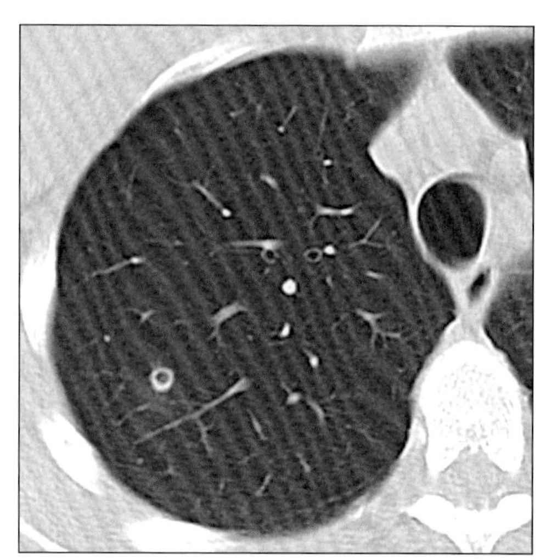

*(**Left**) Axial CECT of a 38-year-old woman with end-stage sarcoidosis and new hemoptysis shows a thick-walled cavitary mass in the left upper lobe with intrinsic heterogeneous content and an air crescent sign. The findings are typical of mycetoma, and aspergilloma was diagnosed on surgical resection. (**Right**) Coronal NECT of a 40-year-old woman shows chronic lung cavities with intrinsic soft tissue nodules consistent with mycetomas or saprophytic aspergillosis ➔.*

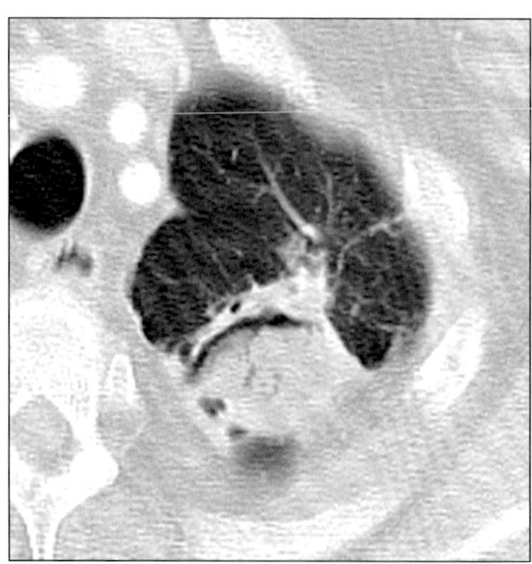

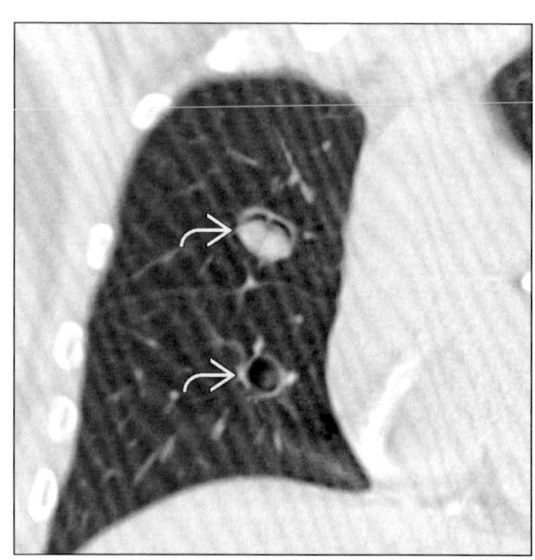

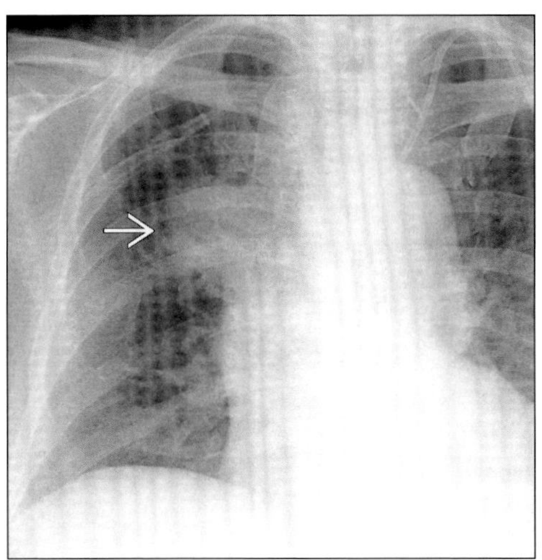

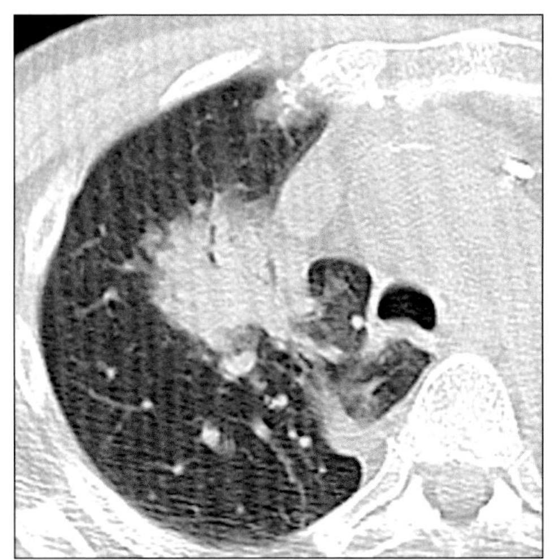

(Left) *AP chest radiograph of a 75-year-old man with acute myelogenous leukemia and neutropenic fever shows a focal right upper lobe mass-like opacity ➔.* ***(Right)*** *Axial NECT of the same patient confirms a 5 cm mass with intrinsic air bronchograms. CT-guided percutaneous biopsy demonstrated invasive aspergillosis. While the halo sign is helpful in suggesting angioinvasive fungal disease, its absence does not exclude the diagnosis. The diagnosis should be suspected in patients with neutropenic fever.*

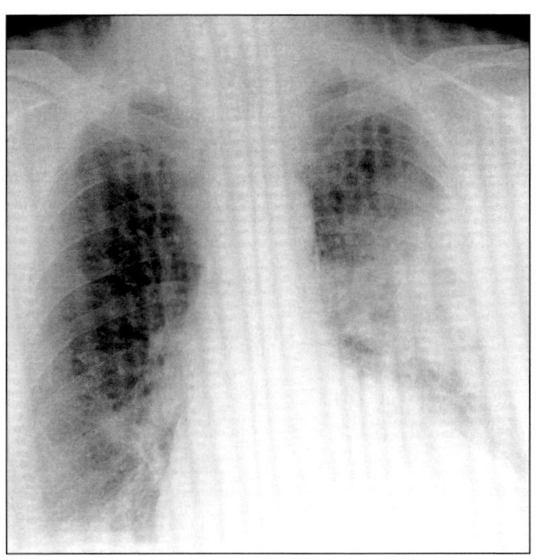

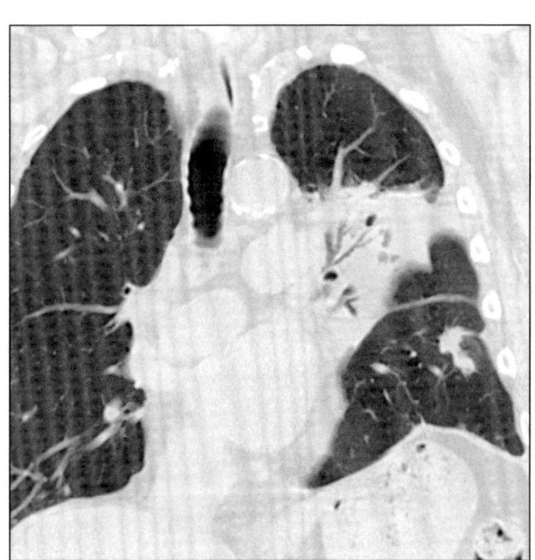

(Left) *PA chest radiograph of an 80-year-old diabetic man with chronic alcoholism shows a large left upper lobe consolidation that progressed in spite of antibiotic treatment.* ***(Right)*** *Coronal NECT of the same patient shows a dominant left upper lobe consolidation. Transbronchial biopsy confirmed semi-invasive aspergillosis. Such abnormalities in the correct clinical setting are highly suspicious for invasive fungal disease, and treatment is often started without biopsy confirmation.*

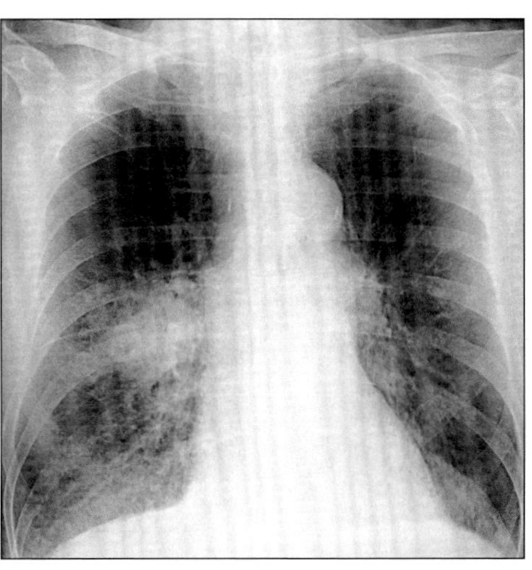

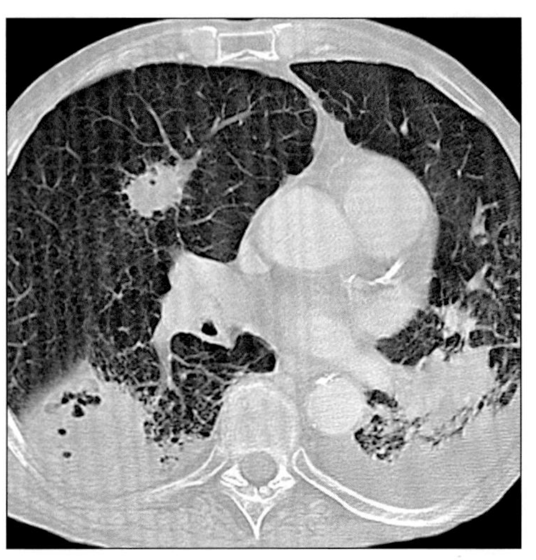

(Left) *PA chest radiograph of a 67-year-old man with head and neck cancer, chronic dyspnea, and cough shows multifocal consolidations with a dominant right perihilar lesion that did not resolve following antibiotic therapy.* ***(Right)*** *Axial NECT of the same patient shows a small left pleural effusion and multifocal nodular cavitary consolidations suggestive of necrotizing pneumonia. CT-guided biopsy confirmed invasive aspergillosis and absence of metastatic disease. Invasive aspergillosis may also affect the pleura.*

ZYGOMYCOSIS

Key Facts

Terminology

- Synonym: Mucormycosis
- Opportunistic infection caused by fungi belonging to *Zygomycetes* class
  - *Rhizopus* & *Mucor* are most common

Imaging

- Radiography
  - Unilateral or bilateral mass-like consolidation
  - Solitary or multiple nodules or masses
  - Pleural effusion
  - Hilar lymphadenopathy
- CT
  - Nodule(s) & mass(es)
  - Ground-glass halo related to hemorrhage
  - Reverse halo sign
  - Cavitation
  - Consolidation; may be mass-like or wedge-shaped

Top Differential Diagnoses

- Aspergillosis
- Bacterial pneumonia

Pathology

- Distinctive hyphae: Branching at 90° angles with rare septations

Clinical Issues

- Risk factors
  - Hematologic malignancy
  - Solid organ or hematopoietic stem cell transplant
  - Diabetic ketoacidosis
  - Steroid treatment
- Treatment
  - Lobectomy for localized disease
  - Amphotericin B
- High mortality: > 60%

*(**Left**) PA chest radiograph of a patient with lung cancer and chemotherapy-induced neutropenia and fever shows a heterogeneous right apical mass. (**Right**) Axial NECT of the same patient shows a right upper lobe mass-like consolidation with internal areas of cavitation. CT-guided percutaneous fine needle aspiration revealed hyphae with right angle branching patterns characteristic of zygomycosis. Given immunosuppression, other fungal infections and tuberculosis would also have to be considered.*

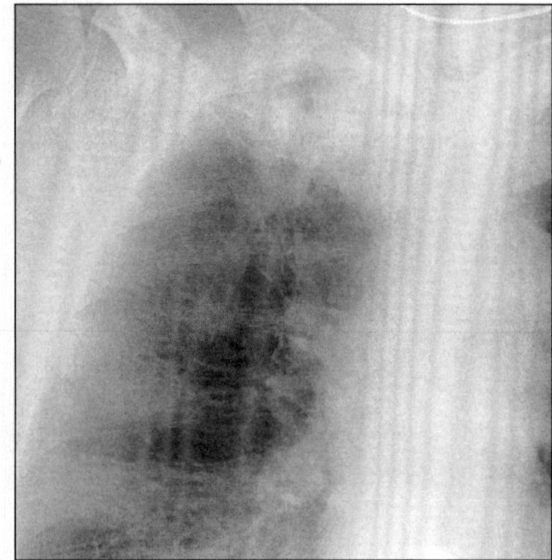

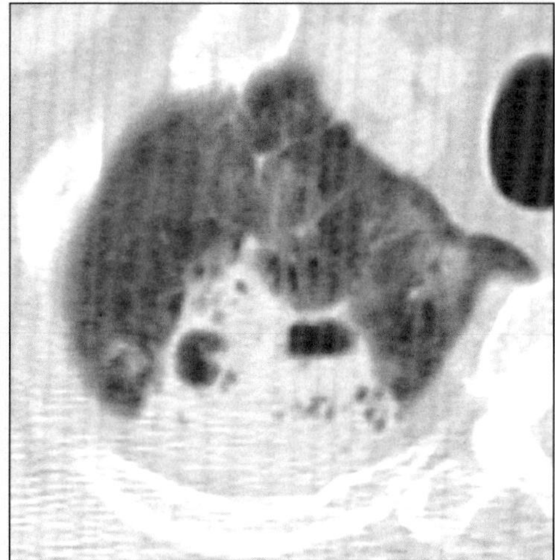

*(**Left**) Axial NECT of a heart and kidney transplant recipient who presented with chest pain shows a large right upper lobe mass abutting the adjacent chest wall with a surrounding ground-glass halo. CT-guided needle biopsy confirmed the diagnosis of zygomycosis. (**Right**) Axial NECT of a patient on steroid therapy for a glioma, who developed rhinocerebral zygomycosis, shows a cavitary right upper lobe nodule. Other cavitary lung nodules (not shown) were also present, consistent with pulmonary zygomycosis.*

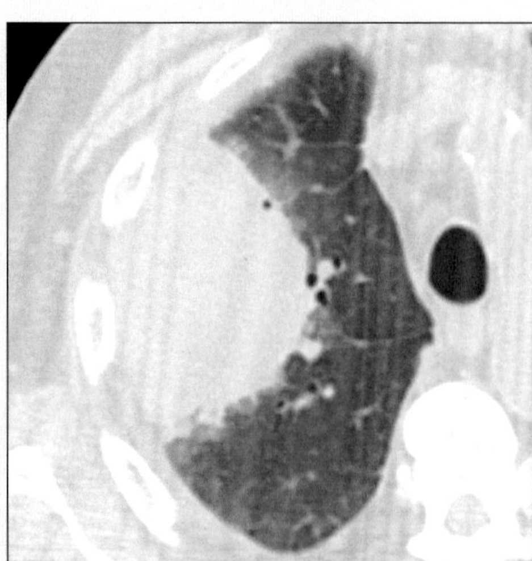

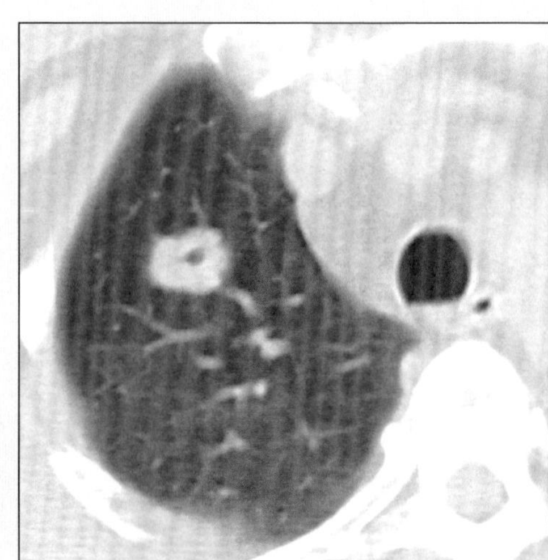

ZYGOMYCOSIS

TERMINOLOGY

Synonyms

- **Mucormycosis**

Definitions

- Opportunistic infection caused by fungi belonging to *Zygomycetes* class, which includes *Rhizopus, Mucor, Rhizomucor, Absidia*, etc.

IMAGING

Radiographic Findings

- Unilateral or bilateral consolidation, may be mass-like
- Solitary or multiple nodules or masses
- Pleural effusion
- Hilar lymphadenopathy

CT Findings

- Nodule(s) & mass(es)
  - Ground-glass halo related to hemorrhage
  - Air crescent sign, central cavitation
  - Reverse halo sign, ground-glass opacity surrounded by peripheral consolidation
    - Most common cause of reverse halo in immunocompromised host
- Consolidation
  - May be wedge-shaped
  - May exhibit internal air bronchograms
- Pulmonary artery pseudoaneurysm (infrequent)
- Direct extension into adjacent mediastinum or heart
- Hypoattenuating hepatic or renal lesions from hematogenous spread

Imaging Recommendations

- Best imaging tool
  - CT helpful for further characterization of radiographic abnormalities & formulation of differential diagnosis
  - CT-guided needle biopsy helpful in identifying organism

DIFFERENTIAL DIAGNOSIS

Aspergillosis

- Difficult to distinguish from zygomycosis clinically & radiographically
- Factors that favor zygomycosis over aspergillosis
  - Concomitant sinusitis
  - > 10 pulmonary nodules on CT
  - Pleural effusion
  - Prior voriconazole prophylaxis

Bacterial Pneumonia

- Lack of response to empiric antibiotic therapy should raise suspicion for atypical organisms

PATHOLOGY

Microscopic Features

- Distinctive hyphae
  - Broad (5-15 μm in diameter)
  - Irregular branching pattern
  - Branches at 90° angles
  - Rare septations
- Vascular wall invasion with resultant vascular necrosis & infarction
- ± granulomatous reaction

CLINICAL ISSUES

Presentation

- Most common signs/symptoms
  - Fever
  - Cough
  - Dyspnea
  - Chest pain
- Other signs/symptoms
  - Hemoptysis

Demographics

- Epidemiology
  - 3rd most common invasive fungal infection, after aspergillosis & candidiasis
  - 8.3-13.0% of all fungal infections in autopsies of patients with hematologic malignancies
  - Pulmonary involvement caused by inhalation of spores or hematogenous spread
    - Ubiquitous in nature: Decaying vegetation & soil
  - Risk factors
    - Leukemia, lymphoma
    - Diabetes, particularly those with ketoacidosis
    - Solid organ & hematopoietic stem cell transplant
    - Intravenous drug user
    - Deferoxamine therapy (for treatment of iron overload)
      - Deferoxamine-iron chelate stimulates fungal growth
    - Steroid treatment
    - Neutropenia

Natural History & Prognosis

- Rapid progression & tissue destruction
- Mortality 60-100% in immunocompromised patients

Treatment

- Surgical resection
  - Lobectomy for localized disease
- Antibiotics
  - Intravenous amphotericin B
  - Oral posaconazole
    - After patient has responded to amphotericin B
    - Second-line therapy for patients who cannot tolerate or do not respond to amphotericin B
  - Voriconazole, used to treat *Aspergillus*, is not effective against zygomycosis
- Control of underlying risk factors, such as diabetes or neutropenia

SELECTED REFERENCES

1. Severo CB et al: Chapter 7: zygomycosis. J Bras Pneumol. 36(1):134-41, 2010
2. Mantadakis E et al: Clinical presentation of zygomycosis. Clin Microbiol Infect. 15 Suppl 5:15-20, 2009
3. Brown J: Zygomycosis: an emerging fungal infection. Am J Health Syst Pharm. 62(24):2593-6, 2005

PNEUMOCYSTIS JIROVECI PNEUMONIA

Key Facts

Terminology
- Pneumocystis pneumonia (PCP)
- Opportunistic fungal infection often affecting individuals with T-cell immunodeficiency

Imaging
- Radiography
  - May be normal, diffuse bilateral airspace disease
  - Spontaneous pneumothorax in HIV(+) patient is virtually diagnostic of PCP
- CT
  - Ground-glass opacity is dominant finding
  - "Crazy-paving" pattern less common
  - Cysts (30%)
  - Atypical patterns (5-10%): Multiple small nodules, asymmetric ground-glass, & consolidation
  - Lymphadenopathy uncommon (10%)
  - Pleural effusion rare

Top Differential Diagnoses
- Hypersensitivity pneumonitis
- Lymphocytic interstitial pneumonia
- Diffuse alveolar hemorrhage
- Cytomegalovirus pneumonia
- Pulmonary alveolar proteinosis

Clinical Issues
- Most prevalent opportunistic infection in AIDS
- HIV(+) patients: Subacute fever, cough, dyspnea
- Non-HIV patients: Fulminant respiratory failure with fever & cough
- Treatment: Trimethoprim-sulfamethoxazole, IV pentamidine

Diagnostic Checklist
- Consider PCP in immunocompromised patient with diffuse bilateral ground-glass opacities

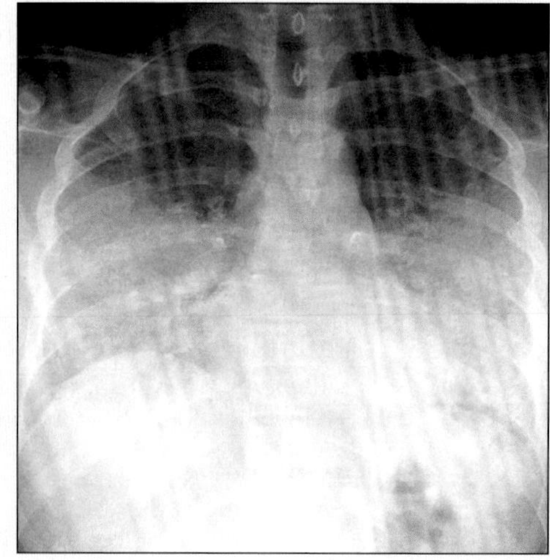
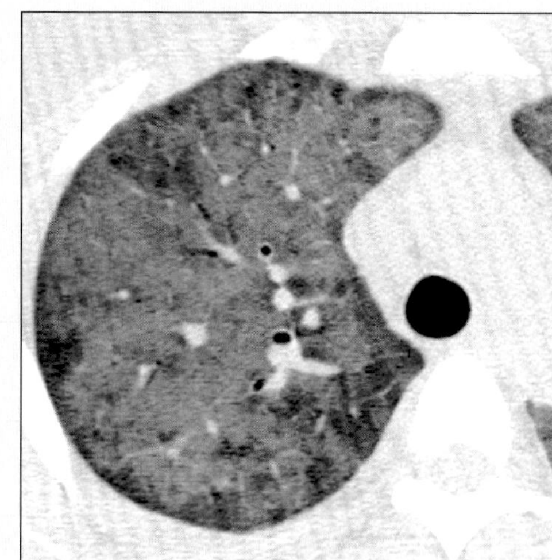

(Left) *PA chest radiograph of a 30-year-old woman, who presented with progressive cough and dyspnea for several weeks, shows diffuse bilateral hazy airspace disease.* ***(Right)*** *Axial NECT of the same patient shows diffuse ground-glass opacities with relative subpleural sparing, which affected the lungs bilaterally. Once neutropenia was detected, HIV infection was suspected and PCP was diagnosed with bronchial washings. PCP is the most prevalent opportunistic infection in patients with HIV infection.*

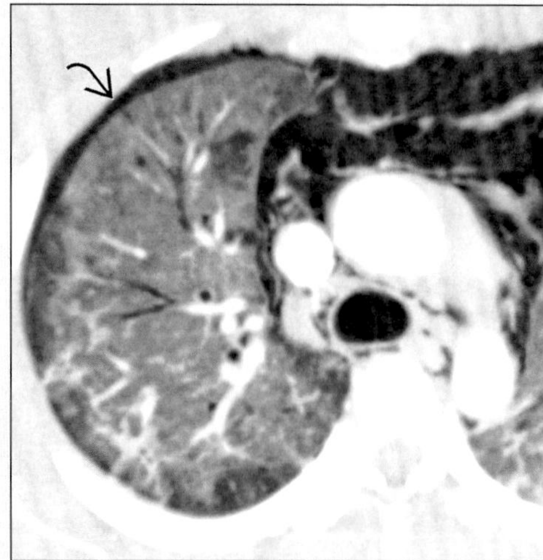
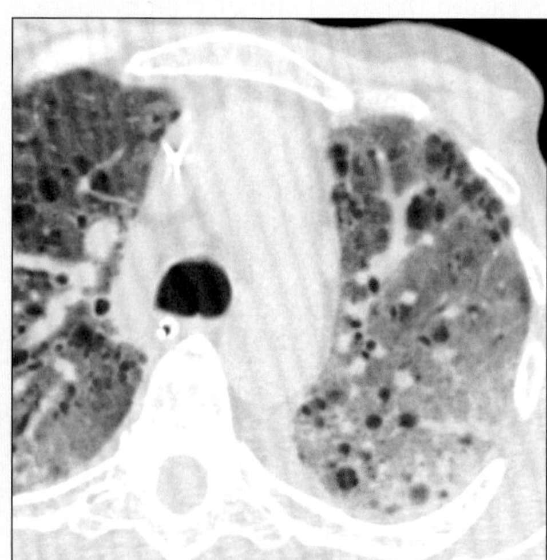

(Left) *Axial CECT of the same patient obtained 4 weeks after a prolonged hospitalization shows a small right pneumothorax ⇒ and a large pneumomediastinum. The patient required intubation and expired a few days later. Spontaneous pneumothorax in an HIV(+) patient represents PCP until proven otherwise.* ***(Right)*** *Axial NECT of a 55-year-old man who developed PCP following stem cell transplantation shows diffuse ground-glass opacities and numerous lung cysts not present on a prior CT scan (not shown).*

PNEUMOCYSTIS JIROVECI PNEUMONIA

TERMINOLOGY

Abbreviations

- **Pneumocystis pneumonia (PCP)**

Definitions

- Opportunistic fungal infection often affecting individuals with T-cell immunodeficiency
  - *Pneumocystis jiroveci*

IMAGING

General Features

- Best diagnostic clue
  - Diffuse symmetric ground-glass opacities in hypoxic immunocompromised patient
- Location
  - Diffuse perihilar involvement with sparing of peripheral subpleural lung
  - Less commonly upper lobe predominant disease with thin-walled cysts
- Morphology
  - Ground-glass opacities with cysts (30%)

Radiographic Findings

- Chest radiograph may be normal
- Spontaneous pneumothorax in patients with AIDS
  - Highly suggestive of PCP

CT Findings

- Morphology
  - **Ground-glass opacity** is dominant finding
    - Superimposed intralobular lines & smooth interlobular septal thickening ("crazy-paving" pattern) less common
  - **Cysts (30%)**
    - Thin walled, usually with ground-glass opacities
    - Typical upper lobe distribution
    - Predisposition to pneumothorax
    - Resolution over 5 months with successful treatment
    - Rarely described in non-AIDS PCP
  - **Atypical patterns (5-10%)**
    - Multiple small nodules (may cavitate)
    - Asymmetric ground-glass or consolidation
    - Reticular (interlobular & intralobular) opacities rarely dominant finding
- Distribution
  - HIV(+)
    - Diffuse symmetric ground-glass opacities
    - Sparing of lung periphery (40%)
    - Mosaic attenuation (30%)
    - Upper lobe distribution may be associated with aerosolized pentamidine prophylaxis
  - Non-HIV
    - Often spares 1 lung zone (upper, middle, lower)
  - Prior irradiated lung protected: PCP develops only outside radiation ports
- Other
  - Lymphadenopathy uncommon (10%), short axis diameter > 1 cm
    - More common with other fungal or tuberculous infections
  - Pleural effusion rare
- Confident diagnosis in 95% of patients with AIDS

Nuclear Medicine Findings

- Historically, gallium scan used for problem cases
  - Widespread lung activity in PCP
- Largely replaced by CT; long imaging times (24 hours)

Imaging Recommendations

- Best imaging tool
  - HRCT is imaging modality of choice

DIFFERENTIAL DIAGNOSIS

Hypersensitivity Pneumonitis

- Antigen source identified with detailed history
  - More subacute or chronic onset of dyspnea & nonproductive cough
  - Hypoxia often less severe, fever less common
- Diffuse ground-glass opacities, most common imaging manifestation
- Ill-defined centrilobular nodules more common than in PCP
- Air-trapping common at expiratory CT, uncommon with PCP
- May also exhibit lung cysts

Lymphocytic Interstitial Pneumonia

- Increased frequency in AIDS, especially in children
- Thin-walled cysts, ground-glass opacities, centrilobular nodules
- Lymph nodes may be enlarged, uncommon with PCP

Diffuse Alveolar Hemorrhage (DAH)

- Anemia common
- Clinical history, tissue sampling, & laboratory investigation required to differentiate various etiologies of DAH
- Diffuse or extensive bilateral ground-glass opacities & consolidations similar to PCP

Cytomegalovirus Pneumonia

- Similar predisposition (cell-mediated immunodeficiency): Most common associated infection with PCP
- Bilateral diffuse ground-glass opacities most frequent finding
- Centrilobular nodules (often admixed with ground-glass opacities) more common than in PCP

Noncardiogenic Edema

- Usually predisposing etiology (sepsis, toxic fume inhalation, surgery, aspiration)
- Gradient of findings: Normal nondependent lung to ground-glass opacities to consolidated dependent lung
- Severely hypoxic patients

Pulmonary Alveolar Proteinosis

- More indolent symptoms (often over months), except rare patients with hematological malignancy
- Fever & severe hypoxia uncommon (33% are asymptomatic)
- Ground-glass with concurrent intra-, interlobular reticulation ("crazy-paving" pattern)
  - "Crazy-paving" pattern less common with PCP

PNEUMOCYSTIS JIROVECI PNEUMONIA

PATHOLOGY

General Features

- Etiology
  - Patients with impaired cell-mediated immunity are predisposed to PCP
    - **AIDS, especially patients with CD4 counts < 200/mm³**
    - **Long-term corticosteroid therapy**, particularly during tapering phase
    - Organ transplantation, bone marrow transplantation (BMT), chemotherapy
    - Monoclonal antibodies: Adalimumab, infliximab, etanercept, rituximab used in autoimmune diseases & malignancy
    - Congenital immunodeficiency, such as thymic aplasia, bare lymphocyte syndrome, combined immunodeficiency syndrome
    - Prematurity & malnutrition
- Initially classified as protozoan
  - RNA ribosomal sequencing phylogenetically reclassified as fungus

Gross Pathologic & Surgical Features

- Opportunistic infection caused by *Pneumocystis jiroveci*
  - 2 fungal forms: Trophozoites & cysts
- Organism is difficult to culture

Microscopic Features

- Intraalveolar foamy exudate, fungus usually seen in tiny bubble-like areas
  - Gomori methenamine silver (GMS) or calcofluor white (CW) stains excellent for detecting cysts
  - Giemsa stain useful to demonstrate trophozoites
- Radiologic-pathologic correlation
  - Ground-glass opacities: Alveolar filling by foamy exudates (surfactant, fibrin, cellular debris)
  - Inter-, intralobular reticular opacities: Interstitial edema or cellular infiltration
  - Nodules: Granulomatous inflammation

CLINICAL ISSUES

Presentation

- Most common signs/symptoms
  - HIV(+) patients
    - Fever, cough, dyspnea; often **subacute**, gradually worsening over 2-6 weeks
  - Non-HIV patients
    - Symptoms of **fulminant** respiratory failure with fever & cough usually presenting over 4-10 days
- Other signs/symptoms
  - Hypoxia on room air: Common & important clinical feature, particularly during minimal exercise
    - Absence of hypoxia favors entities other than PCP
  - White blood cell count usually not elevated
  - Patients with AIDS usually develop infection when CD4 count < 200/mm³
    - 90% have elevated LDH
    - Rising LDH level despite therapy predicts poor outcome

Demographics

- Age
  - Any age, dependent on risk factors
- Epidemiology
  - Organism can be found in normal lungs
  - Airborne transmission
  - Even with highly active antiretroviral therapy (HAART), PCP remains most prevalent opportunistic infection in AIDS
  - Develops in up to 15% patients after bone marrow or solid organ transplant (without prophylaxis)

Natural History & Prognosis

- Prophylaxis in patients with AIDS indicated when CD4 count < 200/mm³
  - Those with CD4 < 200/mm³ who are not receiving prophylaxis are 9x more likely to develop infection
  - Consider in patients on prolonged corticosteroid therapy or monoclonal antibodies
  - Main prophylactic medications: Oral trimethoprim-sulfamethoxazole or, if allergic, oral dapsone
- HIV
  - Diagnosis: Bronchoscopy with bronchoalveolar lavage (BAL) is procedure of choice
    - Sensitivity: 90-98%
- Non-HIV: PCP more difficult to diagnose
  - Less fungal load, greater inflammatory component
  - Delayed diagnosis: Negative sputum &/or BAL may lead to consideration of another diagnosis
    - High clinical suspicion required
    - Transbronchial biopsy may be needed for diagnosis
- Mortality rate in affected patients with AIDS currently 6%, higher in non-AIDS patients

Treatment

- Appropriately treated PCP has very good prognosis
  - Trimethoprim-sulfamethoxazole or intravenous (IV) pentamidine effective in most
    - Common progression of radiographic abnormalities during early course of therapy since medications require large amount of IV fluid for administration
  - After initiation of treatment, clinical improvement in 80% of cases (mean: 5 days)
    - Radiographic improvement lags by 5 days
  - In patients with PCP & severe hypoxia, early adjunctive treatment with corticosteroids has significantly decreased rate of respiratory failure

DIAGNOSTIC CHECKLIST

Consider

- PCP in immunocompromised patient with diffuse bilateral ground-glass opacities

SELECTED REFERENCES

1. Hardak E et al: Radiological features of Pneumocystis jirovecii Pneumonia in immunocompromised patients with and without AIDS. Lung. 188(2):159-63, 2010
2. Tasaka S et al: Comparison of clinical and radiological features of pneumocystis pneumonia between malignancy cases and acquired immunodeficiency syndrome cases: a multicenter study. Intern Med. 49(4):273-81, 2010
3. D'Avignon LC et al: Pneumocystis pneumonia. Semin Respir Crit Care Med. 29(2):132-40, 2008

PNEUMOCYSTIS JIROVECI PNEUMONIA

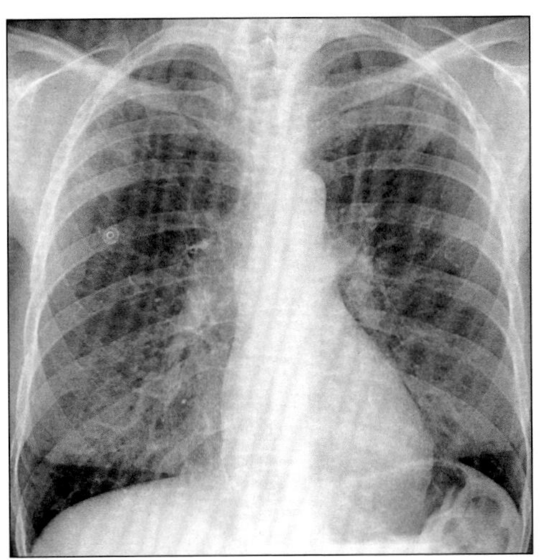

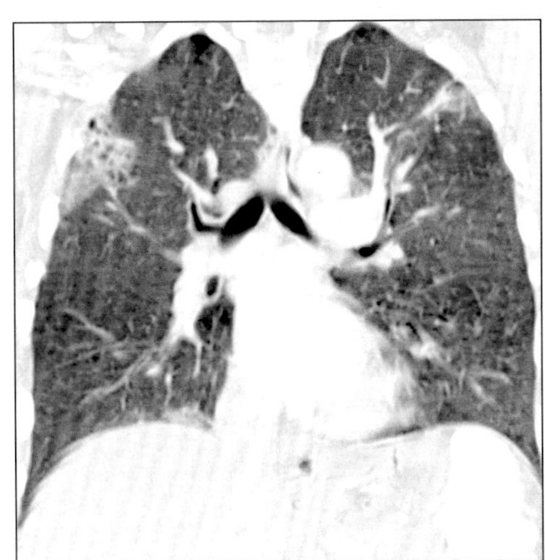

(Left) *PA chest radiograph of a 44-year-old woman with HIV infection and increasing dyspnea shows patchy bilateral upper lobe airspace opacities.* ***(Right)*** *Coronal CECT of the same patient shows diffuse bilateral ground-glass opacities with bilateral focal upper lobe peripheral consolidations. Sputum samples were positive for P. jiroveci, and the patient recovered following a course of trimethoprim-sulfamethoxazole.*

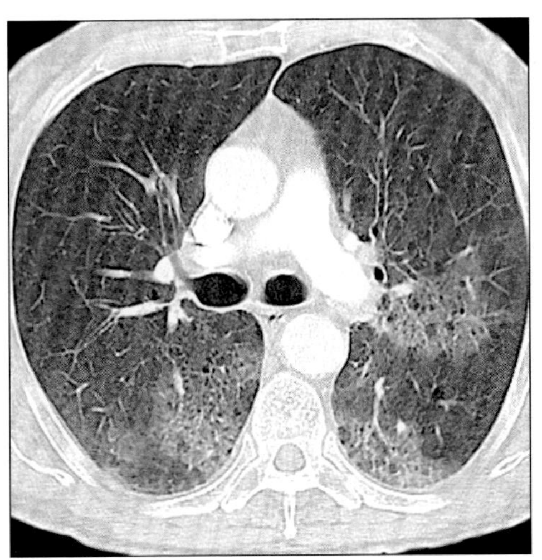

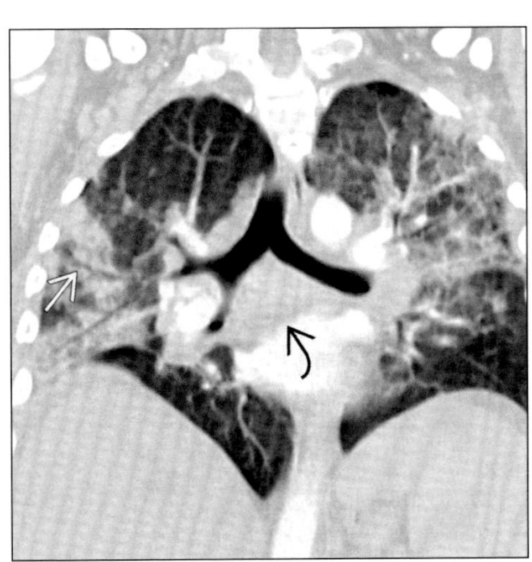

(Left) *Axial CECT of a 72-year-old man who was receiving chemotherapy for lymphoma and presented with cough and fever shows multifocal geographic areas of ground-glass attenuation. PCP was detected on sputum analysis.* ***(Right)*** *Coronal CECT of a 53-year-old man with neutropenic fever and PCP shows patchy bilateral ground-glass opacities and consolidations with intrinsic air bronchograms ➔ and mediastinal lymphadenopathy ➔ related to known lymphoma.*

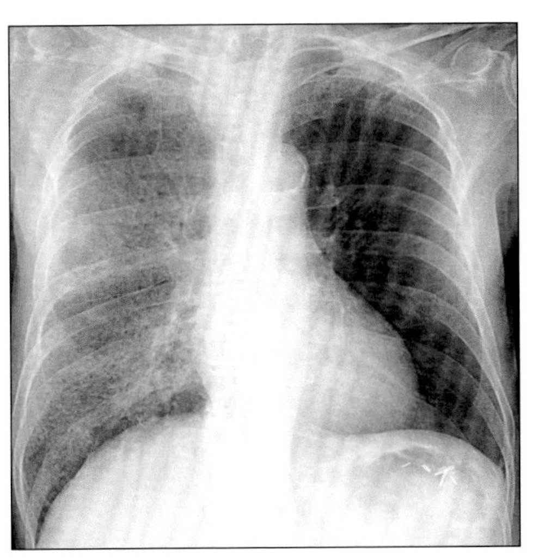

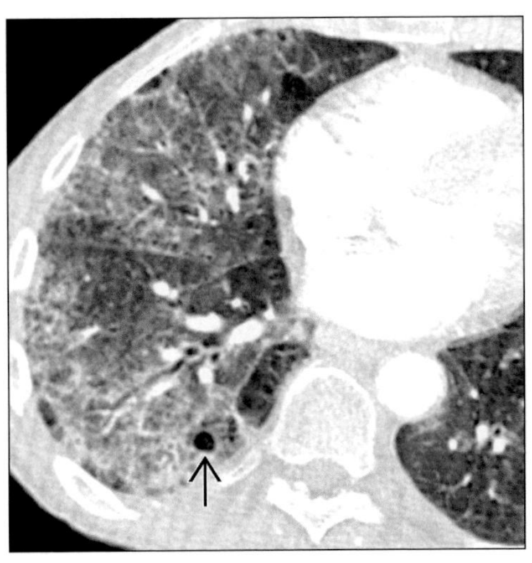

(Left) *PA chest radiograph of a 40-year-old man with HIV infection noncompliant with highly active antiretroviral therapy (HAART) shows PCP manifesting with diffuse, hazy, and reticular opacities throughout the right lung.* ***(Right)*** *Axial CECT of the same patient shows asymmetric right lung ground-glass opacity, thickening of the peribronchovascular interstitium, and a small thin-walled cyst ➔ in the right lower lobe. Asymmetric involvement is an atypical manifestation of PCP.*

DIROFILARIASIS

Key Facts

Terminology
- *Dirofilaria immitis* (dog "heartworm")
- Filarial nematode found commonly in dog heart

Imaging
- Radiography
  - Solitary pulmonary nodule
  - Well-circumscribed, noncalcified lung nodule
  - Typically subpleural (68%)
  - Right lower lobe (76%)
  - < 3 cm in diameter
- CT
  - Solitary/multiple nodules
  - Typically subpleural
  - Eccentric calcification (rare)
  - Air crescent sign (rare)
  - Invasion of chest wall & mediastinum (rare)
  - Pleural effusion (rare)

Top Differential Diagnoses
- Fungal infection
- Lung cancer
- Metastasis

Clinical Issues
- Usually asymptomatic
- Subcutaneous or lung parenchymal nodule(s)
- M:F = 2:1 (USA patients)

Diagnostic Checklist
- Lack of characteristic symptoms, laboratory, or radiographic findings
- Serology using ELISA: Positive in 75% of cases
- Consider dirofilariasis in patient with solitary lung nodule & close association with domestic dogs
- *D. immitis* increasingly recognized as inadvertent human pathogen

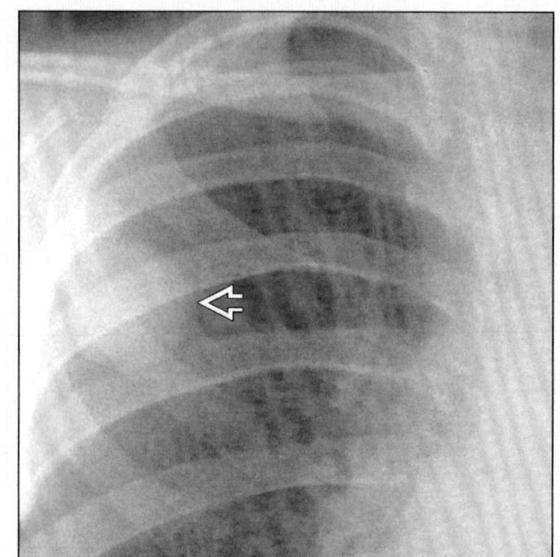

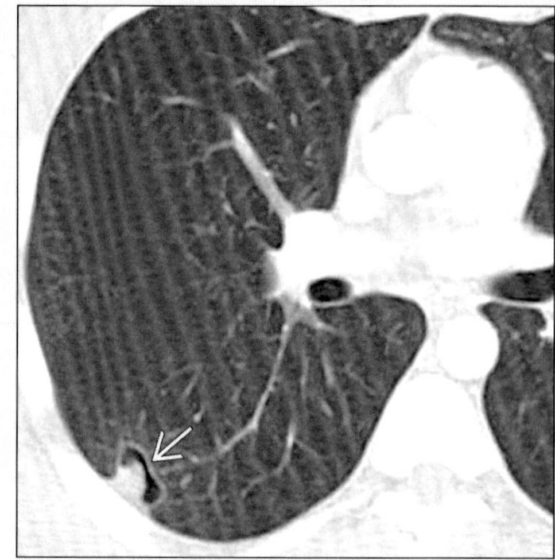

(Left) *PA chest radiograph of an asymptomatic 14-year-old girl with dirofilariasis shows a solitary lung nodule ➡ in the right upper lobe. Histopathologic analysis demonstrated an infarcted peripheral vessel containing remnants of the parasite. Surgical excision is usually required for definitive diagnosis.* ***(Right)*** *Axial CECT of a patient with dirofilariasis shows a peripheral lung nodule with a surrounding air crescent ➡. CT findings may mimic angioinvasive fungal infection. (Courtesy P. Boiselle, MD.)*

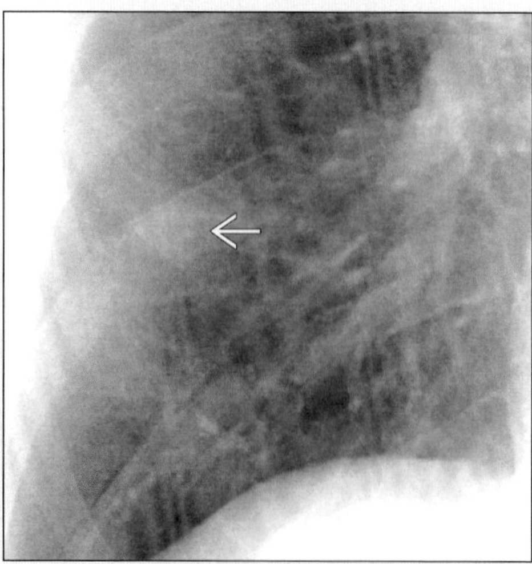

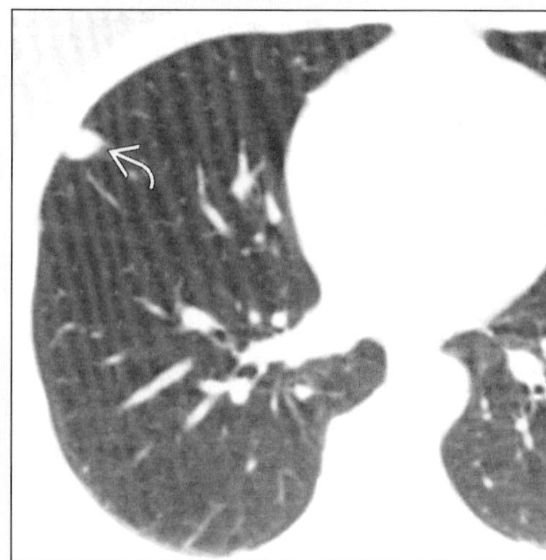

(Left) *PA chest radiograph of a patient with dirofilariasis shows a faint nodular opacity ➡ in the right middle lobe.* ***(Right)*** *Axial NECT of the same patient shows a solitary well-defined middle lobe nodule ➡. Primary lung cancer should be excluded, particularly if the patient is a smoker. Definitive diagnosis is usually made histologically or sporadically, with aspiration of the nodule and demonstration of fragments of the parasite. (Courtesy N. Patz, MD.)*

DIROFILARIASIS

TERMINOLOGY

Synonyms

- *Dirofilaria immitis* **(dog "heartworm")**

Definitions

- Filarial nematode found commonly in dog heart
- Man: Dead-end host

IMAGING

General Features

- Best diagnostic clue
  - **Solitary pulmonary nodule**
  - Endemic areas
- Location
  - Right lower lobe
- Morphology
  - Spherical, wedge-shaped

Radiographic Findings

- Radiography
  - Well-circumscribed, noncalcified lung nodule
  - Typically subpleural (68%)
  - Right lower lobe in 76% of cases
  - < 3 cm in diameter

CT Findings

- NECT
  - Solitary/multiple lung nodules
    - Typically subpleural (68%)
    - Eccentric calcification (rare)
    - Air crescent sign (rare)
  - Pleural thickening or effusion

DIFFERENTIAL DIAGNOSIS

Fungal Infection

- Histoplasmosis; coccidioidomycosis

Lung Cancer

- May manifest as solid or subsolid lung nodule

Metastasis

- Typically multiple, solitary metastasis rare

PATHOLOGY

General Features

- Etiology
  - *Dirofilaria immitis* (dog "heartworm")

Gross Pathologic & Surgical Features

- Solitary (90%) or multiple (10%) pulmonary nodules
- **Lung nodule**: End-stage lesion resulting from death of parasite in pulmonary vascular bed
  - Well-circumscribed, grayish-yellow rounded nodule
  - Surrounded by granulomatous zone of epithelial cells, plasma cells, lymphocytes, & fibrous capsule rich in eosinophils
  - Calcification & caseous necrosis
  - Dead parasite within thrombotic pulmonary artery
  - Peripheral fibrosis
  - Overlying pleura usually inflamed & fibrotic (75%)

CLINICAL ISSUES

Presentation

- Most common signs/symptoms
  - Usually asymptomatic
  - Subcutaneous or lung parenchymal nodule(s)
- Other signs/symptoms
  - Cough & hemoptysis
  - Blood eosinophilia (10-20%)

Demographics

- Gender
  - M:F = 2:1 (USA patients)
- Epidemiology
  - Related to prevalence of canine dirofilariasis & suitable mosquito vectors
  - Temperate climates: East Coast & Southern United States; sporadic cases worldwide
  - Should be included in differential diagnosis of solitary lung nodule, especially in endemic areas

Natural History & Prognosis

- Usually infects dogs
- Transferred to humans by mosquito bites
  - Pulmonary embolization: Granulomatous reaction & infarct
- Dirofilaria stop developing at temperatures below 14°C
  - Predominant occurrence in warmer climates

DIAGNOSTIC CHECKLIST

Consider

- Dirofilariasis in patient with solitary pulmonary nodule & close association with domestic dogs at time of diagnosis

Image Interpretation Pearls

- *D. immitis* increasingly recognized as inadvertent human pathogen

Reporting Tips

- Preoperative diagnosis is difficult
- Pulmonary lesions initially misidentified as malignancy
  - Lack of characteristic symptoms, laboratory, or radiographic findings
  - Serologic studies using ELISA: Positive in 75% of cases
  - Fine-needle aspiration of peripheral pulmonary lesions (few cases)

SELECTED REFERENCES

1. Martínez S et al: Thoracic manifestations of tropical parasitic infections: a pictorial review. Radiographics. 25(1):135-55, 2005
2. Oshiro Y et al: Pulmonary dirofilariasis: computed tomography findings and correlation with pathologic features. J Comput Assist Tomogr. 28(6):796-800, 2004
3. Flieder DB et al: Pulmonary dirofilariasis: a clinicopathologic study of 41 lesions in 39 patients. Hum Pathol. 30(3):251-6, 1999

HYDATIDOSIS

Key Facts

Terminology

- Parasitic disease caused by larvae of class *Cestoda*: *E. granulosus* & *E. multilocularis*
- Hydatidosis: Human infection by metacestodes

Imaging

- Radiography
  - Solitary or multiple spherical or ovoid masses with well-defined borders
  - Variable size (1 cm to > 20 cm in diameter)
  - Tracheobronchial communication (rupture): Meniscus/crescent sign or water lily/camalote sign
  - Pleural effusion; hydropneumothorax
- CT
  - Spherical or ovoid fluid-filled cyst
  - Cyst wall enhancement
  - May involve mediastinum, heart, chest wall, pulmonary artery, diaphragm

Top Differential Diagnoses

- Metastases
  - Sarcoma; colonic & renal adenocarcinoma; benign metastasizing leiomyoma
- Rare neoplasms
  - Lung cancer: Large cell neuroendocrine carcinoma
  - Localized fibrous tumor of pleura

Clinical Issues

- Usually asymptomatic: Incidental imaging finding
- Compression of adjacent structures
- Cyst rupture (tracheobronchial tree or pleura)
- Serologic test: ELISA AgB (antigen B-rich fraction)

Diagnostic Checklist

- Consider hydatid cyst in patients from endemic sheep-raising areas with solitary or multiple, well-defined pulmonary nodule(s) or mass(es)

*(**Left**) PA chest radiograph of a 54-year-old man with pulmonary hydatid disease shows a large, sharply marginated lobular mass in the left upper lung zone. (**Right**) Axial CECT of the same patient shows a mass of homogeneous fluid attenuation surrounded by an enhancing peripheral soft tissue rim ➔. E. granulosus was identified at pathologic analysis. In endemic areas, a large solitary spherical or ovoid fluid-filled cystic lung mass with well-marginated borders is characteristic of hydatid disease.*

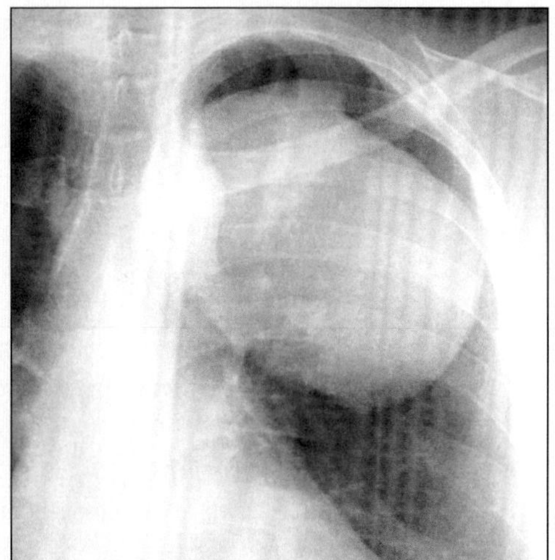

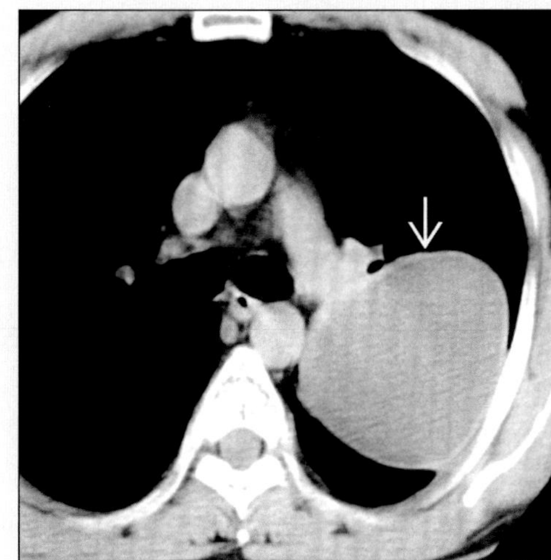

*(**Left**) PA chest radiograph of a patient with a complicated hydatid cyst shows air between the pericyst ➔ and exocyst ➔, resulting in a "crescent" sign. (**Right**) PA chest radiograph of a patient with a ruptured hydatid cyst in the right lower lung shows a cavitary lesion with lobular contents ➔ floating in fluid within the pericyst ➔. This appearance represents the "water lilly" sign. Both signs, in the appropriate clinical setting, are highly characteristic of hydatidosis.*

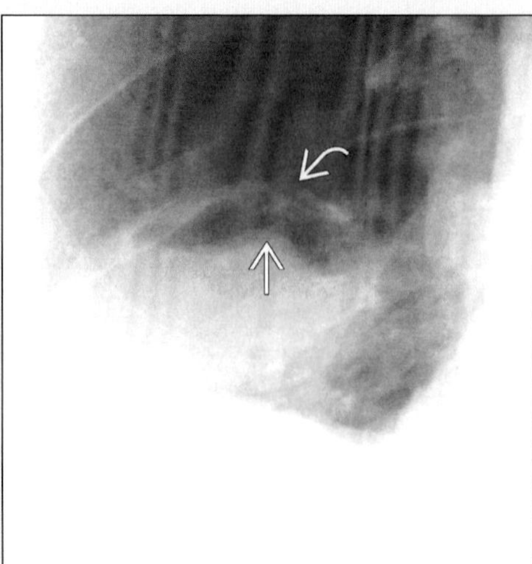

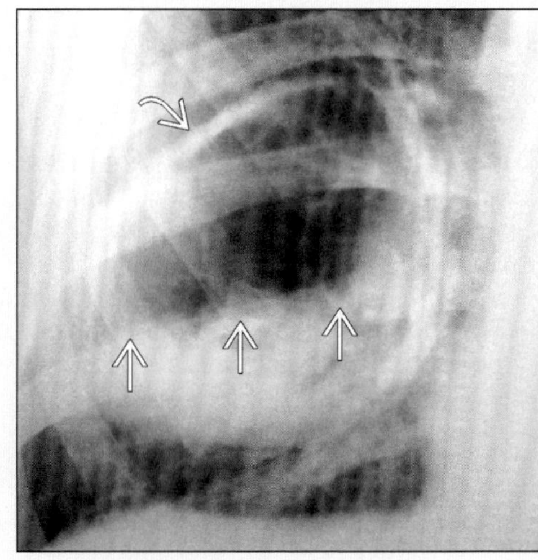

HYDATIDOSIS

TERMINOLOGY

Synonyms

- Hydatid disease
- Echinococcosis

Definitions

- Parasitic disease caused by larvae of class *Cestoda*: *E. granulosus* & *E. multilocularis*
  - Pastoral form (*E. granulosus*): More common, wider distribution, endemic in sheep-raising areas (Australia, Mediterranean region, South America, Middle East, & New Zealand)
    - Unilocular cystic hydatidosis
  - Sylvatic form (*E. multilocularis*): Associated with animals in wild ecosystems, especially foxes, wolves, mice
    - Alveolar hydatidosis
- **Hydatidosis**: Human infection by metacestodes
- **Echinococcosis**: Term more appropriately used for infection of nonhuman carnivores by adult parasite

IMAGING

Radiographic Findings

- Radiography
  - Solitary or multiple spherical or ovoid masses with well-defined borders
    - Multiple in 30% of cases, bilateral in 20%, lower lobe location in 60%
  - Variable size (1 cm to > 20 cm)
  - Complications
    - Tracheobronchial tree communication (rupture)
      - **Meniscus or crescent sign**: Cyst communication with bronchus (air between pericyst & exocyst)
      - **Water lily or camalote sign**: Undulating cyst membranes floating in fluid
      - Hydatid pneumonitis: Aspiration of hydatid material (vomica)
    - Pleural effusion; hydropneumothorax

CT Findings

- NECT
  - Spherical or ovoid fluid-filled cyst (~ 0 HU); smooth, thin walls
  - Calcification extremely rare (0.7%)
- CECT
  - Cyst wall enhancement
  - May involve mediastinum, heart, chest wall, pulmonary artery, diaphragm
  - Complications
    - Acute hydatid pulmonary embolism (rare): Invasion of cardiovascular system

DIFFERENTIAL DIAGNOSIS

Metastases

- Sarcoma; colonic & renal adenocarcinoma; benign metastasizing leiomyoma

Rare Thoracic Neoplasms

- Lung cancer: Large-cell neuroendocrine carcinoma
- Localized fibrous tumor of pleura

PATHOLOGY

Gross Pathologic & Surgical Features

- 3 layers
  - **Pericyst**: Dense & fibrous, host reaction to parasite
  - **Exocyst** (outer laminated cyst membrane): Acellular portion of parasite, permits passage of nutrients
  - **Endocyst** (inner membrane): Germinal layer, produces larval scolices

CLINICAL ISSUES

Presentation

- Most common signs/symptoms
  - Usually asymptomatic: Incidental imaging finding
  - Compression of adjacent structures: Chest pain, cough, hemoptysis
  - Cyst rupture (tracheobronchial tree or pleura)
    - Expectoration of cyst fluid, membranes, scolices ("hydatid vomica")
    - Aspiration pneumonitis
    - Hypersensitivity reaction (antigenic material released by cyst): Fever, wheezing, urticaria; anaphylaxis (rare)
    - Chest pain: Pleural effusion, pneumothorax
- Other signs/symptoms
  - Laboratory
    - Serologic test: ELISA AgB (antigen B-rich fraction)

Natural History & Prognosis

- Dog: Definitive host for *E. granulosus* (harbors adult worm in intestine)
  - Eggs shed in dog feces: Viable for weeks, contaminate food sources of intermediate hosts (sheep, cattle, horses)
- Humans (accidental intermediate hosts): Food contaminated with eggs; eggs migrate from GI tract to circulation & reach liver (primarily affected organ)
  - Hydatid cysts develop over several months or years
- Secondary involvement due to hematogenous dissemination may affect almost any anatomic location

DIAGNOSTIC CHECKLIST

Consider

- Hydatid cyst in patients from endemic sheep-raising areas with solitary or multiple, well-defined pulmonary nodule(s) or mass(es)

Image Interpretation Pearls

- Signs of complicated hydatid cyst: Meniscus or crescent sign, water lily or camalote sign

SELECTED REFERENCES

1. Martínez S et al: Thoracic manifestations of tropical parasitic infections: a pictorial review. Radiographics. 25(1):135-55, 2005
2. Pedrosa I et al: Hydatid disease: radiologic and pathologic features and complications. Radiographics. 20(3):795-817, 2000

STRONGYLOIDIASIS

Key Facts

Terminology

- Infection by *Strongyloides stercoralis*

Imaging

- Autoinfection
  - Diffuse reticular opacities & miliary nodules
  - Bronchopneumonia & patchy airspace opacities that may coalesce
  - Serial radiography may show migratory disease
- Hyperinfection syndrome
  - Diffuse bilateral airspace opacities
  - Diffuse alveolar hemorrhage
  - Imaging findings of ARDS
- Pleural effusions
- Cardiac enlargement
  - Migration of larvae into pericardium
- Secondary infection and abscess formation: Cavitation and air-fluid levels

Top Differential Diagnoses

- Bronchopneumonia
- Diffuse alveolar hemorrhage
- Acute respiratory distress syndrome (ARDS)
- Chronic eosinophilic pneumonia

Pathology

- Autoinfection: Cycle of endogenous reinfection
- Hyperinfection syndrome: High worm burden
- Disseminated strongyloidiasis: Spread to organs outside of normal migration pattern
- Identification of larvae in stool, sputum, ± skin

Clinical Issues

- Hyperinfection syndrome may mimic pulmonary embolism or exacerbation of asthma or COPD
- Treatment: Thiabendazole or mebendazole, hyperinfection syndrome may require intubation

*(**Left**) AP chest radiograph of a patient with strongyloidiasis shows bilateral miliary nodules. Autoinfection may manifest as miliary disease. (**Right**) Composite image with CECT in lung (left) and soft tissue (right) windows shows a right upper lobe abscess ➔ with an intrinsic air-fluid level and adjacent airspace disease ➔. A smaller abscess ➔ is present in the right lower lobe superior segment. Mortality approaches 80% in patients with strongyloidiasis complicated by secondary infection.*

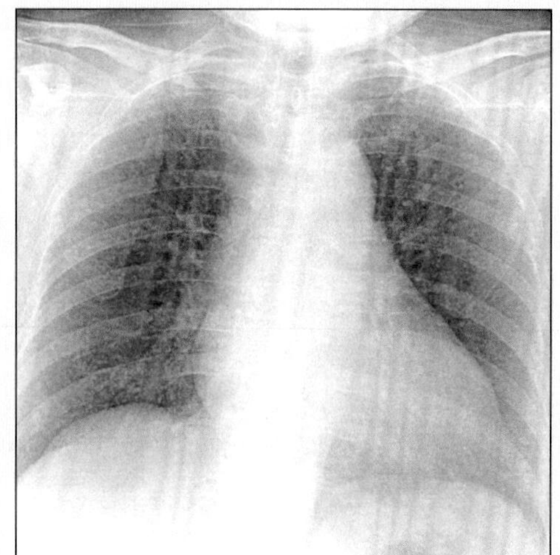

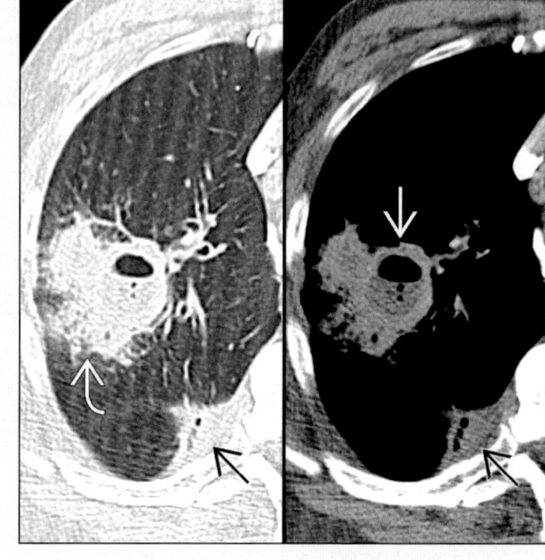

*(**Left**) Axial NECT of a patient with autoinfection shows a left lower lobe mass-like consolidation ➔ with intrinsic air bronchograms. In these patients, coalescent airspace opacities and consolidation indicate progression of disease burden. (**Right**) AP chest radiograph of an intubated patient demonstrates diffuse bilateral airspace opacities. Washings from bronchoalveolar lavage revealed Strongyloides stercoralis organisms in this patient with hyperinfection syndrome.*

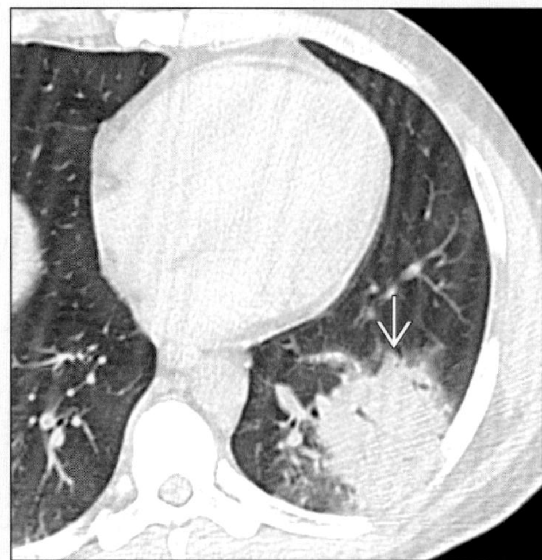

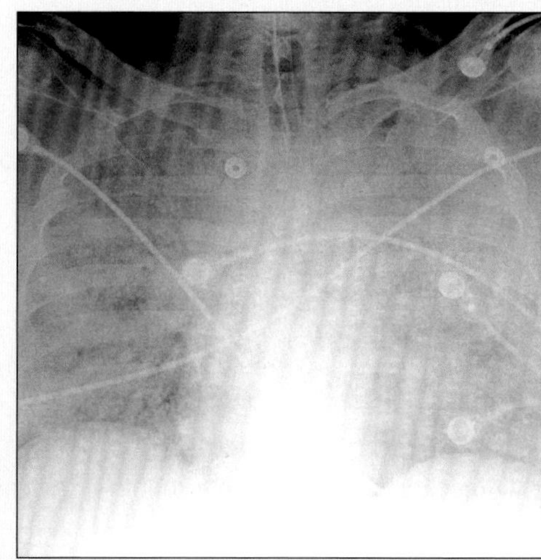

STRONGYLOIDIASIS

TERMINOLOGY

Definitions

- Infection by *Strongyloides stercoralis*

IMAGING

Radiographic Findings

- **Autoinfection**
  - Migration of larvae from capillary bed into alveoli
    - Diffuse reticular opacities
    - Miliary nodules
  - Progression of disease burden
    - Bronchopneumonia
    - Patchy airspace opacities that may coalesce
    - Serial radiography may show migratory involvement
- **Hyperinfection syndrome**
  - Diffuse bilateral airspace opacities
  - Diffuse alveolar hemorrhage
  - Acute respiratory distress syndrome (ARDS)
    - Bilateral airspace opacities & consolidations
- Pleural effusions
- Cardiac enlargement
  - Migration of larvae into pericardium
  - Pericarditis & pericardial effusion

CT Findings

- Identification of findings of secondary infection & abscess formation
  - Cavitation & air-fluid levels

Imaging Recommendations

- Best imaging tool
  - Chest radiography adequate for monitoring disease course
  - CT used as problem-solving tool

DIFFERENTIAL DIAGNOSIS

Bronchopneumonia

- Focal parenchymal abnormality in patient with fever
- Pattern ranges from consolidation to interstitial thickening, may be focal or diffuse (multilobar)

Diffuse Alveolar Hemorrhage

- Diffuse bilateral airspace opacities
- Normal heart size

Acute Respiratory Distress Syndrome (ARDS)

- Radiologic & pathologic findings typically discussed in terms of hours, days, weeks, & months
- Days: Bilateral airspace opacities & consolidation within 24 hours
- Weeks: Consolidation decreases; patchy airspace or reticular opacities persist
- Months: Subpleural reticular opacities & honeycomb lung

Chronic Eosinophilic Pneumonia

- Chronic peripheral upper lobe consolidation
  - Peripheral distribution (outer 2/3) of upper lobes
- Migratory consolidation: Waxing & waning; simultaneous involvement of different lung regions

PATHOLOGY

General Features

- Etiology
  - *Strongyloides stercoralis*: Small nematode
    - **Autoinfection**
      - Cycle of endogenous reinfection within host unique to *S. stercoralis*
      - May lead to chronic infection of 50+ years
    - **Hyperinfection syndrome**
      - Acceleration of nematode life cycle
      - High worm burden; normal migration pattern
      - Affected patients usually immunocompromised
    - **Disseminated strongyloidiasis**
      - Spread to extraintestinal organs outside of normal migration pattern (central nervous system, heart, & urinary tract)

Microscopic Features

- **Identification of larvae** in stool, sputum, ± skin

CLINICAL ISSUES

Presentation

- Most common signs/symptoms
  - **Hyperinfection syndrome**
    - Wheezing, shortness of breath, & chest pain
    - May mimic pulmonary embolism or exacerbation of asthma or COPD
- Other signs/symptoms
  - Gastrointestinal involvement
    - Nausea, vomiting, diarrhea, & abdominal pain
  - Skin involvement: Urticaria & macular rashes
  - Eosinophilia common in chronic infection

Demographics

- Epidemiology
  - Tropical & subtropical climates
  - USA: Southeast & Puerto Rico
  - > 100 million persons with chronic infection worldwide

Natural History & Prognosis

- Mortality from hyperinfection or dissemination: 70%
  - Complicated by secondary infection: 80%

Treatment

- Thiabendazole or mebendazole
  - Duration depends on disease severity
  - Multidrug therapy in cases of resistance
- Patients with hyperinfection syndrome may require intubation & mechanical ventilation

DIAGNOSTIC CHECKLIST

Consider

- Strongyloidiasis in patients with focal or diffuse airspace disease in endemic locations

SELECTED REFERENCES

1. Martínez S et al: Thoracic manifestations of tropical parasitic infections: a pictorial review. Radiographics. 25(1):135-55, 2005

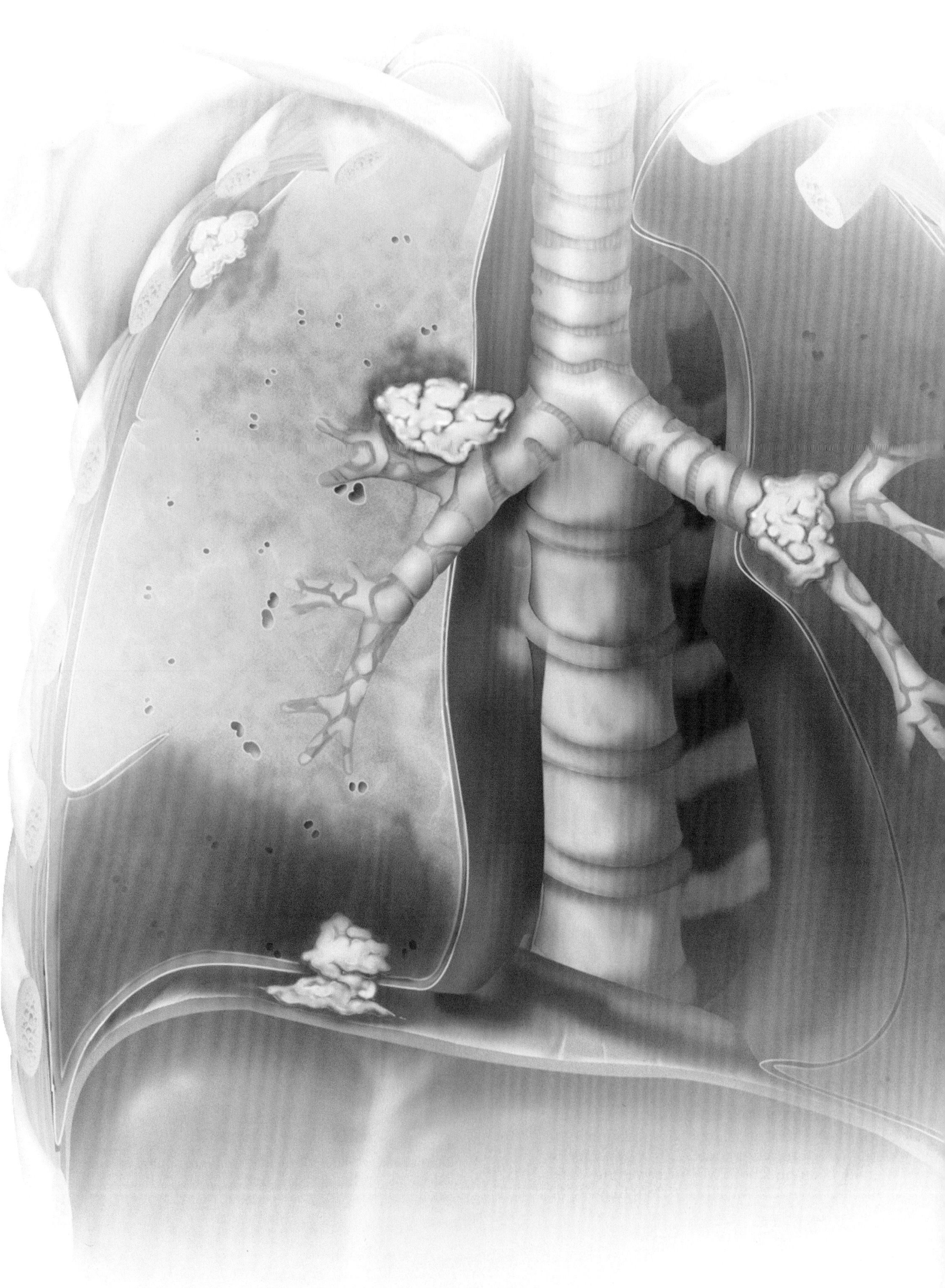

SECTION 5
Pulmonary Neoplasms

Introduction and Overview

Lung Cancer

Uncommon Neoplasms

Lymphoma and Lymphoproliferative Disorders

Metastatic Disease

APPROACH TO PULMONARY NEOPLASMS

Introduction

Pulmonary neoplasms are a heterogeneous group of lesions with variable morphologic and imaging features. The most common neoplasm of the lung is metastatic disease, and the most common primary pulmonary neoplasm is lung cancer. Other primary malignant lung neoplasms are rare. Lymphoma may result in either primary or secondary lung involvement. Although benign lung neoplasms are also rare, establishing a prospective diagnosis of benignity in a lung lesion is important in order to avoid unnecessary invasive procedures.

The radiologist plays a critical role in the detection, diagnosis, and management of lung neoplasms. A major challenge is the prospective distinction of various tumor-like nonneoplastic infectious and inflammatory conditions from pulmonary neoplasia. In some cases, lung lesions resolve on imaging follow-up after medical treatment, allowing a confident diagnosis of benignity.

Pulmonary Metastases

Metastases, the most common pulmonary neoplasms, characteristically manifest with multifocal lung nodules or masses that typically exhibit spherical shapes, well-defined borders, and a basilar-predominant distribution. Hemorrhagic metastases may exhibit ill-defined borders secondary to surrounding alveolar hemorrhage. Atypical manifestations of metastatic disease include solitary nodule, cavitation, and calcification. Metastatic disease may also manifest as lymphangitic carcinomatosis with patchy reticular opacities that represent interlobular septal thickening. Lung metastases characteristically disseminate via hematogenous routes, but lymphatic and tracheobronchial dissemination and direct lung invasion may also occur.

Many patients with metastatic disease have a known malignancy. However, some affected patients present with pulmonary metastases of unknown origin. In these cases, the primary malignancy may not be found on imaging studies, by physical exam, or at autopsy. Although these patients have a very poor prognosis, it is important to obtain tissue diagnosis to identify the cell type of the malignancy and determine the most appropriate therapy.

Lung Cancer

Lung cancers are primary malignant lung neoplasms that comprise a wide range of histologic cell types, including adenocarcinoma, squamous cell carcinoma, small cell carcinoma, large cell carcinoma, and neoplasms of mixed histology. These lesions exhibit variable morphologic features and biologic behavior. Lung cancer is associated with inhaled carcinogens and is intimately related to cigarette smoking. Other carcinogens that play a role in the development of lung cancer include asbestos, arsenic, radon, and polycyclic aromatic hydrocarbons. Affected patients may be occupationally exposed to these substances. The term "bronchogenic carcinoma" was traditionally used to refer to these neoplasms, but it has now been established that many lung cancers arise in the lung periphery beyond a recognizable bronchus.

Epidemiology

In 2008, lung cancer was the most frequently diagnosed malignancy and the leading cause of cancer mortality in men worldwide and the second leading cause of cancer mortality in women. The highest rates of lung cancer in men are found in eastern and southern Europe, North America, Micronesia, Polynesia, and eastern Asia, while in women the highest incidence rates are in North America, Northern Europe, and Australia/New Zealand. In the United States, it is estimated that in 2011 there will be over 200,000 new cases of lung cancer and approximately 155,000 lung cancer deaths. In spite of this, lung cancer mortality rates in men in the United States have been decreasing and, for the first time in recent history, have started to decrease in women.

Clinical Presentation

Patients with lung cancer characteristically present with symptoms. Presenting complaints may be related to central neoplasms that produce bronchial obstruction or local invasion of thoracic structures. Some patients present with symptoms related to metastatic disease or paraneoplastic syndromes. While a large number of patients with lung cancer present with advanced stage disease, an increasing number of affected patients are asymptomatic and diagnosed because of an incidentally discovered imaging abnormality.

Imaging Features

Lung cancer exhibits a wide range of imaging findings. Peripheral lung cancer often manifests as a pulmonary nodule, mass, or consolidation. Such lesions may invade extrapulmonary structures including the chest wall, diaphragm, and mediastinum. Central lung cancer often manifests as a hilar or perihilar mass, which may be obscured by surrounding pneumonia &/or atelectasis. Thus, unexplained atelectasis should be investigated and consolidations in adults should be followed to complete resolution to exclude underlying malignancy. Some lung cancers, specifically adenocarcinomas, may manifest as multifocal lung nodules, masses, or consolidations that mimic metastases. Advanced lung cancer may manifest with extensive intrathoracic lymphadenopathy and may mimic lymphoma and metastatic disease. In some cases, patients with lung cancer are initially diagnosed because of distant metastases to the abdomen, brain, skeleton, or extrathoracic lymph nodes.

Although radiologists are often the first health care providers to suggest the diagnosis of lung cancer, interpretation of chest radiographs is fraught with pitfalls related to superimposition of numerous structures of various size and radiographic opacity and to the poor conspicuity and small size of many lung cancers. Observer error, technical factors, failure to compare to prior imaging, and incomplete clinical information may further exacerbate the problem. In fact, missed lung cancer on radiography constitutes the second leading cause of malpractice actions against radiologists. Radiologists interpreting chest imaging studies must have in-depth knowledge of normal imaging anatomy, evaluate imaging studies in a systematic manner, and consistently compare current to prior studies. When suspicious abnormalities are found, the radiologist must directly communicate unexpected findings to the referring clinician and outline management recommendations, which may include further imaging &/or tissue sampling.

Diagnosis

Although imaging features may be highly suggestive of lung cancer, microscopic analysis of tissue samples is required for a specific and definitive diagnosis. A careful evaluation of the anatomic location of the lesion &/or its metastases and identification of affected extrapulmonary structures allows the radiologist to suggest the most appropriate site and method of tissue sampling, including image-guided biopsy, bronchoscopy, or more invasive surgical procedures such as mediastinoscopy, mediastinotomy, video-assisted thoracoscopic surgery, or thoracotomy. In some cases, the radiologist may both diagnose and stage lung cancer by performing image-guided biopsy of metastatic foci.

Histologic Classification

The most common cell type of lung cancer is adenocarcinoma, which is characterized by glandular differentiation or mucin production. Adenocarcinomas are typically peripheral lung neoplasms and may be multicentric. They typically grow slowly but metastasize early. A new classification of adenocarcinoma was recently introduced and advocates a multidisciplinary approach to the diagnosis of lung cancer in which the radiologist plays a crucial role. Squamous cell carcinoma is characterized by flattened cells and is typically a central neoplasm that manifests with an irregular polypoid endoluminal lesion in a central bronchus. Squamous cell carcinoma exhibits rapid growth and a strong association with cigarette smoking. Small cell carcinoma is a highly aggressive lung cancer that is almost universally metastatic at presentation. It has an irrefutable association with cigarette smoking, and affected patients have a very poor prognosis.

Staging

In 2009, a revised TNM (tumor, node, metastasis) staging system for lung cancer was proposed by the International Association for the Study of Lung Cancer and accepted by the Union Internationale Contre le Cancer and the American Joint Committee on Cancer. The revisions were based on over 81,000 cases of lung cancer collected in 20 countries and four continents. Clinical stage is determined by combining all information about the tumor prior to any treatment and includes imaging findings. Pathologic stage is determined after the tumor has been resected. Although pathologic staging is preferable, management decisions are made shortly after diagnosis and are often based on imaging findings. Radiologists can significantly contribute to patient management by prospectively identifying patients with advanced unresectable disease in order to avoid futile thoracotomies.

Treatment

Identification of the lung cancer cell type allows treatment planning, which may traditionally include surgery, chemotherapy, &/or radiation but may also include ablation procedures, laser therapy, and photodynamic therapy. Resectable lung cancer is typically treated surgically. Advanced lung cancer may be treated with combination chemotherapy to achieve maximal disease control. This may be followed by single-agent maintenance (consolidation) therapy with novel chemotherapeutic and molecularly targeted agents, with reports of improvement in progression-free survival and possible survival benefits. Despite advances in lung cancer therapy, the prognosis of affected patients remains poor.

Screening

The National Lung Screening Trial (NLST) recently reported a 20% decrease in death from lung cancer in high-risk persons undergoing screening with low-dose chest CT. Initial reports document detection of more cases of early stage lung cancer and fewer cases of advanced lung cancer. This implies the ability to diagnose affected patients at an early stage when curative surgical treatment may still be employed. Although lung cancer screening is not currently recommended or reimbursed by insurance companies (even in patients at high risk), several authors advocate screening, when requested by informed patients, with CT studies to be performed at centers with expertise in thoracic imaging. It should be noted that the NLST has not yet sufficiently evaluated the potential morbidity from CT screening. If screening for lung cancer is endorsed by the scientific and medical communities, guidelines and inclusion criteria for screening the general population will be needed as will expert thoracic imagers to interpret the studies.

Uncommon Primary Pulmonary Neoplasms

Most pulmonary neoplasms are metastases and primary lung cancers. Other primary pulmonary neoplasms are rare. Bronchial carcinoid is an important lung malignancy with a favorable prognosis. Affected patients are generally younger than patients with lung cancer. Bronchial carcinoid typically manifests as a central lung nodule or mass that exhibits a bronchial relationship and may enhance intensely. Affected patients typically present with symptoms related to the endoluminal neoplasm, including wheezing, hemoptysis, recurrent pneumonia, &/or atelectasis.

Lymphoproliferative disorders may also affect the lung. While most thoracic lymphomas are lymph node malignancies primarily affecting the mediastinum, both Hodgkin and non-Hodgkin lymphomas can affect the lung with primary or secondary involvement. These lesions may manifest with lung nodules, masses, or consolidations and may exhibit a multifocal distribution mimicking lung cancer and metastatic disease. These tumors may exhibit intrinsic air bronchograms and may simulate pulmonary infections and other nonneoplastic processes. A series of nonneoplastic lymphoproliferative disorders may also affect the lung, including nodular lymphoid hyperplasia, lymphocytic interstitial pneumonia, and follicular bronchiolitis. While these conditions are not neoplastic, affected patients typically have altered immunity and may progress to develop lymphoma.

Pulmonary hamartoma is a rare benign lung neoplasm characterized by intrinsic heterogeneous tissues in varying proportions, including cartilage, fat, connective tissue, and smooth muscle. Most hamartomas are peripheral tumors, and affected patients are often asymptomatic and diagnosed because of the incidental discovery of an indeterminate pulmonary nodule. Identification of fat and chondroid calcification within these lesions allows a confident prospective diagnosis of hamartoma. In these cases, excision is generally not warranted in the absence of symptoms.

APPROACH TO PULMONARY NEOPLASMS

(Left) PA chest radiograph of an asymptomatic 45-year-old man with an incidentally discovered radiographic abnormality shows a subtle right upper lobe indeterminate nodule ➡. **(Right)** Axial CECT of the same patient shows the right upper lobe nodule, which exhibits pleural tags, part-solid attenuation, a dominant solid component, and intrinsic air bronchiolograms. Such features are characteristic of invasive adenocarcinoma, and excisional biopsy is recommended.

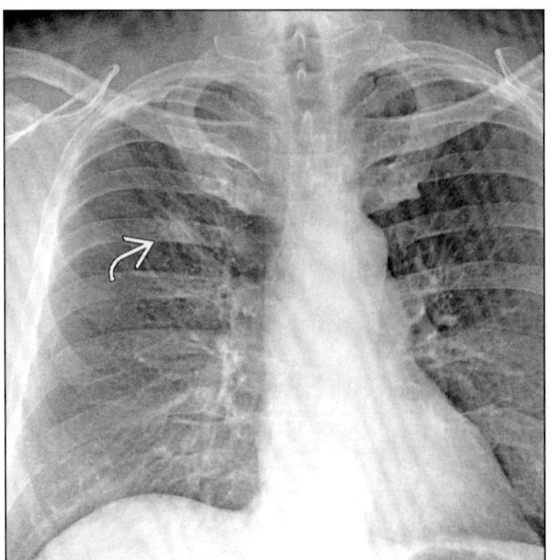

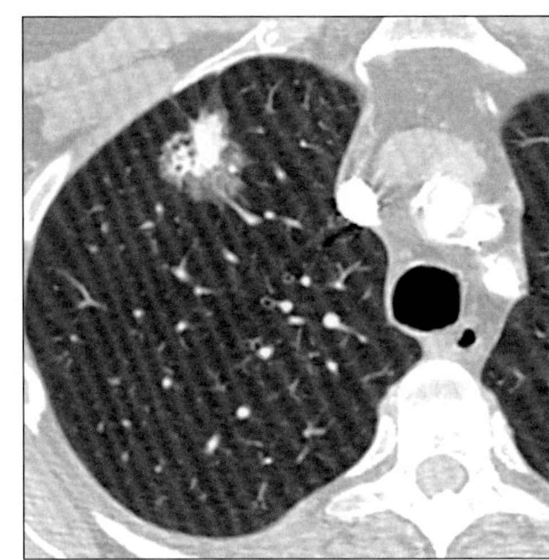

(Left) PA chest radiograph of a 60-year-old woman who presented with hemoptysis shows a large right upper lobe pulmonary mass that is highly suspicious for primary lung cancer given its large size. **(Right)** Axial CECT of the same patient shows the large lobular right upper lobe mass, which involves the lumen of the right upper lobe anterior segmental bronchus. Endoluminal involvement by the neoplasm ➡ likely contributed to hemoptysis. Note surrounding centrilobular emphysema.

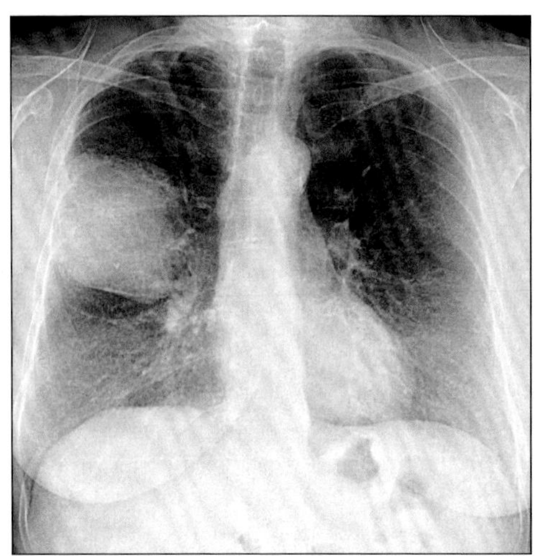

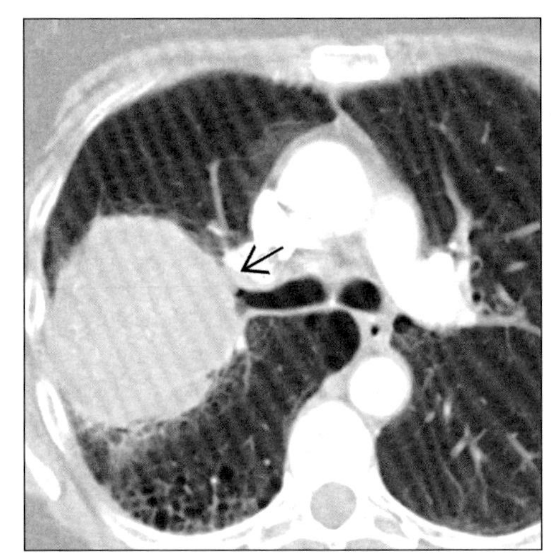

(Left) PA chest radiograph of a smoker who presented with weight loss and hemoptysis shows marked volume loss of the middle and right lower lobes with associated inferior displacement of the minor fissure ➡ secondary to a right hilar mass ➡. **(Right)** Axial CECT of the same patient shows complete right lower lobe atelectasis ➡ and displacement of the minor fissure ➡ from middle lobe volume loss secondary to a centrally obstructing tumor. Small cell carcinoma was diagnosed at bronchoscopy.

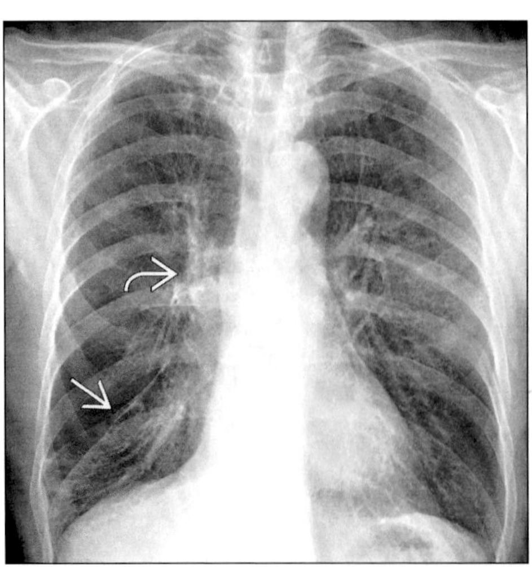

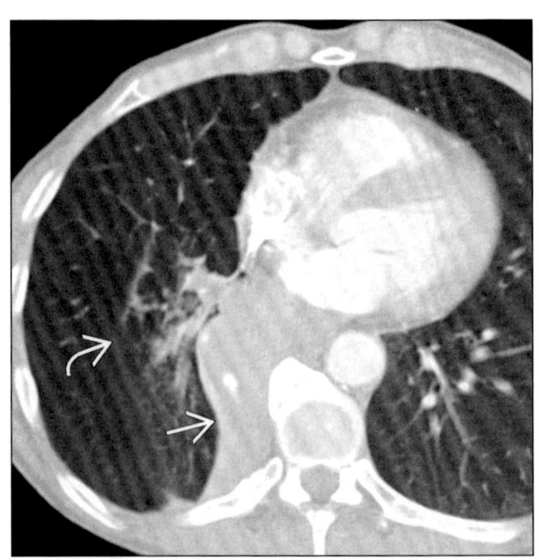

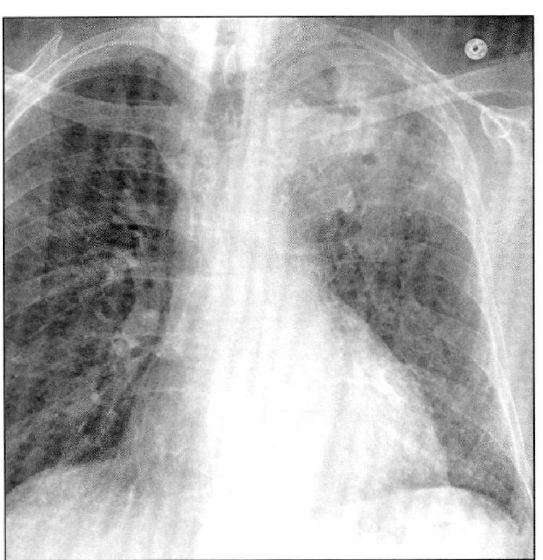

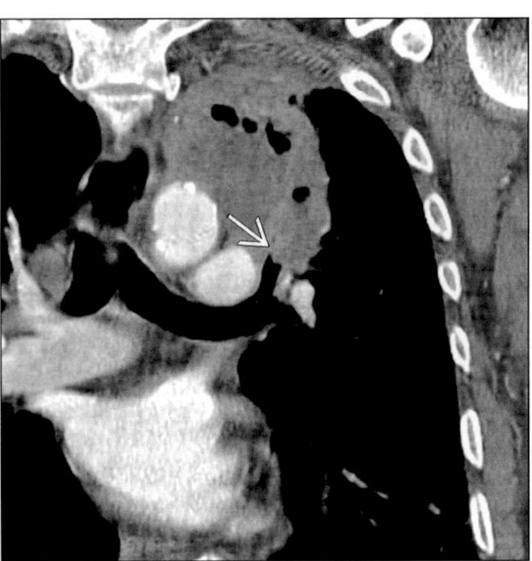

*(**Left**) PA chest radiograph of a patient with squamous cell carcinoma who presented with cough and hemoptysis shows a left apical consolidation with intrinsic cavitation. Lung cancer may manifest as pulmonary consolidation. (**Right**) Coronal CECT of the same patient shows that the lesion corresponds to a large, heterogeneous, centrally necrotic cavitary mass that directly invades the mediastinum and produces luminal obstruction of the left upper lobe apicoposterior segmental bronchus ➡.*

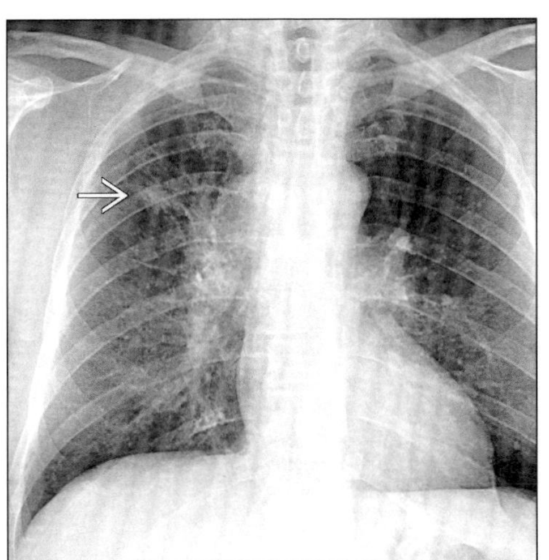

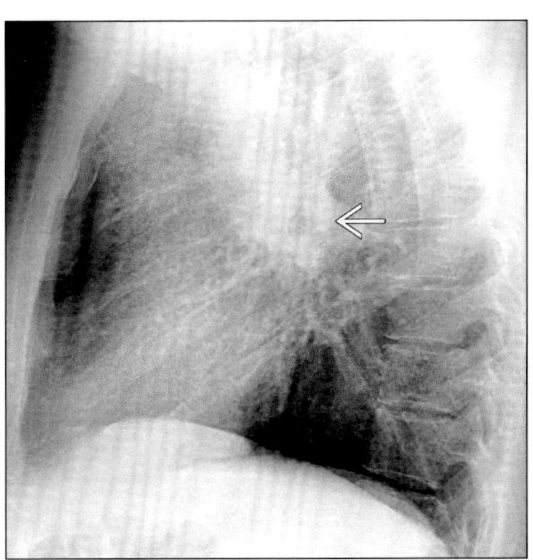

*(**Left**) PA chest radiograph of a 52-year-old smoker who presented with advanced lung adenocarcinoma shows a right upper lobe nodule ➡ and ipsilateral right hilar and mediastinal lymphadenopathy. (**Right**) Lateral chest radiograph of the same patient shows thickening of the intermediate stem line ➡ produced by locally invasive tumor. Skeletal metastases (not shown) were also present. Adenocarcinoma is characterized by slow growth and early distant metastases.*

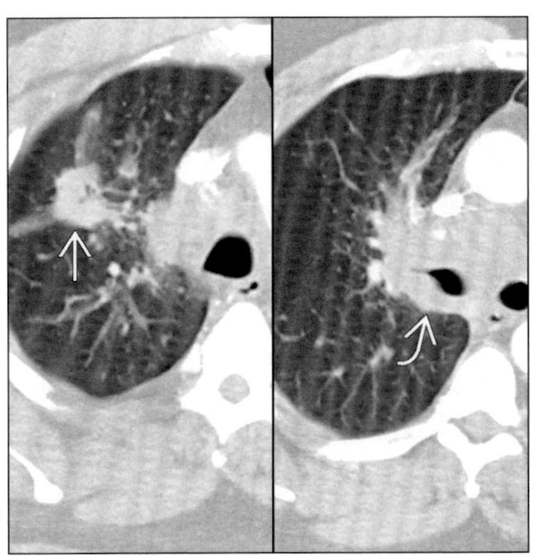

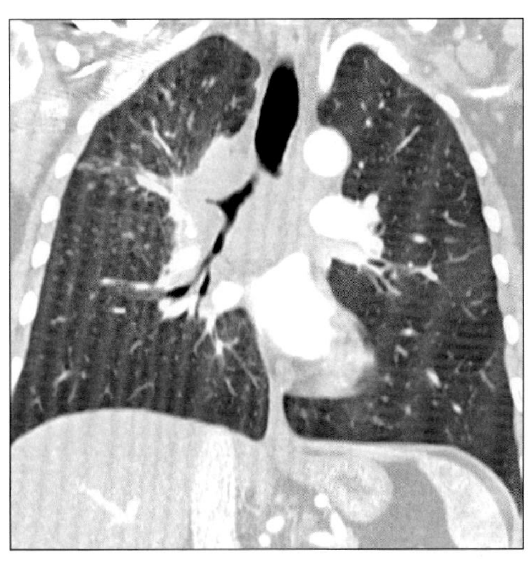

*(**Left**) Composite image with axial CECT of the same patient shows an irregular right upper lobe nodule ➡ and ipsiaxial hilar and mediastinal lymphadenopathy with encasement and narrowing of the right central tracheobronchial tree and thickening of the posterior wall of the right mainstem bronchus ➡. (**Right**) Coronal CECT of the same patient shows encasement and narrowing of the right tracheobronchial tree by coalescent mediastinal and hilar lymphadenopathy.*

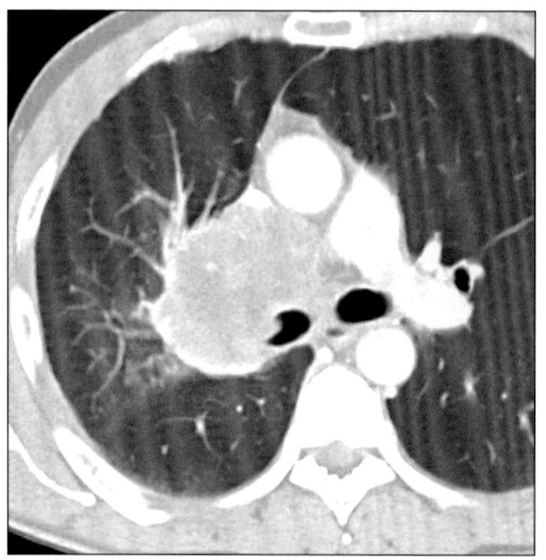

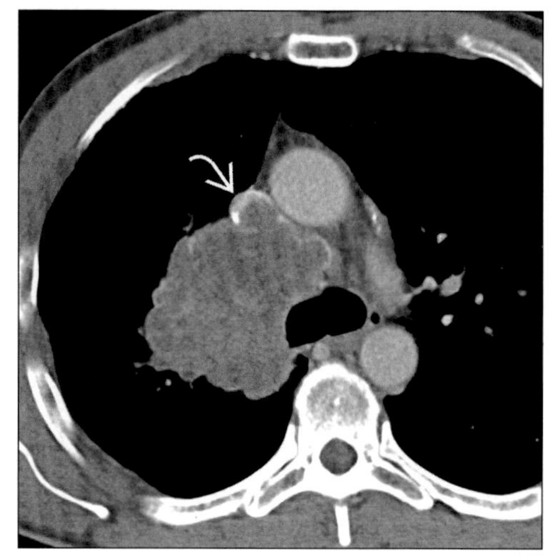

(Left) *Axial CECT of a patient with advanced lung cancer shows a large right hilar mass with associated endoluminal tumor within the right mainstem bronchus.* ***(Right)*** *Axial CECT of the same patient shows a large, heterogeneous tumor that directly invades the mediastinum and the lumen of the superior vena cava . Central low attenuation with peripheral enhancement suggests extensive central necrosis. Central lung cancer typically produces symptoms and may manifest as a hilar or perihilar mass.*

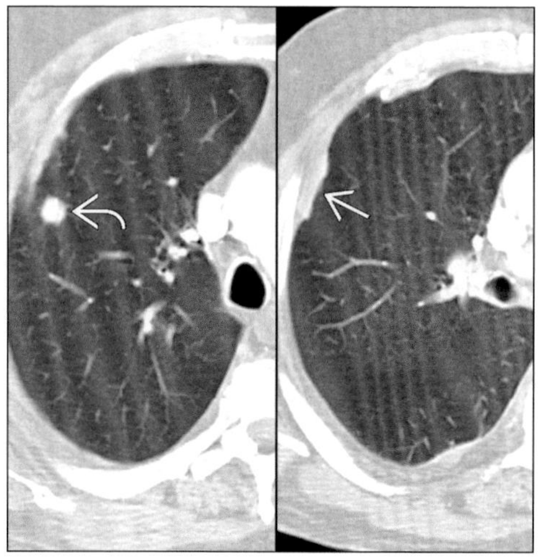

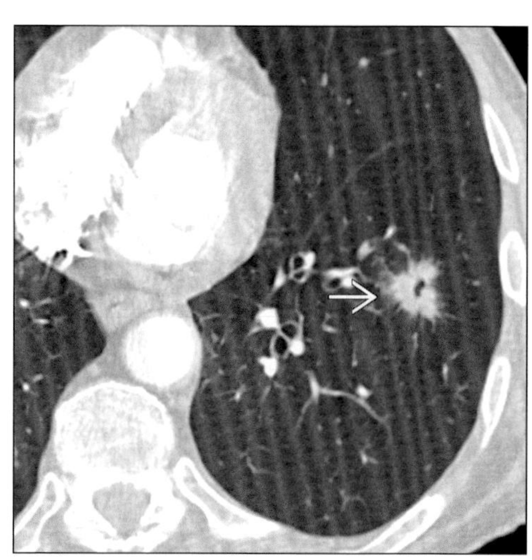

(Left) *Composite image with axial CECT of an asymptomatic smoker shows a small right upper lobe spiculated nodule and multifocal discontinuous pleural plaques , consistent with prior asbestos exposure. Smokers occupationally exposed to asbestos have a high risk for developing lung cancer.* ***(Right)*** *Axial CECT of a patient with lung cancer shows a polylobular spiculated cavitary nodule . Spiculation and polylobular morphology are highly suspicious features for primary lung cancer.*

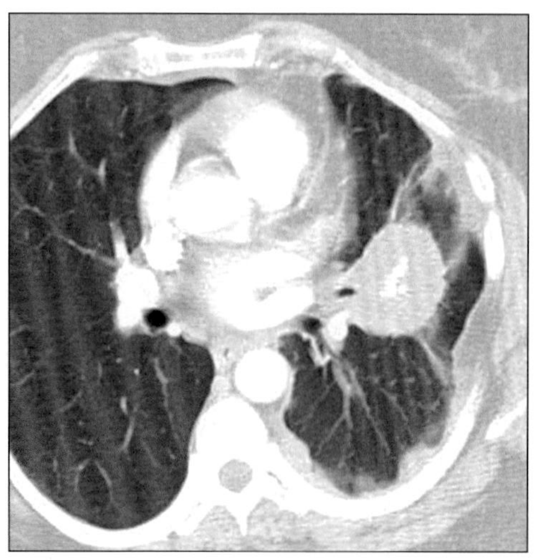

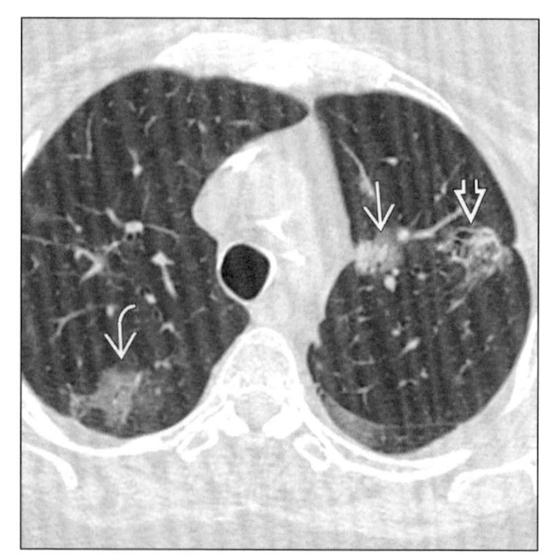

(Left) *Axial CECT of a patient with advanced lung cancer shows a left lower lobe mass with irregular borders and pleural tags and multifocal left pleural nodules consistent with pleural metastases. The findings are consistent with M1a, stage IV lung cancer.* ***(Right)*** *Axial NECT of a patient with biopsy-proven multifocal adenocarcinoma shows lesions in every lung lobe exhibiting a spectrum of morphologic features, including ground-glass opacity , part-solid attenuation , and bubbly appearance .*

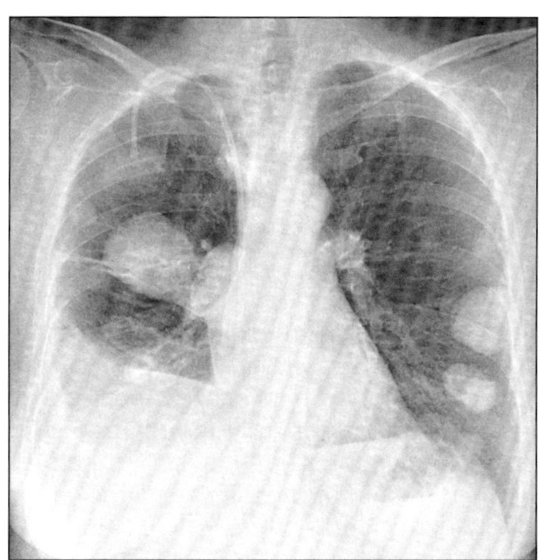

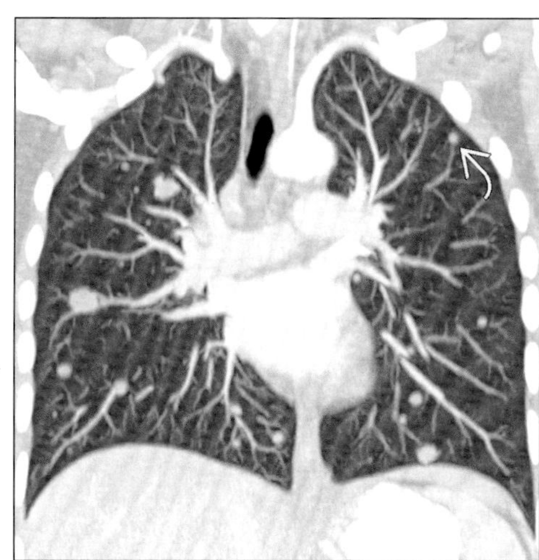

(Left) *PA chest radiograph of a patient with metastatic cervical cancer shows bilateral well-defined lung nodules and masses and a right pleural effusion. The lesions are most numerous in the mid and lower lung zones, consistent with the distribution of the pulmonary circulation.* ***(Right)*** *Coronal CECT MIP image of a patient with metastatic carcinoma of unknown primary shows multifocal well-defined lung nodules, some with an angiocentric distribution ➦, consistent with hematogenous metastases.*

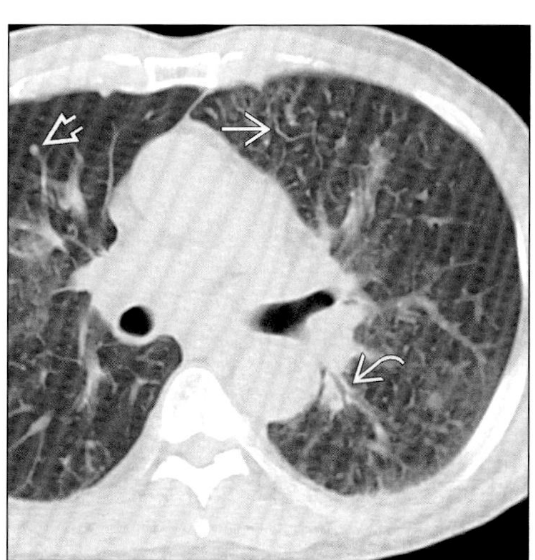

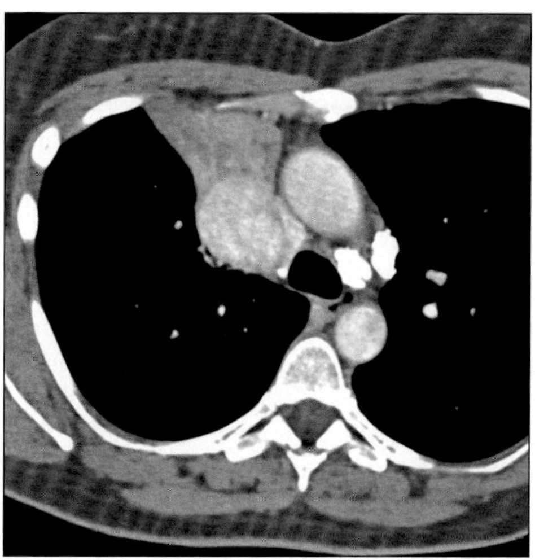

(Left) *Axial NECT of a patient with lymphangitic carcinomatosis shows bilateral patchy interlobular septal thickening ➔ and bronchial wall thickening ➦. Small pulmonary nodules ➪ represent hematogenous metastases.* ***(Right)*** *Axial CECT of a patient with hemoptysis shows a bronchial carcinoid tumor manifesting as a central, spherical, enhancing mass that produces right upper lobe atelectasis with intrinsic mucus-filled dilated bronchi from bronchial obstruction.*

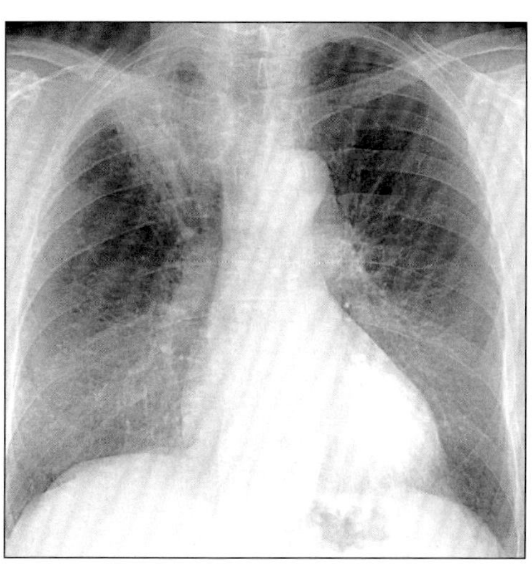

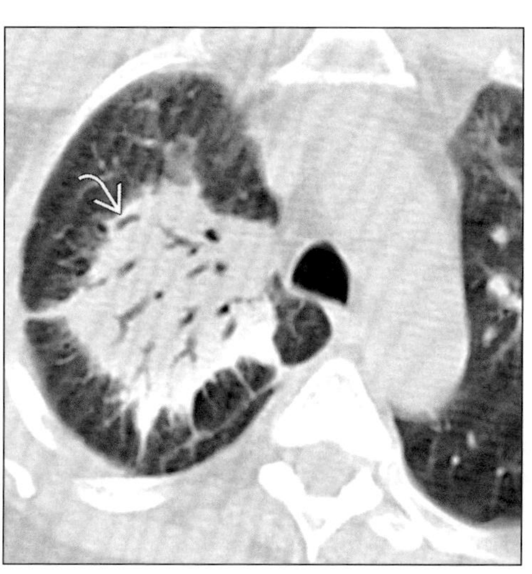

(Left) *PA chest radiograph of a 79-year-old man with cough and malaise shows a right upper lobe consolidation with intrinsic air bronchograms that did not respond to antibiotic therapy.* ***(Right)*** *Axial NECT of the same patient shows a right upper lobe mass-like consolidation with spiculated borders and intrinsic air bronchograms ➦. CT-guided lung biopsy revealed primary B-cell pulmonary non-Hodgkin lymphoma. Pulmonary lymphoma may exhibit air bronchograms and mimic pulmonary infection.*

Differential Diagnosis of the Solitary Pulmonary Nodule

Common

- Granuloma
- Lung cancer
- Intrapulmonary lymph node

Less Common

- Hamartoma
- Carcinoid
- Solitary metastasis
- Nodule mimics (pseudonodules)
- Infectious/inflammatory process

Rare but Important

- Arteriovenous malformation

Introduction

Solitary pulmonary nodules (SPNs) are frequent incidental findings on chest radiographs and chest CT studies performed for various indications. Solitary nodules found on radiography in North American patients are often related to remote granulomatous infection. The presence of a benign pattern of nodule calcification &/or documentation of stability allows the radiologist to make the presumptive diagnosis of benignity, obviating further imaging or intervention. When a prospective determination of benignity cannot be made with certainty, further imaging is typically required. Guidelines for the evaluation and management of lung nodules have been published, but it has been shown that radiologists in practice may be unaware of such guidelines or may fail to apply them consistently. Some lung nodules are malignant, including lung cancer, bronchial carcinoid tumor, and metastatic disease. The utilization of a multidisciplinary approach to the diagnosis and management of patients with malignancy allows the radiologist to make a positive impact on patient care.

Radiologists must thus gain expertise in the assessment and imaging follow-up of patients with lung nodules in order to identify benign and malignant imaging features and to make recommendations regarding further imaging or appropriate management.

Terminology

A solitary pulmonary nodule is defined as a single, focal, spherical or ovoid opacity measuring ≤ 3 cm. Larger lesions (> 3 cm) are referred to as pulmonary masses. This differs from the terminology used in other organ systems in which a lesion as small as 2 cm may be referred to as a mass. The proper use of these terms is important in helping to communicate the likelihood of malignancy. As a pulmonary nodule enlarges, the likelihood of malignancy increases, and malignancy must be suspected and excluded in any case of a pulmonary mass.

Detection of SPN

Radiography

Solitary pulmonary nodules are found on up to 2% of chest radiographs. In such cases, nodule assessment and characterization is of critical importance to exclude malignancy. Most SPNs measuring < 9 mm on radiography are likely to represent calcified pulmonary granulomas. Interestingly, observers have a 50-50 chance of seeing or detecting such a nodule, typically due to poor conspicuity. Thus, when a small nodule exhibits growth and is subsequently confirmed to represent malignancy, it is often visible retrospectively on prior chest radiographs.

Dual-energy radiography is a technique in which the chest radiographic image is optimized by obtaining two radiographs at different x-ray mean beam energies. Subtraction of overlying ribs allows improved visualization of lung nodules that may otherwise be missed and improves detection of calcification.

Computed Tomography

CT is superior to radiography in its ability to identify lung nodules. In addition, CT allows identification of intrinsic calcium or fat within lung nodules, which may allow a prospective diagnosis of benignity. Concurrent assessment of thin-section, multiplanar reformatted, and maximum intensity projection (MIP) images is helpful in increasing conspicuity and optimizing visualization of lung nodules and in identifying intrinsic calcification.

In spite of the advantages of CT, lung nodules are still missed with this imaging modality. Computer-aided detection (CAD) is a promising technique for the detection of subtle nodules. It has been shown that this technique increases radiologists' sensitivity for detecting lung nodules without compromising interpretation time. It should be noted that MIP images may be as sensitive as CAD for the detection of lung nodules.

Characterization of SPN

Imaging Assessment

The **chest radiograph** is a very useful tool in the assessment of patients with thoracic complaints. However, chest radiographic interpretation is fraught with pitfalls, including the superimposition of numerous normal structures of various radiographic densities and the relative subtlety of some lung nodules. One of the first steps in the assessment of pulmonary nodules is the exclusion of so-called pseudonodules, which are generally related to lesions that mimic the appearance of a pulmonary nodule. These usually include chest wall skeletal and soft tissue lesions such as nipples, moles, skin tags or other cutaneous lesions and skeletal lesions such as bone islands and healing or healed rib fractures.

CT allows optimal characterization of pulmonary nodules. Identification of characteristic patterns of calcification may allow the radiologist to make the diagnosis of benignity. Alternatively, some SPNs exhibit morphologic features that may raise suspicion for malignancy, such as lobular contours, spiculated borders, and heterogeneous attenuation, including subsolid attenuation, intrinsic air bronchograms, and pseudocavitation.

Positron emission tomography (PET)/CT is not routinely used for the assessment of lung nodules. However, it may be used when lung cancer is suspected in order to determine the metabolic activity of the nodule. In general, increased metabolic activity as measured by fluorodeoxyglucose (FDG) activity that is higher than background activity in a SPN generally correlates with malignancy but is also noted in infection and inflammation.

Systematic characterization of imaging features allows the radiologist to stratify SPNs into three different categories including benign, indeterminate, and possibly malignant SPNs. Patients with a benign SPN require no further imaging follow-up and no treatment. Patients with a possibly malignant SPN require further imaging assessment &/or image-guided or excisional biopsy for definitive diagnosis. Finally, a very important category of SPN is the indeterminate nodule, which requires imaging follow-up to document resolution, stability, or growth in accordance with published guidelines.

Specific SPN Features

Size, morphology, and border characteristics: Although immense time and resources are expended in the follow-up of SPN, it should be noted that 90% of lung nodules under 2 cm are benign lesions. Larger lesions have a higher likelihood of malignancy. Although not pathognomonic of benignity, spherical shapes are more characteristic of benign lesions. Lobular borders imply histologic heterogeneity and are seen in approximately 40% of malignant nodules. However, benign neoplasms such as hamartomas, which contain heterogeneous tissues, may also exhibit lobular borders. The presence of spiculation is highly suggestive of malignancy but can also be seen in inflammatory processes. Pleural tags are linear opacities that extend from a lung lesion to the visceral pleural surface and are seen in 60-80% of peripheral lung cancers. Spiculation and pleural tags may also correlate with fibrosis, which could be a response to inflammation or represent desmoplastic reaction to the presence of tumor, as in cases of adenocarcinoma.

Attenuation: SPN attenuation should be characterized as solid or subsolid. Solid nodules exhibit soft tissue attenuation. Subsolid nodules are subdivided into nonsolid (ground-glass) nodules and part-solid (semisolid) nodules. Part-solid nodules exhibit both ground-glass and soft tissue attenuation. Although most lung cancers exhibit solid attenuation, solid SPNs are less likely to be malignant than subsolid SPNs. Approximately 40-50% of part-solid nodules measuring less than 1.5 cm are malignant, and the risk of malignancy increases with size. Approximately 34% of ground-glass nodules are malignant, particularly if the nodule is larger than 1.5 cm. SPNs may also be heterogeneous by virtue of intrinsic air bronchograms or air bronchiolograms, which are more common in malignant lesions. Cavitation may occur in both benign and malignant SPNs, but irregular, nodular cavity walls > 16 mm thick should suggest malignancy.

Calcification: Nodules may exhibit intrinsic calcification &/or fat attenuation on CT. The presence of calcification within a pulmonary nodule does not necessarily imply benignity, and patterns of calcification must be carefully analyzed in order to identify benign calcification. In general, central, laminar, and complete calcification imply benignity. However, complete calcification may also be seen in bone-forming malignant lesions such as metastatic osteosarcoma. Stippled calcification may be seen in malignancies such as lung cancer and bronchial carcinoid tumors. Fat within a nodule is virtually diagnostic of benignity.

Enhancement: In many centers, CT evaluation of pulmonary nodules does not include the use of intravenous contrast. However, it has been demonstrated that dynamic contrast-enhanced CT may be a useful tool in the evaluation of SPNs. Dynamic CT is based on the hypothesis that malignant tumor vascularity in a nodule can be assessed and quantified on enhanced CT. This technique has shown significantly greater enhancement in malignant than in benign nodules. In addition, it has been shown that nodule enhancement of less than 15 Hounsfield units (HU) is strongly indicative of benignity, whereas enhancement of more than 15 HU is sensitive but not specific for malignancy. Indeed, not all enhancing nodules represent lung malignancy. Benign vascular lesions, such as arteriovenous malformations, may enhance intensely and are usually diagnosed on CT after identification of a feeding artery and draining vein.

Metabolic activity: PET is increasingly used in the assessment and staging of malignancy. However, this technique is also used in the assessment of an indeterminate SPN. PET/CT allows correlation of increased metabolic activity with specific anatomic locations. PET relies on 18F-fluorodeoxyglucose (FDG) activity within a lesion to determine metabolic activity, which is quantitated as maximum standard uptake values (SUV). In general, PET-positive lung nodules detected in patients over 60 years of age have a 90% likelihood of malignancy. Unfortunately, inflammatory nodules may yield false-positive results, and indolent and low-grade malignancies such as some adenocarcinomas and carcinoid tumors may yield false-negative results. In addition, lung nodules < 1 cm may also yield false-negative results. In general, FDG activity higher than background in a SPN < 1.5 cm and SUV > 2.5 in any nodule are highly suspicious features for malignancy.

Imaging Follow-Up

Nodules are often followed with radiography or CT to detect lesion growth. In many cases, retrieval of prior radiographs or CT studies allows the prospective diagnosis of benignity through documentation of stability of a solid nodule for two years or longer. However, it should be noted that indolent, slow-growing malignancies occur and that benign neoplasms and granulomas may also exhibit growth. Lesion doubling times of less than seven days or more than 465 days suggest benignity. Most nodules are evaluated with bidimensional measurements on axial CT images. Nodule growth does not necessarily occur along the axial plane and may only be detected as craniocaudal growth on sagittal or coronal reformatted images. Volumetric assessment of solid nodules may also provide documentation of growth.

Suspicion of Malignancy

Nodule assessment must also take into consideration patient characteristics and risk factors for malignancy. Lung cancer is the most common primary lung malignancy. Patients with lung cancer are typically older than forty years of age. Carcinoid tumor is an uncommon low-grade malignant neoplasm that affects patients who are typically decades younger than those affected by lung cancer. Exposure to a variety of carcinogens, including cigarette smoke and asbestos (but also other agents to which the patient may be occupationally exposed), increases the likelihood of malignancy in a lung nodule. History of prior malignancy, pulmonary fibrosis, or lung cancer in a first-degree relative also increases a given patient's risk for developing primary lung cancer.

Fleischner Society Recommendations for Nodules Detected Incidentally at Nonscreening CT

Nodule Size	*Low-Risk Patient*	*High-Risk Patient*
≤ 4 mm	No follow-up	Follow-up CT at 12 months; if unchanged, no further follow-up
> 4-6 mm	Follow-up CT at 12 months; if unchanged, no further follow-up	Follow-up CT at 6-12 months, then at 18-24 months if no change
> 6-8 mm	Follow-up CT at 6-12 months, then at 18-24 months if no change	Follow-up CT at 3-6 months, then at 9-12 months and 24 months if no change
> 8 mm	Follow-up CT at 3, 9, and 24 months; dynamic contrast CT, PET, &/or biopsy	Same as for low-risk patient

Applicable to patients ≥ 35 years; size based on average of axial length & width. High risk: History of smoking, exposure to carcinogens, or lung cancer in 1st-degree relative.

Interim Guidelines for Assessment and Management of Subsolid Lung Nodules

Nodule Type/Size	*Management Recommendation*
Solitary GGO, < 5 mm	No follow-up
Solitary GGO, 5-10 mm	Follow-up CT in 3-6 months; if no resolution, annual CT x 3 years
Solitary GGO, > 10 mm	Follow up-CT in 3-6 months; if no resolution, surgical biopsy
Solitary part solid, any size	Follow up CT in 3-6 months, if no resolution, PET/CT followed by image-guided biopsy of solid component or surgical biopsy
Multiple GGO, < 5 mm	Long-term annual CT follow-up for minimum of 3 years
Multiple GGO, 5-10 mm	Follow-up CT in 3-6 months; if no resolution, annual CT x minimum of 3 years
Multiple GGO with dominant lesion(s)	Consider limited surgical resection, PET/CT, or biopsy

GGO: Ground-glass opacity. Adapted from Godoy MC et al: Subsolid pulmonary nodules and the spectrum of peripheral adenocarcinomas of the lung: recommended interim guidelines for assessment and management. Radiology. 253(3):606-22, 2009.

Differential Diagnosis

Granulomas

Granulomas are very common causes of SPN in the United States and are frequently encountered in daily practice. They are typically solid nodules of spherical morphology that exhibit stability over time. Granulomas often exhibit satellite nodules on CT. Granulomas are often the sequela of endemic fungal pulmonary infections in United States patients, typically histoplasmosis. However, tuberculosis is a common cause of granulomatous disease worldwide. Granulomas may exhibit characteristic patterns of calcification including laminar and concentric types, which are most predictive of benignity. Diffuse and central patterns of calcification (the latter involving > 10% of the SPN cross section) are also characteristic. However, diffuse and stippled calcification can also be seen in malignancy (metastatic osteosarcoma and carcinoid tumor).

Lung Cancer

Lung cancer is a common cause of an SPN and predominantly occurs in the upper lobes, specifically the right upper lobe. Peripheral and basilar lung cancers have a tendency to occur in patients with preexisting pulmonary fibrosis. Lung cancer typically manifests as an SPN > 1 cm with doubling times between 1-18 months. Irregular, spiculated, and lobular borders are characteristic. Calcification may occur in 13% of lung cancers, but it is usually eccentric or stippled.

Intrapulmonary Lymph Node

Intrapulmonary lymph nodes are a common finding on thin-section multidetector CT and are often small, well defined, and solitary. They are usually located in the lung periphery caudal to the level of the carina, exhibit an elongate morphology and a fissural location, and are within 20 mm from the pleura. These lesions may exhibit an increase &/or a decrease in size over time.

Hamartoma

Hamartomas are benign lung neoplasms characterized by slow growth and well-defined lobular borders. In almost 50% of cases, CT may help establish the prospective diagnosis through identification of intralesional fat or calcification. Calcification, when present, may exhibit a speckled or popcorn morphology representing calcification of cartilaginous elements within the lesion.

Carcinoid

Carcinoid tumor is a low-grade primary malignant lung neoplasm that frequently exhibits well-defined borders and a relationship to an airway. These lesions may be completely or partially endoluminal or may abut a bronchus. They may exhibit contrast enhancement and stippled or coarse calcification.

Metastasis

Solitary metastases are rare and typically result from sarcomas, melanomas, and testicular cancers. They are characterized by their peripheral location and angiocentricity, often manifested with a feeding vessel coursing into the lesion. A new nodule in an adult with known extrapulmonary malignancy is more likely to represent primary lung cancer than a solitary metastasis.

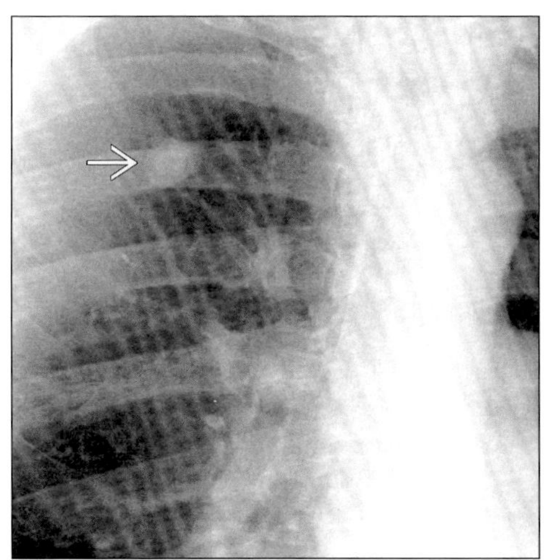

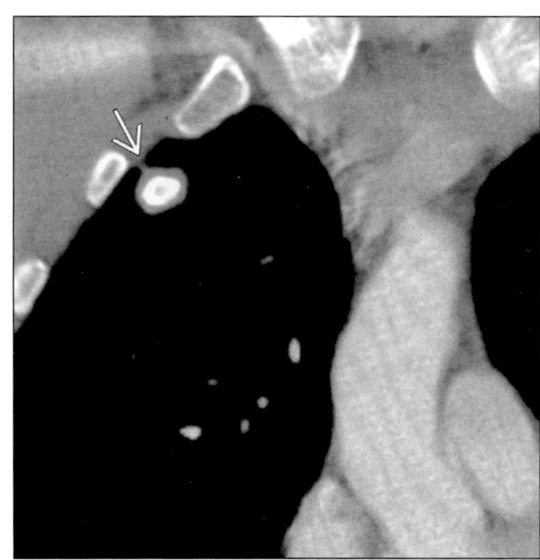

(Left) *PA chest radiograph shows a right upper lobe ovoid solitary pulmonary nodule (SPN) ➔ with intrinsic central calcification that occupies the majority of the visualized nodule area.* ***(Right)*** *Coronal CECT (soft tissue window) of the same patient confirms dense laminar calcification within the nodule, surrounded by a thin soft tissue rim and associated with a small pleural tag ➔. The findings are diagnostic of granuloma.*

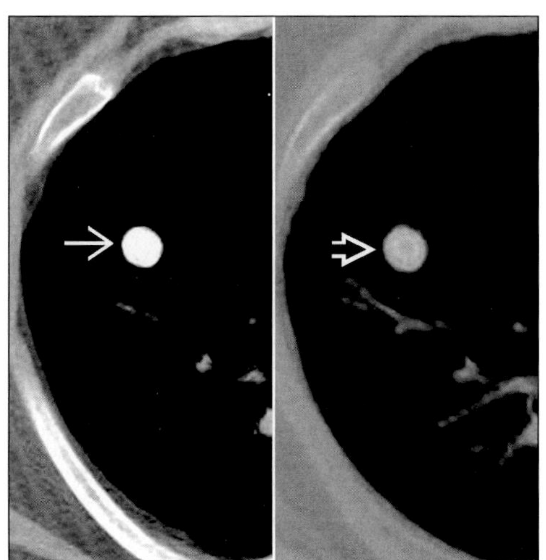

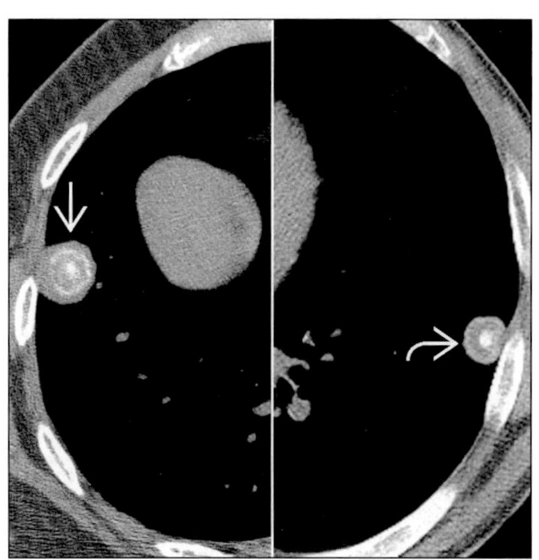

(Left) *Composite image with axial NECT in soft tissue (left) and bone (right) window shows a completely calcified solitary nodule ➔ that exhibits concentric or laminar calcifications ➲, characteristic of granuloma.* ***(Right)*** *Composite image with axial NECT of 2 different patients with histoplasmosis shows laminar calcification in a right lower lobe SPN ➔ and central rounded calcification surrounded by low attenuation in a left lung SPN ➚. The CT findings are diagnostic of granuloma.*

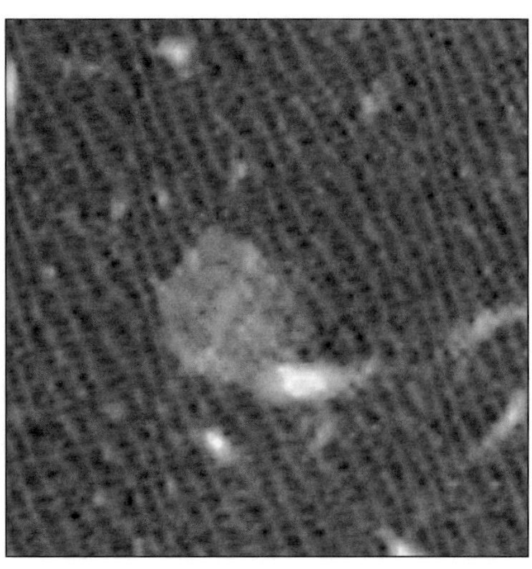

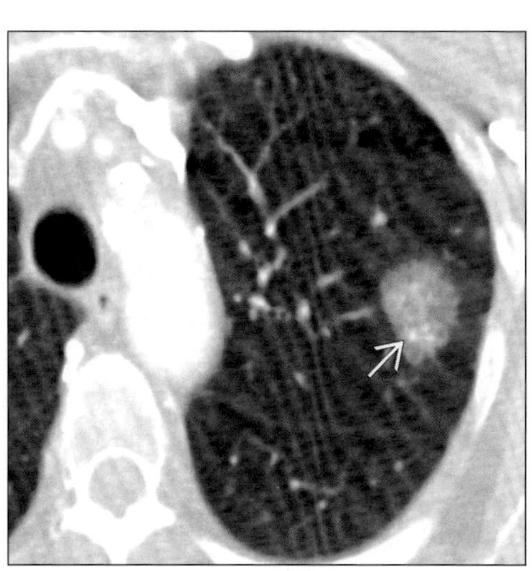

(Left) *Axial NECT shows a small ground-glass SPN with visualization of normal underlying pulmonary architecture. The differential diagnosis includes atypical adenomatous hyperplasia, adenocarcinoma in situ, and minimally invasive adenocarcinoma.* ***(Right)*** *Axial CECT shows a left upper lobe part-solid SPN with predominant ground-glass opacity and intrinsic small nodular soft tissue ➔ components. The CT features and lesion size are highly suspicious for invasive adenocarcinoma.*

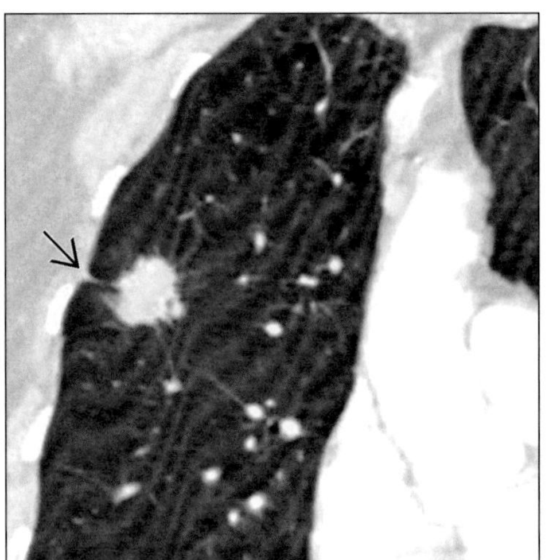

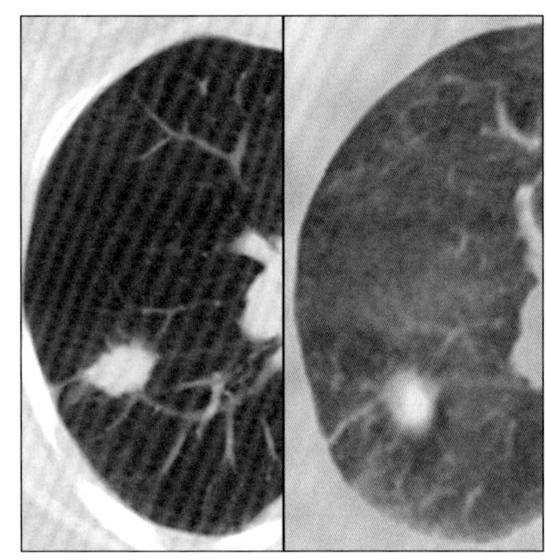

*(**Left**) Coronal CECT shows a solid right upper lobe SPN with spiculated and lobular borders and a pleural tag ⇨. The nodule morphology is characteristic of primary lung cancer. (**Right**) Composite image with axial NECT (left) and axial fused PET/CT of a patient with invasive adenocarcinoma shows a spiculated right lower lobe nodule that exhibits intense FDG uptake. The morphologic features of the lesion and the documentation of increased metabolic activity are highly suspicious for primary lung cancer.*

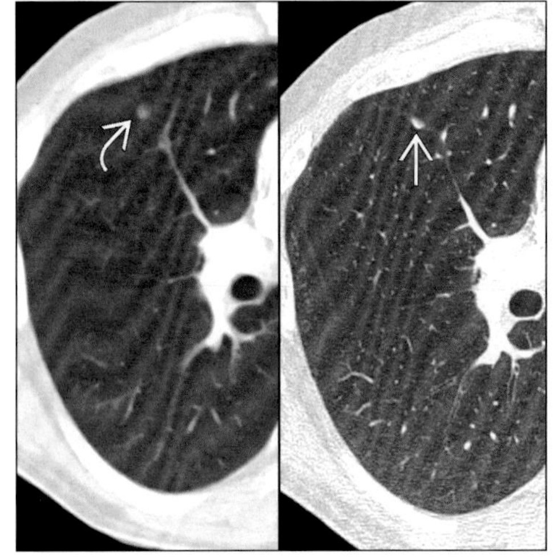

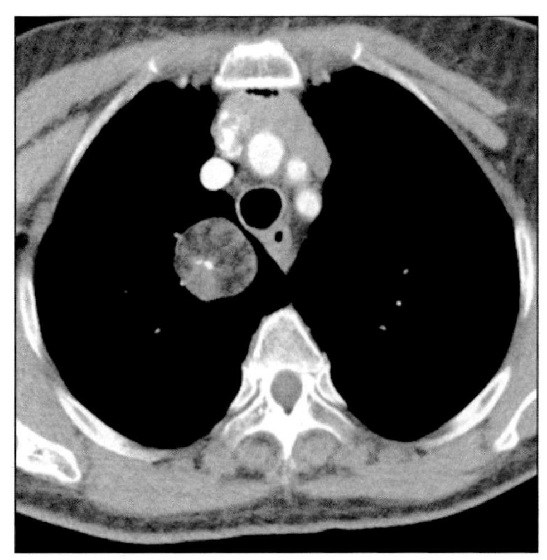

*(**Left**) Composite image with axial CECT (left) and HRCT (right) shows a tiny SPN near the minor fissure ➡ that exhibits an elongate morphology oriented along the fissure ➡ on HRCT, typical of intrapulmonary lymphoid tissue. (**Right**) Axial CECT of a patient with a right upper lobe hamartoma shows a well-defined lung nodule with internal calcification, fat, and soft tissue attenuation. The presence of fat and calcification in a well-defined lung nodule is diagnostic of hamartoma.*

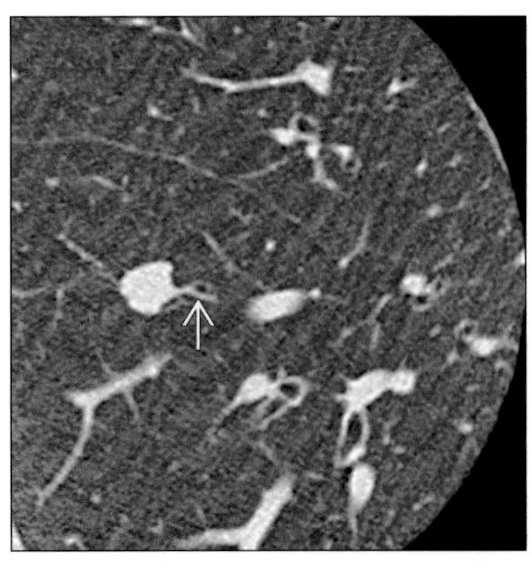

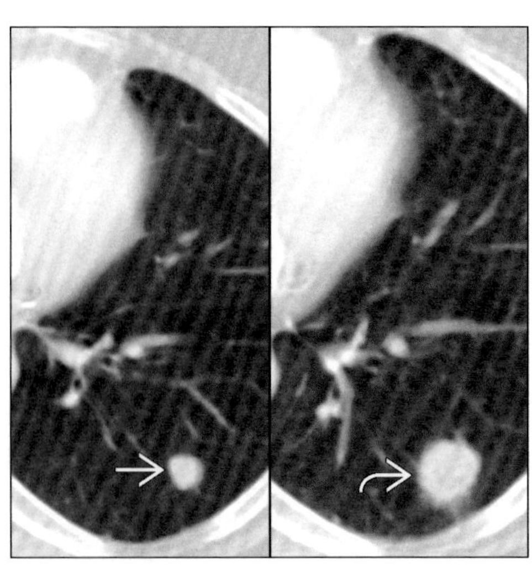

*(**Left**) Axial HRCT of a patient with carcinoid tumor shows a small SPN with well-defined lobular margins. The nodule is intimately related to an adjacent airway ➡, a characteristic feature of bronchial carcinoid tumor. (**Right**) Composite image with axial CECT of a left lower lobe SPN ➡ demonstrates interval growth ➡, spiculated borders, and a pleural tag on the axial CECT obtained 3 months later (right). Although this lesion was a solitary metastasis, primary lung cancer should also be considered.*

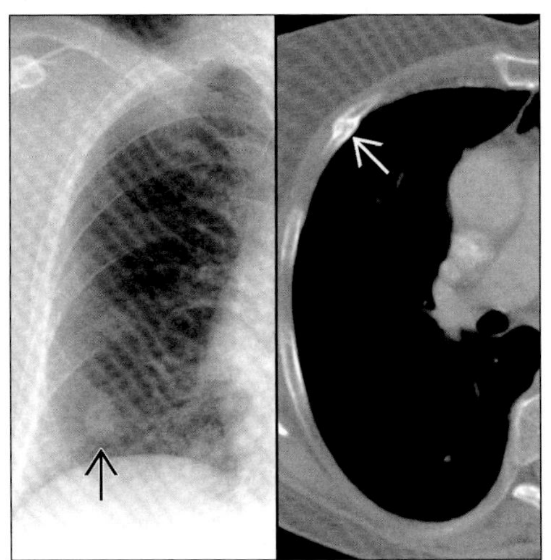

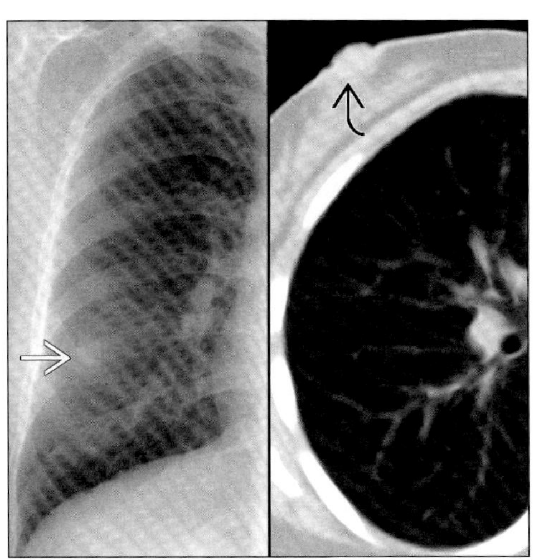

(Left) *Composite image with PA chest radiograph (left) and axial CECT (right) shows a nodular opacity projecting over the right anterior 4th rib. The lesion corresponds to a mildly displaced healed rib fracture on axial CECT (bone window).* ***(Right)*** *Composite image with PA chest radiograph (left) and axial CECT (right) shows a nodular opacity with a sharp outer margin and an indistinct inner margin typical of a nipple shadow, confirmed on CT.*

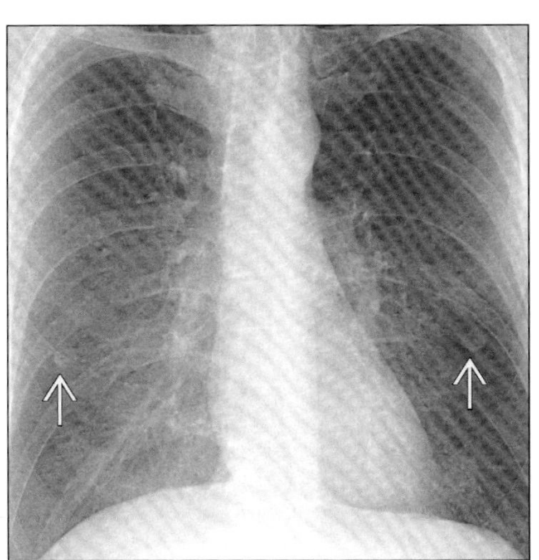

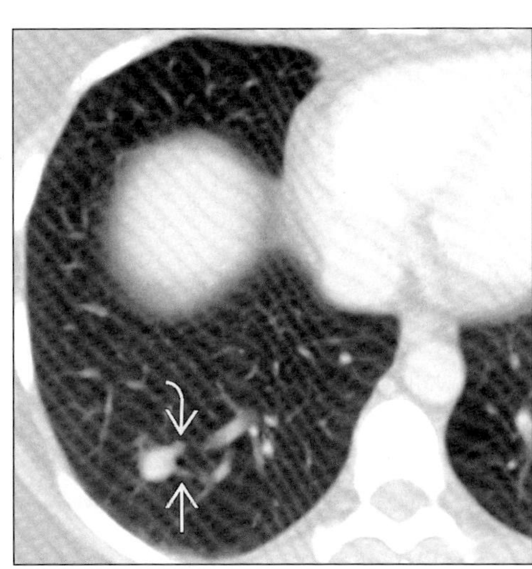

(Left) *PA chest radiograph shows bilateral symmetric nodular opacities that project over the mid lung zones, exhibit the incomplete border sign, and are consistent with nipple shadows.* ***(Right)*** *Axial CECT of a patient with a solitary arteriovenous malformation shows a right lower lobe enhancing nodule with 2 associated tubular opacities that represent a feeding artery and a draining vein. The CT findings are diagnostic of pulmonary arteriovenous malformation.*

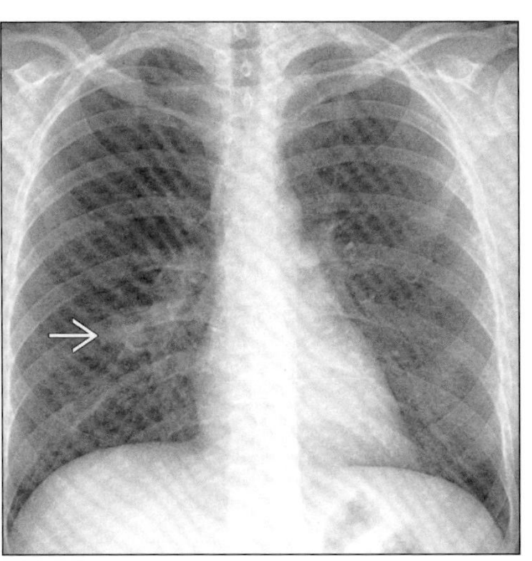

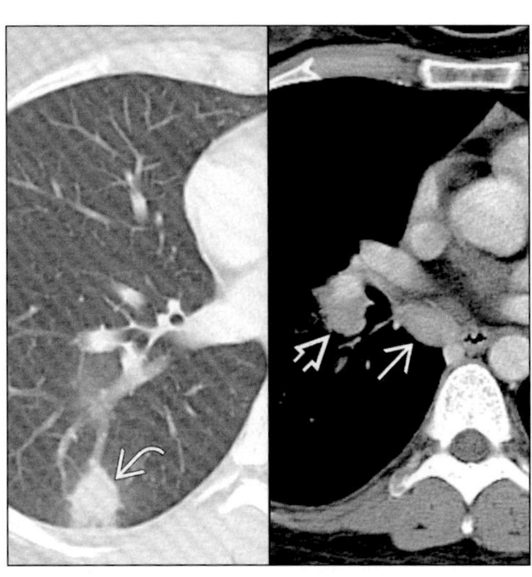

(Left) *PA chest radiograph of a patient with acute histoplasmosis (who presented with malaise and fever) shows an ill-defined right mid lung zone SPN and ipsilateral hilar lymphadenopathy.* ***(Right)*** *Composite image with axial CECT in lung (left) and soft tissue (right) window of the same patient shows a peripheral right lower lobe nodule and ipsilateral right hilar and mediastinal lymphadenopathy. Fungal infections may manifest with lung nodules that mimic primary lung cancer.*

ADENOCARCINOMA

Key Facts

Terminology
- Spectrum of malignant epithelial neoplasms with glandular differentiation or mucin production
  - Range from preinvasive to invasive lesions

Imaging
- Radiography
  - Solitary nodule/mass, consolidation
  - Multifocal nodules, masses, consolidations
  - Central lesion: Postobstructive atelectasis/ pneumonia
  - Local invasion, lymphadenopathy, pleural effusion
- CT
  - Solid or subsolid nodule or mass
  - Irregular, lobular, or spiculated borders
  - Local invasion, lymphadenopathy, metastases
  - Pleural effusion, nodular pleural thickening
- PET: Staging & restaging

Top Differential Diagnoses
- Other non-small cell lung cancers
- Pulmonary metastases
- Pulmonary lymphoma
- Bacterial pneumonia
- Cryptogenic organizing pneumonia
- Chronic eosinophilic pneumonia

Pathology
- Excisional biopsy favored over percutaneous biopsy for ground-glass & part-solid nodules

Clinical Issues
- Asymptomatic lesions
  - Cough, chest pain, dyspnea

Diagnostic Checklist
- Consider adenocarcinoma in asymptomatic patients with incidentally found subsolid lung nodules

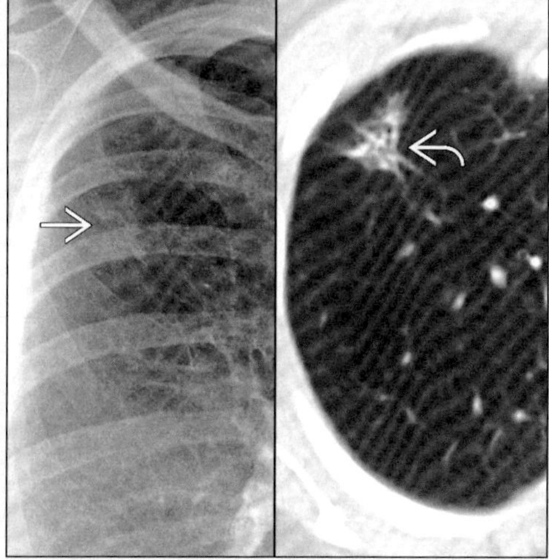

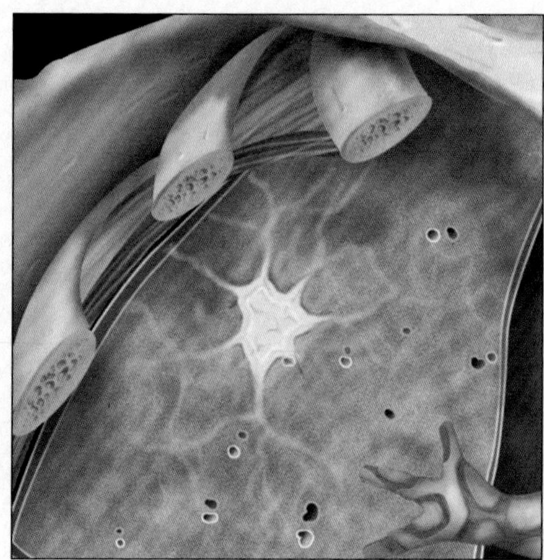

*(**Left**) Composite image with PA chest radiograph (left) and axial NECT (right) of a patient with invasive right upper lobe adenocarcinoma shows an ill-defined peripheral lung nodule ➔ on radiography, which manifests as a spiculated heterogeneous lung nodule ➔ with pleural tags and intrinsic air bronchiolograms on CT. (**Right**) Graphic illustrates the typical morphologic features of invasive adenocarcinoma, which often manifests as a peripheral lung lesion with spiculated margins and pleural tags.*

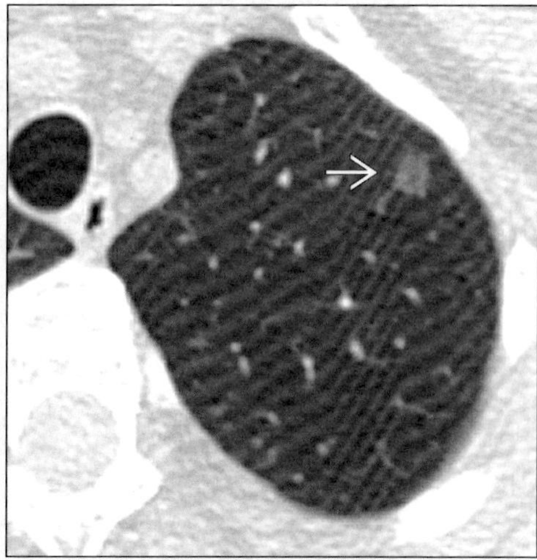

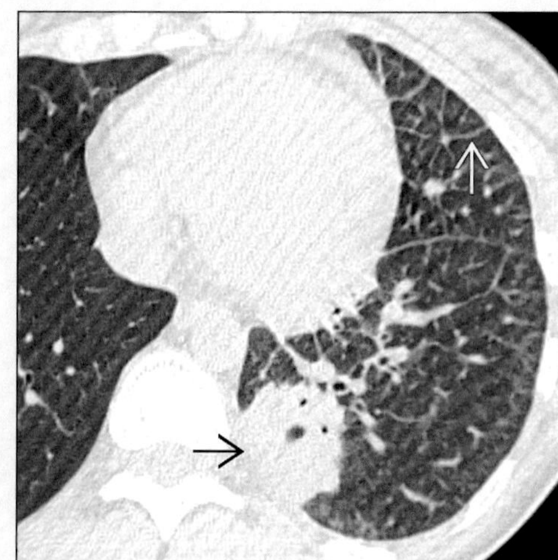

*(**Left**) Axial NECT of a patient evaluated for dyspnea shows an incidentally discovered nodule of pure ground-glass opacity ➔, histologically proven to represent atypical adenomatous hyperplasia. Although the nodule is clearly visible, underlying vascular structures can also be identified. (**Right**) Axial NECT of a patient with advanced adenocarcinoma shows a left lower lobe polylobular cavitary mass ➔ with associated interlobular septal thickening ➔ from lymphangitic carcinomatosis.*

ADENOCARCINOMA

TERMINOLOGY

Abbreviations

- **Atypical adenomatous hyperplasia (AAH)**
- **Adenocarcinoma in situ (AIS)**
- **Minimally invasive adenocarcinoma (MIA)**

Definitions

- Spectrum of malignant epithelial neoplasms with glandular differentiation or mucin production
  - Range from preinvasive lesions (AAH, AIS) to invasive adenocarcinoma
- **Use of former term bronchioloalveolar carcinoma (BAC) no longer recommended**
- Lung nodules
  - **Solid nodule**: Spherical soft tissue density, obscures normal underlying structures
  - **Subsolid nodule**
    - **Ground-glass (nonsolid)**: Spherical lung density, normal underlying structures visible
    - **Part-solid**: Solid & ground-glass components

IMAGING

General Features

- Best diagnostic clue
  - Solitary lung nodule or mass ± lymphadenopathy &/ or metastases
- Location
  - Typically peripheral
- Size
  - **AAH**: ≤ 5 mm
  - **AIS**: ≤ 3 cm
  - **MIA**: ≤ 3 cm
  - **Invasive adenocarcinoma**: Variable size
- Morphology
  - Shape: Spherical, ovoid
  - Margin: Smooth, polylobular, spiculated

Radiographic Findings

- Preinvasive lesions often not visible
- Invasive adenocarcinoma
  - Solitary nodule/mass
  - Local invasion
  - Central lesions: Postobstructive atelectasis/ consolidation
  - Hilar/mediastinal lymphadenopathy
  - Multifocal nodules, masses, consolidations

CT Findings

- Imaging features often overlap
- **AAH**
  - Ground-glass nodule ≤ 5 mm (but up to 12 mm)
- **AIS**
  - Ground-glass, part-solid, or solid nodule
  - May exhibit slightly higher attenuation than AAH
  - ≤ 3 cm (typically < 2 cm)
- **MIA**
  - Part-solid nodule: Predominant ground-glass component & small solid component ≤ 5 mm
  - Imaging features not yet well defined
- **Invasive adenocarcinoma**
  - Lung nodule or mass
    - Predominant solid component in part-solid nodule
    - Polylobular or spiculated borders, pleural tags
    - Internal air bronchograms, bubbly lucencies
    - Mass-like consolidation
    - Local invasion: Pleura, chest wall, diaphragm
  - Multifocal nodules, masses, consolidations
  - Central lesions: Endobronchial component, postobstructive pneumonia/atelectasis
  - Smooth or nodular interlobular septal thickening from lymphangitic carcinomatosis
  - Hilar/mediastinal lymphadenopathy
  - Pleural effusion, pleural nodules

Nuclear Medicine Findings

- PET
  - Not recommended in preinvasive lesions
  - Used for staging prior to resection of stable or growing part-solid nodules
  - Staging & restaging of invasive adenocarcinoma

MR Findings

- DWI
  - Preinvasive lesions tend to have less diffusion restriction signal compared to invasive adenocarcinoma

Imaging Recommendations

- Best imaging tool
  - CT for detection, characterization, & surveillance
  - PET/CT for preoperative staging

DIFFERENTIAL DIAGNOSIS

Other Non-Small Cell Lung Cancer (NSCLC)

- Squamous cell carcinoma: Central mass, frequent cavitation
- Large cell carcinoma: Peripheral, large mass
- Local invasion, lymphadenopathy, metastases

Small Cell Lung Cancer (SCLC)

- Large central mass with hilar/mediastinal lymphadenopathy
- Typically metastatic at presentation

Pulmonary Metastases

- Multifocal lung nodules/masses, consolidations
- Lower lobe predominance
- ± lymphadenopathy &/or pleural effusion

Pulmonary Lymphoma

- Multifocal lung nodules/masses, consolidations

Bacterial Pneumonia

- Mass-like consolidations may mimic lung cancer
- Leukocytosis, fever
- Responsive to antibiotics

Cryptogenic Organizing Pneumonia

- Chronic multifocal peripheral consolidations
  - May exhibit reverse halo sign
- Unresponsive to antibiotics, responsive to steroids

Chronic Eosinophilic Pneumonia

- Peripheral consolidations & ground-glass opacities
- Migratory opacities

ADENOCARCINOMA

PATHOLOGY

General Features

- Genetics
  - Molecular markers
    - *EGFR* (epidermal growth factor receptor) mutation
      - Good response to tyrosine kinase inhibitor therapy
    - *KRAS* mutation
      - Suggests poor response to tyrosine kinase inhibitor therapy

Staging, Grading, & Classification

- AAH
  - Small (≤ 5 mm) proliferation of atypical type II pneumocytes, Clara cells, & occasional respiratory bronchioles
- AIS
  - Adenocarcinoma (≤ 3 cm) with pure lepidic growth (restricted to alveolar framework)
  - No stromal, vascular, or pleural invasion
  - No nuclear atypia
  - Nonmucinous (vast majority)
    - Type II pneumocytes &/or Clara cells
  - Mucinous (rare)
    - Tall columnar cells
- MIA
  - Adenocarcinoma (≤ 3 cm) with predominant lepidic growth
  - Invasion of ≤ 5 mm
  - Solitary & discrete
  - Nonmucinous (majority) & mucinous (rare) types
  - Lepidic-predominant adenocarcinoma (LPA)
    - Invasion of lymphatics, vessels, pleura
    - Tumor necrosis
    - > 5 mm nonlepidic growth
- Invasive adenocarcinoma
  - Complex mixture of heterogeneous subtypes, classified by predominant feature
  - Lepidic, acinar, papillary, micropapillary, solid with mucin production, & other variants

Microscopic Features

- Small biopsy or cytology: Noninvasive pattern referred to as "lepidic growth" instead of AIS & MIA due to possibility of sampling errors
- Lepidic pattern on histology generally corresponds to ground-glass opacity on CT; invasive pattern generally corresponds to solid opacity

Tissue Processing/Diagnosis

- Excisional biopsy recommended over percutaneous biopsy for ground-glass & part-solid nodules to avoid sampling errors
- Should be tested for *EGFR* mutation: If positive, eligible for tyrosine-kinase inhibitor (TKI) therapy

CLINICAL ISSUES

Presentation

- Most common signs/symptoms
  - Preinvasive lesions typically asymptomatic
    - Incidental finding
  - Cough, chest pain, hemoptysis, dyspnea

Demographics

- Gender
  - More common in women
- Epidemiology
  - Associated with smoking (46%)
  - Adenocarcinoma: Most common type of NSCLC

Natural History & Prognosis

- Preinvasive lesions by definition: Near 100% disease-specific survival if resected
- AAH & AIS: Very slow growth
  - Long-term (≥ 3 years) follow-up at 6-12 month intervals
- If not resected, will likely progress to invasive adenocarcinoma (may take several years)

Treatment

- Lobectomy is standard of care for solid & part-solid lesions ≤ 2 cm
- Sublobar resection considered in selected patients with ground-glass nodules
- Multiple lesions
  - Excision of dominant/growing lesions
  - No contraindication to surgical exploration in absence of lymphadenopathy
  - Treatment not standardized

DIAGNOSTIC CHECKLIST

Consider

- Adenocarcinoma in patients with chronic or growing subsolid nodules

Image Interpretation Pearls

- Intratumoral air bronchogram suggests well-differentiated tumor
- Notches or concave cuts in solid lesions suggest poor differentiation & poor outcome

Reporting Tips

- Recommendation to discontinue use of term "bronchioloalveolar carcinoma"
- Recommendations for CT follow-up of nonsolid nodules
  - < 5 mm: No follow-up
  - 5-10 mm: 3-6 months, then yearly for ≥ 3 years
  - > 10 mm: 3-6 months; if persistent, consider excisional biopsy
- Recommendation for CT follow-up of part-solid nodules
  - 3-6 month CT follow-up
  - If persistent, excisional biopsy after staging PET/CT

SELECTED REFERENCES

1. Nair A et al: Revisions to the TNM staging of non-small cell lung cancer: rationale, clinicoradiologic implications, and persistent limitations. Radiographics. 31(1):215-38, 2011
2. Travis WD et al: International association for the study of lung cancer/american thoracic society/european respiratory society international multidisciplinary classification of lung adenocarcinoma. J Thorac Oncol. 6(2):244-85, 2011
3. Godoy MC et al: Subsolid pulmonary nodules and the spectrum of peripheral adenocarcinomas of the lung: recommended interim guidelines for assessment and management. Radiology. 253(3):606-22, 2009

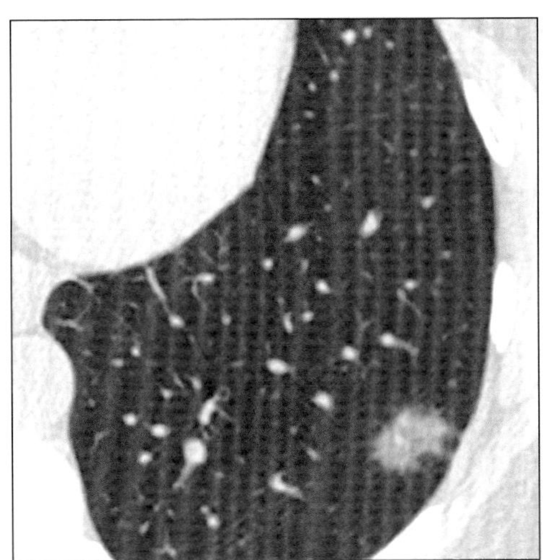

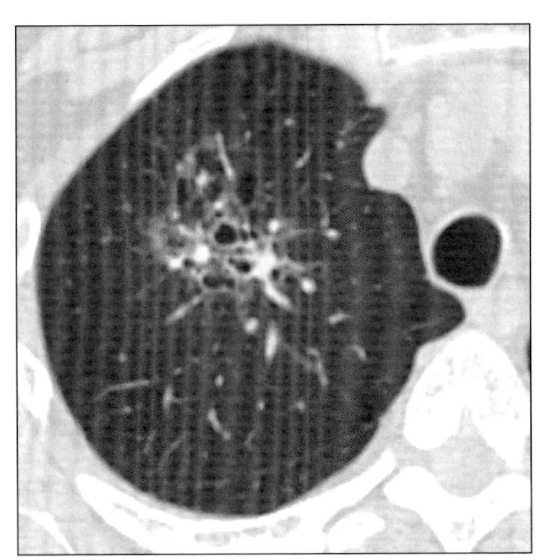

(Left) *Axial NECT shows an adenocarcinoma manifesting as a pure ground-glass opacity (nonsolid) nodule. Excisional biopsy should be considered for nonsolid nodules larger than 10 mm that grow or persist at 3-6 month CT follow-up.* ***(Right)*** *Axial NECT shows an invasive right upper lobe adenocarcinoma manifesting as a heterogeneous lung mass with an internal "bubbly" appearance that typically correlates with intrinsic airway distortion.*

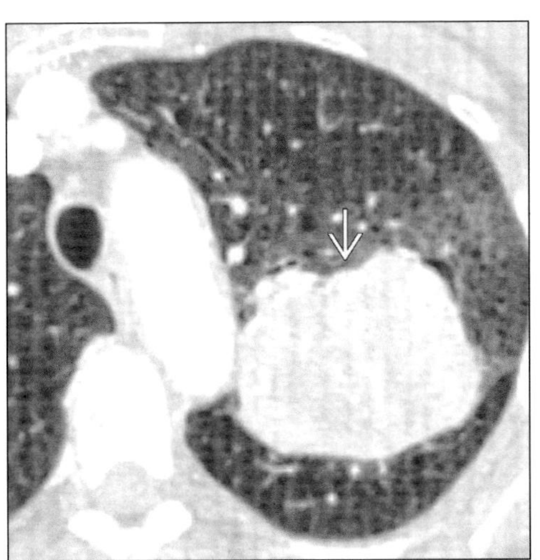

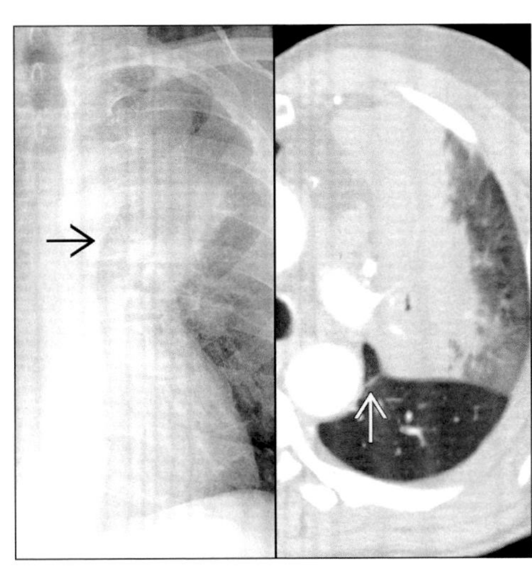

(Left) *Axial NECT of a patient with invasive adenocarcinoma shows a large polylobular left upper lobe mass ➔ and surrounding centrilobular emphysema.* ***(Right)*** *Composite image with PA chest radiograph (left) and axial CECT (right) shows an invasive adenocarcinoma manifesting as a large central mass that causes left upper lobe atelectasis and exhibits the luftsichel sign ➔, which is produced by interposition of the aerated left lower lobe ➔ between the atelectatic left upper lobe and the aorta.*

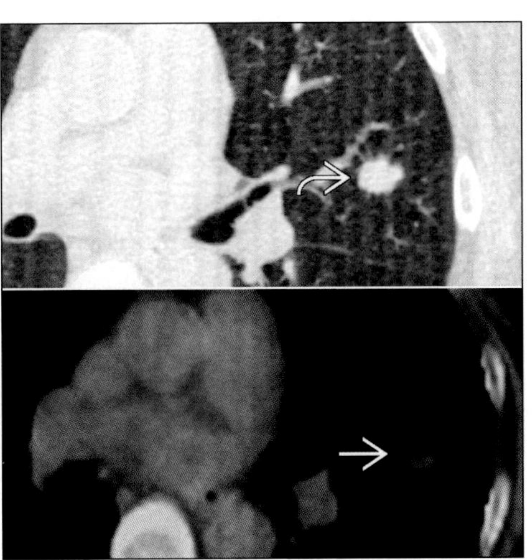

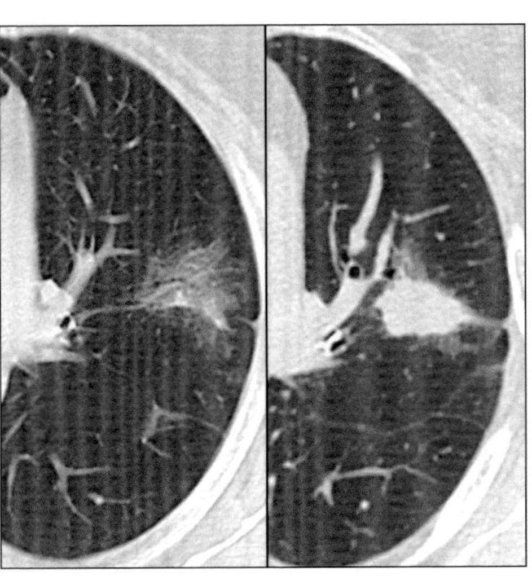

(Left) *Composite image with axial NECT (top) and fused PET/CT (bottom) shows a left upper lobe polylobular nodule ➔ that exhibits FDG avidity ➔. PET/CT is useful for evaluating and staging solid lung nodules.* ***(Right)*** *Composite image with axial NECT in a patient with adenocarcinoma shows a predominantly ground-glass nodule with intrinsic air bronchograms (left). Six years later, the nodule exhibits growth of the solid component (right), illustrating the need for long term follow-up of such lesions.*

SQUAMOUS CELL CARCINOMA

Key Facts

Terminology
- Squamous cell carcinoma (SCC)

Imaging
- Radiography
  - Central hilar/perihilar mass
  - Bronchial obstruction with postobstructive atelectasis/pneumonia
  - Mediastinal/hilar lymphadenopathy
  - Peripheral lung nodule or mass
- CT
  - Central nodule/mass ± postobstructive effects
  - Assessment of lymphadenopathy, local invasion
  - Peripheral nodule/mass, assessment of morphologic features, local invasion
- MR: Complementary to CT, assessment of brachial plexus, mediastinum, chest wall
- PET/CT: Staging & restaging

Top Differential Diagnoses
- Adenocarcinoma
- Small cell carcinoma
- Mediastinal metastases from other primary
- Bronchial carcinoid

Pathology
- Irregular endobronchial lesion, may be polypoid
- Cells with irregular nuclei, large nucleoli, & intercellular bridges

Clinical Issues
- Symptoms/signs: Cough, hemoptysis, dyspnea
- Pancoast syndrome, paraneoplastic hypercalcemia

Diagnostic Checklist
- Consider SCC in a smoker with a central lung mass ± postobstructive atelectasis/pneumonia

(Left) *PA chest radiograph of a patient with SCC shows left upper lobe atelectasis manifesting with obscuration of the left heart border and the luftsichel sign ➡, a crescentic lucency that represents the aerated left lower lobe adjacent to the aortic arch.* ***(Right)*** *Lateral chest radiograph of the same patient confirms left upper lobe atelectasis outlining the margins of the left major fissure ➡. SCC is typically a central lesion and may manifest with postobstructive atelectasis.*

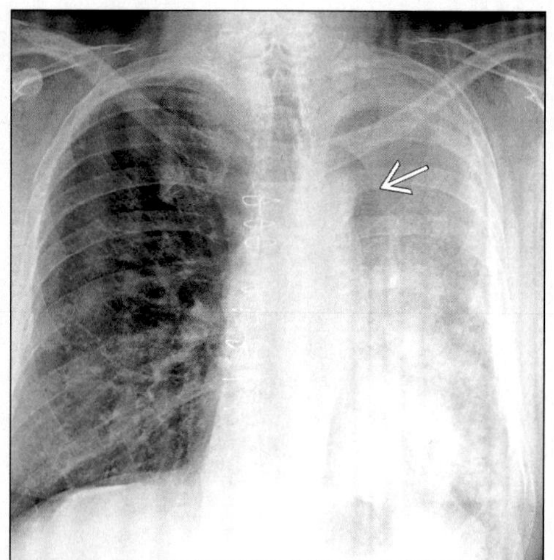

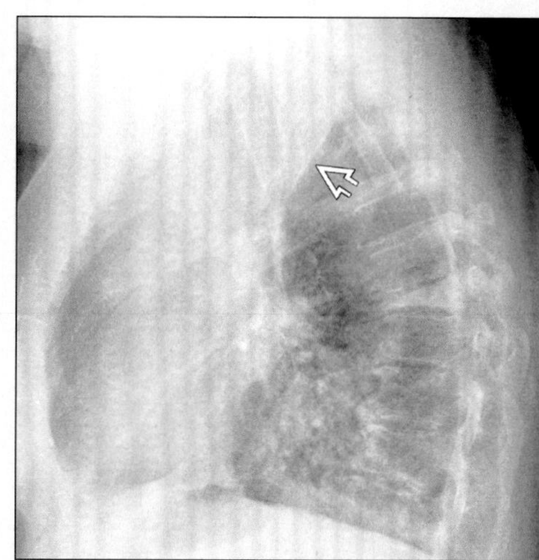

(Left) *PA chest radiograph shows left lower lobe atelectasis manifesting with left retrocardiac opacity ➡ and obscuration of the left hemidiaphragm and the left paraaortic interface.* ***(Right)*** *Composite image with coronal CECT in lung (left) and soft tissue (right) window in the same patient confirms left lower lobe atelectasis ➡ secondary to a central low-attenuation obstructing mass ➡ with an endoluminal component ➡. SCC may manifest with postobstructive atelectasis or consolidation.*

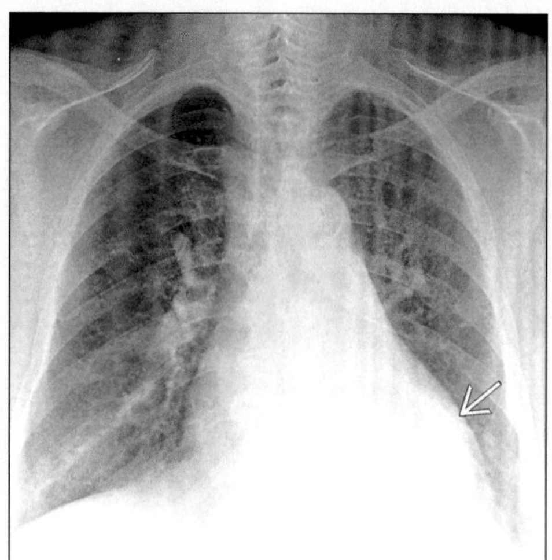

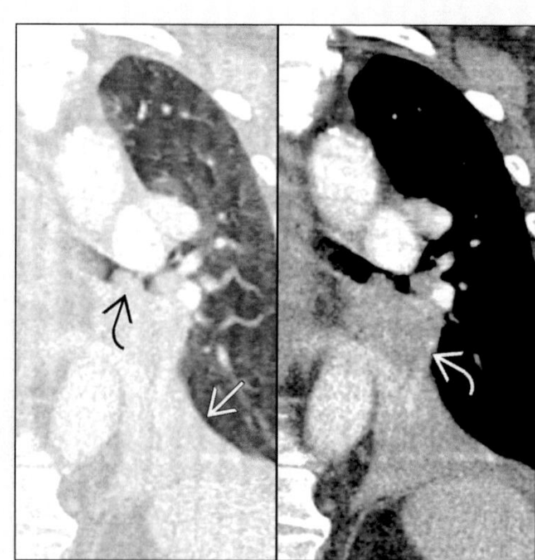

SQUAMOUS CELL CARCINOMA

TERMINOLOGY

Abbreviations

- **Squamous cell carcinoma (SCC)**

Definitions

- Primary lung malignancy thought to evolve from squamous metaplasia (preinvasive lesion)
- "Squamous" means "flat" when describing tumor cell morphology

IMAGING

General Features

- Best diagnostic clue
  - Endoluminal obstructing lesion with postobstructive atelectasis/pneumonia
- Location
  - Typically central
    - 2/3 in mainstem, lobar, or segmental bronchi
- Size
  - Average: ~ 2.5 cm on radiography
  - Incidentally detected lesions: ~ 0.8-1.5 cm on CT
- Morphology
  - Borders: Spiculated, lobular, smooth
  - Attenuation: Homogeneous or heterogeneous, may exhibit necrosis/cavitation or calcification

Radiographic Findings

- **Central hilar/perihilar mass**
  - **Atelectasis**: Sublobar, lobar, complete
    - **S-sign of Golden**: Atelectasis associated with central mass, S-shaped morphology of aerated/ atelectatic lung interface
    - Central bronchial stenosis or cut-off
  - **Postobstructive pneumonia**
    - May obscure underlying lesion
  - Regional hyperlucency
    - Endobronchial obstruction reduces ventilation
    - Hypoxic vasoconstriction reduces lung density
- **Mediastinal/hilar lymphadenopathy**
  - Wide mediastinum, splaying of carina, absence of AP window concavity, unilateral or bilateral hilar enlargement
- Pulmonary nodule or mass, 1-10 cm
  - Nodules < 1 cm rarely detected on radiography
  - Cavitation (15%)

CT Findings

- NECT
  - Disadvantages: Difficult assessment of hilar lymphadenopathy, local invasion, & liver lesions
  - Advantages: No contrast side effects, better characterization of adrenal nodules
- CECT
  - **Central nodule/mass**
    - Increased conspicuity of endobronchial lesion
    - Assessment of bronchial obstruction, particularly if surrounding atelectasis/pneumonia
    - Assessment of local invasion
  - **Peripheral nodule/mass**
    - Assessment of border characteristics
      - Lobulation, spiculation, pleural tags
    - Central necrosis, cavitation, assessment of cavity wall thickness & morphology
      - Cavitation more frequent in larger lesions
      - Wall thickness typically > 1.5 cm
    - Calcification in approximately 13%
  - **Assessment of local invasion**
    - Mediastinal structures: Heart, pericardium, great vessels, aerodigestive tract
    - Pleura
    - Chest wall: Factors favoring invasion
      - > 3 cm tumor-pleura contact
      - Obtuse angle of tumor-pleura interface
    - Diaphragm
  - **Lymphadenopathy**
    - Lymph node enlargement with increased probability of metastases: > 1 cm short axis
    - Subcarinal lymph nodes: > 1.2 cm short axis
    - Retrocrural, paraaortic, juxtapericardial lymph nodes: > 0.8 cm short axis
  - **Pleural/pericardial effusion**
    - Identification of associated soft tissue nodules/ masses
  - Identification of pulmonary metastases
  - Adrenal gland
    - Malignancy favored with mass > 3 cm, poorly defined margins, irregular rim enhancement, invasion of adjacent structures
    - Benign etiology favored if attenuation < 10 HU

MR Findings

- Problem-solving in selected cases
  - Assessment of local invasion
  - Brachial plexus evaluation in Pancoast tumors
- Brain assessment for suspected metastases

Nuclear Medicine Findings

- PET/CT
  - Activity > mediastinal background, standard uptake value (SUV) > 2.5: Greater likelihood of malignancy
    - False-positives: Infection, granulomatous disease
    - False-negatives: Lesions < 1 cm
  - Mediastinum: Activity > background or SUV > 2.5 considered abnormal
    - Specificity 80%; positive result requires pathologic confirmation
  - Prevention of futile thoracotomy in 20% of patients by detection of metastases

Imaging Recommendations

- Best imaging tool
  - CT & whole body PET/CT for diagnosis, staging, & surveillance
- Protocol advice
  - CT for clinical staging
    - Thorax to adrenal glands
    - Evaluation of primary tumor, thoracic lymph nodes, metastases
    - Image-guided biopsy planning
  - Contrast-enhanced CT for optimal evaluation of hilar lymphadenopathy

DIFFERENTIAL DIAGNOSIS

Adenocarcinoma

- Solid, part-solid, ground-glass nodule or mass
- Spiculated or lobular lesion border

SQUAMOUS CELL CARCINOMA

Small Cell Carcinoma
- Central, locally invasive mass, lymphadenopathy

Bronchial Carcinoid
- Central nodule/mass with endoluminal component

Mediastinal Metastases from Other Primary
- May mimic advanced primary lung cancer

PATHOLOGY

General Features
- Etiology
  - Postulated progression: Squamous metaplasia → dysplasia → carcinoma in situ → invasive carcinoma
  - **Strong association with cigarette smoking**
    - 50% of lung cancers develop in smokers or former smokers
    - Lung cancer risk directly related to number of cigarettes smoked, length of smoking history, & tar/nicotine content
    - Cessation of smoking reduces lung cancer risk

Staging, Grading, & Classification
- CT & PET/CT for clinical staging
- Thoracentesis
  - Malignant pleural effusion upstages to M1a
  - May provide therapeutic relief in large effusions

Gross Pathologic & Surgical Features
- Irregular endobronchial lesion, may be polypoid
  - Near universal bronchial wall invasion
  - May grow along bronchial mucosa
  - May produce bronchial obstruction
  - May directly invade adjacent lymph nodes
- Large tumors may exhibit cavitation

Microscopic Features
- Cells with irregular nuclei, large nucleoli, & intercellular bridges; stain positive for keratin
- Keratin pearls: Laminated whorls of eosinophilic cells in well-differentiated tumors
- High mitotic rates, necrosis
- Positive stains for TTF-1 and napsin A favor diagnosis

CLINICAL ISSUES

Presentation
- Most common signs/symptoms
  - Asymptomatic in 7-10%
    - Incidental imaging diagnosis
  - Cough, hemoptysis, dyspnea, fever
    - Symptoms more common with central lesions & advanced disease
- Other signs/symptoms
  - Postobstructive pneumonia/atelectasis from bronchial stenosis
  - Chest pain from chest wall invasion
  - **Pancoast syndrome**
    - Neuropathic pain or atrophy of ipsilateral upper extremity due to brachial plexus involvement
    - **Horner syndrome**: Sympathetic chain & stellate ganglion involvement
  - Paraneoplastic syndromes: Hypercalcemia due to secretion of parathyroid hormone-like substance by tumor

Demographics
- Age
  - Risk of lung cancer increases with age
    - Highest rate of smoking-related cancer in patients over 70 years
- Gender
  - Tobacco-related cancer incidence higher in men
- Ethnicity
  - Higher incidence of lung cancer in African-Americans compared with other racial groups
- Epidemiology
  - 203,536 people in USA diagnosed with lung cancer (all types) in 2007
  - Estimated 150,000 deaths from lung cancer (all types) in USA in 2010

Natural History & Prognosis
- Lifetime risk of developing lung cancer: 1 in 14 persons (6.95%)
- Survival decreases with increasing TNM stage
  - 5-year survival of 3.6% with distant metastases (all lung cancer subtypes)

Diagnosis
- Sputum cytology for identification of malignant cells
- Bronchoscopy
  - Diagnosis of central tumors; false-negative rate: 40%
  - Bronchial washing cytology for malignant cells
- Image-guided biopsy

Treatment
- Stage I-II: Surgical resection with adjuvant chemotherapy in select cases
- Stage IIIA: Surgery, chemotherapy, radiation therapy, or combination
- Stage IIIB: Chemotherapy & radiation therapy
- Stage IV: Chemotherapy with palliative radiation therapy in select cases
  - Resection of solitary brain metastasis in selected cases
- Multidisciplinary approach recommended

DIAGNOSTIC CHECKLIST

Consider
- SCC in smoker with central lung mass ± postobstructive atelectasis/pneumonia

Reporting Tips
- Consolidations in adults should be followed to resolution to exclude underlying malignancy
- Lesions suspicious for lung cancer should be biopsied even if PET/CT is negative

SELECTED REFERENCES

1. Nair A et al: Revisions to the TNM staging of non-small cell lung cancer: rationale, clinicoradiologic implications, and persistent limitations. Radiographics. 31(1):215-38, 2011
2. Almeida FA et al: Initial evaluation of the nonsmall cell lung cancer patient: diagnosis and staging. Curr Opin Pulm Med. 16(4):307-14, 2010

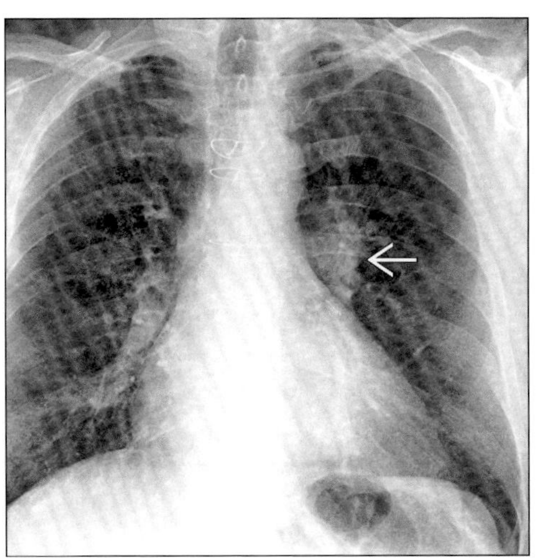

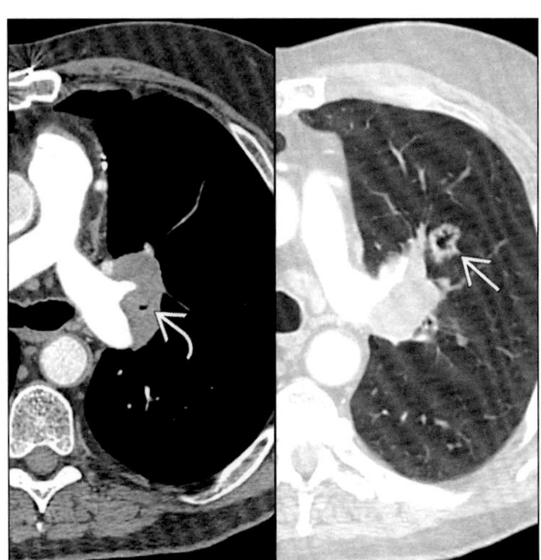

(Left) *PA chest radiograph of a 62-year-old smoker who presented with hemoptysis shows a left hilar mass ➡. Chest CT is indicated in smokers over the age of 40 years who present with hemoptysis.* ***(Right)*** *Composite image with axial CECT in soft tissue (left) and lung (right) windows shows a left hilar mass that nearly obliterates the apicoposterior left upper lobe bronchus ➡ and an adjacent polylobular cavitary lung nodule ➡ not visible on radiography. Bronchoscopic biopsy revealed SCC.*

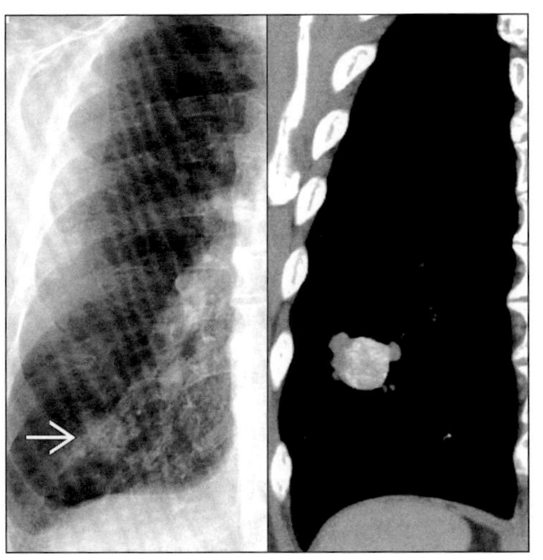

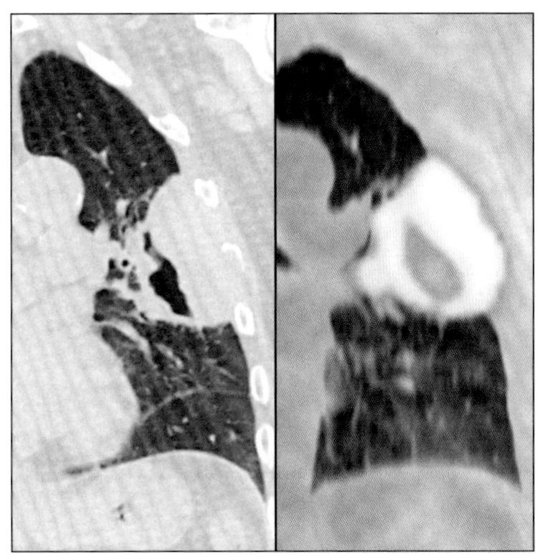

(Left) *Composite image with PA chest radiograph (left) and coronal NECT (right) of a patient with SCC shows a polylobular right lower lobe nodule ➡ with diffuse calcification. Approximately 13% of lung cancers exhibit calcification.* ***(Right)*** *Composite image with coronal CECT (left) and coronal fused PET/CT (right) of a patient with SCC shows a large left upper lobe cavitary mass with thick nodular cavity walls and intense FDG uptake with a maximum SUV of 16.8 and central photopenia from necrosis.*

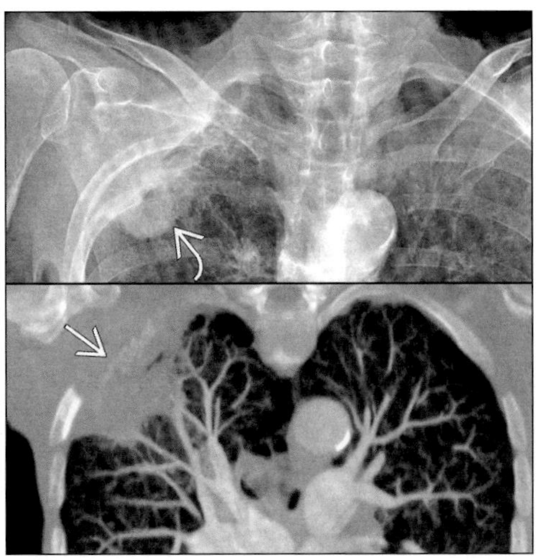

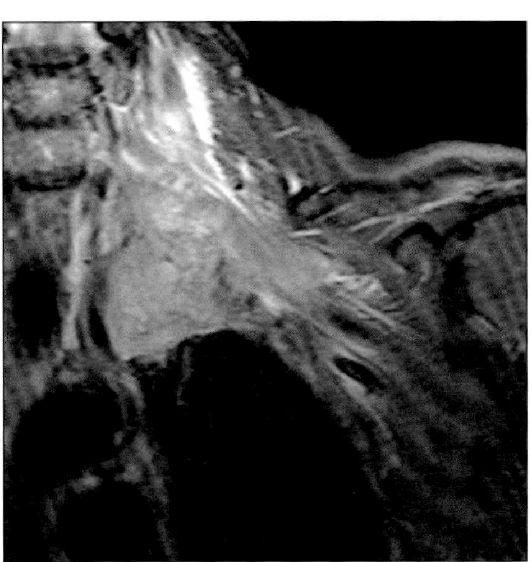

(Left) *Composite image with PA chest radiograph (top) and coronal CECT (bottom) of an elderly woman with right shoulder pain shows a peripheral lung mass ➡ with direct chest wall invasion and rib destruction ➡, consistent with a Pancoast tumor.* ***(Right)*** *Coronal T2WI MR of a patient with a Pancoast tumor shows direct tumor invasion of the left apical chest wall. SCC is the most common type of lung cancer to manifest as a Pancoast tumor, and MR is useful for evaluating extent of invasion in affected patients.*

SMALL CELL CARCINOMA

Key Facts

Terminology

- Small cell lung cancer (SCLC)
- Highly malignant neuroendocrine lung cancer thought to arise from Kulchitsky cells

Imaging

- Radiography
  - Large central/mediastinal mass
  - Hilar mass ± postobstructive effects
  - Elevated hemidiaphragm from phrenic nerve involvement
  - Solitary nodule or mass
- CT
  - Large hilar/mediastinal mass/lymphadenopathy
  - Encasement/invasion of mediastinal structures
  - Bronchial encasement/obstruction & postobstructive effects
  - Metastases to adrenal gland, liver, skeleton

Top Differential Diagnoses

- Lymphoma
- Non-small cell lung cancer (NSCLC)
- Mediastinal metastases

Pathology

- Small blue cells, high mitotic rates, frequent necrosis

Clinical Issues

- Cough, chest pain, hemoptysis, dyspnea
- Paraneoplastic syndromes
- Metastatic disease at presentation
- Overall poor prognosis
  - 1-2% 5-year survival with advanced disease

Diagnostic Checklist

- Consider small cell carcinoma in smoker with large central mass & paraneoplastic syndrome

*(**Left**) PA chest radiograph of a patient with small cell carcinoma shows typical imaging features at presentation including bulky mediastinal ➲ and hilar ➔ lymphadenopathy. (**Right**) Axial CECT of the same patient shows bulky coalescent mediastinal and hilar lymphadenopathy producing near complete obstruction of the superior vena cava ➔. SCLC is typically metastatic at presentation and is a common cause of SVC syndrome.*

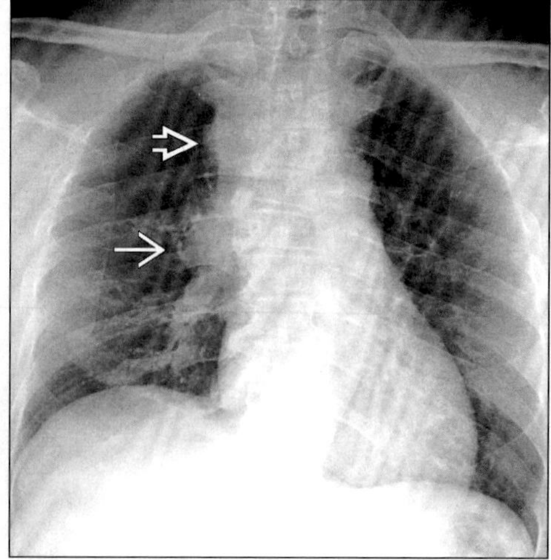

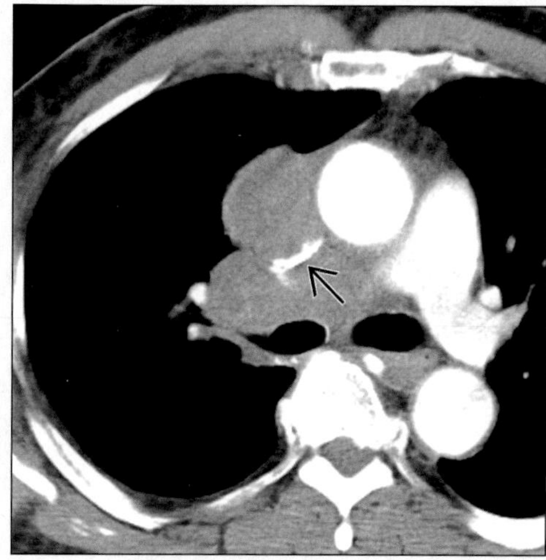

*(**Left**) PA chest radiograph of a patient with SCLC shows a large polylobular right perihilar lung mass ➔ with associated right paratracheal convexity ➲ from mediastinal lymphadenopathy. SCLC commonly exhibits mediastinal lymphadenopathy. (**Right**) Coronal CECT maximum intensity projection (MIP) image of the same patient confirms a right central mass ➔ with hilar, mediastinal, and subcarinal lymphadenopathy ➔. These are typical imaging findings at presentation in patients with SCLC.*

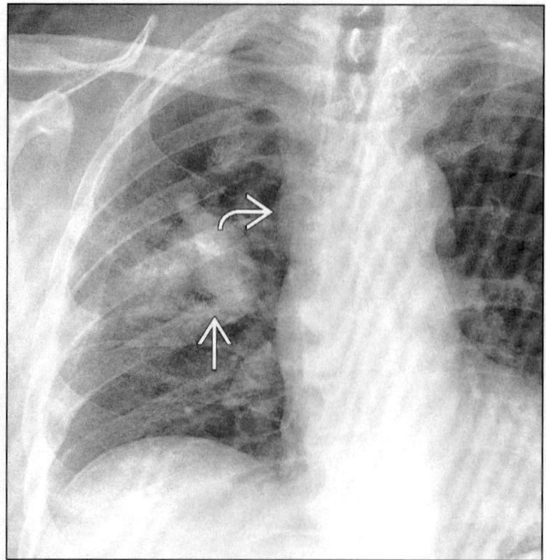

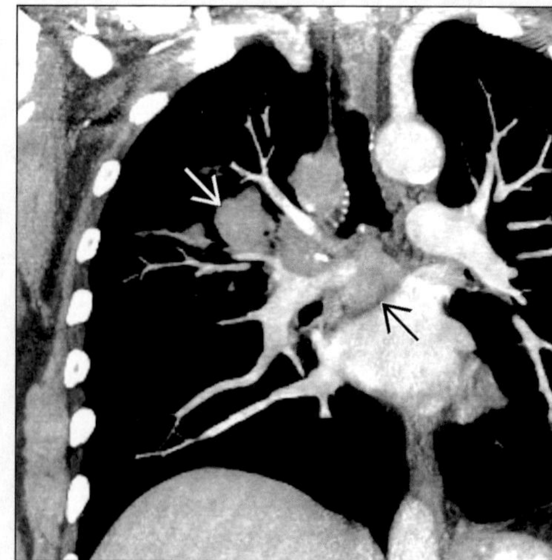

SMALL CELL CARCINOMA

TERMINOLOGY

Abbreviations

- **Small cell lung cancer** (SCLC)

Definitions

- Highly malignant neuroendocrine lung cancer thought to arise from Kulchitsky cells
  - Distinct from non-small cell lung cancers for treatment purposes

IMAGING

General Features

- Best diagnostic clue
  - Large locally invasive central mass with hilar/mediastinal lymphadenopathy
- Location
  - Origin from lobar or main stem bronchi (up to 95%)
  - Endoluminal lesion typically not visible
- Size
  - Usually large at presentation
- Morphology
  - Bulky central mass &/or lymphadenopathy
  - Solitary nodule/mass (5-10%)
  - Distant (hematogenous) metastases (70%)
    - Abdomen, especially adrenal gland & liver (60%)
    - Bone (35%)
    - Brain (10%)

Radiographic Findings

- **Large central/mediastinal mass** involving at least 1 hilum (85%)
- Bronchial obstruction
  - Sublobar, lobar, or complete lung atelectasis
  - Bronchial cut-off sign
- Solitary nodule or mass
  - Less frequent manifestation
  - Variable lesion size
  - No cavitation or calcification
- Elevated hemidiaphragm: Phrenic nerve involvement
- Pleural effusion
- Visualization of metastases

CT Findings

- CECT
  - **Large hilar/mediastinal mass &/or lymphadenopathy**
    - ± contralateral, supraclavicular, cervical lymphadenopathy
  - **Encasement/invasion of mediastinal structures**
    - Invasion of heart & great vessels
    - SVC compression/invasion in 10-15%
      - 25% of SVC syndrome cases are caused by SCLC
    - Encasement/invasion of aerodigestive tract
  - Bronchial encasement with compression/obstruction & resultant atelectasis, postobstructive pneumonia
    - Endoluminal neoplasm typically not apparent
  - Solitary nodule or mass
  - Pleural effusion, nodular pleural thickening
  - Metastases: Adrenal, liver, skeleton

MR Findings

- Rarely used for evaluation of intrathoracic disease
- Modality of choice for imaging brain metastases
- Consider liver, adrenal, skeletal MR in selected cases

Nuclear Medicine Findings

- Bone scan
  - High sensitivity for skeletal metastases
- PET/CT
  - Staging & restaging
  - May result in upstaging of clinical CT stage
  - Very high SUV indicates poorer prognosis

Imaging Recommendations

- Best imaging tool
  - CECT to determine extent of disease
  - MR with gadolinium for brain metastases
  - Skeletal scintigraphy for osseous metastases
  - FDG PET for identification of distant metastases

DIFFERENTIAL DIAGNOSIS

Other Malignant Neoplasms

- Lymphoma
  - Mediastinal/hilar lymphadenopathy
- Non-small cell lung cancer (NSCLC)
  - Primary tumor usually visible, less bulky mediastinal disease
- Mediastinal metastases
  - Breast, head & neck, renal/testicular, & thyroid cancers, melanoma

Nonneoplastic Lymphadenopathy

- Tuberculosis
  - Smaller, discrete lymph nodes with central necrosis
- Sarcoidosis
  - Symmetric lymphadenopathy
- Mediastinal fibrosis
  - Partially calcified locally invasive mediastinal mass

Solitary Pulmonary Nodule

- Non-small cell lung cancer
  - Indistinguishable from SCLC
  - May exhibit cavitation (rare in untreated SCLC)
- Solitary metastasis
  - Indistinguishable from SCLC
  - Rare manifestation of metastatic disease

PATHOLOGY

General Features

- Etiology
  - **Irrefutable relationship to tobacco use**
    - Occurs almost exclusively in smokers
  - Radiation exposure, synergistic effect with tobacco
    - Uranium mining
    - Radon exposure
  - Bis-chloromethyl ether exposure (industrial liquid, use highly restricted)
- Aggressive behavior: Rapid growth & early metastases

Staging, Grading, & Classification

- Tumor, node, metastasis (TNM) classification use advocated
  - Particularly appropriate when considering resection
- Limited vs. extensive stage SCLC often used to determine therapy
  - **Limited stage**

SMALL CELL CARCINOMA

- Confined to ipsilateral hemithorax, within single radiation port
- Includes mediastinum & supraclavicular lymph nodes
- **Extensive stage**: All others
  - Disease not confined to single radiation port
  - Malignant pleural effusion

Gross Pathologic & Surgical Features

- Coalescent hilar & mediastinal mass
  - Lymphatic & vascular invasion
  - Hematogenous metastases to lung, adrenal, liver, kidney, brain, bone

Microscopic Features

- Small blue cells 2x size of lymphocytes
  - Finely stippled chromatin, scant cytoplasm, small or absent nucleoli, crush artifact
- High mitotic rates, necrosis common
- May exhibit non-small cell carcinoma cell populations

CLINICAL ISSUES

Presentation

- Most common signs/symptoms
  - Cough, chest pain, hemoptysis, dyspnea
- Other signs/symptoms
  - Typically systemic disease at presentation including bone marrow suppression
    - Weight loss, anorexia
  - Hypertrophic osteoarthropathy rare compared to NSCLC
  - **Compression of mediastinal structures**
    - **Superior vena cava syndrome**
    - Dysphagia from esophageal compression
    - Hoarseness from recurrent laryngeal nerve involvement
  - **Symptoms of metastatic disease**
    - Headache, mental status change, seizure, ataxia from brain metastases
    - Bone pain
    - Pruritus, jaundice from liver metastases
  - **Nonendocrine paraneoplastic syndromes**
    - Eaton-Lambert-Myasthenia syndrome
    - Limbic encephalitis
    - Cerebellar degeneration
    - Anti-Hu encephalomyelitis
    - Dermatomyositis/polymyositis
  - **Endocrine paraneoplastic syndromes**
    - Syndrome of inappropriate antidiuretic hormone secretion
    - Ectopic ACTH causing Cushing syndrome
    - Hypercalcemic hyperparathyroidism

Demographics

- Age
  - 5th to 7th decades of life
- Gender
  - M > F
- Epidemiology
  - 14% of all primary lung cancers

Natural History & Prognosis

- Rapidly growing malignant neoplasm
- Usually fatal within 4 months without treatment
- Often complete response to treatment, but recurrence in < 2 years
- Overall poor prognosis
  - **Limited stage**
    - Median survival: 15-20 months
    - 5-year survival: 10-13%
  - **Extensive stage**
    - Median survival: 8-13 months
    - 5-year survival: 1-2%
  - Screening not proven to decrease mortality from SCLC

Treatment

- Limited disease
  - Combination chemotherapy & radiation therapy
  - Prophylactic cranial irradiation
  - Surgery considered in selected solitary lesions
- Extensive disease
  - Chemotherapy
  - Radiation reserved for palliation
  - Cerebral metastases usually treated with radiation, occasionally with surgery

DIAGNOSTIC CHECKLIST

Consider

- Small cell carcinoma in smoker with large central mass, lymphadenopathy, & paraneoplastic syndrome

Image Interpretation Pearls

- SCLC produces extensive mediastinal/hilar lymphadenopathy & may mimic lymphoma or metastatic disease
- Evaluate extrathoracic sites, particularly adrenal glands, liver, & brain for metastatic disease
- Osteoblastic healing response to chemotherapy may mimic sclerotic metastases & disease progression

SELECTED REFERENCES

1. Cuffe S et al: Characteristics and outcomes of small cell lung cancer patients diagnosed during two lung cancer computed tomographic screening programs in heavy smokers. J Thorac Oncol. 6(4):818-22, 2011
2. Thomson D et al: The role of positron emission tomography in management of small cell lung cancer. Lung Cancer. 73(2):121-6, 2011
3. Stattaus J et al: Osteoblastic response as a healing reaction to chemotherapy mimicking progressive disease in patients with small cell lung cancer. Eur Radiol. 19(1):193-200, 2009
4. Vallières E et al: The IASLC Lung Cancer Staging Project: proposals regarding the relevance of TNM in the pathologic staging of small cell lung cancer in the forthcoming (seventh) edition of the TNM classification for lung cancer. J Thorac Oncol. 4(9):1049-59, 2009
5. Chong S et al: Neuroendocrine tumors of the lung: clinical, pathologic, and imaging findings. Radiographics. 26(1):41-57; discussion 57-8, 2006

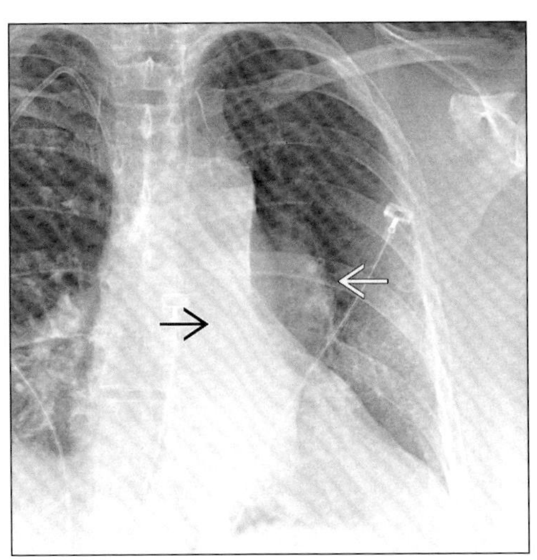

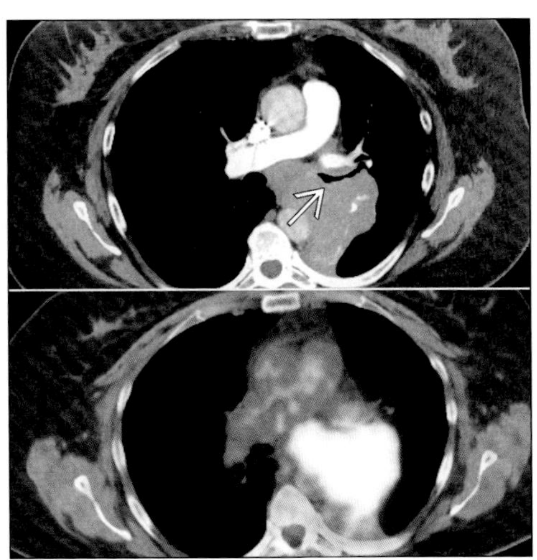

(Left) *PA chest radiograph of a patient with SCLC shows a left hilar mass ➡ that produces cut-off of the left lower lobe bronchus ⇨ and left lower lobe atelectasis.* ***(Right)*** *Composite image with axial CECT (top) and fused PET/CT (bottom) of the same patient shows a large central soft tissue mass that encases and obstructs the left lower lobe bronchus ➡ with resultant left lower lobe atelectasis. The mass exhibits intense activity (maximum SUV = 11).*

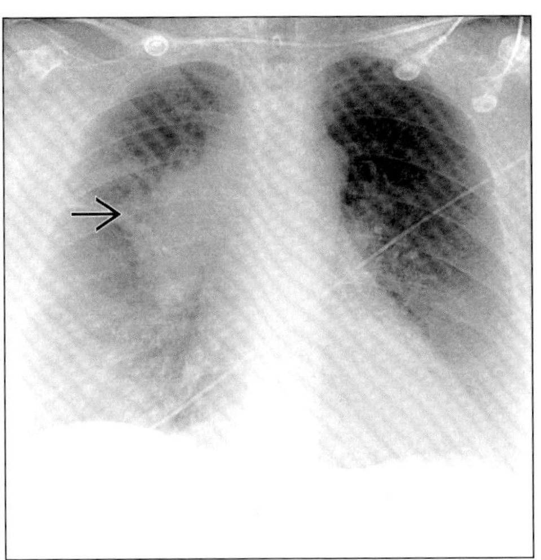

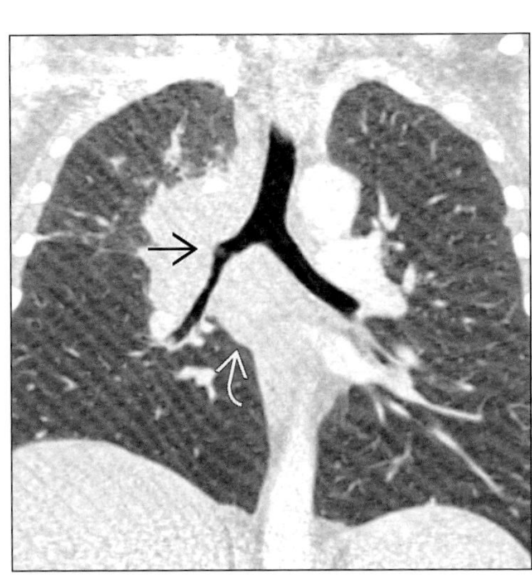

(Left) *PA chest radiograph of a patient with SCLC who presented with dyspnea shows a large right hilar/perihilar mass ⇨ with ill-defined lobular borders.* ***(Right)*** *Coronal CECT of the same patient shows the right hilar mass, which obliterates the lumen of the right upper lobe bronchus ⇨, and adjacent subcarinal lymphadenopathy ➦. SCLC typically manifests as a central mass representing the primary neoplasm &/or metastatic lymphadenopathy.*

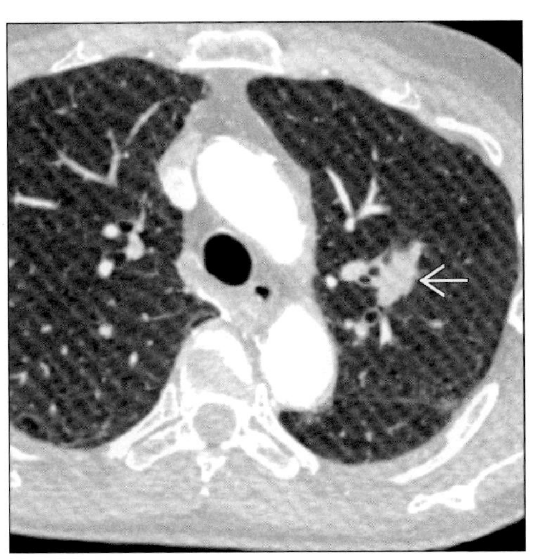

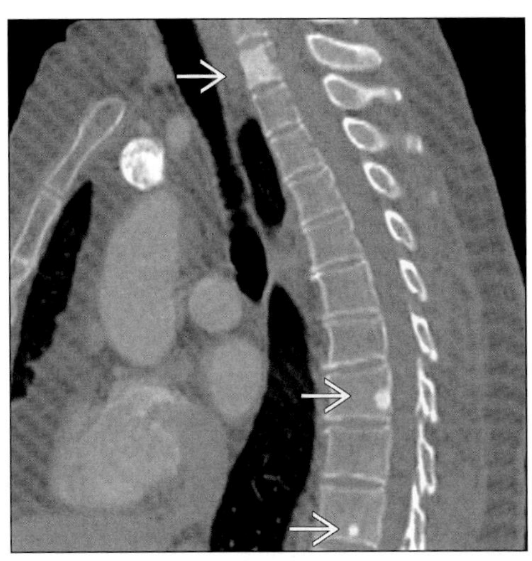

(Left) *Axial CECT of a patient with SCLC shows a small polylobular left upper lobe nodule ➡ and surrounding centrilobular emphysema. Solitary pulmonary nodule is an unusual manifestation of SCLC. In the absence of metastatic disease, surgical resection may be contemplated.* ***(Right)*** *Sagittal CECT of a patient with SCLC shows sclerotic metastases ➡ affecting multiple vertebral bodies. It should be noted that "flare phenomenon" may mimic progression of skeletal metastases.*

MULTIFOCAL LUNG CANCER

Key Facts

Terminology

- Synchronous lung cancers: 2 or more lung cancers detected simultaneously, without metastases
- Metachronous: 2 or more lung cancers detected at different times, without metastases
- Primary lung cancer with satellite lesion(s)
- 1° lung cancer with metastases of same histology

Imaging

- Radiography
  - Multiple nodules, masses, consolidations
- CT
  - Multiple lung nodules, masses, consolidations
  - Solid &/or subsolid attenuation
  - Dominant lesion may occur
- PET/CT
  - Clinical staging/restaging of malignancy
  - Evaluation of extrathoracic disease

Top Differential Diagnoses

- Primary lung cancer & benign lung nodule
- Extrapulmonary malignancy with hematogenous metastases

Pathology

- Synchronous lung cancers differentiated based on histology or molecular analysis

Clinical Issues

- Cough, hemoptysis, dyspnea
  - May be asymptomatic
- Survival: Synchronous lung cancers (18-76%)
- Multiple biopsies may be required for diagnosis

Diagnostic Checklist

- Consider multifocal lung cancer in patients with multiple lung lesions without lymphadenopathy or distant metastases

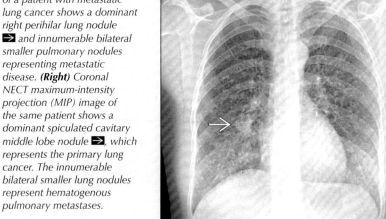

*(**Left**) PA chest radiograph of a patient with metastatic lung cancer shows a dominant right perihilar lung nodule ➔ and innumerable bilateral smaller pulmonary nodules representing metastatic disease. (**Right**) Coronal NECT maximum-intensity projection (MIP) image of the same patient shows a dominant spiculated cavitary middle lobe nodule ➔, which represents the primary lung cancer. The innumerable bilateral smaller lung nodules represent hematogenous pulmonary metastases.*

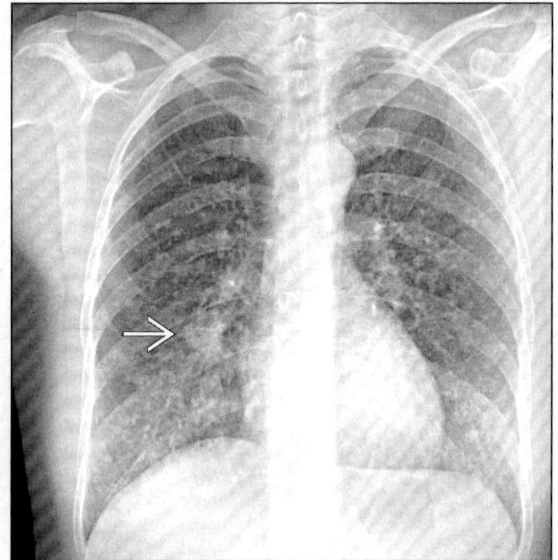

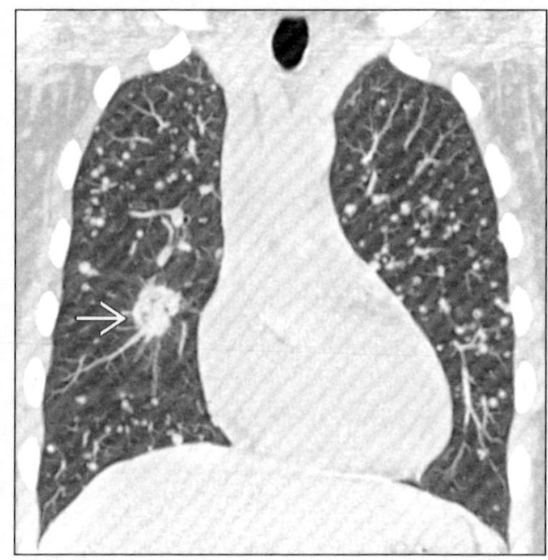

*(**Left**) Composite image with axial CECT shows a left apical spiculated lung nodule (top) & a left upper lobe polylobular cavitary lung mass (bottom). In the absence of metastases or lymphadenopathy, these may represent synchronous primary lung cancers. Histologic and molecular analysis may be required for confirmation. (**Right**) Axial NECT of a patient with multifocal adenocarcinomas shows multiple nonsolid and part-solid nodules ➔. Biopsy of one of the nodules confirmed adenocarcinoma with acinar pattern.*

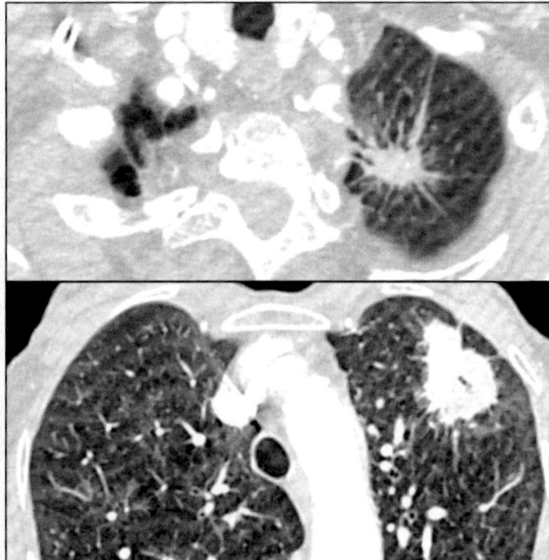

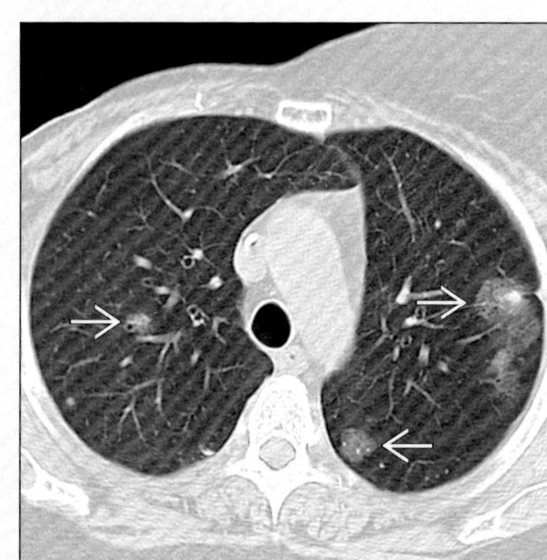

MULTIFOCAL LUNG CANCER

TERMINOLOGY

Definitions

- Multiple primary lung cancers, clinical criteria
  - **Synchronous**: 2 or more separate lung cancers detected simultaneously, without systemic metastases
    - If same histology, should be in different lobes, without N2 or N3 disease
  - **Metachronous**: Detection of 2 or more lung cancers separated by time, without systemic metastases
    - If same histology, ≥ 2 year interval
- Primary lung cancer with satellite lesion(s)
  - Lesions of same histology within same lobe regardless of size, without systemic metastases
- **Hematogenous metastases**
  - Lung cancer with multiple lung metastases of same histology
  - Lesions of same histology in different lobes with N2 or N3 disease

IMAGING

Radiographic Findings

- Radiography
  - ≥ 2 lung nodules, masses, consolidations
  - Dominant lesion may occur
  - ± lymphadenopathy in metastatic disease
  - ± pleural effusion

CT Findings

- 2 or more lung nodules, masses, consolidations
- Solid & subsolid attenuation
- Dominant lesion may occur
- ± lymphadenopathy in cases of metastatic disease
- Pleural effusion, pleural nodules

Nuclear Medicine Findings

- PET
  - Optimal imaging modality for clinical staging
  - Evaluation of extrathoracic disease
  - Does not differentiate between multiple primary neoplasms & pulmonary metastases

Imaging Recommendations

- Protocol advice
  - NECT with thin slices for evaluation of subsolid nodules

DIFFERENTIAL DIAGNOSIS

Primary Lung Cancer & Benign Lung Nodule

- Majority of lung nodules detected in association with lung cancer are benign (57-86%)
- Atypical adenomatous hyperplasia in patients with adenocarcinoma

Extrapulmonary Malignancy with Hematogenous Metastases

- Clinical history & biopsy critical for diagnosis
- Spherical well-defined nodules with peripheral/basilar predominance

PATHOLOGY

Staging, Grading, & Classification

- Synchronous lung cancers differentiated with histology or molecular analysis
- Same histology: Molecular markers for optimal differentiation of satellite/metastatic lesions from synchronous primaries
- 7th edition of TNM staging system: Primary lung cancer with satellite malignant lesions
  - T3: Satellite lesions in same lobe as primary tumor
  - T4: Satellite lesions in different ipsilateral lobe as primary tumor
  - M1a: Contralateral satellite lesions
- Synchronous lesions: Size of largest tumor may be most important factor in surgical decision making

CLINICAL ISSUES

Presentation

- Most common signs/symptoms
  - Cough, hemoptysis, dyspnea
  - May be asymptomatic

Natural History & Prognosis

- Survival: Synchronous lung cancers (18-76%)
- Differentiation between multiple primary lesions & metastatic disease important for patient management

Evaluation

- Multiple biopsies may be required to exclude multiple primary lung cancers
- Core needle biopsy recommended
  - Cytologic accuracy for determining lung cancer cell type only 60-80%
  - Improved accuracy with larger specimens
- Careful staging of synchronous lung cancers
  - Brain contrast-enhanced MR
  - Whole body PET/CT
  - Mediastinoscopy

Treatment

- Single primary lung cancer with satellite lesion in same lobe
  - Lobectomy
- Multiple primary lung cancers
  - Resection if no lymph node involvement or distant metastases

DIAGNOSTIC CHECKLIST

Consider

- Multiple primary lung cancers in patients with multiple lung lesions without lymphadenopathy or distant metastases
- Multifocal adenocarcinomas in patients with slow growing part-solid & nonsolid nodules

SELECTED REFERENCES

1. Shen KR et al: Special treatment issues in lung cancer: ACCP evidence-based clinical practice guidelines (2nd edition). Chest. 132(3 Suppl):290S-305S, 2007

RESECTABLE LUNG CANCER

Key Facts

Terminology

- Non-small cell lung cancer (NSCLC)
- Small cell lung cancer (SCLC)
- Lung cancer potentially curable with complete surgical resection

Imaging

- Clinical stage I-IIIA may be resectable
- CT for evaluation of size, morphology, & location in relation to pleura, mediastinum, & carina
  - Lymph nodes > 1 cm in mediastinum or > 1.2 cm in subcarinal region suspicious for metastases
  - Evaluation of pleura for nodules & effusions
  - Evaluation for distant metastases
- CT is modality of choice in initial evaluation of pulmonary nodule
- PET/CT is modality of choice for initial clinical staging

Top Differential Diagnoses

- Adenocarcinoma
- Squamous cell carcinoma
- Small cell carcinoma
- Large cell carcinoma
- Carcinoid

Clinical Issues

- Functional status of patient is critical part of evaluation to determine surgical clearance
- NSCLC: 5-year survival stage IA: 50%; stage IIIA: 19%
- SCLC: 5-year survival 13% at best

Diagnostic Checklist

- Consider lung cancer in differential diagnosis of incidentally discovered lung nodules as disease is common & deadly, especially with advanced stage

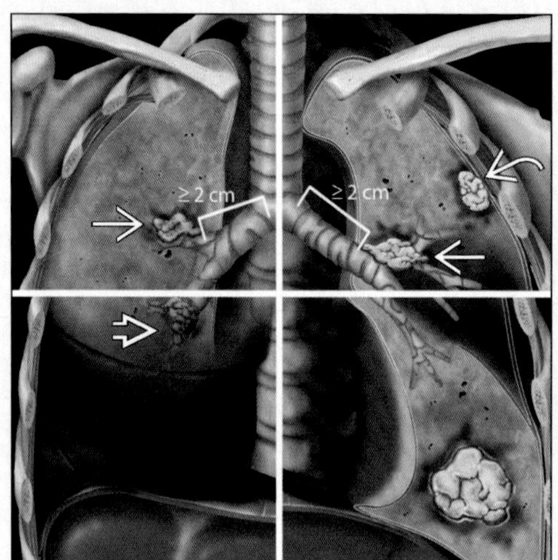

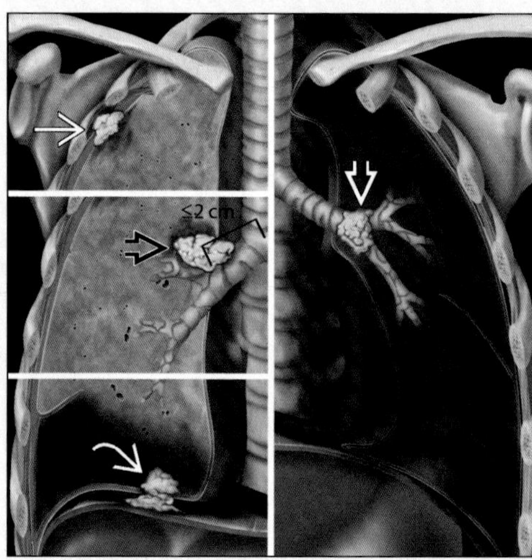

*(**Left**) Graphic illustrates T2 tumors involving the bronchus ≥ 2 cm from the carina ➡, invading the visceral pleura ➡, and associated with partial atelectasis/pneumonitis ➡. T2a applies to masses > 3 cm but ≤ 5 cm. T2b applies to masses > 5 cm but ≤ 7 cm. (**Right**) Graphic depicts T3 tumor invading the chest wall ➡, invading the main stem bronchus < 2 cm from the carina ➡, invading the diaphragm ➡, and causing atelectasis or pneumonitis of an entire lung ➡.*

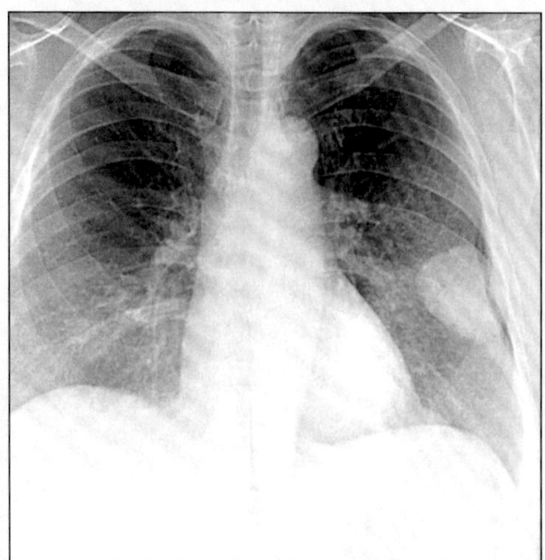

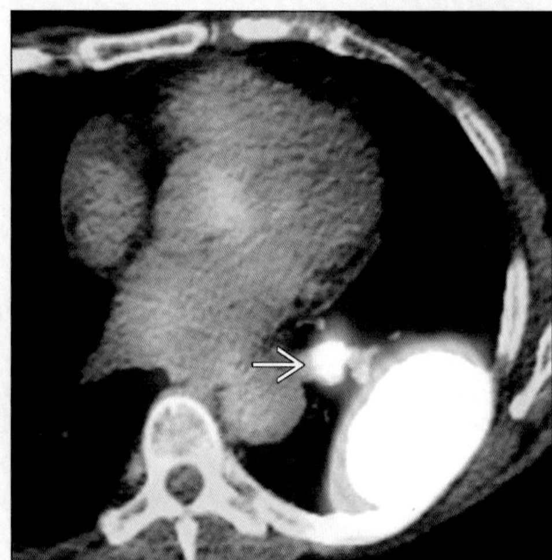

*(**Left**) PA chest radiograph of a 56-year-old female smoker with cough and chest pain shows a 5 cm left lower lobe mass with an adjacent loculated left pneumothorax. (**Right**) Axial fused PET/CT of the same patient shows marked FDG uptake in the mass and an ipsilateral left hilar lymph node ➡. More than 3 cm of pleural contact and associated loculated pneumothorax suggest invasion of the visceral pleura, consistent with clinical stage IIB (T2 N1). Adenocarcinoma was confirmed at surgery.*

RESECTABLE LUNG CANCER

TERMINOLOGY

Abbreviations

- **Non-small cell lung cancer** (NSCLC)
- **Small cell lung cancer** (SCLC)

Definitions

- Lung cancer potentially curable with complete surgical resection

IMAGING

General Features

- Best diagnostic clue
  - Clinical stages I-IIIA may be resectable
- Size
  - Size alone does not exclude surgical excision

Radiographic Findings

- Radiography
  - Solitary nodule (< 3 cm) or mass (≥ 3 cm)
  - Ipsilateral hilar & mediastinal lymphadenopathy
    - Thickening of paratracheal stripe, abnormal AP window or subcarinal region, wide mediastinum
  - Recurrent postobstructive pneumonia
  - Lobar collapse may be due to bronchial invasion or mass effect from adjacent lymphadenopathy

CT Findings

- CECT
  - Tumor size measured in 3 dimensions with assessment of intrinsic attenuation (ground-glass, solid, part-solid, calcium, fat)
  - Description of tumor location with respect to pleura, mediastinum, & carina
  - Evaluation of lymph nodes
    - Short axis > 1 cm in mediastinum or > 1.2 cm in subcarinal region are suspicious for metastasis
  - Evaluation of pleura for nodules & effusions
    - Suspect pleural invasion in masses with > 3 cm of pleural contact
  - Consider chest wall or mediastinal involvement when normal fat planes are obliterated
  - Evaluation for distant metastases
    - Adrenal (40%), liver (30%), bone (20%), brain (10%)

Nuclear Medicine Findings

- PET/CT
  - Frequently performed for detection of extrapulmonary disease & mediastinal staging
    - Occult metastases in 24% of patients with "surgical disease" based on initial staging
  - Used postoperatively to detect local recurrence
  - False-positive findings with inflammatory processes

MR Findings

- May be used for evaluation of suspected myocardial or chest wall invasion
- Modality of choice to evaluate for brain metastasis

Imaging Recommendations

- Best imaging tool
  - CT is modality of choice in initial evaluation of pulmonary nodule
  - PET/CT is modality of choice for initial clinical staging of lung cancer

DIFFERENTIAL DIAGNOSIS

Adenocarcinoma

- Ground-glass, solid, or part-solid nodule/mass
- Spiculated, irregular, or lobular margins

Squamous Cell Carcinoma

- Centrally located mass
- Peripheral lesions may exhibit cavitation

Small Cell Carcinoma

- Large central mass invading hilum & mediastinum with frequent metastases

Large Cell Carcinoma

- Peripherally located large mass with central necrosis

Bronchial Carcinoid

- Well-defined central nodule or mass, frequent endoluminal component

PATHOLOGY

Staging, Grading, & Classification

- Applicable to non-small cell & small cell lung cancers & bronchial carcinoids
- Factors preventing operative management
  - N3 lymph node &/or distant metastasis (including contralateral pulmonary nodules, pleural or pericardial involvement)

Microscopic Features

- Classification based on histologic type
- Bronchioloalveolar carcinoma no longer a recognized cell type of adenocarcinoma

CLINICAL ISSUES

Presentation

- Most common signs/symptoms
  - Often incidentally detected on imaging studies
  - CT screening of high-risk patients aged 55-75 may decrease mortality by 20%
- Other signs/symptoms
  - Cough, dyspnea, atelectasis, wheezing, recurrent postobstructive pneumonia
  - Paraneoplastic syndromes
    - Syndrome of inappropriate antidiuretic hormone production (SIADH), hypertrophic osteoarthropathy, Cushing syndrome
- Clinical profile
  - Functional status of patient is critical part of initial evaluation & ultimately determines surgical clearance
    - Only 33% of patients who present with surgical disease are medically cleared for surgery
  - Current or former smokers account for majority of affected patients (> 85%)
  - Asbestos exposure increases risk of lung cancer 5x
    - Tobacco smoke increases risk synergistically
  - Other carcinogens
    - Exposure to beryllium, nickel, copper, chromium, & cadmium associated with lung cancer risk

Demographics

- Gender
  - M > F

Lung Carcinoma, AJCC Staging

TNM	*Definitions*
(T) Primary Tumor	
TX	Primary tumor cannot be assessed
T0	No primary tumor
Tis	Carcinoma in situ
T1	Tumor ≤ 3 cm in largest dimension, surrounded by lung or visceral pleura, not proximal to lobar bronchus (i.e., not in main stem bronchus)[1]
T1a	Tumor ≤ 2 cm in greatest dimension
T1b	Tumor > 2 cm but ≤ 3 cm in greatest dimension
T2	Tumor > 3 cm but ≤ 7 cm or with any of the following features: Invades visceral pleura, involves main stem bronchus ≥ 2 cm distal to carina, atelectasis or obstructive pneumonia extending to hilum but not involving entire lung
T2a	Tumor > 3 cm but ≤ 5 cm in greatest dimension
T2b	Tumor > 5 cm but ≤ 7 cm in greatest dimension
T3	Tumor > 7 cm, tumor directly invading chest wall, diaphragm, phrenic nerve, mediastinal pleura, parietal pericardium; tumor in main stem bronchus < 2 cm distal to carina, atelectasis or obstructive pneumonia of entire lung, separate tumor nodule(s) in same lobe
T4	Tumor of any size invading heart, great vessels, trachea, recurrent laryngeal nerve, esophagus, vertebral body, carina, or separate tumor nodule(s) in different ipsilateral lobe
(N) Regional Lymph Nodes	
NX	Regional lymph nodes cannot be assessed
N0	No regional lymph node metastases
N1	Metastasis in ipsilateral peribronchial &/or perihilar lymph nodes & intrapulmonary lymph nodes, including involvement by direct extension
N2	Metastasis in ipsilateral mediastinal &/or subcarinal lymph node(s)
N3	Metastasis in contralateral mediastinal, contralateral hilar, ipsilateral or contralateral scalene, or supraclavicular lymph node(s)
(M) Distant Metastasis	
M0	No distant metastasis
M1	Distant metastasis
M1a	Separate tumor nodule(s) in contralateral lobe, tumor with pleural nodules, or malignant pleural dissemination[2]
M1b	Distant metastasis

[1]The uncommon superficial spreading tumor of any size with invasive component limited to the bronchial wall, which may extend proximal to the main stem bronchus, is also classified as T1a. [2]Most pleural (& pericardial) effusions in lung cancer are due to tumors. In a few patients, multiple cytopathologic examinations of pleural (pericardial) fluid are negative for tumors, and the fluid is not bloody and is not an exudate. Where these elements and clinical judgment dictate that the effusion is not related to a tumor, the effusion should be excluded as a staging element and the disease should be classified as M0. Adapted from AJCC Cancer Staging Forms, 7th ed., 2010.

- Epidemiology
  - Most common cause of cancer deaths worldwide
  - Kills more people per year in USA than cancers of breast, colon, prostate, & lymphomas combined
  - 226,000 new cases and 157,00 deaths per year in USA (2010)

Natural History & Prognosis

- NSCLC: 5-year survival
  - Stage IA: 50%
  - Stage IIIA: 19%
- SCLC: 5-year survival 13% at best

Treatment

- NSCLC stage I or II: Surgical resection with mediastinal lymph node dissection & adjuvant chemoradiation therapy in selected patients
  - Lobectomy preferable, but sublobar resection may be performed if limited pulmonary reserve
    - May be performed by video-assisted thoracoscopic surgery (VATS)
  - T3 tumors often require pneumonectomy
  - Radiation or percutaneous ablation if medically nonoperative candidate
- NSCLC stage IIIA: Surgical resection usually combined with chemoradiation
- SCLC: Usually widespread at diagnosis; systemic therapy, surgery plays small role

DIAGNOSTIC CHECKLIST

Consider

- Lung cancer in cases of incidentally discovered indeterminate lung nodules as disease is common & deadly, especially with advanced stage

SELECTED REFERENCES

1. American Joint Committee on Cancer: AJCC Cancer Staging Manual. 7th ed. New York: Springer. 253-70, 2010
2. Kligerman S et al: A radiologic review of the new TNM classification for lung cancer. AJR Am J Roentgenol. 2010 Mar;194(3):562-73. Review. Erratum in: AJR Am J Roentgenol. 194(5):1404, 2010
3. Detterbeck FC et al: The new lung cancer staging system. Chest. 136(1):260-71, 2009

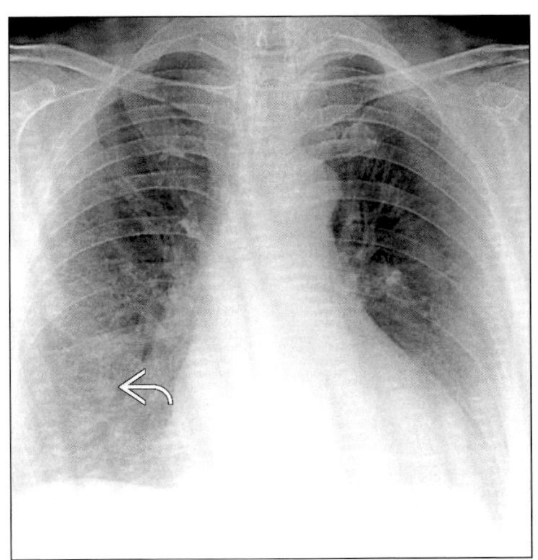

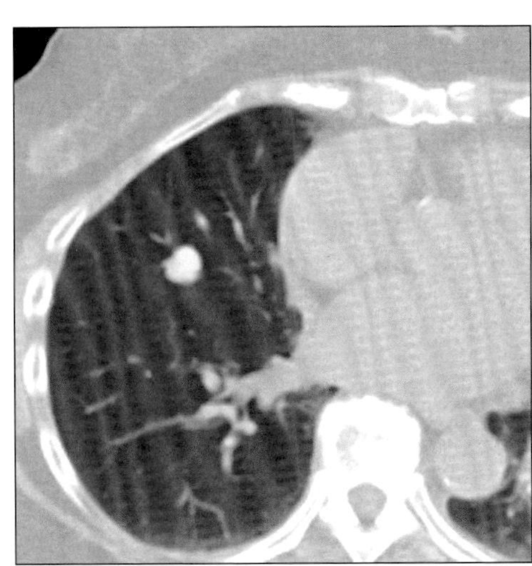

(Left) *AP chest radiograph of an asymptomatic 60-year-old woman shows a 1.4 cm indeterminate nodule in the right mid lung ➔.* ***(Right)*** *Axial NECT of the same patient confirms the presence of a middle lobe nodule and shows its polylobular borders to better advantage. Subsequent PET/CT (not shown) demonstrated focal FDG uptake without evidence of metastatic disease, suggesting clinical stage IA (T1a N0 M0). Right middle lobectomy confirmed the diagnosis of adenocarcinoma.*

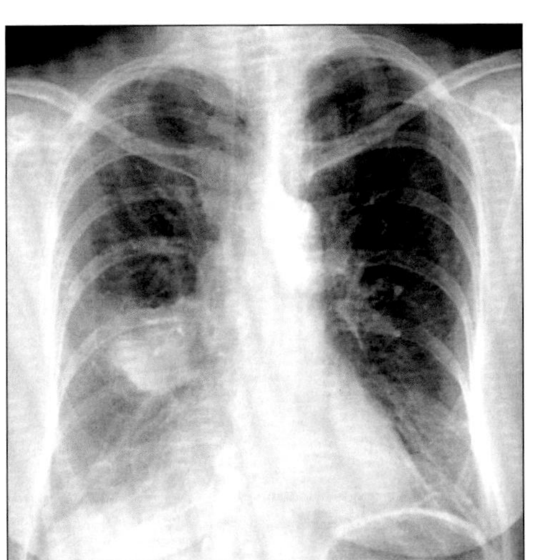

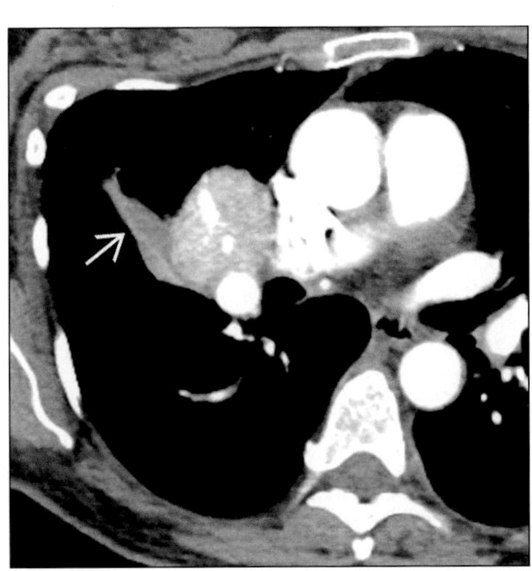

(Left) *PA chest radiograph of a 52-year-old woman (never a smoker) who presented with massive hemoptysis shows a central polylobular 5 cm mass in the right mid lung.* ***(Right)*** *Axial CECT of the same patient shows a lobular 5 cm mass containing intrinsic calcifications and producing middle lobe atelectasis ➔. Transbronchial biopsy confirmed the diagnosis of carcinoid tumor, which was characterized as T2 N0 M0 disease and treated with a right middle lobectomy.*

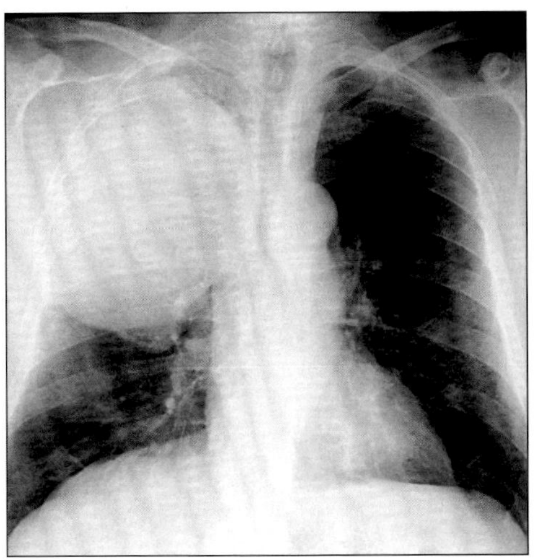

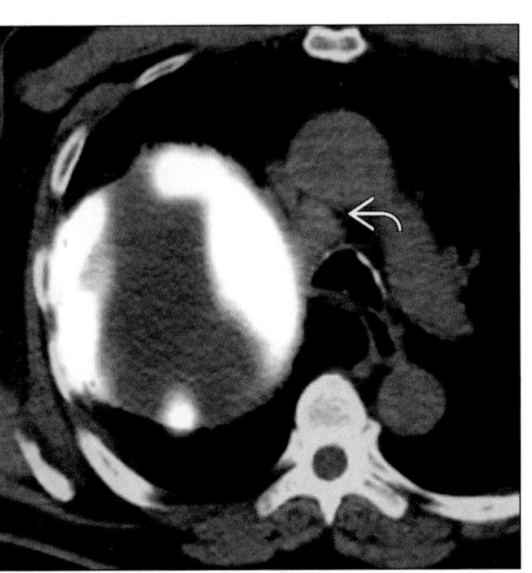

(Left) *PA chest radiograph of a 70-year-old smoker with weight loss shows an 11 cm mass occupying the upper right hemithorax.* ***(Right)*** *Axial PET/CT of the same patient shows marked peripheral FDG uptake and central necrosis in this squamous cell carcinoma. Note mild FDG uptake in a right paratracheal lymph node (4R) ➔. These findings are consistent with a clinical stage IIIA (T3 N2) lung cancer. The patient is doing well 3 years post right upper lobectomy, lymph node dissection, and chemotherapy.*

UNRESECTABLE LUNG CANCER

Key Facts

Terminology

- Non-small cell lung cancer (NSCLC)
- Small cell lung cancer (SCLC)
- Lung cancer for which surgery does not provide survival benefit: Clinical stages IIIB & IV

Imaging

- T4: Invasion of mediastinal structures, vertebral body, tumor nodule(s) in separate ipsilateral lung lobe
- N3: Metastases to scalene, supraclavicular, contralateral mediastinal, or contralateral nodes
  - N3: Lymph nodes or distant metastases preclude operative management
- M1: Nodules in contralateral lobe, malignant pleural effusion/nodule, malignant pericardial effusion
- CECT: Modality of choice for initial characterization
- PET/CT & MR: Optimal for detecting metastases

Top Differential Diagnoses

- Adenocarcinoma
- Squamous cell carcinoma
- Small cell carcinoma
- Large cell carcinoma

Clinical Issues

- Symptoms/signs
  - Cough, dyspnea, hemoptysis, weight loss
  - Pancoast syndrome, superior vena cava syndrome
  - Mental status change or seizure from brain metastasis
- NSCLC 5-year survival: Stage IIIB = 7%; stage IV = 2%
- SCLC: Rare survival over 6 months

Diagnostic Checklist

- Radiologist plays crucial role in identifying patients with potentially unresectable disease

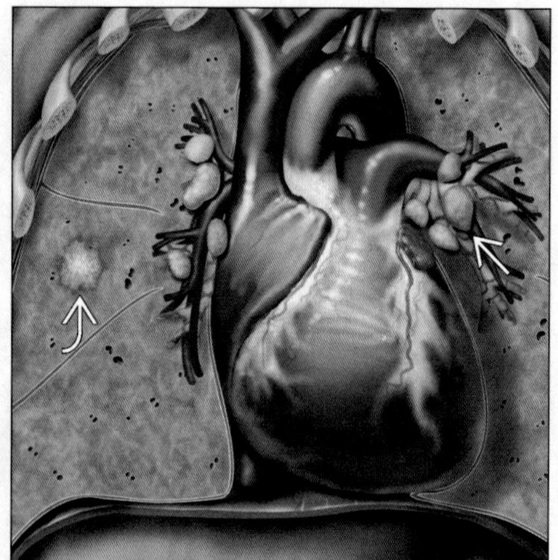

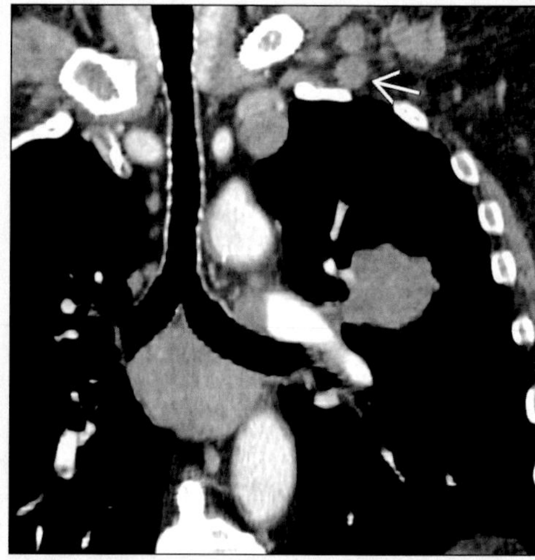

(Left) *Graphic shows a middle lobe unresectable lung cancer ➡ with bilateral metastatic hilar lymphadenopathy. Involvement of contralateral hilar lymph nodes ➡ (or ipsilateral scalene/supraclavicular or contralateral mediastinal lymph nodes) is considered N3 unresectable disease.* ***(Right)*** *Coronal CECT of a 56-year-old male smoker shows a 3 cm left upper lobe lung cancer with subcarinal, mediastinal, and left supraclavicular ➡ lymphadenopathy. N3 disease upstages a patient to unresectable stage IIIB.*

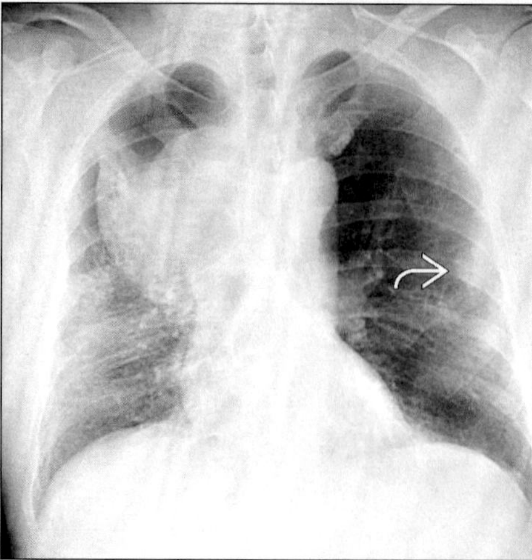

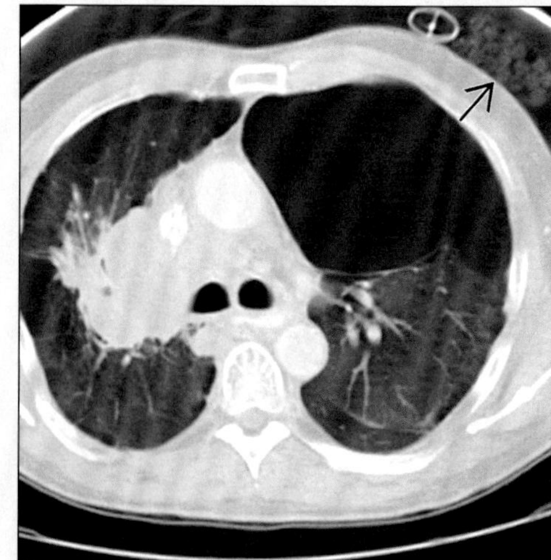

(Left) *PA chest radiograph of a 55-year-old man with dyspnea shows a large right suprahilar mass producing right upper lobe atelectasis and a 1.5 cm left upper lobe nodule ➡.* ***(Right)*** *Axial CECT of the same patient shows a large right upper lobe central mass with mediastinal invasion and lymphadenopathy, severe left upper lobe bullae, and a pack of cigarettes ➡ in the patient's pocket, which confirms an active smoking status. Direct mediastinal invasion and contralateral malignancy make this patient unresectable.*

UNRESECTABLE LUNG CANCER

TERMINOLOGY

Abbreviations

- **Non-small cell lung cancer (NSCLC)**
- **Small cell lung cancer (SCLC)**

Definitions

- Lung cancer for which surgery does not provide survival benefit: Clinical stages IIIB & IV

IMAGING

General Features

- Best diagnostic clue
  - N3 lymph node or distant metastasis precludes operative management

Radiographic Findings

- Radiography
  - Pulmonary nodule (< 3 cm) or mass (≥ 3 cm)
  - Hilar & mediastinal lymphadenopathy (contralateral)
    - Thickening of paratracheal stripe, abnormal AP window or subcarinal region, wide mediastinum
  - Osseous metastasis
  - Pleural effusion

CT Findings

- CECT
  - **T4 lesions**: Invasion of mediastinal structures, vertebral body, tumor nodule(s) in separate ipsilateral lung lobe
  - **N3 lymph nodes**: Scalene, supraclavicular, contralateral mediastinal, contralateral hilar, > 1 cm in short axis
  - **M1 disease**: Tumor nodule(s) in contralateral lobe, malignant pleural effusion, solid pleural metastases
    - Lesion biopsy or fluid analysis required for definitive diagnosis
    - Distant metastases: Adrenal (40%), liver (30%), bone (20%), brain (10%)

Nuclear Medicine Findings

- PET/CT
  - Modality of choice for **detection of extrapulmonary disease & mediastinal staging**
    - 24% of operative patients upstaged to inoperable
    - Not sensitive in detection of brain metastases
  - Used to monitor response to therapy

MR Findings

- Modality of choice in diagnosis of brain metastases
  - Ring-enhancing lesion(s)
- Used for evaluation of myocardial, mediastinal, vascular, brachial plexus, or vertebral body invasion

Ultrasonographic Findings

- Used to guide thoracentesis or lesion biopsy

Imaging Recommendations

- Best imaging tool
  - CECT is imaging modality of choice for initial lesion characterization & initial staging
  - PET/CT & MR optimal modalities for detection of metastases

DIFFERENTIAL DIAGNOSIS

Adenocarcinoma

- Ground-glass, solid or part-solid nodule/mass
- Spiculated, irregular, or lobulated margins

Squamous Cell Carcinoma

- Centrally located mass, often with cavitation

Small Cell Lung Cancer

- Large central mass with hilar/mediastinal invasion & frequent lymphadenopathy

Large Cell Carcinoma

- Peripherally located large mass with central necrosis

PATHOLOGY

General Features

- Genetics
  - Lifelong nonsmokers more likely to have mutation in epidermal growth factor gene (*EGFR*)
    - High response rate to tyrosine kinase inhibitors

Staging, Grading, & Classification

- Applicable for staging NSCLC

Microscopic Features

- Adenocarcinoma
  - Mucinous or nonmucinous with gland formation; acinar &/or lepidic growth pattern
- Squamous cell carcinoma
  - Keratin pearls, intercellular desmosome bridges
- Small cell carcinoma
  - Small round cells, scant cytoplasm, frequent mitoses
- Large cell carcinoma
  - Large cells, pale cytoplasm, prominent nucleoli

CLINICAL ISSUES

Presentation

- Most common signs/symptoms
  - Cough, dyspnea, hemoptysis, weight loss, recurrent pneumonia
- Other signs/symptoms
  - Pain from chest wall invasion
  - Mental status change or seizure from brain metastases
  - Superior vena cava syndrome
  - Hoarseness from invasion of recurrent laryngeal nerve
  - Pancoast syndrome: Upper extremity neuropathic pain, ptosis, myosis, enophthalmos, anhydrosis
  - Paraneoplastic syndromes, most common with SCLC
    - Syndrome of inappropriate antidiuretic hormone production (SIADH), hypertrophic osteoarthropathy (HOA), Cushing syndrome
- Clinical profile
  - Current or former smokers account for > 85% of patients with lung cancer

Demographics

- Gender
  - M:F = 2:1

Natural History & Prognosis

- NSCLC: 5-year survival by clinical stage
  - Stage IIIB: 7%

UNRESECTABLE LUNG CANCER

AJCC Stages/Prognostic Groups

Stage	T	N	M
Occult carcinoma	TX	N0	M0
0	Tis	N0	M0
IA	T1a	N0	M0
	T1b	N0	M0
IB	T2a	N0	M0
IIA	T2b	N0	M0
	T1a	N1	M0
	T1b	N1	M0
	T2a	N1	M0
IIB	T2b	N1	M0
	T3	N0	M0
IIIA	T1a	N2	M0
	T1b	N2	M0
	T2a	N2	M0
	T2b	N2	M0
	T3	N1	M0
	T3	N2	M0
	T4	N0	M0
	T4	N1	M0
IIIB	T1a	N3	M0
	T1b	N3	M0
	T2a	N3	M0
	T2b	N3	M0
	T3	N3	M0
	T4	N2	M0
	T4	N3	M0
IV	Any T	Any N	M1a
	Any T	Any N	M1b

Adapted from 7th edition AJCC Cancer Staging Forms.

 - Stage IV: 2%
- SCLC: Rapidly progressive with rare survival over 6 months

Treatment

- **NSCLC stage IIIB**
  - Concurrent chemoradiation therapy improved survival compared to sequential therapy; current treatment of choice
    - Optimal chemotherapy regimen not yet determined; combinations of cisplatin, etoposide, carboplatin, &/or paclitaxel reported
- **NSCLC stage IV**
  - Solitary brain metastasis may be treated with surgical resection or radiosurgery
  - Palliative treatment with any combination of chemotherapy, radiation, or ablation
- **SCLC**: Chemotherapy & radiation therapy
  - 14-month median survival with limited stage disease, 5-year survival 10%
  - Several drug combinations using cisplatin, carboplatin, etoposide, cyclophosphamide, doxorubicin, paclitaxel, & vincristine have shown efficacy

DIAGNOSTIC CHECKLIST

Reporting Tips

- Radiologist plays crucial role in identifying patients with potentially unresectable disease & confirming unresectability through image-guided biopsy

SELECTED REFERENCES

1. Reungwetwattana T et al: Chemotherapy for non-small-cell lung carcinoma: from a blanket approach to individual therapy. Semin Respir Crit Care Med. 32(1):78-93, 2011
2. Kligerman S et al: A radiologic review of the new TNM classification for lung cancer. AJR Am J Roentgenol. 2010 Mar;194(3):562-73. Review. Erratum in: AJR Am J Roentgenol. 194(5):1404, 2010
3. Paesmans M et al: Primary tumor standardized uptake value measured on fluorodeoxyglucose positron emission tomography is of prognostic value for survival in non-small cell lung cancer: update of a systematic review and meta-analysis by the European Lung Cancer Working Party for the International Association for the Study of Lung Cancer Staging Project. J Thorac Oncol. 5(5):612-9, 2010
4. UyBico SJ et al: Lung cancer staging essentials: the new TNM staging system and potential imaging pitfalls. Radiographics. 30(5):1163-81, 2010
5. Detterbeck FC et al: The new lung cancer staging system. Chest. 136(1):260-71, 2009

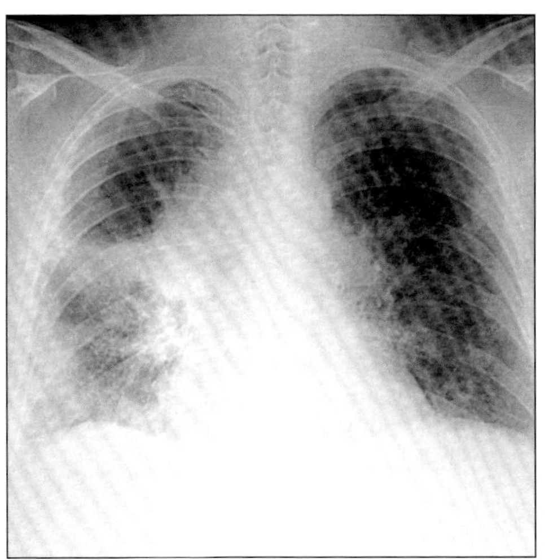

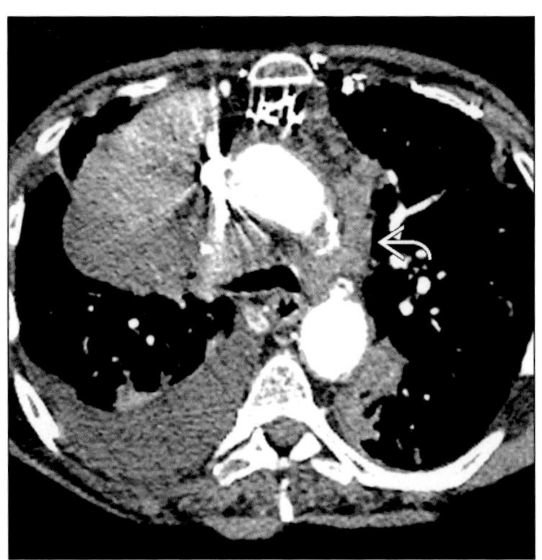

*(**Left**) PA chest radiograph of a 73-year-old former smoker with increasing dyspnea shows a wide mediastinum and bilateral hilar enlargement, consistent with lymphadenopathy. (**Right**) Axial CECT of the same patient shows a 12 cm lobulated right perihilar mass, contralateral mediastinal lymphadenopathy ➔, and a right pleural effusion cytologically proven to be malignant. Contralateral nodules and a brain mass were also detected, consistent with clinical stage IV disease (T4 N3 M1b).*

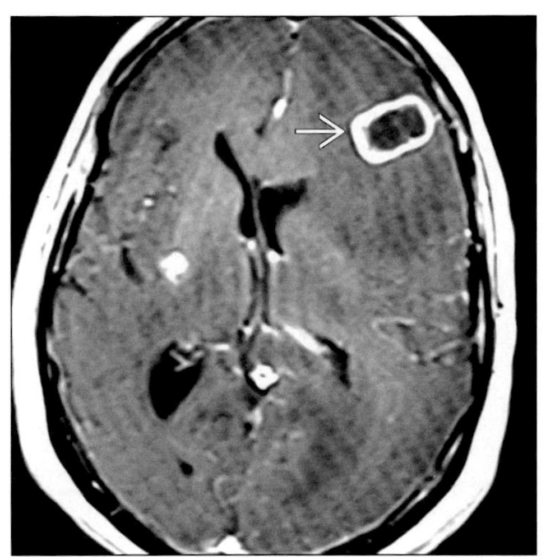

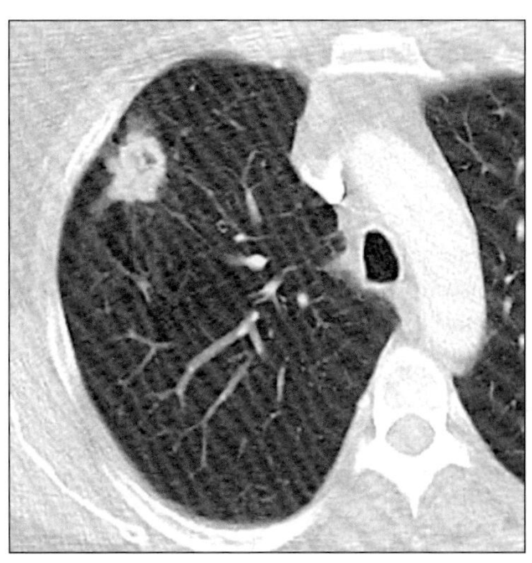

*(**Left**) Axial T1WI C+ brain MR of a 45-year-old woman with headache shows multiple bilateral lesions (one with ring enhancement ➔), surrounding edema, and mass effect. (**Right**) Axial CECT of the same patient shows a 3 cm polylobular right upper lobe mass. An indeterminate adrenal nodule was detected (not shown) and biopsy proven to represent metastatic lung adenocarcinoma stage IV (T1b N0 M1b). The patient was treated with chemoradiation therapy but survived only 2 months.*

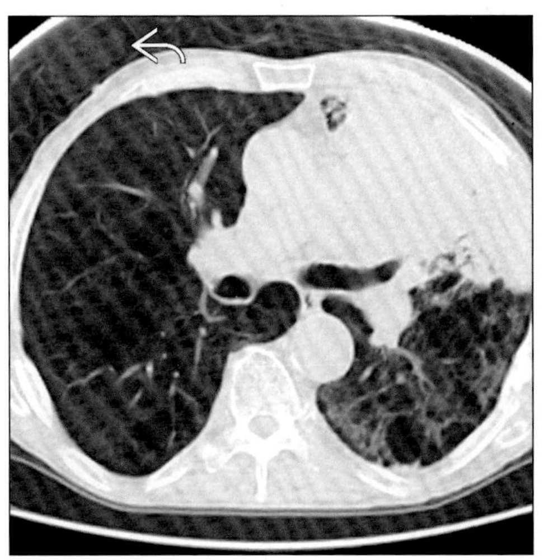

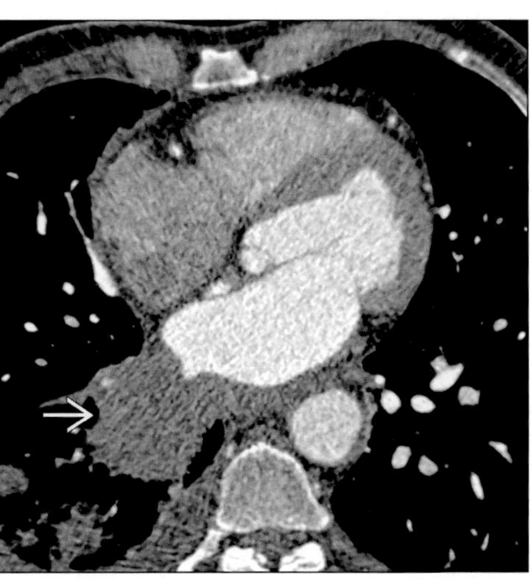

*(**Left**) Axial NECT of a 66-year-old man with cough shows a 12 cm mass obstructing the left upper lobe bronchus with mediastinal and pleural invasion. Cigarettes in the patient's pocket ➔ confirm current smoking status. CT-guided biopsy showed a small cell carcinoma. (**Right**) Axial cardiac CT of a 44-year-old man with squamous cell cancer performed to exclude cardiac invasion shows a large right lower lobe mass ➔ with myocardial invasion, consistent with unresectable disease.*

PULMONARY HAMARTOMA

Key Facts

Terminology

- Benign pulmonary neoplasm containing variety of tissues
- Varying amounts of cartilage, fat, connective tissue, smooth muscle, epithelial-lined clefts

Imaging

- Radiography
  - Solitary pulmonary nodule or mass
  - Calcification in up to 15%
- CT
  - Solitary nodule or mass, smooth or lobular borders
  - Calcification more common in larger hamartomas
  - Classic "popcorn" calcification in only 10-15%
  - Fat attenuation in up to 60%
  - Intrinsic fat & calcium virtually diagnostic
- FDG PET
  - Up to 20% show FDG uptake

Top Differential Diagnoses

- Lung cancer
- Carcinoid
- Solitary metastasis
- Lipoid pneumonia

Pathology

- Most common benign lung tumor (75%)
- 6% of all solitary pulmonary nodules

Clinical Issues

- Typically detected incidentally on radiography or CT of asymptomatic patients

Diagnostic Checklist

- Always evaluate thin-section CT images of newly detected lung nodules or masses since visualization of calcium & fat is considered diagnostic of hamartoma

(Left) Graphic demonstrates the characteristic morphologic features of pulmonary hamartoma, which typically manifests as a well-defined polylobular pulmonary nodule composed of heterogeneous elements, often including fat and cartilage. (Right) Axial NECT (bone window) of a patient with a pulmonary hamartoma shows a polylobular right upper lobe nodule with "popcorn" calcification, a finding considered pathognomonic for pulmonary hamartoma. Only 10-15% of hamartomas exhibit "popcorn" calcification.

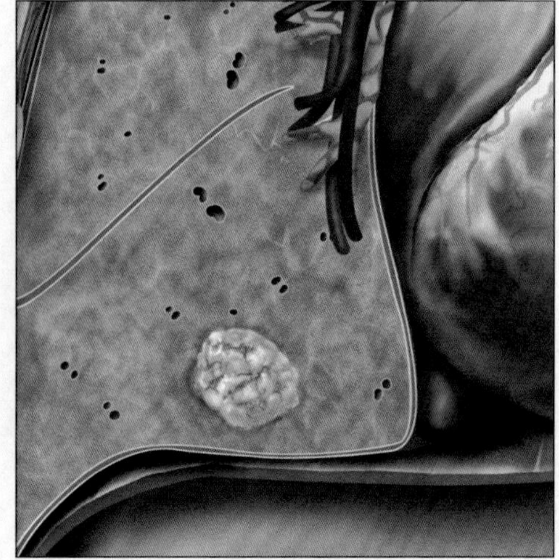

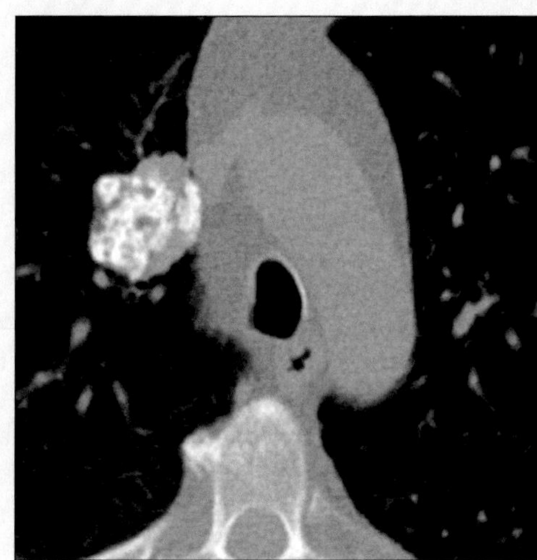

(Left) Axial NECT of a 65-year-old woman with a right lower lobe paravertebral pulmonary hamartoma shows a well-circumscribed lung nodule ➔ containing both fat and calcium. These imaging features are diagnostic for pulmonary hamartoma. (Right) Axial NECT shows an incidentally discovered right lower lobe pulmonary hamartoma manifesting as a well-defined lung nodule ➔ with predominant soft tissue attenuation and intrinsic foci of fat attenuation.

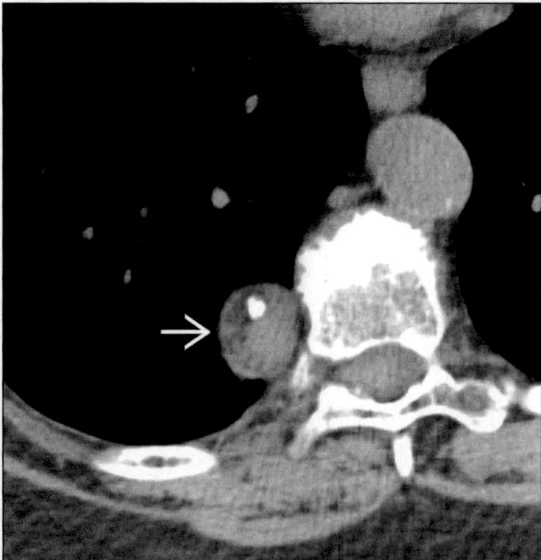

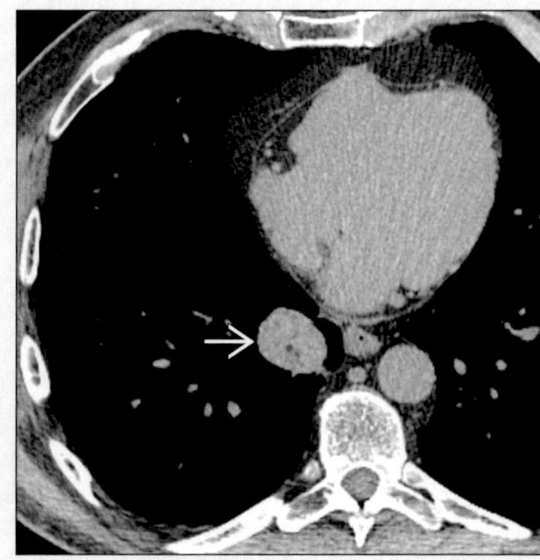

PULMONARY HAMARTOMA

TERMINOLOGY

Synonyms

- Chondromatous hamartoma
- Mesenchymoma

Definitions

- Derived from "hamartia," Greek work for "error"
- Benign pulmonary neoplasm containing variety of tissues
  - Varying amounts of cartilage, fat, connective tissue, smooth muscle, epithelial-lined clefts

IMAGING

General Features

- Best diagnostic clue
  - Solitary pulmonary nodule or mass with **intrinsic calcium & fat**
- Location
  - Majority located in lung periphery
  - Endobronchial location ~ 20%
    - Central lesions may produce postobstructive effects
  - No lobar predilection
- Size
  - Typically < 4 cm, may be > 10 cm
- Morphology
  - Well-circumscribed, smooth or lobular borders

Radiographic Findings

- Radiography
  - **Solitary pulmonary nodule or mass with smooth or lobular borders**
  - Calcification in up to 15%
    - Characteristic "**popcorn**" calcification
  - Central lesions
    - Postobstructive effects: Atelectasis, consolidation

CT Findings

- NECT
  - Solitary pulmonary nodule or mass with smooth or lobular margins
    - Rarely multiple
  - 10x more sensitive than radiography in detecting calcifications
    - Hounsfield units (HU) > 200 considered calcium
  - Calcification more common as hamartoma increases in size
    - Up to 75% in nodules > 5 cm vs. only 10% in nodules < 2 cm
    - **Classic "popcorn" cartilaginous calcification seen in only 10-15%**
  - **Fat attenuation in up to 60%**
    - **-40 to -120 HU**
    - Volume averaging often problematic when measuring regions of interest (ROI) on 5 mm CT sections
    - Better visualized with thin-section (0.6-1.2 cm) images
  - Visualization of **intrinsic fat & calcium considered diagnostic**
- CECT
  - Heterogeneous enhancement is typical
  - Enhancing internal septations correlate with epithelial-lined clefts

MR Findings

- T1WI
  - Intermediate-signal intensity
- T2WI
  - High signal intensity
- T1WI C+
  - Enhancement of capsule & peripheral epithelial-lined clefts
- Not necessary as part of evaluation
- May be incidentally found on spine MR

Nuclear Medicine Findings

- PET/CT
  - Up to 20% show FDG uptake
  - Larger masses more likely to be FDG avid
  - Not necessary with typical CT features

Imaging Recommendations

- Best imaging tool
  - CT is imaging modality of choice, contrast typically not helpful
- Protocol advice
  - NECT with thin sections through nodule for optimal visualization of intratumoral fat

DIFFERENTIAL DIAGNOSIS

Lung Cancer

- Solitary pulmonary nodule, may exhibit spiculated margins
- Does not contain fat & calcium
- 2% of cancers < 3 cm in size contain calcification
- Highly FDG avid on PET/CT
- Coexisting emphysema and history of cigarette smoking

Carcinoid

- Hypervascular mass with well-defined lobular margins
- Frequent endobronchial component, which may result in postobstructive changes
- 30% contain calcifications
- Low-grade malignancy with metastatic potential
  - Surgical resection is treatment of choice

Solitary Metastasis

- Metastases typically manifest with multiple nodules/ masses in patient with known malignancy
- Calcified nodules of metastatic osteosarcoma may mimic multifocal hamartomas
  - Affected patients may present with pneumothorax
- Solitary pulmonary metastases: Colon, breast, renal, & testicular primary malignancies, osteosarcoma, melanoma

Lipoid Pneumonia

- Fat-containing consolidation or spiculated mass in patient who uses mineral oil (usually for constipation)
- Calcifications are not typical
- Can be FDG avid on PET/CT

Liposarcoma

- Exceedingly rare aggressive neoplasm containing fat & soft tissue
- Typically in chest wall or mediastinum

PULMONARY HAMARTOMA

PATHOLOGY

General Features

- Etiology
  - Unknown
- Genetics
  - Recombination of chromosomal bands 6p21 & 14q24 supports pulmonary hamartoma being **benign mesenchymal neoplasm** rather than embryologic rest
- Associated abnormalities
  - **Carney triad**: Multiple pulmonary chondromas, gastric epithelioid leiomyosarcoma, & functional extraadrenal paraganglioma
    - Chondromas considered histologically distinct from hamartomas
  - Association with lung cancer suggested in 1980s, but contemporary studies fail to show association

Staging, Grading, & Classification

- Benign neoplasm without staging or grading system

Gross Pathologic & Surgical Features

- Well circumscribed, firm mass, usually easily resected from surrounding pulmonary parenchyma
- May be densely calcified

Microscopic Features

- Encapsulated mass composed of myxomatous connective tissue containing cartilage with varying amounts of fat, smooth muscle, bone, & lymphovascular structures
- Double-layered epithelial cell-lined clefts typically seen in lesion periphery

CLINICAL ISSUES

Presentation

- Most common signs/symptoms
  - Usually incidentally detected on radiography or CT of asymptomatic patients
  - Often identified on screening CT scans
- Other signs/symptoms
  - Rarely cough, hemoptysis, or recurrent pneumonia

Demographics

- Age
  - Adults in 6th decade of life
  - Rarely seen in pediatric patients
- Gender
  - Men have 2-3x higher incidence than women
- Epidemiology
  - Most common benign lung tumor (75%)
  - Represents 6% of all solitary pulmonary nodules
  - Affects 0.025-0.32% of population

Natural History & Prognosis

- Malignant transformation exceedingly rare & reportable
- Slow growth is typical

Diagnosis

- CT imaging may be diagnostic
- CT-guided biopsy for diagnosis if CT findings are not diagnostic

Treatment

- Watchful waiting in most patients
- Surgical resection if symptomatic or rapidly enlarging
  - Curative with only rare case reports describing local recurrence
- Endobronchial hamartoma may be resected bronchoscopically

DIAGNOSTIC CHECKLIST

Consider

- Other etiologies of solitary pulmonary nodules since only 6% will be hamartomas

Image Interpretation Pearls

- Always evaluate thin-section CT images of newly detected lung nodules or masses since visualization of calcium & fat is virtually diagnostic of pulmonary hamartoma

Reporting Tips

- Hamartomas often grow slowly; slight interval enlargement in asymptomatic patient does not necessarily mandate excision

SELECTED REFERENCES

1. Khan AN et al: The calcified lung nodule: What does it mean? Ann Thorac Med. 5(2):67-79, 2010
2. Kim SA et al: Bronchoscopic features and bronchoscopic intervention for endobronchial hamartoma. Respirology. 15(1):150-4, 2010
3. Park CM et al: Images in clinical medicine. "Popcorn" calcifications in a pulmonary chondroid hamartoma. N Engl J Med. 360(12):e17, 2009
4. De Cicco C et al: Imaging of lung hamartomas by multidetector computed tomography and positron emission tomography. Ann Thorac Surg. 86(6):1769-72, 2008
5. Guo W et al: Surgical treatment and outcome of pulmonary hamartoma: a retrospective study of 20-year experience. J Exp Clin Cancer Res. 27:8, 2008
6. Park KY et al: Diagnostic efficacy and characteristic feature of MRI in pulmonary hamartoma: comparison with CT, specimen MRI, and pathology. J Comput Assist Tomogr. 32(6):919-25, 2008
7. Wood B et al: Diagnosis of pulmonary hamartoma by fine needle biopsy. Acta Cytol. 52(4):412-7, 2008
8. Ludwig C et al: Recurrent hamartoma at the trocar incision site after video-assisted thoracic surgical resection. J Thorac Cardiovasc Surg. 130(2):609-10, 2005
9. Gaerte SC et al: Fat-containing lesions of the chest. Radiographics. 22 Spec No:S61-78, 2002
10. Siegelman SS et al: Pulmonary hamartoma: CT findings. Radiology. 160(2):313-7, 1986

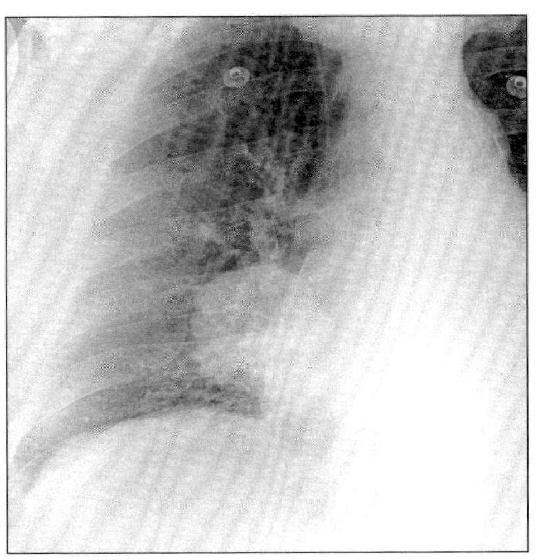

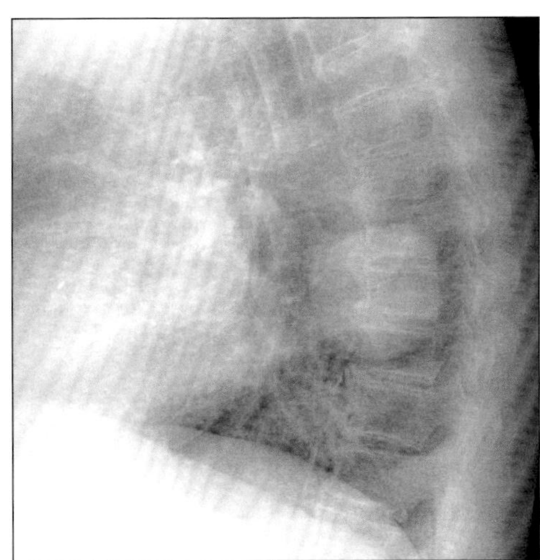

(Left) *PA chest radiograph of a 44-year-old man with an incidentally discovered right lower lobe pulmonary hamartoma shows a large well-defined pulmonary mass.* ***(Right)*** *Lateral chest radiograph of the same patient shows a 6 cm well-circumscribed right lower lobe mass with well-defined lobular margins. There are no radiographically detectable calcifications to suggest the correct diagnosis.*

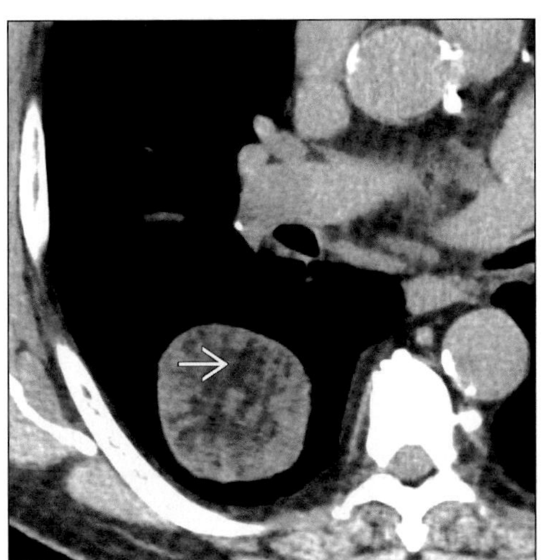

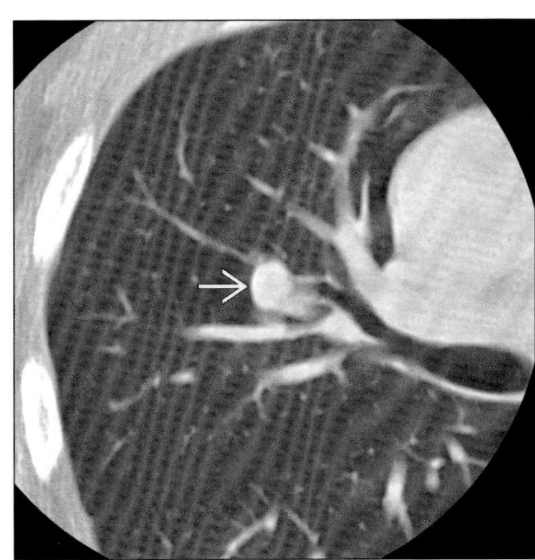

(Left) *Axial NECT of the same patient shows a spherical right lower lobe mass of well-defined borders and heterogeneous attenuation. Region of interest measurements of the low-attenuation areas ➔ were -85 HU, consistent with fat and diagnostic of pulmonary hamartoma.* ***(Right)*** *Axial NECT of a 56-year-old man with recurrent pneumonia shows a lung nodule ➔ that partially occludes a branch of the anterior segment right upper lobe bronchus. Surgical pathology confirmed the diagnosis of hamartoma.*

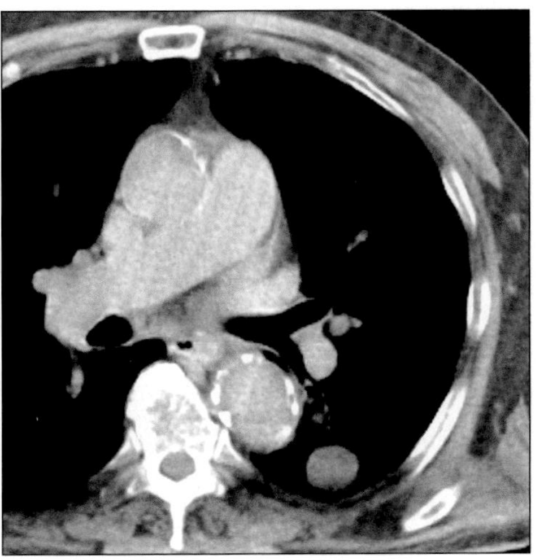

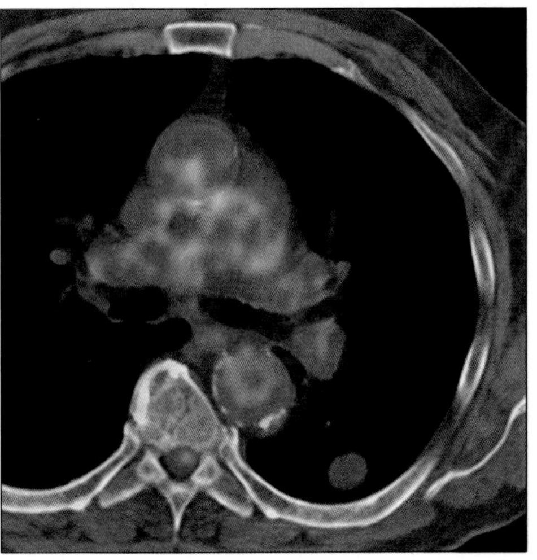

(Left) *Axial NECT of an asymptomatic man shows a well-defined left lower lobe indeterminate lung nodule. The lesion had grown from 1.9 x 1.7 cm to 2.6 x 2.3 cm when compared to a chest CT obtained 3 years earlier.* ***(Right)*** *Axial fused PET/CT of the same patient shows low-level metabolic activity in the nodule with a maximum SUV of 1.6. Sublobar resection following an inconclusive needle biopsy revealed a pulmonary hamartoma. Hamartomas are benign neoplasms that may exhibit slow growth.*

BRONCHIAL CARCINOID

Key Facts

Terminology

- Low-grade malignant neuroendocrine neoplasm with metastatic potential

Imaging

- Radiography
  - Central hilar or perihilar nodule or mass
  - Solitary peripheral lung nodule
  - Postobstructive atelectasis, pneumonia
- CT
  - Avidly enhancing central nodule or mass
  - Calcification/ossification in 30%
  - Endobronchial, partially endobronchial, abutting bronchus, peripheral
  - Postobstructive effects: Atelectasis, consolidation bronchiectasis
- Nuclear medicine
  - FDG PET: Frequent false-negative results

Top Differential Diagnoses

- Adenoid cystic carcinoma
- Hamartoma
- Lung cancer

Pathology

- Smooth, red, polypoid endobronchial nodule/mass
- Typical & atypical subtypes

Clinical Issues

- Symptoms/signs: Cough, hemoptysis, wheezing, recurrent pneumonia
- Treatment: Surgical resection

Diagnostic Checklist

- Consider carcinoid tumor in symptomatic young/ middle-aged patients with well-defined central nodule or mass with endoluminal component

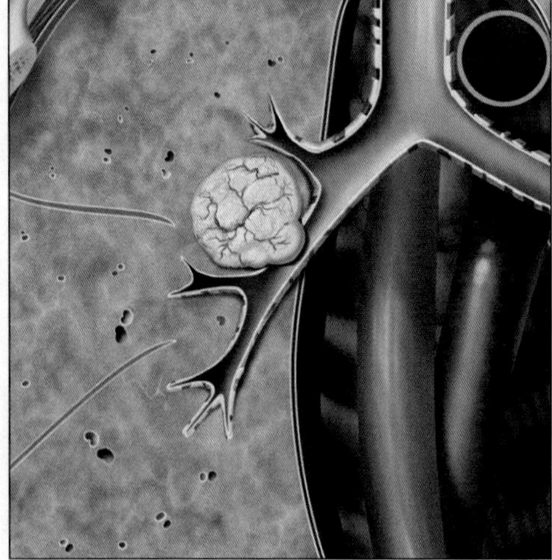

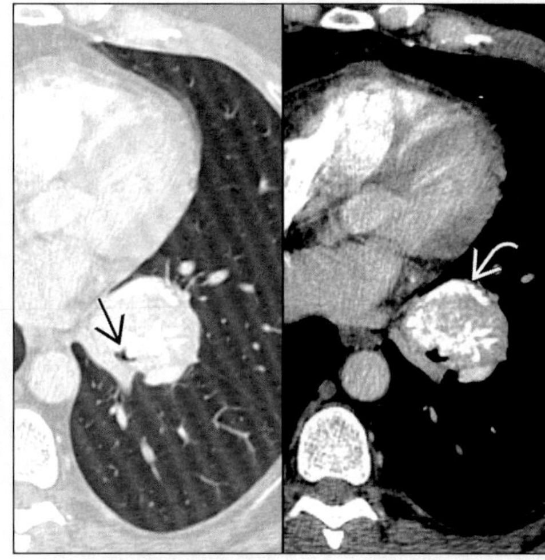

(Left) *Graphic shows the typical morphologic features of bronchial carcinoid, which characteristically manifests as a central polylobular nodule with an endoluminal component. Blood vessels in the tumor stroma may result in intense contrast enhancement.* ***(Right)*** *Composite image with CECT in lung (left) and soft tissue (right) window of a 48-year-old man who presented with wheezing shows a central bronchial carcinoid with a large endoluminal component ➔ and multifocal intrinsic calcifications ➔.*

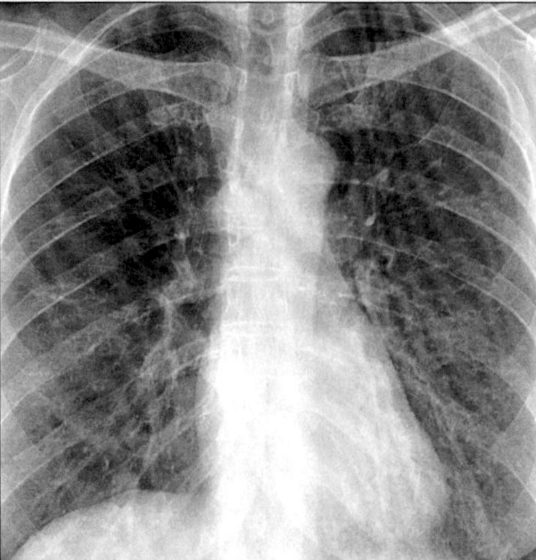

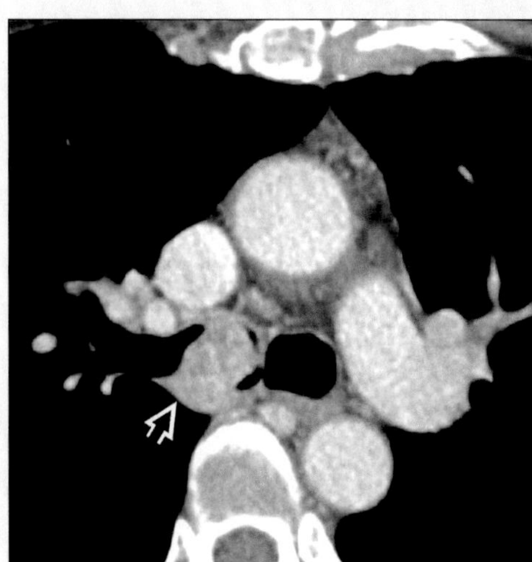

(Left) *PA chest radiograph of a patient with "adult-onset asthma" and hemoptysis shows a central nodule with an endoluminal component in the distal trachea and proximal right mainstem bronchus.* ***(Right)*** *Axial CECT of the same patient confirms an enhancing endobronchial nodule partially occluding the proximal right mainstem bronchus ➔. Bronchoscopic biopsy revealed typical bronchial carcinoid, which was successfully treated with sleeve resection and right mainstem bronchus reconstruction.*

BRONCHIAL CARCINOID

TERMINOLOGY

Synonyms

- "Bronchial adenoma" formerly used to describe tumors arising in central airways (trachea & main bronchi)
  - Encompassed several central airway malignant neoplasms
    - Bronchial carcinoid
    - Adenoid cystic carcinoma
    - Mucoepidermoid carcinoma
    - Other central airway neoplasms
  - All carcinoid tumors are malignant; therefore term "adenoma" should not be used

Definitions

- Low-grade malignant neuroendocrine neoplasm with metastatic potential
  - Arises from neuroendocrine cells normally scattered throughout tracheobronchial epithelium
  - Lung is 2nd most common location
    - Gastrointestinal tract carcinoids account for approximately 90% of all carcinoids

IMAGING

General Features

- Best diagnostic clue
  - Well-defined hilar/perihilar mass ± associated postobstructive atelectasis, pneumonia, or mucus plugging
- Location
  - **Typical carcinoid**
    - **85% in main, lobar, or segmental bronchi**
    - 15-20% peripheral in location (subsegmental bronchi & beyond)
    - Tracheal location very rare
  - **Atypical carcinoid**
    - Most develop in lung periphery
    - Enlarged hilar/mediastinal lymph nodes secondary to metastases more commonly seen
  - Metastases (15% of bronchial carcinoids)
    - Liver, bone (sclerotic), adrenal glands, brain
- Size
  - Usually 1-5 cm
  - Atypical carcinoids tend to be larger
- Morphology
  - Well-marginated central nodule or mass
  - Lobular borders
  - Bronchial relationship: Partially or completely endoluminal or close bronchial relationship

Radiographic Findings

- Central hilar or perihilar well-defined mass
- 4% exhibit calcification/ossification on radiography
- Effects of central airway obstruction
  - Atelectasis
  - Air-trapping
  - Mucoid impaction, bronchiectasis
    - "Finger in glove" sign
      - V- or Y-shaped opacities radiating from hilum
  - Postobstructive pneumonia, may be recurrent
- Peripheral indeterminate solitary lung nodule

CT Findings

- **Typical bronchial carcinoid**
  - **Lung nodule or mass**
    - **Endobronchial**
      - **"Iceberg" lesion**: Small endoluminal tumor with dominant extraluminal component
      - May be entirely endoluminal
      - May abut bronchus
    - 30% of central carcinoids exhibit variable amounts of calcification/ossification
    - Marked, homogeneous contrast enhancement
    - 20% are solitary peripheral lung nodules
      - Well-defined smooth or lobulated borders
      - Slow growing
  - **Hilar &/or mediastinal lymphadenopathy**
    - Metastases
    - Reactive lymph nodes from recurrent pneumonia
  - **Bronchial obstruction**
    - Air-trapping due to ball-valve obstruction
    - Atelectasis
    - **Postobstructive pneumonia**
      - Bronchiectasis
      - Lung abscess
    - Mucoid impaction
      - Fluid-filled (< 20 HU) branching structures
      - Peripheral hyperlucency due to air-trapping
- **Atypical carcinoid**
  - **Lung nodule or mass**
    - **Lobular or irregular contours**
    - Less uniform enhancement
    - More likely to be peripheral
  - Lymph node metastases more common
- Multiple carcinoid tumors & tumorlets (DIPNECH)
  - Multiple, bilateral pulmonary nodules
  - Mosaic attenuation
    - Air-trapping on expiratory images

MR Findings

- Hyperintense on T2WI

Nuclear Medicine Findings

- PET
  - FDG PET often falsely negative due to relative low metabolism of carcinoid tumors
- Octreotide scan (somatostatin analogue) successfully used to diagnose & locate occult carcinoid tumors
  - Utilizes tumor somatostatin-binding sites

Imaging Recommendations

- Best imaging tool
  - Contrast-enhanced CT with thin collimation
- Protocol advice
  - IV contrast: Carcinoid tumors are vascular & typically (but not universally) exhibit avid enhancement

DIFFERENTIAL DIAGNOSIS

Adenoid Cystic Carcinoma

- Salivary gland malignancy, often arises in trachea or main bronchi
  - 10% in lung periphery
- Locally aggressive, requires careful evaluation for extraluminal or mediastinal growth

Hamartoma

- Lung nodule with macroscopic fat on CT

BRONCHIAL CARCINOID

- Calcification common; less enhancement than carcinoid tumors
- Endobronchial location in 4%

Mucoepidermoid Carcinoma

- Rare salivary gland tumor arising in lobar or segmental bronchi
- Ovoid, polypoid, or lobular lesion, well-defined margins, calcification in 50%

Lung Cancer

- Margins usually ill-defined, lobular, or spiculated
- Affected patients tend to be older than those with carcinoid
- History of cigarette smoking

Broncholithiasis

- Small endobronchial calcified nodule

Pulmonary Metastases

- Multiple carcinoid tumors & tumorlets mimic lung metastases

PATHOLOGY

General Features

- Etiology
  - No association with cigarette smoking or inhalation of carcinogens
- Associated abnormalities
  - Small pulmonary tumorlets occasionally associated with carcinoid tumors
    - Tumorlets represent benign neuroendocrine hyperplastic growths

Gross Pathologic & Surgical Features

- Smooth, red, polypoid endobronchial nodule/mass
- Most arise within central bronchi

Microscopic Features

- **Neuroendocrine neoplasm** in spectrum of more aggressive large cell neuroendocrine & small cell carcinomas
- **Typical carcinoid** (80-90%)
  - Uniform cells in sheets, trabeculae or gland-like structures, separated by thin fibrovascular stroma
  - Moderate cytoplasm with numerous neurosecretory granules
  - Rare mitotic figures
  - Dystrophic calcification, ossification
- **Atypical carcinoid** (10-20%)
  - Tumor necrosis
  - Loss of typical architecture with increased cellularity
  - 2-10 mitoses per 10 high-power fields
  - Increased nuclear:cytoplasmic ratio or nuclear pleomorphism

CLINICAL ISSUES

Presentation

- Most common signs/symptoms
  - Cough
  - Hemoptysis in 50% (vascular neoplasm)
  - Recurrent pneumonia
  - Adult onset "asthma," wheezing
- Other signs/symptoms
  - Cushing syndrome: Ectopic production of ACTH
    - 2% of bronchial carcinoids
  - Carcinoid syndrome
    - Rare with thoracic carcinoid tumors
    - Almost all affected patients have hepatic metastases

Demographics

- Age
  - Typical carcinoid: 30-60 years of age
    - Atypical carcinoid: Decade older
  - Most frequent primary pulmonary neoplasm in childhood
- Gender
  - Bronchial carcinoid: Roughly equal distribution
  - Multiple carcinoid tumors & tumorlets: Predominantly affect women
- Epidemiology
  - Bronchial carcinoid: 1-2% of all lung neoplasms

Natural History & Prognosis

- Typical carcinoid: 5% have lymph node metastases at presentation
  - 5-year survival
    - 90-95% without lymph node involvement
    - 76-88% with lymph node metastases
- Atypical carcinoid: 50-60% have lymph node metastases at presentation
  - 5-year survival
    - 40-70%, depending on stage at presentation
- Multiple carcinoid tumors & tumorlets
  - Limited data: Generally good prognosis, stable disease even without treatment

Treatment

- Complete surgical excision most effective

DIAGNOSTIC CHECKLIST

Consider

- Carcinoid tumor in symptomatic young/middle-aged patients with well-defined central nodule or mass with endoluminal component

SELECTED REFERENCES

1. Aubry MC et al: Significance of multiple carcinoid tumors and tumorlets in surgical lung specimens: analysis of 28 patients. Chest. 131(6):1635-43, 2007
2. Davies SJ et al: Diffuse idiopathic pulmonary neuroendocrine cell hyperplasia: an under-recognised spectrum of disease. Thorax. 62(3):248-52, 2007
3. Divisi D et al: Carcinoid tumors of the lung and multimodal therapy. Thorac Cardiovasc Surg. 53(3):168-72, 2005
4. Jeung MY et al: Bronchial carcinoid tumors of the thorax: spectrum of radiologic findings. Radiographics. 22(2):351-65, 2002
5. Rosado de Christenson ML et al: Thoracic carcinoids: radiologic-pathologic correlation. Radiographics. 19(3):707-36, 1999

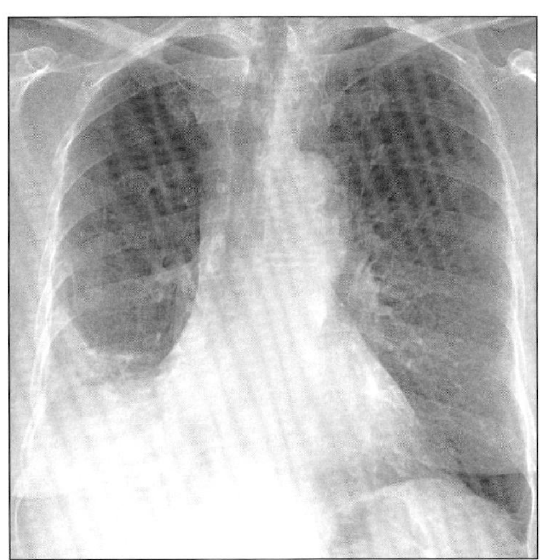

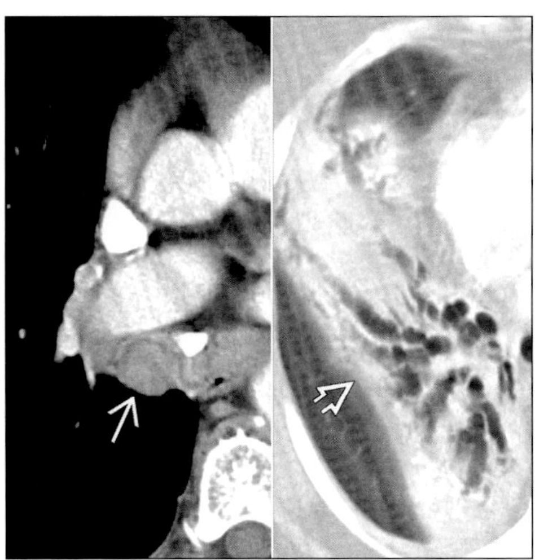

(Left) *PA chest radiograph shows right middle and lower lobe airspace disease and volume loss in this patient with recurrent pneumonia.* ***(Right)*** *Composite image with axial CECT in soft tissue (left) and lung (right) window shows a mildly enhancing endoluminal lesion occluding the bronchus intermedius and an incidental calcified subcarinal granulomatous lymph node. The lesion produces middle and right lower lobe atelectasis with intrinsic bronchiectasis distal to the endoluminal obstruction.*

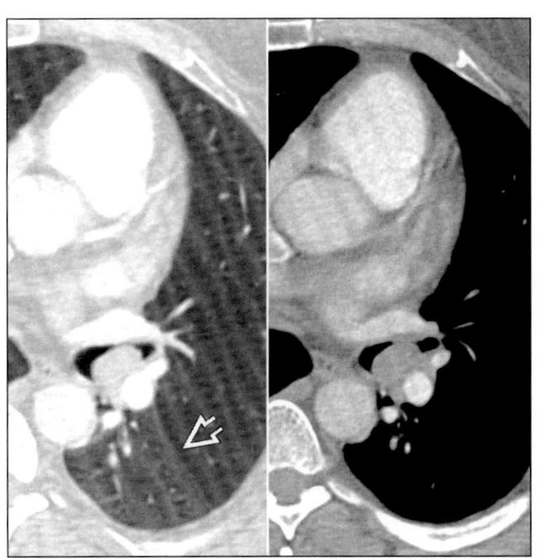

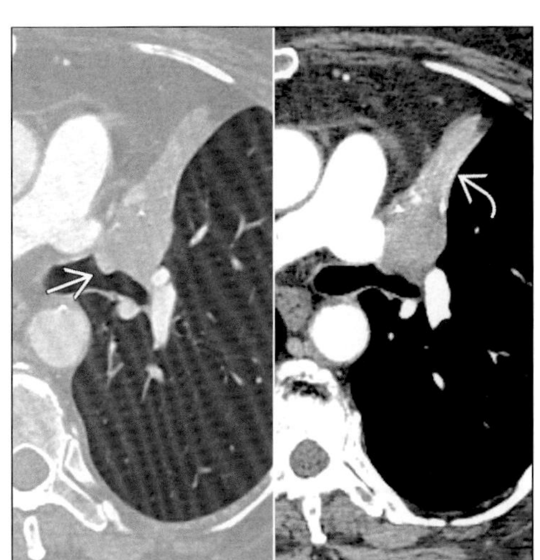

(Left) *Composite image with axial CECT in lung (left) and soft tissue (right) window shows a completely endoluminal carcinoid that partially obstructs the left lower lobe bronchial lumen with resultant left lower lobe volume loss manifesting with posterior displacement of the left major fissure.* ***(Right)*** *Composite image with axial CECT in lung (left) and soft tissue (right) window shows a central carcinoid with an endoluminal component and marked left upper lobe atelectasis.*

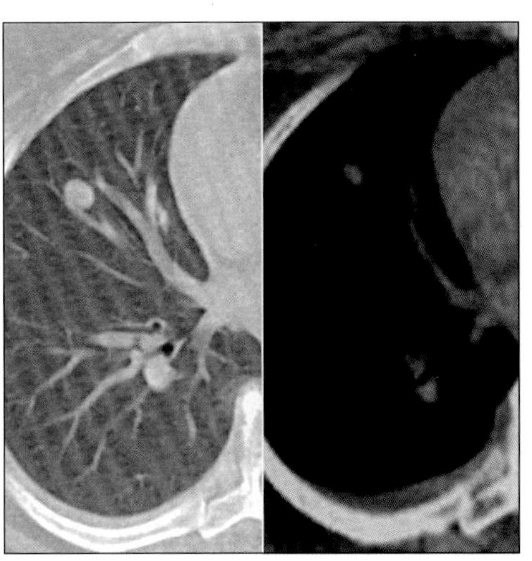

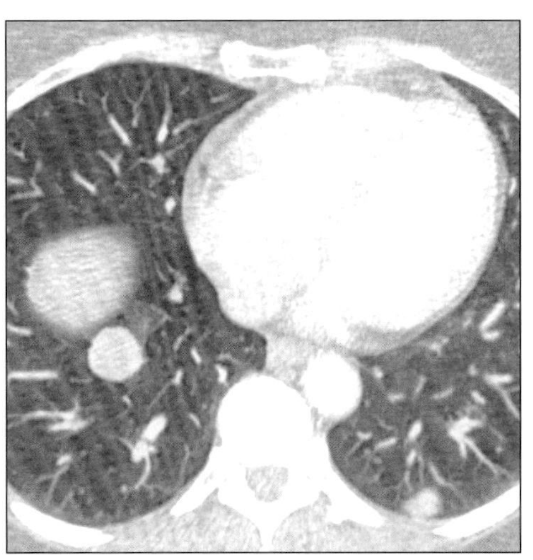

(Left) *Composite image with axial NECT (left) and fused FDG PET/CT of an asymptomatic patient with an incidentally discovered peripheral carcinoid. The lesion exhibited only minimal FDG uptake. PET/CT of carcinoid tumors is often false-negative.* ***(Right)*** *Axial CECT MIP image of an asymptomatic patient shows multiple well-defined nodules of various sizes. Sublobar resection confirmed multiple carcinoid tumors and tumorlets, an unusual entity that mimics pulmonary metastases.*

NEUROENDOCRINE CARCINOMA

Key Facts

Terminology

- Typical carcinoid (TC), atypical carcinoid (AC)
- Large cell neuroendocrine carcinoma (LCNEC)
- Small cell lung cancer (SCLC)
- Malignant tumors of neuroendocrine origin

Imaging

- Radiography
  - Carcinoid: Central nodule ± endoluminal lesion
  - SCLC: Large hilar/mediastinal mass
- CT
  - TC & AC: Enhancing nodule ± endobronchial component
  - LCNEC: Discrete or irregular necrotic mass
  - SCLC: Invasive hilar or mediastinal mass (95%)
- FDG PET
  - TC: Little or no activity
  - LCNEC & SCLC: Staging & restaging

Top Differential Diagnoses

- DDx of TC & AC
  - Other lung neoplasm, metastasis
  - Bronchial atresia with mucous plugging
- DDx of SCLC
  - Non-small cell lung cancer
  - Lymphoma, thymic carcinoma, metastases

Clinical Issues

- Symptoms/signs
  - Cough, wheezing, hemoptysis, pneumonia
  - SCLC: SVC syndrome, vocal cord paralysis, paraneoplastic syndrome
- Age
  - TC & AC: Mean is 45 years
  - LCNEC & SCLC: Mean is > 60 years
- 10-year survival: TC 85%; AC 35%
- LCNEC & SCLC: Poor prognosis

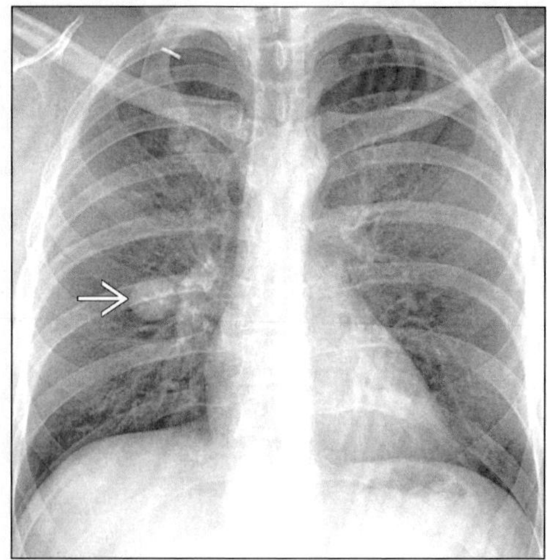

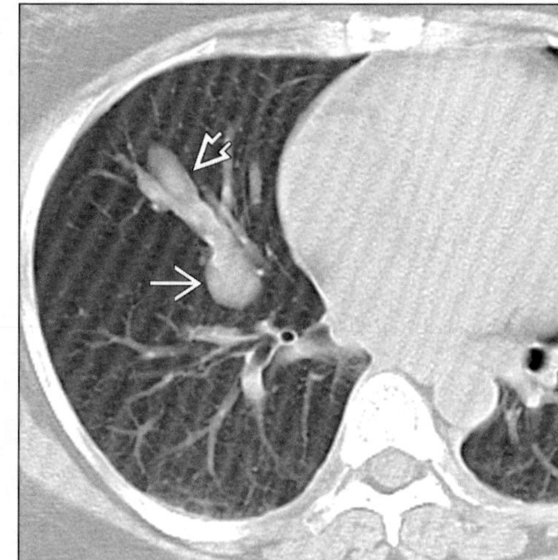

(Left) *PA chest radiograph of a patient with typical carcinoid shows a well-marginated middle lobe solitary pulmonary nodule ➡. Typical and atypical carcinoid are low- to intermediate-grade malignancies and are incidentally detected in 25% of cases.* ***(Right)*** *Axial NECT of the same patient shows a discrete middle lobe lung nodule ➡ with associated mucoid impaction ⇨ in the lateral segmental middle lobe bronchi. Bronchial obstruction from carcinoid may also cause distal atelectasis, consolidation, or air-trapping.*

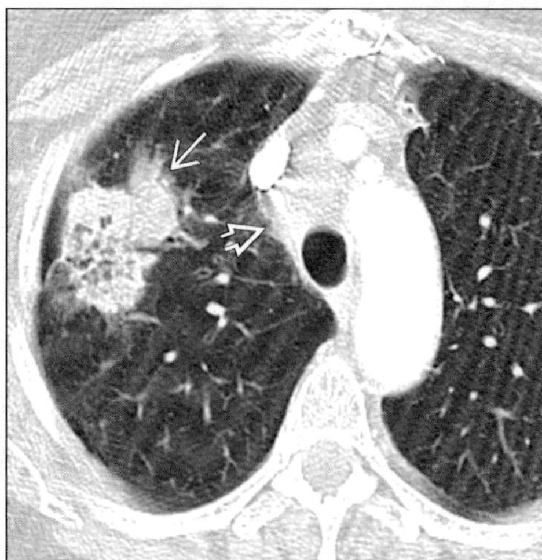

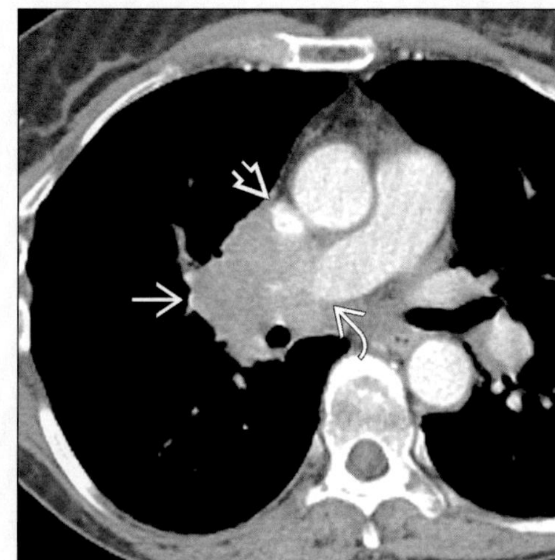

(Left) *Axial CECT of a patient with large cell neuroendocrine carcinoma (LCNEC) shows an irregular bubbly peripheral right upper lobe mass ➡ and ipsilateral mediastinal lymph node metastases ⇨. LCNEC is typically a large and aggressive neoplasm that may be metastatic at presentation.* ***(Right)*** *Axial CECT shows SCLC manifesting as an aggressive right hilar mass ➡ that invades the SVC ⇨ and the right pulmonary artery ↪ and encases the bronchus intermedius. SCLC often manifests with intrathoracic metastatic lymphadenopathy.*

NEUROENDOCRINE CARCINOMA

TERMINOLOGY

Abbreviations

- **Typical carcinoid** (TC)
- **Atypical carcinoid** (AC)
- **Large cell neuroendocrine carcinoma** (LCNEC)
- **Small cell lung cancer** (SCLC)

Definitions

- Malignant neoplasms of **neuroendocrine origin**
  - Derived from endodermal cells, not neural crest cells
    - Arise from Kulchitsky cells of bronchial mucosa
- Spectrum: Low grade (TC) to aggressive (SCLC)

IMAGING

General Features

- Best diagnostic clue
  - TC: Enhancing nodule ± endobronchial component
  - SCLC: Invasive necrotic hilar or mediastinal mass
- Size
  - TC & AC: 5-30 mm
  - LCNEC & SCLC: Typically large
- Morphology
  - TC & AC: Spherical or oblong nodule
  - LCNEC: Discrete or irregular mass
  - SCLC: Invasive central necrotic mass

Radiographic Findings

- Carcinoid: Central lung nodule ± endoluminal lesion
- SCLC: Large hilar/mediastinal mass

CT Findings

- CECT
  - TC & AC: Discrete pulmonary nodule
    - Intense enhancement
    - Endobronchial component ± obstruction
      - Distal mucous plugging, atelectasis, air-trapping
    - 30% exhibit calcification or ossification
  - LCNEC: Discrete or irregular necrotic mass ± metastases
  - SCLC: Large necrotic hilar or perihilar mass (95%)
    - Mediastinal lymphadenopathy
    - Distant metastases at presentation
    - Primary tumor rarely evident
    - Cavitation extremely rare

Nuclear Medicine Findings

- FDG PET
  - TC: Little or no activity
  - LCNEC & SCLC: Staging & restaging
- Radio-labeled octreotide (somatostatin analog)
  - Detection of occult neuroendocrine neoplasm

Imaging Recommendations

- Best imaging tool
  - CT is optimal modality for initial assessment
- Protocol advice
  - IV contrast
    - Useful for distinguishing central tumor from adjacent mucous plug, atelectasis
    - Assessment of mediastinal invasion & lymph node metastases

DIFFERENTIAL DIAGNOSIS

DDx of Carcinoid

- Other primary lung neoplasm or metastasis
- Bronchial atresia with mucous plugging

DDx of Small Cell Lung Cancer

- Non-small cell lung cancer
- Lymphoma, thymic carcinoma
- Metastases

PATHOLOGY

Staging, Grading, & Classification

- TC & AC
  - Low to intermediate grade & mitotic rates
- SCLC
  - Limited stage (confined to 1 hemithorax) vs. advanced (70%)

Gross Pathologic & Surgical Features

- TC & AC
  - Discrete nodule, endoluminal component
- LCNEC
  - Large, necrotic, bulky, > 3 cm mass
  - Rapid growth & early metastases
- SCLC
  - Proximal growth along central bronchial submucosa
  - External compression, but no endobronchial lesion
  - Extensive necrosis & hemorrhage

CLINICAL ISSUES

Presentation

- Most common signs/symptoms
  - Cough, wheezing, hemoptysis, postobstructive pneumonia
  - SCLC: SVC syndrome, vocal cord paralysis
- Other signs/symptoms
  - Multiple endocrine neoplasia type 1 (TC & AC)
  - Ectopic Cushing syndrome
  - Secretion of inappropriate antidiuretic hormone
  - Eaton-Lambert syndrome, muscle weakness

Demographics

- Age
  - TC & AC: Mean is 45 years
  - LCNEC & SCLC: Mean is > 60 years
- Epidemiology
  - LCNEC & SCLC: Strong association with smoking

Natural History & Prognosis

- 10-year survival: TC 85%; AC 35%
- LCNEC & SCLC: Poor prognosis

Treatment

- TC & AC: Surgical resection ± chemoradiation
- SCLC: Chemotherapy & radiation

SELECTED REFERENCES

1. Franks TJ et al: Lung tumors with neuroendocrine morphology: essential radiologic and pathologic features. Arch Pathol Lab Med. 132(7):1055-61, 2008

KAPOSI SARCOMA

Key Facts

Terminology

- Kaposi sarcoma (KS)
- Acquired immunodeficiency syndrome-Kaposi sarcoma (AIDS-KS)
- Iatrogenic-Kaposi sarcoma (I-KS)
- Low-grade mesenchymal neoplasm of blood & lymphatic vessels, primarily affecting skin

Imaging

- AIDS-KS: Poorly marginated peribronchovascular nodules, lymphadenopathy, & bilateral pleural effusions
- Nodules
  - Flame-shaped, > 1 cm in diameter
  - Peribronchovascular with tendency to coalesce
  - CT halo sign
- Lymphadenopathy: Mediastinal, hilar, axillary
- Pleural effusions (common)

Top Differential Diagnoses

- Sarcoidosis
- Lymphoma
- Lymphangitic carcinomatosis
- Bacillary angiomatosis

Pathology

- Human herpes virus type 8

Clinical Issues

- Symptoms/signs: Dyspnea, cough, CD4 lymphocyte count (< 150-200 cells/mm^3)
- Demographics
  - Classic-KS: M:F, 10-15:1
  - AIDS-KS: Homosexual/bisexual men with AIDS
- Treatment
  - AIDS-KS: HAART ± chemotherapy
  - I-KS: Decrease in immunosuppressive therapy

__(Left)__ Axial graphic shows the typical morphologic features of pulmonary Kaposi sarcoma with noncontiguous tumor infiltrating along bronchovascular bundles, extending from the hilum to the lung periphery. __(Right)__ PA chest radiograph of a patient with AIDS-KS shows extensive bilateral perihilar and basilar heterogeneous nodular opacities. In this case, AIDS-KS mimics pulmonary edema or infection, and the diagnosis can only be suggested based on clinical information.

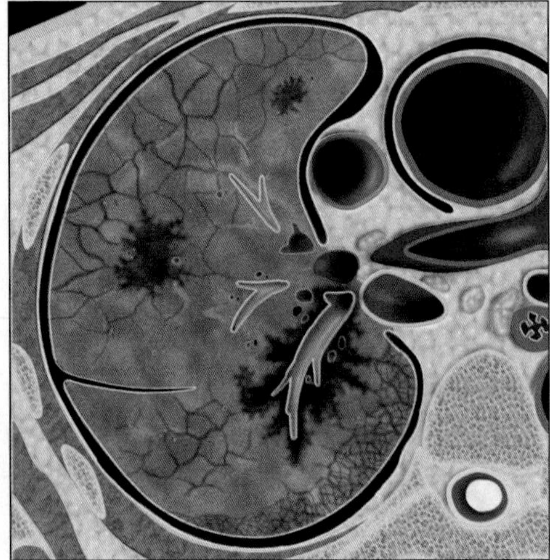

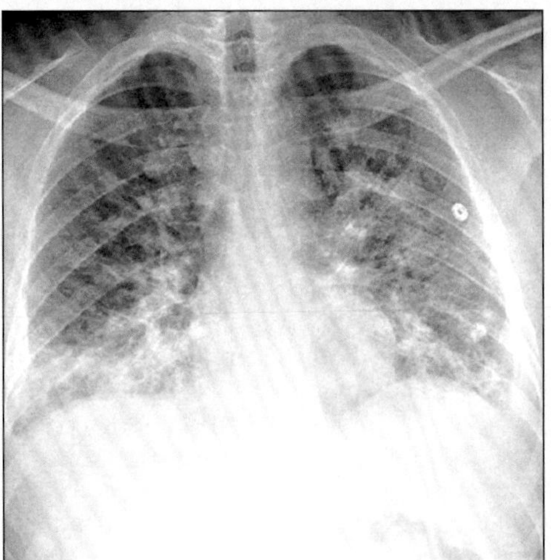

__(Left)__ PA chest radiograph of a patient with AIDS-KS demonstrates extensive bilateral heterogeneous irregular mass-like opacities and consolidations with central distribution. __(Right)__ Axial NECT of a patient with AIDS-KS shows a polylobular middle lobe mass with irregular borders and surrounding ground-glass opacities. Irregular nodules or masses with a peribronchovascular distribution are often referred to as flame-shaped lesions and are very characteristic of this type of malignancy.

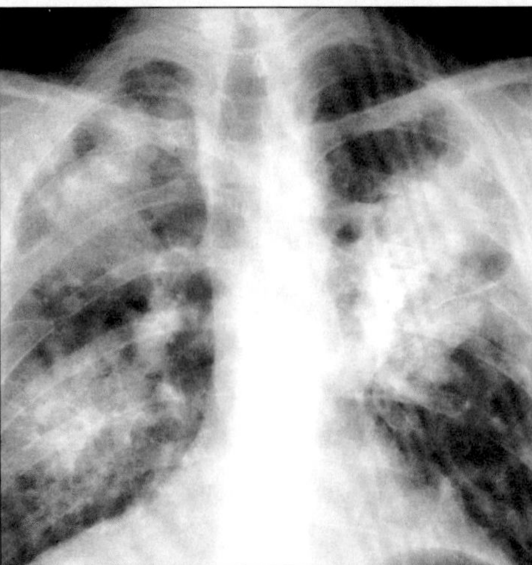

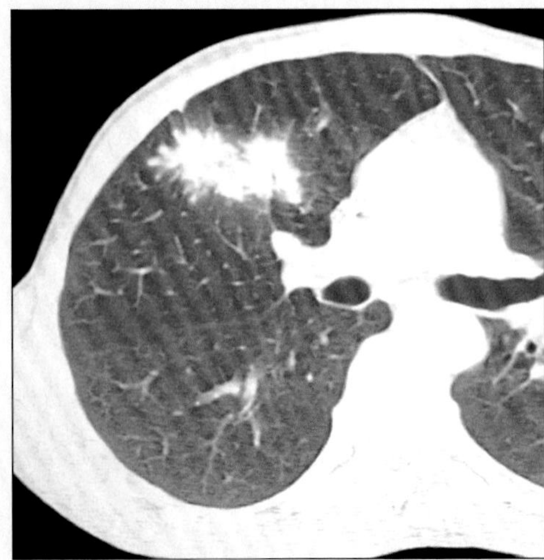

KAPOSI SARCOMA

TERMINOLOGY

Abbreviations

- **Kaposi sarcoma (KS)**
- Acquired immunodeficiency syndrome-Kaposi sarcoma (AIDS-KS): **Epidemic-KS**
- **Iatrogenic-Kaposi sarcoma (I-KS)**

Definitions

- **Low-grade mesenchymal neoplasm of blood & lymphatic vessels, primarily affecting skin**
- Can cause disseminated disease in a variety of organs: Lymphatic system, lungs, airways, abdominal viscera, etc.
- **AIDS-KS:** KS related to HIV/AIDS
- **I-KS:** KS related to immunosuppression

IMAGING

General Features

- Best diagnostic clue
  - AIDS-KS: Coexistence of poorly marginated peribronchovascular nodules, lymphadenopathy, & bilateral pleural effusions

Radiographic Findings

- **AIDS-KS**
  - Middle to lower lung zone reticular opacities & parenchymal nodules
  - Granular opacities: More diffuse/apical distribution or cavitation with concomitant opportunistic infection
- **I-KS**
  - Scattered, well-defined pulmonary nodules
  - Reticular opacities

CT Findings

- **AIDS-KS**
  - **Nodules**
    - Bilateral, symmetric, poorly marginated, emanating from hila (**flame-shaped**)
    - **Peribronchovascular** with tendency to coalesce, usually > 1 cm in diameter
    - Ground-glass opacities surrounding nodules (**halo sign**)
    - Cavitary nodules often associated with opportunistic infection, such as *Pneumocystis* pneumonia
  - **Peribronchovascular & interlobular septal thickening**
  - Fissural nodularity
  - **Lymphadenopathy**
    - Axillary, mediastinal, hilar
    - Often enhances with contrast
  - **Pleural effusions (common)**
  - Pleural implants (rare)
  - Osseous lytic lesions: Sternum, thoracic spine
  - Cutaneous & subcutaneous soft tissue thickening
- **I-KS**
  - Scattered pulmonary nodules
  - Lymphadenopathy
  - Pleural effusions

MR Findings

- Rarely used, but may be useful for assessment of osseous & soft tissue involvement
- T1WI: Hyperintense
- T2WI: Markedly reduced signal
- Strong tumoral enhancement after gadolinium

Nuclear Medicine Findings

- PET/CT
  - AIDS-KS
    - Foci of AIDS-KS are FDG avid
    - Useful for detection of occult lesions
  - I-KS
    - FDG-avid lung nodules & lymphadenopathy
- Gallium-67 & thallium scintigraphy
  - Combined approach helpful to differentiate epidemic-KS, infection, & lymphoma
  - Ga-67 negative in epidemic-KS, but positive for infection & lymphoma
  - Thallium: Positive in epidemic-KS & lymphoma

DIFFERENTIAL DIAGNOSIS

Pulmonary Edema

- Difficult differentiation from non-nodular KS
- History of AIDS or transplant & presence of skin lesions may be helpful

Sarcoidosis

- Bronchovascular bundle thickening, lung nodules, & septal thickening (often nodular) may mimic KS
- Lymphadenopathy more symmetric than KS, does not typically enhance

Lymphoma

- Peribronchovascular bundle thickening & lung nodules may mimic KS
- Lung nodules vary in size, but often larger than KS nodules
- Air bronchograms more common in lymphoma than in KS nodules

Lymphangitic Carcinomatosis

- Peribronchovascular bundle & septal thickening (often nodular), may mimic AIDS-KS
- Unilateral distribution favors lymphangitic carcinomatosis from primary lung cancer over KS

Infectious Bronchiolitis

- Mycobacterial & bacterial infections
- Nodules < 1 cm
- More centrilobular than peribronchovascular, often with frank tree-in-bud appearance

Bacillary Angiomatosis

- Rare infection due to *Bartonella henselae*
- Skin lesions, enhancing lymph nodes, & lung nodules mimic KS
- Peribronchovascular thickening not as common
- Consider in heterosexual patients with AIDS being evaluated for AIDS-KS

PATHOLOGY

General Features

- Etiology
  - **Human herpes virus type 8** (HHV8 or KS-associated herpes virus)

KAPOSI SARCOMA

- Also associated with primary effusion lymphoma & multicentric Castleman disease
  - Other cofactors
    - Tumor necrosis factor A
    - Interleukin 6
    - Basic fibroblast growth factor
    - Vascular endothelial growth factor
  - Mode of transmission
    - Not completely understood
    - Adult homosexual male contact (North America)
    - Mother-to-child & child-to-child (Africa & southern Europe)
    - Reactivation may have role in I-KS
- Genetics
  - Classic-KS
    - Patients of European or Mediterranean origin & Ashkenazi Jews
  - African-KS
    - East & Central Africa
    - 9% of all cancer in Uganda

Staging, Grading, & Classification

- 4 different types
  - Classic, sporadic, or Mediterranean KS (first described)
  - Endemic or African KS
  - AIDS-KS (most common)
  - I-KS
- AIDS-KS staging
  - **Extent of tumor (T)**
    - T0 (good risk): Localized tumor (i.e., KS only in skin &/or lymph nodes, small amount of disease on palate, flat lesions in mouth)
    - T1 (poor risk): Widespread KS
      - 1 or more of the following: Edema, extensive oral KS, lesions in organs other than lymph nodes
      - KS of lungs carries poor prognosis
  - **Immune status (I)**
    - I0 (good risk): CD4 cell count ≥ 200 cells/mm³
    - I1 (poor risk): CD4 cell count < 200 cells/mm³
  - **Systemic illness status (S)**
    - S0 (good risk): No systemic illness present
      - No history of opportunistic infections or thrush
      - No B symptoms (i.e., unexplained fever, night sweats, weight loss, diarrhea)
      - Karnofsky performance status score ≥ 70
    - S1 (poor risk): Systemic illness present with 1 or more of the following
      - History of opportunistic infections or thrush
      - 1 or more B symptoms present
      - Karnofsky performance status score < 70
      - Other HIV-related illness is present, such as neurological disease or lymphoma

Gross Pathologic & Surgical Features

- AIDS-KS
  - Skin lesions frequently absent
  - Visceral organs affected in AIDS-KS
    - Lymph nodes (72%)
    - Lung (51%)
    - GI tract (48%), liver (34%), spleen (27%)
  - Thorax affected in 45% of all cases

Microscopic Features

- Spindle-shaped stromal cells
- Abnormal endothelial lining of vascular channels
- Slit-like spaces of extravasated red cells

CLINICAL ISSUES

Presentation

- Most common signs/symptoms
  - Dyspnea, cough
  - CD4 lymphocyte count (< 150-200 cells/mm³)
- Other signs/symptoms
  - Hemoptysis

Demographics

- Age
  - Classic-KS: 50-80 years
  - African-KS: 4th decade
- Gender
  - Classic-KS: M:F = 10-15:1
  - African-KS: Male predominance
  - AIDS-KS: Homosexual or bisexual male AIDS patients
- Epidemiology
  - Most common AIDS-related neoplasm, but decreased prevalence in current era of highly active antiretroviral therapy

Natural History & Prognosis

- AIDS-KS indicators of shorter survival
  - White homosexual male, better survival than black, female IV drug user
  - Prior or coexistent opportunistic infection
  - Systemic symptoms (e.g., unexplained fever > 2 weeks, weight loss > 10%, diarrhea, or night sweats)
  - CD4 lymphocyte count (< 100-300 cells/mm³)
  - Pleural effusions
- Opportunistic infections cause of death in 80% of patients with AIDS-KS

Treatment

- AIDS-KS: Highly active antiretroviral therapy (HAART) ± chemotherapy
- I-KS: Decrease in immunosuppressive therapy

DIAGNOSTIC CHECKLIST

Image Interpretation Pearls

- Flame-shaped nodules on CT are highly suggestive of AIDS/KS in appropriate clinical setting

SELECTED REFERENCES

1. Martinez S et al: Kaposi sarcoma after bilateral lung transplantation. J Thorac Imaging. 23(1):50-3, 2008
2. Restrepo CS et al: Imaging manifestations of Kaposi sarcoma. Radiographics. 26(4):1169-85, 2006
3. Cheung MC et al: AIDS-Related Malignancies: Emerging Challenges in the Era of Highly Active Antiretroviral Therapy. Oncologist. 10(6):412-26, 2005

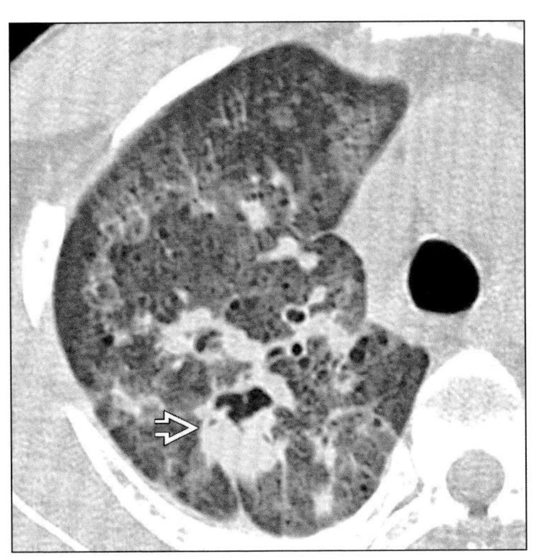

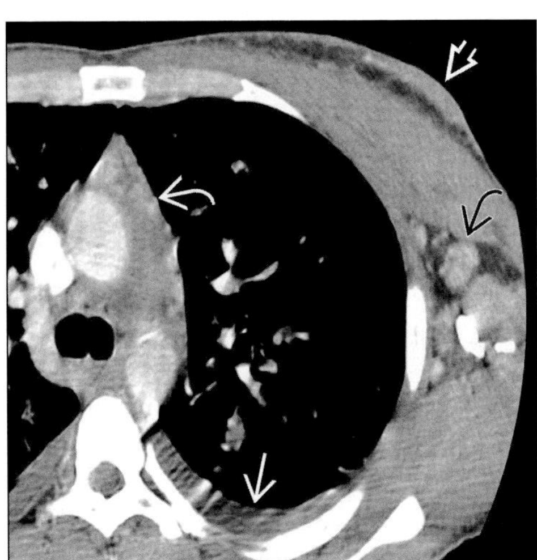

(Left) *Axial NECT of a patient with AIDS-KS and coexistent Pneumocystis pneumonia shows a cavitary right upper lobe nodule ⮚. Cavitary lesions in these patients are almost always related to superimposed infection.* ***(Right)*** *Axial CECT shows a patient with AIDS-KS manifesting with bilateral pleural effusions ⮚, conspicuous mediastinal ⮚ and axillary ⮚ enhancing lymph nodes, and left pectoral skin thickening ⮚. All these findings are characteristic of AIDS-KS.*

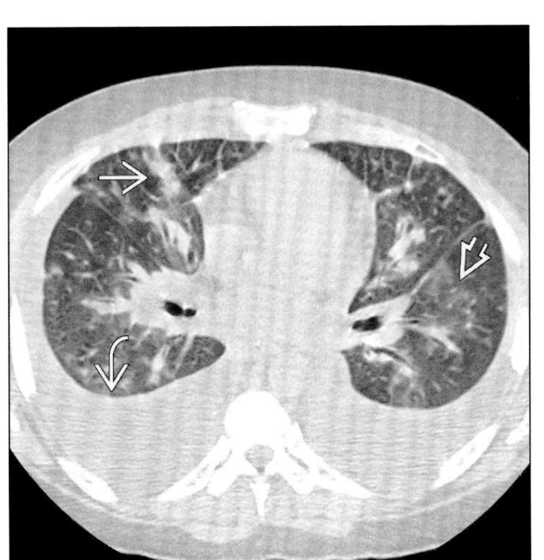

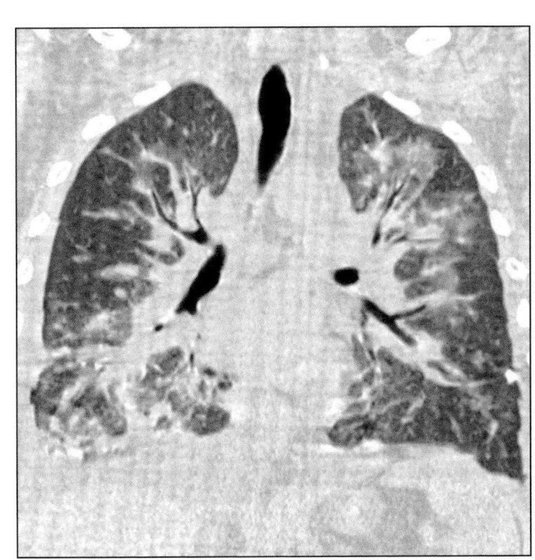

(Left) *Axial NECT of the same patient shows moderate bilateral pleural effusions ⮚, peribronchovascular nodular consolidations ⮚, and ground-glass opacities ⮚.* ***(Right)*** *Coronal NECT of the same patient shows extensive bilateral peribronchovascular opacities. Pleural effusions, lower lobe predominant abnormalities, and interlobular septal thickening suggest pulmonary edema. Infection would also be difficult to exclude based solely on the imaging abnormalities.*

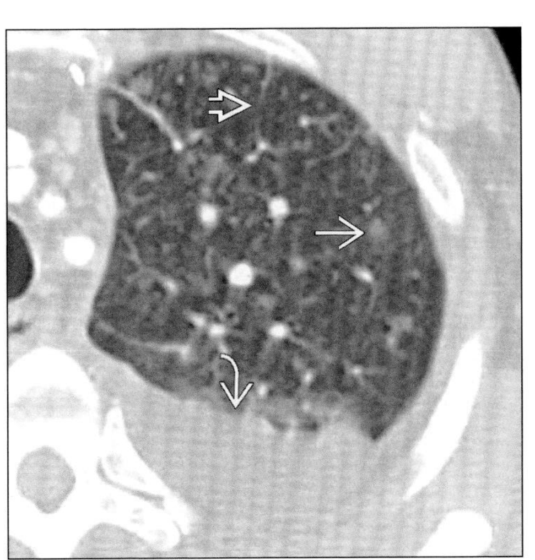

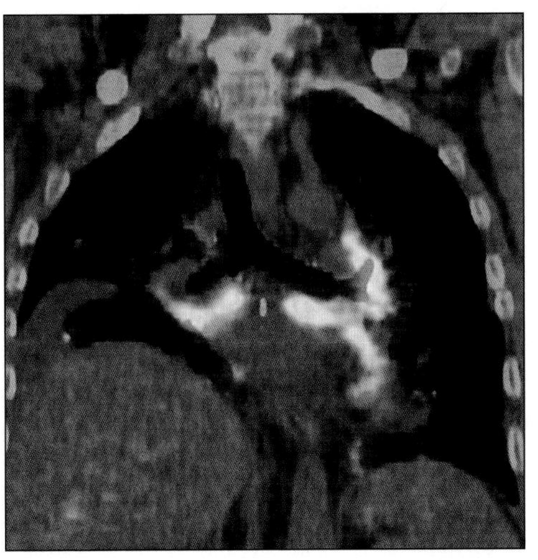

(Left) *Axial CECT of a patient with I-KS following bilateral lung transplants shows profuse small ground-glass nodules ⮚, thick interlobular septa ⮚, and a moderate left pleural effusion ⮚.* ***(Right)*** *Coronal fused PET/CT of a patient with I-KS following bilateral lung transplants shows extensive FDG uptake in mediastinal and bilateral hilar lymph nodes. Also note FDG uptake in scattered pulmonary nodules. Foci of both AIDS-KS and I-KS have been reported to exhibit FDG avidity.*

FOLLICULAR BRONCHIOLITIS

Key Facts

Terminology

- Follicular bronchiolitis (FB)
- Proliferation of polyclonal lymphoid follicles in small airway walls & peribronchiolar interstitium

Imaging

- Radiography
  - Normal chest radiographs or subtle abnormalities
  - Diffuse reticular or reticulonodular opacities
- CT
  - Centrilobular & peribronchovascular micronodules (1-3 mm)
  - Tree-in-bud opacities less common
  - Nodular ground-glass opacities & lung cysts similar to findings of lymphocytic interstitial pneumonia
- HRCT most sensitive for demonstration of abnormalities & their distribution

Top Differential Diagnoses

- Lymphocytic interstitial pneumonia
- Respiratory bronchiolitis & respiratory bronchiolitis-interstitial lung disease
- Hypersensitivity pneumonitis
- Diffuse panbronchiolitis

Clinical Issues

- Associated with collagen vascular disease & immunodeficiency
- Symptoms/signs: Dyspnea, wheezing, crackles

Diagnostic Checklist

- Consider FB in patients with chronic cellular bronchiolitis in association with collagen vascular disease or immunodeficiency
- Overlap of imaging findings of follicular bronchiolitis & lymphocytic interstitial pneumonia

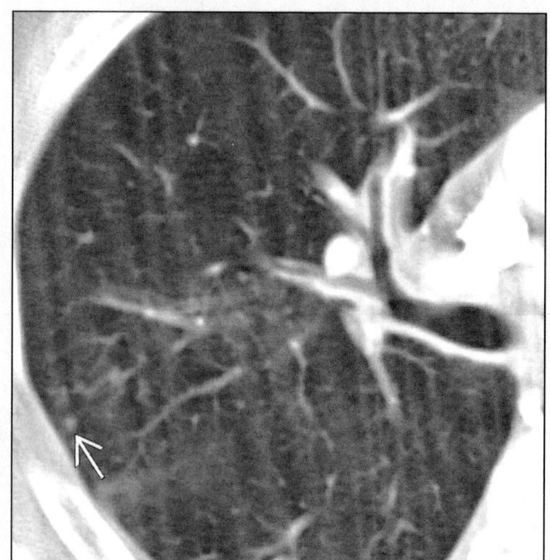

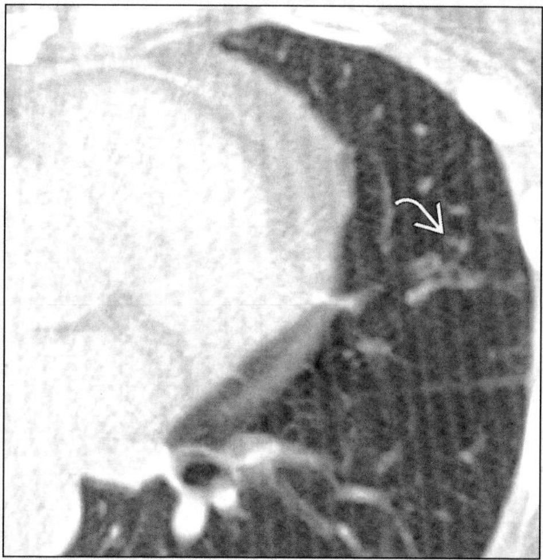

(Left) *Axial CECT of a 64-year-old man with yellow nail syndrome and follicular bronchiolitis (FB) shows centrilobular nodules ➡ in the right upper lobe. Centrilobular nodules are the most common imaging manifestation of FB.* ***(Right)*** *Axial NECT of a 51-year-old woman with Sjögren syndrome and FB shows focal tree-in-bud opacities ➡ in the lingula, an uncommon imaging manifestation of FB. FB is associated with collagen vascular diseases and AIDS.*

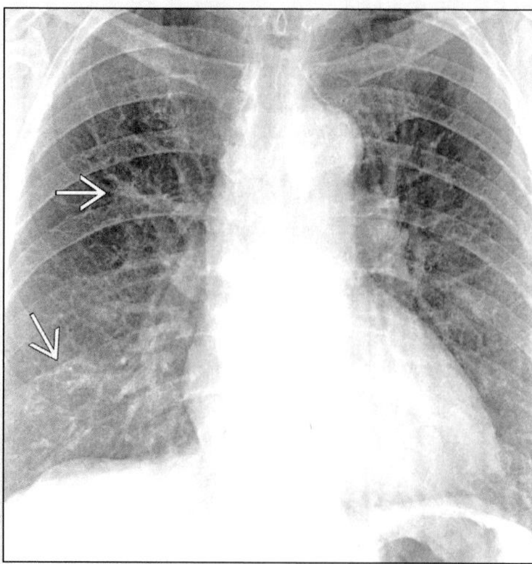

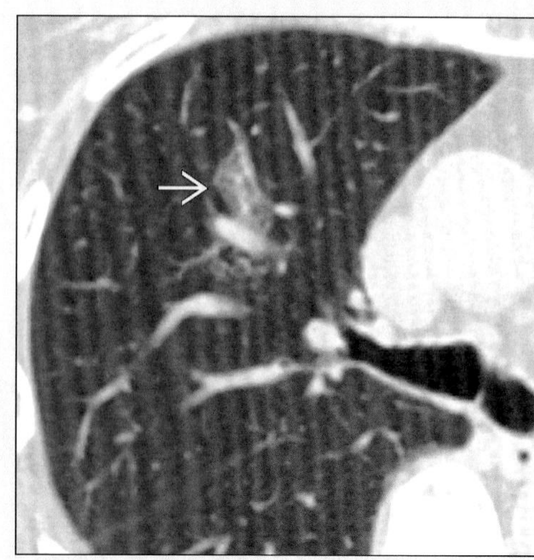

(Left) *PA chest radiograph of a 68-year-old woman with follicular bronchiolitis shows patchy reticulonodular opacities ➡ in the right lung. Reticular and reticulonodular opacities may be subtle and are the most common radiographic finding of follicular bronchiolitis.* ***(Right)*** *Axial CECT of the same patient shows peribronchovascular ground-glass opacities ➡. Ground-glass opacities and lung cysts are also seen in lymphocytic interstitial pneumonia, and these entities may represent a disease continuum.*

FOLLICULAR BRONCHIOLITIS

TERMINOLOGY

Abbreviations

- **Follicular bronchiolitis (FB)**

Definitions

- Proliferation of polyclonal lymphoid follicles in small airway walls & peribronchiolar interstitium

IMAGING

General Features

- Best diagnostic clue
  - Small centrilobular nodules in the setting of chronic airways disease
- Location
  - Centrilobular & peribronchovascular distribution most common
- Size
  - Small nodules, 1-3 mm

Radiographic Findings

- Normal chest radiographs or subtle abnormalities
- Diffuse reticular or reticulonodular opacities

CT Findings

- HRCT
  - Centrilobular & peribronchovascular micronodules (1-3 mm)
  - Tree-in-bud opacities less common
  - Nodular ground-glass opacities & lung cysts similar to findings of lymphocytic interstitial pneumonia

Imaging Recommendations

- Best imaging tool
  - HRCT most sensitive for demonstration of lung abnormalities & their distribution

DIFFERENTIAL DIAGNOSIS

Lymphocytic Interstitial Pneumonia

- Ground-glass opacity is predominant feature
- Poorly defined centrilobular nodules
- Thin-walled cysts in 70%
- Significant overlap with FB, continuum of bronchus associated lymphoid tissue (BALT) hyperplasia

Respiratory Bronchiolitis & Respiratory Bronchiolitis-Interstitial Lung Disease

- Upper lobe predominant centrilobular micronodules
- Reticular opacities primarily in lower lobes
- Smoking history

Hypersensitivity Pneumonitis

- Faint centrilobular nodules & ground-glass opacities
- Air-trapping, "head cheese" sign
- Almost exclusively in nonsmokers

Diffuse Panbronchiolitis

- Patients mainly in Asia (Japan, Korea)
- Centrilobular nodules & tree-in-bud opacities
- Basal & peripheral predominance

PATHOLOGY

General Features

- Etiology
  - Present in chronic airways diseases such as bronchiectasis
  - Secondary FB occurs in inflammation or infection
  - Bronchus-associated lymphoid tissue (BALT) hyperplasia
- Associated abnormalities
  - Middle lobe syndrome
  - Lymphoproliferative disorders
    - Mucosa-associated lymphoid tissue (MALT) lymphoma (MALToma)
- Subtype of chronic cellular bronchiolitis

Microscopic Features

- Lymphocytic infiltrate in small airway walls
- Peribronchiolar reactive lymphoid follicles & chronic inflammatory cells

CLINICAL ISSUES

Presentation

- Most common signs/symptoms
  - Dyspnea, often progressive
  - Wheezing, crackles
- May occur in
  - Collagen vascular diseases (e.g., rheumatoid arthritis, Sjögren syndrome)
  - Immunodeficiency (e.g., AIDS)
  - Hypersensitivity pneumonitis
  - Workers exposed to nylon or polyethylene flock

Demographics

- Age
  - Young adults

Treatment

- Corticosteroids variably effective

DIAGNOSTIC CHECKLIST

Consider

- FB in patients with chronic cellular bronchiolitis in association with collagen vascular disease or immunodeficiency

Image Interpretation Pearls

- Overlap of imaging findings of follicular bronchiolitis & lymphocytic interstitial pneumonia

SELECTED REFERENCES

1. Kang EY et al: Bronchiolitis: classification, computed tomographic and histopathologic features, and radiologic approach. J Comput Assist Tomogr. 33(1):32-41, 2009
2. Lynch DA: Imaging of small airways disease and chronic obstructive pulmonary disease. Clin Chest Med. 29(1):165-79, vii, 2008
3. Pipavath SJ et al: Radiologic and pathologic features of bronchiolitis. AJR Am J Roentgenol. 185(2):354-63, 2005
4. Howling SJ et al: Follicular bronchiolitis: thin-section CT and histologic findings. Radiology. 212(3):637-42, 1999

LYMPHOCYTIC INTERSTITIAL PNEUMONIA

Key Facts

Terminology

- Lymphocytic interstitial pneumonia (LIP)
- Diffuse polyclonal lymphocytic infiltration of alveolar septa
  - Part of spectrum of lymphoproliferative disorders
- Included in ATS/ERS 2001 classification of idiopathic interstitial pneumonias

Imaging

- Radiography
  - Basal reticular/reticulonodular opacities
- CT
  - Bilateral ground-glass opacities
  - Poorly defined centrilobular nodules
  - Small subpleural nodules (~ 85%)
  - Bronchovascular bundle thickening (~ 85%)
  - Mild interlobular septal thickening (~ 85%)
  - Thin-walled cysts (~ 70%)

Top Differential Diagnoses

- Nonspecific interstitial pneumonia (NSIP)
- Pulmonary Langerhans cell histiocytosis (PLCH)
- Hypersensitivity pneumonitis
- Lymphangioleiomyomatosis (LAM)
- Birt-Hogg-Dubé syndrome

Pathology

- Most patients with LIP have autoimmune disease or immunodeficiency
  - Adults: Sjögren syndrome most common
  - Children: HIV infection most common

Diagnostic Checklist

- Perivascular distribution of cysts in correct clinical setting very suggestive of LIP
- Ground-glass opacities & centrilobular nodules suggestive of LIP in patients with Sjögren syndrome

__(Left)__ Axial HRCT of a patient with LIP and Sjögren syndrome shows thin-walled lung cysts ➡ ranging in size from a few millimeters to a few centimeters. LIP cysts are fewer than those of lymphangioleiomyomatosis (LAM). __(Right)__ Coronal NECT of the same patient shows the basal predominance of LIP cysts in contrast to the upper lobe predominance of pulmonary Langerhans cell histiocytosis cysts and the diffuse distribution of LAM cysts. Many cysts have a blood vessel ⇨ coursing along their walls.

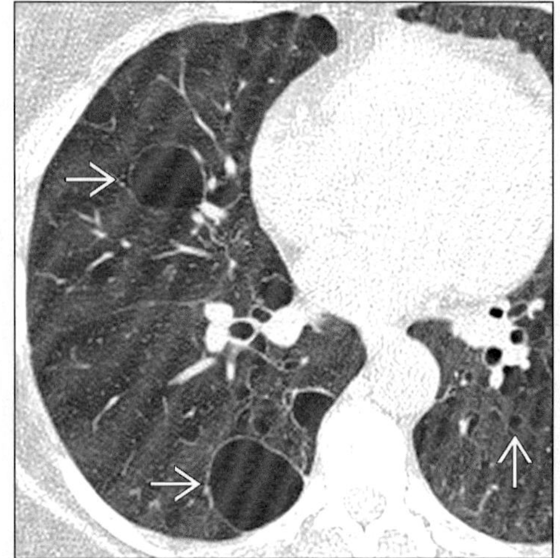

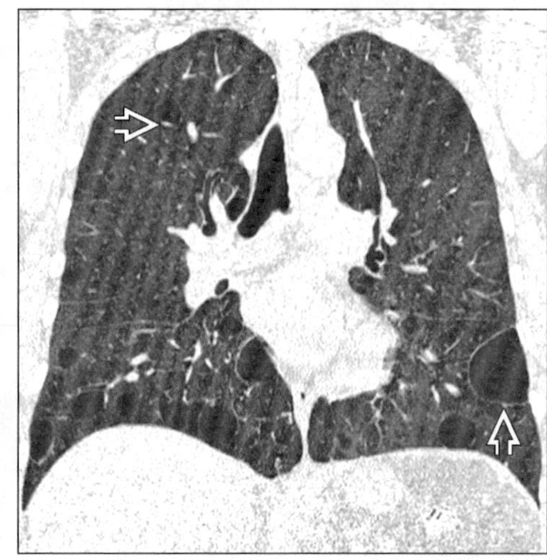

__(Left)__ Axial CECT of a patient with LIP and Sjögren syndrome shows multiple tiny thin-walled cysts ➡ and patchy ground-glass opacities ⇨. __(Right)__ Axial HRCT of a patient with LIP shows the typical combination of diffuse ground-glass opacities ⇨ and thin-walled cysts ➡. Note the vessels coursing along some cyst walls ↪, reflecting the perivascular distribution of many cysts. Ground-glass opacity is not a common finding in patients with lymphangioleiomyomatosis.

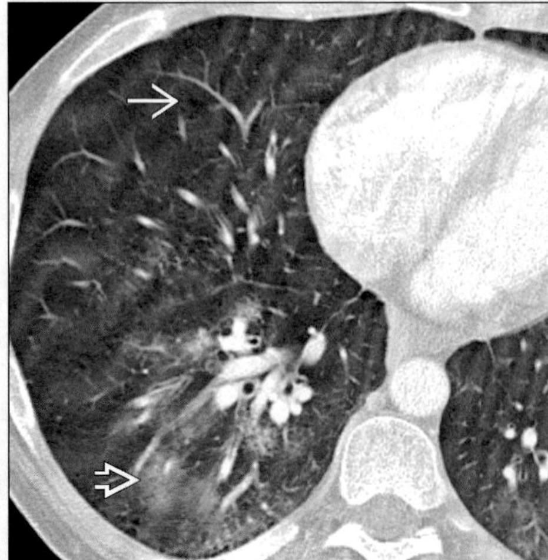

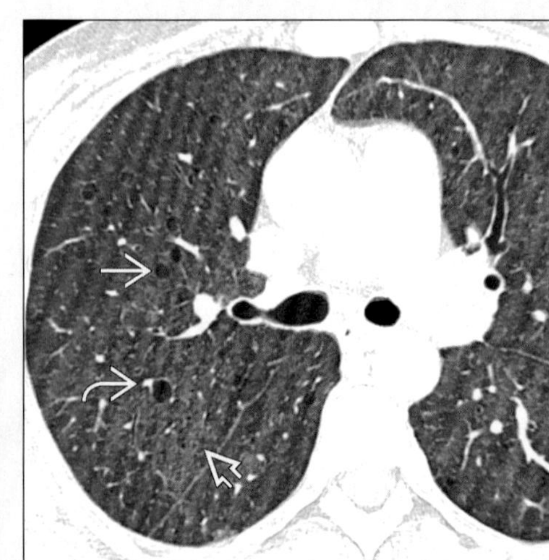

LYMPHOCYTIC INTERSTITIAL PNEUMONIA

TERMINOLOGY

Abbreviations

- **Lymphocytic interstitial pneumonia (LIP)**

Synonyms

- Lymphoid interstitial pneumonia

Definitions

- Diffuse polyclonal lymphocytic infiltration of alveolar septa
- Part of spectrum of lymphoproliferative disorders
  - Follicular bronchiolitis (lymphoid hyperplasia) to lymphoma
- Included in ATS/ERS 2001 classification of idiopathic interstitial pneumonias

IMAGING

General Features

- Best diagnostic clue
  - Basal predominant pulmonary involvement
  - Perivascular thin-walled cysts, ground-glass opacities, & centrilobular nodules
- Location
  - Basal predominant
- Size
  - Cysts usually up to 30 mm in diameter
  - Nodules usually few mm in diameter
- Morphology
  - Cysts have thin walls
  - Nodules with poorly defined borders

Radiographic Findings

- Radiography
  - Basal predominant reticular or reticulonodular opacities most common
    - Can be primarily nodular
  - Less common
    - Diffuse or patchy ground-glass opacities
    - Patchy lung consolidation
  - Cysts may be apparent on radiography
  - Pleural effusions conspicuously absent

CT Findings

- HRCT
  - Predominant findings
    - Bilateral ground-glass opacities
    - Poorly defined centrilobular nodules
  - Other common findings
    - Small subpleural nodules (~ 85%)
    - Bronchovascular bundle thickening (~ 85%)
    - Mild interlobular septal thickening (~ 85%)
    - Thin-walled cysts (~ 70%)
      - Range from 1-30 mm in diameter
      - Perivascular & subpleural distribution
      - Isolated to diffuse lung involvement
    - Mild mediastinal lymphadenopathy (70%)
      - Usually not apparent on radiography
    - Less common findings
      - Larger nodules (1-2 cm)
      - Consolidation
      - Bronchiectasis
      - Honeycomb lung
    - Pleural effusions characteristically absent
  - Evolution
    - Ground-glass opacities & nodules tend to decrease or resolve with treatment
    - Cysts remain & may gradually enlarge
    - Honeycomb lung in small number of patients

Imaging Recommendations

- Best imaging tool
  - HRCT for optimal characterization of lung & mediastinal abnormalities
- Protocol advice
  - Unenhanced volumetric HRCT in inspiration
    - Prone & expiratory imaging not required

DIFFERENTIAL DIAGNOSIS

Nonspecific Interstitial Pneumonia (NSIP)

- Cellular or fibrotic, temporally homogeneous histology
- Idiopathic or associated with collagen vascular disease
- Diffuse or basal predominant ground-glass opacities
- Cysts & nodules not characteristic findings

Pulmonary Langerhans Cell Histiocytosis (PLCH)

- Smoking-related interstitial lung disease
- Upper lobe predominant cysts & nodules
  - Cysts become irregular as they enlarge
  - Nodules may cavitate & become cysts
- Characteristic basal sparing

Hypersensitivity Pneumonitis

- History of antigenic exposure
  - Common: Birds, fungi, agriculture, low molecular weight inorganic compounds
- Diffuse ground-glass opacities & poorly defined centrilobular nodules
- Lobular air-trapping
- Cysts may be present, but are few in number
- Interstitial fibrosis often mid & upper lung zone predominant

Lymphangioleiomyomatosis (LAM)

- Diffuse thin-walled cysts
- Nodules far less common
- Chylous pleural effusions
- Mediastinal & retroperitoneal lymphangioleiomyomas
- Renal angiomyolipomas
- Women with tuberous sclerosis complex (TSC)
  - Spontaneous LAM less common
  - Rare in men with TSC

Birt-Hogg-Dubé Syndrome

- Autosomal dominant inheritance
- Associated with fibrofolliculomas of face & upper trunk
- Renal neoplasms ranging from oncocytoma to chromophobe renal cell carcinoma
- Lung cysts
  - Few in number
  - Perivenous or septopleural junctions
  - Spherical or ovoid with thin walls

PATHOLOGY

General Features

- Etiology
  - Exact disease mechanism unknown

LYMPHOCYTIC INTERSTITIAL PNEUMONIA

- Associated abnormalities
  - Most patients have autoimmune disease or immunodeficiency
    - Adults: Sjögren syndrome most common
    - Children: HIV infection most common
  - Idiopathic LIP extremely rare

Microscopic Features

- Diffuse alveolar septal infiltration by lymphocytes
  - Variable number of plasma cells
  - Polyclonal lymphoproliferative disorder
- Localized proliferation, germinal centers sometimes present
- Fibrosis absent or mild
  - May be associated with microscopic honeycomb lung
- Airspaces usually spared
- Must be distinguished from lymphoma
  - Readily accomplished by immunohistochemical staining
  - Correlation with HRCT findings helpful (presence of cysts & absence of pleural effusions)

CLINICAL ISSUES

Presentation

- Most common signs/symptoms
  - Onset usually gradual over several years
  - Cough, dyspnea
  - Fatigue
  - Other symptoms related to predisposing diseases
    - Sjögren syndrome
      - Sicca syndrome (dry eyes, dry mouth)
      - Parotid gland enlargement
    - Immunodeficiency
      - Recurrent infections
- Other signs/symptoms
  - Dysproteinemia (~ 80%)
    - Polyclonal hypergammaglobulinemia most common
  - Rheumatoid factor usually positive in Sjögren
  - Pulmonary function tests
    - Restrictive defect with decreased diffusion capacity
  - Bronchoalveolar lavage often shows lymphocytosis
  - Definitive diagnosis usually requires surgical lung biopsy
    - Yield of transbronchial biopsy low

Demographics

- Age
  - Most adults present between 50-60 years of age
- Gender
  - M:F = 1:2
    - Sjögren syndrome M:F = 1:9
- Epidemiology
  - Most cases in HIV-positive children
  - Sjögren syndrome
    - 25% of adults with Sjögren syndrome have LIP

Natural History & Prognosis

- Variable
  - Usually dictated by underlying disease
  - High risk of lymphoma in patients with Sjögren syndrome
- Median survival of 11 years

Treatment

- Steroids (most commonly used), cytotoxic drugs
  - Most patients have good initial response
  - Some patients progress despite therapy
    - Interstitial fibrosis & honeycomb lung may develop

DIAGNOSTIC CHECKLIST

Consider

- Other causes of diffuse lung disease in patients with autoimmune disorders
  - Especially nonspecific interstitial pneumonia (NSIP)
    - Cysts not typical feature

Image Interpretation Pearls

- Perivascular distribution of cysts in correct clinical setting very suggestive of LIP
- Ground-glass opacities & poorly defined centrilobular nodules very suggestive of LIP in patients with Sjögren syndrome

SELECTED REFERENCES

1. Kanne JP: Idiopathic interstitial pneumonias. Semin Roentgenol. 45(1):8-21, 2010
2. Silva CI et al: Idiopathic interstitial pneumonias. J Thorac Imaging. 24(4):260-73, 2009
3. Cha SI et al: Lymphoid interstitial pneumonia: clinical features, associations and prognosis. Eur Respir J. 28(2):364-9, 2006
4. Silva CI et al: Diffuse lung cysts in lymphoid interstitial pneumonia: high-resolution CT and pathologic findings. J Thorac Imaging. 21(3):241-4, 2006
5. Do KH et al: Pulmonary parenchymal involvement of low-grade lymphoproliferative disorders. J Comput Assist Tomogr. 29(6):825-30, 2005
6. American Thoracic Society; European Respiratory Society: American Thoracic Society/European Respiratory Society International Multidisciplinary Consensus Classification of the Idiopathic Interstitial Pneumonias. This joint statement of the American Thoracic Society (ATS) and the European Respiratory Society (ERS) was adopted by the ATS board of directors, June 2001 and by the ERS Executive Committee, June 2001. Am J Respir Crit Care Med. 165(2):277-304, 2002
7. Swigris JJ et al: Lymphoid interstitial pneumonia: a narrative review. Chest. 122(6):2150-64, 2002
8. Nicholson AG: Lymphocytic interstitial pneumonia and other lymphoproliferative disorders in the lung. Semin Respir Crit Care Med. 22(4):409-22, 2001
9. Travis WD et al: Non-neoplastic pulmonary lymphoid lesions. Thorax. 56(12):964-71, 2001
10. Johkoh T et al: Lymphocytic interstitial pneumonia: follow-up CT findings in 14 patients. J Thorac Imaging. 15(3):162-7, 2000

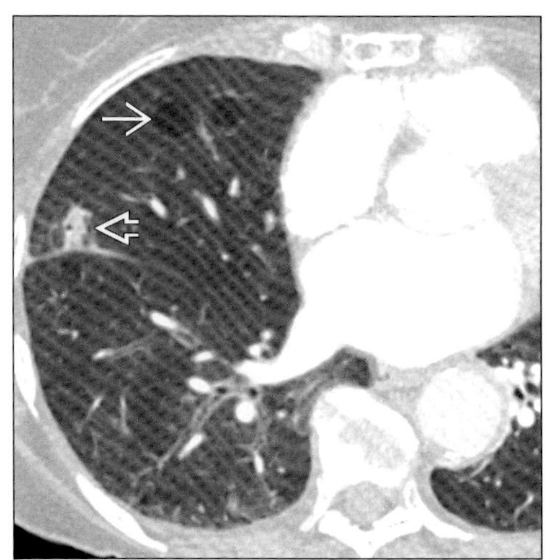

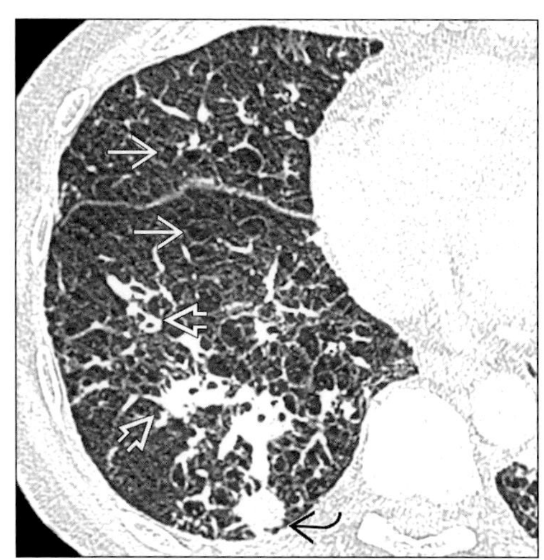

(Left) *Axial CECT of a patient with LIP and Sjögren syndrome shows a small number of thin-walled cysts ➔. While poorly defined centrilobular nodules are more common, large discrete nodules ➔ are occasionally present in patients with LIP.* ***(Right)*** *Axial HRCT of a patient with LIP shows extensive bronchovascular bundle thickening ➔, especially in the right lower lobe, multiple thin-walled cysts ➔, and a large nodule ➔ in the posterior aspect of the right lower lobe.*

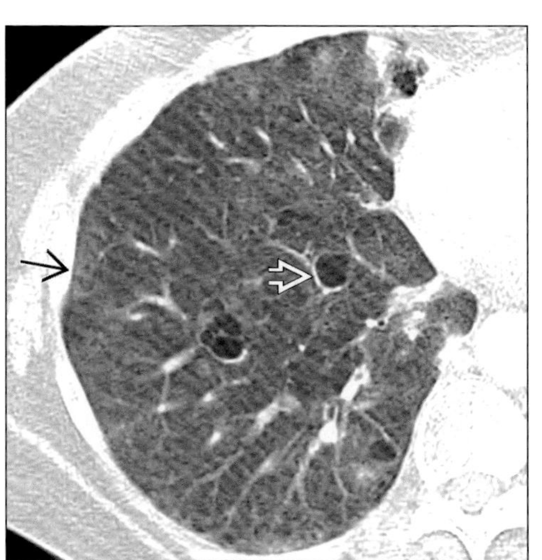

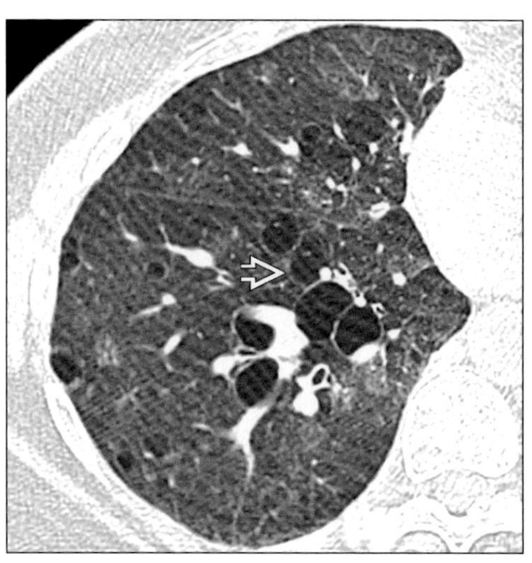

(Left) *Axial CECT of a patient with LIP and Sjögren syndrome shows ground-glass opacity, ill-defined centrilobular nodules ➔, & scattered thin-walled perivascular cysts ➔. This constellation of findings is highly specific for LIP.* ***(Right)*** *Axial HRCT of the same patient obtained 3 years later shows near resolution of ground-glass opacities & centrilobular nodules, but increased cyst sizes and numbers ➔. Nodules & ground-glass opacities usually clear with treatment, while cysts remain & may enlarge.*

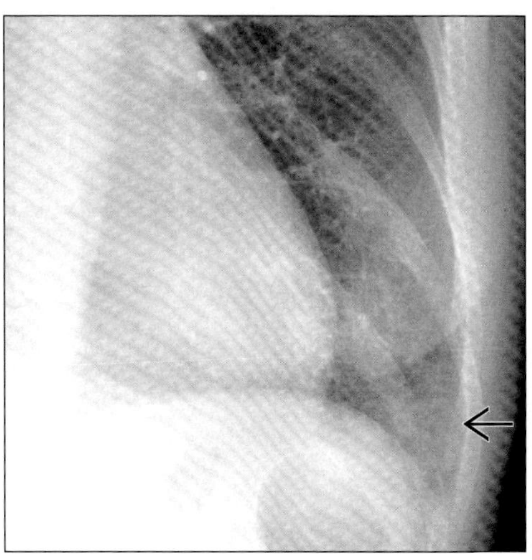

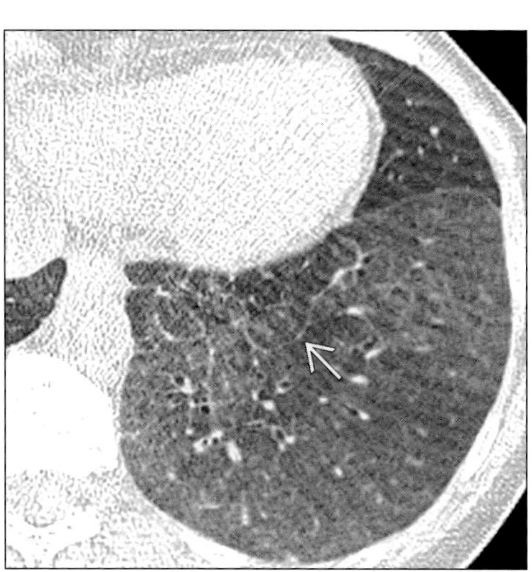

(Left) *PA chest radiograph (coned-down to the left lower lobe) of a patient with Sjögren syndrome and LIP shows fine linear opacities ➔ in the left lung base.* ***(Right)*** *Axial HRCT of the same patient shows diffuse left lower lobe ground-glass opacity with mild superimposed smooth interlobular septal thickening ➔. LIP is typically a diffuse process affecting both lungs. Septal and bronchovascular bundle thickening occur in approximately 85% of affected patients.*

NODULAR LYMPHOID HYPERPLASIA

Key Facts

Terminology

- Nodular lymphoid hyperplasia (NLH)
- Reactive nodular lymphoid proliferation manifesting with pulmonary nodule(s)/mass(es)

Imaging

- Radiography
  - Pulmonary nodule(s): Discrete or ill-defined, solitary (65%), multiple (35%)
  - May exhibit air bronchograms
- CT
  - Pulmonary nodule with solid or ground-glass attenuation
  - Nodule may exhibit air bronchograms
  - Lymphadenopathy (rare)
  - Pleural effusion (rare)
- PET/CT
  - Nodule(s) may exhibit FDG uptake (SUV = 2.5)

Top Differential Diagnoses

- Low-grade B-cell lymphoma
- Lymphocytic interstitial pneumonia
- Follicular bronchiolitis

Pathology

- Well-circumscribed gray to white-tan nodule(s)
- Abundant reactive germinal centers with sheets of interfollicular plasma cells
- Interfollicular fibrosis of variable degree often present

Clinical Issues

- Symptoms/signs
  - Asymptomatic (most)
  - Cough, dyspnea, pleuritic chest pain
- Good prognosis
  - Surgical resection curative
  - May regress without treatment

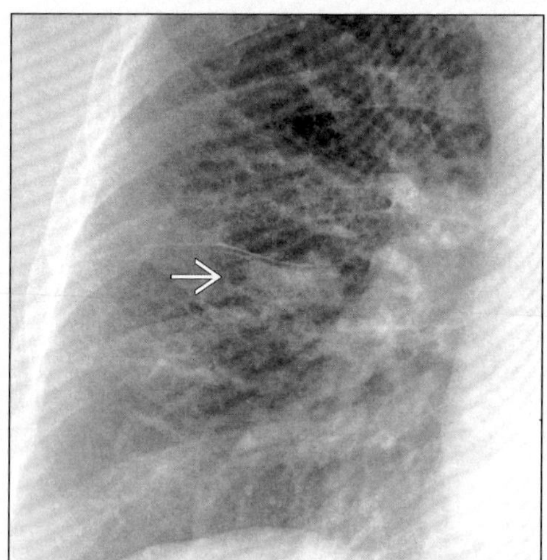

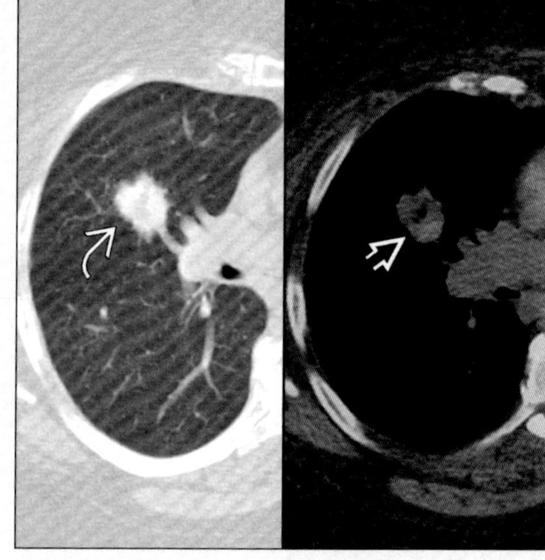

(Left) *PA chest radiograph of an asymptomatic patient with nodular lymphoid hyperplasia (NLH) shows an ill-defined soft tissue nodule ➔ in the middle lobe.* ***(Right)*** *Composite image with axial NECT (left) and fused PET/CT (right) of the same patient shows a slightly spiculated peribronchovascular middle lobe nodule ➔ that exhibits moderate FDG avidity ➔ on fused PET/CT. A solitary pulmonary nodule is the most common imaging manifestation of this lymphoproliferative process.*

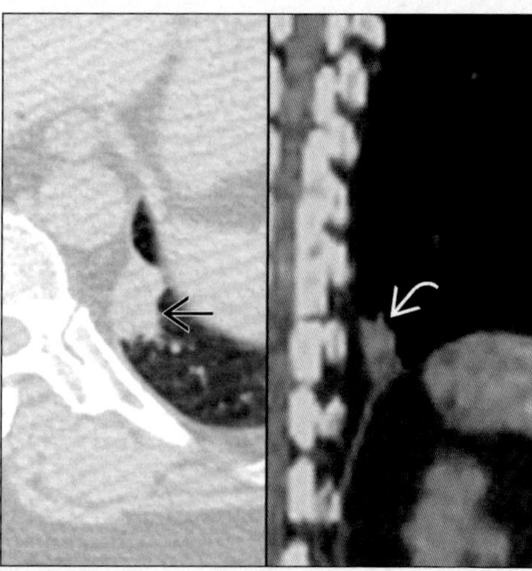

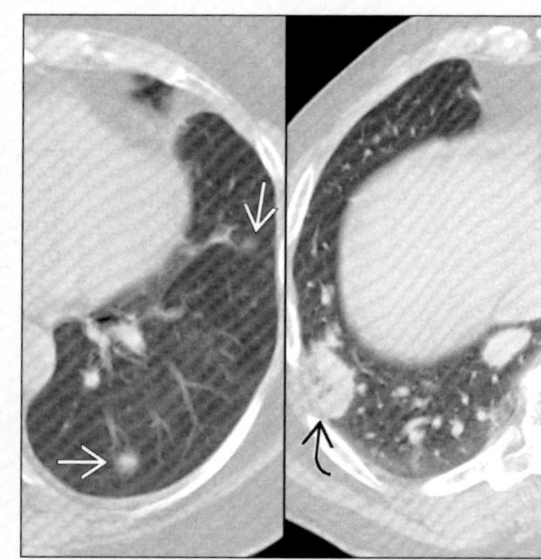

(Left) *Composite image with axial NECT (left) and coronal fused PET/CT (right) of a patient with NLH shows a subpleural left lower lobe nodule ➔ with moderate FDG uptake ➔.* ***(Right)*** *Composite image with axial NECT of 2 different patients with NLH shows small solid and ground-glass left basilar nodules ➔ and multiple larger discrete right lower lobe nodules ➔ with intrinsic air bronchograms. Multiple nodules with or without air bronchograms are common imaging manifestations of NLH.*

NODULAR LYMPHOID HYPERPLASIA

TERMINOLOGY

Abbreviations

- **Nodular lymphoid hyperplasia (NLH)**

Definitions

- Reactive nodular lymphoid proliferation manifesting with pulmonary nodule(s)/mass(es)

IMAGING

General Features

- Location
  - Subpleural or peribronchial location
- Size
  - 2-4 cm nodules
- Morphology
  - Discrete or ill-defined nodule(s)/mass(es)

Radiographic Findings

- Pulmonary nodule(s)
  - Solitary pulmonary nodule (65%)
  - Multiple nodules (35%)
  - Air bronchograms within lung nodules

CT Findings

- Pulmonary nodule
  - Solid or ground-glass attenuation
  - Intrinsic air bronchograms
- Lymphadenopathy (rare)
- Pleural effusion (rare)

Nuclear Medicine Findings

- PET/CT
  - Nodule(s) may exhibit FDG uptake (SUV = 2.5)

DIFFERENTIAL DIAGNOSIS

Low-grade B-cell Lymphoma

- Similar imaging findings
- Histological, immunohistochemical, & molecular characterization allows differentiation

Lymphocytic Interstitial Pneumonia (LIP)

- Imaging: Cysts & ground-glass opacities on CT
- Pathology: Diffuse reticulonodular or small nodular infiltrates

Follicular Bronchiolitis

- Imaging: Centrilobular micronodules on CT
- Pathology: Peribronchial or peribronchiolar lymphocytic infiltrate

PATHOLOGY

General Features

- Etiology
  - Unknown
  - Most cases not associated with autoimmune disease, immunodeficiency, or prior viral infection
    - Common associations with these entities in follicular bronchiolitis & LIP
- Formerly known as pseudolymphoma
  - Some cases of pseudolymphoma may have represented low-grade B-cell lymphoma of BALT
  - NLH considered reactive condition with specific histologic, immunophenotypic, & genotypic criteria
    - Immunohistochemical & molecular studies may be necessary for definitive diagnosis

Gross Pathologic & Surgical Features

- Well-circumscribed gray to white-tan nodule(s)
- Multiple nodules (~ 30%)
- Subpleural or peribronchial distribution
- Mediastinal &/or hilar lymphadenopathy (~ 30%)

Microscopic Features

- Abundant reactive germinal centers with sheets of interfollicular plasma cells
  - Reactive germinal centers may occur along alveolar septa
- Lymphoepithelial lesions
- Interfollicular fibrosis of variable degree often present
- Occasional giant cells (rare)
- Plaque-like pleural involvement

Immunohistochemical and Molecular Studies

- Reactive lymphoid follicles stain positive for B-cell markers (CD20, CD79-a)
- Intrafollicular lymphocytes stain positive for T-cell markers (CD3, CD43, CD5)
- Plasma cells are polyclonal on PCR analysis & stain positive for κ and λ light chains
- No coexpression of CD20 & CD43 by lymphocytes, unlike in cases of low-grade B-cell lymphoma

CLINICAL ISSUES

Presentation

- Most common signs/symptoms
  - Asymptomatic (most) with incidental lung nodule found on imaging
  - Cough
  - Dyspnea
  - Pleuritic chest pain

Demographics

- Age
  - Average: 60 years (range: 19-80 years)
- Gender
  - F:M = 4:3

Natural History & Prognosis

- Good prognosis

Treatment

- Surgical resection curative
- May regress without treatment

SELECTED REFERENCES

1. Guinee DG Jr: Update on nonneoplastic pulmonary lymphoproliferative disorders and related entities. Arch Pathol Lab Med. 134(5):691-701, 2010
2. Miyoshi S et al: A case of pulmonary nodular lymphoid hyperplasia with a resected cavity, followed by spontaneous regression of the remaining lesions. Intern Med. 49(15):1617-21, 2010
3. Kajiwara S et al: Multifocal nodular lymphoid hyperplasia of the lung. J Thorac Imaging. 20(3):239-41, 2005

POST-TRANSPLANT LYMPHOPROLIFERATIVE DISEASE (PTLD)

Key Facts

Terminology

- Post-transplant lymphoproliferative disease (PTLD)
- Disorder of B or T cells usually related to Ebstein-Barr virus (EBV) infection

Imaging

- Radiography
  - Nodule(s) (50%), may be multiple
  - Consolidations
  - Hilar & mediastinal lymphadenopathy (50%)
  - Associated pleural effusion
- CT
  - Identification of nodules & lymphadenopathy not visible on radiography
  - Nodules with low-density centers or CT halo sign
  - Mediastinal lymphadenopathy (50%)
- Nodules & consolidations, but most PTLD is either primarily nodular or primarily consolidative

Top Differential Diagnoses

- Fungal pneumonia
- Cryptogenic organizing pneumonia
- Lung cancer

Pathology

- Related to EBV infection: Immunosuppression allows proliferation of EBV-infected cells, may become monoclonal & malignant

Clinical Issues

- Intrathoracic involvement in 70%
- Most common in 1st year post transplantation
- Treatment: Reduction of immunosuppression (especially decreased cyclosporine dose)

Diagnostic Checklist

- Consider infection & lung cancer in transplant recipients with new lung masses/consolidations

*(**Left**) Axial CECT of a renal transplant recipient shows PTLD manifesting as borderline enlarged mediastinal lymph nodes. PTLD is limited to lymph nodes in approximately 1/3 of affected patients. (**Right**) Axial CECT of a double lung transplant recipient shows a large, low-attenuation mediastinal mass that produces mass effect on the ascending aorta and invades the right ventricular outflow tract. Mediastinal PTLD can range from focal or generalized lymphadenopathy to a large, infiltrating mass.*

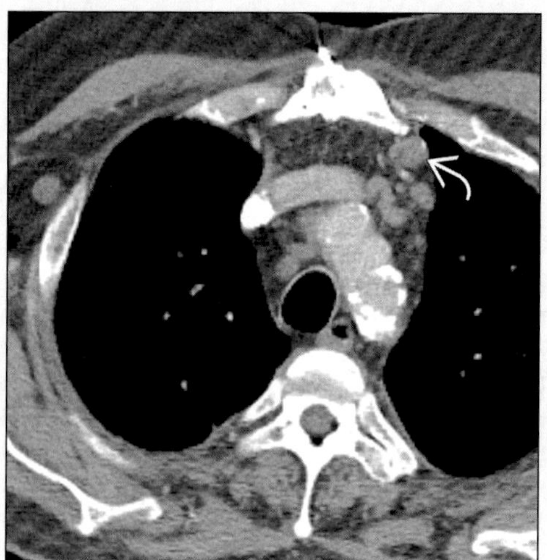

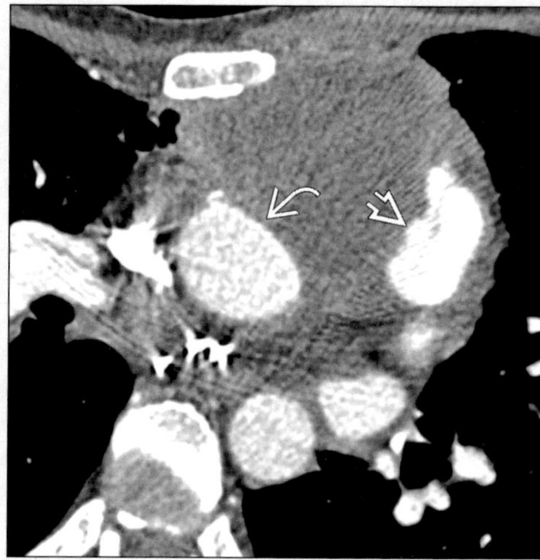

*(**Left**) Axial HRCT of a double lung transplant recipient shows a subpleural focus of nodular consolidation. Thoracic involvement is very common in patients with PTLD, with approximately 50% of affected patients having solitary or multiple lung nodules. (**Right**) Axial HRCT of a lung transplant recipient shows left lower lobe peripheral nodular consolidations. Other causes of lung consolidation, such as infection and organizing pneumonia, should also be considered in transplant recipients.*

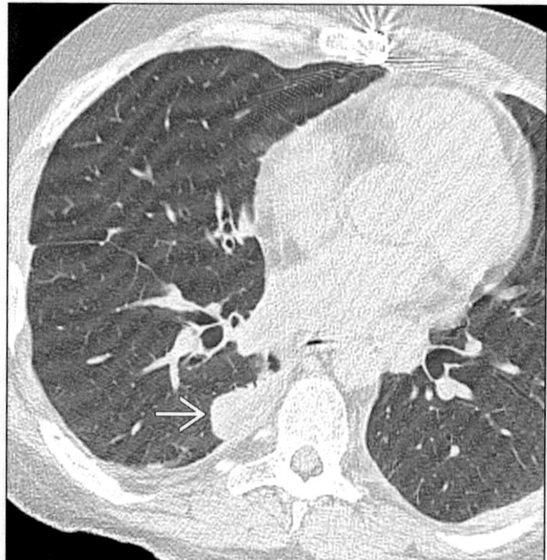

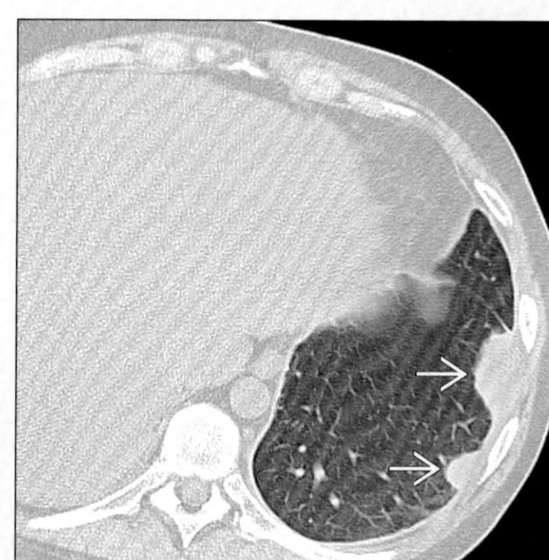

POST-TRANSPLANT LYMPHOPROLIFERATIVE DISEASE (PTLD)

TERMINOLOGY

Abbreviations

- **Post-transplant lymphoproliferative disease (PTLD)**

Definitions

- Post-transplantation **disorder of B or T cells** usually related to **Ebstein-Barr virus (EBV) infection**

IMAGING

General Features

- Best diagnostic clue
  - Lung nodules or consolidations & hilar/mediastinal lymphadenopathy
- Location
  - Lung & mediastinum most commonly affected
  - Other locations
    - Thymus, pericardium
    - Esophagus, abdominal organs
    - Tonsils, lymph nodes
- Size
  - Nodule(s) average 2 cm in size
- Morphology
  - Well-defined nodule(s), rarely cavitate

Radiographic Findings

- Radiography
  - **Nodule(s)**
    - **Solitary pulmonary nodule (50%)**
      - Well-circumscribed
      - 3 mm to 5 cm in size (average 2 cm)
      - Rarely cavitary
      - Variable distribution
      - Variable rate of growth, usually slow progression
    - **Multiple pulmonary nodules (50%)**
      - Similar features as solitary pulmonary nodule
- **Consolidation**
  - Multifocal consolidation (8%)
  - Usually subsegmental
  - Bronchovascular location with air bronchograms
  - Nodules & consolidation may coexist
    - Typically PTLD is either primarily nodular or primarily consolidative
- Thoracic lymph node involvement
  - Hilar & mediastinal lymphadenopathy (50%)
    - Typically paratracheal, anterior mediastinal, aortopulmonary window lymph nodes
    - Average size: 4 cm in diameter
    - Rarely large mass (10%) that encases mediastinal vessels
  - Lymph node involvement of bronchus-associated lymphoid tissue (BALT), airway narrowing
- Combination of lung nodules/consolidations & lymphadenopathy highly suggestive of PTLD
- Pleural involvement
  - Pleural effusions may accompany other forms of intrathoracic involvement
    - Not seen as isolated finding
- Resolution after treatment
  - Slowly over a period of weeks
  - Rarely rapidly over a few days

CT Findings

- CECT
  - Usually shows nodules & lymphadenopathy not apparent on radiography
  - **Nodules**
    - May exhibit low-density centers & occasionally CT halo sign
    - Usually located along peribronchovascular or subpleural regions
  - **Mediastinal lymphadenopathy (50%)**
    - Usually associated with either pulmonary nodules or consolidations
  - Ground-glass opacities, centrilobular nodules, & thin-walled cysts suggest lymphocytic interstitial pneumonia (LIP)
  - Thymic involvement rare, but relatively specific for PTLD
  - Pericardial thickening or effusion (10%)
  - Esophageal wall thickening

Nuclear Medicine Findings

- PET
  - Especially useful for evaluation of occult extranodal involvement

Imaging Recommendations

- Best imaging tool
  - CT useful for characterization of both lung abnormalities & extent of lymphadenopathy
- Protocol advice
  - CECT of neck, chest, abdomen, & pelvis: Widespread disease commonly involving multiple nodal & extranodal sites

DIFFERENTIAL DIAGNOSIS

Fungal Pneumonia

- Clinical symptoms of infection
- Commonly associated with pleural effusion
- Nodules less well defined & more commonly cavitary than in PTLD

Cryptogenic Organizing Pneumonia

- Often peripheral, peribronchial, & basilar distribution
- Focal rounded areas of parenchymal consolidation
- Air bronchograms common
- Good response to steroids

Lung Cancer

- Heterogeneously enhancing soft tissue mass on CECT
- May be indistinguishable from PTLD
- Biopsy often required to establish diagnosis

Diffuse Alveolar Hemorrhage

- Widespread parenchymal opacity, usually not nodular
- May be associated with hemoptysis & anemia

PATHOLOGY

General Features

- Etiology
  - Related to EBV infection
    - Immunosuppression with cyclosporine allows unrestricted proliferation of EBV-infected cells
    - May become monoclonal & malignant
  - EBV virus is a herpes virus
    - Nearly 100% of adult population seropositive

POST-TRANSPLANT LYMPHOPROLIFERATIVE DISEASE (PTLD)

- Causes clinical syndrome of infectious mononucleosis in adolescents & adults
- EBV seropositivity is most important risk factor for development of PTLD
- Risk of developing PTLD in EBV-positive donor & EBV-negative recipient, 25-50%

- PTLD thought to be stepwise progression from benign lymphoid polyclonal hyperplasia to frank lymphoma
  - Early diagnosis important before disease evolves into aggressive form
- **Extranodal (2/3 of patients)**
  - Head & neck: Waldeyer ring (nasopharyngeal, oropharyngeal, tonsils)
  - Esophageal/bowel wall thickening
  - Splenomegaly
  - Liver: Focal low-attenuation masses (1-4 cm in diameter) or diffuse hepatic infiltration
  - Central nervous system: Focal intraaxial masses
- Nodal (1/3 of patients)
  - Lymphadenopathy in any lymph node group: Retroperitoneal, mesenteric, axillary

Staging, Grading, & Classification

- Classification
  - Early (reactive hyperplasia)
  - Polymorphic (polyclonal)
  - Monomorphic (monoclonal B-cell or T-cell)
  - Lymphoma
    - Classic Hodgkin lymphoma
    - B-cell non-Hodgkin lymphoma
    - T-cell non-Hodgkin lymphoma

Gross Pathologic & Surgical Features

- Single organ or site (50%)
  - Brain (60%)
  - Individual abdominal organs (20%)
- Multiple sites (50%)

Microscopic Features

- Categories
  - Plasmacytic hyperplasia
    - Most common in oropharynx or lymph nodes
    - Usually polyclonal
  - Polymorphic B-cell hyperplasia & lymphoma
    - Lymph nodes or extranodal sites
    - Usually monoclonal
  - Immunoblastic lymphoma or multiple myeloma
    - Widespread disease
    - Monoclonal

CLINICAL ISSUES

Presentation

- Most common signs/symptoms
  - Infectious mononucleosis-like syndrome (20%)
  - Tonsillitis, sinusitis, otitis media
  - Lymphadenopathy
- Other signs/symptoms
  - Asymptomatic: Incidental finding on follow-up imaging

Demographics

- Age
  - Can occur at any age
    - Highest incidence in children
- Epidemiology
  - Intrathoracic involvement in 70%
  - Incidence varies based on type of transplant
    - Heart-lung & intestinal transplant (20%)
    - Heart, lung, pancreas, or liver transplants (3-8%)
    - Blood stem cell transplantation (donor B cells) or kidney transplants (< 1%)

Natural History & Prognosis

- Most common within 1st year after transplantation (60%)
- Uncommon 5 years after transplantation (< 10%)
- Lethal if untreated
  - Mortality 20%
- Poor prognostic factors
  - Early onset
  - Infectious mononucleosis presentation
  - Extent of disease
  - CNS involvement
  - Monoclonal tumor
  - T-cell origin (90% are of B-cell origin)

Treatment

- Reduction of immunosuppression (especially decreased cyclosporine dose)
  - May develop graft rejection with treatment of PTLD
  - May have to be retransplanted
- Rituximab if reduction in immunosuppression fails
- Antiviral drugs controversial
- Chemotherapy ± radiation therapy for aggressive disease

DIAGNOSTIC CHECKLIST

Consider

- Infection & lung cancer in transplant recipients with new lung masses/consolidations or intrathoracic lymphadenopathy

SELECTED REFERENCES

1. Blaes AH et al: Post-transplant lymphoproliferative disorders following solid-organ transplantation. Expert Rev Hematol. 3(1):35-44, 2010
2. DiNardo CD et al: Treatment advances in posttransplant lymphoproliferative disease. Curr Opin Hematol. 17(4):368-74, 2010
3. Evens AM et al: Post-transplantation lymphoproliferative disorders: diagnosis, prognosis, and current approaches to therapy. Curr Oncol Rep. 12(6):383-94, 2010
4. Borhani AA et al: Imaging of posttransplantation lymphoproliferative disorder after solid organ transplantation. Radiographics. 29(4):981-1000; discussion 1000-2, 2009
5. Scarsbrook AF et al: Post-transplantation lymphoproliferative disorder: the spectrum of imaging appearances. Clin Radiol. 60(1):47-55, 2005

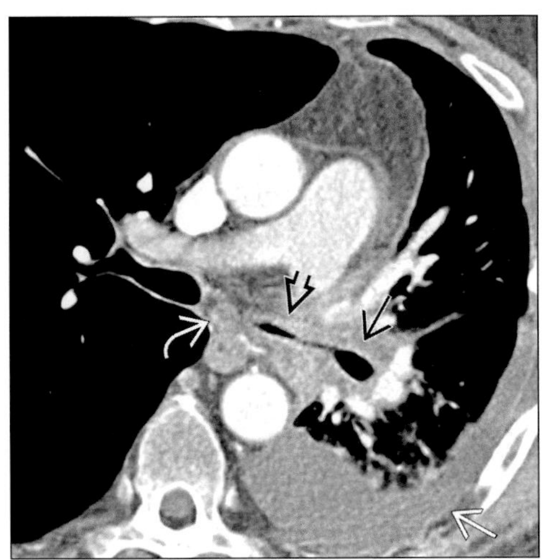

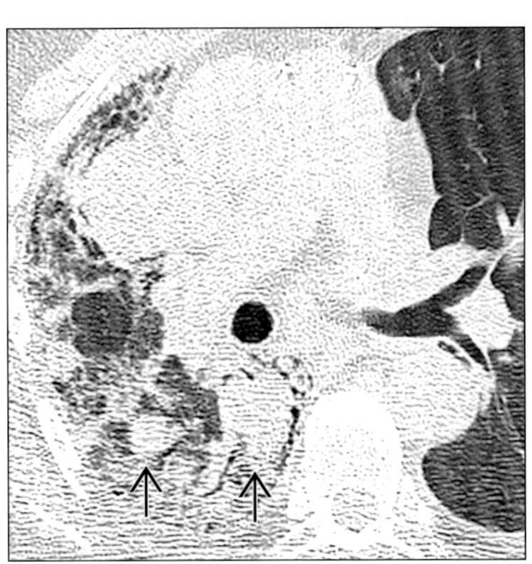

(Left) *Axial CECT of a lung transplant recipient shows PTLD manifesting as infiltrating soft tissue encasing the left main stem* ➪ *and lower lobe* ➔ *bronchi. Note the small right paraesophageal lymph node* ➦ *and the left pleural effusion* ➔*, which resulted from central pulmonary venous obstruction.* ***(Right)*** *Axial HRCT of a left lung transplant recipient shows PTLD manifesting as several large nodules* ➔ *in the native fibrotic right lung. Opportunistic fungal infection should also be considered.*

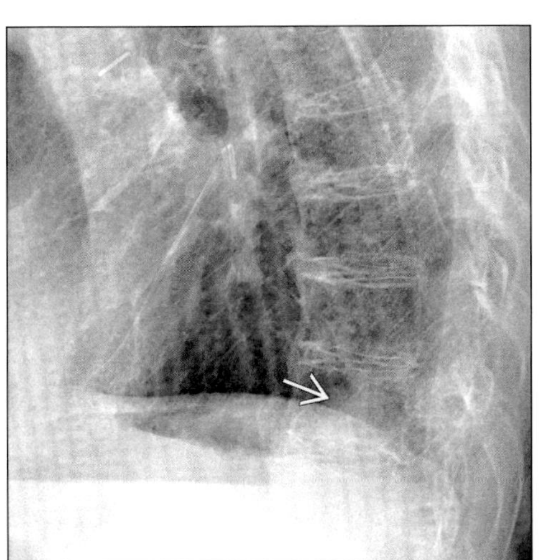

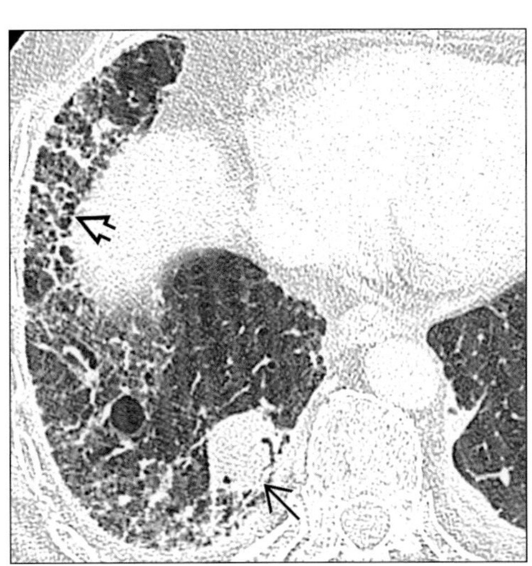

(Left) *Lateral chest radiograph of a patient who underwent single left lung transplantation for idiopathic pulmonary fibrosis shows a poorly defined lower lobe nodule* ➔*.* ***(Right)*** *Axial HRCT of the same patient shows PTLD manifesting as a large right lower lobe soft tissue nodule* ➔ *with intrinsic air bronchograms. Note subpleural honeycomb lung* ➪ *from end-stage fibrosis. Primary lung cancer and fungal infection should also be considered in this patient.*

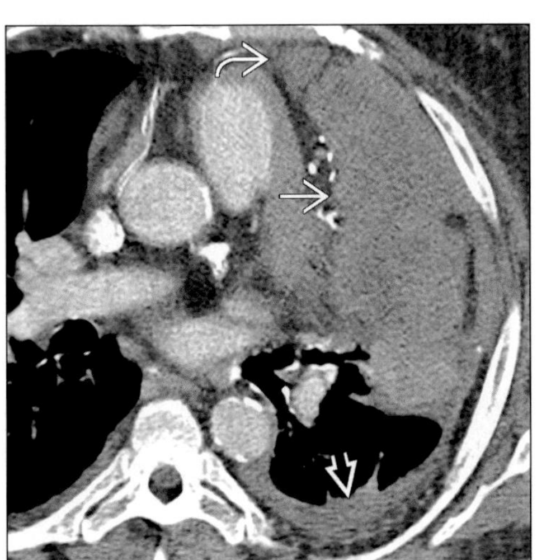

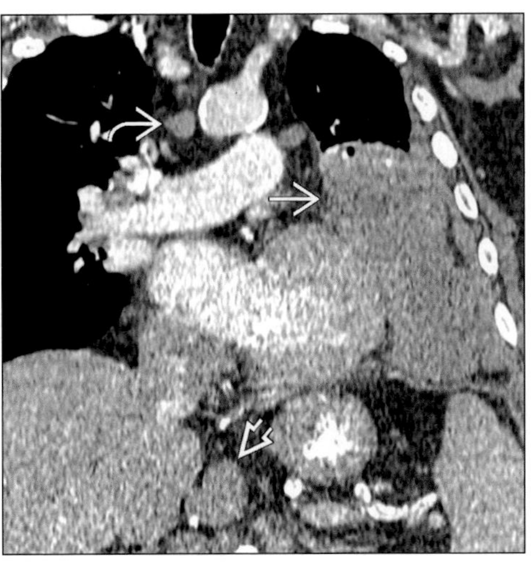

(Left) *Axial CECT of a renal transplant recipient shows PTLD manifesting as a large, heterogeneous soft tissue mass* ➔ *in the left hemithorax. Note the large left pericardiophrenic lymph node* ➦ *and the small left pleural effusion* ➪*.* ***(Right)*** *Coronal CECT of the same patient shows the large left hemithorax soft tissue mass* ➔ *as well as mediastinal* ➦ *and retroperitoneal* ➪ *lymphadenopathy. The anatomic extent of PTLD significantly affects the prognosis.*

PULMONARY NON-HODGKIN LYMPHOMA

Key Facts

Terminology
- Non-Hodgkin lymphoma (NHL)
- Pulmonary involvement by NHL: Hematogenous, contiguous invasion, primary pulmonary lymphoma

Imaging
- Radiography
  - Single or multiple nodules & masses
  - Consolidation or ground-glass opacities
- CT
  - Single or multiple nodules & masses
  - Airspace consolidation, ground-glass opacity
  - Peribronchovascular and subpleural distribution
  - ± air bronchogram
  - ± cavitation
- PET
  - Staging & monitoring response to treatment
  - Low-grade lymphoma not always FDG avid

Top Differential Diagnoses
- Pulmonary nodules
  - Septic emboli, fungal infection, metastases
- Peribronchovascular, subpleural opacities
  - Sarcoidosis, organizing pneumonia
- Consolidation
  - Pneumonia, organizing pneumonia, lung cancer

Clinical Issues
- Treatment
  - Pulmonary resection for localized disease
  - Chemotherapy
- Presentation & prognosis widely variable

Diagnostic Checklist
- Consider pulmonary lymphoma in patients with chronic multifocal nodules, masses, or consolidations not responsive to antimicrobials

__(Left)__ PA chest radiograph of a patient who presented with chest tightness shows bilateral consolidations that persisted despite antibiotic therapy. __(Right)__ Axial CECT of the same patient confirms middle and right lower lobe consolidations with intrinsic air bronchograms. Surgical biopsy revealed MALT lymphoma, which was treated with combination chemotherapy. The patient remains disease free 8 years later. Airway dilatation within lymphoma lesions on CT is considered a good prognostic sign for MALT lymphoma.

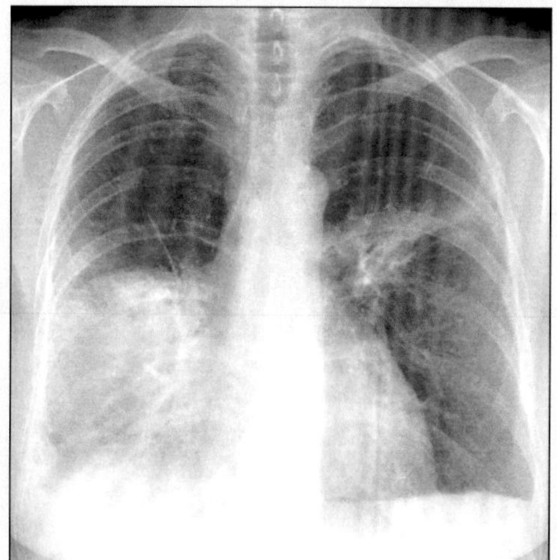

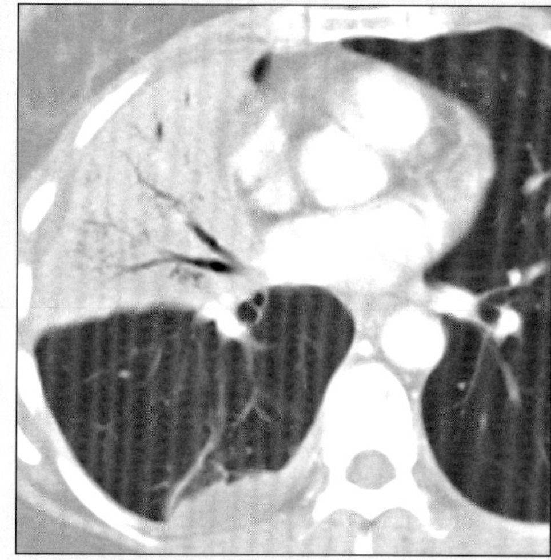

__(Left)__ Axial CECT of a patient with relapsed gastric MALT lymphoma shows bilateral dense consolidations with intrinsic air bronchograms ⇒, ground-glass opacities, and interlobular septal thickening. __(Right)__ Axial CECT of a patient with relapsed angioimmunoblastic T-cell lymphoma shows multiple bilateral subpleural and peribronchovascular lung nodules ➡. Pulmonary involvement as part of disseminated or recurrent lymphoma is more common than primary pulmonary lymphoma.

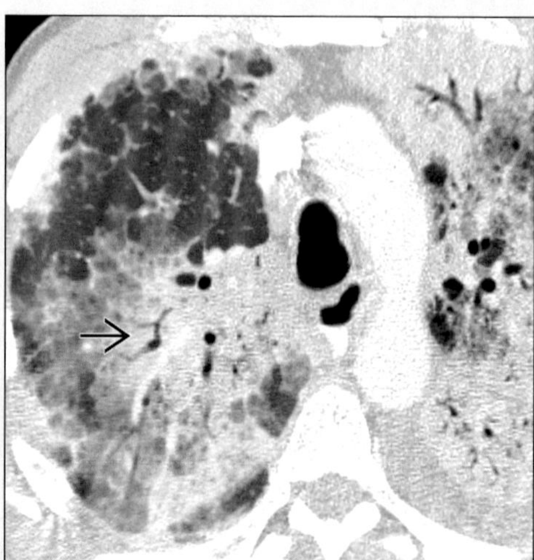

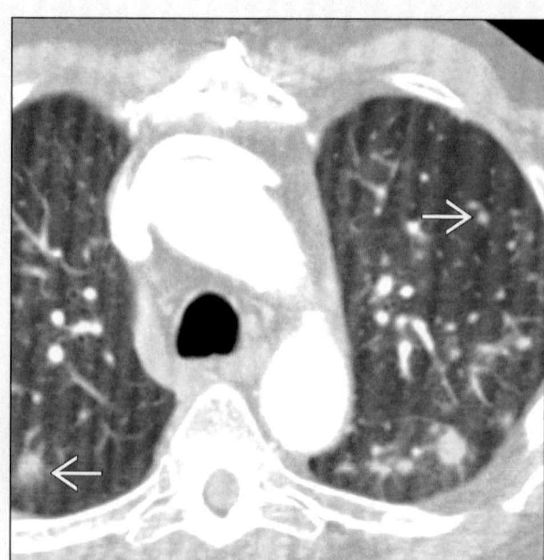

PULMONARY NON-HODGKIN LYMPHOMA

TERMINOLOGY

Abbreviations

- **Non-Hodgkin lymphoma (NHL)**
- **Primary pulmonary lymphoma (PPL)**
- **Mucosa-associated lymphoid tissue (MALT)**
- **Lymphomatoid granulomatosis (LG)**

Synonyms

- Low-grade primary pulmonary B-cell lymphoma
- Formerly called "pseudolymphoma"

Definitions

- NHL accounts for 85-90% of all lymphomas & 40-45% of patients with NHL have intrathoracic disease at presentation
- NHL can involve lungs in 3 ways
  - Hematogenous dissemination of NHL
  - Contiguous invasion from hilar or mediastinal lymph nodes
  - **Primary pulmonary NHL** (0.4% of all lymphomas): Clonal lymphoid proliferation affecting 1 or both lungs in patient with no detectable extrapulmonary involvement at diagnosis or during subsequent 3 months

IMAGING

General Features

- Location
  - Pulmonary involvement more often represents disseminated or recurrent disease than primary lymphoma
  - Reflects distribution of pulmonary lymphatics: Along bronchovascular bundles, interlobular septa, & subpleural regions

Radiographic Findings

- Radiography
  - Single or multiple lung nodules & masses
  - Consolidations or ground-glass opacities
  - Associated mediastinal or hilar lymphadenopathy
  - Pleural effusions

CT Findings

- Solitary or multiple **pulmonary nodules/masses**
  - Well-defined or ill-defined margins
  - ± cavitation
  - ± air bronchograms
- **Airspace opacity**
  - **Consolidation with air bronchogram**
  - Ground-glass opacities ± interlobular septal thickening
  - Ill-defined opacities along bronchovascular bundles & interlobular septa
  - Atelectasis or postobstructive pneumonia due to airway obstruction/compression by adjacent lymphadenopathy
- Endobronchial tumor (rarely)
  - Lobar collapse
- Enlarged lymph nodes or mediastinal mass
- Pleural effusion
- Features of specific subtypes of primary pulmonary lymphoma; in addition to imaging findings described above
  - **MALT lymphoma**
    - Bilateral, multiple nodular opacities
    - Dilated bronchi; considered good prognostic sign
    - Reticular opacities
  - **High-grade B-cell lymphoma**
    - Subpleural, peribronchial opacities
  - **Primary pulmonary plasmacytoma**
    - Solitary pulmonary nodule most common
  - **Pulmonary intravascular lymphoma**
    - Normal-appearing CT
    - Mild ground-glass or reticular opacities
  - **Lymphomatoid granulomatosis**
    - Multiple lower lobe predominant nodules or masses
      - Central low attenuation or cavitation
      - Peripheral enhancement
      - Halo sign

Imaging Recommendations

- Best imaging tool
  - PET/CT provides comprehensive assessment of disease extent during staging & restaging

Nuclear Medicine Findings

- PET
  - Increased FDG uptake at sites of lymphoma involvement
    - Detection of lymphoma in normal-sized lymph nodes
    - Detection of extranodal disease
      - Particularly helpful in detecting pulmonary intravascular lymphoma where CT findings can be minimal or absent
    - Monitor treatment response
      - Better than CT in differentiating viable tumor from post-treatment necrosis & fibrosis
  - Variable uptake, some low-grade lymphomas are not FDG avid

DIFFERENTIAL DIAGNOSIS

Pulmonary Nodules

- Fungal infection
- Septic emboli
- Metastatic disease
- Wegener granulomatosis
  - May mimic lymphomatoid granulomatosis

Peribronchovascular, Subpleural Opacities

- Sarcoidosis
- Organizing pneumonia
  - Reverse halo sign seen in both organizing pneumonia & lymphoma & alveolar sarcoidosis
- Nonspecific interstitial pneumonia
  - Traction bronchiectasis helpful if present

Consolidation

- Pneumonia
  - Persistence of consolidation after appropriate antibiotic treatment should prompt further diagnostic work-up
- Organizing pneumonia
- Pulmonary hemorrhage
- Lung cancer

PULMONARY NON-HODGKIN LYMPHOMA

PATHOLOGY

General Features

- Etiology
  - **Bronchial MALT lymphoma**: Chronic antigenic stimulation in autoimmune disorders
    - Sjögren syndrome
    - Systemic lupus erythematosus
    - Multiple sclerosis
  - High-grade B-cell primary pulmonary NHL
    - Solid organ transplantation with immunosuppression
    - Human immunodeficiency virus (HIV) infection
    - Sjögren syndrome
    - Epstein-Barr virus (EBV) infection

Staging, Grading, & Classification

- Low-grade B-cell NHL: 58-87% of PPL
  - Bronchial MALT lymphoma accounts for 90%
  - Follicular lymphoma
  - Mantle lymphocytic lymphoma
- High-grade B-cell NHL: 11-19% of PPL
  - Diffuse large B-cell NHL most common
- Primary pulmonary plasmocytoma: Extremely rare
- Pulmonary intravascular lymphoma: Extremely rare
- Lymphomatoid granulomatosis (LG)
  - Rare, angiocentric, Epstein-Barr virus (EBV)-positive B-cell lymphoproliferative disease with reactive T cells

Microscopic Features

- Absence of Reed-Sternberg cells
- **Clonal proliferation of either T- or B-cell origin**
- Immunohistochemical analysis helpful for confirmation & classification
- Low-grade B-cell NHL
  - Proliferation of small lymphoid cells analogous to marginal zone cells of Peyer patches or spleen follicles
- High-grade B-cell NHL
  - Blast-like lymphoid cells with strong mitotic activity
- Primary pulmonary plasmacytoma
  - Plasmacytes with variable cytologic anomalies
- Pulmonary intravascular lymphoma
  - Atypical lymphoid cells within capillaries, arterioles, venules, & lymph ducts with little or no invasion of adjacent lung
- Lymphomatoid granulomatosis
  - Angioinvasive lymphoid infiltration composed of lymphocytes, plasma cells, & histiocytes
  - Grading based on number of neoplastic large B cells & degree of cytological atypia
  - Grade 3 lesion treated as large B-cell lymphoma

CLINICAL ISSUES

Low-grade B-cell NHL

- Nearly 1/2 asymptomatic, incidental imaging abnormality
- Cough, mild dyspnea
- Age at diagnosis: 50-60 years
- Diagnosis: Transbronchial biopsy + bronchoalveolar lavage, transthoracic needle biopsy, or surgery
- Treatment
  - Surgical resection for localized disease
  - Chemotherapy: 1 or multiple agents
- 5-year survival > 80%, mean survival > 10 years

High-grade B-cell NHL

- Dyspnea, fever, weight loss
- Age at onset ~ 60 years
- Diagnosis: Transbronchial or transthoracic biopsy
- Treatment
  - Surgical resection
  - Combination chemotherapy
- Mean survival ~ 8-10 years, lower in transplant recipients & patients with HIV

Primary Pulmonary Plasmacytoma

- Usually asymptomatic
- Age at onset ~ 40 years
- Diagnosis: Usually requires surgical resection
- Treatment
  - Surgery
  - If surgery contraindicated, radiation therapy
- 5-year survival: 40%
  - 15-30% develop multiple myeloma

Pulmonary Intravascular Lymphoma

- Fever & hypoxemia
- Diagnosis: Transbronchial or surgical biopsy
- Treatment: Combination chemotherapy
- Complete response rate ~ 50%

Lymphomatoid Granulomatosis

- Fever, weight loss, cough, dyspnea
- Age ~ 30-50 years
- Can also involve skin, nervous system
- Diagnosis: Requires surgical biopsy
- Treatment: Chemotherapy
- Prognosis widely variable; poor for high-grade lesions

DIAGNOSTIC CHECKLIST

Consider

- Pulmonary lymphoma in patients with chronic multifocal nodules, masses, or consolidations not responsive to antimicrobials

SELECTED REFERENCES

1. Niida T et al: Pulmonary intravascular lymphoma diagnosed by 18-fluorodeoxyglucose positron emission tomography-guided transbronchial lung biopsy in a man with long-term survival: a case report. J Med Case Reports. 5(1):295, 2011
2. Katzenstein AL et al: Lymphomatoid granulomatosis: insights gained over 4 decades. Am J Surg Pathol. 34(12):e35-48, 2010
3. Chua SC et al: Imaging features of primary extranodal lymphomas. Clin Radiol. 64(6):574-88, 2009
4. Bae YA et al: Cross-sectional evaluation of thoracic lymphoma. Radiol Clin North Am. 46(2):253-64, viii, 2008

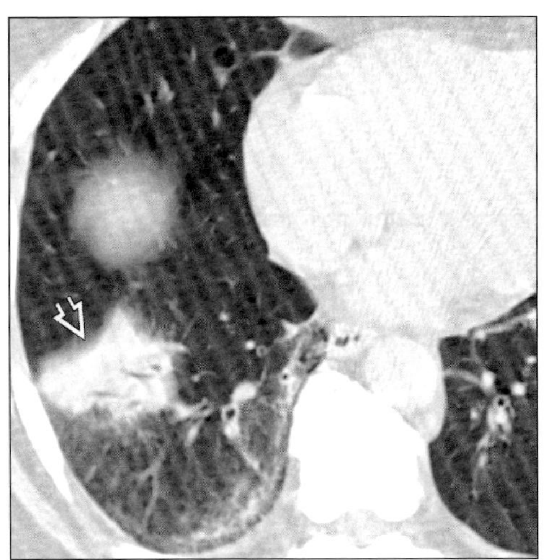

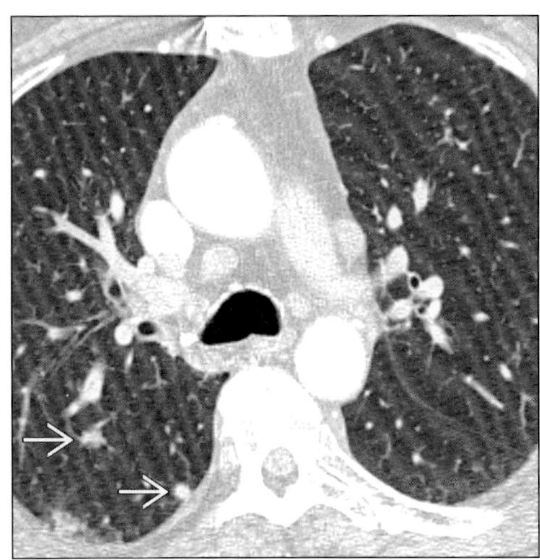

(Left) *Axial NECT of a patient with dry cough shows a nodular consolidation ➡ in the right lower lobe proven to represent a MALT lymphoma. The patient was treated with a right lower lobectomy.* ***(Right)*** *Axial CECT performed for melanoma staging shows bilateral peribronchovascular and subpleural nodules ➡ proven to represent MALT lymphoma. The nodules remained stable without treatment for over 7 years. Primary pulmonary MALT lymphoma has a variable clinical presentation and course.*

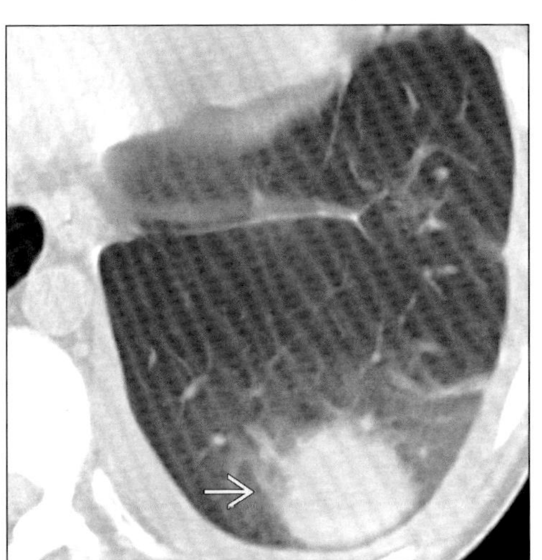

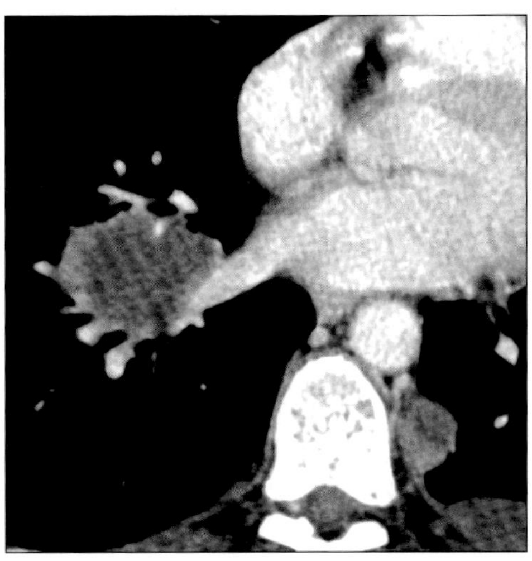

(Left) *Axial NECT of a lung transplant recipient shows multiple nodules and a dominant left lower lobe mass with a peripheral ground-glass halo ➡. Surgical biopsy revealed a high-grade B-cell lymphoma, which is more commonly seen in immunosuppressed patients.* ***(Right)*** *Axial CECT of a patient with lymphomatoid granulomatosis shows a right peribronchovascular mass and a left lower lobe subpleural nodule that exhibit peripheral enhancement and central low attenuation.*

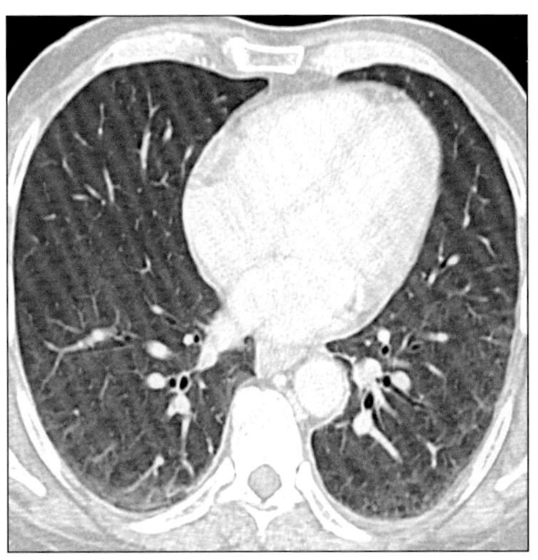

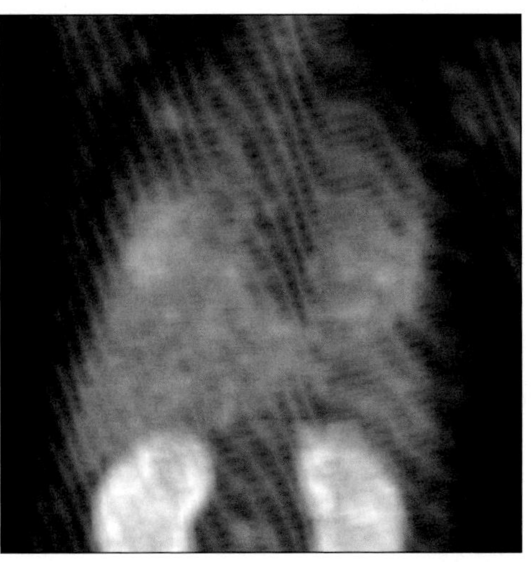

(Left) *Axial CECT of a patient who presented with fever and progressive dyspnea shows mild bilateral diffuse ground-glass opacities.* ***(Right)*** *Coronal FDG PET of same patient shows diffuse uptake in both lungs. Surgical wedge biopsy revealed pulmonary intravascular lymphoma. CT of patients with pulmonary intravascular NHL is frequently normal or may show only minimal abnormality. PET is helpful for detection of abnormal FDG uptake within the lungs and for directing biopsy.*

PULMONARY HODGKIN LYMPHOMA

Key Facts

Terminology
- Hodgkin lymphoma (HL)
- Cancer of lymphatic system: Systemic disease

Imaging
- Radiography
  - 65-75% of affected patients have abnormal chest radiographs at presentation
  - Most common: Multiple nodules & masses
  - Lobar consolidation
  - Reticulation & bronchovascular thickening
  - Pleural effusions (15%)
- CT
  - Ill- or well-defined lung nodules: Unilateral or bilateral
  - Cavitary nodules (10-20%)
  - Almost always associated with mediastinal &/or hilar lymphadenopathy

Top Differential Diagnoses
- Pulmonary metastases
- Pneumonia
- Wegener granulomatosis
- Septic emboli

Pathology
- Reed-Sternberg cell
- Staging: Ann Arbor classification

Clinical Issues
- Presentation
  - Asymptomatic cervical or supraclavicular lymphadenopathy
  - Splenomegaly
  - B symptoms
- Bimodal age distribution: 3rd & 6th decades
- Good prognosis generally

__(Left)__ PA chest radiograph of a patient with Hodgkin lymphoma shows multiple pulmonary nodular and mass-like opacities ➔. __(Right)__ Axial CECT of the same patient shows bilateral lung nodules and masses, some of which exhibit cavitation ➔. Cavitary nodules and masses occur in a minority of patients with pulmonary HL and are a nonspecific finding, as they may also occur in patients with fungal pneumonia, septic emboli, pulmonary metastases, and pulmonary vasculitis.

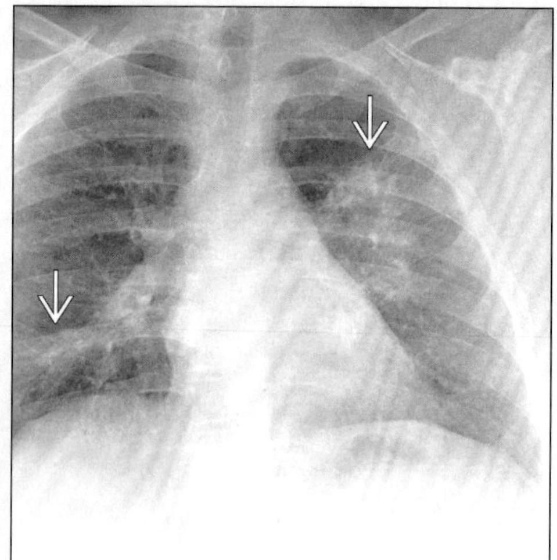

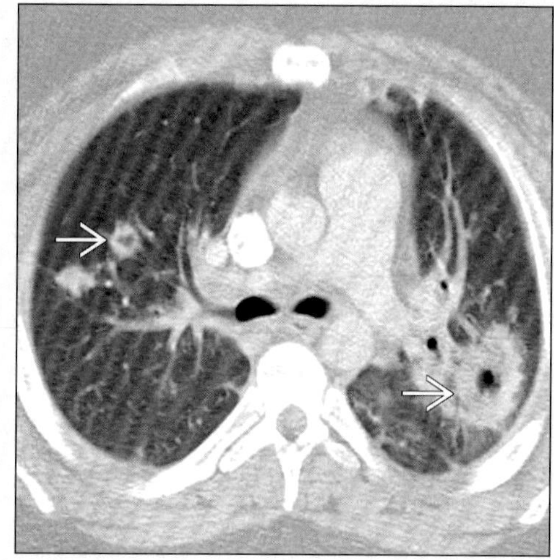

__(Left)__ Axial CECT of a patient with pulmonary Hodgkin lymphoma shows bilateral lung nodules, one of which exhibits intrinsic cavitation ➔. Note associated mediastinal lymphadenopathy ➔. __(Right)__ Axial CECT of the same patient shows hilar ➔ and mediastinal → lymphadenopathy and a dominant left upper lobe pulmonary nodule ➔ with irregular margins. Pulmonary Hodgkin lymphoma occurs almost exclusively in association with mediastinal or hilar lymphadenopathy.

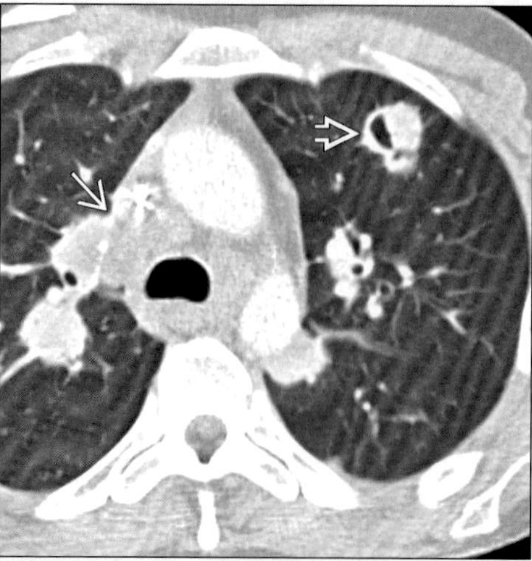

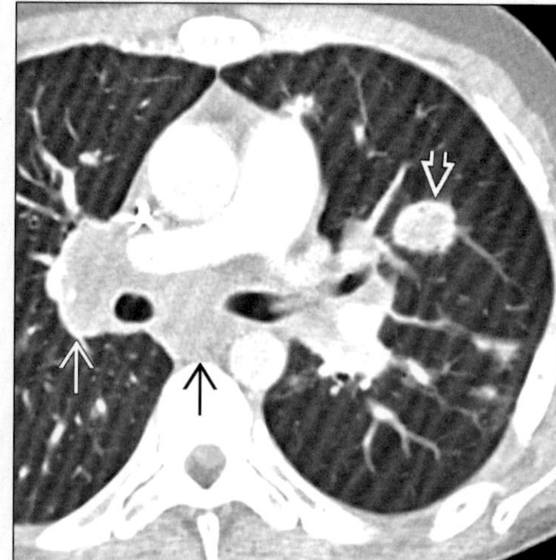

PULMONARY HODGKIN LYMPHOMA

TERMINOLOGY

Abbreviations

- **Hodgkin lymphoma** (HL)

Definitions

- Cancer of lymphatic system: Systemic disease

IMAGING

General Features

- Best diagnostic clue
  - Multiple pulmonary nodules or masses
    - Often irregularly marginated

Radiographic Findings

- Radiography
  - 65-75% of patients with HL have abnormal chest radiographs (typically lymph node involvement)
  - Most common pattern of lung involvement: **Multiple pulmonary nodules & masses**
  - Lobar **consolidation**
  - Reticulation & bronchovascular thickening
    - Obstruction of lymphatic or pulmonary veins from central nodal disease
    - Direct lymphomatous infiltration of pulmonary lymphatics
  - Pleural effusions (15%)

CT Findings

- CECT
  - Ill-defined or well-defined **pulmonary nodules or masses: Unilateral or bilateral**
    - Cavitary nodules (10-20%)
    - Almost always associated with mediastinal &/or hilar lymphadenopathy
  - Lobar consolidation
  - Endobronchial nodule or mass
    - Postobstructive volume loss
    - Postobstructive pneumonia
  - Reticulation & bronchovascular thickening
  - Miliary or perilymphatic pattern (rare)

Nuclear Medicine Findings

- PET
  - Variable FDG uptake
  - In cases of avid FDG uptake, degree of FDG uptake decreases with successful treatment

Imaging Recommendations

- Best imaging tool
  - PET/CT is modality of choice for initial staging & follow-up of patients with HL

DIFFERENTIAL DIAGNOSIS

Pulmonary Nodules

- Wide differential diagnosis
- Pulmonary metastases
  - Cavitary: Squamous cell carcinoma, sarcoma, transitional cell carcinoma
- Infection
- Wegener granulomatosis
- Septic emboli

Consolidation

- Pneumonia
- Organizing pneumonia
- Pulmonary hemorrhage
- Low-grade adenocarcinoma in setting of chronic disease

Reticulation & Bronchovascular Thickening

- Lymphangitic carcinomatosis
- Sarcoidosis

PATHOLOGY

Staging, Grading, & Classification

- Hodgkin lymphoma: Nodular sclerosis (70%); mixed cellularity (20%); lymphocytic predominant (5%); lymphocytic depleted (5%)
- Staging: Ann Arbor classification

Microscopic Features

- Reed-Sternberg cell

CLINICAL ISSUES

Presentation

- Most common signs/symptoms
  - Asymptomatic cervical or supraclavicular lymphadenopathy
- Other signs/symptoms
  - Cough or chest pain from mediastinal involvement
  - Splenomegaly, B symptoms

Demographics

- Age
  - Bimodal distribution
    - In industrialized nations: 1st peak is 20 years of age, while 2nd peak is 55 years or older
- Epidemiology
  - Link between HL & certain viral illnesses: Epstein-Barr virus, human herpes virus 6

Natural History & Prognosis

- Prognosis generally good

Treatment

- Treatment depends on histologic subtype, stage of disease, & age of patient
  - Standard treatment of early stage Hodgkin lymphoma: Chemotherapy & irradiation
- Bone marrow transplant

DIAGNOSTIC CHECKLIST

Image Interpretation Pearls

- Intrathoracic HL is usually associated with mediastinal lymph node involvement

SELECTED REFERENCES

1. Bae YA et al: Cross-sectional evaluation of thoracic lymphoma. Radiol Clin North Am. 46(2):253-64, viii, 2008

HEMATOGENOUS METASTASES

Key Facts

Terminology

- Distant spread of cancer hematogenously to lungs
- Lung most common site of metastases: 50% at autopsy

Imaging

- Radiography
  - Multiple well-defined lung nodules/masses
  - Variably sized: Miliary to "cannonball"
  - Preferential involvement of lung bases & periphery
- CT
  - Highly sensitive (> 90%) for nodules
  - Multifocal, well-defined lung nodules/masses
  - Most metastases in outer 1/3 of lung
  - Hematogenous nodules often have feeding artery
  - Halo sign in hemorrhagic metastases
  - Beaded, enlarged vessels & branching opacities suggest tumor emboli

Top Differential Diagnoses

- Multiple pulmonary nodules
  - Granulomas
  - Infection
  - Arteriovenous malformations (AVMs)
  - Wegener granulomatosis
- Chronic consolidation
  - Adenocarcinoma
  - Organizing pneumonia

Clinical Issues

- Symptoms/signs: Variable, may be asymptomatic
- Generally poor prognosis

Diagnostic Checklist

- Consider metastatic disease in differential diagnosis of multifocal lung nodules, masses, or consolidations in patients with malignancy

(Left) PA chest radiograph of a 49-year-old woman with metastatic breast cancer shows innumerable lower lobe predominant small pulmonary nodules. Hematogenous metastases are often lower lobe predominant due to the dominant blood flow in the lung. *(Right)* Coronal CECT of the same patient shows innumerable well-defined and coalescent lung nodules of various sizes with lower lobe predominance. Breast and colon cancers are the most common primary tumors that produce hematogenous metastases.

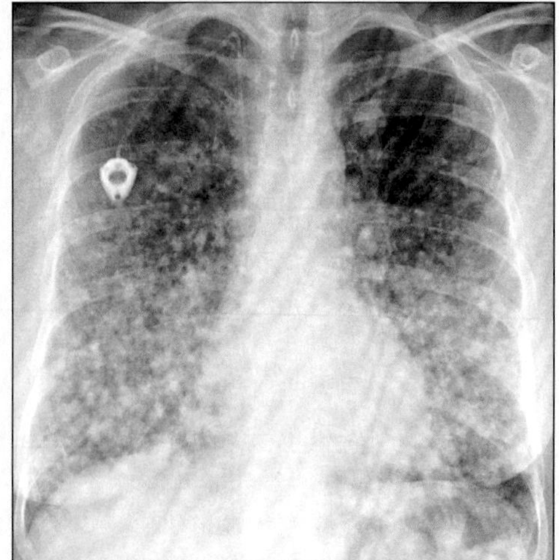

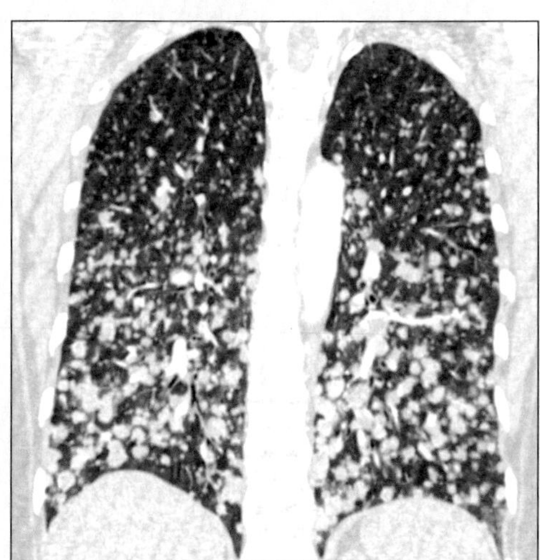

(Left) Graphic shows typical morphologic features of hematogenous pulmonary metastases with multifocal pulmonary nodules of various sizes predominantly affecting the peripheral lower lung zones. *(Right)* PA chest radiograph of a 34-year-old woman with metastatic alveolar soft part sarcoma shows multiple well-circumscribed masses ➡ in the left mid and lower lung zones, consistent with "cannonball" metastases. This patient also has metastatic disease to the heart and pericardium ➡.

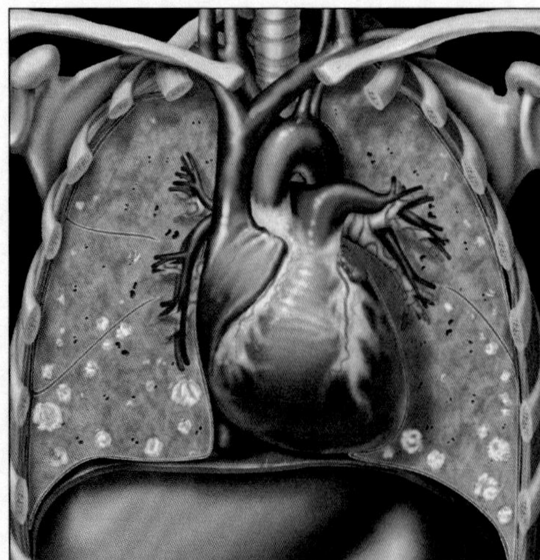

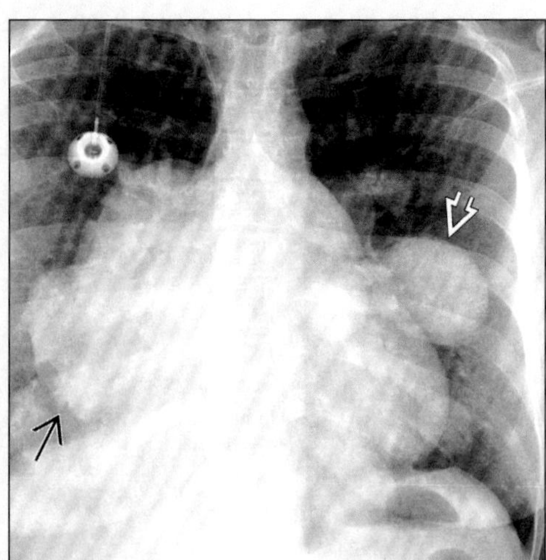

HEMATOGENOUS METASTASES

TERMINOLOGY

Definitions

- Distant spread of cancer hematogenously to lungs
- Lung most common site of metastases: 50% at autopsy

IMAGING

General Features

- Best diagnostic clue
  - Variably sized, sharply defined multiple pulmonary nodules
- Location
  - Hematogenous metastases most common in lung bases & lung periphery
  - Branching opacities & peribronchovascular irregular nodularity suggest tumor emboli

Radiographic Findings

- Multifocal lung nodules, masses, or consolidations
  - Rarely, focal disease or solitary nodule
- Variable sizes; well- or ill-defined borders
- Preferential involvement of lower lung zones
- May exhibit cavitation
- Endobronchial metastases may manifest with post-obstructive atelectasis or consolidation
- May exhibit associated mediastinal/hilar lymphadenopathy &/or pleural effusion

CT Findings

- Multifocal, well-defined pulmonary nodules/masses
  - Solitary metastasis: Renal cell, colon, & breast cancers, sarcoma, melanoma
- Most metastases in outer 1/3 of lung
- **Vascular pattern**
  - Hematogenous spread
  - Sharply defined, variably sized, spherical lung nodules
  - Ill-defined margins in hemorrhagic metastases (choriocarcinoma, renal cell carcinoma, melanoma)
    - May exhibit halo sign (solid nodule surrounded by ground-glass opacity)
  - Preferential lower lobe involvement due to gravitational forces & dominant blood flow
  - 80% located within 2 cm of pleura
  - Cavitation common in squamous cell cancers & sarcomas
  - **Miliary pattern**: Medullary thyroid carcinoma, melanoma, renal cell carcinoma, ovarian carcinoma
  - **"Cannonball" metastases**: Colorectal carcinoma, renal cell carcinoma, sarcoma, melanoma
  - Some metastases may **calcify** (osteosarcoma, chondrosarcoma, thyroid) & may mimic granulomas
  - Occasionally associated with spontaneous pneumothorax, especially in sarcomas
  - Hematogenous nodules often exhibit feeding artery
- **Endobronchial pattern**
  - Bronchogenic airway seeding or hematogenous dissemination to airway wall
  - Lung, lobar, or segmental atelectasis
  - Post-obstructive pneumonia: Segmental, lobar, lung
  - Adenocarcinoma, basal cell carcinoma of head/neck, breast & renal cancers, sarcoma
- **Pleural pattern**
  - Lymphangitic or hematogenous spread
  - Pleural effusion may be massive, free, or loculated
  - Discrete pleural nodules/masses
- **Consolidative pattern**
  - Hematogenous spread
  - Mimics pneumonia, peripheral consolidation with air-bronchograms
  - Lepidic growth of adenocarcinoma
- **Tumor embolus pattern**
  - Hematogenous spread
  - **Beaded, enlarged vessels or irregular, nodular opacities along bronchovascular structures**
  - Mass conforming to vascular shape or branching
  - Pulmonary infarction
- **Lymph node involvement**: Mediastinal or hilar mass
  - Hematogenous or lymphangitic spread
  - Common in genitourinary (prostate, renal, ovarian, testicular, transitional cell), head/neck, breast cancers & melanoma

Nuclear Medicine Findings

- PET/CT
  - CT highly sensitive (> 90%) for nodules & findings of metastatic disease

Imaging Recommendations

- Best imaging tool
  - **PET/CT most sensitive examination; optimally characterizes pattern & extent of disease**

DIFFERENTIAL DIAGNOSIS

Multiple Pulmonary Nodules

- Granulomas
  - Often exhibit benign patterns of calcification
  - Associated with calcifications in liver & spleen
  - Bone-forming primary tumor metastases may mimic granulomas
- Infection
  - Miliary tuberculosis, viral pneumonia
  - Septic emboli often cavitate
- Arteriovenous malformations (AVMs)
  - Feeding arteries & draining veins
- Wegener granulomatosis
  - Usually cavitary
  - May be associated with subglottic stenosis & pulmonary hemorrhage

Endobronchial Mass

- Lung cancer
  - Associated with regional lymphadenopathy
  - More common than endobronchial metastasis
  - Smoking history
- Broncholith
  - Calcified endobronchial nodule
- Foreign body
  - Most common endobronchial lesion in children

Interstitial Lung Disease

- Sarcoidosis
  - Perilymphatic micronodules
  - Frequent lymphadenopathy
  - Miliary nodules described
- Silicosis
  - May exhibit multiple pulmonary nodules
- Scleroderma & other collagen vascular diseases
  - Septa smooth, not beaded

HEMATOGENOUS METASTASES

- Associated bone changes (rheumatoid) or esophageal dilatation (scleroderma)

Chronic Consolidation

- Adenocarcinoma
  - Septa usually not involved
  - Lobular ground-glass pattern in multiple lobes coalescing to frank consolidation
- Organizing pneumonia
  - Subpleural basilar distribution
- Pulmonary alveolar proteinosis
  - Geographic distribution of ground-glass opacities, interlobular & intralobular lines (crazy-paving pattern)

Primary Malignancies

- Lung cancer
  - Large solitary mass, may obstruct airways & vascular structures
- Lymphoma
  - Multifocal pulmonary nodules ± lymphadenopathy
  - Common in patients with HIV

Pulmonary Embolus

- Transient, acute symptoms
- Will not significantly distend vessel if acute

Pulmonary Artery Sarcoma

- Common location in pulmonary trunk
- Solitary, not multiple

PATHOLOGY

General Features

- Etiology
  - Pathology reflects metastatic route
  - Metastatic models
    - Mechanical anatomic model: Metastases filtered in first draining organ, commonly the lung
    - Environmental model: Metastases preferentially find target sites due to favorable molecular or cellular environments, "seed & soil" hypothesis
  - Most likely extrathoracic malignancies: Breast, colon, uterine
  - **Highest rate of lung metastases: Choriocarcinoma, osteosarcoma, testicular tumors, melanoma**
- Associated abnormalities
  - Frequent lytic or sclerotic skeletal metastases depending on tumor extent & cell type

Staging, Grading, & Classification

- Generally regarded as stage IV for most tumor staging

Gross Pathologic & Surgical Features

- Lepidic growth
  - Distal arteriole seeding, growth in interstitium & alveoli
  - No architectural distortion
  - Tumor uses lung as a scaffolding to grow
  - Typical of adenocarcinoma
- Hilic growth
  - Tumor replaces normal lung
  - Typical of hematogenous metastases

Microscopic Features

- Tumor cells invade draining venules, enter venous circulation
- Typical of primary tumor

CLINICAL ISSUES

Presentation

- Most common signs/symptoms
  - Variable, depends on pattern of spread
  - May be asymptomatic

Demographics

- Age
  - Any age but more common in adults
- Epidemiology
  - **Metastasis most common lung neoplasm**
  - Vascular pattern typical of carcinomas (lung, breast, gastrointestinal tract tumors) & sarcomas
  - Pleural pattern typical of adenocarcinomas, especially lung & breast
  - Consolidative pattern typical of gastrointestinal adenocarcinoma & lymphoma
  - Pulmonary embolus pattern typical of hepatocellular, breast, & renal cell carcinomas, choriocarcinoma, angiosarcoma
  - Bronchogenic pattern typical of adenocarcinoma (consolidation), basal cell carcinoma of head & neck (endobronchial)
  - Mediastinal spread typical of nasopharyngeal, genitourinary (renal, prostate, testicular, transitional cell, ovarian), & breast cancers & melanoma

Natural History & Prognosis

- Generally poor, but depends on treatments available for primary tumor type

Treatment

- Depends on histology of primary tumors, generally palliative radiation or chemotherapy
- If lung only site, consider metastasectomy, especially if interval from primary resection to metastases > 1 month
  - Resection of osteosarcomas, solitary metastases, & slow-growing metastases
- Percutaneous ablation promising palliative therapy

DIAGNOSTIC CHECKLIST

Consider

- Metastatic disease in differential diagnosis of multifocal lung nodules, masses, or consolidations in patients with malignancy

SELECTED REFERENCES

1. Aquino SL: Imaging of metastatic disease to the thorax. Radiol Clin North Am. 43(3):481-95, vii, 2005
2. Seo JB et al: Atypical pulmonary metastases: spectrum of radiologic findings. Radiographics. 21(2):403-17, 2001

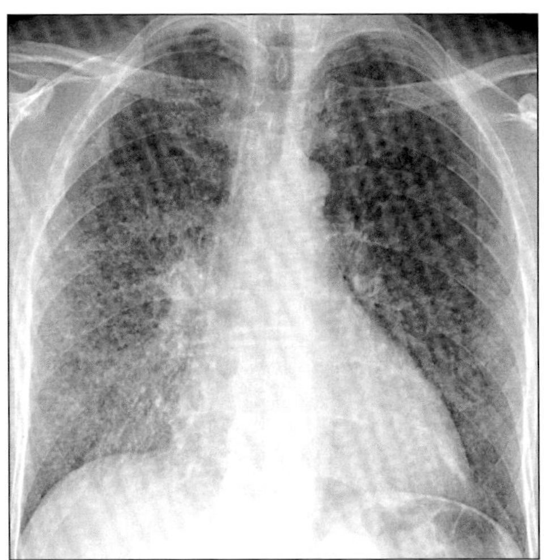

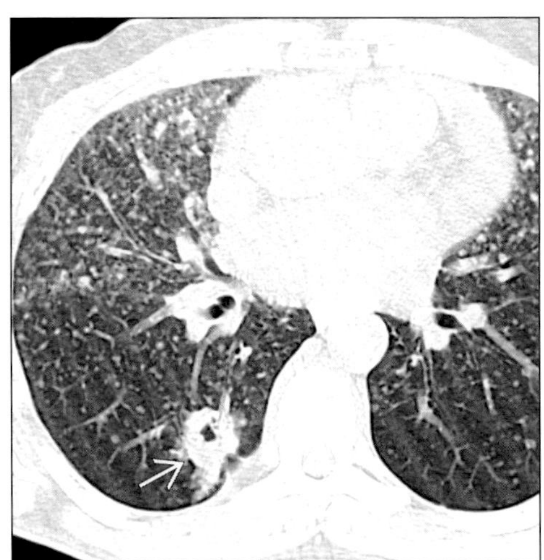

(Left) *PA chest radiograph of a patient with metastatic lung adenocarcinoma shows innumerable bilateral tiny pulmonary nodules consistent with miliary metastases.* ***(Right)*** *Axial NECT of the same patient shows multiple tiny pulmonary nodules consistent with hematogenous spread of adenocarcinoma. The primary lung adenocarcinoma ➔ is also visible. Common extrathoracic primaries causing miliary metastases include medullary thyroid carcinoma, renal cell carcinoma, and melanoma.*

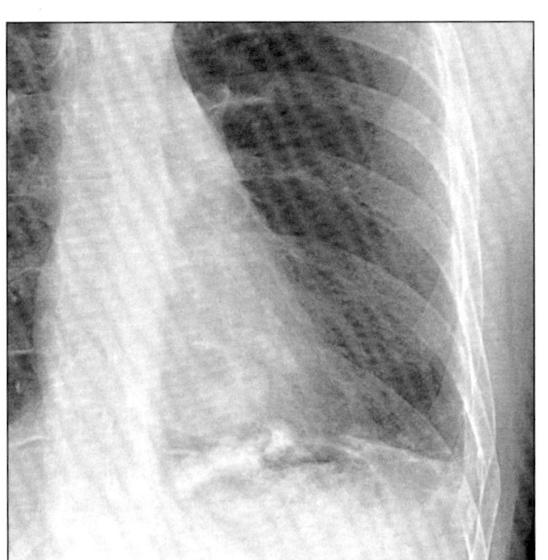

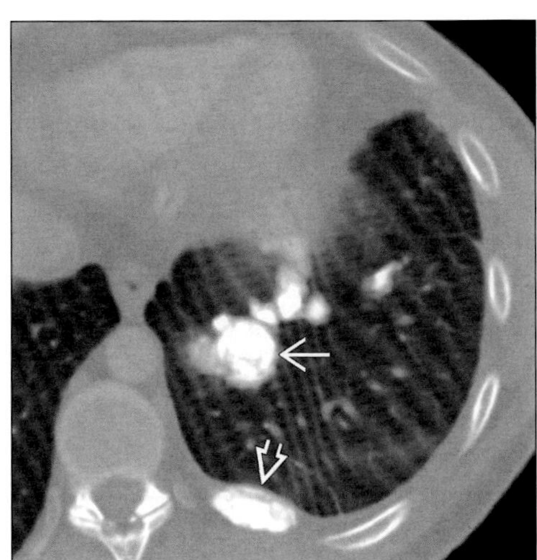

(Left) *PA chest radiograph of a 30-year-old man with metastatic osteosarcoma shows multiple dense nodules in the left lower lobe that represented calcified metastases.* ***(Right)*** *Axial CECT (bone window) of the same patient shows multiple calcified left lower lobe ➔ and pleural ➯ metastases. Metastases that calcify include those from osteosarcoma, chondrosarcoma, thyroid carcinoma, and occasionally treated metastases.*

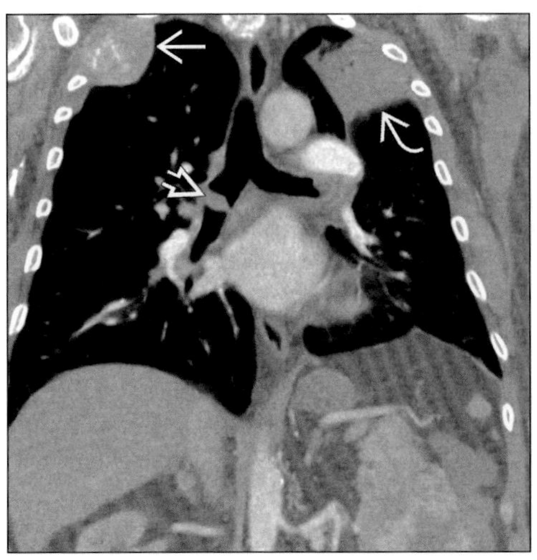

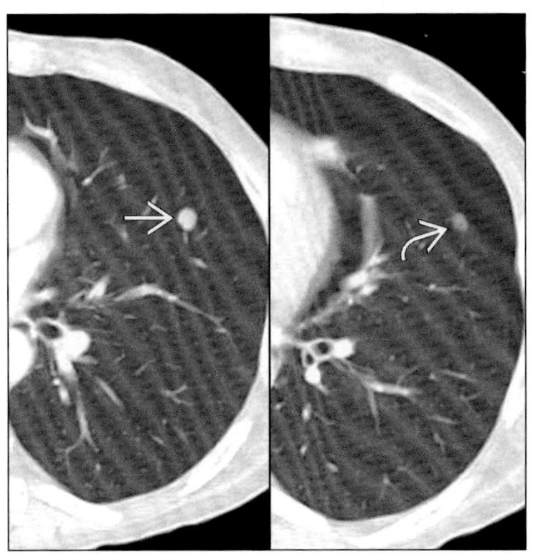

(Left) *Coronal CECT of a 71-year-old woman with metastatic renal cell carcinoma shows an endobronchial metastasis ➯ and chest wall ➔ and pulmonary ➦ metastases.* ***(Right)*** *Composite image with axial CECT of a patient with left chest pain shows a spontaneous left pneumothorax secondary to pulmonary metastases ➔ of unknown primary. Subpleural metastases ➦ are a cause of secondary spontaneous pneumothorax, typically in patients with metastatic osteosarcoma.*

LYMPHANGITIC CARCINOMATOSIS

Key Facts

Terminology
- Permeation of lymphatics by neoplastic cells

Imaging
- Radiography
  - Chest radiograph may be normal
  - Reticulonodular opacities, septal thickening, Kerley B lines
  - Fissural thickening from subpleural edema
  - Mimics interstitial edema, unresponsive to diuretics
- HRCT
  - Frequency of involvement: Axial (75%) > axial + peripheral (20%) > peripheral (5%)
  - Smooth or nodular thickening of interlobular septa &/or bronchovascular bundles
  - Lung architecture preserved
- Pleural effusion
- Lymphadenopathy

Top Differential Diagnoses
- Pulmonary edema
- Idiopathic pulmonary fibrosis
- Scleroderma
- Lymphoma
- Sarcoidosis

Pathology
- Interlobular septal thickening by tumor cells, desmoplastic reaction, & dilated lymphatics

Clinical Issues
- Insidious progressive dyspnea & cough
- Poor prognosis: 15% survive 6 months

Diagnostic Checklist
- Consider lymphangitic carcinomatosis in patients with malignancy & nodular septal thickening on CT

(Left) Graphic illustrates the morphologic features of lymphangitic carcinomatosis characterized by irregular and nodular interlobular septal thickening ➔ and asymmetric involvement. Lymphangitic carcinomatosis more commonly involves the right lung. (Right) Gross lung specimen shows the morphologic features of lymphangitic carcinomatosis with nodular thickening of the visceral pleura, interlobular septa ➔, and bronchovascular bundles ➔ secondary to tumor dissemination in pulmonary lymphatics.

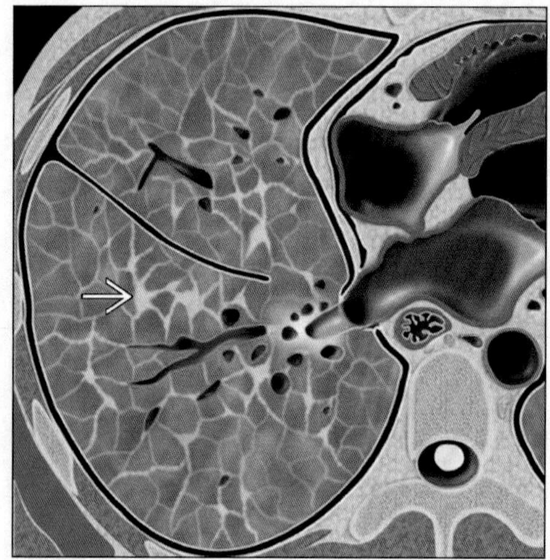

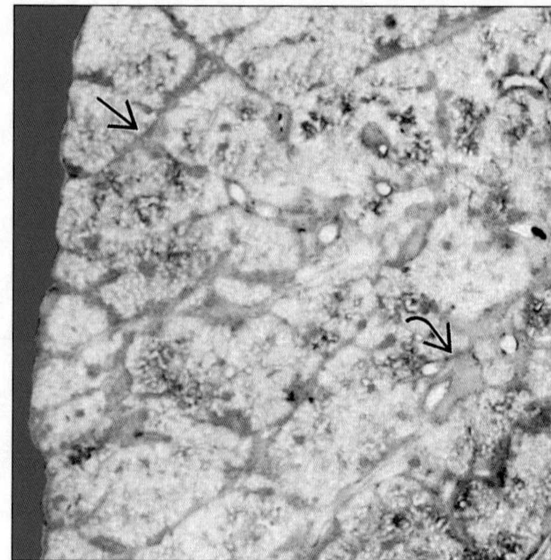

(Left) PA chest radiograph of a 68-year-old man with advanced lung cancer who presented with hemoptysis and weight loss shows a cavitary left upper lobe mass ➔ and diffuse reticular and nodular opacities ➔, most pronounced in the right lung. (Right) Axial CECT of the same patient shows scattered nodular interstitial thickening ➔, central bronchial wall thickening, hilar and mediastinal lymphadenopathy, and a right pleural effusion, consistent with advanced lung cancer and lymphangitic carcinomatosis.

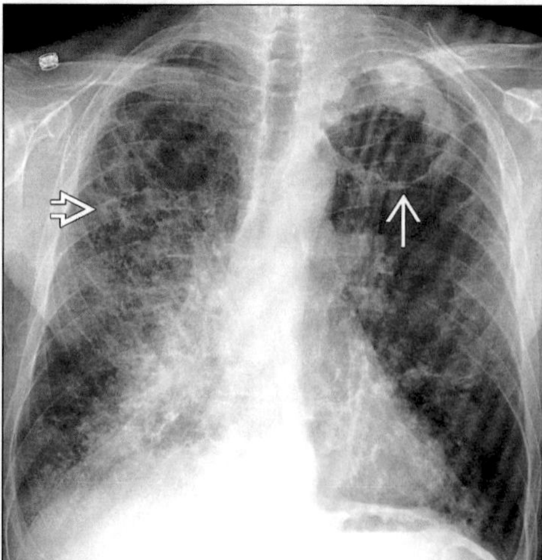

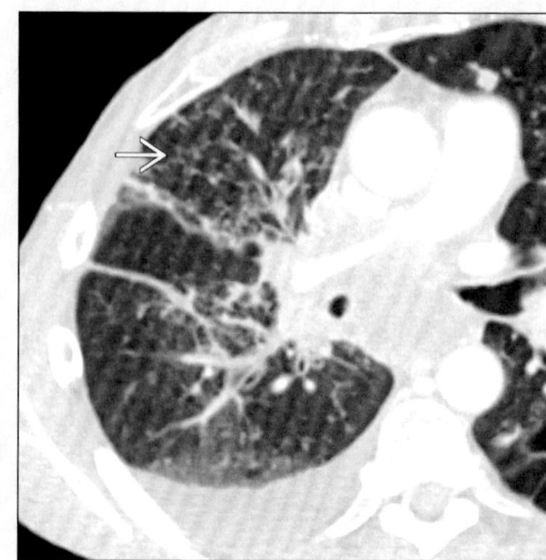

LYMPHANGITIC CARCINOMATOSIS

TERMINOLOGY

Synonyms

- **Lymphangitic tumor/metastases**

Definitions

- **Permeation of lymphatics by neoplastic cells**
- Tumor emboli or direct spread to lungs from hilar lymph nodes or central lung cancer
  - Common malignancies
    - Lung cancer
    - Breast cancer
    - Carcinomas of pancreas, stomach, colon, prostate, cervix, thyroid
  - Typically **adenocarcinomas**

IMAGING

General Features

- Best diagnostic clue
  - Nodular or beaded interlobular septal thickening
- Location
  - Usually diffuse, confined to 1 lung or lobe in 30%
- Size
  - Interstitial thickening, up to 10 mm
- Morphology
  - Irregular or beaded interlobular septa
  - Nodular bronchovascular thickening

Radiographic Findings

- Radiography
  - **Chest radiograph may be normal (30-50%)**
  - **Abnormal interstitium**
    - **Reticulonodular opacities**
    - **Coarse bronchovascular markings**
    - **Septal lines**
    - **Fissural thickening** from subpleural edema
    - **Kerley B lines** common
    - May resemble interstitial edema, but chronic & unresponsive to diuretics
  - Distribution
    - Confined to 1 lung or lobe in 30%, more common on right
    - Unilateral disease: Most commonly due to lung cancer
    - Bilateral symmetric disease: Commonly due to extrathoracic primary tumor
  - Associated findings
    - Hilar & mediastinal lymphadenopathy (30%)
    - Pleural effusion (50%)

CT Findings

- HRCT
  - **Abnormal secondary pulmonary lobule**
    - Peripheral or axial distribution within lobular interstitium
    - Frequency of involvement: Axial (75%) > axial + peripheral (20%) > peripheral (5%)
    - **Nodular or beaded thickening of interlobular septa &/or bronchovascular bundles**
    - **Smooth septal thickening** (may be due to edema rather than tumor)
    - **Small centrilobular nodules**, thick centrilobular bronchovascular bundles
    - Smooth or nodular thickening of interlobar fissures
  - **Pulmonary nodules**
    - Various sizes
    - May exhibit angiocentric distribution
    - May represent hematogenous metastases
  - Lung architecture preserved
  - Patchy ground-glass & airspace opacities, nonspecific
    - Airways may be narrowed from lymphatic permeation leading to atelectasis or obstructive pneumonitis
  - Distribution
    - Basilar predominance
    - Commonly asymmetric, may spare lobes or 1 lung (50%)
  - Associated findings
    - Pleural effusion
    - Hilar/mediastinal lymphadenopathy
    - Primary tumor may be visible in cases of lung cancer
    - Metastatic disease: Bone, liver

Imaging Recommendations

- Best imaging tool
  - HRCT is optimal imaging modality to evaluate for lymphangitic carcinomatosis; more sensitive & accurate than chest radiography
    - Confident diagnosis in 50% of those with lymphangitic tumor

Nuclear Medicine Findings

- PET/CT
  - Highly sensitive & specific with diffuse involvement; may miss focal disease adjacent to primary tumor

DIFFERENTIAL DIAGNOSIS

Pulmonary Edema

- Smooth interlobular septal thickening
- Bilateral pleural effusions common
- Gravity-dependent ground-glass opacities: Alveolar edema
- Cardiomegaly common
- Rapid resolution with treatment

Idiopathic Pulmonary Fibrosis

- Linear interstitial thickening, not nodular
- Bilateral basilar subpleural distribution
- Slow progression
- No lymphadenopathy or pleural effusion
- Honeycomb lung & architectural distortion

Scleroderma

- Dilated esophagus
- Linear interstitial thickening, not nodular
- Subpleural bilateral basilar distribution
- Honeycomb lung & architectural distortion

Lymphoma

- Nodules usually larger (> 1 cm)
- Frequent lymphadenopathy
- Usually secondary or recurrent disease in patient with known lymphoma

Drug Reaction

- Drug history, especially patients on chemotherapy
- Linear interstitial thickening, not nodular

LYMPHANGITIC CARCINOMATOSIS

- Honeycomb lung & architectural distortion more common

Sarcoidosis

- May exhibit similar imaging features
- Upper lung zone predominant abnormalities
- No pleural effusions

Asbestosis

- Pleural plaques
- Linear interstitial thickening, not nodular
- Honeycomb lung & architectural distortion more common
- No pleural effusion or lymphadenopathy

Hypersensitivity Pneumonitis

- Antigen exposure
- Diffuse or centrilobular ground-glass opacities
- Air-trapping common
- Linear interstitial thickening when present, not nodular
- No lymphadenopathy or pleural effusion

DDx for Unilateral Lung Disease (PEARL)

- Pneumonia
- Edema
- Aspiration
- Radiation
- Lymphangitic tumor

PATHOLOGY

General Features

- Etiology
  - Hematogenous metastases: Tumor emboli to small pulmonary artery branches with subsequent spread along lymphatics
  - Some tumors, such as lymphoma, may spread retrograde from hilar nodes to pulmonary lymphatics
  - Lung cancer may spread to adjacent lung along lymphatics
- **Frequent form of tumor spread** found in 33-50% of patients with solid tumors at autopsy
- Permeation of lymphatics by neoplastic cells
- Common tumors: **Cancers of breast, stomach, pancreas, prostate, lung**
  - Typically **adenocarcinomas**

Staging, Grading, & Classification

- Lymphangitic carcinomatosis denotes end-stage unresectable disease

Gross Pathologic & Surgical Features

- Thickening of interlobular septa due to tumor cells, desmoplastic reaction, & dilated lymphatics
- Hilar & mediastinal lymph nodes may or may not be involved

Microscopic Features

- Nests of tumor cells within lymphatics; may be associated with fibrosis
  - Tumor emboli in small adjacent arterioles also common
  - Occluded lymphatics may also be edematous or fibrotic

CLINICAL ISSUES

Presentation

- Most common signs/symptoms
  - **Insidious progressive dyspnea**
  - **Cough**
  - Usually not first manifestation of malignancy, typically in patients with known malignancy
- Other signs/symptoms
  - Progressive dyspnea in young adults often from occult gastric carcinoma
  - May present with asthma

Demographics

- Age
  - Incidence increases with age, reflects age at which tumors develop in population

Natural History & Prognosis

- Poor; 15% survive 6 months

Treatment

- Aimed at underlying malignancy
  - With successful chemotherapy, lymphangitic tumor may regress
- Hospice care

Diagnosis

- Diagnosis may be inferred from imaging abnormalities
- No known malignancy
  - Sputum cytology
  - Transbronchial biopsy
  - Image-guided biopsy
  - Open lung biopsy

DIAGNOSTIC CHECKLIST

Consider

- Lymphangitic carcinomatosis in patients with known malignancy & nodular septal thickening on CT or HRCT

SELECTED REFERENCES

1. Prakash P et al: FDG PET/CT in assessment of pulmonary lymphangitic carcinomatosis. AJR Am J Roentgenol. 194(1):231-6, 2010
2. Acikgoz G et al: Pulmonary lymphangitic carcinomatosis (PLC): spectrum of FDG-PET findings. Clin Nucl Med. 31(11):673-8, 2006
3. Castaner E et al: Diseases affecting the peribronchovascular interstitium: CT findings and pathologic correlation. Curr Probl Diagn Radiol. 34(2):63-75, 2005
4. Honda O et al: Comparison of high resolution CT findings of sarcoidosis, lymphoma, and lymphangitic carcinoma: is there any difference of involved interstitium? J Comput Assist Tomogr. 23(3):374-9, 1999

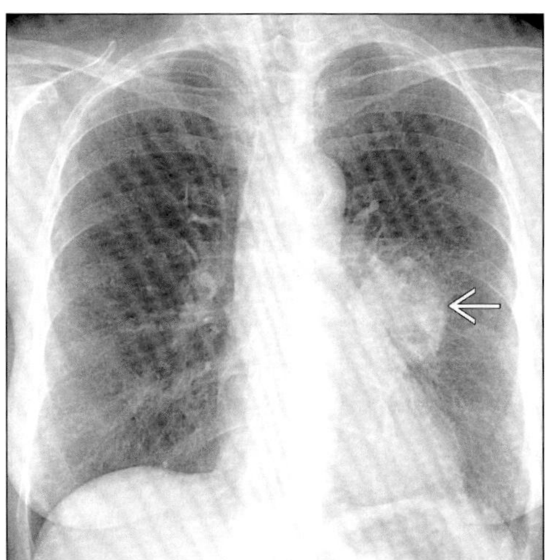

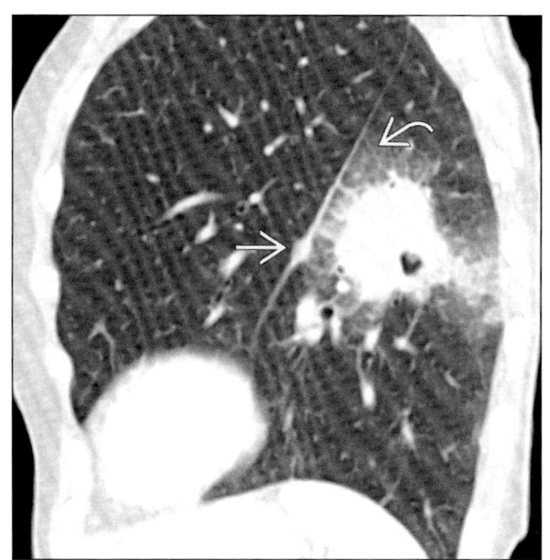

(Left) *PA chest radiograph of a 44-year-old woman with newly diagnosed lung cancer shows a dominant left lower lobe perihilar mass ➔ with surrounding reticular opacities.* ***(Right)*** *Sagittal CECT shows the large left lower lobe mass, which exhibits focal central cavitation and surrounding thick interlobular septa ↷ and nodular thickening of the adjacent major fissure ➔. CT is superior to radiography in detecting findings of lymphangitic carcinomatosis.*

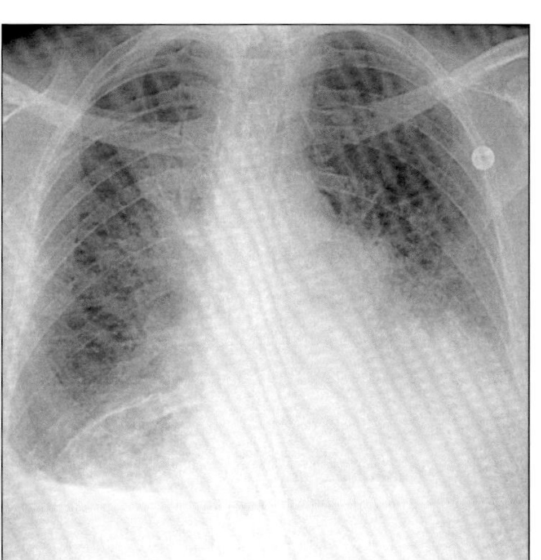

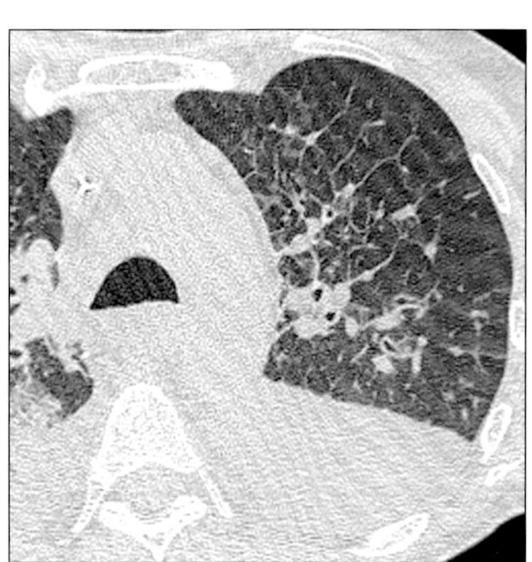

(Left) *PA chest radiograph of a 57-year-old woman with breast cancer shows cardiomegaly, bilateral pleural effusions, and diffuse bilateral reticular opacities. Although the presumptive diagnosis was pulmonary edema, symptoms did not improve with diuresis.* ***(Right)*** *Axial HRCT of the same patient shows smooth and nodular thickening of interlobular septa, bronchial wall thickening, and moderate bilateral pleural effusions. Transbronchial biopsy confirmed lymphangitic carcinomatosis.*

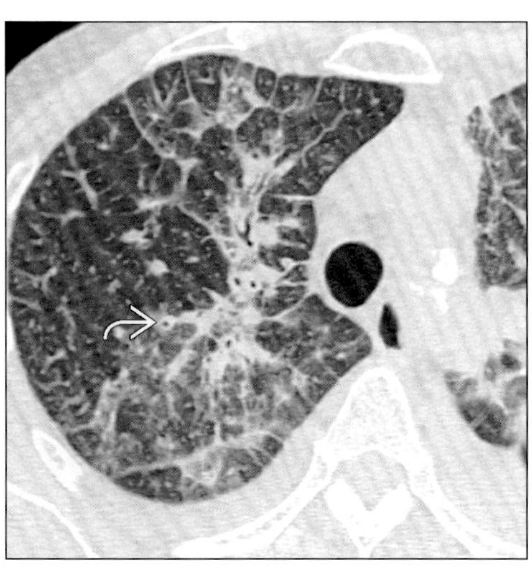

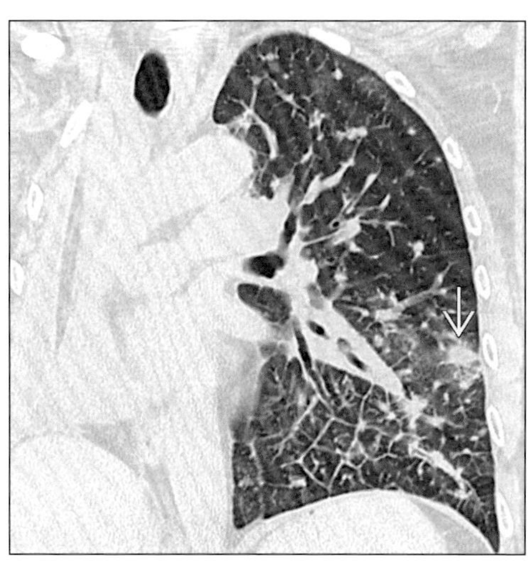

(Left) *Axial NECT shows lymphangitic carcinomatosis manifesting with bilateral pleural effusions and typical patchy ground-glass opacities, smooth interlobular septal thickening, and central bronchial wall thickening ↷.* ***(Right)*** *Coronal NECT shows lymphangitic carcinomatosis post right pneumonectomy for lung cancer manifesting with basilar interlobular septal thickening and lung nodules ➔. Lymphangitic carcinomatosis may result from hematogenous metastases. (Courtesy S. Rossi, MD.)*

TUMOR EMBOLI

Key Facts

Terminology

- Pulmonary vascular occlusion by tumor cells

Imaging

- Radiography
  - Chest radiograph often normal
  - Focal or diffuse heterogeneous opacities
  - May mimic lymphangitic carcinomatosis
  - Cardiomegaly
  - Pulmonary hypertension
- CT
  - Right heart & pulmonary trunk enlargement
  - Visualization of IVC or right atrial tumor
- HRCT
  - Focal/multifocal, unilateral/bilateral involvement
  - Dilated, beaded peripheral pulmonary arteries
  - Tree-in-bud opacities
  - Centrilobular or miliary nodules ± halo sign

Top Differential Diagnoses

- Pulmonary emboli
- Pulmonary artery sarcoma
- Behçet syndrome
- Metastases with extravascular involvement

Pathology

- Primary neoplasms include hepatocellular carcinoma, renal cell carcinoma, and angiosarcoma
- Tumor emboli within large central to small peripheral arteries

Clinical Issues

- Progressive dyspnea, cough
- Diagnosis: Rarely diagnosed antemortem
  - 2-26% of autopsies
- Treatment: Anticoagulation, chemotherapy
- Prognosis: Grave

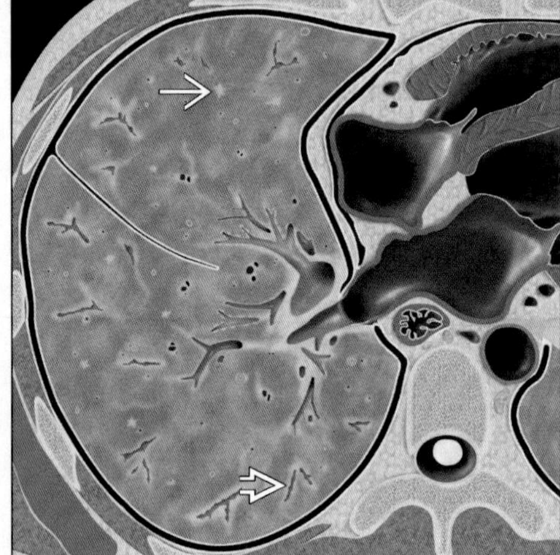

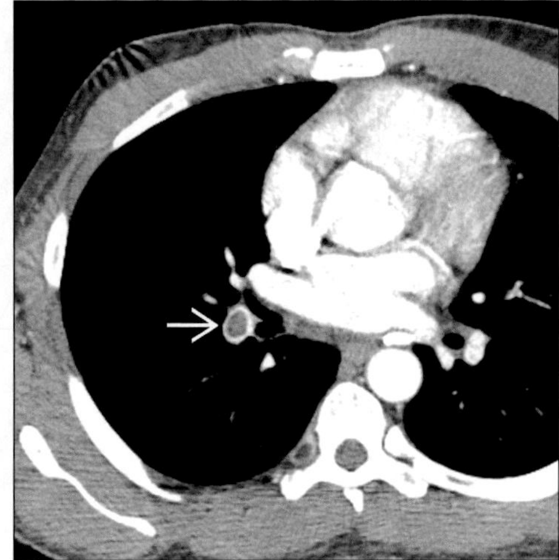

(Left) *Graphic depicts the morphologic features of tumor emboli, which may affect pulmonary arteries of various sizes. Tumor emboli may manifest with filling defects in central arteries, centrilobular nodules ➔, tree-in-bud opacities, and beaded pulmonary arteries ⇨.* ***(Right)*** *Axial CTA of a patient with hepatocellular carcinoma that invaded the inferior vena cava shows a filling defect in a right lower lobe pulmonary artery ➔. The defect resulted from tumor embolization from the inferior vena cava mass.*

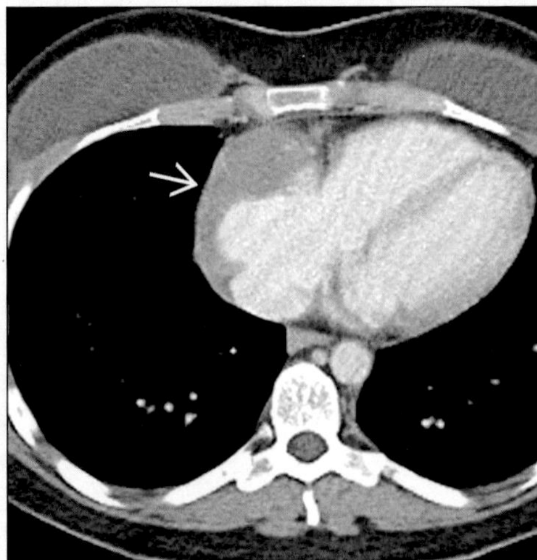

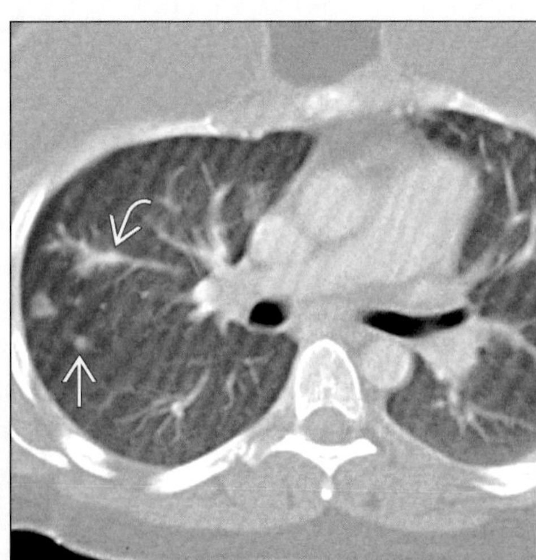

(Left) *Axial CECT of a 26-year-old woman with a cardiac angiosarcoma shows a low-attenuation mass ➔ that invades and thickens the right atrial wall.* ***(Right)*** *Axial CECT of the same patient shows multifocal ill-defined pulmonary nodules ➔ as well as dilatation and beading of a pulmonary artery branch ↙, which was filled with tumor emboli from the right atrial mass. Malignant neoplasms that involve the vena cava and the right cardiac chambers may produce pulmonary arterial tumor emboli.*

TUMOR EMBOLI

TERMINOLOGY

Definitions

- Occlusion of pulmonary vasculature by tumor cells
  - Nonthrombotic embolism

IMAGING

General Features

- Best diagnostic clue
  - Normal chest radiograph with progressive hypoxia in patient with malignancy
- Location
  - Variable: From central to centrilobular pulmonary arteries
    - Typically medium to small arteries
- Size
  - Variably sized filling defects or vascular beading
- Morphology
  - Endoluminal soft tissue, no extravascular proliferation

Radiographic Findings

- Nonspecific appearance
  - Normal radiograph, common
  - Focal or diffuse heterogeneous opacities
    - Miliary nodules
  - May mimic lymphangitic carcinomatosis
    - Reticular opacities
  - Cardiomegaly
  - Pulmonary artery hypertension
    - Enlarged pulmonary trunk & central pulmonary arteries with peripheral pruning

CT Findings

- CECT
  - Normal CT, not uncommon
  - Right heart enlargement
  - Pulmonary trunk > 3 cm
- HRCT
  - Focal or multifocal, unilateral or bilateral involvement
  - **Dilated & beaded peripheral pulmonary arteries**
  - **Tree-in-bud opacities**
    - Filling of centrilobular arteries with tumor cells
  - **Centrilobular nodules**
    - Arteriolar involvement
  - Miliary nodules
    - Diffuse hematogenous intravascular dissemination
  - Nodule surrounded by halo of ground-glass opacity
    - Ill-defined margins
    - Peritumoral hemorrhage
- CTA
  - Large **filling defects** in central, lobar, & segmental pulmonary arteries
  - **Peripheral wedge-shaped opacities**
    - Pulmonary infarction
  - **Filling defect or mass in right atrium or ventricle**
  - Mosaic perfusion
    - Small vessel occlusion, decreased vascular caliber in hyperlucent lung
    - No air-trapping

Angiographic Findings

- Angiography rarely performed
  - Poor sensitivity & specificity
- Pruning & tortuosity of 3rd- to 5th-order arteries
- Delayed filling of segmental pulmonary arteries
- Subsegmental pulmonary artery filling defects
- Large filling defects
  - Central, lobar, & segmental pulmonary arteries
- Variant
  - Lung cancer with systemic arterial tumor emboli
  - Filling defect or occlusion of medium-sized or small arteries

Nuclear Medicine Findings

- V/Q scan
  - Ventilation perfusion mismatched defects
    - Multiple, small peripheral subsegmental perfusion defects
    - Visualization of interlobar fissures

Imaging Recommendations

- Best imaging tool
  - No imaging feature is pathognomonic
  - HRCT or ventilation perfusion scintigraphy may suggest diagnosis
  - CTA for detection of large vessel emboli
- Protocol advice
  - Ventilation perfusion scintigraphy
    - Reduce number of particles to 100,000-200,000 in patients with pulmonary hypertension
      - Macroaggregated albumin may further occlude small vessels
      - Potential for cardiac arrest due to right heart failure

DIFFERENTIAL DIAGNOSIS

Pulmonary Emboli

- Increased frequency in patients with cancer
- Difficult to distinguish from tumor emboli
- Most cases respond to treatment & do not progress

Pulmonary Artery Sarcoma

- Solid intraarterial lobulated filling defect/mass
- May enhance with intravenous contrast
- May expand artery, typically central location

Behçet Syndrome

- Pulmonary artery aneurysms with in situ thromboses

Infection

- Tree-in-bud opacities from small airways bronchiolitis
- Mosaic attenuation with air-trapping on expiration
- No pulmonary artery hypertension

Metastases with Extravascular Involvement

- HRCT or CTA to show pulmonary, lymphatic, or airway spread

Lesions with CT Halo Sign

- Invasive aspergillosis
  - Usually hematopoietic malignancy, not solid organ
  - Neutropenic, usually febrile patient
  - Fulminant, rapid progression
- Candidiasis
  - Immunocompromised, acutely ill, sepsis
  - Usually on broad spectrum antibiotics with central lines in place
- Wegener granulomatosis
  - Renal failure, upper airway disease

TUMOR EMBOLI

- Multiple cavitary nodules or consolidations
- Tuberculosis
  - Upper lobe location
- Adenocarcinoma
  - Airways involvement, not intravascular
  - No extrapulmonary source for emboli

Treatment-related Pulmonary Disease

- Hypersensitivity pneumonitis
  - May be secondary to chemotherapeutic drugs, especially methotrexate
  - Centrilobular fuzzy nodules
  - Diffuse ground-glass opacities
  - Response to steroids
- Cryptogenic organizing pneumonia
  - Multifocal consolidations
  - Small centrilobular nodules
  - Peripheral wedge-shaped opacities that may resemble infarcts
  - Responds to steroids

PATHOLOGY

General Features

- Etiology
  - Occlusion of pulmonary microvasculature by tumor cells
  - Primary tumors
    - Hepatocellular carcinoma
    - Renal cell carcinoma
    - Angiosarcoma
    - Breast cancer
    - Gastric carcinoma
    - Lung cancer
    - Prostate carcinoma
    - Pancreas carcinoma
    - Osteosarcoma, chondrosarcoma
    - Choriocarcinoma
    - Thyroid carcinoma
  - Tumors that tend to invade systemic veins
    - Hepatocellular carcinoma invading hepatic veins
    - Renal cell carcinoma invading renal vein & inferior vena cava
    - Angiosarcomas that invade systemic veins or right heart

Gross Pathologic & Surgical Features

- Tumor emboli within large central to small peripheral arteries

Microscopic Features

- Involves multiple levels of microscopic pulmonary vasculature
  - From elastic arteries to alveolar septal capillaries
- Thrombotic microangiopathy of pulmonary tumors
  - Extensive fibrocellular intimal hyperplasia of small pulmonary arteries
  - Initiated by tumor microemboli
- Progressive & irreversible obstruction of vascular bed
- Peritumoral halo: Hemorrhage due to rupture of fragile vessels

CLINICAL ISSUES

Presentation

- Most common signs/symptoms
  - Progressive dyspnea, cough
  - Chest & abdominal pain
  - Hypoxia
  - Acute right heart failure
  - Progressive cor pulmonale over weeks or months
  - Ascites
- Other signs/symptoms
  - Tumor thrombi may produce subacute & progressive clinical symptoms

Demographics

- Age
  - Childhood to elderly
- Gender
  - M = F
- Epidemiology
  - 2-26% of autopsies

Diagnosis

- Cytology of blood aspirated from wedged Swan-Ganz catheter
- Biopsy
- Autopsy

Treatment

- Anticoagulation
- Chemotherapy

Natural History & Prognosis

- Prognosis: Grave
  - Dependent on response to therapy
- Rarely identified antemortem

DIAGNOSTIC CHECKLIST

Consider

- Tumor emboli in dyspneic patients with malignancy involving vena cava or right heart chambers & distended beaded pulmonary arteries

SELECTED REFERENCES

1. Han D et al: Thrombotic and nonthrombotic pulmonary arterial embolism: spectrum of imaging findings. Radiographics. 23(6):1521-39, 2003
2. Roberts KE et al: Pulmonary tumor embolism: a review of the literature. Am J Med. 115(3):228-32, 2003
3. Seo JB et al: Atypical pulmonary metastases: spectrum of radiologic findings. Radiographics. 21(2):403-17, 2001
4. Kim AE et al: Pulmonary tumor embolism presenting as infarcts on computed tomography. J Thorac Imaging. 14(2):135-7, 1999
5. Moores LK et al: Diffuse tumor microembolism: a rare cause of a high-probability perfusion scan. Chest. 111(4):1122-5, 1997

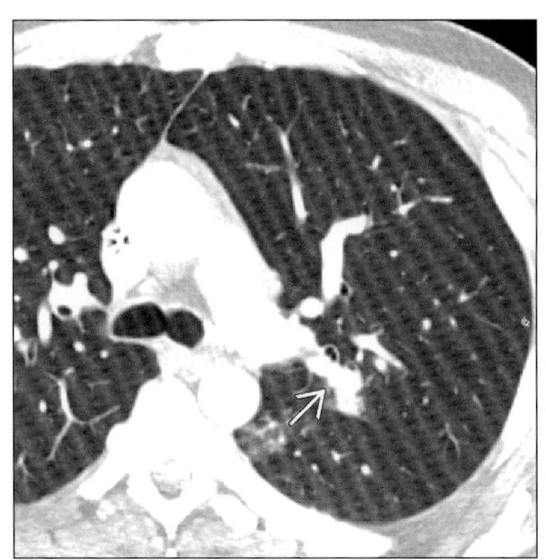

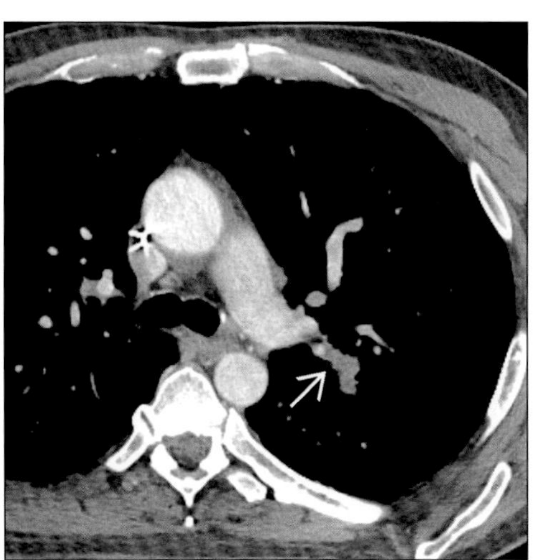

(Left) *Axial CECT of a patient with papillary thyroid carcinoma shows a dilated left upper lobe tubular structure* ➡ *contiguous with the pulmonary arteries.* ***(Right)*** *Axial CECT of the same patient shows a low-attenuation pulmonary artery filling defect* ➡ *that represented a tumor embolus. Tumor emboli are indistinguishable from pulmonary thromboembolic disease, and the diagnosis is rarely made antemortem. Visualization of vena cava or right heart endoluminal tumor should raise suspicion.*

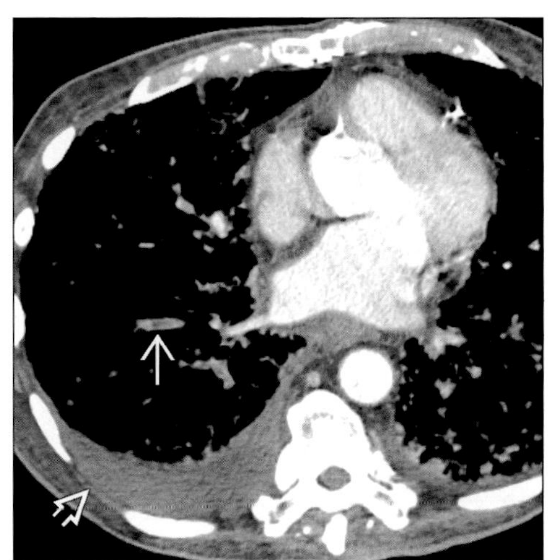

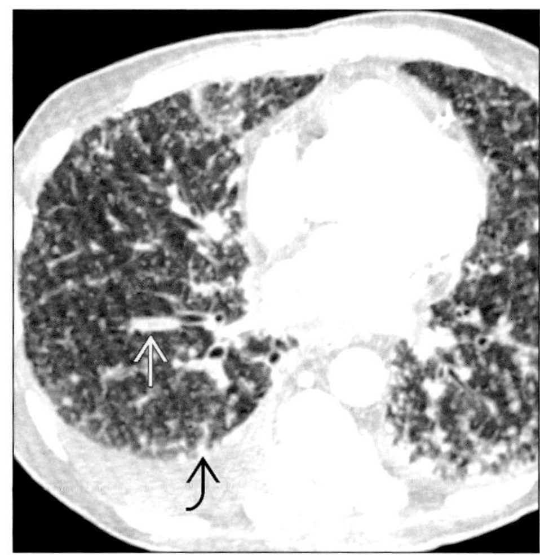

(Left) *Axial CECT of a patient with hepatocellular carcinoma shows a filling defect in a right lower lobe pulmonary artery branch* ➡ *and a small right pleural effusion* ⇨. ***(Right)*** *Axial CECT of the same patient shows the pulmonary artery branch dilated by tumor embolus* ➡. *A perilymphatic pattern of metastatic disease suggestive of lymphangitic carcinomatosis is also present, manifesting with multiple tiny centrilobular, fissural, and septal micronodules* ↪.

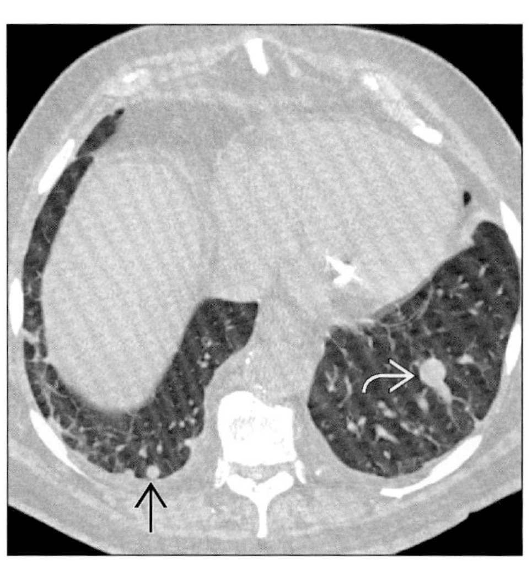

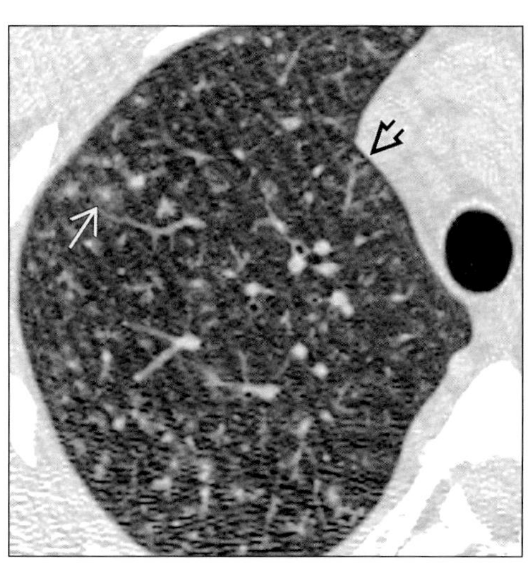

(Left) *Axial CECT of a patient with renal cell carcinoma shows a left lower lobe tubular structure* ↪ *representing a tumor-filled pulmonary artery. Note the right lower lobe pulmonary metastases* →. ***(Right)*** *Axial HRCT of a patient with right atrial rhabdomyosarcoma shows multiple tiny tumor emboli manifesting with tree-in-bud opacities* ⇨. *Ground-glass opacity halos* ➡ *surrounding small lung nodules represent hemorrhage due to fragile neovascular tissue.*

SECTION 6
Interstitial, Diffuse, and Inhalational Lung Disease

Introduction and Overview

Idiopathic Interstitial Lung Diseases

Smoking-related Diseases

Pneumoconiosis

Other Inhalational Disorders

Eosinophilic Lung Disease

Metabolic Diseases and Miscellaneous Conditions

APPROACH TO INTERSTITIAL, DIFFUSE, AND INHALATIONAL LUNG DISEASE

Background

The category of "interstitial lung disease" refers to diffuse parenchymal lung diseases included in a list of some 200 entities. Most of these involve not only the pulmonary interstitium but also other anatomic elements of the lung, including bronchi, bronchioles, epithelial and vascular cells of the alveoli, and the pleura. These diseases typically affect both lungs in an acute, subacute, or chronic manner. Moreover, many of these entities overlap in their clinical, imaging, physiologic, and pathologic manifestations.

Idiopathic Interstitial Pneumonias

The most common group of diseases producing diffuse parenchymal lung disease are the idiopathic interstitial pneumonias, currently classified by a joint effort of the American Thoracic Society (ATS) and the European Respiratory Society (ERS). Currently, this classification includes idiopathic pulmonary fibrosis (IPF), nonspecific interstitial pneumonia (NSIP), cryptogenic organizing pneumonia (COP), acute interstitial pneumonia (AIP), respiratory bronchiolitis-associated interstitial lung disease (RB-ILD), desquamative interstitial pneumonia (DIP), and lymphoid interstitial pneumonia (LIP). Future revisions may include the syndrome of combined pulmonary fibrosis and emphysema and acute exacerbations of pulmonary fibrosis, as well as incorporating recently reported genetic and pathophysiologic findings.

Other Disease Entities

Occupational and environmental exposures are common causes of diffuse parenchymal lung disease. Other causes include granulomatous disorders (e.g., sarcoidosis), inhalational diseases, eosinophilic lung disease, and various metabolic and miscellaneous disorders.

Imaging Modalities

The chest radiograph is typically the first imaging study utilized in evaluating patients with diffuse parenchymal lung disease, often prompted by the frequent complaint of dyspnea. In some disease entities (e.g., sarcoidosis, silicosis, pulmonary Langerhans cell histiocytosis) patients may be relatively asymptomatic in the early course of their disease, despite the presence of extensive parenchymal abnormalities on chest radiographs.

Chest radiography may be normal in 10% of affected patients. In other cases, radiographs may demonstrate characteristic patterns (e.g., the usual interstitial pneumonia [UIP] pattern of idiopathic pulmonary fibrosis). In other instances, the radiographic appearances of different disease entities may overlap (e.g., sarcoidosis, silicosis, pulmonary Langerhans cell histiocytosis) and require HRCT/CT analysis to narrow the list of differential diagnostic considerations.

With the advent of the clinical use of HRCT in 1989, the imaging evaluation of patients with diffuse parenchymal lung disease made a quantum leap in diagnostic accuracy. Thin-section images obtained with a small field-of-view and using a high spatial frequency algorithm have enabled radiologists to function in a similar manner to macroscopic pathologists. Indeed, grayscale images of the lungs obtained with HRCT rival the macroscopic appearances evaluated by pathologists when examining gross specimens of sectioned lungs. Despite the increased accuracy that can be achieved with HRCT, imaging findings must be correlated with clinical and pathologic features of the disease in order to achieve a multidisciplinary assessment regarded as the most accurate and effective manner of evaluating these patients.

Anatomic Distribution of Imaging Patterns

Abnormalities detected on HRCT should be analyzed for their relationship to the secondary pulmonary lobule (SPL). Such findings may involve the interlobular septa or the intralobular structures or may be centrilobular in distribution. A perilymphatic distribution of abnormalities manifests with findings along the axial peribronchovascular interstitium &/or the peripheral, subpleural interstitium (including interlobar fissures), with or without involvement of the interlobular septa of the SPL.

HRCT may reveal specific imaging patterns of various diseases (e.g., nodules, reticulation, ground-glass opacity, consolidation, traction bronchiectasis) and delineate their anatomic distribution. Combining pattern recognition with disease distribution may enable radiologists to form a concise list of differential diagnostic possibilities.

For example, reticular opacities in a subpleural and bibasilar distribution suggest the UIP pattern; ancillary findings may include traction bronchiectasis and reduced lung volumes. Correlation with clinical findings may lead to an imaging differential diagnosis of idiopathic pulmonary fibrosis, connective tissue disease, or occupational lung disease. In another instance, detection of small nodules in a perilymphatic distribution with predominant involvement of the mid and upper lung zones is very suggestive of sarcoidosis, with or without the presence of hilar and mediastinal lymphadenopathy. Smooth thickening along the same perilymphatic pathways is characteristic of pulmonary edema (typically bilateral and symmetric), although the same finding may be a manifestation of lymphangitic carcinomatosis, a process that may be focal or multifocal, unilateral or bilateral. Associated clinical findings and temporal considerations are useful factors in narrowing the list of differential diagnostic possibilities.

Physiologic Considerations

Diseases related to inhalation of various agents often manifest with upper &/or mid lung predominant findings. Because of ventilation and perfusion gradients in the human lung and related enhanced clearing in the lower lung zones (more effective coughing), there is less effective clearance of inhaled agents from the upper lung zones. Sarcoidosis (postulated inhaled unknown etiologic agent), silicosis (inhaled silicates), and Langerhans cell histiocytosis (inhaled cigarette smoke) may produce very similar radiographic findings (reticulonodular opacities that predominantly involve the mid and upper lung zones).

An exception to this is the retention of asbestos fibers in the lower lung zones. Asbestos fibers penetrate deeply into lung tissues and are often resistant to normal clearing mechanisms.

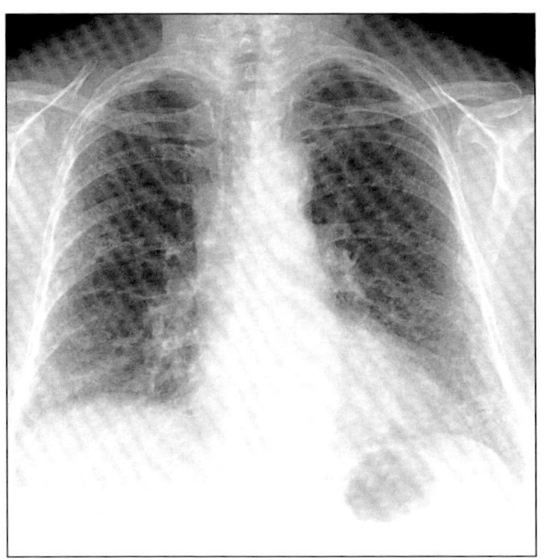

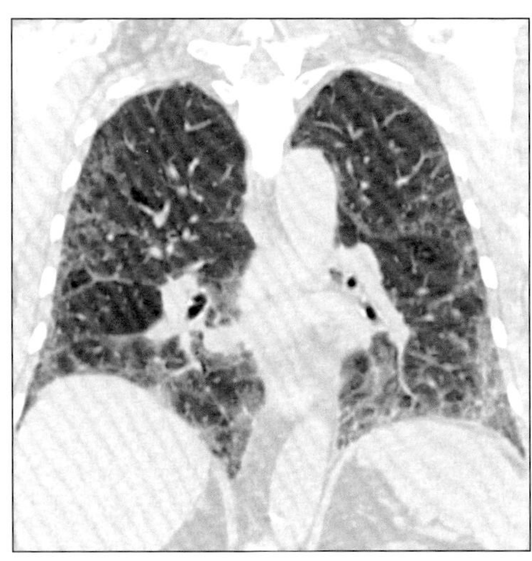

(Left) *PA chest radiograph of a patient with idiopathic pulmonary fibrosis (IPF) shows reduced lung volumes and peripheral and predominantly bibasilar reticular opacities, representing the usual interstitial pneumonia (UIP) pattern of pulmonary fibrosis.* ***(Right)*** *Coronal NECT of the same patient confirms the presence of peripheral and bibasilar reticular opacities with associated architectural distortion and decreased lung volumes. The findings in this case were idiopathic (IPF).*

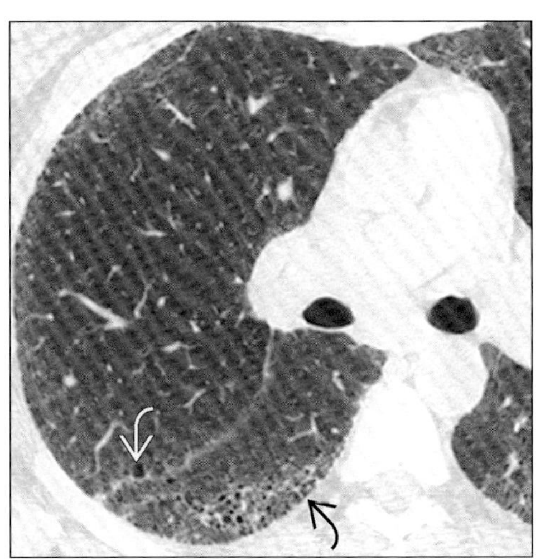

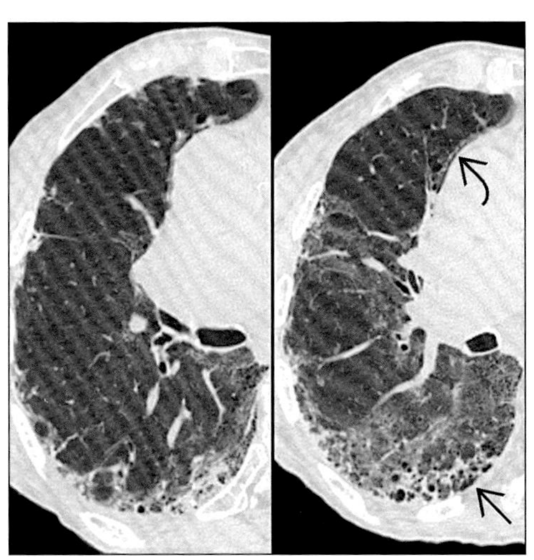

(Left) *Axial HRCT of a patient with IPF demonstrates peripheral reticular opacities and fine honeycombing →. Subpleural reticulation also extends along the right major fissure →.* ***(Right)*** *Composite image with axial HRCT of a patient with moderately advanced IPF and reduced lung volumes demonstrates coarse peripheral reticular opacities, architectural distortion, and moderate honeycombing →. Note irregular interfaces along the mediastinal pleural surfaces →.*

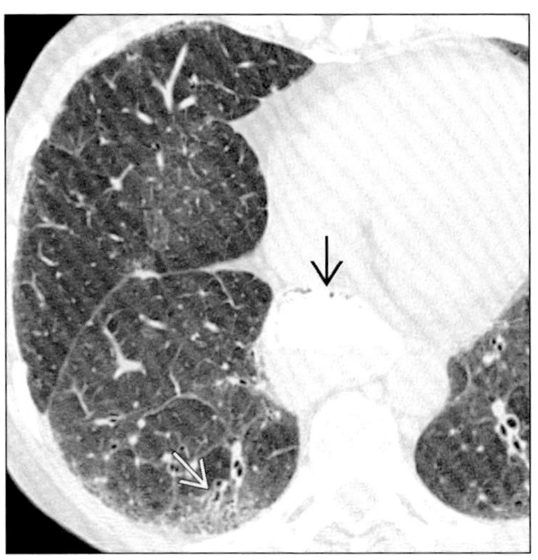

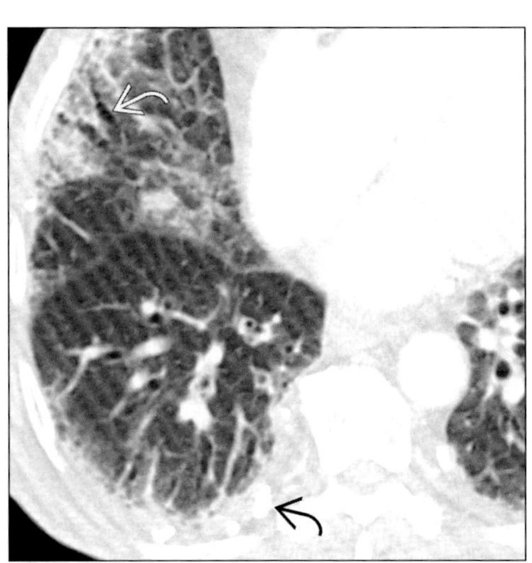

(Left) *Axial CECT of a patient with NSIP related to scleroderma shows peripheral ground-glass and reticular opacities, traction bronchiectasis →, and esophageal dilatation →.* ***(Right)*** *Axial CECT of a patient with asbestosis shows peripheral ground-glass and reticular opacities and traction bronchiectasis →. Pleural plaques → indicating asbestos exposure provide an important clue to the diagnosis. The latency period between the time of asbestos exposure and development of asbestosis is 20-30 years.*

*(**Left**) Axial CECT of a patient with nonspecific interstitial pneumonia (NSIP) demonstrates patchy ground-glass opacities with underlying reticulation and focal areas of traction bronchiolectasis ➚. (**Right**) Coronal NECT of a patient with NSIP demonstrates peripheral bibasilar ground-glass opacities with underlying reticulation, traction bronchiectasis ➡, and relative subpleural sparing ➚ along the juxtadiaphragmatic lung surfaces.*

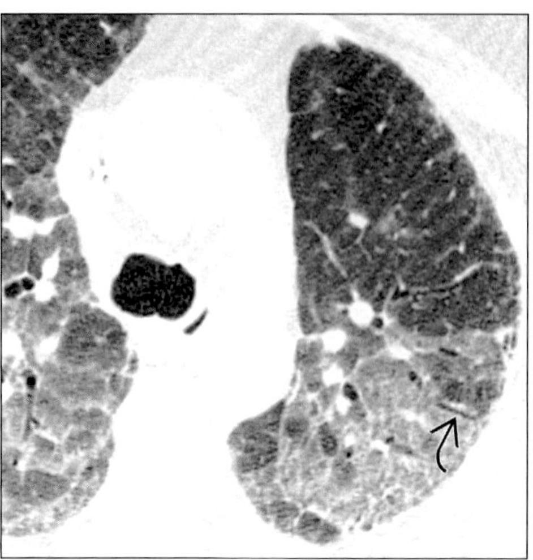

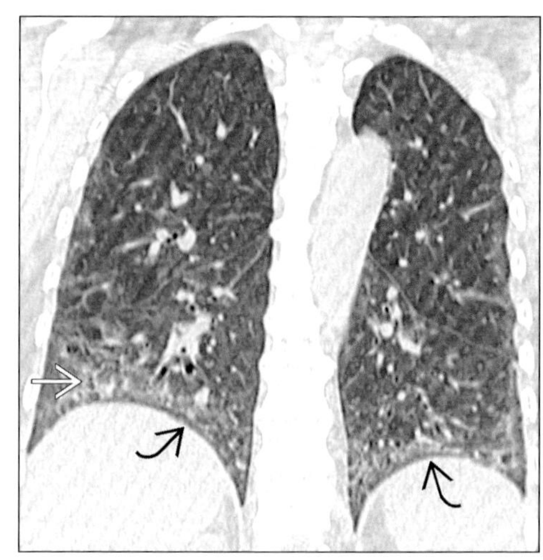

*(**Left**) PA chest radiograph of a patient with sarcoidosis demonstrates diffuse bilateral reticulonodular opacities predominantly involving the mid and upper lung zones as well as bilateral hilar lymphadenopathy. (**Right**) HRCT of the same patient shows small nodules in a perilymphatic distribution, extending along bronchovascular structures ➚, in subpleural lung, and along interlobular septa ➡. Small nodules were also demonstrated along the interlobar fissures (not shown).*

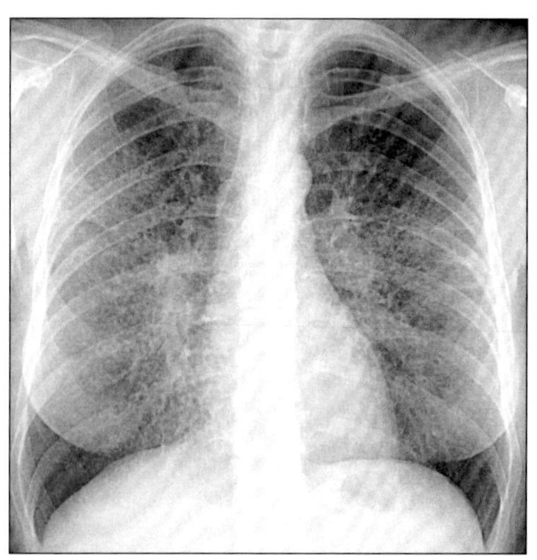

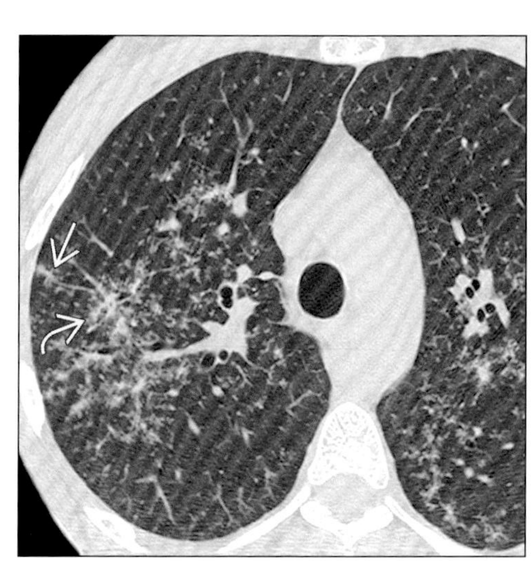

*(**Left**) PA chest radiograph of a stone quarry worker with silicosis shows nodules and reticulonodular opacities predominantly involving the upper and mid lung zones, with relative sparing of the lower lung zones. Some nodules have coalesced over time into conglomerate opacities ➚ (progressive massive fibrosis). (**Right**) HRCT of the same patient shows well-defined small nodules, some along the interlobular septa ➡ (i.e., perilymphatic). Note the right upper lobe conglomerate mass ➚.*

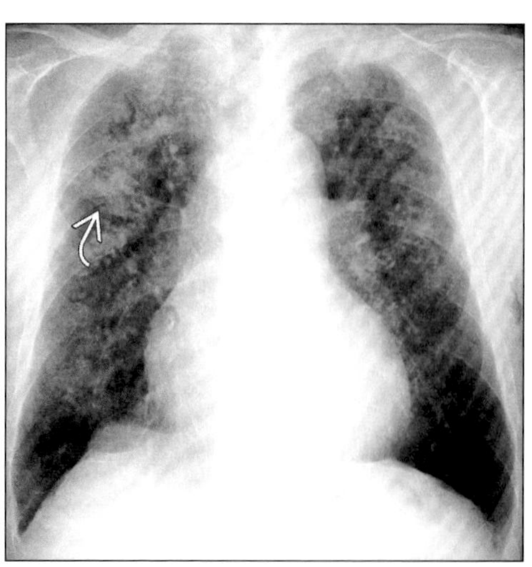

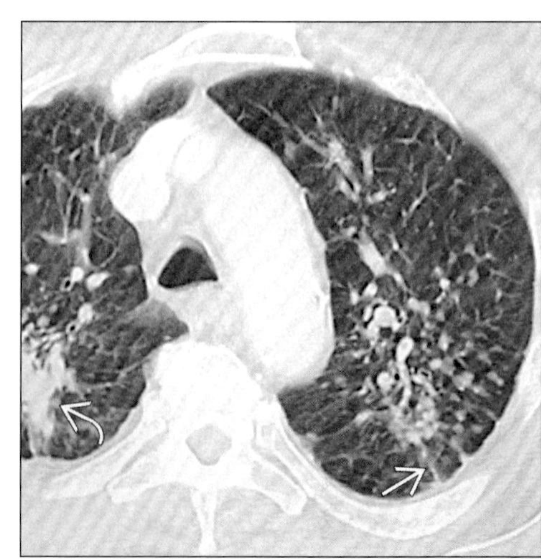

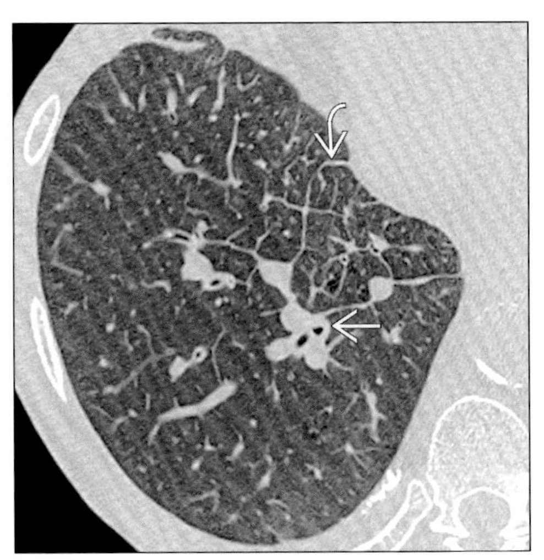

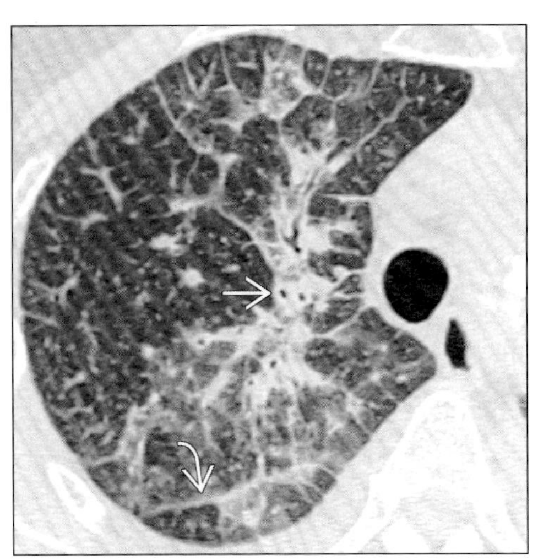

(Left) Axial HRCT of a patient with lymphangitic carcinomatosis shows smooth thickening of the interlobular septa ➔ and peribronchovascular interstitium ➔. *(Right)* Axial HRCT of a patient with lymphangitic carcinomatosis shows smooth thickening of interlobular septa and the peribronchovascular ➔ and subpleural interstitium along the major fissure ➔. Although the distribution of disease is also perilymphatic, lymphangitic carcinomatosis should not be confused with sarcoidosis or silicosis.

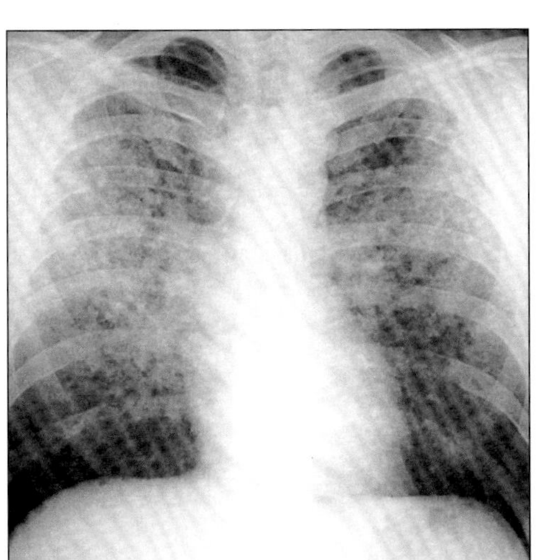

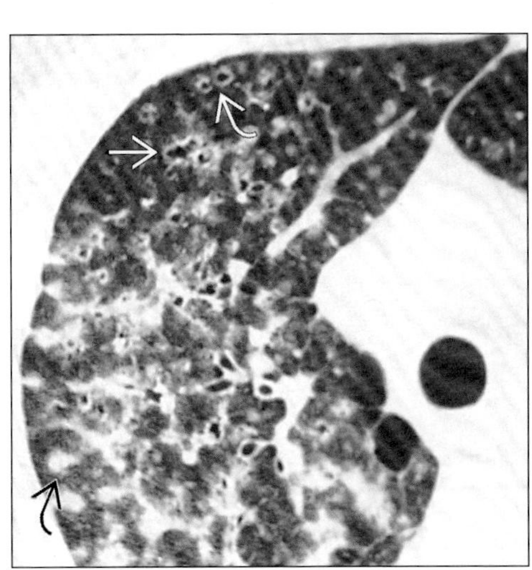

(Left) PA chest radiograph of a cigarette smoker with pulmonary Langerhans cell histiocytosis (PLCH) shows coarse reticulonodular opacities distributed predominantly in the mid and upper lung zones, with relative sparing of the lung bases. *(Right)* HRCT of the same patient shows irregular nodules in a centrilobular ➔ distribution, with thick and thin-walled cavitary nodules ➔ and an irregular cyst ➔. The abnormalities spared the lung bases, a characteristic feature of PLCH.

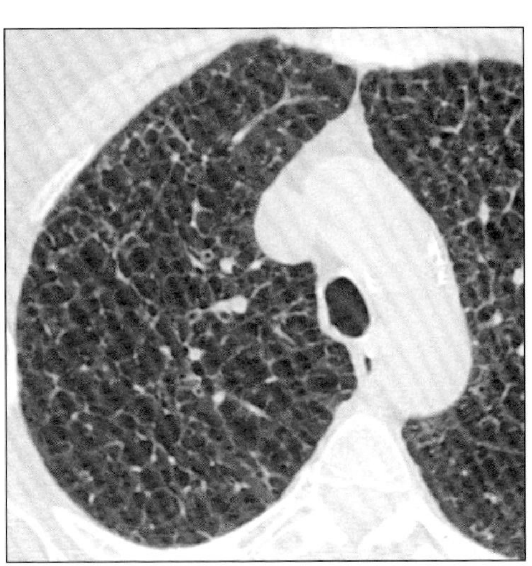

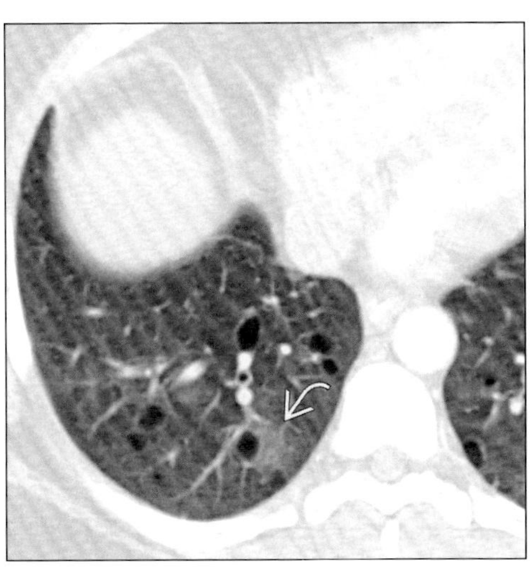

(Left) Axial HRCT of a patient with lymphangioleiomyomatosis (LAM) demonstrates numerous thin-walled cysts that were diffusely distributed throughout both lungs. The diffuse bilateral involvement is characteristic of LAM, whether the cysts are small and mildly profuse, as in the early stage of the disease, or large and extensive, as in more advanced cases. *(Right)* Axial CECT of a patient with lymphoid interstitial pneumonia (LIP) shows thin-walled cysts with surrounding ground-glass opacity ➔.

ACUTE RESPIRATORY DISTRESS SYNDROME (ARDS)

Key Facts

Terminology
- Acute respiratory distress syndrome (ARDS)

Imaging
- Imaging & pathologic findings discussed in terms of hours, days, weeks, & months
- Radiography/CT
  - Hours: May be normal in initial 12-24 hours
  - Days: Bilateral airspace opacities & consolidation within 24 hours
  - Weeks: Decreasing consolidation, persistent reticular opacities
  - Months: Subpleural reticular opacities & honeycombing
- Pulmonary injury: Consolidation & ground-glass opacity equally common, asymmetric
- Extrapulmonary injury: Ground-glass opacity more common than consolidation, symmetric

Top Differential Diagnoses
- Acute interstitial pneumonia
- Cardiogenic pulmonary edema
- Noncardiogenic pulmonary edema
- Pulmonary hemorrhage

Pathology
- Characterized by diffuse alveolar damage (DAD)

Clinical Issues
- ARDS may be complicated by pneumonia
- Survivors may develop fibrosis & honeycombing
- Treatment: Mechanical ventilation with high peak end-expiratory pressure

Diagnostic Checklist
- Consider ARDS in intubated patients who develop bilateral airspace opacities & consolidation

*(**Left**) AP chest radiograph of a patient with ARDS shows bilateral mid and lower lung zone consolidations, more pronounced on the right, and an appropriately positioned endotracheal tube ➔. Bilateral airspace opacities and consolidations are the most common imaging feature of ARDS. (**Right**) Axial CECT of the same patient shows dense consolidations ➚ in the posterior aspects of the upper lobes with intrinsic air bronchograms ➔ and ground-glass opacities ➪ in the nondependent aspects of the lungs.*

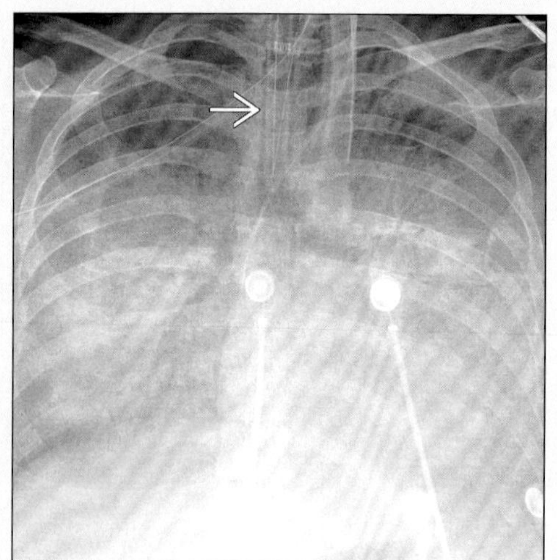

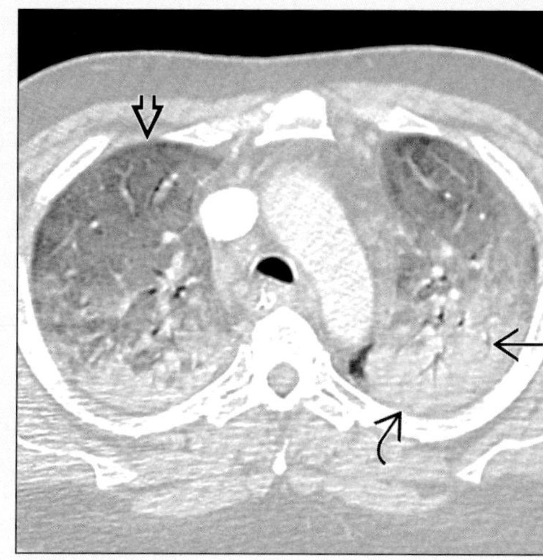

*(**Left**) Axial CECT of a patient with ARDS shows bilateral ground-glass opacities ➔, consolidations ➚, and a left pleural effusion ➔. Ground-glass opacity is more prevalent than consolidation in cases of ARDS from extrapulmonary etiologies. (**Right**) Axial CECT of a patient with lung fibrosis secondary to previous ARDS shows bilateral anterior architectural distortion and reticular opacities ➔. Note sparing of the posterior lung parenchyma, which may have been "protected" by prior atelectasis and consolidation.*

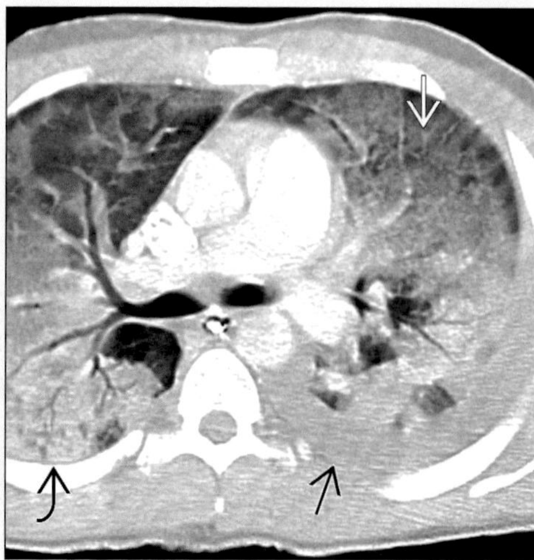

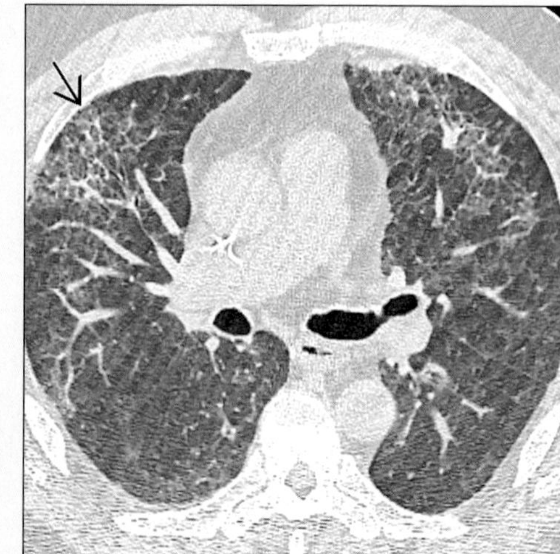

ACUTE RESPIRATORY DISTRESS SYNDROME (ARDS)

TERMINOLOGY

Abbreviations

- **Acute respiratory distress syndrome** (ARDS)

Synonyms

- Adult respiratory distress syndrome

IMAGING

General Features

- Best diagnostic clue
  - Bilateral airspace opacities & consolidations
- Radiologic & pathologic findings typically discussed in stages based on hours, days, weeks, & months

Radiographic Findings

- Radiography
  - Hours: May be normal 12-24 hours after injury
  - Days: Bilateral airspace opacities & consolidations within 24 hours
    - Dependent atelectasis
  - Weeks: Decreasing consolidation
    - Patchy airspace or reticular opacities persist
  - Months: Reticular opacities

CT Findings

- HRCT
  - Hours: May be normal 12-24 hours after injury
  - Days
    - General
      - Bilateral airspace opacities & consolidations within 24 hours
      - Dependent atelectasis
      - Interlobular septal thickening & pleural effusions less common than in cardiogenic pulmonary edema
    - Pulmonary injury
      - Consolidations & ground-glass opacities equally common
      - Asymmetric lung involvement
    - Extrapulmonary injury
      - Ground-glass opacities more common than consolidations
      - Symmetric lung involvement
  - Weeks: Consolidation decreases
    - Patchy airspace or reticular opacities persist
    - Ground-glass opacities
  - Months: Subpleural reticular opacities & honeycombing
    - May exhibit anterior predominance
    - Atelectasis/consolidation may "protect" posterior lungs from effects of mechanical ventilation

Imaging Recommendations

- Best imaging tool
  - Chest radiography adequate for monitoring disease
  - CT used as problem-solving tool

DIFFERENTIAL DIAGNOSIS

Acute Interstitial Pneumonia

- Idiopathic acute respiratory distress syndrome
- Imaging findings indistinguishable from ARDS

Cardiogenic Pulmonary Edema

- Central > peripheral opacities (bat-wing distribution)
- Kerley B lines, peribronchial cuffing, & pleural effusions
- Increased heart size

Noncardiogenic Pulmonary Edema

- Peripheral > central opacities
- Kerley B lines, peribronchial cuffing, & pleural effusion less common than in cardiogenic pulmonary edema
- Normal heart size

Pulmonary Hemorrhage

- Diffuse bilateral airspace opacities
- Normal heart size

PATHOLOGY

General Features

- Etiology
  - Pulmonary injury: Pneumonia, aspiration, inhalational injury, & trauma
  - Extrapulmonary injury: Sepsis & nonthoracic trauma

Microscopic Features

- Characterized by diffuse alveolar damage (DAD)
  - Early exudative stage (hours after precipitating event): Endothelial cell edema, capillary congestion, & minimal interstitial hemorrhage/edema
  - Late exudative stage (1 day to 1 week): Necrosis of type I pneumocytes, pulmonary edema, hemorrhage
  - Proliferative or reparative stage (1 week to 1 month): Proliferation of type II pneumocytes, fibroblast proliferation, collagen deposition
  - Fibrotic stage (months): Interstitial fibrosis

CLINICAL ISSUES

Presentation

- Most common signs/symptoms
  - Shortness of breath, tachypnea, hypoxia

Natural History & Prognosis

- ARDS may be complicated by pneumonia
  - Dense consolidation in nondependent location
- Survivors may develop fibrosis & honeycombing

Treatment

- Mechanical ventilation with high peak end-expiratory pressure

DIAGNOSTIC CHECKLIST

Consider

- ARDS in intubated patients who develop bilateral airspace opacities & consolidation

SELECTED REFERENCES

1. Goodman LR et al: Adult respiratory distress syndrome due to pulmonary and extrapulmonary causes: CT, clinical, and functional correlations. Radiology. 213(2):545-52, 1999

ACUTE INTERSTITIAL PNEUMONIA

Key Facts

Terminology

- Acute interstitial pneumonia (AIP)
- Rapidly progressive respiratory failure of unknown etiology in patients without preexisting lung disease

Imaging

- Radiography
  - Diffuse bilateral symmetric pulmonary opacities without zonal predilection
  - Usually on mechanical ventilation
  - Septal lines & small pleural effusions
- CT
  - Ground-glass opacity (± crazy-paving)
  - Consolidation, typically in dependent lung
  - Small pleural effusions in 30%
  - Mild mediastinal lymphadenopathy in 5-10%
  - Traction bronchiectasis & bronchiolectasis
  - Honeycomb lung develops in 10-26%

Top Differential Diagnoses

- Acute respiratory distress syndrome (ARDS)
- Pneumocystis pneumonia
- Diffuse alveolar hemorrhage
- Hydrostatic pulmonary edema
- Connective tissue disease

Pathology

- Diffuse alveolar damage (not specific to AIP)

Clinical Issues

- Acute onset (over 1-3 weeks)
- Poor prognosis
  - Mortality rate ≥ 50%
  - Most deaths within 2 months of onset
- Treatment
  - No known effective treatment
  - Supportive care

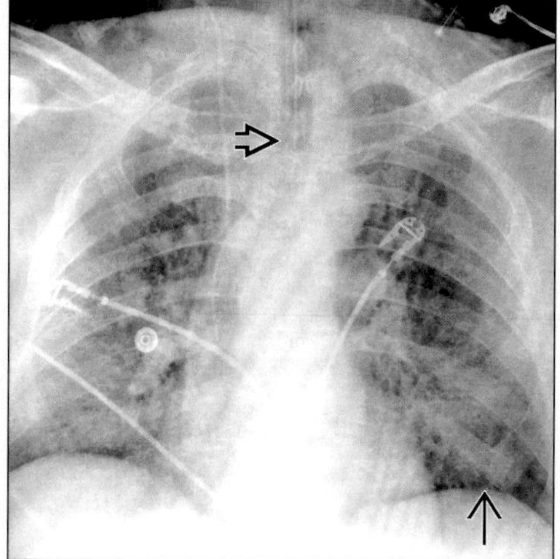

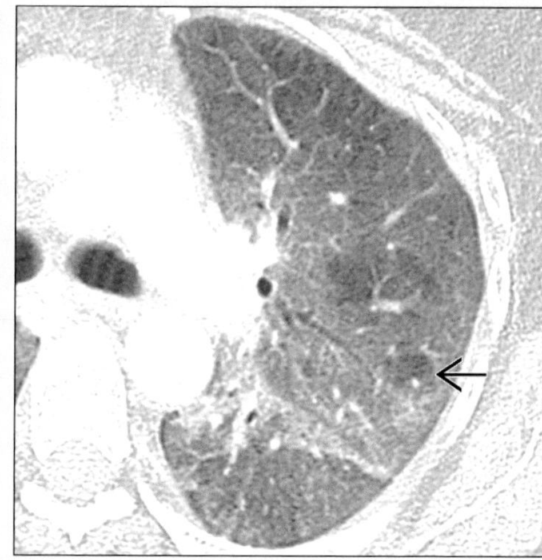

*(**Left**) AP chest radiograph of a patient with AIP shows diffuse bilateral hazy opacities with patchy foci of denser opacity ➡ in the lower zones and an endotracheal tube ➡ in place. Note relatively normal cardiac size and absence of pleural effusions. (**Right**) Axial NECT of a patient with AIP shows diffuse ground-glass opacity with sparing of some secondary pulmonary lobules ➡. As the disease progresses, ground-glass opacity and lung consolidation usually become more extensive and confluent.*

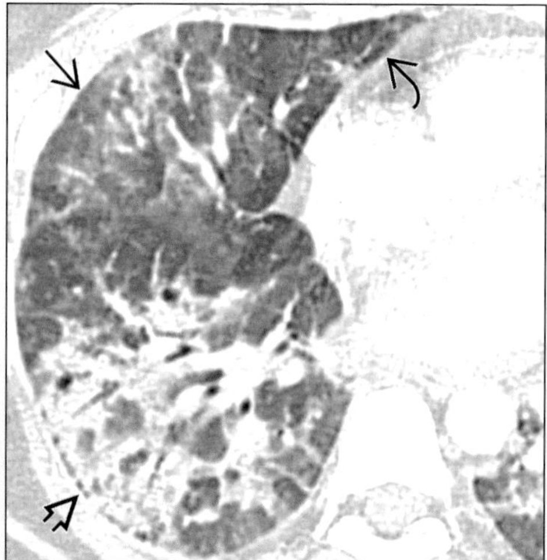

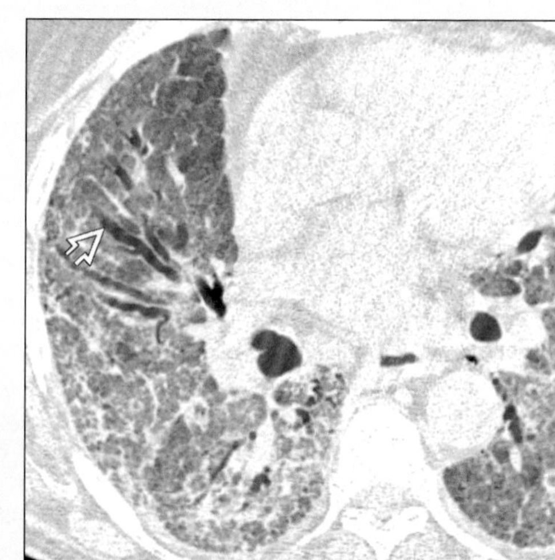

*(**Left**) Axial HRCT of a patient with AIP shows patchy consolidation ➡ in the dependent lung and patchy ground-glass opacity ➡ in the nondependent lung. Note sparing of several secondary pulmonary lobules ➡. (**Right**) Axial HRCT of a patient with AIP in the organizing phase of the disease shows diffuse ground-glass opacity with superimposed reticulation and traction bronchiectasis ➡. Interstitial fibrosis may leave surviving patients who have AIP with residual restrictive pulmonary dysfunction.*

ACUTE INTERSTITIAL PNEUMONIA

TERMINOLOGY

Abbreviations

- **Acute interstitial pneumonia (AIP)**

Synonyms

- Hamman-Rich syndrome
- Diffuse alveolar damage (DAD)
- Idiopathic acute respiratory distress syndrome (ARDS)

Definitions

- Rapidly progressive respiratory failure of unknown etiology in patients without preexisting lung disease

IMAGING

General Features

- Best diagnostic clue
  - Radiography: Diffuse symmetric airspace opacification
  - CT: Extensive ground-glass opacity & consolidation

Radiographic Findings

- Radiography
  - Diffuse bilateral symmetric lung opacities
    - Usually on mechanical ventilation
    - No particular zonal predilection
    - Septal lines & small pleural effusions

CT Findings

- **Ground-glass opacity**
  - Initially patchy, becoming more diffuse with disease progression
  - Geographic appearance from focal lobular sparing
  - Superimposed septal lines common: Crazy-paving pattern
- **Consolidation**
  - Present in most patients
  - Patchy or confluent, predominantly in dependent lung
  - Peripheral predominance in 10-20%
- Small pleural effusions in 30%
- Mild mediastinal lymphadenopathy in 5-10%
- Traction bronchiectasis & bronchiolectasis
  - Late proliferative & fibrotic phases
- Honeycomb lung develops in 10-26%

Imaging Recommendations

- Protocol advice
  - CT can be performed without contrast

DIFFERENTIAL DIAGNOSIS

Acute Respiratory Distress Syndrome (ARDS)

- Associated with a known cause
- Imaging findings indistinguishable from AIP

Pneumocystis Pneumonia

- Typically bilateral ground-glass opacity
- Immunocompromised host

Diffuse Alveolar Hemorrhage

- Diffuse ground-glass opacity, often evolves to reticular opacities
- Features of pulmonary fibrosis with repeated episodes

Hydrostatic Pulmonary Edema

- Septal lines ± airspace opacities
- Cardiomegaly
- Pleural effusion

Connective Tissue Disease

- Typically systemic lupus erythematosus (acute lupus pneumonitis)
- DAD is an uncommon complication

PATHOLOGY

General Features

- Etiology
  - Temporal uniformity suggests single (overwhelming) injury
- Diffuse alveolar damage (not specific to AIP)
  - Acute hypersensitivity pneumonitis
  - ARDS
  - Connective tissue disease
  - Drug reaction
  - Infection
  - Toxins: Nitrogen dioxide, oxygen toxicity, paraquat, chlorine gas

CLINICAL ISSUES

Presentation

- Most common signs/symptoms
  - Acute onset (over 1-3 weeks)
    - Rapid progression to respiratory failure requiring mechanical ventilation
    - Similar to ARDS in presentation, but no identifiable etiologic factor
  - Flu-like prodrome in majority of patients: Headache, myalgia, sore throat, malaise, dry cough

Demographics

- Age
  - Mean age of 50; range from children to adults
- Gender
  - M = F

Natural History & Prognosis

- Poor prognosis: Mortality rate ≥ 50%, most deaths within 2 months of symptom onset
- Survivors may completely recover lung function
  - Persistent, stable, restrictive physiology also common
  - Recurrence seen but extremely rare

Treatment

- No known effective treatment
- Supportive care is mainstay of treatment

SELECTED REFERENCES

1. Kim DS et al: Classification and natural history of the idiopathic interstitial pneumonias. Proc Am Thorac Soc. 3(4):285-92, 2006
2. Swigris JJ et al: Acute interstitial pneumonia and acute exacerbations of idiopathic pulmonary fibrosis. Semin Respir Crit Care Med. 27(6):659-67, 2006
3. Lynch DA et al: Idiopathic interstitial pneumonias: CT features. Radiology. 236(1):10-21, 2005

IDIOPATHIC PULMONARY FIBROSIS

Key Facts

Terminology

- Idiopathic pulmonary fibrosis (IPF)
- Idiopathic usual interstitial pneumonia (UIP)
- Fibrosing idiopathic interstitial pneumonia with histologic pattern of UIP on surgical biopsy
- ~ 40% of all idiopathic interstitial pneumonias

Imaging

- Radiography
  - Basilar reticular opacities
  - Low lung volume
  - Pulmonary arterial hypertension
- HRCT
  - Basilar predominant reticulation
  - Traction bronchiectasis or bronchiolectasis
  - Honeycomb lung
  - Ground-glass less extensive than reticulation
  - Dominant nodule/mass suggests lung cancer

Top Differential Diagnoses

- Asbestosis
- Chronic hypersensitivity pneumonitis
- Rheumatoid arthritis
- Systemic sclerosis
- Drug reaction

Pathology

- Usual interstitial pneumonia

Clinical Issues

- Symptoms: Dyspnea, nonproductive cough
- Age: 55-70 years; M:F ≈ 2:1
- Inexorable progression with poor prognosis

Diagnostic Checklist

- Idiopathic subpleural & basal reticulation with honeycombing enables HRCT diagnosis of IPF

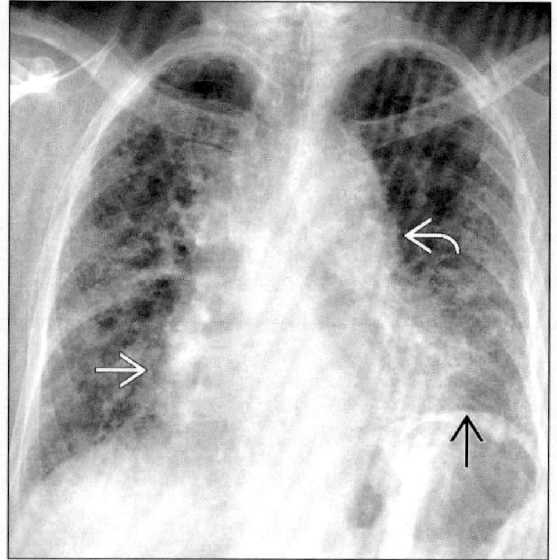

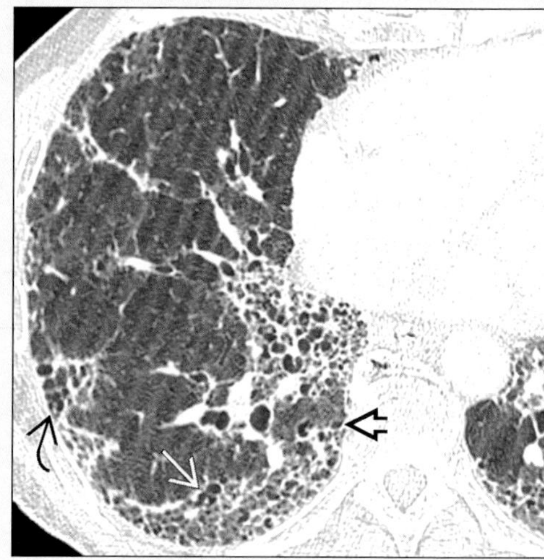

(Left) *PA chest radiograph of a patient with IPF shows extensive peripheral basal predominant reticulation ⇨ with enlargement of the pulmonary trunk ➡ and right atrium ➡, suggestive of pulmonary arterial hypertension (a known complication of IPF).* ***(Right)*** *Axial HRCT of a patient with IPF shows subpleural predominant reticulation and honeycomb lung ⇨ with traction bronchiectasis ➡ and traction bronchiolectasis ⇨. Note relative sparing of the central portions of the lung.*

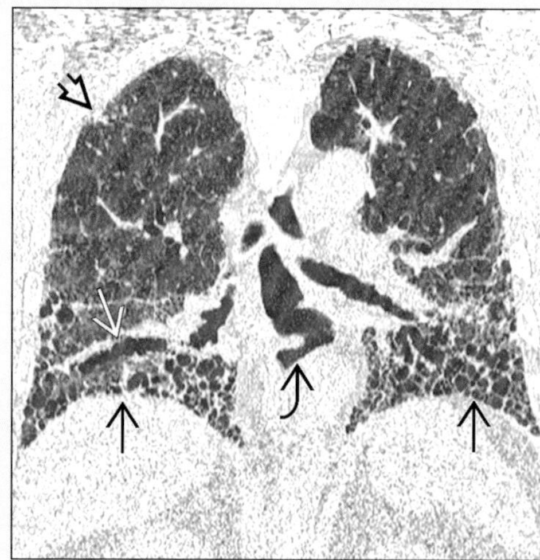

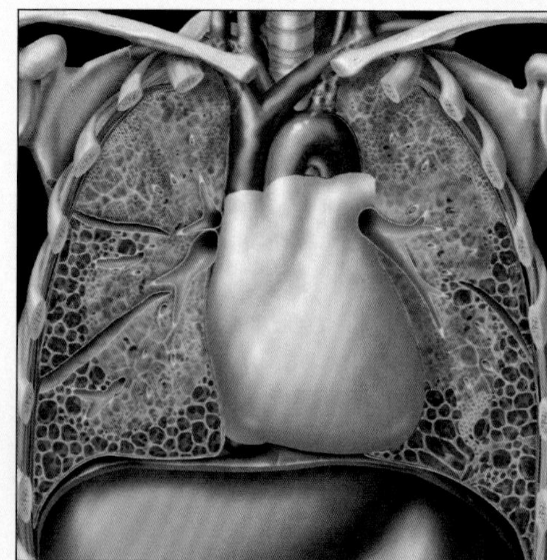

(Left) *Coronal NECT shows peripheral and basal predominant honeycomb lung ⇨, traction bronchiectasis ➡, and subpleural reticulation ⇨ in the upper lobes. Although IPF primarily affects the lower lobes, upper lobe involvement is usually evident, but to a lesser degree. Esophageal gas ⇨ is presumably from presbyesophagus in this patient with no known connective tissue disease.* ***(Right)*** *Graphic illustrates the characteristic subpleural and basal distribution of fibrosis and honeycombing in IPF.*

IDIOPATHIC PULMONARY FIBROSIS

TERMINOLOGY

Abbreviations

- **Idiopathic pulmonary fibrosis (IPF)**

Synonyms

- **Cryptogenic fibrosing alveolitis (CFA)**
- Idiopathic usual interstitial pneumonia (UIP)

Definitions

- Distinct form of fibrosing idiopathic interstitial pneumonia associated with histologic pattern of UIP on surgical biopsy
- Accounts for approximately 40% of all idiopathic interstitial pneumonias

IMAGING

General Features

- Best diagnostic clue
  - Subpleural & basal reticulation with traction bronchiectasis, architectural distortion, & honeycomb lung
  - Absence of atypical features: Micronodules, basal sparing, extensive lobular air-trapping, consolidation, &/or ground-glass opacity
- Location
  - Mid & lower lung zone subpleural lung
- Morphology
  - Reticulation, traction bronchiectasis/bronchiolectasis, honeycomb lung

Radiographic Findings

- Radiography
  - Reticular or reticulonodular opacities
  - Mid/lower zone peripheral lung parenchyma
  - Lower zone volume loss
    - Persistent low lung volume
  - Pulmonary trunk & right heart chamber enlargement
    - Secondary pulmonary arterial hypertension

CT Findings

- HRCT
  - More sensitive & specific than radiography for diagnosis of IPF
  - Clinical & HRCT findings sufficient to establish diagnosis of IPF in 50-70% of patients with > 90% specificity
  - **Reticulation**
    - Basal & subpleural predominance
    - Usually also present in upper lobes, but to lesser extent
  - **Traction bronchiectasis or bronchiolectasis**
    - Basal & peripheral predominance
    - Usually associated with areas of reticulation
  - **Honeycombing**
    - Most specific finding of IPF
    - Subpleural lung cysts, usually in clusters or rows
  - Ground-glass opacity
    - Less extensive than reticular opacities
      - Exuberant ground-glass opacity suggests alternate diagnosis (hypersensitivity pneumonitis or NSIP)
      - May reflect acute exacerbation of IPF in patients with acute respiratory illness
  - Volume loss in advanced disease
  - Coexistent centrilobular or paraseptal emphysema in ~ 30%
  - **Persistent or growing dominant lung nodule/mass should raise suspicion for lung cancer**
  - Mediastinal lymph node enlargement in ~ 70%
    - Usually mild (occult on radiography)

Imaging Recommendations

- Best imaging tool
  - HRCT to detect & characterize interstitial lung disease

DIFFERENTIAL DIAGNOSIS

Asbestosis

- Subpleural reticular opacities with honeycomb lung
  - Subpleural lines not pathognomonic
- Ill-defined subpleural "dots"
  - Thought to represent peribronchial fibrosis
- Fibrosis in asbestosis may be coarser than in IPF
- Associated findings
  - Calcified and noncalcified pleural plaques
  - Parenchymal bands
  - Subpleural curvilinear opacities

Chronic Hypersensitivity Pneumonitis

- Relative sparing of extreme bases in most patients
  - Bases usually most severely involved in IPF
- Lobular areas of apparent sparing (due to associated bronchiolitis & resultant air-trapping)
  - "Head cheese" sign: Mosaic of ground-glass attenuation, normal & hypoattenuating (air-trapping) pulmonary lobules
- Poorly defined centrilobular nodules suggest chronic hypersensitivity pneumonitis
- May be indistinguishable from IPF

Rheumatoid Arthritis

- UIP pattern may be seen more frequently than nonspecific interstitial pneumonia (NSIP) pattern
  - HRCT findings indistinguishable from UIP & NSIP from other causes
  - May progress more slowly than IPF
- Other features of rheumatoid arthritis
  - Joint erosions
  - Serum markers (e.g., rheumatoid factor)
  - Pleural effusion
  - Rheumatoid nodules

Systemic Sclerosis

- NSIP pattern much more common than UIP pattern
  - Ground-glass predominant
  - Honeycomb lung uncommon except in advanced, longstanding disease
- Patulous esophagus common in systemic sclerosis
- Cutaneous findings of systemic sclerosis usually readily apparent

Drug Reaction

- Can cause similar radiographic abnormalities
- Typical drugs: Nitrofurantoin or chemotherapy drugs

Sarcoidosis

- Typically causes bronchocentric fibrosis in upper lung zones
- Small proportion exhibit imaging pattern indistinguishable from IPF

IDIOPATHIC PULMONARY FIBROSIS

PATHOLOGY

General Features

- Etiology
  - Unknown etiology
    - Suspected but unproven association with cigarette smoking
  - Unproven associations
    - Chronic aspiration
    - Infections (e.g., Epstein-Barr, influenza, Cytomegalovirus)
    - Inorganic dusts & solvents
- Genetics
  - Familial cases of IPF reported (probably autosomal dominant inheritance)
  - No genetic markers yet identified
- Key features: Patchy fibrosis & architectural distortion

Gross Pathologic & Surgical Features

- **Usual interstitial pneumonia**
  - **Spatial & temporal heterogeneity** (key finding)
    - Varying proportions of fibrosis, inflammation, & honeycomb lung interspersed with normal lung

Microscopic Features

- **Fibrosis**
  - Subpleural predominant distribution
  - Characteristic fibroblastic foci
    - Not feature of other idiopathic interstitial pneumonias
  - Dense acellular collagen
- **Mild to moderate interstitial inflammation**
- **Honeycomb lung**
  - Honeycomb cysts lined by bronchiolar epithelium
- **Regions of normal lung**

CLINICAL ISSUES

Presentation

- Most common signs/symptoms
  - Insidious onset of dyspnea on exertion
    - Usually present for months prior to clinical presentation
  - Nonproductive cough
- Other signs/symptoms
  - Digital clubbing
  - Fine inspiratory ("Velcro®") crackles
  - Signs of right heart failure
  - Pulmonary function tests
    - Restrictive abnormalities with decreased diffusion capacity (DLCO)

Demographics

- Age
  - 55-70 years
- Gender
  - M:F ≈ 2:1

Natural History & Prognosis

- **Inexorable progression, poor prognosis**
- Median survival following diagnosis ~ 3.5 years
- Rarely, rapid decline & death after period of relatively slower progression
  - Acute exacerbation of IPF
- **Lung cancer in ~ 10% of patients with IPF**
  - Most patients current or former smokers

Treatment

- To date no treatment regimen of proven benefit in improving survival of patients with IPF
- Lung transplantation for progressive functional decline
  - Mean survival at 5-years only 50%

DIAGNOSTIC CHECKLIST

Consider

- Drug reaction in any patient with IPF pattern of imaging abnormalities
- Undocumented or unsuspected connective tissue disease (especially rheumatoid arthritis) in patients with IPF

Image Interpretation Pearls

- Subpleural & basal predominant reticulation with honeycombing in absence of any known cause of pulmonary fibrosis should enable confident HRCT diagnosis of IPF

Reporting Tips

- Degree of confidence should be stated in report
  - "Definite UIP/IPF"
    - May obviate need for surgical biopsy
  - "Possible UIP/IPF"
    - Typical features of UIP/IPF without definitive honeycomb lung
  - "Inconsistent with UIP/IPF"
    - Atypical features, including basal sparing, significant air-trapping, micronodules, extensive ground-glass opacity

SELECTED REFERENCES

1. Edey AJ et al: Fibrotic idiopathic interstitial pneumonias: HRCT findings that predict mortality. Eur Radiol. Epub ahead of print, 2011
2. Raghu G et al: An Official ATS/ERS/JRS/ALAT Statement: Idiopathic Pulmonary Fibrosis: Evidence-based Guidelines for Diagnosis and Management. Am J Respir Crit Care Med. 183(6):788-824, 2011
3. Kanne JP: Idiopathic interstitial pneumonias. Semin Roentgenol. 45(1):8-21, 2010
4. Silva CI et al: Idiopathic interstitial pneumonias. J Thorac Imaging. 24(4):260-73, 2009
5. Misumi S et al: Idiopathic pulmonary fibrosis/usual interstitial pneumonia: imaging diagnosis, spectrum of abnormalities, and temporal progression. Proc Am Thorac Soc. 3(4):307-14, 2006
6. Lynch DA et al: High-resolution computed tomography in idiopathic pulmonary fibrosis: diagnosis and prognosis. Am J Respir Crit Care Med. 172(4):488-93, 2005
7. Souza CA et al: Idiopathic pulmonary fibrosis: spectrum of high-resolution CT findings. AJR Am J Roentgenol. 185(6):1531-9, 2005

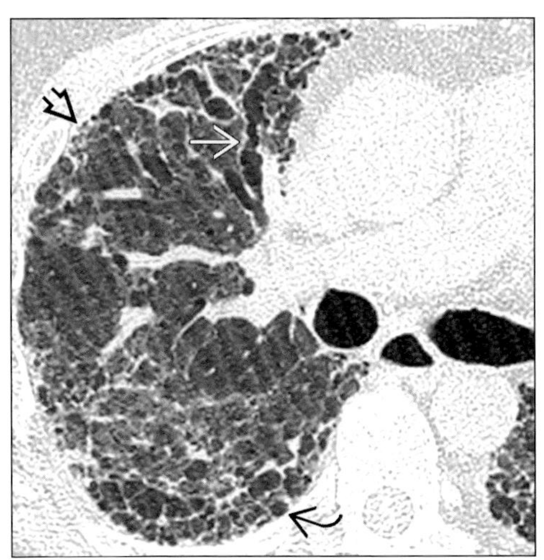

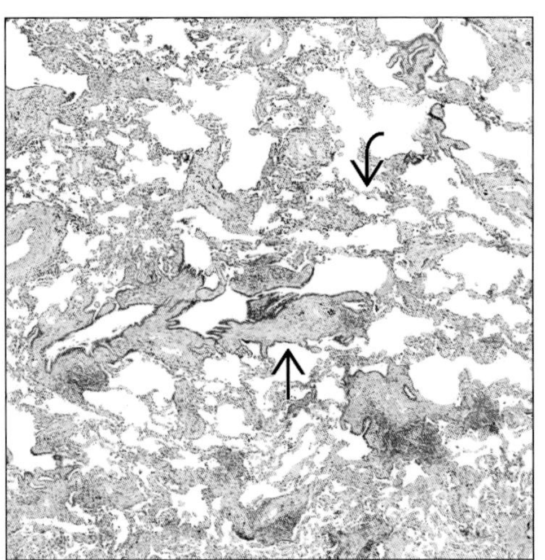

(Left) *Axial HRCT of a patient with IPF shows subpleural honeycombing and reticulation with traction bronchiectasis and scattered foci of normal lung.* ***(Right)*** *Low-power photomicrograph (H&E stain) shows the typical histology of usual interstitial pneumonia with foci of interstitial fibrosis amid normal lung parenchyma. The coexistence of lesions in different stages of organization has been described as "temporal heterogeneity." (Courtesy S. Suster, MD.)*

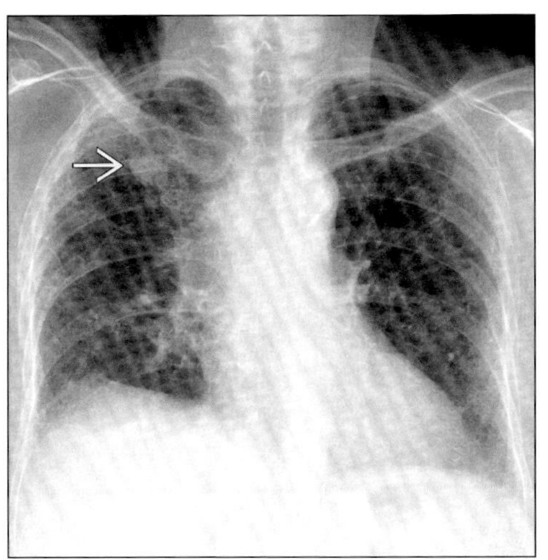

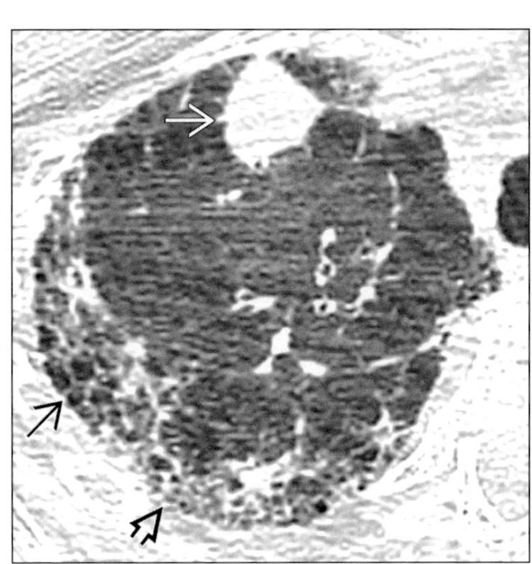

(Left) *PA chest radiograph of a patient with IPF shows peripheral and basal predominant reticulation and low lung volumes. A well-defined indeterminate nodule is present in the right upper lobe.* ***(Right)*** *Axial HRCT of the same patient shows subpleural honeycomb lung, reticulation, and traction bronchiolectasis. The dominant right upper lobe nodule was proven to be an adenocarcinoma. Patients with pulmonary fibrosis are at increased risk of developing lung cancer.*

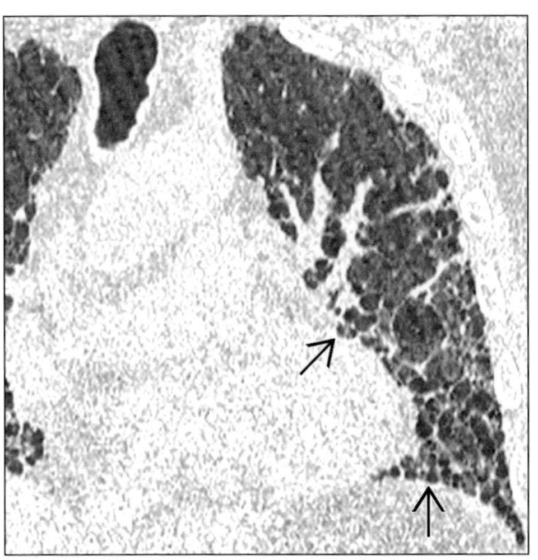

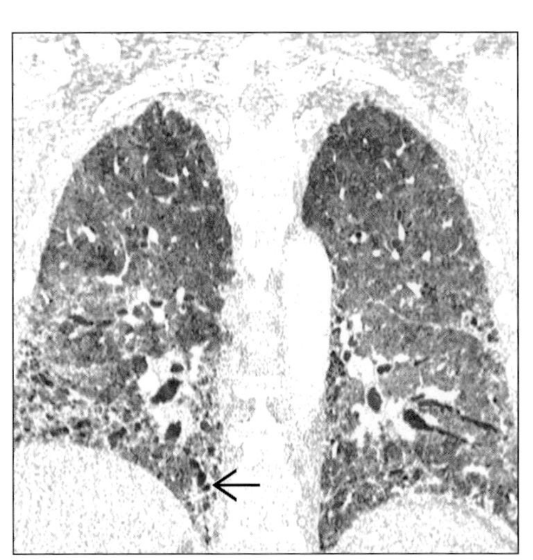

(Left) *Coronal NECT of a patient with IPF shows subpleural basal predominant honeycombing. The presence of honeycomb lung is a strong predictor of a UIP pattern of interstitial fibrosis.* ***(Right)*** *Coronal NECT of a patient with an acute exacerbation of IPF shows patchy ground-glass opacities superimposed on interstitial fibrosis manifesting with basal peripheral architectural distortion and traction bronchiectasis. Honeycombing may not be evident in patients with proven or presumed IPF.*

NONSPECIFIC INTERSTITIAL PNEUMONIA

Key Facts

Terminology
- Nonspecific interstitial pneumonia (NSIP)
- Idiopathic interstitial pneumonia
- Cellular & fibrotic subtypes

Imaging
- Radiography
  - Lower lobe volume loss
  - Bilateral basilar reticular opacities
- HRCT
  - Symmetric lower lobe volume loss
  - Ground-glass opacities
  - Reticular opacities
  - Traction bronchiectasis/bronchiolectasis
  - Peripheral distribution, may exhibit subpleural sparing & peribronchovascular distribution
- Overlapping imaging features of cellular & fibrotic NSIP; no reliable differentiation on imaging

Top Differential Diagnoses
- Idiopathic pulmonary fibrosis
- Cryptogenic organizing pneumonia
- Hypersensitivity pneumonitis
- Desquamative interstitial pneumonia

Pathology
- Spatial & temporal homogeneity of interstitial inflammation &/or fibrosis

Clinical Issues
- Gradual onset of symptoms: Dyspnea, cough, malaise, fatigue
- Important distinction of NSIP from UIP
  - Better prognosis with NSIP

Diagnostic Checklist
- Consider open lung biopsy when clinical & HRCT findings are discordant

*(**Left**) PA chest radiograph of a patient with NSIP shows low lung volumes and subtle fine reticular opacities involving the bilateral lung bases. Patients with NSIP may exhibit volume loss that is most prevalent in the lower lobes. (**Right**) Lateral chest radiograph of the same patient shows mild basilar reticular opacities with associated volume loss ➡. Although nonspecific, these are the 2 most common radiographic findings seen in patients with NSIP.*

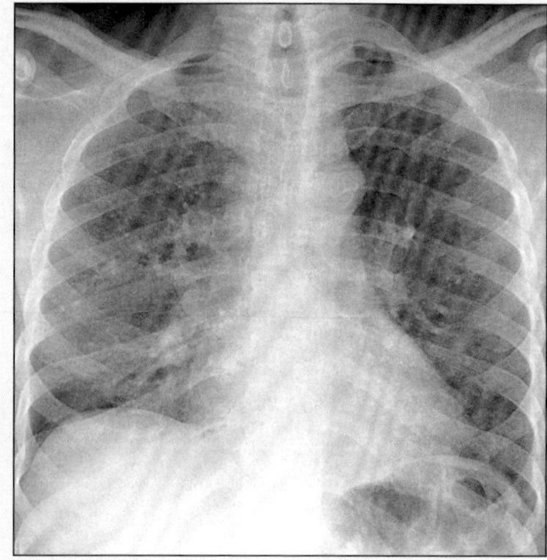

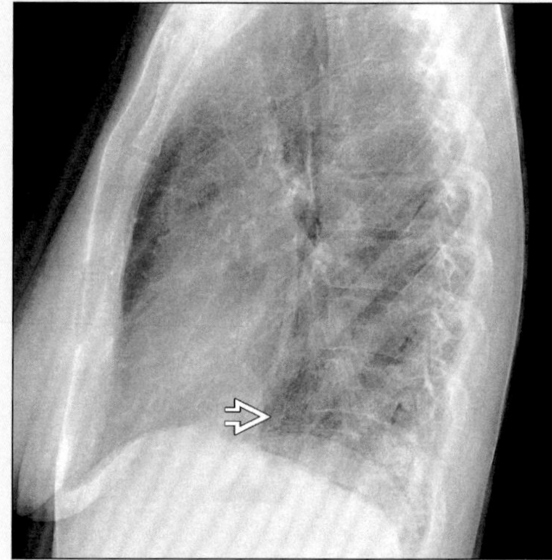

*(**Left**) Axial HRCT of a patient with NSIP shows scattered peripheral fine reticular opacities ➡ associated with mild, patchy, ground-glass opacities and mild traction bronchiolectasis ➡. The imaging features are characteristic of NSIP. (**Right**) Axial prone HRCT of a patient with NSIP shows subpleural reticulation ➡ and mild traction bronchiolectasis ➡ without evidence of honeycombing. The presence of honeycomb lung should suggest the alternative diagnosis of idiopathic pulmonary fibrosis.*

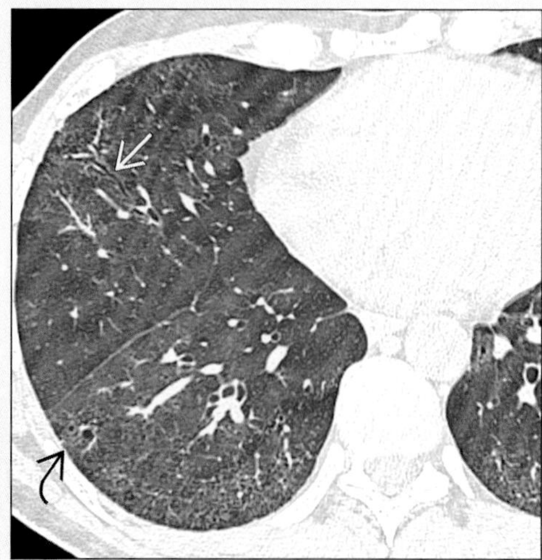

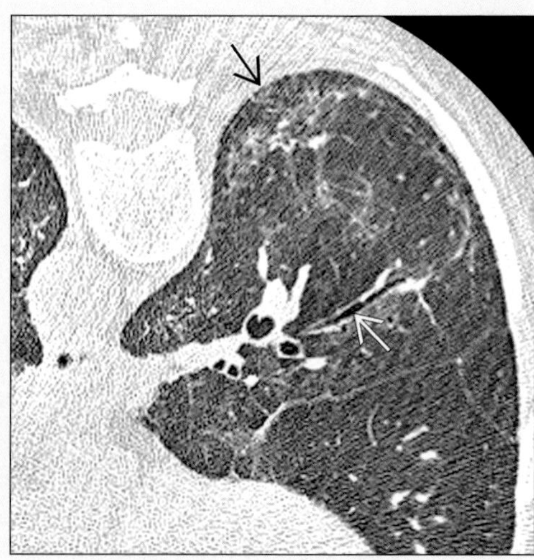

NONSPECIFIC INTERSTITIAL PNEUMONIA

TERMINOLOGY

Abbreviations

- **Nonspecific interstitial pneumonia (NSIP)**

Definitions

- 2nd most common idiopathic interstitial pneumonia
- Subtypes
  - Cellular
  - Fibrotic

IMAGING

General Features

- Best diagnostic clue
  - HRCT: Bibasilar symmetric ground-glass opacities with reticulation & traction bronchiectasis
- Location
  - Lower lobe predominance
  - Classically peripheral, but may exhibit peribronchovascular distribution & subpleural sparing

Radiographic Findings

- Abnormal radiographs in 90% of cases, but typically nonspecific radiographic abnormalities
- **Lower lobe volume loss**
- **Bilateral basilar reticular opacities**
- No pleural effusion

CT Findings

- HRCT
  - **Symmetric lower lobe volume loss**
  - **Ground-glass opacities**
    - Very common in early disease
    - Basilar predominant
    - Upper lobe predominant abnormalities should suggest other entities
  - **Reticular opacities**
    - More prevalent in fibrotic NSIP
    - May coexist with ground-glass opacities
  - **Traction bronchiectasis/bronchiolectasis**
    - Most conspicuous in lower lobes
    - Suggests fibrotic NSIP
  - Consolidation
    - Often in association with bronchiectasis
    - Should not be predominant abnormality
  - Honeycomb lung
    - Varying reports, but probably rare (5%)
    - Honeycomb lung suggests idiopathic pulmonary fibrosis (IPF)
  - Cellular & fibrotic NSIP exhibit overlapping imaging features; no reliable way of differentiation
    - **Cellular**
      - Bibasilar symmetric ground-glass opacities
      - Reticular opacities
      - Absence of fibrosis or honeycomb lung
      - Subpleural sparing more common
    - **Fibrotic**
      - Reticulation more common
      - Architectural distortion, traction bronchiectasis/bronchiolectasis, & honeycomb lung more common
      - Subpleural distribution more common

Imaging Recommendations

- Best imaging tool
  - HRCT is optimal imaging modality for characterization & assessment of disease extent
- Protocol advice
  - Supine & prone HRCT for optimal demonstration of basilar abnormalities & fibrosis

DIFFERENTIAL DIAGNOSIS

Idiopathic Pulmonary Fibrosis (IPF)

- May resemble fibrotic NSIP on HRCT
- Basilar subpleural location
- Honeycomb lung much more common
- Open lung biopsy may not be required if HRCT findings characteristic
- Much poorer prognosis than NSIP

Cryptogenic Organizing Pneumonia

- Greater degree of consolidation
- Peribronchovascular opacities
- Reticular opacities less common
- Steroid responsive

Hypersensitivity Pneumonitis

- Geographic ground-glass opacities, centrilobular nodules
- Mosaic attenuation
  - Due to small airway inflammation
  - Air-trapping on expiratory HRCT
- History of exposure important for diagnosis

Desquamative Interstitial Pneumonia

- Smoking-related lung disease
- Basilar ground-glass opacities, often with associated small thin-walled cysts
- Steroid responsive

Pulmonary Alveolar Proteinosis

- "Crazy-paving" pattern
- Ground-glass opacities
- Interlobular septal thickening & intralobular lines

Sarcoidosis

- Classic findings of perilymphatic micronodules & symmetric lymphadenopathy
- Upper lobe predominance

Lipoid Pneumonia

- Inhalation or aspiration of lipid (e.g., mineral oil)
- Airspace disease may exhibit fat attenuation on CT
- Mass-like opacities, may mimic neoplasia
- Airspace disease resembling pneumonia
- "Crazy-paving" pattern on HRCT

PATHOLOGY

General Features

- Etiology
  - Idiopathic
  - Collagen vascular diseases can cause NSIP pattern
    - Systemic sclerosis, polymyositis/dermatomyositis, Sjögren syndrome, rheumatoid arthritis
  - Hypersensitivity pneumonitis
  - Drug-induced lung disease

- Amiodarone, nitrofurantoin, gold salts, methotrexate, vincristine, fludarabine
  - Radiation toxicity
  - Does not represent early form of IPF
- Associated abnormalities
  - Not associated with cigarette smoking

Microscopic Features

- **Spatial & temporal homogeneity**
  - Important for distinguishing NSIP from UIP
- Varying degrees of interstitial inflammation &/or fibrosis
- Cellular & fibrotic subtypes
- Cellular (less common)
  - Interstitial infiltrate: Lymphocytes, plasma cells
  - Hyperplasia of alveolar lining cells
  - Minimal fibrosis
- Fibrotic
  - Interstitial collagen deposition
  - Marked alveolar septal thickening
  - Derangement of lung architecture
  - May be difficult to distinguish from UIP

CLINICAL ISSUES

Presentation

- Most common signs/symptoms
  - Gradual onset of symptoms
    - **Dyspnea**
    - **Cough**
    - **Malaise**
    - **Fatigue**
    - **Anorexia, weight loss**
    - Fever is uncommon
  - Symptoms for 6-18 months prior to presentation
    - Range: 1 week to 5 years
  - Signs
    - **Crackles**
    - Digital clubbing < 35%
- **Pulmonary function tests**
  - Restrictive ventilatory defect
  - Mild reduction of FEV_1
  - Reduced diffusion capacity (DLco)
  - Extent of disease on HRCT correlates significantly with pulmonary function

Demographics

- Age
  - 40-50 years; mean age: 49 years
    - Younger age than patients with UIP
- Gender
  - M = F for idiopathic NSIP
  - NSIP related to collagen vascular disease, more common in women

Natural History & Prognosis

- Potentially reversible features
  - Ground-glass opacities
  - Reticular opacities
- Greater the proportion of fibrosis, worse the prognosis
  - Even with fibrosis, better prognosis than UIP
  - Fibrotic NSIP worse prognosis than cellular NSIP
- NSIP
  - Complete recovery (45%)
  - Stability or improvement (42%)
  - Mortality (11%)
- Important distinction of NSIP from UIP
  - Better prognosis with NSIP
  - Median survivals
    - NSIP: > 13 years
    - UIP: 2-4 years

Diagnosis

- Transbronchial biopsy may provide incorrect diagnosis, e.g., cryptogenic organizing pneumonia
- Bronchoalveolar lavage: Increased lymphocytes
- Definitive diagnosis: Open lung biopsy

Treatment

- Corticosteroids

DIAGNOSTIC CHECKLIST

Consider

- Open lung biopsy when clinical & HRCT findings are discordant

Image Interpretation Pearls

- Nodules, cysts, low-attenuation areas, & unilateral disease should suggest alternate diagnosis
- Look for imaging findings of collagen vascular disease: Esophageal dilatation, pleural/pericardial effusion, pulmonary artery enlargement, musculoskeletal involvement

Reporting Tips

- Interdisciplinary consensus between clinicians, radiologists, & pathologists strongly encouraged to make diagnosis

SELECTED REFERENCES

1. Akira M et al: Usual interstitial pneumonia and nonspecific interstitial pneumonia with and without concurrent emphysema: thin-section CT findings. Radiology. 251(1):271-9, 2009
2. Kligerman SJ et al: Nonspecific interstitial pneumonia: radiologic, clinical, and pathologic considerations. Radiographics. 29(1):73-87, 2009
3. Silva CI et al: Nonspecific interstitial pneumonia and idiopathic pulmonary fibrosis: changes in pattern and distribution of disease over time. Radiology. 247(1):251-9, 2008
4. Travis WD et al: Idiopathic nonspecific interstitial pneumonia: report of an American Thoracic Society project. Am J Respir Crit Care Med. 2008 Jun 15;177(12):1338-47. Epub 2008 Apr 3. Review. Erratum in: Am J Respir Crit Care Med. 178(2): 211, 2008
5. Lynch DA et al: Idiopathic interstitial pneumonias: CT features. Radiology. 236(1):10-21, 2005
6. Ellis SM et al: Idiopathic interstitial pneumonias: imaging-pathology correlation. Eur Radiol. 12(3):610-26, 2002
7. Coche E et al: Non-specific interstitial pneumonia showing a "crazy paving" pattern on high resolution CT. Br J Radiol. 74(878):189-91, 2001
8. Nishiyama O et al: Serial high resolution CT findings in nonspecific interstitial pneumonia/fibrosis. J Comput Assist Tomogr. 24(1):41-6, 2000

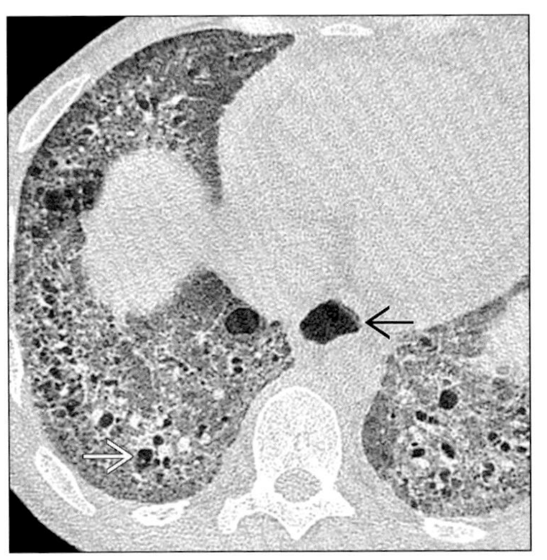

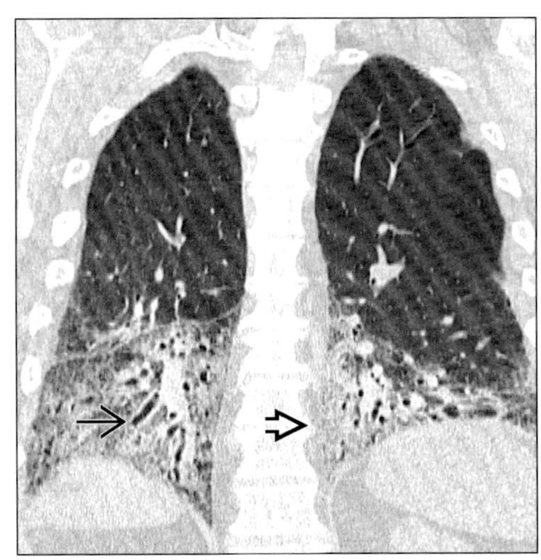

(Left) *Axial HRCT of a patient with NSIP secondary to scleroderma shows basilar ground-glass opacities with associated fine reticulation, bronchiectasis ➔, and bronchiolectasis. The dilated esophagus → is consistent with the known diagnosis of scleroderma.* ***(Right)*** *Coronal NECT of a patient with NSIP shows basilar ground-glass opacities ⇨ with intrinsic traction bronchiectasis → and bronchiolectasis and upper lung sparing. NSIP abnormalities typically exhibit a predilection for the lung bases.*

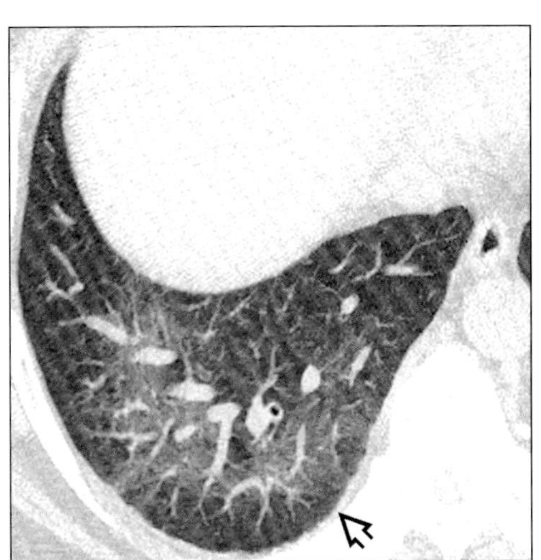

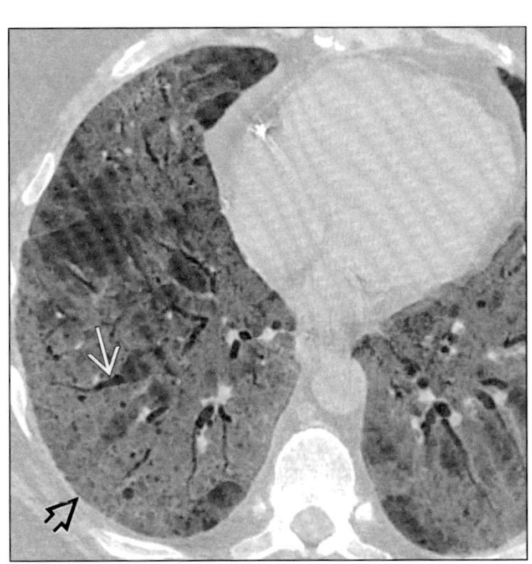

(Left) *Axial NECT of a patient with NSIP shows basilar predominant ground-glass opacities with characteristic sparing of the subpleural lung parenchyma ⇨. Absence of reticulation and bronchiectasis is consistent with cellular NSIP.* ***(Right)*** *Axial NECT minimum-intensity projection (minIP) image of a patient with NSIP shows diffuse bilateral ground-glass opacities ⇨ with scattered areas of lung sparing. The minIP highlights the multifocal associated bronchiectasis ➔ in this case.*

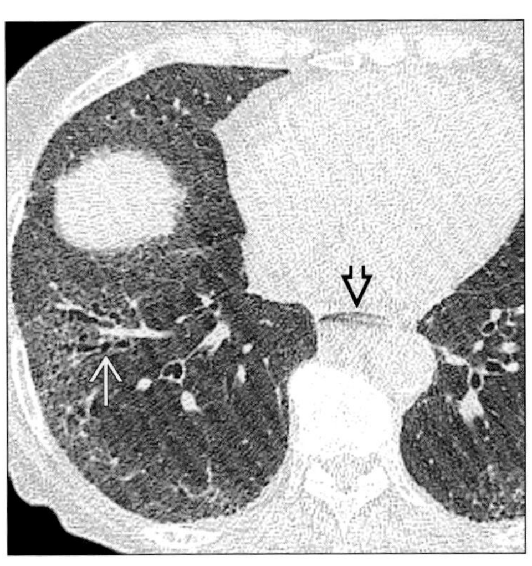

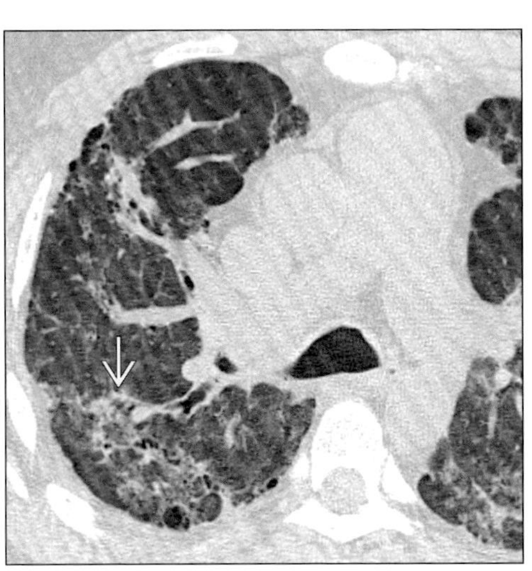

(Left) *Axial NECT of a patient with scleroderma and NSIP shows patchy ground-glass and fine reticular opacities and peripheral traction bronchiectasis ➔. The dilated distal esophagus ⇨ provides a clue to the diagnosis of scleroderma.* ***(Right)*** *Axial HRCT of a patient with fibrotic NSIP shows patchy peribronchovascular architectural distortion ➔ and ground-glass and reticular opacities. NSIP may exhibit a peribronchovascular distribution of CT abnormalities.*

CRYPTOGENIC ORGANIZING PNEUMONIA

Key Facts

Terminology
- Cryptogenic organizing pneumonia (COP)
- Clinicopathological entity characterized by polypoid plugs of loose granulation tissue within airspaces

Imaging
- Radiography
  - Bilateral consolidations ± ground-glass opacity
  - Patchy distribution, preserved lung volume
  - Often waxing & waning/fleeting evolution
- HRCT
  - Consolidation ± ground-glass opacity
  - Subpleural &/or bronchovascular
  - Mid & lower lung zones
  - Reverse halo sign: Central ground-glass opacity with surrounding rim of consolidation
  - Perilobular pattern: Linear opacities along interlobular septa

Top Differential Diagnoses
- Pulmonary lymphoma
- Low-grade adenocarcinoma
- Sarcoidosis
- Chronic eosinophilic pneumonia
- Lipoid pneumonia

Pathology
- Loosely organized intraalveolar granulation tissue extending through collateral pathways
- Exclusion of other causes of organizing pneumonia

Clinical Issues
- Corticosteroid treatment; good prognosis

Diagnostic Checklist
- COP is diagnosis of exclusion; consider other causes of chronic multifocal air space disease

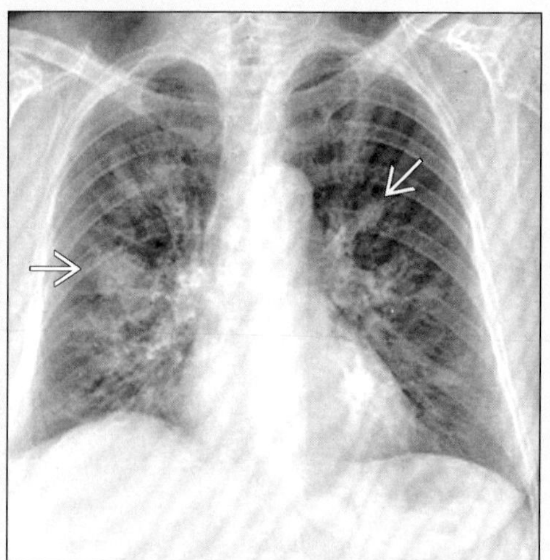

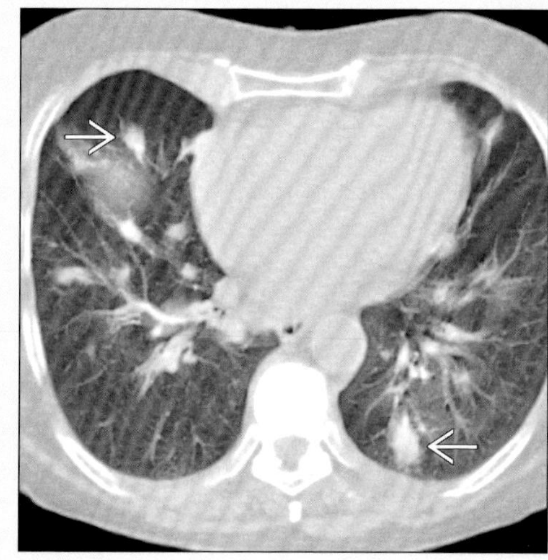

(Left) *PA chest radiograph of a patient with cryptogenic organizing pneumonia shows multifocal bilateral nodular consolidations ➡.* ***(Right)*** *Axial HRCT of the same patient shows peribronchovascular nodular opacities ➡. These findings, if chronic, are consistent with organizing pneumonia. However, the differential diagnosis is broad. In the acute setting, bacterial or fungal pneumonia as well as aspiration should first be excluded.*

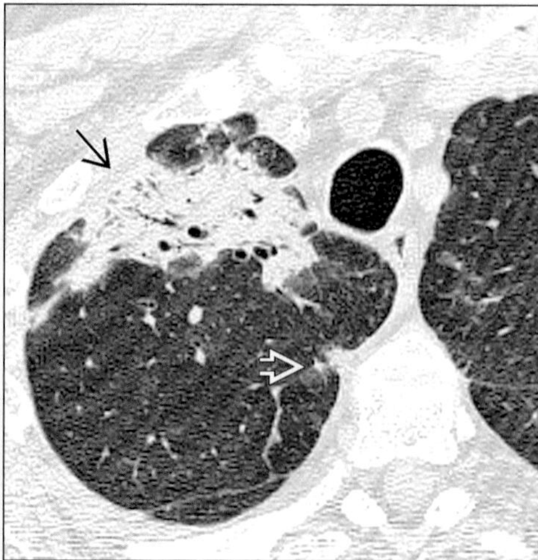

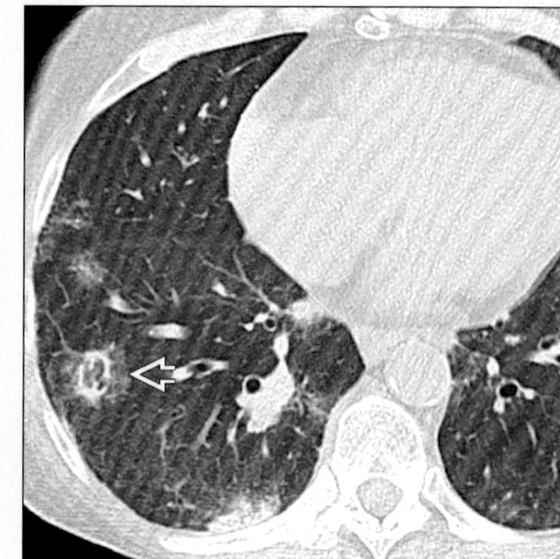

(Left) *Axial HRCT of a patient with cryptogenic organizing pneumonia shows a dominant, dense, mass-like consolidation → in the right upper lobe and a smaller subpleural nodular opacity ⇨. Given the overlap of the imaging appearances of malignancy and organizing pneumonia, close imaging follow-up after treatment is mandatory.* ***(Right)*** *Axial HRCT of a patient with organizing pneumonia shows peripheral nodular opacities, one of which exhibits the reverse halo sign ⇨.*

CRYPTOGENIC ORGANIZING PNEUMONIA

TERMINOLOGY

Abbreviations

- **Cryptogenic organizing pneumonia (COP)**
- Bronchiolitis obliterans organizing pneumonia (BOOP)

Definitions

- Clinicopathological entity characterized by polypoid plugs of loose granulation tissue within airspaces

IMAGING

General Features

- Best diagnostic clue
  - Bilateral, peripheral, basal, patchy consolidation
  - Often exhibits waxing & waning or fleeting evolution
- Location
  - Typically mid & lower zones

Radiographic Findings

- Radiography
  - Bilateral consolidations ± ground-glass opacity
    - May be migratory
    - Rarely unilateral
  - Usually patchy distribution
  - Preserved lung volume
  - Rare findings
    - Micronodules
    - Large nodules (may mimic metastases)
    - Reticulonodular opacities
    - Solitary pulmonary nodule/mass (may mimic primary lung cancer)

CT Findings

- HRCT
  - **Consolidation**
    - Isolated or associated with ground-glass opacity
    - Predominantly subpleural &/or bronchovascular
    - Typically in mid & lower zones
    - More common in immunocompetent than in immunocompromised patients
    - Presence of consolidation associated with greater likelihood of partial or complete response to treatment
  - **Ground-glass opacity**
    - Variable distribution
  - **Reverse halo sign/atoll sign**
    - **Central ground-glass opacity with surrounding rim of consolidation**
    - Minority of patients (20%)
    - Suggestive but not pathognomonic
      - Also occurs in fungal pneumonia, tuberculosis, Wegener granulomatosis, pulmonary infarct, alveolar sarcoid
  - **Perilobular pattern**
    - Linear opacities along interlobular septa thicker & less well-defined than septal thickening
    - Characteristic of COP
    - 60% of cases
  - **Nodules**
    - Variable distribution
  - **Reticular opacities**
    - Associated with increased risk of persistent or progressive disease
    - Not as prevalent as consolidation or ground-glass opacity
  - Other less common CT patterns
    - Bronchial wall thickening
    - Bronchial dilatation
    - Solitary pulmonary mass simulating malignancy
    - Honeycomb lung
    - Small pleural effusions

Imaging Recommendations

- Best imaging tool
  - HRCT for detection & characterization of airspace disease
- Protocol advice
  - Standard HRCT technique
  - Chest radiographs usually sufficient for follow-up
  - CT useful for characterization of pulmonary disease
  - CTA for exclusion of pulmonary embolism

DIFFERENTIAL DIAGNOSIS

Pulmonary Lymphoma

- Usually secondary to systemic lymphoma
- Lymphadenopathy
- No peripheral predominance, often centered on bronchi with air bronchograms

Low-grade Adenocarcinoma

- Not predominantly subpleural
- Subsolid lung nodule

Sarcoidosis

- No peripheral predominance, follows bronchovascular bundles
- Alveolar sarcoidosis: Few large airspace masses with air bronchograms
- Preferential involvement of upper lung zones
- Associated with symmetric hilar/mediastinal lymphadenopathy

Chronic Eosinophilic Pneumonia

- Usually upper lung zone predominant
- Nodules, nonseptal linear opacities, reticulation, & peribronchiolar distribution are more common in COP
- Septal lines more common in chronic eosinophilic pneumonia
- Eosinophilia suggests eosinophilic pneumonia

Lung Cancer (Solitary Mass)

- No distinguishing features, tissue diagnosis
- Relatively uncommon pattern for COP

Lipoid Pneumonia

- May exhibit fat attenuation within pulmonary consolidations at CT
- May manifest with "crazy-paving" appearance on CT
- History of lipid ingestion: Oily-nose drops, mineral oil

Pulmonary Infarcts

- Peripheral location in lung bases (identical to COP)
- May also exhibit reverse halo sign
- Tend to resolve centripetally ("iceberg" sign)
- Usually associated with pleural effusions
- Known risk factors for thromboembolism

CRYPTOGENIC ORGANIZING PNEUMONIA

PATHOLOGY

General Features

- Etiology
  - Idiopathic (by definition)
  - Exclusion of other causes of organizing pneumonia
    - Infection
      - Bacteria
      - Fungi
      - Viruses
      - Parasites
    - Drugs: Amiodarone, bleomycin, busulphan, gold salts, sulfasalazine, tacrolimus, cocaine
    - Connective tissue disease: Rheumatoid arthritis, dermatomyositis, Sjögren syndrome, polymyalgia rheumatica
    - Transplantation: Lung, bone marrow, liver
    - Inflammatory bowel disease: Ulcerative colitis, Crohn disease
    - Hematologic disorder: Myelodysplastic syndrome, leukemia
    - Immunologic/inflammatory disorder: Behçet disease, common variable immunodeficiency
    - Radiation therapy
      - Not limited to irradiated portions of lungs
      - Most often described in setting of breast cancer
    - Aspiration
- Primary pathology located in alveolus with secondary extension into small airways

Gross Pathologic & Surgical Features

- Preserved lung architecture (no fibrosis)
- Granulation tissue extends into airway lumen (bronchiolitis component)

Microscopic Features

- Buds of loosely organized granulation tissue extend through pores of Kohn to next alveolus ("butterfly" pattern)
- Mononuclear cell interstitial infiltration admixed with other inflammatory cells (nonspecific feature)

Laboratory Findings

- Pulmonary function tests
  - Usually restrictive
  - May be mixed restrictive & obstructive

CLINICAL ISSUES

Presentation

- Most common signs/symptoms
  - Symptoms generally develop over period of a few weeks
  - Common clinical features
    - Nonproductive cough
    - Malaise
    - Weight loss
    - Anorexia
    - Mild exertional dyspnea
- Other signs/symptoms
  - Less common clinical features
    - Hemoptysis
    - Chest pain
    - Arthralgia
    - Night sweats
    - Bronchorrhea

Demographics

- Age
  - Typically 50-60 years
    - Wide range: 20-80 years
- Gender
  - M = F
- Epidemiology
  - Most patients are nonsmokers or ex-smokers
  - Very rare seasonal cases (associated with biochemical cholestasis)

Natural History & Prognosis

- Waxing & waning course
- Often treated for months for "recurrent" pneumonia
- Good prognosis with treatment, but may relapse off corticosteroids

Treatment

- Corticosteroids are mainstay of treatment
  - Response to steroids generally striking
  - Less dramatic response than eosinophilic pneumonia
  - Symptomatic improvement usually in 24-48 hours
  - Complete radiographic resolution may take weeks
- Relapses (despite treatment) in over 50%
  - Relapse associated with delay in initiation of treatment, presence of mild cholestasis, & rapid withdrawal of therapy
  - Prolonged treatment not needed to suppress relapses
  - Prognosis not influenced by relapse

DIAGNOSTIC CHECKLIST

Image Interpretation Pearls

- COP is diagnosis of exclusion after other potential causes of chronic multifocal airspace disease are excluded

SELECTED REFERENCES

1. Lynch DA: Lung disease related to collagen vascular disease. J Thorac Imaging. 24(4):299-309, 2009
2. Silva CI et al: Idiopathic interstitial pneumonias. J Thorac Imaging. 24(4):260-73, 2009
3. Mueller-Mang C et al: What every radiologist should know about idiopathic interstitial pneumonias. Radiographics. 27(3):595-615, 2007
4. Lynch DA et al: Idiopathic interstitial pneumonias: CT features. Radiology. 236(1):10-21, 2005
5. Oymak FS et al: Bronchiolitis obliterans organizing pneumonia. Clinical and roentgenological features in 26 cases. Respiration. 72(3):254-62, 2005
6. Takada H et al: Bronchiolitis obliterans organizing pneumonia as an initial manifestation in systemic lupus erythematosus. Pediatr Pulmonol. 2005
7. Cordier JF: Cryptogenic organizing pneumonia. Clin Chest Med. 25(4):727-38, vi-vii, 2004
8. Epler GR: Drug-induced bronchiolitis obliterans organizing pneumonia. Clin Chest Med. 25(1):89-94, 2004
9. Pipavath S et al: Imaging of the chest: idiopathic interstitial pneumonia. Clin Chest Med. 25(4):651-6, v-vi, 2004

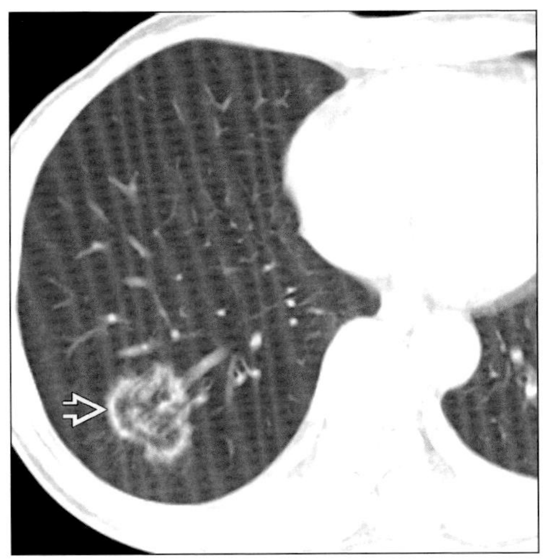

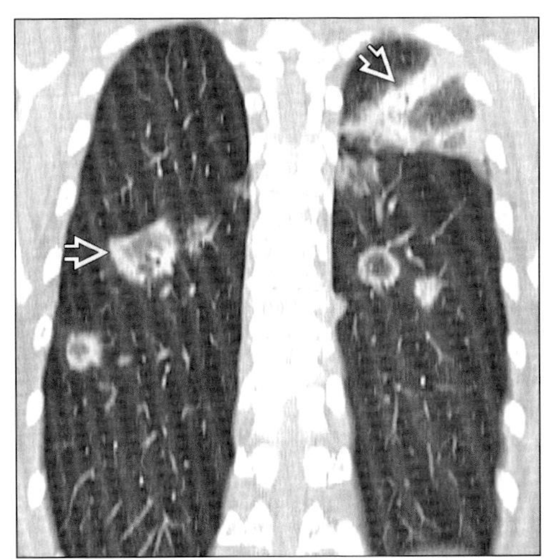

(Left) *Axial NECT of a patient with organizing pneumonia shows a focal lesion characterized by central ground-glass opacity with a peripheral rim of consolidation (reverse halo sign) ⇨.* ***(Right)*** *Coronal HRCT of a patient with organizing pneumonia shows multiple nodular consolidations that exhibit the reverse halo sign ⇨. The reverse halo sign is nonspecific, but is suggestive of organizing pneumonia in patients with a chronic or subacute presentation.*

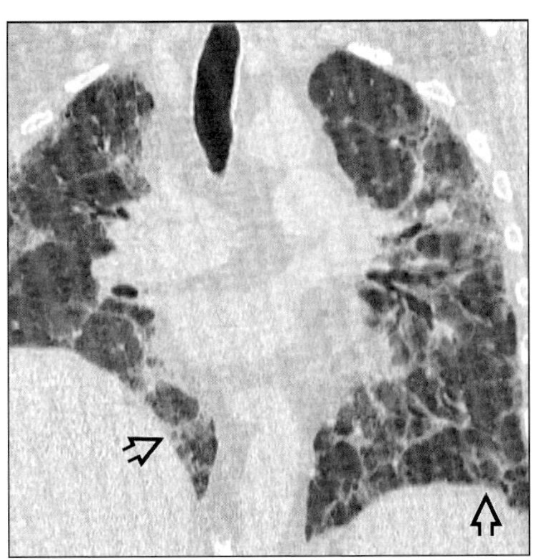

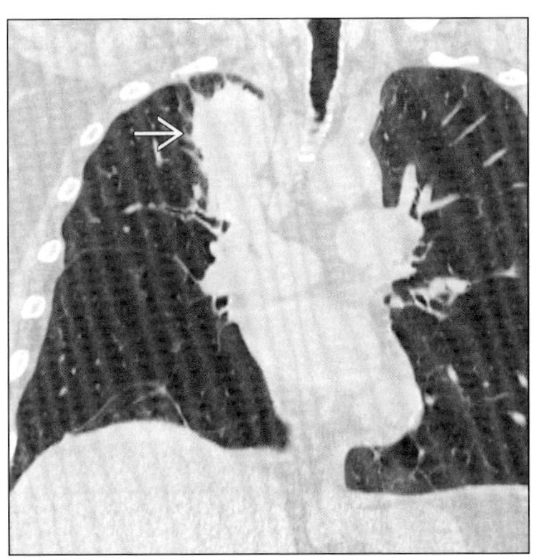

(Left) *Coronal HRCT shows a perilobular distribution of ground-glass opacities ⇨, typical for cryptogenic organizing pneumonia.* ***(Right)*** *Coronal CECT shows a right upper lobe mass-like consolidation ➡, highly suspicious for bronchogenic carcinoma. However, follow-up studies (not shown) demonstrated interval decrease in the size of the lesion, which was eventually shown to represent organizing pneumonia.*

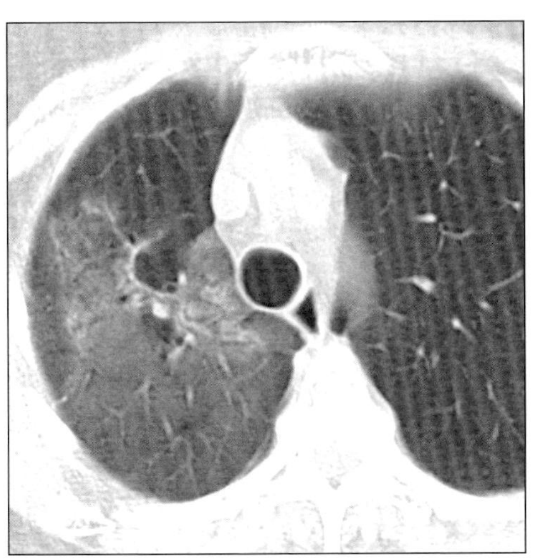

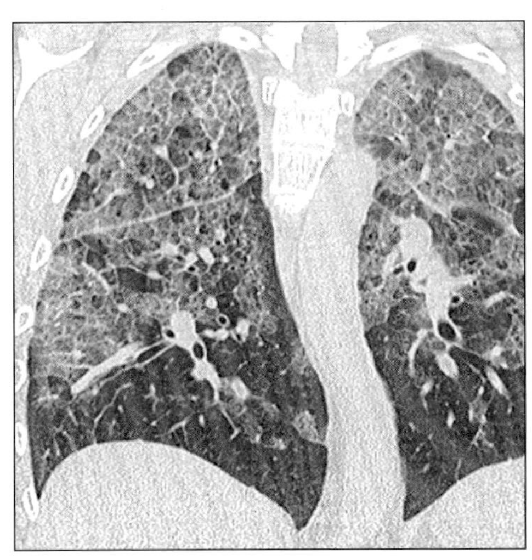

(Left) *Axial NECT of a patient with organizing pneumonia shows right upper lobe ground-glass opacity. Although organizing pneumonia typically manifests with consolidation, isolated ground-glass opacity may also occur.* ***(Right)*** *Coronal HRCT of a patient with cryptogenic organizing pneumonia shows bilateral mid and upper lung ground-glass opacities and reticulation ("crazy-paving" pattern), a less common but recognized HRCT manifestation of cryptogenic organizing pneumonia.*

SARCOIDOSIS

Key Facts

Terminology

- Systemic granulomatous disease of unknown etiology; affects young & middle-aged adults
- Frequent hilar/mediastinal lymphadenopathy, pulmonary involvement, eye & skin lesions

Imaging

- Radiography: Abnormal in up to 90% of cases
  - Lymphadenopathy (75-90%)
  - Upper/mid lung small nodular/reticular opacities
  - Large nodules/consolidations ± air bronchograms
  - Upper lung zone fibrosis (stage IV)
- CT/HRCT
  - Bilateral upper/mid lung zone perilymphatic micronodules
  - Nodular sarcoidosis: Large lung nodules/masses
  - Airway involvement: Stenosis, small airway disease
  - Pulmonary fibrosis (20%), mycetoma formation

Top Differential Diagnoses

- Silicosis
- Lymphangitic carcinomatosis

Pathology

- Noncaseating epithelioid granulomas
- Diagnosis of exclusion

Clinical Issues

- Symptoms/signs
  - Asymptomatic (30-50% of patients)
  - Dyspnea, cough, chest pain, wheezing
  - Fatigue, fever, weight loss, sweats, arthralgias
- Affected patients typically < 40 years
- Prognosis
  - Stability or remission in 2/3 of patients
  - Chronic disease & lung fibrosis in 20%
- Treatment: Corticosteroids, immunosuppressants

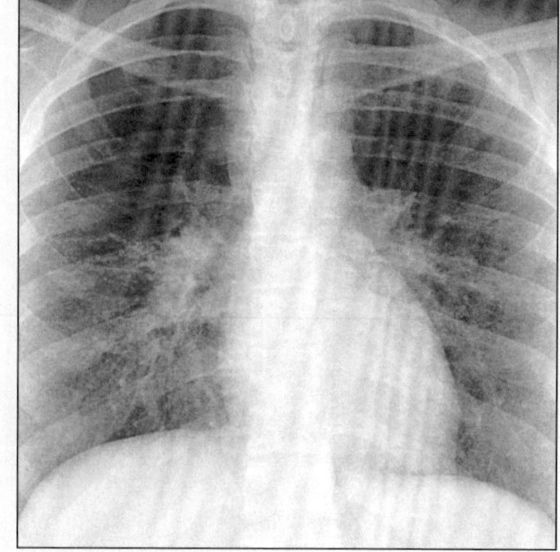

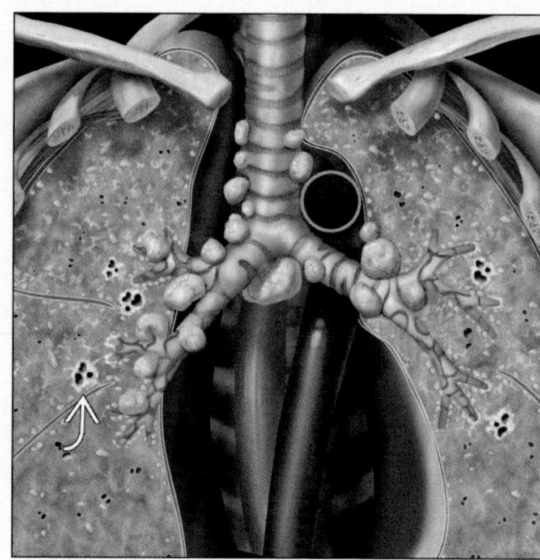

(Left) *PA chest radiograph of a young woman with stage II sarcoidosis shows bilateral hilar and right paratracheal lymphadenopathy and profuse bilateral pulmonary micronodules predominantly affecting the perihilar lung parenchyma.* ***(Right)*** *Graphic shows the characteristic imaging features of sarcoidosis, including symmetric bilateral hilar and mediastinal lymphadenopathy, upper and mid lung predominant perilymphatic micronodules, and nodular thickening of the axial bronchoarterial interstitium ➔.*

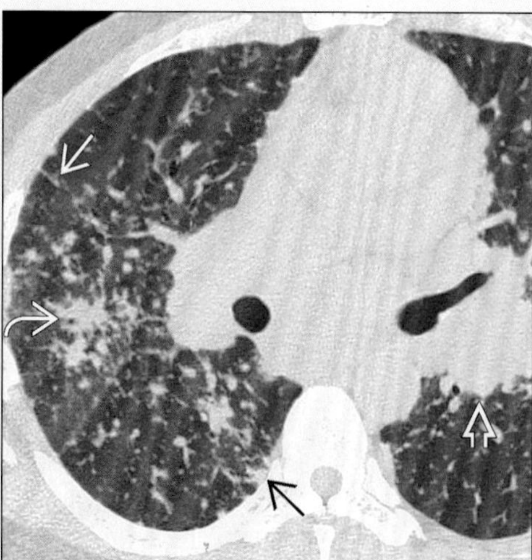

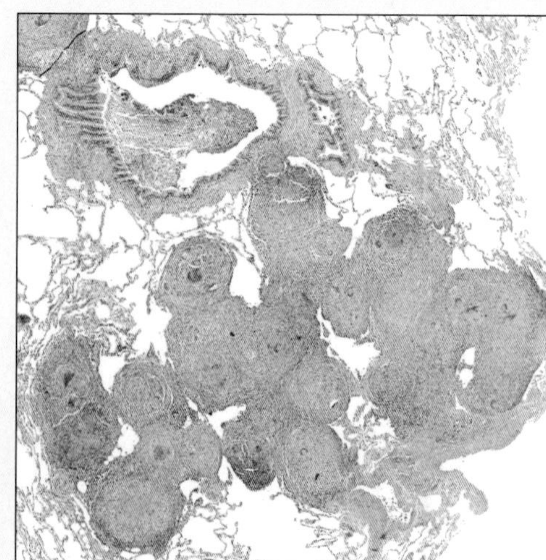

(Left) *Axial NECT of a patient with sarcoidosis shows profuse clustered perilymphatic micronodules along the pleura ⇒, the peribronchovascular regions ➔, and the interlobular septa ➔, as well as symmetric bilateral hilar and subcarinal lymphadenopathy ➔.* ***(Right)*** *Low-power photomicrograph (H&E stain) shows typical histologic features of sarcoidosis. Epithelioid granulomas along bronchovascular bundles correlate with the nodular peribronchovascular thickening seen on HRCT. (Courtesy S. Suster, MD.)*

SARCOIDOSIS

TERMINOLOGY

Definitions

- **American Thoracic Society definition**
  - Multisystem granulomatous disorder of unknown etiology; affects young & middle-aged adults
  - Frequent hilar lymphadenopathy, pulmonary involvement, eye & skin lesions
  - Typical clinical & imaging findings supported by histology: Noncaseating epithelioid granulomas
  - Exclusion of other granulomatous diseases or local sarcoid reactions

IMAGING

General Features

- Best diagnostic clue
  - Bilateral hilar/mediastinal lymphadenopathy ± perilymphatic micronodules
- Location
  - Pulmonary involvement: Upper/mid lung zones
  - Lymphadenopathy: Hilar, paratracheal, AP window, subcarinal
- Size
  - Lung lesions: Small nodules to large masses
  - Lymphadenopathy: Variable, may be bulky

Radiographic Findings

- Abnormal chest radiograph in up to 90% of cases
- Lymphadenopathy (75-90%)
  - Bilateral hilar & right paratracheal: **Garland triad**
- Pulmonary involvement
  - Lungs may appear normal
  - Upper/mid lung small nodular/reticular opacities
  - Large nodules/masses ± air bronchograms
  - Pulmonary fibrosis (stage IV)
    - Upper lung architectural distortion, volume loss, cystic changes
    - Mycetoma formation: Air-crescent sign, adjacent pleural thickening
- Radiographic staging
  - Stage 0: Normal chest radiograph
  - Stage I: Lymphadenopathy, no pulmonary disease
  - Stage II: Lymphadenopathy & pulmonary disease
  - Stage III: Pulmonary disease, no lymphadenopathy
  - Stage IV: Pulmonary fibrosis

CT Findings

- Lung
  - Distribution: Bilateral upper & mid lung zones
  - **Perilymphatic (axial & peripheral interstitium) micronodules** (90-100% of patients with lung involvement)
    - Typically small (1-4 mm), range from miliary to large nodules
    - Axial interstitium
      - Centrilobular nodules
      - Nodular thickening of vessel & airway walls
    - Peripheral interstitium
      - Subpleural & fissural nodules
      - Nodular interlobular septal thickening
  - Nodular sarcoidosis (1-10 cm)
    - Nodular & mass-like opacities
    - Nummular or "alveolar" sarcoidosis: Nodular consolidations ± air bronchograms, irregular borders
    - **Galaxy sign**: Large nodules with irregular borders consisting of satellite micronodules; coalescent sarcoid granulomas
    - **Reversed halo sign**: Crescentic/ring-shaped opacities with central ground-glass attenuation
    - Patchy ground-glass opacities
- Airway involvement
  - Mosaic attenuation, expiratory air-trapping
  - Airway distortion/stenosis; may lead to atelectasis
  - Nodular thickening of airway wall
- Lymphadenopathy
  - All lymph node stations may be affected
    - **Symmetric**: Bilateral hilar, paratracheal, AP window, subcarinal lymph nodes
    - Lymph node calcification with chronic disease
- Complications
  - Pulmonary fibrosis (20%)
    - Upper & mid lung zone architectural distortion & traction bronchiectasis
    - Irregular linear opacities
    - Mass-like fibrosis with irregular borders
    - Posterior displacement of main & upper bronchi with volume loss
    - Cystic changes
      - Cysts, bullae, honeycomb lung
      - Rarely cavitation
    - Mycetoma formation
      - Stage IV sarcoidosis; intracystic soft tissue, air-crescent sign, adjacent pleural thickening
    - Pulmonary arterial hypertension
- Rare manifestations
  - Solitary/dominant nodule or mass
  - Pleural effusion, pleural thickening, spontaneous pneumothorax

Imaging Recommendations

- Best imaging tool
  - CT more sensitive & specific than radiography in assessment of diffuse lung disease & complications
- Protocol advice
  - HRCT evaluation of pulmonary sarcoidosis
- Indications for CT/HRCT
  - Atypical clinical or radiographic findings
  - Evaluation of pulmonary complications
  - Normal chest radiograph & suspected sarcoidosis

Nuclear Medicine Findings

- Gallium-67 scintigraphy: Nonspecific
  - Increased uptake in infection & inflammation
  - Characteristic uptake patterns in sarcoidosis
    - **"Lambda" sign**: Paratracheal & hilar uptake
    - **"Panda" sign**: Lacrimal & parotid uptake
- FDG PET: Nonspecific uptake pattern & intensity

DIFFERENTIAL DIAGNOSIS

Lymphangitic Carcinomatosis

- Known malignancy, typically adenocarcinoma
- Smooth or nodular interstitial thickening
  - Nodules typically septal & peribronchovascular
- Asymmetric lymphadenopathy, pleural effusion

SARCOIDOSIS

Silicosis

- History of exposure, elderly men
- Posterior centrilobular/subpleural small nodules
- Lymphadenopathy ± "eggshell" calcification

PATHOLOGY

General Features

- Etiology
  - Unknown

Microscopic Features

- Diagnosis of exclusion
  - Sarcoid-like reactions: Infection, neoplasia, pneumoconiosis, hypersensitivity pneumonitis
- Noncaseating epithelioid granulomas
  - Mononuclear phagocytes (epithelioid & giant cells), peripheral lymphocytes, no extensive necrosis
- Fibrosis

CLINICAL ISSUES

Presentation

- Most common signs/symptoms
  - Asymptomatic (30-50% of patients)
  - Dyspnea, cough
  - Chest pain
  - Wheezing
  - Fatigue, fever, weight loss, sweats, arthralgias, muscle weakness
- Other signs/symptoms
  - Skin, eye, lymph node involvement in up to 30%
  - Hemoptysis from mycetoma formation (stage IV)
- Clinical profile
  - Acute presentation
    - **Löfgren syndrome**: Bilateral hilar lymphadenopathy, erythema nodosum, fever, arthralgias/arthritis
  - **Heerfordt syndrome**: Uveitis, parotitis, fever
  - Insidious onset
    - **Lupus pernio**: Chronic cutaneous induration & purple discoloration of central face & hands
    - Chronic uveitis, hypercalcemia/nephrocalcinosis, involvement of nasal mucosa, cystic skeletal lesions, neurosarcoidosis, cardiac sarcoidosis
- Laboratory abnormalities
  - ↑ angiotensin-converting enzyme (ACE), derived from granuloma
  - ↑ lysozyme, derived from macrophage
  - Not sensitive or specific for diagnosis
- Pulmonary function
  - Restriction
    - ↓ volume, vital capacity, & total lung capacity
  - ↓ diffusing capacity for carbon monoxide (DLCO)
  - Obstruction from endobronchial sarcoidosis

Demographics

- Age
  - Affected patients typically < 40 years
    - Peak incidence: 20-29 years
- Gender
  - Slightly higher disease rate in women
- Ethnicity
  - Highest prevalence in African-Americans, Scandinavians, Japanese
- Epidemiology
  - Prevalence in United States
    - African-Americans: 35.5/100,000 people
    - Caucasians: 10.9/100,000 people

Natural History & Prognosis

- **Diagnosis**
  - Typical imaging features in asymptomatic patient
  - Clinical & imaging findings supported by histologic evidence of noncaseating epithelioid granulomas
  - Typical clinical syndromes (Löfgren or Heerfordt) after exclusion of other diagnoses
  - Biopsy methods
    - Transbronchial biopsy; diagnostic accuracy 70%
    - Transesophageal endoscopic ultrasound-guided fine needle aspiration (EUS-FNA)
      - Diagnostic yield: 82-86%
    - Endobronchial ultrasound-guided transbronchial needle aspiration (EBUS-TBNA)
      - Diagnostic yield: 85-93%
    - Mediastinoscopy, open lung biopsy
- Prognosis
  - Stability or remission in 2/3 of patients
    - Löfgren syndrome: Excellent prognosis, spontaneous remission
  - Chronic disease & lung fibrosis in 20%
  - Good prognosis: Low stage
  - Poor prognosis: High stage, onset after 40 years, extrapulmonary involvement, hypercalcemia, lupus pernio
  - Mortality: < 5%
    - Respiratory failure, cardiac sarcoidosis, neurosarcoidosis

Treatment

- Corticosteroids: Severe or progressive disease, extrapulmonary disease, symptomatic patients
- Immunosuppressive & cytotoxic agents: Nonresponders or adverse effects from steroids
- Infliximab: Tumor necrosis factor-α inhibitor

DIAGNOSTIC CHECKLIST

Consider

- Sarcoidosis in asymptomatic young patients with typical lymphadenopathy ± small upper/mid lung predominant nodules

Image Interpretation Pearls

- Perilymphatic micronodules & typical distribution of lymphadenopathy are virtually pathognomonic in appropriate clinical setting
- Nodular consolidations with lymphadenopathy should suggest sarcoidosis

SELECTED REFERENCES

1. Criado E et al: Pulmonary sarcoidosis: typical and atypical manifestations at high-resolution CT with pathologic correlation. Radiographics. 30(6):1567-86, 2010
2. Hawtin KE et al: Pulmonary sarcoidosis: the 'Great Pretender'. Clin Radiol. 65(8):642-50, 2010
3. Hoang DQ et al: Sarcoidosis. Semin Roentgenol. 45(1):36-42, 2010

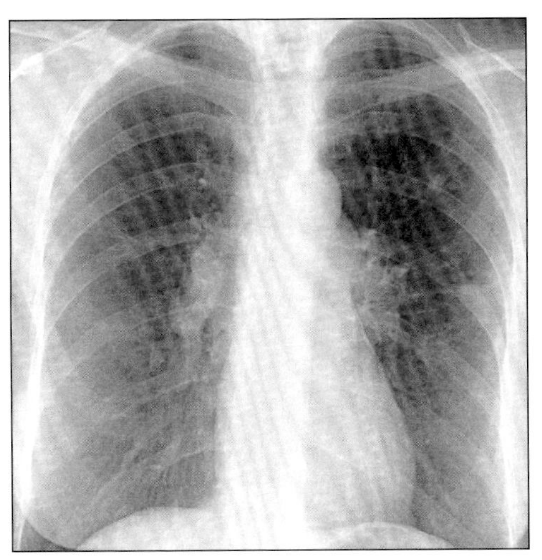

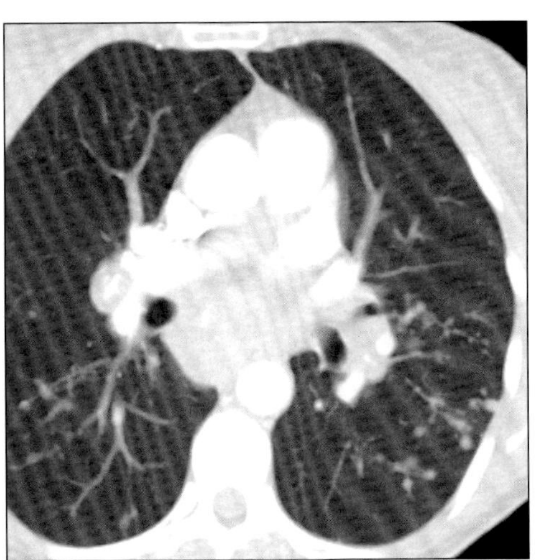

(Left) *PA chest radiograph of a patient with sarcoidosis shows bilateral hilar and AP window lymphadenopathy and left lung predominant nodules.* ***(Right)*** *Axial CECT of the same patient shows bilateral hilar and subcarinal lymphadenopathy and bilateral small pulmonary nodules along bronchovascular bundles, interlobular septa, and subpleural regions. The combination of perilymphatic micronodules and symmetric lymphadenopathy strongly suggests the diagnosis of sarcoidosis.*

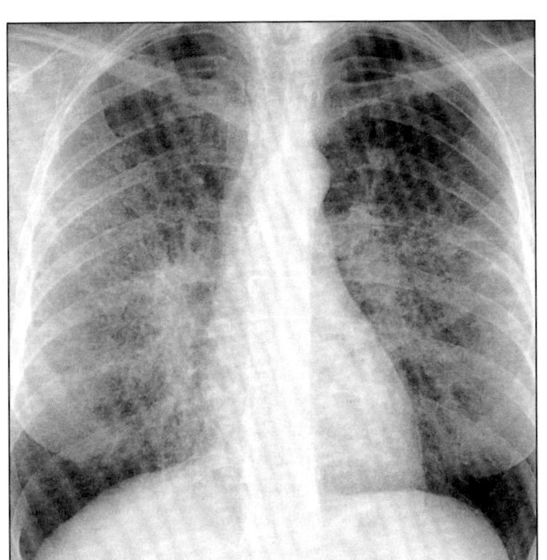

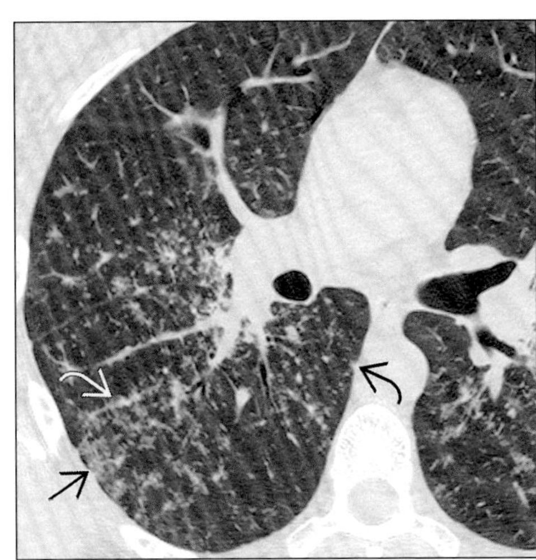

(Left) *PA chest radiograph of a young woman with sarcoidosis shows bilateral mid and upper lung zone fine nodular and reticular opacities with sparing of the lung bases and bilateral hilar lymphadenopathy.* ***(Right)*** *Axial NECT of the same patient shows multifocal bilateral clustered perilymphatic micronodules with centrilobular ⇨ and peribronchovascular ➯ distribution. Scattered subpleural micronodules ⇨ help confirm the perilymphatic location of the sarcoid granulomas.*

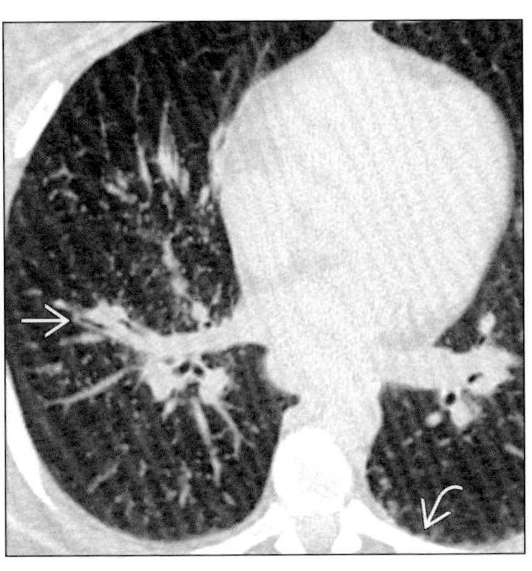

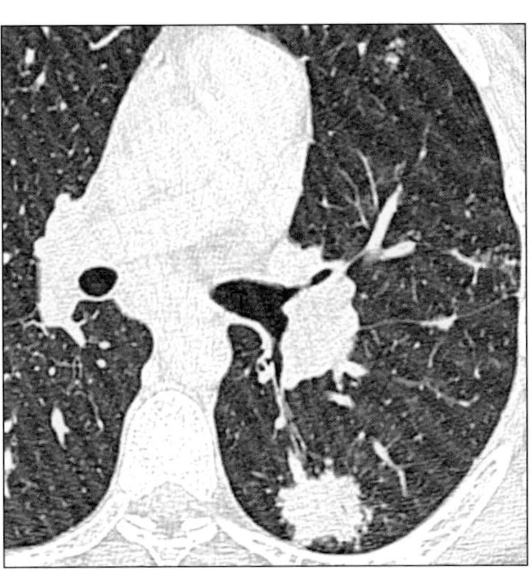

(Left) *Axial NECT of a patient with sarcoidosis shows peribronchovascular nodular thickening ➔ and scattered miliary micronodules. The clustered non-random nodule distribution and the subpleural nodularity ➯ help localize the nodules to the perilymphatic regions of the lung.* ***(Right)*** *Axial NECT of a patient with sarcoidosis shows a dominant left lower lobe nodule with irregular borders formed by surrounding micronodules, the so-called sarcoid galaxy sign that results from coalescence of granulomas.*

*(**Left**) Coronal CECT of a patient with nodular sarcoidosis shows bilateral large nodules, some with intrinsic air bronchograms →. This "alveolar" or nodular form of sarcoidosis may mimic metastatic disease and multifocal infection. (**Right**) Axial CECT of a patient with "alveolar" sarcoidosis shows bilateral consolidations with intrinsic air bronchograms →. Note micronodules associated with the left lower lobe airspace disease and bilateral hilar ⇨ and subcarinal lymphadenopathy.*

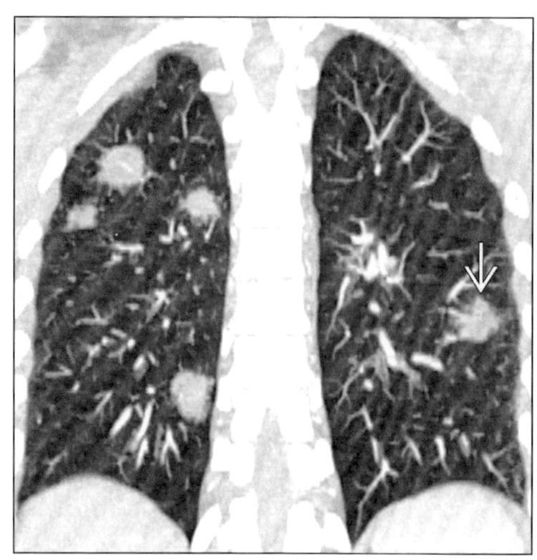

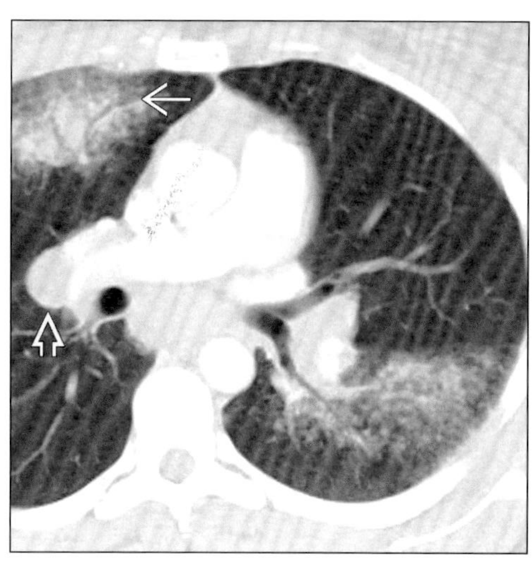

*(**Left**) Coronal volume-rendered surface-shaded CT image of a patient with sarcoidosis shows focal stenosis of the left mainstem bronchus ↪ secondary to bronchial involvement by sarcoidosis. Note scattered bilateral clustered small lung nodules →. (**Right**) Axial NECT of a patient with sarcoidosis shows middle lobe atelectasis secondary to airway stenosis, multifocal areas of air-trapping secondary to small airway obstruction, and scattered bilateral perilymphatic micronodules.*

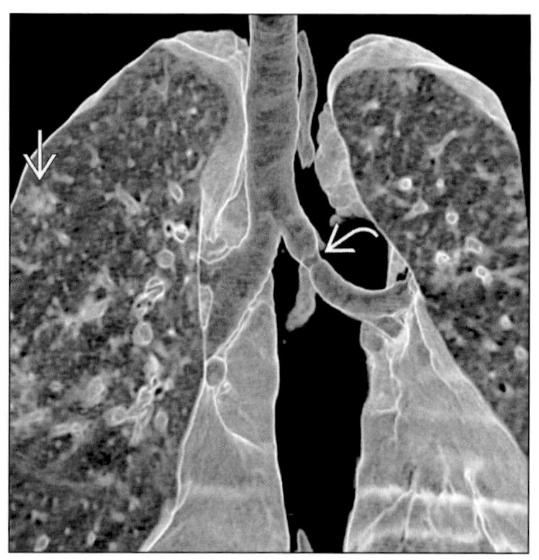

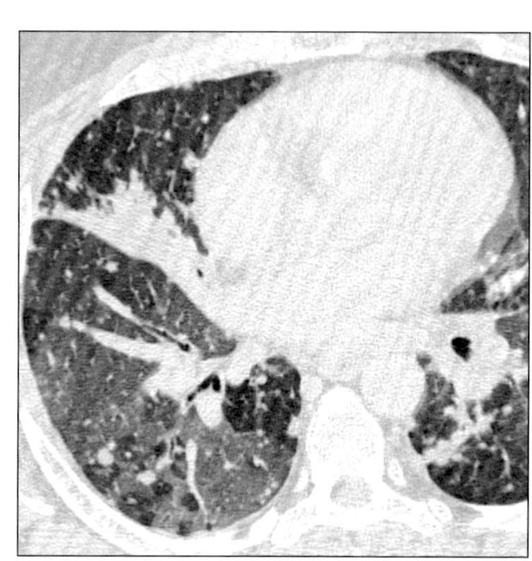

*(**Left**) PA chest radiograph of a patient with stage IV sarcoidosis shows low lung volumes and bilateral perihilar reticular opacities and architectural distortion. (**Right**) Axial NECT of the same patient shows mosaic attenuation of the lung, fine intralobular reticular opacities, and bilateral lower lobe peribronchovascular architectural distortion and traction bronchiectasis ↪. Unlike idiopathic pulmonary fibrosis, fibrosis from sarcoidosis typically affects the peribronchovascular regions.*

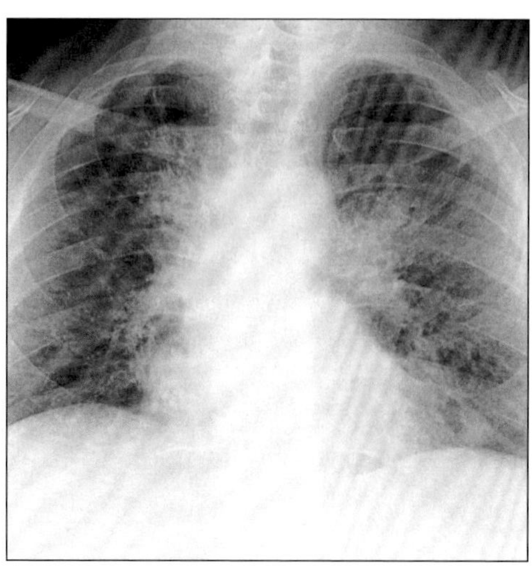

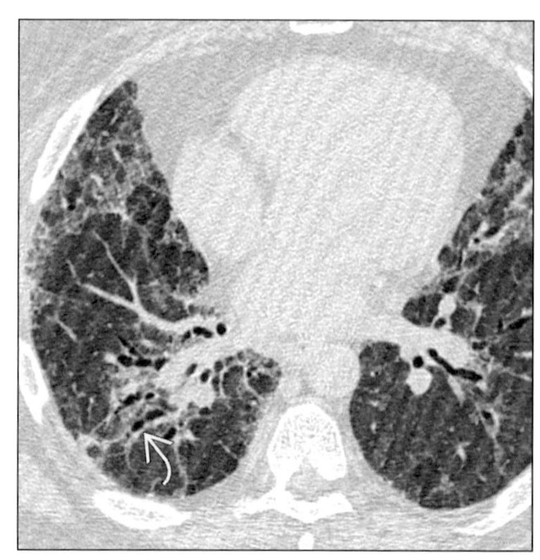

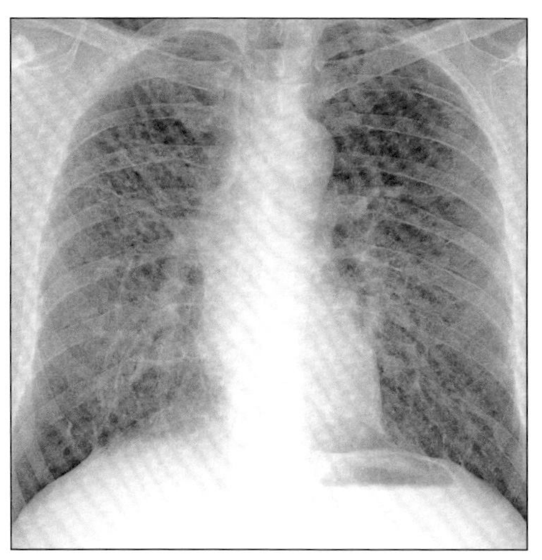

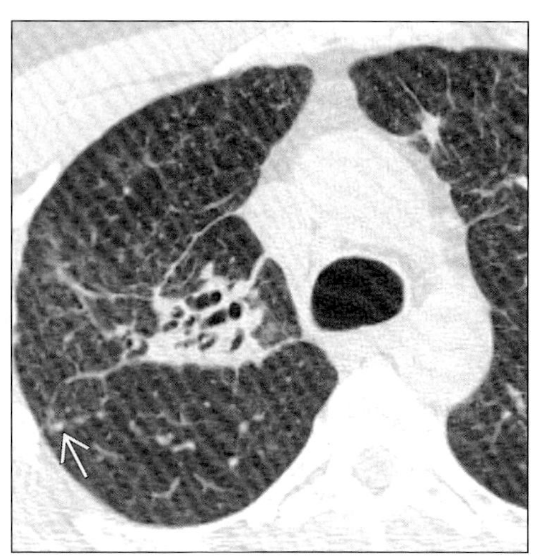

(Left) *PA chest radiograph of a patient with end-stage sarcoidosis shows bilateral perihilar architectural distortion and fine reticular opacities. Although the lung volumes are mostly preserved, there is right upper lobe volume loss with ipsilateral right hilar retraction.* ***(Right)*** *Axial HRCT of the same patient shows focal right upper lobe architectural distortion with intrinsic traction bronchiectasis resembling progressive massive fibrosis and nodular thickening of interlobular septa ➔.*

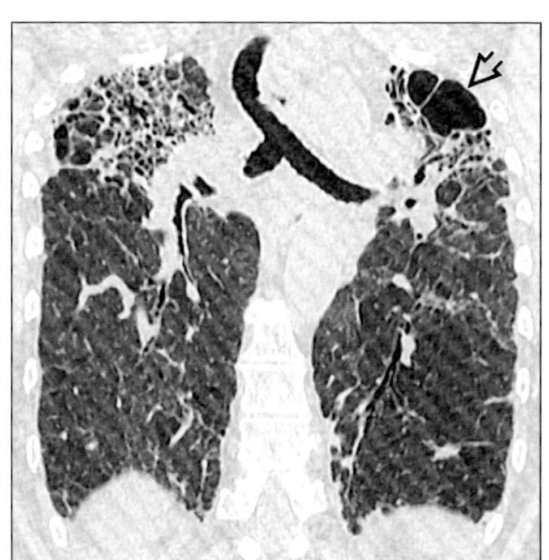

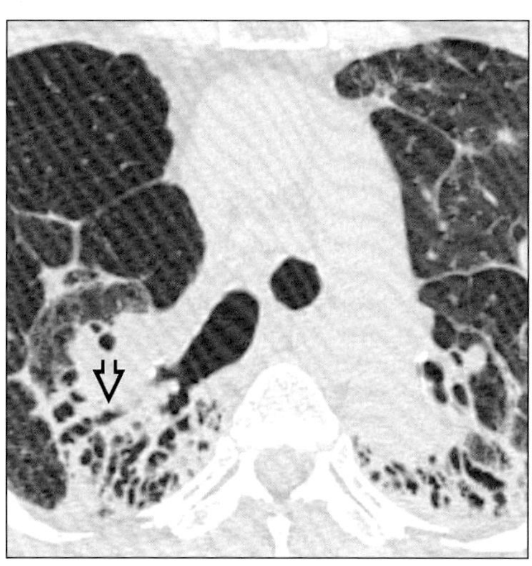

(Left) *Coronal HRCT of a patient with stage IV sarcoidosis shows marked upper lobe volume loss and hilar retraction with extensive upper lobe architectural distortion, traction bronchiectasis, honeycomb lung, and cystic changes ⇨ with relative sparing of the lung bases.* ***(Right)*** *Axial NECT of a patient with end-stage sarcoidosis shows bilateral upper lobe volume loss, architectural distortion, and traction bronchiectasis ⇨ with typical posterior hilar displacement.*

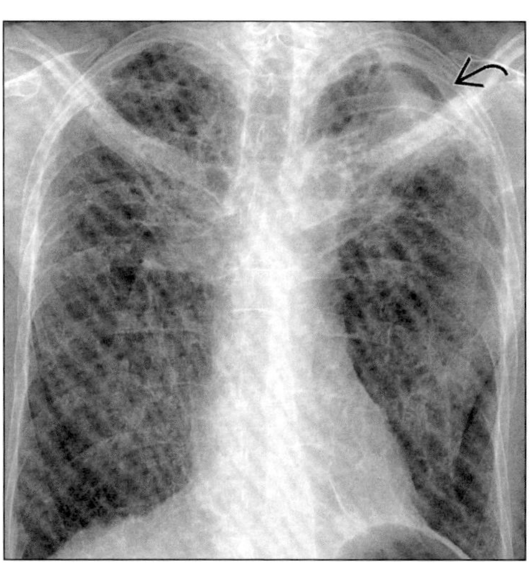

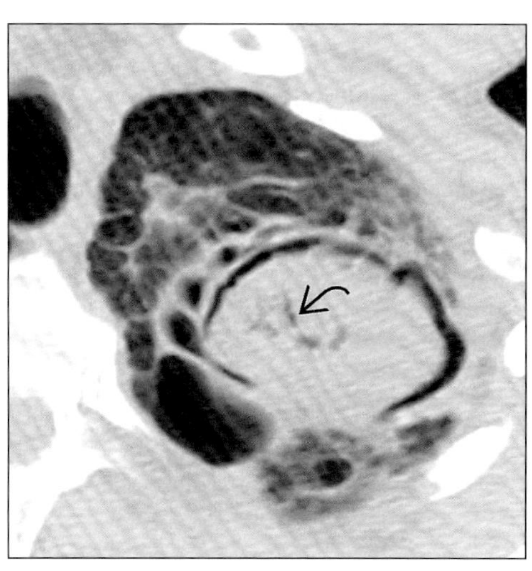

(Left) *PA chest radiograph of a patient with stage IV sarcoidosis who presented with hemoptysis shows severe upper lobe volume loss, bilateral hilar retraction, and architectural distortion. A left apical cystic space contains a mass and exhibits an air-crescent sign and adjacent pleural thickening ⇗, consistent with mycetoma.* ***(Right)*** *Axial NECT of the same patient shows an intracavitary mycetoma with intrinsic air-containing clefts ⇗ and a nondependent crescent of air.*

RESPIRATORY BRONCHIOLITIS AND RBILD

Key Facts

Terminology

- Respiratory bronchiolitis (RB)
- Respiratory bronchiolitis-associated interstitial lung disease (RB-ILD)
- RB: Histologic reaction to cigarette smoke
- RB-ILD & desquamative interstitial pneumonia regarded as spectrum of smoking-related lung disease

Imaging

- Respiratory bronchiolitis
  - HRCT often normal (sensitivity 25%)
  - Subtle micronodular centrilobular opacities
  - Patchy ground-glass opacities
- Respiratory bronchiolitis-interstitial lung disease
  - Upper lobe centrilobular nodules more pronounced
  - Distinct reticular opacities (from mild fibrosis) primarily in lower lobes

Top Differential Diagnoses

- Desquamative interstitial pneumonia (DIP)
- Hypersensitivity pneumonitis

Pathology

- Respiratory bronchioles filled with pigmented macrophages
- Macrophages may spill into surrounding alveoli

Clinical Issues

- RB: Universal histologic response in smokers
- RB: Asymptomatic
- RB-ILD: Cough, dyspnea

Diagnostic Checklist

- Consider RB in smokers with upper lung centrilobular ground-glass nodules on CT & RB-ILD in symptomatic smokers with similar findings

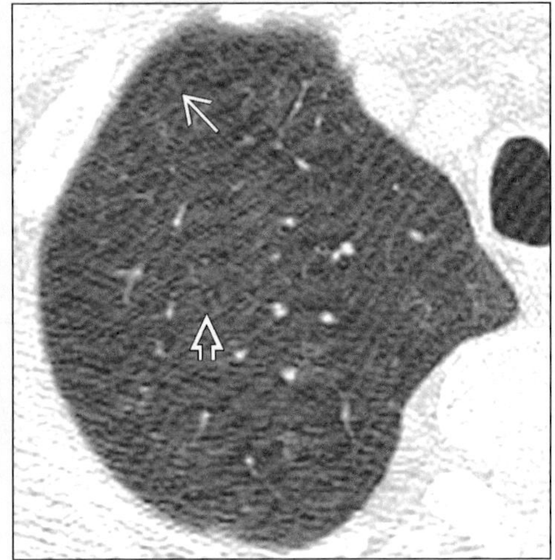

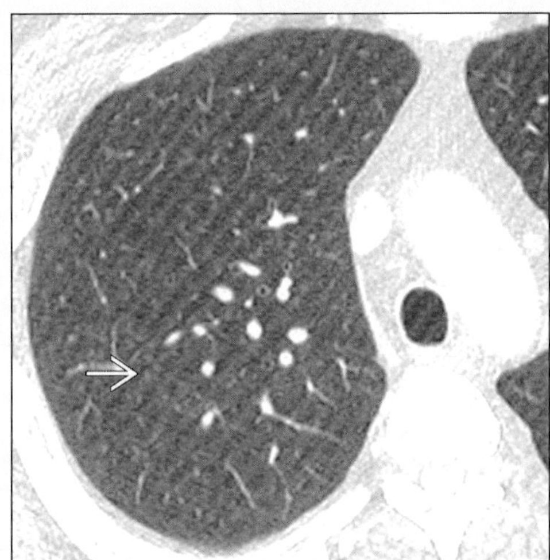

(Left) *Axial HRCT of a patient with respiratory bronchiolitis shows scattered ground-glass centrilobular nodules ➡, characteristic of smoking-related respiratory bronchiolitis, and mild centrilobular emphysema ⮕.* ***(Right)*** *Axial HRCT of a cigarette smoker with respiratory bronchiolitis shows scattered right upper lobe ground-glass attenuation centrilobular micronodules ➡. These nodules are often apparent on thin-section CT and MIP images of asymptomatic cigarette smokers.*

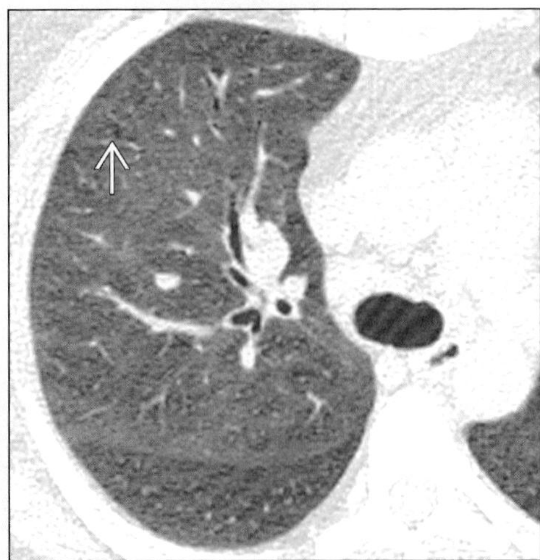

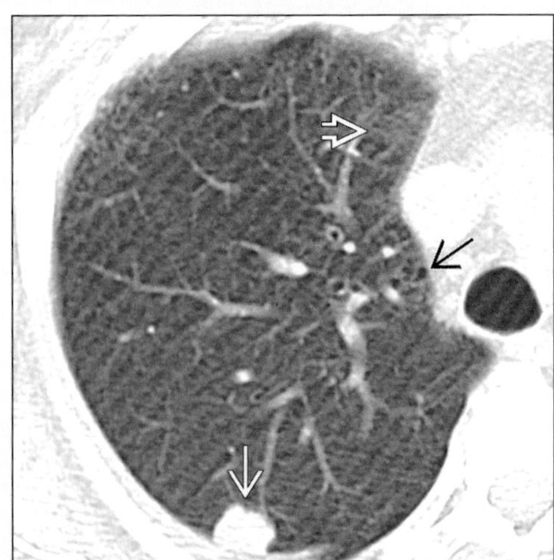

(Left) *Axial HRCT of a smoker with respiratory bronchiolitis shows extensive but patchy ground-glass opacities in the right upper lobe and a tiny focus of centrilobular emphysema ➡. RB is a common histologic finding on surgical specimens of cigarette smokers.* ***(Right)*** *Axial NECT of a smoker shows a non-small cell lung cancer manifesting as a large subpleural right upper lobe polylobular nodule ➡, with associated patchy ground-glass opacities ⮕ (representing RB) and mild emphysema ⇨.*

RESPIRATORY BRONCHIOLITIS AND RBILD

TERMINOLOGY

Abbreviations

- **Respiratory bronchiolitis (RB)**
- **Respiratory bronchiolitis-associated interstitial lung disease (RB-ILD)**

Definitions

- RB: Histologic reaction to cigarette smoke
- RB-ILD & desquamative interstitial pneumonia (DIP) regarded as spectrum of smoking-related interstitial lung disease
  - DIP: More extensive form of pigmented alveolar macrophage accumulation in bronchioles & alveoli

IMAGING

General Features

- Best diagnostic clue
  - Centrilobular ground-glass opacities in upper lobes
- Location
  - Gradient: More predominant in upper lung zone diminishing toward lung bases
- Size
  - Centrilobular nodules 3-5 mm in diameter

Radiographic Findings

- Respiratory bronchiolitis: **Chest radiograph normal**
- Respiratory bronchiolitis-interstitial lung disease
  - **Chest radiograph normal** in up to 50% of patients
  - Normal lung volumes
  - Poorly defined hazy areas of increased opacity
  - Bronchial wall thickening
  - Fine reticular or reticulonodular opacities (rare)
  - Small peripheral ring opacities

CT Findings

- HRCT
  - **Respiratory bronchiolitis**
    - HRCT often normal (sensitivity 25%)
    - **Faint micronodular centrilobular opacities**
    - Patchy distribution of ground-glass opacities
      - Abnormal-attenuation lobules adjacent to normal-attenuation lobules
    - **Ground-glass opacities** may be widespread
    - Upper lung zone predominant involvement
    - May exhibit associated centrilobular emphysema, particularly in older patients
  - **Respiratory bronchiolitis-associated interstitial lung disease**
    - Upper lobe centrilobular nodules are more pronounced than in RB
    - Distinct reticular opacities (from mild pulmonary fibrosis) primarily in lower lobes
    - **Centrilobular emphysema** more common
    - Mild bronchial wall thickening
  - May be combined with other manifestations of cigarette smoking (lung cancer)

Imaging Recommendations

- Best imaging tool
  - HRCT is most sensitive imaging modality for RB & RB-ILD
    - Expiratory HRCT may demonstrate air-trapping
    - Subtle bronchocentric & nodular centrilobular ground-glass opacities may be difficult to detect
  - MIP images increase conspicuity of pulmonary micronodules

DIFFERENTIAL DIAGNOSIS

Desquamative Interstitial Pneumonia (DIP)

- Ground-glass opacities are more diffuse
- Opacities usually more subpleural or patchy
- Not as bronchocentric as RB-ILD
- Intervening alveolar spaces between bronchioles are diffusely filled with macrophages
- Subtle signs of fibrosis in advanced cases (e.g., reticulation)
- Part of spectrum of smoking-related lung disease

Hypersensitivity Pneumonitis

- Similar radiographic & CT findings
- More widespread than bronchocentric
- Opacities less subtle than in RB-ILD
- Chronic hypersensitivity pneumonitis exhibits more features of fibrosis
- Importance of documenting history of contact with inhalational allergen
- Incidence of hypersensitivity pneumonitis decreased in smokers

Pulmonary Langerhans Cell Histiocytosis

- Most adult patients are heavy smokers
- Often bronchocentric-like RB-ILD
- More conspicuous & profuse irregularly shaped micronodules
- Similar upper lung zone predominance
- Micronodules may cavitate & exhibit cystic transformation
- May progress to severe pulmonary fibrosis
- Typical Langerhans cells in biopsy specimens

Acute Pneumonia

- Ground-glass opacities are either more diffuse or localized
- May affect all portions of lung
- More widespread than bronchocentric
- May be associated with pleural effusion
- Typical clinical presentation with fever & cough

PATHOLOGY

General Features

- Etiology
  - Airflow dynamics for small particulate material
    - Air flows rapidly down conducting airways (trachea to terminal bronchioles)
    - Velocity rapidly decreases distally to allow gas exchange
    - Small particles included in smoke (< 5 μ) escape impacting into larger airways
    - Particles deposited in respiratory bronchioles
- Insults to respiratory bronchioles ("small airways")
  - Contents of cigarette smoke
  - Other inhaled fumes (less common)
- Reactive accumulation of macrophages within respiratory bronchiole lumina (2nd order) & surrounding alveoli

RESPIRATORY BRONCHIOLITIS AND RBILD

Gross Pathologic & Surgical Features

- Associated centrilobular emphysema in smokers
- Mild bronchial wall thickening

Microscopic Features

- RB commonly encountered as incidental histologic finding in lung specimens from cigarette smokers
- Respiratory bronchioles filled with pigmented macrophages
  - Macrophages may spill into surrounding alveoli
- Macrophages typically exhibit brown cytoplasm with some black particles
- Bronchiolar walls may exhibit mild chronic inflammation
- Advanced cases
  - Bronchial wall remodeling
  - Interstitial fibrosis extending along surrounding alveolar walls
- Epithelial lining ranges from cuboidal to bronchiolar-type, pseudostratified ciliated respiratory epithelium
- Bronchiolar epithelial cells may exhibit goblet cell metaplasia
- Cuboidal cell hyperplasia may be seen along neighboring bronchioles, alveolar ducts, & alveoli
- If alveolar macrophages absent, alveolar parenchyma between bronchioles is relatively normal without interstitial fibrosis

CLINICAL ISSUES

Presentation

- Most common signs/symptoms
  - **RB: Asymptomatic**
  - **RB-ILD: Cough, dyspnea**
    - Fine bibasilar end-expiratory crackles
- Other signs/symptoms
  - Clubbing (rare)
  - Mild hypoxia may be present at rest or with exercise
- Pulmonary function tests may be normal (especially in respiratory bronchiolitis)
  - When abnormal: Mixed restrictive-obstructive pattern
  - When abnormal: Isolated increase of residual volume
  - Slightly reduced diffusing capacity common

Demographics

- Age
  - Mean age at onset: 36 years (range: 22-53 years)
- Epidemiology
  - RB: Histologic reaction to inhaled dusts, especially cigarette smoke
    - **RB: Universal histologic response in smokers**
    - Virtually all patients with RB-ILD are heavy smokers
  - When functional alterations cause symptomatic disease, referred to as RB-ILD

Natural History & Prognosis

- Respiratory bronchiolitis may be precursor to centrilobular emphysema
  - Respiratory bronchiolitis occurs early after smoking
  - Location in 2nd-order respiratory bronchioles
  - Evolution of centrilobular nodules (presumed RB) to centrilobular emphysema demonstrated in longitudinal studies performed at 5-10 year intervals

Treatment

- Smoking cessation
  - Histologic abnormalities reversible with cessation of smoking
- Effectiveness of steroids questionable

DIAGNOSTIC CHECKLIST

Consider

- RB in patients with upper lung zone centrilobular nodules & ground-glass opacities on CT, particularly if centrilobular emphysema is also present
- RB-ILD in symptomatic smokers with upper lung zone centrilobular micronodules & ground-glass opacity on CT

Image Interpretation Pearls

- HRCT
  - Small centrilobular ground-glass nodules
  - Upper lobe predominance
  - Smoking history mandatory, usually heavy smoking history in patients with RB-ILD
  - Usually no signs of fibrosis

SELECTED REFERENCES

1. Tazelaar HD et al: Desquamative interstitial pneumonia. Histopathology. 58(4):509-16, 2011
2. Beasley MB: Smoking-related Small airway disease--a review and update. Adv Anat Pathol. 17(4):270-6, 2010
3. Chung JH et al: Smoking-related interstitial lung diseases. Semin Roentgenol. 45(1):29-35, 2010
4. Galvin JR et al: Smoking-related lung disease. J Thorac Imaging. 24(4):274-84, 2009
5. Kanne JP et al: Smoking-related emphysema and interstitial lung diseases. J Thorac Imaging. 2007 Aug;22(3):286-91. Review. Erratum in: J Thorac Imaging. 23(2):144, 2008
6. Lynch DA et al: Idiopathic interstitial pneumonias: CT features. Radiology. 236(1):10-21, 2005
7. Davies G et al: Respiratory bronchiolitis associated with interstitial lung disease and desquamative interstitial pneumonia. Clin Chest Med. 25(4):717-26, vi, 2004
8. Wittram C: The idiopathic interstitial pneumonias. Curr Probl Diagn Radiol. 33(5):189-99, 2004
9. Desai SR et al: Smoking-related interstitial lung diseases: histopathological and imaging perspectives. Clin Radiol. 58(4):259-68, 2003
10. Ryu JH et al: Bronchiolar disorders. Am J Respir Crit Care Med. 168(11):1277-92, 2003
11. Wittram C et al: CT-histologic correlation of the ATS/ERS 2002 classification of idiopathic interstitial pneumonias. Radiographics. 23(5):1057-71, 2003
12. American Thoracic Society; European Respiratory Society: American Thoracic Society/European Respiratory Society International Multidisciplinary Consensus Classification of the Idiopathic Interstitial Pneumonias. This joint statement of the American Thoracic Society (ATS), and the European Respiratory Society (ERS) was adopted by the ATS board of directors, June 2001 and by the ERS Executive Committee, June 2001. Am J Respir Crit Care Med. 165(2):277-304, 2002

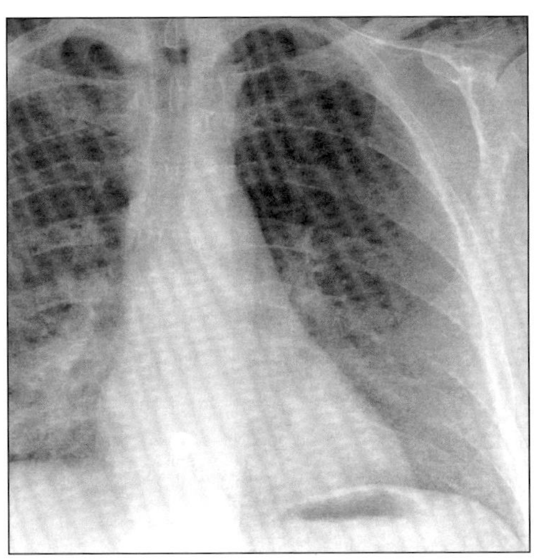

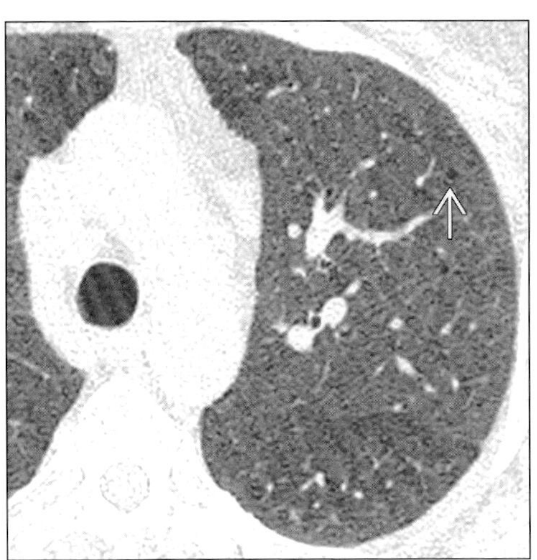

(Left) *PA chest radiograph of a heavy cigarette smoker with dyspnea shows faint, poorly defined opacities that give the lung a "dirty appearance," but no discrete pulmonary nodules.* ***(Right)*** *Axial HRCT of the same patient shows patchy ground-glass opacities and a tiny focus of centrilobular emphysema →. Transbronchial biopsy showed respiratory bronchiolitis. A diagnosis of RB-ILD was rendered based on the combined clinical, radiologic, and histopathologic findings.*

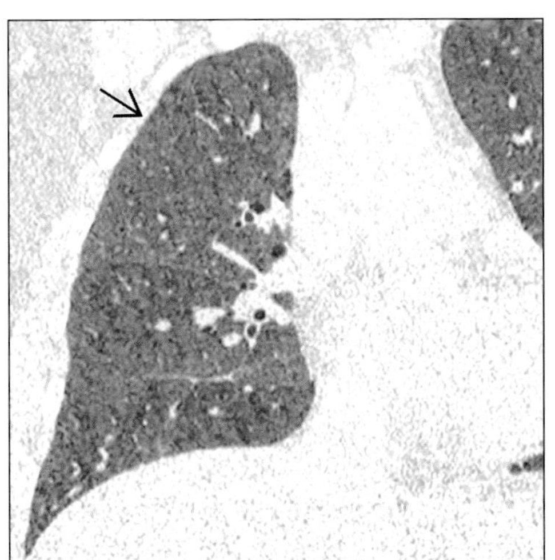

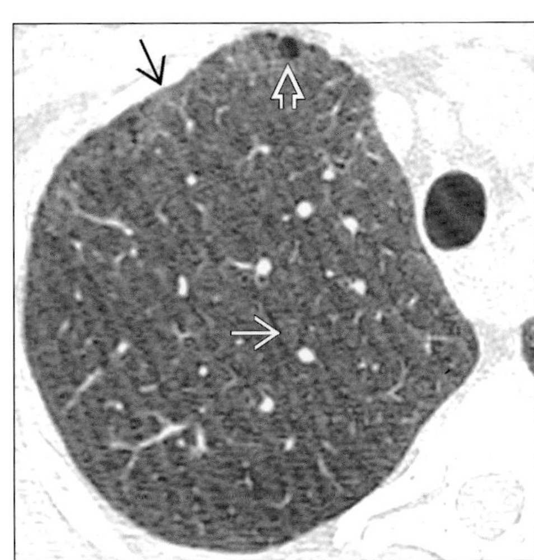

(Left) *Coronal NECT shows extensive ground-glass opacity →, most conspicuous in the upper lobes. While RB-ILD is a clinical diagnosis, the extent of RB on histopathologic specimens is typically greater in symptomatic patients with respiratory dysfunction.* ***(Right)*** *Axial HRCT of a cigarette smoker with RB-ILD who presented with dyspnea and cough shows patchy ground-glass opacities →, subtle centrilobular ground-glass nodules →, and mild centrilobular and paraseptal emphysema →.*

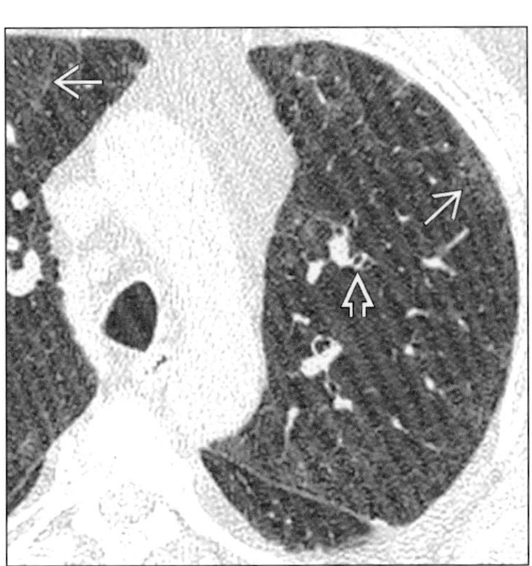

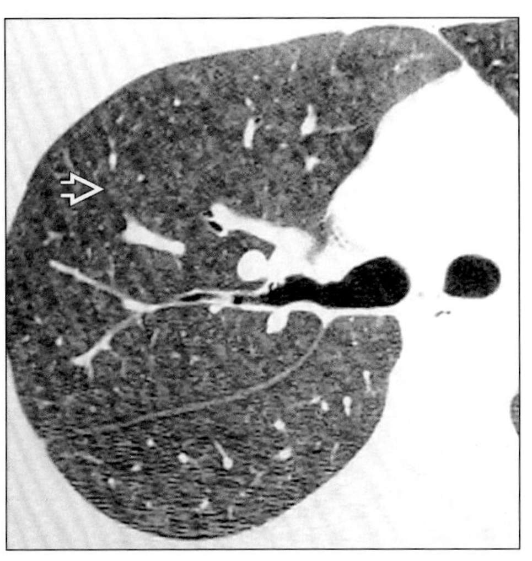

(Left) *Axial HRCT of a heavy cigarette smoker diagnosed with RB-ILD shows patchy ground-glass opacity → in the upper lobes and bronchial wall thickening →. The latter is a nonspecific finding, but is often present in smokers.* ***(Right)*** *Axial HRCT of a cigarette smoker with respiratory bronchiolitis shows extensive centrilobular ground-glass nodules →, an appearance nearly identical to that encountered in hypersensitivity pneumonitis (HP). However, the incidence of HP is lower in cigarette smokers.*

DESQUAMATIVE INTERSTITIAL PNEUMONIA

Key Facts

Terminology

- Desquamative interstitial pneumonia (DIP)
- Chronic interstitial pneumonia characterized by macrophage filling of alveolar spaces & strongly associated with cigarette smoking
- Continuum of smoking-related lung injury: Respiratory bronchiolitis → respiratory bronchiolitis-associated interstitial lung disease (RB-ILD) → DIP

Imaging

- Radiography
  - Basilar reticulation & ill-defined airspace opacities
  - Variable lung volume: May be mildly reduced
- HRCT
  - Ground-glass opacity (80%): Basilar, peripheral
  - Basilar reticular opacities (60%)
  - Small, well-defined cysts
  - Honeycomb lung unusual (10%)

Top Differential Diagnoses

- RB-ILD
- Cryptogenic organizing pneumonia
- Drug reaction
- Hypersensitivity pneumonitis
- Nonspecific interstitial pneumonia
- Lymphoid interstitial pneumonia
- *Pneumocystis jiroveci* pneumonia

Clinical Issues

- History of smoking (up to 90%)
- Insidious onset dyspnea, dry cough, digital clubbing
- Diagnosis
  - Transbronchial biopsy to exclude other etiologies
  - Surgical biopsy when HRCT not typical for IPF
- Treatment: Smoking cessation, corticosteroids
- Prognosis: DIP worse prognosis than RB-ILD

*(**Left**) PA chest radiograph of a smoker with desquamative interstitial pneumonia shows basilar predominant fine reticular and ground-glass opacities and mildly decreased lung volumes. (**Right**) Coronal HRCT maximum-intensity projection (MIP) image shows diffuse patchy bilateral ground-glass opacities ⇨ and scattered small thin-walled pulmonary cysts →. Associated findings of other smoking-related diseases, such as centrilobular emphysema, may also be identified in patients with DIP.*

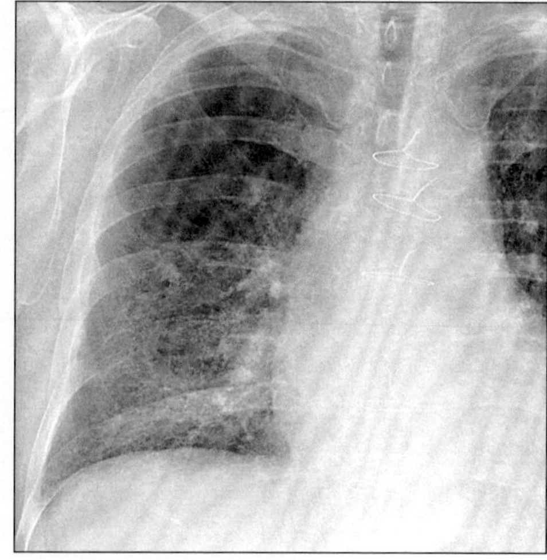

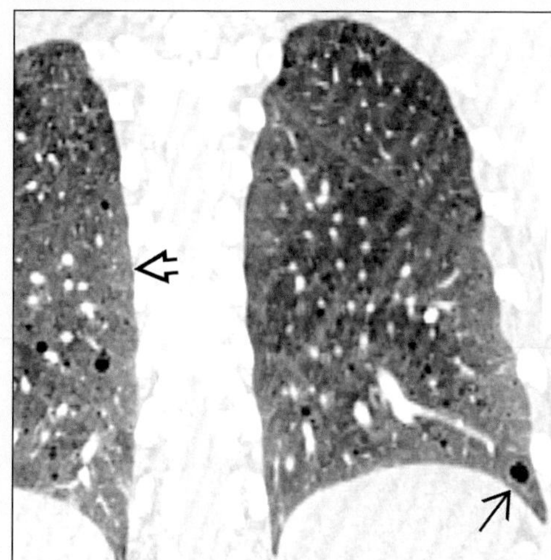

*(**Left**) Axial HRCT of a patient with biopsy-proven DIP shows scattered patchy ground-glass opacities → and numerous small thin-walled lung cysts ➡. DIP falls within the spectrum of smoking-related lung diseases and may exhibit features of respiratory bronchiolitis and emphysema. (**Right**) Axial HRCT of the same patient shows more extensive bilateral ground-glass opacities ➡, basilar reticulation →, and multiple small pulmonary cysts. The findings of DIP are most pronounced in the lung bases.*

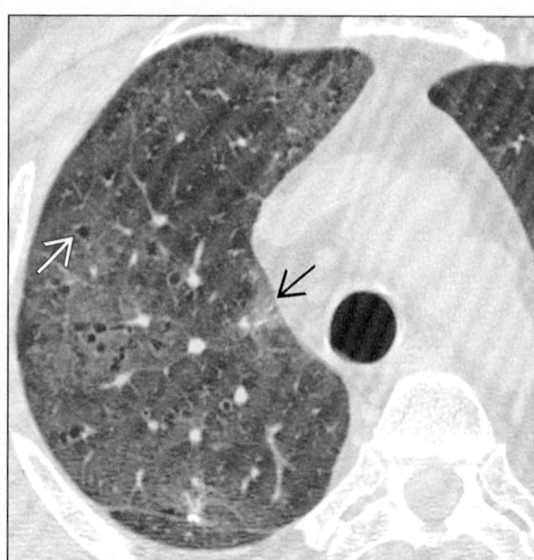

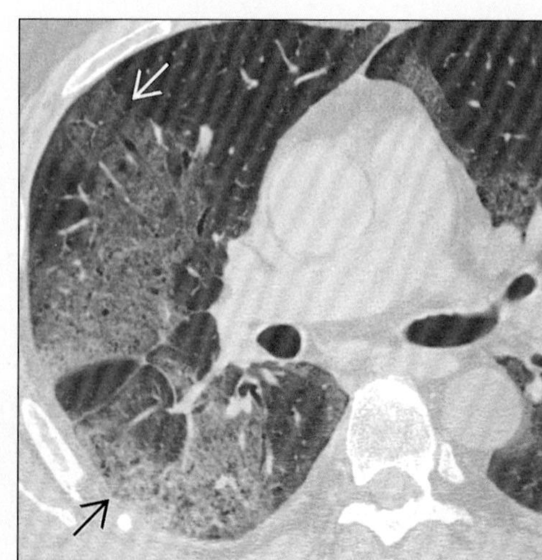

DESQUAMATIVE INTERSTITIAL PNEUMONIA

TERMINOLOGY

Abbreviations

- **Desquamative interstitial pneumonia (DIP)**

Definitions

- Chronic interstitial pneumonia characterized by macrophage filling of alveolar spaces & strongly associated with cigarette smoking
  - "Desquamative" a misnomer: Intraalveolar macrophages originally thought to represent desquamated alveolar lining cells
- Continuum of smoking-related lung injury: Respiratory bronchiolitis → respiratory bronchiolitis-associated interstitial lung disease (RB-ILD) → DIP

IMAGING

General Features

- Best diagnostic clue
  - Smoker with basilar peripheral ground-glass opacities on HRCT

Radiographic Findings

- Radiography
  - Variable nonspecific abnormalities
  - Basilar reticulation & ill-defined airspace opacities
  - Variable lung volume: Mildly reduced from DIP, may be increased with coexistent emphysema

CT Findings

- HRCT
  - **Ground-glass opacity (80%)**
    - **Basilar (70%)** & peripheral (60%) predominance
  - **Reticular opacities (60%)**
    - Bibasilar irregular linear opacities
  - Small, well-defined lung cysts
    - Round, thin-walled, < 2 cm in diameter
  - Honeycomb lung unusual (10%)

DIFFERENTIAL DIAGNOSIS

Respiratory Bronchiolitis-associated Interstitial Lung Disease (RB-ILD)

- Smoking-related disease
- Abnormalities centered on respiratory bronchiole
- Centrilobular ground-glass opacities

Cryptogenic Organizing Pneumonia

- Not related to smoking
- Subpleural ground-glass opacities or consolidation
- No honeycomb lung

Drug Reaction

- Bleomycin, nitrofurantoin
- May exhibit identical imaging findings

Hypersensitivity Pneumonitis

- Uncommon in smokers
- Diffuse ground-glass opacities
- Ill-defined centrilobular nodules
- Mosaic attenuation & air-trapping, common

Nonspecific Interstitial Pneumonia

- May exhibit identical imaging appearance
- Cellular & fibrosing types

Lymphocytic Interstitial Pneumonia

- Associated with collagen vascular disease, immunodeficiency, & Sjögren syndrome
- May exhibit identical imaging appearance

Pneumocystis jiroveci Pneumonia

- History of immunosuppression
- Diffuse ground-glass opacities, pneumatoceles

PATHOLOGY

General Features

- Etiology
  - Association with cigarette smoking (up to 90%)
  - Concept that DIP evolves to UIP now discredited

Microscopic Features

- Intraalveolar & alveolar duct pigmented macrophages
- Mild interstitial chronic inflammation
- Distinction of DIP from RB-ILD
  - RB-ILD: Bronchiolocentric macrophage accumulation
  - DIP: More uniform & widespread involvement

CLINICAL ISSUES

Presentation

- Most common signs/symptoms
  - Insidious onset dyspnea, dry cough, digital clubbing
- Pulmonary function tests: Decreased diffusion capacity (DLCO), restrictive abnormality

Demographics

- Age
  - 4th & 5th decades of life
- Gender
  - M:F = 2:1

Natural History & Prognosis

- HRCT useful for predicting prognosis
  - Ground-glass opacities: Favorable prognosis
  - Honeycomb lung & traction bronchiectasis: Decreased survival
- Evolution
  - May remit spontaneously
  - May progress despite steroids or lung transplantation
- 30% mortality at 10 years

Diagnosis

- Transbronchial lung biopsies generally not diagnostic, but used to exclude other etiologies
- Surgical biopsy when HRCT not typical for IPF

Treatment

- Smoking cessation, corticosteroids

SELECTED REFERENCES

1. Galvin JR et al: Smoking-related lung disease. J Thorac Imaging. 24(4):274-84, 2009
2. Attili AK et al: Smoking-related interstitial lung disease: radiologic-clinical-pathologic correlation. Radiographics. 28(5):1383-96; discussion 1396-8, 2008

PULMONARY LANGERHANS CELL HISTIOCYTOSIS

Key Facts

Terminology
- Pulmonary Langerhans cell histiocytosis (PLCH)
- Peribronchiolar infiltration by stellate nodules that contain Langerhans cells

Imaging
- Radiography
  - Normal or increased lung volume
  - Symmetric upper lung zone predominant reticulonodular opacities, nodules, cysts
  - Spares lung bases
- HRCT
  - Irregular, small nodules & cysts with upper/mid lung zone predominance
  - Bronchiolocentric nodules, irregular/stellate borders, 1-10 mm in size
  - Cysts: Variable sizes & bizarre shapes, thin or thick/nodular irregular walls

Top Differential Diagnoses
- Lymphangioleiomyomatosis (LAM)
- *Pneumocystis jiroveci* pneumonia
- Silicosis
- Sarcoidosis

Pathology
- Bronchiolocentric proliferation of Langerhans cells

Clinical Issues
- Symptoms & signs: Cough, dyspnea, chest pain, fever, weight loss; asymptomatic in 25%
- M = F; 20-40 years of age
- 95% of affected patients are cigarette smokers

Diagnostic Checklist
- Consider PLCH in adult smokers with upper lung predominant small nodular &/or cystic lung disease

*(**Left**) Graphic shows the distribution and morphology of lung abnormalities in patients with PLCH. The disease manifests with upper lobe predominant small nodules, cysts, or both and exhibits relative sparing of the basilar lung parenchyma near the costophrenic angles. (**Right**) PA chest radiograph of a 35-year-old female smoker with PLCH who presented with cough and dyspnea demonstrates upper and mid lung zone predominant small irregular nodules, some of which exhibit central lucency ➔.*

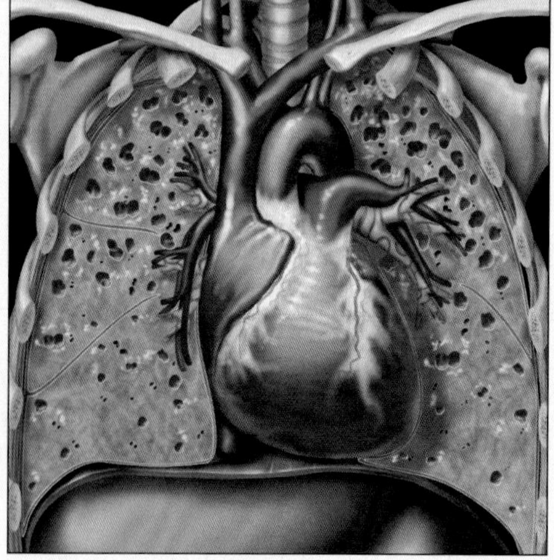

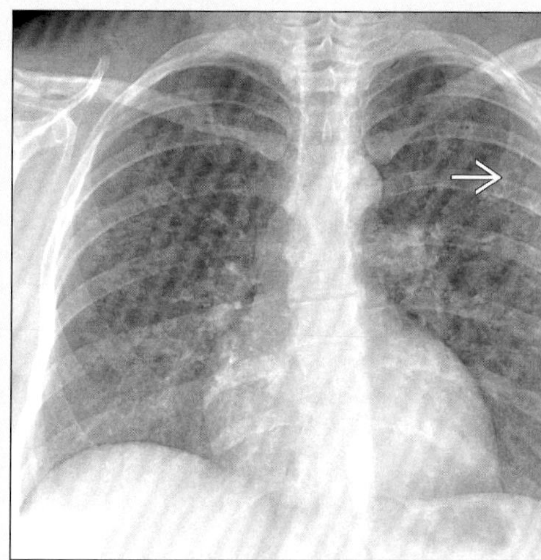

*(**Left**) Axial NECT of the same patient demonstrates upper lung zone predominant small cavitary and noncavitary nodules with normal-appearing intervening lung parenchyma. Some of the noncavitary nodules ➔ exhibit a stellate morphology characteristic of PLCH lesions. (**Right**) Axial NECT of the same patient demonstrates relative sparing of the lung bases manifesting with decreased profusion of lung nodules ➔. The morphology and distribution of the abnormalities are characteristic of PLCH.*

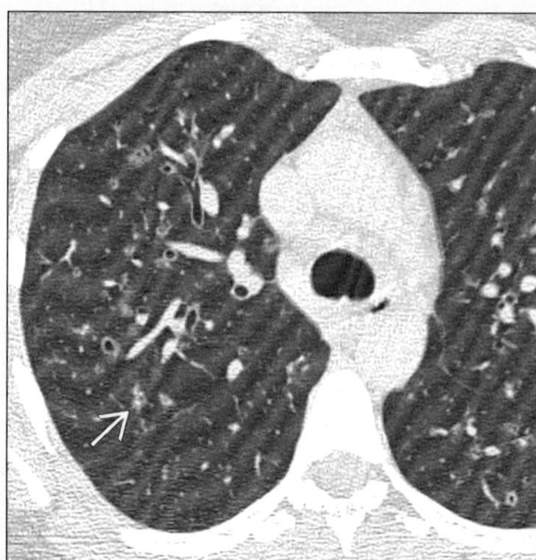

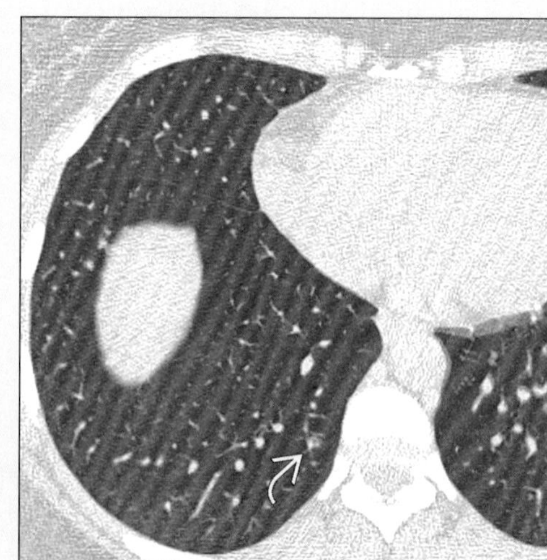

PULMONARY LANGERHANS CELL HISTIOCYTOSIS

TERMINOLOGY

Abbreviations

- **Pulmonary Langerhans cell histiocytosis (PLCH)**

Definitions

- Peribronchiolar infiltration of stellate nodules that contain Langerhans cells

IMAGING

General Features

- Best diagnostic clue
  - HRCT: Nodules & bizarre-shaped pulmonary cysts in upper & mid lung zones in cigarette smokers
- Location
  - Upper & mid lung
  - Bilateral symmetrical involvement
  - Spares basilar lung near costophrenic angle
- Size
  - Nodules,1-10 mm in diameter
  - Cysts 1-3 cm in diameter
- Morphology
  - HRCT: Irregular stellate nodules
  - Cysts with variable wall thickness & shape

Radiographic Findings

- Radiography
  - **Normal or increased lung volume**
  - Diffuse symmetric **reticulonodular opacities**
  - Multiple ill-defined **nodules** 1-10 mm in diameter
  - **Cysts** 1-3 cm in diameter
    - Cysts may not be evident on radiography
  - Upper & mid lung predominant involvement
    - Spare basilar lung near costophrenic angles
  - Secondary spontaneous pneumothorax
    - Recurrent, unilateral or bilateral
  - Uncommon features
    - Skeletal involvement: Lytic or expansile lesion(s)
    - Lymphadenopathy
    - Airspace disease
    - Solitary nodule
    - Pleural effusion
    - Normal chest radiograph

CT Findings

- NECT
  - Upper & mid lung predominance
  - Relative sparing of lung bases
- HRCT
  - Irregular, small nodules & cysts with intervening normal lung
  - **Nodules**
    - Centrilobular, peribronchial, peribronchiolar
    - Typically **irregular/stellate** borders, 1-10 mm, occasionally > 1 cm
    - Cavitary nodules with thick walls
    - Range from few to innumerable lung nodules
    - Nodules may progress to cavitary nodules & cysts
  - **Cysts**
    - **More common than nodules**
    - 1-10 mm, may be > 1 cm
    - Variable shape, may exhibit bizarre shapes
    - Thin or thick nodular/irregular walls
    - Cysts may occur ± nodules
  - Ground-glass opacities, reticular opacities, septal lines, irregular bronchovascular bundles
  - Coalescent cysts, fibrosis, honeycomb lung in late disease

Imaging Recommendations

- Best imaging tool
  - HRCT is optimal imaging modality for assessment of PLCH

DIFFERENTIAL DIAGNOSIS

Lymphangioleiomyomatosis

- Unique to females, unless related to tuberous sclerosis
- Spherical cysts, thin-walled, uniformly distributed
- Normal intervening lung
- Nodules uncommon
- Chylothorax may occur (pleural effusion rare in LCH)
- Secondary spontaneous pneumothorax

Pneumocystis jiroveci Pneumonia

- Pneumatoceles may manifest as lung cysts
- Cysts associated with ground-glass opacities

Silicosis & Coal Worker's Pneumoconiosis

- Upper lobe, perilymphatic nodules
- Eggshell lymph node calcifications
- Progressive massive fibrosis, peripheral emphysema
- No pulmonary cysts

Sarcoidosis

- Upper lobe predominant perilymphatic micronodules; cavitation very rare
- Hilar/mediastinal lymphadenopathy
- End-stage disease: Upper lobe fibrosis, cysts, honeycomb lung
  - May resemble end-stage PLCH

Laryngeal Papillomatosis

- Laryngeal & tracheal mural nodules
- Pulmonary nodules typically cavitate
- Cystic lesions typically in lower lobes & dorsal lungs

Hypersensitivity Pneumonitis

- Upper lobe predominant involvement
- Ground-glass centrilobular nodules
- May exhibit cysts, but usually few in number

Bullous Emphysema

- Lung destruction with imperceptible walls & central lobular artery
- May mimic end-stage PLCH

PATHOLOGY

General Features

- Etiology
  - Pathogenesis incompletely understood
    - Childhood PLCH: Clonal cellular process unrelated to smoking
    - Adult PLCH: Immune-mediated nonclonal proliferation related to smoking
      - Postulated to be allergic reaction to constituent of cigarette smoke

- Smoke postulated to stimulate cytokine production, causing activation of Langerhans cells
- Associated abnormalities
  - Rarely reported following radiation or chemotherapy for Hodgkin lymphoma

Gross Pathologic & Surgical Features

- Majority of affected adults have disease limited to lung
- Cellular & fibrotic lesions with variable cyst formation
  - Well-defined, airway-centered nodules with irregular stellate borders
- End-stage: Fibrosis, honeycomb lung, cysts, emphysema

Microscopic Features

- Bronchiolocentric proliferation of Langerhans cells
- Nodules
  - Bronchiolocentric (terminal & respiratory bronchioles), stellate shaped
  - Typically < 1 cm in diameter, may be 1.5-2 cm
  - Intervening relatively normal or somewhat distorted lung
  - "Cavitary" nodules: Cavity represents enlarged airway lumen
  - Thick- & thin-walled lung cysts
- Desquamative interstitial pneumonia (DIP), cryptogenic organizing pneumonia (COP), & respiratory bronchiolitis (RB) may occur in adjacent lung
- Progression from dense cellular nodules to cavitary nodules to increasing fibrosis
  - Fibrotic scars surrounded by enlarged distorted airspaces

CLINICAL ISSUES

Presentation

- Most common signs/symptoms
  - Nonproductive cough, dyspnea, fatigue, chest pain, fever, weight loss
  - Asymptomatic (25%)
  - Pneumothorax in 25% during course of disease
    - Unilateral, bilateral may recur
- Other signs/symptoms
  - **Former terms referring to variants of LCH; usage now discouraged**
    - Hand-Schüller-Christian disease: Young adults & adolescents with lung, bone, & pituitary involvement (diabetes insipidus)
    - Letterer-Siwe: Infants, multiorgan involvement, malignant Langerhans cells, poor prognosis
    - Eosinophilic granuloma: Single organ involvement of LCH
      - PLCH preferred term for isolated pulmonary involvement
- Pulmonary function tests
  - Reduced carbon monoxide diffusing capacity
  - Normal total lung capacity

Demographics

- Age
  - Typically 20-40 years of age; wide range
- Gender
  - M = F
- Ethnicity
  - Caucasian adults, less common in African-Americans
- Epidemiology
  - Smoking-related lung disease (95% in smokers)
    - Only small percentage of smokers develop LCH
  - Bone involvement, skin lesions, & diabetes insipidus (< 15%)

Diagnosis

- Transbronchial lung biopsy
- Bronchoalveolar lavage: > 5% CD1a(+) Langerhans cells
- Open lung biopsy may be required

Natural History & Prognosis

- Early phase predominantly nodular, later phase predominantly cystic
- Disease may regress or resolve, become stable, or progress to advanced cystic disease
  - 75% of patients with eventual resolution or stability
- May recur up to 7 years after presentation, even with smoking cessation
- May recur in transplanted lung
- End-stage disease may mimic panlobular emphysema or honeycomb lung
- Pulmonary artery hypertension (33%)
- Prognosis is variable
  - Complete remission to respiratory failure
  - Mortality < 5%; worse in men, elderly, & patients with recurrent pneumothoraces

Treatment

- Smoking cessation
- Corticosteroids for progressive disease
- Lung transplantation for advanced disease

DIAGNOSTIC CHECKLIST

Consider

- PLCH in adult smokers with upper lung predominant small nodular &/or cystic lung disease

Image Interpretation Pearls

- Characteristic HRCT appearance may be diagnostic in appropriate setting

SELECTED REFERENCES

1. Seaman DM et al: Diffuse cystic lung disease at high-resolution CT. AJR Am J Roentgenol. 196(6):1305-11, 2011
2. Galvin JR et al: Smoking-related lung disease. J Thorac Imaging. 24(4):274-84, 2009
3. Abbott GF et al: From the archives of the AFIP: pulmonary Langerhans cell histiocytosis. Radiographics. 24(3):821-41, 2004
4. Vassallo R et al: Pulmonary Langerhans'-cell histiocytosis. N Engl J Med. 342(26):1969-78, 2000
5. Brauner MW et al: Pulmonary Langerhans cell histiocytosis: evolution of lesions on CT scans. Radiology. 204(2):497-502, 1997

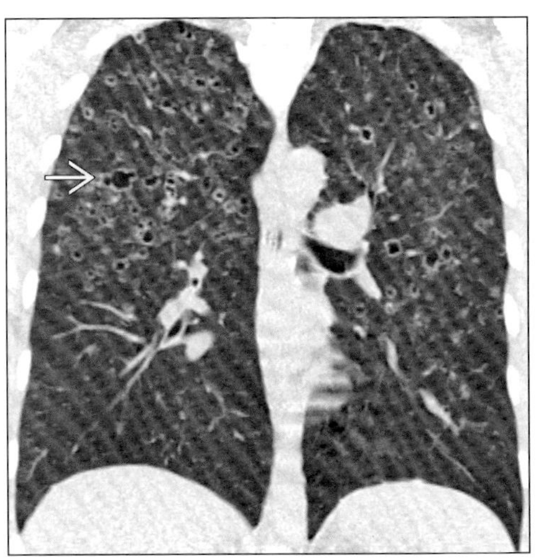

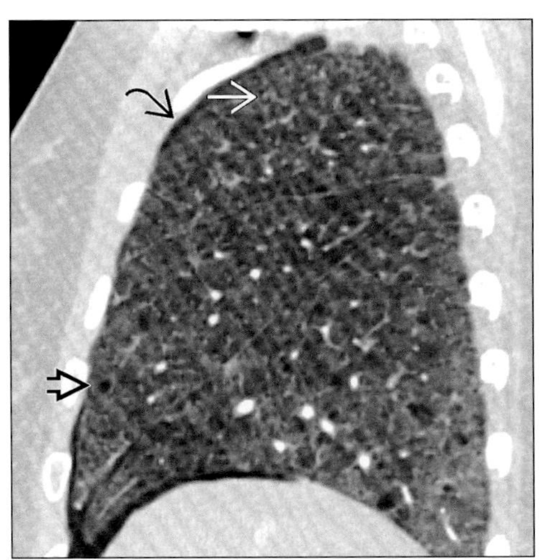

(Left) *Coronal NECT of a patient with PLCH shows the typical distribution of pulmonary abnormalities. Multiple small cysts, some with bizarre shapes, predominantly affect the upper lungs and spare the bases.* ***(Right)*** *Sagittal NECT of a patient with PLCH who presented with acute chest pain shows profuse involvement of the lung with cysts, small nodules, and a small anterior right-sided pneumothorax. PLCH is a recognized cause of secondary spontaneous pneumothorax.*

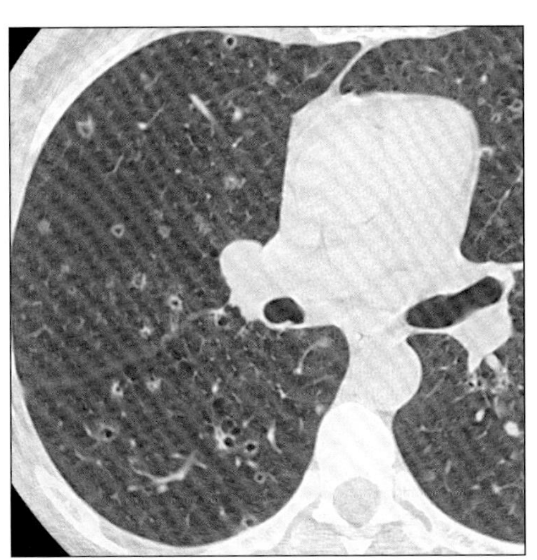

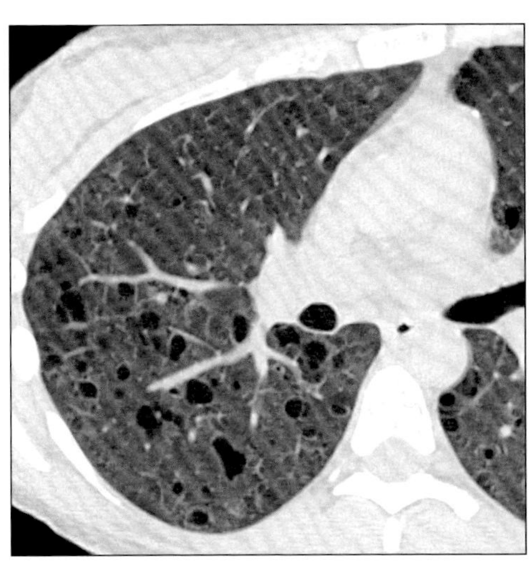

(Left) *Axial NECT of a patient with PLCH shows multifocal bilateral small pulmonary cysts with thick irregular walls associated with centrilobular emphysema. As PLCH is a smoking-related lung disease, it is not surprising that it can occur in association with other smoking-related diseases.* ***(Right)*** *Axial NECT of a patient with PLCH demonstrates thin-walled pulmonary cysts of varying sizes, some with bizarre shapes. PLCH cysts may exhibit smooth or irregular cyst walls and may mimic other cystic lung diseases.*

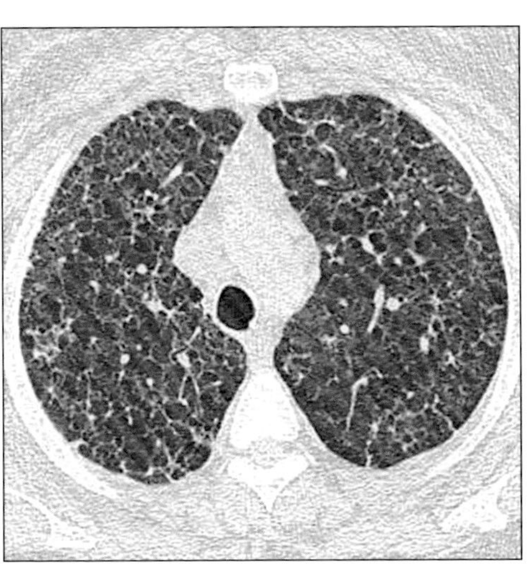

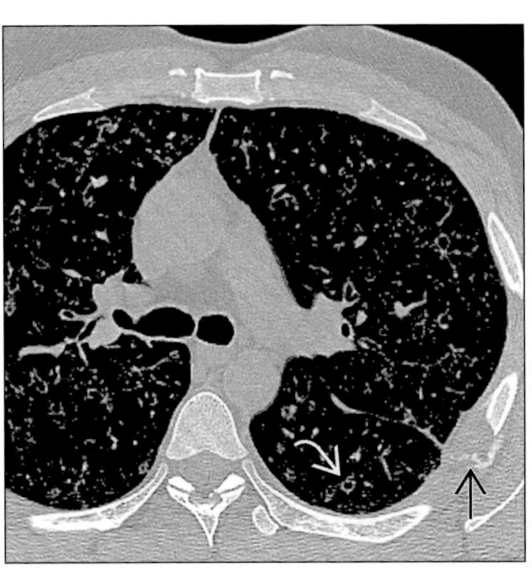

(Left) *Axial HRCT of a female smoker with end-stage PLCH shows profusion and coalescence of upper lung predominant pulmonary cysts. PLCH lesions may exhibit regression, stability, or progression on serial imaging studies.* ***(Right)*** *Axial NECT (bone window) of a patient with PLCH shows multifocal pulmonary cysts with irregular walls and a sharply beveled lytic bone lesion affecting a left-sided rib. Skeletal lesions are an uncommon but recognized manifestation of PLCH.*

PULMONARY FIBROSIS ASSOCIATED WITH SMOKING

Key Facts

Terminology

- Pulmonary fibrosis associated with cigarette smoking
  - End-stage of smoking-related interstitial lung disease

Imaging

- Radiography
  - Volume loss
  - Reticular & reticulonodular opacities
  - Pulmonary arterial hypertension
- CT
  - Reticular & reticulonodular interstitial opacities
  - Honeycomb lung (in idiopathic pulmonary fibrosis)
  - Traction bronchiectasis
- Findings of other smoking-related lung diseases
  - Centrilobular emphysema
  - Respiratory bronchiolitis
- HRCT for optimal characterization of lung disease related to smoking, including pulmonary fibrosis

Top Differential Diagnoses

- Idiopathic pulmonary fibrosis
- Respiratory bronchiolitis-interstitial lung disease
- Desquamative interstitial pneumonia
- Pulmonary Langerhans cell histiocytosis
- Hypersensitivity pneumonitis

Pathology

- Fibrosis
- Interstitial inflammation
- Honeycomb lung in cases of usual interstitial pneumonia

Diagnostic Checklist

- Indeterminate lung nodules must be identified & managed appropriately in these patients, given that smoking is risk factor for lung cancer

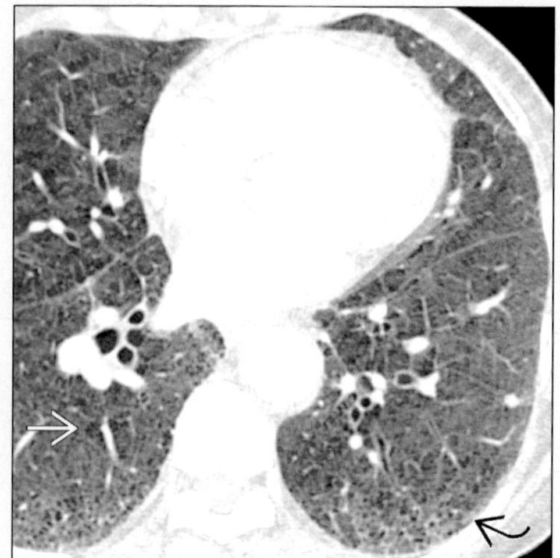

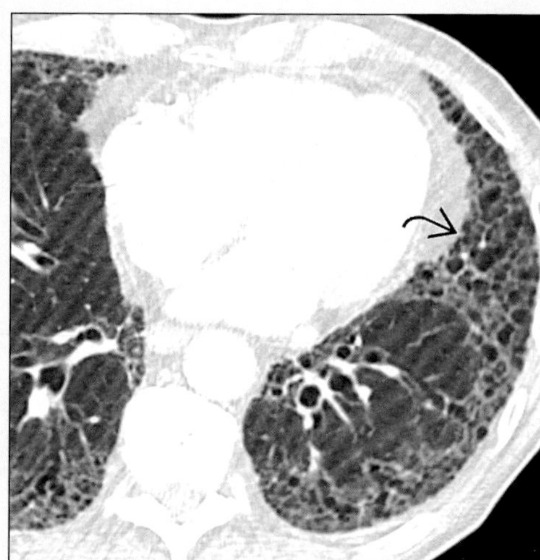

(Left) *Axial CECT of a smoker with emphysema and idiopathic pulmonary fibrosis (IPF) shows centrilobular emphysema ➔ and subpleural reticular opacities ➔. HRCT is the imaging modality of choice for detecting pulmonary fibrosis, which manifests with reticular and reticulonodular opacities, traction bronchiectasis, and honeycombing.* ***(Right)*** *Axial CECT of a smoker with IPF shows subpleural cystic spaces ➔, consistent with honeycomb lung on a background of reticular opacities.*

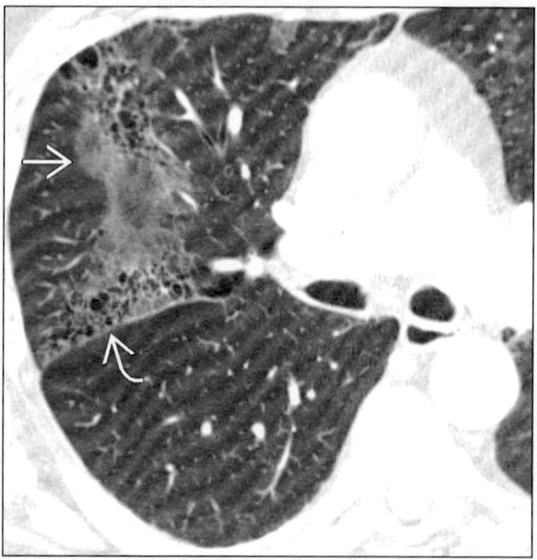

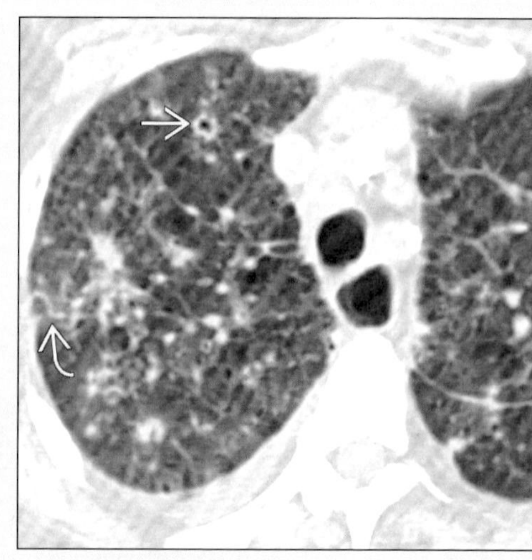

(Left) *Axial CECT of a 59-year-old smoker with desquamative interstitial pneumonia (DIP) shows middle lobe ground-glass opacity ➔ with subpleural reticular opacities and cystic spaces ➔, consistent with pulmonary fibrosis. Honeycomb lung may be present in advanced cases of DIP.* ***(Right)*** *Axial NECT of an adult smoker with pulmonary Langerhans cell histiocytosis shows right upper lobe pulmonary nodules, some of which have cavitated ➔. Reticular opacities ➔ indicate pulmonary fibrosis.*

PULMONARY FIBROSIS ASSOCIATED WITH SMOKING

TERMINOLOGY

Definitions

- Pulmonary fibrosis associated with cigarette smoking
  - End-stage of smoking-related interstitial lung disease

IMAGING

General Features

- Best diagnostic clue
  - Volume loss, architectural distortion, honeycomb lung, traction bronchiectasis

Radiographic Findings

- Fibrosis characterized by **volume loss**
  - May be combined with emphysema, resulting in mixed pattern of hyperinflation & regional volume loss
- **Reticular & reticulonodular opacities**
- Pulmonary arterial hypertension
  - Central pulmonary artery enlargement
  - Right heart enlargement

CT Findings

- HRCT
  - **Pulmonary fibrosis**
    - Reticular & reticulonodular interstitial opacities
    - Honeycomb lung (idiopathic pulmonary fibrosis)
    - Traction bronchiectasis
  - **Pulmonary arterial hypertension**
  - Other smoking-associated lung diseases
    - **Centrilobular emphysema**
    - Respiratory bronchiolitis: Centrilobular micronodular opacities & patchy ground-glass opacities

Imaging Recommendations

- Best imaging tool
  - HRCT for optimal characterization of lung disease related to smoking, including pulmonary fibrosis

DIFFERENTIAL DIAGNOSIS

Idiopathic Pulmonary Fibrosis (IPF)

- Suspected association with cigarette smoking
- Mid & lower lung zone predominant
- Subpleural reticulation, traction bronchiectasis, & honeycomb lung

Respiratory Bronchiolitis-associated Interstitial Lung Disease (RB-ILD)

- Upper lobe predominant centrilobular & peribronchial nodules
- Subpleural reticular opacities indicating fibrosis, lower lobe predominant
- Mild bronchial wall thickening

Desquamative Interstitial Pneumonia (DIP)

- Ground-glass opacities, typically diffuse
- Fibrosis, honeycombing in advanced cases

Pulmonary Langerhans Cell Histiocytosis (PLCH)

- Upper lobe predominant micronodules & cysts
- Adults, heavy smokers

Hypersensitivity Pneumonitis

- Diffuse centrilobular ground-glass opacities
- History of exposure to allergen
- Decreased incidence in smokers

Drug Reaction

- Including chemotherapy agents, nitrofurantoin
- May progress to interstitial fibrosis

Collagen Vascular Disease

- Rheumatoid arthritis, systemic sclerosis
- May exhibit honeycomb lung

PATHOLOGY

General Features

- Etiology
  - Smoking-related interstitial lung diseases (ILD), which may result in fibrosis
    - RB-ILD, DIP, PLCH
  - IPF may be associated with smoking
- Pathology based on underlying interstitial lung disease

Gross Pathologic & Surgical Features

- Fibrosis, interstitial inflammation
- Honeycombing in usual interstitial pneumonia

CLINICAL ISSUES

Presentation

- Most common signs/symptoms
  - Chronic dyspnea, nonproductive cough
- Other signs/symptoms
  - Clubbing
  - Restrictive pulmonary function tests
    - Usually with decreased diffusion capacity

Natural History & Prognosis

- Based on underlying interstitial lung disease

Treatment

- Fibrosis represents irreversible lung damage
  - Most other smoking-related interstitial lung diseases reversible with smoking cessation
  - Corticosteroids may be beneficial in some forms of smoking-related ILD

DIAGNOSTIC CHECKLIST

Image Interpretation Pearls

- Imaging signs of pulmonary fibrosis have important clinical & prognostic significance

Reporting Tips

- Indeterminate lung nodules must be identified & managed appropriately in these patients, given that smoking is risk factor for lung cancer

SELECTED REFERENCES

1. Chung JH et al: Smoking-related interstitial lung diseases. Semin Roentgenol. 45(1):29-35, 2010
2. Attili AK et al: Smoking-related interstitial lung disease: radiologic-clinical-pathologic correlation. Radiographics. 28(5):1383-96; discussion 1396-8, 2008

ASBESTOSIS

Key Facts

Terminology

- Interstitial lung disease due to asbestos fiber inhalation

Imaging

- Radiography
  - May be normal (10-20%)
  - Peripheral lower zone predominant abnormalities
  - Irregular reticular or small nodular opacities
  - "Shaggy" cardiac borders in advanced disease
  - Late: End-stage honeycomb lung
- HRCT
  - Early: Peripheral posterior basilar reticular opacities, centrilobular nodules, & branching opacities are most common abnormalities
  - Late: More severe reticulation, traction bronchiectasis, honeycomb lung (similar to UIP)
  - Pleural plaques in 80%

Top Differential Diagnoses

- Idiopathic pulmonary fibrosis
- Scleroderma
- Rheumatoid arthritis
- Chronic hypersensitivity pneumonitis

Pathology

- Fibrosis + asbestos bodies = asbestosis
- Increased deposition of fibers in lower lung zones

Clinical Issues

- Gradual dyspnea on exertion, nonproductive cough
- Men more often affected, occupational exposure
- No known treatment

Diagnostic Checklist

- Consider asbestosis in patients with basilar interstitial lung disease & pleural plaques

(Left) Graphic shows features of asbestosis characterized by abnormal reticulation predominantly involving the periphery of the lower lobes. Pleural plaques ➔ are helpful in suggesting the diagnosis, but may be absent in up to 20% of affected patients. (Right) Coronal HRCT of a patient with asbestosis shows peripheral reticular opacities ⇨ and mild honeycomb lung with associated traction bronchiectasis/bronchiolectasis in a pattern similar to that of usual interstitial pneumonia.

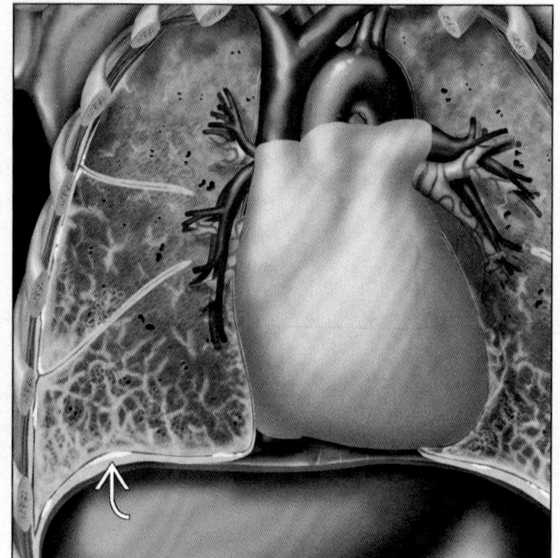

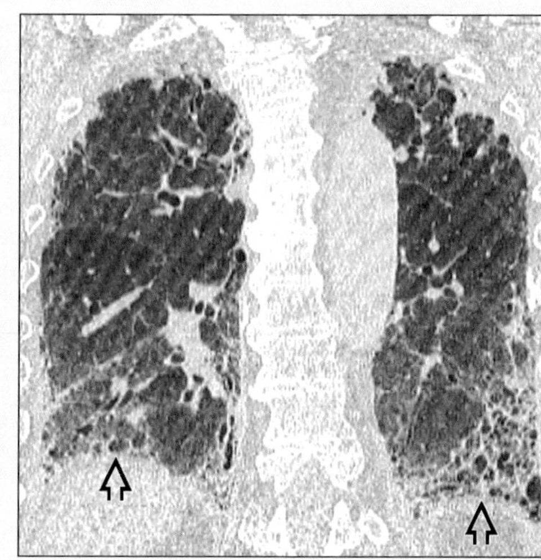

(Left) Axial CECT of a patient with asbestosis shows bilateral subpleural reticulation and posterior pleural plaques ⇨. (Right) Axial CECT of a patient with asbestosis shows subpleural reticulation and mild honeycombing ➔. Discontinuous foci of pleural calcification ➔ are consistent with asbestos-related pleural disease, indicative of asbestos exposure, and provide a clue to the etiology and diagnosis of the pulmonary disease.

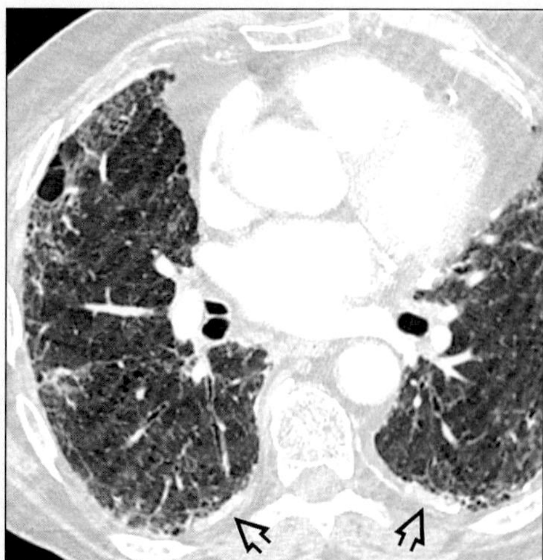

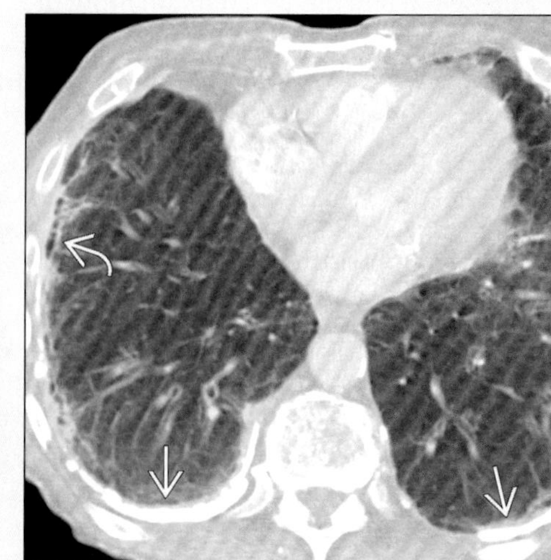

ASBESTOSIS

TERMINOLOGY

Definitions

- Interstitial lung disease due to asbestos fiber inhalation
- Asbestosis is **not** synonymous with asbestos-related pleural disease

IMAGING

General Features

- Best diagnostic clue
  - Basilar interstitial fibrosis & pleural plaques
- Location
  - Posterior basilar subpleural lung
- Morphology
  - Fibrosis centered on respiratory bronchioles

Radiographic Findings

- Radiography
  - May be normal (10-20%)
  - **Peripheral basilar abnormalities**
  - **Irregular reticular or small nodular opacities**
  - "Shaggy" cardiac border in advanced disease
  - Late disease: End-stage honeycomb lung
  - Pleural plaques (25%)
  - Pleural thickening
  - **Lung cancer**: Lower zone predominance in contrast to upper zone predominance in smokers
  - Progressive massive fibrosis extremely rare
  - "B" reading: International Labor Office (ILO) classification compared to standard radiographs
    - Asbestosis generally exhibits s, t, or u opacities

CT Findings

- CECT
  - Useful to differentiate lung nodules from pleural plaques, round atelectasis, & lung fibrosis
- HRCT
  - More sensitive than chest radiography
  - Screening of asbestos-exposed workers
    - Chest radiography of patients with clinical asbestosis, abnormal in 80%; HRCT abnormal in 96%
    - 33% of patients without clinical or radiographic evidence of asbestosis have abnormal HRCT
    - False negatives for early asbestosis in 25%
  - **Early**: Peripheral posterior basilar reticular opacities, centrilobular nodules, & branching opacities most common abnormalities
  - **Late**: More severe reticulation, traction bronchiectasis, honeycomb lung (similar to UIP)
  - **Subpleural curvilinear lines** early sign
    - Parallel chest wall within 1 cm of pleura, 5-10 cm long
    - Peribronchial confluent fibrosis or atelectasis associated with obstructed respiratory bronchioles
  - **Parenchymal bands** project from pleura
    - 2-5 cm long
    - Fibrosis along interlobular septa or bronchovascular bundles
  - Nonspecific ground-glass opacities
  - Mosaic attenuation from air-trapping
  - **Pleural plaques in 80%**
    - Indicative of previous asbestos exposure

Nuclear Medicine Findings

- Ga-67 scintigraphy
  - Usually positive in asbestosis, but rarely used today

Imaging Recommendations

- Best imaging tool
  - HRCT to characterize lung & pleural disease
- Protocol advice
  - Prone HRCT essential to differentiate mild interstitial lung disease from dependent atelectasis

DIFFERENTIAL DIAGNOSIS

Idiopathic Pulmonary Fibrosis

- No pleural plaques
- Traction bronchiolectasis & honeycomb lung more common (less common in asbestosis)
- Band-like opacities less common
- Mosaic perfusion less common (no airway obstruction)

Scleroderma

- No pleural plaques, but pleural thickening & pseudoplaques common
- Dilated esophagus
- Fine reticular opacities with similar distribution
- Ground-glass opacity more common than in asbestosis
- Honeycomb lung less common

Rheumatoid Arthritis

- No pleural plaques
- Skeletal abnormalities
- Similar interstitial fibrosis

Chronic Hypersensitivity Pneumonitis

- No pleural plaques
- Pulmonary fibrosis less severe in lung bases, more severe in mid & upper lungs
- Superimposed subacute hypersensitivity pneumonitis (ground-glass opacity, often centrilobular)
- Mosaic perfusion from air-trapping more common

Lymphangitic Carcinomatosis

- Asymmetric nodular thickening of interlobular septa & core bronchovascular structures
- No pleural plaques, but pleural effusion common

Drug Reaction

- Prototypical drug: Methotrexate
- No pleural plaques
- Similar interstitial fibrosis

PATHOLOGY

General Features

- Associated abnormalities
  - Asbestos-related pleural disease
    - Benign exudative pleural effusion
    - Pleural plaques
    - Diffuse pleural thickening
  - Rounded atelectasis
  - Malignant mesothelioma
  - Lung cancer
- Asbestos
  - Fibrous mineral properties: Heat resistant, high tensile strength, flexible, durable

ASBESTOSIS

- 2 types of fibers: Serpentine & amphibole
  - Serpentine (chrysotile or white asbestos): 90% of commercial asbestos
    - Curly, wavy fiber
    - Long (> 100 μm)
    - Diameter (20-40 μm)
  - Amphibole
    - Crocidolite (blue asbestos), amosite (brown asbestos), anthophyllite, tremolite, actinolite
    - Straight, rigid fiber
    - Aspect ratio (length/width) > 3:1
- Retention: Long thin fibers > short thick fibers

- Pathophysiology
  - Increased deposition of fibers in lower lung zones from gravitational ventilatory gradient
  - Fibers deposit in respiratory bronchioles
  - No lymphatic removal, largest & most harmful fibers too large for removal by macrophages

Staging, Grading, & Classification

- American College of Pathology
  - Grade 1: Fibrosis in respiratory bronchiole wall
  - Grade 2 & 3: Extension into alveoli
  - Grade 4: Alveolar & septal fibrosis with spaces larger than alveoli (honeycomb lung)

Gross Pathologic & Surgical Features

- Coarse honeycomb lung & volume loss, particularly in lower lobes
- Transbronchial biopsy: Poor yield, of little value

Microscopic Features

- **Fibrosis + asbestos bodies = asbestosis**
- Early fibrosis: Centered on respiratory bronchioles, centrifugal spread
  - Important pathologic difference from idiopathic interstitial fibrosis where fibrosis generally distorts airways (traction bronchiolectasis)
- Patchy distribution, severe honeycomb lung uncommon
- Fibrosis associated with > 1 million fibers/gm lung tissue
- **Asbestos (ferruginous) bodies**
  - Hemosiderin-coated fiber (typically amphibole)
    - Coated fibers fewer than uncoated fibers
  - Incompletely phagocytized by macrophages
  - May be retrieved with bronchoalveolar lavage (BAL)
    - Not pathognomonic for asbestosis
    - Does not correlate with fibrosis

CLINICAL ISSUES

Presentation

- Most common signs/symptoms
  - Gradual onset dyspnea on exertion, nonproductive cough
  - Rales (end-inspiratory crackles)
  - Clubbing in 1/3
  - American Thoracic Society (AST) general criteria for diagnosis of asbestosis (2003)
    - Evidence of structural pathology consistent with asbestosis as documented by imaging or histology
    - Evidence of causation as documented by occupational & exposure history (including pleural plaques & asbestos bodies)
    - Exclusion of alternative plausible causes for findings
- Pulmonary function tests
  - Restriction & decreased diffusion capacity
  - Decreased small airway flow rates

Demographics

- Gender
  - Men due to occupational exposure
    - Spouse of occupationally exposed (nonoccupational exposure)
- Epidemiology
  - Long-term exposure to asbestos fibers: Asbestos mills, insulation, shipyards, construction
  - Dose-response relationship
    - Usually requires high dust concentrations
    - Typically 20 years following initial exposure, but could be as short as 3 years
    - 1% risk of asbestosis after cumulative dose of 10 fiber-year/ml tissue

Natural History & Prognosis

- **Latency period 20-30 years**
- Does not regress, slowly progresses
- Asbestos as carcinogen: Multiplicative risk factor for lung cancer
  - **High proportion die of lung cancer (1 in 4)**

Treatment

- No known treatment
- Smoking cessation
- Consider lung cancer screening
- Control & regulation of asbestos in workplace
- Eligible for worker compensation
  - Pathologic tissue not required to gain compensation

DIAGNOSTIC CHECKLIST

Consider

- Asbestosis in patients with basilar interstitial lung disease & pleural plaques

Image Interpretation Pearls

- Pulmonary fibrosis without pleural plaques does not exclude asbestosis

Reporting Tips

- Asbestosis may be reportable disease in some states

SELECTED REFERENCES

1. Chong S et al: Pneumoconiosis: comparison of imaging and pathologic findings. Radiographics. 26(1):59-77, 2006
2. Akira M et al: High-resolution CT of asbestosis and idiopathic pulmonary fibrosis. AJR Am J Roentgenol. 181(1):163-9, 2003
3. Roach HD et al: Asbestos: when the dust settles an imaging review of asbestos-related disease. Radiographics. 22 Spec No:S167-84, 2002
4. Kim KI et al: Imaging of occupational lung disease. Radiographics. 21(6):1371-91, 2001

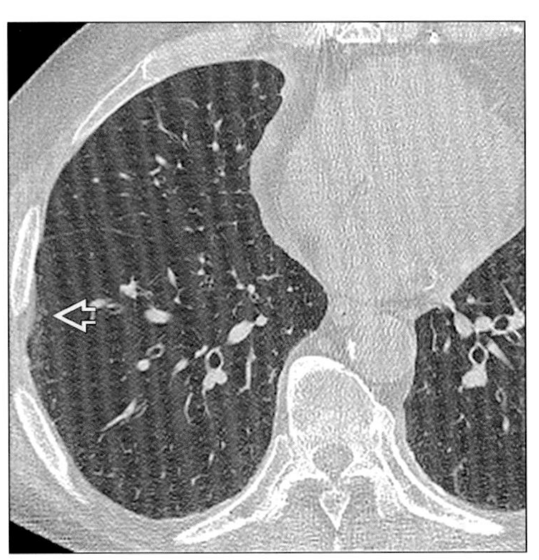

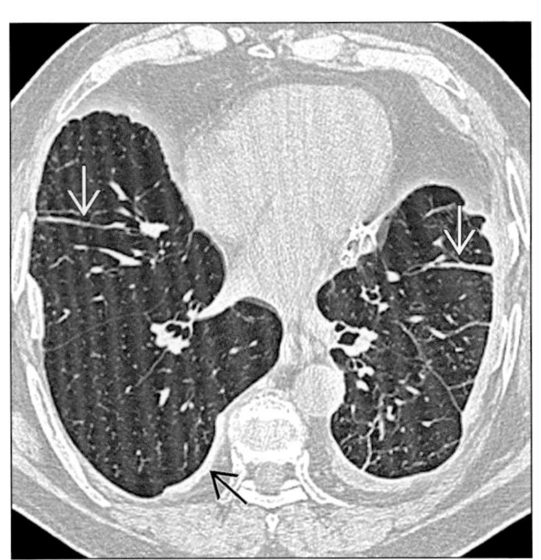

(Left) *Axial HRCT of a patient with asbestosis shows subtle lower lobe subpleural short branching linear opacities* ➡ *indicative of early disease. Other images (not shown) showed multiple pleural plaques indicative of asbestos exposure.* ***(Right)*** *Axial HRCT of a patient with asbestosis shows long parenchymal bands* ➡ *and multifocal discontinuous calcified pleural plaques* ➡, *indicative of asbestos exposure. Parenchymal bands correlate with fibrosis along interlobular septa in patients with asbestosis.*

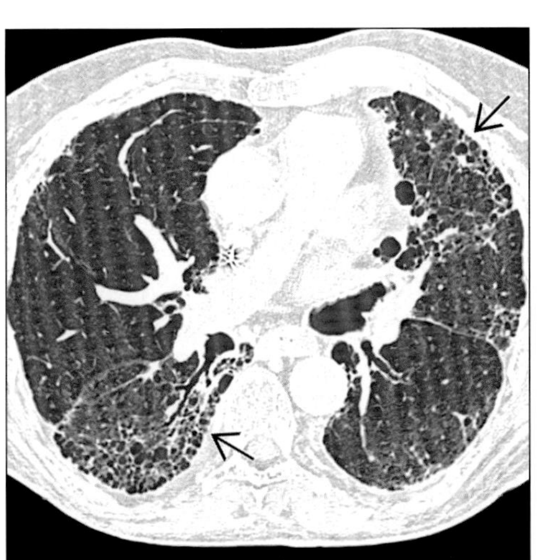

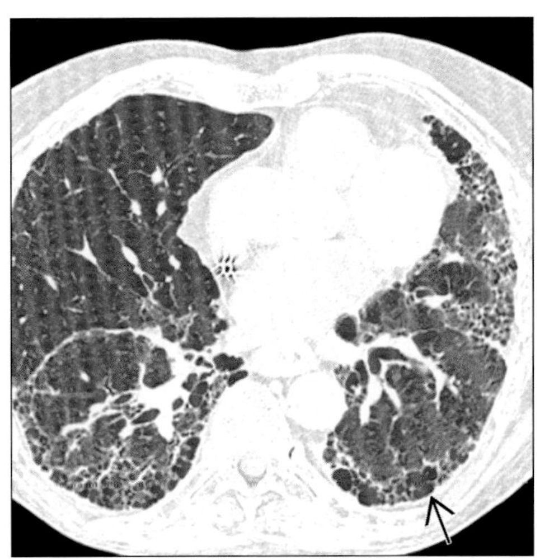

(Left) *Axial HRCT of a patient with asbestosis shows subpleural reticulation, traction bronchiolectasis, and honeycomb lung* ➡. ***(Right)*** *Axial HRCT of the same patient shows honeycombing* ➡, *reticulation, and traction bronchiolectasis. Asbestosis is often indistinguishable from usual interstitial pneumonia (UIP), as in this case. Documentation of a history of asbestos exposure is critical in establishing the correct diagnosis, especially in the absence of asbestos-related pleural disease.*

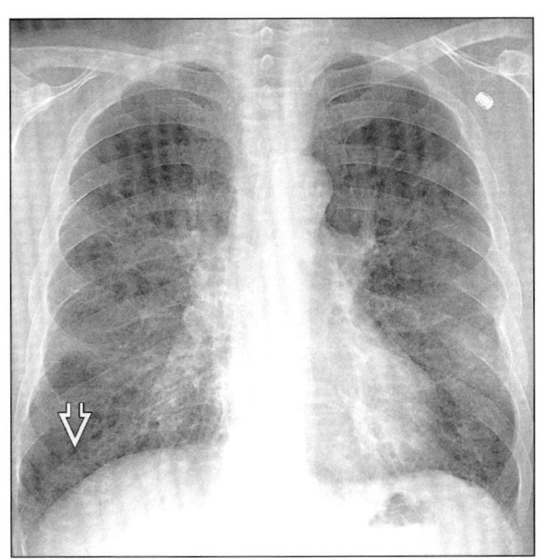

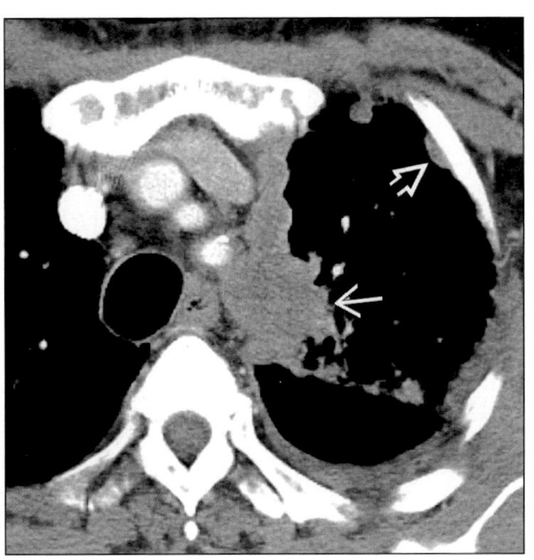

(Left) *PA chest radiograph of a patient with asbestosis shows mild basilar reticulation* ➡ *suggestive of interstitial lung disease. Further evaluation with HRCT is mandatory to fully characterize the lung abnormality.* ***(Right)*** *Axial CECT of a patient with asbestosis shows a small cell carcinoma manifesting as a left upper lobe mass* ➡ *abutting the mediastinum and pleural metastases* ➡. *Patients with asbestos exposure and asbestosis are at an increased risk of developing lung cancer.*

SILICOSIS AND COAL WORKER'S PNEUMOCONIOSIS

Key Facts

Terminology

- Coal worker's pneumoconiosis (CWP)
- Progressive massive fibrosis (PMF)
- Silicosis & CWP: Lung diseases due to inorganic mineral dust inhalation

Imaging

- Radiograph
  - 1-3 mm round nodules, may calcify
  - Predominantly upper & dorsal lung zones
  - Complicated pneumoconiosis or PMF: Aggregation of nodules into masses
  - Acute silicoproteinosis: Central alveolar opacities with air bronchograms
- HRCT
  - Centrilobular & juxtapleural micronodules
  - Dorsal upper lobes, right > left
  - Hilar/mediastinal lymphadenopathy, may calcify

Top Differential Diagnoses

- Sarcoidosis
- Tuberculosis
- Pulmonary Langerhans cell histiocytosis
- Hypersensitivity pneumonitis
- Talcosis

Clinical Issues

- Simple silicosis, asymptomatic; PMF, symptomatic
- Occupations: Sandblasting, quarrying, mining, glassblowing, pottery
- Complicated PMF, death from respiratory failure, pneumothorax, tuberculosis

Diagnostic Checklist

- Consider a thorough review of occupational history in any patient with upper lobe nodular interstitial lung disease

*(**Left**) Axial HRCT of a patient with simple silicosis shows subpleural and centrilobular pulmonary micronodules ⇨. As opposed to sarcoidosis, silicosis typically spares the bronchovascular and septal regions of the lung. (**Right**) Axial HRCT of a patient with simple silicosis shows multiple small upper lobe nodules ➡, many with a centrilobular distribution. As in many patients with simple silicosis, there is concomitant emphysema ➡, likely from cigarette smoking.*

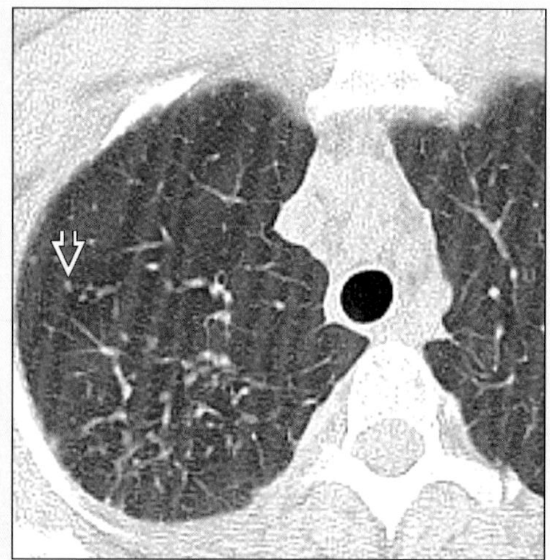

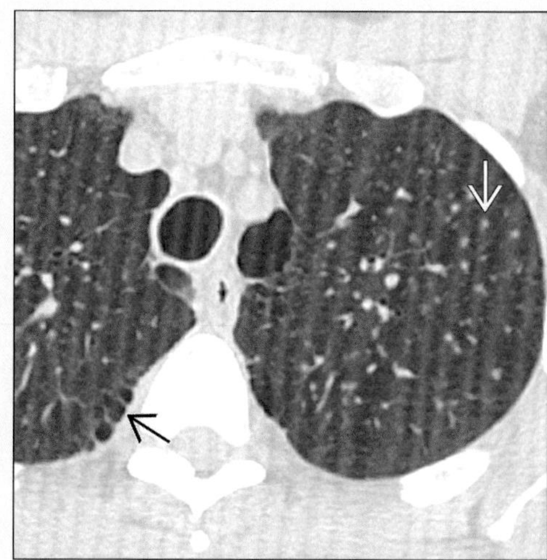

*(**Left**) PA chest radiograph of a patient with silicosis shows subtle upper lobe predominant small nodules. The patient had a history of working in a foundry for the previous 20 years. (**Right**) PA chest radiograph of the same patient obtained many years later shows development of progressive massive fibrosis manifesting with bilateral upper lung masses with associated volume loss and hilar retraction. The lateral margins of the mass-like lesions are relatively well defined.*

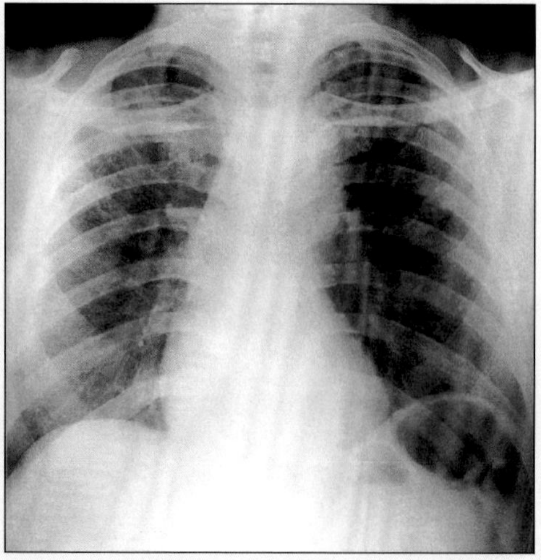

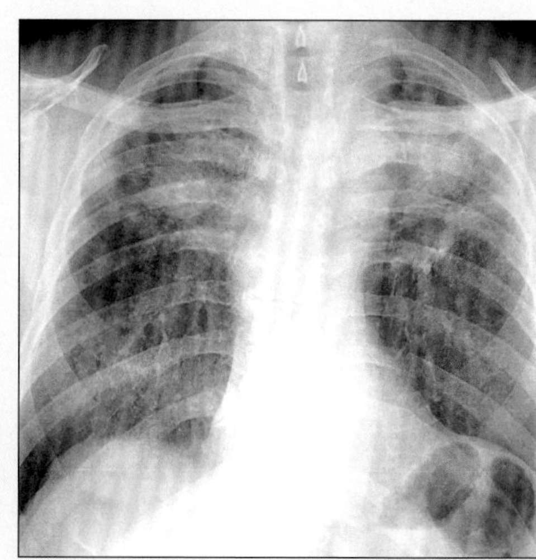

SILICOSIS AND COAL WORKER'S PNEUMOCONIOSIS

TERMINOLOGY

Abbreviations

- **Coal worker's pneumoconiosis (CWP)**

Synonyms

- Simple pneumoconiosis, complicated pneumoconiosis, **progressive massive fibrosis (PMF)**, anthracosis, anthracosilicosis

Definitions

- **Silicosis & CWP**: Lung diseases due to inhalation of inorganic mineral dusts
- **Simple or chronic pneumoconiosis**: Lung nodules < 1 cm, more profuse in upper lung zones, often with hilar/ mediastinal lymphadenopathy
- **Complicated pneumoconiosis** (progressive massive fibrosis): Aggregation of nodules into large masses > 1 cm in diameter
- **Acute silicoproteinosis**: Resembles alveolar proteinosis, develops within weeks after heavy dust exposure
- **Caplan syndrome**: CWP + rheumatoid arthritis + necrobiotic nodules

IMAGING

General Features

- Best diagnostic clue
  - Small solid centrilobular & subpleural upper lung zone nodules ± PMF
- Location
  - Rounded dusts predominately affect upper lung zones
  - Coal dust accumulates about respiratory bronchioles
  - Silica accumulates along lymphatics in centriacinar & peripheral portions of lobule
- Size
  - Nodules range from 1-3 mm in diameter

Radiographic Findings

- Findings seen 10-20 years after exposure
- Silicosis & CWP similar, lung disease usually less severe in CWP
- Hilar & mediastinal lymphadenopathy, may calcify
- **Simple pneumoconiosis**
  - 1-3 mm round nodules, may calcify
  - Predominantly affects upper lung zones, particularly dorsal aspects
- **Complicated pneumoconiosis or PMF**
  - Nodules coalesce, > 1 cm in diameter
  - Usually bilateral, right > left, located in dorsal lung
  - PMF: May be lenticular (wide on PA, narrow on lateral radiography)
  - Lateral margin of PMF coarsely parallels chest wall, sharply defined; medial inner edge less well defined
  - Overall profusion of nodules decreases due to aggregation into PMF
  - May exhibit foci of amorphous calcification
  - May cavitate
  - Central migration with time
  - Emphysema peripheral to PMF: Risk for pneumothorax
- Acute silicoproteinosis
  - Central "butterfly" alveolar opacities with air bronchograms
  - Common hilar/mediastinal lymphadenopathy
  - Rapid progression over months
  - Evolution to fibrosis with severe architectural distortion, bullae, pneumothorax
- Caplan syndrome
  - Multiple large nodules/masses, < 5 cm in diameter (may cavitate or calcify)
  - Nodules are peripheral & subpleural
  - Nodule cavitation may lead to pneumothorax
  - May evolve quickly or may disappear
  - Nodules enlarge faster than silicotic PMF
  - Skeletal findings of rheumatoid arthritis: Humeral or clavicular erosions, lung abnormalities may precede bone disease

CT Findings

- HRCT
  - More sensitive than chest radiography
  - **Micronodules < 7 mm, centrilobular & subpleural distribution**
    - More profuse in **dorsal aspects of upper lobes**, right > left
    - Silicotic nodules tend to be more sharply defined than CWP
    - Calcification in 3%
    - Aggregate subpleural nodules produce pseudoplaques
  - Intralobular or interlobular lines uncommon
  - Detection of aggregation of nodules into PMF
    - Irregularly elliptical shape with emphysema peripheral to mass
    - Masses > 4 cm characteristically have low-attenuation areas from necrosis
  - **Hilar & mediastinal lymphadenopathy, may calcify** (eggshell calcification: 5%)

Imaging Recommendations

- Best imaging tool
  - HRCT more sensitive than radiography for detection of lung disease & detection/evaluation of PMF

DIFFERENTIAL DIAGNOSIS

Sarcoidosis

- No occupational exposure, PMF less likely
- Nodules tend to cluster (galaxy sign)

Tuberculosis (TB)

- Nodules do not aggregate as masses, nodules less profuse

Pulmonary Langerhans Cell Histiocytosis

- Subpleural nodules unusual, no PMF
- Cysts, often irregular in shape; absent in pneumoconiosis

Hypersensitivity Pneumonitis

- Ground-glass centrilobular nodules, no PMF, primarily mid lung involvement
- Air-trapping common at HRCT, less likely in patients with pneumoconiosis

Talcosis

- Nodules generally smaller, < 1 mm in diameter
- Panacinar emphysema, more common in lower lobes

SILICOSIS AND COAL WORKER'S PNEUMOCONIOSIS

PATHOLOGY

General Features

- Etiology
  - Inhaled silica dust, silicon dioxide (SiO_2) or coal dust deposited in respiratory bronchioles, removed by macrophages & lymphatics
  - Slow removal, half-time of single dust burden on order of 100 days
- Silica more fibrogenic than coal
- Increased risk of tuberculosis

Gross Pathologic & Surgical Features

- Primarily involves upper lung zones, PMF may progress to end-stage lung
- Silicotic lung content generally 2-3% (up to 20%), normal silica content of dried lung 0.1%

Microscopic Features

- **Silica**
  - Silica particles centered within concentric lamellae of collagen located along bronchioles, small vessels, lymphatics
  - Birefringent silicate crystals (1-3 μ) in nodules on polarized microscopy
  - Silica-laden macrophages carry particles to hilar/ mediastinal lymph nodes & form granulomas
  - **Silicoproteinosis**: High silica concentrations, alveoli filled by lipoproteinaceous material, similar to alveolar proteinosis
- **Coal**
  - **Coal macule**: Stellate collection of macrophages containing black particles (1-5 μ), in terminal/ respiratory bronchioles & pleural lymphatics, little or no collagen
  - Macule surrounded by focal emphysema

CLINICAL ISSUES

Presentation

- Most common signs/symptoms
  - Symptoms
    - None with simple silicosis
    - Miners commonly smoke & may have bronchitis or emphysema
    - Cough, dyspnea, increased sputum in complicated disease
    - Black sputum in coal workers
- Other signs/symptoms
  - Cor pulmonale in advanced disease
  - Caplan syndrome
    - Clinical features of rheumatoid arthritis
- Clinical profile
  - Typical occupations: Sandblasting, quarrying, mining, glassblowing, pottery
  - Coal mines usually contain silica (most common element of earth's crust)
  - Acute silicoproteinosis
    - Massive exposure to silica dust, usually seen in sandblasters
- Pulmonary function tests
  - **Simple pneumoconiosis**: Usually normal
  - **Complicated pneumoconiosis**: Decreased diffusion capacity, decreased lung volumes, restrictive defect
  - Often with mixed obstruction & restriction due to combined effects of smoking & interstitial fibrosis
  - Functional impairment more closely associated with degree of emphysema (as determined by CT) than profusion of nodules

Demographics

- Age
  - Simple & complicated pneumoconiosis is rare under age 50 years
- Gender
  - More common in men due to occupational exposure
- Epidemiology
  - Risk related to both dose (intensity of exposure) & time (length of exposure)
  - Up to 15% of miners may exhibit disease progreession to interstitial fibrosis

Natural History & Prognosis

- **Usually requires > 20 years exposure**
- Simple pneumoconiosis, normal longevity
- Complicated PMF, death from respiratory failure, pneumothorax, TB
- Silicoproteinosis: Death within 2-3 years
- **Debatable increased risk of lung cancer**

Treatment

- Prevention: Respirators in dusty environment, dust control to reduce ambient dust concentrations
- Removal from work environment or transfer to less dusty environment
- Smoking cessation
- No specific treatment for pneumoconiosis available
- At risk for TB: Cavitation in PMF requires culture
  - TB skin tests important

DIAGNOSTIC CHECKLIST

Consider

- Thorough review of occupational history in any patient with upper lobe nodular interstitial lung disease

SELECTED REFERENCES

1. Sirajuddin A et al: Occupational lung disease. J Thorac Imaging. 24(4):310-20, 2009
2. Chong S et al: Pneumoconiosis: comparison of imaging and pathologic findings. Radiographics. 26(1):59-77, 2006
3. Remy-Jardin M et al: Computed tomographic evaluation of silicosis and coal workers' pneumoconiosis. Radiol Clin North Am. 30(6):1155-76, 1992
4. Remy-Jardin M et al: Coal worker's pneumoconiosis: CT assessment in exposed workers and correlation with radiographic findings. Radiology. 177(2):363-71, 1990

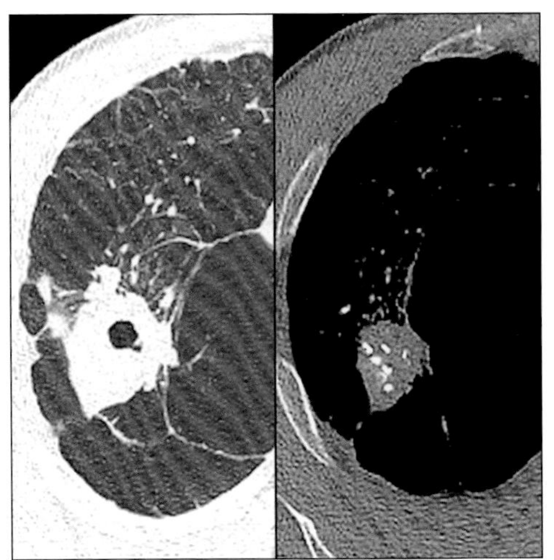

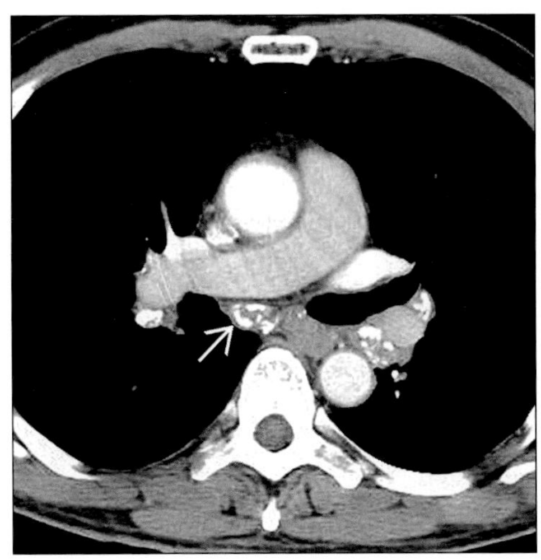

(Left) *Composite image with axial HRCT in lung (left) and bone (right) window shows PMF with cavitation, punctate calcifications, and adjacent small nodules. Emphysema is likely paracicatricial and related to smoking. Symmetric upper lung masses with adjacent small nodules in the setting of known occupational exposure usually obviates tissue diagnosis.* ***(Right)*** *Axial CECT shows enlarged hilar and mediastinal calcified lymph nodes, some with eggshell calcification* ➡ *characteristic of silicosis.*

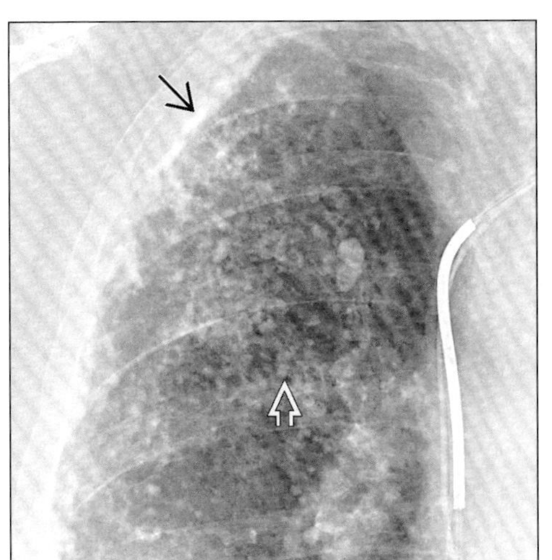

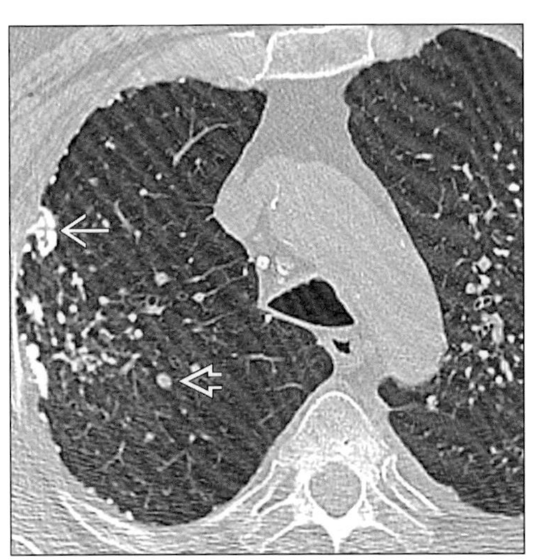

(Left) *PA chest radiograph (coned-down to the right upper lobe) shows calcified lung nodules* ⇨*. Apparent pleural calcification* → *is seen in the right hemithorax.* ***(Right)*** *Axial HRCT of a patient with silicosis shows calcified centrilobular* ⇨ *and subpleural nodules* ➡ *forming pseudoplaques. Rarely, as in this case, silicosis pseudoplaques may mimic asbestos-related pleural plaques on radiography. HRCT is helpful in demonstrating the discrete nodules in the juxtapleural lung.*

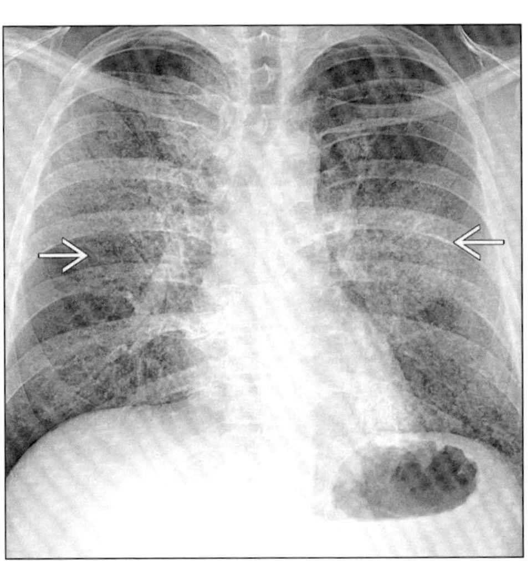

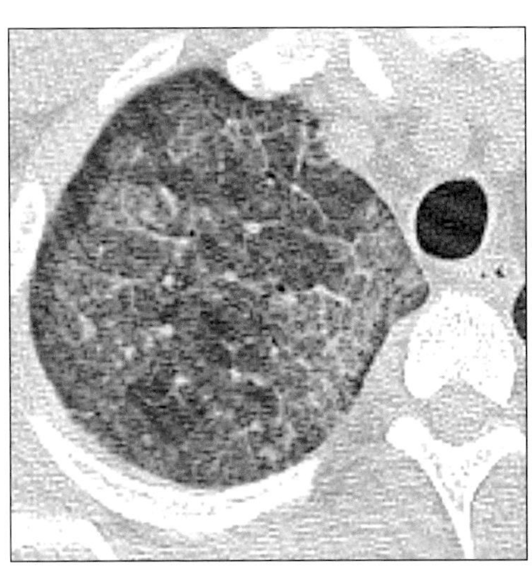

(Left) *PA chest radiograph of a patient with massive silica dust inhalation shows perihilar opacities* ➡*.* ***(Right)*** *Axial HRCT of the same patient shows bilateral ground-glass opacities with interlobular and intralobular lines producing a crazy-paving pattern consistent with silicoproteinosis, given history. Silicoproteinosis is one of the many causes of secondary pulmonary alveolar proteinosis and should be differentiated from primary disease, given treatment ramifications.*

HARD METAL PNEUMOCONIOSIS

Key Facts

Terminology

- Hard metal pneumoconiosis (HMP)
- Rare occupational lung disease from inhalation of hard metal or diamond-cobalt dust
- Hard metal lung disease, cobalt lung, giant cell interstitial pneumonitis

Imaging

- Radiography
  - May be normal in early or mild disease
  - Patchy irregular opacities in mid/lower lungs
  - Nodular or reticulonodular opacities
- HRCT
  - Ground-glass opacity & consolidation
  - Linear opacities & reticulation
  - Subpleural bullae
  - Long-term exposure: Fibrosis, architectural distortion, bronchiectasis, honeycomb lung

Top Differential Diagnoses

- Hypersensitivity pneumonitis
- Usual interstitial pneumonia
- Nonspecific interstitial pneumonia

Pathology

- Inhalational exposure to hard metal (tungsten carbide and cobalt) or diamond-cobalt
- Not clearly related to total dust burden, individual susceptibility

Clinical Issues

- Symptoms & signs
  - Upper airway & conjunctival symptoms
  - Cough, dyspnea, wheezing, chest tightness
- Symptom decrease/resolution away from exposure
- Very good prognosis with removal from exposure
- Treatment: Removal from exposure paramount

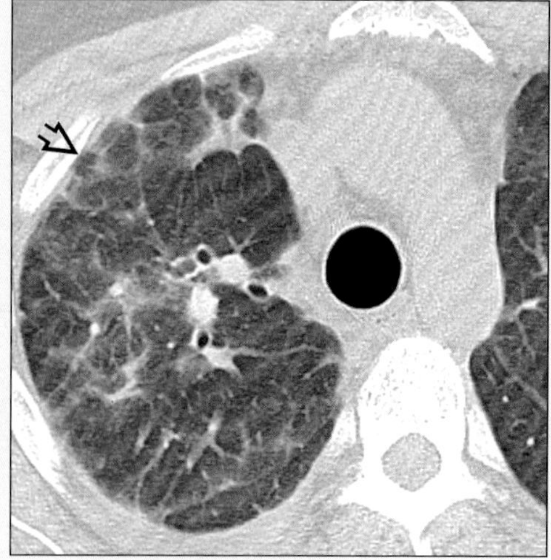
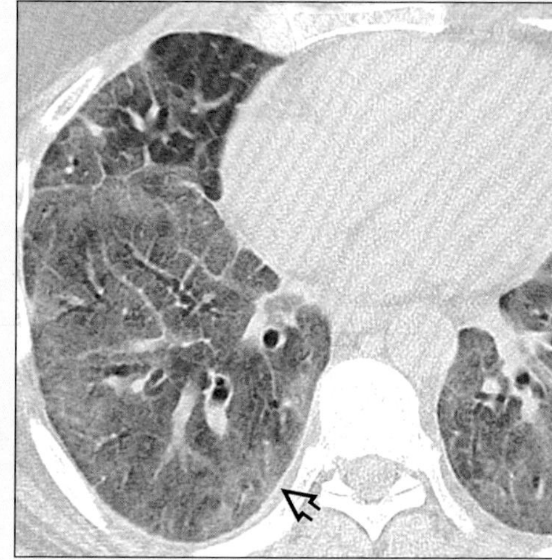

(Left) *Axial HRCT of a patient with hard metal pneumoconiosis shows patchy bilateral ground-glass opacities ⇨ in a perilobular configuration.* ***(Right)*** *Axial HRCT of the same patient obtained near the lung bases shows a more diffuse pattern of ground-glass opacity ⇨. Imaging abnormalities in patients with hard metal pneumoconiosis are often nonspecific. Thus, a detailed work history is essential in order to suggest the diagnosis of all occupational lung diseases, including hard metal lung disease.*

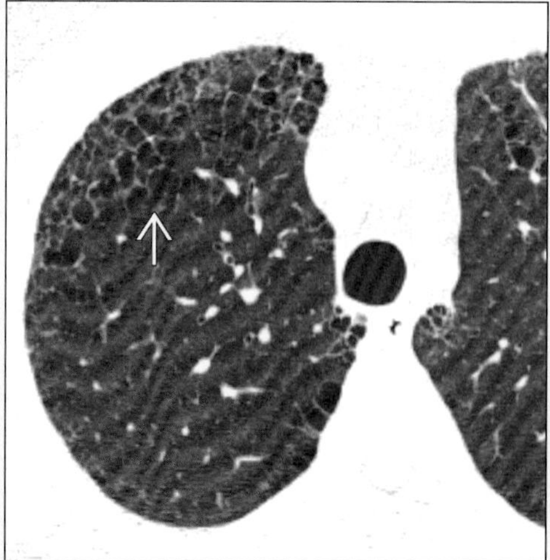
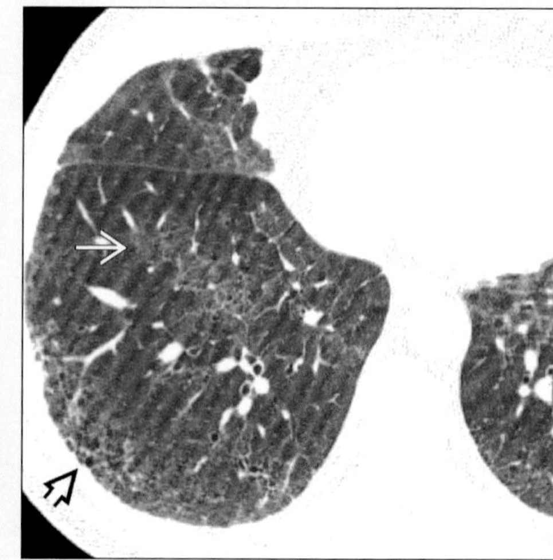

(Left) *Axial HRCT of a patient with hard metal pneumoconiosis shows upper lobe bullae and mild reticulation ➡.* ***(Right)*** *Axial HRCT of the same patient obtained more inferiorly shows patchy ground-glass opacities ➡, reticulation, and traction bronchiolectasis ⇨. The presence of reticulation and traction bronchiolectasis is suggestive of fibrosis, indicating chronic exposure in this patient with hard metal lung disease.*

HARD METAL PNEUMOCONIOSIS

TERMINOLOGY

Abbreviations

- **Hard metal pneumoconiosis (HMP)**

Synonyms

- Hard metal lung disease, cobalt lung, giant cell interstitial pneumonitis

Definitions

- Rare occupational lung disease from inhalation of hard metal or diamond-cobalt dust

IMAGING

General Features

- Best diagnostic clue
  - Ground-glass opacity & consolidation ± fibrosis with exposure to hard metal dust
- Location
  - Typically, mid & lower lung zones

Radiographic Findings

- May be normal in early or mild disease
- Patchy irregular opacities in mid & lower lung zones
- Nodular or reticulonodular opacities

CT Findings

- HRCT
  - **Ground-glass opacity** & **consolidation**
  - Linear opacities & reticulation
  - Subpleural bullae
  - **Long-term exposure**: **Fibrosis** with architectural distortion, traction bronchiectasis, honeycomb lung

DIFFERENTIAL DIAGNOSIS

Hypersensitivity Pneumonitis (HP)

- Upper lung predominant ground-glass opacity
- Centrilobular (characteristic), patchy, diffuse
- Mosaic attenuation from air-trapping
- Chronic HP may result in pulmonary fibrosis

Usual Interstitial Pneumonia

- Basilar & peripheral pulmonary fibrosis
- Honeycomb lung, reticulation, traction bronchiectasis
- Paucity of ground-glass opacity

Nonspecific Interstitial Pneumonia

- Basilar predominant ground-glass opacity, reticulation, traction bronchiectasis
- Paucity of honeycomb lung
- Usually secondary to collagen vascular disease, chronic HP, or drugs

PATHOLOGY

General Features

- Etiology
  - Inhalational exposure to hard metal (tungsten carbide, cobalt) or diamond-cobalt
    - Hard metal derives name from extremely high heat & wear resistance as well as hardness
  - Cobalt likely main cause of lung disease
  - Not clearly related to total dust burden, individual susceptibility
  - May be TGF-β 1 &/or TNF-α mediated
- Genetics
  - Associated with glutamate at position 69 of HLA-DP β-chain

Staging, Grading, & Classification

- 3 main respiratory complications from hard metal exposure
  - **Asthma, hypersensitivity pneumonitis, pulmonary fibrosis**
  - Acute respiratory distress is less common

Microscopic Features

- Cobalt rapidly excreted from body through urine; rarely detected in tissue
- 2 histological patterns
  - Centrilobular interstitial inflammation & fibrosis with desquamative interstitial pneumonia pattern
  - **Giant cell interstitial pneumonitis**: Combination of large giant cells & macrophages in air spaces
    - Usually indicates HMP but can occur in other settings
  - End-stage fibrosis in honeycomb lung

CLINICAL ISSUES

Presentation

- Most common signs/symptoms
  - Upper airway & conjunctival symptoms
    - Sneezing, rhinorrhea, sore throat
  - Cough, dyspnea, wheezing, chest tightness
  - Asthenia, fatigue, weight loss
  - Pruritus or rash from airborne dermatitis
  - Cyanosis, clubbing
  - Symptoms may decrease or resolve while away from occupational exposure
  - Pulmonary function tests: Nonspecific; restrictive pattern with decreased DLCO is most common

Demographics

- Epidemiology
  - Rare; prevalence estimated at 0.7-13% of hard metal plant workers
  - Work history
    - Hard metal manufacturing or maintenance
    - Diamond tool production or use

Natural History & Prognosis

- **Very good prognosis with early detection & removal from exposure**
- Respiratory insufficiency & cor pulmonale in fibrotic stage

Treatment

- Removal from exposure paramount
- Corticosteroids or cyclophosphamide may be helpful

SELECTED REFERENCES

1. Fontenot AP et al: Metal-induced diffuse lung disease. Semin Respir Crit Care Med. 29(6):662-9, 2008

BERYLLIOSIS

Key Facts

Terminology

- Inhalational lung disease with 2 pulmonary syndromes: Acute chemical pneumonitis & chronic granulomatous lung disease

Imaging

- Radiography
  - Acute: Noncardiogenic pulmonary edema within 72 hours of exposure
  - Chronic: Symmetric bilateral hilar lymphadenopathy & diffuse reticulonodular opacities
- HRCT
  - Identical to sarcoidosis
  - Thick nodular bronchovascular bundles & nodular interlobular septal thickening (50%)
  - Hilar or mediastinal lymphadenopathy (40%), always associated with lung disease

Top Differential Diagnoses

- Sarcoidosis
- Pulmonary Langerhans cell histiocytosis
- Silicosis

Pathology

- Noncaseating granulomas indistinguishable from sarcoid granulomas in chronic disease

Clinical Issues

- Signs & symptoms
  - Dyspnea (95%)
  - Cough, chest pain, arthralgia, fatigue, weight loss
- Progression relatively slow; survival of 15-20 years is common
- Treatment
  - Removal from workplace environment
  - Steroids & possibly methotrexate

(Left) *Graphic shows hilar and mediastinal lymphadenopathy and upper lung predominant perilymphatic micronodules. Lymph node involvement of berylliosis usually occurs in association with pulmonary involvement.* ***(Right)*** *PA chest radiograph shows symmetric bilateral hilar lymphadenopathy and mid lung zone nodules consistent with sarcoidosis or berylliosis. A detailed history and physical examination were essential to establish the diagnosis of berylliosis, as in most cases of occupational lung disease.*

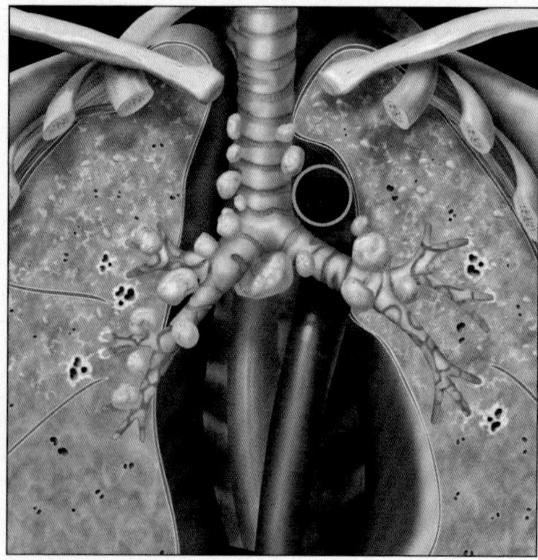

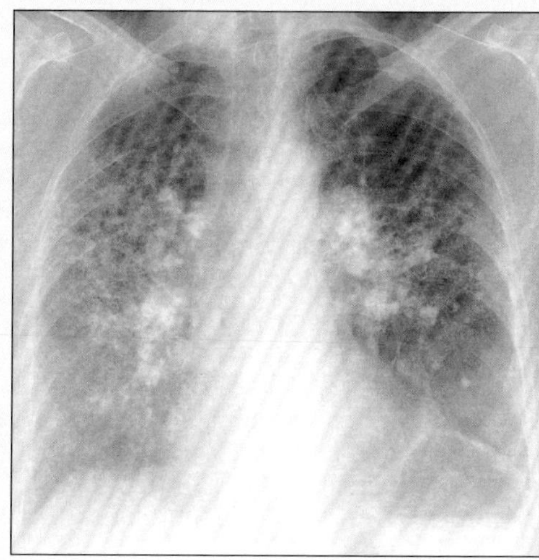

(Left) *Axial HRCT of a patient with berylliosis shows peribronchovascular micronodules ➔ in the mid lung zones as well as nodules along interlobular septa, which is consistent with a perilymphatic anatomic distribution.* ***(Right)*** *Axial NECT of the same patient shows mediastinal ➔ and hilar ➲ lymphadenopathy. In patients with berylliosis, significant lymphadenopathy typically does not occur in the absence of lung disease, a distinguishing feature from sarcoidosis.*

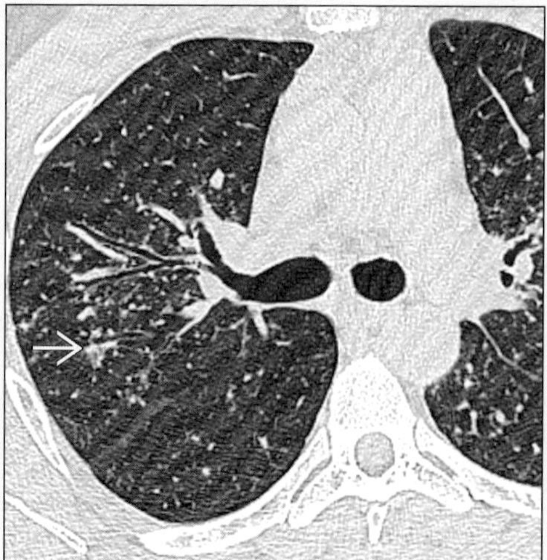

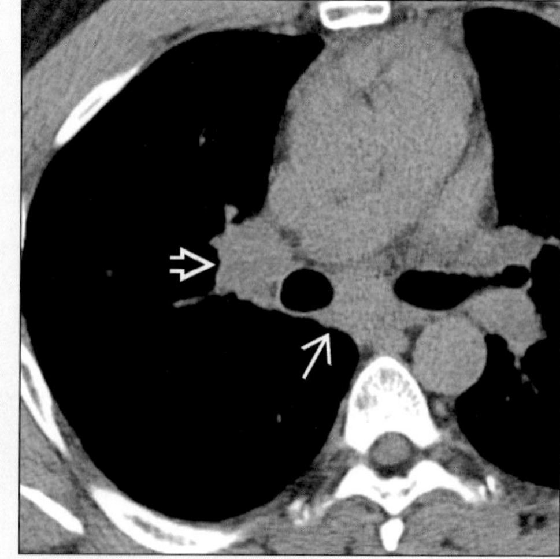

BERYLLIOSIS

TERMINOLOGY

Definitions

- Inhalational lung disease exhibiting 2 pulmonary syndromes
  - Acute chemical pneumonitis
  - Chronic granulomatous lung disease

IMAGING

General Features

- Best diagnostic clue
  - **Findings of sarcoidosis in patient with beryllium exposure**
- Location
  - Primarily mid lung involvement; upper lobe predilection in chronic fibrosis

Radiographic Findings

- Radiography
  - Acute
    - Associated with large exposures
    - Noncardiogenic pulmonary edema within 72 hours of exposure
  - Chronic
    - Normal radiographs in 50%
    - Symmetric bilateral hilar lymphadenopathy & diffuse reticulonodular opacities
    - Large bullae in 10%

CT Findings

- HRCT
  - Normal in 25% of subjects with proven disease
  - Findings identical to those of sarcoidosis
  - Nodules (65%) > ground-glass opacities (55%) > septal lines (50%)
  - Nodules may aggregate as progressive massive fibrosis (5%)
  - Thick nodular bronchovascular bundles & nodular interlobular septal thickening (50%)
  - Hilar or mediastinal lymphadenopathy (40%), always associated with lung disease
    - Lymph nodes may exhibit diffuse or eggshell calcification
  - Honeycomb lung in advanced disease (5%), typically worse in upper lung zones
  - Upper zonal pleural thickening due to pseudoplaques (aggregation of subpleural nodules)

DIFFERENTIAL DIAGNOSIS

Sarcoidosis

- Hilar lymphadenopathy may occur without lung disease
- Lymphadenopathy typically regresses as lung disease worsens, unlike berylliosis
- Diffuse ground-glass opacities less common than in berylliosis
- Extra-thoracic involvement suggestive of sarcoidosis

Pulmonary Langerhans Cell Histiocytosis

- Upper lobe predominant centrilobular nodules &/or cysts
- Bizarre-shaped cysts in chronic disease

Silicosis

- Exposure history
- Perilymphatic nodules, progressive massive fibrosis
- Nodules & lymph nodes may also calcify

PATHOLOGY

General Features

- Etiology
  - Delayed-type hypersensitivity reaction: Beryllium functions as hapten leading to granulomatous reaction
- Genetics
  - Genotype HLA-DPb1 (Glu 69) marker of susceptibility to disease

Microscopic Features

- Noncaseating granulomas indistinguishable from sarcoid granulomas in chronic disease
- Diffuse alveolar damage in patients with acute pneumonitis

CLINICAL ISSUES

Presentation

- Most common signs/symptoms
  - Dyspnea (95%)
  - Cough, chest pain, arthralgia, fatigue, weight loss
- Clinical profile
  - Pulmonary function tests
    - Obstructive pattern in 40%
    - Restrictive pattern in 20%
    - Decreased diffusing capacity in 15%, good marker of disease progression

Demographics

- Epidemiology
  - 1-15% of exposed persons develop beryllium hypersensitivity & chronic disease

Natural History & Prognosis

- Criteria for diagnosis
  - History of beryllium exposure: Latency of 1 month to 40 years (average: 10-15 years)
  - Positive blood or bronchoalveolar lavage **beryllium lymphocyte proliferation test**
  - **Noncaseating granulomas** on lung biopsy
- High-risk occupations
  - Nuclear power, aerospace, & electronics industries
  - Used in x-ray tubes, rocket engines, ceramics, computers, dental alloys; older fluorescent tubes
- **Relatively slow disease progression**
- **Survival of 15-20 years is common**

Treatment

- Removal from workplace environment
- Steroids & possibly methotrexate for symptomatic disease; may relapse off therapy

SELECTED REFERENCES

1. Flors L et al: Uncommon occupational lung diseases: high-resolution CT findings. AJR Am J Roentgenol. 194(1):W20-6, 2010

SILO-FILLER'S DISEASE

Key Facts

Terminology

- Occupational lung disease resulting from exposure to nitrogen oxides
- Inhalation of toxic gases from freshly stored silage

Imaging

- Radiography
  - Initial chest radiograph may be normal
  - Early findings: Noncardiogenic pulmonary edema, normal heart size, pleural effusions uncommon
  - Late findings: Hyperinflation from constrictive bronchiolitis, diffuse ill-defined small/miliary nodules
- HRCT
  - Early: Bilateral consolidations & ground-glass opacities, cryptogenic organizing pneumonia
  - Late: Constrictive bronchiolitis
- Chest radiography for assessment & monitoring

Top Differential Diagnoses

- Agricultural lung diseases
  - Dung lung, anhydrous ammonia inhalation
  - Organic dust toxicity syndrome
  - Pesticide exposure
- Hypersensitivity pneumonitis (farmer's lung)
- Smoke inhalation

Clinical Issues

- Symptoms/signs
  - Cough, lightheadedness, dyspnea, fatigue
  - Severity based on exposure duration/concentration
  - Late: Relapse of dyspnea & cough
- Presentation usually in September & October

Diagnostic Checklist

- Consider silo-filler's disease in any breathless farmer presenting at harvest time

*(**Left**) PA chest radiograph of a patient who developed acute dyspnea within hours of working in a freshly filled silo shows dense bilateral perihilar consolidations consistent with pulmonary edema. Note the absence of cardiomegaly or pleural effusion. (**Right**) PA chest radiograph of a man with silo-filler's disease who presented with chronic dyspnea shows numerous bilateral small pulmonary nodules. Silo-filler's disease should be suspected in farmers presenting with dyspnea, particularly during harvest time.*

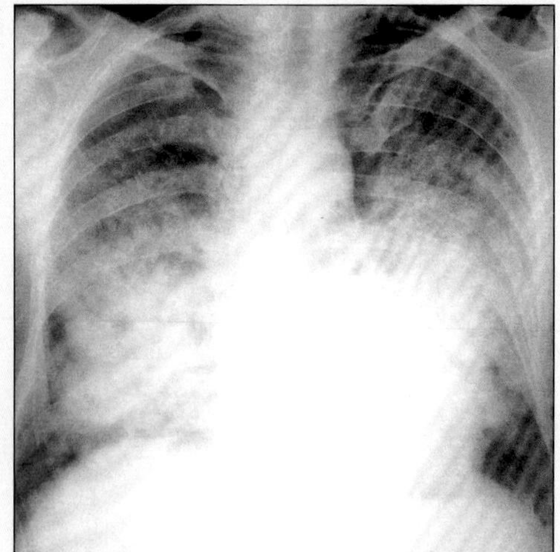

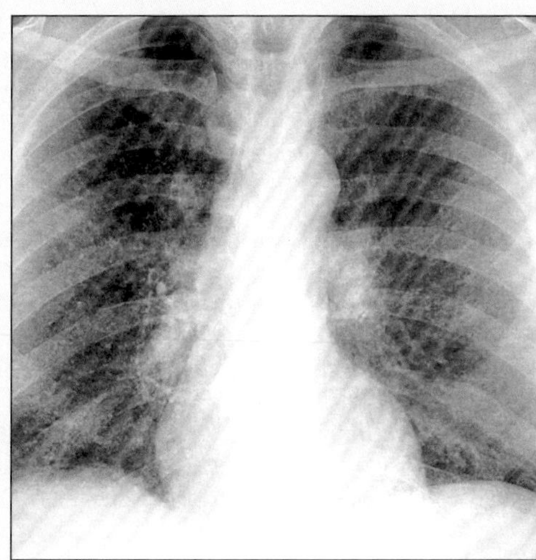

*(**Left**) Axial CECT of a patient with silo-filler's disease who presented with dyspnea shows patchy bilateral ground-glass opacities and findings of mild paraseptal emphysema. (**Right**) HRCT of a patient with late-stage silo-filler's disease shows mosaic attenuation from constrictive bronchiolitis. Note paucity of vascular structures in areas of lung hyperlucency and dilated airways with mildly thickened walls ➔. Silo-filler's disease is a recognized etiology of constrictive bronchiolitis.*

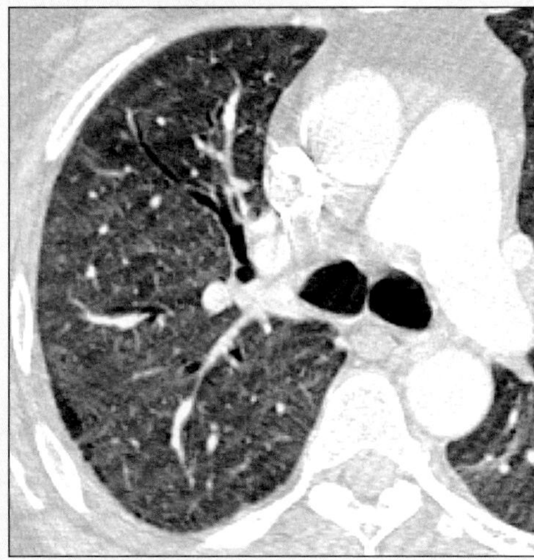

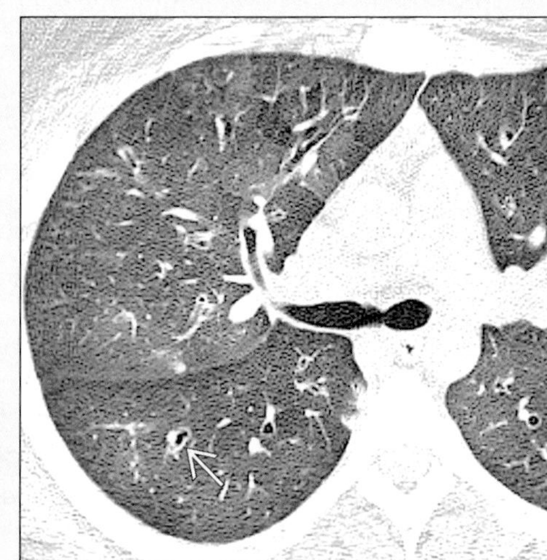

SILO-FILLER'S DISEASE

TERMINOLOGY

Definitions

- Occupational lung disease resulting from exposure to nitrogen oxides
- Inhalation of toxic gases from freshly stored silage

IMAGING

General Features

- Best diagnostic clue
  - Early: Pulmonary edema within hours of inhalation
  - Late: Mosaic attenuation on HRCT from constrictive bronchiolitis

Radiographic Findings

- Initial chest radiograph may be normal
- Early findings
  - Parenchymal injury immediately within 1st 48 hours
  - Noncardiogenic pulmonary edema (sometimes hemorrhagic)
    - 6-12 hours after exposure
    - Ill-defined, alveolar opacities, nonspecific pulmonary edema pattern
  - Resolution over 3-5 days
    - Progression of consolidation after 1st 48 hours should be considered superinfection
  - Normal heart size
  - Pleural effusions uncommon
- Late findings
  - 2-4 weeks after exposure (range: Weeks to months)
  - Hyperinflation from constrictive bronchiolitis
  - Diffuse ill-defined small or miliary nodules

CT Findings

- HRCT
  - Early: Bilateral airspace & ground-glass opacities, patchy or diffuse
  - Cryptogenic organizing pneumonia (COP)
  - Late: Constrictive bronchiolitis
    - Mosaic attenuation

Imaging Recommendations

- Best imaging tool
  - Chest radiographs suffice for initial assessment & monitoring of disease course
- Protocol advice
  - Early: Serial radiography
  - Late: HRCT

DIFFERENTIAL DIAGNOSIS

Agricultural Lung Diseases

- Other toxic gases: Hydrogen sulfide (H_2S), ammonia, carbon dioxide, methane
  - Toxic swine & dairy manure exposure (dung lung)
  - Anhydrous ammonia inhalation
- Organic dust toxicity syndrome
  - Usually seen in spring from moldy dust silage (silo-filler's disease occurs in autumn)
- Pesticide exposure
  - Paraquat lung: Usually absorbed through skin
  - Rapid pulmonary fibrosis, often fatal

Hypersensitivity Pneumonitis (Farmer's Lung)

- Exposure to dust (not gas)
  - Allergic reaction to fungi (typically *Actinomycetes*) in hay
- CT: Centrilobular ground-glass nodules, mosaic attenuation

Smoke Inhalation

- Acutely, bronchial wall thickening & subglottic edema
- Perihilar & upper lung zone pulmonary edema

PATHOLOGY

General Features

- Etiology
  - Nitrogen dioxide production in top-unloading silo
    - Silage is product of anaerobic bacterial fermentation of grass crops, used to feed livestock
    - NO_2 heavier than air, settles on top of silage, orange color with bleach-like odor
  - Inhalation of NO_2 leads to cellular damage

Microscopic Features

- Acute: Diffuse alveolar damage with hyaline membrane formation
- Late: Small airway damage, constrictive bronchiolitis

CLINICAL ISSUES

Presentation

- Most common signs/symptoms
  - Severity based on duration of exposure & concentration of gas
  - Acute: Minutes to hours after exposure
    - Most symptomatic exposures mild/self-limited
      - Cough, lightheadedness, dyspnea, fatigue
    - Sudden death if high concentration
    - Pulmonary edema due to cellular damage
  - Late: Relapse of dyspnea, cough

Demographics

- Epidemiology
  - 5 cases/100,000 silo-associated farm workers/year
  - September & October (harvest months)

Natural History & Prognosis

- Variable, depends on extent of initial injury
- 1/3 with severe exposure die from pulmonary edema or constrictive bronchiolitis

Treatment

- Preventive: Avoid freshly filled silo for 14 days
- Monitor those exposed for 48 hours, steroids

DIAGNOSTIC CHECKLIST

Consider

- Silo-filler's disease in any breathless farmer presenting at harvest time

SELECTED REFERENCES

1. Leavey JF et al: Silo-Filler's disease, the acute respiratory distress syndrome, and oxides of nitrogen. Ann Intern Med. 141(5):410-1, 2004

HYPERSENSITIVITY PNEUMONITIS

Key Facts

Terminology
- Hypersensitivity pneumonitis (HP)
- Diffuse granulomatous interstitial lung disease caused by inhalation of various antigenic particles

Imaging
- Radiography
  - Acute/subacute: Normal or mid & lower lung zone nodularity
  - Chronic: Mid & upper lung fibrosis (architectural distortion, volume loss)
- HRCT
  - Ground-glass opacity (100%)
  - Centrilobular ground-glass nodules (70%)
  - Expiratory air-trapping (95%)
  - Head cheese sign: Geographic areas of ground-glass opacity, normal lung, air-trapping
  - Chronic: Mid & upper lung zone fibrosis

Top Differential Diagnoses
- Idiopathic pulmonary fibrosis
- Nonspecific interstitial pneumonia
- Respiratory bronchiolitis
- Pulmonary Langerhans cell histiocytosis

Pathology
- Classic triad: Cellular bronchiolitis, lymphocytic interstitial infiltrate, nonnecrotizing granulomas

Clinical Issues
- 95% of cases in nonsmokers; nonspecific symptoms
- Treatment: Avoid antigen exposure; corticosteroids

Diagnostic Checklist
- Consider HP in symptomatic patients with bilateral ground-glass opacities, centrilobular ground-glass nodules, & lobular air-trapping

*(**Left**) Graphic shows the typical features of hypersensitivity pneumonitis, which manifests with chronic multifocal, bilateral, diffuse centrilobular, ill-defined ground-glass nodules. The differential diagnosis also includes respiratory bronchiolitis. (**Right**) Axial HRCT of a patient with dyspnea shows centrilobular ground-glass nodular opacities ➡, suggestive of hypersensitivity pneumonitis. Correlation with a detailed history and physical exam is essential to establish the diagnosis.*

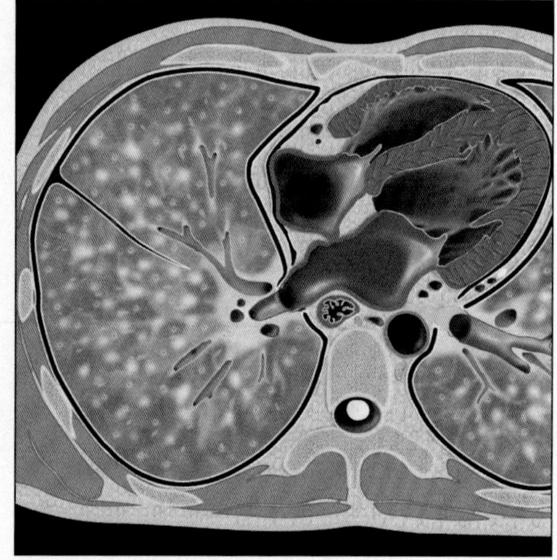

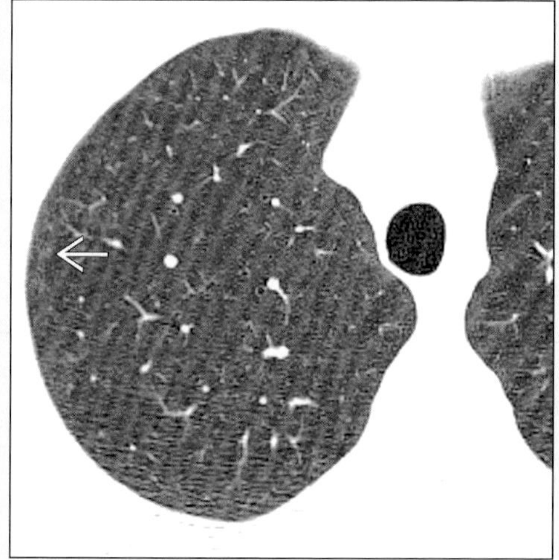

*(**Left**) Axial HRCT of a patient with acute hypersensitivity pneumonitis shows diffuse bilateral ground-glass opacities and a small pneumatocele ➡ in the left upper lobe. (**Right**) Axial expiratory HRCT of a patient with hypersensitivity pneumonitis shows lobular areas of air trapping ➡ bilaterally. Air trapping in combination with patchy ground-glass opacities (in a centrilobular distribution) is highly suggestive of hypersensitivity pneumonitis.*

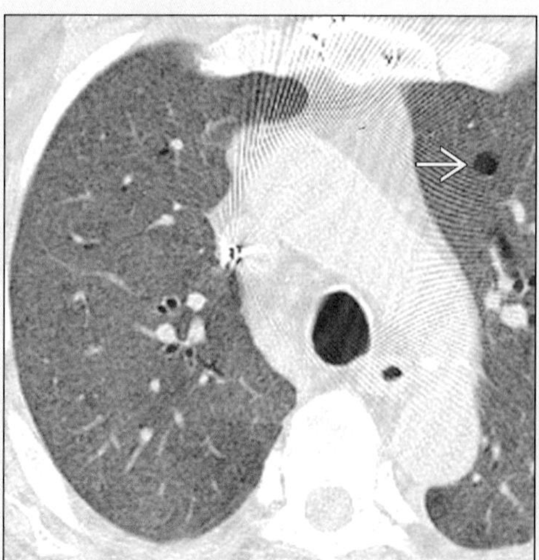

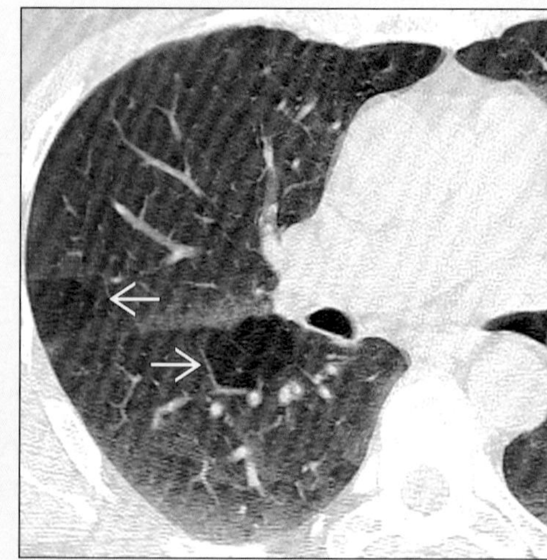

HYPERSENSITIVITY PNEUMONITIS

TERMINOLOGY

Abbreviations

- **Hypersensitivity pneumonitis (HP)**

Synonyms

- **Extrinsic allergic alveolitis (EAA)**

Definitions

- Diffuse granulomatous interstitial lung disease caused by inhalation of various antigenic particles
  - Microbes, animal proteins, low-molecular weight chemicals
  - Farmer's lung & bird fancier's lung most common forms

IMAGING

General Features

- Best diagnostic clue
  - Ground-glass centrilobular nodules with mosaic attenuation (air-trapping) on HRCT
- Location
  - Mid & lower lung zones most commonly affected, spares lung bases
- Morphology
  - Ground-glass opacity & ground-glass centrilobular nodules

Radiographic Findings

- Radiography
  - **Acute stage**
    - **Chest radiographs usually normal (90%)**
    - Fine miliary nodules
    - Consolidation rare
  - **Subacute stage**
    - **Chest radiographs usually abnormal (90%)**
    - Poorly defined small nodules
    - Diffuse or middle & lower lung increased opacity
  - **Chronic stage**
    - Findings of **fibrosis**: Architectural distortion, volume loss
    - Mid & upper lung zone predominant
    - No pleural disease or lymphadenopathy
    - Sparing of or less severe findings in lung bases
  - Absent
    - Pleural effusion
    - Cavitation
    - Hilar/mediastinal lymphadenopathy

CT Findings

- General features
  - **Ground-glass opacity (100%)**
    - Geographic distribution in central & peripheral lung
  - Faint, **ill-defined centrilobular nodules** < 5 mm in diameter (70%)
  - **Mosaic attenuation** (variable lung attenuation & vessel size) (80%)
  - **Expiratory air-trapping (95%)**
  - Combined findings
    - **Head cheese sign**: Geographic ground-glass opacity, normal lung, & air-trapping
      - Considered pathognomonic
    - Ground-glass centrilobular nodules + mosaic attenuation (air-trapping)
  - Mediastinal lymphadenopathy in 50% (lymph nodes typically < 2 cm short axis diameter)
- **Acute stage**
  - Small, ill-defined centrilobular ground-glass nodules
  - Bilateral ground-glass opacity
- **Subacute stage**
  - **Mosaic attenuation** (air-trapping)
  - **Ground-glass opacity** (patchy distribution)
  - Small, ill-defined **centrilobular ground-glass nodules**
  - Mid & lower lung predominance
  - Lung cysts (10%)
    - Few in number, 3-25 mm diameter, usually associated with ground-glass opacity
- **Chronic stage**
  - **Fibrosis**: Honeycomb lung, traction bronchiectasis, architectural distortion
  - Mid & upper lung zone predominance
  - Lung bases less severely involved
  - Superimposed subacute findings: Ground-glass opacity & small, ill-defined, centrilobular nodules
- Resolution
  - Ground-glass opacities, centrilobular nodules, mosaic attenuation, & air-trapping may resolve with treatment
  - Fibrosis persists

Imaging Recommendations

- Best imaging tool
  - HRCT: More sensitive than radiography for subtle findings of hypersensitivity pneumonitis

DIFFERENTIAL DIAGNOSIS

Idiopathic Pulmonary Fibrosis

- HRCT: Honeycomb lung, bibasilar reticular opacities, traction bronchiectasis
- Anatomic distribution: Peripheral, subpleural, bibasilar
  - Lung bases usually severely involved
- Mild or absent ground-glass opacity
- Centrilobular nodules uncommon
- Air-trapping absent

Nonspecific Interstitial Pneumonia (NSIP)

- 2 histologic patterns: Cellular & fibrotic
- HRCT: Ground-glass opacity > reticular opacities
- Honeycomb lung absent or minimal
- Peribronchovascular distribution
- Centrilobular nodules uncommon
- Air-trapping not a feature

Respiratory Bronchiolitis

- Smokers (smoking protects from hypersensitivity pneumonitis)
- Centrilobular nodules, fewer in number
- Upper lung zone predominant
- Associated centrilobular emphysema

Pulmonary Langerhans Cell Histiocytosis

- Smokers
- Centrilobular irregular nodules, often cavitate
- Upper lung zone predominant

HYPERSENSITIVITY PNEUMONITIS

Sarcoidosis
- Solid micronodules rather than ground-glass
- Typically bronchovascular & subpleural distribution
  - Subpleural perilymphatic deposits rare in HP
- Upper lung zone predominant

Silicosis
- Occupational history
- Solid nodules, may calcify
- Typically centrilobular & subpleural distribution
  - Subpleural perilymphatic deposits rare in HP
- Lymphadenopathy, ± calcification (eggshell)
- Air-trapping not a feature

PATHOLOGY

General Features
- Etiology
  - Microbes: **Thermophilic actinomyces** grow in moldy hay; principal cause of farmer's lung, bagassosis, & mushroom worker's lung
    - **Nontuberculous atypical mycobacteria** principal cause of **hot tub lung**
  - **Animal proteins**: Avian proteins, principal cause of **bird fancier's lung**
  - Low-molecular weight chemicals: Isocyanates (production of foams, paints) principal cause of occupational asthma
  - Pathophysiology
    - Small particles deposit in bronchioles, incite allergic granulomatous reaction
- Allergic reaction to airborne organic particles (1-5 μm)
  - More than 200 different organic antigens from variety of sources
  - 40% of offending agents not identified
- **95% of cases in nonsmokers**
- Regardless of antigen, < 1% of exposed develop hypersensitivity reaction

Microscopic Features
- Histologic features not pathognomonic
  - Classic triad: Cellular bronchiolitis, lymphocytic interstitial infiltrate, poorly formed nonnecrotizing granulomas
- Acute: Neutrophilic infiltration of respiratory bronchioles & alveoli
- Subacute: Cellular bronchiolitis, noncaseating granulomas, bronchiolocentric interstitial lymphocytic pneumonitis
  - Granulomas may be few & difficult to find, often loosely organized (in contrast to tightly organized granulomas of sarcoidosis)
- Chronic: Various fibrotic patterns; 50% NSIP, 40% usual interstitial pneumonia, 10% cryptogenic organizing pneumonia

CLINICAL ISSUES

Presentation
- Most common signs/symptoms
  - Considerable overlap of acute, subacute, chronic forms
  - **Acute**: Sudden onset of flu-like syndrome
    - Fever, chills, malaise
    - Pulmonary symptoms: Severe dyspnea, chest tightness, dry or mildly productive cough
    - Peak intensity of symptoms: 3-6 hours after initial exposure
    - Signs/symptoms gradually clear over 24-48 hours
    - Often mistaken for pneumonia
  - **Subacute**: Insidious onset of nonspecific symptoms, malaise, fatigue, weight loss
    - Hemoptysis in up to 1/4
  - **Chronic**: Dyspnea
    - Indistinguishable from other chronic interstitial lung diseases
- Pulmonary function tests
  - Restrictive pattern, diminished DLCO
  - Air-trapping: Increased ratio of residual volume to total lung capacity

Demographics
- Epidemiology
  - Uncommon: Farmer's lung (2-8%); bird fancier's lung (1-10%)
  - Less common in smokers

Natural History & Prognosis
- Acute: May completely return to normal
- Subacute/chronic: May progress even after eliminating antigen exposure
- Mortality rates variable: 1-10%

Treatment
- Avoid exposure to antigen
  - Quandary for farmers whose livelihood at risk
  - Quandary for bird breeders who develop emotional attachment to birds
- Corticosteroids

DIAGNOSTIC CHECKLIST

Consider
- HP in symptomatic nonsmokers with bilateral ground-glass opacities, centrilobular ground-glass nodules, & lobular air-trapping
- Chronic hypersensitivity pneumonitis in NSIP
  - Chronic HP may result in secondary NSIP

Image Interpretation Pearls
- Centrilobular nodules & air-trapping are characteristic of acute-subacute HP
- Upper lung predominant fibrosis & honeycomb lung are characteristic of chronic HP

SELECTED REFERENCES

1. Hirschmann JV et al: Hypersensitivity pneumonitis: a historical, clinical, and radiologic review. Radiographics. 29(7):1921-38, 2009
2. Sirajuddin A et al: Occupational lung disease. J Thorac Imaging. 24(4):310-20, 2009
3. Silva CI et al: Hypersensitivity pneumonitis: spectrum of high-resolution CT and pathologic findings. AJR Am J Roentgenol. 188(2):334-44, 2007
4. Pipavath S et al: Imaging of interstitial lung disease. Clin Chest Med. 25(3):455-65, v-vi, 2004

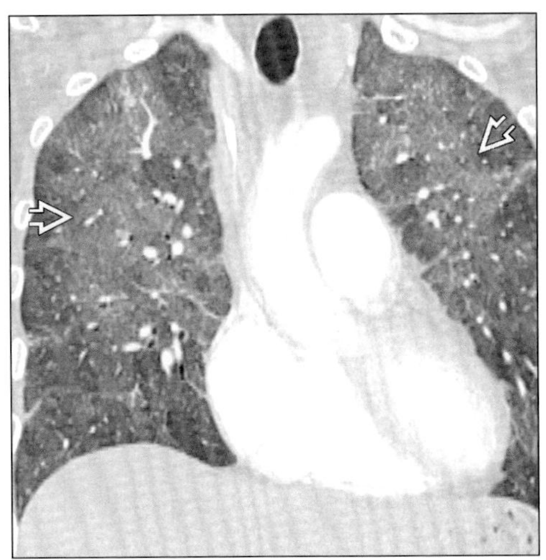

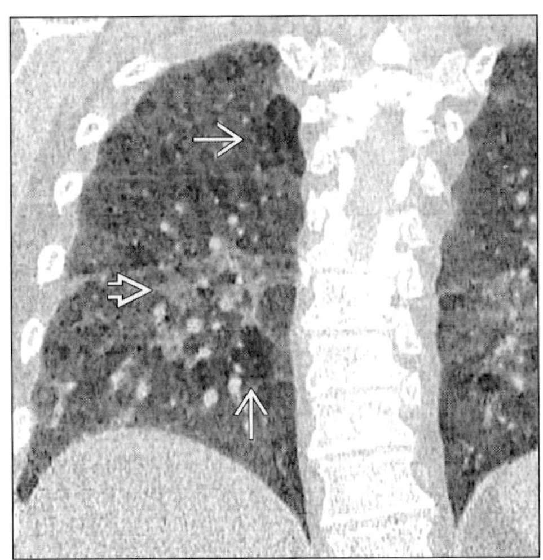

(Left) *Coronal CECT of a patient with hypersensitivity pneumonitis shows diffuse bilateral patchy ground-glass opacities ➾ and scattered low-attenuation areas.* ***(Right)*** *Coronal expiratory HRCT of a patient with HP shows lobular air-trapping ➡ and areas of hyperattenuation ➾ relative to the normal background lung density. The coexistence of these 3 different lung densities (usually with geographic margination) has been termed the head cheese sign and is highly suggestive of hypersensitivity pneumonitis.*

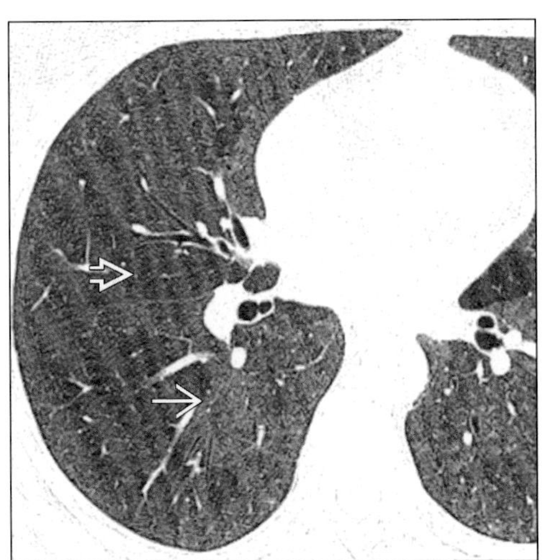

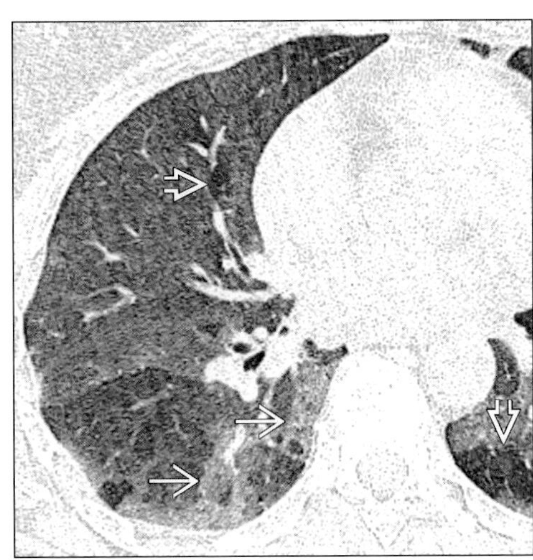

(Left) *Axial HRCT shows centrilobular and confluent ground-glass opacities ➡ and subtle areas of lobular hypoattenuation ➾.* ***(Right)*** *Axial expiratory HRCT of the same patient (obtained at the same location) shows lobular air-trapping ➾, areas of hyperattenuation ➡, and areas of normal expiratory attenuation, consistent with the head cheese sign. Correlation with clinical history is paramount to identify the culprit antigenic exposure in patients with hypersensitivity pneumonitis.*

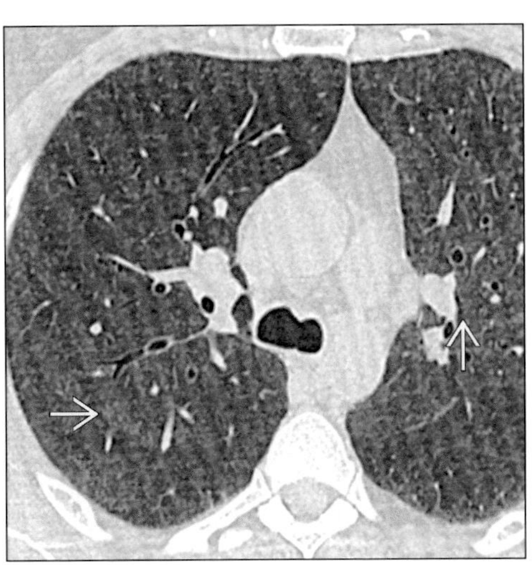

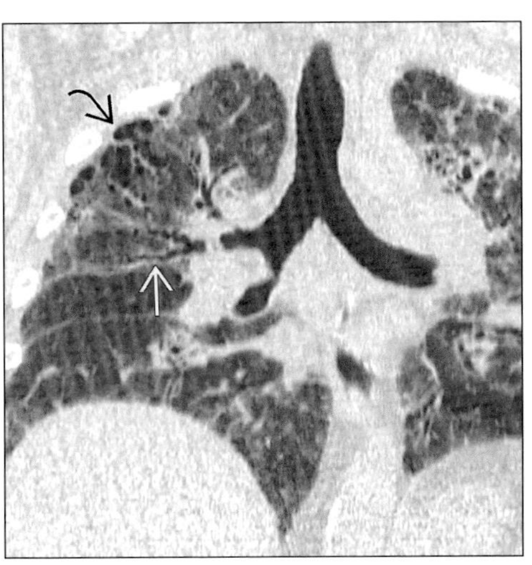

(Left) *Axial HRCT of a patient with HP shows faint centrilobular ground-glass opacities ➡. Smoking-related respiratory bronchiolitis should also be considered in the differential diagnosis.* ***(Right)*** *Coronal HRCT of a patient with chronic HP shows upper lobe predominant fibrosis manifesting with reticulation, architectural distortion, traction bronchiectasis ➡, and honeycombing ➚. Patchy areas of ground-glass opacity likely represent residual abnormalities from subacute HP.*

SMOKE INHALATION

Key Facts

Terminology

- Inhalation injury to upper & lower respiratory tract due to thermal, chemical, & particulate matter from products of combustion

Imaging

- Severity of injury dependent on concentration & length of exposure: Airways primarily affected on 1st day, lung affected over next 2 days
- Acute: Up to 48 hours
  - Initial radiograph often normal
  - Diffuse bronchial wall thickening (85%)
  - Conical narrowing of subglottic trachea
- Subacute: 3 days to end of hospitalization
  - Superimposed pneumonia
  - Cardiogenic edema, large IV fluid volumes
- Delayed: Weeks to months after hospital discharge
  - Bronchiectasis, mosaic attenuation, air-trapping

Top Differential Diagnoses

- Hydrostatic pulmonary edema
- Pneumonia
- Aspiration
- Neurogenic pulmonary edema

Pathology

- Friable airway mucosa with ulceration & charring
- Acute: Diffuse alveolar damage with hyaline membrane formation
- Delayed: Constrictive bronchiolitis

Clinical Issues

- Symptoms & signs
  - Dyspnea, wheezing, carbonaceous sputum
  - Singed nasal hairs, burns
- Smoke inhalation is primary cause of death in 75% of patients with burn injuries

__(Left)__ AP chest radiograph of a 52-year-old man with acute exposure to an industrial smoke fire shows mildly decreased lung volumes and diffuse bilateral reticular opacities. __(Right)__ Axial NECT of the same patient shows mild bronchial wall thickening and diffuse patchy ground-glass opacity. Scattered areas of centrilobular and paraseptal emphysema are also present and are related to chronic history of cigarette smoking.

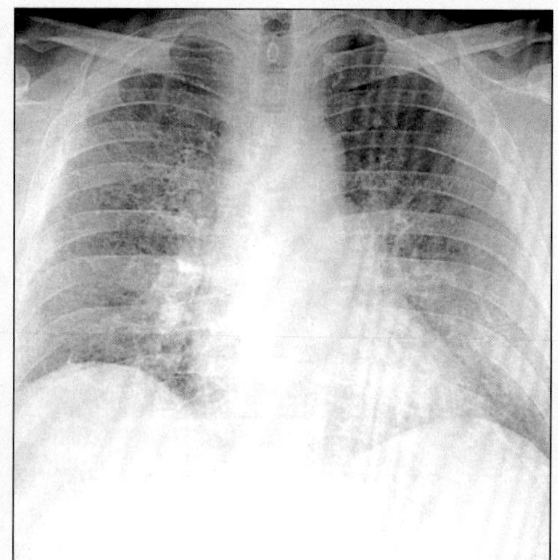

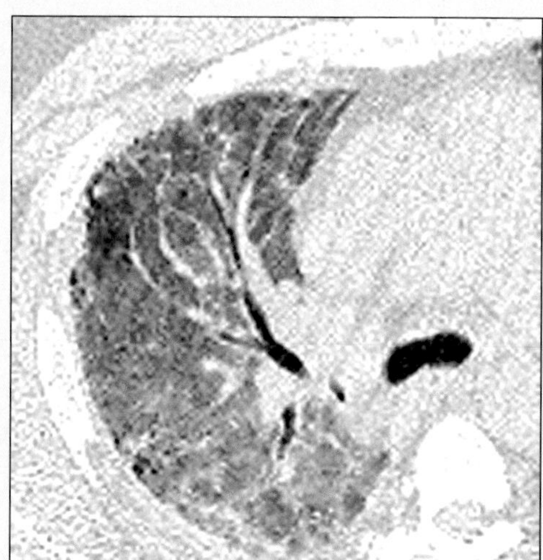

__(Left)__ AP chest radiograph of a 28-year-old man who was intubated on admission following smoke inhalation during a house fire shows multifocal bilateral airspace disease with dense right upper lobe consolidation. __(Right)__ Axial CECT of the same patient obtained 5 years later shows mosaic attenuation with areas of hyperlucency, scattered areas of bronchiectasis, and mild bronchial wall thickening. The central airway abnormalities are distributed in regions of prior inhalational injury.

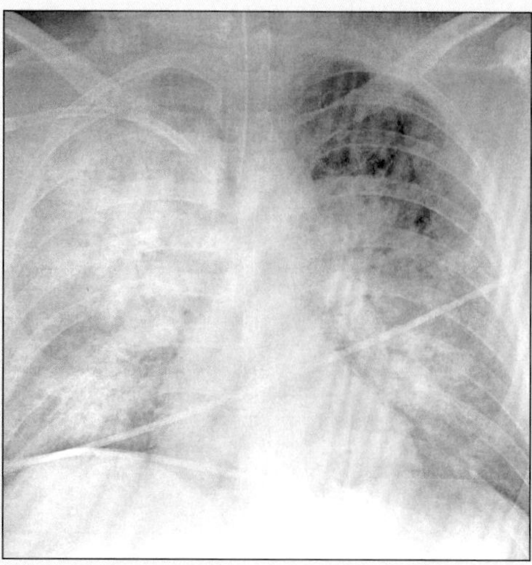

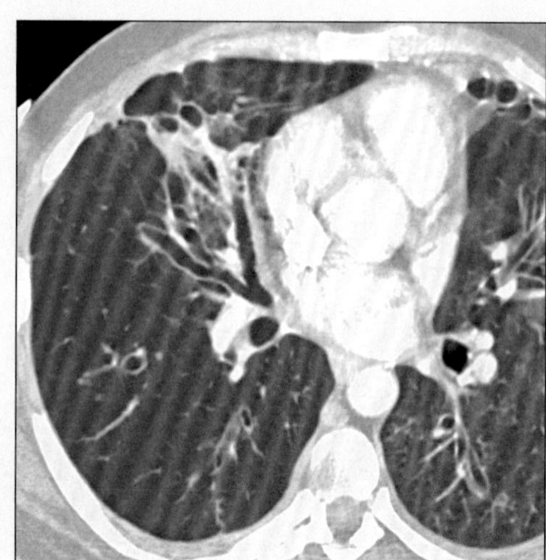

SMOKE INHALATION

TERMINOLOGY

Definitions

- Inhalation injury to upper & lower respiratory tract due to thermal, chemical, & particulate matter from products of combustion

IMAGING

General Features

- Best diagnostic clue
  - Upper zone predominant multifocal airspace disease & subglottic tracheal narrowing in patient with appropriate history

Radiographic Findings

- Radiography
  - Severity of injury dependent on concentration & length of exposure
    - Airways primarily affected on 1st day
    - Pulmonary parenchyma affected over next 2 days
  - **Acute**: Up to 48 hours
    - Initial radiograph often normal
    - Diffuse bronchial wall thickening (85%)
    - Conical narrowing of subglottic trachea from edema
    - Subsegmental atelectasis: Airway lumina narrowed by mucosal edema
    - Consolidation predominantly in perihilar & upper lung zones
  - **Subacute**: 3 days to end of hospitalization
    - Barotrauma due to positive pressure ventilation common
    - Superimposed pneumonia common, especially in those with cutaneous burns
      - Suspect pneumonia if parenchymal abnormalities progress after 1st 48 hours
      - Pneumonia develops in up to 40%
    - Cardiogenic pulmonary edema commonly superimposed
      - Large volumes of administered fluid, especially in patients with cutaneous burns
    - Acute respiratory distress syndrome (ARDS), severe complication with high mortality
  - **Delayed**: Weeks to months after hospital discharge
    - Hyperinflation & small nodules in previously affected lung due to constrictive bronchiolitis

CT Findings

- Acute
  - Bronchial wall thickening
  - Ground-glass opacities due to edema or mosaic attenuation from small airway edema
- Subacute
  - CT evaluation of suspected complications, such as pulmonary embolus
  - CT assessment of parenchymal abnormalities, especially in patients with complicated clinical course
- Delayed
  - Mosaic attenuation
  - Bronchiectasis
  - Expiratory air-trapping

Other Modality Findings

- Xenon-133 ventilation scanning
  - Delayed washout, incomplete washout within 120 seconds, or segmental hang-up
  - May be abnormal when chest radiograph normal, rarely used today

Imaging Recommendations

- Best imaging tool
  - Chest radiography for initial assessment & for monitoring disease course
  - CT used as problem-solving tool or to evaluate unexplained radiographic abnormalities

DIFFERENTIAL DIAGNOSIS

Hydrostatic Pulmonary Edema

- Smoke inhalation has proclivity for upper lung zones
- Fluid overload common in smoke inhalation due to massive fluid administration for burns

Pneumonia

- Similar imaging findings, however clinical history suggests proper diagnosis
- Superimposed pneumonia common in smoke inhalation, develops > 48 hours after admission

Aspiration

- Similar radiographic findings
- Hypoxic neurologically impaired victim of smoke inhalation at high risk for aspiration

Neurogenic Pulmonary Edema

- Requires central nervous system insult that will raise intracranial pressure
- Hypoxic neurologically impaired victim often requires head CT to exclude intracranial pathology

Mitral Regurgitant Pulmonary Edema

- Pulmonary edema due to heart failure in patient with incompetent mitral valve
- Diffuse involvement, but more severe in right upper lobe due to directional backflow through right superior pulmonary vein
- Enlarged heart, usually normal in smoke inhalation
- Responds quickly to diuretic and inotropic support

PATHOLOGY

General Features

- Etiology
  - Nitric oxide (NO)
    - Smoke-induced release from epithelial cells & alveolar macrophages
    - NO causes loss of hypoxic vasoconstriction & increased vascular permeability
  - Bronchial blood flow markedly increased (up to 20x)
    - May contribute to pulmonary edema
    - In animal models, bronchial artery occlusion lessens severity of smoke injury
- Smoke consists of gases & fine particulate material
  - Carbonaceous particles (soot) absorb noxious substances in gas & act as delivery vehicles to respiratory mucosa
- Water solubility of combustion products determines site of action

- Highly water-soluble products are irritating & affect upper airways
  - Ammonia, hydrogen chloride, sulfur dioxide
- Less water-soluble products are nonirritating & primarily affect distal airway
  - Chlorine, nitrogen oxides, phosgene
- Severity of chemical pneumonitis dependent on composition & concentration of smoke & length of exposure
  - Injury may occur from upper airways to pulmonary capillary bed
- Airway wall
  - Spectrum of findings beginning with edema & inflammatory cells, proceeding to hemorrhage, necrosis, ulceration, & charring
- Airway casts commonly cause widespread bronchial plugging
  - Casts composed of neutrophils shed bronchial epithelium, mucin, & fibrin
  - Mean reduction in cross-sectional area: Bronchi (30%), bronchioles (10%) 48 hours after injury

Pathophysiology

- General
  - Gas concentrations in lung determined by ventilation perfusion ratio (V/Q)
  - Normal upright lung, V/Q ratio highest in upper lung zone, therefore inhaled gas concentrated in nondependent lung
- Thermal injury
  - Rare, inhaled gases rapidly cooled by upper respiratory tract
  - Injury limited to upper respiratory tract & larynx
  - Seen primarily with superheated steam & explosions
- Asphyxiation due to carbon monoxide & carbon dioxide
  - Carbon monoxide displaces oxygen, produces profound hypoxemia, accounts for 50% of fire-related fatalities
  - Carbon dioxide reduces ambient oxygen concentration
- Pyrolysis
  - Cyanide gas from natural & synthetic fabric & plastics (especially polyvinyl chloride-PVC)
  - Hydrogen chloride from PVC combustion combines with water to produce hydrochloric acid

Gross Pathologic & Surgical Features

- Diffusely friable airway mucosa with ulceration & charring

Microscopic Features

- Acute: Diffuse alveolar damage with hyaline membrane formation
- Delayed: Constrictive bronchiolitis

CLINICAL ISSUES

Presentation

- Most common signs/symptoms
  - Dyspnea
  - Wheezing
  - Carbonaceous sputum
  - Singed nasal hairs
  - Burns
- Other signs/symptoms
  - Elevated carboxyhemoglobin (from carbon monoxide inhalation)
    - Increased mixed venous PO_2 & decreased arteriovenous oxygen difference suggests either carbon monoxide or hydrogen cyanide poisoning
  - Wheezing common due to airway narrowing
- Bronchoscopy findings (typically used acutely for diagnosis)
  - Laryngeal edema, airway ulceration, charring
- Delayed symptoms months later: Dyspnea, nonproductive cough

Demographics

- Epidemiology
  - 23,000 injuries & 5,000 deaths per year in USA
- Firefighters
  - Long-term risk of obstructive lung disease

Natural History & Prognosis

- Smoke inhalation is primary cause of death in 75% of patients with burn injuries
- Mortality rate ranges: 50-80%
- Abnormal chest radiograph within 48 hours of exposure is poor prognostic sign
- Despite advances in cutaneous burn care, mortality from smoke inhalation has not improved over past 2 decades

Treatment

- Supportive, intubation & ventilation with supplemental oxygen to counter hypoxia
- Fluid management critical to support cardiac & urine output
- Steroids may be detrimental, prophylactic antibiotics do not influence survival
- Promising: Aerosolized acetylcysteine & heparin

DIAGNOSTIC CHECKLIST

Consider

- Hydrogen cyanide exposure in patients with unexplained respiratory failure or persistent anion gap metabolic acidosis

SELECTED REFERENCES

1. Toon MH et al: Management of acute smoke inhalation injury. Crit Care Resusc. 12(1):53-61, 2010
2. Weiden MD et al: Obstructive airways disease with air trapping among firefighters exposed to World Trade Center dust. Chest. 137(3):566-74, 2010
3. Rehberg S et al: Pathophysiology, management and treatment of smoke inhalation injury. Expert Rev Respir Med. 3(3):283-297, 2009
4. Koljonen V et al: Multi-detector computed tomography demonstrates smoke inhalation injury at early stage. Emerg Radiol. 14(2):113-6, 2007
5. Reske A et al: Computed tomography--a possible aid in the diagnosis of smoke inhalation injury? Acta Anaesthesiol Scand. 49(2):257-60, 2005
6. Latenser BA et al: Smoke inhalation injury. Semin Respir Crit Care Med. 22(1):13-22, 2001
7. Teixidor HS et al: Smoke inhalation: radiologic manifestations. Radiology. 149(2):383-7, 1983

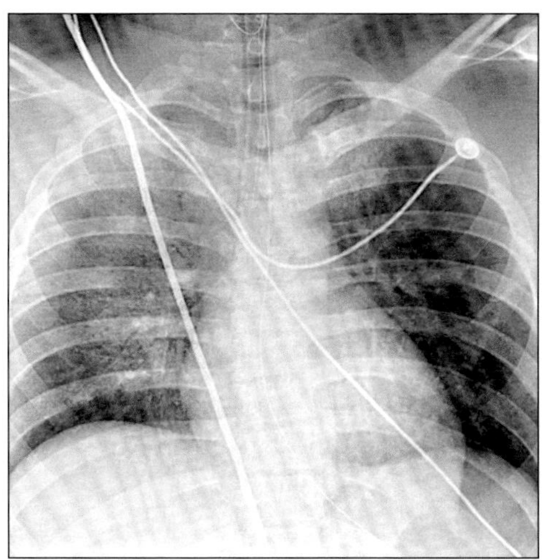

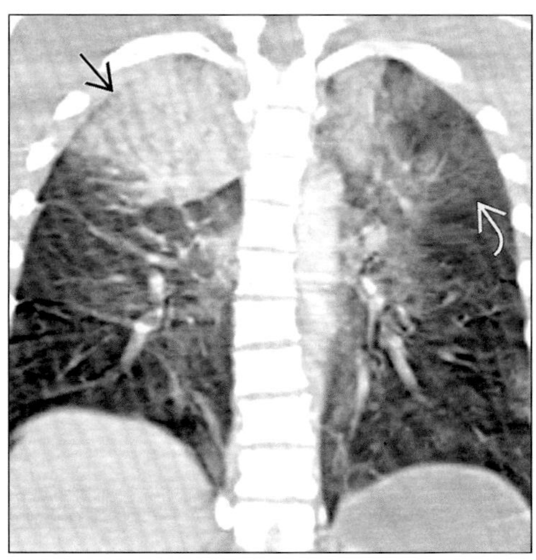

(Left) *AP chest radiograph of a 21-year-old man who sustained 30% skin burns and smoke inhalation injury during a house fire shows multifocal upper lung zone predominant airspace opacities with confluent right upper lung and perihilar consolidations.* ***(Right)*** *Coronal CECT of the same patient shows bilateral upper lobe consolidations → and patchy ground-glass opacities ➔. Bronchoscopy revealed tracheal edema, erythema, and ulceration, consistent with smoke inhalation injury.*

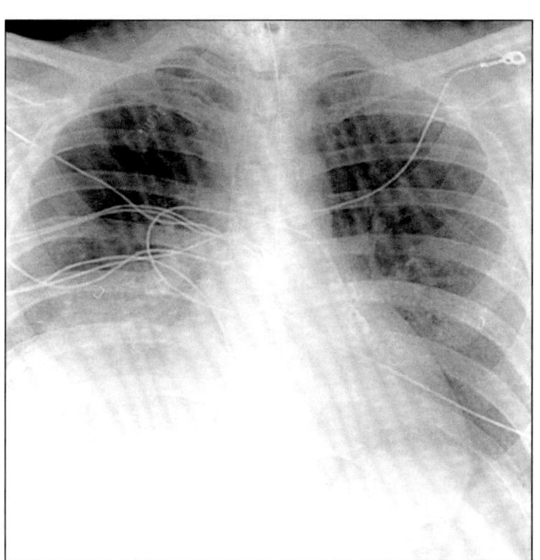

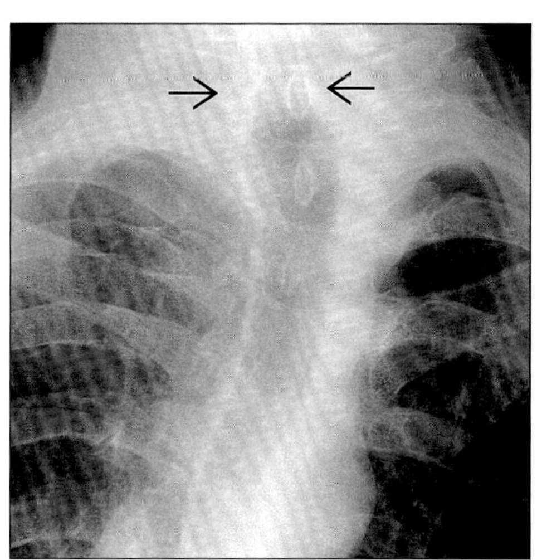

(Left) *AP chest radiograph of the same patient 4 weeks later shows clearing of the upper lobe airspace disease and new right lower lobe consolidation. Pneumonia commonly develops in patients with smoke inhalation injury, which is the cause of death in 75% of burn patients.* ***(Right)*** *AP chest radiograph (coned down to the trachea) of a patient who sustained 70% skin burns in a house fire shows subglottic narrowing → that required intubation for airway protection.*

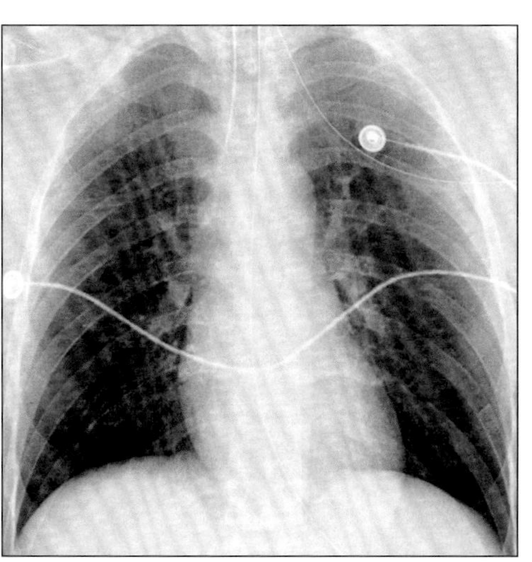

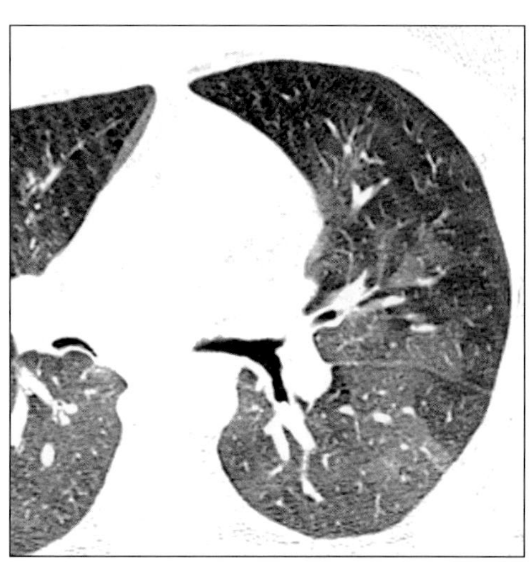

(Left) *AP chest radiograph of a 35-year-old man trapped in a nightclub fire shows hyperinflated but clear lungs. A normal initial chest radiograph is commonly seen in patients with smoke inhalation injury.* ***(Right)*** *Axial expiratory HRCT of a patient who was trapped in a nightclub fire 4 years previously shows diffuse mosaic attenuation due to air-trapping. Chronic dyspnea related to smoke inhalation may be the result of constrictive bronchiolitis or asthma.*

ASPIRATION

Key Facts

Terminology
- Synonyms
  - Aspiration pneumonia, aspiration pneumonitis, aspiration bronchiolitis

Imaging
- Chest radiography
  - Unilateral or bilateral consolidation (gravitational)
  - Atelectasis (segmental/lobar)
- NECT
  - Focal/multifocal consolidation; gravitational
  - Atelectasis: Endobronchial aspirated material
  - Centrilobular nodules & tree-in-bud opacities
  - Pneumatoceles
- CECT
  - Evaluation of complications: Necrotizing pneumonia, abscess, empyema, pulmonary embolus

Top Differential Diagnoses
- Multifocal consolidations
  - Organizing/eosinophilic pneumonia
  - Tuberculosis
- Atelectasis
  - Endobronchial tumor
  - Broncholithiasis
- Focal mass
  - Lipoid pneumonia
  - Organizing pneumonia
  - Lung cancer

Clinical Issues
- Symptoms relate to amount/type of aspirated material, frequency, & host response
- Acute: Cough, wheezing, cyanosis, tachypnea
- Subacute/chronic aspiration may mimic asthma
- Common cause of hospital-acquired infections

*(**Left**) Axial NECT of a 68-year-old woman with achalasia shows a dilated esophagus with an air-fluid level ➔ and patchy left upper lobe ground-glass and tree-in-bud opacities. Aspirative cellular bronchiolitis is a common complication of achalasia. (**Right**) Coronal NECT of a patient with acute aspiration pneumonia shows bilateral perihilar alveolar opacities and a distended stomach containing heterogeneous material ⇨. Aspiration pneumonia is the etiology of most hospital-acquired infections.*

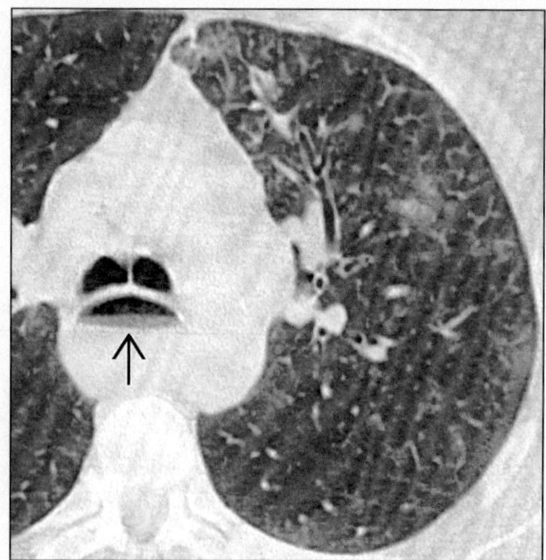

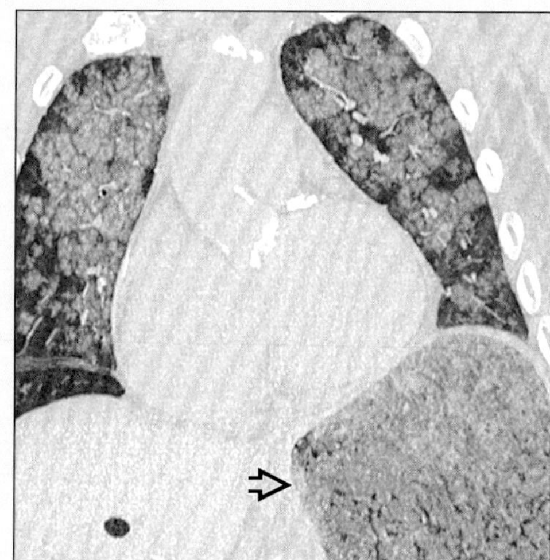

*(**Left**) Axial NECT of a 46-year-old man with severe periodontal disease shows a left lower lobe cavitary mass ➔ with ill-defined borders. Aspiration-related lung abscess may occur in patients with poor oral hygiene. (**Right**) AP chest radiograph obtained 24 hours after surgery shows extensive bilateral consolidations secondary to aspiration while under anesthesia. Acute pneumonitis due to aspiration of sterile gastric content (Mendelson syndrome) is associated with a high mortality rate.*

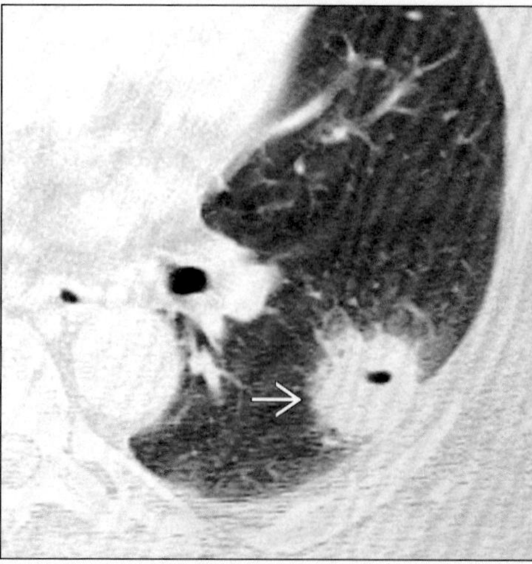

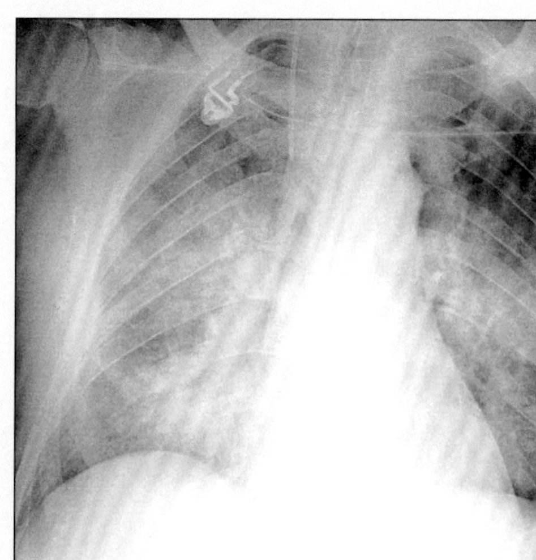

ASPIRATION

TERMINOLOGY

Synonyms

- **Aspiration pneumonia**: Lung infection caused by aspiration of colonized oropharyngeal secretions
- **Aspiration pneumonitis**: Acute lung injury caused by aspiration of material inherently toxic to lungs
- **Aspiration bronchiolitis**: Chronic inflammatory reaction to recurrent aspirated foreign particles in bronchioles

Definitions

- Aspiration syndromes
  - **Aspiration pneumonia**: Most hospital-acquired infections
    - **Lentil aspiration pneumonia**: Leguminous material (lentils, beans, peas)
    - Fistulas between esophagus & trachea, bronchi or lung: Congenital tracheoesophageal fistula; esophageal cancer (5-10%)
  - **Aspiration pneumonitis**
    - **Mendelson syndrome**: Sterile gastric contents (peripartum, anesthesia)
    - **Exogenous lipoid pneumonia**: Mineral oil or related substances
    - **Hydrocarbon aspiration pneumonia**
      - Children: Accidental poisoning
      - Fire-eaters: Hydrocarbon-containing fluids (petroleum)
  - Aspiration of inert fluids or particulates
    - Foreign bodies: Food particles (children); tooth fragments (elderly)
    - Near drowning: Massive amount of fresh or salt water
  - **Aspiration bronchiolitis**: Obliterative bronchiolitis & gastroesophageal reflux (mimics asthma)

IMAGING

General Features

- Best diagnostic clue
  - Gravity-dependent opacities
  - Radiopaque material within airways
- Location
  - Recumbent patients: Diffuse perihilar consolidation (upper lobe superior segments, lower lobe posterior basal segments)
  - Upright patients: Lower lobe basal segments

Radiographic Findings

- Radiography
  - Unilateral or bilateral air-space consolidation (gravitational distribution)
  - Focal/multifocal consolidation; hyperdense (Barium)
  - Abscess
  - Atelectasis (segmental/lobar): Endobronchial radiopaque material

CT Findings

- NECT
  - Air-space consolidation, solitary or multiple; gravitational distribution
  - Atelectasis: Endobronchial aspirated material
  - Centrilobular ill-defined nodules & tree-in-bud opacities
  - Pneumatoceles
- CECT
  - Evaluation of complications: Necrotizing pneumonia, abscess, empyema, pulmonary embolus

Imaging Recommendations

- Best imaging tool
  - Chest radiography for initial diagnosis & follow-up
  - Chest CT for assessment of complications

DIFFERENTIAL DIAGNOSIS

Multifocal Consolidation

- Organizing/eosinophilic pneumonia
- Tuberculosis

Atelectasis

- Endobronchial tumor: Lung cancer, carcinoid, metastases
- Broncholithiasis

Focal Mass

- Lipoid pneumonia
- Organizing pneumonia
- Lung cancer

PATHOLOGY

General Features

- Etiology
  - Common cause of hospital-acquired infections
  - Causes of aspiration: Alcoholism, loss of consciousness, neuromuscular disorder, poor dental hygiene or advanced periodontal disease

Gross Pathologic & Surgical Features

- **Necrotizing acute bronchopneumonia**: Alveolar edema, hemorrhage, numerous polymorphonuclear leukocytes, foreign body granulomas
- **Obliterative bronchiolitis**: Bronchiolar mucosal injury & subsequent airflow obstruction

CLINICAL ISSUES

Presentation

- Most common signs/symptoms
  - Variable: Amount/type of aspirated material, frequency, & host response
  - Acute
    - Cough, wheezing, cyanosis, tachypnea
    - After acute meat aspiration: "Cafe coronary syndrome" (mimics myocardial infarction)
    - Pneumonia: Fever, cough, purulent sputum
  - Subacute/chronic
    - Mimics asthma
- Other signs/symptoms
  - Pleuritic chest pain; occasionally hemoptysis

SELECTED REFERENCES

1. Marik PE: Aspiration pneumonitis and aspiration pneumonia. N Engl J Med. 344(9):665-71, 2001

TALCOSIS

Key Facts

Terminology

- 4 forms: 3 inhalational, 1 intravenous
  - Inhalation of pure talc (talcosis)
  - Inhalation of talc & silica (talco-silicosis)
  - Inhalation of talc & asbestos (talco-asbestosis)
  - Intravenous (IV) illicit drug use

Imaging

- Multiple punctate lung nodules
  - Predominantly in upper lung zones
- May evolve into progressive massive fibrosis (PMF)
  - PMF may exhibit high attenuation
  - Architectural distortion adjacent to PMF
- Basilar panlobular emphysema in intravenous methylphenidate (Ritalin) abusers
- Lower zone reticular opacities & pleural plaques or thickening in talco-asbestosis

Top Differential Diagnoses

- Sarcoidosis
- Metastatic pulmonary calcification
- Silicosis
- Amyloidosis
- Amiodarone toxicity

Pathology

- Inhalational
  - Occupational exposure in mining, milling, packaging of talc
- Intravenous
  - Talc (& cellulose) common filler in oral medication

Clinical Issues

- Inhalational: Dry cough & chronic dyspnea progressing to cor pulmonale in end-stage disease
- Intravenous: Progressive dyspnea & COPD

*(**Left**) PA chest radiograph of a patient with pulmonary talcosis shows diffuse punctate lung nodules and central consolidations ➔. Conglomerate fibrosis in talcosis exhibits a more perihilar distribution than PMF in silicosis. Calcification is usually not evident on chest radiography. (**Right**) Axial HRCT of a patient with pulmonary talcosis shows diffuse, poorly defined punctate lung nodules. Lung nodules in silicosis and coal worker's pneumoconiosis tend to be slightly larger and better defined.*

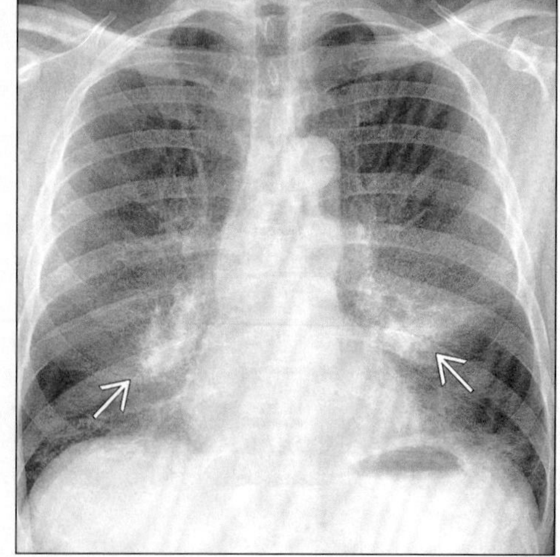

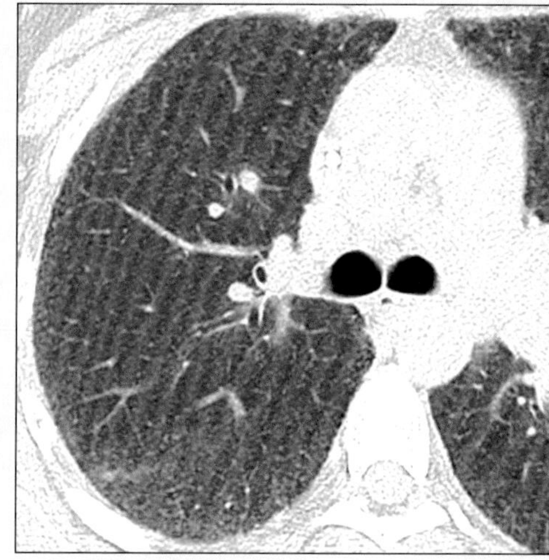

*(**Left**) PA chest radiograph of a patient with talcosis shows bilateral perihilar mass-like consolidations with bilateral upward hilar retraction, reflecting progressive massive fibrosis. The imaging features are similar to those of silicosis with PMF from coalescence of pneumoconiotic nodules. (**Right**) Axial CECT of the same patient shows dense mass-like perihilar upper lobe consolidations ➔. As in silicosis, development of progressive massive fibrosis in talcosis can occur despite cessation of exposure.*

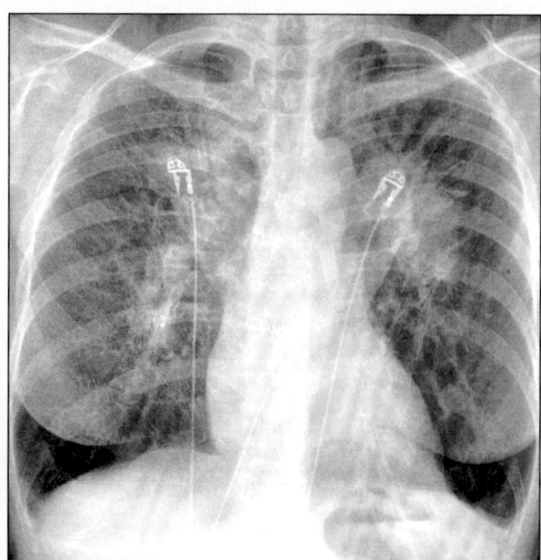

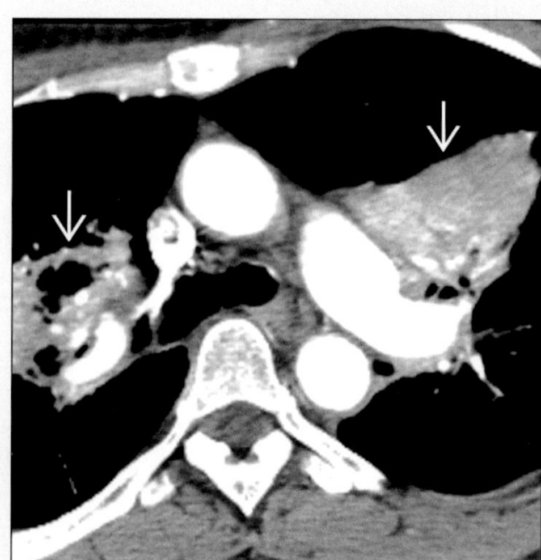

TALCOSIS

TERMINOLOGY

Definitions

- 4 forms: 3 inhalational, 1 intravenous
  - Inhalation of pure talc (talcosis)
  - Inhalation of talc & silica (talco-silicosis)
  - Inhalation of talc & asbestos (talco-asbestosis)
  - Intravenous (IV) illicit drug use

IMAGING

General Features

- Best diagnostic clue
  - Diffuse fine punctate nodularity & high-attenuation perihilar conglomeration
  - Basilar panlobular emphysema in intravenous methylphenidate (Ritalin) abusers
- Morphology
  - Diffuse punctate micronodules with perihilar progressive massive fibrosis (PMF) & emphysema

Radiographic Findings

- Radiography
  - **Inhalational**
    - Multiple punctate lung nodules
    - Upper lung zone predominant
    - May evolve into PMF (may progress rapidly over 12 months)
    - Lower zone reticular opacities & pleural plaques or thickening in talco-asbestosis
    - Enlarged hilar lymph nodes with eggshell calcification (especially in silico-talcosis)
  - **Intravenous**
    - Multifocal punctate lung nodules
    - Occasional lymphadenopathy
    - Perihilar PMF
    - Emphysema, either centrilobular (upper lung zone) or panacinar (lower lung zone)

CT Findings

- HRCT
  - **Inhalational**
    - Centrilobular & subpleural nodules, may calcify
    - Aggregation of nodules into PMF (identical to silicosis)
    - Architectural distortion adjacent to PMF
    - Pleural & diaphragmatic plaques identical to asbestos-related pleural disease
      - Pleural thickening may be dramatic
  - **Intravenous**
    - Emphysema may be upper or lower lung zone predominant (even in absence of smoking)
    - Methylphenidate: Special proclivity for severe lower lobe panacinar emphysema
      - May result in severe isolated lower lung zone panacinar emphysema (without nodularity)
    - Centrilobular (punctate) nodules & tree-in-bud opacities
    - PMF in perihilar distribution with high attenuation (highly suggestive of talcosis)
    - PMF superimposed on punctate nodular opacities

DIFFERENTIAL DIAGNOSIS

Sarcoidosis

- No occupational exposure, PMF less likely
- Nodules usually larger & clustered (galaxy sign)
- Peribronchovascular distribution of nodules
- Affected lymph nodes may exhibit eggshell calcification, nodules rarely calcify

Metastatic Pulmonary Calcification

- No PMF
- Emphysema, if present, admixed with ground-glass opacities or consolidation
- Large, mulberry-shaped centrilobular nodules with a tendency to cluster
- Typically affects upper lungs

Silicosis

- Occupational history
- Nodules tend to be larger than those of talcosis
- PMF usually more cephalad & peripheral in upper lung zones & not of high attenuation
- Affected lymph nodes may exhibit eggshell calcification
- Talc & silica may be admixed together

Amyloidosis

- May also relate to IV drug abuse
- Nodular form: Multiple small scattered pulmonary nodules
- May calcify, but calcification in small nodules rare

Amiodarone Toxicity

- Accumulates in lung & liver
- Focal areas of consolidation randomly distributed

PATHOLOGY

General Features

- Etiology
  - Inhalational
    - Occupational exposure in mining, milling, packaging of talc
  - Intravenous
    - Talc (& cellulose) common filler in oral medication

CLINICAL ISSUES

Presentation

- Most common signs/symptoms
  - Inhalational
    - Dry cough & chronic dyspnea progressing to cor pulmonale in end-stage disease
  - Intravenous
    - Progressive dyspnea & COPD

SELECTED REFERENCES

1. Marchiori E et al: Pulmonary talcosis: imaging findings. Lung. 188(2):165-71, 2010
2. Chong S et al: Pneumoconiosis: comparison of imaging and pathologic findings. Radiographics. 26(1):59-77, 2006

ACUTE EOSINOPHILIC PNEUMONIA

Key Facts

Terminology

- Acute eosinophilic pneumonia (AEP)
- Idiopathic acute febrile illness with rapid onset respiratory failure due to pulmonary eosinophilia
  - Peripheral eosinophilia usually absent

Imaging

- Mimics cardiogenic pulmonary edema
  - Earliest findings: Septal lines & reticular opacities
  - Rapid progression to extensive bilateral ground-glass opacities & confluent consolidations
  - Small bilateral pleural effusions common
  - Heart size usually normal
  - No lymphadenopathy or pericardial effusion
- Presence of bilateral effusions helps distinguish AEP from other eosinophilic lung diseases
- Chest radiography often sufficient for diagnosis & follow-up

Top Differential Diagnoses

- Cardiogenic edema
- Acute interstitial pneumonia & ARDS
- Other causes of eosinophilic lung disease

Pathology

- Etiology unknown: Associated with recent onset or binge cigarette smoking
- Microscopic findings: Eosinophilic pneumonia with diffuse alveolar damage

Clinical Issues

- Bronchoalveolar lavage is diagnostic test of choice
- Rapid clearance with corticosteroids

Diagnostic Checklist

- Consider AEP in patients with suspected hydrostatic edema nonresponsive to diuresis

*(**Left**) AP chest radiograph of a patient with AEP shows diffuse bilateral interlobular septal thickening that mimics pulmonary interstitial edema. Note the normal heart size. (**Right**) Axial HRCT of a patient with AEP shows patchy ground-glass opacities, interlobular septal thickening ⇨, and small bilateral pleural effusions →. While the findings mimic cardiogenic pulmonary edema, the nongravitationally dependent distribution of airspace disease in this patient should suggest other possibilities.*

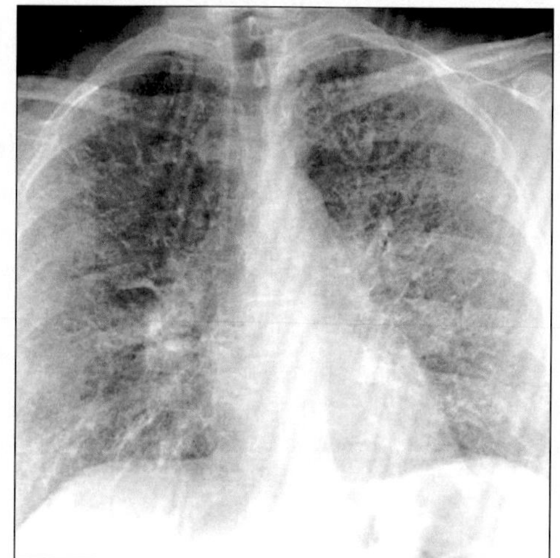

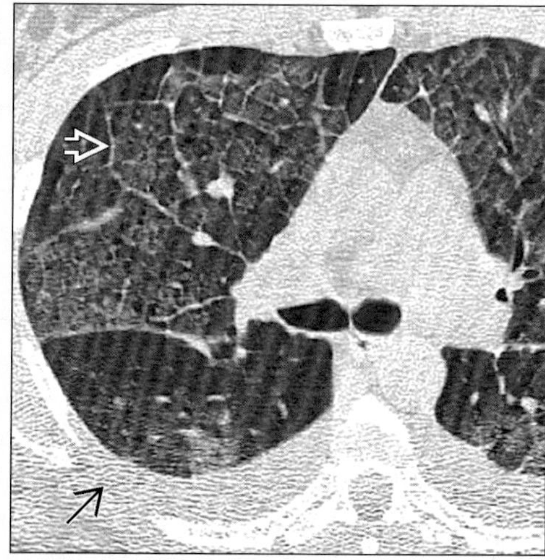

*(**Left**) Axial HRCT of a young woman who recently started smoking cigarettes and developed AEP shows smooth interlobular septal thickening →, patchy consolidations ⇨, and trace right pleural effusion. Although there was no peripheral blood eosinophilia, bronchoalveolar lavage showed extensive pulmonary eosinophilia. (**Right**) Axial CECT of a patient with AEP shows smooth interlobular septal thickening →, a few foci of peripheral lung consolidation ↪, and a small right pleural effusion.*

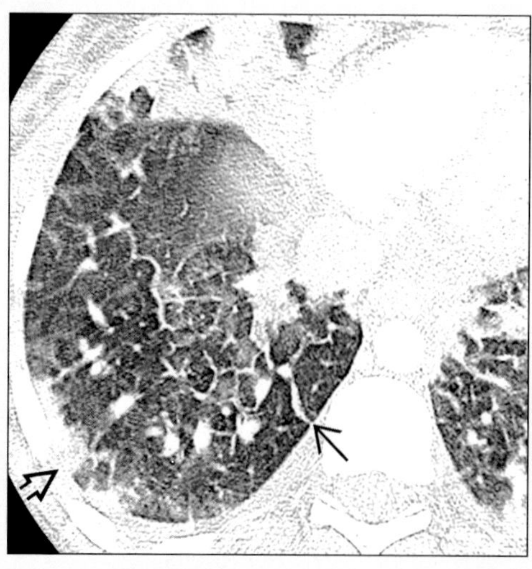

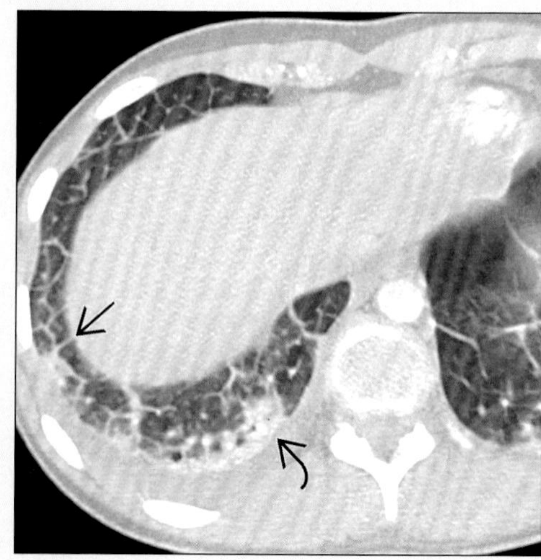

ACUTE EOSINOPHILIC PNEUMONIA

TERMINOLOGY

Abbreviations

- Acute eosinophilic pneumonia (AEP)

Definitions

- Idiopathic **acute febrile illness** with rapid onset **respiratory failure** due to **pulmonary eosinophilia**
  - Peripheral eosinophilia usually absent

IMAGING

General Features

- Best diagnostic clue
  - Mimics cardiogenic pulmonary edema on imaging
  - Presence of bilateral pleural effusions may help distinguish AEP from other eosinophilic lung diseases
- Location
  - Variable distribution of abnormalities in cephalocaudal & axial planes

Radiographic Findings

- Radiography
  - **Mimics cardiogenic pulmonary edema**
    - Earliest findings: Septal lines & reticular opacities
    - Rapid progression (hours to days) to extensive bilateral ground-glass opacities & confluent consolidations
    - Small bilateral pleural effusions common
    - Heart size usually normal

CT Findings

- Mimics cardiogenic pulmonary edema
- Morphology
  - **Ground-glass opacities most common (100%)**
    - May exhibit "crazy-paving" pattern or mosaic attenuation
  - **Smooth interlobular septal thickening (90%)**
  - Consolidation (55%)
  - Poorly defined centrilobular nodules (30%)
  - Bronchovascular thickening (66%)
- Distribution
  - Ground-glass opacities often centered on bronchovascular bundles
  - Craniocaudal
    - Variable (60%)
    - Lower lung zone (20%)
    - Upper lung zone (15%)
  - Axial
    - Variable (60%)
    - Peripheral (30%)
    - Central (5%)
- Pleura
  - **Effusions (80%)**, nearly always **bilateral (95%)**
  - Small to moderate in size
- Pertinent absent findings
  - Lymphadenopathy
  - Pericardial effusion

Imaging Recommendations

- Best imaging tool
  - Chest radiography usually sufficient for diagnosis & follow-up

DIFFERENTIAL DIAGNOSIS

Cardiogenic Edema

- May be indistinguishable from AEP on imaging
  - Heart size normal in AEP
  - Edema usually gravity-dependent compared to variable distribution of AEP

Acute Interstitial Pneumonia & ARDS

- Early exudative phase may mimic AEP
- Later organizing phase shows parenchymal distortion not seen with AEP

Other Causes of Eosinophilic Lung Disease

- Drug-induced eosinophilic lung disease
  - More commonly associated with rash than AEP
  - CT findings nearly identical
    - Consolidation > ground-glass in drug reactions
    - Peripheral distribution more common with drugs
    - Upper lung zone distribution more common with drugs
    - Bilateral pleural effusions less common
  - Common drugs
    - Antibiotics
    - Nonsteroidal anti-inflammatory agents & aspirin
    - Agents used for treatment of inflammatory bowel disease: Sulfasalazine
    - Inhaled illicit drugs including cocaine & heroin
    - Most chemotherapy drugs: Methotrexate
- Parasitic infection
  - Must be excluded in patients with eosinophilic lung disease
  - Common parasites
    - *Ascaris lumbricoides*
    - *Strongyloides stercoralis*
    - *Ancylostoma duodenale*
- Allergic bronchopulmonary aspergillosis
  - Central bronchiectasis more conspicuous in upper lobes
  - High-attenuation mucous plugging on CT
  - Common history of asthma
- Churg-Strauss syndrome
  - Pleural effusions, less common than in AEP
  - Systemic disease (unlike AEP)
    - Neuropathy more common
    - Paranasal sinus disease more common
- Hypereosinophilic syndrome
  - Systemic disease (unlike AEP)
    - Multiorgan involvement, especially cardiac
  - Persistent eosinophilia > 6 months
  - Eosinophil count often > 1.5 x 10^8
  - Transient consolidations
- Chronic eosinophilic pneumonia
  - Insidious onset of symptoms, usually present for 1 month before diagnosis
  - Peripheral upper lobe consolidations should help distinguish from AEP
  - Relapse after steroid discontinuation common

Diffuse Alveolar Hemorrhage

- Similar radiographic abnormalities
- Patients commonly anemic (uncommon in AEP)
- History of renal disease common
- Absence of pleural effusion distinguishes from AEP

ACUTE EOSINOPHILIC PNEUMONIA

PATHOLOGY

General Features

- Etiology
  - Pathogenesis unknown
    - Proposed hypothesis: Exposure to smoke or other environmental agents may give rise to hypersensitivity reaction
    - Associated with recent onset of cigarette smoking or binge smoking
      - Given high incidence of smoking & rarity of AEP, unlikely that smoking is single inciting factor
    - Single case report of New York City fireman developing AEP with acute heavy exposure to World Trade Center dust during rescue operations after September 11, 2001 attack
  - Important to distinguish from eosinophilic responses secondary to drug reactions or fungal/parasitic infection
- Eosinophils derived from bone marrow; when released into circulation, last for 13-18 hours

Staging, Grading, & Classification

- Diagnostic criteria
  - Acute febrile illness of < 1 month duration (often < 7 days)
  - Hypoxemia
  - Diffuse ground-glass, reticular, & consolidative opacities on imaging
  - Bronchoalveolar lavage (BAL) fluid with > 25% eosinophils
    - No fungi, parasites, or infectious agents identified on stains
  - Prompt & complete response to corticosteroids with no relapse after cessation

Microscopic Features

- Eosinophilic pneumonia with diffuse alveolar damage

CLINICAL ISSUES

Presentation

- Most common signs/symptoms
  - AEP
    - Acute onset of fever (often high) & rapidly progressing shortness of breath
    - Myalgias in 50%
    - Pleuritic chest pain in 75%
  - Often history of recent intense exposure to dust, smoke, or fumes
- Other signs/symptoms
  - Pulmonary function: Decreased diffusion capacity & restrictive pattern

Demographics

- Age
  - AEP is most common in young adults, mean age of 29 years
- Gender
  - No gender predominance
- Epidemiology
  - Incidence: 9 per 100,000 person-years
    - Based on study of AEP in military personnel

Laboratory Data

- Marked increase in eosinophils on BAL: > 25% eosinophils, (normal is < 1%)
- Peripheral eosinophil count usually normal at presentation, may become elevated with disease progression

Diagnosis

- **BAL diagnostic test of choice**
  - Eosinophilia in absence of infectious agents after careful medical history should preclude lung biopsy

Natural History & Prognosis

- Rapid clearing with steroids over days (usually complete resolution in a week)
- AEP may be associated with hemodynamic instability
  - True hemodynamic shock rare
  - Absence of multiple organ failure (as may be seen with ARDS)

Treatment

- **Rapid response to corticosteroid therapy**, sometimes within hours of 1st dose
  - May spontaneously resolve
- Mechanical ventilation may be required in up to 2/3 of patients
- Relapse rare

DIAGNOSTIC CHECKLIST

Consider

- AEP in patients with suspected hydrostatic edema nonresponsive to diuresis
- Always consider & exclude specific causes of eosinophilic lung disease: Drugs, parasitic infestation, fungal infection

Image Interpretation Pearls

- AEP mimics pulmonary edema

SELECTED REFERENCES

1. Galvin JR et al: Smoking-related lung disease. J Thorac Imaging. 24(4):274-84, 2009
2. Vassallo R et al: Tobacco smoke-related diffuse lung diseases. Semin Respir Crit Care Med. 29(6):643-50, 2008
3. Jeong YJ et al: Eosinophilic lung diseases: a clinical, radiologic, and pathologic overview. Radiographics. 27(3):617-37; discussion 637-9, 2007
4. Kanne JP et al: Smoking-related emphysema and interstitial lung diseases. J Thorac Imaging. 22(3):286-91, 2007
5. Wechsler ME: Pulmonary eosinophilic syndromes. Immunol Allergy Clin North Am. 27(3):477-92, 2007
6. Lynch DA et al: Idiopathic interstitial pneumonias: CT features. Radiology. 236(1):10-21, 2005
7. Philit F et al: Idiopathic acute eosinophilic pneumonia: a study of 22 patients. Am J Respir Crit Care Med. 166(9):1235-9, 2002
8. Rom WN et al: Acute eosinophilic pneumonia in a New York City firefighter exposed to World Trade Center dust. Am J Respir Crit Care Med. 166(6):797-800, 2002
9. Johkoh T et al: Eosinophilic lung diseases: diagnostic accuracy of thin-section CT in 111 patients. Radiology. 216(3):773-80, 2000

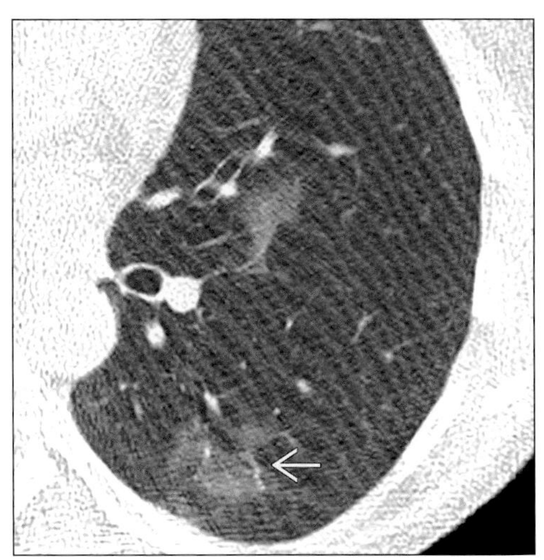

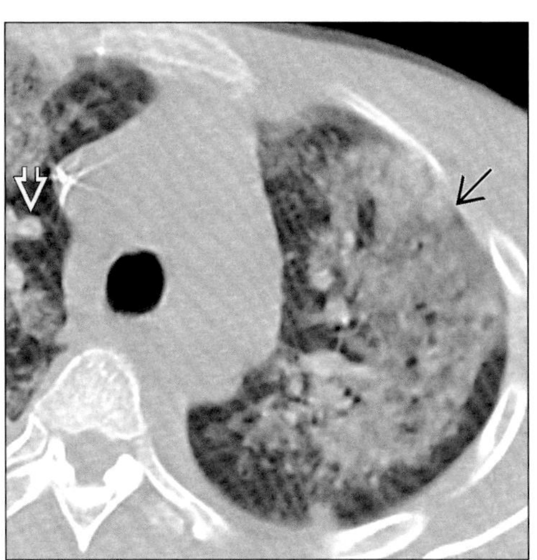

(Left) Axial HRCT of a patient with AEP shows scattered foci of ground-glass opacity ➔. The degree of pulmonary involvement by ground-glass opacity can be mild, as in this patient, or can be quite extensive. *(Right)* Axial NECT of a patient with AEP shows nodules ➔ and geographic nonsegmental ground-glass opacity and consolidation ➔ resulting from leishmaniasis. Parasitic infection must be considered and excluded in patients presenting with eosinophilic pneumonia.

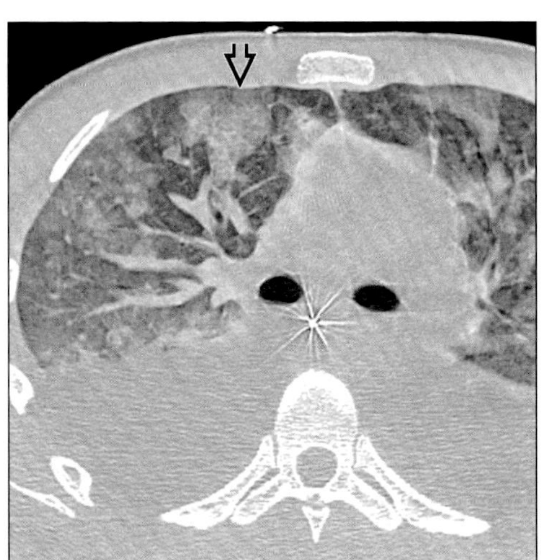

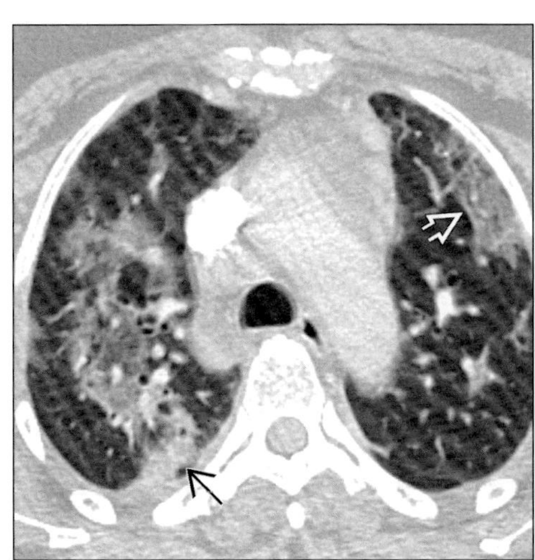

(Left) Axial HRCT of a patient with AEP shows multifocal ground-glass opacities and consolidations ➔ with some lobular sparing and moderate to large bilateral pleural effusions. Pleural effusions occur in the majority of patients with AEP and are almost always bilateral. *(Right)* Axial CECT of a patient with AEP shows patchy bilateral nonsegmental ground-glass opacities ➔ and a few small foci of consolidation ➔. A nonsegmental distribution of pulmonary opacities is typical of AEP.

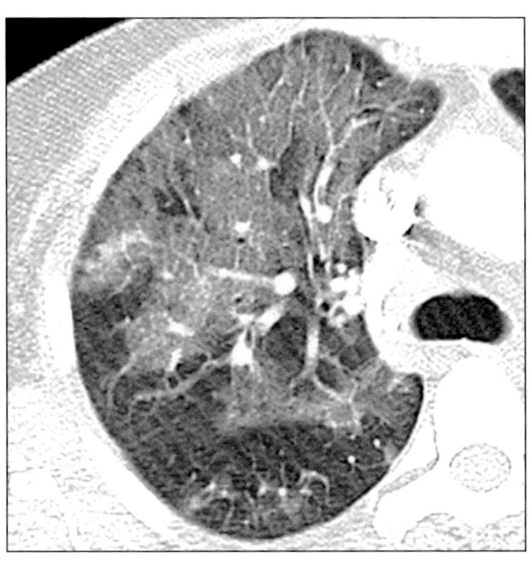

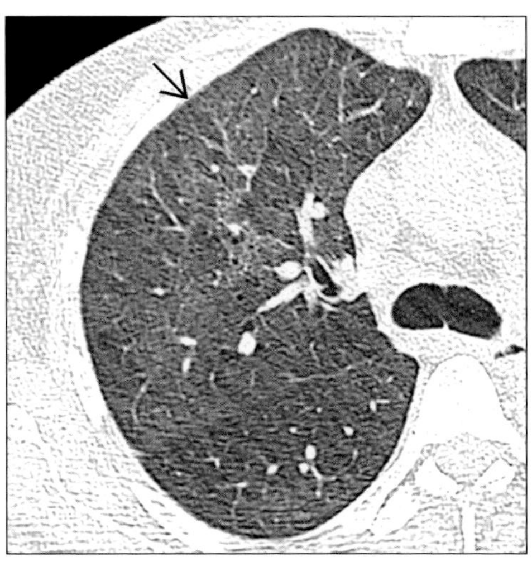

(Left) Axial CECT of a patient with AEP who presented with cough, fever, and dyspnea shows extensive ground-glass opacity in the right upper lobe. Bronchoalveolar lavage showed marked eosinophilia. *(Right)* Axial HRCT of the same patient 6 days later shows a dramatic response to corticosteroid therapy with mild residual ground-glass opacity ➔ in the right upper lobe. Patients with acute eosinophilic pneumonia typically exhibit a rapid clinical and imaging response to corticosteroid therapy.

CHRONIC EOSINOPHILIC PNEUMONIA

Key Facts

Terminology

- Chronic eosinophilic pneumonia (CEP)
- Idiopathic chronic condition characterized by alveolar filling & inflammatory infiltrate consisting largely of eosinophils

Imaging

- Radiography
  - Chronic peripheral upper lobe consolidations
- HRCT
  - Upper lobe predominant peripheral consolidations & ground-glass opacity
  - Nodular consolidation
  - "Crazy-paving" pattern (8%)
  - Small pleural effusions (10%)
- Evolution
  - Migratory consolidation (waxing & waning)
  - Recurrence: Same place, size, shape

Top Differential Diagnoses

- Cryptogenic organizing pneumonia (COP)
- Simple pulmonary eosinophilia (Löffler syndrome)
- Churg-Strauss syndrome
- Community-acquired pneumonia
- Adenocarcinoma
- Sarcoidosis
- Pulmonary infarcts
- Pulmonary alveolar proteinosis

Clinical Issues

- Blood eosinophilia common (90%)
- Rapid dramatic response to corticosteroids

Diagnostic Checklist

- Consider CEP in patient with chronic symptoms & peripheral upper lung zone consolidations

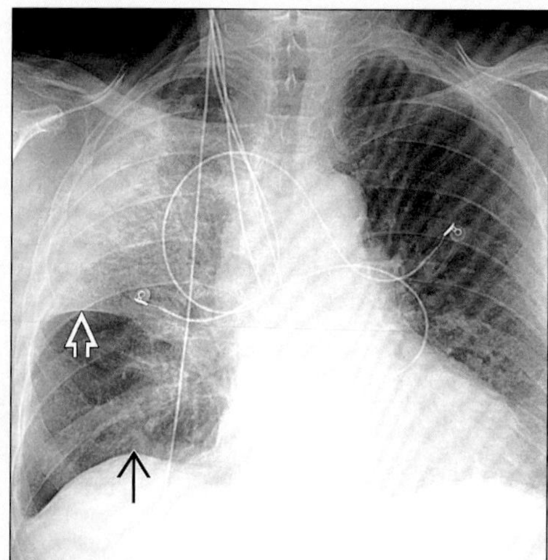

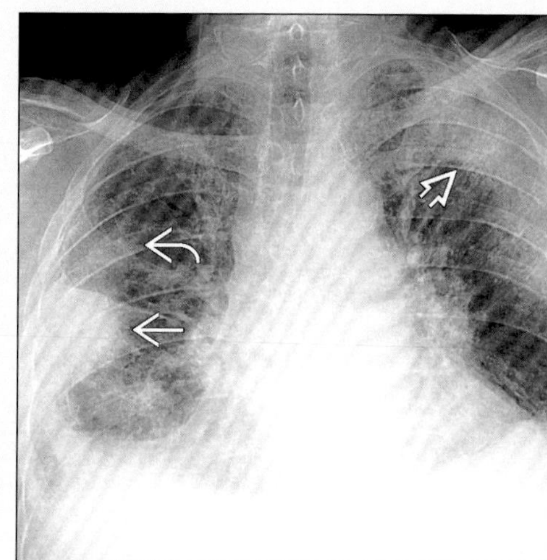

(Left) *AP chest radiograph of a patient with CEP shows a peripheral right upper lobe consolidation ➡ with medial hazy opacity and bibasilar ill-defined opacities →.* ***(Right)*** *AP chest radiograph of the same patient obtained several days later shows a new dense middle lobe consolidation ➡, and hazy left upper lobe ➡, and right basilar opacities. Note residual hazy opacity ➡ in the right upper lobe. The peripheral distribution and migratory nature of the airspace disease suggest CEP.*

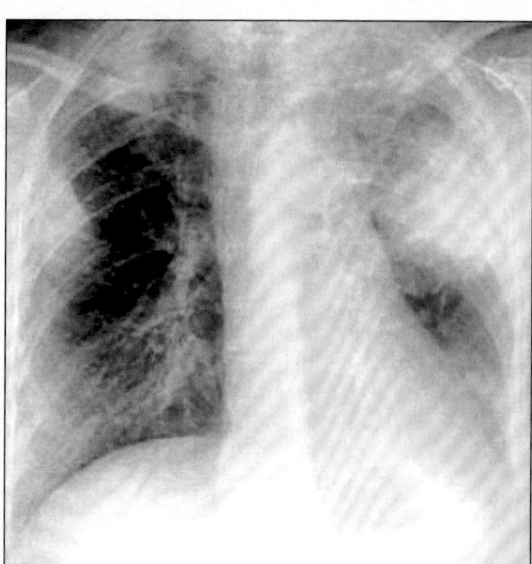

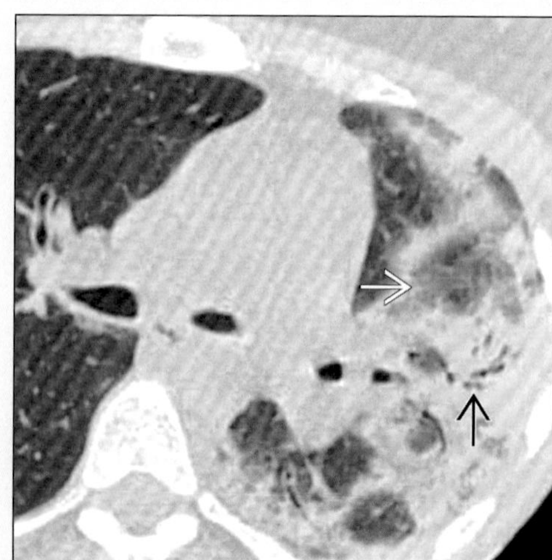

(Left) *AP chest radiograph of a patient with CEP shows bilateral peripheral mass-like consolidations predominantly affecting the upper lungs.* ***(Right)*** *Axial HRCT of the same patient shows a heterogeneous left lung consolidation with air bronchograms → and surrounding ground-glass opacity ➡. Consolidation is the primary radiographic and CT finding of CEP, but ground-glass opacity is a frequent associated feature. Ground-glass opacity may persist as consolidation begins to clear after initiation of therapy.*

CHRONIC EOSINOPHILIC PNEUMONIA

TERMINOLOGY

Abbreviations

- **Chronic eosinophilic pneumonia** (CEP)

Definitions

- Idiopathic chronic condition characterized by alveolar filling with **mixed inflammatory infiltrate** consisting largely of **eosinophils**

IMAGING

General Features

- Best diagnostic clue
  - Chronic peripheral upper lobe consolidation
- Location
  - Peripheral distribution (outer 2/3) of upper lobes
- Morphology
  - Consolidation predominates, often admixed with ground-glass opacities

Radiographic Findings

- Classic: Bilateral, nonsegmental, symmetric consolidations with peripheral & upper lobe distribution (25-50% of patients)

CT Findings

- Morphology
  - **Homogeneous consolidations** (100%)
  - **Ground-glass opacities** (90%)
  - Typically a **combination of both findings** (**consolidation > ground-glass opacity**)
    - May manifest as peripheral band-like opacities
    - May spare the subpleural lung parenchyma
  - Nodular consolidation (40%)
    - May exhibit peribronchovascular distribution
  - Interlobular septal thickening (20%)
  - "Crazy-paving" pattern (8%)
  - Rarely
    - Cavitation
    - Emphysema (affected patients are usually nonsmokers)
- Distribution
  - Bilateral (75%)
  - Craniocaudal
    - Upper lung zones (40%)
    - Lower lung zones (20%)
    - Variable (40%)
  - Axial
    - Peripheral (85%)
    - Variable (15%)
    - Central (0%)
- Associated findings
  - Small pleural effusions (10%)
  - Mediastinal lymphadenopathy
    - < 2 cm short axis diameter (10%)
- **Evolution**
  - Migratory consolidation with waxing & waning in different lung regions simultaneously (25%)
  - Early (< 1 month duration) consolidation tends to be peripheral
  - Late (> 1 month duration) consolidation becomes patchy & may spare lung edge
  - **Resolution** (or natural evolution) of consolidations tends to be from lateral to medial
    - Last portion of consolidation to resolve is medial border of peripheral consolidation, leaves bands or lines of consolidated lung that parallel chest wall ("wisp of smoke")
  - Relapse or recurrence: Same place, same size, same shape

Imaging Recommendations

- Best imaging tool
  - Chest radiography usually sufficient for initial evaluation & follow-up
  - CT may be helpful in cases lacking classic radiographic features
    - Characteristic peripheral distribution more frequently detected with CT (85-100%) than with radiography (60%)
- Protocol advice
  - Unenhanced thin-section chest CT

DIFFERENTIAL DIAGNOSIS

Cryptogenic Organizing Pneumonia (COP)

- May exhibit identical imaging appearance
- Distribution
  - More often peribronchial & peribronchovascular in distribution than CEP
  - Both peripheral, but lower lobe distribution in COP, upper lobe in CEP
- Morphology
  - COP more likely to exhibit nodules, masses, or predominant reticular opacities
  - Bronchial dilatation more common in COP
  - Reverse halo sign uncommon in CEP
- Responsive to steroid therapy, but slower resolution than CEP; also prone to relapse after discontinuation of steroids
- Not as strongly associated with peripheral eosinophilia as CEP
  - Bronchoalveolar lavage fluid usually shows preponderance of lymphocytes

Simple Pulmonary Eosinophilia (Löffler Syndrome)

- Fleeting opacities that change over days
- Opacities also peripheral in distribution
- Usually self-limited process

Churg-Strauss Syndrome

- Systemic symptoms: Asthma, skin lesions, peripheral neuropathy
- Less strongly associated with peripheral consolidation than CEP

Community-acquired Pneumonia

- Patient often treated for pneumonia before CEP suspected clinically or radiographically
- White blood cell differential & sputum cultures important

Adenocarcinoma

- Can exhibit identical imaging appearance
- Consolidation does not improve, continues to worsen
- Not associated with eosinophilia

CHRONIC EOSINOPHILIC PNEUMONIA

Sarcoidosis

- Can occasionally mimic CEP with predominantly peripheral distribution
- Not associated with eosinophilia
- Nodularity, typically centrilobular & peribronchovascular
- Large mass-like areas of consolidation, also typically upper lobe predominant

Pulmonary Infarcts

- Peripheral distribution may mimic CEP, but infarcts are usually more discrete & less confluent than CEP
- Lower lobe predominant & often wedge-shaped with central ground-glass opacity

Pulmonary Alveolar Proteinosis

- May manifest with chronic consolidation
- Distribution central, not peripheral
- More likely to exhibit "crazy-paving" pattern

PATHOLOGY

General Features

- Etiology
  - Pathogenesis unknown but speculated to represent hypersensitivity reaction to unknown antigen
    - History of asthma or atopy in 50% of patients
    - 90% of patients are nonsmokers (smoking may be protective)
  - Important to exclude eosinophilic response from drug reactions or parasitic infections
- Associated abnormalities
  - May precede rheumatoid arthritis
  - May be associated with cutaneous T-cell lymphoma
  - May develop following radiation therapy for breast cancer

Microscopic Features

- Eosinophil derived from bone marrow; transient half-life of 18 hours
- Alveolar flooding with inflammatory infiltrate containing preponderance of eosinophils
  - Infiltration of alveolar septa
  - Eosinophilic microabscesses common
- Mild inflammatory infiltrate may also be seen in perivascular spaces
- Bronchial abnormalities indicative of coexistent asthma may be present

Laboratory Findings

- **Blood eosinophilia common (90%)**, although its absence does not exclude diagnosis
- Increased eosinophils (> 25%) in bronchoalveolar lavage fluid, often > 40%
- Pulmonary function tests
  - Obstructive pattern (33%)
  - Restrictive pattern (33%)
  - Normal (33%)

CLINICAL ISSUES

Presentation

- Most common signs/symptoms
  - Insidious onset of fever (often nocturnal), malaise, weight loss, dyspnea, & dry cough
  - Asthma (50%), chronic sinusitis (20%)
  - Hemoptysis & chest pain uncommon
  - Much less fulminant presentation than that observed with acute eosinophilic pneumonia
  - Average duration of symptoms 7.7 months before diagnosis
    - Usually at least 1 month
- Clinical profile
  - 90% of affected patients are nonsmokers
  - Diagnosis of CEP often not suspected clinically or radiographically before peripheral eosinophilia detected
  - Clinician often suspects & treats pneumonia (multiple times) before diagnosis of CEP made
  - Bronchoalveolar lavage fluid demonstrating increased eosinophils may be helpful in difficult cases
  - Lung biopsy rarely indicated

Demographics

- Age
  - Peak incidence in 5th decade
    - Wide age range (18-80 years)
- Gender
  - M:F = 1:2
- Epidemiology
  - CEP accounts for approximately 2.5% of cases of chronic diffuse lung disease

Natural History & Prognosis

- Symptoms usually present months before diagnosis
- Rapid & dramatic response to corticosteroid therapy
- Most patients relapse after steroid withdrawal (80%)

Treatment

- < 10% have spontaneous resolution
- **Rapid response to corticosteroid therapy**
  - Resolution in 1 week (70%)
- Relapse extremely common once steroids tapered
  - Within 4 years (50%)
  - Within 6 years (70%)
  - Within 10 years (80%)
  - May require prolonged treatment: Months or years

DIAGNOSTIC CHECKLIST

Consider

- CEP in patient with chronic symptoms & peripheral upper lung zone consolidations

Image Interpretation Pearls

- Review of prior imaging studies often suggests diagnosis: Chronic slowly evolving consolidation unchanged for weeks to months

SELECTED REFERENCES

1. Katz U et al: Pulmonary eosinophilia. Clin Rev Allergy Immunol. 34(3):367-71, 2008
2. Alam M et al: Chronic eosinophilic pneumonia: a review. South Med J. 100(1):49-53, 2007
3. Marchand E et al: Idiopathic chronic eosinophilic pneumonia. Semin Respir Crit Care Med. 27(2):134-41, 2006

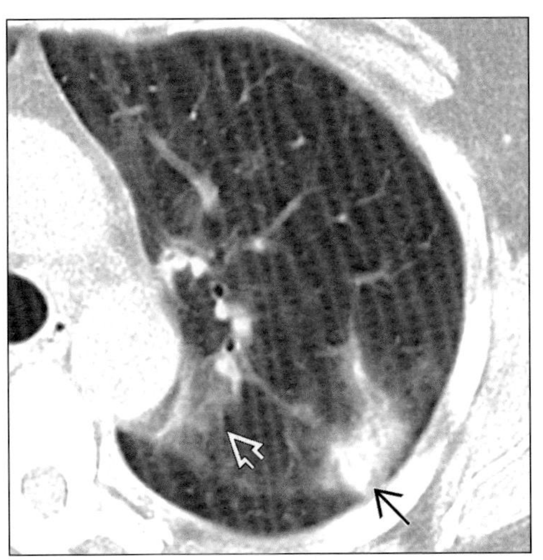

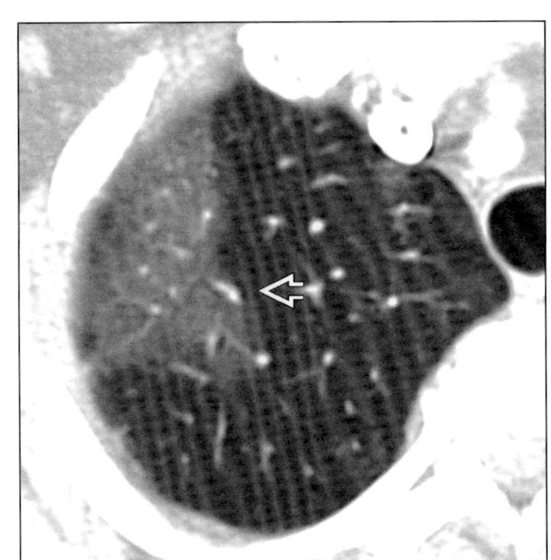

(Left) *Axial HRCT of a patient with CEP shows a peripheral nodular left upper lobe consolidation ➔ and adjacent patchy ground-glass opacities ➔. Consolidation in CEP may be focal, nodular, or diffuse and extensive.* ***(Right)*** *Axial HRCT of a patient with CEP shows peripheral ground-glass opacity ➔ in the right upper lobe. Note visualization and preservation of underlying pulmonary architecture. Ground-glass opacity in CEP may reflect developing or clearing pulmonary consolidation.*

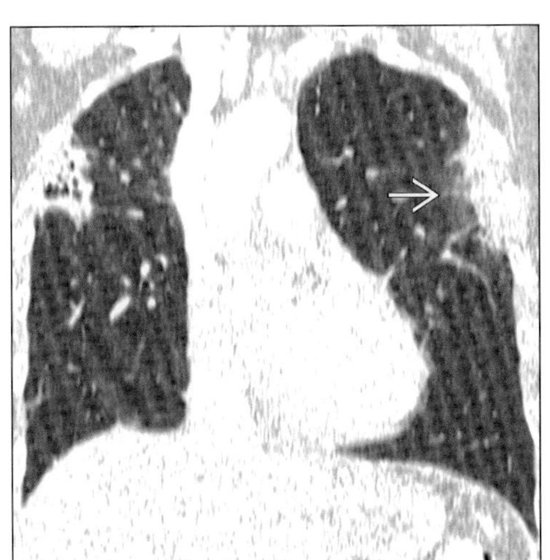

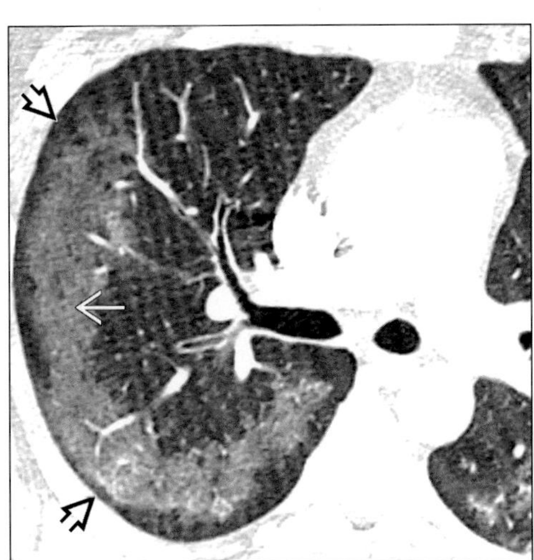

(Left) *Coronal NECT of a patient with CEP shows bilateral peripheral upper lung zone consolidations with a small amount of adjacent ground-glass opacity ➔. CEP is typically bilateral but may be asymmetric as in this patient.* ***(Right)*** *Axial CECT of a patient with CEP shows bilateral peripheral ground-glass opacities ➔ with exquisite demonstration of subpleural sparing ➔, a finding that can also be seen in nonspecific interstitial pneumonia and alveolar hemorrhage.*

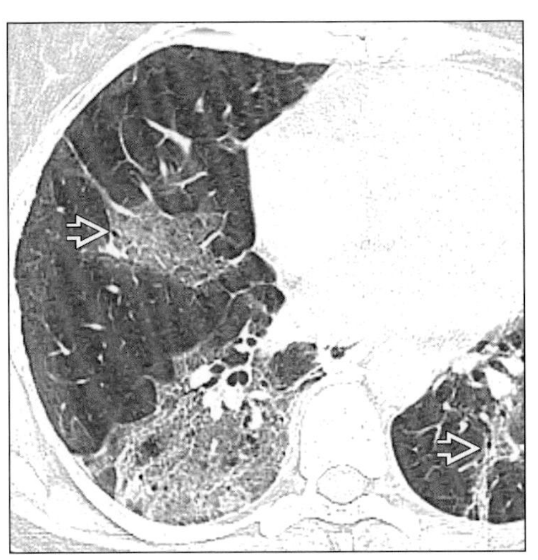

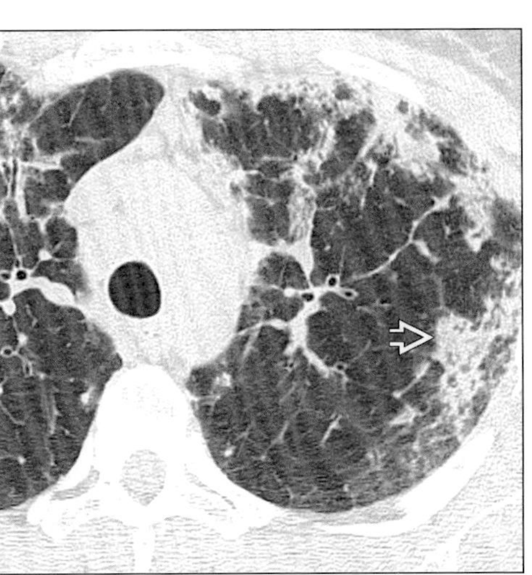

(Left) *Axial HRCT of a patient with CEP shows bilateral patchy ground-glass opacities with superimposed septal thickening, resulting in a "crazy-paving" pattern ➔. This finding is much less commonly seen in patients with CEP than consolidation and ground-glass opacity.* ***(Right)*** *Axial NECT of a patient with CEP shows bilateral upper lobe peribronchial peripheral consolidations ➔. Peribronchial distribution of airspace disease may mimic CT findings of cryptogenic organizing pneumonia.*

HYPEREOSINOPHILIC SYNDROME

Key Facts

Terminology

- Hypereosinophilic syndrome (HES)
- Rare idiopathic disorder characterized by overproduction of eosinophils with subsequent infiltration of & damage to multiple organs
- Diagnostic criteria
  - Sustained absolute eosinophil count ≥ 1,500 cells/mL for at least 6 months
  - Evidence of end-organ damage
  - Exclusion of other causes of eosinophilia
- Lungs involved in approximately 40% of patients

Imaging

- Transient hazy opacities or consolidations
- Small nodules: Few mm to 1 cm, most exhibit ground-glass opacity halos, peripheral predominance
- Septal thickening
- Pleural effusion in < 50%

Top Differential Diagnoses

- Eosinophilic pneumonia
- Restrictive cardiomyopathy
- Cardiogenic pulmonary edema

Pathology

- Eosinophilic infiltration of lung
- Tissue necrosis

Clinical Issues

- Symptoms/signs
  - Cough, dyspnea, wheezing
- Most patients between 20-50 years (mean: 33 years)
- M:F = 7:1
- Cardiac involvement is main cause of morbidity & mortality
- Overall prognosis poor
- Treatment: Corticosteroids initial treatment of choice

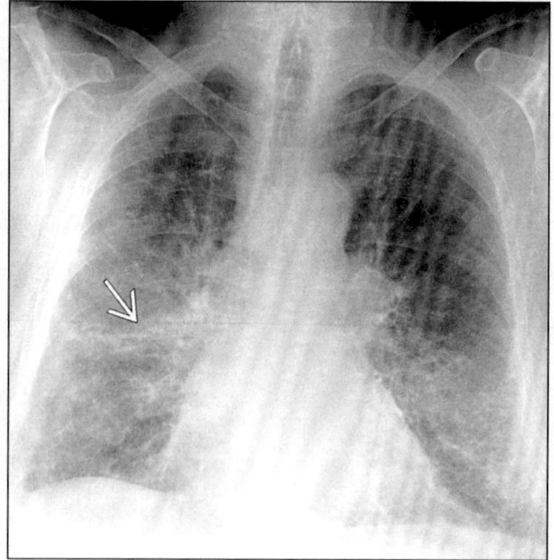

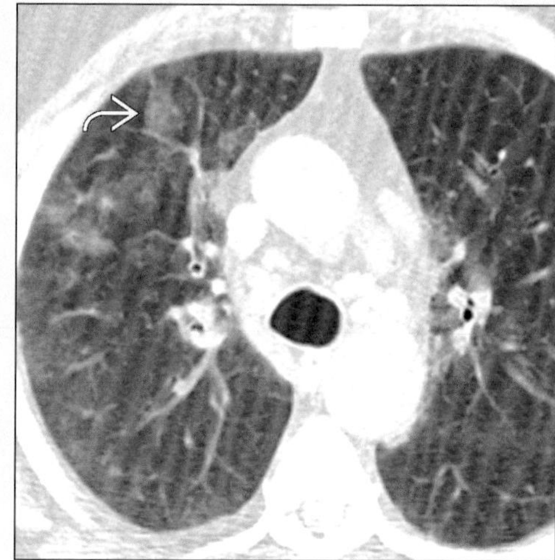

(Left) *PA chest radiograph of a patient with HES shows patchy peribronchial → and peripheral opacities. The radiographic findings of hypereosinophilic syndrome are very nonspecific and frequently mimic those of cardiogenic pulmonary edema.* ***(Right)*** *Axial NECT of a patient with HES shows patchy bilateral foci of ground-glass opacity →. Ground-glass opacities in patients with hypereosinophilic syndrome usually exhibit a variable distribution throughout the lungs.*

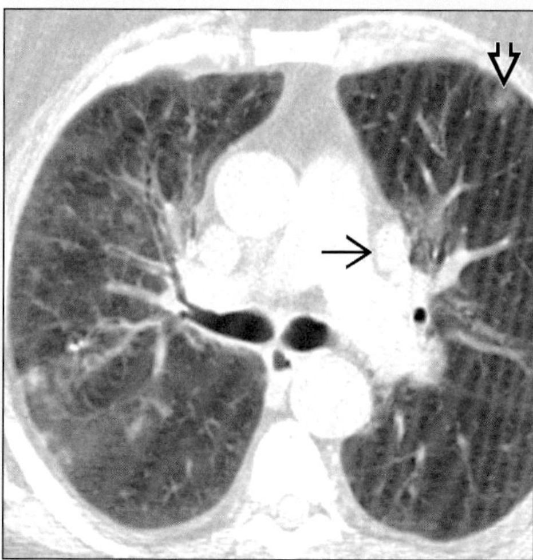

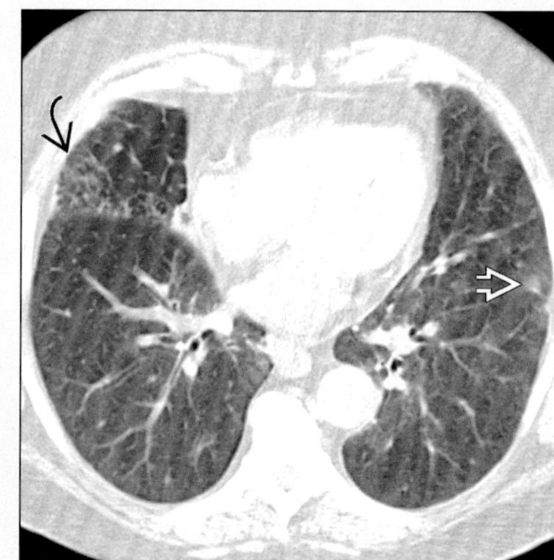

(Left) *Axial NECT of a patient with HES shows scattered small lung nodules → surrounded by halos of ground-glass opacity and a few scattered ground-glass opacities. There is also mild mediastinal lymph node enlargement →.* ***(Right)*** *Axial NECT of a patient with HES shows peripheral reticulation → in the right middle lobe, a poorly defined nodule → in the left lower lobe, and scattered ground-glass opacities. CT manifestations of HES are typically nonspecific.*

HYPEREOSINOPHILIC SYNDROME

TERMINOLOGY

Abbreviations

- **Hypereosinophilic syndrome (HES)**

Synonyms

- Hypereosinophilia, acquired hypereosinophilia

Definitions

- Rare idiopathic disorder characterized by **overproduction of eosinophils** with subsequent **infiltration of & damage to multiple organs**
  - **Diagnostic criteria**
    - Sustained absolute eosinophil count ≥ 1,500 cells/mL for at least 6 months
    - Evidence of end-organ damage
    - Exclusion of other causes of eosinophilia
- Heart & CNS most commonly involved
- Lungs involved in approximately 40% of patients

IMAGING

General Features

- Best diagnostic clue
  - **Chronic blood eosinophilia with lung nodules & ground-glass opacities**

Radiographic Findings

- Radiography
  - Transient hazy opacities or consolidations
  - Cardiac involvement
    - Cardiomegaly
    - Pulmonary edema
    - Pleural effusion

CT Findings

- HRCT
  - **Small nodules**
    - Few mm to 1 cm
    - Most exhibit ground-glass opacity halos
    - Peripheral predominance
  - **Ground-glass opacities**
    - Variable distribution
  - Septal thickening
    - Variable distribution
  - Pleural effusion in < 50%

Imaging Recommendations

- Best imaging tool
  - Chest radiographs usually show findings of pulmonary edema with extensive heart involvement

DIFFERENTIAL DIAGNOSIS

Eosinophilic Pneumonia

- May exhibit blood eosinophilia
  - Does not meet criteria for HES
- Often associated with asthma
- Acute eosinophilic pneumonia associated with drug reaction or cigarette smoking
- May be manifestation of parasitic infection

Restrictive Cardiomyopathy

- May exhibit radiographic findings of heart failure
- Other causes of myocardial infiltration
- Does not meet criteria for HES

Cardiogenic Pulmonary Edema

- No blood eosinophilia
- Ischemic heart disease most common cause
- CT: Small lung nodules not typical

PATHOLOGY

Gross Pathologic & Surgical Features

- Endocardial fibrosis
  - Valvular damage leading to regurgitation
  - Mural thrombosis from akinetic or hypokinetic segments

Microscopic Features

- **Eosinophilic infiltration of lung**
- Tissue necrosis
- Bronchoalveolar lavage: Eosinophils may exceed 70%

CLINICAL ISSUES

Presentation

- Most common signs/symptoms
  - Cough
  - Dyspnea
  - Wheezing
- Other signs/symptoms
  - Congestive heart failure
    - Decreased breath sounds & dullness to percussion
    - Peripheral edema

Demographics

- Age
  - Most patients between 20-50 years (mean: 33 years)
- Gender
  - M:F = 7:1

Natural History & Prognosis

- Cardiac involvement is main cause of morbidity & mortality
- Overall prognosis poor

Treatment

- Corticosteroids are initial treatment of choice
  - 50-70% of patients initially respond
  - High rate of relapse while on treatment
- Interferon-α & hydroxyurea: 2nd-line agents
- Cytotoxic drugs reserved for patients failing other treatments

SELECTED REFERENCES

1. Peros-Golubicić T et al: Hypereosinophilic syndrome: diagnosis and treatment. Curr Opin Pulm Med. 13(5):422-7, 2007
2. Kang EY et al: Pulmonary involvement of idiopathic hypereosinophilic syndrome: CT findings in five patients. J Comput Assist Tomogr. 21(4):612-5, 1997
3. Slabbynck H et al: Idiopathic hypereosinophilic syndrome-related pulmonary involvement diagnosed by bronchoalveolar lavage. Chest. 101(4):1178-80, 1992
4. Spry CJ et al: Clinical features of fifteen patients with the hypereosinophilic syndrome. Q J Med. 52(205):1-22, 1983

ALVEOLAR MICROLITHIASIS

Key Facts

Terminology

- Rare idiopathic disorder characterized by diffuse deposition of intraalveolar microliths

Imaging

- Dense lungs, out of proportion to symptoms
- Radiography
  - Dense lungs, obscure heart borders & diaphragm
  - Diffuse miliary calcifications: Alveolar microliths
  - "Black" pleura: Small subpleural cysts (5-10 mm)
- CT/HRCT
  - Micronodular discrete calcifications superimposed on ground-glass opacity
  - Calcifications more numerous along pleura, interlobular septa, & bronchovascular bundles
  - "Black" pleura correlates with subpleural cysts
  - Small apical bullae occasionally present
  - No lymphadenopathy

Top Differential Diagnoses

- Metastatic pulmonary calcification
- Dendritiform pulmonary ossification
- Silicosis
- Sarcoidosis

Pathology

- Up to 80% of alveoli contain calcospherites
- Interstitial fibrosis & pleural thickening

Clinical Issues

- Often asymptomatic (70%)
- Slow progression, may result in respiratory or cardiac failure

Diagnostic Checklist

- Consider microlithiasis in patients with dense or calcified lungs & mild symptoms

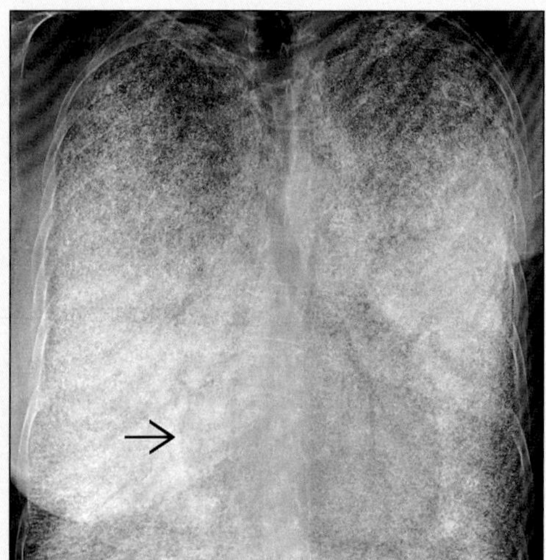

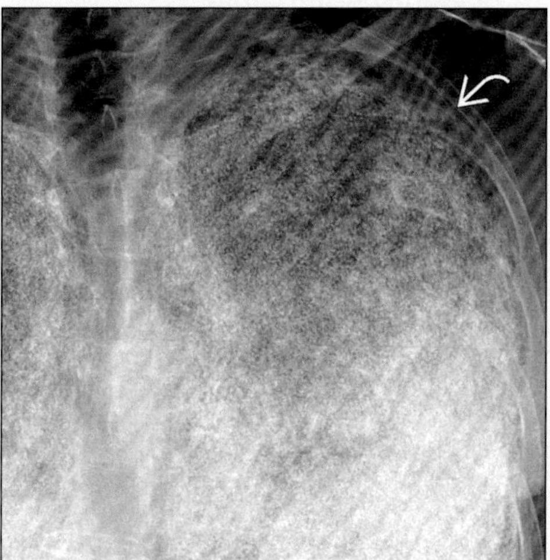

(Left) *PA chest radiograph of a patient with pulmonary alveolar microlithiasis shows diffuse bilateral pulmonary calcification and a "lucent" mediastinum ⇒ produced by surrounding alveolar calcification. (Courtesy J. Donohoo, MD.)* ***(Right)*** *PA chest radiograph (coned to the left upper lobe) of the same patient shows characteristic sandstorm calcification, visualization of individual calcospherites, and the black pleura sign ➡ thought to result from subpleural lung cysts. (Courtesy J. Donohoo, MD.)*

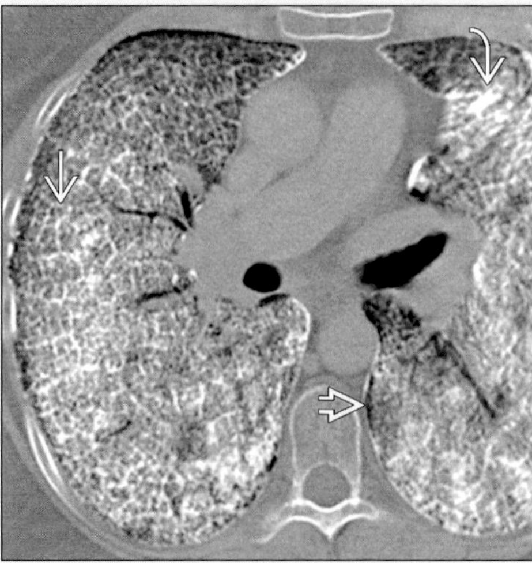

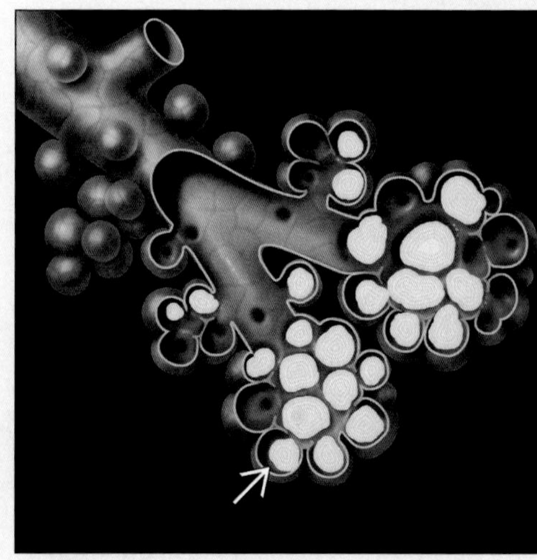

(Left) *Axial NECT (bone window) of the same patient shows diffuse pulmonary ground-glass opacity, dense calcification ➡ in the right lower and left upper lobes, and small subpleural lung cysts ➡. Typical distribution of calcification results in interlobular septal thickening and intralobular reticulation ➡. (Courtesy J. Donohoo, MD.)* ***(Right)*** *Graphic shows laminated calcospherites ➡ in the alveolar spaces. Individual calcospherites stay confined to the alveolar space and do not aggregate.*

ALVEOLAR MICROLITHIASIS

TERMINOLOGY

Synonyms

- Pulmonary alveolar microlithiasis

Definitions

- Rare disorder of unknown etiology characterized by diffuse bilateral deposition of intraalveolar microliths

IMAGING

General Features

- Best diagnostic clue
  - Dense lungs, out of proportion to symptoms
- Location
  - Diffuse but more pronounced in dorsal & inferior aspects of lung

Radiographic Findings

- Radiography
  - Lungs extremely dense: May obscure mediastinum & diaphragm or result in **"lucent" mediastinum**
  - **Diffuse miliary calcifications** (so-called "sandstorm") due to **individual microliths**
    - Symmetric increased density at lung bases; often obscures diaphragm & mediastinal borders
  - **"Black" pleura sign**: Small subpleural cysts (5-10 mm)

CT Findings

- HRCT
  - Ground-glass opacity early
  - Micronodular discrete calcifications superimposed on ground-glass opacity
  - Distribution of micronodular calcifications
    - Peripheral & basilar
    - Anterolateral lingula & middle lobe, anterior aspects of upper lobes
  - **Calcifications** more numerous along **pleura**, **interlobular septa**, & **bronchovascular bundles**
  - Small apical bullae occasionally present
  - **"Black" pleura** correlates with subpleural cysts
  - No lymphadenopathy

Other Modality Findings

- Bone scan
  - Variable uptake with bone-seeking radionuclides

DIFFERENTIAL DIAGNOSIS

Metastatic Pulmonary Calcification

- Associated with hypercalcemia
- Upper lung centrilobular ground-glass or calcification; less sharply defined than microlithiasis

Dendritiform Pulmonary Ossification

- Associated with pulmonary fibrosis
- Dendritic ossification in lower lobes

Silicosis

- Silicotic nodules may calcify
- Nodules more profuse in upper lung zones, may lead to progressive massive fibrosis
- Lymphadenopathy absent in microlithiasis

Sarcoidosis

- Perilymphatic micronodules, rarely calcify
- Nodules more profuse in upper lung zones, may lead to peribronchial fibrosis
- Lymphadenopathy absent in microlithiasis

PATHOLOGY

General Features

- Etiology
  - Increased alkalinity in intraalveolar secretions may promote precipitation of calcium phosphates & carbonates
- Genetics
  - Familial autosomal recessive (50%)
- Associated abnormalities
  - Microliths also reported in lumbar sympathetic chain & testes

Microscopic Features

- Up to 80% of alveoli contain calcospherites
- Interstitial fibrosis & pleural thickening

CLINICAL ISSUES

Presentation

- Most common signs/symptoms
  - **Often asymptomatic (70%) in spite of severe imaging abnormalities**
  - **Normal serum calcium & phosphorus**
- Other signs/symptoms
  - Microliths may be recovered from bronchoalveolar lavage fluid or transbronchial biopsy
  - Pulmonary function tests
    - Normal or mild restriction early

Demographics

- Age
  - All ages (average: 35 years)
- Gender
  - Slight female predominance in familial cases
  - Slight male predominance in sporadic cases
- Epidemiology
  - **More prevalent in Turkey (33% of world's cases)**

Natural History & Prognosis

- Slow progression may eventually result in respiratory or cardiac failure

Treatment

- No known treatment
- Lung transplantation for end-stage lung disease

DIAGNOSTIC CHECKLIST

Consider

- Microlithiasis in patients with dense or calcified lungs & mild symptoms

SELECTED REFERENCES

1. Siddiqui NA et al: Best cases from the AFIP: pulmonary alveolar microlithiasis. Radiographics. 31(2):585-90, 2011

METASTATIC PULMONARY CALCIFICATION

Key Facts

Imaging

- Best clue: High density or calcified upper lung zone opacities in patient with chronic renal failure
- Radiography
  - Low sensitivity unless severe involvement
  - Diffuse or focal, ill-defined, nodular & linear opacities that may mimic infection or edema
  - Upper lobes most commonly involved
  - Findings of renal failure: Cardiomegaly, renal osteodystrophy
- CT/HRCT
  - Centrilobular mulberry-shaped, amorphous calcifications (3-10 mm)
  - Nonspecific ground-glass opacities/consolidations
  - Small vessel calcification: Chest wall, heart, lung
- Nuclear medicine
  - Bone scan: Uptake in pulmonary opacities confirmatory

Top Differential Diagnoses

- Silicosis
- Sarcoidosis
- Alveolar microlithiasis
- Dendritiform pulmonary ossification

Pathology

- Most commonly due to chronic renal failure

Clinical Issues

- Gradual onset dyspnea; occasional sudden onset of symptoms with rapid fulminant course
- Prognosis: Varies from stable incidental finding to fulminant life-threatening course

Diagnostic Checklist

- Suspect metastatic calcification in hemodialysis patients with chronic upper lung zone opacities

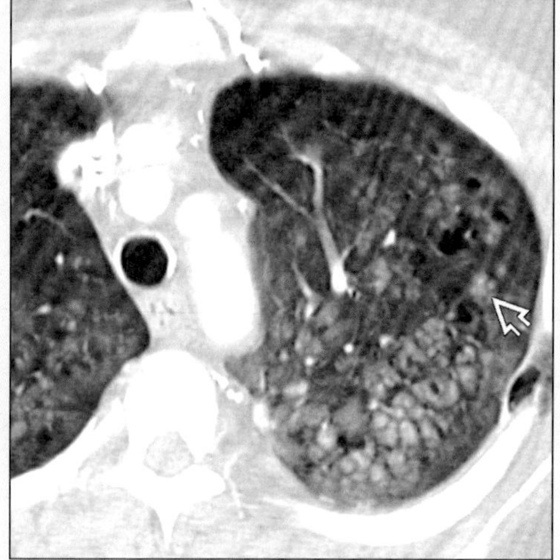
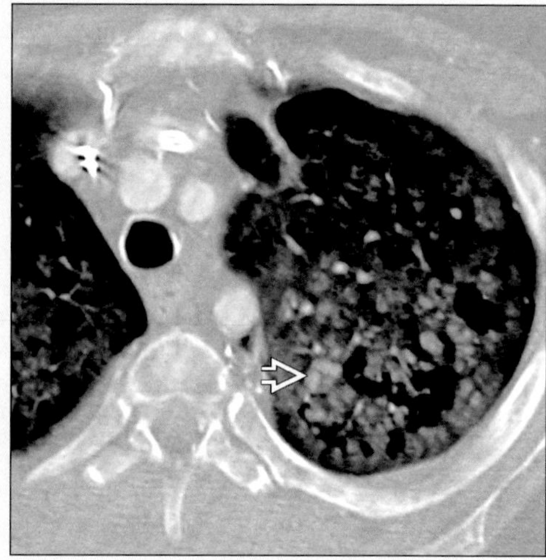

(Left) *Axial CECT of a patient with metastatic pulmonary calcification shows centrilobular mulberry-like opacities ➲ related to parenchymal calcification and scattered areas of centrilobular emphysema.* ***(Right)*** *Axial CECT (bone window) of the same patient show the high-attenuation nodules ➲, consistent with calcification. The centrilobular location of metastatic pulmonary calcification is typical. Upper lung predominance is common, likely due to the alkaline environment in the lung apices.*

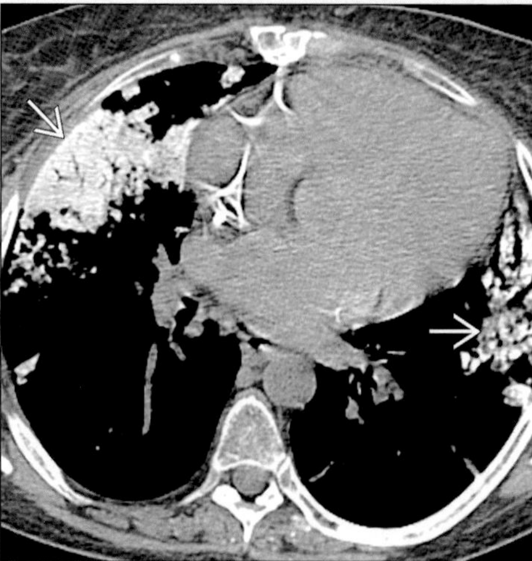
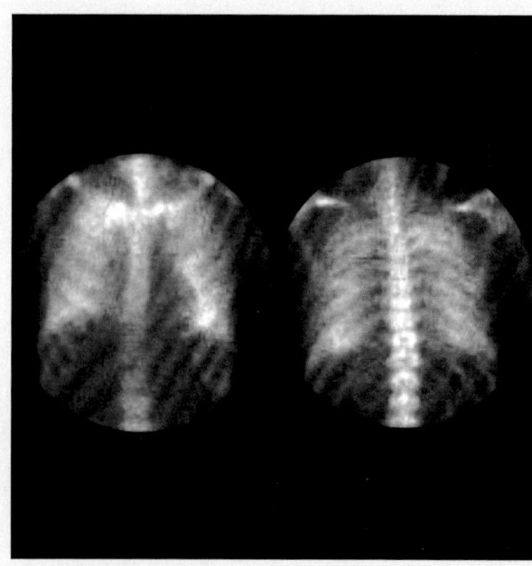

(Left) *Axial NECT of a patient with metastatic calcification shows densely calcified consolidations ➔ in the anterior aspects of the lungs.* ***(Right)*** *Frontal and posterior images from a bone scan of a patient with metastatic calcification show diffuse uptake in the lungs. Skeletal nuclear scintigraphy is helpful for establishing the diagnosis of metastatic calcification in cases in which HRCT findings are indeterminate.*

METASTATIC PULMONARY CALCIFICATION

TERMINOLOGY

Synonyms

- Pulmonary calcinosis

Definitions

- Calcium deposition in normal lung tissue

IMAGING

General Features

- Best diagnostic clue
  - High density or calcified opacities in upper lung zones in patient with chronic renal failure
- Location
  - Tropism for tissues with relatively alkaline pH
    - Upper lung zones, stomach, renal medulla

Radiographic Findings

- Radiography
  - **Low sensitivity** unless severe
  - Diffuse or focal, ill-defined, nodular & linear opacities
    - May mimic pneumonia, aspiration, or edema
  - Upper lobes most commonly involved
  - Cardiomegaly from fluid overload
  - Renal osteodystrophy
  - Lytic brown tumors from hyperparathyroidism

CT Findings

- HRCT
  - More sensitive than chest radiography for detection of pulmonary opacities & calcification
  - **Centrilobular mulberry-shaped, amorphous calcifications (3-10 mm)**
  - Nonspecific ground-glass opacities or consolidations
  - Small vessel calcification: Chest wall, heart, lung

Nuclear Medicine Findings

- Bone scan
  - **Uptake in pulmonary opacities confirmatory**

Imaging Recommendations

- Best imaging tool
  - CT & bone scan sensitive for detection of calcium; CT useful for characterization of distribution

DIFFERENTIAL DIAGNOSIS

Silicosis

- Upper lobe nodules, better defined than in metastatic calcification
- Subpleural nodules, rare in metastatic calcification
- Occupational exposure history
- Calcified mediastinal & hilar lymphadenopathy, not seen in metastatic calcification

Sarcoidosis

- Nodules occasionally calcify, upper lobe predominant
- Peribronchial/subpleural distribution, not seen in metastatic calcification
- Lymphadenopathy not seen in metastatic calcification
- Sarcoidosis associated with hypercalcemia may result in metastatic pulmonary calcification

Alveolar Microlithiasis

- Smaller calcified nodules (1 mm)
- Diffuse disease, more severe in lower lobes
- Paraseptal emphysema

Dendritiform Pulmonary Ossification

- Dendritic ossification in lower lobes
  - Usually associated with pulmonary fibrosis

PATHOLOGY

General Features

- Etiology
  - **Hypercalcemic conditions**
    - Chronic renal failure (most common)
    - Hyperparathyroidism, hypervitaminosis D, milk-alkali syndrome, sarcoidosis
  - Physiology: Normally high V/Q ratio in upper lobes leads to alkaline pH (7.51)
    - Calcium less soluble in alkaline environment
- Associated abnormalities
  - Lungs, stomach, kidney, & heart most frequently involved

Microscopic Features

- Alveolar septal & vascular calcium deposition
- Fibrosis develops in more severe or longstanding cases

CLINICAL ISSUES

Presentation

- Most common signs/symptoms
  - Asymptomatic to slowly progressive respiratory failure
  - Gradual onset of dyspnea; occasional sudden onset of symptoms with rapid fulminant course
- Other signs/symptoms
  - With severe disease, restrictive pulmonary function & decreased DLCO

Natural History & Prognosis

- Varies from incidental finding that remains stable for years to fulminant life-threatening course
- May be reversible with correction of hypercalcemia
- Death usually due to cardiac involvement

Treatment

- Correction of hypercalcemia
- Treatment of underlying cause

DIAGNOSTIC CHECKLIST

Image Interpretation Pearls

- Suspect metastatic calcification in hemodialysis patients with chronic upper lung zone opacities
- Confirm diagnosis with HRCT or bone scan

SELECTED REFERENCES

1. Marchiori E et al: Consolidation with diffuse or focal high attenuation: computed tomography findings. J Thorac Imaging. 23(4):298-304, 2008

LYMPHANGIOLEIOMYOMATOSIS

Key Facts

Terminology
- Lymphangioleiomyomatosis (LAM)
- Rare interstitial lung disease characterized by proliferation of smooth muscle cells

Imaging
- Best clue: Diffuse, thin-walled lung cysts
- Radiography
  - Lung volumes normal to increased
  - Bilateral reticular or reticulonodular opacities
  - Interlobular septal thickening
- HRCT
  - Diffuse, thin-walled parenchymal cysts
  - Interlobular septal thickening
  - Patchy ground-glass opacities
  - Hilar & mediastinal lymphadenopathy
- LAM & TSC are indistinguishable on imaging
- Complications: Pneumothorax & chylous effusion

Top Differential Diagnoses
- Centrilobular emphysema
- Pulmonary Langerhans cell histiocytosis
- Lymphocytic interstitial pneumonia
- Idiopathic pulmonary fibrosis

Pathology
- Cysts & atypical smooth muscle (LAM) cells

Clinical Issues
- Symptoms/signs
  - Dyspnea, pneumothorax, cough
  - Chest pain, hemoptysis, wheezing
- Women of childbearing age

Diagnostic Checklist
- Consider LAM in women of childbearing age with numerous thin-walled lung cysts on HRCT

*(**Left**) PA chest radiograph of a woman with LAM shows bilateral basilar reticular opacities ➡. Reticular or reticulonodular opacities are present in 80-90% of patients with LAM. Radiographic abnormalities increase in conspicuity with progression of disease. (**Right**) Axial CECT of a patient with LAM demonstrates bilateral thin-walled lung cysts ➡ with normal intervening lung parenchyma. LAM cysts may be round, polygonal, or ovoid in morphology and are usually surrounded by normal lung.*

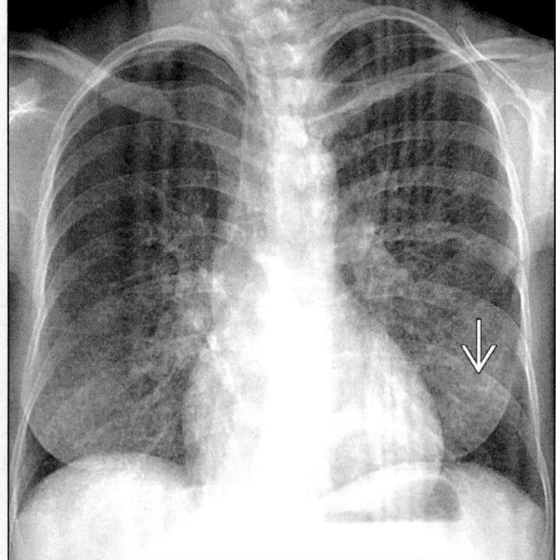

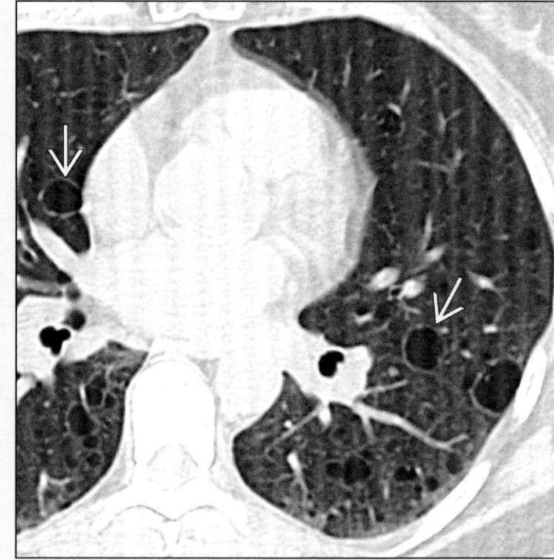

*(**Left**) Axial HRCT of a patient with LAM demonstrates diffuse bilateral thin-walled parenchymal cysts ➡ in the right lung and the visualized left lung. Although LAM cysts may be of different sizes, most range in size from 2-5 mm. (**Right**) Coronal HRCT of the same patient shows cysts ➡ in all lung zones. Although LAM cysts typically exhibit no zonal predominance, preferential involvement of the upper or lower lung zones has been reported.*

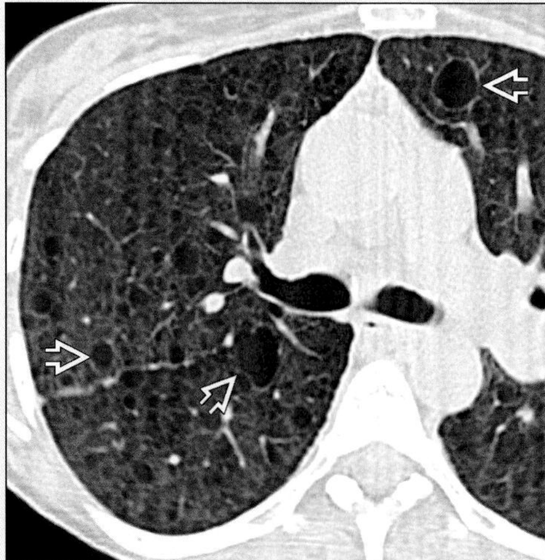

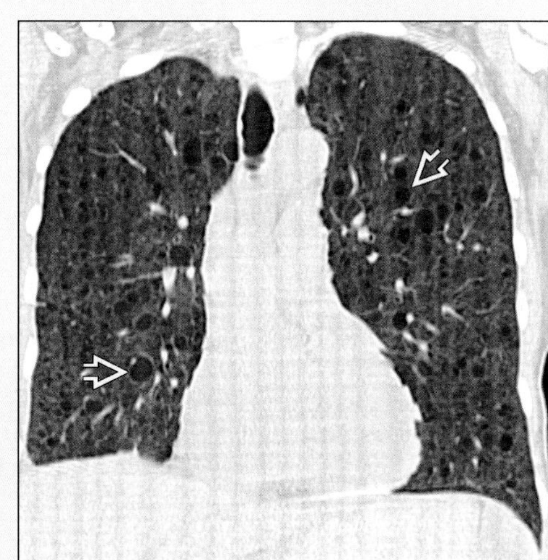

LYMPHANGIOLEIOMYOMATOSIS

TERMINOLOGY

Abbreviations

- Lymphangioleiomyomatosis (LAM)
- Tuberous sclerosis complex (TSC)

Definitions

- Rare interstitial lung disease characterized by **proliferation of smooth muscle cells** in lungs & lymphatic systems of the chest & retroperitoneum

IMAGING

General Features

- Best diagnostic clue
  - Diffuse, thin-walled lung cysts
- Size
  - Most 2-5 mm on HRCT
    - Cysts as large as 30 mm reported
- Morphology
  - Round, polygonal, ovoid

Radiographic Findings

- Radiography
  - May be normal in early disease
  - **Lung volumes normal to increased**
  - Bilateral **reticular or reticulonodular opacities**
    - 80-90% of cases
    - Visualization of superimposed cyst walls
    - Radiographic abnormalities become more conspicuous with progressive clinical deterioration
    - Various distributions described
      - No zonal predominance
      - Upper or lower lung zone predominance
  - Interlobular septal thickening
    - Likely represents dilated lymphatics
  - Pneumothorax
  - Chylous pleural effusions: Unilateral or bilateral

CT Findings

- NECT
  - **Pneumothorax**
    - Usually in combination with lung cysts
  - **Chylous pleural effusions**
    - Unilateral or bilateral
    - May exhibit low (fat) or high (proteinaceous material) attenuation
  - Hilar & mediastinal **lymphadenopathy**
  - Pericardial effusion
- HRCT
  - **Diffuse parenchymal cysts**
    - Thin walled
    - Most are uniform in size
    - Various morphologies
    - Various distributions described
      - No zonal predominance
      - Upper or lower lung zone predominance
    - **Normal intervening lung**
    - Increase in size & number of cysts with disease progression, may replace entire lung
  - Interlobular septal thickening
  - Patchy ground-glass opacities
    - May represent pulmonary hemorrhage
  - Occasional small nodules
  - LAM & TSC are indistinguishable on imaging

Imaging Recommendations

- Best imaging tool
  - HRCT to evaluate morphology, extent, & distribution of lung cysts
  - More sensitive than chest radiography for determination of extent of disease

DIFFERENTIAL DIAGNOSIS

Centrilobular Emphysema

- Preserved or increased lung volumes
- Reticular opacities on chest radiography
- Cystic changes
  - Irregular shapes
  - Imperceptible walls
  - Predominantly located in upper lung zones
- Affects men & women

Pulmonary Langerhans Cell Histiocytosis

- Preserved or increased lung volumes
- Reticular opacities on chest radiography
- Nodules & cysts
  - Predominantly located in upper lung zones
  - Spare lower lung zones
  - Cysts irregular in appearance
- Affects men & women

Lymphocytic Interstitial Pneumonia

- Normal lung volumes
- Basilar interlobular septal thickening on chest radiography
- Thin-walled cysts characteristic
- Nonspecific ground-glass opacity or consolidation
- Centrilobular & subpleural nodules
- Primarily affects women

Idiopathic Pulmonary Fibrosis

- Progressive decrease in lung volumes
- Bilateral basilar & subpleural reticular opacities, honeycomb lung
  - Adjacent lung parenchyma abnormal & distorted
- Affects men & women

PATHOLOGY

General Features

- Genetics
  - TSC results from mutation in 1 of 2 genes
    - *TSC1* or *TSC2* (chromosomes 9 & 16)
- Associated abnormalities
  - Small percentage of cases associated with TSC
  - Extrathoracic findings
    - Renal angiomyolipomas
    - Chylous ascites
    - Abdomen & pelvis lymphangioleiomyomas
    - Uterine leiomyomas
    - Lymphaticoureteric & lymphaticovenous connections

Staging, Grading, & Classification

- LAM histologic scoring system (LHS)
  - Total percentage of parenchyma affected by cysts & LAM cells
  - Strong correlation with overall patient survival
  - Survival at 10 years

- LHS-1 (1-25% involvement): 100%
- LHS-2 (25-50%): 75%
- LHS-3 (> 50%): < 53%

Gross Pathologic & Surgical Features

- Enlarged lungs
- Numerous cysts along visceral pleura & homogeneously throughout lung parenchyma
  - Cysts typically range in size from 0.5-2.0 cm
  - Parenchymal cysts may be filled with air or chylous/ serosanguineous fluid
- Involved lymph nodes appear white or pale tan
- Enlargement of thoracic duct & lymphatics

Microscopic Features

- Characterized by cysts & atypical smooth muscle cells (LAM cells)
- LAM cells are morphologically heterogeneous
  - Small & round, large & spindle-shaped, epithelioid
  - Varying amounts of eosinophilic cytoplasm
- LAM cells present in cyst walls & along pulmonary lymphatics
  - Infiltration of distal airways leads to narrowing, air-trapping, bullae, & pneumothoraces
  - Obstruction of lymphatics leads to chylous pleural effusions
  - Involvement of pulmonary vessels leads to hemosiderosis & hemoptysis
- Histologic features of sporadic LAM & LAM associated with TSC are almost indistinguishable
  - Multifocal micronodular pneumocyte hyperplasia (MMNPH) is only unique feature of TSC
    - Pathognomonic for TSC in patients with LAM
    - Nodules consisting of type 2 pneumocytes that proliferate along alveolar walls

CLINICAL ISSUES

Presentation

- Most common signs/symptoms
  - Dyspnea
  - Cough
  - Spontaneous pneumothorax
- Other signs/symptoms
  - Chest pain, hemoptysis, wheezing
  - Chylothorax, chyloptysis, chylous pericardial effusion

Demographics

- Age
  - Reproductive years
    - Mean age: 34 years
  - Postmenopausal
    - Hormonal replacement therapy
- Gender
  - Women exclusively
    - Few cases reported in men were in setting of TSC
- Epidemiology
  - 100 cases/year worldwide incidence
  - **1 case/1,000,000 persons prevalence** in United Kingdom, France, & United States

Natural History & Prognosis

- Pulmonary function & imaging findings determine progression
- Progressive deterioration of pulmonary function typical
  - Respiratory failure & cor pulmonale
- Recent studies have shown improved survival
  - 91% survival rate at 10 years
- Greater likelihood of more rapid disease progression
  - Cigarette smoking
  - Pregnancy following onset of symptoms
  - Progesterone treatment
- Predominant finding of cysts in biopsy specimens associated with poor prognosis

Treatment

- Pneumothorax
  - Higher recurrence rates with aspiration or intercostal drainage
  - Lower recurrence rates with pleural abrasion, pleurodesis, pleurectomy, thoracoscopic pleurodesis with long-term drainage, or bullectomy with pleurodesis
- Chylous pleural effusions
  - Thoracentesis, chemical pleurodesis, or parietal pleurectomy
- Hormonal therapy controversial
- **Lung transplantation**
  - Recent studies have shown improved survivals
    - 1 year: 100%
    - 2 years: 90%
    - 5 years: 69%

DIAGNOSTIC CHECKLIST

Consider

- LAM in women of childbearing age with numerous thin-walled lung cysts on HRCT

Image Interpretation Pearls

- Consider imaging abdomen & pelvis in patients with LAM to identify additional abnormalities associated with LAM & TSC

SELECTED REFERENCES

1. Avila NA et al: Imaging features of lymphangioleiomyomatosis: diagnostic pitfalls. AJR Am J Roentgenol. 196(4):982-6, 2011
2. Abbott GF et al: From the archives of the AFIP: lymphangioleiomyomatosis: radiologic-pathologic correlation. Radiographics. 25(3):803-28, 2005
3. Kirchner J et al: Pulmonary lymphangioleiomyomatosis: high-resolution CT findings. Eur Radiol. 9(1):49-54, 1999
4. Rappaport DC et al: Pulmonary lymphangioleiomyomatosis: high-resolution CT findings in four cases. AJR Am J Roentgenol. 152(5):961-4, 1989

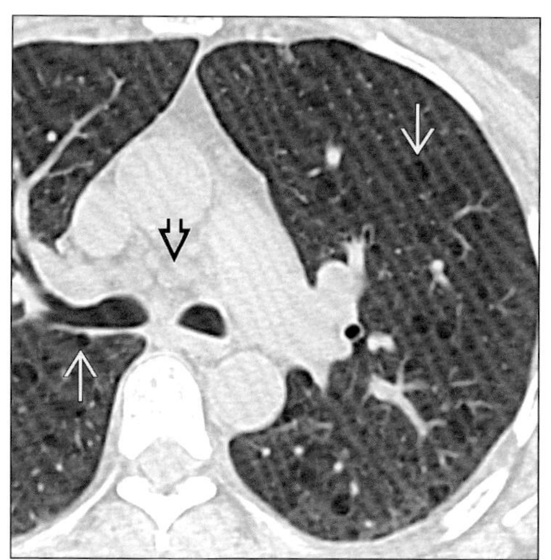

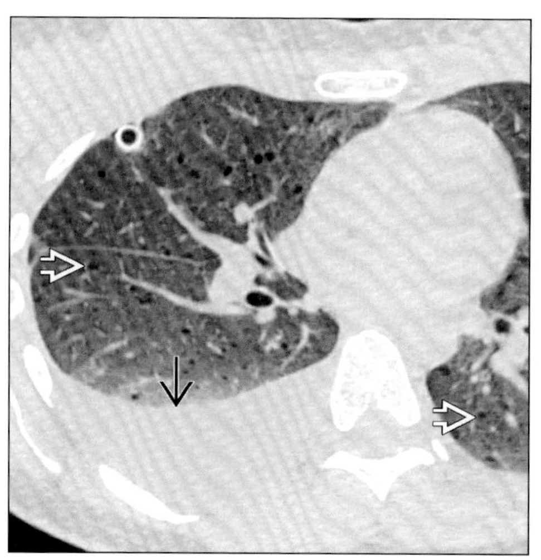

(Left) *Axial NECT of a patient with LAM shows diffuse thin-walled lung cysts ➔ and multiple conspicuous mediastinal lymph nodes ⇨. Lymphadenopathy is not an uncommon finding in patients with LAM.* ***(Right)*** *Axial NECT of a patient with LAM shows small thin-walled cysts ➔ in the right lung and visualized left lung and a moderate right chylous pleural effusion ⇨. Chylous pleural effusions may be hyperdense (secondary to proteinaceous material) or hypodense (secondary to fat) on CT.*

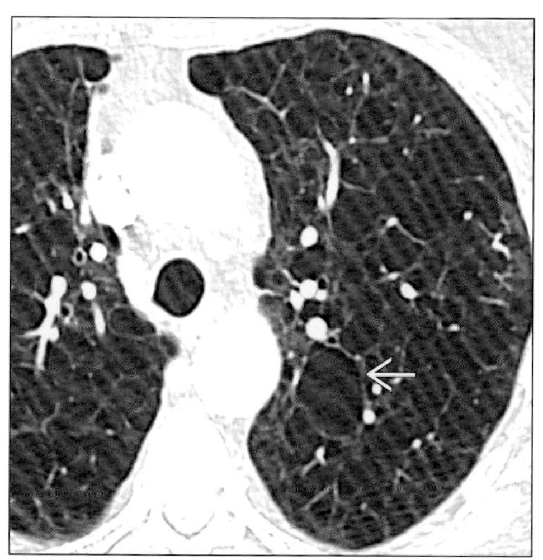

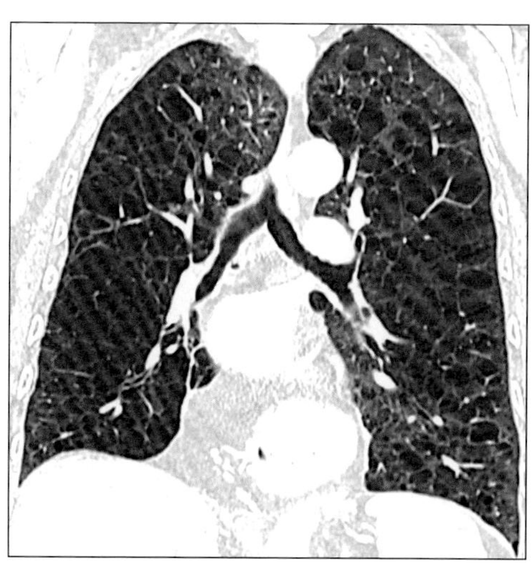

(Left) *Axial CECT of a patient with LAM demonstrates large thin-walled cysts ➔ throughout both lungs, with little normal intervening lung parenchyma identified.* ***(Right)*** *Coronal CECT of the same patient shows that the diffuse lung cysts have replaced a large amount of the normal lung parenchyma. LAM cysts typically increase in size and number with disease progression.*

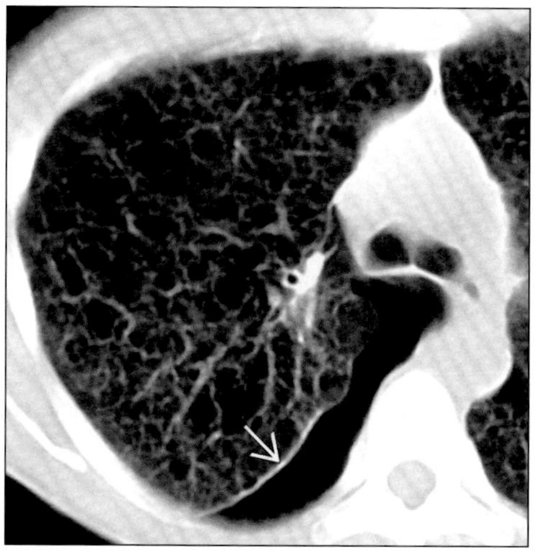

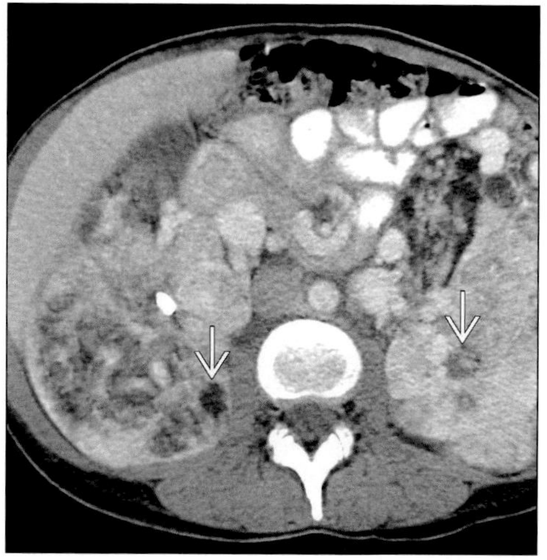

(Left) *Axial NECT of a patient with LAM demonstrates a small right pneumothorax ➔. Pneumothorax, a known potential complication of LAM, typically occurs in association with diffuse parenchymal cysts.* ***(Right)*** *Axial CECT through the upper abdomen of a patient with LAM demonstrates bilateral heterogeneous renal masses with multiple fat attenuation foci ➔. These lesions are consistent with angiomyolipomas, which are often associated with LAM.*

PULMONARY AMYLOIDOSIS

Key Facts

Terminology

- Heterogeneous group of disorders characterized by abnormal extracellular accumulation of insoluble fibrillar proteins

Imaging

- Tracheobronchial abnormalities
  - Airway wall thickening, mural/intraluminal nodules, submucosal calcification
- Parenchymal abnormalities
  - Nodules: Single or multiple, 0.5-5 cm, 20% calcify
  - Interstitial disease: Fine linear or reticulonodular opacities; honeycomb lung (uncommon); miliary nodules
- Lymphadenopathy
  - Stippled, diffuse, or eggshell calcifications
- Other: Cardiomegaly, pleural effusion/thickening, soft tissue deposition

Top Differential Diagnoses

- Tracheobronchial: Neoplasms, tracheobronchopathia osteochondroplastica, relapsing polychondritis
- Nodular: Lung cancer, metastases, granulomatous disease
- Interstitial lung disease: Idiopathic pulmonary fibrosis, scleroderma, rheumatoid arthritis
- Diffuse or multifocal lung calcification: Granulomatous disease, silicosis
- Lymphadenopathy: Sarcoidosis, tuberculosis
- Pleural thickening: Mesothelioma, metastases

Clinical Issues

- Amyloid light chain (AL): 10% of patients with multiple myeloma develop amyloidosis
- Amyloid A chain (AA): Familial Mediterranean fever & age-related (senile)
- Poor prognosis for diffuse disease: Survival < 2 years

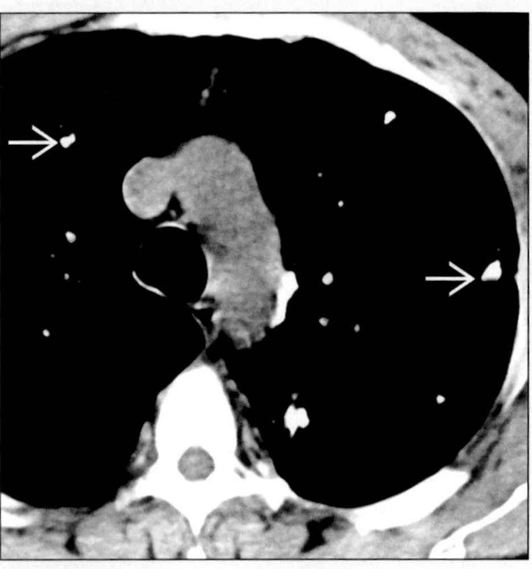

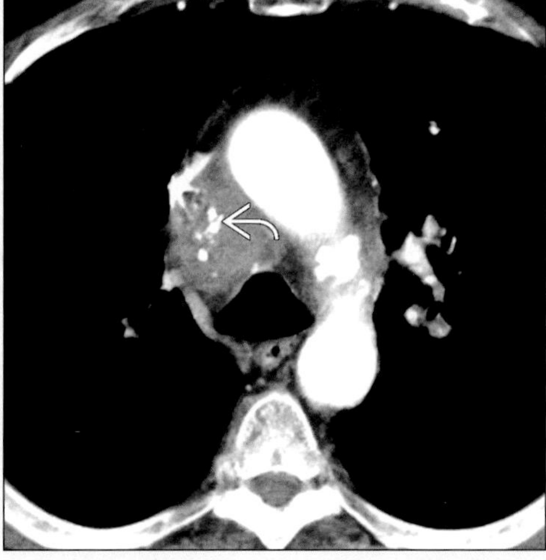

*(**Left**) Axial NECT of a patient with primary amyloidosis (AL) shows multiple randomly distributed calcified lung nodules ➡ of different sizes and lobulated borders. Calcified pulmonary nodules are present in 20% of cases of amyloidosis. (Courtesy E. Marchiori, MD.) (**Right**) Axial CECT of a 68-year-old patient with multiple myeloma shows right paratracheal lymphadenopathy containing multiple punctate calcifications ⮫. Lymphadenopathy is common in AL type amyloidosis with systemic disease.*

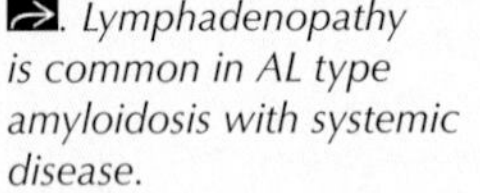

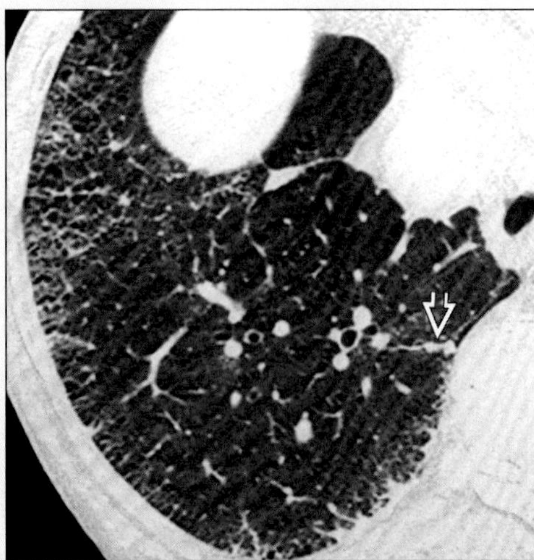

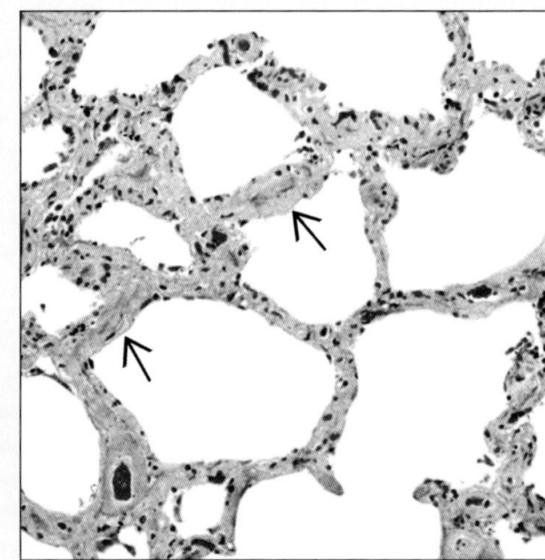

*(**Left**) Axial NECT of a 54-year-old woman with monoclonal gammopathy shows diffuse pulmonary involvement with peripheral smooth interlobular septal thickening and reticulation. Note that small nodules ⇨ are also seen. (**Right**) High-power photomicrograph (H&E stain) from the biopsy specimen of the same patient shows diffuse smooth interstitial thickening ➡ produced by amyloid accumulation. Diffuse interstitial amyloidosis is the least common form of pulmonary amyloidosis.*

PULMONARY AMYLOIDOSIS

TERMINOLOGY

Definitions

- Generic term for heterogeneous group of disorders characterized by abnormal extracellular accumulation of insoluble fibrillar proteins
  - **Amyloid light chain (AL)** (primary amyloidosis): Widespread deposition of amyloid fibrils derived from monoclonal immunoglobulin light chains (monoclonal gammopathy or multiple myeloma)
  - **Amyloid A chain (AA)** (secondary amyloidosis): Extracellular protein deposition caused by underlying chronic inflammatory disease such as, infection, bronchiectasis, rheumatic disease, neoplasms, age-related (senile) & familial Mediterranean fever
- **Major clinical forms**: Systemic & localized
- **Thoracic amyloidosis**: Cardiac > tracheobronchial > parenchymal > lymph nodes > pleura

IMAGING

General Features

- Best diagnostic clue
  - Multiple tracheal or pulmonary nodules (± calcification) + diffuse septal thickening + lymphadenopathy (± calcification)

Radiographic Findings

- Radiography
  - **Tracheobronchial abnormalities**: Mural nodules & diffuse thickening (± calcification)
  - **Parenchymal abnormalities**
    - Nodules: Single or multiple, 0.5-5 cm, calcification in 20%
    - Interstitial disease: Fine linear or reticulonodular opacities; honeycomb lung (uncommon); miliary nodules
  - **Lymphadenopathy**: Isolated finding or associated with interstitial disease
    - May exhibit stippled, diffuse, or eggshell calcification
  - **Other**: Cardiomegaly, pleural effusion, irregular pleural thickening (± calcification)

CT Findings

- NECT
  - **Tracheobronchial abnormalities**: Airway wall thickening, mural/intraluminal nodules, submucosal calcification
  - **Parenchymal abnormalities**
    - Diffuse micronodular (± calcification), reticulonodular, or linear opacities
    - Ground-glass opacities, honeycomb lung, thick bronchovascular bundles
  - **Lymphadenopathy**: Stippled, diffuse, or eggshell calcifications
  - **Other**: Soft tissue deposition

Imaging Recommendations

- Best imaging tool
  - Chest radiography sufficient for documentation of extent of thoracic involvement
  - HRCT: More sensitive in detecting tracheobronchial involvement & subtle parenchymal abnormalities

DIFFERENTIAL DIAGNOSIS

Tracheobronchial

- Primary benign & malignant neoplasms, tracheobronchopathia osteochondroplastica, relapsing polychondritis

Nodular

- Lung cancer, pulmonary metastases, granulomatous disease, rheumatoid nodules

Interstitial Lung Disease

- Idiopathic pulmonary fibrosis, scleroderma, rheumatoid arthritis, drug toxicity

Diffuse or Multifocal Lung Calcification

- Granulomatous infection, alveolar microlithiasis, metastatic calcification, silicosis, sarcoidosis, dendritic calcification, healed varicella

Lymphadenopathy

- Sarcoidosis, tuberculosis

Pleural Thickening

- Mesothelioma, pleural metastases

PATHOLOGY

General Features

- Extracellular protein deposition
- Vascular deposition leads to fragility & bleeding

Microscopic Features

- Amyloid in small blood vessel media, interstitium, & airways (uniform & linear or multiple small nodules)
- Calcification & foreign body giant cell reaction may be present
- Apple-green birefringence under polarized light after Congo red staining

CLINICAL ISSUES

Presentation

- Tracheobronchial form: Simulates asthma
- Nodular & interstitial form: Usually asymptomatic

Demographics

- Epidemiology
  - **Amyloid light chain (AL)**: 10% of patients with multiple myeloma develop amyloidosis
  - **Amyloid A chain (AA)**: Familial Mediterranean fever & age-related (senile)

Natural History & Prognosis

- Poor prognosis for diffuse disease: Survival < 2 years

Treatment

- No therapy is uniformly effective

SELECTED REFERENCES

1. Aylwin AC et al: Imaging appearance of thoracic amyloidosis. J Thorac Imaging. 20(1):41-6, 2005
2. Chung MJ et al: Metabolic lung disease: imaging and histopathologic findings. Eur J Radiol. 54(2):233-45, 2005
3. Pickford HA et al: Thoracic cross-sectional imaging of amyloidosis. AJR Am J Roentgenol. 168(2):351-5, 1997

PULMONARY ALVEOLAR PROTEINOSIS

Key Facts

Terminology
- Pulmonary alveolar proteinosis (PAP)
- Alveolar accumulation of proteinaceous & lipid-rich surfactant-like material

Imaging
- Radiography
  - Bilateral central & symmetric reticular, reticulonodular, or heterogeneous opacities
  - Relative sparing of lung apices & bases; may affect lung diffusely
  - Abnormalities appear more severe than clinical status; "clinicoradiologic discrepancy"
  - May mimic pulmonary edema
- HRCT
  - Autoimmune PAP: "Crazy-paving" pattern (75%)
  - Secondary PAP: Evenly distributed diffuse ground-glass opacities

Top Differential Diagnoses
- Pulmonary edema
- *Pneumocystis jiroveci* pneumonia
- Diffuse alveolar hemorrhage

Pathology
- Firm lung with yellow surface
- Alveolar lipoproteinaceous material

Clinical Issues
- Symptoms/signs
  - Asymptomatic, dyspnea, cough
  - Opportunistic pneumonia
- Treatment: Whole lung lavage

Diagnostic Checklist
- Consider PAP in patient with chronic multifocal airspace or mixed airspace-interstitial processes

__(Left)__ Graphic depicts findings of pulmonary alveolar proteinosis. Lipid and proteinaceous-rich material resembling surfactant fill the alveoli. __(Right)__ Composite image with sagittal macroscopic lung section (right) and fluid obtained after bronchoalveolar lavage (left) shows areas of yellowish discoloration ⇒ representing lipid-rich material and "milky" appearance of lavage fluid secondary to lipoproteinaceous components characteristic of PAP.

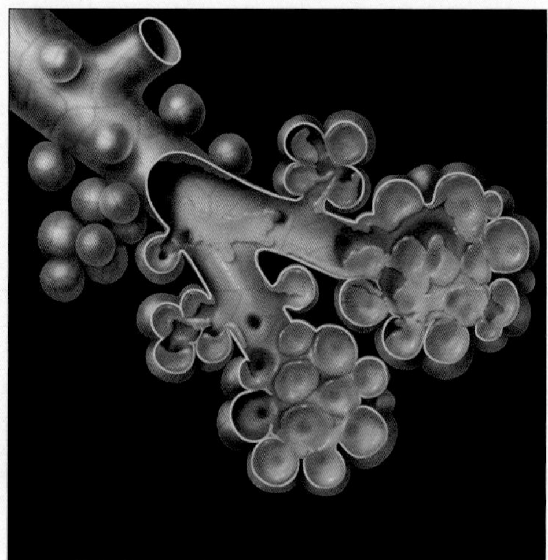

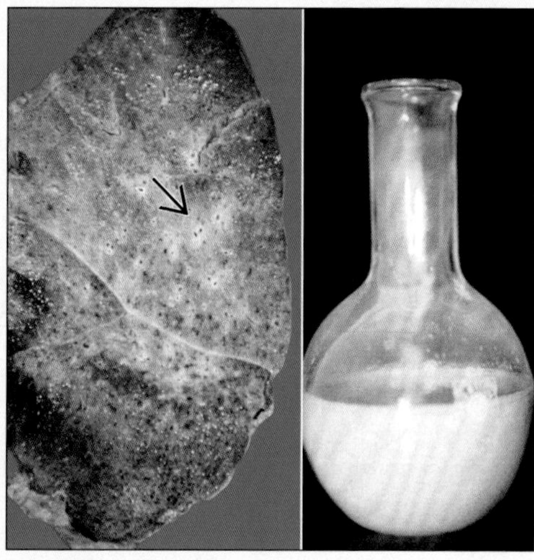

__(Left)__ PA chest radiograph of a patient with autoimmune PAP demonstrates characteristic radiographic findings with bilateral central symmetric heterogeneous airspace disease. __(Right)__ PA chest radiograph of a patient with autoimmune PAP demonstrates subtle diffuse bilateral reticular opacities prior to treatment with whole lung lavage. Most patients experience significant improvement after the initial lavage procedure, although additional lavage treatments may be required.

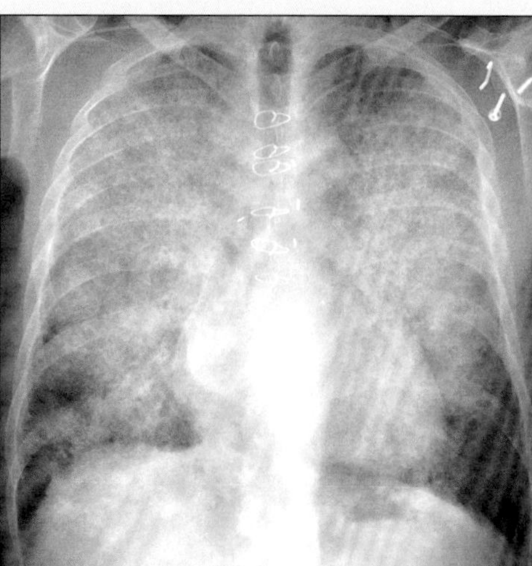

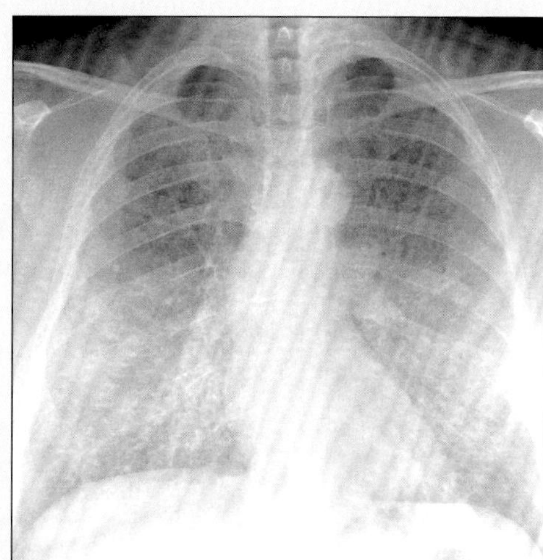

PULMONARY ALVEOLAR PROTEINOSIS

TERMINOLOGY

Abbreviations

- **Pulmonary alveolar proteinosis (PAP)**

Synonyms

- Pulmonary alveolar phospholipoproteinosis, lipoproteinosis

Definitions

- Alveolar accumulation of proteinaceous & lipid-rich surfactant-like material

IMAGING

General Features

- Best diagnostic clue
  - Radiography: **Mimics pulmonary edema** without pleural effusion or cardiomegaly
  - CT: **"Crazy-paving" pattern**

Radiographic Findings

- Radiography
  - Bilateral central & symmetric reticular, reticulonodular, or heterogeneous opacities
    - Air bronchograms may be present
    - Mimics pulmonary edema without pleural effusions or cardiomegaly
    - Radiographic abnormalities often appear more severe than clinical status (i.e., "**clinicoradiologic discrepancy**")
  - Relative sparing of lung apices & bases; may affect lung diffusely
  - Findings suspicious for superimposed infection
    - Pleural effusion
    - Lymphadenopathy
    - Dominant opacity/mass ± cavitation
- Post-treatment (lavage)
  - Acute complications: Pneumothorax, pneumomediastinum
  - ↑ parenchymal opacities due to retained lavage fluid
  - Gradual improvement in 1st week
  - Marked improvement by 6 weeks, with frequent persistent abnormalities

CT Findings

- HRCT
  - **Autoimmune PAP**
    - Random geographic distribution (abnormalities clearly demarcated from adjacent normal lung)
    - **"Crazy-paving" pattern (75%)**
      - Ground-glass opacities with superimposed thick interlobular septa
      - Widespread & bilateral
    - Consolidation
    - Severity of ground-glass opacity & consolidation correlates with severity of functional parameters
    - Mediastinal lymphadenopathy
      - 1-2 lymph nodes > 1 cm short axis diameter
      - More numerous lymph nodes suggest superinfection or underlying hematologic disorder
      - Hilar lymphadenopathy may be seen in silicoproteinosis-related PAP
    - Fibrosis: Central or peripheral, traction bronchiectasis
  - **Secondary PAP**
    - Evenly distributed diffuse ground-glass opacities
    - "Crazy-paving" pattern much less frequent

MR Findings

- MR not indicated
- Lung abnormalities reported to exhibit low signal on T1WI with mild increase in signal intensity on T2WI

Nuclear Medicine Findings

- PET/CT
  - Not indicated
  - Reports of mild & heterogeneous FDG accumulation
- Ga-67 scintigraphy
  - Not needed; anecdotally may show Ga-67 uptake

Imaging Recommendations

- Best imaging tool
  - HRCT for characterization of diffuse lung disease
  - CECT best for detection & characterization of complications, such as opportunistic infection

DIFFERENTIAL DIAGNOSIS

Pulmonary Edema

- May manifest with "crazy-paving" pattern
- Cardiomegaly & pleural effusion in appropriate clinical scenario

Pneumocystis jiroveci Pneumonia

- May manifest with "crazy-paving" pattern
- Appropriate history & acute symptoms

Diffuse Alveolar Hemorrhage

- May manifest with "crazy-paving" pattern
- ↓ hematocrit, sometimes hemoptysis
- More acute onset

Lung Cancer (Invasive Mucinous Adenocarcinoma)

- May manifest with "crazy-paving" pattern
- Constitutional symptoms, such as weight loss
- May exhibit lymphadenopathy

Other Entities with "Crazy-Paving" Pattern

- Sarcoidosis
- Nonspecific interstitial pneumonia
- Organizing pneumonia
- Acute respiratory distress syndrome (ARDS)
- Lipoid pneumonia

PATHOLOGY

General Features

- Etiology
  - Congenital
    - Minority of cases
    - Disorders caused by
      - Homozygous mutation of genes encoding surfactant protein (SP)-B, SP-C, & ABCA3 transporter
      - Absence of granulocyte/macrophage colony stimulating factor (GM-CSF) receptor
  - **Autoimmune**

- **Majority of cases (90%)**
- Adults with high prevalence of anti-granulocyte-macrophage colony-stimulating factor (GM-CSF)

  - Secondary
    - 5-10% of cases
    - **Inhalational exposure**: Silica, cement, aluminum, titanium dioxide, nitrogen dioxide, fiberglass
    - **Hematologic malignancy**: Acute myeloid leukemia, myelodysplastic syndrome, chronic myeloid leukemia
    - **Immunodeficiency**: Immunosuppressive therapy, HIV
- Associated abnormalities
  - Superimposed infection in 13%

Gross Pathologic & Surgical Features

- Firm lung with yellow surface (due to lipid)

Microscopic Features

- Alveolar lipoproteinaceous material; periodic-acid Schiff (PAS)-positive
- Thick alveolar walls due to hyperplasia of type II pneumocytes
- Variable chronic inflammatory cells & fibrosis

CLINICAL ISSUES

Presentation

- Most common signs/symptoms
  - **Asymptomatic (33%)**
  - **Progressive shortness of breath**
  - **Dry or minimally productive cough**
  - Crackles
  - Clubbing
  - Cyanosis
- Other signs/symptoms
  - Fatigue
  - Weight loss
  - Low-grade fever
  - Chest pain
  - Hemoptysis
- Clinical profile
  - **Autoimmune PAP has strong association with cigarette smoking (75% of cases)**
- Laboratory findings
  - ↑ lactate dehydrogenase
  - Arterial blood gases: Hypoxemia, ↑ arterial oxygen tension (PaO_2), ↑ alveolar-arterial oxygen tension ($aAPO_2$)
  - Pulmonary function tests: ↓ diffusion capacity (DLCO), ↓ lung volumes, ↓ compliance
  - Granulocyte-macrophage colony-stimulating factor (GM-CSF) autoantibodies
    - Autoimmune PAP: Positive
    - Secondary: Negative
- Bronchoalveolar lavage (BAL): "Milky" material
- Complications
  - Opportunistic pneumonia (13%): *Nocardia*, *Candida*, *C. neoformans*, *Aspergillus*, Cytomegalovirus, *M. tuberculosis*, nontuberculous mycobacteria, *H. capsulatum*, *P. jiroveci*, *S. pneumoniae*
  - Fibrosis (rare): Unclear whether coincidental finding or end-stage of PAP

Demographics

- Age
  - Autoimmune PAP
    - Average age: 40 years (20-50 years)
    - May affect young children
- Gender
  - Autoimmune PAP
    - Smokers: Men 3x more commonly affected
    - Nonsmokers: No gender predilection
- Epidemiology
  - Autoimmune PAP
    - Incidence: 0.36 new cases/million persons/year
    - Prevalence: 3.7 cases/million persons

Natural History & Prognosis

- Good prognosis
  - Disease-specific survival exceeds 80% at 5 years
  - Marked increase in survival over recent decades due to better treatment
  - BAL techniques have markedly improved prognosis
- Significant pulmonary fibrosis (rare)

Treatment

- **Whole lung lavage**
  - 25-40 liters of saline, both lungs, usually performed sequentially
  - May be repeated several times
  - Most patients experience significant improvement from single thorough lavage
  - After lavage, up to 70% of patients remain symptom-free at 7 years
  - Few patients require annual or biannual therapeutic lavage
- Immunomodulation
  - Subcutaneous administration of GM-CSF for treatment of autoimmune PAP has moderate success
  - Experimental treatment includes plasmapheresis

DIAGNOSTIC CHECKLIST

Consider

- PAP in patient with chronic multifocal airspace or mixed airspace-interstitial processes

Image Interpretation Pearls

- "Crazy-paving" pattern is not specific for PAP
- "Crazy-paving" pattern is classic HRCT finding of pulmonary alveolar proteinosis, but this disease is rare

SELECTED REFERENCES

1. Ishii H et al: Comparative study of high-resolution CT findings between autoimmune and secondary pulmonary alveolar proteinosis. Chest. 136(5):1348-55, 2009
2. Frazier AA et al: From the archives of the AFIP: pulmonary alveolar proteinosis. Radiographics. 28(3):883-99; quiz 915, 2008
3. Inoue Y et al: Characteristics of a large cohort of patients with autoimmune pulmonary alveolar proteinosis in Japan. Am J Respir Crit Care Med. 177(7):752-62, 2008
4. Ioachimescu OC et al: Pulmonary alveolar proteinosis. Chron Respir Dis. 3(3):149-59, 2006

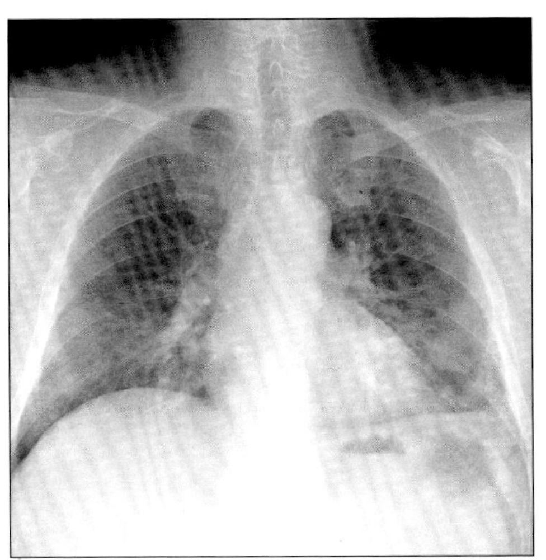

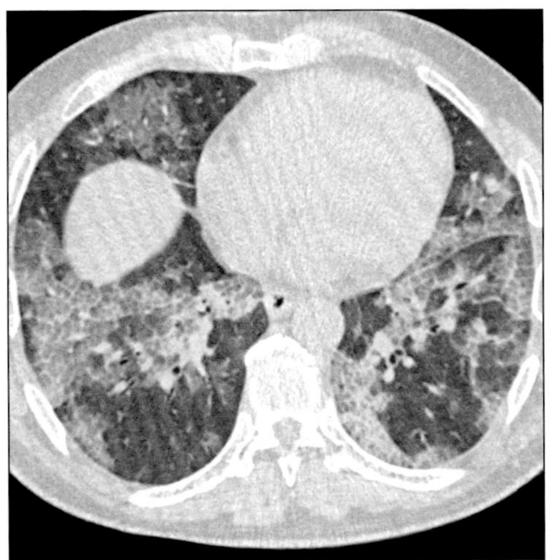

(Left) *PA chest radiograph of a patient with autoimmune PAP shows bilateral scattered, ill-defined, subsegmental, heterogeneous airspace opacities.* ***(Right)*** *Axial HRCT of the same patient shows geographic areas of "crazy-paving" characterized by ground-glass opacity and septal thickening. Histologically, ground-glass opacities correlated with alveolar filling. Superimposed thick septa result from expansion of interlobular septa by edema and massively dilated lymphatic channels.*

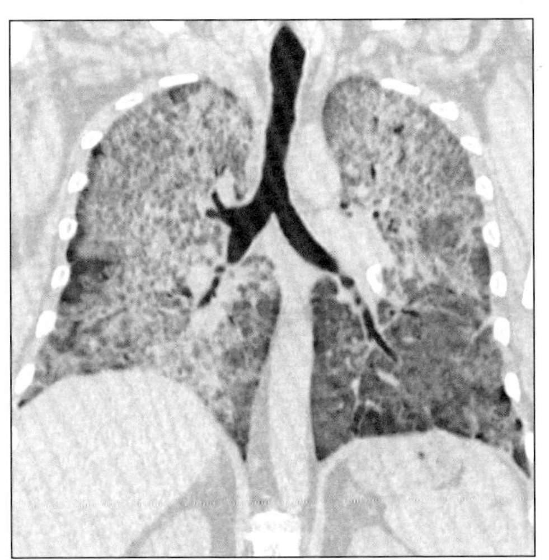

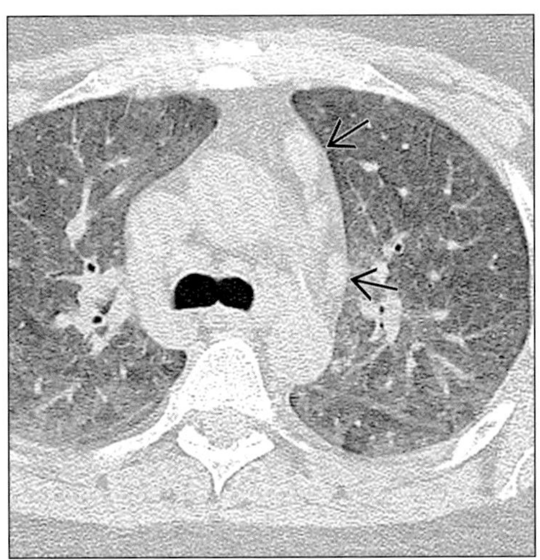

(Left) *Coronal NECT of a patient with autoimmune PAP shows diffuse pulmonary abnormalities with relative sparing of the left lung base near the costophrenic angle.* ***(Right)*** *Axial HRCT of a patient with leukemia and secondary PAP shows characteristic diffuse bilateral ground-glass opacities without thick interlobular septa and mediastinal lymphadenopathy ➔. While the "crazy-paving" pattern can be seen in patients with secondary PAP, it is an uncommon imaging manifestation.*

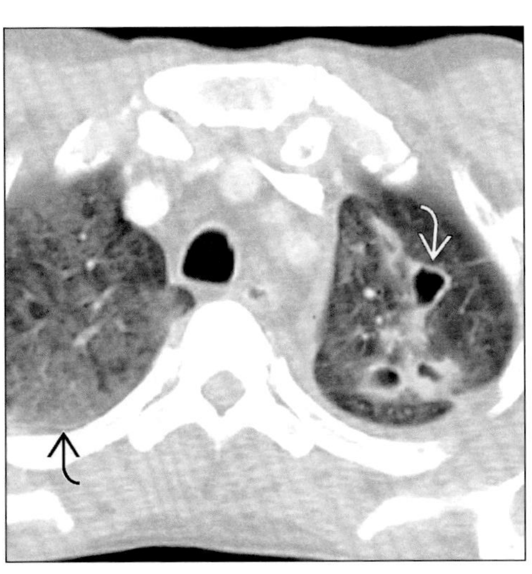

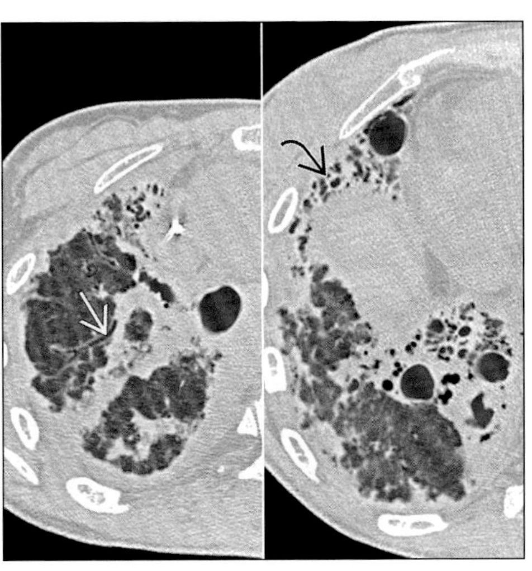

(Left) *Axial CECT of a patient with PAP and nocardiosis shows bilateral diffuse ground-glass opacities ➔ and left upper lobe thick- and thin-walled cavities ➔.* ***(Right)*** *Axial HRCT of a patient with PAP shows heterogeneous consolidation and reticular opacities with traction bronchiectasis/ bronchiolectasis ➔ and honeycomb lung ➔. The patient was treated with bilateral lung transplantation. Histopathological analysis of the native lungs showed pulmonary fibrosis. (Courtesy C. S. Restrepo, MD.)*

LIPOID PNEUMONIA

Key Facts

Terminology
- Endogenous lipoid pneumonia ("golden pneumonia")
  - Accumulation of alveolar macrophages due to airway obstruction or impaired mucociliary clearance
- Exogenous lipoid pneumonia
  - Repetitive aspiration or inhalation of mineral oil

Imaging
- Radiography
  - Acute aspiration: Focal or multifocal consolidations, predilection for lower lobes
  - Chronic aspiration: Mass-like or nodular lesion
- CT
  - Focal/extensive areas of low (fat) attenuation
  - Fat attenuation in nodule or mass-like consolidation
  - "Crazy-paving" pattern on HRCT

Top Differential Diagnoses
- Consolidation
  - Bacterial pneumonia, organizing pneumonia
- Nodule or mass-like consolidation
  - Lung cancer, focal organizing pneumonia
- "Crazy-paving" pattern
  - Alveolar proteinosis, adenocarcinoma, *P. jiroveci* pneumonia, pulmonary hemorrhage

Clinical Issues
- Symptoms/signs
  - Acute: Cough, dyspnea, low-grade fever
  - Subacute/chronic: Asymptomatic, chronic cough

Diagnostic Checklist
- Consider lipoid pneumonia in patients with lung nodule, mass, or consolidation with intrinsic fat attenuation or "crazy-paving" pattern on CT

__(Left)__ AP scout CT of a 26-year-old woman with anorexia, repetitive mineral oil aspiration, and exogenous lipoid pneumonia shows bilateral consolidations with air bronchograms in the middle lobe, lingula, and lower lobes. (Courtesy A. Hidalgo, MD.) __(Right)__ Axial NECT of the same patient shows fat attenuation ➔ within middle lobe and lingular consolidations and small bilateral pleural effusions. Careful clinical history is required to identify the source of the aspirated material. (Courtesy A. Hidalgo, MD.)

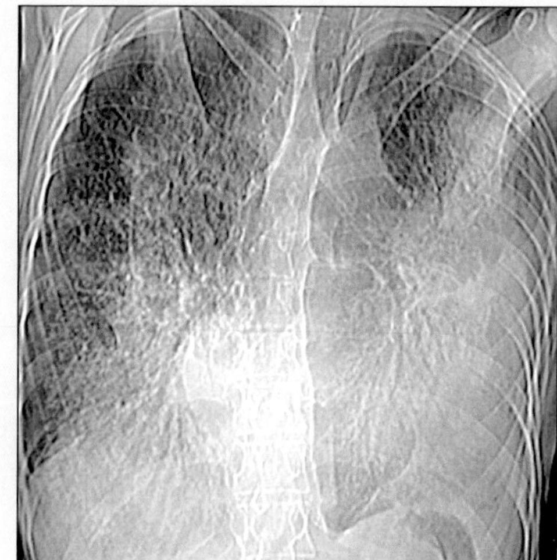

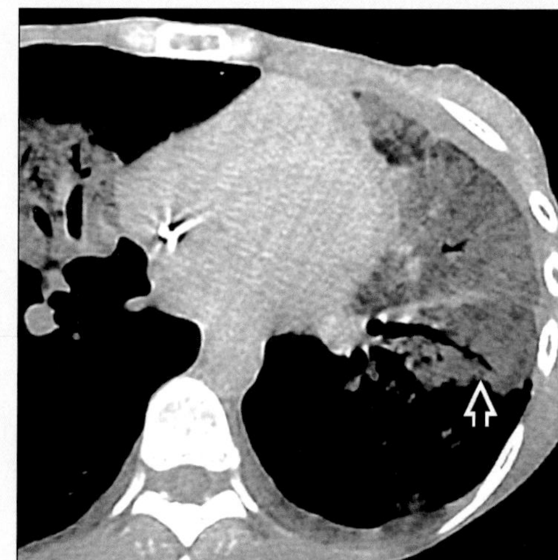

__(Left)__ Composite image shows NECT of lung (left) and mediastinal (right) window of a patient with lipoid pneumonia manifesting as a spiculated mass ➔ with intrinsic fat attenuation ➔ and surrounding bronchiolitis. __(Right)__ HRCT of a 78-year-old man with exogenous lipoid pneumonia due to mineral oil aspiration shows "crazy-paving" pattern characterized by ground-glass opacity with intrinsic interlobular septal thickening ➔ and intralobular lines. This finding has been described in lipoid pneumonia.

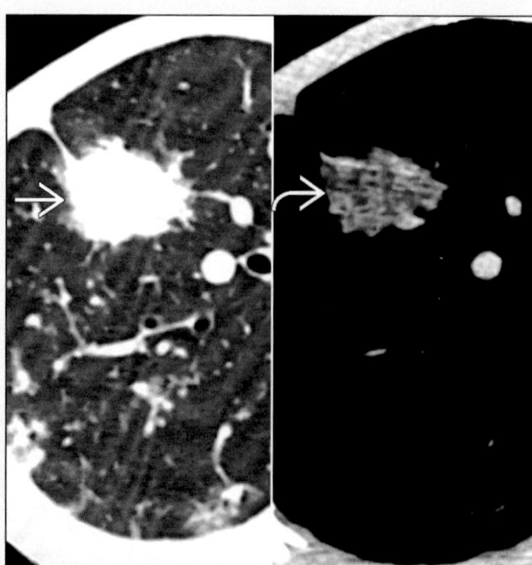

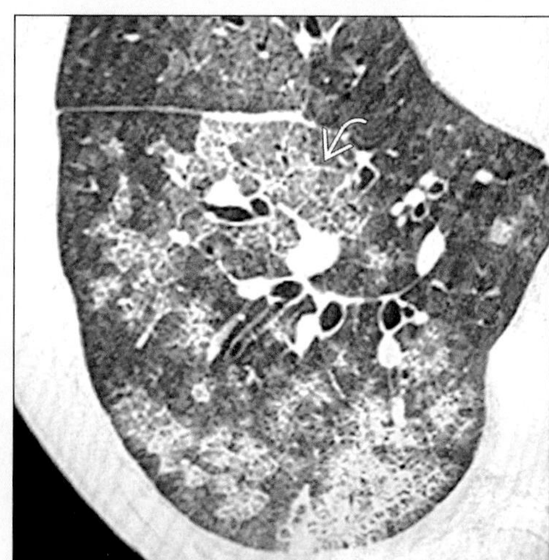

LIPOID PNEUMONIA

TERMINOLOGY

Synonyms

- Endogenous lipoid pneumonia ("golden pneumonia")

Definitions

- **Endogenous lipoid pneumonia**: Accumulation of alveolar macrophages due to airway obstruction or impaired mucociliary clearance
- **Exogenous lipoid pneumonia**: Repetitive aspiration or inhalation of mineral oil or related material into lung
  - Animal or vegetable oils, oral laxatives, oil-based nose drops, liquid paraffin

IMAGING

General Features

- Best diagnostic clue
  - Consolidation with -30 to -150 HU attenuation
- Location
  - Gravity-dependent areas of lung

Radiographic Findings

- Radiography
  - **Acute aspiration**: Radiographically visible within 30 minutes of aspiration or inhalation
    - Bilateral or unilateral diffuse consolidation
    - Focal or multifocal segmental consolidations; predominantly in lower lobes
  - **Chronic aspiration**: Mass-like or nodular lesion with irregular margins; may mimic lung cancer

CT Findings

- Focal/extensive areas of low (fat) attenuation
- Fat attenuation within mass-like consolidation
- **"Crazy-paving" pattern**: Ground-glass opacity with interlobular septal thickening & intralobular lines

MR Findings

- Visualization of fat: High signal on T1WI & T2WI or documentation of fat on chemical shift MR

Imaging Recommendations

- Best imaging tool
  - CT is imaging modality of choice for demonstrating fat attenuation within lipoid pneumonia lesions

DIFFERENTIAL DIAGNOSIS

Consolidation

- Bacterial pneumonia
- Organizing pneumonia

Nodule or Mass-like Consolidation

- Lung cancer (spiculated margins)
- Focal organizing pneumonia

"Crazy-Paving" Pattern

- Alveolar proteinosis
- Adenocarcinoma
- *Pneumocystis jiroveci* pneumonia
- Pulmonary hemorrhage

PATHOLOGY

General Features

- Etiology
  - **Mineral oil** is most common agent
  - Animal & vegetable oils also implicated

Gross Pathologic & Surgical Features

- Chronically, lipid is fibrogenic; may produce architectural distortion

Microscopic Features

- Bronchopneumonia, alveolar lipid-laden macrophages
- Interstitial accumulation of lipid, inflammatory cellular infiltration, variable fibrosis
- Positive Congo red stain

CLINICAL ISSUES

Presentation

- Most common signs/symptoms
  - Acute: Cough, dyspnea, low-grade fever
  - Subacute/chronic (repeated subclinical aspiration): Usually asymptomatic, chronic nonproductive cough
    - Lipid not irritant, silent aspiration while sleeping

Demographics

- Age
  - Any age
- Epidemiology
  - Patients at risk
    - Neonates, infants with feeding problems
    - Elderly
    - Swallowing dysfunction or esophageal abnormality

Natural History & Prognosis

- Directly related to type & extent of aspiration
  - Recurrent aspiration may lead to fibrosis

Treatment

- Discontinuation of use of lipoid agent

Diagnosis

- Transthoracic needle biopsy may be diagnostic

DIAGNOSTIC CHECKLIST

Consider

- Lipoid pneumonia in patients with pulmonary nodule, mass, or consolidation with intrinsic fat attenuation or "crazy-paving" pattern on CT

SELECTED REFERENCES

1. Betancourt SL et al: Lipoid pneumonia: spectrum of clinical and radiologic manifestations. AJR Am J Roentgenol. 194(1):103-9, 2010
2. Franquet T et al: The crazy-paving pattern in exogenous lipoid pneumonia: CT-pathologic correlation. AJR Am J Roentgenol. 170(2):315-7, 1998

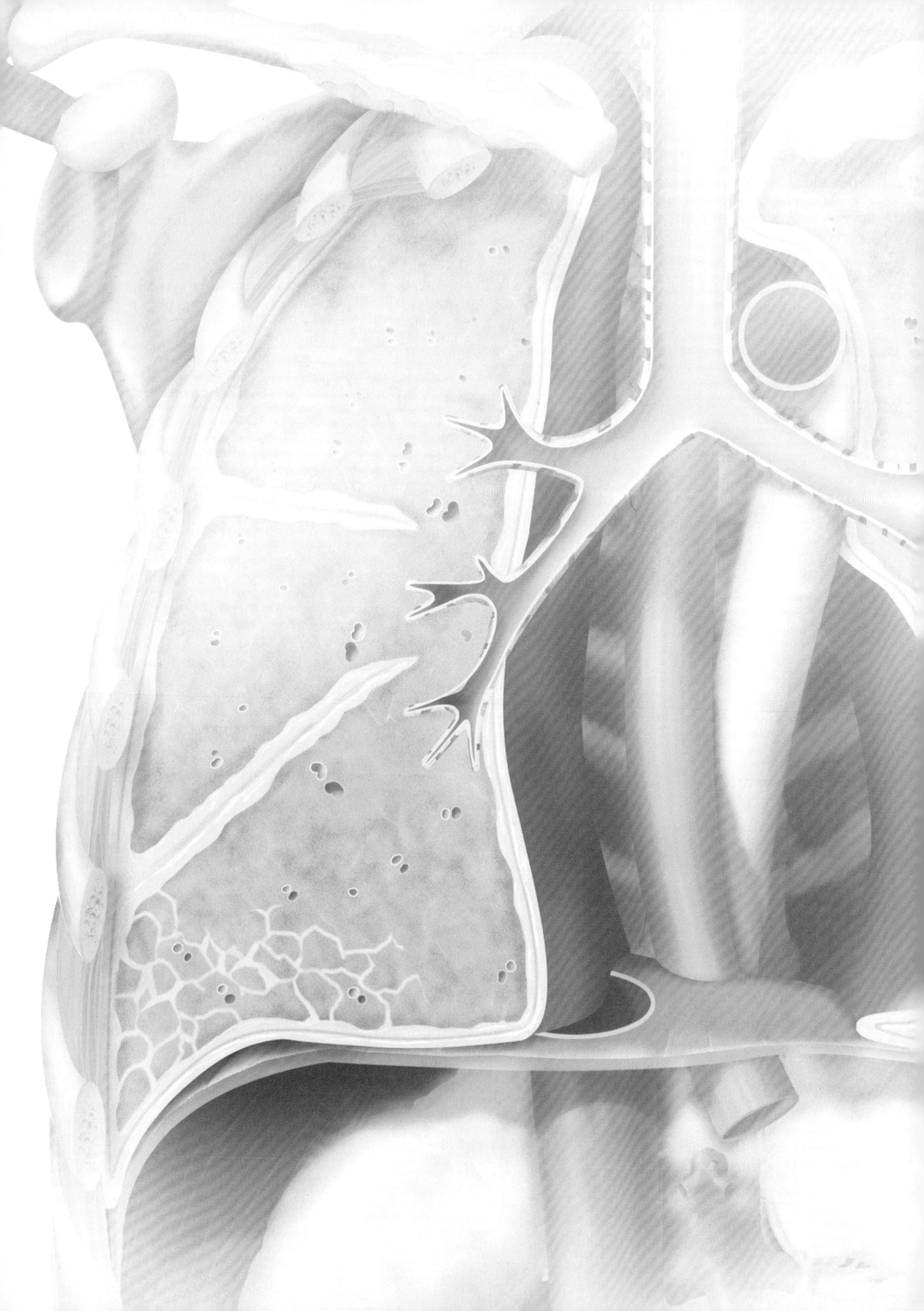

SECTION 7
Connective Tissue Disorders, Immunological Diseases, and Vasculitis

Introduction and Overview

Immunological and Connective Tissue Disorders

Thoracic Complications in Immunocompromised Patients

Pulmonary Hemorrhage and Vasculitis

APPROACH TO CONNECTIVE TISSUE DISORDERS, IMMUNOLOGICAL DISEASES, AND VASCULITIS

Imaging Modalities

For patients with connective tissue disorders, immunological diseases, and vasculitis who have symptoms referable to the thorax, the imaging evaluation typically begins with chest radiography but often requires CT/HRCT studies for accurate detection and characterization of pleuropulmonary abnormalities. In some cases, the pleuropulmonary imaging findings of these disorders are the initial manifestation of the disease, which may not become clinically apparent until months or years later.

Connective Tissue Disease

Connective tissue diseases (also called collagen vascular diseases) comprise a group of autoimmune disorders characterized by damage to connective tissue components at various anatomic locations in the body. These include rheumatoid arthritis, scleroderma, mixed connective tissue disorder, polymyositis and dermatomyositis, systemic lupus erythematosus, Sjögren syndrome, and ankylosing spondylitis. These disease processes may be associated with focal or diffuse pulmonary abnormalities. Diffuse infiltrative pulmonary disease is most commonly detected in patients with rheumatoid arthritis and in those with progressive systemic sclerosis (scleroderma).

The majority of connective tissue diseases have the potential to produce a chronic interstitial lung disease that is indistinguishable from usual interstitial pneumonia (UIP) in its clinical, radiographic, and CT/HRCT manifestations. However, ground-glass opacity is often a predominant CT/HRCT finding in patients with lung disease associated with connective tissue disorders, typically with finer reticulation and less frequent honeycombing than that which characterizes UIP and idiopathic pulmonary fibrosis (IPF). Connective tissue diseases are often associated with pathologic abnormalities other than UIP, including nonspecific interstitial pneumonia (NSIP), bronchiolitis obliterans, bronchiectasis, lymphoid interstitial pneumonia (LIP), and cryptogenic organizing pneumonia (COP).

Because patients with connective tissue disease are at risk for the development of interstitial lung disease, which may progress to end-stage fibrosis and honeycomb lung, they are also at increased risk for the development of primary lung cancer. Thus, radiologists must regard any new pulmonary nodule or mass in such patients with a high index of suspicion for malignancy and should aggressively pursue a definitive diagnosis in these cases.

Immunocompromised Patients

In recent decades, several factors have led to an increased number of immunocompromised patients, including the widespread use of ablative chemotherapy in the management of patients with cancer, an increase in the frequency of solid organ and bone marrow transplantation, and the epidemic of HIV infection. Detection of pleuropulmonary imaging abnormalities in immunocompromised patients should always prompt consideration of infection as an important differential diagnostic possibility. However, many other disease processes that mimic infection must also be excluded, including cytotoxic and noncytotoxic drug reactions, interstitial lung diseases, lymphoproliferative disorders, and malignant neoplasms.

The chest radiograph is an important initial imaging modality in the evaluation of symptomatic immunocompromised patients, but it may be normal in 10% of patients with pulmonary complications. Chest CT and HRCT provide improved accuracy in the demonstration of imaging abnormalities, their patterns, distribution, and the extent of pulmonary involvement. When combined with clinical and epidemiological information, imaging findings may help to narrow the differential diagnostic possibilities and determine the next best steps in the diagnostic process. Comparison with previous chest imaging studies is critical to recognize new abnormalities and determine the temporal sequence of their progression.

The presence or absence of associated findings such as lymphadenopathy and pleural effusion may help to narrow the list of differential diagnostic possibilities. Specific clinical and imaging features may be important clues to the diagnosis. For example, lung nodules, masses, and consolidations detected by CT or HRCT in association with neutropenia should prompt consideration of invasive aspergillosis as a leading diagnostic possibility. In fact, management decisions in the treatment of opportunistic infections in immunocompromised patients are frequently made based on imaging abnormalities and may not require microbiologic confirmation. On the other hand, the finding of ground-glass opacity in patients with HIV/AIDS is highly suggestive of *Pneumocystis jiroveci* pneumonia (PCP).

Pulmonary Hemorrhage and Vasculitis

Pulmonary vasculitis syndromes include several disease entities, some of which frequently affect the lung (e.g., Wegener granulomatosis, Churg-Strauss vasculitis, and microscopic polyangiitis). Pulmonary vasculitis also occurs in miscellaneous systemic disorders, in diffuse pulmonary hemorrhagic syndromes, and in other secondary, localized forms. The pulmonary vasculitis syndromes are clinicopathologic entities; their diagnosis is based not solely on pathologic findings, but rather on a correlation among clinical, imaging, and pathologic features.

Clinical settings in which pulmonary vasculitis may occur are variable and include diffuse pulmonary hemorrhage, pulmonary renal syndromes, pulmonary nodular and/or cavitary disease, and upper airway lesions. When patients present with pulmonary hemorrhage, corroborated by imaging findings and clinical testing, pulmonary vasculitis should be considered as a differential diagnostic possibility, including the most common vasculitis syndrome, Wegener granulomatosis. The diagnosis of idiopathic pulmonary hemorrhage is always a diagnosis of exclusion.

Selected References

1. Hansell DM et al: Idiopathic interstitial pneumonias and immunologic disease of the lungs. In Imaging of Diseases of the Chest. St. Louis: Mosby. 608-39, 2010

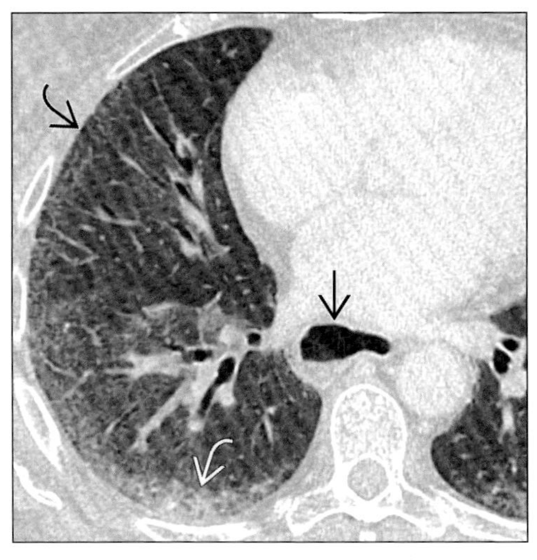

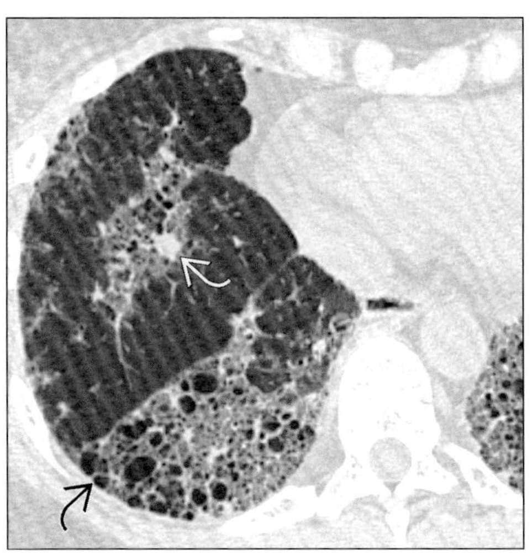

*(**Left**) HRCT of a patient with scleroderma shows esophageal dilatation → and posterior subpleural ground-glass → and reticular opacities →. Connective tissue diseases may exhibit findings indistinguishable from UIP. However, ground-glass opacity is typically the predominant finding in patients with associated NSIP. (**Right**) HRCT of a patient with scleroderma shows pulmonary fibrosis and honeycombing →. A focal nodular lesion → represents associated primary lung cancer.*

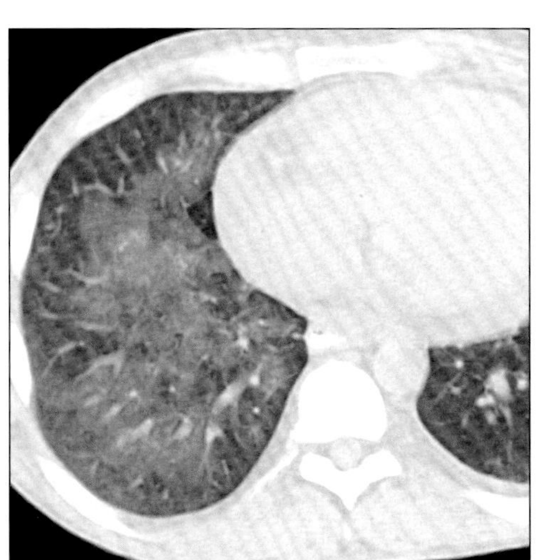

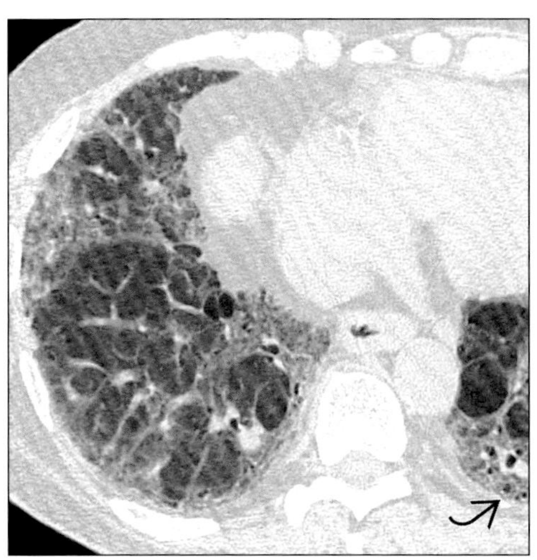

*(**Left**) CECT of a patient with lupus pneumonitis demonstrates patchy ground-glass opacities that involved both lungs. The CT imaging differential diagnosis of ground-glass opacity in patients with lupus also includes pneumonia and pulmonary hemorrhage. (**Right**) CECT of a patient with systemic lupus erythematosus shows bibasilar subpleural reticular opacities, traction bronchiectasis, and early honeycombing →. Patients with lupus may exhibit CT manifestations of usual interstitial pneumonia.*

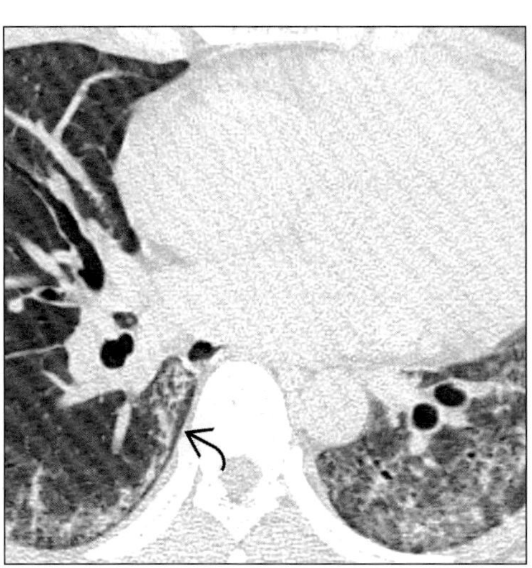

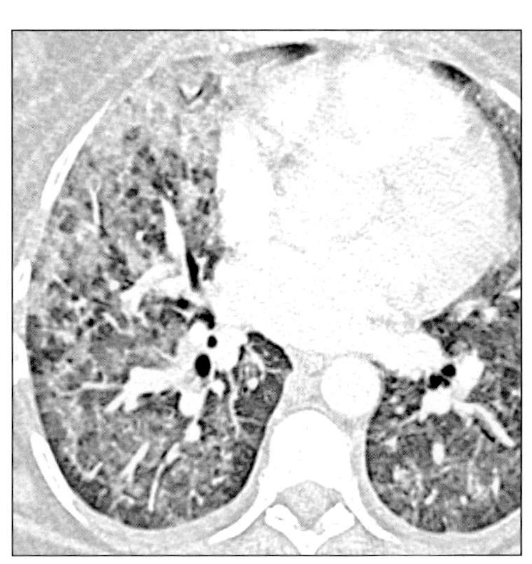

*(**Left**) CECT of a patient with polymyositis shows findings of nonspecific interstitial pneumonia with subpleural reticular and ground-glass opacities. Note the relative sparing of the subpleural lung →, a CT finding that is very suggestive of NSIP. (**Right**) CECT of a patient with idiopathic pulmonary hemorrhage (IPH) shows bilateral multifocal ground-glass opacities. Approximately 25% of patients with IPH will subsequently develop an autoimmune disorder.*

RHEUMATOID ARTHRITIS

Key Facts

Terminology

- Rheumatoid arthritis (RA)
- Subacute or chronic inflammatory polyarthropathy of unknown cause

Imaging

- Radiographs
  - Pleural thickening &/or effusion
  - Reticulonodular & irregular linear opacities, lower lung zones
  - Rheumatoid nodules (< 5%)
- CT/HRCT
  - Evaluation of pleural effusions & thickening
  - Interstitial fibrosis (30-40%): Usual interstitial pneumonia & nonspecific interstitial pneumonia
  - Nodules or masses
  - Bronchiectasis, bronchial wall thickening, constrictive bronchiolitis

Top Differential Diagnoses

- Idiopathic pulmonary fibrosis (IPF)
- Scleroderma
- Cryptogenic organizing pneumonia (COP)
- Asbestosis

Clinical Issues

- Involves synovial membranes & articular structures
- Extraarticular RA: More common in men
- Thoracic RA: Dyspnea, cough, pleuritic pain
  - May be asymptomatic
- 5-year survival 40%: Infection most common cause of death

Diagnostic Checklist

- Consider RA-related lung disease in patient with lung fibrosis & history of RA or polyarthritis (especially distal clavicular resorption)

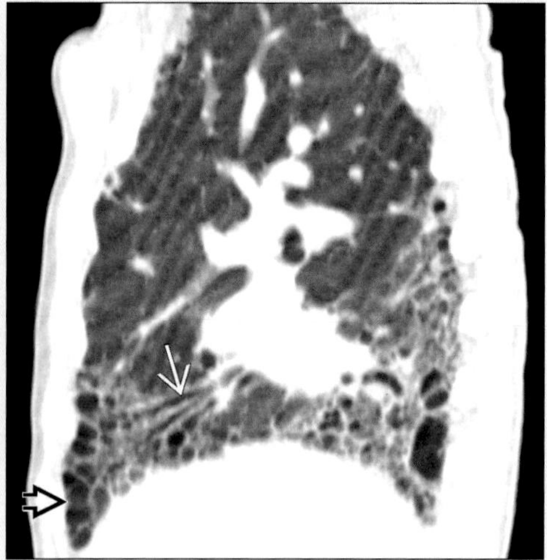
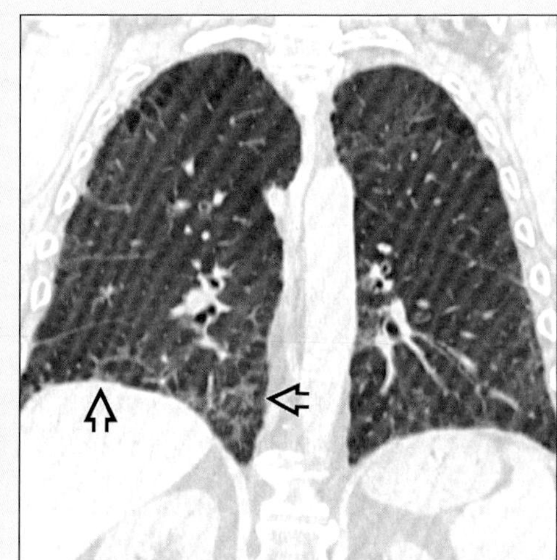

(Left) *Sagittal HRCT of a patient with RA shows basilar and peripheral predominant pulmonary fibrosis with honeycombing, traction bronchiectasis, reticulation, and mild ground-glass opacity, suggestive of usual interstitial pneumonia pattern of disease.* ***(Right)*** *Coronal HRCT of a patient with RA shows mild peripheral subpleural mixed ground-glass and reticular opacities diagnosed as NSIP on lung biopsy. In cases of mild lung fibrosis, tissue sampling is often required for definitive diagnosis.*

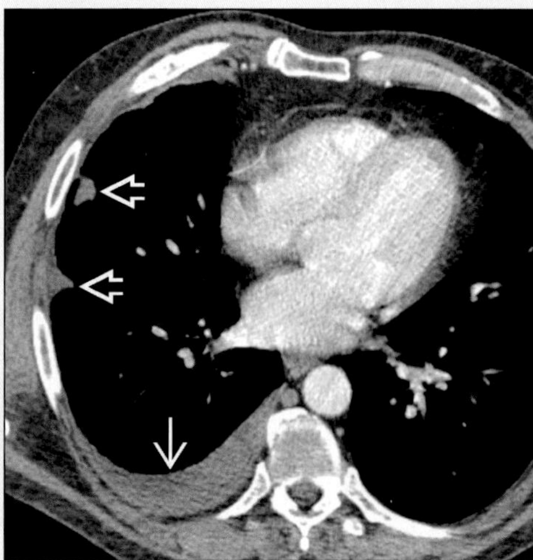
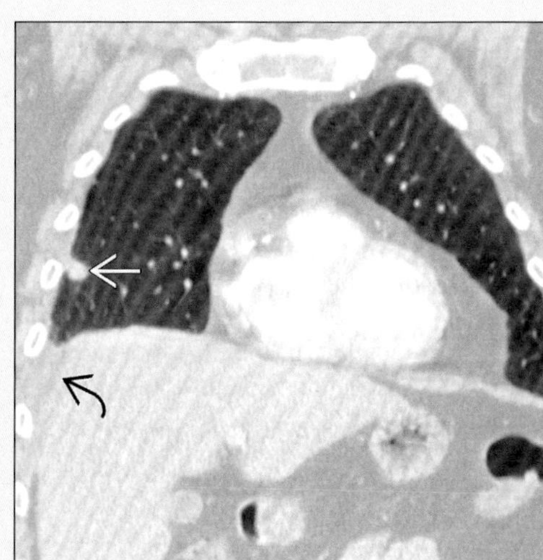

(Left) *Axial CECT of a patient with RA shows a small right pleural effusion and 2 peripheral right lung nodules.* ***(Right)*** *Coronal CECT of a middle-aged man with RA shows a right middle lobe nodule, consistent with a rheumatoid nodule. Note the small right pleural effusion. Thoracic manifestations of RA are much more common in men than in women, although RA is more common in women overall.*

RHEUMATOID ARTHRITIS

TERMINOLOGY

Abbreviations

- **Rheumatoid arthritis (RA)**

Definitions

- Subacute or chronic inflammatory polyarthropathy of unknown cause
  - Associated thoracic findings: Pleural disease, interstitial fibrosis, lung nodules, airway disease
  - Complications: Pneumonia, empyema, drug reaction, amyloidosis, cor pulmonale

IMAGING

General Features

- Best diagnostic clue
  - Interstitial lung disease in patient with polyarthritis (especially distal clavicular resorption)
- Location
  - Interstitial lung disease: Lower lobes

Radiographic Findings

- **Pleural disease**
  - Pleural thickening (20%)
  - Pleural effusion
    - Much more common in men
    - Small to large, usually unilateral, may be bilateral
    - Transient, persistent, or relapsing
    - Susceptibility to empyema
  - Pneumothorax: Rare
    - Associated with rheumatoid nodules
- **Parenchymal disease**
  - Reticulonodular & irregular linear opacities with lower lung zone predominance
    - Interstitial fibrosis in 5% on chest radiography
  - Progressive lower lobe volume loss
  - Rheumatoid nodules (< 5%)
    - Solitary or multiple, 5 mm to 7 cm
    - Peripheral (subpleural)
    - Waxing & waning course
    - May cavitate (50%), thick smooth wall
    - More common in men, especially smokers
  - **Caplan syndrome**: Very rare
    - Multiple lung nodules in coal miners with RA
    - Large rounded nodules (0.5-5 cm)
    - Nodules exhibit peripheral distribution
- Airway disease
  - Hyperinflation
  - Diffuse reticulonodular opacities: Follicular bronchiolitis
  - Bronchiectasis (20%)
    - Isolated or related to traction bronchiectasis
    - Pulmonary micronodules

CT Findings

- HRCT
  - Abnormal in 50%, more sensitive than pulmonary function tests (PFTs)
  - Pleural disease: Common abnormality in RA
    - Pleural effusion
      - Moderate size; often subacute or chronic
      - Often loculated
    - Pleural thickening
      - Fibrothorax
      - Rounded atelectasis
    - May be associated with pericarditis, interstitial fibrosis, interstitial pneumonia, &/or lung nodules
  - Rheumatoid lung disease
    - Much more common in men
    - Interstitial fibrosis in 30-40% by HRCT
    - Typically usual interstitial pneumonia (UIP) & nonspecific interstitial pneumonia (NSIP)
      - UIP: Subpleural & basilar predominant reticulation, traction bronchiolectasis, & honeycomb lung
      - NSIP: Basilar predominant ground-glass opacity & reticulation; may spare subpleural lung
    - Cryptogenic organizing pneumonia (COP): Less common
      - Peripheral or central consolidation & ground-glass opacities; may be mass-like or nodular
  - Nodules or masses
    - May mimic neoplasia: Discrete, rounded or lobulated, subpleural nodules
    - Pleural abnormalities & lung nodules, when present, help distinguish RA-related interstitial lung disease from UIP
  - Airway disease
    - Bronchiectasis & bronchial wall thickening: Earliest thoracic finding
    - Constrictive bronchiolitis
      - Mosaic attenuation/expiratory air-trapping
      - Cylindrical bronchiectasis & bronchial wall thickening
    - Micronodules
      - < 1 cm, centrilobular, subpleural, peribronchial
      - Centrilobular nodules & tree-in-bud opacities in follicular bronchiolitis
    - Bronchocentric granulomatosis: Bronchocentric nodules, similar to rheumatoid nodules
    - Follicular bronchiolitis
      - Rare
      - Caused by lymphoid follicular hyperplasia along airways
      - Centrilobular nodules & peribronchial thickening
  - Drug reaction
    - RA-related treatment may lead to infiltrative lung disease
    - Drug treatment may produce constrictive bronchiolitis
    - Corticosteroids: Opportunistic infection
    - Gold: Ground-glass opacity along bronchovascular bundles; COP
    - Methotrexate: Subacute hypersensitivity pneumonitis; NSIP
    - Anti-tumor necrosis factor-α antibodies: Mycobacterial or fungal pneumonia
  - Other findings
    - Pulmonary hypertension, lymphadenopathy, mediastinal fibrosis, & pericardial effusion or thickening

Imaging Recommendations

- Best imaging tool
  - HRCT useful to characterize pattern & extent of RA-related lung & airway disease
  - CT useful for evaluation of RA-related pleural disease

RHEUMATOID ARTHRITIS

DIFFERENTIAL DIAGNOSIS

Idiopathic Pulmonary Fibrosis (IPF)

- May exhibit identical imaging findings: Peripheral, basilar fibrosis with honeycombing on HRCT
- Absence of pleural, pericardial, & airways disease
- No skeletal erosions

Scleroderma

- May exhibit identical imaging findings: NSIP pattern on HRCT
- Dilated esophagus: Relaxation of lower esophageal sphincter
- No joint erosions as in RA: Hallmark is acroosteolysis (resorption distal phalanx)

Asbestosis

- May exhibit identical imaging findings: UIP pattern on HRCT
- May exhibit pleural plaques (± calcification) or thickening
- Occupational history is of paramount importance
- No skeletal erosions

Cryptogenic Organizing Pneumonia

- Bilateral or unilateral, patchy consolidations, or ground-glass opacities; often subpleural or peribronchial
- Basilar irregular linear opacities

PATHOLOGY

General Features

- Etiology
  - Possible inflammatory, immunologic, hormonal, & genetic factors
- Subacute or chronic inflammatory polyarthropathy of unknown cause
- Interstitial lung disease
  - Usual interstitial pneumonia
  - Nonspecific interstitial pneumonia
  - Cryptogenic organizing pneumonia
- Airways disease
  - Bronchiectasis or bronchitis
  - Constrictive bronchiolitis
  - Follicular bronchiolitis

Microscopic Features

- Pulmonary fibrosis: Usually UIP or NSIP pattern
- Other pulmonary findings: Interstitial pneumonitis, COP, lymphoid follicles, rheumatoid nodules (pathognomonic)
- Pleural biopsy: May show rheumatoid nodules
- Pleural fluid: Lymphocytes, acutely neutrophils & eosinophils

Laboratory Abnormalities

- Pleural fluid: High protein, low glucose, low pH, high LDH, high RF, low complement
- Pulmonary function tests
  - Restrictive pulmonary function, reduced diffusing capacity
  - Obstructive defect if predominant airways disease

CLINICAL ISSUES

Presentation

- Most common signs/symptoms
  - Primary sites of inflammation: Synovial membranes & articular structures
  - Onset usually between 25 & 50 years
  - Insidious onset, with relapses & remissions
- Other signs/symptoms
  - Extraarticular RA: More common in men, age range of 50-60 years
- Thoracic symptoms
  - Thoracic disease may develop before, at onset, or after onset of arthritis
  - May be asymptomatic
  - Dyspnea, cough, pleuritic pain, finger clubbing, hemoptysis, infection, bronchopleural fistula, pneumothorax
  - Most affected patients have arthritis; positive rheumatoid factor (RF) (80%) & cutaneous nodules

Demographics

- Age
  - Any age, but more common in middle aged adults
- Gender
  - 3x more common in women
- Epidemiology
  - Thoracic involvement much more common in men
  - Pleural disease common; 40-75% in postmortem studies

Natural History & Prognosis

- 5-year survival: 40%
- Death from infection, respiratory failure, cor pulmonale, amyloidosis
  - Infection is most common cause of death

Treatment

- Treatment: Corticosteroids, immunosuppressant drugs
- Drugs used to treat RA may cause interstitial lung disease
  - Methotrexate
  - Gold
  - D-penicillamine
  - Anti-tumor necrosis factor-α antibodies

DIAGNOSTIC CHECKLIST

Consider

- RA-related lung disease in patient with lung fibrosis & history of RA or polyarthritis (especially with distal clavicular resorption)

Image Interpretation Pearls

- Hand radiographic abnormalities &/or findings of distal clavicle erosions are useful for differentiating RA from other interstitial lung diseases

SELECTED REFERENCES

1. Lynch DA: Lung disease related to collagen vascular disease. J Thorac Imaging. 24(4):299-309, 2009

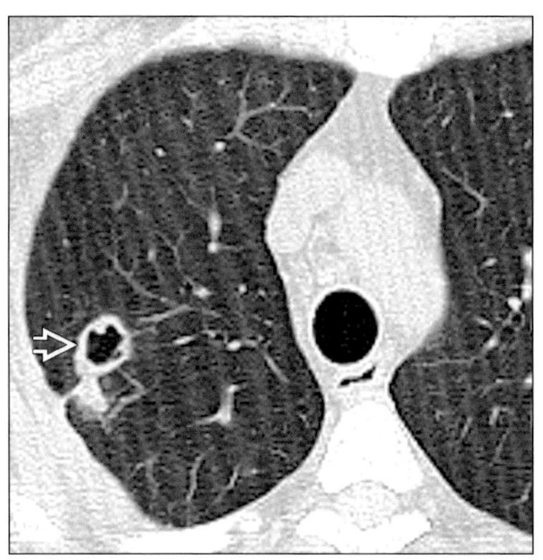

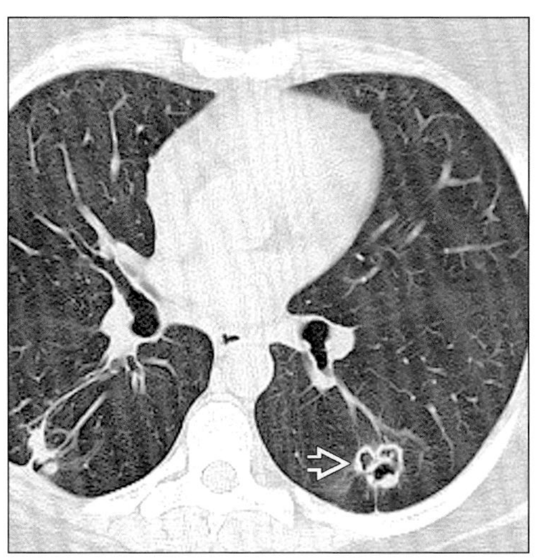

(Left) *Axial NECT of a patient with pulmonary involvement by RA shows 2 adjacent right upper lobe pulmonary nodules, one of which exhibits cavitation ➡ and a thick nodular wall.* ***(Right)*** *Axial NECT of the same patient shows additional bilateral lung nodules, one with cavitation ➡, consistent with rheumatoid nodules. Rheumatoid nodules affect less than 5% of patients with RA. The differential diagnosis includes cavitary metastases, septic emboli, vasculitis, and fungal or necrotizing pneumonia.*

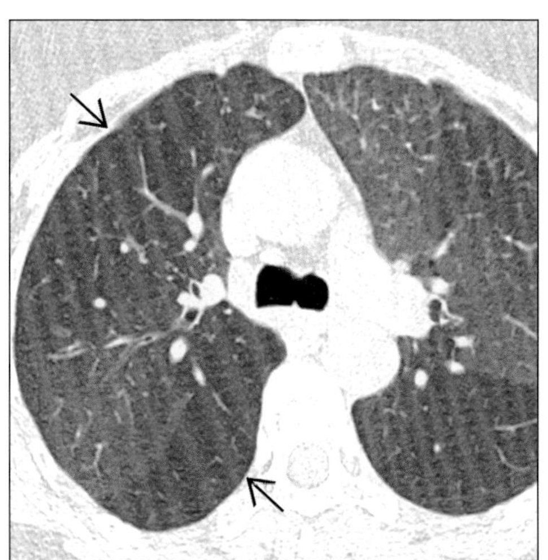

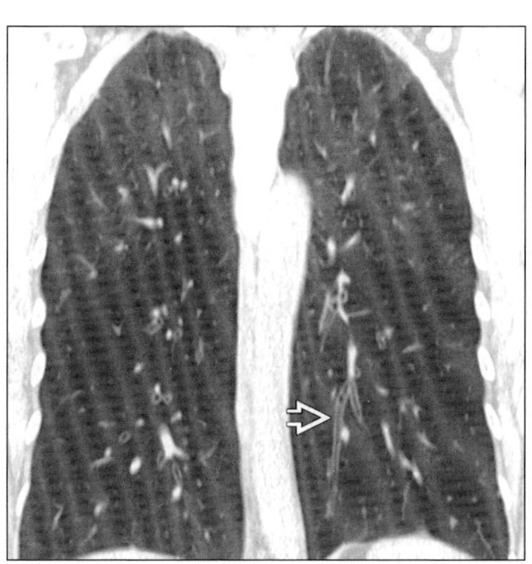

(Left) *Axial expiratory HRCT of a patient with RA shows large regions of air-trapping → secondary to RA-related constrictive bronchiolitis.* ***(Right)*** *Coronal HRCT of the same patient shows bilateral mosaic attenuation and areas of air-trapping with intrinsic cylindrical bronchiectasis ➡ and bronchial wall thickening, consistent with constrictive bronchiolitis. Although there is imaging overlap between constrictive bronchiolitis and asthma, the former produces irreversible airway obstruction.*

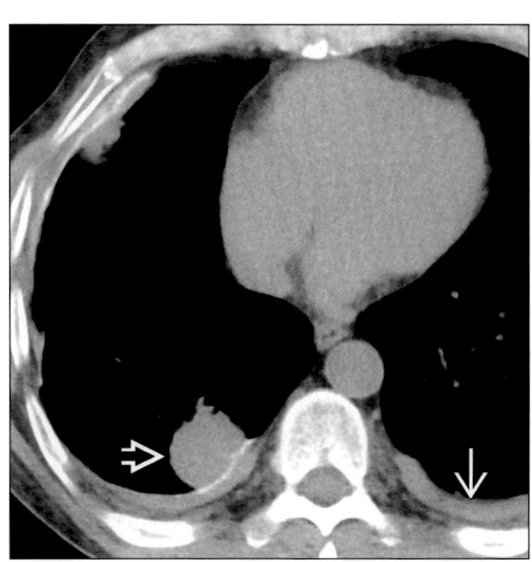

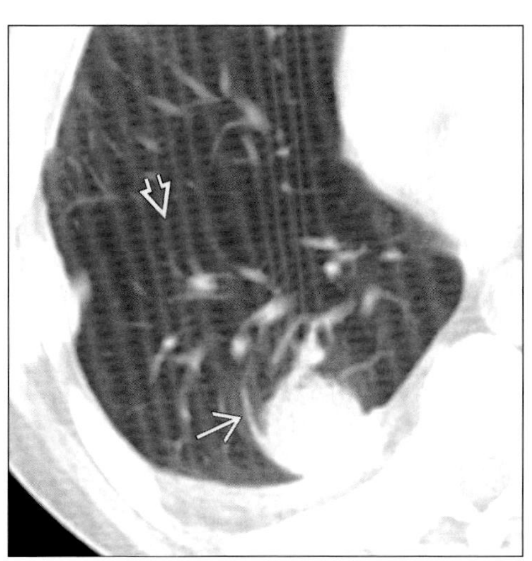

(Left) *Axial NECT of a patient with RA shows bilateral pleural thickening ➡ with partial calcification on the right. There is an adjacent subpleural soft tissue mass in the right lower lobe ➡.* ***(Right)*** *Axial NECT of the same patient shows that the right lower lobe mass abuts the thickened pleura, exhibits the "comet tail" sign ➡, and is associated with right lower lobe volume loss with posterior displacement of the right major fissure ➡. The findings are diagnostic of rounded atelectasis.*

SCLERODERMA

Key Facts

Terminology
- Generalized connective tissue disorder affecting multiple organs, including skin, lungs, heart, & kidneys

Imaging
- Radiography
  - Symmetric basal reticulonodular opacities
  - Decreased lung volumes, sometimes out of proportion to lung disease
  - Dilated, air-filled esophagus best seen on lateral
- CT
  - Interstitial lung disease: Nonspecific interstitial pneumonia > > usual interstitial pneumonia
  - Thin-walled subpleural cysts: 10-30 mm
  - Esophageal dilatation (80%)
  - Pulmonary arterial hypertension
  - Lymphadenopathy (60-70%)

Top Differential Diagnoses
- Idiopathic pulmonary fibrosis
- Aspiration pneumonia
- Nonspecific interstitial pneumonia

Pathology
- Collagen overproduction & deposition in tissue

Clinical Issues
- Pulmonary disease usually follows skin manifestations
- Increased risk of lung cancer, usually in patients with pulmonary fibrosis
- Poor prognosis; death usually from aspiration pneumonia

Diagnostic Checklist
- Consider scleroderma in patient with chronic interstitial lung disease & dilated esophagus

*(**Left**) Axial HRCT of a patient with known scleroderma shows symmetric peripheral ground-glass and reticular opacities with subpleural sparing ⇨ and a dilated distal esophagus →. (**Right**) Coronal NECT minIP image of the same patient shows basilar predominant lung disease ⇨ and debris within a dilated esophagus →, which is highly suggestive of esophageal dysmotility. Esophageal dysmotility is commonly present in patients with scleroderma.*

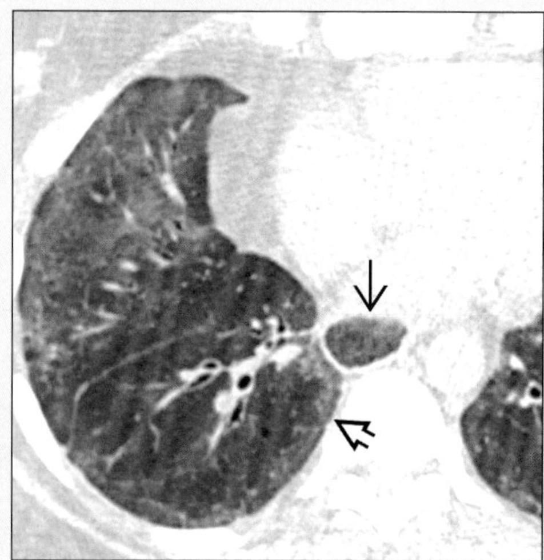

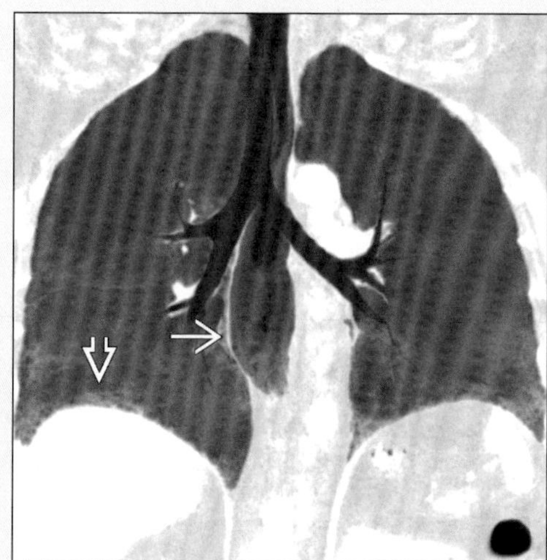

*(**Left**) Axial HRCT of a patient with scleroderma shows peripheral ground-glass and reticular opacities → and a dilated distal esophagus ⇨, consistent with esophageal dysmotility. (**Right**) Frontal hand radiograph of the same patient shows joint space narrowing, osteopenia →, and soft tissue calcifications ⇨. Concomitant imaging findings of skeletal abnormalities and soft tissue calcifications in the setting of collagen vascular disease are helpful in suggesting a specific diagnosis.*

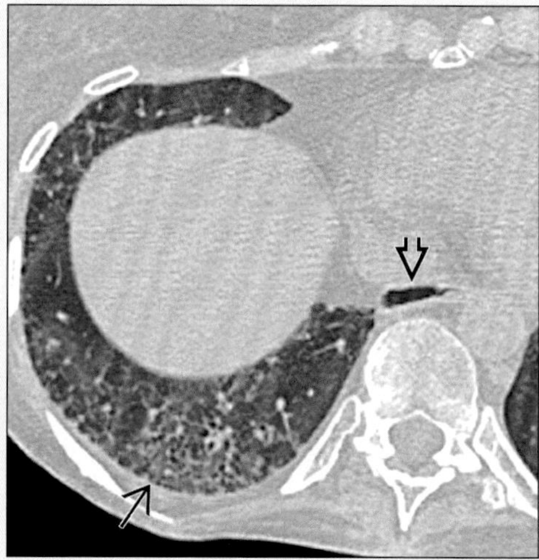

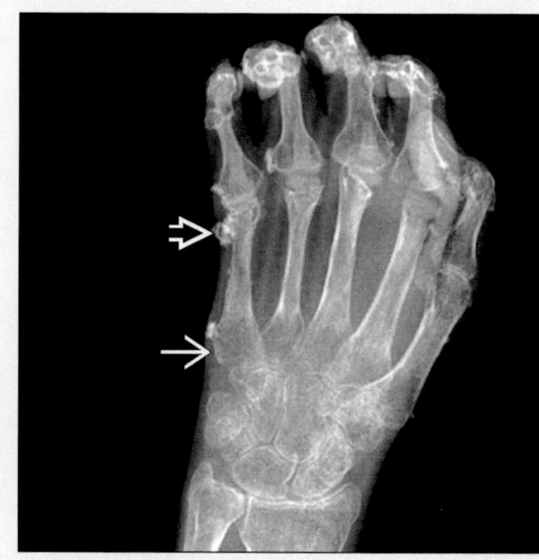

SCLERODERMA

TERMINOLOGY

Synonyms

- Systemic sclerosis

Definitions

- Generalized connective tissue disorder affecting multiple organs, including skin, lungs, heart, & kidneys
- Limited cutaneous systemic sclerosis (60%)
  - Skin involvement of hands, forearms, feet, & face
  - Longstanding Raynaud phenomenon
  - CREST syndrome: **C**alcinosis, **R**aynaud phenomenon, **e**sophageal dysmotility, **s**clerodactyly, **t**elangiectasias
- Diffuse cutaneous systemic sclerosis (40%)
  - Acute onset: Raynaud phenomenon, acral & truncal skin involvement
  - High frequency of interstitial lung disease
- Scleroderma sine scleroderma (rare)
  - Interstitial lung disease without skin manifestations

IMAGING

General Features

- Best diagnostic clue
  - Basilar interstitial thickening with dilated esophagus
- Location
  - Lower lung zones

Radiographic Findings

- Radiography
  - **Abnormal in 20-65% of cases**
  - **Lungs**
    - **Symmetric basal reticulonodular pattern**
    - Progression of **fine basilar reticulation** (lace-like) **to coarse fibrosis**
    - **Decreased lung volumes**, sometimes out of proportion to lung disease
    - Elevated diaphragm; may also be due to diaphragmatic muscle atrophy & fibrosis
  - Associated findings
    - **Dilated, air-filled esophagus** best seen on lateral chest radiography
    - Pleural thickening & effusions rare (< 15%)
    - Superior & posterolateral rib erosion (< 20%)
    - Resorption of distal phalanges, tuft calcification
    - Secondary lung cancer, often adenocarcinoma or adenocarcinoma in situ
  - Cardiomegaly
    - Pericardial effusion
    - Pulmonary arterial hypertension
    - Myocardial ischemia due to small vessel disease
    - Infiltrative cardiomyopathy

CT Findings

- CECT
  - **Esophageal dilatation (80%)**
  - **Lymphadenopathy (60-70%)**
    - Rarely identified on chest radiography
    - Most often reactive
    - Usually seen in those with interstitial lung disease
  - Pulmonary artery enlargement from **pulmonary arterial hypertension**; may occur without interstitial lung disease
  - Pleural thickening (pseudoplaques, 33%)
    - Subpleural micronodules
    - Pseudoplaques (90%): Confluence of subpleural micronodules < 7 mm in width
    - Diffuse pleural thickening (33%)
- HRCT
  - **Abnormal in 60-90% of cases**
  - Interstitial lung disease
    - **Most often nonspecific interstitial pneumonia (NSIP)**
      - Basilar predominant ground-glass opacity
      - Posterior & subpleural reticulation
      - Traction bronchiectasis & bronchiolectasis
      - Bronchovascular distribution with subpleural sparing; highly suggestive of NSIP
      - Often peripheral predominant
      - Absent to mild honeycomb lung
    - Usual interstitial pneumonia (UIP) pattern less common
      - Subpleural & basilar distribution
      - Honeycomb lung should suggest diagnosis
      - Minimal ground-glass opacity: Significant ground-glass opacity in acute exacerbation or superimposed atypical infection
  - Cysts
    - Thin-walled subpleural cysts 10-30 mm in diameter
    - Predominantly in mid & upper lungs

Other Modality Findings

- Esophagram
  - Dilated, aperistaltic esophagus (50-90%)
  - Gastroesophageal reflux
  - Patulous gastroesophageal junction

Imaging Recommendations

- Best imaging tool
  - HRCT more sensitive than radiography for identification of pulmonary involvement
  - Esophagram to assess esophageal motility

DIFFERENTIAL DIAGNOSIS

Idiopathic Pulmonary Fibrosis

- No esophageal dilatation or musculoskeletal changes
- Interstitial lung disease more coarse, honeycomb lung more common
- Ground-glass opacities less common
- Subpleural distribution

Aspiration Pneumonia

- Recurrent dependent opacities & chronic fibrosis
- Known esophageal motility disorder
- Scleroderma patients at risk

Nonspecific Interstitial Pneumonia

- Identical HRCT pattern
- Esophagus not dilated

Asbestosis

- Pleural plaques (80%)
- UIP pattern of pulmonary fibrosis
- No esophageal dilatation

Rheumatoid Arthritis

- No esophageal dilatation
- May exhibit identical HRCT pattern (NSIP or UIP)
- Symmetric articular erosive changes

SCLERODERMA

Drug Reaction
- No esophageal dilatation
- May exhibit identical HRCT pattern

Sarcoidosis
- No esophageal dilatation
- Perilymphatic micronodules predominantly in mid & upper lungs

PATHOLOGY

General Features
- Etiology
  - Reduced circulating T suppressor cells & natural killer cells, which can suppress fibroblast proliferation
  - Antitopoisomerase I (30%), anti-RNA polymerase III, & antihistone antibodies associated with interstitial lung disease
  - Anticentromere antibodies in CREST variant associated with absence of interstitial lung disease
- Genetics
  - Suspect genetic susceptibility &/or environmental factors (silica, industrial solvents)
- Overproduction & tissue deposition of collagen
- Lung is 4th most commonly affected organ after skin, arteries, esophagus

Staging, Grading, & Classification
- **American College of Rheumatology criteria**: Scleroderma requires **1 major or 2 minor criteria**
  - **Major criterion**: Involvement of skin proximal to metacarpophalangeal joints
  - **Minor criteria**: Sclerodactyly, pitting scars, loss of finger tip tufts, bilateral pulmonary basal fibrosis

Microscopic Features
- Pulmonary hypertension
  - Most distinctive finding: Concentric laminar fibrosis with few plexiform lesions
- NSIP: Cellular or fibrotic (80%)
- UIP: Fibroblast proliferation, fibrosis, & architectural distortion (10-20%)

CLINICAL ISSUES

Presentation
- Most common signs/symptoms
  - Pulmonary disease usually follows skin manifestations
    - Most common presentation is Raynaud phenomenon (up to 90%), tendonitis, arthralgia, arthritis
    - Dyspnea (60%), cough, pleuritic chest pain, fever, hemoptysis, dysphagia
- Other signs/symptoms
  - Skin tightening, induration, & thickening
  - Vascular abnormalities
  - Musculoskeletal manifestations
  - Visceral involvement of lungs, heart, & kidneys
  - Esophageal dysmotility, gastroesophageal reflux, esophageal candidiasis, esophageal stricture, weight loss
  - Renal disease: Hypertension, renal failure
  - Antinuclear antibodies (100%)
  - Pulmonary function tests
    - Restrictive or obstructive
    - Decreased diffusion capacity
  - Bronchoalveolar lavage varies from lymphocytic to neutrophilic alveolitis (50%)

Demographics
- Age
  - Usual onset: 30-50 years
- Gender
  - M:F = 1:3
- Epidemiology
  - 1.2 cases/100,000 persons
  - Pulmonary disease in > 80% at autopsy

Natural History & Prognosis
- Lung disease is indolent & progressive
- Increased risk for lung cancer; associated with pulmonary fibrosis
  - Often adenocarcinoma or adenocarcinoma in situ
- Poor prognosis: 70% 5-year survival rate
- Cause of death usually aspiration pneumonia

Treatment
- Directed towards affected organs
- Interstitial lung disease: Cyclophosphamide, corticosteroids
- Aggressive blood pressure control important for prevention of renal failure

DIAGNOSTIC CHECKLIST

Consider
- Scleroderma in patient with chronic interstitial lung disease & dilated esophagus
- Lung carcinoma in patient with scleroderma & dominant solid or subsolid lung nodule

SELECTED REFERENCES

1. Strollo D et al: Imaging lung disease in systemic sclerosis. Curr Rheumatol Rep. 12(2):156-61, 2010
2. Lynch DA: Lung disease related to collagen vascular disease. J Thorac Imaging. 24(4):299-309, 2009
3. de Azevedo AB et al: Prevalence of pulmonary hypertension in systemic sclerosis. Clin Exp Rheumatol. 23(4):447-54, 2005
4. Galie N et al: Pulmonary arterial hypertension associated to connective tissue diseases. Lupus. 14(9):713-7, 2005
5. Highland KB et al: New Developments in Scleroderma Interstitial Lung Disease. Curr Opin Rheumatol. 17(6):737-45, 2005
6. Desai SR et al: CT features of lung disease in patients with systemic sclerosis: comparison with idiopathic pulmonary fibrosis and nonspecific interstitial pneumonia. Radiology. 232(2):560-7, 2004

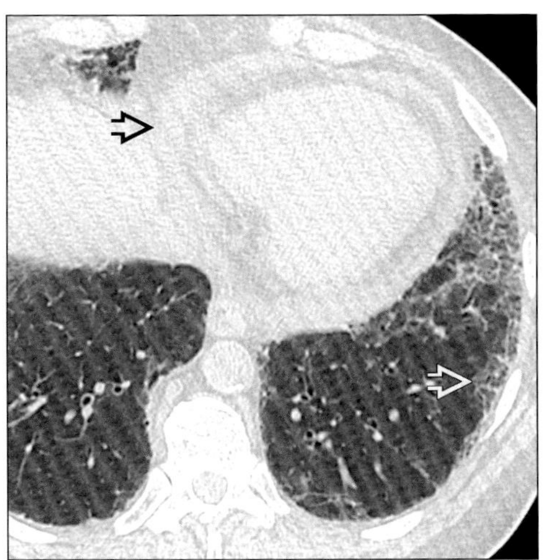

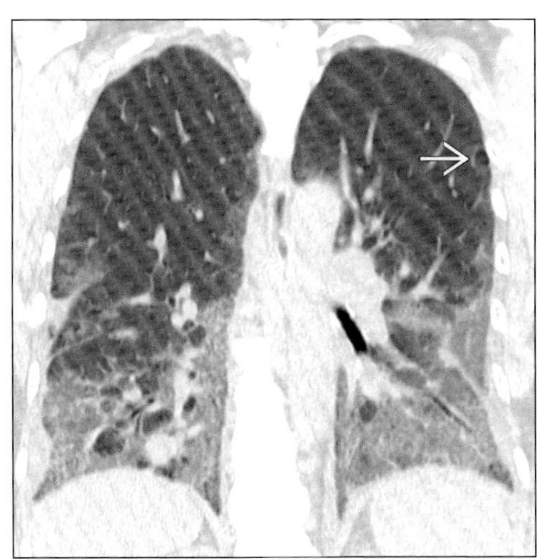

(Left) *Axial HRCT of a patient with scleroderma shows peripheral ground-glass opacities and reticulation with mild traction bronchiolectasis. Pericardial effusion in the setting of scleroderma without an alternative explanation suggests pulmonary hypertension.* ***(Right)*** *Coronal NECT of a patient with NSIP related to scleroderma shows striking basilar predominant ground-glass opacities and reticulation. A small subpleural air cyst is present in the left upper lung zone.*

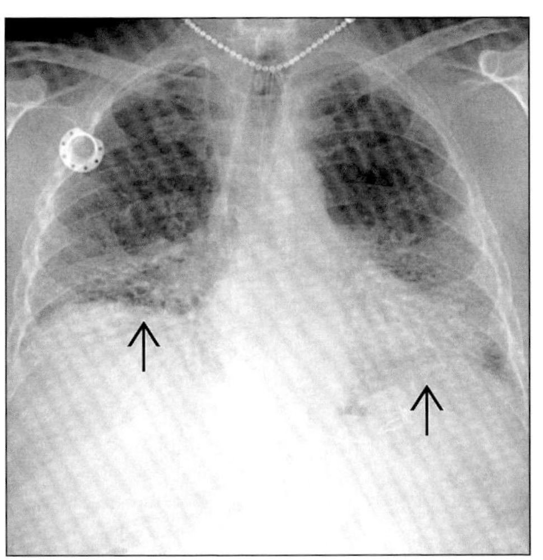

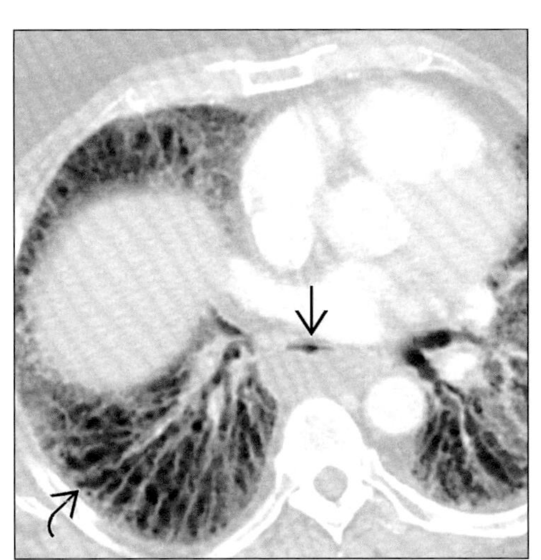

(Left) *PA chest radiograph of a patient with scleroderma shows low lung volumes and basilar reticular opacities. In suspected interstitial lung disease, further evaluation with HRCT is mandatory.* ***(Right)*** *Axial NECT of a patient with scleroderma shows bilateral basilar lower lobe bronchiectasis, ground-glass opacity, and reticulation with associated crowding of vessels and airways, suggestive of volume loss. Note dilated distal esophagus with intrinsic air-fluid level.*

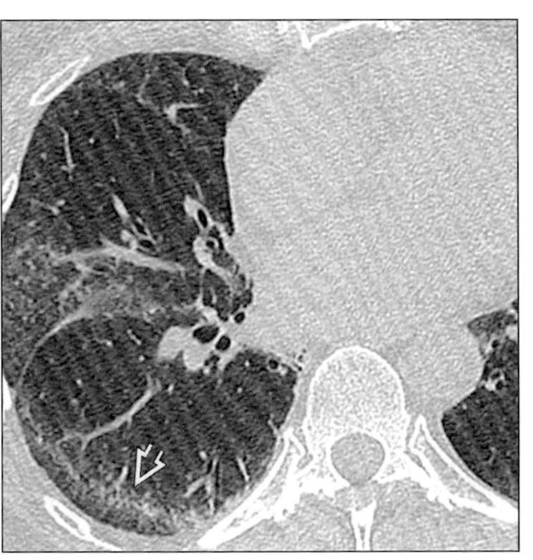

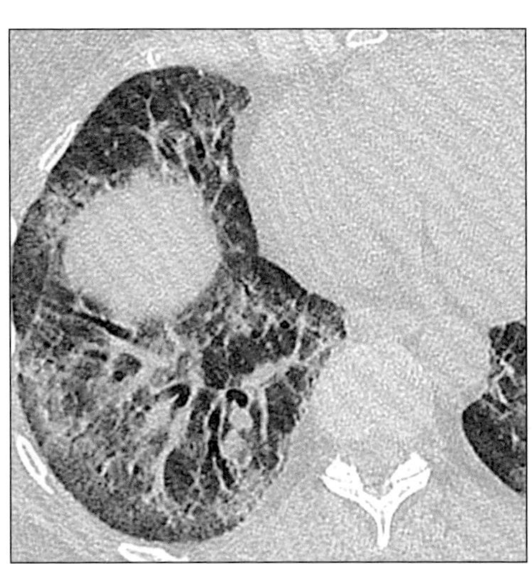

(Left) *Axial HRCT of a patient with scleroderma shows NSIP manifesting with peripheral predominant ground-glass and reticular opacities and subpleural sparing.* ***(Right)*** *Axial HRCT of the same patient shows a bronchovascular distribution of the lung disease with traction bronchiectasis and subpleural sparing. The basilar and bronchovascular distribution of ground-glass opacity and pulmonary fibrosis in association with subpleural sparing is highly suggestive of NSIP, which is common in scleroderma.*

MIXED CONNECTIVE TISSUE DISEASE

Key Facts

Terminology
- Syndrome with overlapping features of systemic sclerosis, SLE, and polymyositis/dermatomyositis
- Overlap syndrome; similar to MCTD without anti-RNP antibodies

Imaging
- Radiography
  - Basilar reticular opacities
  - Pleural effusion or thickening in 10%
- CT
  - Pulmonary disease in majority of patients
  - NSIP: Basilar ground-glass opacity ± reticulation
  - Consolidation, honeycomb lung, bronchiectasis
  - Pulmonary cysts less common
  - Pulmonary hypertension: Enlarged pulmonary trunk and central pulmonary arteries, pulmonary mosaic attenuation

Top Differential Diagnoses
- Systemic lupus erythematosus (SLE)
- Scleroderma
- Polymyositis; dermatomyositis
- Rheumatoid arthritis (RA)
- Primary pulmonary artery hypertension

Clinical Issues
- High titer of anti-RNP antibodies
- Arthritis and arthralgia; myositis
- Heartburn and dysphagia from esophageal dysmotility
- Skin: Raynaud phenomenon, sclerodactyly, scleroderma, malar rash, photosensitivity

Diagnostic Checklist
- Consider MCTD in undefined connective tissue disease with NSIP or pulmonary hypertension

*(**Left**) Axial HRCT of a patient with mixed connective tissue disease shows bilateral lower lobe ground-glass opacity with associated mild airway dilatation ⇗, which is suggestive of early traction bronchiectasis. (**Right**) Coronal NECT of the same patient shows lower lung predominant ground-glass opacity ➡. The findings are consistent with cellular nonspecific interstitial pneumonia (NSIP). Paucity of reticulation and architectural distortion suggests a favorable response to corticosteroid therapy.*

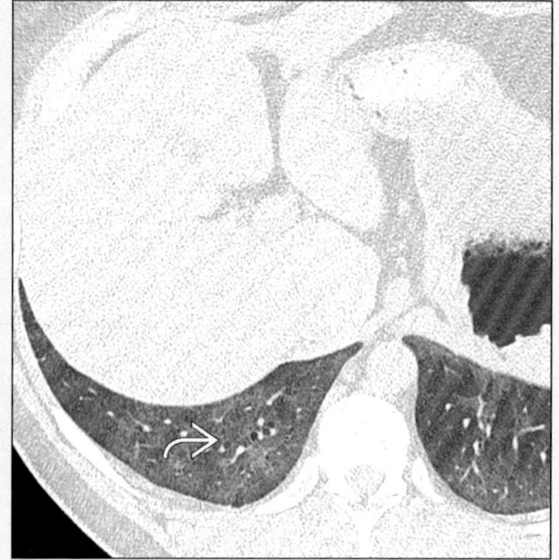

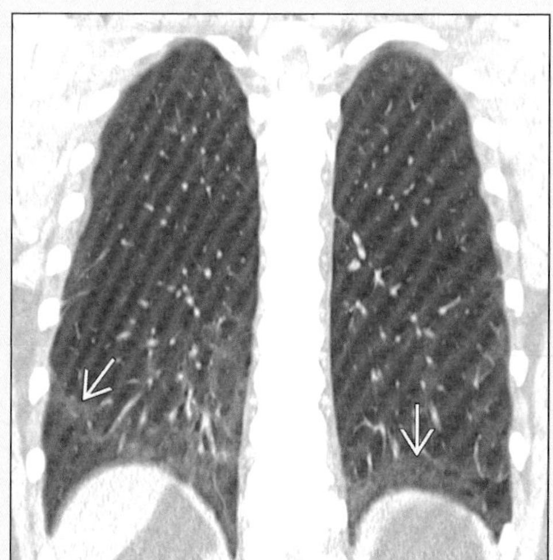

*(**Left**) Axial HRCT of a patient with mixed connective tissue disease shows patchy bilateral ground-glass opacities and associated interlobular and intralobular reticulations ⇨, consistent with interstitial lung disease. (**Right**) Axial NECT of a patient with mixed connective tissue disease shows dilation of the pulmonary artery ➡, consistent with pulmonary arterial hypertension. Pulmonary hypertension in mixed connective tissue disease may occur without significant associated lung disease.*

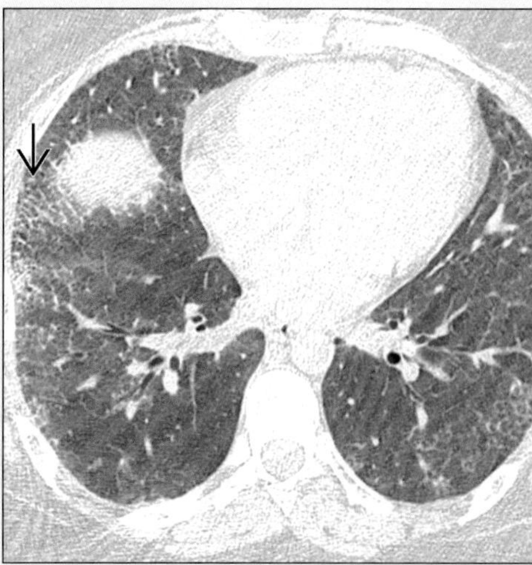

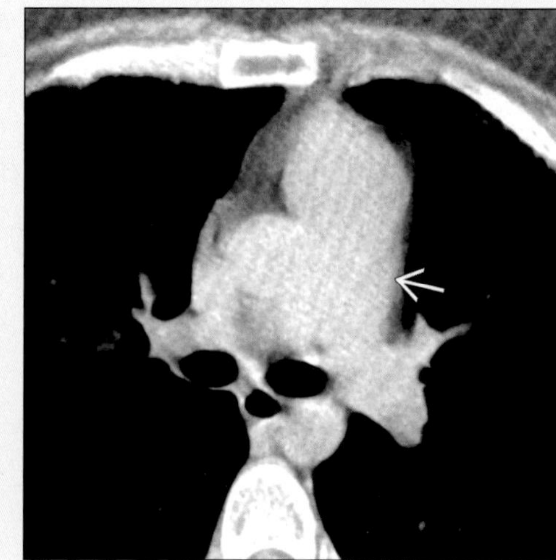

MIXED CONNECTIVE TISSUE DISEASE

TERMINOLOGY

Abbreviations

- **Mixed connective tissue disease (MCTD)**
- **Anti-ribonucleic protein (anti-RNP)** antibody

Synonyms

- **Overlap syndrome**; disease similar to MCTD without anti-RNP antibodies
  - Undifferentiated connective tissue disease not synonymous with MCTD
  - Does not fulfill criteria for defined connective tissue disease

Definitions

- Syndrome of combined features of systemic sclerosis, systemic lupus erythematosus (SLE), and polymyositis/dermatomyositis

IMAGING

General Features

- Best diagnostic clue
  - Interstitial lung disease with pattern of nonspecific interstitial pneumonia (NSIP) in patient with elevated anti-RNP antibodies
- Location
  - Lung bases
- Morphology
  - Ground-glass opacity ± reticulation

Radiographic Findings

- Basilar reticular opacities
- Pleural effusion or pleural thickening in 10%
  - Pleural effusions usually small and self-limited
- Cardiac enlargement: Pericardial effusion or volume overload from renal failure

CT Findings

- **Pulmonary disease** in majority of patients
- **NSIP pattern**: Basilar ground-glass opacity ± reticulation
- Subpleural micronodules
- Small pleural or pericardial effusion
- Consolidation, honeycomb lung, bronchiectasis, pulmonary cysts less common
- Pulmonary hypertension: Enlarged pulmonary trunk and central pulmonary arteries, mosaic lung attenuation
- Esophageal dysmotility: Dilated esophagus ± gas/fluid level

Imaging Recommendations

- Best imaging tool
  - HRCT superior to radiography in detection and characterization of interstitial lung disease

DIFFERENTIAL DIAGNOSIS

Systemic Lupus Erythematosus (SLE)

- Pleurisy in 40-60%; pleural effusion
- Pulmonary hemorrhage: Opacities sparing lung periphery
- Fibrotic lung disease less common

Scleroderma

- Lung fibrosis common
  - Typically NSIP
  - Usual interstitial pneumonia (UIP) less common
- Pulmonary hypertension ± lung disease

Polymyositis/Dermatomyositis

- Lower lung predominant NSIP
- Organizing pneumonia; confluent airspace disease with reticulation and traction bronchiectasis

Rheumatoid Arthritis (RA)

- Airways disease early
  - Bronchiolitis obliterans: Bronchial wall-thickening and air-trapping
  - Mild cylindrical bronchiectasis
  - Follicular bronchiolitis: Faint centrilobular nodules
- UIP or NSIP lung fibrosis pattern; men > women

Primary Pulmonary Artery Hypertension

- Enlarged pulmonary artery with peripheral tapering
- Mosaic lung attenuation

CLINICAL ISSUES

Presentation

- Most common signs/symptoms
  - **High titer of anti-RNP antibodies** requisite
  - Arthritis and arthralgia; myositis
  - Heartburn and dysphagia from esophageal dysmotility
  - Serositis: Pleuritis or pericarditis
  - Pulmonary arterial hypertension
  - Skin: Raynaud phenomenon, sclerodactyly, scleroderma, malar rash, photosensitivity, dermatomyositis
  - Decreased lung diffusion

Demographics

- Epidemiology
  - 1/10,000 people; average age: 37 years
  - Women affected 9x more often than men
  - Lung involvement in 80%; may be asymptomatic

Natural History & Prognosis

- Poor prognosis
- Death most often from pulmonary hypertension

Treatment

- **No specific treatment**
- Dependent on pattern of involvement
- Analgesics and nonsteroidal anti-inflammatory drugs
- Corticosteroids and cytotoxic agents

DIAGNOSTIC CHECKLIST

Consider

- MCTD in patients with undefined connective tissue disease and NSIP or pulmonary hypertension

SELECTED REFERENCES

1. Lynch DA: Lung disease related to collagen vascular disease. J Thorac Imaging. 24(4):299-309, 2009

POLYMYOSITIS/DERMATOMYOSITIS

Key Facts

Terminology
- Polymyositis: Inflammatory myopathy of limbs & anterior neck muscles
- Dermatomyositis: Myopathy & characteristic rash

Imaging
- Radiography
  - Frequently normal
  - Peripheral & basilar reticular opacities
  - Honeycomb lung may be present
  - Consolidation corresponds to cryptogenic organizing pneumonia (COP) or diffuse alveolar damage (DAD) histologic patterns
- HRCT
  - Reticular opacities, consolidation & ground-glass
  - Consolidation ± ground-glass opacity
  - Ground-glass opacity
  - Subpleural reticular opacities ± honeycomb lung

Top Differential Diagnoses
- Drug reaction
- Nonspecific interstitial pneumonia (NSIP)
- Cryptogenic organizing pneumonia
- Idiopathic pulmonary fibrosis (IPF)

Pathology
- Autoimmune disease
- Histologic patterns: NSIP (most common), COP, usual interstitial pneumonia, & DAD

Clinical Issues
- Women affected 2x as often as men
- Treatment: Corticosteroids

Diagnostic Checklist
- Consider polymyositis/dermatomyositis in patient with lung abnormalities & myositis or skin rash

*(**Left**) PA chest radiograph of a patient with dermatomyositis shows reticular ➔ opacities in the peripheral and basilar aspects of both lungs. (**Right**) Axial CECT of the same patient demonstrates extensive peripheral subpleural reticular opacities ➔, intrinsic traction bronchiolectasis, and subtle scattered areas of honeycomb lung ➔. These findings are most consistent with a histologic pattern of usual interstitial pneumonia.*

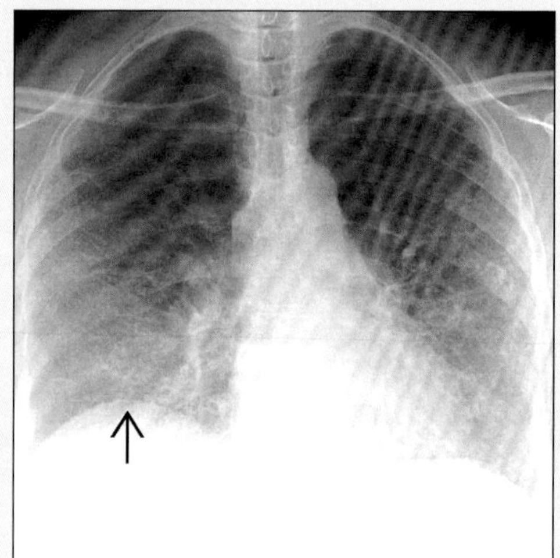

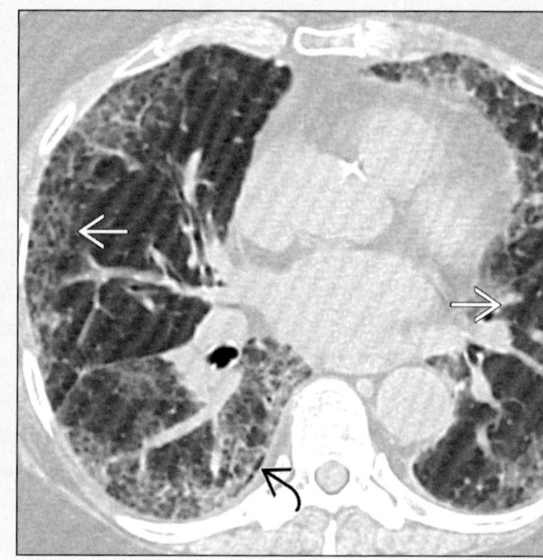

*(**Left**) Axial CECT of a patient with polymyositis shows bibasilar ground-glass opacities ➔ with intrinsic traction bronchiectasis ➔, an NSIP pattern of diffuse lung disease. (**Right**) Axial CECT of a patient with polymyositis shows basilar ground-glass opacities ➔ and associated traction bronchiectasis ➔. This NSIP pattern of lung disease is the most common of the 4 histologic patterns that may be seen in patients with polymyositis/dermatomyositis-related lung disease.*

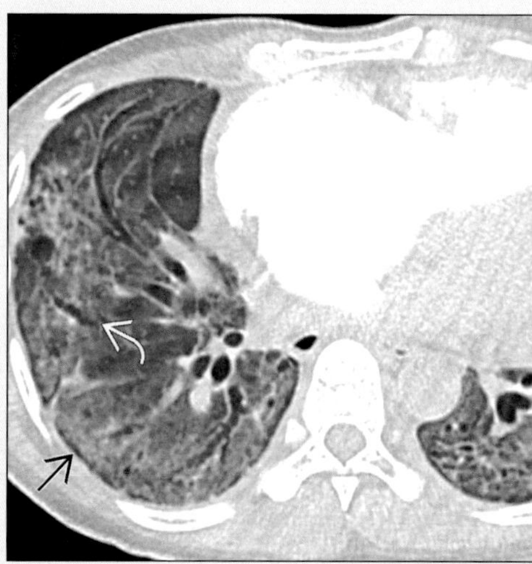

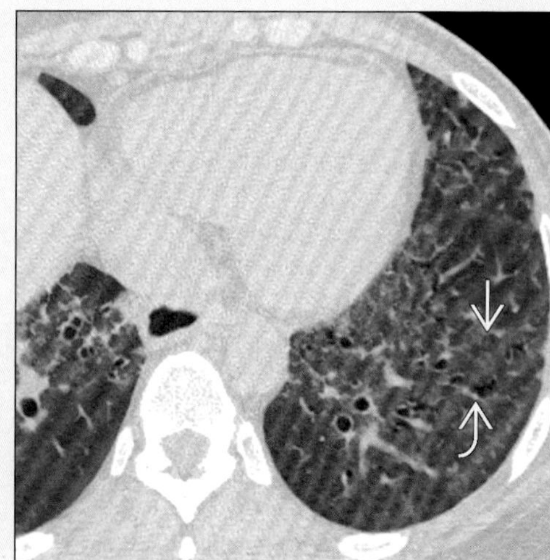

POLYMYOSITIS/DERMATOMYOSITIS

TERMINOLOGY

Definitions

- **Polymyositis**: Inflammatory myopathy of limbs & anterior neck muscles
- **Dermatomyositis**: Myopathy & characteristic rash

IMAGING

General Features

- Best diagnostic clue
  - Reticular opacities with areas of consolidation & ground-glass opacity in patient with inflammatory myopathy/rash

Radiographic Findings

- Chest radiographs are frequently normal
- Peripheral & basilar reticular opacities
- Honeycomb lung may be present
- Consolidation corresponds to cryptogenic organizing pneumonia (COP) or diffuse alveolar damage (DAD) histologic patterns

CT Findings

- HRCT
  - Most commonly reticular opacities with areas of consolidation & ground-glass opacity
  - Consolidation ± ground-glass opacity
    - Corresponds to COP or DAD histologic patterns
  - Ground-glass opacity
    - Corresponds to nonspecific interstitial pneumonia (NSIP) histologic pattern
  - Subpleural reticular opacities ± honeycomb lung
    - Corresponds to usual interstitial pneumonia (UIP) histologic pattern

Imaging Recommendations

- Best imaging tool
  - HRCT is optimal imaging modality for assessment of interstitial lung disease

DIFFERENTIAL DIAGNOSIS

Drug Reaction

- Multiple HRCT patterns, including DAD, NSIP, COP, & UIP

Nonspecific Interstitial Pneumonia

- Ground-glass opacity is most common finding
- Bronchiolectasis & bronchiectasis
- Fibrosis & honeycomb lung in fibrotic NSIP
- Etiologies: Idiopathic, collagen vascular disease, drug reaction

Cryptogenic Organizing Pneumonia

- Idiopathic (by definition)
- Subpleural consolidation ± ground-glass opacity
- Reverse halo sign: Central ground-glass opacity with surrounding rim of consolidation

Idiopathic Pulmonary Fibrosis

- Subpleural & basilar reticular opacities
- Traction bronchiectasis, architectural distortion, & honeycomb lung

UIP Pattern of Lung Disease

- Imaging findings identical to IPF
- Etiologies: Asbestosis, collagen vascular disease, drug reaction

PATHOLOGY

General Features

- Etiology
  - Autoimmune disease

Microscopic Features

- NSIP (most common), COP, UIP, & DAD patterns

Types of Thoracic Involvement

- Hypoventilation & respiratory failure
  - Secondary to involvement of respiratory muscles
- Interstitial pneumonia
- Aspiration pneumonia
  - Secondary to pharyngeal muscle weakness

CLINICAL ISSUES

Presentation

- Most common signs/symptoms
  - 3 groups classified by clinical presentation
    - **Acute onset of symptoms**
      - Fever & rapidly progressive dyspnea
    - **Slowly progressive dyspnea on exertion**
    - **Asymptomatic** with abnormal chest radiographs or pulmonary function tests

Demographics

- Age
  - Bimodal peaks: Childhood & middle adulthood
- Gender
  - Women affected 2x as often as men

Natural History & Prognosis

- Factors predictive of favorable prognosis
  - Younger age (< 50 years) at presentation
  - Slowly progressive dyspnea on exertion
  - COP & NSIP histologic patterns
- Factors predictive of poor prognosis
  - Acute onset of symptoms
  - DAD & UIP histologic patterns
- Respiratory failure is most common cause of death

Treatment

- Corticosteroids

DIAGNOSTIC CHECKLIST

Consider

- Polymyositis/dermatomyositis in patients with lung parenchymal abnormalities & history of myositis or skin rash

SELECTED REFERENCES

1. Bonnefoy O et al: Serial chest CT findings in interstitial lung disease associated with polymyositis-dermatomyositis. Eur J Radiol. 49(3):235-44, 2004

Key Facts

Terminology
- Systemic lupus erythematosus (SLE), lupus, lupus erythematosus (LE)
- Chronic collagen vascular disease with frequent thoracic manifestations

Imaging
- Radiography
  - Pleural effusion or pleural thickening
  - Consolidation: Pneumonia, hemorrhage, lupus pneumonitis
  - Low lung volume, atelectasis
  - Cardiomegaly
- HRCT
  - Interstitial lung disease
  - Centrilobular nodules
  - Bronchiectasis, bronchial wall thickening
  - Lymphadenopathy

Top Differential Diagnoses
- Cardiogenic pulmonary edema
- Pneumonia
- Goodpasture syndrome
- Usual interstitial pneumonia (UIP)
- Nonspecific interstitial pneumonia (NSIP)
- Drug toxicity

Clinical Issues
- Symptoms/signs
  - Pleuritic chest pain
  - Pulmonary hemorrhage
  - Acute lupus pneumonitis
- Most patients present between 15-50 years of age
  - M:F = 1:10
- Treatment
  - Steroids
  - Immunosuppressants

__(Left)__ Axial CECT of a patient with SLE who presented with pleurisy shows a large right pleural effusion that produces right lower lobe relaxation atelectasis ➡. Note small pericardial effusion ➡ and left ventricular hypertrophy ➡, which can develop from hypertension and chronic renal disease. __(Right)__ Axial CECT of a patient with SLE and alveolar hemorrhage shows "acinar" opacities coalescing to form a left lower lobe consolidation with surrounding ground-glass opacity.

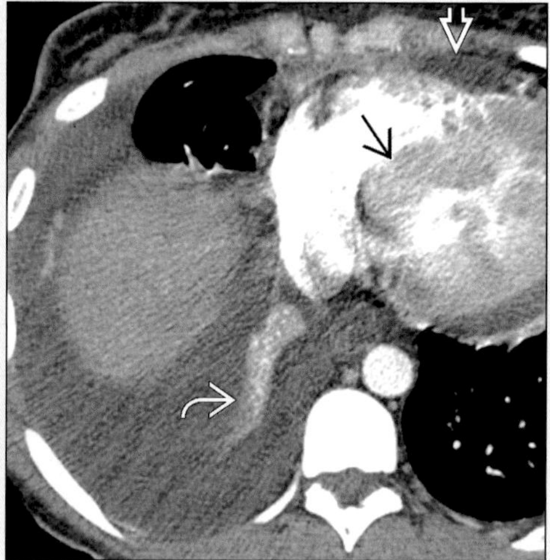

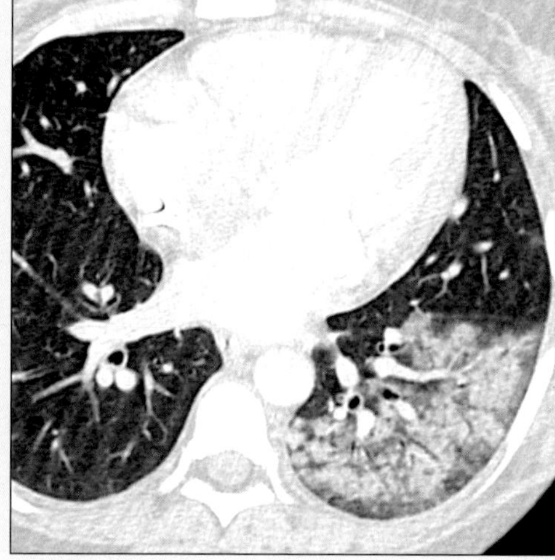

__(Left)__ PA chest radiograph of a patient with SLE shows multiple bilateral, poorly defined nodular consolidations ➡ that predominantly affect the lower lungs. __(Right)__ Axial HRCT of the same patient shows solid ➡, ground-glass ➡, and part-solid ➡ right lung nodules. Patchy ground-glass opacity ➡ is also present. Transbronchial biopsy revealed organizing pneumonia, which can be both a primary manifestation of SLE and a manifestation of drug reaction or infection.

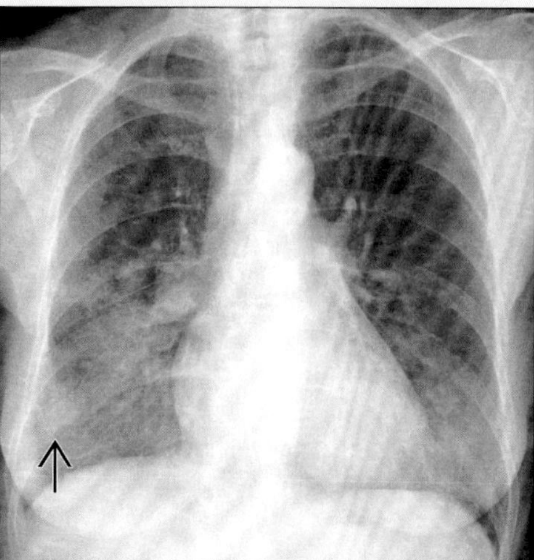

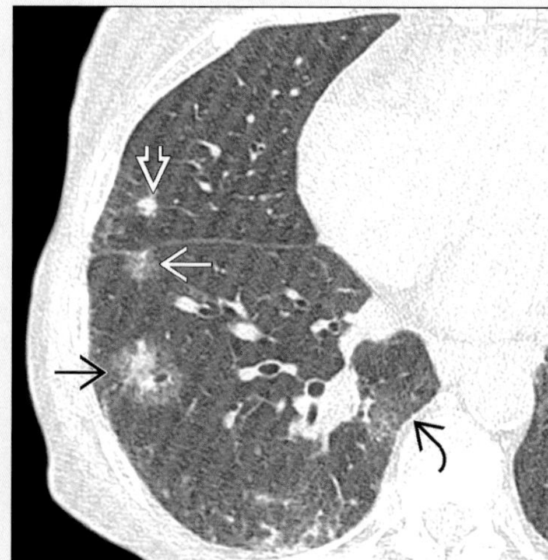

SYSTEMIC LUPUS ERYTHEMATOSUS

TERMINOLOGY

Synonyms

- **Systemic lupus erythematosus (SLE), lupus, lupus erythematosus (LE)**

Definitions

- **Chronic collagen vascular disease**
  - May manifest with cough, dyspnea, & pleuritic chest pain
  - **Thoracic manifestations in 70%**
  - Other manifestations: Arthritis, serositis, photosensitivity; renal, hematologic, central nervous system involvement

IMAGING

General Features

- Best diagnostic clue
  - Pleural thickening or effusion most common
    - Unexplained small bilateral pleural effusions or pleural thickening in young women

Radiographic Findings

- Radiography
  - **Pleural effusion or pleural thickening (50%)**
    - Usually small, unilateral or bilateral
  - **Consolidation**
    - Pneumonia (conventional or opportunistic)
    - Alveolar hemorrhage
    - Acute lupus pneumonitis (1-4%)
    - Infarcts from thromboembolism
    - Organizing pneumonia
  - Elevated diaphragm or atelectasis (20%)
    - Related to respiratory muscle & diaphragmatic dysfunction
    - "Shrinking lung syndrome"
  - **Cardiac enlargement**
    - Pericardial effusion
    - Renal failure
  - Only 1-6% have chest radiographic or clinical findings of interstitial lung disease

CT Findings

- HRCT
  - More sensitive than chest radiography or pulmonary function tests
    - Findings of **intersitial lung disease in 60%** of symptomatic patients
    - 38% of symptomatic patients have normal chest radiograph
  - May exhibit usual interstitial pneumonia (UIP) pattern
    - Bibasilar subpleural reticular opacities
    - Traction bronchiectasis
    - Honeycomb lung
  - Centrilobular nodules (20%)
  - Bronchiectasis or bronchial wall thickening (33%)
  - Findings of chronic interstitial pneumonia (3-13%)
    - Extensive ground-glass opacities, especially with nonspecific interstitial pneumonia (NSIP)
    - Coarse linear bands
    - Honeycomb cysts
- Other CT findings
  - Mild lymphadenopathy < 2 cm (20%)
  - Pulmonary embolism
    - Thromboembolic disease resulting from antiphospholipid antibodies
  - Ground-glass opacity
    - Pneumonia
    - Acute lupus pneumonitis
    - Alveolar hemorrhage
  - Pulmonary artery enlargement from pulmonary hypertension (5-14%)
    - Usually primary
    - May be secondary to chronic pulmonary thromboembolism
  - Cavitary pulmonary nodules
    - May be secondary to infarction

DIFFERENTIAL DIAGNOSIS

Cardiogenic Pulmonary Edema

- Interstitial thickening less common with SLE
- History helps in diagnosis

Pneumonia

- Identical radiographic findings, often seen with SLE

Goodpasture Syndrome

- Extent of parenchymal findings more severe than SLE

Usual Interstitial Pneumonia (UIP)

- Interstitial lung disease with honeycomb lung (rare with SLE)

Nonspecific Interstitial Pneumonia (NSIP)

- Cellular NSIP, fibrotic NSIP; honeycomb lung uncommon

Drug Toxicity

- Many drugs produce SLE pattern

Rheumatoid Arthritis

- Interstitial thickening less common with SLE

Viral Pleuropericarditis

- Identical appearance, but limited course

PATHOLOGY

General Features

- Etiology
  - Collagen vascular disease involving
    - Blood vessels (vasculitis)
    - Serosal surfaces & joints
    - Kidneys, central nervous system, skin
  - **Immune system**
    - SLE affects complement system, T suppressor cells, & cytokine production
    - Results in generation of **autoantibodies**
  - Unknown: Majority of cases
  - **Drug-induced lupus**
    - **90%** of drug-induced SLE associated with
      - Procainamide
      - Hydralazine
      - Isoniazid
      - Phenytoin
      - Thyroid blockers
      - Antiarrhythmic drugs
      - Anticonvulsants

- Antibiotics
  - Renal & central nervous system disease usually absent
    - Anti-DNA antibodies absent

Gross Pathologic & Surgical Features

- Pulmonary pathology nonspecific
  - Vasculitis, hemorrhage, organizing pneumonia

Microscopic Features

- **Hematoxylin bodies pathognomonic**
  - Rare in lung (< 1%)
- Alveolar hemorrhage reflects diffuse endothelial injury
- Diffuse alveolar damage seen with acute lupus pneumonitis
- Pleural findings are nonspecific
  - Lymphocytic & plasma cell infiltration, fibrosis, fibrinous pleuritis

CLINICAL ISSUES

Presentation

- Most common signs/symptoms
  - **Pleuritic pain in 15-60% of patients**, may occur ± pleural effusion
- **11 diagnostic criteria**; presence of any 4 for diagnosis of SLE
  - Skin (80%): Malar rash, photosensitivity, discoid lesions
  - Oral ulceration (15%)
  - Arthropathy (85%) (nonerosive)
  - Serositis (pericardial or pleural) (50%)
  - Renal proteinuria or casts (50%)
  - Neurologic epilepsy or psychosis (40%)
  - Hematologic anemia or pancytopenia
  - Immunologic abnormalities
  - Positive antinuclear antibody test
- Pleural disease, usually painful
  - Antinuclear antibody (ANA), anti-DNA antibodies, & LE cells found in pleural fluid
  - Exudative effusion with higher glucose & lower lactate than pleural effusion in rheumatoid arthritis
- Pulmonary hemorrhage may not result in hemoptysis
  - Mortality: 50-90%
  - Often associated with glomerulonephritis
- **Thromboembolic disease**
  - Related to **anticardiolipin antibody**
  - May require lifelong anticoagulation
- **Antiphospholipid antibodies (40%)**
- Pulmonary function: Restrictive with normal diffusion capacity reflects diaphragm dysfunction
- Acute lupus pneumonitis
  - Rare, life-threatening, immune complex disease
  - Fever, cough, & hypoxia requiring mechanical ventilation
- Constrictive bronchiolitis rarely reported with SLE
  - ± organizing pneumonia
- Respiratory muscle dysfunction seen in up to 25% of SLE patients

Demographics

- Age
  - Most patients present between 15-50 years
- Gender
  - M:F = 1:10
- Epidemiology
  - **50 cases per 100,000 persons**

Natural History & Prognosis

- Chronic disease (> 10 years) except in acute lupus pneumonitis
- Risk for thromboembolic disease & opportunistic infections
- Acute lupus pneumonitis & hemorrhage associated with high mortality
- Most common causes of death: Sepsis, renal disease

Treatment

- Steroids or immunosuppressants
- Nonsteroidal antiinflammatory drugs (NSAIDs) may be effective for mildly symptomatic pleurisy

SELECTED REFERENCES

1. Kocheril SV et al: Comparison of disease progression and mortality of connective tissue disease-related interstitial lung disease and idiopathic interstitial pneumonia. Arthritis Rheum. 53(4):549-57, 2005
2. Filipek MS et al: Lymphocytic interstitial pneumonitis in a patient with systemic lupus erythematosus: radiographic and high-resolution CT findings. J Thorac Imaging. 19(3):200-3, 2004
3. Lalani TA et al: Imaging findings in systemic lupus erythematosus. Radiographics. 24(4):1069-86, 2004
4. Najjar M et al: Cavitary lung masses in SLE patients: an unusual manifestation of CMV infection. Eur Respir J. 24(1):182-4, 2004
5. Paran D et al: Pulmonary disease in systemic lupus erythematosus and the antiphospholpid syndrome. Autoimmun Rev. 3(1):70-5, 2004
6. Nomura A et al: Unusual lung consolidation in SLE. Thorax. 58(4):367, 2003
7. Saito Y et al: Pulmonary involvement in mixed connective tissue disease: comparison with other collagen vascular diseases using high resolution CT. J Comput Assist Tomogr. 26(3):349-57, 2002
8. Cheema GS et al: Interstitial lung disease in systemic sclerosis. Curr Opin Pulm Med. 7(5):283-90, 2001
9. Rockall AG et al: Imaging of the pulmonary manifestations of systemic disease. Postgrad Med J. 77(912):621-38, 2001
10. Keane MP et al: Pleuropulmonary manifestations of systemic lupus erythematosus. Thorax. 55(2):159-66, 2000
11. Mayberry JP et al: Thoracic manifestations of systemic autoimmune diseases: radiographic and high-resolution CT findings. Radiographics. 20(6):1623-35, 2000
12. Warrington KJ et al: The shrinking lungs syndrome in systemic lupus erythematosus. Mayo Clin Proc. 75(5):467-72, 2000
13. Murin S et al: Pulmonary manifestations of systemic lupus erythematosus. Clin Chest Med. 19(4):641-65, viii, 1998
14. Ooi GC et al: Systemic lupus erythematosus patients with respiratory symptoms: the value of HRCT. Clin Radiol. 52(10):775-81, 1997
15. Sant SM et al: Pleuropulmonary abnormalities in patients with systemic lupus erythematosus: assessment with high resolution computed tomography, chest radiography and pulmonary function tests. Clin Exp Rheumatol. 15(5):507-13, 1997
16. Fenlon HM et al: High-resolution chest CT in systemic lupus erythematosus. AJR Am J Roentgenol. 166(2):301-7, 1996
17. Bankier AA et al: Discrete lung involvement in systemic lupus erythematosus: CT assessment. Radiology. 196(3):835-40, 1995

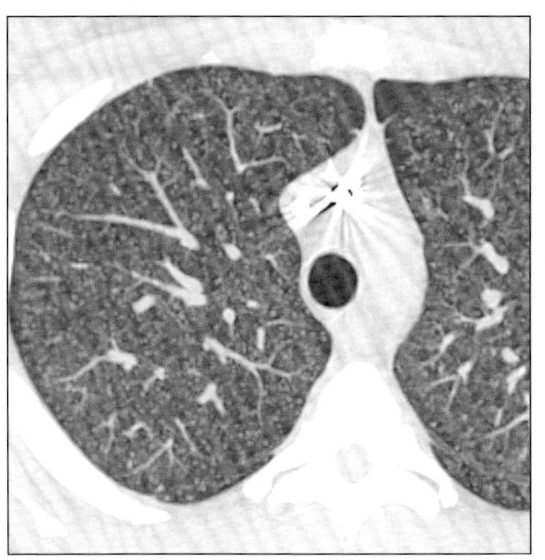

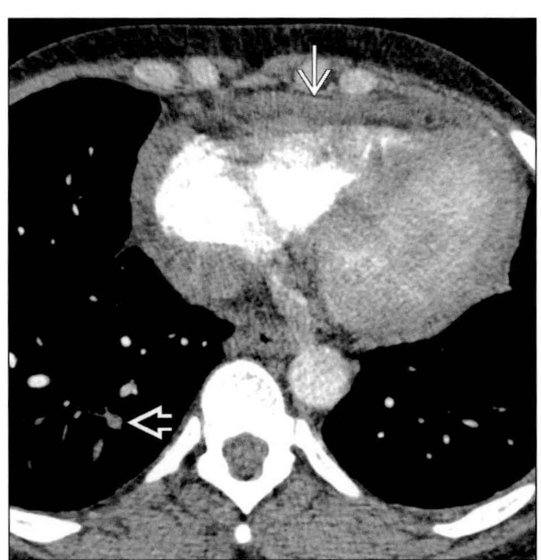

(Left) *Axial HRCT MIP of a patient with SLE and tuberculosis shows diffuse miliary lung nodules. SLE predisposes affected patients to pulmonary infection secondary to immune dysfunction and immunosuppressive drugs. Tuberculosis and nocardiosis are common opportunistic infections.* ***(Right)*** *Axial CECT of a patient with SLE and antiphospholipid antibody syndrome shows acute pulmonary emboli ⇨ in the right lower lobe and a moderate pericardial effusion →.*

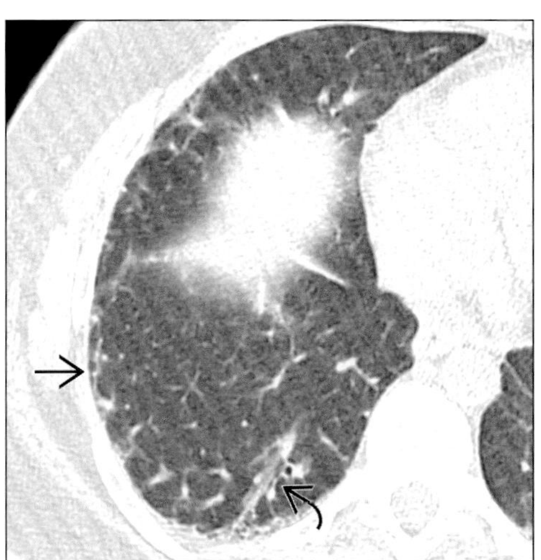

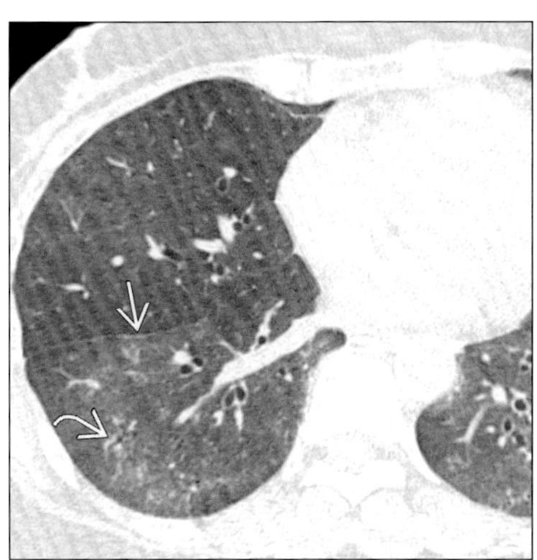

(Left) *Axial HRCT of a patient with SLE shows subpleural reticulation → and traction bronchiolectasis ↷, consistent with interstitial fibrosis. Interstitial pneumonia is far less common in patients with SLE than in those with other connective tissue diseases.* ***(Right)*** *Axial HRCT of a patient with SLE shows patchy basilar predominant ground-glass opacity →, mild subpleural reticulation, and mild traction bronchiolectasis ↷, proven to represent NSIP on open lung biopsy.*

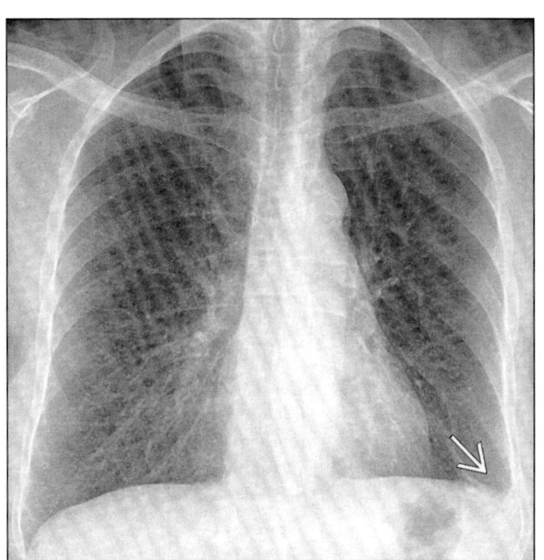

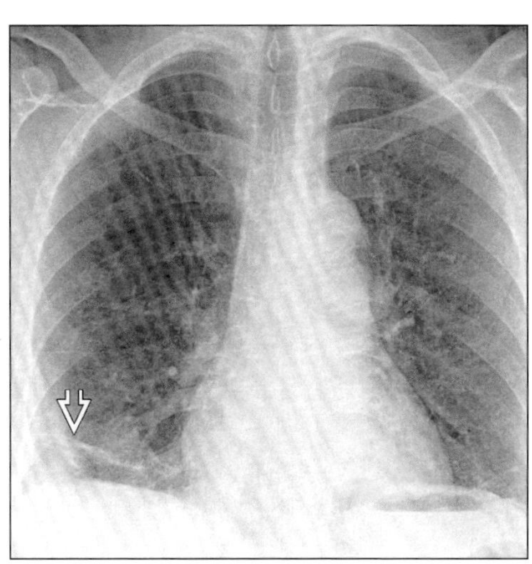

(Left) *PA chest radiograph of a patient with SLE shows normal lung volumes and blunting of the left costophrenic sulcus → from a small pleural effusion.* ***(Right)*** *PA chest radiograph of the same patient obtained 4 years later shows low lung volumes, bilateral pleural thickening, and bibasilar atelectasis ⇨. "Shrinking lung syndrome" can result from chronic diaphragmatic dysfunction and progressive pleural thickening. Rounded atelectasis can develop adjacent to areas of pleural thickening.*

SJÖGREN SYNDROME

Key Facts

Terminology
- Sjögren syndrome (SS)
- Immunologic disease defined primarily by dry eyes (keratoconjunctivitis sicca) & dry mouth (xerostomia)
  - Primary & secondary Sjögren syndrome

Imaging
- Radiography
  - LIP: Reticulonodular & ground-glass opacities, pulmonary cysts
- CT
  - Follicular bronchiolitis: Centrilobular nodules
  - Lymphocytic interstitial pneumonia (LIP): Cysts & septal thickening
  - Nonspecific interstitial pneumonia (NSIP): Basilar ground-glass opacity with superimposed reticular opacities & bronchiolectasis
  - Lymphoma: Mass-like consolidations with air bronchograms ± mediastinal & hilar lymphadenopathy

Top Differential Diagnoses
- Amyloidosis
- Cystic lung disease
- Scleroderma
- Rheumatoid arthritis

Clinical Issues
- Symptoms/signs
  - Xerostomia
  - Keratoconjunctivitis sicca
  - Respiratory symptoms ~ 10%

Diagnostic Checklist
- Consider pulmonary lymphoma in patient with Sjögren syndrome & new mass/consolidation

*(**Left**) PA chest radiograph of a patient with lymphocytic interstitial pneumonia and Sjögren syndrome shows multiple thin-walled cysts ➔ in the lower lung zones. (**Right**) Axial HRCT of the same patient shows multiple thin-walled cysts, some of which are perivascular with a vessel ➡ coursing along the cyst wall. Scattered centrilobular ground-glass opacities ➦ are also present. The cysts in LIP are basal predominant and typically fewer than those associated with lymphangioleiomyomatosis.*

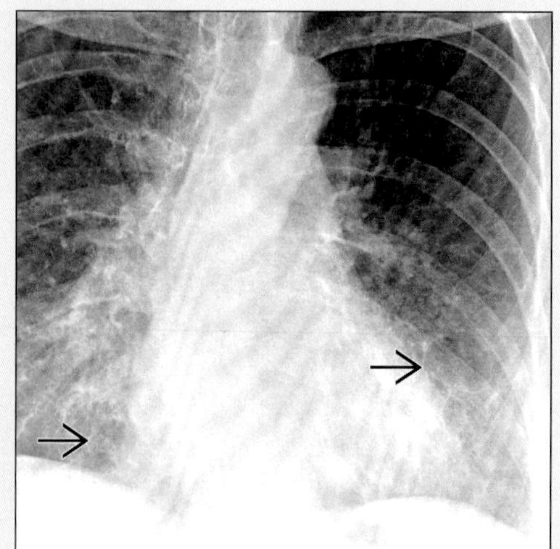

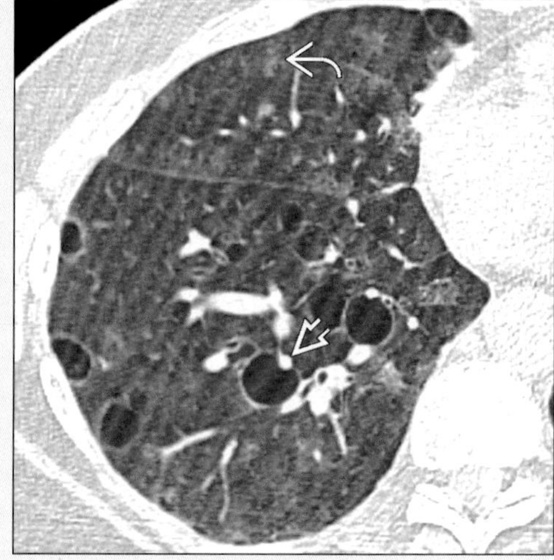

*(**Left**) Axial HRCT of a patient with LIP and Sjögren syndrome shows scattered thin-walled cysts of varying sizes. Note the perivascular distribution of many cysts, characterized by a vessel ➦ coursing along the cyst wall. (**Right**) Axial HRCT of a patient with Sjögren syndrome and LIP shows a single thin-walled cyst ➡ in the right middle lobe. Fine peripheral and basal predominant reticular opacities ➔ are also present without evidence of honeycomb lung.*

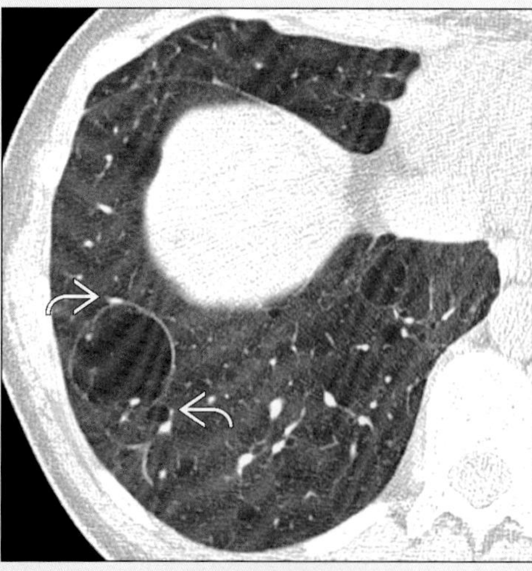

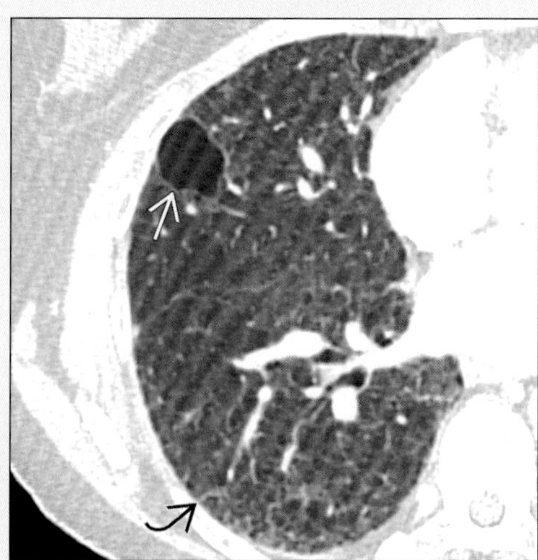

SJÖGREN SYNDROME

TERMINOLOGY

Abbreviations

- **Sjögren syndrome (SS)**

Synonyms

- Sicca syndrome, Mikulicz syndrome

Definitions

- Immunologic disease defined primarily by dry eyes (keratoconjunctivitis sicca) & dry mouth (xerostomia)
- **Primary Sjögren syndrome**
  - Occurs in absence of other autoimmune disease
- **Secondary Sjögren syndrome**
  - Associated with other autoimmune disease
    - Especially rheumatoid arthritis, systemic sclerosis, & primary biliary cirrhosis
  - Associated with chronic liver disease
    - Evidence of liver disease in approximately 10% of patients with Sjögren syndrome
    - Possible link between hepatitis C & Sjögren syndrome

IMAGING

General Features

- Best diagnostic clue
  - Lung cysts in setting of sicca syndrome
- Location
  - Lungs
    - Basal predominant
- Size
  - 1-30 mm
- Morphology
  - Thin walls
  - Perivascular

Radiographic Findings

- Radiography
  - **Lymphocytic interstitial pneumonia (LIP)**
    - Reticular or reticulonodular opacities & ground-glass opacities
      - Bilateral, basal predominant
    - Pleural disease rare in primary Sjögren syndrome
  - **Lymphoma**
    - Mediastinal & hilar lymphadenopathy
    - Primary pulmonary lymphoma: Persistent focal or multifocal mass/consolidation

CT Findings

- HRCT
  - **Follicular bronchiolitis**
    - **Small centrilobular nodules**
    - Varying degree of peribronchial nodules & ground-glass opacities
    - Mild bronchial dilatation
    - Few small, thin-walled cysts
  - **Lymphocytic interstitial pneumonia**
    - **Cysts (in approximately 2/3 of patients)**
      - Range from 1-30 mm (mean: 6 mm)
      - Bilateral, basal predominant
      - Perivascular
      - Affect < 10% of lung parenchyma
    - Poorly defined centrilobular nodules
    - Smooth interlobular septal thickening
  - **Nonspecific interstitial pneumonia (NSIP)**
    - **Ground-glass opacity**
      - Basal predominant (90%), diffuse (10%)
      - Superimposed reticulation, traction bronchiectasis, & bronchiolectasis
      - Honeycomb lung uncommon
  - **Lymphoma**
    - **Mediastinal & hilar lymphadenopathy**
      - Anterior mediastinal & paratracheal lymph nodes most commonly involved
    - Primary pulmonary lymphoma
      - Focal or multifocal lung mass/consolidation
      - Air bronchograms common
      - Mediastinal lymphadenopathy uncommon with primary pulmonary mucosa-associated lymphoid tissue (MALT) lymphoma (MALToma)
  - Bronchiectasis
    - Up to 1/3 of patients with Sjögren syndrome
    - May be associated with air-trapping

Imaging Recommendations

- Best imaging tool
  - HRCT is optimal imaging modality for evaluation of interstitial lung & small airway diseases

DIFFERENTIAL DIAGNOSIS

Amyloidosis

- May manifest with cysts & nodules
  - Calcification frequent
- No clinical manifestations of sicca syndrome

Cystic Lung Disease

- Lymphangioleiomyomatosis (LAM): Diffuse lung cysts
- Pulmonary Langerhans cell histiocytosis (PLCH): Irregular, upper lobe predominant cysts
- Birt-Hogg-Dubé syndrome: Facial fibrofolliculomas, renal neoplasms

Scleroderma

- Cutaneous features: Sclerodactyly, taught facial skin
- Calcinosis cutis
- Esophageal dysmotility

Rheumatoid Arthritis

- Synovitis, arthritis
- Rheumatoid factor positivity

AIDS

- LIP: More common in children with AIDS
- HIV seropositivity

Castleman Disease

- Lymphadenopathy/lymphoid mass
  - Often hypervascular (hyalinizing vascular subtype)

PATHOLOGY

General Features

- Etiology
  - Incompletely understood
  - Environmental factors activate HLA-DR-dependent immune system
    - Affects vascular endothelium of exocrine glands
- Genetics
  - Associated with *HLA-DR3* & some *HLA-DQ* alleles

SJÖGREN SYNDROME

- Associated abnormalities
  - Antibody to Sjögren-syndrome-related antigen A (anti-SS-A) or B (anti-SS-B)
    - Not specific for Sjögren syndrome: Occurs in subset of patients with systemic lupus erythematosus

Microscopic Features

- Lymphocytic infiltration of exocrine glands
- **LIP**
  - Proliferation of lymphocytes & plasma cells in pulmonary interstitium
- **Follicular bronchiolitis**
  - Infiltration of lymphocytes & plasma cells in bronchial walls & peribronchial interstitium
- **NSIP**
  - Temporally homogeneous expansion of alveolar interstitium
    - Fibrosis, inflammation, or both
  - Absent or inconspicuous fibroblastic foci

CLINICAL ISSUES

Presentation

- Most common signs/symptoms
  - **Xerostomia**
    - Dysphagia
    - Dysphonia
  - **Keratoconjunctivitis sicca**
    - Irritation
    - Photophobia
    - Loss of corneal integrity
  - **Salivary gland swelling**
    - Acute: Infection
    - Slowly progressive: Lymphoma
- Other signs/symptoms
  - Respiratory symptoms (~ 10%)
  - Cutaneous vasculitis (~ 10%)
  - Raynaud phenomenon (~ 30%)
  - Myalgia & arthralgia
    - Frank arthritis uncommon

Demographics

- Age
  - Develops at any age (mean: 59 years)
    - Peaks in decades after menarche & menopause
- Gender
  - M:F = 1:9
- Epidemiology
  - Prevalence
    - 14.4 cases per 100,000 persons

Natural History & Prognosis

- Lymphoma major cause of morbidity & mortality
  - 44x increased risk of non-Hodgkin lymphoma

Treatment

- Sicca syndrome
  - Keratoconjunctivitis sicca
    - Topical drops
    - Punctal occlusion
      - Temporary or permanent obstruction of tear ducts
  - Xerostomia
    - Pilocarpine & cevimeline to increase saliva production
- Systemic
  - Hydroxychloroquine
  - Immunosuppressive agents
    - Methotrexate
    - Cyclosporine
- Lymphoma
  - Chemotherapy &/or radiation therapy

DIAGNOSTIC CHECKLIST

Consider

- Lymphoma
  - New or progressive mediastinal lymphadenopathy
  - Persistent or slowly enlarging single or multifocal lung mass or consolidation
- LIP
  - Basal predominant perivascular lung cysts
  - Centrilobular nodules or ground-glass opacities
- NSIP
  - Basal predominant ground-glass opacities with superimposed reticulation

SELECTED REFERENCES

1. Nikolov NP et al: Pathogenesis of Sjögren's syndrome. Curr Opin Rheumatol. 21(5):465-70, 2009
2. Parambil JG et al: Interstitial lung disease in primary Sjögren syndrome. Chest. 130(5):1489-95, 2006
3. Fox RI: Sjögren's syndrome. Lancet. 366(9482):321-31, 2005
4. Ito I et al: Pulmonary manifestations of primary Sjogren's syndrome: a clinical, radiologic, and pathologic study. Am J Respir Crit Care Med. 171(6):632-8, 2005
5. Lazarus MN et al: Development of additional autoimmune diseases in a population of patients with primary Sjögren's syndrome. Ann Rheum Dis. 64(7):1062-4, 2005
6. Jeong YJ et al: Amyloidosis and lymphoproliferative disease in Sjögren syndrome: thin-section computed tomography findings and histopathologic comparisons. J Comput Assist Tomogr. 28(6):776-81, 2004
7. Kim EA et al: Interstitial lung diseases associated with collagen vascular diseases: radiologic and histopathologic findings. Radiographics. 2002 Oct;22 Spec No:S151-65. Review. Erratum in: Radiographics. 23(5):1340, 2003
8. Tonami H et al: Clinical and imaging findings of lymphoma in patients with Sjögren syndrome. J Comput Assist Tomogr. 27(4):517-24, 2003
9. Vitali C et al: Classification criteria for Sjögren's syndrome: a revised version of the European criteria proposed by the American-European Consensus Group. Ann Rheum Dis. 61(6):554-8, 2002
10. Uffmann M et al: Lung manifestation in asymptomatic patients with primary Sjögren syndrome: assessment with high resolution CT and pulmonary function tests. J Thorac Imaging. 16(4):282-9, 2001

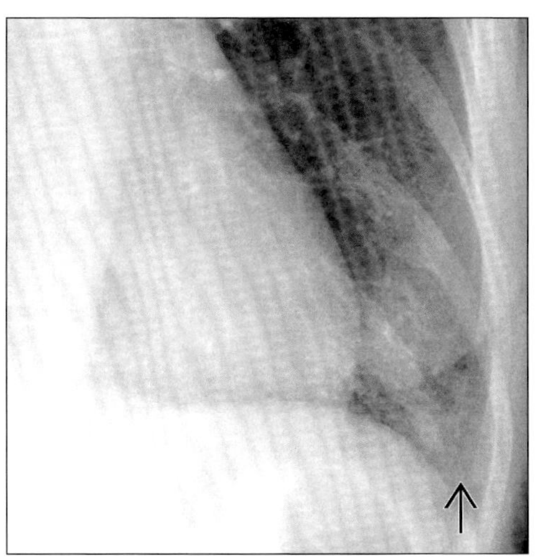

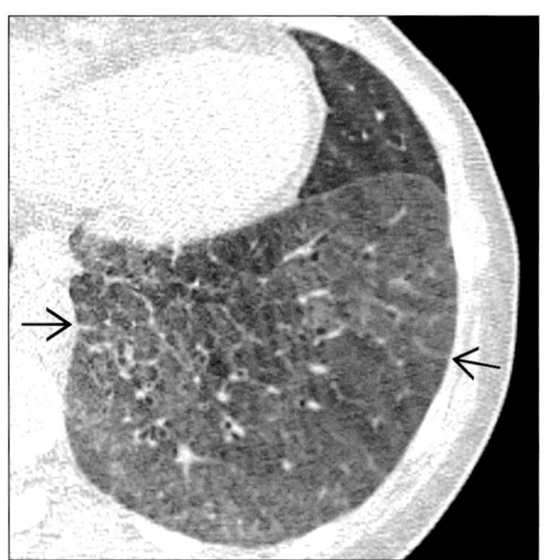

***(Left)** PA chest radiograph of a patient with LIP and Sjögren syndrome shows fine left basilar reticular opacities →. **(Right)** Axial HRCT of the same patient shows diffuse left lower lobe ground-glass opacity with superimposed interlobular septal thickening →. While typically bilateral, on occasion LIP can be a more localized process, as in this patient. Furthermore, pulmonary cysts are not always present in patients with LIP.*

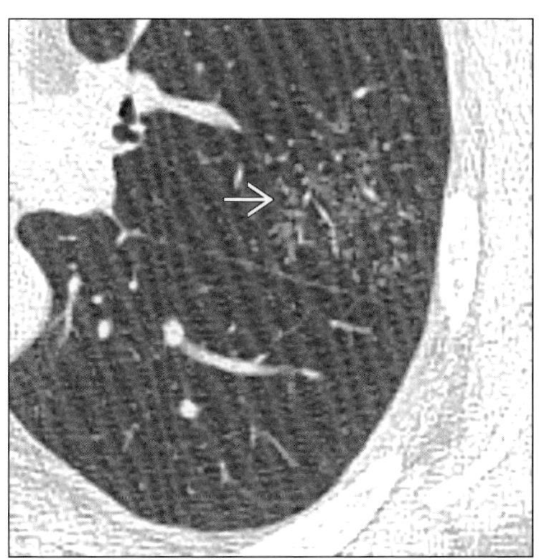

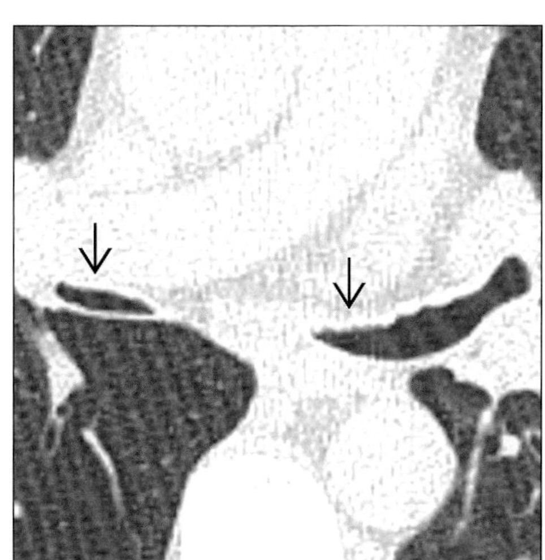

***(Left)** Axial HRCT of a patient with Sjögren syndrome and follicular bronchiolitis shows clustered centrilobular micronodules ➡ in the left upper lobe. Like LIP, follicular bronchiolitis is more often diffuse but can be limited in extent. **(Right)** Axial HRCT of the same patient shows flattening of the anterior walls → of the bronchus intermedius and left mainstem bronchus from bronchomalacia related to lymphocytic infiltration of the bronchial walls.*

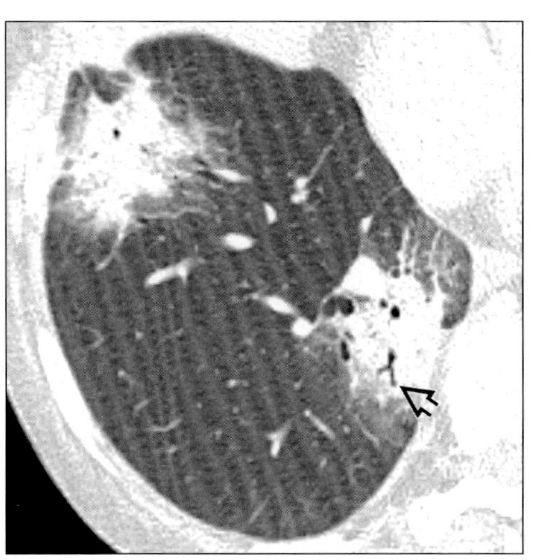

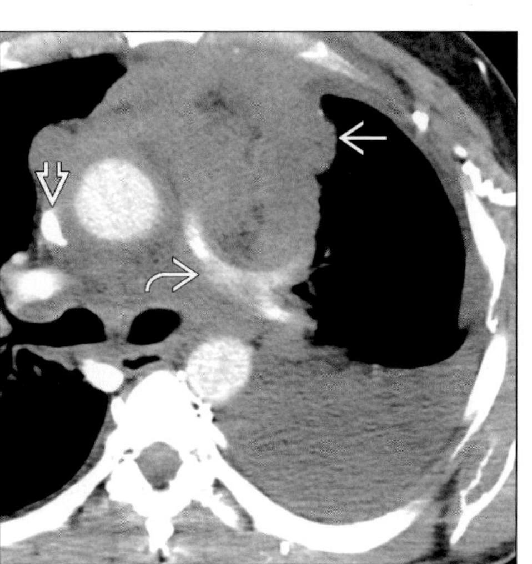

***(Left)** Axial HRCT of a patient with Sjögren syndrome shows MALT lymphoma manifesting as 2 mass-like consolidations in the right lower lobe with intrinsic air bronchograms ⇨. **(Right)** Axial CECT of a patient with Sjögren syndrome and non-Hodgkin lymphoma shows a bulky infiltrative mediastinal mass ➡ that produces narrowing of the superior vena cava ⇨ and the left pulmonary artery ↗. The left pleural effusion is caused by left pulmonary vein obstruction.*

ANKYLOSING SPONDYLITIS

Key Facts

Terminology
- Ankylosing spondylitis (AS)
- Chronic seronegative arthritis primarily involving axial skeleton

Imaging
- Radiography
  - Upper lobe symmetric fibrobullous disease (rare)
  - Spinal ankylosis
  - Squared vertebrae
  - Bamboo spine
- HRCT
  - Apical fibrobullous disease
  - Traction bronchiectasis from interstitial fibrosis
  - Paraseptal emphysema, cicatricial fibrosis, cavities
  - Mycetoma formation in cysts or cavities
  - Nonapical interstitial lung disease (5%): Ground-glass, thick interlobular septa, honeycombing

Top Differential Diagnoses
- Tuberculosis
- Sarcoidosis
- Silicosis & coal worker's pneumoconiosis

Pathology
- Strong association with inflammatory bowel disease
- Correlation with HLA-B27

Clinical Issues
- Symptoms/signs
  - Insidious back pain before age of 40: Sacroiliac joint involvement progressing up spine
  - Hemoptysis from mycetomas

Diagnostic Checklist
- Consider AS in patients with apical fibrobullous disease & spinal ankylosis

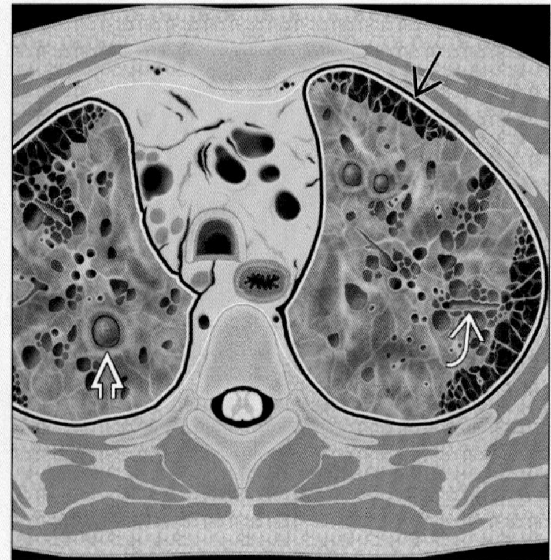

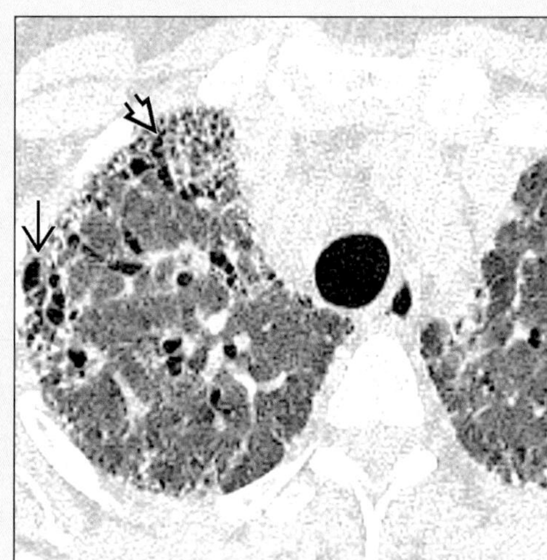

(Left) Graphic shows typical pulmonary involvement in AS, consisting of apical subpleural bullous and cystic lesions ⇒, with interstitial thickening and mild traction bronchiectasis ⇒, and a propensity for mycetoma ⇒ formation. (Right) Axial HRCT shows corresponding alterations in a patient with advanced AS and pulmonary involvement characterized by cysts ⇒, reticular opacities, and traction bronchiectasis ⇒. AS is a rare cause of upper lobe preponderant fibrosis.

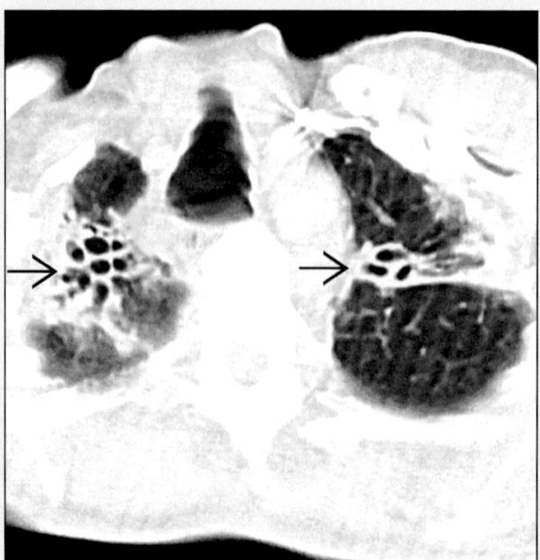

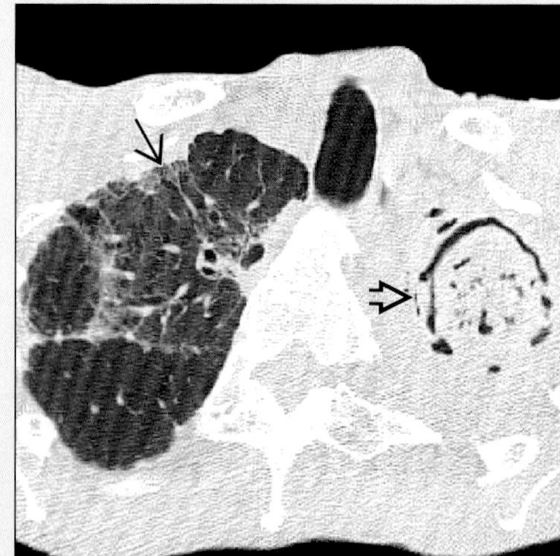

(Left) HRCT of a patient with AS shows bilateral pulmonary fibrosis characterized by airspace disease with intrinsic traction bronchiectasis ⇒ in the apical aspects of the upper lobes. (Right) Axial HRCT of a patient with AS shows reticular opacities in the right upper lobe ⇒, volume loss consistent with pulmonary fibrosis, and a left upper lobe mycetoma ⇒. Mycetomas are not uncommon in AS-associated cavitary or cystic lung disease, and affected patients may present with hemoptysis.

ANKYLOSING SPONDYLITIS

TERMINOLOGY

Abbreviations

- **Ankylosing spondylitis (AS)**

Definitions

- Chronic seronegative arthritis primarily involving axial skeleton

IMAGING

General Features

- Best diagnostic clue
  - **Upper lobe fibrobullous disease with spinal ankylosis**

Radiographic Findings

- Lung
  - Upper lobe symmetric fibrobullous disease (rare)
- Skeletal changes
  - **Ankylosis (nearly always precedes lung disease)**
  - "Shiny corner" sign: Small erosions at corners of vertebral bodies surrounded by reactive sclerosis
  - Squared vertebral body: Combination of corner erosions & periosteal new bone along anterior vertebral body
  - Complete spinal fusion: Bamboo spine

CT Findings

- HRCT
  - **Apical fibrobullous disease**
    - Nonspecific appearance similar to post primary tuberculosis
    - Traction bronchiectasis from interstitial fibrosis
    - Cystic disease from paraseptal emphysema, cicatricial fibrosis, cavities
    - **Mycetomas common in cysts or cavities**
  - Nonapical interstitial lung disease (5%)
    - Ground-glass opacity, thick interlobular septa, honeycomb lung
  - Aortic insufficiency: Dilated aorta

Imaging Recommendations

- Best imaging tool
  - CT may reveal subtle apical alterations undetected on chest radiography
  - CTA or MRA to evaluate aorta

DIFFERENTIAL DIAGNOSIS

Tuberculosis

- Apical fibrocavitary disease identical to AS
- Culture required for diagnosis

Sarcoidosis

- Perilymphatic nodularity & lymphadenopathy
- Chronic upper lobe fibrosis

Silicosis & Coal Worker's Pneumoconiosis

- Simple: Centrilobular & subpleural nodules
- Complicated: Progressive massive fibrosis
- Eggshell calcification in mediastinal/hilar lymph nodes

PATHOLOGY

General Features

- Genetics
  - Strong association with histocompatibility antigen **HLA-B27**
- Associated abnormalities
  - Strong association with inflammatory bowel disease

Staging, Grading, & Classification

- Diagnosis based on
  - History of inflammatory back pain
  - Limited lumbar motion & chest expansion
  - Radiographic sacroiliitis

CLINICAL ISSUES

Presentation

- Most common signs/symptoms
  - Insidious back pain before age 40 years
  - Morning stiffness that improves with exercise or activity
  - Hemoptysis: Mycetomas
- Other signs/symptoms
  - Pulmonary function tests: Mixed restrictive & obstructive pattern
  - Acute anterior uveitis: Most common extraarticular manifestation (25%)

Demographics

- Age
  - 15-35 years of age at presentation
- Gender
  - M:F = 8:1
- Epidemiology
  - Approximately 1 in 2,000 individuals
  - Pleuropulmonary disease, 1-2% of AS
    - Late onset, 15-20 years after spinal disease

Natural History & Prognosis

- Initial involvement of sacroiliac joint with progression up spine
- Mortality: Aortitis, inflammatory bowel disease, nephritis (amyloid)
- Most serious complication: Spinal fracture, most commonly cervical

Treatment

- No definitive treatment
- Local glucocorticoid administration & mydriatic agents for iritis
- Aortic valve replacement for valvulitis
- Bronchial artery embolization for severe hemoptysis

DIAGNOSTIC CHECKLIST

Consider

- AS in patients with apical fibrobullous disease & spinal ankylosis

SELECTED REFERENCES

1. Sampaio-Barros PD et al: Pulmonary involvement in ankylosing spondylitis. Clin Rheumatol. 26(2):225-30, 2007

INFLAMMATORY BOWEL DISEASE

Key Facts

Terminology
- Inflammatory bowel disease (IBD)
- Idiopathic inflammatory diseases of digestive tract: Crohn disease, ulcerative colitis

Imaging
- Radiography
  - Tracheobronchitis, bronchiolitis
  - Intersitial pneumonia
  - Pulmonary hemorrhage
- HRCT
  - Tracheobronchitis, tracheal/bronchial stenosis, bronchiectasis
  - Organizing pneumonia
  - Cellular & constrictive bronchiolitis
  - Interstitial fibrosis
- Expiratory HRCT for confirmation of suspected constrictive bronchiolitis

Top Differential Diagnoses
- Acute tracheobronchitis
- Constrictive bronchiolitis
- Idiopathic pulmonary fibrosis
- Mycobacterial pneumonia
- Drug reaction

Clinical Issues
- Ulcerative colitis
  - Peak incidence: 15-25 years & 55-65 years
- Crohn disease
  - Peak incidence: 15-25 years & 50-80 years

Diagnostic Checklist
- Consider infection, especially if immunosuppressed
- Consider drug reaction; detailed drug history helpful
- Expiratory HRCT useful in demonstrating indirect signs of bronchiolitis

*(**Left**) Axial NECT of a patient with IBD shows smooth circumferential tracheal wall thickening ➔. Airway inflammation in IBD typically affects central bronchi, but the trachea may also be involved. (**Right**) Axial NECT of a patient with active ulcerative colitis who presented with cough shows multifocal bilateral bronchiectasis, bronchial wall thickening, and mild mucus plugging. Airway inflammation is common in patients with IBD and respiratory involvement and typically manifests as bronchiectasis.*

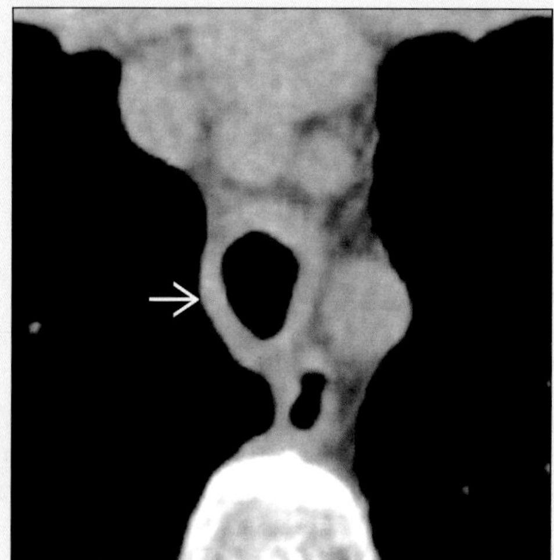

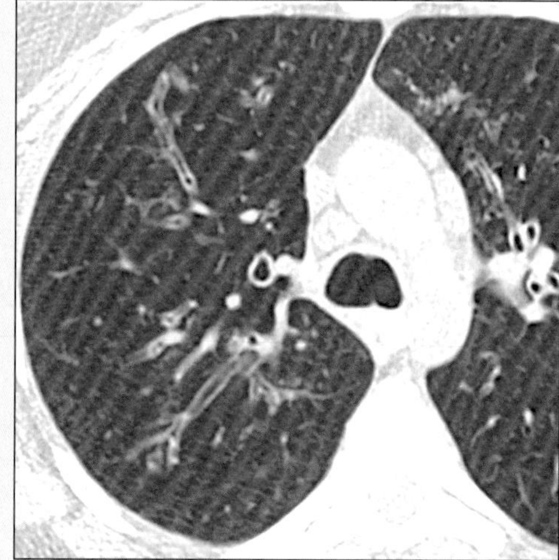

*(**Left**) Coronal HRCT of a patient with Crohn disease-related constrictive bronchiolitis shows hyperinflation, mosaic attenuation, and mild bronchiectasis ➔. Areas of ground-glass attenuation ➔ represent normal lung. Expiratory HRCT helps confirm air-trapping by accentuating abnormalities. (**Right**) Axial HRCT of a patient with Crohn disease shows peripheral basilar ground-glass and reticular opacities ➔, consistent with nonspecific interstitial pneumonia (NSIP).*

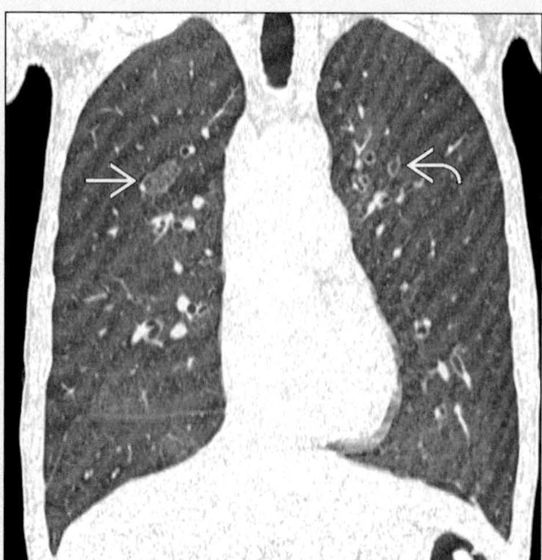

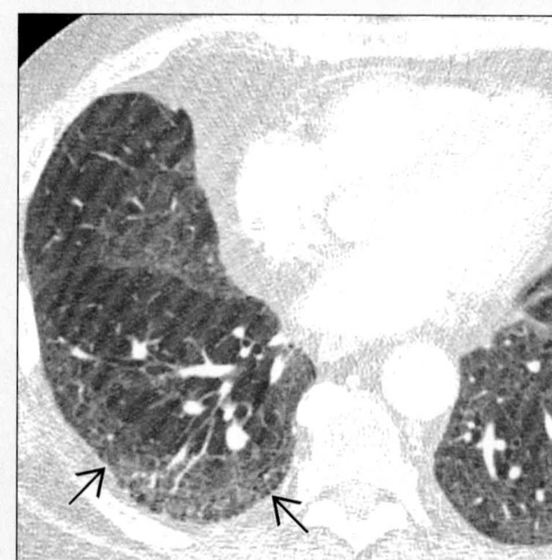

INFLAMMATORY BOWEL DISEASE

TERMINOLOGY

Abbreviations

- **Inflammatory bowel disease (IBD)**

Synonyms

- Crohn disease, ulcerative colitis

Definitions

- Idiopathic inflammatory diseases of digestive tract
  - **Crohn disease**
    - Can involve any site in digestive tract
    - Formation of noncaseating granulomas
  - **Ulcerative colitis**
    - Limited to colon & rectum

IMAGING

General Features

- Best diagnostic clue
  - **Pulmonary disease in patient with established diagnosis of inflammatory bowel disease**
- Location
  - Airways, lung parenchyma

Radiographic Findings

- Findings depend on underlying pathology
  - **Tracheobronchitis**
    - Tracheobronchial wall thickening
    - Bronchiectasis
  - **Bronchiolitis**
    - Centrilobular micronodules, tree-in-bud opacities
    - Hyperinflation
  - **Intersitial pneumonia**
    - Basal predominant reticulation
    - Multifocal lung consolidation
  - **Pulmonary hemorrhage**
    - Focal or multifocal, unilateral or bilateral
    - Ground-glass opacity, consolidation

CT Findings

- HRCT
  - **Tracheobronchitis**
    - Patchy, irregular tracheobronchial wall thickening
  - **Tracheal or bronchial stenosis**
    - Focal or long segment
  - **Bronchiectasis**
    - May be secondary to constrictive bronchiolitis
  - **Organizing pneumonia**
    - Peripheral, perilobular, peribronchial consolidation & ground-glass opacity
    - Nodular ground-glass opacity with peripheral consolidation (reverse halo sign)
  - **Cellular bronchiolitis**
    - Diffuse tree-in-bud opacities, centrilobular nodules; may reflect infectious bronchiolitis
  - **Constrictive bronchiolitis**
    - Mosaic lung attenuation
    - Air-trapping on expiratory CT
  - **Interstitial fibrosis**
    - Basal predominant ground-glass & reticulation
    - Traction bronchiectasis/bronchiolectasis
    - Honeycomb lung uncommon, typically indicates usual interstitial pneumonia (UIP) pattern

Other CT Findings

- Eosinophilic pneumonia
- Necrobiotic nodules
- High incidence of pulmonary thromboembolic disease

Imaging Recommendations

- Best imaging tool
  - HRCT for assessment of airway & lung involvement
- Protocol advice
  - Expiratory HRCT for confirming suspected constrictive bronchiolitis

DIFFERENTIAL DIAGNOSIS

Acute Tracheobronchitis

- Viral infection
- Usually less severe than IBD-related tracheobronchitis

Constrictive Bronchiolitis

- Multiple etiologies
  - Certain drugs (e.g., penicillamine)
  - Inhalational injury (smoke, nitrous oxide)

Idiopathic Pulmonary Fibrosis

- Usually affects older adults (> 60 years)
- Usual interstitial pneumonia (UIP) pattern on HRCT

Mycobacterial Pneumonia

- Involvement of central airways
- Long segment airway stenoses more common

Drug Reaction

- Common with drugs used to treat IBD (e.g., sulfasalazine)

CLINICAL ISSUES

Demographics

- Age
  - Ulcerative colitis
    - Peak incidence: 15-25 years & 55-65 years
  - Crohn disease
    - Peak incidence: 15-25 years & 50-80 years
- Gender
  - Ulcerative colitis more common in women
- Ethnicity
  - Caucasians more commonly affected

DIAGNOSTIC CHECKLIST

Consider

- Infection; especially if immunosuppressed
- Drug reaction; detailed drug history helpful

Image Interpretation Pearls

- Expiratory HRCT useful in demonstrating indirect signs of bronchiolitis: Expiratory air-trapping

SELECTED REFERENCES

1. Betancourt SL et al: Thoracic manifestations of inflammatory bowel disease. AJR Am J Roentgenol. 197(3):W452-6, 2011
2. Black H et al: Thoracic manifestations of inflammatory bowel disease. Chest. 131(2):524-32, 2007

ERDHEIM-CHESTER DISEASE

Key Facts

Terminology

- Erdheim-Chester disease (ECD)
- Non-Langerhans cell histiocytosis of unknown origin

Imaging

- Radiography
  - Diffuse bilateral septal thickening (90%)
  - Mild to moderate pleural thickening (66%)
  - Generalized cardiac enlargement
  - Bilateral symmetric long bone osteosclerosis
- CT
  - Smooth pleural thickening ± effusions
  - Ground-glass opacity & smooth septal thickening
  - Centrilobular nodules
  - Pericardial soft tissue thickening or effusion
  - Right atrial & atrioventricular involvement
  - Soft tissue encasement of aorta & great vessels
  - Renal encasement by soft tissue

Top Differential Diagnoses

- Lung
  - Congestive heart failure
  - Sarcoidosis
  - Lymphangitic carcinomatosis
- Pleura
  - Asbestos-related pleural disease
  - Mesothelioma

Clinical Issues

- Slow onset of cough & dyspnea
- Pulmonary function: Moderate restriction, ↓ DLCO
- Pleuropulmonary involvement: 3-year survival 66%

Diagnostic Checklist

- Combination of pleural or diffuse septal thickening, perirenal soft tissue, aortic wall thickening, & bone sclerosis are considered pathognomonic for ECD

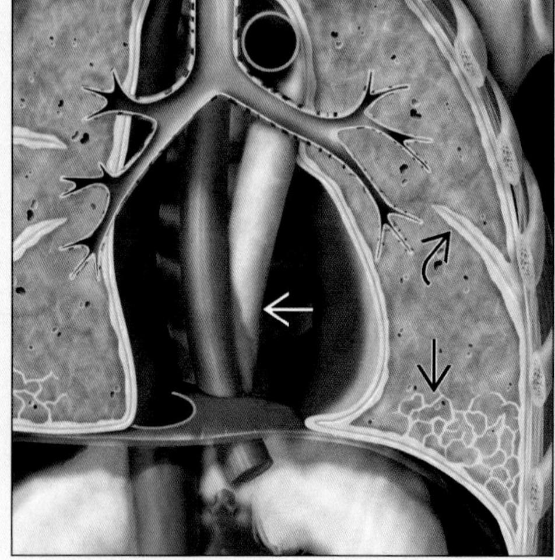

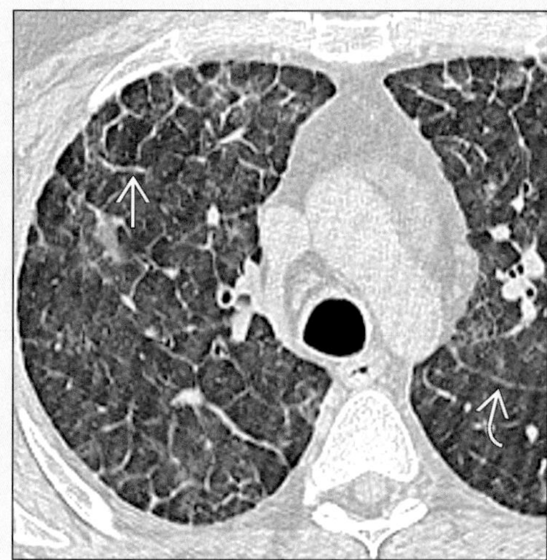

__(Left)__ Graphic shows thoracic features of ECD, including interlobular septal thickening →, pleural thickening ↗, and soft tissue encasement of the aorta ➡ and kidneys. __(Right)__ Axial HRCT of a patient with ECD shows diffuse bilateral interlobular septal thickening ➡, patchy ground-glass opacities, and mild thickening of the left major fissure ➡. Although the findings mimic those of interstitial edema, other findings (skeletal, periaortic, and perirenal) usually suggest the correct diagnosis.

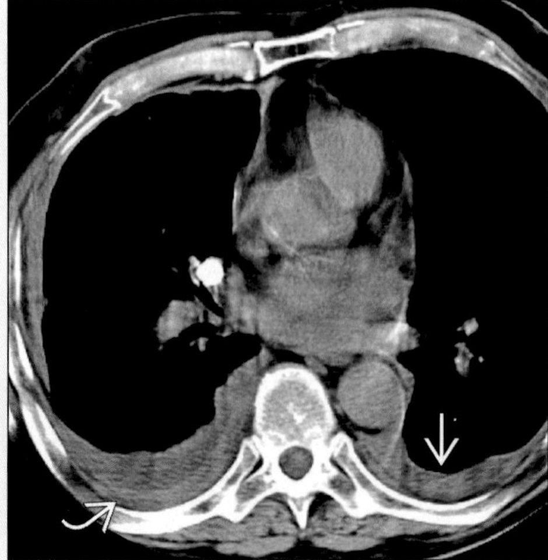

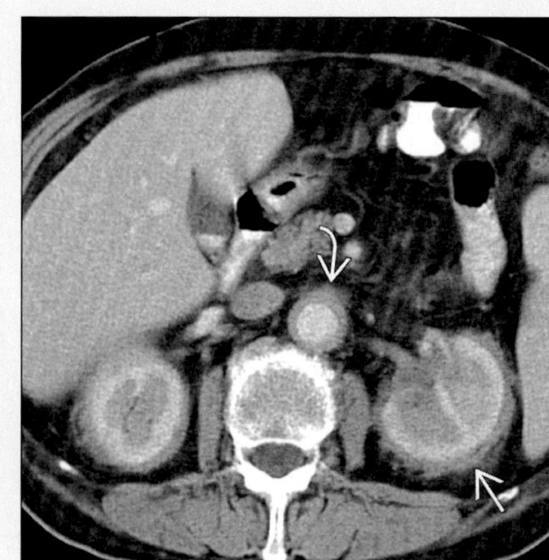

__(Left)__ Axial NECT of a patient with ECD shows bilateral pleural thickening ➡ and small bilateral pleural effusions ➡. __(Right)__ Axial CECT of a patient with ECD shows diffuse hyperdense soft tissue encasement of the aorta ➡ and bilateral kidneys ➡. This constellation of findings combined with interlobular septal thickening and ground-glass opacity in the lung is highly suggestive of Erdheim-Chester disease.

ERDHEIM-CHESTER DISEASE

TERMINOLOGY

Abbreviations

- **Erdheim-Chester disease (ECD)**

Definitions

- Non-Langerhans cell histiocytosis of unknown origin

IMAGING

General Features

- Best diagnostic clue
  - **Triad of osteosclerotic bone lesions, perirenal soft tissue, & pleural or diffuse septal thickening**

Radiographic Findings

- Diffuse lung involvement with thick septal lines (90%)
- Mild to moderate pleural thickening (66%)
- Generalized cardiac enlargement

CT Findings

- CECT
  - **Smooth pleural thickening** extending into fissures, ± pleural effusions
  - Ground-glass opacities & **smooth, uniform interlobular septal thickening**
  - Centrilobular nodules
  - Smooth, long-segment encasement of aorta & great vessels by thick soft tissue
  - Renal encasement by soft tissue
  - Bilateral symmetric osteosclerosis of leg long bone metaphyses & diaphyses: Considered pathognomonic
  - Cardiac
    - Pericardial soft tissue thickening or effusion
    - Right atrial & atrioventricular involvement

Imaging Recommendations

- Best imaging tool
  - CECT & HRCT: Lung, pleural, aortic, & skeletal abnormalities

DIFFERENTIAL DIAGNOSIS

Heart

- Congestive heart failure
  - Enlarged heart, pleural effusion, & septal thickening
  - Responds to diuretic & inotropic therapy

Lung

- Edema
  - Septal thickening
  - Usually gravitationally dependent
- Sarcoidosis
  - Nodular septal thickening, preferentially follows bronchovascular bundles
  - Lymphadenopathy; rare in ECD
- Lymphangitic carcinomatosis
  - Asymmetric nodular septal thickening with areas of sparing

Pleura

- Asbestos-related pleural disease
  - Bilateral discontinuous pleural thickening ± calcification
  - ECD: Diffuse pleural thickening, no calcification
- Mesothelioma
  - Unilateral circumferential nodular pleural thickening
  - Lung encasement & volume loss

Aorta

- Takayasu aortitis
  - Does not involve kidneys, lungs, or pleura
  - ECD usually more extensive, coating entire aorta

PATHOLOGY

Gross Pathologic & Surgical Features

- Symmetric involvement: Long bones, pleura, perirenal, & lung; never unilateral

Microscopic Features

- Lymphangitic expansion by inflammatory cells & fibrosis
  - Inflammatory cells: Large foamy histiocytes, lymphocytes, plasma cells, & Touton giant cells
  - Fibrosis: Fine fibrillary mature collagen without fibroblast proliferation

CLINICAL ISSUES

Presentation

- Most common signs/symptoms
  - Slow onset of cough & dyspnea
  - Pulmonary function tests: Moderate restriction & decreased DLCO
- Other signs/symptoms
  - Diabetes insipidus (20%), exophthalmos (15%), renal failure (15%), xanthomas (10%)

Demographics

- Age
  - > 40 years
- Gender
  - No gender predilection

Natural History & Prognosis

- Slowly progressive disease, prognosis depends on extent of extraosseous disease
- Pleuropulmonary involvement: Significant morbidity & mortality, 3-year survival 66%

Treatment

- Corticosteroids
- Vincristine & related chemotherapeutic agents
- Radiotherapy for focal masses

DIAGNOSTIC CHECKLIST

Image Interpretation Pearls

- Combination of pleural or diffuse septal thickening, perirenal soft tissue, aortic wall thickening, & bone sclerosis are considered pathognomonic for ECD

SELECTED REFERENCES

1. Dion E et al: Imaging of thoracoabdominal involvement in Erdheim-Chester disease. AJR Am J Roentgenol. 183(5):1253-60, 2004

Key Facts

Terminology

- Hematopoietic stem cell transplantation (HSCT)
  - Bone marrow, peripheral blood stem cell, & cord blood stem cell transplantation
- Graft-vs.-host disease (GVHD): Donor T cells attack recipient's organs as foreign bodies

Imaging

- Imaging abnormalities vary depending on time elapsed after HSCT
- Infections vary according to specific host immunodeficiency
- Neutropenic phase: 2-3 weeks after HSCT, profound neutropenia
  - Pulmonary edema: Bilateral perihilar opacities
  - Bacterial pneumonia: Consolidation
  - Fungal infection: Nodules ± cavitation
  - Alveolar hemorrhage: Patchy bilateral opacities
- Early phase: 2-3 weeks to 100 days after HSCT, depressed cellular & humoral immunity
  - Viral pneumonia: Ground-glass opacities
  - Idiopathic pneumonia syndrome: Bilateral opacities with basal predominance
- Late phase: 100 days to 1 year after HSCT, GVHD
  - Constrictive bronchiolitis: Mosaic attenuation, expiratory air-trapping
  - Organizing pneumonia: Peribronchovascular & subpleural opacities

Clinical Issues

- Pulmonary complications in 40-60% of recipients

Diagnostic Checklist

- Consider opportunistic infection in patients who develop fever post HSCT
- Consider time elapsed since HSCT & host immunity to suggest specific organisms & other complications

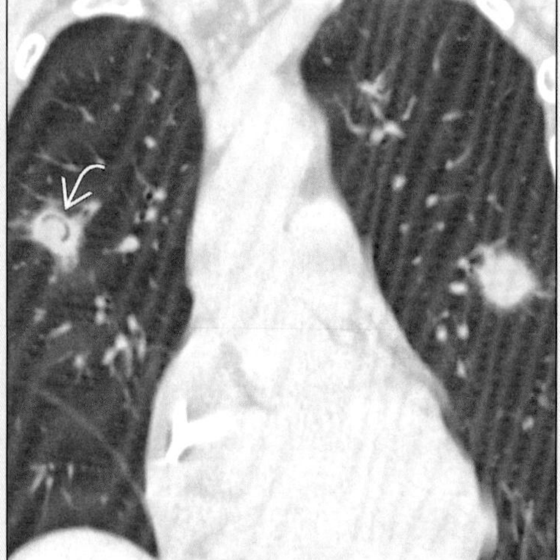
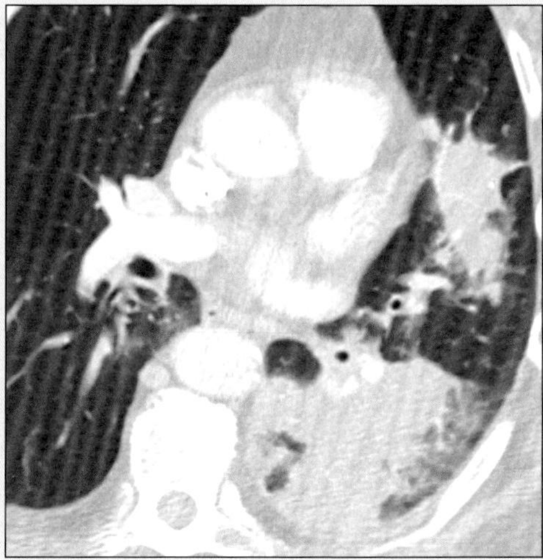

(Left) *Coronal NECT of a patient 13 days post bone marrow transplant for aplastic anemia shows bilateral pulmonary nodules with subtle peripheral ground-glass halos and an air crescent sign ➔, consistent with angioinvasive fungal infection.* ***(Right)*** *Axial CECT of a patient with S. aureus pneumonia developing 20 days post bone marrow transplant shows left upper and lower lobe dense consolidations. Within 2-3 weeks of HSCT patients are particularly susceptible to fungal and bacterial infections.*

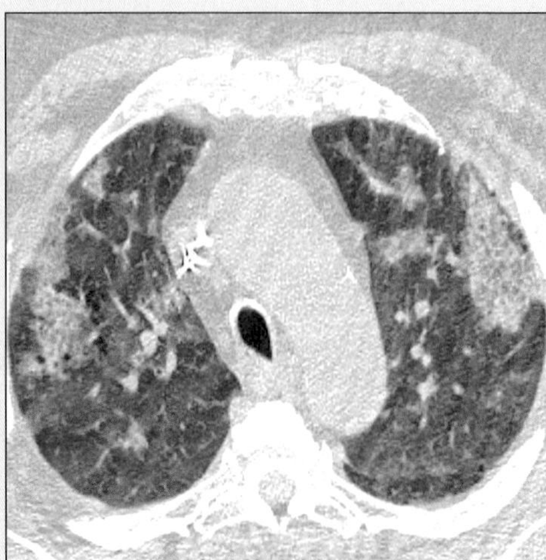
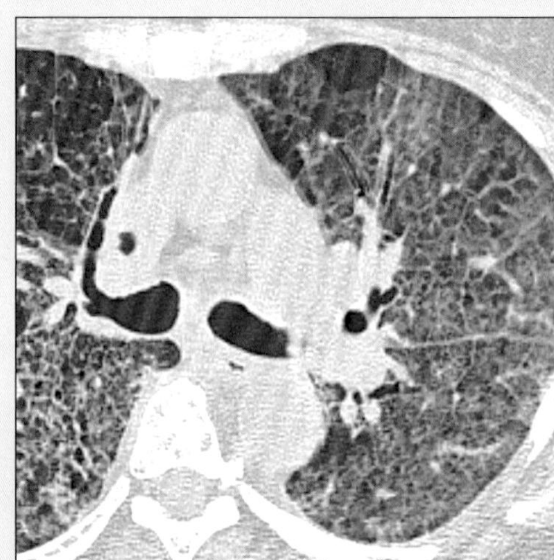

(Left) *Axial NECT of a patient who developed pulmonary alveolar hemorrhage 3 weeks post HSCT shows bilateral patchy ground-glass opacities with intrinsic intralobular reticular opacities.* ***(Right)*** *Axial HRCT of a patient 2 weeks post HSCT shows bilateral diffuse ground-glass opacities and interlobular septal thickening related to busulfan-induced diffuse alveolar damage. Pulmonary hemorrhage and drug toxicity are important differential considerations in the early post-transplant period.*

HEMATOPOIETIC STEM CELL TRANSPLANTATION

TERMINOLOGY

Abbreviations

- **Hematopoietic stem cell transplantation (HSCT)**

Definitions

- HSCT
  - Types
    - **Bone marrow** transplantation, **peripheral blood stem cell** transplantation, **cord blood stem cell** transplantation
    - **Autologous transplantation uses patient's own stem cells**
    - **Allogeneic transplantation uses cells from human leukocyte antigen-consistent donor**
  - Procedure
    - Intensive chemotherapy & total body irradiation (TBI) to eradicate recipient's malignant cells
    - TBI followed by infusion of donor's hematopoietic stem cells
  - Complications
    - **Graft-vs.-host disease** (GVHD): Donor T lymphocytes attack recipient's organs as foreign bodies, occurs with allogeneic transplantation

IMAGING

General Features

- Imaging abnormalities vary depending on time elapsed after HSCT
- Infections vary according to specific host immunodeficiency

Neutropenic (Engraftment) Phase

- General features
  - Time frame
    - 2-3 weeks after HST
  - Host immunity
    - Profound neutropenia
- **Pulmonary edema** from heart failure, fluid overload, or capillary leak
  - Interlobular septal thickening
  - Bilateral ground-glass opacities
  - Perihilar consolidations
  - Pleural effusions
- **Infections**
  - **Bacterial pneumonia**
    - Consolidation
    - Ground-glass opacities
  - **Fungal infection**
    - Invasive pulmonary aspergillosis (IPA)
      - CT halo sign: Nodule surrounded by ground-glass opacity
      - Air crescent sign: Cavitary nodule with soft tissue content surrounded by air
      - Airway IPA: Bronchial & bronchiolar wall thickening, tree-in-bud opacities
    - ***Candida* infection**
      - Patchy opacities
      - Ill-defined nodules
      - Miliary nodules
    - **Zygomyces:** *Mucor* & *Rhizopus*
      - Nodules ± cavitation
      - CT halo sign
- **Diffuse alveolar hemorrhage**
  - Bilateral ground-glass opacities
  - Interlobular septal thickening & intralobular reticulation
- **Drug toxicity**
  - Diffuse alveolar damage
    - Bilateral patchy or diffuse opacities
  - Hypersensitivity pneumonitis
    - Centrilobular ground-glass nodules
    - Mosaic attenuation (head cheese sign)
    - Air-trapping on expiratory images

Early Phase

- General features
  - Time frame
    - 2-3 weeks to 100 days after HSCT
  - Host immunity
    - Depressed cellular & humoral immunity
- *Pneumocystis jiroveci* pneumonia (PCP) now rare with effective prophylaxis
  - Chest radiographs may be normal
  - Diffuse ground-glass opacities
  - Pneumatoceles, cysts
  - Pleural effusion & lymphadenopathy uncommon
- **Cytomegalovirus pneumonia**
  - Patchy or diffuse ground-glass opacities
  - Centrilobular & random nodules
- **Other viral pneumonias** (respiratory syncytial virus, influenza virus, adenovirus)
  - Bilateral ground-glass opacities
  - Centrilobular nodules
  - Bronchial wall thickening
  - Tree-in-bud opacities
- Idiopathic pneumonia syndrome (IPS)
  - Bilateral consolidations or ground-glass opacities
    - Basilar or dorsal predominance
- Engraftment syndrome (capillary leak)
  - Bilateral ground-glass opacities, consolidation

Late Phase

- General features
  - Time frame
    - 100 days to 1 year after HSCT
  - Host immunity
    - GVHD with different pulmonary manifestations
- **Constrictive bronchiolitis** (bronchiolitis obliterans)
  - Mosaic attenuation
  - Bronchiectasis
  - Bronchial wall thickening
  - Air-trapping on expiratory CT
- **Organizing pneumonia**
  - Consolidations or ground-glass opacities
    - Peribronchovascular or subpleural
  - Atoll sign, reverse halo sign
    - Central ground-glass opacity surrounded by denser consolidation
- **Nonspecific interstitial pneumonia (NSIP)**
  - Subpleural reticular & ground-glass opacities
  - Traction bronchiectasis

Imaging Recommendations

- Best imaging tool
  - Chest radiography for evaluation of suspected or documented pulmonary infection

- CT more sensitive & specific than radiography for diagnosis of acute & late complications
  - Helps narrow differential diagnosis
  - Directs further tests, such as bronchoalveolar lavage or lung biopsy

DIFFERENTIAL DIAGNOSIS

Ground-Glass Opacities

- Pulmonary edema
- Diffuse alveolar hemorrhage
- Viral pneumonia
- Drug toxicity
- Engraftment syndrome
- Organizing pneumonia
- Constrictive bronchiolitis

Nodules or Masses

- Septic emboli
- Fungal infection

PATHOLOGY

Microscopic Features

- Idiopathic pneumonia syndrome
  - Diffuse alveolar damage in absence of lower respiratory tract infection
- Constrictive bronchiolitis
  - Chronic inflammatory & fibroproliferative process centered on terminal & respiratory bronchiole
  - Bronchiolar stenosis & scarring
- Organizing pneumonia
  - Granulation tissue, polyps in lumina of alveolar ducts & bronchioles
  - Interstitial inflammation & fibrosis

CLINICAL ISSUES

Demographics

- Epidemiology
  - Pulmonary complications in 40-60% of HSCT recipients
  - Lower incidence of CMV & fungal infections, IPS, GVHD, & constrictive bronchiolitis in autologous transplant recipients
- Indications for HSCT
  - Acute & chronic leukemia
  - Lymphoma
  - Multiple myeloma
  - Myelodysplastic syndrome
  - Thalassemia
  - Sickle cell anemia
  - Aplastic anemia

Engraftment Syndrome

- Fever, erythematous rash, capillary leak
- 7-11% of patients
- Treatment: Corticosteroids

Diffuse Alveolar Hemorrhage

- Up to 21% of HSCT patients
- Mortality: 50-80%
- Within 1st month of HSCT
- Dyspnea, cough, not necessarily hemoptysis
- Diagnosis: Bronchoalveolar lavage
- Treatment
  - Supportive
  - Corticosteroids

CMV Pneumonia

- 10-40% of allogeneic transplant recipients
- Mortality: Up to 85%
- Diagnosis: Bronchoalveolar lavage
- Treatment
  - Ganciclovir
  - Immunoglobulin

Idiopathic Pneumonia Syndrome

- Allogeneic > autologous transplant recipients
- Mortality: > 70%
- Dyspnea, fever
- Diagnosis of exclusion
- Treatment: Immunosuppressive therapy

Graft-vs.-Host Disease (GVHD)

- Up to 50% of allogeneic transplant recipients
- Multiple organs affected
  - Skin: Rash
  - Gastrointestinal tract: Diarrhea
  - Liver: Jaundice
- Chronic GVHD: Develops > 100 days after HSCT
  - Pulmonary manifestations
  - Constrictive bronchiolitis
    - 2-14% of allogeneic recipients who survive > 3 months
    - High mortality rate
    - Nonproductive cough, dyspnea, asymptomatic decline in pulmonary function
    - Diagnosis: Obstructive pattern on pulmonary function tests
    - Treatment: Immunosuppressive therapy
  - Organizing pneumonia
    - Up to 10% of HSCT recipients
    - 1-13 months after HSCT
    - Treatment: Immunosuppressive therapy

DIAGNOSTIC CHECKLIST

Consider

- Opportunistic infection in patients who develop fever post HSCT
- Time elapsed since HSCT & host immunity to suggest specific organisms & other complications

SELECTED REFERENCES

1. Tanaka N et al: High-resolution computed tomography of chest complications in patients treated with hematopoietic stem cell transplantation. Jpn J Radiol. 29(4):229-35, 2011
2. Jagannathan JP et al: Imaging of complications of hematopoietic stem cell transplantation. Radiol Clin North Am. 46(2):397-417, x, 2008
3. Coy DL et al: Imaging evaluation of pulmonary and abdominal complications following hematopoietic stem cell transplantation. Radiographics. 25(2):305-17; discussion 318, 2005
4. Evans A et al: Imaging in haematopoietic stem cell transplantation. Clin Radiol. 58(3):201-14, 2003

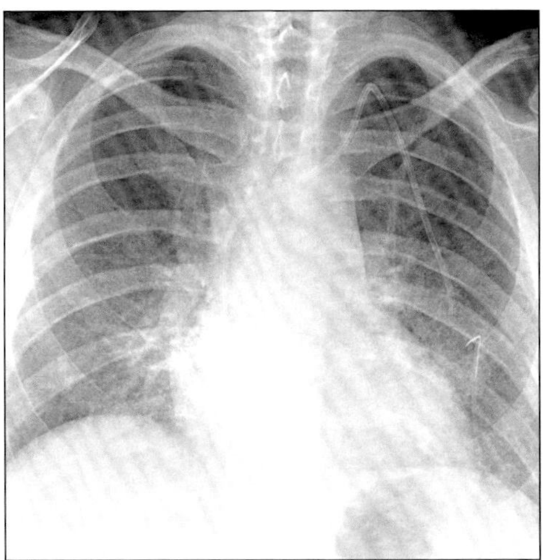

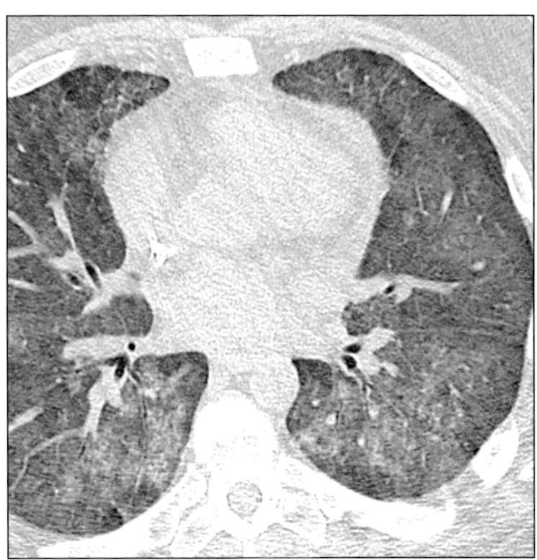

(Left) *AP chest radiograph shows bilateral diffuse hazy ground-glass opacities in a patient who developed dyspnea and fever 3 months post HSCT secondary to Pneumocystis pneumonia.* **(Right)** *Axial NECT of the same patient shows bilateral diffuse ground-glass opacities. Pneumocystis jiroveci pneumonia is no longer a common infection in HSCT recipients due to the effectiveness of prophylactic antibiotic therapy.*

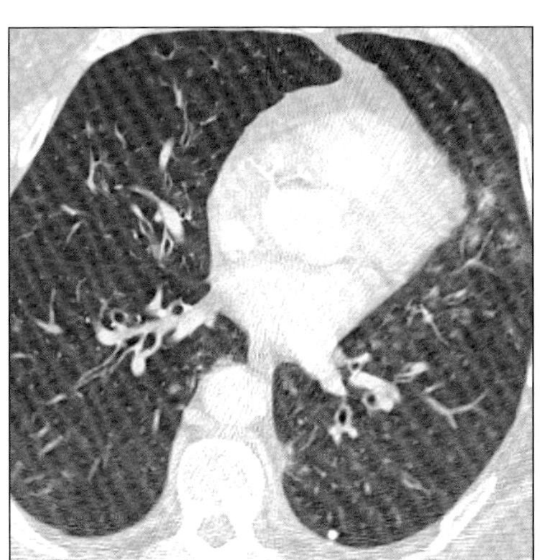

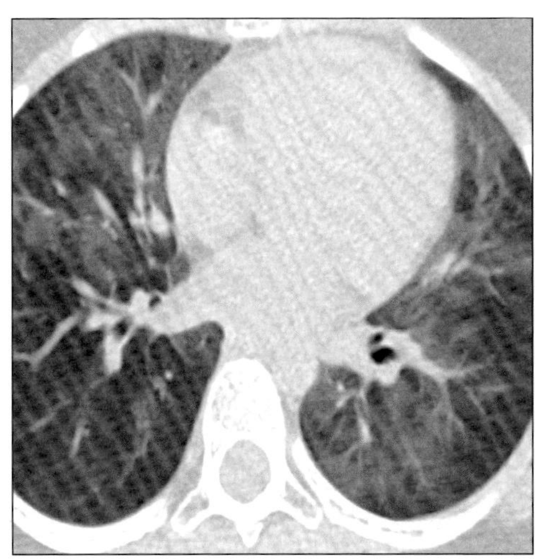

(Left) *Axial CECT of a patient who developed respiratory syncytial virus pneumonia 25 days post HSCT shows bilateral centrilobular ground-glass nodules and lingular tree-in-bud opacities. Viral pneumonia usually occurs 2 weeks to 3 months after HSCT due to compromised cellular host immunity.* **(Right)** *Axial NECT of a patient with chronic graft-vs.-host disease 2 years after HSCT shows bilateral peribronchovascular patchy ground-glass opacities consistent with organizing pneumonia.*

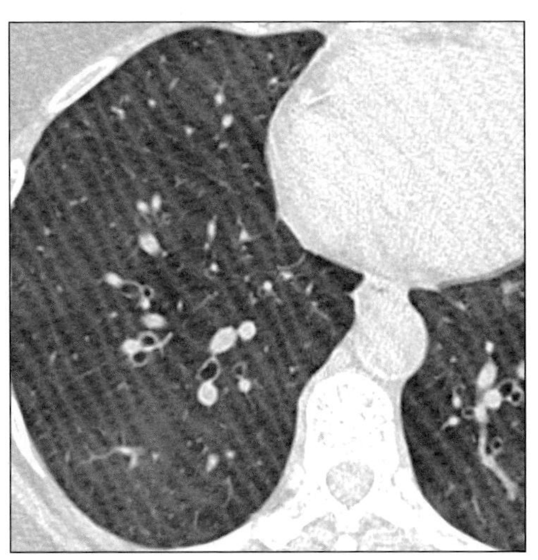

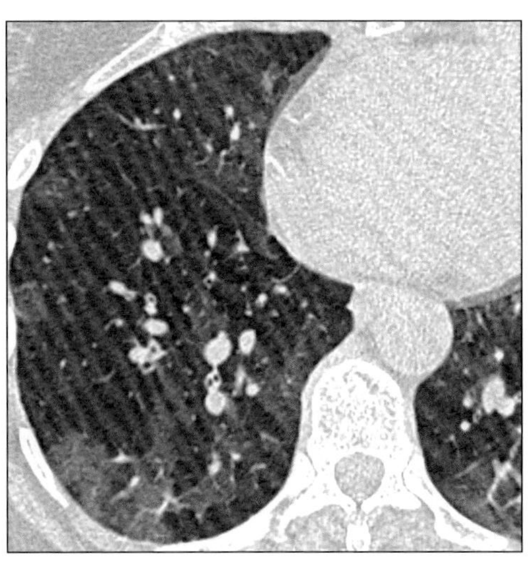

(Left) *Axial NECT of a patient who developed graft-vs.-host disease following HSCT shows mild bronchial wall thickening and dilatation and subtle mosaic attenuation of the pulmonary parenchyma.* **(Right)** *Axial NECT of the same patient performed during expiration shows accentuation of mosaic attenuation due to marked air-trapping consistent with constrictive bronchiolitis. Constrictive bronchiolitis is one of the manifestations of GVHD in allogeneic hematopoietic stem cell transplant recipients.*

Key Facts

Terminology

- Solid organ transplant (SOT)
- Transplantation of heart, lung, liver, kidney, pancreas, small bowel, etc.

Imaging

- Infection
  - Viral: Diffuse or focal ground-glass opacities
  - Fungal: Nodules ± cavitation
- Bronchiolitis obliterans syndrome (BOS)
  - Airtrapping
  - Bronchiectasis
- Post-transplant lymphoproliferative disorder (PTLD)
  - Pulmonary nodules, lymphadenopathy
- Kaposi sarcoma
  - Peribronchovascular nodular opacities
  - Enhancing lymphadenopathy
- Lung cancer
  - Lung nodule/mass ± lymphadenopathy
- Role of Imaging
  - Radiography & CT: Detection of complications, monitoring treatment response
  - CT-guided biopsy for definitive diagnosis
  - PET/CT: Staging & monitoring response of PTLD

Top Differential Diagnoses

- Consolidation
  - Infection
  - Pulmonary edema
- Ground-glass opacities
  - Viral infection
  - Pulmonary edema
  - Drug toxicity
- Pulmonary nodules
  - Septic emboli
  - Fungal or mycobacterial infection
  - Lung cancer
  - PTLD, Kaposi sarcoma

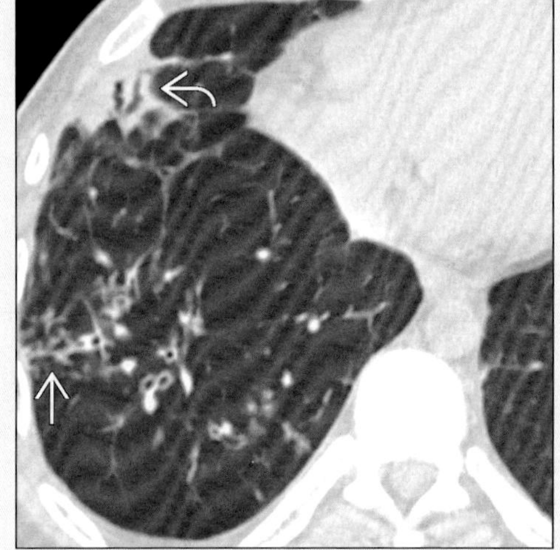

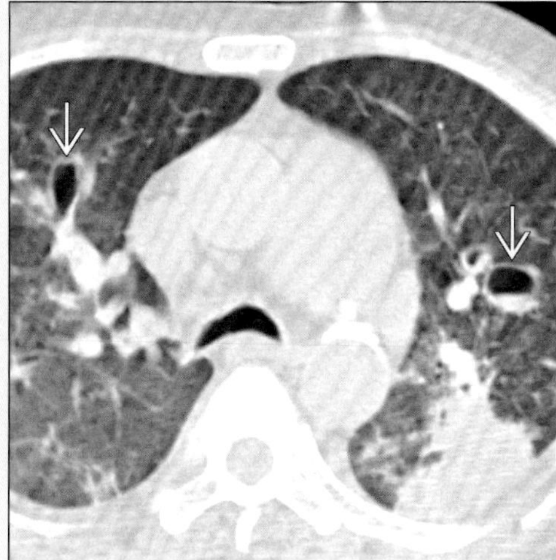

(Left) *Axial NECT of a lung transplant recipient with Pseudomonas pneumonia shows patchy consolidation ➥, bronchial wall thickening, and tree-in-bud opacities ➔ in the right lung.* ***(Right)*** *Axial NECT of a renal transplant recipient with angioinvasive Aspergillus infection shows bilateral cavitary nodules ➔. During the hospitalization, a new left lower lobe consolidation developed due to hospital-acquired Pseudomonas pneumonia. SOT recipients are prone to various infections due to chronic immunosuppression.*

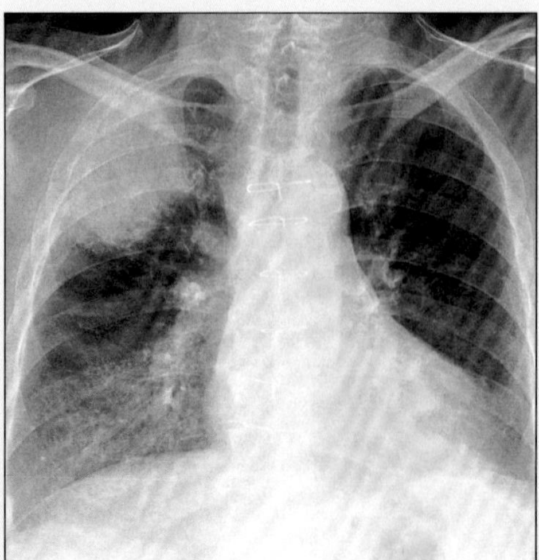

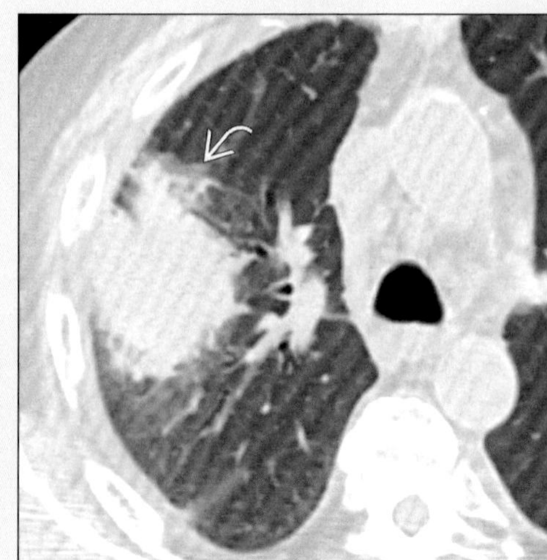

(Left) *PA chest radiograph of a heart and renal transplant recipient who presented with shortness of breath and chest pain shows a right upper lobe mass.* ***(Right)*** *Axial NECT of the same patient shows a right upper lobe mass with a surrounding ground-glass halo ➥. Percutaneous needle biopsy revealed Rhizopus species consistent with pulmonary mucormycosis. A right upper lobectomy was performed and the patient was placed on long-term antifungal maintenance therapy.*

SOLID ORGAN TRANSPLANTATION

TERMINOLOGY

Abbreviations

- **Solid organ transplant (SOT)**

Definitions

- Transplantation of heart, lung, liver, kidney, pancreas, small bowel, etc. (as opposed to hematopoietic stem cell transplant)
- Requires lifelong immunosuppressive therapy to prevent rejection of allografts

IMAGING

General Features

- Imaging frequently used for evaluation of complications
- Correct diagnosis requires high index of suspicion & knowledge of potential complications

Imaging Findings of Specific Complications

- **Infection**
  - **Viral infection**: Cytomegalovirus (CMV) is most important organism
    - Diffuse or focal ground-glass opacities
    - Consolidations
    - Nodules
    - Small pleural effusions
  - **Fungal infection**
    - Nodules ± cavitation
    - Consolidations
    - Pleural effusions
    - Lymphadenopathy
  - **Bacterial pneumonia**
    - Consolidations
    - Cavitation
    - Lung nodules
  - **Mycobacterial infection**
    - Nodules & masses ± cavitation
    - Tree-in-bud opacities
    - Lymphadenopathy
- **Bronchiolitis obliterans syndrome (BOS)**
  - Defined by clinical criteria based on pulmonary function abnormalities of airflow obstruction rather than on histologic diagnosis
    - Clinical BOS does not always correlate with HRCT findings of expiratory air-trapping
  - Air-trapping on expiratory HRCT
    - Most sensitive predictor of BOS in lung transplant recipients
  - Bronchial wall thickening
  - Bronchial dilatation
  - Mosaic attenuation
- **Neoplasm**
  - Post-transplant lymphoproliferative disorder (PTLD)
    - Thoracic involvement less common than abdominal involvement
      - Pulmonary masses & nodules
      - Homogeneous soft tissue nodules
      - CT halo sign or central necrosis may occur
      - Lymphadenopathy
      - Consolidation
      - Pleural or pericardial effusion
      - Thymic enlargement
      - Chest wall soft tissue nodules/masses
    - Gastrointestinal involvement common
      - Bowel wall thickening
      - Dilated bowel loops
      - Eccentric mass
    - Liver involvement
      - Low-attenuation hypovascular nodular lesions
      - Infiltrative pattern
  - **Kaposi sarcoma (KS)**
    - Peribronchovascular nodular opacities
    - Enhancing lymphadenopathy
  - **Lung cancer**
    - Lung nodule/mass ± lymphadenopathy
    - Imaging features similar to those of lung cancer in general population
- **Drug toxicity**
  - Sirolimus: Immunosuppressive agent
    - Organizing pneumonia
      - Patchy peribronchovascular or subpleural opacities
    - Interstitial pneumonia
      - Subpleural reticular opacities with basilar predominance
    - Venous thromboembolism
      - Vascular filling defects
- Cardiac transplant rejection
  - Increase in heart size
  - Pulmonary edema
  - Pericardial & pleural effusions
  - Accelerated atherosclerosis in graft

Imaging Recommendations

- Best imaging tool
  - Chest radiography: Typically used for initial detection of complications & subsequent evaluation of treatment response
  - CT: Useful in symptomatic patients with negative or nonspecific radiographic findings
  - CT-guided aspiration or biopsy: Helpful for establishing definitive diagnosis
  - PET/CT: Staging & monitoring treatment response of PTLD

DIFFERENTIAL DIAGNOSIS

Consolidation

- Infection
- Pulmonary edema
- Acute rejection in lung transplant

Ground-Glass Opacities

- Viral infection
- *Pneumocystis jiroveci* pneumonia
  - Uncommon with use of prophylactic antibiotics
- Pulmonary edema

Pulmonary Nodules

- Septic emboli
- Fungal infection
- Mycobacterial infection
- Lung cancer
- Post-transplant lymphoproliferative disorder
- Kaposi sarcoma

SOLID ORGAN TRANSPLANTATION

CLINICAL ISSUES

Infection

- CMV infection: 8-50% of solid organ transplant recipients
  - Direct effects: Flu-like symptoms
    - 1st 3 months post transplant
  - Indirect effects
    - Immunomodulatory effects → acute & chronic rejection
      - Coronary atherosclerosis in heart transplant recipients
      - Bronchiolitis obliterans in lung transplant recipients
    - Increased risk of opportunistic infections
  - Highest risk for CMV in recipients of CMV(+) organs
  - Treatment & prophylaxis
    - IV ganciclovir or oral valganciclovir
    - CMV-specific immune globulin (CMVIG)
- Fungal infection: Fusarium most common, *Aspergillus*, Zygomycetes, *Scedosporium* & *Blastoschizomyces* with increasing frequency
  - *Aspergillus*
    - Invasive pulmonary aspergillosis (IPA): 2-4% of SOT recipients
    - *Aspergillus* isolated in 33% of lung transplant recipients in 1 study, ranging from colonization to IPA
    - Galactomannan enzyme immunoassay: Sensitive screening test for early detection of invasive *Aspergillus* infection
  - Signs & symptoms
    - Dyspnea, fever, hemoptysis
    - May be asymptomatic
  - Diagnosis
    - Bronchoscopy with bronchoalveolar lavage, transbronchial biopsy
    - CT-guided percutaneous transthoracic biopsy or aspiration
  - Treatment
    - Appropriate antibiotics
    - Surgical resection
- Bacterial pneumonia
  - Incidence highest in heart-lung & liver transplant, lowest in renal transplant
  - 1st month after transplant: Gram-negative rods, gram-positive cocci
- Mycobacterial infection
  - *Mycobacterium tuberculosis*
    - Up to 15% of SOT recipients in endemic regions
    - Most commonly reactivation of latent tuberculosis in previously exposed patients
  - Atypical mycobacterial infection uncommon

Neoplasm

- Nonmelanoma skin cancer in up to 82% of transplant recipients
  - Squamous cell cancer most common
- Post-transplant lymphoproliferative disorder
  - 1-11% of SOT patients
    - Incidence highest in 1st year post transplant
    - Incidence highest in small bowel transplant (20%)
  - Usually B-cell proliferation related to Ebstein-Barr virus (EBV)
  - Wide range of disease: Lymphoid hyperplasia to frank lymphoma
  - Most likely to occur in anatomic location of allograft
    - Pulmonary PTLD preferentially affects lung & heart transplant recipients
  - Symptoms: Fever, lymphadenopathy, weight loss
  - Diagnosis requires tissue sampling
  - Treatment
    - Reduction of immunosuppression
    - Chemotherapy
    - Rituximab: anti-CD20 monoclonal antibody
- Kaposi sarcoma (KS)
  - 6% of SOT recipients
    - Incidence 500x higher in SOT recipients than in general population
  - Median time from transplant to diagnosis of KS: 1.5 years
  - Associated with HHV-8 infection
  - Risk factors: Male gender, older age at transplantation
  - Treatment
    - Immunosuppression reduction
    - Chemotherapy
- Lung cancer
  - Incidence 20-25x higher in SOT recipients than general population
  - Risk factors: Cigarette smoking, advanced age at transplantation

Bronchiolitis Obliterans (Obliterative Bronchiolitis)

- Most important cause of morbidity & mortality in heart-lung & lung transplant recipients after 1 year
  - Accounts for ~ 30% of deaths > 1 year post transplant
  - Develops in ~ 50% of transplant recipients by 5 years post transplant
- Develops 6-18 months after transplant
- Risk factors
  - Acute rejection
  - Lymphocytic bronchitis, bronchiolitis
  - CMV pneumonia
  - Medication noncompliance
- Treatment
  - Increased immunosuppressive therapy

SELECTED REFERENCES

1. Borhani AA et al: Imaging of posttransplantation lymphoproliferative disorder after solid organ transplantation. Radiographics. 29(4):981-1000; discussion 1000-2, 2009
2. Zafar SY et al: Malignancy after solid organ transplantation: an overview. Oncologist. 13(7):769-78, 2008
3. Bellil Y et al: Bronchogenic carcinoma in solid organ transplant recipients. Curr Treat Options Oncol. 7(1):77-81, 2006
4. Chhajed PN et al: Patterns of pulmonary complications associated with sirolimus. Respiration. 73(3):367-74, 2006
5. Yao Z et al: Fungal respiratory disease. Curr Opin Pulm Med. 12(3):222-7, 2006

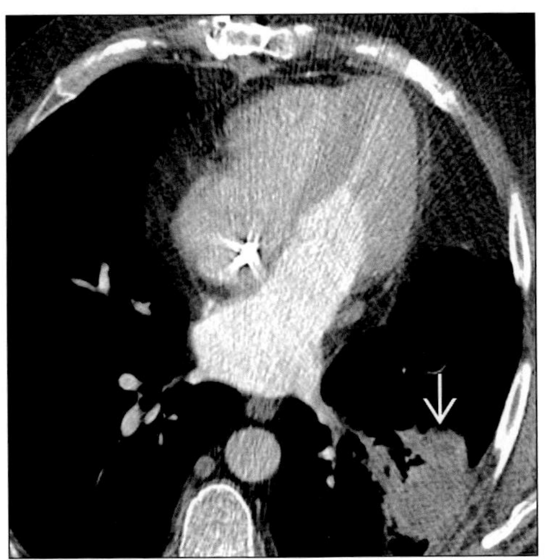

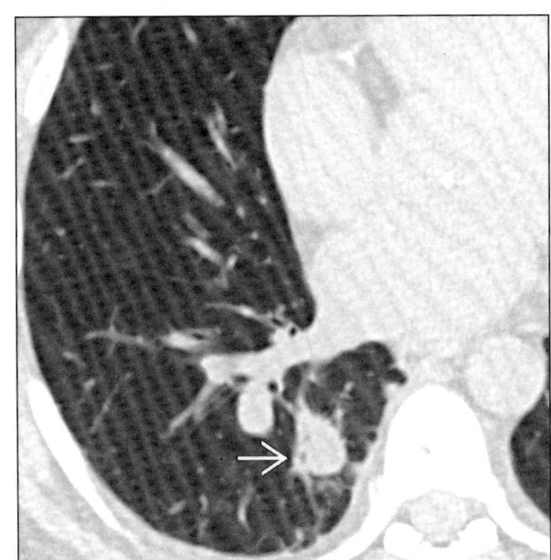

(Left) *Axial CECT of a patient who presented with low-grade fever 13 years post heart transplant shows a Scedosporium apiospermum fungal abscess manifesting as a peripheral heterogeneous left lower lobe mass ➔.* ***(Right)*** *Axial NECT of a renal transplant recipient with Mycobacterium kansasii infection shows a right lower lobe nodule ➔. Atypical fungal and mycobacterial infections must be considered in the differential diagnosis when lung nodules or masses are seen in SOT recipients.*

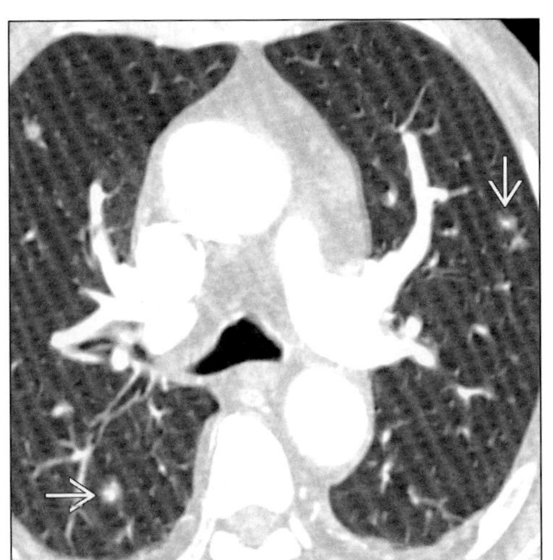

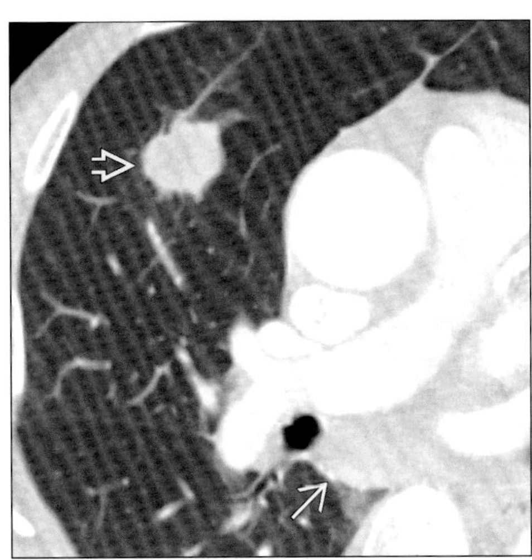

(Left) *Axial CECT of a renal transplant recipient with disseminated Kaposi sarcoma shows bilateral small peribronchovascular nodules ➔ with subtle ground-glass opacity halos.* ***(Right)*** *Axial CECT of a renal transplant recipient shows a right middle lobe squamous cell lung cancer manifesting as a spiculated nodule ⇨ with associated subcarinal lymphadenopathy ➔. Kaposi sarcoma and lung cancer both occur in greater frequency in SOT recipients than in the general population.*

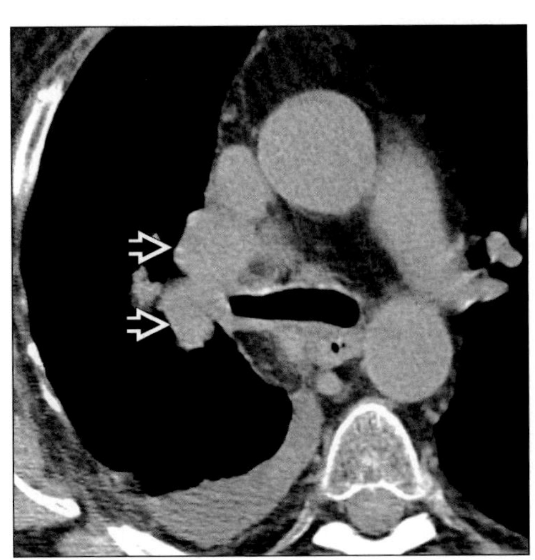

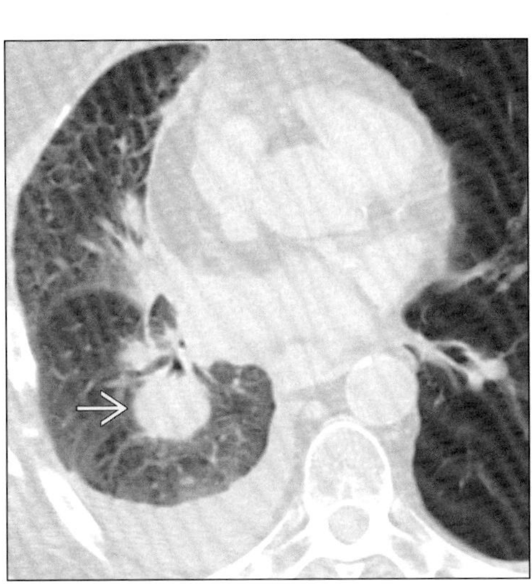

(Left) *Axial NECT of a patient who presented with shortness of breath 3 months following a right single lung transplant for chronic obstructive pulmonary disease shows right hilar lymphadenopathy ⇨ and a small right pleural effusion.* ***(Right)*** *Axial NECT of the same patient shows a right lower lobe nodule ➔ secondary to diffuse large B-cell lymphoma, consistent with post-transplant lymphoproliferative disorder (PTLD). PTLD ranges from lymphoid hyperplasia to frank lymphoma.*

HIV/AIDS

Key Facts

Terminology

- HIV: Retrovirus that infects helper T cells, macrophages, & dendritic cells with ↓ in cell-mediated immunity
- AIDS: HIV(+) patients with CD4 < 200 cells/μL

Imaging

- *Pneumocystis jiroveci* pneumonia (PCP): CD4 < 200
  - Bilateral ground-glass opacities
- Tuberculosis
  - CD4 > 200: Post-primary pattern
  - CD4 < 200: Primary pattern
  - Very low CD4: Negative chest radiograph
- Kaposi sarcoma: CD4 < 200
  - Peribronchovascular flame-shaped lesions
  - Enhancing lymphadenopathy
- Lymphocytic interstitial pneumonia: Any CD4
  - Centrilobular, peribronchovascular nodules
  - Ground-glass opacities, cysts
- Multicentric Castleman disease: Any CD4
  - Lymphadenopathy ± enhancement
- Immune reconstitution inflammatory syndrome: Paradoxical deterioration from recovery of immune function after HAART

Clinical Issues

- Symptoms/signs
  - Cough, fever
  - Weight loss
  - Lymphadenopathy
  - Weakness, malaise
- Prognosis
  - Marked mortality reduction with HAART
  - Poor prognosis for patients without access to or noncompliant with HAART
- Treatment
  - HAART
  - Prophylactic antibiotics

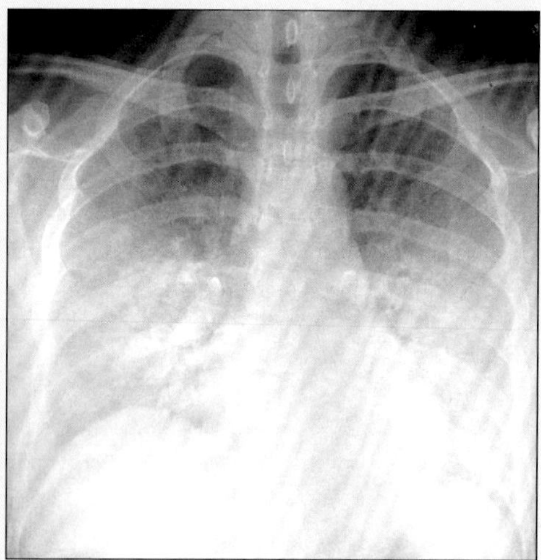

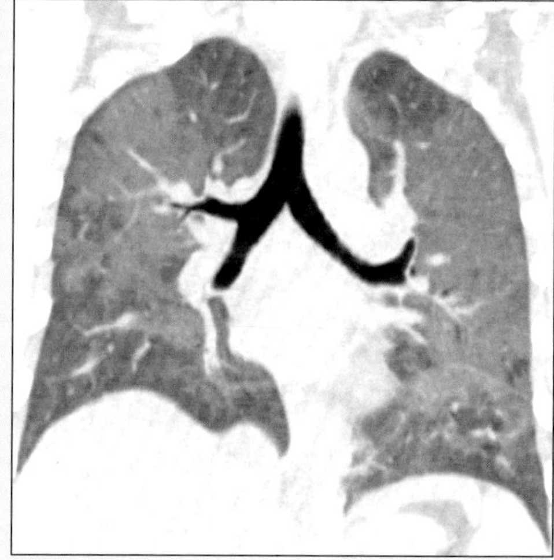

(Left) *PA chest radiograph shows bilateral hazy airspace opacities in an HIV(+) patient who was noncompliant with HAART and had a 2-week history of dyspnea.* ***(Right)*** *Coronal NECT shows diffuse bilateral ground-glass opacities, suspicious for Pneumocystis jiroveci pneumonia (PCP), subsequently confirmed by bronchoalveolar lavage. Bilateral ground-glass opacities in an HIV(+) patient with CD4 count < 200 and subacute onset of symptoms are highly suggestive of PCP.*

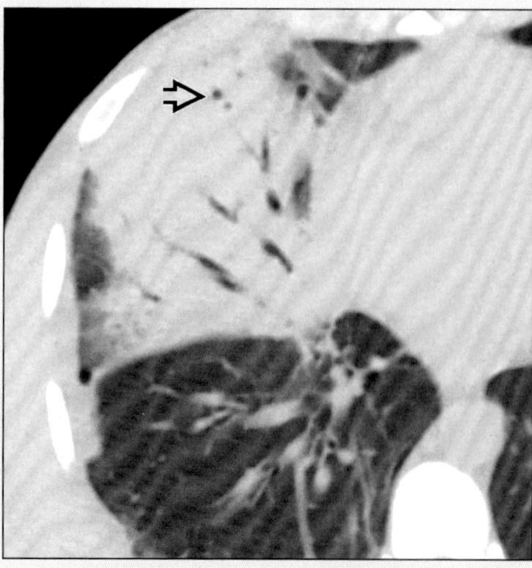

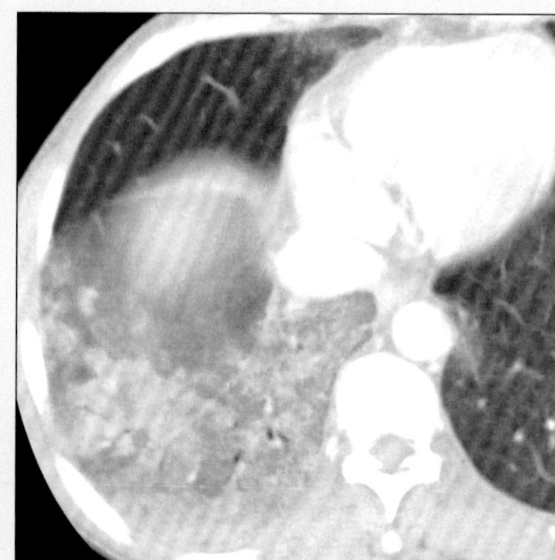

(Left) *Axial NECT of an HIV(+) patient with S. pneumoniae pneumonia shows middle lobe consolidation with tiny intrinsic cavities ⇨. Bacterial bronchitis and pneumonia are the most common causes of respiratory infection in HIV(+) patients with any CD4 count.* ***(Right)*** *Axial CECT of an HIV(+) patient with tuberculosis (TB) shows right lower lobe consolidation and ground-glass opacity; lymphadenopathy was also present but is not shown. HIV(+) adults with low CD4 counts and TB may exhibit the primary pattern of disease.*

HIV/AIDS

TERMINOLOGY

Abbreviations

- **Human immunodeficiency virus (HIV)**
- **Acquired immunodeficiency syndrome (AIDS)**

Definitions

- HIV: Retrovirus that infects helper T cells, macrophages, & dendritic cells → decrease in cell-mediated immunity
- CD4 count: Helper T-cell level
  - Widely accepted measure of immunosuppression in HIV(+) patients
- AIDS: HIV(+) patients with CD4 < 200 cells/μL at risk for opportunistic infections & malignant neoplasms

IMAGING

General Features

- Best diagnostic clue
  - *Pneumocystis jiroveci* pneumonia (PCP): Bilateral, symmetric ground-glass opacities, CD4 < 200
  - Kaposi sarcoma (KS): Flame-shaped lesions, enhancing lymphadenopathy, male patient, CD4 < 200

Complications of HIV/AIDS

- **Infection**
  - **Bacterial pneumonia**: Most common respiratory infection, any CD4 count
    - 50% focal consolidation (segmental or lobar)
    - 50% other patterns: Diffuse opacities, nodules, cavities
  - *Pneumocystis jiroveci* **pneumonia**: Decreased prevalence, still common presenting illness in patients with previously undiagnosed HIV infection; CD4 < 200
    - Chest radiograph normal in > 40% of cases
    - Bilateral, perihilar or diffuse, symmetric fine granular, reticular, or ground-glass opacities
    - Cysts or pneumatoceles in 10-40%
      - Spontaneous pneumothorax
  - **Tuberculosis (TB)**
    - Imaging findings depend on CD4 count
    - CD4 > 200: Post-primary pattern
      - Apical or posterior segments of upper lobes or superior segment of lower lobes
      - Cavitary lesions
      - Tree-in-bud opacities
    - CD4 < 200: Primary pattern
      - Consolidation
      - Lymphadenopathy (peripheral enhancement, central necrosis)
      - Pleural effusion, empyema
      - Miliary nodules
    - Very low CD4: Lack of immune response, minimal findings
      - Normal chest radiograph
      - Tiny & few miliary nodules
  - **Atypical mycobacterial infection**: *Mycobacterium avium complex* (MAC), *Mycobacterium kansasii*, CD4 < 50
    - Radiographic appearance similar to that of TB; miliary nodules uncommon
  - *Cryptococcus* & other disseminated fungal infections (histoplasmosis, coccidioidomycosis), CD4 < 100
    - Nodules ± cavitation
    - Miliary nodules
    - Lymphadenopathy
- **Neoplasm**
  - **Kaposi sarcoma**: Mostly affects men, caused by human herpes virus (HSV)-8, CD4 < 200
    - Flame-shaped lesions: Ill-defined nodules surrounded by ground-glass halo; along bronchovascular bundles
    - Interlobular septal thickening
    - Enhancing lymphadenopathy
  - **Lymphoma**: Decreasing incidence, associated with Epstein-Barr virus, CD4 < 100
    - Lymphadenopathy
    - Solitary or multiple nodules
    - Consolidation
  - **Lung cancer**: Increased risk due to altered immune function, any CD4 count
    - Pulmonary nodule or mass
    - Lymphadenopathy: Same drainage pattern as in general population
- Noninfectious, nonneoplastic conditions
  - **Lymphocytic interstitial pneumonia** (LIP): Lymphoproliferative disorder, children > adults, any CD4 count
    - Centrilobular, peribronchovascular nodules
    - Ground-glass opacities
    - Cysts
  - **Bronchiectasis**
    - More extensive and severe than expected with brief or no history of infection
  - Emphysema: Related to abnormal activity of cytotoxic T cells, 15% of HIV(+) patients
  - **Multicentric Castleman disease**: Lymphoproliferative disorder associated with HSV-8, any CD4 count
    - Lymphadenopathy ± enhancement
    - Peribronchovascular & interlobular septal thickening, nodules
  - **Sarcoidosis**: Increasing incidence in era of highly active antiretroviral therapy (HAART), may be related to drug reaction or alteration in immune regulation
    - Perilymphatic micronodules
    - Lymphadenopathy
- Cardiovascular complications
  - Pulmonary arterial hypertension (PAH)
    - Enlarged pulmonary trunk
    - Dilated right heart chambers
  - Cardiomyopathy
    - Cardiomegaly
    - Pulmonary edema: Septal thickening, perihilar opacities
    - Pleural effusions
  - Premature atherosclerosis
    - Vascular calcification
- Immune reconstitution inflammatory syndrome (IRIS)
  - Paradoxical clinical & imaging deterioration due to recovery of immune function after initiation of HAART
  - Risk factor: Low CD4 (< 50) & high viral load prior to initiation of HAART

- Imaging shows worsening of underlying infections (common with mycobacterial infection) or neoplasms (KS, lymphoma)

Imaging Recommendations

- Best imaging tool
  - Radiography for initial detection of complications & follow-up
  - CT: More sensitive & specific than radiography
    - Assessment of radiographically occult infection (PCP, TB)
    - Characterization of nonspecific radiographic findings
    - Planning or guidance of biopsy or drainage procedures
    - Staging of HIV-related neoplasms

DIFFERENTIAL DIAGNOSIS

Lymphadenopathy

- Diffusely enhancing
  - Kaposi sarcoma
  - Castleman disease
- Peripherally enhancing with necrotic center
  - Tuberculosis
  - Atypical mycobacterial infection
  - Fungal infection
- Soft tissue density
  - Lymphoma
  - Lung cancer
  - Generalized HIV lymphadenopathy
  - Sarcoidosis

Lung Nodules

- Miliary nodules
  - Tuberculosis
  - Disseminated fungal infection
- Peribronchovascular nodules
  - Kaposi sarcoma
  - Lymphoma
  - Sarcoidosis
- Macronodules > 1 cm
  - Lung cancer
  - Pulmonary lymphoma
  - Mycobacterial infection
  - Fungal infection
  - Septic emboli

Cysts

- *Pneumocystis jiroveci* pneumonia
- Lymphocytic interstitial pneumonia

Consolidation

- Bacterial pneumonia
- Tuberculosis
- Atypical mycobacterial infection
- Fungal infection
- Lymphoma

Ground-Glass Opacities

- *Pneumocystis jiroveci* pneumonia
- Viral pneumonia
- Lymphocytic interstitial pneumonia

CLINICAL ISSUES

Presentation

- Most common signs/symptoms
  - Cough, fever
    - Abrupt onset (< 1 week): Bacterial pneumonia
    - Gradual onset (> 1 week): PCP, mycobacterial infection, neoplasm
  - Weight loss
- Other signs/symptoms
  - Lymphadenopathy
  - Weakness, malaise

Demographics

- Epidemiology
  - Spread through close contact with bodily fluids
    - Unsafe sex
    - Contaminated needles, IV drug abuse
    - Perinatal transmission from infected mother to child
    - Blood transfusion no longer common cause in developed countries
  - 33.3 million living with HIV worldwide at end of 2009

Natural History & Prognosis

- Marked reduction in morbidity & mortality with HAART in developed countries
  - Life expectancy: 20-50 years after diagnosis of HIV infection
- Poor prognosis for patients without access to or noncompliant with HAART
  - Survival: 6-19 months after developing AIDS

Treatment

- HAART
- Prophylactic antibiotics (depends on CD4 level) for PCP, toxoplasmosis, TB, atypical mycobacterial infection

DIAGNOSTIC CHECKLIST

Image Interpretation Pearls

- Important to employ an integrated approach combining
  - Radiographic pattern recognition
  - Chronicity of clinical symptoms
  - Immune status
    - CD4 count in HIV(+) patient
    - Risk factors for HIV in those with unknown HIV status
  - Compliance with HAART & prophylactic antibiotic therapy

SELECTED REFERENCES

1. Brecher CW et al: CT and radiography of bacterial respiratory infections in AIDS patients. AJR Am J Roentgenol. 180(5):1203-9, 2003
2. Boiselle PM et al: Update on lung disease in AIDS. Semin Roentgenol. 37(1):54-71, 2002
3. Saurborn DP et al: The imaging spectrum of pulmonary tuberculosis in AIDS. J Thorac Imaging. 17(1):28-33, 2002

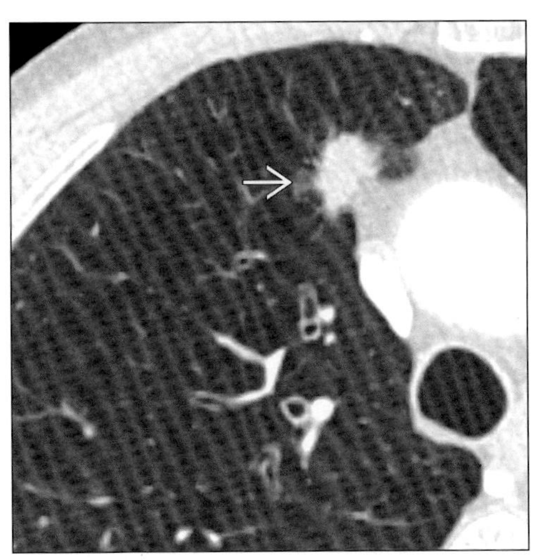

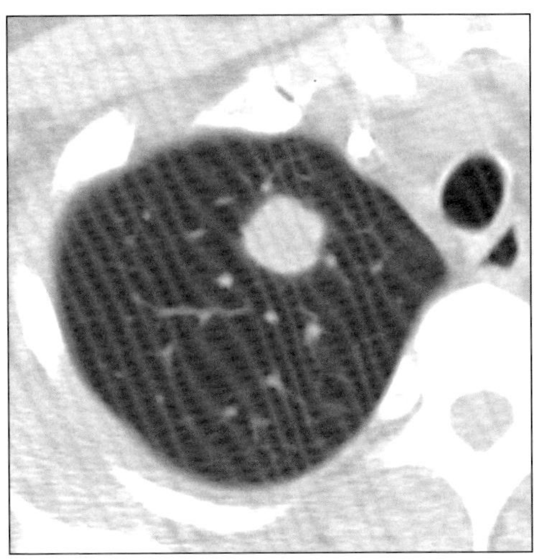

(Left) *Axial CECT of an HIV(+) patient with lung adenocarcinoma shows a spiculated right upper lobe nodule ➔ and centrilobular emphysema. HIV(+) patients are more likely to develop emphysema and lung cancer at a younger age due to immune dysfunction.* ***(Right)*** *Axial NECT of a patient with AIDS and pulmonary B-cell lymphoma shows a right upper lobe pulmonary nodule. Patients with AIDS are at a higher risk of developing pulmonary lymphoma, either primary or disseminated.*

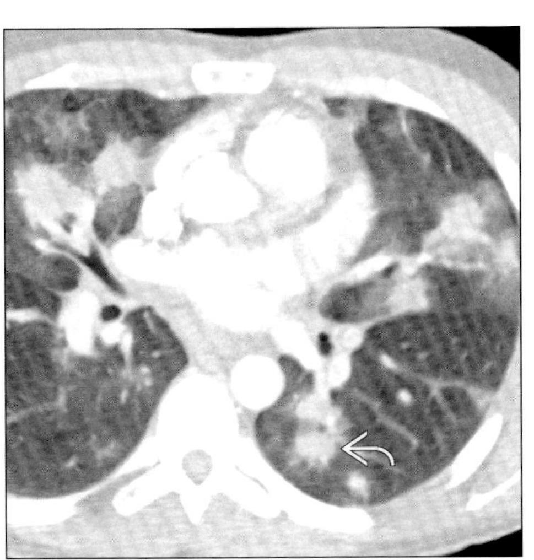

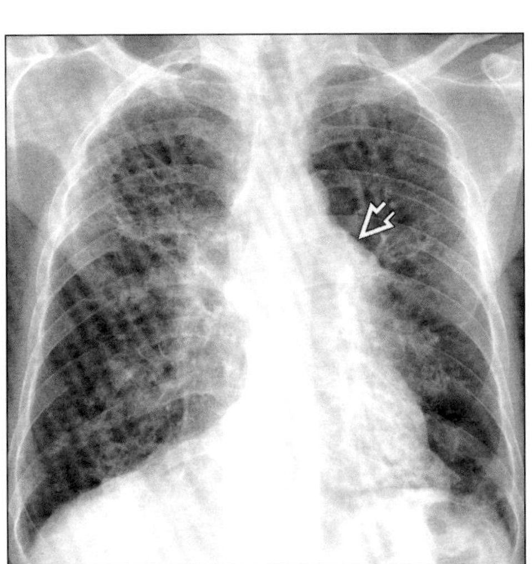

(Left) *Axial CECT of a patient with AIDS and Kaposi sarcoma shows bilateral peribronchovascular nodules with ground-glass opacity halos ↩ or flame-shaped lesions.* ***(Right)*** *PA chest radiograph of an HIV(+) patient with bronchiectasis and pulmonary hypertension shows bilateral cystic bronchiectasis with bronchial wall thickening and enlargement of the pulmonary trunk ⇨. HIV(+) patients are more likely to develop bronchiectasis and pulmonary hypertension than the general population.*

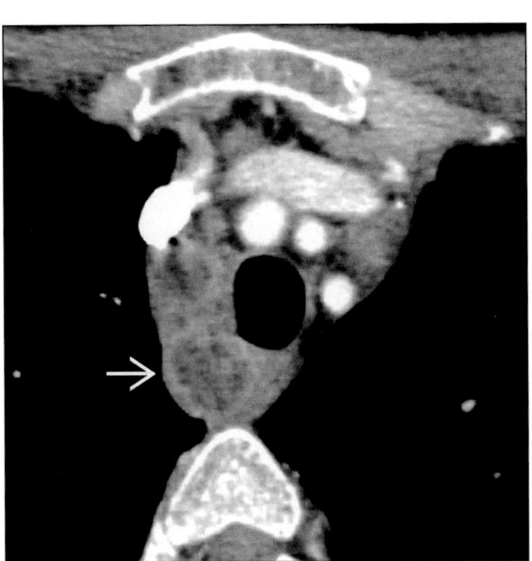

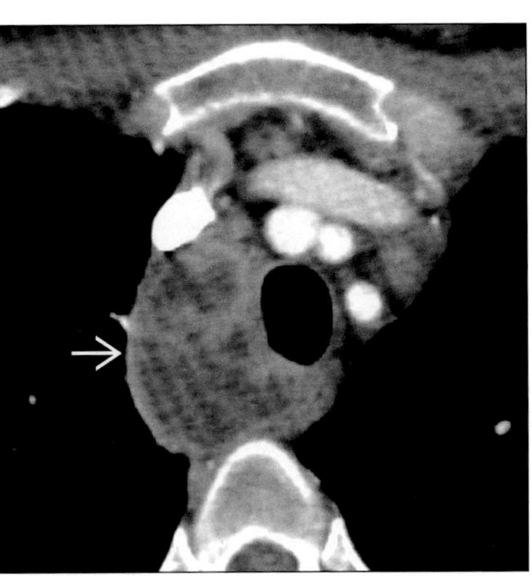

(Left) *Axial CECT of an HIV(+) patient with biopsy-proven Mycobacterium avium infection shows right paratracheal lymphadenopathy ➔ with central low attenuation and peripheral enhancement characteristic of mycobacterial and fungal infection.* ***(Right)*** *Axial CECT of the same patient 6 weeks after initiation of HAART shows further enlargement of right paratracheal lymphadenopathy ➔ thought to be related to immune reconstitution inflammatory syndrome (IRIS).*

NEUTROPENIA

Key Facts

Terminology

- Neutropenia: Absolute neutrophil count (ANC) of < 1,500/microliter of blood

Imaging

- Radiography
  - Often negative or nonspecific in neutropenic febrile patients
- CT
  - Invasive pulmonary aspergillosis (IPA): Nodules with halo or air crescent sign
  - Mucormycosis: Solitary or multiple nodules
  - *Pneumocystis jiroveci* pneumonia (PCP): Bilateral ground-glass opacities
  - Viral pneumonia: Ground-glass opacities, consolidations, tree-in-bud opacities
- Chest CT should be considered in early evaluation of febrile neutropenia

Top Differential Diagnoses

- Nodular opacities
  - IPA, fungal & mycobacterial infections
  - Septic emboli
  - Neoplasm
  - Cryptogenic organizing pneumonia
- Ground-glass opacities
  - PCP, viral pneumonia
  - Pulmonary hemorrhage
  - Pulmonary edema

Clinical Issues

- Symptoms/signs: Malaise, chills, fever
- Infection-related mortality rate: Up to 38%

Diagnostic Checklist

- Early imaging diagnosis of infection in febrile neutropenia crucial for prompt therapy

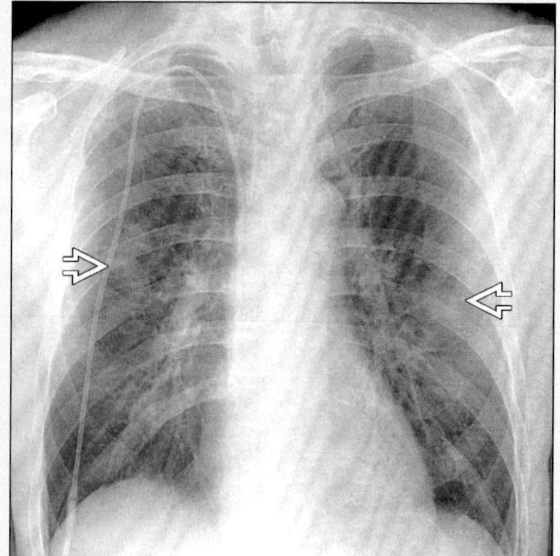

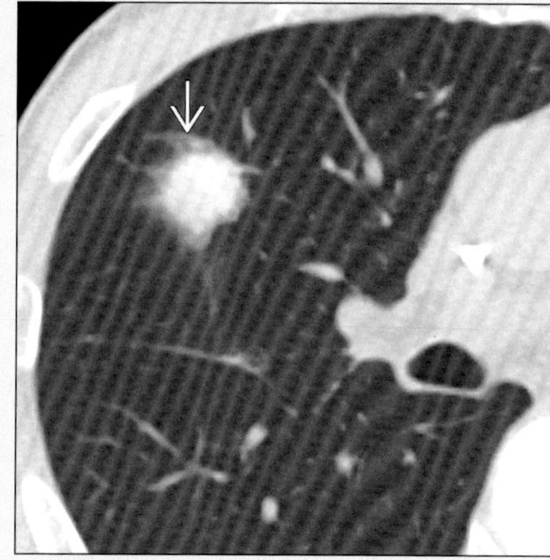

(Left) *PA chest radiograph of a febrile neutropenic patient status post bone marrow transplant shows bilateral nonspecific pulmonary nodular opacities ⇨.* ***(Right)*** *Axial NECT of the same patient shows a right upper lobe nodule with a ground-glass halo →, which in this clinical setting is highly suspicious for angioinvasive fungal infection. The CT halo sign appears early in the disease course. Recognition of this sign helps suggest the diagnosis and allows early initiation of antifungal therapy.*

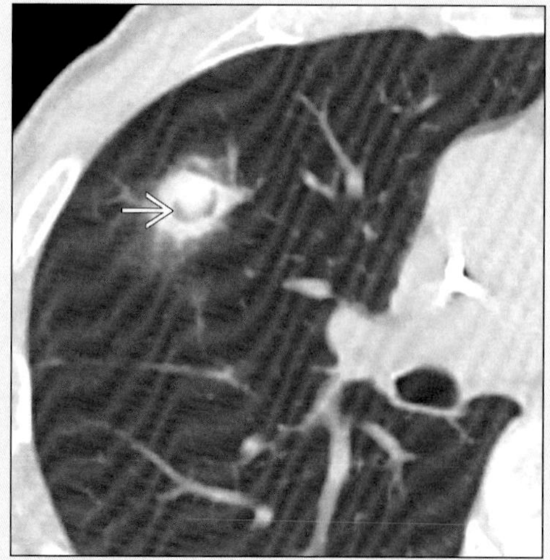

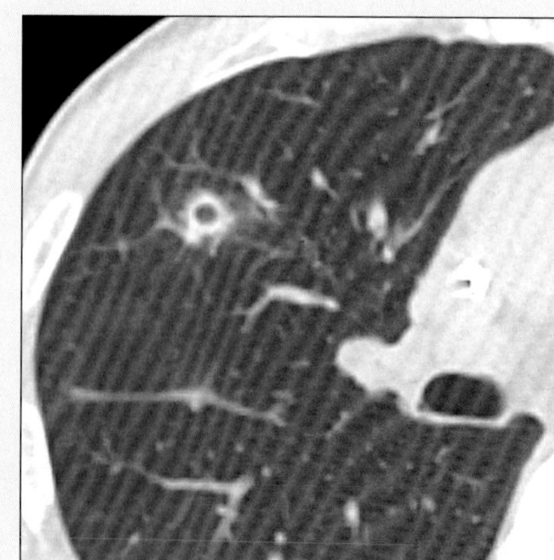

(Left) *Axial NECT of the same patient obtained 3 days later demonstrates the air crescent sign →. Intracavitary opacities in invasive aspergillosis are typically nondependent in contrast to fungus balls or mycetomas. The air crescent sign occurs later in the disease course and is considered a good prognostic factor.* ***(Right)*** *Axial NECT of the same patient 10 days later shows near resolution of the surrounding ground-glass halo and decrease in the size of the nodule, consistent with response to treatment.*

NEUTROPENIA

TERMINOLOGY

Definitions

- Neutrophil: Type of white blood cell that kills & digests microorganisms via phagocytosis
- Neutropenia
  - Abnormally low level of neutrophils in blood
  - Absolute neutrophil count (ANC) of < 1,500/ microliter of blood

IMAGING

General Concepts

- Chest radiography in febrile neutropenic patients
  - Significant number of chest radiographs are normal
  - Significant number of chest radiographs show nonspecific abnormalities

Radiographic Findings

- Radiography
  - Ground-glass opacity
  - Consolidation
  - Lung nodule/mass: May exhibit cavitation
  - Reticular opacities
  - Pleural effusion

CT Findings

- **Invasive pulmonary aspergillosis** (IPA)
  - **CT halo sign**: Central nodule or mass surrounded by ground-glass attenuation rim
    - Highly sensitive finding in early stage IPA
    - Ground-glass opacity related to angioinvasive nature of disease, producing perilesional hemorrhage
    - Empiric initiation of targeted antibiotic treatment for IPA at detection of CT halo sign in neutropenic patients improves survival
  - Hypodense sign
    - Early imaging manifestation
    - Visualization of central hypodensity in lung consolidation, mass, or nodule
    - May be seen without intravenous contrast
  - **Air crescent sign**: Cavity with intracavitary mass
    - Occurs later in course of IPA
    - Coincident with resolution of neutropenia; favorable sign
    - Central "mass" is due to necrotic lung, usually adherent to cavity wall, not gravity-dependent
  - CTA of IPA
    - Interruption of pulmonary artery branch at border of focal lesion, nonvisualization of vessel within or peripheral to lesion
  - Airway-invasive aspergillosis
    - Centrilobular nodules
    - Bronchial wall thickening
    - Peribronchiolar ground-glass opacity or consolidation
  - Pulmonary opacities may remain stable 1-2 weeks after initiation of appropriate treatment
    - Postulated immunological phenomenon due to recovery of neutrophil count
  - Lesion size & number may increase after institution of appropriate treatment
- **Mucormycosis**
  - Solitary or multiple nodules ± ground-glass halo
- **Bacterial infection**
  - Bacterial pneumonia
    - Ground-glass opacities
    - Consolidations
    - Pleural effusions
  - Septic emboli
    - Multiple nodules ± cavitation
    - Peripheral & lower lobe distribution
- **Pneumocystis jiroveci pneumonia** (PCP)
  - Bilateral ground-glass opacities
  - Interlobular septal thickening
- **Viral pneumonia**: CMV, RSV, adenovirus
  - Bilateral ground-glass opacities
  - Consolidations
  - Tree-in-bud opacities
  - Bronchial wall thickening
- **Drug toxicity**
  - General concepts
    - Many chemotherapeutic agents may induce neutropenia
    - Drug toxicity may produce variety of pulmonary abnormalities on imaging
  - Diffuse alveolar damage
    - Bilateral consolidations or ground-glass opacities
  - Organizing pneumonia
    - Patchy opacities with peribronchial & subpleural distribution & lower lobe predominance
    - Atoll or reverse halo sign
      - Central ground-glass opacity with rim of consolidation
  - Interstitial fibrosis: Usual interstitial pneumonia (UIP) or nonspecific interstitial pneumonia (NSIP) patterns
    - Subpleural reticular opacities
    - Traction bronchiectasis
    - Ground-glass opacities (NSIP)
    - Honeycomb lung (UIP)
- **Radiation pneumonitis**
  - Radiation &/or concurrent chemotherapy may cause neutropenia
  - Geographic consolidations or ground-glass opacities in radiation port distribution
- **Pulmonary hemorrhage**
  - Neutropenic patients may exhibit concurrent thrombocytopenia or coagulopathy
  - Patchy or diffuse ground-glass opacities or consolidations

MR Findings

- IPA
  - Hypointense on T1WI
  - Hyperintense on T2WI
  - Uniform gadolinium enhancement during early stage
  - Peripheral gadolinium enhancement in late stage

Imaging Recommendations

- Best imaging tool
  - Chest radiography: Initial imaging modality for evaluation of febrile neutropenic patient
  - **Consider chest CT early in evaluation of febrile neutropenic patient** with normal or nonspecific chest radiographic findings
    - 50% of patients with normal radiographs have findings suggestive of pneumonia on CT
    - CT helps narrow differential diagnosis & guide work-up & therapy

NEUTROPENIA

Image-Guided Biopsy

- CT-guided percutaneous needle aspiration or biopsy helpful in obtaining samples for pathologic diagnosis or microbiology culture

DIFFERENTIAL DIAGNOSIS

Nodular Opacities

- Invasive pulmonary aspergillosis
- Septic emboli
- Mycobacterial infection
- Fungal infection
- Neoplasm
  - Lung cancer
  - Pulmonary metastases
  - Lymphoma
- Cryptogenic organizing pneumonia

Ground-Glass Opacities

- *Pneumocystis jiroveci* pneumonia
- Viral infection
- Pulmonary hemorrhage
- Pulmonary edema
- Pulmonary alveolar proteinosis
  - Associated with hematologic malignancy

PATHOLOGY

General Features

- Etiology
  - Inadequate or ineffective granulopoiesis
    - Aplastic anemia
    - Leukemia
    - Chemotherapy
    - Drug toxicity
      - Chloramphenicol
      - Sulfonamides
      - Chlorpromazine
    - Radiation
  - Accelerated removal or destruction of neutrophils
    - Overwhelming bacterial or fungal infections
    - Splenomegaly

CLINICAL ISSUES

Presentation

- Most common signs/symptoms
  - Malaise
  - Chills
  - Fever
- Other signs/symptoms
  - Weakness
  - Ulcerating, necrotizing lesions of oral cavity

Demographics

- Epidemiology
  - Incidence of pneumonia in neutropenic cancer patients: 17-24%
  - Bacterial infection responsible for ≈ 90% of infections in early neutropenia

Natural History & Prognosis

- Infection-related mortality rate: Up to 38%
- Survival rates in patients with IPA undergoing chemotherapy and bone marrow or stem cell transplant: < 10%
- Viral pneumonia: Mortality 50% in neutropenic host

Treatment

- Removal of offending drug
- Control of infections
  - Antibiotics
  - Surgical drainage
  - Surgical resection
- Recombinant hematopoietic growth factors
  - Granulocyte colony-stimulating factor (G-CSF)
  - Granulocyte-macrophage colony-stimulating factor (GM-CSF)

DIAGNOSTIC CHECKLIST

Consider

- Early imaging diagnosis of opportunistic infections in febrile neutropenic patients is crucial for prompt institution of appropriate antimicrobial therapy

SELECTED REFERENCES

1. Shiley KT et al: Chest CT features of community-acquired respiratory viral infections in adult inpatients with lower respiratory tract infections. J Thorac Imaging. 25(1):68-75, 2010
2. Greene RE et al: Imaging findings in acute invasive pulmonary aspergillosis: clinical significance of the halo sign. Clin Infect Dis. 44(3):373-9, 2007
3. Brodoefel H et al: Long-term CT follow-up in 40 non-HIV immunocompromised patients with invasive pulmonary aspergillosis: kinetics of CT morphology and correlation with clinical findings and outcome. AJR Am J Roentgenol. 187(2):404-13, 2006
4. Horger M et al: Invasive pulmonary aspergillosis: frequency and meaning of the "hypodense sign" on unenhanced CT. Br J Radiol. 78(932):697-703, 2005
5. Sonnet S et al: Direct detection of angioinvasive pulmonary aspergillosis in immunosuppressed patients: preliminary results with high-resolution 16-MDCT angiography. AJR Am J Roentgenol. 184(3):746-51, 2005
6. Heussel CP et al: Pneumonia in neutropenic patients. Eur Radiol. 14(2):256-71, 2004
7. Maschmeyer G: Pneumonia in febrile neutropenic patients: radiologic diagnosis. Curr Opin Oncol. 13(4):229-35, 2001

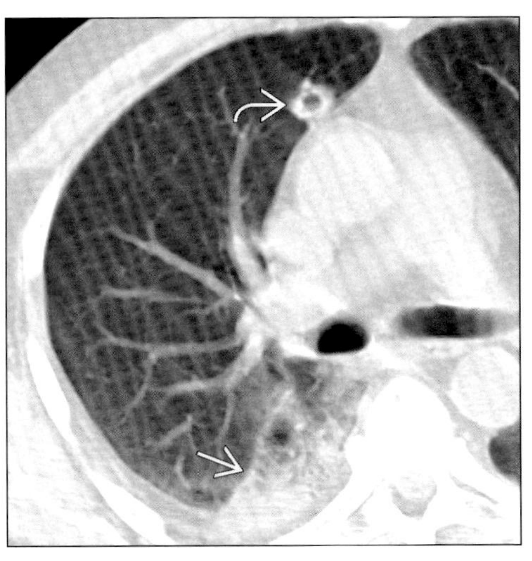
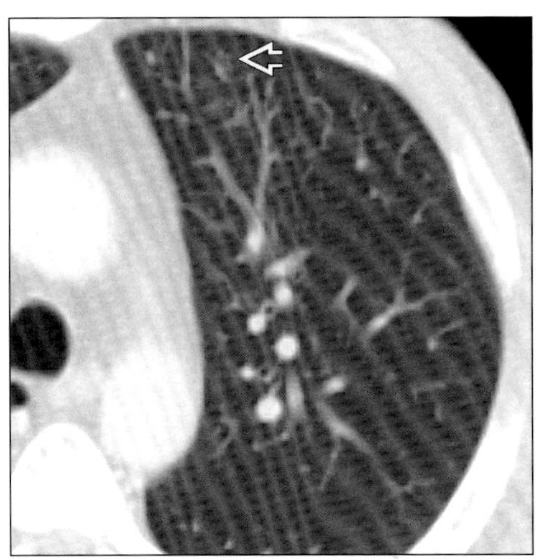

(Left) *Axial NECT of a patient with chemotherapy-induced neutropenia complicated by infection with mucormycosis (diagnosed by bronchoalveolar lavage) shows a right upper lobe cavitary nodule* ➔ *and a right lower lobe consolidation* ➔. *Opportunistic fungal infections can manifest with nodules, masses, or consolidations.* ***(Right)*** *Axial CECT of a febrile neutropenic patient with Cytomegalovirus (CMV) pneumonia shows tree-in-bud opacities* ➔ *in the left upper lobe.*

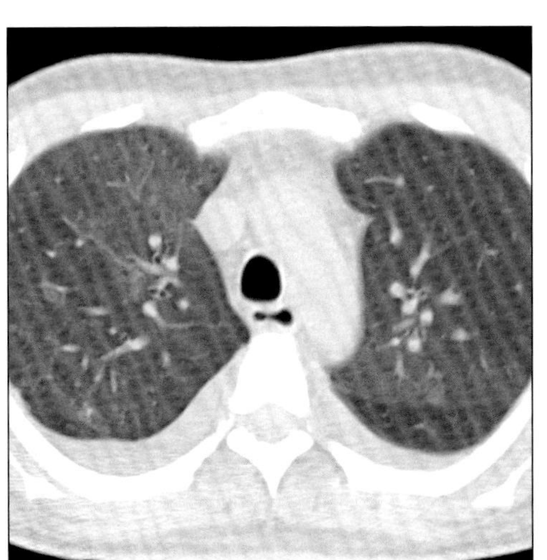
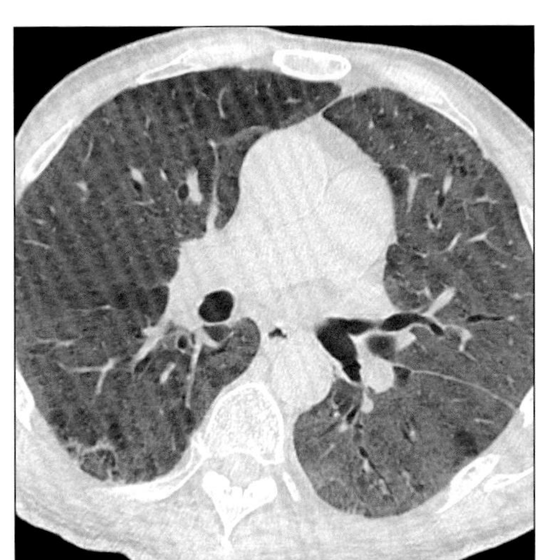

(Left) *Axial NECT of a neutropenic patient with respiratory syncytial virus (RSV) shows bilateral diffuse ground-glass opacities and bilateral pleural effusions.* ***(Right)*** *Axial NECT of a febrile neutropenic patient with Pneumocystis jiroveci pneumonia (PCP) (diagnosed by bronchoalveolar lavage) shows bilateral diffuse ground-glass attenuation. The main differential diagnostic considerations for diffuse ground-glass opacity in febrile neutropenic patients are PCP and viral pneumonia.*

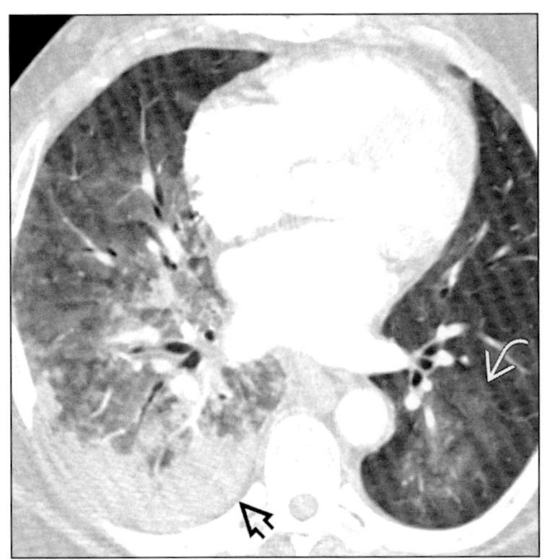
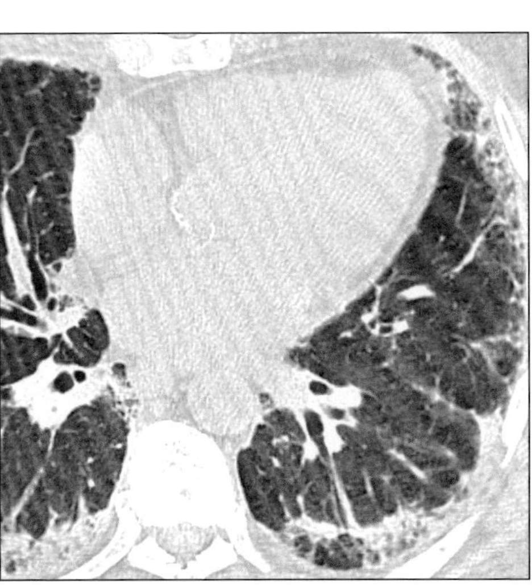

(Left) *Axial CECT of a neutropenic, thrombocytopenic patient undergoing chemotherapy shows bilateral ground-glass opacities* ➔ *and a right lower lobe consolidation* ➔. *Bronchoalveolar lavage confirmed pulmonary hemorrhage and excluded infection.* ***(Right)*** *Axial HRCT of a neutropenic patient undergoing chemotherapy shows bilateral subpleural reticular opacities and subtle traction bronchiolectasis secondary to bleomycin-induced interstitial fibrosis.*

IDIOPATHIC PULMONARY HEMORRHAGE

Key Facts

Terminology
- Idiopathic pulmonary hemorrhage (IPH)
- Synonym: Idiopathic pulmonary hemosiderosis
- Recurrent diffuse alveolar hemorrhage without underlying cause; diagnosis of exclusion

Imaging
- Radiography
  - Bilateral airspace disease
- CT/HRCT
  - Multifocal bilateral ground-glass opacities
  - Development of reticulation & honeycomb lung

Top Differential Diagnoses
- Pulmonary edema
- Pneumonia
- Wegener granulomatosis
- Goodpasture syndrome

Pathology
- Lungs are diffusely brown
- Hemosiderin-laden alveolar macrophages
- Absence of vasculitis, capillaritis, granulomas, or immunoglobulin deposition

Clinical Issues
- Symptoms/signs
  - Dyspnea, nonproductive cough, hemoptysis
  - Dyspnea on exertion & fatigue
  - Hemoptysis may be absent
- 80% of cases in children, typically < 10 years
- 25% subsequently develop autoimmune disorder
- Treatment: Glucocorticoids

Diagnostic Checklist
- Consider IPH in patient with hemoptysis, anemia, & bilateral airspace disease of unknown etiology

*(**Left**) AP chest radiograph of a 33-year-old man with iron deficiency anemia and chronic recurrent hemoptysis shows diffuse bilateral reticular opacities and bilateral lower zone airspace opacities. (**Right**) Axial HRCT of the same patient shows lower lung zone predominant centrilobular ground-glass opacities ➔ and subpleural reticular opacities ⇨. Transbronchial biopsy confirmed the diagnosis of pulmonary hemosiderosis. The diagnosis of IPH was made after exclusion of other potential etiologies.*

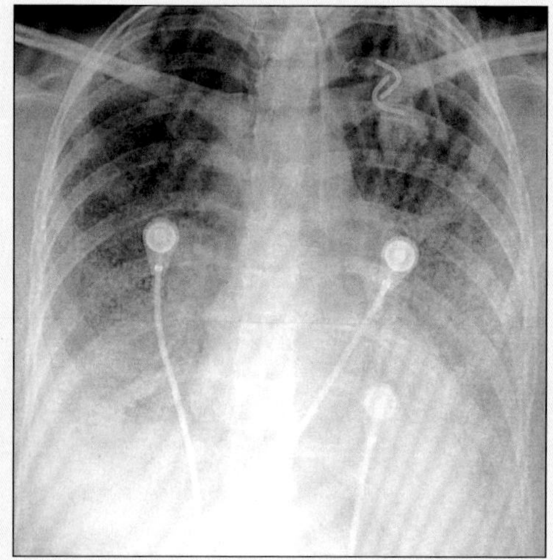

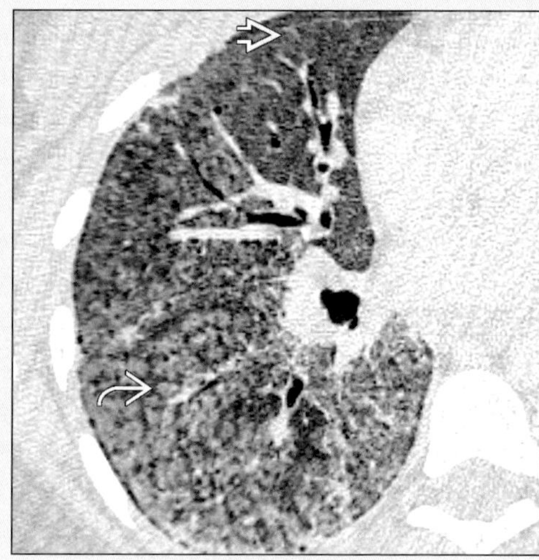

*(**Left**) PA chest radiograph of a 26-year-old woman with hemoptysis and a history of idiopathic pulmonary hemorrhage since childhood shows a patchy airspace opacity in the right lower lung. (**Right**) Axial NECT of the same patient shows diffuse ground-glass opacity in the right lower lobe and a small right pleural effusion. IPH is a diagnosis of exclusion that should be considered in the appropriate clinical setting. Histologic documentation of intraalveolar hemosiderin-laden macrophages helps confirm the diagnosis.*

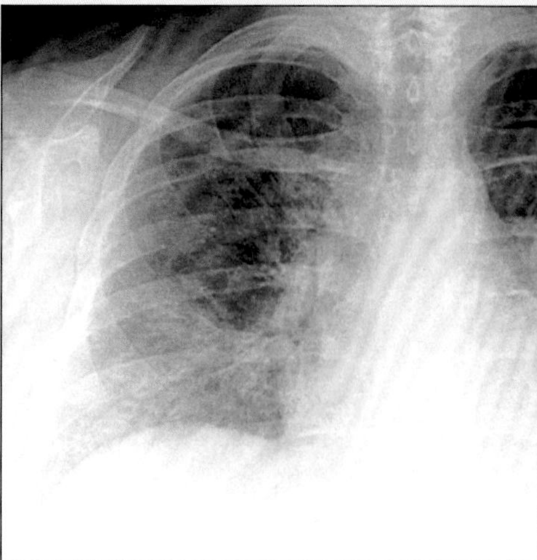

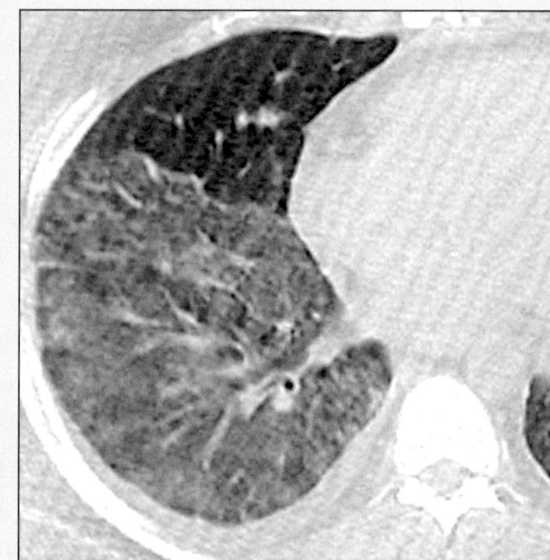

IDIOPATHIC PULMONARY HEMORRHAGE

TERMINOLOGY

Abbreviations

- **Idiopathic pulmonary hemorrhage (IPH)**

Synonyms

- Idiopathic pulmonary hemosiderosis

Definitions

- Recurrent diffuse alveolar hemorrhage without underlying cause; diagnosis of exclusion

IMAGING

General Features

- Best diagnostic clue
  - Bilateral airspace disease in patient with hemoptysis & iron deficiency anemia
- Location
  - Lower lobes more commonly affected, may be diffuse

Radiographic Findings

- Multifocal airspace disease

CT Findings

- HRCT
  - Multifocal bilateral ground-glass opacities: Centrilobular, geographic, or diffuse
  - Subpleural reticulation & honeycomb cystic change may develop with recurrent episodes of hemorrhage

Imaging Recommendations

- Best imaging tool
  - HRCT is imaging modality of choice

DIFFERENTIAL DIAGNOSIS

Pulmonary Edema

- Cardiomegaly, bilateral pleural effusions, bilateral reticular opacities/airspace disease

Pneumonia

- Focal or multifocal pulmonary consolidation
- Fever, productive cough, & leukocytosis

Wegener Granulomatosis

- Systemic vasculitis often involving kidneys; c-ANCA
- Affected patients may present with airspace disease secondary to pulmonary hemorrhage

Goodpasture Syndrome

- Antibasement membrane antibodies
- May be complicated by pulmonary hemorrhage with resultant airspace disease

Acute Respiratory Distress Syndrome (ARDS)

- Typically associated with known cause of lung injury
- Diffuse bilateral airspace disease

Churg-Strauss Syndrome

- Systemic vasculitis & peripheral eosinophilia in patient with asthma
- Peripheral, transient consolidations & small pleural effusions

PATHOLOGY

General Features

- Etiology
  - Unknown, but clinical response to immunosuppression suggests immune process
- Genetics
  - Familial clustering reported, but no gene has been identified

Gross Pathologic & Surgical Features

- Lungs are diffusely brown

Microscopic Features

- Hemosiderin-laden alveolar macrophages
- Free iron within pulmonary tissue results in fibrosis
- Swollen vacuolated endothelial cells
- Absence of vasculitis, capillaritis, granulomas, or immunoglobulin deposition

CLINICAL ISSUES

Presentation

- Most common signs/symptoms
  - Dyspnea & nonproductive cough progresses to hemoptysis
  - Dyspnea on exertion & fatigue may be due to iron deficiency anemia
  - Hemoptysis may be absent
- Other signs/symptoms
  - 20% have hepatomegaly or splenomegaly

Demographics

- Age
  - 80% of cases in children, typically < 10 years
- Epidemiology
  - Extremely rare: < 1 per million

Natural History & Prognosis

- 25% subsequently develop autoimmune disorder
- Lane-Hamilton syndrome = IPH & celiac disease
  - Pulmonary symptoms improve with gluten-free diet
- Massive acute pulmonary hemorrhage or chronic pulmonary fibrosis are most frequent causes of death

Treatment

- Sparse data, but glucocorticoids are drugs of choice
  - Azathioprine, hydroxychloroquine, cyclophosphamide, & 6-mercaptopurine have been added in some cases
- IPH may recur following lung transplantation

DIAGNOSTIC CHECKLIST

Consider

- IPH in patient with hemoptysis, anemia, & bilateral airspace disease of unknown etiology

SELECTED REFERENCES

1. Fishbein GA et al: Lung vasculitis and alveolar hemorrhage: pathology. Semin Respir Crit Care Med. 32(3):254-63, 2011
2. Pedersen FM et al: [Idiopathic pulmonary hemosiderosis.] Ugeskr Laeger. 158(7):902-4, 1996

GOODPASTURE SYNDROME

Key Facts

Terminology

- Anti-glomerular basement membrane (Anti-GBM) disease
- Glomerulonephritis & diffuse alveolar hemorrhage (DAH) caused by anti-GBM antibodies

Imaging

- Acute: Onset < 24 hours
  - Bilateral, often asymmetric opacities
  - Characteristic sparing of lung periphery
- Subacute
  - CT: Ground-glass opacities & consolidations with interlobular septal thickening
  - Pulmonary opacities tend to resolve within 2 weeks
- Recurrent/chronic: Pulmonary fibrosis, reticular opacities, & architectural distortion
- Pleural effusion rare

Top Differential Diagnoses

- Wegener granulomatosis
- Systemic lupus erythematosus vasculitis
- Microscopic polyangiitis
- Noncardiogenic pulmonary edema

Clinical Issues

- Symptoms/signs
  - Acute dyspnea, hemoptysis (80% of patients)
  - Renal & lung involvement in 60-80% of cases
- Bimodal distribution: Young men, older women

Diagnostic Checklist

- Consider Goodpasture syndrome in patient with renal disease & imaging findings of pulmonary hemorrhage
- Evolution of pulmonary opacities is important in diagnosis of pulmonary hemorrhage

*(**Left**) PA chest radiograph of a patient with Goodpasture syndrome and acute hemoptysis shows bilateral patchy airspace disease ➔ representing pulmonary hemorrhage. The distribution is central, with sparing of the lung bases and apices. Given this clinical history, absence of pleural effusions further supports pulmonary hemorrhage. (**Right**) Axial CECT of the same patient shows centrilobular ground-glass opacities and patchy nodular consolidations that are characteristic of acute pulmonary hemorrhage.*

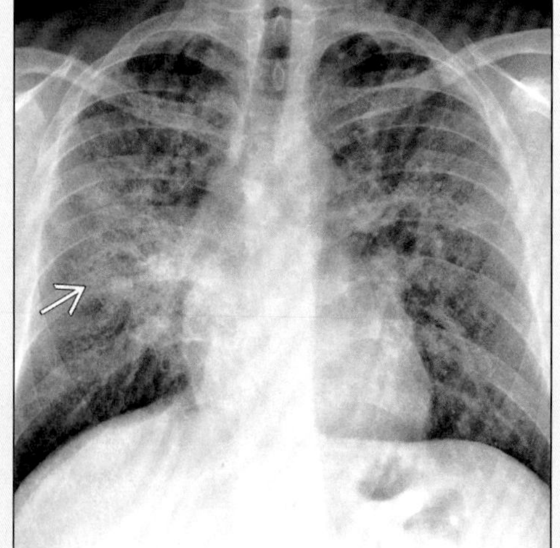

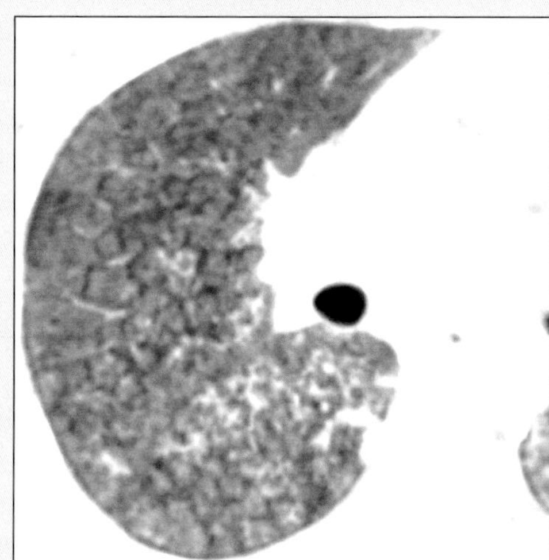

*(**Left**) Coronal CECT of the same patient shows patchy bilateral centrilobular ground-glass opacities with relative apical sparing. (**Right**) Coronal NECT of a patient with Goodpasture syndrome shows ground-glass opacities in the lower lobes with relative sparing of the left lung base near the costophrenic angle. Nearly 20% of patients with pulmonary hemorrhage lack hemoptysis, and these imaging findings may be the only diagnostic clue to the etiology of the pulmonary abnormalities.*

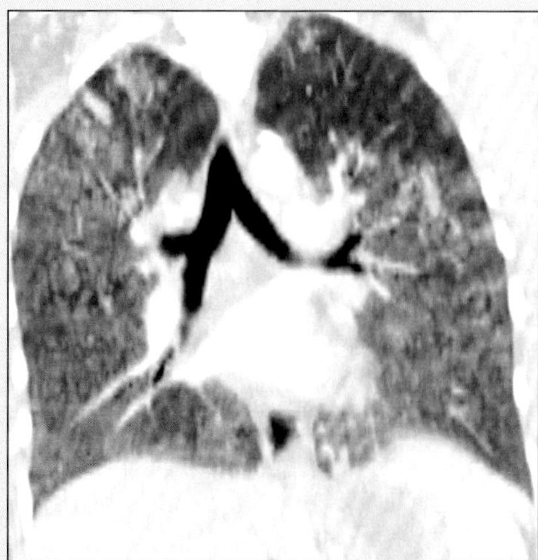

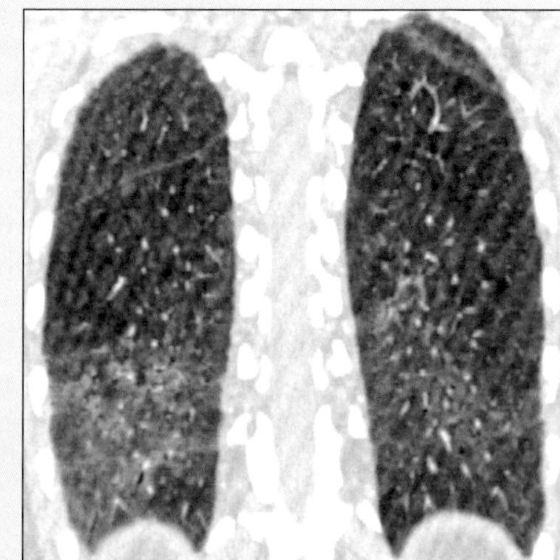

GOODPASTURE SYNDROME

TERMINOLOGY

Abbreviations

- **Anti-glomerular basement membrane (anti-GBM) disease**

Definitions

- **Goodpasture syndrome**: Described initially as combination glomerulonephritis & diffuse alveolar hemorrhage (DAH)
  - Caused by antibodies directed against glomerular basement membranes, cross-react with alveolar basement membranes
  - **Anti-GBM disease: Circulating antiglomerular basement membrane antibodies, glomerulonephritis & DAH**

IMAGING

General Features

- Best diagnostic clue
  - Acute, diffuse ground-glass opacities & consolidation in patient with hemoptysis & renal disease

Radiographic Findings

- **Radiographic findings vary depending on chronicity of hemorrhagic episodes**
  - **Acute: Onset < 24 hours**
    - Bilateral, often asymmetric opacities
    - Lung periphery & bases near costophrenic angles usually spared
      - Involvement of periphery or lung base should suggest another diagnosis
    - Unilateral involvement rare
  - **Subacute**
    - Opacities gradually decrease after single episode of hemorrhage
    - Pulmonary opacities resolve within 2 weeks
  - **Recurrent/chronic**
    - Architectural distortion from fibrosis
    - Reticular opacities in areas of prior hemorrhage
- **Pleural effusion rare**; should suggest another diagnosis or concurrent cardiac failure

CT Findings

- HRCT
  - **Acute**
    - Bilateral patchy ground-glass opacities & consolidations
    - Usually without interlobular septal thickening
    - Characteristic sparing of periphery, apices, & basilar lungs near costophrenic angles
  - **Subacute**
    - Ground-glass opacities & consolidations with interlobular septal thickening & intralobular reticulation
    - Near complete clearing of airspace opacities within 2 weeks of single episode
  - **Recurrent/chronic**
    - Pulmonary fibrosis, reticular opacities, & architectural distortion
    - Lobular sparing

MR Findings

- Role of MR in Goodpasture syndrome not defined
- Low signal in lungs secondary to paramagnetic properties of hemosiderin
  - Pulmonary edema & pneumonia demonstrate high signal intensity on T2WI
- Low signal intensity in reticuloendothelial system: Important clue for hemosiderosis

Imaging Recommendations

- Best imaging tool
  - CT to characterize distribution & extent of disease

DIFFERENTIAL DIAGNOSIS

Wegener Granulomatosis

- Systemic vasculitis, typically affects kidneys, upper & lower respiratory tracts
- Peripheral wedge-shaped consolidations &/or cavitary nodules
  - Less common: Acute diffuse bilateral consolidation, often seen early or in younger patients
  - DAH likely represents capillaritis form of Wegener
- c-ANCA positive in 85-98% of patients with active disease
- Systemic symptoms: Fever, weight loss, arthralgias, peripheral neuropathy

Systemic Lupus Erythematosus Vasculitis

- Immune complex-mediated microvasculitis
- Most common collagen vascular disease associated with DAH, although only 2% of patients with SLE develop DAH
  - May present with DAH, closely resembling anti-GBM disease or idiopathic pulmonary hemorrhage
  - Renal involvement in 60-90%
- Pleural effusion in 50% of cases

Microscopic Polyangiitis

- Necrotizing vasculitis involving small vessels (arterioles, venules, capillaries) & no immune deposits
- Involvement: Kidneys in > 95%, lung in about 50%
- Onset may be rapid with fever, myalgia, arthralgia & ear, nose, or throat symptoms
  - Extensive bilateral consolidations common; usually with lower lobe distribution
- > 80% with positive ANCA, usually p-ANCA

Noncardiogenic Pulmonary Edema

- Common: Acute onset of diffuse ground-glass opacities & consolidations
- Pleural effusion common
- Hemoptysis rare

Churg-Strauss Syndrome

- Multisystem disorder: Asthma/history of allergy, peripheral blood eosinophilia, & systemic vasculitis
  - Diagnosis based on clinical criteria
- Multifocal & evolving consolidations: 1 of 6 criteria
  - Consolidation not diffuse, tends to involve lung periphery

Pneumocystis jiroveci Pneumonia

- Cell-mediated immunodeficiency, especially AIDS
- Subacute onset of dyspnea, fever, & hypoxia
- Common: Perihilar or diffuse ground-glass opacities & consolidations of insidious onset
  - No renal involvement or hemoptysis

GOODPASTURE SYNDROME

Idiopathic Pulmonary Hemorrhage

- Diffuse pulmonary hemorrhage syndrome without identifiable cause
- Recurrent episodes of diffuse pulmonary hemorrhage, usually in young patients (< 10 years)
- Hemoptysis very common, may be quite severe
- No renal involvement; ANCAs & antibasement membrane antibodies absent

PATHOLOGY

General Features

- Etiology
  - Type II antibody reaction to glomerular basement membrane, also affects alveolar basement membrane
    - Combination of glomerulonephritis & pulmonary hemorrhage
  - Anti-GBM antibodies detected by serum radioimmunoassay in > 90%
    - Antibodies directed at type IV collagen alpha-3 chain
- Genetics
  - Anti-GBM disease reported in siblings & identical twins; supports genetic predisposition
    - *HLA-DR2* seen in majority of patients
- Associated abnormalities
  - 30% have positive serum c- or p-ANCA

Microscopic Features

- Renal biopsy demonstrates linear deposition of IgG along glomerular basement membranes by immunofluorescence
  - Renal biopsy is most common method to establish diagnosis
- Lung biopsy not common, but similar findings of linear IgG found along alveolar basement membranes
  - Distribution more patchy & more difficult to interpret than renal biopsy specimens
  - Intraalveolar hemorrhage & hemosiderin
  - Occasional neutrophilic capillaritis present, but extensive vasculitis not present

CLINICAL ISSUES

Presentation

- Most common signs/symptoms
  - **Acute shortness of breath, hemoptysis (80%)**
    - Anemia, pallor
  - Renal & lung involvement in 60-80%
    - Renal involvement alone in 20-40%
    - Lung involvement alone in < 10%
  - Pulmonary hemorrhage may precede renal disease by up to several months
- Other signs/symptoms
  - Hematuria, proteinuria, & elevated serum creatine
    - Glomerulonephritis is usually rapidly progressive
  - Renal failure
  - **History of recent viral illness common**

Demographics

- Age
  - **Bimodal distribution**
    - Most common: Young white males with lung & renal disease, usually > 15 years
    - Less common: Older women with predominant renal involvement
- Gender
  - M:F at least 2:1, but may be as high as 9:1 in younger patients
- Epidemiology
  - Rare, occurs in 0.5 people per million per year
  - Associated with influenza A & various inhalational exposures, such as hydrocarbons

Natural History & Prognosis

- Diagnosis made by enzyme-linked immunosorbent assay (ELISA) or radioimmunoassay for anti-GBM antibodies
- Recurrent episodes of pulmonary hemorrhage common
  - May lead to progressive pulmonary hypertension & fibrosis
  - Progressive renal insufficiency common
- Untreated Goodpasture syndrome often has fulminant course leading to death
- Early therapy results in remission of both renal & lung disease

Treatment

- Combination of corticosteroids & immunosuppressive therapy
  - Plasmapheresis removes circulating antibodies
  - Immunosuppression with corticosteroids & cytotoxic drugs
- End-stage renal failure may necessitate renal transplant

DIAGNOSTIC CHECKLIST

Consider

- **Goodpasture syndrome in patient with renal disease & imaging findings of pulmonary hemorrhage**

Image Interpretation Pearls

- Evolution of pulmonary opacities is important for diagnosis of pulmonary hemorrhage

SELECTED REFERENCES

1. Chung MP et al: Imaging of pulmonary vasculitis. Radiology. 255(2):322-41, 2010
2. Lara AR et al: Diffuse alveolar hemorrhage. Chest. 137(5):1164-71, 2010
3. Travis WD et al: Non-neoplastic disorders of the lower respiratory tract. AFIP Atlas of Nontumor Pathology, 1st ed. Washington, D.C.: 184-5, 2002
4. Primack SL et al: Diffuse pulmonary hemorrhage: clinical, pathologic, and imaging features. AJR Am J Roentgenol. 164(2):295-300, 1995

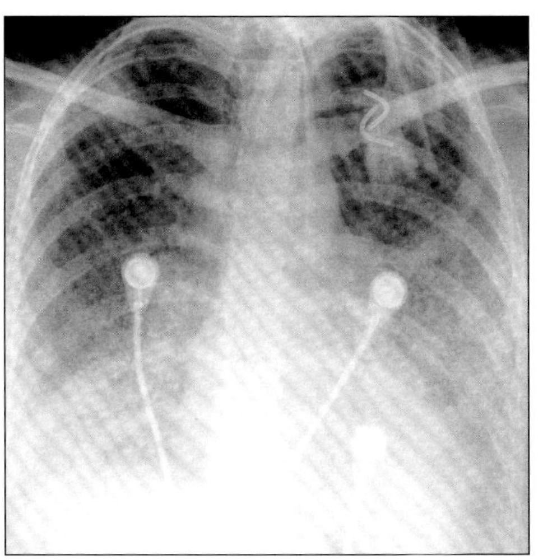

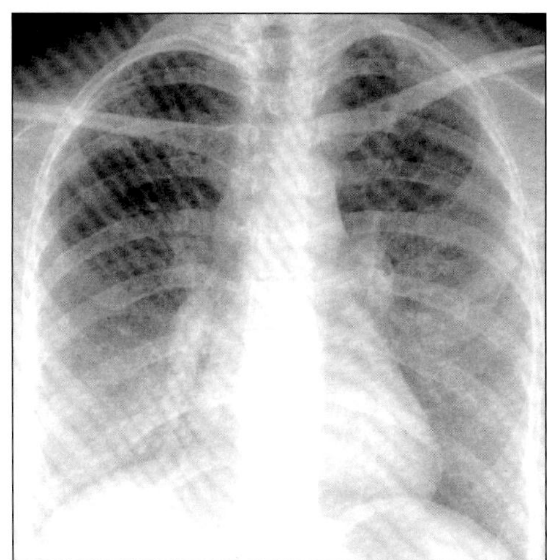

(Left) *AP chest radiograph of a patient with hemoptysis and Goodpasture syndrome shows patchy lower lobe opacities with relative sparing of the lung apices and absence of pleural effusions, which is consistent with acute pulmonary hemorrhage.* ***(Right)*** *PA chest radiograph of the same patient obtained 2 weeks later shows replacement of previous basilar opacities by fine reticular opacities. Subacute pulmonary hemorrhage is characterized by septal thickening and improving airspace disease.*

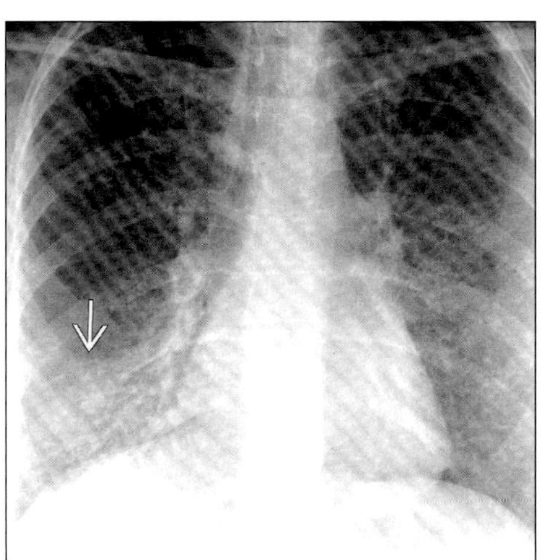

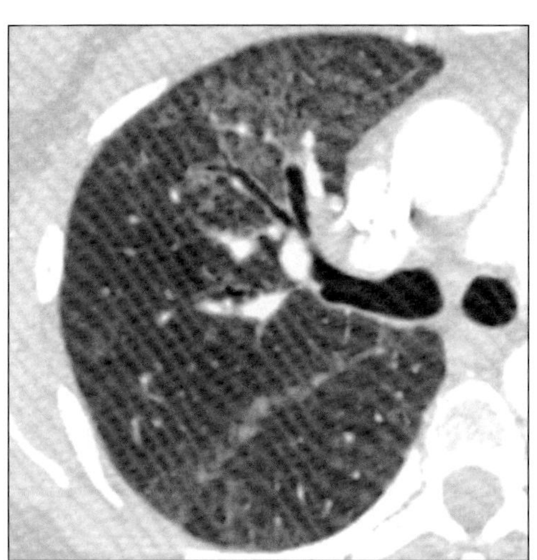

(Left) *PA chest radiograph of a patient with Goodpasture syndrome and cough shows patchy airspace disease ➔ in the right lower lung zone.* ***(Right)*** *Axial CECT of the same patient shows patchy ground-glass and reticular opacities, consistent with subacute pulmonary hemorrhage. Pulmonary hemorrhage in Goodpasture syndrome is usually bilateral, but can be predominantly unilateral, as in this case.*

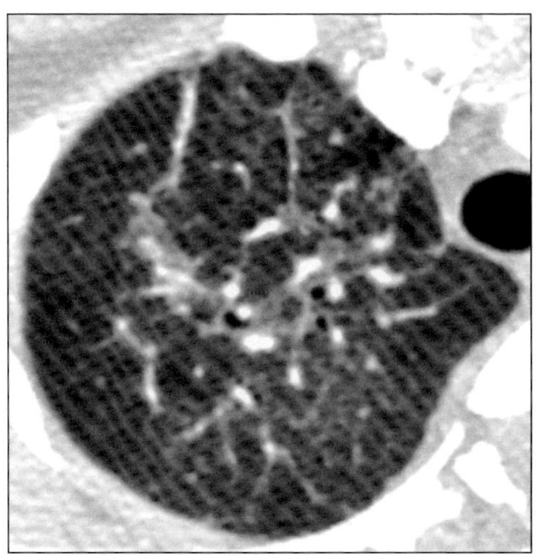

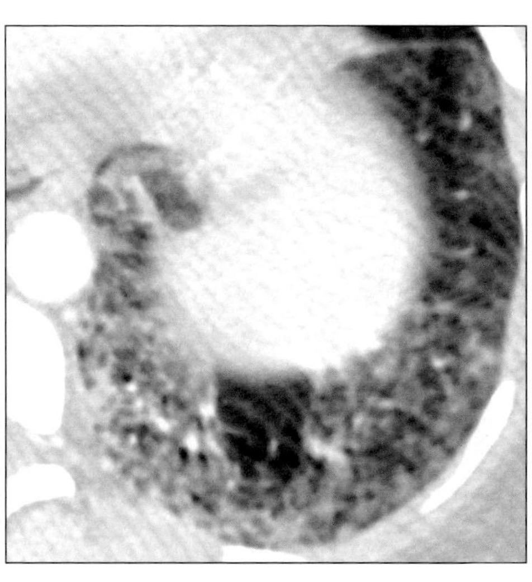

(Left) *Axial CECT of a patient with longstanding Goodpasture syndrome shows reticular and linear opacities in the right apex with associated traction bronchiectasis. Fibrosis is a complication of recurrent or chronic pulmonary hemorrhage.* ***(Right)*** *Axial CECT of a patient with Goodpasture syndrome shows basilar ground-glass opacities with lobular sparing, which can be present in recurrent or chronic pulmonary hemorrhage.*

PULMONARY WEGENER GRANULOMATOSIS

Key Facts

Terminology
- Wegener granulomatosis (WG)
- Multisystem necrotizing granulomatous vasculitis of small to medium-sized vessels

Imaging
- Radiography
  - Multiple lung nodules/masses ± cavitation
  - Multifocal consolidation, may represent hemorrhage
- CT
  - Ground-glass opacity from hemorrhage
  - Multifocal lung nodules/masses/consolidations
  - Cavitation more common in larger nodules
  - Air-fluid levels suggest secondary infection
  - Halo sign, reverse halo sign, feeding vessel sign
  - Pulmonary fibrosis may occur
  - Pleural effusion

Top Differential Diagnoses
- Pulmonary metastases
- Septic emboli
- Lung abscess

Clinical Issues
- Symptoms/signs: Cough, hemoptysis, dyspnea
- Laboratory: Cytoplasmic antineutrophil cytoplasmic antibody (c-ANCA)
- Diagnosis: Nasal, paranasal sinus, lung, or renal biopsy
- Treatment: Corticosteroids, cyclophosphamide
  - Remission in approximately 90% with treatment

Diagnostic Checklist
- Consider Wegener granulomatosis in patients with multiple cavitary lung nodules or masses & in those presenting with pulmonary hemorrhage

*(**Left**) AP chest radiograph of a patient with Wegener granulomatosis shows multiple bilateral pulmonary nodules ➡. The largest nodule in the right mid lung zone exhibits central lucency. (**Right**) Axial NECT of the same patient shows multifocal nodular lesions with central ground-glass opacity and a rim of peripheral consolidation ➡, the reverse halo sign, consistent with an organizing pneumonia-type reaction in the peripheral aspects of areas of pulmonary hemorrhage.*

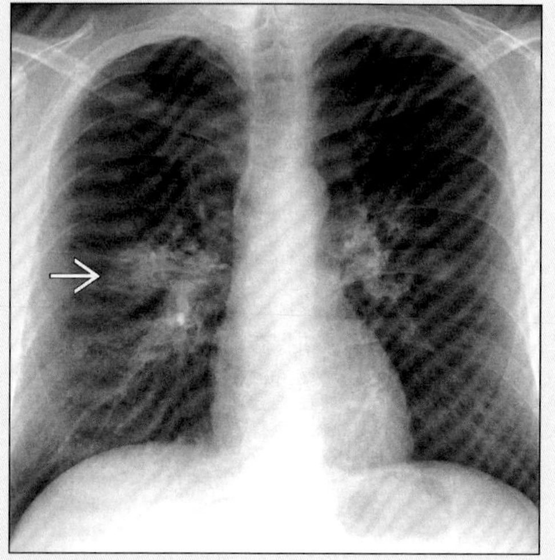

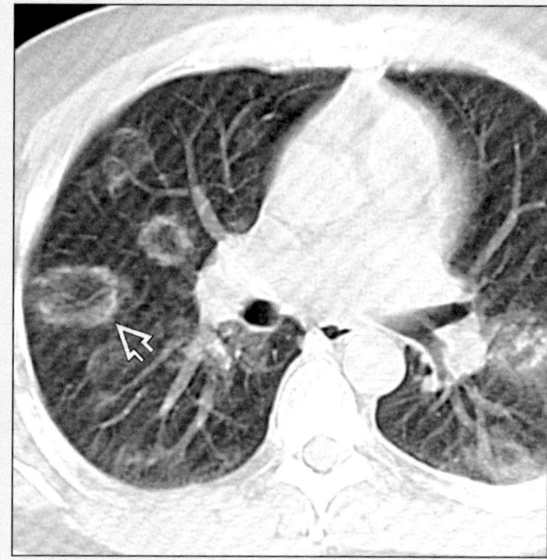

*(**Left**) PA chest radiograph of a 30-year-old man with Wegener granulomatosis shows 2 cavitary right lower lobe masses with air-fluid levels ➡ and an ill-defined left perihilar lung nodule ➡. (**Right**) Composite image with axial (left) and coronal (right) CECT of the same patient shows 2 right lower lobe cavitary masses with nodular walls and surrounding ground-glass opacity ➡, consistent with the CT halo sign and characteristic of WG. Visualization of air-fluid levels suggests superimposed infection.*

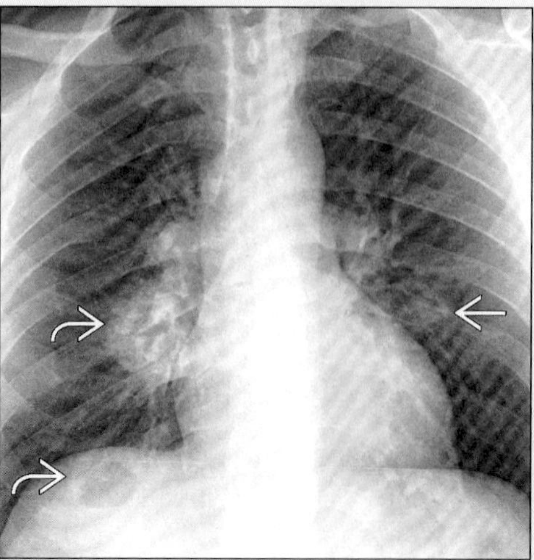

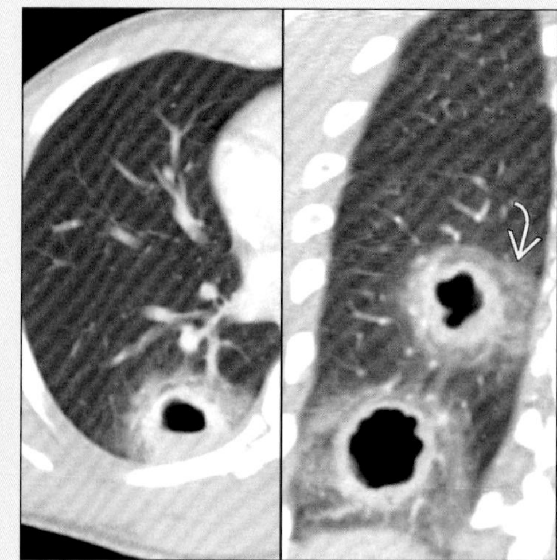

PULMONARY WEGENER GRANULOMATOSIS

TERMINOLOGY

Abbreviations

- **Wegener granulomatosis (WG)**

Synonyms

- **Granulomatosis with polyangiitis (GPA)**

Definitions

- Multisystem necrotizing granulomatous vasculitis of small to medium-sized blood vessels

IMAGING

General Features

- Best diagnostic clue
  - Multiple cavitary lung nodules or masses
- Location
  - Bilateral
  - No zonal predilection, but apices tend to be spared
- Size
  - Range: Few mm-10 cm; most lesions are 2-4 cm
- Morphology
  - Nodules & masses typically well circumscribed
    - Irregular borders suggest positive response to treatment

Radiographic Findings

- Radiography
  - **Radiographs may be normal** (20%)
  - **Multiple nodules or masses**
    - Most common abnormality
    - Present in 40-70% of patients
    - **Cavitation** more common in larger nodules
      - Present in up to 50% of patients
      - Occurs in 25% of nodules > 2 cm
      - Walls may be thin or thick & nodular
      - Intracavitary air-fluid levels suggest secondary infection
  - **Airspace opacities**
    - Reflect pulmonary hemorrhage, infarction, or organizing pneumonia
    - Wedge-shaped consolidation abutting pleura
    - Central necrosis may be present
    - Often initially characterized as pneumonia, does not resolve with treatment
    - May evolve into cavitary lesions
  - Less common manifestations
    - Atelectasis
    - Reticular opacities
- Radiographs used to monitor response to treatment
  - Findings suggestive of relapse/recurrence
    - Increase in size &/or number of parenchymal findings
  - Findings suggestive of favorable response/improvement
    - Decrease in nodule size
    - Increased wall thickness of cavitary lesions
    - Progression of lesion margin irregularity

CT Findings

- **Pulmonary nodules or masses**
  - Usually multiple
  - Well circumscribed
  - **Cavitation** more common in larger nodules
- **Ground-glass opacity**
  - **Diffuse alveolar hemorrhage**
    - Occurs in approximately 10%
    - Diffuse with subpleural sparing
    - Interlobular septal thickening
      - Lymphatic congestion
      - Hemosiderin-laden macrophages
  - Mosaic perfusion
    - Arteriolar involvement
- **Halo sign**
  - Ground-glass opacity surrounding nodules or consolidations
    - Reflects adjacent alveolar hemorrhage
- **Reverse halo sign**
  - Consolidation rim surrounding central ground-glass opacity
    - Reflects organizing pneumonia-type reaction in peripheral aspect of pulmonary hemorrhage
- **Feeding vessel sign**
  - Pulmonary vessel coursing directly into pulmonary nodule
  - Described in 88% of cases in 1 series
- **Tree-in-bud opacities**
  - Arteriolar involvement
- **Pulmonary fibrosis**
  - Subpleural reticular opacities & honeycomb lung
    - Peripheral & lower lung zone distribution
  - Mimics idiopathic pulmonary fibrosis
- Other pulmonary abnormalities
  - Parenchymal bands
  - Interlobular septal thickening
  - Bronchial wall thickening
- Pleural abnormalities
  - Pleural effusion is most common
  - Pleural thickening, empyema, & pneumothorax rare
- Mediastinal lymphadenopathy
  - Occurs in up to 15% of cases
  - Always concomitant with pulmonary abnormalities

Nuclear Medicine Findings

- Ga-67 scintigraphy
  - Lesions are typically gallium-avid
  - May be used to monitor disease activity

DIFFERENTIAL DIAGNOSIS

Pulmonary Metastases

- Well-formed pulmonary nodules or masses
- Hemorrhagic metastases may exhibit irregular margins & surrounding ground-glass opacity
  - Renal cell carcinoma, melanoma, & choriocarcinoma
- Squamous cell carcinomas & sarcomas may cavitate

Septic Emboli

- Poorly defined pulmonary nodules or masses
- Varying degrees of cavitation

Lung Abscess

- Cavitary mass most common finding
- Air-fluid levels may be present
- Consolidation or ground-glass opacity may be present in adjacent lung parenchyma

PULMONARY WEGENER GRANULOMATOSIS

PATHOLOGY

General Features

- Etiology
  - Autoimmune syndrome of unknown etiology
  - Lung most commonly affected (94%)
    - Paranasal sinuses (91%)
    - Kidneys (85%)

Staging, Grading, & Classification

- Classical & limited types have been described
- **Classical**
  - Involvement of upper & lower respiratory tract & kidneys
  - Small vessel vasculitis
- **Limited**
  - Confined to lung
  - Upper airway not involved
  - No evidence of systemic vasculitis or glomerulonephritis

Gross Pathologic & Surgical Features

- Gray-white, solid or cavitary nodules
  - May coalesce as large areas of brown-red necrosis
  - Adjacent discolored areas of consolidation or hemorrhage
- Isolated parenchymal involvement may be seen
  - Up to 25% of cases
  - Reddish pulmonary hemorrhage
  - Tan fibrosis
  - Yellow consolidation
    - Endogenous lipoid pneumonia

Microscopic Features

- 3 major histologic features
  - Vasculitis
  - Necrosis
  - Granulomatous inflammation
    - Accompanying mixed cellular infiltrate composed of neutrophils, lymphocytes, plasma cells, histiocytes, & eosinophils
- Interpretation may be complicated by interstitial fibrosis or opportunistic infection

CLINICAL ISSUES

Presentation

- Most common signs/symptoms
  - **Classical**
    - Triad of pulmonary disease, febrile sinusitis, & glomerulonephritis
  - Most common symptoms related to upper airway involvement
    - Rhinitis, sinusitis
    - Otitis media
  - Variable onset of symptoms related to bronchopulmonary involvement
    - Cough, fever, dyspnea, hemoptysis, & chest pain
- Other signs/symptoms
  - Cardiac involvement
    - Coronary vasculitis, pancarditis, & valvular lesions
    - Acute pericarditis, dilated cardiomyopathy, acute valvular insufficiency with pulmonary edema, & cardiac arrest secondary to ventricular arrhythmias
- Laboratory findings
  - Cytoplasmic antineutrophil cytoplasmic antibody (c-ANCA)
    - Detected by indirect immunofluorescence
    - Suggestive of diagnosis, but not singularly sufficient
    - Levels of c-ANCA correlate with disease activity
    - Sensitivity
      - Active generalized WG: 96%
      - Active localized disease: 67%
    - Specificity: 99%

Demographics

- Age
  - Classical
    - Peak incidence: 4th & 5th decades
- Gender
  - Classical: M > F
  - Limited: F > M
- Epidemiology
  - Affects 3 per 100,000 in USA

Diagnosis

- Nasal, paranasal sinus, lung, or renal biopsy for diagnosis

Treatment

- Immunosuppressive drugs
  - Systemic corticosteroids & cyclophosphamide
- Complications of therapy: Pneumonia, sepsis, hemorrhagic cystitis

Natural History & Prognosis

- Nodules/masses increase in size & number with disease progression
- Remission rate approximately 90% with treatment
- Limited WG carries more favorable prognosis
- Mean 5-year survival rate: 90-95%
  - Renal failure most common cause of death in untreated patients

DIAGNOSTIC CHECKLIST

Consider

- Wegener granulomatosis in patients with multiple cavitary lung nodules or masses

Image Interpretation Pearls

- Pulmonary hemorrhage may be initial manifestation of Wegener granulomatosis

SELECTED REFERENCES

1. Castañer E et al: When to suspect pulmonary vasculitis: radiologic and clinical clues. Radiographics. 30(1):33-53, 2010
2. Ananthakrishnan L et al: Wegener's granulomatosis in the chest: high-resolution CT findings. AJR Am J Roentgenol. 192(3):676-82, 2009
3. Sheehan RE et al: Computed tomography features of the thoracic manifestations of Wegener granulomatosis. J Thorac Imaging. 18(1):34-41, 2003

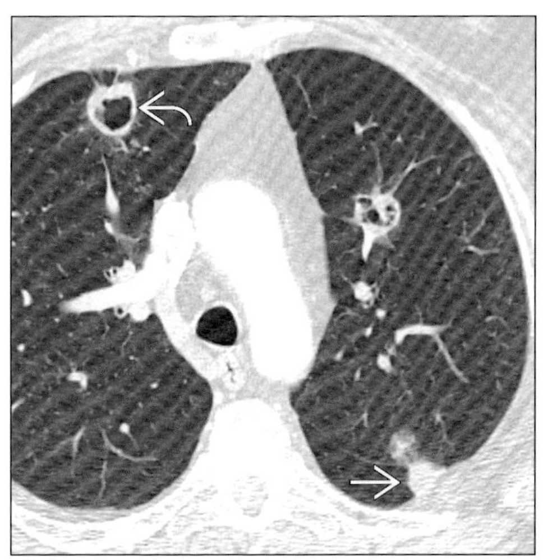

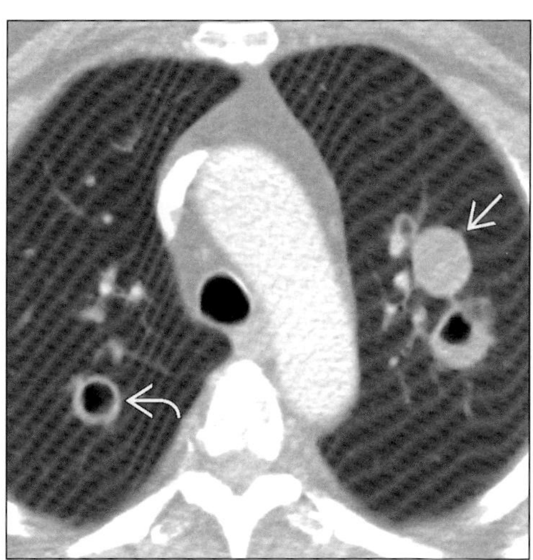

*(**Left**) Axial CECT of a 58-year-old man with WG shows multifocal bilateral lung nodules, some with intrinsic cavitation and nodular cavity walls ➲, and a wedge-shaped nodular lesion ➡ abutting the pleura, suggestive of an infarct. (**Right**) Axial CECT of a patient with Wegener granulomatosis shows multiple pulmonary nodules, 2 of which are cavitary ➲ and 1 of which is solid ➡. The most common imaging feature of Wegener granulomatosis is multiple cavitary nodules or masses.*

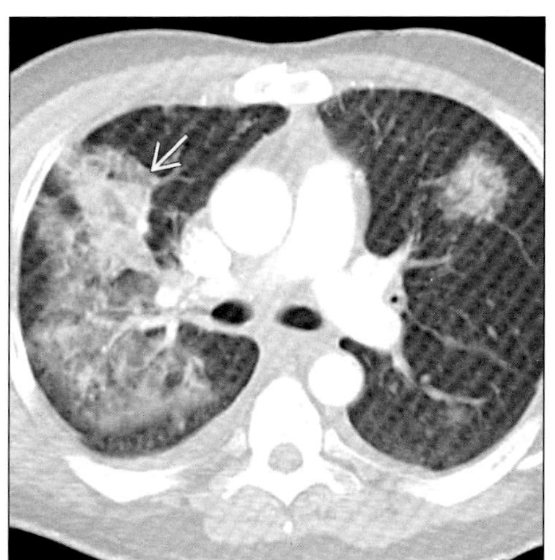

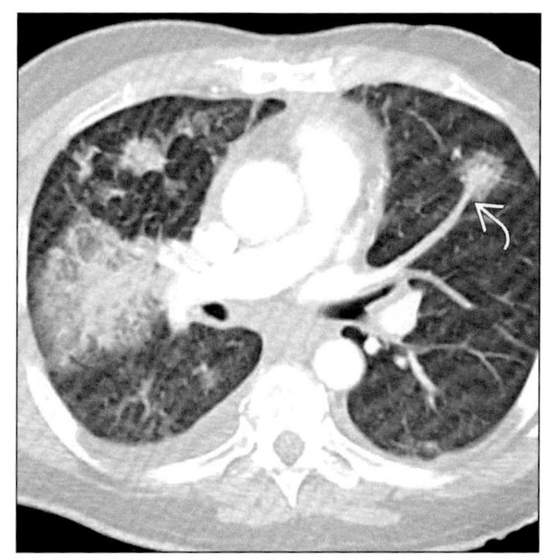

*(**Left**) Axial CECT of a patient with WG shows a right upper lobe consolidation ➡ with surrounding ground-glass opacity and a left upper lobe nodule. (**Right**) Axial CECT of the same patient shows a right perihilar consolidation with peripheral ground-glass opacity, a small right pleural effusion, and bilateral lung nodules. One of the nodules exhibits the feeding vessel sign ➲ described in angiocentric lesions, including pulmonary vasculitis. Ground-glass opacity likely relates to pulmonary hemorrhage.*

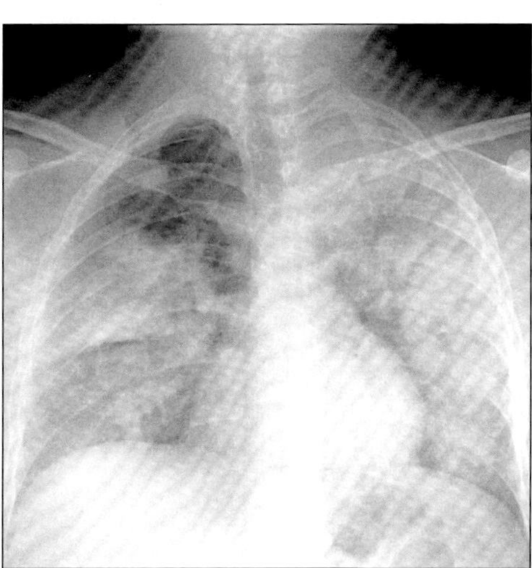

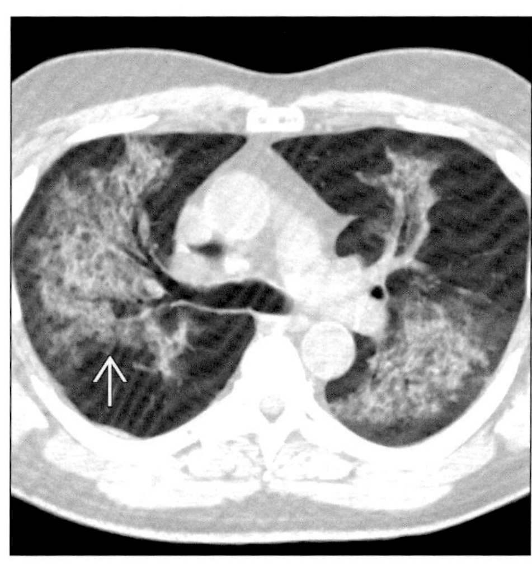

*(**Left**) AP chest radiograph of a patient with WG who presented with hemoptysis demonstrates extensive bilateral consolidations, consistent with diffuse alveolar hemorrhage. (**Right**) Axial NECT of a patient with Wegener granulomatosis demonstrates bilateral central heterogeneous consolidations with surrounding ground-glass opacity ➡ and characteristic subpleural sparing secondary to diffuse alveolar hemorrhage. Alveolar hemorrhage may be the presenting imaging manifestation of WG.*

CHURG-STRAUSS SYNDROME

Key Facts

Terminology

- Synonyms: Allergic granulomatosis, allergic granulomatous angiitis

Imaging

- Radiography
  - Peripheral, transient consolidation
  - Mimics eosinophilic pneumonia
- CT/HRCT
  - Peripheral consolidations & ground-glass opacities, often transient or migratory
  - Interlobular septal thickening
  - Pulmonary nodules & masses are less common
  - Small pleural effusions
  - Bronchial wall thickening/dilatation, air-trapping
- Cardiac CTA
  - Cardiomegaly
  - Regional hypo- or akinesis; arteritis

Top Differential Diagnoses

- Eosinophilic pneumonia
- Allergic bronchopulmonary aspergillosis
- Bacterial pneumonia
- Wegener granulomatosis
- Cryptogenic organizing pneumonia

Pathology

- Small vessel vasculitis

Clinical Issues

- Affected patients mostly middle-aged at diagnosis
- 5-year survival 60-80%; mortality typically from cardiac involvement

Diagnostic Checklist

- Consider Churg-Strauss in patient with asthma, transient consolidations, & positive p-ANCA

*(**Left**) Axial HRCT of a patient with Churg-Strauss syndrome who presented with asthma shows asymmetric bilateral ground-glass opacities ➡ with superimposed interlobular septal thickening. The patient met diagnostic criteria for Churg-Strauss syndrome. (**Right**) Coronal NECT of the same patient shows peripheral and upper lung predominant ground-glass opacities ➡, interlobular septal thickening, and mild bronchial wall thickening ➡, suggestive of asthma-related large airways disease.*

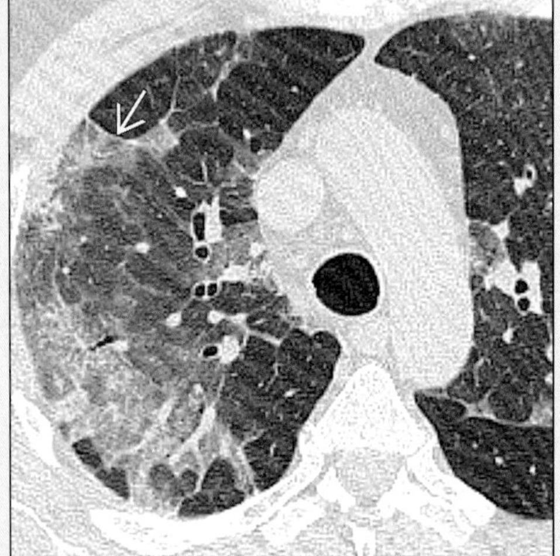

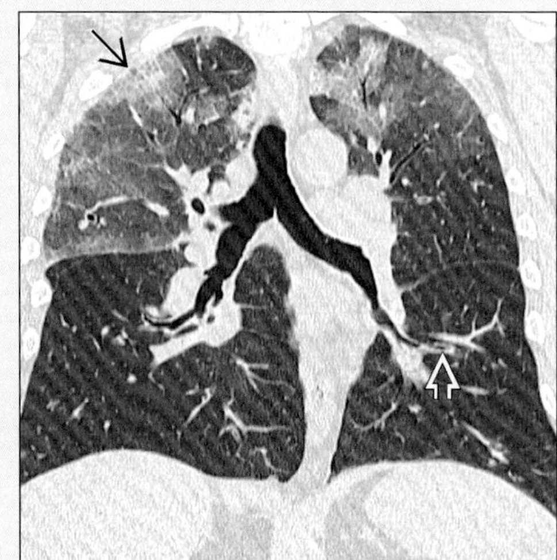

*(**Left**) Axial HRCT of a patient with Churg-Strauss syndrome shows ground-glass opacities and consolidations ➡ in the lung periphery. Associated interlobular septal thickening ➡ may be related to eosinophilic infiltration or left-sided heart failure due to cardiac involvement. (**Right**) Axial CECT of a patient with Churg-Strauss syndrome shows asymmetric bilateral patchy ground-glass opacities with more confluent involvement of the left lung.*

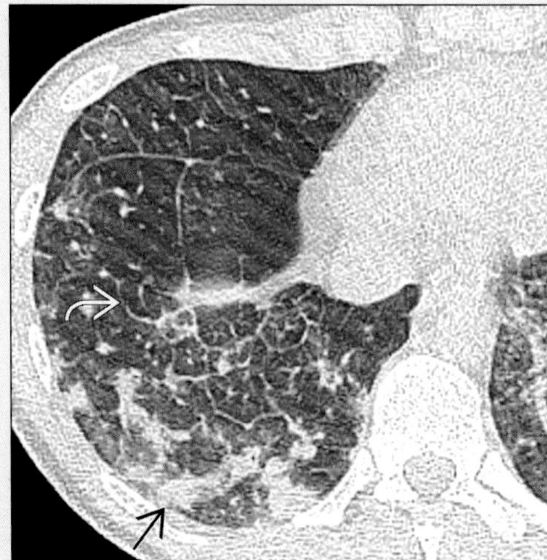

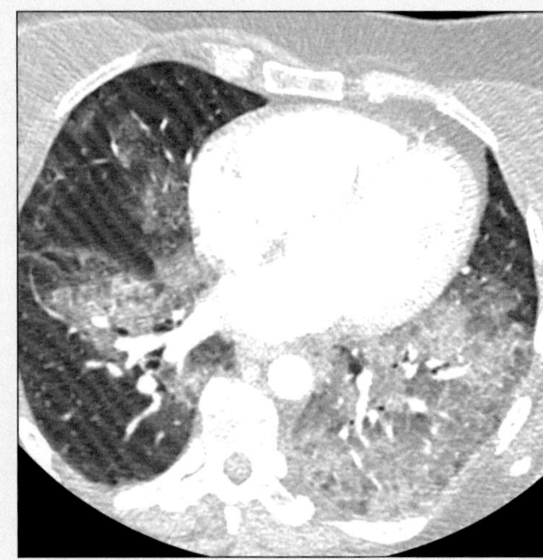

CHURG-STRAUSS SYNDROME

TERMINOLOGY

Synonyms

- **Allergic granulomatosis, allergic granulomatous angiitis**

IMAGING

General Features

- Best diagnostic clue
  - Transient, peripheral consolidation in patient with asthma & positive p-ANCA

Radiographic Findings

- Radiography
  - Peripheral, transient consolidations
  - Mimics eosinophilic pneumonia

CT Findings

- HRCT
  - Peripheral predominant consolidations & ground-glass opacities, often transient or migratory; no zonal predilection
  - Interlobular septal thickening either from heart failure or eosinophilic infiltration
  - Pulmonary nodules & masses are less common; cavitation extremely rare as compared to Wegener granulomatosis
  - Bronchial wall thickening/dilatation, air-trapping
  - Small pleural effusions
- Cardiac gated CTA
  - Cardiomegaly
  - Regional hypo- or akinesis; arteritis

MR Findings

- Delayed Enhancement
  - Abnormal focal delayed enhancement either representing scar or active inflammation
  - Myocardial infarct: Subendocardial to transmural delayed enhancement in coronary artery territory

DIFFERENTIAL DIAGNOSIS

Eosinophilic Pneumonia

- Simple: Fleeting, peripheral pulmonary opacities, self-limited, rapidly changing (days)
- Chronic: Fleeting peripheral consolidations & ground-glass opacities, evolution over weeks, centripetal resolution

Allergic Bronchopulmonary Aspergillosis

- Central & upper lung predominant bronchiectasis & mucous plugging in patient with asthma
- Migratory pulmonary opacities may be seen before development of bronchiectasis

Bacterial Pneumonia

- Focal or multifocal consolidation
- Cough, fever, chills, ↑ white blood cell count

Wegener Granulomatosis

- Positive c-ANCA
- Cavitary nodules & masses > consolidations as compared to Churg-Strauss syndrome

Cryptogenic Organizing Pneumonia

- May have identical imaging appearance
- Reversed halo sign: Central ground-glass opacities with surrounding rim of consolidation

PATHOLOGY

General Features

- Etiology
  - Small vessel vasculitis
  - Majority exhibit positive p-ANCA
- Associated abnormalities
  - Typically **asthma**; marked **peripheral eosinophilia**

Microscopic Features

- 3 key findings, but unusual to find all 3 (20%)
  - Vasculitis, necrotizing extravascular granulomas, tissue eosinophilia

CLINICAL ISSUES

Presentation

- Most common signs/symptoms
  - **Diagnostic criteria** proposed by American College or Rheumatology (4 of 6 required)
    - Asthma
    - Blood eosinophilia > 10%
    - Poly- or mononeuropathy
    - Migratory or fleeting pulmonary opacities
    - Paranasal sinus disease
    - Extravascular eosinophilia on biopsy
  - Cardiac involvement common (up to 1/2 of patients): Myocardial infarction (coronary arteritis), myocarditis, heart failure, pericarditis
  - Skin, renal, & gastrointestinal involvement

Demographics

- Age
  - Mostly middle-aged patients
- Gender
  - Men slightly more commonly affected than women
- Epidemiology
  - Rare, 1-3 per million people

Natural History & Prognosis

- 5-year survival of 60-80%
- Cardiac involvement leading cause of mortality

DIAGNOSTIC CHECKLIST

Consider

- Churg-Strauss syndrome in patient with asthma, transient, peripheral consolidation, & positive p-ANCA

SELECTED REFERENCES

1. Castaner E et al: When to suspect pulmonary vasculitis: radiologic and clinical clues. Radiographics. 30(1):33-53, 2010
2. Chung MP et al: Imaging of pulmonary vasculitis. Radiology. 255(2):322-41, 2010

BEHÇET SYNDROME

Key Facts

Terminology

- Chronic systemic inflammatory disease characterized by oral & genital mucosal ulcers & uveitis
- Thoracic disease includes
  - Vascular aneurysms ± luminal thrombus
  - Lung & airway disease

Imaging

- Radiography
  - Aneurysms of thoracic aorta & pulmonary artery
  - Pleural effusion
- CT
  - Pulmonary artery aneurysm ± thrombus
  - Subpleural, wedge-shaped or ill-defined opacities
  - Pleural nodules & effusions
- CT for optimal evaluation of extent of disease & pulmonary involvement
- MR for optimal evaluation of intracardiac thrombus

Top Differential Diagnoses

- Pulmonary vasculitis
- Sarcoidosis
- Tuberculosis
- Hughes-Stovin syndrome

Clinical Issues

- Symptoms/signs
  - Oral & genital ulcers
  - Ocular lesions, skin lesions
- Most prevalent in Mediterranean region, especially Turkey
- Mean age: 20-30 years
- Males 2-5x more commonly affected

Diagnostic Checklist

- Consider Behçet syndrome in patients with pulmonary artery aneurysms, particularly young men of Mediterranean ethnicity

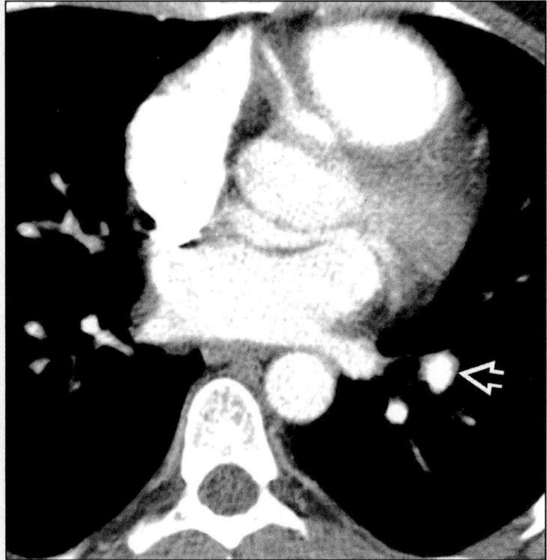

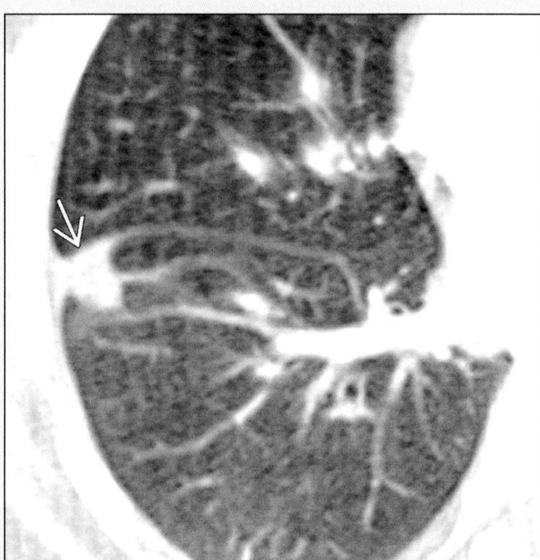

(Left) *Axial CECT of a 33-year-old man with Behçet syndrome shows focal dilatation of a left lower lobe pulmonary artery ➡. Behçet syndrome is the most common cause of pulmonary artery aneurysm. Behçet syndrome typically affects young males of Mediterranean ethnicity.* ***(Right)*** *Axial CECT of the same patient shows a peripheral wedge-shaped opacity ➡ in the right lower lobe, consistent with a pulmonary infarct.*

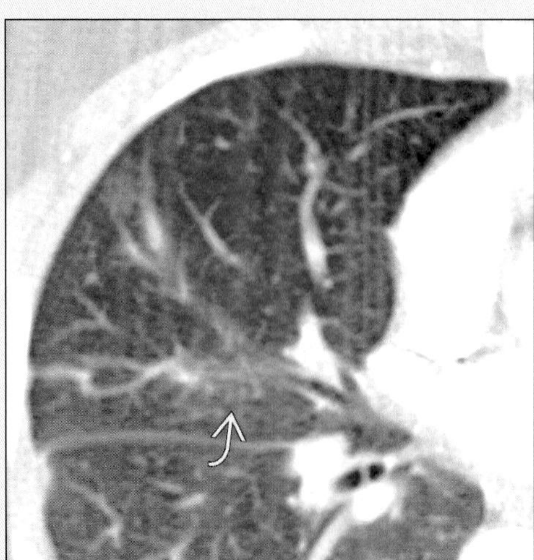

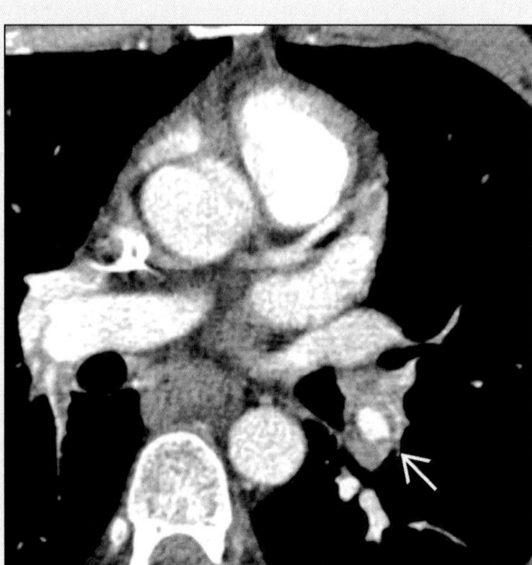

(Left) *Axial CECT of the same patient shows patchy middle lobe ground-glass opacities ➡ in a peribronchovascular distribution secondary to pulmonary hemorrhage.* ***(Right)*** *Axial CECT of a 29-year-old man with Behçet syndrome shows an aneurysm ➡ of the left interlobar pulmonary artery. Peripheral low attenuation in this aneurysm represents endoluminal thrombus. Pulmonary artery thrombus in these aneurysms is thought to occur in situ rather than as the result of thromboembolic disease.*

BEHÇET SYNDROME

TERMINOLOGY

Synonyms

- Behçet disease, Silk Road disease

Definitions

- Chronic systemic inflammatory disease characterized by oral & genital mucosal ulcers & uveitis
  - Thoracic disease includes
    - Vascular aneurysms ± luminal thrombus
    - Lung & airway disease
    - Pleural nodules & effusions
    - Mediastinal lymphadenopathy, fibrosis

IMAGING

Radiographic Findings

- Aneurysmal dilation of thoracic aorta, pulmonary artery
  - May cause mediastinal widening, hilar enlargement
- Pleural effusion
- Mediastinal widening/lymphadenopathy

CT Findings

- Thoracic vasculature
  - Venous thrombosis (SVC, mediastinal veins), thrombophlebitis
  - Pulmonary artery aneurysm ± thrombus
    - **Behçet syndrome is most common cause of pulmonary artery aneurysms**
  - Thoracic aortic aneurysm or vessel wall thickening
- Lungs
  - Subpleural, wedge-shaped or ill-defined opacities
  - Ground-glass opacities & interlobular septal thickening from pulmonary hemorrhage
  - Consolidation from organizing pneumonia or eosinophilic pneumonia
  - Tracheobronchial ulcers/stenosis
  - Mosaic attenuation/perfusion
  - Expiratory air-trapping, small airways disease
  - Pulmonary fibrosis in chronic disease
- Pleural nodules & effusions
- Mediastinum
  - Lymphadenopathy
  - Focal or diffuse fibrosing mediastinitis
  - Pericardial effusion
  - Intracardiac thrombus

MR Findings

- MR for optimal evaluation of suspected intracardiac thrombus
- May be used for surveillance of known aneurysms

Imaging Recommendations

- Best imaging tool
  - CT for optimal evaluation of extent of disease & pulmonary involvement

DIFFERENTIAL DIAGNOSIS

Pulmonary Vasculitis

- RA & SLE associated with organizing pneumonia
- Pulmonary hemorrhage: Microscopic polyangiitis, Wegener granulomatosis, Goodpasture syndrome

Sarcoidosis

- Subpleural opacities may be similar
- Calcified lymph nodes may help differentiate

Tuberculosis

- "Rasmussen" pulmonary artery aneurysms are rare
- Cavitary lesions & apical distribution characteristic

Hughes-Stovin Syndrome

- Similar radiologic & histopathologic findings
- No oral or genital ulcers

PATHOLOGY

General Features

- Genetics
  - Predisposition in patients with *HLA-B51*
- Associated abnormalities
  - Superior vena cava syndrome

Microscopic Features

- Vasculitis & perivascular infiltration, inflammation of vasa vasorum, destruction of elastic fibers

CLINICAL ISSUES

Presentation

- Most common signs/symptoms
  - Oral & genital ulcers
  - Ocular lesions including uveitis, retinal vasculitis
  - Skin lesions: Folliculitis, erythema nodosum
- Other signs/symptoms
  - Hemoptysis

Demographics

- Age
  - Mean age: 20-30 years
- Gender
  - Males 2-5x more commonly affected
- Ethnicity
  - Most prevalent in Mediterranean region, especially in Turkey
- Epidemiology
  - Vascular involvement discovered in 25% of patients
    - Most common cause of mortality

Natural History & Prognosis

- Pulmonary artery aneurysm carries poor prognosis

Treatment

- Corticosteroids, cyclophosphamide

DIAGNOSTIC CHECKLIST

Consider

- Behçet syndrome in patients with pulmonary artery aneurysms, particularly young men of Mediterranean ethnicity

SELECTED REFERENCES

1. Ceylan N et al: Pulmonary and vascular manifestations of Behcet disease: imaging findings. AJR Am J Roentgenol. 194(2):W158-64, 2010

Key Facts

Terminology
- Noncaseating granulomatous disease characterized by extensive areas of necrosis & vasculitis

Imaging
- Radiography
  - Multiple, bilateral, well-defined pulmonary nodules & masses with cavitation
  - Hilar lymphadenopathy variable
- CT
  - Subpleural & peribronchovascular nodules
  - Lung nodules often cavitary

Top Differential Diagnoses
- Wegener granulomatosis
- Pulmonary metastases
- Infection
- Churg-Strauss syndrome

Pathology
- Noncaseating granulomas similar to sarcoidosis
- Pulmonary vasculitis, often with vascular occlusion
- Widespread coagulative necrosis

Clinical Issues
- Symptoms/signs
  - Pleuritic chest pain, dyspnea
  - Cough, hemoptysis
  - Fever, weight loss, fatigue
- M:F = 1:2.2
- Clinical course typically benign

Diagnostic Checklist
- Consider necrotizing sarcoid granulomatosis in patients with multiple cavitary nodules in perilymphatic distribution
- Infection & metastatic disease must be excluded

*(**Left**) PA chest radiograph of a 53-year-old man with necrotizing sarcoid granulomatosis shows multifocal perihilar nodular opacities. (**Right**) Axial NECT of the same patient shows a cavitary mass in the right lower lobe ➔ and peribronchovascular nodular opacities ➔ in the left lower lobe. Associated lower lobe ground-glass opacity may be secondary to surrounding pulmonary hemorrhage.*

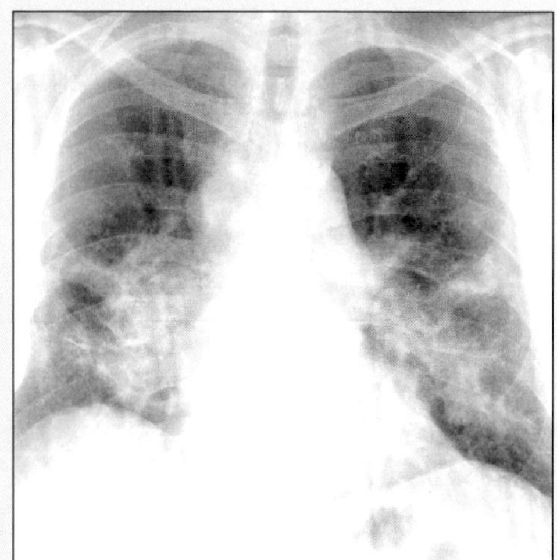

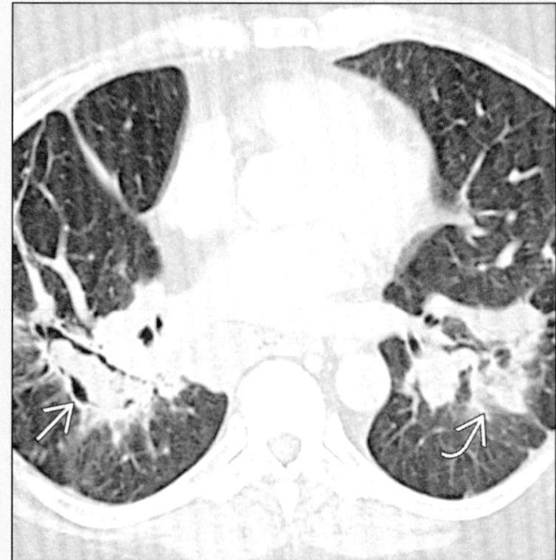

*(**Left**) Coronal NECT of the same patient shows the right lower lobe cavitary mass as well as right lateral pleural thickening and irregularity ➔. Pleural nodules, fibrosis, and adhesions may be present in necrotizing sarcoid granulomatosis. (**Right**) Axial CECT of a 64-year-old man with necrotizing sarcoid granulomatosis shows a cavitary mass in the right upper lobe ➔ located along the central bronchovascular bundles and subpleural nodular opacities ➔.*

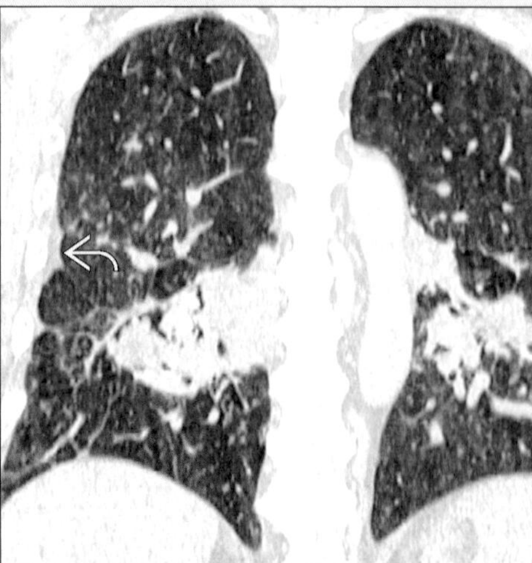

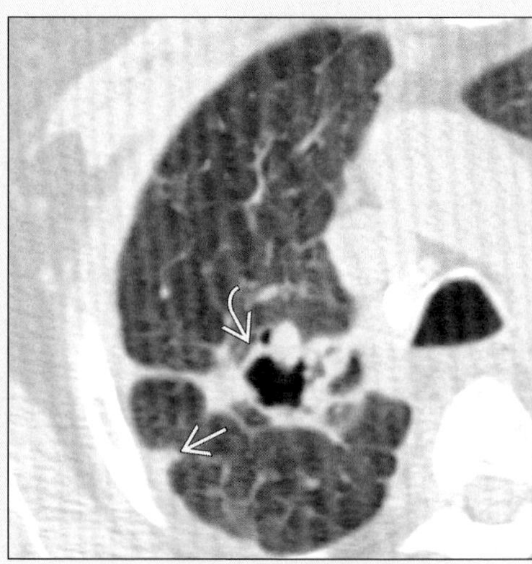

NECROTIZING SARCOID GRANULOMATOSIS

TERMINOLOGY

Definitions

- Noncaseating granulomatous disease characterized by extensive areas of lung necrosis & vasculitis

IMAGING

General Features

- Best diagnostic clue
  - Multiple, bilateral pulmonary nodules
    - Subpleural & peribronchovascular distribution

Radiographic Findings

- Multiple, bilateral, well-defined pulmonary nodules & masses with cavitation
- Hilar lymphadenopathy variable
- Pleural effusion uncommon

CT Findings

- Subpleural & peribronchovascular nodules
  - Often cavitary
  - Often demonstrate heterogeneous enhancement indicative of central necrosis
- Parenchymal opacities in same distribution
- Hilar lymphadenopathy variable

Nuclear Medicine Findings

- PET/CT
  - Evaluation of extent of disease & active lesions

Imaging Recommendations

- Best imaging tool
  - CT for optimal evaluation of lung involvement

DIFFERENTIAL DIAGNOSIS

Wegener Granulomatosis

- Reticular or nodular opacities early, then multifocal nodules & masses (cavitary in 25-50%)
- May present with pulmonary hemorrhage
- Associated with renal disease
- Upper airway disease, systemic vasculitis

Pulmonary Metastases

- Multifocal lung nodules/masses, may be cavitary
- Cavitary metastases: Squamous cell carcinoma, sarcomas

Infection

- May cause multifocal opacities
- Cavitary infection: Tuberculosis, fungal disease
- Septic abscesses: Subpleural, frequently cavitary

Churg-Strauss Syndrome

- Nodules or ill-defined opacities
  - May be asynchronous & migratory
- Associated with asthma, peripheral eosinophilia

Lymphomatoid Granulomatosis

- Lymphoproliferative disorder most common in middle-aged men
- Subpleural nodules or masses with coalescence & cavitation (30%)

Bronchocentric Granulomatosis

- Granulomatosis involving bronchi & bronchioles
- Upper lobe predominant nodules & masses
  - Commonly unilateral
- Associated with mucoid impaction & ABPA

PATHOLOGY

General Features

- Noncaseating granulomas similar to sarcoidosis
  - Subpleural & peribronchovascular distribution
  - Nodules & conglomerate masses
- Pulmonary vasculitis, often with vascular occlusion
- Widespread coagulative necrosis

Gross Pathologic & Surgical Features

- Pleural nodules with fibrosis & adhesions

Microscopic Features

- 3 patterns of pulmonary vasculitis
  - Necrotizing granulomas, giant cell vasculitis, chronic inflammatory cell infiltration

CLINICAL ISSUES

Presentation

- Most common signs/symptoms
  - Pleuritic chest pain, dyspnea
  - Cough, hemoptysis
  - Fever, weight loss, fatigue
- Other signs/symptoms
  - 25% of patients asymptomatic
  - Extrapulmonary manifestations are infrequent

Demographics

- Age
  - 3rd to 7th decades of life; mean age 49 years
- Gender
  - M:F = 1:2.2

Natural History & Prognosis

- Clinical course typically benign

Treatment

- Corticosteroids

DIAGNOSTIC CHECKLIST

Consider

- Necrotizing sarcoid granulomatosis in patients with multiple cavitary nodules in perilymphatic distribution

Image Interpretation Pearls

- Metastatic disease & infectious etiologies must be excluded

SELECTED REFERENCES

1. Arfi J et al: F-18 FDG PET/CT findings in pulmonary necrotizing sarcoid granulomatosis. Clin Nucl Med. 35(9):697-700, 2010
2. Frazier AA et al: Pulmonary angiitis and granulomatosis: radiologic-pathologic correlation. Radiographics. 18(3):687-710; quiz 727, 1998

SECTION 8
Mediastinal Abnormalities

Introduction and Overview

Primary Neoplasms

Lymphadenopathy

Cysts

Vascular Lesions

Glandular Enlargement

Diseases of the Esophagus

Miscellaneous Conditions

Introduction

The mediastinum is an intrathoracic space located between the pleural surfaces, bound anteriorly by the sternum and posteriorly by the spine. It extends from the thoracic inlet to the diaphragm and contains the thymus, heart and pericardium, thoracic great vessels, central airways, and esophagus. In addition, the mediastinum contains lymph nodes, the thoracic duct, various nerves, including the phrenic and vagus nerves, and mesenchymal tissues mostly composed of mediastinal fat. Although often included in the mediastinum, the bilateral paravertebral regions are not truly part of the mediastinum. Thus, although neurogenic neoplasms are often referred to as posterior mediastinal tumors, they are more correctly regarded as lesions of the paravertebral regions.

The many tissues and organs contained within the mediastinum may be affected by primary benign and malignant neoplasms. In addition, both thoracic and extrathoracic malignancies may metastasize to the mediastinum and manifest with mediastinal lymphadenopathy or coalescent lymph node masses. Vascular malformations, proliferations, and aneurysms as well as normal variants may produce mediastinal contour abnormalities on radiography. Enlargement of the thyroid and thymus glands and intrathoracic herniation of abdominal contents may also manifest as mediastinal masses.

The diagnosis of mediastinal abnormalities requires understanding of and familiarity with normal mediastinal anatomy. Knowledge of the normal mediastinal contours and the normal mediastinal lines, stripes, and interfaces demonstrated on chest radiographs is crucial for the detection of subtle abnormalities and differentiation of these lesions from normal variants.

The Mediastinal Compartments

Various mediastinal compartments have been described. However, it should be noted that such compartments are not typically bound by existing mediastinal tissue planes. Rather, mediastinal compartmentalization is usually undertaken for the purpose of formulating a differential diagnosis and varies from specialty to specialty with separate anatomic, surgical, and radiologic mediastinal divisions.

Anatomic Mediastinal Compartments

Anatomists divide the mediastinum into four different compartments: Superior, anterior, middle, and posterior. The anatomic superior mediastinum contains structures and tissues located above an imaginary horizontal line that connects the manubriosternal joint and the inferior aspect of the T4 vertebral body. The mediastinum below this imaginary line is divided into anterior, middle, and posterior compartments. The middle mediastinum is defined by the tissue planes of the fibrous pericardium, which contains within it the serous pericardium, the heart, and portions of the inferior and superior vena cava, pulmonary trunk, and ascending aorta. The anterior mediastinum is located anterior to the middle mediastinum and posterior to the sternum. The posterior mediastinum is located posterior to the middle mediastinum and anterior to the vertebral bodies. Thus, the anatomic mediastinal compartments are confined to the mediastinum proper and do not include the paravertebral regions.

Surgical Mediastinal Compartments

Surgeons also divide the mediastinum into four compartments: Superior, anterior, middle, and posterior. The surgical superior and anterior mediastinal compartments are identical to the corresponding anatomic mediastinal compartments. However, the surgical middle mediastinum includes the heart and extends posteriorly to the anterior aspects of the thoracic vertebral bodies. The paravertebral regions are considered the surgical posterior mediastinum.

Mediastinal Compartments According to Felson

The radiographic mediastinal compartments were introduced by Benjamin Felson. The Felson classification uses normal landmarks visible on lateral chest radiography to compartmentalize the mediastinum. Radiographic localization of mediastinal abnormalities to a particular compartment is performed in order to formulate a differential diagnosis.

The Felson method divides the mediastinum into anterior, middle, and posterior compartments. The anterior mediastinum is located between the sternum and a line drawn along the anterior trachea and continued along the posterior aspect of the heart. The posterior mediastinum includes the paravertebral region and is located posterior to a line drawn vertically along the anterior thirds of the thoracic vertebral bodies. The middle mediastinum is located between the anterior and posterior mediastinal compartments.

Mediastinal Compartments According to Fraser and Paré

The Fraser and Paré mediastinal compartmentalization is also based on the lateral chest radiograph; however, it recognizes that the paravertebral region is not located in the mediastinum proper. It also addresses the fact that mediastinal masses may occupy more than one mediastinal compartment. Thus, mediastinal lesions are described as occurring predominantly within a specific compartment or region.

Lesions are localized within anterior or middle-posterior mediastinal compartments or paravertebral regions. The anterior mediastinal compartment is identical to that described by Felson. The paravertebral region includes lesions occurring posterior to a line drawn along the anterior margins of the vertebral bodies. The middle-posterior mediastinal compartment is situated between the anterior mediastinum and the paravertebral region.

Difficulties in Mediastinal Compartmentalization

Localization of a lesion in a radiographic mediastinal compartment allows the radiologist to formulate a focused differential diagnosis and to recommend the most appropriate next imaging study to further evaluate the abnormality. Although most mediastinal abnormalities are assessed with chest CT, MR, angiography, ultrasonography, &/or echocardiography may also be used. Unfortunately, confusion may arise when descriptions of lesion location use radiographic, surgical, and anatomic mediastinal compartments interchangeably. In addition, because the imaging mediastinal compartments are based on radiography, radiologists may find it difficult to describe the location of a lesion on cross-sectional imaging. It should also be noted that mediastinal masses may be large enough to occupy more than one mediastinal compartment and may exhibit mobility within the thorax. In fact, radiographic localization of a lesion may not correlate with the cross-sectional imaging localization as the patient is imaged in the upright and supine positions, respectively.

Cross-sectional Imaging

Cross-sectional imaging is used to further localize mediastinal lesions and to describe their relationship or proximity to adjacent normal structures. Thus, lesions are localized within various mediastinal spaces, including the aorticopulmonary window and the supraaortic, prevascular, pretracheal, paratracheal, paraesophageal (azygoesophageal), and paracardial spaces. Lesions may also be localized in the paravertebral and retrocrural regions. This allows a more precise description of lesion location. The radiologist should also comment on the effects mediastinal lesions produce on adjacent structures, including mass effect, local invasion, encasement, &/or obstruction.

Cross-sectional imaging studies provide important information regarding the morphologic features and tissue composition of mediastinal masses. Associated findings such as lymphadenopathy and local invasion are helpful in formulating a differential diagnosis. In addition, unsuspected associated findings in the lung, pleura, chest wall, and diaphragm may be identified and are useful for refining the differential diagnosis, staging malignancy, and guiding management, including image-guided endoscopic or surgical biopsy &/or surgical excision.

Imaging Evaluation of the Abnormal Mediastinum

PA and lateral chest radiography is widely used for the initial evaluation of thoracic disorders. Although patients with mediastinal abnormalities may present with symptoms, their lesions are often discovered incidentally because of an abnormality found on radiographs obtained for other reasons (preoperative, employment). Thus, radiologists must recognize early subtle mediastinal abnormalities to ensure appropriate imaging follow-up and timely diagnosis and management.

Radiographic analysis should include a description of lesion localization and morphology, including the radiographic mediastinal compartment affected and whether the lesion manifests as a focal contour abnormality or as diffuse mediastinal enlargement. The former suggests a primary mediastinal lesion, while the latter suggests lymphadenopathy, including primary and secondary malignant neoplasia. Visualization and characterization of calcification may be helpful in suggesting granulomatous lymphadenopathy, mediastinal teratoma, mediastinal goiter, neurogenic neoplasm, or aneurysm. Benign skeletal pressure erosion associated with a paravertebral lesion suggests a neurogenic etiology, which includes neurogenic neoplasm and lateral thoracic meningocele. Likewise, identification of skeletal and cardiopulmonary findings of chronic anemia in association with a paravertebral mass suggests extramedullary hematopoiesis.

Most patients with a radiographic mediastinal abnormality are evaluated with chest CT, typically performed with intravenous contrast. Contrast allows evaluation of vascular lesions and may optimize visualization of soft tissue elements and areas of necrosis. In patients with paravertebral lesions, the most appropriate next imaging study is MR to assess for the intraspinal involvement that may occur in neurogenic neoplasms.

Differential Diagnosis by Location and Demographics

Approximately 20% of primary mediastinal lesions are thymomas, 20% are cysts, and 20% are neurogenic neoplasms occurring in the anterior mediastinum, middle-posterior mediastinum, and paravertebral regions, respectively. Teratomas, lymphomas, granulomas, and thyroid lesions comprise another 30% of cases. Knowledge of patient demographics and presenting symptoms is helpful in narrowing the differential diagnosis. For example, thymomas and mature teratomas are both anterior mediastinal masses but typically affect patients over or under the age of 40 years, respectively.

General Cross-sectional Imaging Features

Cross-sectional imaging allows morphologic characterization of mediastinal masses and the surrounding tissues. Identification of lymphadenopathy suggests metastatic disease or lymphoma, and lymph node calcification suggests benign lymphadenopathy. Visualization of intact tissue planes is helpful in predicting resectability, and locally invasive behavior suggests an aggressive biological behavior.

Cystic change is frequently seen in mediastinal lesions. Careful analysis for identification of mural nodules and septations allows differentiation of a congenital cyst from a vascular malformation or a cystic neoplasm. Congenital cysts are characteristically unilocular lesions, vascular malformations are usually multilocular and cystic, and mural nodules are typically associated with neoplasms.

Identification of fat within a mediastinal mass may allow the prospective diagnosis of lipomatosis, thymolipoma, Morgagni hernia, or extramedullary hematopoiesis. Likewise, identification of fat within a cystic anterior mediastinal mass is virtually pathognomonic of mature teratoma.

It should be noted that approximately 10% of mediastinal abnormalities are related to vascular lesions. Continuity with a vessel lumen or a vascular pattern of enhancement allows a confident diagnosis of aneurysms and paraesophageal varices. Intense contrast enhancement is typical of mediastinal goiter, Castleman disease, hemangioma, paraganglioma, and metastases from vascular malignant neoplasms.

The Radiologist's Role

Radiologists play a crucial role in the evaluation and management of mediastinal abnormalities. Radiographic localization of a lesion in a specific mediastinal compartment allows the formulation of a prospective differential diagnosis and helps guide further imaging and management.

Differentiation between neoplastic and nonneoplastic lesions, and between surgical and nonsurgical lesions, should be attempted. Image-guided biopsy should be considered in nonsurgical lesions such as lymphomas and malignant germ cell tumors. In some cases, imaging findings are pathognomonic and the radiologist can provide a definitive diagnosis.

APPROACH TO MEDIASTINAL ABNORMALITIES

*(**Left**) Graphic shows a cross section of the mediastinum. The mediastinum is the space between the pleural surfaces, bound anteriorly by the sternum and posteriorly by the spine. It contains tissues, structures, and organs that may be affected by various disease processes. Mediastinal divisions are arbitrary and not based on existing tissue planes. (**Right**) Graphic shows a sagittal view of the mediastinum, which extends from the thoracic inlet superiorly to the diaphragm inferiorly.*

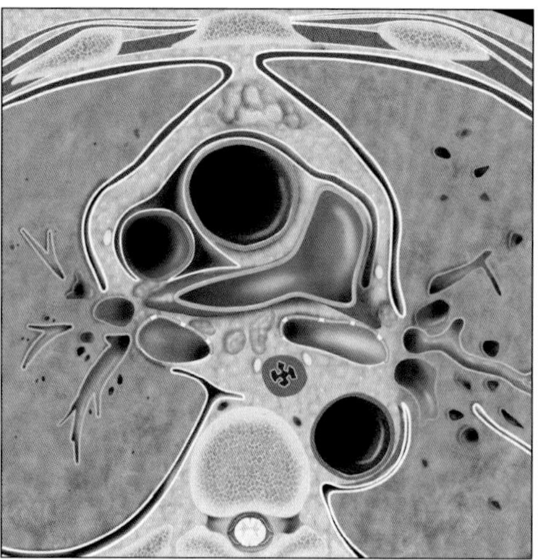

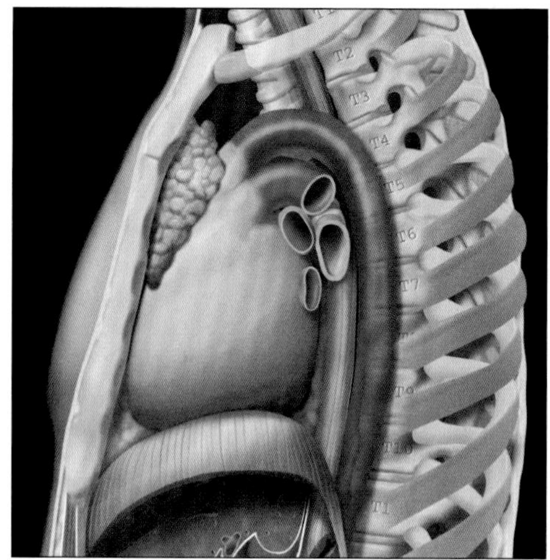

*(**Left**) Graphic shows the mediastinum proper (in color), which does not include the paravertebral regions. The paravertebral regions are included in the posterior mediastinal compartment in the surgical and the Felson mediastinal divisions. (**Right**) Graphic illustrates the anatomic mediastinal compartments: Superior (green), anterior (yellow), middle (red), and posterior (blue). The anatomic mediastinal compartments do not include the paravertebral regions.*

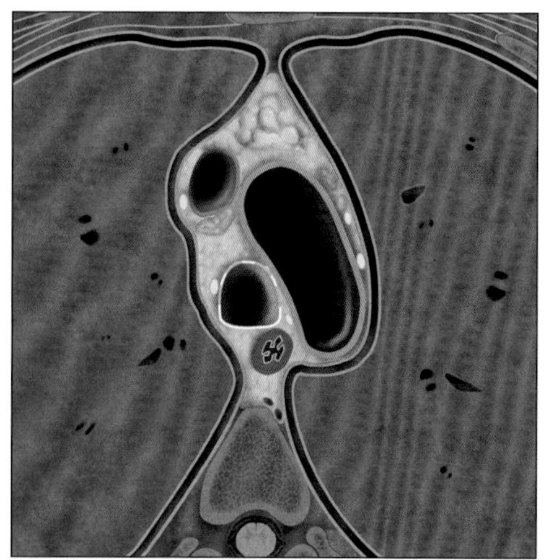

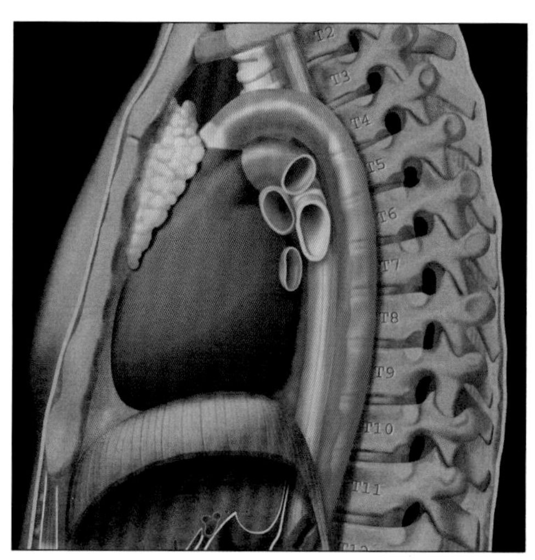

*(**Left**) Lateral chest radiograph shows the Felson divisions. The anterior mediastinum is situated anterior to a line (blue) drawn along the anterior trachea and posterior heart. The posterior mediastinum is posterior to a line (magenta) drawn 1 cm posterior to the anterior vertebral margins. The middle mediastinum is between the anterior and posterior compartments. (**Right**) Graphic shows the Felson mediastinal divisions: Anterior (yellow), middle (red), and posterior (blue) compartments.*

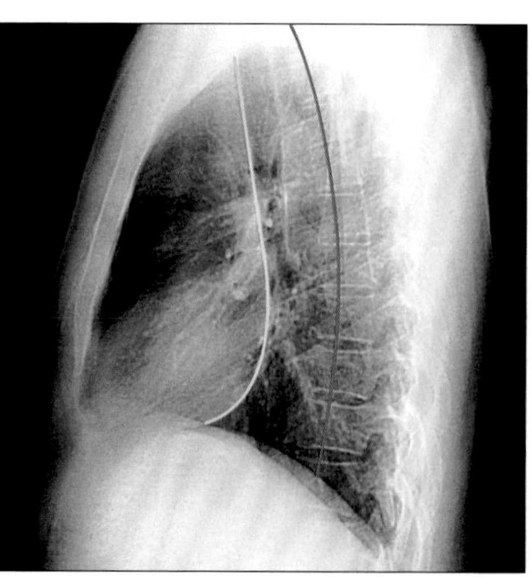

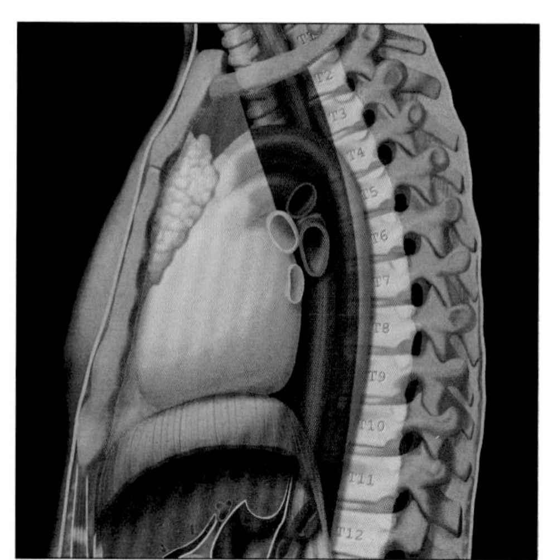

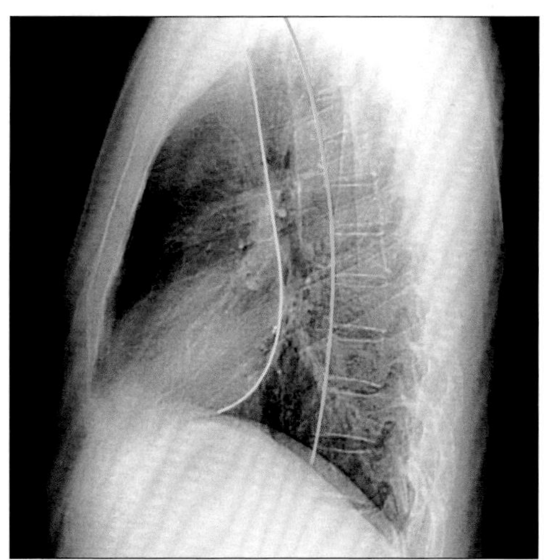

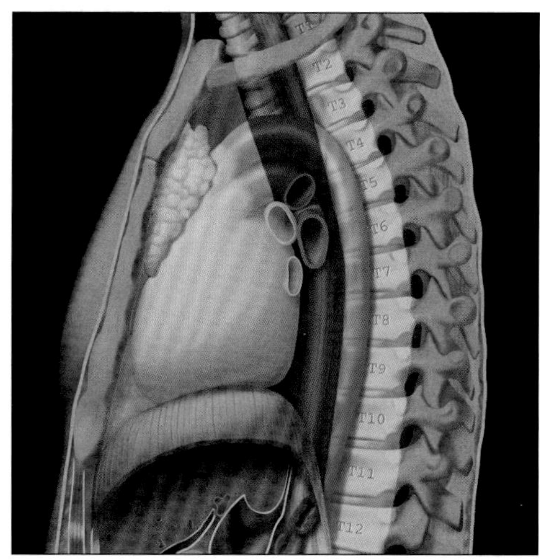

(Left) *Lateral chest radiograph shows the Fraser and Paré mediastinal compartments. The anterior mediastinum is the same as in the Felson division. The paravertebral region is posterior to the (green) line drawn along the anterior vertebral margins. The middle-posterior mediastinum is between the anterior mediastinum and the paravertebral region.* ***(Right)*** *Graphic shows the Fraser and Paré compartments: Anterior mediastinum (yellow), middle-posterior mediastinum (red), and paravertebral (blue) regions.*

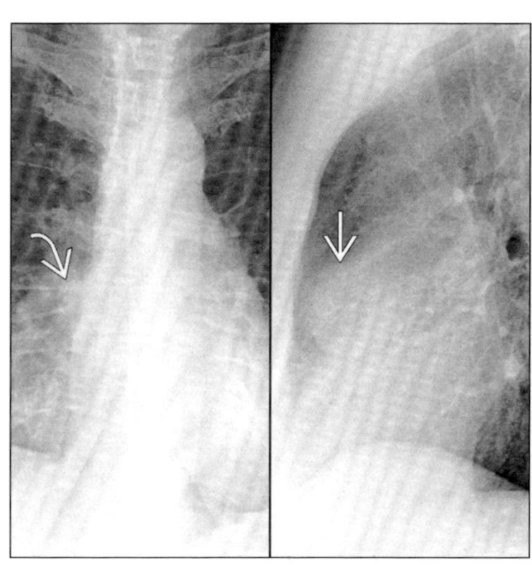

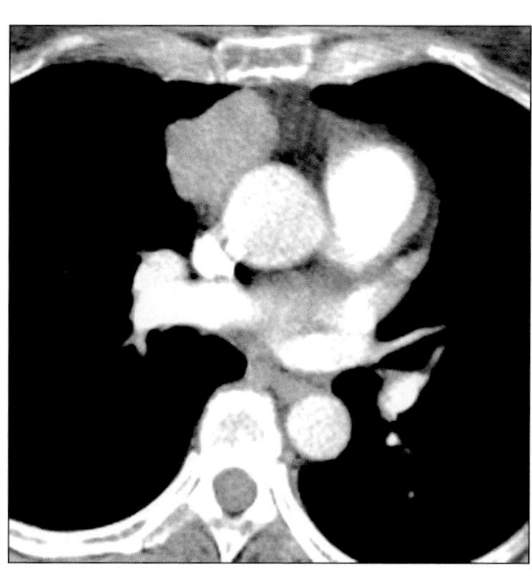

(Left) *Composite image with PA (left) and lateral (right) chest radiographs of an asymptomatic 54-year-old woman shows a subtle right mediastinal contour abnormality on the PA radiograph and an ill-defined mass that projects over the radiographic anterior mediastinum on the lateral.* ***(Right)*** *CECT of the same patient shows a focal lobular right anterior mediastinal mass abutting the ascending aorta. Thymoma is the most likely diagnosis given the demographic information and imaging features.*

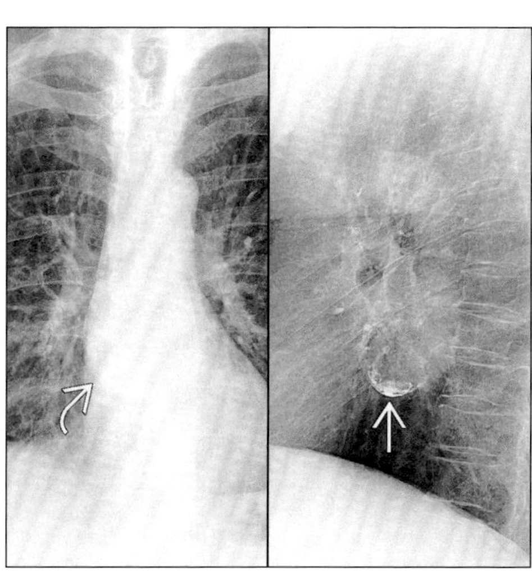

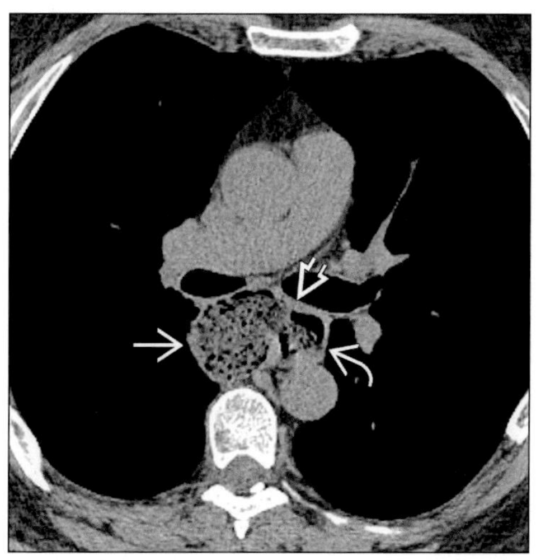

(Left) *Composite image with PA (left) and lateral (right) chest radiographs demonstrates a subcarinal mediastinal mass with intrinsic dependent contrast. The lesion projects over the radiographic middle-posterior mediastinum of Fraser and Paré.* ***(Right)*** *Axial NECT of the same patient shows a heterogeneous mediastinal mass containing air and debris, consistent with a large diverticulum with a wide neck arising from the mid portion of the esophagus.*

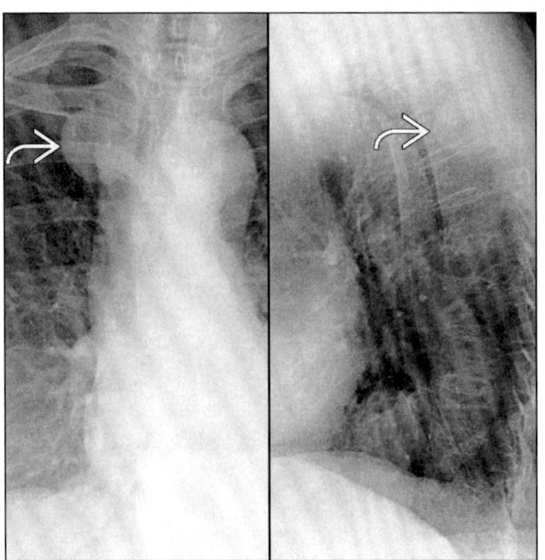

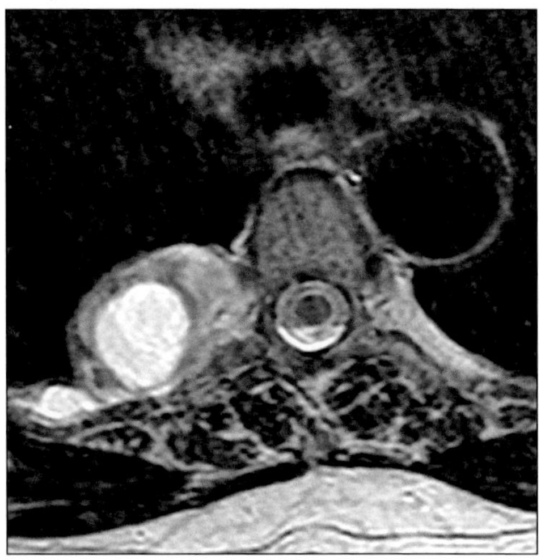

(Left) *Composite image with PA (left) and lateral (right) chest radiographs of an asymptomatic elderly woman with a schwannoma shows a right paravertebral spherical mass ➔. The spherical morphology of the lesion and its anatomic location are consistent with a benign neurogenic neoplasm of nerve sheath origin.* ***(Right)*** *Axial T2WI MR shows a heterogeneous spherical paravertebral lesion with internal cystic change and without evidence of intraspinal growth.*

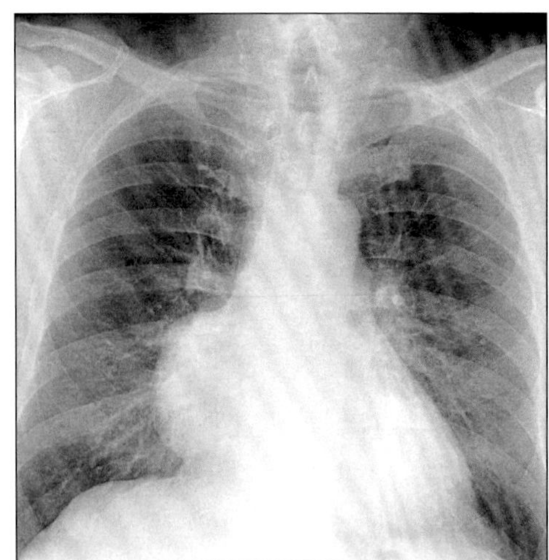

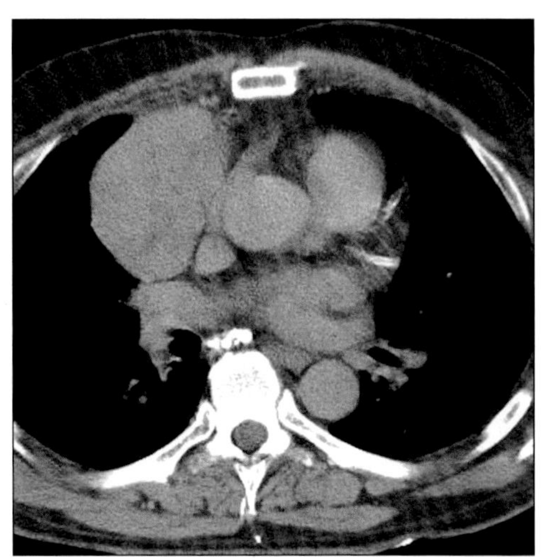

(Left) *PA chest radiograph of an asymptomatic patient shows a focal right-sided mediastinal mass located in the anterior compartment on the lateral radiograph (not shown). The focal nature of the lesion suggests a primary mediastinal neoplasm, and thymoma would be most likely given the demographic and clinical information.* ***(Right)*** *Axial CECT of the same patient shows a polylobular right anterior mediastinal soft tissue mass without associated lymphadenopathy.*

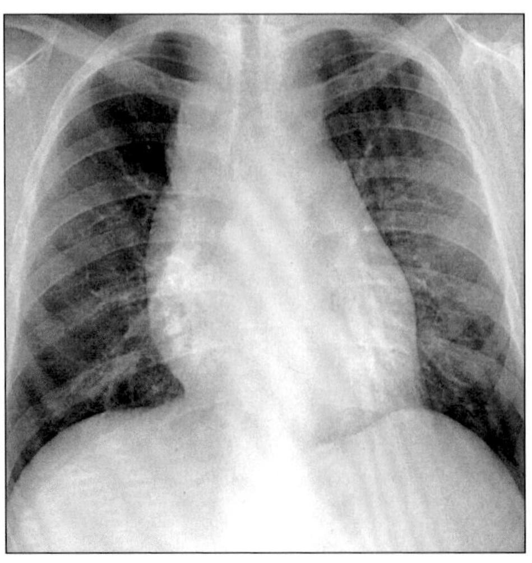

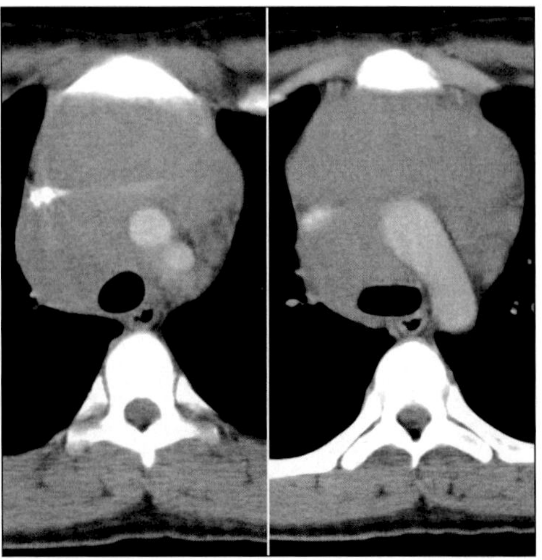

(Left) *PA chest radiograph of a 16-year-old boy shows diffuse mediastinal enlargement consistent with lymphadenopathy and likely related to lymphoma given demographic and imaging features.* ***(Right)*** *Composite image with axial CECT of the same patient shows homogeneous mediastinal soft tissue involving multiple lymph node stations and encasing the vascular structures, consistent with coalescent lymphadenopathy. Hodgkin lymphoma was confirmed at biopsy.*

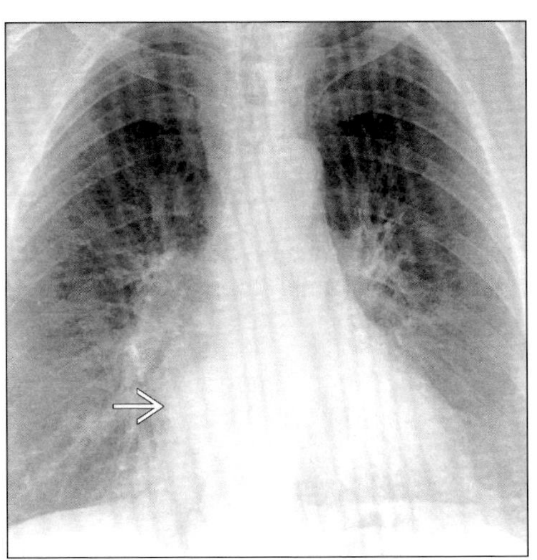

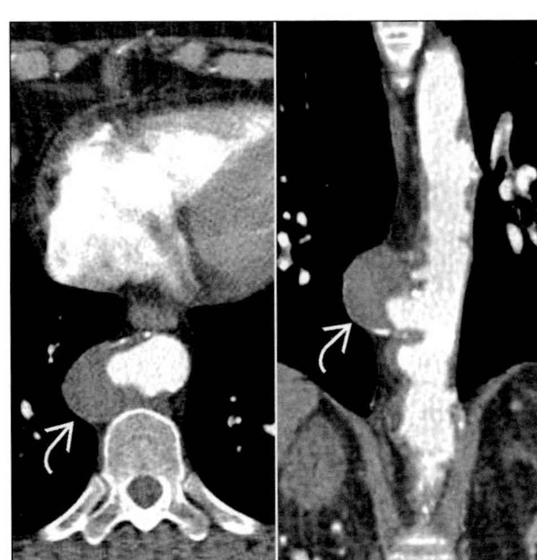

(Left) *PA chest radiograph of a 72-year-old woman who presented with chest pain shows a focal right inferior mediastinal contour abnormality ➡ that was not visible on the lateral chest radiograph (not shown).* ***(Right)*** *Composite image with axial (left) and coronal (right) CECT of the same patient shows that the mediastinal contour abnormality corresponds to a right-sided saccular aneurysm ↪ of the descending aorta. Approximately 10% of mediastinal abnormalities are related to vascular lesions.*

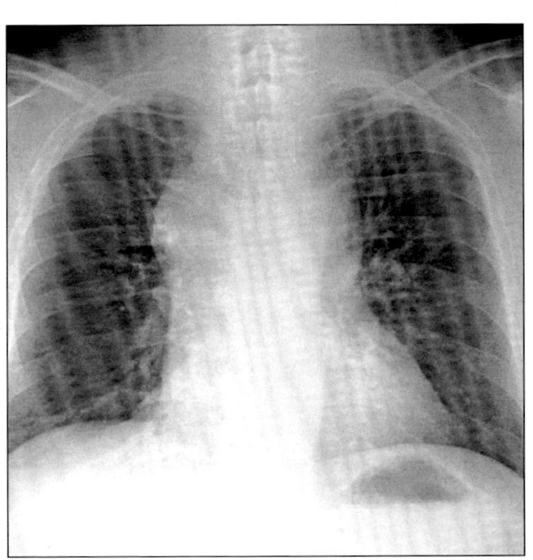

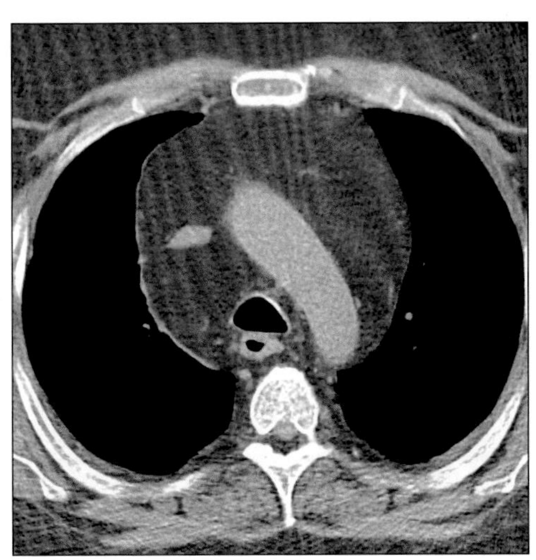

(Left) *PA chest radiograph of a 43-year-old man on chronic corticosteroid therapy shows diffuse mediastinal widening suspicious for lymphadenopathy.* ***(Right)*** *Axial NECT of the same patient shows mediastinal lipomatosis manifesting with diffuse fat attenuation tissue surrounding the mediastinal vascular structures, trachea, and esophagus without obstruction or invasion. Mediastinal lipomatosis is unencapsulated fat, secondary to exogenous hypercortisolism in this case.*

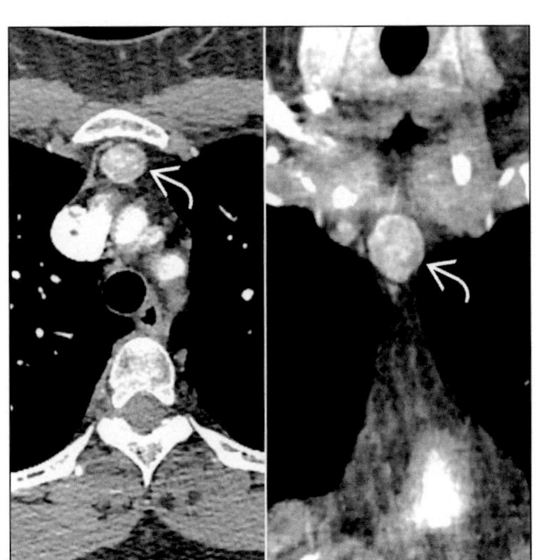

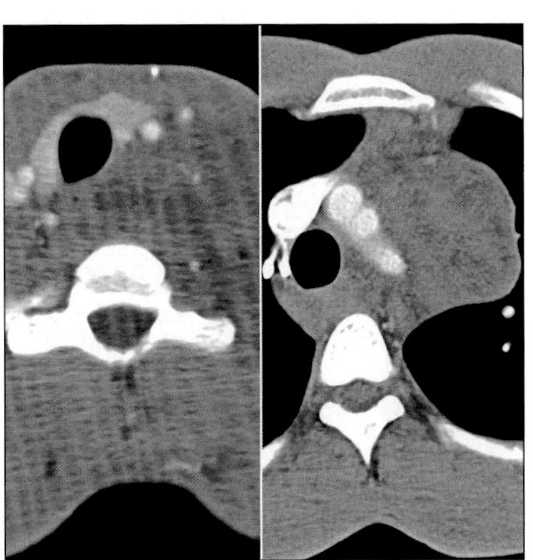

(Left) *Composite image with axial (left) and oblique coronal (right) CECT of an asymptomatic patient with ectopic mediastinal thyroid shows an anterior mediastinal nodule ↪ with intense contrast enhancement. The differential diagnosis should also include Castleman disease and paraganglioma.* ***(Right)*** *Composite image with axial CECT of a young man with lymphangioma shows typical findings of a heterogeneous mediastinal mass that extends into the neck and exhibits internal foci of water attenuation.*

THYMOMA

Key Facts

Terminology

- Most common primary anterior mediastinal neoplasm

Imaging

- Radiography
  - Anterior mediastinal mass with well-defined smooth or lobular borders, typically unilateral
  - Invasive thymoma: Irregular borders, elevated hemidiaphragm, pleural nodules
- CT
  - Anterior mediastinal, spherical/ovoid, unilateral soft tissue mass, smooth or lobular borders
  - No lymphadenopathy
  - Invasive thymoma: Local invasion, pleural nodules
- MR
  - T1WI: Low to intermediate signal intensity
  - T2WI: Hyperintense

Top Differential Diagnoses

- Thymic malignancy
  - Thymic carcinoma & carcinoid
- Lymphoma
- Malignant germ cell neoplasm

Clinical Issues

- 70% present in 5th & 6th decades, M = F
- Symptoms
  - Asymptomatic, incidental diagnosis
  - Compression/invasion of adjacent structures
  - Paraneoplastic syndromes
- Treatment
  - Stage I & II: Complete surgical excision
  - Stage III & IVa: Neoadjuvant chemotherapy & complete excision
  - Stage IVb: Palliative chemotherapy

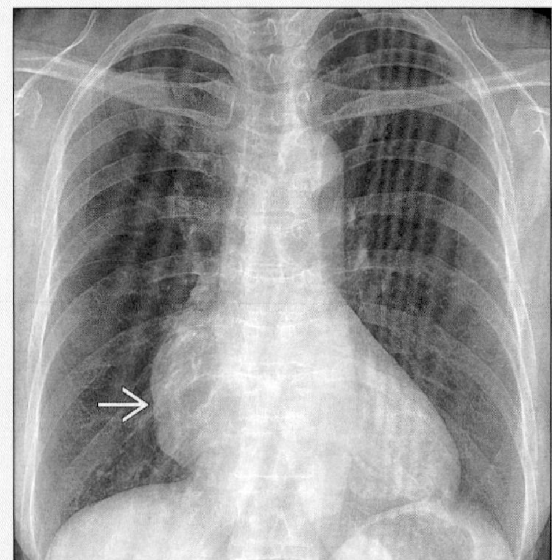

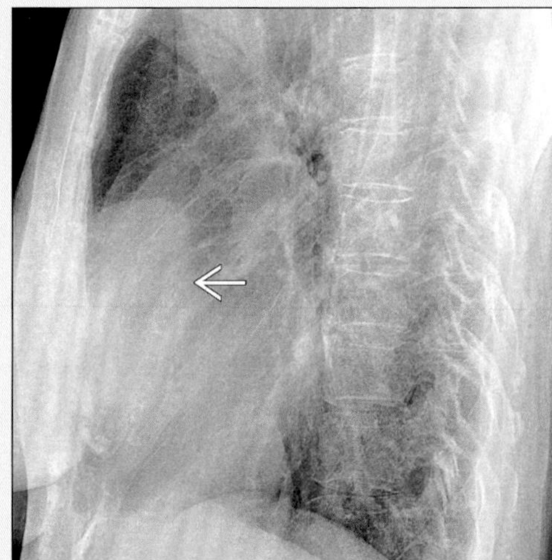

(Left) *PA chest radiograph of a patient with thymoma shows a right mediastinal mass ➔ with well-defined lobular borders. Thymomas often manifest as an abnormal mediastinal contour on frontal chest radiography.* ***(Right)*** *Lateral chest radiograph of the same patient shows the anterior mediastinal location of the mass ➔. The lateral chest radiograph allows localization of mediastinal masses in 1 of the radiographic mediastinal compartments.*

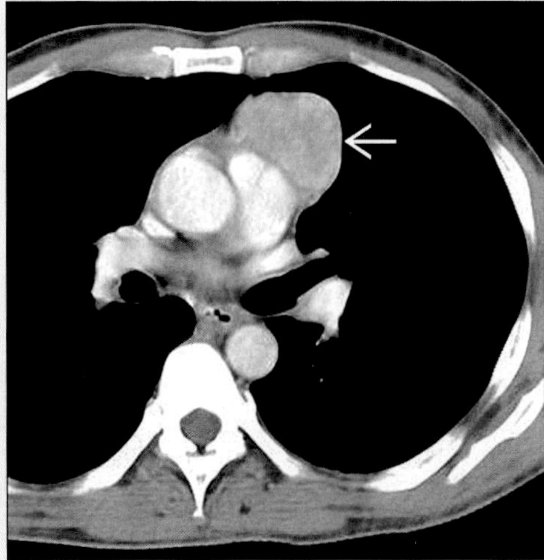

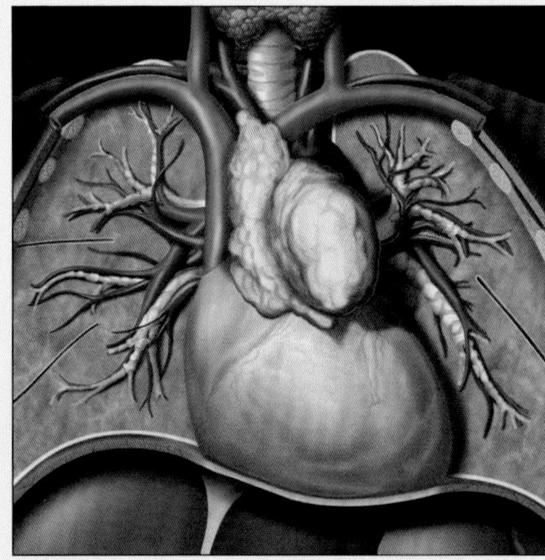

(Left) *CECT of a patient with thymoma shows an anterior mediastinal mass ➔ that exhibits heterogeneous contrast enhancement. The lesion is located in the left anterior mediastinum and abuts the adjacent pulmonary trunk without gross evidence of vascular invasion. Absence of a tissue plane on chest CT does not reliably indicate local invasion.* ***(Right)*** *Graphic shows the morphologic features of thymoma, a primary neoplasm that typically arises in 1 of the thymic lobes and usually exhibits unilateral growth.*

THYMOMA

TERMINOLOGY

Definitions

- Thymic epithelial neoplasm
  - Considered malignant, may metastasize at any stage
- Most common primary thymic & anterior mediastinal neoplasm

IMAGING

General Features

- Best diagnostic clue
  - Spherical or ovoid anterior mediastinal mass
- Location
  - Anterior mediastinum, typically unilateral
- Size
  - Variable: 1-10 cm at diagnosis (mean: 5 cm)
- Morphology
  - Spherical or ovoid, smooth or lobular borders

Radiographic Findings

- Normal radiographs in small or occult thymomas
- **Focal anterior mediastinal mass**
  - May occur anywhere from thoracic inlet to cardiophrenic angle
  - Nodular thickening of anterior junction line
  - Contour abnormality on frontal chest radiograph
  - Well-marginated, smooth or lobular borders
  - Typically unilateral, less frequently bilateral
  - May exhibit calcification
    - Peripheral, curvilinear, thin
    - Focal, multifocal, punctate, coarse
- Anterior mediastinal nodule/mass on lateral radiograph
- **Large thymoma**: **Mass effect** on adjacent structures
- **Invasive thymoma**
  - Lung invasion: Irregular or spiculated margins
  - Phrenic nerve invasion: Diaphragmatic elevation/ paralysis
  - Pleural metastases: Pleural nodules; may progress to circumferential nodular pleural thickening

CT Findings

- CECT
  - **Anterior superior mediastinal soft tissue mass**
    - Abuts superior pericardium & great vessels
    - From thoracic inlet to cardiophrenic angle
    - Rarely in other mediastinal compartments
  - Typically **unilateral**; origin in thymic lobe
  - Variable size
  - **Spherical or ovoid**
  - Smooth or lobular well-defined borders
  - Often homogeneous attenuation
  - Heterogeneous attenuation with
    - Low attenuation from necrosis or hemorrhage
    - Calcification
      - Curvilinear, peripheral, along capsule or septa
      - Coarse or punctate within tumor substance
    - Cystic thymoma
      - Peripheral soft tissue capsule
      - Fluid attenuation content
      - Mural soft tissue nodule(s) of variable size
  - Typically **no associated lymphadenopathy**
  - Exclusion of local invasion of mediastinal fat, vessels, pericardium, heart, pleura, lung
  - **Invasive thymoma** (30-60%)
    - Tissue plane obliteration does not denote invasion
    - Higher frequency of
      - Low-attenuation areas from tumor necrosis
      - Lobular or irregular tumor contours
      - Infiltration of surrounding fat
      - Multifocal calcification in tumor substance
      - Size ≥ 7 cm
    - **Direct signs of invasion**
      - **Vascular invasion**: Irregular vessel contour, encasement/obliteration, endoluminal tumor
      - Single or multiple pleural nodules, typically ipsilateral to thymoma, may be bilateral, may involve pleura diffusely
      - Pericardial thickening, invasion, nodules
      - Pulmonary involvement: Endobronchial involvement may occur

MR Findings

- T1WI
  - Ovoid/spherical anterior mediastinal mass
  - Low to intermediate signal intensity
  - Isointense or higher signal than skeletal muscle
  - Low signal in cystic regions
- T1WI FS
  - No signal decrease on opposed phase imaging; differentiation from thymic hyperplasia
- T2WI
  - Hyperintense, higher signal in cystic components
- Advantages of MR
  - Assessment of invasive tumors; particularly if intravenous contrast contraindicated
  - Visualization of tumor capsule & septa: Low signal thin peripheral rim (capsule) & internal septa
  - Identification of tumor hemorrhage
    - High signal on T1WI & T2WI; hemosiderin
  - Identification of mural nodules in cystic thymoma

Nuclear Medicine Findings

- PET/CT
  - Role of FDG PET not defined: FDG uptake by normal thymus & thymic hyperplasia
  - Used for detection & monitoring of metastases

Imaging Recommendations

- Best imaging tool
  - CECT is modality of choice; assessment of invasion
- Follow-up imaging of completely resected thymoma
  - Annual CECT for 5 years post resection, then annual CT alternating with chest radiography until year 11, then annual chest radiography
- Follow-up imaging of resected stage III or IVa thymoma or incompletely resected thymoma
  - CECT every 6 months for 3 years
- Reporting recommendations: Report should include
  - Tumor size: Axial short & long axes, craniocaudad
  - Lesion location, borders, attenuation, calcification
  - Description of features of invasion
    - Fat infiltration, adjacent lung abnormality
    - Tumor abutting ≥ 50% of adjacent structure
    - Vessel/heart invasion, lymphadenopathy
    - Diaphragm elevation, pleural effusion/nodules
    - Distant metastases

THYMOMA

DIFFERENTIAL DIAGNOSIS

Thymic Malignancy

- Thymic carcinoma
  - Similar demographic distribution to thymoma
  - Histologic features of malignancy
  - Dominant anterior mediastinal mass
    - Lymphadenopathy, local invasion
- Thymic carcinoid
  - Similar demographic distribution to thymoma
    - Clinical hormone syndrome: ACTH
    - Multiple endocrine neoplasia (MEN1) (Wermer)
  - Histologic features of atypical carcinoid
  - Dominant anterior mediastinal mass
    - Lymphadenopathy, local invasion

Lymphoma

- Hodgkin & non-Hodgkin lymphoma
- Anterior mediastinal mass with lymphadenopathy
- Local invasion, central necrosis, cystic change

Malignant Germ Cell Neoplasm

- Symptomatic men, younger than 40 years
- Seminoma & nonseminomatous malignant germ cell neoplasms
  - Seminoma: Homogeneous anterior mediastinal mass
  - Nonseminomatous germ cell neoplasm: Heterogeneous mass with central low attenuation
- Dominant locally invasive mass & lymphadenopathy

Thymic Hyperplasia

- Diffuse or focal nodular thymic enlargement
- Chemical shift MR for differentiation from thymoma

PATHOLOGY

Staging, Grading, & Classification

- **Masaoka-Koga staging**
  - Stage I: Encapsulated thymoma
  - Stage IIa: Microscopic capsular invasion
  - Stage IIb: Invasion of surrounding mediastinal fat
  - Stage III: Invasion of adjacent structure/organ
  - Stage IVa: Pleural or pericardial tumor nodules
  - Stage IVb: Distant metastases

Gross Pathologic & Surgical Features

- Encapsulated thymoma
  - Spherical/ovoid mass surrounded by fibrous capsule
  - Intrinsic fibrous septa connected to capsule
- Necrosis, hemorrhage, cystic change (30-40%)
- Invasive thymoma
  - Invasion of tumor cells through tumor capsule
  - Invasion of mediastinal fat, cardiovascular structures, pleura, lung

Microscopic Features

- Epithelial cells & lymphocytes in varying proportions
- WHO histologic classification of thymoma
  - Based on epithelial cell morphology, cellular atypia, & proportions of epithelial cells to lymphocytes
  - Type A histology: Round/epithelioid tumor cells
  - Type B histology: Oval/spindle tumor cells
  - WHO histologic classification
    - Types A, AB, B1, B2, B3
  - Poor reproducibility & clinical predictive value

CLINICAL ISSUES

Presentation

- Most common signs/symptoms
  - Asymptomatic, incidental diagnosis
  - Symptoms of compression or invasion of adjacent structures
    - Dysphagia, diaphragm paralysis, SVC syndrome
    - Chest pain, dyspnea, cough
  - Paraneoplastic syndrome
    - Myasthenia gravis (MG) (30-50%)
      - 15% of patients with MG have thymoma
    - Hypogammaglobulinemia (10%)
    - Pure red cell aplasia (5%)

Demographics

- Age
  - 70% of patients in 5th & 6th decades
- Gender
  - M = F

Natural History & Prognosis

- Prognosis affected by stage & completeness of excision
- 5-year survival: 65-80%

Treatment

- Stage I: Extended thymectomy
  - Excision of thymus & surrounding fat
- Stage II: Extended thymectomy
  - Stage IIb: Adjuvant radiation therapy
- Stage III: Neoadjuvant chemotherapy & complete excision
  - Postoperative radiation or chemotherapy for incompletely resected thymoma
- Stage IVa: Same as for stage III thymoma
- Stage IVb: Palliative chemotherapy

DIAGNOSTIC CHECKLIST

Image Interpretation Pearls

- Pleural involvement by thymoma rarely produces pleural effusion

Reporting Tips

- Imaging distinction of stage I/II thymoma from stage III/IV thymoma is crucial to identify candidates for neoadjuvant therapy

SELECTED REFERENCES

1. Marom EM et al: Computed tomography findings predicting invasiveness of thymoma. J Thorac Oncol. 6(7):1274-81, 2011
2. Marom EM et al: Standard report terms for chest computed tomography reports of anterior mediastinal masses suspicious for thymoma. J Thorac Oncol. 6(7 Suppl 3):S1717-23, 2011
3. Marom EM: Imaging thymoma. J Thorac Oncol. 5(10 Suppl 4):S296-303, 2010
4. Rosado-de-Christenson ML et al: Imaging of thymic epithelial neoplasms. Hematol Oncol Clin North Am. 22(3):409-31, 2008
5. Maher MM et al: Imaging of thymoma. Semin Thorac Cardiovasc Surg. 17(1):12-9, 2005
6. Jeong YJ et al: Does CT of thymic epithelial tumors enable us to differentiate histologic subtypes and predict prognosis? AJR Am J Roentgenol. 183(2):283-9, 2004

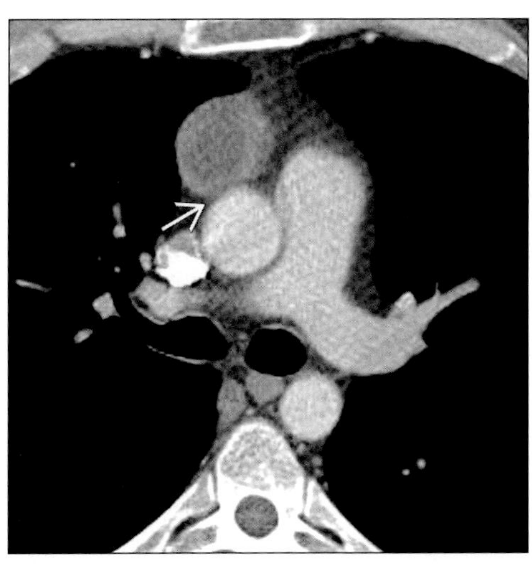

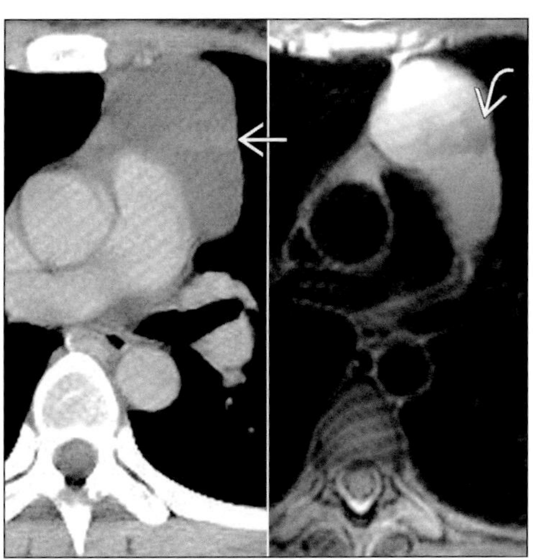

(Left) *CECT of a patient with an encapsulated thymoma shows a spherical right anterior mediastinal mass with central low attenuation due to necrosis. Note intact tissue plane ➔ with adjacent ascending aorta.* ***(Right)*** *Composite image with CECT (left) and axial T2WI MR (right) shows a left anterior mediastinal cystic thymoma with a nodular soft tissue septum ➔, which is more conspicuous ↪ on MR. Mural nodules in a mediastinal cyst should suggest the diagnosis of cystic neoplasm.*

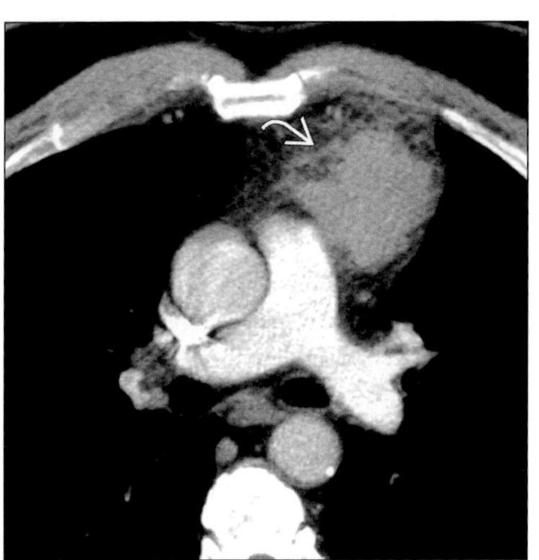

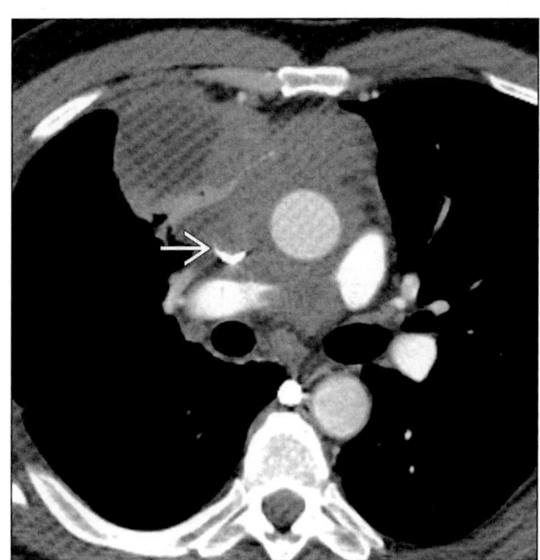

(Left) *Axial CECT shows a left anterior mediastinal thymoma with irregular borders and infiltration of the adjacent mediastinal fat ↪. Mediastinal fat invasion (stage IIa) was confirmed at surgery.* ***(Right)*** *Axial CECT of a patient with invasive thymoma shows a large, polylobular mass encasing the mediastinal vessels and invading the superior vena cava ➔. The patient should receive preoperative neoadjuvant chemotherapy, given imaging documentation of stage III disease. (Courtesy E. Marom, MD.)*

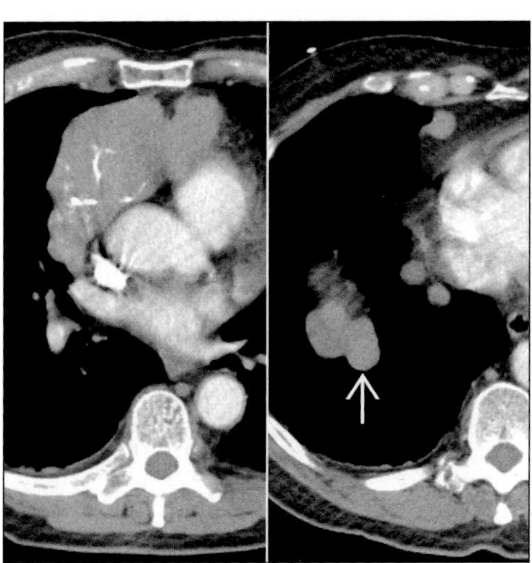

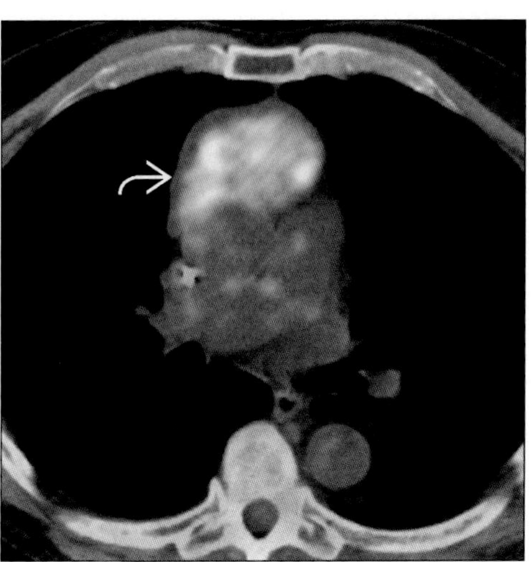

(Left) *Composite image with axial CECT of a patient with invasive thymoma shows a large right polylobular anterior mediastinal mass with coarse calcifications (left) and multifocal ipsilateral diaphragmatic ➔ and medial pleural metastases (right), consistent with stage IVa disease.* ***(Right)*** *Axial fused PET/CT of the same patient shows FDG avidity ↪ in the lesion (SUV of 4.5). While the role of PET/CT in the evaluation of thymoma is not defined, it may be useful in identifying metastases in selected cases.*

THYMIC MALIGNANCY

Key Facts

Terminology

- Malignant neoplasms arising in thymus
  - Thymic carcinoma: Malignant thymic epithelial neoplasm
  - Thymic carcinoid: Malignant neoplasm derived from thymic cells of neural crest origin

Imaging

- Radiography
  - Dominant anterior mediastinal mass
- CT
  - Anterior mediastinal mass ± calcification &/or local invasion
  - Identification of lymphadenopathy & metastases
  - Pleural metastases less common than in thymoma
  - Thymic carcinoid often hyperenhancing on CT
- MR: May mimic thymoma, local invasion
- PET/CT: Detection of metastases & surveillance

Top Differential Diagnoses

- Thymoma
- Malignant germ cell neoplasm
- Mediastinal Hodgkin lymphoma
- Mediastinal metastatic lymphadenopathy

Clinical Issues

- Symptoms/signs
  - May relate to mass effect/invasion; SVC syndrome
  - Thymic carcinoid: Cushing syndrome in ~ 40%
- Thymic carcinoma: Average age 50; M = F
- Thymic carcinoid: Average age 45; M:F = 3:1

Diagnostic Checklist

- Thymic carcinoma, thymic carcinoid, & thymoma not reliably differentiated on imaging
- Distant metastases & lymphadenopathy more common in thymic carcinoma/carcinoid

*(**Left**) PA chest radiograph of a patient with thymic carcinoma shows a soft tissue mass ⇨ widening the superior mediastinum. (**Right**) Axial CECT of the same patient shows an irregular, heterogeneously enhancing anterior mediastinal mass ➔ with surrounding soft tissue stranding and adjacent enhancing mediastinal lymph nodes ⮫. While thymic malignancy is difficult to distinguish from thymoma on imaging, lymphadenopathy and distant metastases suggest thymic carcinoma or thymic carcinoid.*

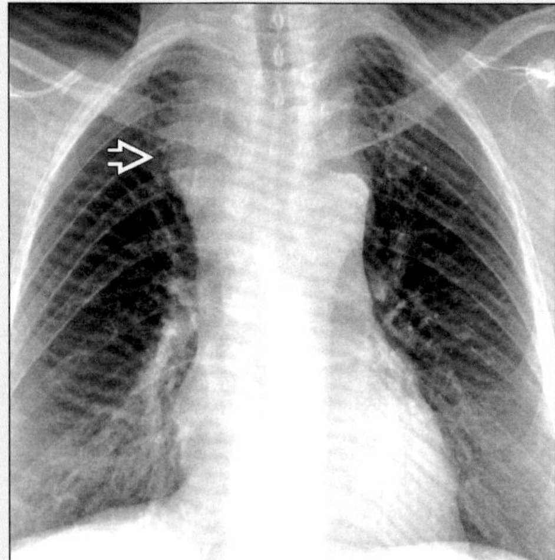

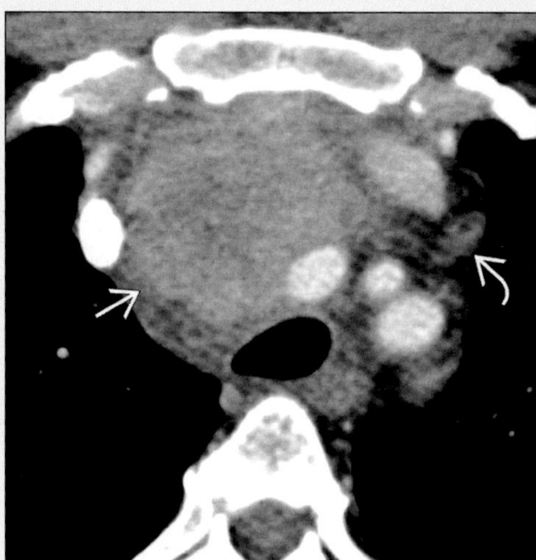

*(**Left**) Axial CECT of a patient with thymic carcinoma shows a large, heterogeneously enhancing anterior mediastinal mass that invades the left anterior chest wall ⇨ and produces mass effect on mediastinal vessels ⮫. Pleural metastases may occur in thymic malignancy but are characteristic of invasive thymoma. (**Right**) Composite image with axial CECT (left) and PET/CT (right) of a patient with thymic carcinoid shows a left anterior mediastinal mass ➔ with calcification, hyperenhancement, and FDG avidity on PET/CT ⮫.*

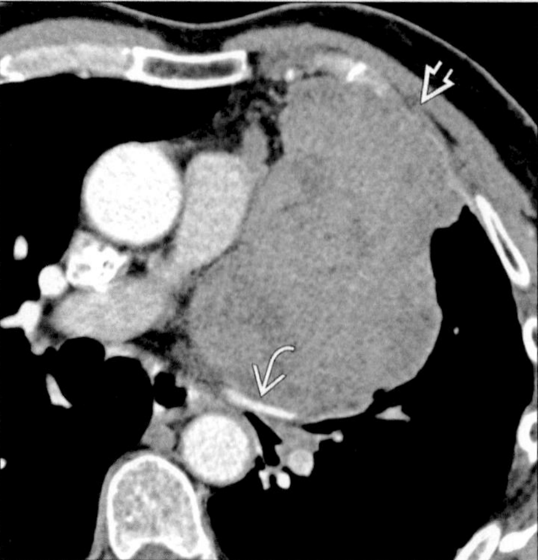

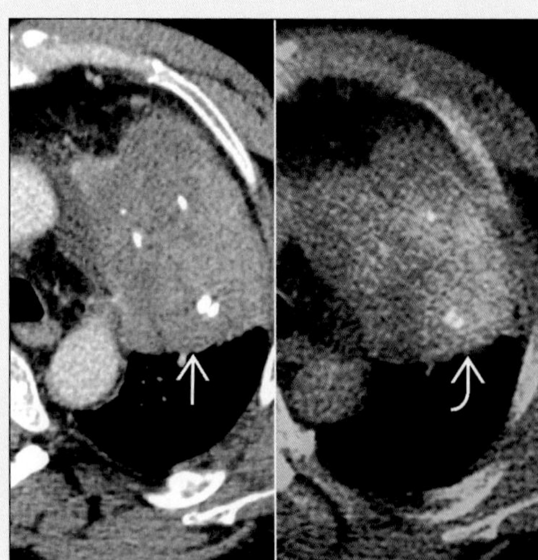

THYMIC MALIGNANCY

TERMINOLOGY

Definitions

- Malignant neoplasms arising in thymus
  - **Thymic carcinoma**: Malignant thymic epithelial neoplasm
  - **Thymic carcinoid**: Malignant neoplasm derived from thymic cells of neural crest origin
- Thymoma: No histologic features of malignancy, but often considered thymic malignancy due to unpredictable biologic behavior

IMAGING

General Features

- Best diagnostic clue
  - Thymic carcinoma/carcinoid not reliably distinguished from thymoma on imaging
    - Lymphadenopathy &/or distant metastases favor thymic malignancy
- Location
  - Metastases more common than in thymoma
    - 50-65% of patients
    - Common sites: Lung, liver, brain, bone
- Size
  - Thymic carcinoma: 5-15 cm in diameter
- Morphology
  - Frequent invasion of mediastinal structures

Radiographic Findings

- Dominant anterior mediastinal mass

CT Findings

- **Thymic carcinoma**
  - **Anterior mediastinal mass** ± calcification &/or local invasion
  - Identification of **lymphadenopathy & metastases**
  - Pleural metastases less common than in thymoma
- **Thymic carcinoid**
  - Anterior mediastinal mass, lymphadenopathy, local invasion
  - Often **hyperenhancing**

MR Findings

- Thymic carcinoma & thymic carcinoid similar to thymoma on MR
- Thymic carcinoma: Hyperintense relative to muscle on T1WI & T2WI
  - Necrosis, cystic change, hemorrhage may result in heterogeneous signal intensity

Nuclear Medicine Findings

- PET/CT
  - Useful for detection of metastases & surveillance

DIFFERENTIAL DIAGNOSIS

Thymoma

- Most common primary anterior mediastinal neoplasm
- Most common primary thymic neoplasm
- Imaging & demographics do not reliably differentiate thymoma from other thymic malignancies
- No lymphadenopathy
- Paraneoplastic syndromes more common

Malignant Germ Cell Neoplasm

- Symptomatic men, usually younger than 40
- Dominant locally invasive mass, lymphadenopathy

Mediastinal Hodgkin Lymphoma

- Hodgkin lymphoma more commonly involves thymus than non-Hodgkin lymphoma
- May calcify with treatment

Mediastinal Metastatic Lymphadenopathy

- Discrete lymph node enlargement, nodal coalescence
- Lung, breast, head & neck, & GU cancers

PATHOLOGY

General Features

- Associated abnormalities
  - Up to 20% of thymic carcinoids associated with multiple endocrine neoplasia (MEN) syndromes

Staging, Grading, & Classification

- Histologic diagnosis of malignancy in thymic carcinoma
- Thymic carcinoid thought to arise from amine precursor uptake & decarboxylase cells (APUD)

CLINICAL ISSUES

Presentation

- Most common signs/symptoms
  - Symptoms of mediastinal mass effect/invasion
  - Superior vena cava syndrome
  - Up to **40% of patients with thymic carcinoid** have **Cushing syndrome**
- Other signs/symptoms
  - Paraneoplastic syndromes rare in thymic carcinoma
    - Myasthenia gravis, pure red cell aplasia, hypogammaglobulinemia

Demographics

- Epidemiology
  - Thymic malignancy accounts for approximately 20% of thymic epithelial neoplasms
- Thymic carcinoma: Average age 50; M = F
- Thymic carcinoid: Average age 45; M:F = 3:1

Natural History & Prognosis

- Thymic carcinoma: 5-year survival rate 30%
- Thymic carcinoid: 5-year survival rate 65%

DIAGNOSTIC CHECKLIST

Image Interpretation Pearls

- Thymic carcinoma, thymic carcinoid, & thymoma not reliably differentiated on imaging
- Distant metastases & lymphadenopathy more common in thymic malignancy

SELECTED REFERENCES

1. Rosado-de-Christenson ML et al: Imaging of thymic epithelial neoplasms. Hematol Oncol Clin North Am. 22(3):409-31, 2008
2. Nishino M et al: The thymus: a comprehensive review. Radiographics. 26(2):335-48, 2006

THYMOLIPOMA

Key Facts

Terminology
- Rare, benign primary thymic neoplasm

Imaging
- Radiography
  - Large anterior mediastinal mass
  - Involvement of anterior inferior mediastinum
  - Smooth or lobular, well-defined borders
  - May mimic cardiomegaly & hemidiaphragm elevation
- CT
  - Fat attenuation mass with soft tissue elements
  - Rarely predominant soft tissue or fat attenuation
  - Anatomic connection to thymus
- MR
  - T1 hyperintense fat components
  - Intermediate signal intensity soft tissue components on T1WI & T2WI

Top Differential Diagnoses
- Lipoma
- Mediastinal lipomatosis
- Teratoma
- Mediastinal fat pad
- Morgagni hernia
- Liposarcoma

Clinical Issues
- Symptoms/signs
  - Most patients asymptomatic
  - Symptoms from mass effect
- Mean age: 22 years
- Surgical resection curative

Diagnostic Checklist
- Consider thymolipoma in young patient with large, pliable, fatty, noninvasive anterior mediastinal mass

*(**Left**) PA chest radiograph of a 17-year-old patient with thymolipoma shows a left anterior mediastinal mass ➡ that exhibits the hilum overlay sign. Thymolipoma typically affects young asymptomatic patients. (**Right**) Axial CECT of a patient with thymolipoma shows a left anterior mediastinal mass ➡ of predominant fat attenuation with internal soft tissue strands and nodules in the anatomic location of the thymus, a well-described CT appearance of this rare neoplasm.*

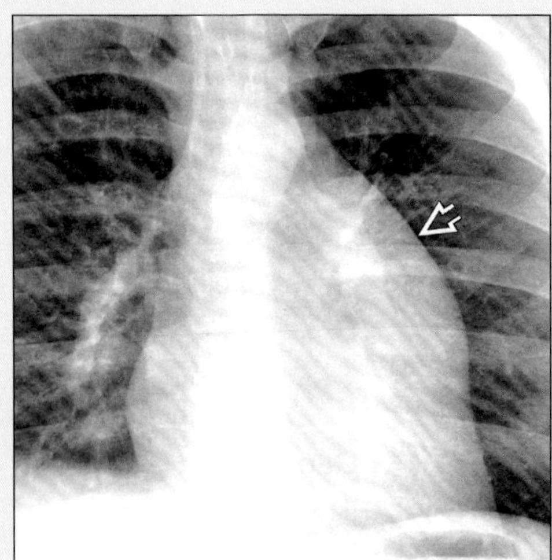

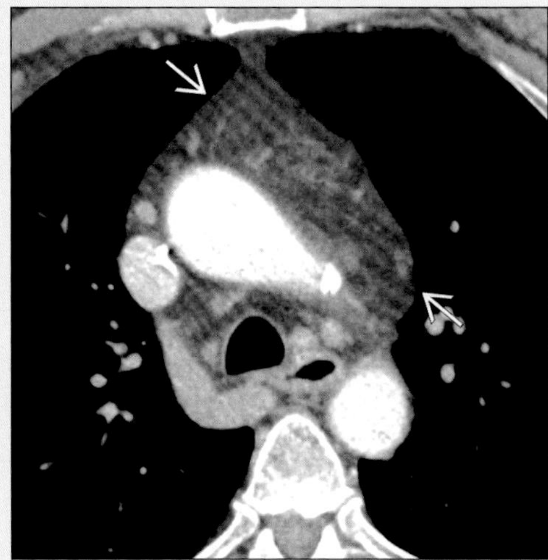

*(**Left**) PA chest radiograph of an asymptomatic 50-year-old woman with thymolipoma shows a mass located at the right cardiophrenic angle ➡. (**Right**) Axial NECT of the same patient shows a mass ➡ of predominant fat attenuation with an atypical dominant central soft tissue nodule. In this case, visualization of an anatomic connection of the lesion to the region of the thymus (not shown) suggested the diagnosis of thymolipoma. Thymolipomas frequently affect the inferior aspect of the anterior mediastinum.*

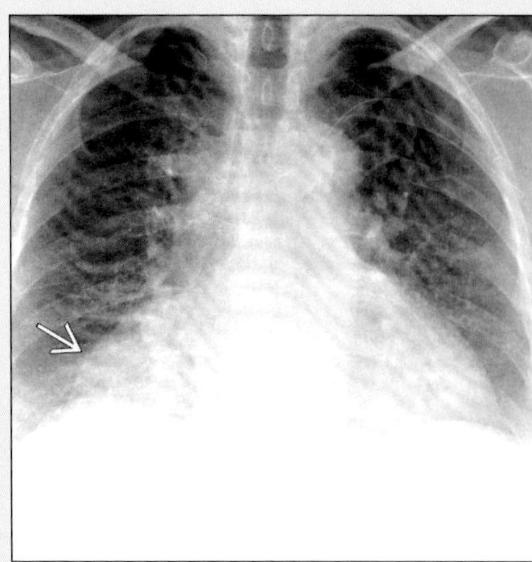

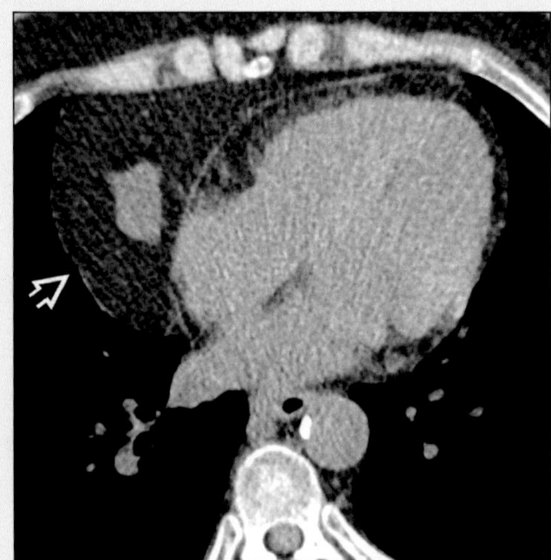

THYMOLIPOMA

TERMINOLOGY

Definitions

- Rare, benign primary thymic neoplasm

IMAGING

General Features

- Best diagnostic clue
  - Anterior mediastinal mass with **fat & soft tissue components**
- Location
  - Anterior mediastinum, typically inferior aspect of anterior mediastinum
- Size
  - Typically large, averaging 20 cm in diameter
- Morphology
  - Well circumscribed
  - Pliable mass, conforms to adjacent organs
  - May exhibit positional changes in shape

Radiographic Findings

- Large unilateral or bilateral anterior mediastinal mass
- Preferential involvement of **inferior aspect of anterior mediastinum**
- Smooth or lobular, well-defined borders
- Conforms to adjacent structures, may mimic cardiomegaly & hemidiaphragm elevation

CT Findings

- Well-defined fat attenuation mass with intrinsic soft tissue elements
- Rarely predominant soft tissue or fat attenuation
- Anatomic connection to thymus

MR Findings

- T1 hyperintense fat components
- Intermediate signal intensity soft tissue components on T1WI & T2WI

Imaging Recommendations

- Best imaging tool
  - CT for determination of extent of disease & surgical planning
  - MR may help confirm fat components

DIFFERENTIAL DIAGNOSIS

Lipoma

- Homogeneous, well-circumscribed fat attenuation
- Absent or small linear soft tissue components
- 2% of primary mediastinal neoplasms

Mediastinal Lipomatosis

- Unencapsulated mediastinal fat
- Associated with obesity & steroid use

Teratoma

- Typically exhibits cystic components &/or calcification

Mediastinal Fat Pad

- Located at cardiophrenic angle
- Associated with obesity, steroids, Cushing syndrome

Morgagni Hernia

- Herniation of abdominal contents through anteromedial diaphragmatic defect
- May contain omental fat, liver, colon
- Omental vessels are important clue

Liposarcoma

- Conspicuous irregular soft tissue components
- Most commonly in middle-posterior mediastinum
- Aggressive features: Local invasion, lymphadenopathy, metastases
- Thymic liposarcoma has been reported
- Rapid growth suggests malignancy

PATHOLOGY

Gross Pathologic & Surgical Features

- Encapsulated soft, yellow tumor

Microscopic Features

- Admixture of mature adipose tissue & thymic tissue

CLINICAL ISSUES

Presentation

- Most common signs/symptoms
  - Most patients **asymptomatic**
- Other signs/symptoms
  - Symptoms from local mass effect on heart & lungs
    - Dyspnea, cough, paroxysmal tachycardia
  - Reported cases of associated myasthenia gravis, aplastic anemia, & Graves disease

Demographics

- Age
  - Mean: 22 years; wide age range
  - Most patients < 50 years
- Gender
  - No gender predilection
- Epidemiology
  - < 5% of primary thymic neoplasms

Treatment

- Surgical resection curative in symptomatic or enlarging lesions

DIAGNOSTIC CHECKLIST

Consider

- Thymolipoma in young patient with large, pliable, fatty, noninvasive anterior mediastinal mass

Image Interpretation Pearls

- Cross-sectional imaging for documentation of anatomic connection of mass to thymic bed

SELECTED REFERENCES

1. Rosado-de-Christenson ML et al: Imaging of thymic epithelial neoplasms. Hematol Oncol Clin North Am. 22(3):409-31, 2008
2. Gaerte SC et al: Fat-containing lesions of the chest. Radiographics. 22 Spec No:S61-78, 2002
3. Boiselle PM et al: Fat attenuation lesions of the mediastinum. J Comput Assist Tomogr. 25(6):881-9, 2001

MEDIASTINAL TERATOMA

Key Facts

Terminology

- Primary germ cell neoplasm (GCN) containing tissues derived from ≥ 2 germinal layers

Imaging

- Radiography
  - Well-defined spherical or ovoid anterior mediastinal mass with smooth or lobular borders
  - Radiographic calcification (20%)
- CT
  - Heterogeneous multilocular cystic anterior mediastinal mass
  - Smooth or lobular borders
  - Fluid attenuation cysts (90%)
  - Fat (75%); fat-fluid levels (10%)
  - Calcification (50%)
- MR superior for tissue characterization & for confirmation of intrinsic fat

Top Differential Diagnoses

- Thymic cyst
- Cystic thymic neoplasm
- Mediastinal lymphangioma

Pathology

- Macroscopic cysts in majority of cases
- Lipid-rich sebaceous material

Clinical Issues

- Symptoms/signs
  - Most patients asymptomatic
  - Cough, dyspnea, chest pain
- Excellent prognosis
  - Nearly 100% 5-year survival

Diagnostic Checklist

- Cystic anterior mediastinal mass containing fat is considered diagnostic of mature teratoma

*(**Left**) PA chest radiograph of a 25-year-old man with a mature cystic teratoma shows a smoothly marginated right anterior mediastinal mass ➡ that exhibits the hilum overlay sign with visualization of the right interlobar pulmonary artery through the lesion. (**Right**) Lateral chest radiograph of the same patient shows that the mass projects over the heart, confirming the anterior mediastinal location of the lesion ➡. Patients with mature teratoma are typically young men or women in the 1st to 4th decades of life.*

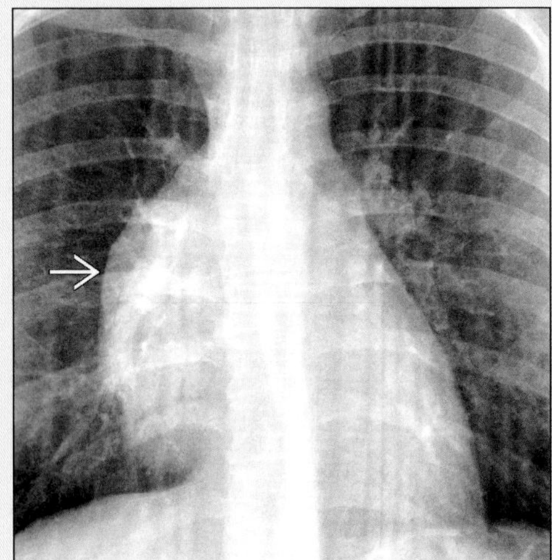

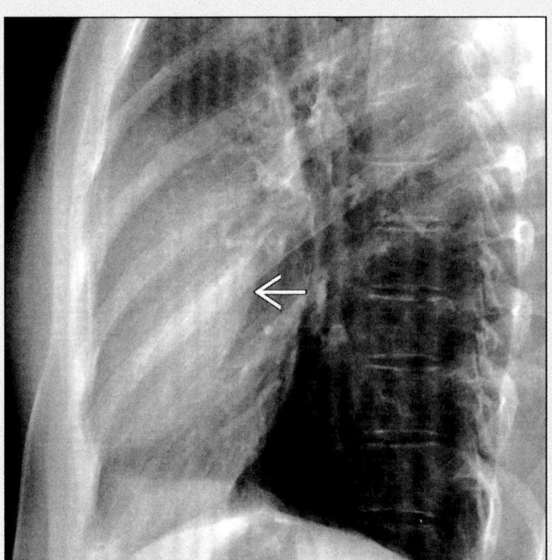

*(**Left**) Axial CECT of a 16-year-old boy with a mature cystic teratoma shows a right anterior mediastinal mass with soft tissue, fluid, and fat attenuation components. Mature teratomas are typically cystic, and 75% exhibit fat attenuation. (**Right**) Cut section of a mature teratoma shows multiple cystic areas ➡ intermixed with solid soft tissue components. The heterogeneous nature of these neoplasms results in characteristic findings on cross-sectional imaging studies. (Courtesy C. Moran, MD.)*

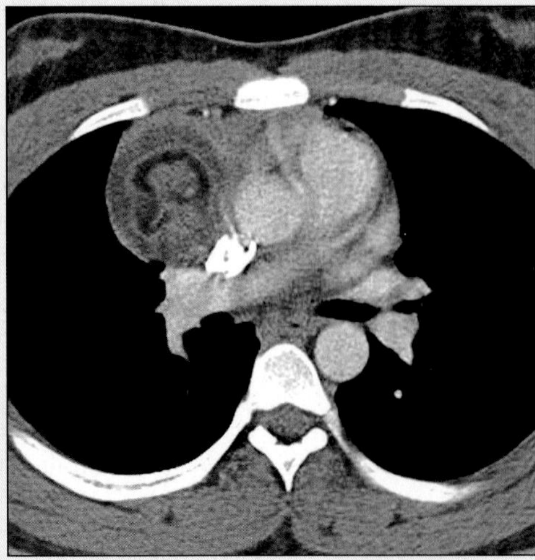

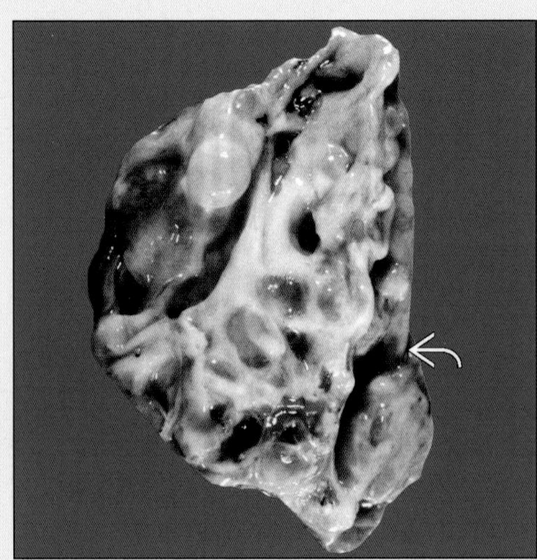

MEDIASTINAL TERATOMA

TERMINOLOGY

Synonyms

- **Germ cell neoplasm** (GCN)

Definitions

- Primary germ cell neoplasm containing tissues derived from at least 2 germinal layers

IMAGING

General Features

- Best diagnostic clue
  - Multilocular cystic anterior mediastinal mass
    - Fluid, fat, soft tissue, & calcification
  - Fat-fluid level in 10% of cases
  - Formed teeth & bone diagnostic, but rare
- Location
  - Anterior mediastinum, prevascular space
  - Other mediastinal compartment (5%)
- Size
  - May be large & multicompartmental
- Morphology
  - Spherical, well circumscribed
  - Most exhibit multilocular cystic components

Radiographic Findings

- Anterior mediastinal mass
  - Mediastinal widening
  - May mimic cardiomegaly
- Well-defined smooth or lobular margins
- Spherical or ovoid shape
- Radiographic calcification in 20%
  - Linear, rim-like, coarse
- Difficult to identify fat on radiographs
- Adjacent airspace disease: Atelectasis &/or consolidation
- Pleural effusion

CT Findings

- Well-defined, unilateral, anterior mediastinal mass
- Smooth or lobular borders
- Unilocular or multilocular cystic lesion
- Heterogeneous attenuation
  - **Fluid attenuation cysts (90%)**
    - Typically thin walled
  - Soft tissue components including cyst walls & septa
    - May exhibit contrast enhancement
  - **Fat attenuation cyst content (75%)**
    - Fat-fluid level diagnostic (10%)
  - **Calcification best detected on CT (50%)**
    - Rim-like or coarse
    - Rarely teeth or bone
- No lymphadenopathy
- Adjacent atelectasis, consolidation
- Pleural &/or pericardial effusion
- Teratoma with malignant component
  - Dominant solid soft tissue components
  - Thick, enhancing cyst capsule
  - Poorly defined margins
  - Mass effect, local invasion
  - Lymphadenopathy & metastatic disease
  - Less frequent fat contents

MR Findings

- T1WI
  - Fat components are T1 hyperintense
  - Proteinaceous fluid & hemorrhage may be T1 hyperintense
- T1WI FS
  - Confirmation of fat components
- Heterogeneous anterior mediastinal mass
- Cystic components exhibit low signal intensity on T1WI & high signal intensity on T2WI

Ultrasonographic Findings

- Encapsulated mass with heterogeneously echogenic components

Imaging Recommendations

- Best imaging tool
  - CT optimally demonstrates multicompartmental extension & calcification
  - MR superior for tissue characterization & for confirmation of fat

DIFFERENTIAL DIAGNOSIS

Thymic Cyst

- Cyst with fluid attenuation, unilocular or multilocular
- High-attenuation content from hemorrhage, infection

Cystic Thymic Neoplasm

- Cystic thymoma
  - Anterior mediastinal cystic lesion with mural nodule(s)
- Thymic carcinoma or carcinoid
  - Lymphadenopathy, local invasion

Mediastinal Lymphangioma

- Multilocular cystic mass
- Involvement of neck, chest wall, axilla

Other Germ Cell Neoplasms

- 10% of primary mediastinal masses
- Seminoma, embryonal carcinoma, endodermal sinus (yolk sac) tumor, choriocarcinoma, mixed types
  - Seminoma typically homogeneous
  - Nonseminomatous germ cell neoplasms are typically heterogeneous from central necrosis & hemorrhage
- Serum tumor markers
  - β-human chorionic gonadotropin, α-fetoprotein

Lipoma

- Homogeneous, encapsulated mass of adipose tissue
- Fat attenuation with soft tissue wisps & vessels

Mediastinal Lipomatosis

- Unencapsulated fat infiltration of mediastinum
- Associated with obesity & steroid use

Mediastinal Fat Pad

- Associated with obesity, steroids, Cushing syndrome
- Cardiophrenic angle fat, no soft tissue or calcification

Morgagni Hernia

- Herniation of abdominal contents through anterior diaphragmatic foramen
- May contain omental fat, liver, bowel

MEDIASTINAL TERATOMA

Thymolipoma

- Rare, benign primary thymic neoplasm
- Typically large, averaging 20 cm
- Soft, pliable tumor without aggressive features
- Anatomic connection to thymus

Liposarcoma

- Most commonly in middle-posterior mediastinum
- Aggressive features: Local invasion, lymphadenopathy, metastases
- May exhibit rapid growth

Metastatic Disease

- Malignant teratoma may metastasize to mediastinum
- Gonadal source usually excluded when malignant teratoma diagnosed in mediastinum

PATHOLOGY

General Features

- Etiology
  - Postulated origin in rests of primitive germ cells left in mediastinum during migration of yolk sac endoderm to urogenital ridge
  - Mediastinum most common location of extragonadal germ cell neoplasms
- Tissues derived from ≥ 2 germinal layers
  - Ectoderm
    - Typically predominates
    - Includes hair, skin, teeth
  - Mesoderm
    - Cartilage, bone, muscle
  - Endoderm
    - Bronchial or gastrointestinal epithelium, mucus glands
    - Pancreatic tissue

Staging, Grading, & Classification

- Pathologic classification
  - **Mature teratoma**
    - Most common; 70% of mediastinal germ cell neoplasms
    - Well-differentiated tissues
  - **Immature teratoma**
    - Contain immature elements (neuroectoderm)
    - Typically benign course in children, more aggressive in adults
  - Teratoma with malignant component
    - Seminoma
    - Yolk sac tumor
    - Embryonal carcinoma
    - Other malignant epithelial component
    - More common in men
  - Teratoma with malignant mesenchymal component
    - Angiosarcoma
    - Rhabdomyosarcoma
    - Osteosarcoma
    - Chondrosarcoma

Gross Pathologic & Surgical Features

- Macroscopic cysts in majority of cases
- Lipid-rich sebaceous material
- Soft tissue components
- Hair, bone, teeth

CLINICAL ISSUES

Presentation

- Most common signs/symptoms
  - Most patients asymptomatic unless lesions are large
  - Teratoma with malignant component is more likely to cause symptoms
- Other signs/symptoms
  - Cough, dyspnea, chest pain
  - Upper respiratory complaints, fever
  - Rupture & infection reported
    - Fistulous tract from digestive enzymes reported

Demographics

- Age
  - Most common in children & young adults
- Gender
  - M = F

Natural History & Prognosis

- Mature teratomas are benign & slow growing
  - Nearly 100% 5-year survival
- Malignant teratoma carries very poor prognosis

Treatment

- Options, risks, complications
  - Rupture into adjacent pleural or pericardial space in up to 30% of cases
    - May also rupture into lung/bronchi
- Mature teratoma
  - Surgical excision curative
- **Mediastinal growing teratoma syndrome**
  - Continued slow growth of benign mature teratoma components after chemotherapy for malignant component

DIAGNOSTIC CHECKLIST

Consider

- Teratoma in patients with cystic anterior mediastinal masses without fat or calcification
- Malignant GCN if dominant solid component, local invasion, &/or lymphadenopathy
- Exclusion of metastasis from gonadal source in cases of mediastinal teratoma with malignant component

Image Interpretation Pearls

- Unilocular or multilocular cystic anterior mediastinal mass with fat is considered diagnostic of mature teratoma
- Fat-fluid levels & teeth are rare but diagnostic of mature teratoma

SELECTED REFERENCES

1. Takahashi K et al: Computed tomography and magnetic resonance imaging of mediastinal tumors. J Magn Reson Imaging. 32(6):1325-39, 2010
2. Moeller KH et al: Mediastinal mature teratoma: imaging features. AJR Am J Roentgenol. 169(4):985-90, 1997
3. Moran CA et al: Primary germ cell tumors of the mediastinum: I. Analysis of 322 cases with special emphasis on teratomatous lesions and a proposal for histopathologic classification and clinical staging. Cancer. 80(4):681-90, 1997

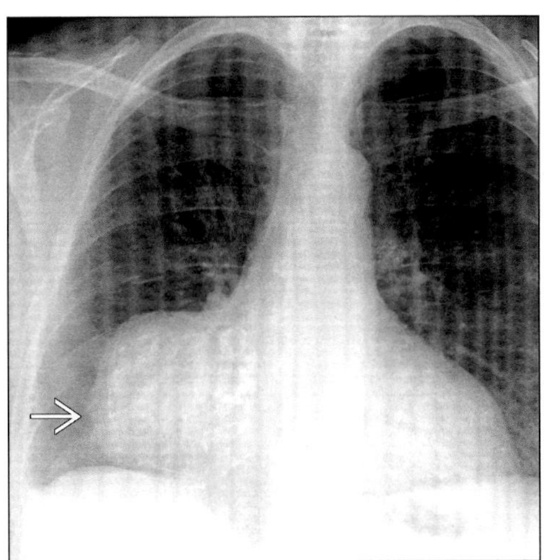

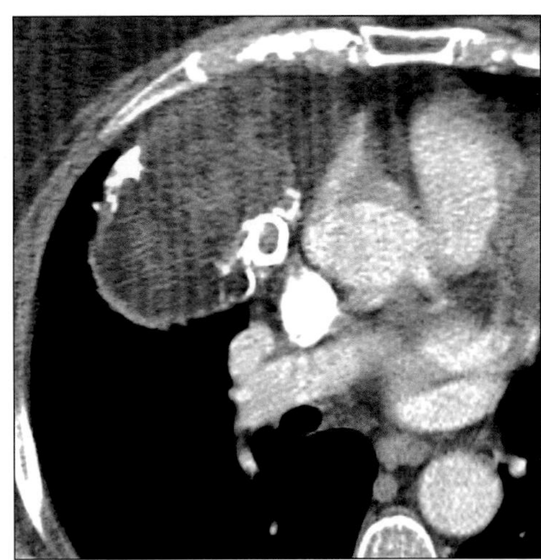

(Left) *PA chest radiograph of a patient with mature teratoma shows a spherical right cardiophrenic angle mass ➡ with intrinsic curvilinear and rounded calcifications. Because of radiographically evident calcification, mature teratoma should be considered in the differential diagnosis.* **(Right)** *Axial CECT of the same patient shows a right cardiophrenic angle mass with internal fat, fluid, soft tissue, and calcification. Calcification in mediastinal teratomas is typically rim-like, linear, or coarse.*

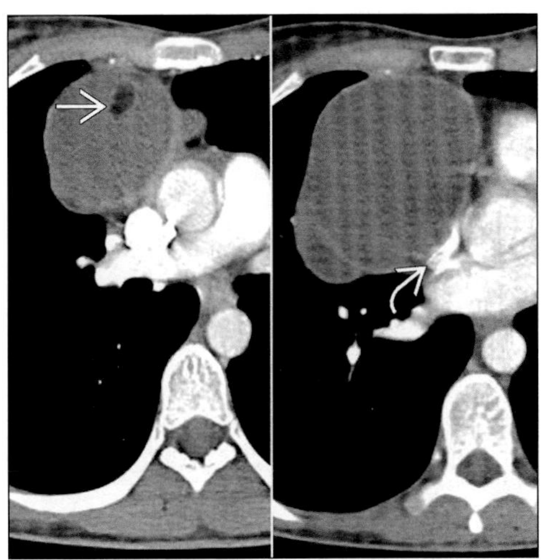

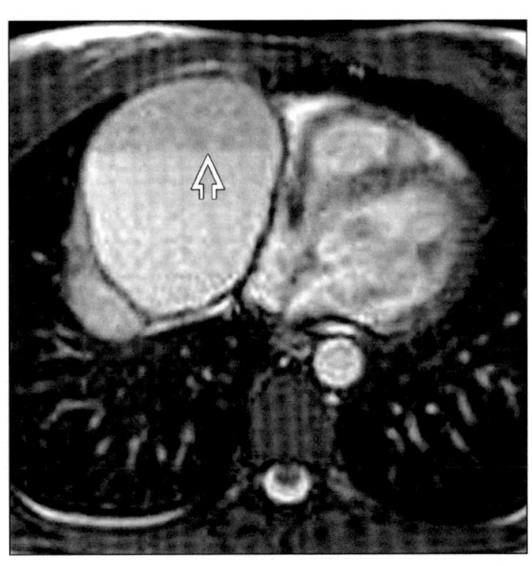

(Left) *Composite image with axial CECT of a young woman with mature teratoma shows a multilocular cystic right anterior mediastinal mass that produces mass effect on the superior vena cava ➡. Although the lesion exhibits predominant fluid attenuation, focal fat attenuation ➡ allows a confident prospective diagnosis of mature teratoma.* **(Right)** *Axial T2WI MR confirms the multilocular cystic nature of the mature teratoma and demonstrates an intrinsic fluid-fluid level ➡ that was not visible on CT.*

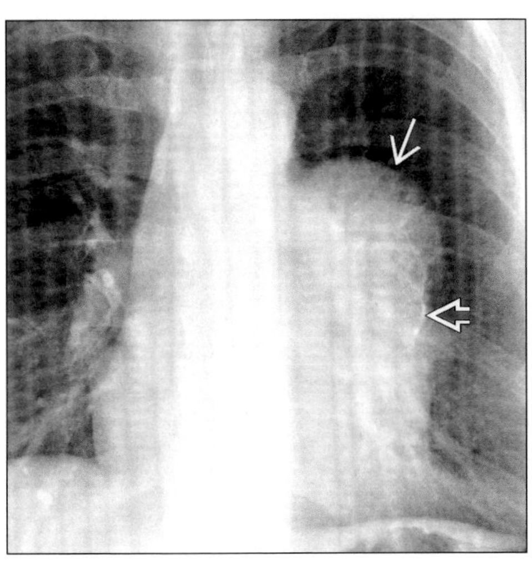

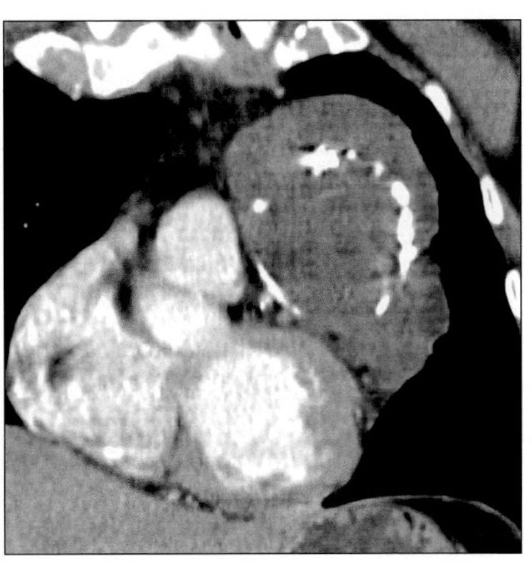

(Left) *PA chest radiograph of a patient with mature teratoma shows a polylobular left anterior mediastinal mass ➡ with curvilinear calcification ➡. Calcifications are detected radiographically in 20% of mature teratomas.* **(Right)** *Coronal CECT of the same patient shows an ovoid polylobular mass with curvilinear calcifications and heterogeneous attenuation. Although fat is not visible, mature teratoma should be considered based on the morphologic features of the lesion and the pattern of calcification.*

MEDIASTINAL SEMINOMA

Key Facts

Terminology

- Malignant germ cell neoplasm (MGCN)
- Definition
  - Primary malignant mediastinal germ cell neoplasm

Imaging

- Radiography
  - Large, lobular anterior mediastinal mass
- CT
  - Large, lobular, mildly enhancing anterior mediastinal soft tissue mass; rare cysts or calcification
  - Mass effect on adjacent mediastinal structures
  - Mediastinal lymphadenopathy
- MR
  - Homogeneous anterior mediastinal mass
  - T2 hypointense, T1 C+ enhancing septa
- PET/CT: FDG-avid mass in anterior mediastinum

Top Differential Diagnoses

- Thymoma
- Lymphoma
- Teratoma

Pathology

- Sheets of uniform round or polyhedral cells

Clinical Issues

- Symptoms/signs
  - Chest pain, dyspnea, cough
  - Fever, weakness, weight loss
- 90% occur in men aged 20-40 years
- Prognosis: 90% 5-year survival without metastases

Diagnostic Checklist

- Consider seminoma in symptomatic male patient with homogeneous anterior mediastinal mass

*(**Left**) PA chest radiograph of a middle-aged man who presented with chest pain shows a lobular mass ➔ in the left anterior mediastinum. The lesion does not obscure the aortic arch. (**Right**) Axial CECT of the same patient shows a polylobular anterior mediastinal mass extending to both sides of the midline. The lesion exhibits mild contrast enhancement. Mediastinal seminoma may mimic mediastinal Hodgkin and non-Hodgkin lymphomas with nodal coalescence.*

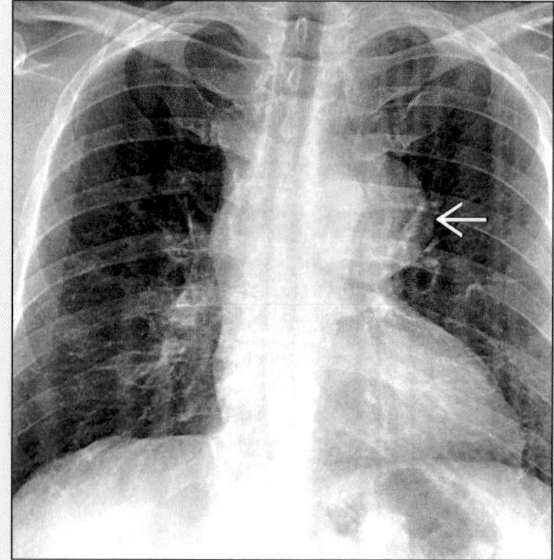

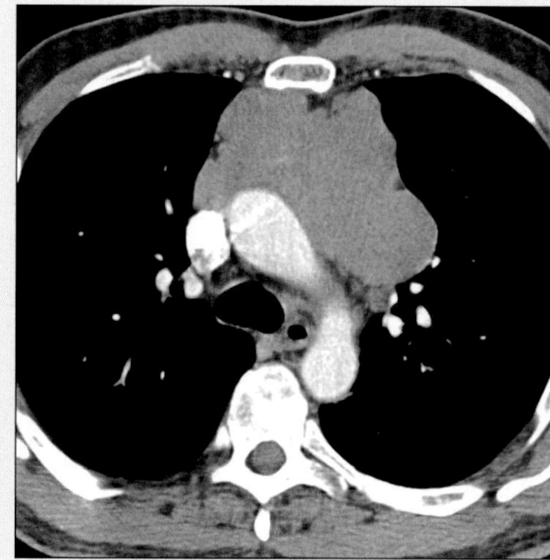

*(**Left**) Axial fused FDG PET/CT of a 39-year-old man shows marked uptake within an incidentally discovered anterior mediastinal mass. An intrathymic seminoma was diagnosed on biopsy. (**Right**) Axial CECT of a 42-year-old man 4 years after chemotherapy for a 6 cm mediastinal seminoma shows stable, nonenhancing mediastinal soft tissue ➔. Follow-up PET/CT showed no evidence of metabolic activity. Residual soft tissue masses are frequently seen following chemotherapy or radiation for mediastinal seminoma.*

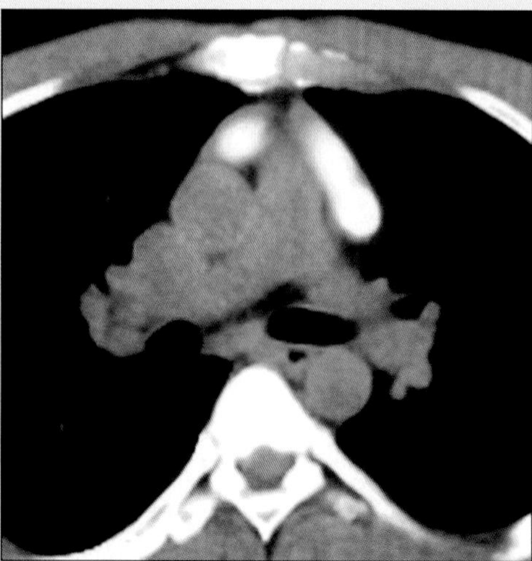

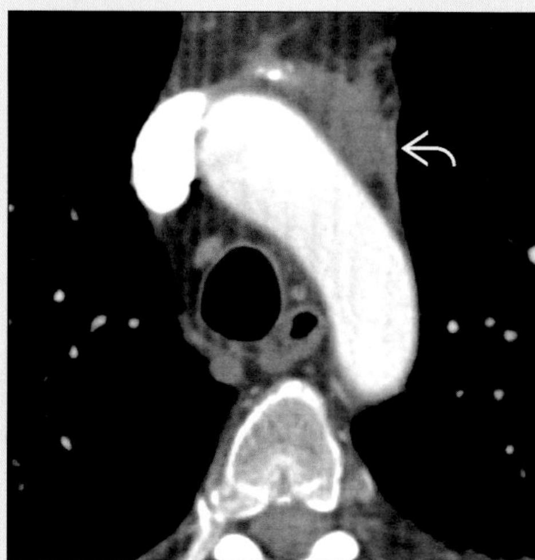

MEDIASTINAL SEMINOMA

TERMINOLOGY

Synonyms

- **Germinoma**
- **Dysgerminoma**

Definitions

- **Primary mediastinal malignant germ cell neoplasm (MGCN)**

IMAGING

General Features

- Best diagnostic clue
  - Large anterior mediastinal mass in young man
- Location
  - Anterior mediastinum
- Size
  - Typically large (> 5 cm)
- Morphology
  - Homogeneous, lobular borders

Radiographic Findings

- Radiography
  - **Large, lobular anterior mediastinal mass**

CT Findings

- CECT
  - Large, lobular, mildly enhancing **anterior mediastinal soft tissue mass**; rare cysts or calcification
  - Mass effect on adjacent mediastinal structures is typical
  - Mediastinal lymphadenopathy

MR Findings

- Homogeneous mass with T2 hypointense, T1 C+ enhancing septa

Nuclear Medicine Findings

- PET/CT
  - FDG-avid mass in anterior mediastinum
  - Detection of residual disease following initial treatment

Imaging Recommendations

- Best imaging tool
  - Contrast-enhanced CT is imaging modality of choice

DIFFERENTIAL DIAGNOSIS

Thymoma

- Anterior mediastinal lobular mass; cysts & necrosis more frequent
- Patients typically > 40 years

Lymphoma

- Multiple lymph node groups & mediastinal compartments involved
- Rarely calcifies prior to treatment

Teratoma

- Multilocular cystic mass with fat, calcium, &/or soft tissue attenuation

Goiter

- Direct connection to thyroid gland
- Tracheal deviation & coarse calcifications are common

PATHOLOGY

General Features

- Associated abnormalities
  - 30% have elevated serum β-human chorionic gonadotropin

Gross Pathologic & Surgical Features

- Large, unencapsulated, well-circumscribed mass
- Hemorrhage, necrosis, cysts rare
- May be located entirely within thymus

Microscopic Features

- Uniform round or polyhedral cells

CLINICAL ISSUES

Presentation

- Most common signs/symptoms
  - Chest pain, dyspnea, cough
  - Fever, weakness, weight loss
  - 25% asymptomatic
  - 10% present with superior vena cava syndrome

Demographics

- Age
  - 90% in men aged 20-40 years
- Epidemiology
  - Most common primary mediastinal MGCN of a single histology (25-50% of all MGCN)
  - 2-4% of all mediastinal masses

Natural History & Prognosis

- Majority are metastatic at diagnosis
  - Regional lymph nodes, lung, bone, liver
- 90% 5-year survival in absence of extrapulmonary metastases
  - Extrapulmonary metastases portend poor prognosis
- Residual mass common on CT following treatment
  - Typically necrotic tissue or desmoplastic reaction
  - PET/CT may play a role in surveillance for recurrent disease

Treatment

- Cisplatin, etoposide, & bleomycin (3 or 4 cycles)
- External beam radiation therapy (35-50 Gy)

DIAGNOSTIC CHECKLIST

Consider

- Seminoma in symptomatic male patient with homogeneous anterior mediastinal mass

SELECTED REFERENCES

1. Strollo DC et al: Primary mediastinal malignant germ cell neoplasms: imaging features. Chest Surg Clin N Am. 12(4):645-58, 2002
2. Rosado-de-Christenson ML et al: From the archives of the AFIP. Mediastinal germ cell tumors: radiologic and pathologic correlation. Radiographics. 12(5):1013-30, 1992

NONSEMINOMATOUS MALIGNANT GERM CELL NEOPLASM

Key Facts

Terminology
- Malignant germ cell neoplasm (MGCN)
- Primary mediastinal yolk sac tumor, choriocarcinoma, embryonal carcinoma, mixed type germ cell neoplasm

Imaging
- Radiography
  - Large anterior mediastinal mass
  - Mass effect on adjacent structures
- CT
  - Large, heterogeneous anterior mediastinal mass
  - Nodular peripheral enhancement
  - Central low attenuation: Hemorrhage & necrosis
  - Lymphadenopathy
- MR
  - Large, heterogeneously enhancing anterior mediastinal mass

Top Differential Diagnoses
- Seminoma
- Thymoma
- Lymphoma

Pathology
- Large necrotic locally invasive mass
- Elevated serum β-human chorionic gonadotropin &/ or α-fetoprotein in 85%

Clinical Issues
- Symptoms/signs: Chest pain, dyspnea, weight loss
- Treatment: Chemotherapy & resection of residual mass

Diagnostic Checklist
- Consider nonseminomatous MGCN in male patient with large, locally invasive, heterogeneous anterior mediastinal mass

*(**Left**) PA chest radiograph of a 30-year-old man with mixed-type mediastinal malignant germ cell neoplasm shows a polylobular left anterior mediastinal mass and several pulmonary nodules, consistent with metastases. (**Right**) Axial CECT of the same patient shows a heterogeneously enhancing soft tissue mass in the left anterior mediastinum and a left posterior pleural metastasis. Primary mediastinal MGCN are highly aggressive lesions and are usually metastatic at the time of diagnosis.*

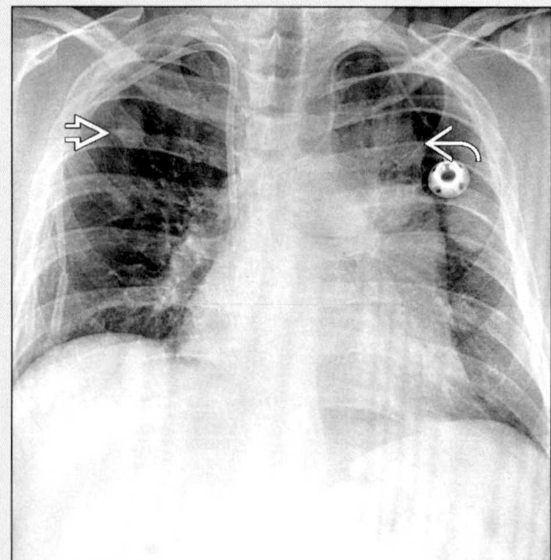

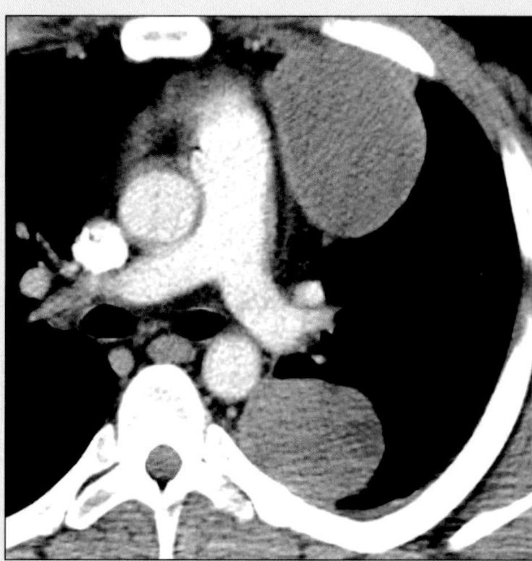

*(**Left**) Coronal CECT of a 41-year-old man with mediastinal yolk sac tumor shows a large heterogeneous anterior mediastinal mass displacing the heart caudally, soft tissue thickening of the pericardium, pericardial effusion, and a right lung metastasis. (**Right**) Axial CECT of a 31-year-old man shows large, heterogeneous mediastinal masses with mass effect upon or invasion of the pulmonary trunk. Although biopsy confirmed embryonal carcinoma, the presence of fat suggests mixed-type MGCN.*

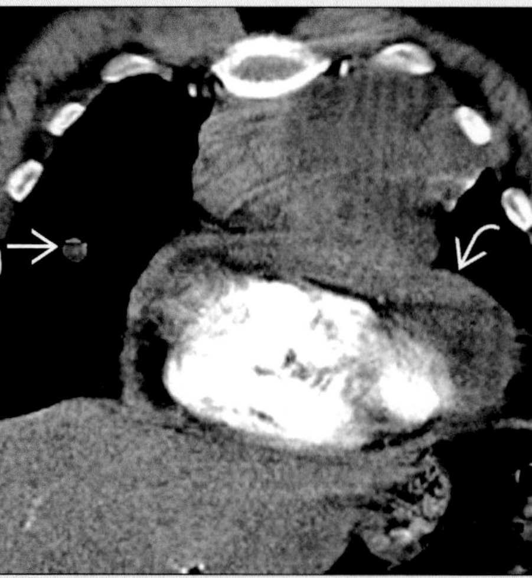

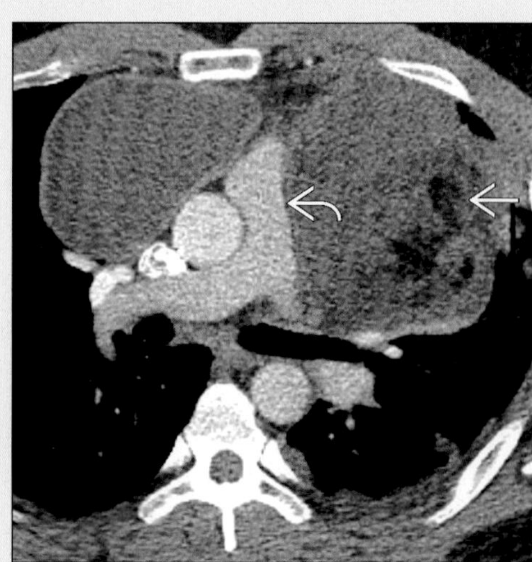

NONSEMINOMATOUS MALIGNANT GERM CELL NEOPLASM

TERMINOLOGY

Abbreviations

- **Malignant germ cell neoplasm (MGCN)**

Definitions

- **Primary mediastinal MGCN**
  - Yolk sac (endodermal sinus) tumor
  - Choriocarcinoma
  - Embryonal carcinoma
  - Mixed type germ cell neoplasm

IMAGING

General Features

- Best diagnostic clue
  - Large, heterogeneous anterior mediastinal mass in young male patient

Radiographic Findings

- Large anterior mediastinal mass
- Mass effect on adjacent structures
- Pleural effusion

CT Findings

- Large, **heterogeneous anterior mediastinal mass**
- **Nodular peripheral enhancement**
- **Central low attenuation** from hemorrhage & necrosis
- May invade adjacent structures, including lung
- Lymphadenopathy
- Pleural/pericardial effusion
- Pleural/pericardial thickening/nodules
- Pulmonary metastases

MR Findings

- Large, heterogeneously enhancing anterior mediastinal mass
- T1 hyperintense foci corresponding to hemorrhage

Imaging Recommendations

- Best imaging tool
  - CECT is imaging modality of choice

DIFFERENTIAL DIAGNOSIS

Seminoma

- Large, homogeneous anterior mediastinal mass
- Rarely cystic or necrotic

Thymoma

- Unilateral anterior mediastinal mass
- May exhibit cystic change & central necrosis
  - Serum tumor markers for differentiation from MGCN

Lymphoma

- Involves multiple nodal groups & mediastinal compartments

Teratoma

- Multilocular cystic mass with fat, calcium, soft tissue

Goiter

- Direct mediastinal extension from thyroid gland
- Intense & sustained contrast enhancement

PATHOLOGY

General Features

- Associated abnormalities
  - Elevated serum β-human chorionic gonadotropin (HCG) &/or α-fetoprotein (AFP) in 85%
  - Association with Klinefelter syndrome

Gross Pathologic & Surgical Features

- Large, necrotic, locally invasive mass

Microscopic Features

- Yolk sac tumor
- Embryonal carcinoma
- Choriocarcinoma
- Mixed type germ cell neoplasms contain at least 2 types of GCN

CLINICAL ISSUES

Presentation

- Most common signs/symptoms
  - Chest pain, dyspnea
  - Weight loss, fever, chills
- Other signs/symptoms
  - Gynecomastia due to elevated serum β-human chorionic gonadotropin

Demographics

- Age
  - Typically 20-40 years
- Gender
  - Males almost exclusively affected
- Epidemiology
  - Less common than seminoma & teratoma

Natural History & Prognosis

- Biopsy required for definitive diagnosis
- Metastases usually present at diagnosis
- Increased risk of developing metachronous testicular GCN (10% at 10 years)
- High incidence of hematologic disorders: Acute myelogenous leukemia, myelodysplasia, malignant mastocytosis, malignant histiocytosis

Treatment

- Etoposide, Ifosfamide, cisplatin (VIP): Chemotherapy followed by surgical resection of residual mass
  - 45% 5-year progression-free survival

DIAGNOSTIC CHECKLIST

Consider

- Nonseminomatous germ cell neoplasm in male patient with large, locally invasive, heterogeneous anterior mediastinal mass

Image Interpretation Pearls

- Testicular ultrasound used to exclude testicular primary MGCN

SELECTED REFERENCES

1. Ueno T et al: Spectrum of germ cell tumors: from head to toe. Radiographics. 24(2):387-404, 2004

NEUROGENIC NEOPLASMS OF THE NERVE SHEATH

Key Facts

Terminology

- Peripheral nerve sheath tumors (PNST)
  - Schwannoma & neurofibroma
- Malignant peripheral nerve sheath tumor (MPNST)

Imaging

- Radiography
  - Spherical paravertebral mass
  - Wide neural foramen
  - Benign pressure erosion of adjacent skeleton
  - Neurofibromatosis: Multifocal neurogenic neoplasms
- CT
  - Spherical paravertebral mass
  - Dumbbell tumor extension into spinal canal (10%)
  - Variable contrast enhancement
- MR for optimal assessment of intraspinal/extradural extension & spinal cord involvement

Top Differential Diagnoses

- Sympathetic ganglion tumor
- Paraganglioma
- Lateral thoracic meningocele

Clinical Issues

- Often asymptomatic
- Demographics: M = F
  - Schwannoma: Average age in 5th decade
  - Neurofibroma: Usually 2nd-4th decades
- Treatment: Surgical excision
- Prognosis
  - Indolent slow growth
  - 5-year survival of patients with MPNST: 35%

Diagnostic Checklist

- Consider PNST in adult patient with spherical paravertebral mass & skeletal pressure erosion

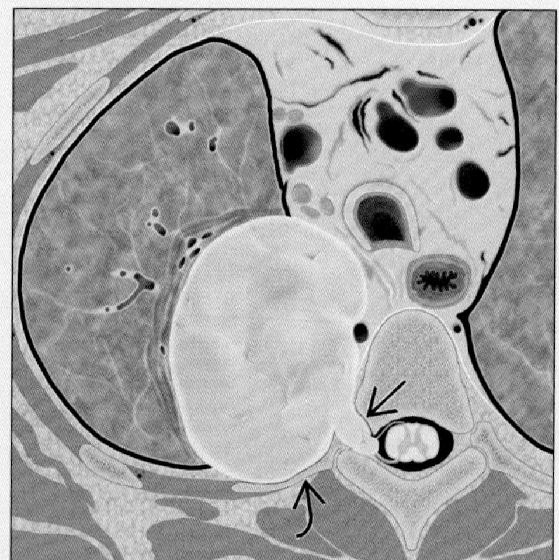

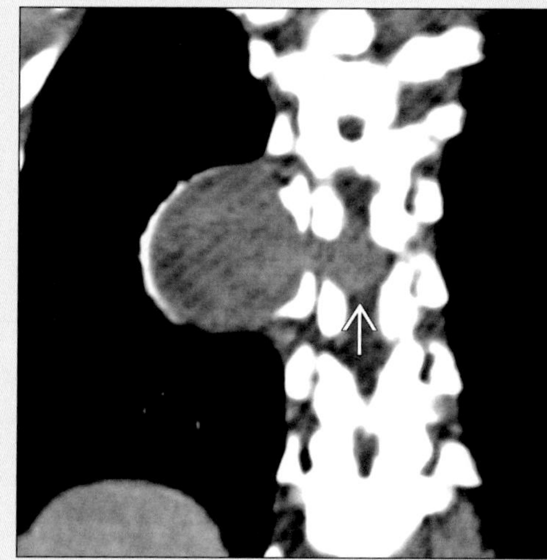

(Left) *Graphic shows the morphologic features of PNST, which manifests as a spherical paravertebral soft tissue mass that may produce benign skeletal pressure erosion ⇨ and widening of the neural foramen ⇨.* ***(Right)*** *Coronal CTA of a 33-year-old woman evaluated for suspected pulmonary embolism shows an incidental heterogeneously enhancing right paravertebral soft tissue mass that grows into the spinal canal ➡ and expands the T8 neural foramen. Ultrasound-guided biopsy confirmed the diagnosis of schwannoma.*

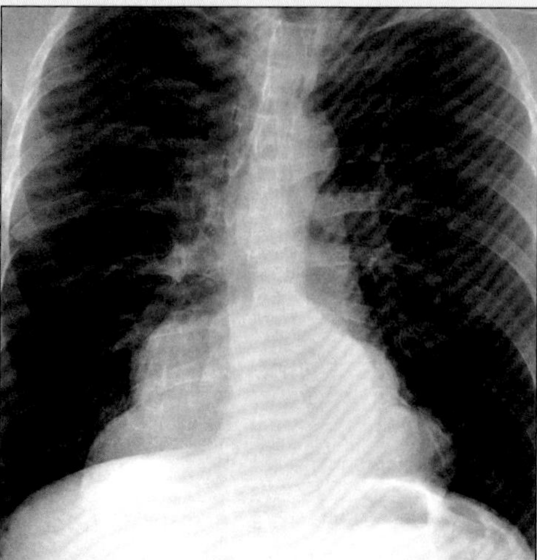

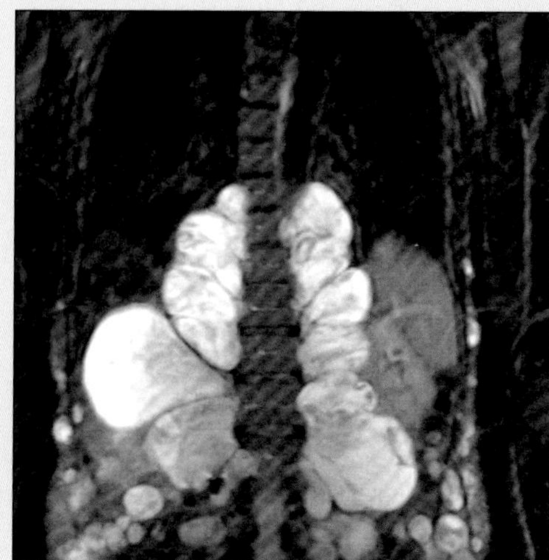

(Left) *PA chest radiograph of a 56-year-old man with neurofibromatosis type 1 (NF1) shows multiple bilateral paravertebral soft tissue masses with well-circumscribed lateral borders and nonvisualization of their medial margins.* ***(Right)*** *Coronal STIR MR shows numerous bilateral high signal intensity paravertebral masses arising from the posterior thoracic nerve roots. Plexiform neurofibromas are seen in 25% of patients with NF1, are difficult to treat, and undergo malignant degeneration in 4%.*

NEUROGENIC NEOPLASMS OF THE NERVE SHEATH

TERMINOLOGY

Definitions

- **Peripheral nerve sheath tumor (PNST)**
  - Schwannoma
  - Neurofibroma
- **Malignant peripheral nerve sheath tumor (MPNST)**
  - Spindle cell sarcoma of nerve sheath origin

IMAGING

General Features

- Best diagnostic clue
  - Spherical paravertebral mass with widened neural foramen
- Location
  - May occur along any peripheral nerve
    - Most commonly intercostal nerve; growth along undersurface of rib
    - May be centered on neural foramen & grow into spinal canal
    - Involvement of phrenic & vagus nerves less common
- Morphology
  - Spherical shape & horizontal axis

Radiographic Findings

- **Spherical or oblong well-marginated paravertebral mass** spanning 1-2 rib interspaces
  - Often centered at neural foramen, may widen neural foramen on lateral radiograph
  - Benign pressure erosion of adjacent skeleton: Posterior ribs, vertebrae
- May follow axis of involved nerve
  - Horizontal extension along intercostal nerve
- **Incomplete border** due to extrapulmonary location
- **Cervicothoracic sign**: Air-soft tissue interface extends above clavicle indicating posterior (paravertebral) location
- **Neurofibromatosis**: Multifocal neurogenic neoplasms
  - Skeletal abnormalities: Benign pressure erosion, skeletal dysplasia, scoliosis

CT Findings

- NECT
  - **Spherical or elongate paravertebral soft tissue mass**
    - Decreased attenuation on CT due to lipid or cystic degeneration
    - **Calcification in 10% of schwannomas**
  - **Evaluation of skeletal findings**: Benign pressure erosion of rib &/or vertebrae
  - **Dumbbell morphology** with extension into spinal canal (**10%**)
  - **Split fat sign**: Fat attenuation surrounding soft tissue neoplasm
  - **Neurofibromatosis**
    - **Multifocal neurogenic neoplasms**
    - Cutaneous nodules: Often multiple, well circumscribed
    - Skeletal manifestations
      - Well-marginated rib erosions from plexiform neurofibromas
      - Rib deformity from associated osseous dysplasia
      - Short segment, acute angle scoliosis
      - Posterior scalloping of vertebral bodies from dural ectasia
    - **Pulmonary manifestations**
      - Thin-walled upper lobe bullae associated with bilateral symmetric basal predominant fibrosis (rare)
      - Pulmonary metastases following malignant degeneration
- CECT
  - Decreased attenuation due to lipid, cystic degeneration
  - Variable contrast enhancement (homogeneous, heterogeneous)
    - Neurofibroma
      - More commonly enhances homogeneously
      - May exhibit early central contrast blush
    - Heterogeneity related to regions of cellular & acellular (myxoid) components
  - Local invasion, osseous destruction, & pleural effusion suggest MPNST
    - Low-attenuation regions due to hemorrhage & hyaline degeneration

MR Findings

- T1WI
  - Variable signal intensity, often isointense to spinal cord
  - Neurofibromas may exhibit central high signal
- T2WI
  - Intermediate to high T2 signal intensity
  - Tumor may be obscured by high signal intensity cerebrospinal fluid
  - Neurofibroma: May exhibit low central signal due to collagen deposition
    - **Target sign**: Central low signal surrounded by peripheral high signal intensity
  - Schwannoma: **Fascicular sign**, multiple hypointense small ring-like structures, correspond to histologic fascicular bundles
- T1WI C+ FS
  - Enhancement pattern mimics that of CECT
  - Neurofibromas may exhibit target appearance

Imaging Recommendations

- Best imaging tool
  - MR for optimal assessment of intraspinal/extradural extension & spinal cord involvement
- Protocol advice
  - Gadolinium helpful for delineating intradural neoplasm

DIFFERENTIAL DIAGNOSIS

Sympathetic Ganglion Tumor

- Oval shape & vertical axis; spans 3-5 interspaces
- More often calcified

Lateral Thoracic Meningocele

- Fluid attenuation lesion contiguous with thecal sac
- May coexist with neurofibroma in patients with neurofibromatosis

Paraganglioma

- Intense contrast enhancement

NEUROGENIC NEOPLASMS OF THE NERVE SHEATH

Neurenteric Cyst

- Rare; fluid attenuation lesion
- Associated with congenital vertebral body anomalies

Paraspinal Abscess

- Centered on disc rather than on neural foramen
- May surround spine

Paraspinal Hematoma

- Occurs following trauma; associated with spinal fracture

PATHOLOGY

General Features

- Genetics
  - 30% of neurofibromas associated with neurofibromatosis 1 (von Recklinghausen disease)
    - Deletion on chromosome 17
  - Neurofibromatosis 2
    - Chromosome 22q deletion
- **90% of all paravertebral masses are of neurogenic origin**
  - **40% are nerve sheath tumors**
  - Schwannoma to neurofibroma ratio of 3:1

Gross Pathologic & Surgical Features

- **Schwannoma**
  - Encapsulated nerve sheath tumor; eccentric growth, nerve compression
  - Frequent cystic degeneration & hemorrhage
- **Neurofibroma**
  - Unencapsulated disorganized proliferation of all nerve elements, centrally positioned in nerve
  - Cystic degeneration & hypocellularity uncommon
  - May be localized, diffuse, or plexiform
- **MPNST**
  - May arise de novo or within preexisting plexiform neurofibroma
  - Rare in preexisting schwannoma
  - Usually > 5 cm

Microscopic Features

- Schwannoma
  - Antoni A (hypercellular spindle cells organized in bundles or interlacing fascicles)
  - Antoni B (hypocellular myxoid tissue)
  - Stain positive for protein S100
- Neurofibroma: Myelinated & unmyelinated axons, collagen, reticulin
- MPNST: Highly cellular with pleomorphic spindle cells; difficult differentiation from sarcoma

CLINICAL ISSUES

Presentation

- Most common signs/symptoms
  - Often asymptomatic
- Other signs/symptoms
  - Symptoms of mass effect or nerve entrapment
  - Pain raises suspicion for malignant degeneration
    - Higher incidence of malignant degeneration in neurofibromatosis 1

Demographics

- Age
  - **Schwannoma**: Average in 5th decade
  - **Neurofibroma**: Usually 2nd-4th decades
  - **MPNST**: Usually 2nd-4th decades
- Gender
  - M = F
- Epidemiology
  - Most common cause of paravertebral mass
  - **90% of PNST are solitary**
    - Solitary PNSTs rarely undergo malignant degeneration
  - Neurofibromatosis: Malignant degeneration in approximately 4%
    - Neurofibromatosis 1: Prevalence of 1 in 3,000
      - Multiple neurogenic tumors or single plexiform neurofibroma
      - Other neoplasms: Pheochromocytoma, chronic myelogenous leukemia, optic nerve glioma, astrocytoma
    - Neurofibromatosis 2: Prevalence of 1 in 1,000,000
  - MPNSTs account for 5-10% of all soft tissue sarcomas

Natural History & Prognosis

- Indolent slow growth
  - Recurrence rare following surgical resection
- 5-year survival of patients with MPNST is 35%

Treatment

- Surgical excision
- Radiation not indicated, may induce malignant degeneration

DIAGNOSTIC CHECKLIST

Consider

- PNST in patient with spherical paravertebral mass & benign skeletal pressure erosion
- MPNST in paravertebral mass with locally aggressive behavior, rapid enlargement, or ill-defined margins
- MPNST when patient develops new symptom of pain related to known nerve sheath tumor

Image Interpretation Pearls

- **Split fat sign**: Fat attenuation/signal surrounding neurovascular bundle; circumscribed tumor surrounded by fat suggests neurogenic tumor
- **Target sign**: Central low signal & peripheral high signal on T2WI, typical of neurofibroma; similar signs described on CT & US
- **Fascicular sign**: Multiple, high signal, small, ring-like structures on T2WI, more common in schwannomas

SELECTED REFERENCES

1. Abreu E et al: Peripheral tumor and tumor-like neurogenic lesions. Eur J Radiol. Epub ahead of print, 2011
2. Nam SJ et al: Imaging of primary chest wall tumors with radiologic-pathologic correlation. Radiographics. 31(3):749-70, 2011
3. Kang J et al: Manifestations of systemic diseases on thoracic imaging. Curr Probl Diagn Radiol. 39(6):247-61, 2010
4. Woertler K: Tumors and tumor-like lesions of peripheral nerves. Semin Musculoskelet Radiol. 14(5):547-58, 2010

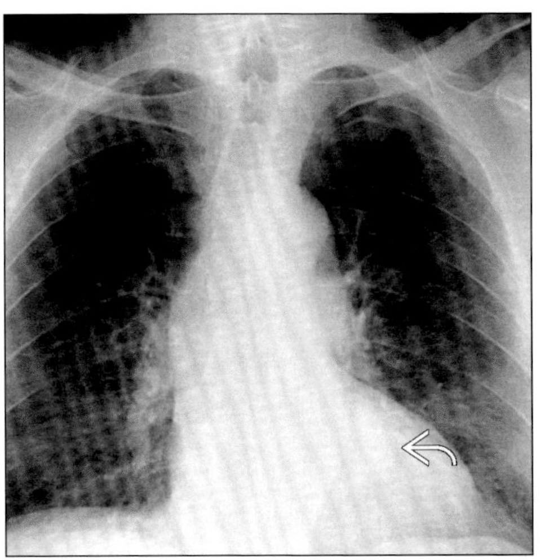

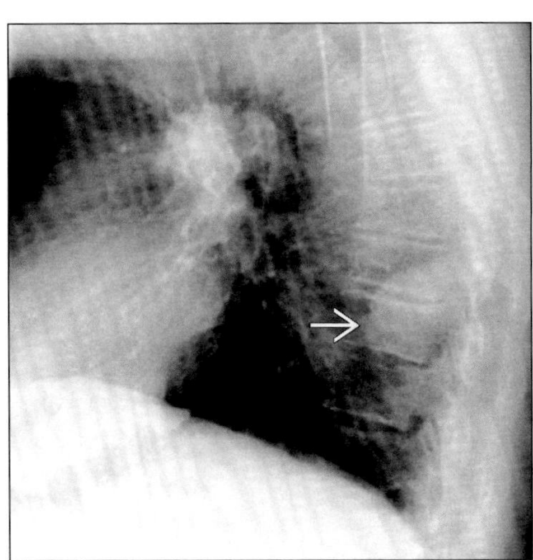

(Left) *PA chest radiograph of an asymptomatic 82-year-old man with a paravertebral schwannoma shows a subtle left retrocardiac mediastinal contour abnormality ➡.* ***(Right)*** *Lateral chest radiograph of the same patient shows that the mass ➡ is paravertebral and exhibits the incomplete border sign due to its extrapulmonary location. The findings are highly suggestive of PNST, and further evaluation with MR is indicated to exclude intraspinal growth.*

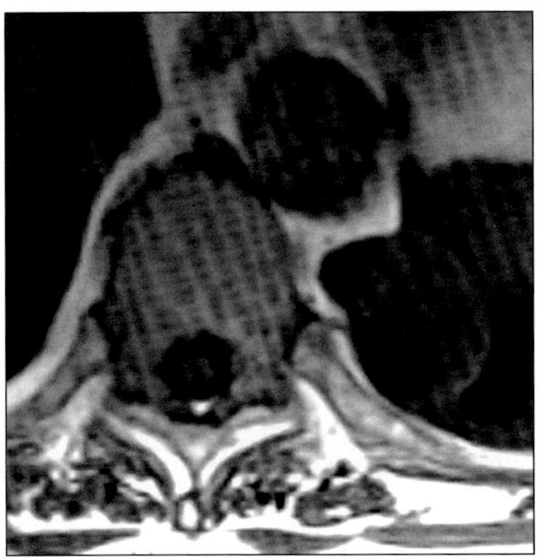

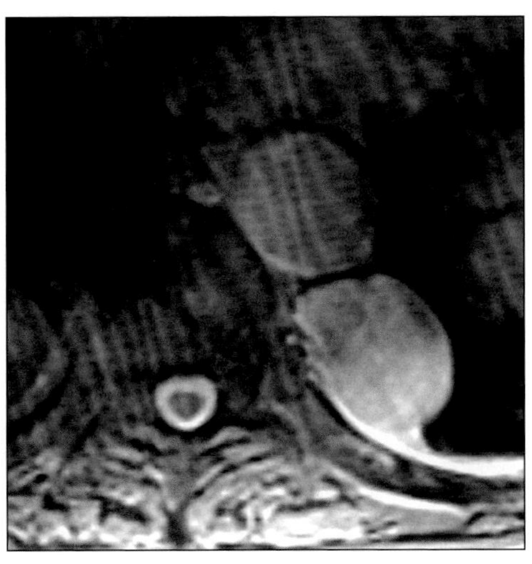

(Left) *Axial T1WI MR of the same patient shows a well-marginated ovoid mass of homogeneous low signal intensity.* ***(Right)*** *Axial T2WI MR of the same patient shows homogeneous high signal intensity throughout the mass. There was no evidence of intraspinal growth. CT-guided biopsy confirmed the diagnosis of schwannoma. Peripheral nerve sheath tumors are often asymptomatic and may be detected incidentally on radiographs obtained for other reasons.*

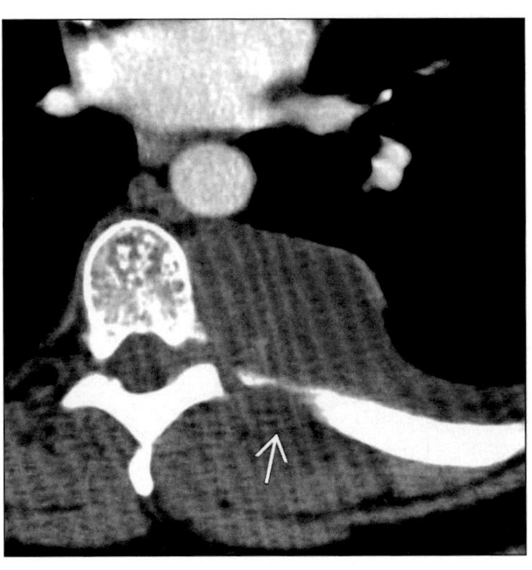

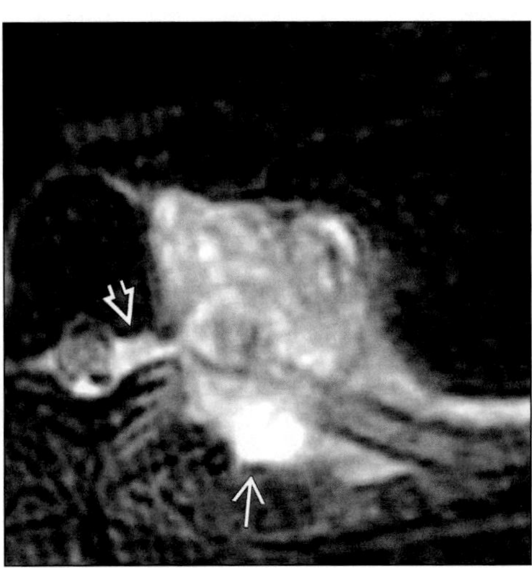

(Left) *Axial CECT of a 39-year-old man with severe back pain shows a soft tissue mass in the left paravertebral region that encases and invades the adjacent left posterior rib ➡ and expands the adjacent neural foramen.* ***(Right)*** *Axial T2WI MR of the same patient shows a heterogeneous high signal intensity mass with ill-defined margins and optimally demonstrates chest wall invasion ➡ and expansion of the adjacent left neural foramen ➡. Ultrasound-guided biopsy confirmed MPNST.*

NEUROGENIC NEOPLASMS OF THE SYMPATHETIC GANGLIA

Key Facts

Terminology
- Ganglioneuroma: Benign neoplasm of sympathetic ganglia
- Ganglioneuroblastoma, neuroblastoma: Malignant neoplasms of sympathetic ganglia
- Paraganglioma: Neoplasm of paraganglion cells in sympathetic or parasympathetic chains

Imaging
- Radiography
  - Elongate paravertebral mass
  - Rib displacement, skeletal pressure erosion
- CT
  - Homogeneous or heterogeneous paravertebral mass
  - Paragangliomas exhibit intense contrast enhancement
- MR
  - Optimal evaluation of intraspinal extension

Top Differential Diagnoses
- Neurogenic neoplasm of nerve sheath
- Neuroenteric cyst
- Lateral thoracic meningocele
- Extramedullary hematopoiesis
- Paraspinal abscess or hematoma

Clinical Issues
- Neuroblastoma: Children < 3 years
- Ganglioneuroblastoma: Children < 10 years
- Ganglioneuroma: Adolescents & young adults

Diagnostic Checklist
- Consider ganglioneuroma in adolescent or young adult with elongate paravertebral mass ± skeletal pressure erosion
- Consider neuroblastoma in infant with paravertebral soft tissue mass ± calcification

*(**Left**) PA chest radiograph of a 30-year-old woman with a right ganglioneuroma shows a large, vertically oriented paravertebral mass that produces splaying of the right posterior 5th and 6th ribs. Note the hilum overlay sign. (**Right**) Lateral chest radiograph of the same patient confirms the paravertebral location of the mass. Ganglioneuromas are benign neoplasms that commonly affect asymptomatic adolescents and young adults, and many are incidentally discovered on imaging.*

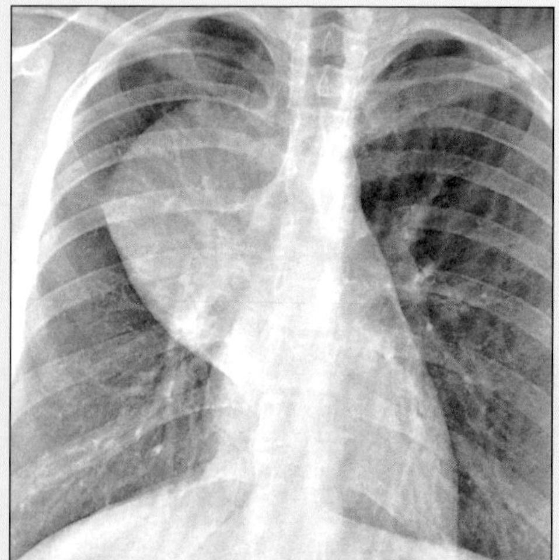

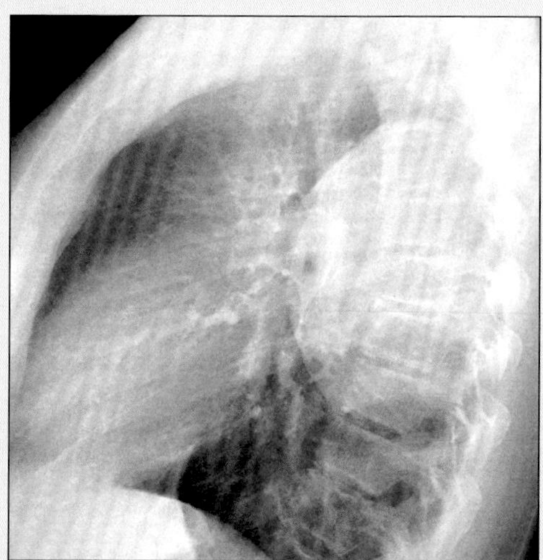

*(**Left**) Composite image with axial (left) and coronal (right) CECT of a 27-year-old man with paraganglioma shows an enhancing left paravertebral mass ➔ that exhibits an elongated morphology on coronal imaging spanning at least 3 vertebral levels. (**Right**) Composite image with axial T2W MR (left top), axial T1 C+ FS MR (left bottom), and posterior view MIBG scintigram (right) of the same patient shows a T2 hyperintense soft tissue mass with flow voids ➔ that exhibits avid enhancement ➔ and intense MIBG uptake ➔.*

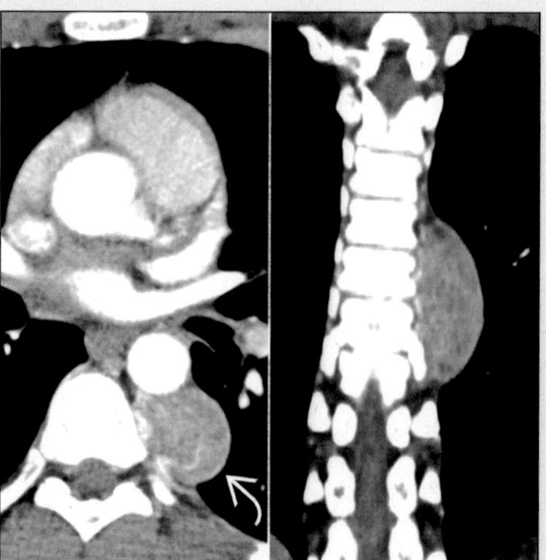

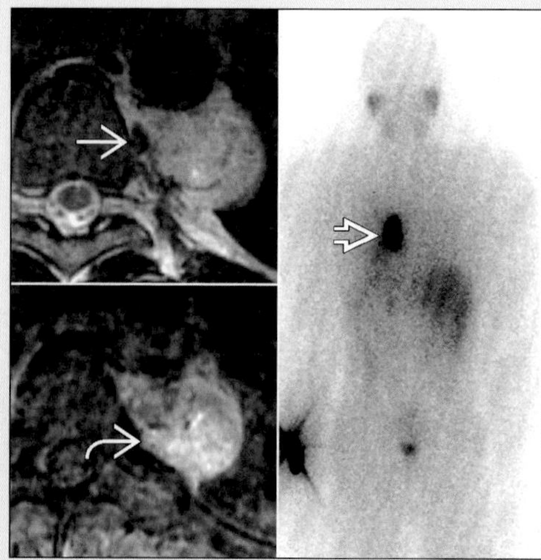

NEUROGENIC NEOPLASMS OF THE SYMPATHETIC GANGLIA

TERMINOLOGY

Definitions

- **Ganglioneuroma**: Benign neoplasm of sympathetic ganglia
- **Ganglioneuroblastoma, neuroblastoma**: Malignant neoplasms of sympathetic ganglia
- **Paraganglioma**: Neoplasm of paraganglion cells in sympathetic or parasympathetic chains

IMAGING

General Features

- Best diagnostic clue
  - **Elongated**, vertically oriented paravertebral mass
- Location
  - Sympathetic chains run vertically near the costovertebral junction
  - Paragangliomas may be located along sympathetic chain, vagus nerve, or within heart
- Morphology
  - Well-circumscribed or lobular soft tissue mass

Radiographic Findings

- Elongate paravertebral mass spanning 2-5 vertebrae
- Rib displacement, pressure erosion of ribs & vertebrae
- Radiographic calcification in 10% of neuroblastomas

CT Findings

- Elongate paravertebral soft tissue mass
  - Homogeneous or heterogeneous
  - Neuroblastoma: Hemorrhage, cystic degeneration, necrosis
  - Approximately 85% of neuroblastomas exhibit calcification on CT
- Paragangliomas exhibit intense contrast enhancement

MR Findings

- Optimal evaluation of intraspinal extension
- Neuroblastoma: Heterogeneous signal intensity
- Ganglioneuroblastoma & ganglioneuroma: Homogeneous intermediate T1 & T2 signal
  - Homogeneous enhancement
- Paraganglioma: Intense gadolinium enhancement
  - Relatively high T1 signal with flow voids

Nuclear Medicine Findings

- PET
  - FDG-PET: Moderate sensitivity for paragangliomas
- MIBG scintigraphy
  - Assessment of disease extent &/or surveillance
  - Up to 30% of neuroblastomas are not MIBG avid

Imaging Recommendations

- Best imaging tool
  - MR optimal modality for evaluation of intraspinal growth of neurogenic neoplasms

DIFFERENTIAL DIAGNOSIS

Neurogenic Neoplasm of Nerve Sheath

- Schwannoma, neurofibroma
- Horizontal axis, round, centered on neural foramen

Neuroenteric Cyst

- Fluid characteristics at MR &/or CT

Lateral Thoracic Meningocele

- Fluid attenuation; contiguous with thecal sac

PATHOLOGY

General Features

- Etiology
  - Neuroblastoma: Derived from neural crest cells
  - Paraganglioma: Neuroendocrine tumor of chromaffin cell origin
- Genetics
  - Paragangliomas may be associated with multiple endocrine neoplasia & von Hippel-Lindau

Staging, Grading, & Classification

- Staging: Neuroblastoma (Evans anatomic staging)
  - 1: Confined to organ of origin
  - 2: Growth beyond organ of origin without crossing midline
  - 3: Growth across midline
  - 4: Distant metastases
    - 4S: Age < 1 year, metastases confined to skin, liver, bone marrow

CLINICAL ISSUES

Presentation

- Most common signs/symptoms
  - Neuroblastoma: Painless mass, paraneoplastic syndrome
  - Ganglioneuroblastoma & ganglioneuroma: May be asymptomatic
  - Paraganglioma: Hypertension, blushing, headaches due to circulating catecholamines

Demographics

- Age
  - Neuroblastoma: Children < 3 years
  - Ganglioneuroblastoma: Children < 10 years
  - Ganglioneuroma: Adolescents & young adults

Natural History & Prognosis

- Ganglioneuroma: Favorable prognosis
- Chest neuroblastoma: Better prognosis than other sites

Treatment

- Surgical resection ± adjuvant chemotherapy & radiation

DIAGNOSTIC CHECKLIST

Consider

- Ganglioneuroma in adolescent or young adult with elongate paravertebral mass ± skeletal erosion
- Neuroblastoma in infant with paravertebral soft tissue mass ± calcification

SELECTED REFERENCES

1. Woo OH et al: Wide spectrum of thoracic neurogenic tumours: a pictorial review of CT and pathological findings. Br J Radiol. 81(968):668-76, 2008

NEUROFIBROMATOSIS

Key Facts

Terminology

- Neurofibromatosis type 1 (NF1) characterized by focal or diffuse benign nerve sheath tumors
- Plexiform neurofibromas considered pathognomonic for NF1

Imaging

- Best diagnostic clue: Multiple subcutaneous & intrathoracic neurofibromas
- Radiography
  - Subcutaneous neurofibromas
  - Rib separation & "ribbon rib" deformities
  - Scoliosis & posterior vertebral body scalloping
- HRCT: Fibrosis, honeycomb lung, bullae, apical neurofibromas, nodules
- CECT
  - Lateral thoracic meningocele: Water attenuation, nonenhancing paravertebral mass
  - Neurofibroma: Paravertebral mass extending into spinal canal & widening neural foramen
- MR
  - Lateral thoracic meningocele: T1 hypointense, T2 hyperintense, no enhancement
  - Neurofibroma: Variable T1, "target" sign on T2, homogeneous enhancement
- PET/CT: Variable ability to differentiate between benign & malignant lesions

Top Differential Diagnoses

- Other neurogenic neoplasms
- Neurenteric cyst
- Extramedullary hematopoiesis
- Lymphadenopathy

Diagnostic Checklist

- Consider NF1 in patient with multiple subcutaneous & intrathoracic soft tissue nodules/masses

*(**Left**) PA chest radiograph of a patient with neurofibromatosis type 1 (NF1) demonstrates typical skeletal manifestations, including dysplastic ribs, some with scalloping and "ribbon rib" deformities ➔. Note the dextroconvex scoliosis of the upper thoracic spine ⇨. (**Right**) Axial NECT of the same patient shows extensive bullae ➔ within the visualized upper lobes, more severe on the right than on the left. Pulmonary manifestations are present in approximately 20% of adult patients with NF1.*

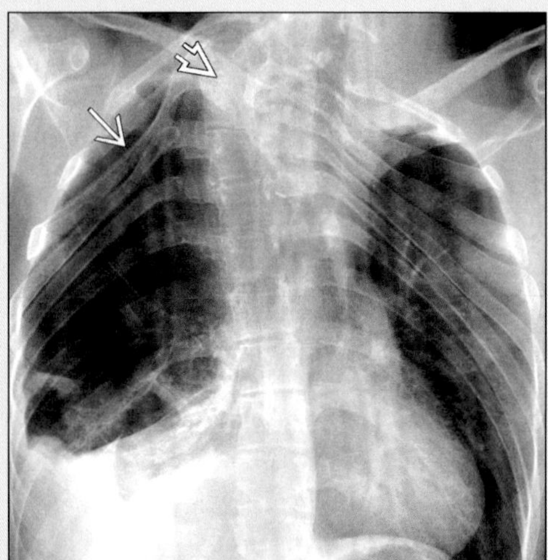

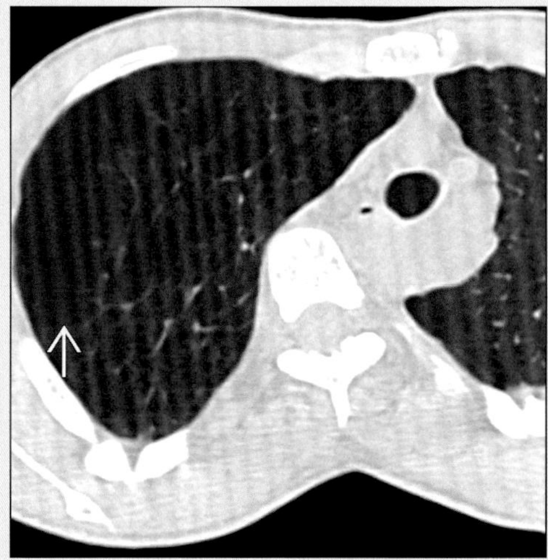

*(**Left**) Axial CECT of a patient with NF1 shows numerous neurofibromas (the largest in the paravertebral regions ➔) and multiple subcutaneous neurofibromas ⮌. (**Right**) Coronal T2WI MR of the same patient demonstrates innumerable neurofibromas ➔ in the subcutaneous and deep soft tissues of the head, neck, upper extremities, and thorax. Most neurofibromas exhibit a "target "sign on T2WI MR, in which the central portion is hypointense and the peripheral portion is hyperintense.*

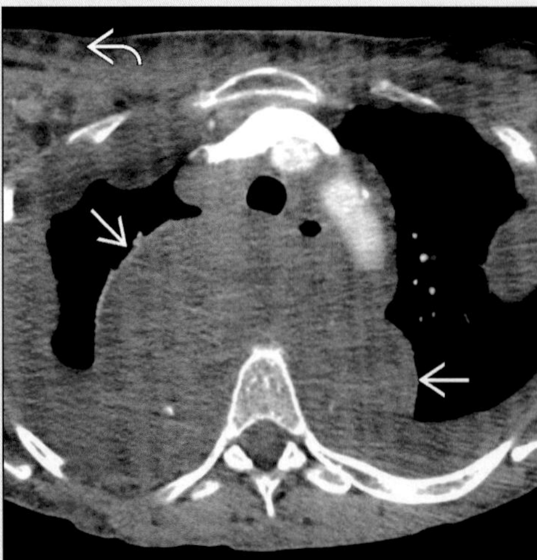

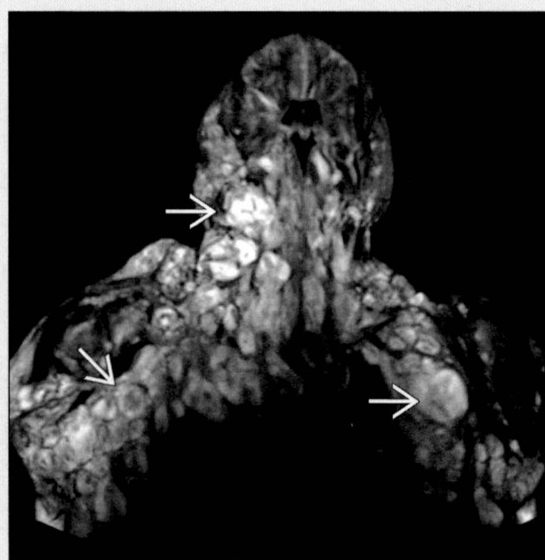

NEUROFIBROMATOSIS

TERMINOLOGY

Abbreviations

- **Neurofibromatosis type 1 (NF1)**

Synonyms

- von Recklinghausen disease

Definitions

- Most common phakomatosis
- Characterized by focal or diffuse benign peripheral nerve sheath tumors
  - Focal: Neurofibromas
  - Diffuse: Plexiform neurofibromas
- **Plexiform neurofibromas considered pathognomonic for NF1**

IMAGING

General Features

- Best diagnostic clue
  - Multiple subcutaneous & intrathoracic neurofibromas (soft tissue nodules/masses)
- Location
  - Chest wall, lung, mediastinum, paravertebral

Radiographic Findings

- Radiography
  - Subcutaneous tissues
    - Neurofibromas
      - Nodular opacities projecting over thorax
      - May mimic pulmonary nodules
  - Ribs
    - Superior or inferior rib erosion
    - Separation of adjacent ribs by neurofibromas
    - "Ribbon rib" deformity
      - Associated primary osseous dysplasia
      - Erosion by adjacent neurofibromas
  - Spine
    - Scoliosis
    - Posterior scalloping of vertebral bodies
    - Lateral thoracic meningocele
      - Well-circumscribed paravertebral mass
  - Peripheral nerves
    - Plexiform neurofibromas
      - Diffuse mediastinal widening or focal mediastinal mass
      - May mimic lymphadenopathy
  - Lungs
    - Bilateral basal fibrosis
    - Honeycomb lung
    - Upper lobe bullae
    - Apical neurofibromas
      - Apical nodular opacity

CT Findings

- CECT
  - Subcutaneous tissues
    - Neurofibromas
  - Spine
    - Enlargement of neural foramina
      - Dural ectasia
      - Extension of neurofibroma
    - Lateral thoracic meningocele
      - Well-circumscribed paravertebral mass
      - Usually fluid attenuation
      - May be difficult to distinguish from hypodense neurofibroma
      - No enhancement
      - Contrast fill-in after intrathecal administration
  - Peripheral nerves
    - Neurofibromas
      - Paravertebral masses extending into spinal canal
      - Dumbbell-shaped
      - Widening of neural foramina
      - Usually hypodense
      - May exhibit calcification
  - Tracheobronchial tree
    - Endoluminal neurofibroma
- HRCT
  - Lungs
    - Bilateral basal fibrosis
    - Honeycomb lung
    - Upper lobe bullae
    - Apical neurofibromas
    - Lung nodules
      - Consider metastatic disease from malignant peripheral nerve sheath tumor (MPNST)

MR Findings

- T1WI
  - Lateral thoracic meningocele: Hypointense
  - Neurofibroma: Variable signal intensity
- T2WI
  - Lateral thoracic meningocele: Hyperintense
  - Neurofibroma: **"Target" sign**
    - Central hypointensity
    - Peripheral hyperintensity
- T1WI C+
  - Lateral meningocele: No enhancement
  - Neurofibroma: Homogeneous enhancement

Nuclear Medicine Findings

- PET/CT
  - Variable ability to differentiate between benign neurogenic neoplasms & MPNST
  - Detection of recurrent or metastatic disease
  - Prognostic implications
    - Reports of better prognosis with SUV < 3
      - Reported mean survival of 52 vs. 13 months
    - Accuracy of 94%

DIFFERENTIAL DIAGNOSIS

Other Neurogenic Neoplasms

- Ganglioneuroma, ganglioneuroblastoma, neuroblastoma, paraganglioma
  - Neuroblastoma: Heterogeneous
  - Ganglioneuroma & ganglioneuroblastoma: Typically homogeneous
  - Paraganglioma: Intense enhancement
- MR useful to evaluate intraspinal growth

Neurenteric Cyst

- Water attenuation mediastinal mass
- Cyst wall may enhance
- Vertebral anomalies cephalad to cyst
  - Hemivertebrae & clefts

NEUROFIBROMATOSIS

Extramedullary Hematopoiesis

- Proliferation of hematopoietic cells outside marrow
- Well-circumscribed paravertebral mass
- Heterogeneous
- Mild contrast enhancement

Lymphadenopathy

- Mediastinal widening on chest radiography
- Low-attenuation or nonenhancing lymph nodes may mimic neurofibromas
- Lymphoma, sarcoidosis, infection, metastatic disease

PATHOLOGY

General Features

- Genetics
  - **Chromosome 17**
    - **Autosomal dominant**
    - **Spontaneous mutation in 50% of cases**

Staging, Grading, & Classification

- **NIH criteria for diagnosis: 2 of 7 required**
  - ≥ 6 café au lait macules
    - > 5 mm in prepubertal individuals
    - > 15 mm in postpubertal individuals
  - ≥ 2 neurofibromas or 1 plexiform neurofibroma
  - Axillary or inguinal freckling
  - Optic glioma
  - ≥ 2 Lisch nodules (hamartomas of iris)
  - Distinctive osseous lesion
    - Sphenoid dysplasia
    - Cortical thinning of long bone ± pseudarthrosis
  - 1st-degree relative with NF1 by above criteria

Microscopic Features

- Diffuse fusiform enlargement of nerves
- Neuronal axons surrounded & displaced by disorganized Schwann cells & matrix
  - Differentiates plexiform neurofibromas from neurofibromas
- MPNST
  - "Marbleized" pattern
    - Dense cellular fascicles & myxoid regions
  - Cells may be spindle-shaped, rounded, or fusiform

CLINICAL ISSUES

Presentation

- Most common signs/symptoms
  - Most benign neurogenic tumors are asymptomatic
  - Pain may indicate malignant degeneration

Demographics

- Age
  - Most patients present in childhood
  - 10% present later in life with forme fruste or atypical findings
- Epidemiology
  - Incidence of 1:2,000 to 1:3,000
  - Neurogenic neoplasms
    - 30% of primary mediastinal tumors in children
    - 9% of primary mediastinal masses in adults
    - 30% of patients with solitary neurofibroma have NF1

Natural History & Prognosis

- Malignant degeneration or MPNST
  - 10% lifetime risk
  - Leading cause of cancer-related death in patients with NF1
  - Imaging findings of degeneration
    - Sudden change in mass size
    - Heterogeneous attenuation & signal intensity from hemorrhage & necrosis
    - Invasion of fat planes
  - 5-year survival: 16-52%
  - Local recurrence rate: 40-65%
  - Distant recurrence rate: 40-68%
  - Improved survival
    - Complete surgical excision
    - Small tumor size (< 5 cm)
    - Low-grade component

Treatment

- Genetic counseling
- Surgical resection
  - Symptomatic benign masses
  - MPNST
    - Resection has best outcome with regards to recurrence & distant metastases
- Radiation therapy
  - Radiation of benign neurofibromas predisposes to malignant degeneration
  - MPNST
    - Allows limb-salvage surgery when combined with wide excision
    - Reduces rate of local disease recurrence
    - No reduction in distant metastases or survival
- Chemotherapy
  - MPNST
    - Limited to high-grade disease with metastases

DIAGNOSTIC CHECKLIST

Consider

- NF1 in patient with multiple subcutaneous & intrathoracic soft tissue nodules/masses (neurofibromas) in appropriate clinical setting

SELECTED REFERENCES

1. Irion KL et al: Neurofibromatosis type 1 with tracheobronchial neurofibromas: case report with emphasis on tomographic findings. J Thorac Imaging. 23(3):194-6, 2008
2. Brenner W et al: Prognostic relevance of FDG PET in patients with neurofibromatosis type-1 and malignant peripheral nerve sheath tumours. Eur J Nucl Med Mol Imaging. 33(4):428-32, 2006
3. Arazi-Kleinmann T et al: Neurofibromatosis diagnosed on CT with MR correlation. Eur J Radiol. 42(1):69-73, 2002
4. Evans DG et al: Malignant peripheral nerve sheath tumours in neurofibromatosis 1. J Med Genet. 39(5):311-4, 2002
5. Fortman BJ et al: Neurofibromatosis type 1: a diagnostic mimicker at CT. Radiographics. 21(3):601-12, 2001
6. Rossi SE et al: Thoracic manifestations of neurofibromatosis-I. AJR Am J Roentgenol. 173(6):1631-8, 1999

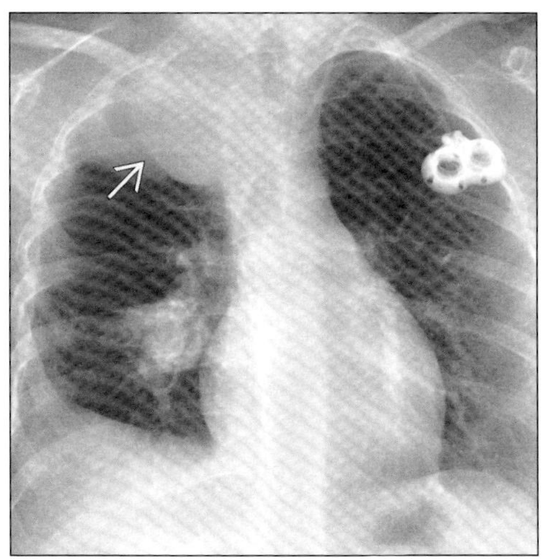

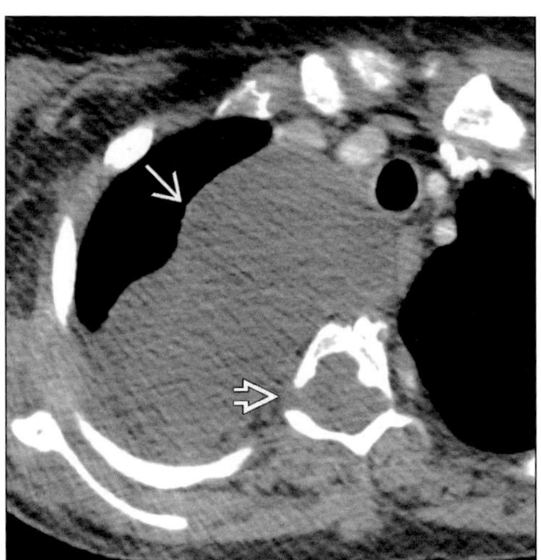

(Left) *AP chest radiograph of a patient with NF1 demonstrates a soft tissue mass ➔ projecting over the right superior mediastinum and medial right upper lung zone.* **(Right)** *Axial CECT of the same patient shows a large nonenhancing water attenuation mass ➔ occupying the majority of the right hemithorax at a level slightly above the aortic arch. The mass expands an adjacent right neural foramen ⇨ and the spinal canal. These findings are consistent with a lateral thoracic meningocele.*

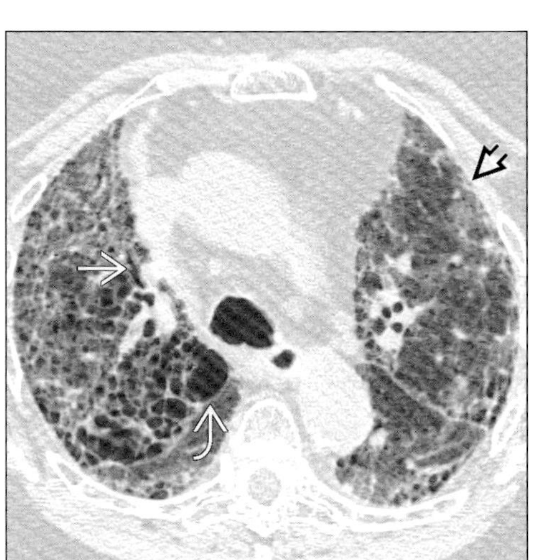

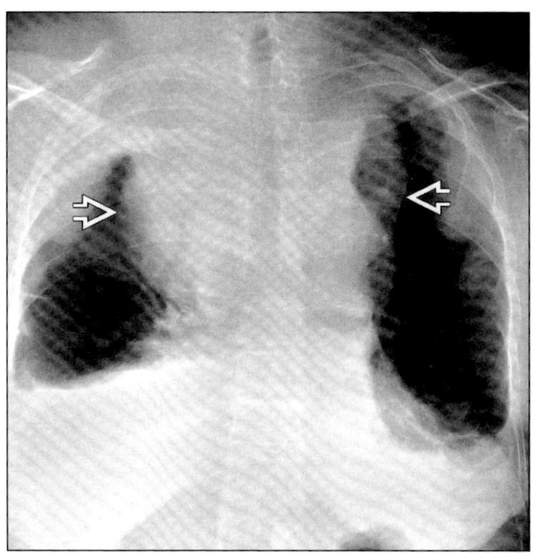

(Left) *Axial HRCT of a patient with NF1 shows subpleural reticular opacities ⇨, bronchiectasis ➔, and honeycomb lung ↪.* **(Right)** *PA chest radiograph of a patient with NF1 demonstrates numerous large bilateral extrapulmonary masses ⇨ that represent neurofibromas and produce mediastinal widening. These findings may mimic lymphadenopathy and other mediastinal masses on chest radiography.*

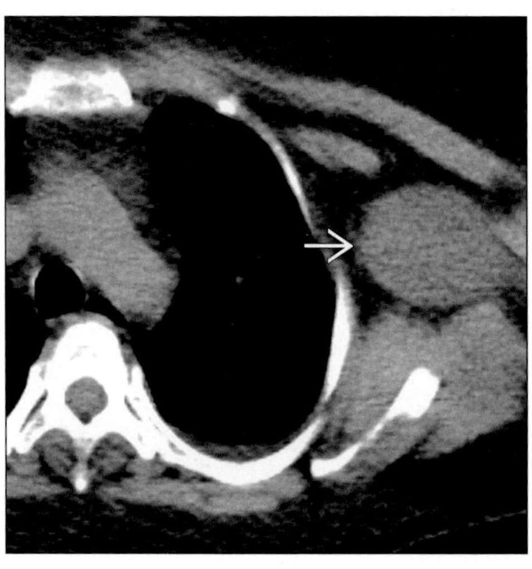

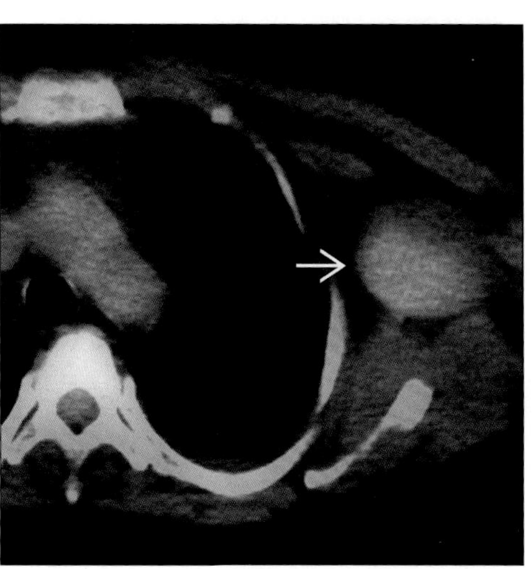

(Left) *Axial NECT of a patient with NF1 demonstrates a hypodense mass ➔ within the left axilla.* **(Right)** *Axial fused PET/CT of the same patient shows intense FDG uptake within the left axillary mass ➔, which is suggestive of malignant degeneration of a neurogenic tumor or a malignant peripheral nerve sheath tumor (MPNST). PET/CT is most useful for detecting recurrent or metastatic disease in patients with known MPNST.*

METASTATIC DISEASE, LYMPHADENOPATHY

Key Facts

Imaging

- Best diagnostic clue: Thoracic lymph nodes ≥ 10 mm on CT with FDG uptake on PET/CT
- Radiography
  - Abnormal mediastinal contours
  - Abnormal lines, stripes, & interfaces
- CT
  - Most common finding is lymph node enlargement
  - Abnormal when most lymph nodes ≥ 10 mm
  - Hypoattenuation, enhancement, &/or calcification
  - Specific lymphatic drainage pathways for intrathoracic & some extrathoracic malignancies
- PET/CT: FDG uptake within lymph nodes
  - Improved detection of lymph node metastases in lung cancer & regional lymph node metastases in esophageal cancer
  - False-positives: Granulomatous diseases & infectious/inflammatory processes

Top Differential Diagnoses

- Lymphoma
- Sarcoidosis

Pathology

- Lymph node metastases more common from intrathoracic than extrathoracic malignancies

Clinical Issues

- Lymph node staging in intrathoracic & extrathoracic malignancy important for prognosis & treatment
  - Lung cancer: Advanced nodal disease precludes surgical resection
  - Breast cancer: Advanced nodal disease necessitates preoperative chemotherapy

Diagnostic Checklist

- Consider metastatic disease in patients with cancer & intrathoracic lymphadenopathy

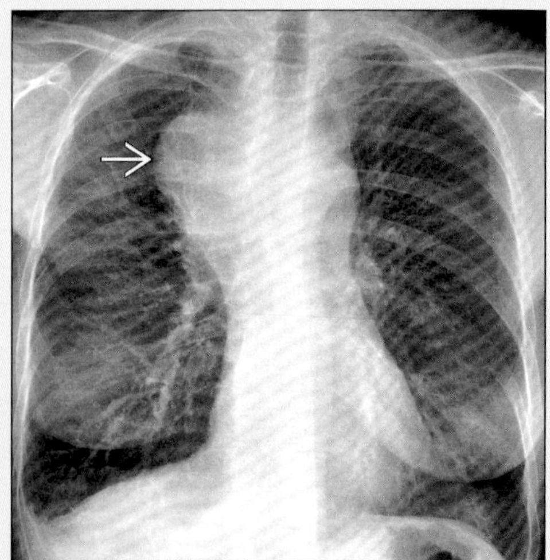

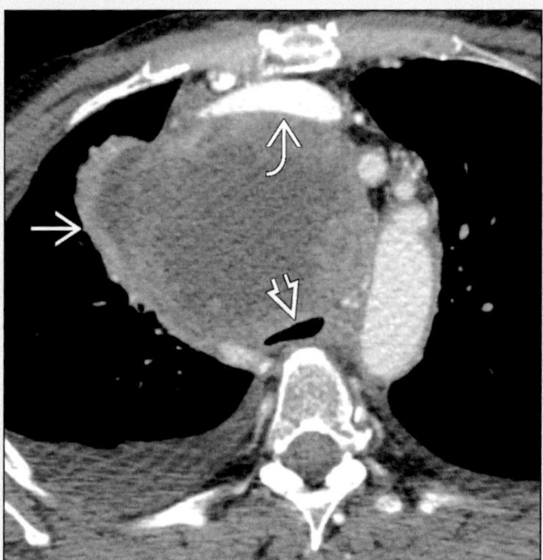

(Left) *PA chest radiograph of a patient with metastatic melanoma shows a large right-sided mediastinal soft tissue mass ➔.* ***(Right)*** *Axial CECT of the same patient demonstrates a large soft tissue mass ➔ of heterogeneous attenuation in the pretracheal region of the mediastinum. It produces severe compression of the trachea ⇨ and displacement of and mass effect on mediastinal vessels ↪. This mass represents extensive coalescent metastatic mediastinal lymphadenopathy.*

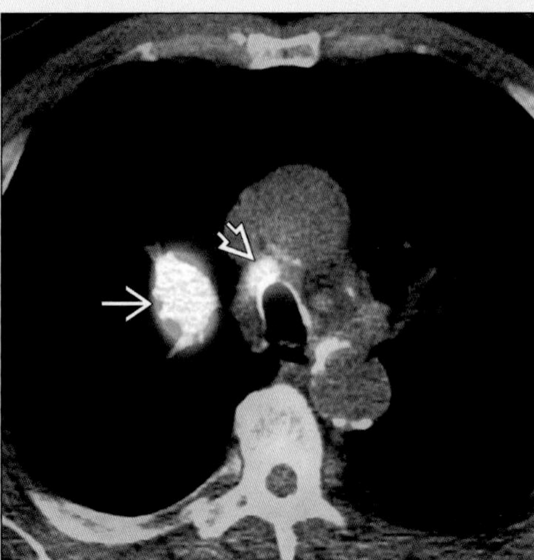

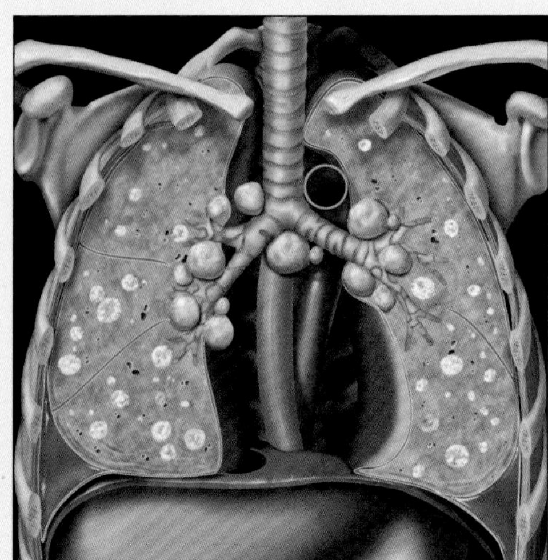

(Left) *Axial fused PET/CT of a patient with primary lung cancer and metastatic mediastinal lymphadenopathy demonstrates an FDG-avid right lung nodule ➔ and an FDG-avid right paratracheal lymph node ⇨ corresponding to primary and metastatic lung cancer, respectively.* ***(Right)*** *Graphic demonstrates typical features of advanced malignancy with multifocal bilateral pulmonary nodules representing metastases, bilateral malignant pleural effusions, and metastatic disease to hilar and mediastinal lymph nodes.*

IMAGING

General Features

- Best diagnostic clue
  - Intrathoracic lymph nodes ≥ 10 mm on CT
  - FDG uptake within lymph nodes on FDG PET/CT
- Location
  - Most commonly involves mediastinal lymph nodes
- Morphology
  - Hypoattenuation, enhancement, &/or calcification

Radiographic Findings

- Radiography
  - Enlarged lymph nodes may produce **abnormal mediastinal contours**
    - General
      - Loss of normal contours or interfaces
      - Thickening of normal stripes & lines
    - Right paratracheal lymph nodes
      - Thickening of right paratracheal stripe
      - Convexity of superior vena cava interface
    - Left paratracheal lymph nodes
      - Thickening of left paratracheal stripe
      - Convexity of left subclavian artery interface
    - Prevascular lymph nodes
      - Anterior mediastinal mass
      - Thickening of anterior junction line
    - Subcarinal lymph nodes
      - Convexity of upper azygoesophageal recess
    - Hilar lymph nodes
      - Hilar enlargement & lobulation
    - Aortopulmonary lymph nodes
      - Convexity of aortopulmonary window

CT Findings

- Lymph node enlargement, most common finding
  - Short-axis lymph node diameter is most reproducible measurement
    - Low paratracheal & subcarinal: > 11 mm
    - High paratracheal & superior mediastinal: > 7 mm
    - Right hilar & paraesophageal: > 10 mm
    - Left hilar & paraesophageal: > 7 mm
    - Peridiaphragmatic: > 5 mm
  - General
    - Paratracheal, hilar, subcarinal, paraesophageal, paraaortic, & subaortic lymph nodes: ≥ 10 mm
    - Internal mammary, retrocrural, & extrapleural lymph nodes: No size criteria
      - Visualization is considered abnormal
  - Nodal size is not always reliable
    - 13% of lymph nodes measuring < 10 mm contain metastatic foci
    - Meta-analysis for lung cancer
      - Sensitivity: 57%
      - Specificity: 82%
      - Positive predictive value (PPV): 56%
      - Negative predictive value (NPV): 83%
  - Sensitivity for axillary metastases: 50-60%
- Various imaging appearances based on primary tumor of origin
  - Hypoattenuation
    - Lung cancer
    - Extrathoracic malignancy: Seminoma & ovarian, thyroid, & gastric cancers
  - Enhancement
    - Lung cancer
    - Extrathoracic malignancy: Renal cell & thyroid cancers, melanoma, sarcoma
  - Calcification
    - Mucinous adenocarcinomas of colon & ovary, thyroid cancer, osteosarcoma
- Intrathoracic malignancy may spread along specific lymphatic drainage pathways
  - Lung cancer
    - Most tumors initially drain to hilar lymph nodes
    - Subsequent spread depends on lobe of origin
    - Right upper lobe
      - Right paratracheal & anterior mediastinal lymph nodes
    - Right middle & lower lobes
      - Subcarinal, right paratracheal, & anterior mediastinal lymph nodes
    - Left upper lobe
      - Subaortic & paraaortic lymph nodes
    - Left lower lobe
      - Subcarinal & subaortic lymph nodes
  - Esophageal cancer
    - Upper & middle esophagus
      - Lymphatics drain cephalad
      - Paratracheal lymph nodes
    - Lower esophagus
      - Lymphatics drain toward abdomen
      - Gastrohepatic ligament lymph nodes
    - Nodal disease may be extensive at time of presentation
    - "Skip" metastases are common
      - Direct communication between esophageal lymphatics & thoracic duct
  - Malignant pleural mesothelioma
    - Drainage pathways differ by location of pleural & diaphragmatic involvement
    - Pleura
      - Anterior: Internal mammary (upper & middle thorax) & peridiaphragmatic lymph nodes (lower thorax)
      - Posterior: Extrapleural lymph nodes
    - Diaphragm
      - Anterior & lateral: Internal mammary & anterior peridiaphragmatic lymph nodes
      - Posterior: Paraaortic & posterior mediastinal lymph nodes
- Some extrathoracic malignancies may spread along specific lymphatic drainage pathways
  - Breast cancer
    - 3 primary routes of spread: Axillary, transpectoral, & internal mammary pathways

Nuclear Medicine Findings

- PET/CT
  - FDG uptake within lymph nodes
    - Improved detection of metastatic lymph nodes in lung cancer
      - Sensitivity: 84%
      - Specificity: 89%
      - PPV: 79%
      - NPV: 93%
    - Improved detection of metastatic regional lymph nodes in esophageal cancer

METASTATIC DISEASE, LYMPHADENOPATHY

Clinical Lymph Node Staging	
Lung Cancer	
N0	No regional lymph nodes
N1	Ipsilateral peribronchial &/or ipsilateral hilar & intrapulmonary lymph nodes
N2	Ipsilateral mediastinal &/or subcarinal lymph nodes
N3	Contralateral mediastinal, contralateral hilar, ipsilateral or contralateral scalene, or supraclavicular lymph nodes
Esophageal Cancer	
N0	No regional lymph nodes
N1	Metastasis in 1-2 regional lymph nodes
N2	Metastasis in 3-6 regional lymph nodes
N3	Metastasis in ≥ 7 regional lymph nodes
Malignant Mesothelioma	
N0	No regional lymph nodes
N1	Ipsilateral bronchopulmonary or hilar lymph nodes
N2	Subcarinal or ipsilateral mediastinal lymph nodes including ipsilateral internal mammary & peridiaphragmatic lymph nodes
N3	Contralateral mediastinal, contralateral internal mammary, ipsilateral or contralateral supraclavicular lymph nodes
Breast Cancer	
N0	No regional lymph nodes
N1	Movable ipsilateral axillary lymph nodes
N2a	Fixed ipsilateral axillary lymph nodes
N2b	Internal mammary lymph nodes with involvement of axillary lymph nodes
N3a	Ipsilateral infraclavicular lymph nodes
N3b	Ipsilateral internal mammary lymph nodes & axillary lymph nodes
N3c	Ipsilateral supraclavicular lymph nodes

- PPV of regional lymph nodes: 93.8% (vs. 62.5-73.7% for CT)
- False-positive findings
  - Granulomatous disease
  - Infectious &/or inflammatory processes

MR Findings

- Accuracy similar to that of CT
- Gadolinium contrast administration improves staging accuracy

Imaging Recommendations

- Best imaging tool
  - CT optimal for identifying lymphadenopathy
    - Nodal size not always reliable indicator of metastatic disease
  - FDG PET/CT improves accuracy

DIFFERENTIAL DIAGNOSIS

Lymphoma

- Enlarged lymph nodes; may or may not enhance
- Untreated lymphoma does not calcify
- Treated lymphoma may calcify
- Hodgkin lymphoma more commonly involves thorax than non-Hodgkin lymphoma

Sarcoidosis

- Multisystem chronic inflammatory disorder characterized by noncaseating granulomas
- Bilateral symmetric hilar & right paratracheal lymphadenopathy
- Calcified lymph nodes may be present
- FDG PET/CT may be used to assess treatment response
  - False-positive in evaluation of intrathoracic metastatic lymphadenopathy

PATHOLOGY

General Features

- Etiology
  - Lymph node metastases more common from intrathoracic than extrathoracic malignancies
    - Intrathoracic: Lung & esophageal cancers, malignant pleural mesothelioma
    - Extrathoracic: Head & neck, genitourinary tract, & breast cancers, melanoma

CLINICAL ISSUES

Treatment

- Lung cancer
  - N1: Resectable in absence of mediastinal tumor invasion, malignant pleural effusion, satellite nodules, or metastases
  - N2: Possibly amenable to surgery; chemotherapy & radiation also used
  - N3: Not amenable to surgery
- Malignant pleural mesothelioma
  - Most patients have advanced disease at presentation
  - Some may benefit from surgery & chemotherapy
    - Epithelioid histology
    - No evidence of extrapleural lymph nodes
- Breast cancer
  - N1: Surgery & chemotherapy ± hormone therapy
  - N2: Surgery, chemotherapy, radiation therapy
  - N3: Preoperative chemotherapy

SELECTED REFERENCES

1. Sharma A et al: Patterns of lymphadenopathy in thoracic malignancies. Radiographics. 24(2):419-34, 2004

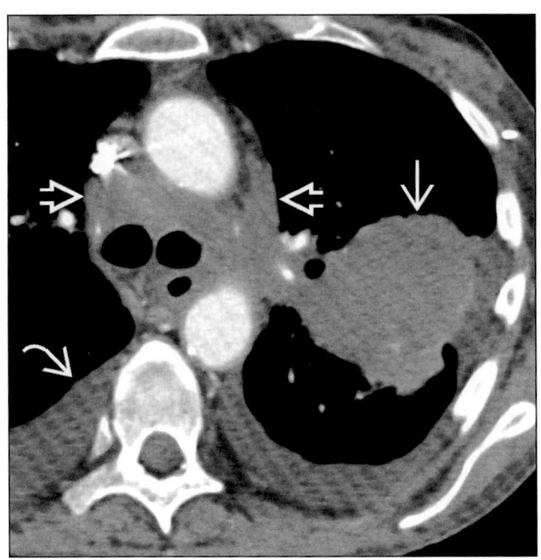

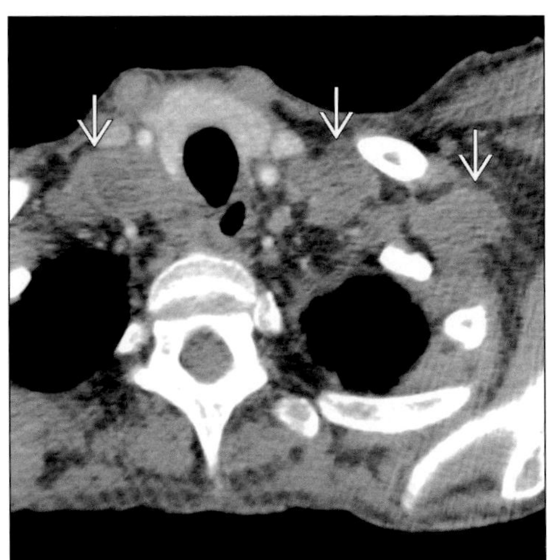

(Left) *Axial CECT of a patient with lung cancer shows a large hypodense left lung mass ➡ and coalescent soft tissue ➡ within the mediastinum in the right and left paratracheal and aortopulmonary window regions. Small bilateral pleural effusions ➡ are also present.* ***(Right)*** *Axial CECT of the same patient demonstrates bilateral supraclavicular lymphadenopathy ➡, which is classified as N3 disease, stage IIIB, and precludes surgical resection.*

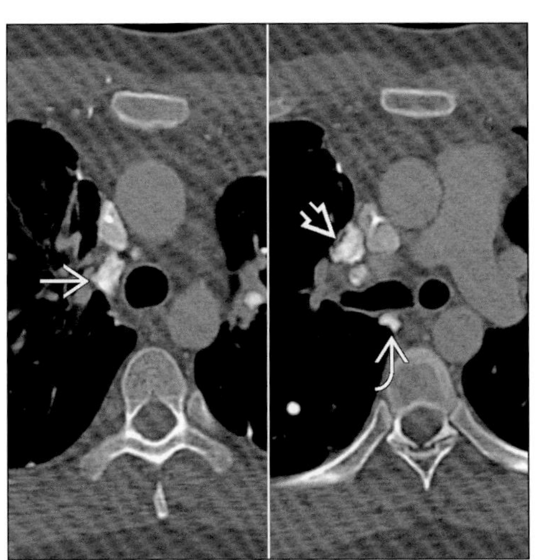

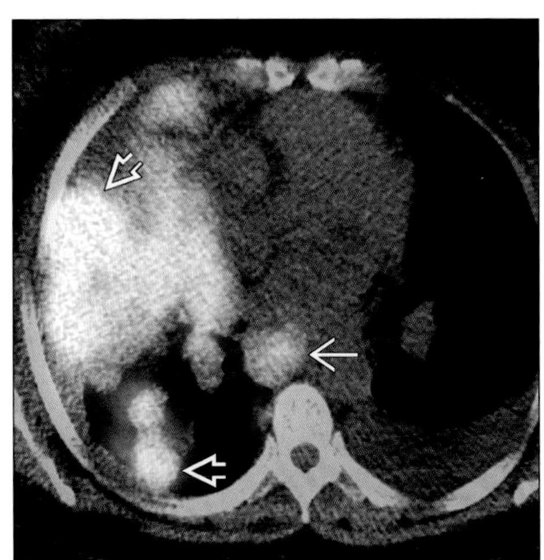

(Left) *Composite image with axial CECT of a patient with osteosarcoma shows calcified right paratracheal ➡, right hilar ➡, and subcarinal ➡ lymph nodes. Mucinous adenocarcinomas of the colon and ovary, thyroid cancer, and osteosarcoma may produce calcified lymph node metastases.* ***(Right)*** *Axial fused PET/CT of a patient with metastatic breast cancer demonstrates FDG uptake within a subcarinal lymph node ➡ and intensely FDG-avid pleural metastatic disease in the right hemithorax ➡.*

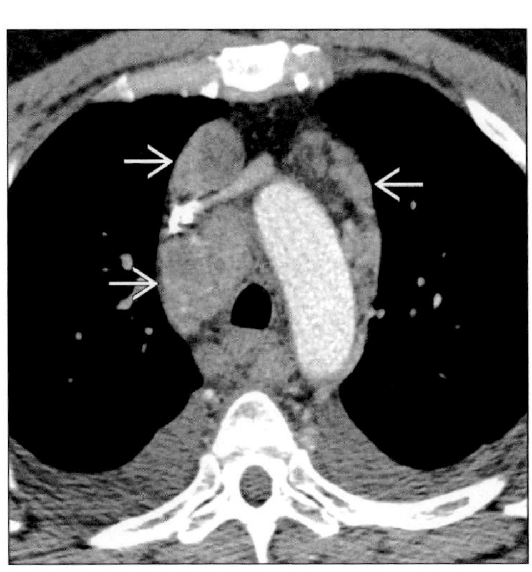

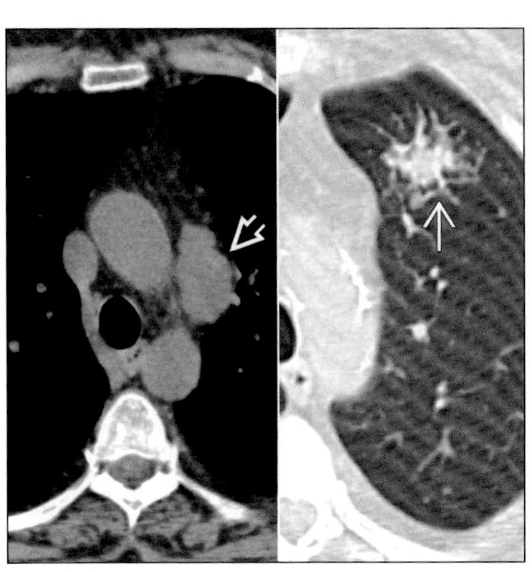

(Left) *Axial CECT of a patient with metastatic hepatocellular carcinoma demonstrates multiple enlarged heterogeneous mediastinal lymph node metastases ➡. Lymph node metastases from extrathoracic malignancies are much less common than those from intrathoracic malignancies.* ***(Right)*** *Composite image with axial NECT in soft tissue (left) and lung window (right) shows a metastatic aortopulmonary window node ➡ from a primary left upper lobe lung cancer ➡.*

MEDIASTINAL HODGKIN LYMPHOMA

Key Facts

Terminology
- Hodgkin lymphoma (HL)
- Lymphoid neoplasm arising from germinal center or post-germinal center B cells

Imaging
- Radiography
  - Lobular/elongated mediastinal mass
  - Bulky lymphadenopathy: > 1/3 maximum intrathoracic diameter
- CT
  - Multiple lymph node groups involved
  - Prevascular, paratracheal, aortopulmonary
  - Cannot detect active disease in residual masses
- PET/CT
  - Standard modality for staging & restaging HL
  - Greater sensitivity for extranodal disease

Top Differential Diagnoses
- Germ cell neoplasm
- Thymic malignancy
- Mediastinal goiter

Clinical Issues
- Symptoms
  - Asymptomatic lymphadenopathy
  - Chest pain, dyspnea, cough
  - B symptoms: Fever, weight loss, sweats
- Treatment
  - Stage I-II: Chemotherapy & radiation
  - Stage II-IV: Combination chemotherapy; radiation in selected patients

Diagnostic Checklist
- Consider Hodgkin lymphoma in patients with multifocal intrathoracic lymphadenopathy

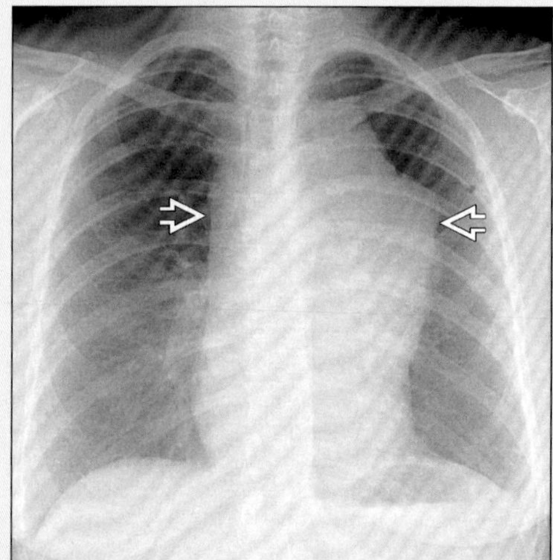

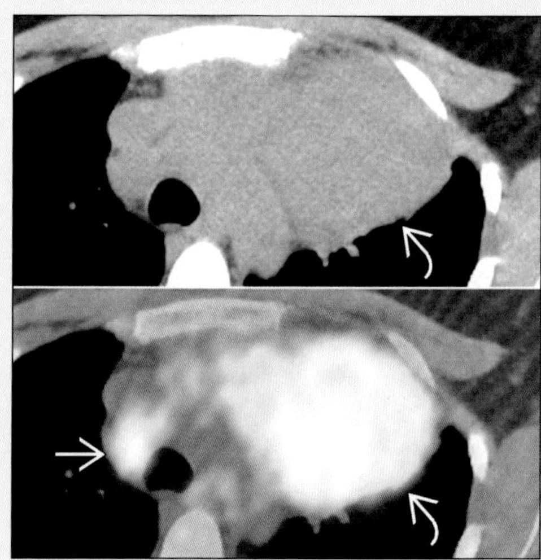

(Left) *PA chest radiograph of a patient with Hodgkin lymphoma shows diffuse bilateral anterior mediastinal enlargement ➔ greater than 1/3 of the transverse thoracic diameter, consistent with bulky lymphadenopathy and implying a poor prognosis.* ***(Right)*** *Composite image with axial NECT (top) and PET/CT (bottom) of the same patient shows a homogeneous FDG-avid anterior mediastinal mass ➔ and right paratracheal lymph node involvement ➔.*

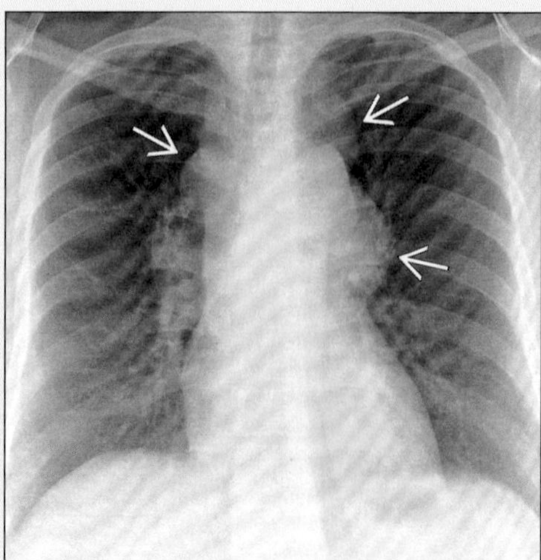

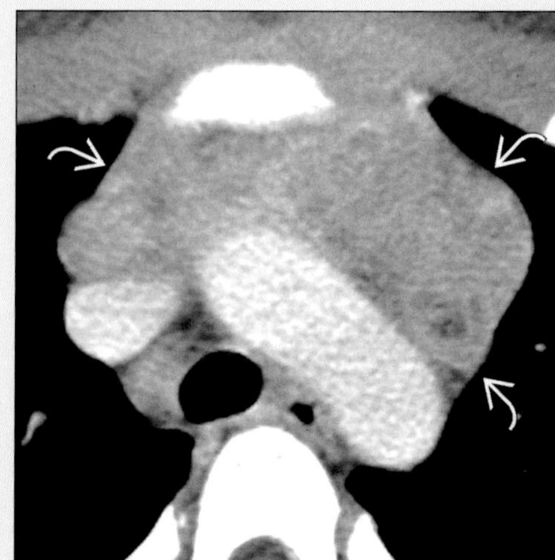

(Left) *PA chest radiograph of a patient with nodular sclerosis classical Hodgkin lymphoma shows bilateral lobular mediastinal widening ➔.* ***(Right)*** *Axial CECT of the same patient shows a large heterogeneous anterior mediastinal mass ➔. Areas of hypodensity often correlate with cystic or necrotic changes. However, this finding is not related to stage, disease distribution or extent, cell type, presence or absence of bulky lymphadenopathy, or prognosis.*

MEDIASTINAL HODGKIN LYMPHOMA

TERMINOLOGY

Abbreviations

- **Hodgkin lymphoma (HL)**

Definitions

- Lymphoid neoplasm arising from germinal center or post-germinal center B cells

IMAGING

General Features

- Location
  - **Mediastinal lymphadenopathy** (most common finding at presentation)
    - Multiple nodal groups involved in 85% of HL with thoracic involvement
    - Prevascular, paratracheal, & aortopulmonary lymphadenopathy (85% of HL & 98% of HL with thoracic involvement)
    - Other groups: Hilar (35%), subcarinal (25%), paracardiac (10%), internal mammary (5%), paravertebral/paraaortic/retrocrural (5%)

Radiographic Findings

- **Lymphadenopathy**
  - Lobular/elongated anterior mediastinal mass
  - **Bulky lymphadenopathy** (PA chest radiography)
    - Mediastinal mass > 1/3 of maximum intrathoracic diameter
    - Implies increased risk of disease progression & recurrence
  - Subtle lymphadenopathy may be missed on chest radiography (~ 10%)
  - Calcification is very rare before treatment
- Primary pulmonary involvement rare; lung invasion from adjacent lymph nodes not uncommon (15-40%)
- Pulmonary HL often manifests as
  - Ill-defined nodule
  - Single or multiple pulmonary nodules
  - Consolidation
- Pleural effusion
- Skeletal lesions: Mixed, lytic, &/or blastic

CT Findings

- **Lymphadenopathy**: > 1.0 cm in short axis on CT
  - Optimal identification of affected lymph node stations; especially helpful in subcarinal, internal mammary, & aortopulmonary stations
  - Homogeneous (most common) or heterogeneous soft tissue attenuation
  - Discrete, matted, or diffuse mediastinal infiltration with well- or ill-defined margins
  - Typical spread following contiguous nodal stations
  - Calcification uncommon but occasionally present before treatment; diffuse, eggshell, or irregular after treatment
  - **Bulky lymphadenopathy**: Mass > 10 cm
  - Invasion of adjacent lung often manifests with poorly defined margins
  - Cannot detect active disease in residual masses
- CECT
  - Minor or moderate contrast enhancement
  - Low attenuation often indicates necrosis (10-20%)
- Thymus involvement (30-40%) is difficult to differentiate from lymphadenopathy

MR Findings

- Evaluation of vascular or cardiac invasion
- Lymphadenopathy
  - Usually homogeneous
  - T1WI: Low signal, similar to muscle
  - T2WI: High signal, equal or higher than fat
  - Residual soft tissue masses after treatment: MR unreliable for differentiation between tumor & fibrous tissue

Nuclear Medicine Findings

- PET/CT
  - Staging of lymphoma
    - **Standard modality for staging** with better accuracy than CT
    - Greater sensitivity for extranodal disease
    - Metabolic activity level correlates with tumor aggressiveness
    - PET/CT improves accuracy by 9% compared to PET alone
  - Role after treatment
    - Detection of active disease in residual lymphadenopathy/mass
      - Signifies early relapse & poor clinical outcome
      - Negative FDG PET generally indicates long-term disease-free survival
    - FDG-avid (> background tissue) lymph node < 2 cm is positive for active disease
    - FDG-avid (> mediastinal blood pool) lymph node > 2 cm is positive for active disease
- Ga-67 scintigraphy
  - Accurately demonstrates viable tumor within residual soft tissue mass after therapy

DIFFERENTIAL DIAGNOSIS

Germ Cell Neoplasms

- Difficult to differentiate from lymphoma on imaging
- Often limited to anterior mediastinum at diagnosis
- Mature teratoma is often cystic with fat & calcification
- Nonseminomatous germ cell neoplasms may be associated with positive serum markers
  - β-human chorionic gonadotropin (choriocarcinoma, embryonal carcinoma)
  - α-fetoprotein (endodermal sinus tumor, embryonal carcinoma)
- Seminoma: May exhibit elevated β-human chorionic gonadotropin, unlikely to exhibit elevated α-fetoprotein

Thymic Malignancy

- Difficult to differentiate from lymphoma on imaging
- Thymoma manifests as focal anterior mediastinal mass without lymphadenopathy
- Invasive thymoma & thymic carcinoma often mimic lymphoma

Mediastinal Goiter

- Often contiguous with cervical thyroid
- Marked contrast enhancement
- Heterogeneous with areas of high attenuation, cystic change, & coarse calcification

MEDIASTINAL HODGKIN LYMPHOMA

PATHOLOGY

Staging, Grading, & Classification

- Lymph nodes divided into anatomic regions encompassed by a single radiation field for staging purposes
  - Waldeyer ring: Tonsils, base of tongue, nasopharynx
  - Ipsilateral cervical, supraclavicular, occipital, & preauricular
  - Infraclavicular
  - Axillary & pectoral
  - Mediastinal: Thymus, prevascular, aortopulmonary, paratracheal, pretracheal, subcarinal, & posterior mediastinal
  - Hilar
  - Paraaortic
- Histologic subtypes (WHO/R.E.A.L classifications): Fail to express genes & gene products that define normal germinal center B cells
  - **Classical HL** (90-95%): Defined by presence of Reed-Sternberg cells
    - Nodular sclerosis classical HL (70%)
    - Mixed cellularity classical HL (20-25%)
    - Lymphocyte-rich classical HL (5%)
    - Lymphocyte-depleted classical HL (< 1%)
  - Nodular lymphocyte-predominant HL (5-10%): Immunophenotypic features of germinal center B cells
- Staging: Ann Arbor Staging (adopted by WHO) with Cotswolds modifications takes into account extent of nodal disease, presence of extranodal disease, & clinical symptoms
  - Stage I: Single lymph node region
  - Stage IE: Single extranodal organ or site
  - Stage II: ≥ 2 lymph node regions on same side of diaphragm
  - Stage IIE: Localized extranodal extension + criteria for stage II
  - Stage III: Lymph node regions on both sides of diaphragm
  - Stage IIIE: Localized extralymphatic extension + criteria for stage III
  - Stage IIIS: Splenic involvement + criteria for stage III
  - Stage IV: Diffuse or disseminated involvement of ≥ 1 extralymphatic organs or tissues, with or without associated lymphatic involvement
  - All cases subclassified based on absence (A) or presence (B) of ≥ 1 of the following systemic symptoms: Significant unexplained fever, night sweats, unexplained weight loss (> 10% of body weight) during 6 months prior to diagnosis
  - Subscript "X" used when bulky disease is present
  - Subscript "E" used if limited extranodal extension is proved

CLINICAL ISSUES

Presentation

- Most common signs/symptoms
  - Asymptomatic lymphadenopathy
  - Mediastinal mass
    - Asymptomatic or associated with chest pain, dyspnea, & cough
  - Systemic symptoms (B symptoms): Fever, weight loss, & sweats
  - Pruritus

Demographics

- Age
  - All ages; peak incidence in 3rd & 7th decades
- Epidemiology
  - 0.5-1% of all new malignancies
  - 10% of all lymphomas
  - Increased incidence among immunosuppressed patients (i.e., solid organ & bone marrow transplantation, immunosuppressive drugs, & HIV infection)
  - Increased incidence among patients with autoimmune diseases
    - Personal history of rheumatoid arthritis, systemic lupus erythematosus, or sarcoidosis
    - Family history of sarcoidosis or ulcerative colitis
  - Increased incidence in relatives of patients with HL

Natural History & Prognosis

- Favorable vs. unfavorable disease
  - Adverse factors influencing outcome
    - Early stage disease (I-II)
      - Age > 30 years at diagnosis
      - ESR > 50 mm/h without B symptoms, ESR > 30 mm/h with B symptoms
      - Bulky mediastinal involvement
      - Involvement of ≥ 4 lymph node regions
    - Advanced disease (III-IV)
      - Age > 45 years at diagnosis
      - Male
      - Stage IV
      - Hemoglobin < 10.5 g/dL
      - Albumin concentration < 40 g/L
      - Lymphocyte count < 0.6 x 10^9/L or < 8%
      - WBC count > 15 x 10^9/L
  - Favorable features lead to reduction of chemo- and radiotherapy in patients with stage I & II HL

Treatment

- Stage I-II: Chemotherapy & radiation
- Stage III-IV: Combination chemotherapy; radiation in selected patients

DIAGNOSTIC CHECKLIST

Consider

- Hodgkin lymphoma in patients with multifocal intrathoracic lymphadenopathy

SELECTED REFERENCES

1. Das P et al: ACR Appropriateness Criteria® on Hodgkin's lymphoma-unfavorable clinical stage I and II. J Am Coll Radiol. 8(5):302-8, 2011
2. Cronin CG et al: Clinical utility of PET/CT in lymphoma. AJR Am J Roentgenol. 194(1):W91-W103, 2010
3. Israel O et al: Positron emission tomography in the evaluation of lymphoma. Semin Nucl Med. 34(3):166-79, 2004
4. Gambhir SS et al: A tabulated summary of the FDG PET literature. J Nucl Med. 42(5 Suppl):1S-93S, 2001
5. Au V et al: Radiologic manifestations of lymphoma in the thorax. AJR Am J Roentgenol. 168(1):93-8, 1997

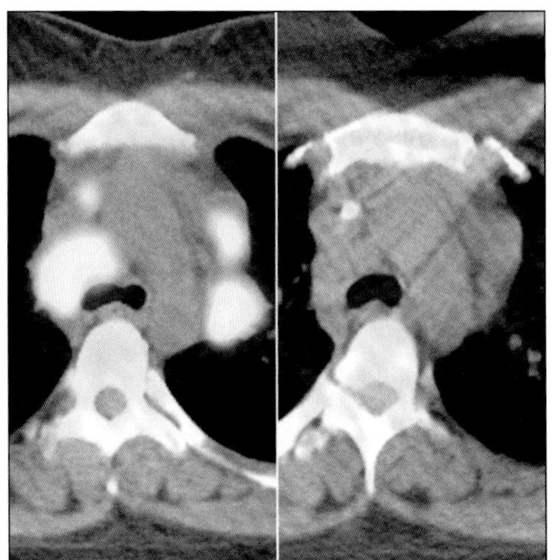

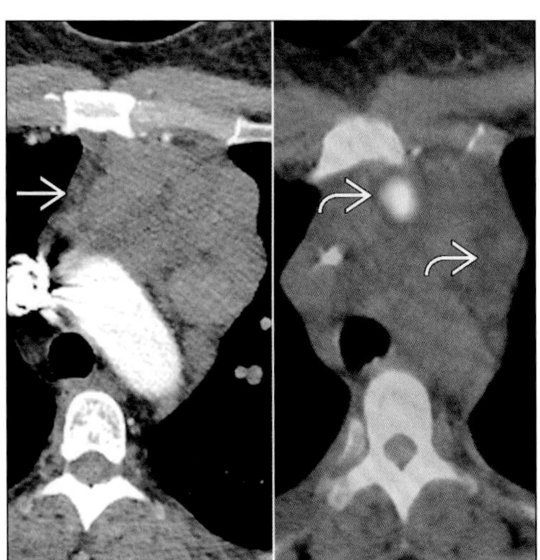

(Left) *Composite image with axial PET/CT shows a patient with nodular sclerosis HL before (left) and after (right) treatment. Note resolution of FDG avidity after treatment in spite of residual mediastinal lymphadenopathy.* ***(Right)*** *Composite image with axial CECT and PET/CT of a patient with nodular sclerosis HL before (left) and after (right) chemotherapy shows extensive anterior mediastinal lymphadenopathy ➔ and residual HL manifesting with areas of avid FDG uptake ➔ in residual mediastinal soft tissue.*

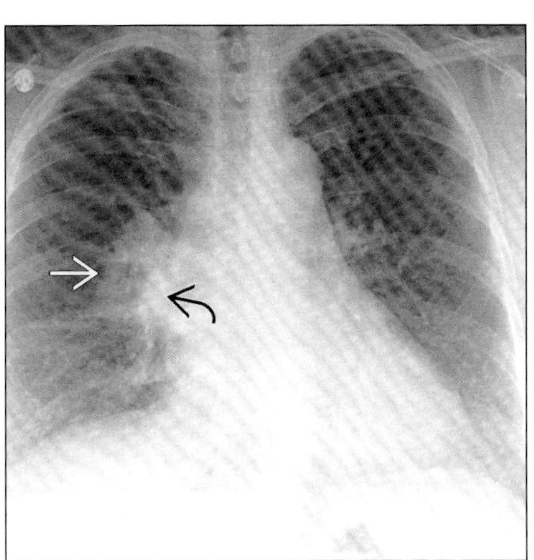

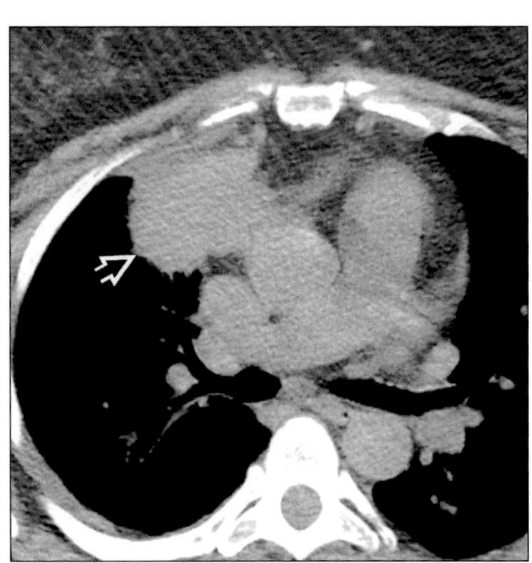

(Left) *PA chest radiograph of a patient with nodular sclerosis HL shows a right anterior mediastinal mass ➔ demonstrating the hilum overlay sign ➔.* ***(Right)*** *Axial NECT of the same patient shows an isolated spiculated right anterior mediastinal mass ➔ abutting the adjacent lung. In this particular case, it is difficult to discern whether the mass arises from or extends into the lung parenchyma. Mediastinotomy was necessary to establish the diagnosis and exact lesion location.*

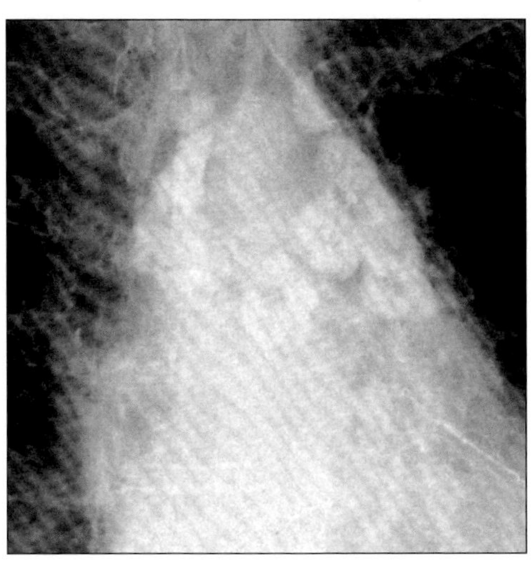

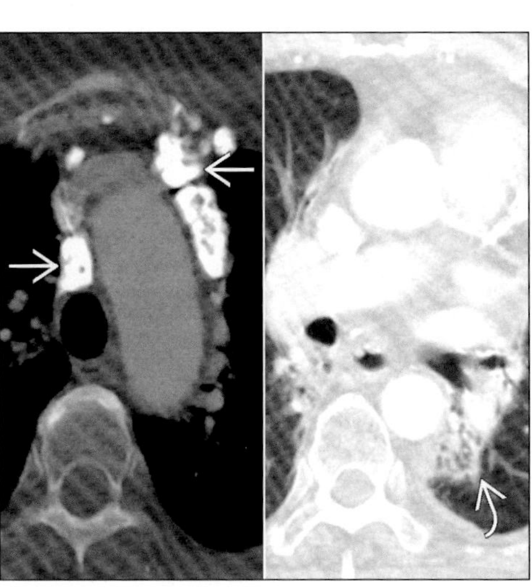

(Left) *PA chest radiograph of a patient with HL treated with radiotherapy shows multiple extensively calcified mediastinal lymph nodes.* ***(Right)*** *Composite image with axial CECT in soft tissue (left) and lung (right) window of the same patient shows densely calcified mediastinal lymph nodes ➔ within the radiation portal and bilateral lower lobe radiation fibrosis ➔. Lymph node calcification in HL typically occurs after treatment and may exhibit diffuse, irregular, or eggshell morphology.*

MEDIASTINAL NON-HODGKIN LYMPHOMA

Key Facts

Terminology

- Group of malignant solid neoplasms of lymphoid tissue derived from B cells, T cells, NK cells
  - Systemic diffuse large B-cell non-Hodgkin lymphoma (NHL) with mediastinal involvement
  - Primary mediastinal large B-cell NHL
  - Primary mediastinal T-cell lymphoblastic NHL

Imaging

- Mediastinal lymphadenopathy: Prevascular, paratracheal, subcarinal, posterior mediastinal, paravertebral/retrocrural, paracardiac lymph nodes
- Primary mediastinal large B-cell NHL: Confined to mediastinum without extrathoracic disease
- Primary mediastinal T-cell lymphoblastic NHL: Cervical, supraclavicular, axillary lymphadenopathy
- PET/CT: Staging, assessment of response to therapy, detection of active disease in residual soft tissue

Top Differential Diagnoses

- Mediastinal Hodgkin lymphoma
- Thymoma
- Germ cell neoplasm

Pathology

- Diffuse large B-cell NHL: Most common type (~ 30%)
- Follicular lymphoma (20%)

Clinical Issues

- Indolent NHL: Slow-growing lymphadenopathy, hepatosplenomegaly
- Aggressive NHL: Rapidly growing mass
- Treatment: Chemotherapy ± radiotherapy

Diagnostic Checklist

- Consider primary mediastinal NHL in classic differential diagnosis of anterior mediastinal masses

*(**Left**) PA chest radiograph of a patient with primary mediastinal large B-cell NHL and SVC syndrome shows diffuse bilateral mediastinal enlargement ⇨ with lobular contours. (**Right**) Axial CECT of the same patient shows a bulky homogeneous (> 10 cm) anterior mediastinal mass with marked mass effect on lung ➡ and mediastinum and a slit-like superior vena cava with an intraluminal tumor ➡ producing SVC syndrome. Despite a large size at diagnosis, these tumors tend to initially manifest with early stage disease.*

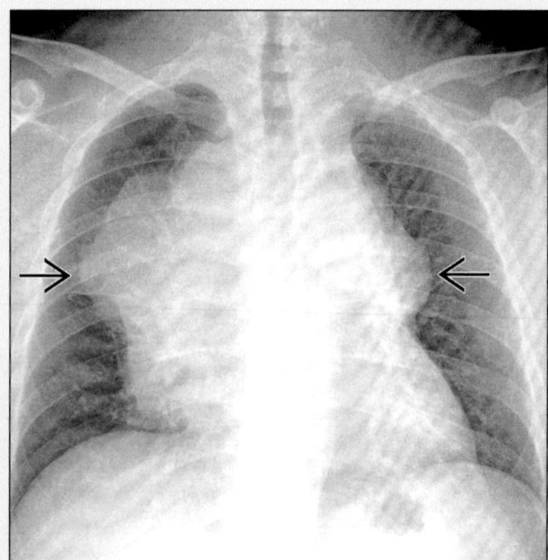

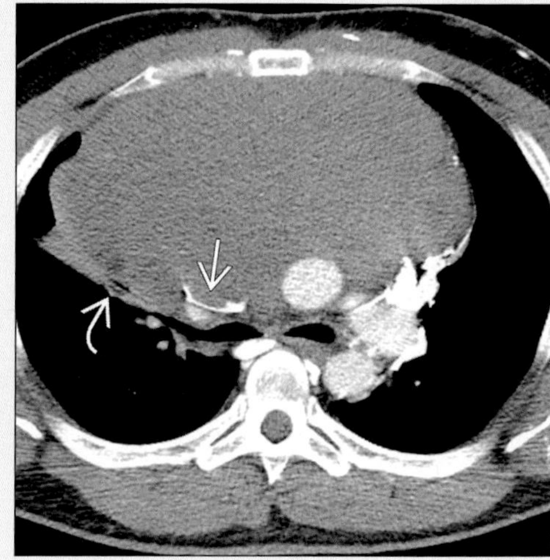

*(**Left**) PA chest radiograph shows a primary mediastinal large B-cell NHL manifesting as a large anterior mediastinal mass ➡ with lobular borders. (**Right**) Coronal fused PET/CT of the same patient shows marked FDG uptake in the anterior mediastinal mass, central photopenic areas ➡ from necrosis, and bilateral supraclavicular lymphadenopathy ➡. While contiguous lymph node involvement occurs, distant lymph node involvement suggests diffuse rather than primary mediastinal large B-cell NHL.*

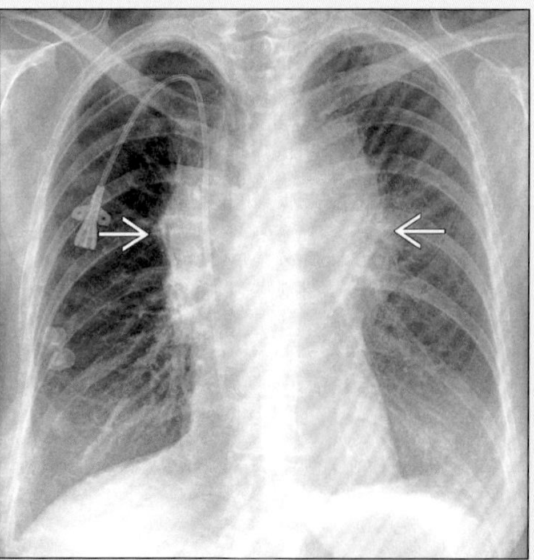

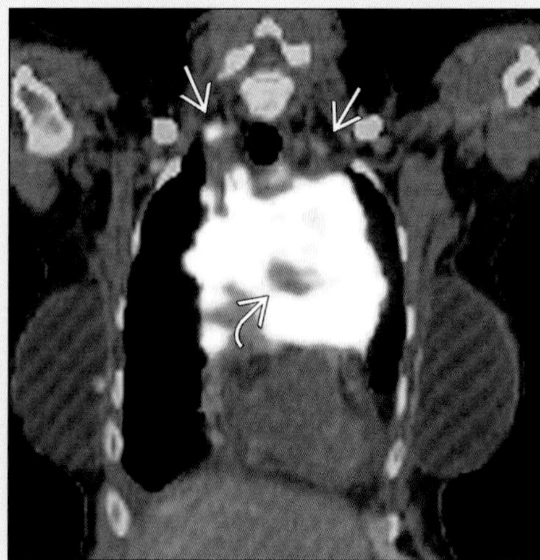

MEDIASTINAL NON-HODGKIN LYMPHOMA

TERMINOLOGY

Abbreviations

- **Non-Hodgkin lymphoma (NHL)**

Definitions

- Group of malignant solid neoplasms of lymphoid tissue derived from B cells, T cells, natural killer (NK) cells, or their precursors
  - **Systemic diffuse large B-cell NHL with mediastinal involvement**
  - **Primary mediastinal NHL**
    - **Primary mediastinal large B-cell NHL**
    - **Primary mediastinal T-cell lymphoblastic NHL/** leukemia

IMAGING

Radiographic Findings

- **Mediastinal & hilar lymphadenopathy**
  - Most common thoracic manifestation of NHL
- Mediastinal mass
- Pleural effusion

CT Findings

- CT more sensitive than radiography for detection of lymphadenopathy (subcarinal, posterior mediastinal, & paracardiac lymph nodes)
- Lymphadenopathy: > 1.0 cm in short axis on CT
- **Diffuse large B-cell lymphoma with mediastinal involvement**
  - **Lymphadenopathy** (most common)
  - Only 1 lymph node group affected (40%)
  - Location: Prevascular & pretracheal (75%), subcarinal (30%), hilar (20%), posterior mediastinal paraaortic, paravertebral, & retrocrural (20%), paracardiac (10%)
  - Hypodense lymphadenopathy often indicates necrosis or cystic change
  - Calcification, rare before treatment
  - Pleural effusion & masses
  - Pericardial effusion & masses
- **Primary mediastinal lymphoma** (large B-cell lymphoma & T-cell lymphoblastic lymphoma)
  - **Bulky anterior mediastinal mass** (> 10 cm)
  - **Low-attenuation areas of necrosis** (common)
  - Pleural effusion or pericardial effusion (common)
  - SVC obstruction (syndrome): Stenosis &/or intraluminal filling defect
  - Tracheal compression

MR Findings

- Lymphadenopathy
  - T1WI: Homogeneous
  - T2WI & T1WI after gadolinium: Homogeneous or heterogeneous due to necrosis
- Homogeneous signal often indicates better survival in patients with high-grade NHL

Nuclear Medicine Findings

- PET/CT
  - Role in staging
    - **Standard modality for staging NHL**
    - Questionable value in small, lymphocytic, extranodal marginal zone lymphoma & extranodal mucosa-associated lymphoid type lymphoma
  - Role after treatment
    - Standard modality for assessing response to therapy
      - Negative PET does not exclude minimal residual disease, but positive PET is predictive of treatment failure
    - Detection of active disease in residual masses after therapy
  - **Primary mediastinal large B-cell NHL**
    - Commonly confined to mediastinum without extrathoracic disease at initial diagnosis
    - Progression or recurrence of disease with hematogenous spread to kidney, liver, ovary, adrenal gland, GI tract, & CNS
  - **Primary mediastinal T-cell lymphoblastic NHL**
    - Cervical, supraclavicular, & axillary lymphadenopathy common at initial diagnosis
    - Extrathoracic lymphadenopathy (common): Superficial cervical, supraclavicular, submandibular, submental, parotid, mesenteric, inguinal
    - Hepatomegaly & splenomegaly (common)
- Ga-67 scintigraphy
  - High-grade NHL shows intense Ga-67 uptake
  - Positive Ga-67 scan midway through chemotherapy course: Alternate therapy options should be considered
  - Useful in patients with residual mass after treatment to assess for active NHL

Imaging Recommendations

- Best imaging tool
  - **FDG PET/CT is modality of choice for staging**

DIFFERENTIAL DIAGNOSIS

Mediastinal Hodgkin Lymphoma

- Tumoral surface more often lobulated than NHL
- Several mediastinal lymph nodes groups affected at a time
- Posterior mediastinal lymph node involvement relatively uncommon

Thymoma

- Difficult to differentiate from thymic malignancy
- Mediastinal lymphadenopathy more common in lymphoma

Germ Cell Neoplasm

- Difficult to differentiate from thymic malignancy
- Serologic markers can be helpful: β-human-chorionic gonadotropin (choriocarcinoma, embryonal carcinoma, seminoma), α-fetoprotein (endodermal sinus tumor, embryonal carcinoma)

PATHOLOGY

General Features

- Etiology
  - NHL linked to altered immunity (e.g., HIV infection, Epstein-Barr virus), environmental exposure (e.g., pesticides & solvents)

Staging, Grading, & Classification

- Common histologic subtypes
  - Diffuse large B-cell NHL: Most common (~ 30%)
  - Follicular NHL (20%)

MEDIASTINAL NON-HODGKIN LYMPHOMA

International Prognostic Index

IPI Score	*Risk*	*Survival*
0-1	Low	73%
2	Low intermediate	51%
3	High intermediate	43%
4-5	High	26%

The International Prognostic Index (IPI) is calculated by assigning 1 point to each factor correlating with shorter survival/relapse-free survival: Age > 60 years, elevated LDH, ECOG performance status ≥ 2, Ann Arbor clinical stage III or IV, number of involved extranodal disease sites > 1.

- Mantle cell NHL
- Small lymphocytic lymphoma/chronic lymphocytic NHL
- Staging
  - Ann Arbor Staging (adopted by the WHO) with Cotswolds Modifications takes into account extent of nodal disease, presence of extranodal disease, & clinical symptoms
    - Much less useful than in Hodgkin lymphoma
  - International prognostic index (IPI)
  - **Diffuse large B-cell NHL**
    - 30-40%: Limited stage (stages I & II)
    - 60-70%: Advanced stage (stages III & IV)
  - **Primary mediastinal large B-cell NHL**
    - Majority stage I or II at diagnosis; IPI is of limited value due to prevalent age
    - Locally invasive: Lungs, chest wall, pleura, pericardium
    - Frequent extranodal relapse: Liver, GI tract, kidneys, ovaries, & CNS
  - **Primary mediastinal T-cell lymphoblastic NHL**
    - > 80% stage III or IV at initial diagnosis

CLINICAL ISSUES

Presentation

- Most common signs/symptoms
  - Indolent NHL
    - Slow-growing lymphadenopathy, hepatomegaly, splenomegaly
    - Cytopenia
  - Aggressive NHL
    - Rapidly growing mass
    - Systemic B symptoms (fever, night seats, weight loss), ↑ LDH, & ↑ uric acid
  - **Primary mediastinal lymphoma** (primary large B-cell lymphoma & primary T-cell lymphoblastic lymphoma)
    - Systemic B symptoms
    - Superior vena cava syndrome
    - Airway compromise: Dyspnea, dysphagia, &/or hoarseness
- Other signs/symptoms
  - Oncologic thoracic emergencies: Spinal cord compression, pericardial tamponade, superior vena cava syndrome, acute airway obstruction, pulmonary embolism
- Clinical profile
  - **Systemic diffuse large B-cell NHL with mediastinal involvement**
    - 7th decade
    - Disease often not localized exclusively to anterior mediastinum
    - Intermediate & high grades more common in immunodeficiency (congenital immunodeficiency, HIV infection, immunosuppressive therapy)
  - **Primary mediastinal large B-cell NHL**
    - Women, 3rd to 4th decades
    - Often confined within anterior mediastinum
  - **Primary T-cell lymphoblastic NHL**
    - Childhood, adolescence, & young adulthood
    - M:F = 2:1

Demographics

- Epidemiology
  - NHL: 3% of all malignancies in adults
    - 2010 (USA): 65,540 new cases & 20,210 deaths
  - **Primary mediastinal large B-cell NHL**: 2.4% of all NHL & 7% of all diffuse large B-cell NHL
  - **Primary mediastinal T-cell lymphoblastic NHL**: 2% of adult NHL

Natural History & Prognosis

- Aggressive & highly aggressive NHL: Diffuse large B-cell lymphoma, Burkitt lymphoma, adult T-cell leukemia/lymphoma, precursor B & T lymphoblastic leukemia/lymphoma
- Indolent NHL: Follicular lymphoma, chronic lymphocytic leukemia/small lymphocytic lymphoma, splenic marginal zone lymphoma

Treatment

- **Limited stage diffuse large B-cell NHL**
  - Chemotherapy with involved-field radiotherapy
- **Advanced stage diffuse large B-cell NHL**
  - Chemotherapy
- **Primary mediastinal large B-cell NHL**
  - Chemotherapy/immunochemotherapy & consolidation radiotherapy

DIAGNOSTIC CHECKLIST

Consider

- Primary mediastinal NHL in the classic differential diagnosis of anterior mediastinal masses

SELECTED REFERENCES

1. Cronin CG et al: Clinical utility of PET/CT in lymphoma. AJR Am J Roentgenol. 194(1):W91-W103, 2010
2. Johnson PW et al: Primary mediastinal B-cell lymphoma. Hematology Am Soc Hematol Educ Program. 349-58, 2008

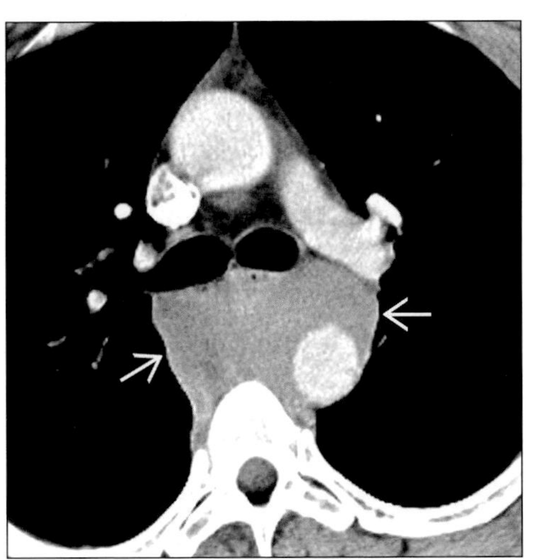

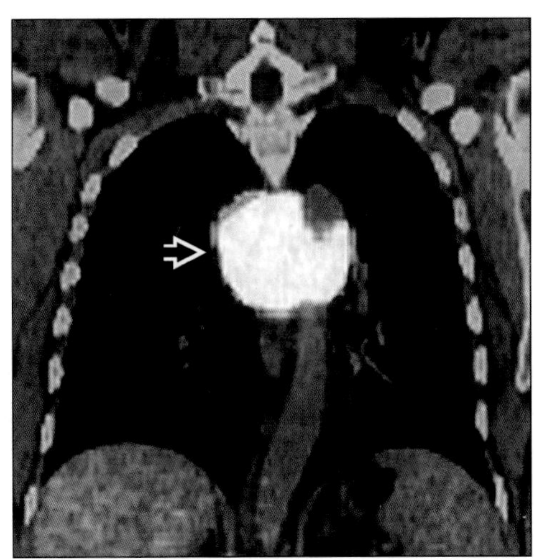

***(Left)** Axial CECT of a patient with follicular NHL shows a mediastinal soft tissue mass → encasing the aorta and adjacent vertebral body and displacing the airways anteriorly. **(Right)** Coronal fused PET/CT of the same patient shows intense FDG uptake ⇨. Follicular lymphoma is the most common indolent NHL. Affected patients are often asymptomatic despite widespread disease. Follicular lymphoma may progress to diffuse large B-cell NHL in 10-70% of patients.*

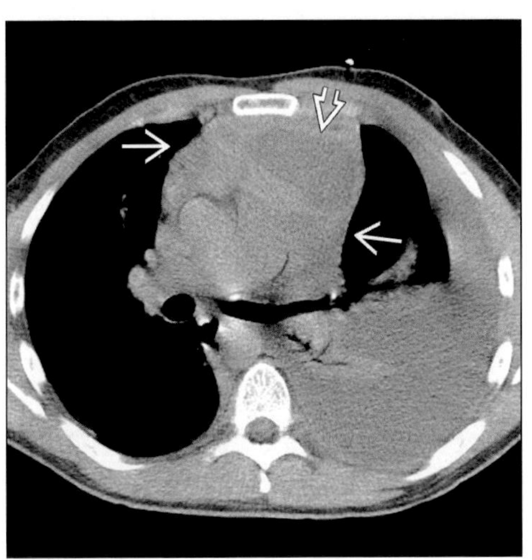

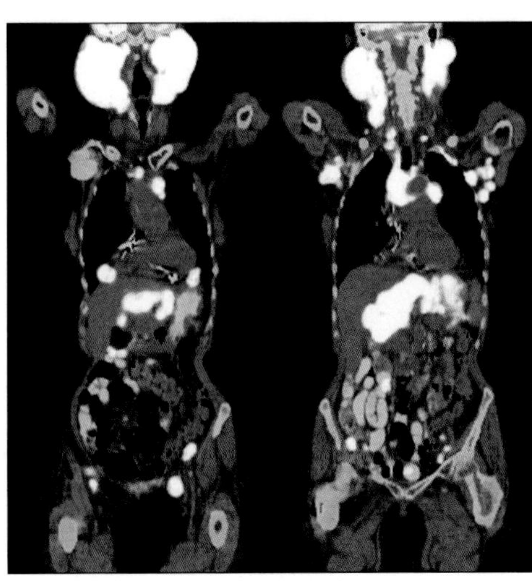

***(Left)** Axial NECT of a patient with primary mediastinal lymphoblastic T-cell NHL demonstrates a large, heterogeneous anterior mediastinal mass → with central necrosis ⇨ and associated left pleural effusion. **(Right)** Coronal fused PET/CT of a patient with diffuse large B-cell NHL with mediastinal involvement shows extensive FDG-avid lymphadenopathy in the neck, chest, abdomen, and pelvis. In comparison to primary mediastinal NHL, diffuse NHL is more likely to exhibit widespread disease.*

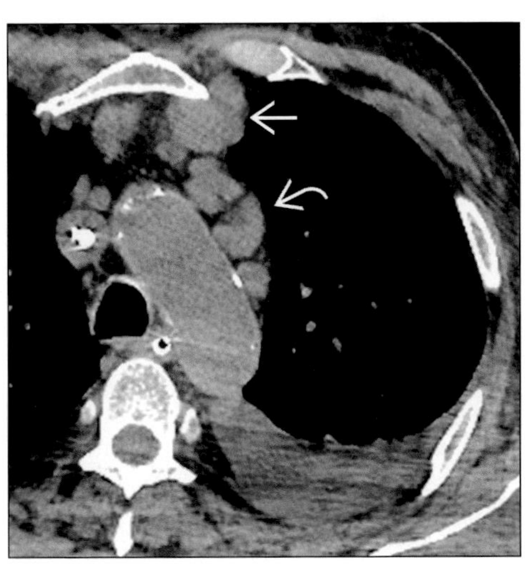

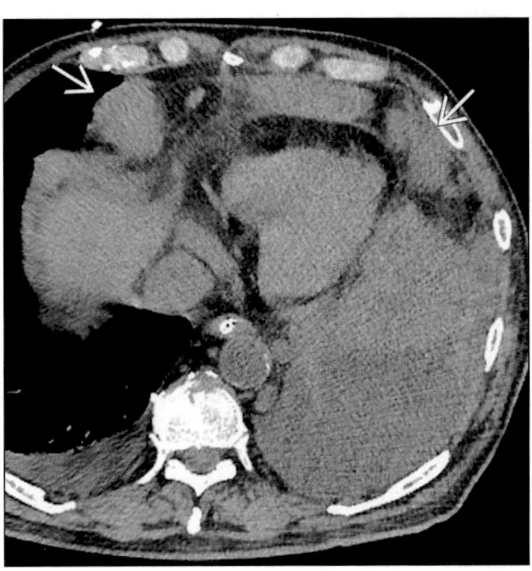

***(Left)** Axial NECT of a patient with diffuse large B-cell NHL with mediastinal involvement shows prevascular ↩ and left internal mammary → lymphadenopathy and a moderate left pleural effusion. **(Right)** Axial NECT of the same patient shows extensive paracardiac lymphadenopathy → and bilateral pleural effusions. Note that, despite extensive disease, the anterior mediastinal lesions in this case are not as significant as those typically seen with primary mediastinal NHL.*

SARCOIDOSIS, LYMPHADENOPATHY

Key Facts

Terminology

- Multisystem chronic inflammatory disorder characterized by noncaseating granulomas

Imaging

- Best diagnostic clue: Bilateral symmetric hilar & right paratracheal lymphadenopathy
- Radiography: Typical & atypical patterns
  - Typical: Bilateral hilar & right paratracheal
  - Atypical: Middle-posterior mediastinal without hilar lymphadenopathy, isolated unilateral hilar lymphadenopathy
- NECT
  - Identification of affected lymph node stations
  - Optimal visualization of lymph node calcification
- CECT: More sensitive than chest radiography for detection of lymphadenopathy
- PET/CT: Can be used to assess treatment response

Top Differential Diagnoses

- Lymphoma
- Metastatic disease
- Infection
- Pneumoconiosis

Pathology

- Staging based on chest radiographic patterns
- Histologic hallmark is noncaseating granuloma

Clinical Issues

- Prognosis
  - 2/3 stable or in remission within a decade
  - 20% progress to pulmonary fibrosis

Diagnostic Checklist

- Consider sarcoidosis in asymptomatic patient with bilateral hilar & right paratracheal lymphadenopathy

(Left) PA chest radiograph of a patient with sarcoidosis shows bilateral hilar enlargement ➔ and thickening of the right paratracheal stripe ⇨, representing lymphadenopathy. (Right) Lateral chest radiograph of the same patient shows bilateral hilar ➔ and subcarinal ↗ lymphadenopathy. Intrathoracic lymphadenopathy occurs in approximately 95% of patients with sarcoidosis. Hilar/mediastinal lymphadenopathy and lung involvement occur in approximately 90% of cases.

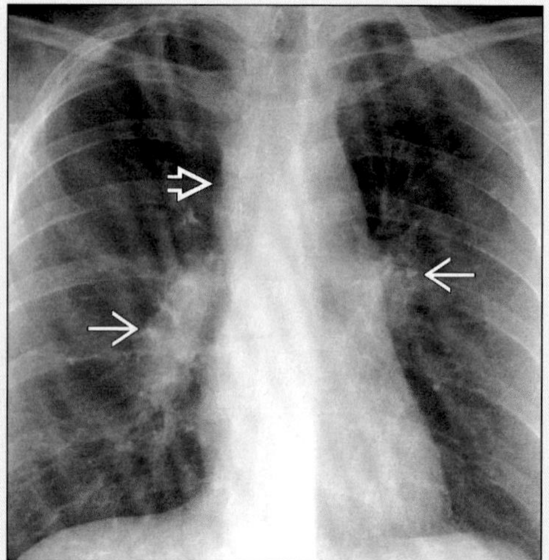

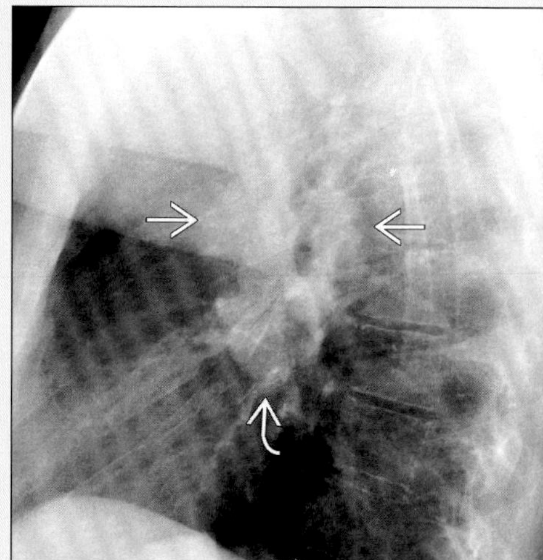

(Left) Graphic shows bilateral and symmetric hilar ⇨, right paratracheal ➔, and subcarinal lymphadenopathy ↗. (Right) Coronal MIP CECT of a patient with stage 2 sarcoidosis shows bilateral hilar, right paratracheal ➔, and subcarinal ↗ lymphadenopathy. The mediastinal and hilar lymph nodes exhibit punctate calcifications. The symmetric distribution of lymphadenopathy is characteristic of sarcoidosis. Bilateral clustered pulmonary nodules ⇨ were also present.

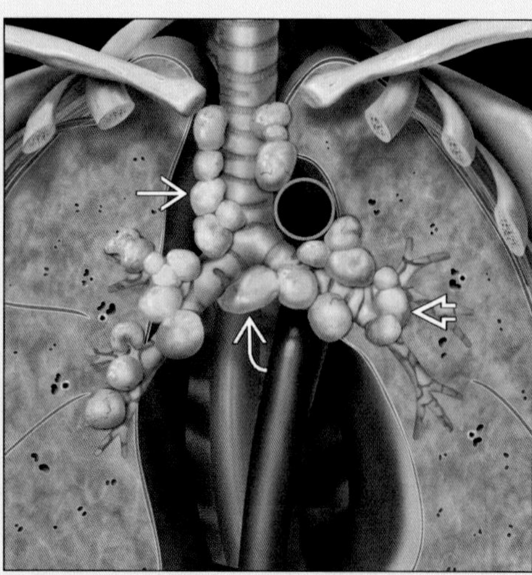

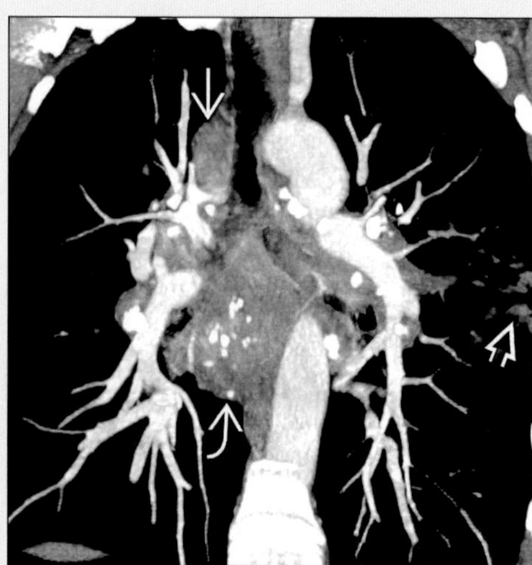

TERMINOLOGY

Definitions

- Multisystem chronic inflammatory disorder characterized by noncaseating granulomas

IMAGING

General Features

- Best diagnostic clue
  - Bilateral symmetric hilar & right paratracheal lymphadenopathy
  - Most common cause of bilateral lymph node enlargement in absence of symptoms
- Location
  - Hila & mediastinum
- Size
  - Variable
    - Subcentimeter to large bulky "potato" lymph nodes

Radiographic Findings

- Radiography
  - Intrathoracic lymphadenopathy is most common finding
    - **Bilateral symmetric hilar ± mediastinal lymphadenopathy in 95% of cases**
    - **Hilar & mediastinal lymphadenopathy + lung involvement in 90% of cases**
    - Middle-posterior mediastinal ± prevascular lymphadenopathy in 50% of cases
  - Typical pattern
    - **Bilateral hilar & right paratracheal lymphadenopathy most common**
      - Bilateral hilar enlargement: Lymph nodes may project over hilar vessels ("hilum overlay" sign)
      - Thickening of right paratracheal stripe > 4 mm
    - Left paratracheal, aortopulmonary window, & prevascular lymphadenopathy less common
      - Less apparent on chest radiography
      - Convexity of aortopulmonary window
  - Atypical pattern
    - Middle-posterior mediastinal lymphadenopathy in absence of hilar lymphadenopathy
      - More common in patients > 50 years
      - Paratracheal, subcarinal, aortopulmonary window, & retroazygos lymph nodes
    - Isolated unilateral hilar lymphadenopathy (1-3%)
    - Anterior mediastinal lymphadenopathy
  - Lymph node calcification
    - Related to duration of disease
      - 5 years: 3% of cases
      - 10 years: 20% of cases
    - Morphology
      - Amorphous, punctate, popcorn-like, & eggshell

CT Findings

- NECT
  - Evaluation of lymphadenopathy & identification of affected lymph node groups
  - Optimal visualization of lymph node calcification
  - Evaluation of parenchymal disease & complications
- CECT
  - More sensitive than chest radiography for detection of lymphadenopathy
  - Left paratracheal, aortopulmonary window, subcarinal, & anterior mediastinal lymphadenopathy readily identified

Nuclear Medicine Findings

- PET/CT
  - Increased FDG uptake within calcified & noncalcified lymph nodes
  - Cannot distinguish between sarcoidosis & other causes of FDG-avid lymphadenopathy
  - Can be used to assess treatment response
- Ga-67 scintigraphy
  - Increased uptake within lymph nodes
    - Nonspecific indicator of active inflammation
    - λ sign
      - Increased uptake within bilateral hilar & right paratracheal lymph nodes
  - Can be used to assess treatment response

Imaging Recommendations

- Best imaging tool
  - Radiography may demonstrate typical pattern of lymphadenopathy
    - Less sensitive for small lymph nodes & atypical pattern of lymphadenopathy
  - CECT best for detecting extent of lymphadenopathy
  - CECT or PET/CT for monitoring treatment response

DIFFERENTIAL DIAGNOSIS

Lymphoma

- Enlarged lymph nodes; may or may not enhance
- Untreated lymphoma does not usually calcify
- Treated lymphoma may calcify
- Both Hodgkin & non-Hodgkin lymphoma may affect thorax

Metastatic Disease

- Enlarged lymph nodes; may or may not enhance
- Most common primary malignancies
  - Head & neck, lung, breast, genitourinary tract cancers, & melanoma
- Calcified lymph node metastases: Thyroid carcinoma & mucinous adenocarcinomas of gastrointestinal & genitourinary tracts

Infection

- Tuberculosis
  - Right paratracheal > bilateral hilar lymphadenopathy
    - May exhibit calcification
- Histoplasmosis
  - Similar distribution of lymphadenopathy
  - May exhibit calcification
- Other fungal infections
  - Coccidioidomycosis
  - Blastomycosis
  - Cryptococcosis

Pneumoconiosis

- Silicosis
  - Hilar & mediastinal lymphadenopathy
    - May exhibit eggshell calcification
- Berylliosis
  - Symmetric bilateral hilar lymphadenopathy
    - Isolated lymphadenopathy less common
    - Diffuse or eggshell calcification

SARCOIDOSIS, LYMPHADENOPATHY

PATHOLOGY

General Features

- Etiology
  - Unknown
  - May be disorder of immune regulation
- Associated abnormalities
  - Increased risk of developing Hodgkin & non-Hodgkin lymphoma
    - "Sarcoidosis-lymphoma syndrome"
    - Estimated 5.5x increased risk of lymphoma compared to others in same age group

Staging, Grading, & Classification

- **Staging based on chest radiography findings**
  - Stage 0: No abnormalities (5-10% at presentation)
  - Stage 1: Lymphadenopathy (50%)
  - Stage 2: Lymphadenopathy & lung opacities (25-30%)
  - Stage 3: Lung opacities (10-12%)
  - Stage 4: Fibrosis (5% at presentation, up to 25% during course of disease)

Gross Pathologic & Surgical Features

- Lymph node enlargement, lung nodules
- Pulmonary fibrosis

Microscopic Features

- Hallmark is **noncaseating granuloma**
  - Central core of histiocytes, epithelioid cells, & multinucleated giant cells
    - Surrounded by lymphocytes, scattered plasma cells, peripheral fibroblasts, & collagen
      - Central lymphocytes express CD4
      - Peripheral lymphocytes express CD8
  - Multinucleated giant cells may demonstrate inclusions, such as asteroid & Schaumann bodies
  - Surrounding fibroblasts, mast cells, collagen, & proteoglycans may lead to fibrosis & end-organ damage
    - Fibrosis spreads from periphery to center
      - Progression to complete fibrosis ± hyalinization
  - May demonstrate coagulative necrosis

CLINICAL ISSUES

Presentation

- Most common signs/symptoms
  - Respiratory symptoms most common
    - Dry cough, dyspnea, bronchial hyperreactivity
  - Fatigue, malaise, fever, night sweats, weight loss, erythema nodosum
  - 50% asymptomatic

Demographics

- Age
  - Any age group may be affected
  - Most commonly affects adults < 40 years
  - Peak incidence: 20-29 years
  - Children rarely affected
- Gender
  - Female > male
- Ethnicity
  - African-Americans, Swedes, & Danes have highest prevalence worldwide
    - Prevalence in other countries may be underestimated secondary to lack of screening programs & misdiagnosis
  - United States: Age-adjusted annual incidence for African-Americans > 3x that for Caucasians
    - 35.5/100,000 vs. 10.9/100,000 persons
- Epidemiology
  - 1-40 cases/100,000 persons

Natural History & Prognosis

- Caucasians often asymptomatic at time of presentation
- African-Americans often present with severe multisystem disease
- African-Americans reported to have higher mortality rate than Caucasians
- 2/3 remain stable or undergo remission within decade
- 20% progress to pulmonary fibrosis
- Course based on chest radiographic patterns
  - Stage 1: Remission in 60-90%
  - Stage 2: Remission in 40-70%
  - Stage 3: Remission in 10-20%
  - Stage 4: Remission in 0%
- Good prognosis
  - Fever, polyarthritis, erythema nodosum, bilateral hilar lymphadenopathy
- Poor prognosis
  - Stage 2 or 3 disease at diagnosis, disease onset after 40 years, African-American race, hypercalcemia, splenomegaly, osseous involvement, chronic uveitis, lupus pernio
- Mortality: 1-5%
  - Causes of death: Respiratory failure, cardiac or neurologic involvement, hemorrhage, infection

Treatment

- Medical therapy
  - Corticosteroids are mainstay of therapy
  - Treatment based on clinical, functional, & radiologic findings

DIAGNOSTIC CHECKLIST

Consider

- Sarcoidosis in asymptomatic patients with symmetric bilateral hilar & right paratracheal lymphadenopathy

SELECTED REFERENCES

1. Criado E et al: Pulmonary sarcoidosis: typical and atypical manifestations at high-resolution CT with pathologic correlation. Radiographics. 30(6):1567-86, 2010
2. Prabhakar HB et al: Imaging features of sarcoidosis on MDCT, FDG PET, and PET/CT. AJR Am J Roentgenol. 190(3 Suppl):S1-6, 2008
3. Miller BH et al: Thoracic sarcoidosis: radiologic-pathologic correlation. Radiographics. 15(2):421-37, 1995

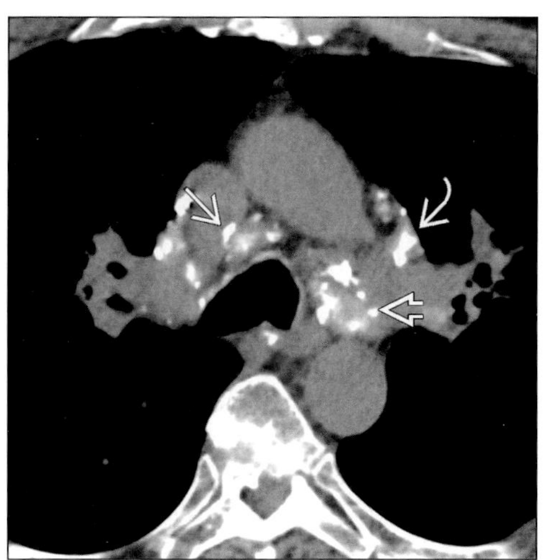

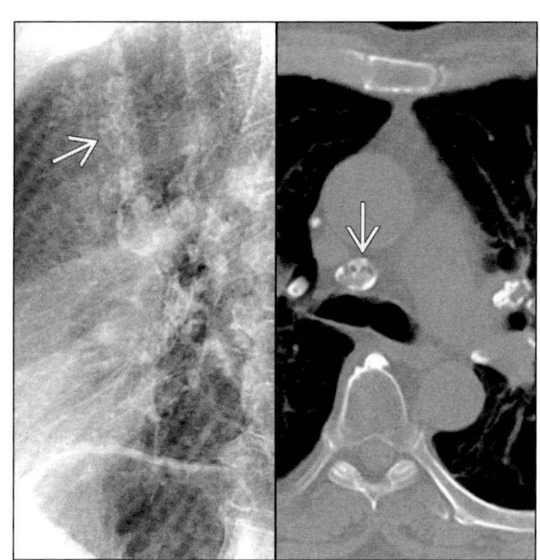

(Left) *Axial NECT of a patient with longstanding sarcoidosis shows numerous calcified pretracheal, left paratracheal, and aortopulmonary window lymph nodes.* ***(Right)*** *Composite image with lateral chest radiograph (left) and axial NECT in bone window (right) of a patient with sarcoidosis shows multifocal mediastinal and hilar lymph nodes with peripheral eggshell calcification nicely demonstrated on chest CT. The prevalence of lymph node calcification increases with disease duration.*

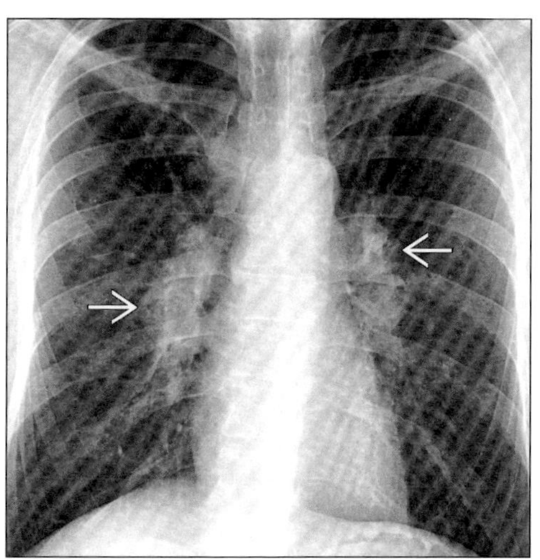

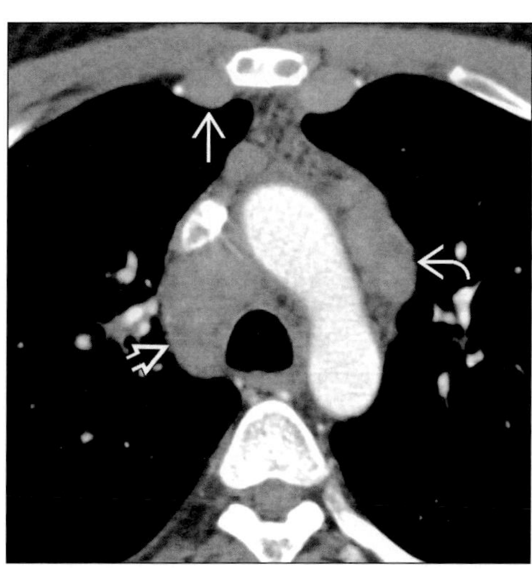

(Left) *Frontal chest radiograph of a patient with sarcoidosis shows bilateral hilar enlargement secondary to bilateral hilar lymphadenopathy.* ***(Right)*** *Axial CECT of a patient with sarcoidosis demonstrates extensive intrathoracic lymphadenopathy affecting right paratracheal, prevascular, anterior mediastinal, and bilateral internal mammary lymph node groups. The enlarged right paratracheal and prevascular lymph nodes demonstrate the characteristic bulky "potato" configuration.*

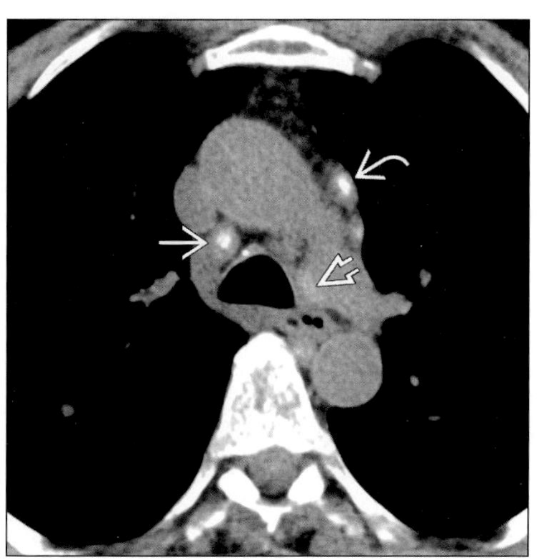

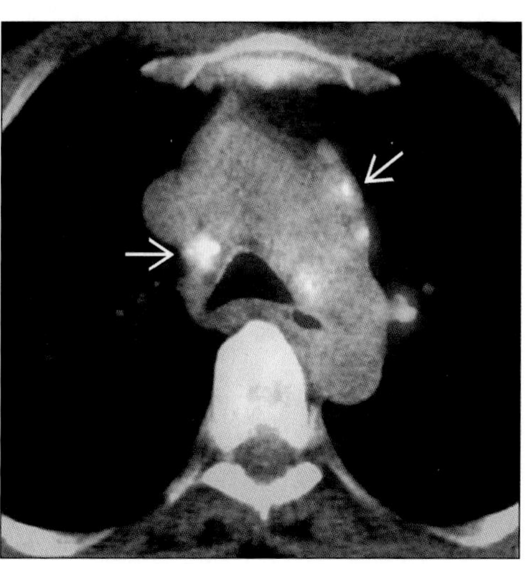

(Left) *Axial NECT demonstrates nonenlarged right and left paratracheal and prevascular lymph nodes that demonstrate calcification.* ***(Right)*** *Axial fused PET/CT of the same patient shows increased FDG uptake within these lymph nodes. PET/CT cannot distinguish between lymphadenopathy related to sarcoidosis and that secondary to lymphoma, metastatic disease, infection, or pneumoconiosis. However, PET/CT can be used to monitor treatment response.*

MEDIASTINAL FIBROSIS

Key Facts

Terminology
- Benign condition characterized by proliferation of dense fibrous tissue in mediastinum

Imaging
- Radiography
  - Mediastinal widening/hilar mass ± calcification
  - Signs of airway or vascular obstruction
- CT
  - Infiltrative mediastinal soft tissue & calcification
  - Surrounds, invades, obstructs structures
  - Focal (calcified) & diffuse (noncalcified) types
- MR
  - Intermediate signal intensity on T1WI
  - Variable signal intensity on T2WI
  - Heterogeneous enhancement
- CECT for optimal evaluation of extent of involvement & complications

Top Differential Diagnoses
- Lymphoma
- Mediastinal carcinomas
- Elastofibroma and fibromatosis

Clinical Issues
- Etiology: *H. capsulatum*, other fungi, tuberculosis
- Symptoms: Cough, dyspnea, infection, hemoptysis, chest pain
- Prognosis: Unpredictable course, 30% mortality
- Treatment
  - Medical: Systemic antifungals & corticosteroids
  - Surgical resection
  - Endobronchial & endovascular stent placement

Diagnostic Checklist
- Consider mediastinal fibrosis in young patients with obstructive mediastinal soft tissue & calcification

*(**Left**) Axial CECT of a patient with mediastinal fibrosis shows a partially calcified precarinal lymph node ➔. (**Right**) Axial CECT of the same patient shows a noncalcified subcarinal soft tissue mass ➔ and a right lung calcified granuloma ↷. Calcified or partially calcified soft tissue masses in the subcarinal, hilar, and paratracheal regions are characteristic of the focal form of mediastinal fibrosis, which is usually secondary to Histoplasma capsulatum infection.*

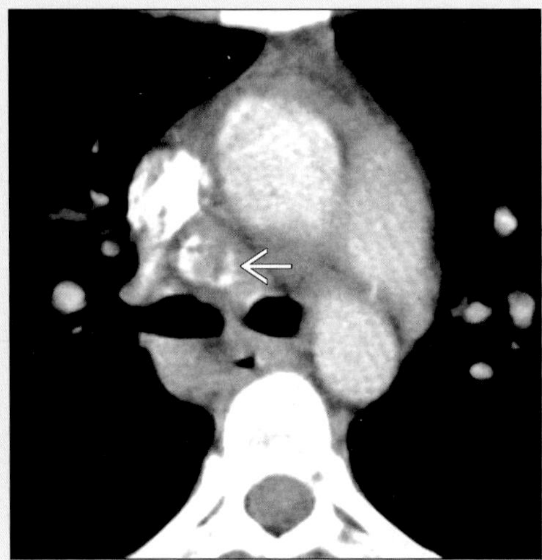

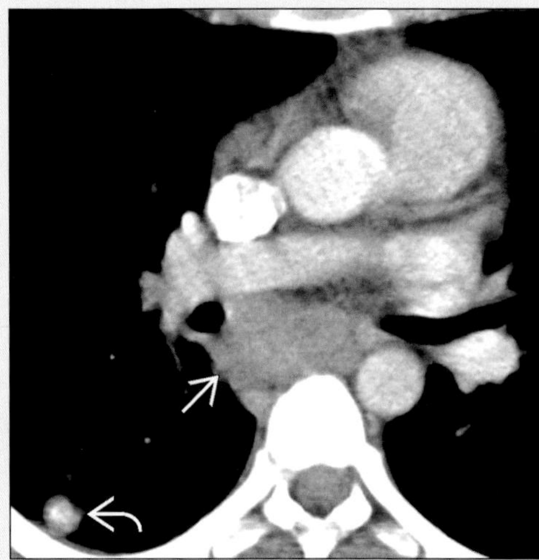

*(**Left**) PA chest radiograph of a patient with mediastinal fibrosis shows bilateral mediastinal widening ➔. A metallic stent ⇩ projects over the expected location of the superior vena cava (SVC). (**Right**) Axial CECT of the same patient demonstrates mediastinal widening and infiltrative soft tissue within the mediastinal fat ➔. A metallic stent ↷ has been placed within the occluded SVC to treat SVC obstruction secondary to mediastinal fibrosis, which can obstruct vessels and airways.*

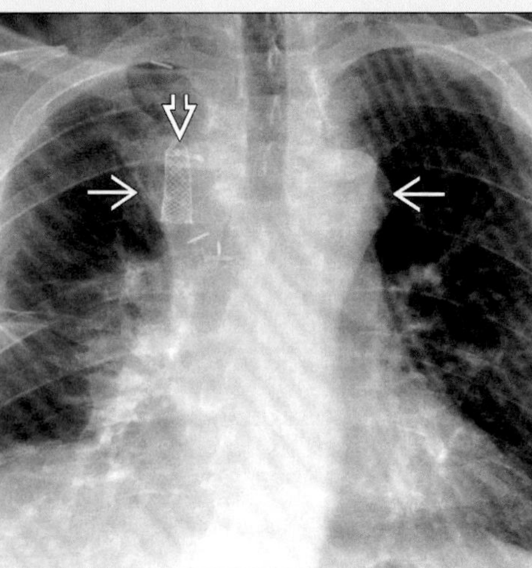

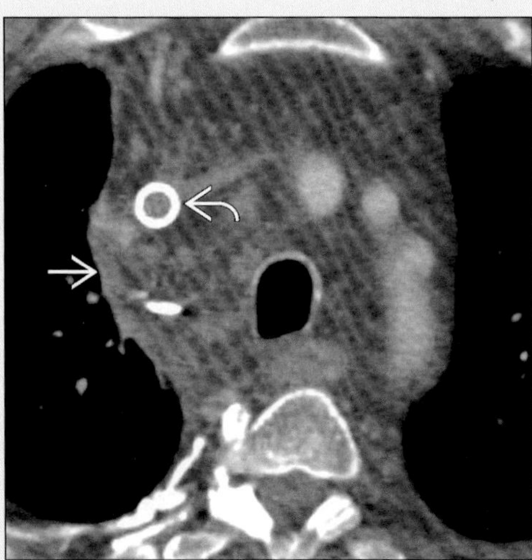

MEDIASTINAL FIBROSIS

TERMINOLOGY

Abbreviations

- **Mediastinal fibrosis (MF)**

Synonyms

- Fibrosing mediastinitis
- Sclerosing mediastinitis

Definitions

- Benign condition characterized by proliferation of dense fibrous tissue in mediastinum

IMAGING

General Features

- Best diagnostic clue
  - Mediastinal soft tissue with calcification
- Location
  - Mediastinum
    - Middle-posterior > anterior
    - Right > left

Radiographic Findings

- Most chest radiographs are abnormal
- Nonspecific mediastinal widening
  - Loss of normal lines, stripes, & interfaces
  - Subcarinal & right paratracheal regions most commonly affected
- Focal hilar mass
- Mediastinal or hilar calcification
- Superior vena cava (SVC) obstruction: Superior mediastinal widening
- Narrowing of tracheobronchial tree
  - Carina & main bronchi most commonly affected
  - Volume loss; atelectasis typically segmental or lobar
  - Recurrent pneumonia
- Obstruction of pulmonary vessels
  - Arteries
    - Decreased size & number of vessels on affected side
  - Veins
    - Localized pulmonary venous hypertension: Peribronchial cuffing, septal thickening, localized pulmonary edema
  - Pulmonary infarction: Peripheral, wedge-shaped opacity

CT Findings

- CECT
  - General
    - Infiltrative mediastinal soft tissue
      - Surrounds or invades mediastinal structures
      - Obliterates mediastinal fat planes
  - 2 patterns
    - **Focal: 82% of cases**
      - Soft tissue mass
      - Usually calcified
      - Variable enhancement
      - Subcarinal, hilar, & paratracheal regions most commonly affected
    - Diffuse: 18% of cases
      - Diffusely infiltrating soft tissue mass
      - Calcification uncommon
      - Variable enhancement
      - Multiple mediastinal compartments affected
  - **SVC obstruction**
    - Nonopacification of SVC
    - Chest wall & mediastinal collateral vessels
  - Narrowing of tracheobronchial tree
    - Delineation of location, extent, & length of airway stenosis
  - Obstruction of pulmonary vessels
    - Arteries
      - Localized oligemia
    - Veins
      - Focal or diffuse hyperattenuation in lung parenchyma
      - Ground-glass opacity
      - Interlobular septal thickening
    - Pulmonary arterial or venous infarction: Peripheral, wedge-shaped opacity

MR Findings

- T1WI
  - Intermediate signal intensity
- T2WI
  - Variable: Regions of hypo- and hyperintensity within soft tissue mass
- T1WI C+
  - Heterogeneous enhancement

Fluoroscopic Findings

- Esophagram
  - Esophageal involvement
    - Junction of upper & middle thirds most commonly affected
    - Involved segment typically adjacent to trachea or mainstem bronchi
    - Typical findings
      - Circumferential narrowing
      - Long segment strictures
      - Esophageal varices in SVC obstruction

Nuclear Medicine Findings

- PET/CT
  - FDG uptake variable; may be present in areas of active inflammation
- V/Q scan
  - Perfusion scintigraphy with Tc-99m-MAA
    - Focal or diffuse perfusion defects
      - Pulmonary arterial or venous obstruction
    - Complete unilateral perfusion defect
      - Focal hilar fibrosis
  - Ventilation scintigraphy with Xe-133 or Tc-99m-DTPA
    - Ventilation defects
      - Lobar or segmental airway occlusion
    - Delayed washout of Xe-133
      - Partial airway obstruction

Angiographic Findings

- Long segment smooth or funnel-shaped vascular stenosis

Imaging Recommendations

- Best imaging tool
  - CECT for optimal evaluation of extent of involvement & complications

MEDIASTINAL FIBROSIS

DIFFERENTIAL DIAGNOSIS

Lymphoma

- Nodal coalescence may form large soft tissue masses
- Untreated lymphoma usually does not calcify
  - Treated lymphoma may calcify

Mediastinal Carcinomas

- Type & imaging appearance depend on mediastinal compartment involved

Elastofibroma and Fibromatosis

- Aggressive fibromatosis
  - Proliferation of fibrous tissue
- Usually homogeneous with similar attenuation to muscle on NECT
- Most demonstrate enhancement on CECT

PATHOLOGY

General Features

- Etiology
  - *Histoplasma capsulatum* infection
    - Most cases of MF occur in regions of endemic infection
    - Patients with positive skin test to specific antigen
    - Evidence of granulomatous disease within tissue
    - *H. capsulatum* organisms may be found in specimens
  - Other fungal infections
    - Aspergillosis
    - Mucormycosis
    - Blastomycosis
    - Cryptococcosis
  - Tuberculosis
  - Uncommon causes
    - Behçet disease
    - Rheumatic fever
    - Radiation therapy
    - Trauma
    - Hodgkin lymphoma
    - Drug reaction
- Genetics
  - Fibroinflammatory response to *H. capsulatum* antigen may occur in genetically susceptible individuals
- Associated abnormalities
  - Other idiopathic fibroinflammatory disorders
    - Retroperitoneal fibrosis
    - Sclerosing cholangitis
    - Riedel thyroiditis
    - Orbital pseudotumor

Staging, Grading, & Classification

- Focal
  - Most common type in United States
  - Fibroinflammatory response to *H. capsulatum* antigen in genetically susceptible individuals
  - Localized mediastinal or hilar fibrosis & extensive calcification
- Diffuse
  - Less common type
  - Idiopathic
  - Related to other fibroinflammatory disorders
  - Multicompartmental fibrosis without calcification

Gross Pathologic & Surgical Features

- Ill-defined mediastinal soft tissue mass
  - Composed of dense, white, fibrous tissue
- Localized mass or diffuse mediastinal infiltration

Microscopic Features

- Infiltration & obliteration of adipose tissue by fibrous tissue & mononuclear cell infiltrate
- Histopathologic spectrum
  - Stage I: Edematous fibromyxoid tissue
  - Stage II: Mediastinal structures infiltrated & surrounded by eosinophilic hyaline material
  - Stage III: Dense paucicellular collagen; classic microscopic features of MF

CLINICAL ISSUES

Presentation

- Most common signs/symptoms
  - Cough, dyspnea, recurrent infection, hemoptysis, pleuritic chest pain
- Other signs/symptoms
  - Fever & weight loss

Demographics

- Age
  - Most patients young at presentation
- Gender
  - M = F

Natural History & Prognosis

- Unpredictable course
  - Spontaneous remission or exacerbation
- Reported mortality as high as 30%
- Causes of death
  - Recurrent infection
  - Hemoptysis
  - Cor pulmonale

Treatment

- Medical therapy
  - Systemic antifungals
  - Corticosteroids
- Surgical resection
  - High morbidity & mortality
- Local therapy for complications
  - Endobronchial & endovascular stent placement

DIAGNOSTIC CHECKLIST

Consider

- Mediastinal fibrosis in young patients with obstructive mediastinal soft tissue & calcification in appropriate clinical setting

SELECTED REFERENCES

1. Kim HY et al: Thoracic sequelae and complications of tuberculosis. Radiographics. 21(4):839-58; discussion 859-60, 2001
2. Rossi SE et al: Fibrosing mediastinitis. Radiographics. 21(3):737-57, 2001

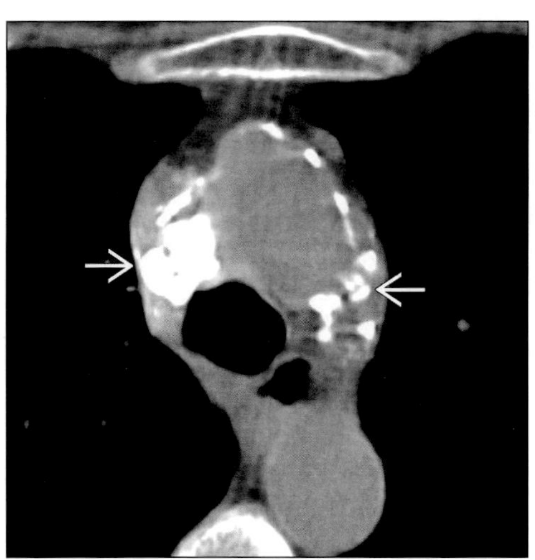

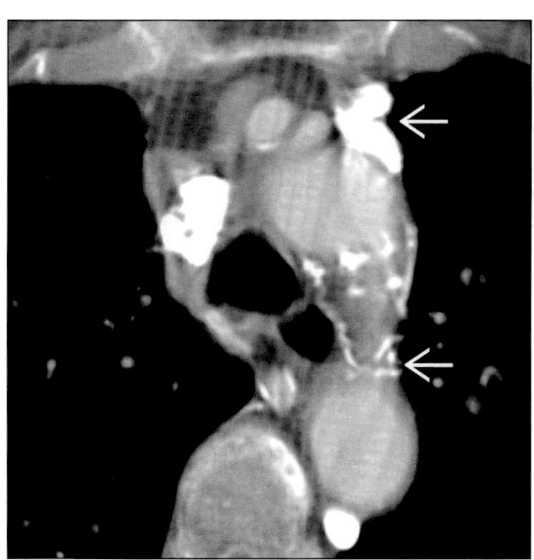

(Left) *Axial NECT of a patient with mediastinal fibrosis shows calcified right paratracheal and aortopulmonary window lymph nodes ➡.* ***(Right)*** *Axial CECT of the same patient shows multiple enhancing mediastinal collateral vessels ➡ secondary to SVC obstruction from mediastinal fibrosis. SVC obstruction may manifest with bilateral mediastinal widening on chest radiography. CECT typically shows nonopacification of the SVC and enhancing mediastinal collateral vessels.*

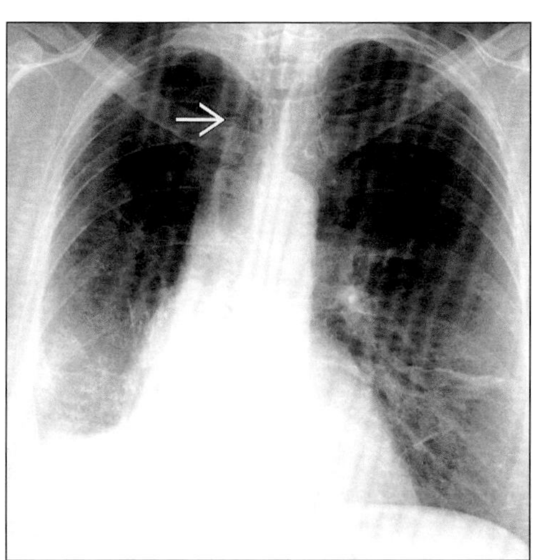

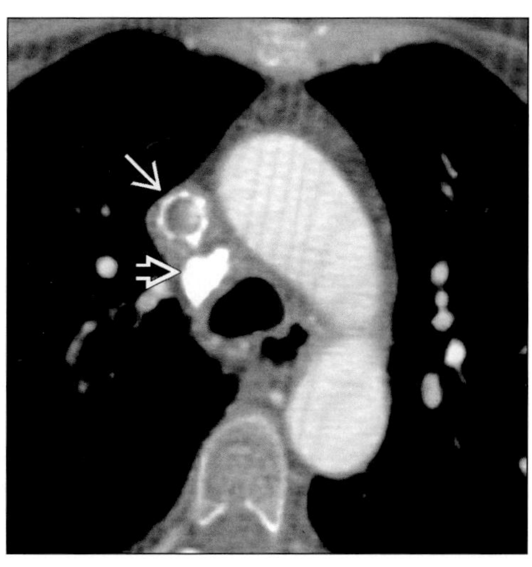

(Left) *PA chest radiograph of a patient with mediastinal fibrosis shows volume loss in the right hemithorax and rightward mediastinal shift ➡. Obscuration of the right heart border and right hemidiaphragm are consistent with adjacent atelectasis secondary to airway narrowing and obstruction.* ***(Right)*** *Axial CECT of a patient with mediastinal fibrosis and SVC obstruction shows a patent SVC stent ➡. Note the calcified right paratracheal lymph node ➡.*

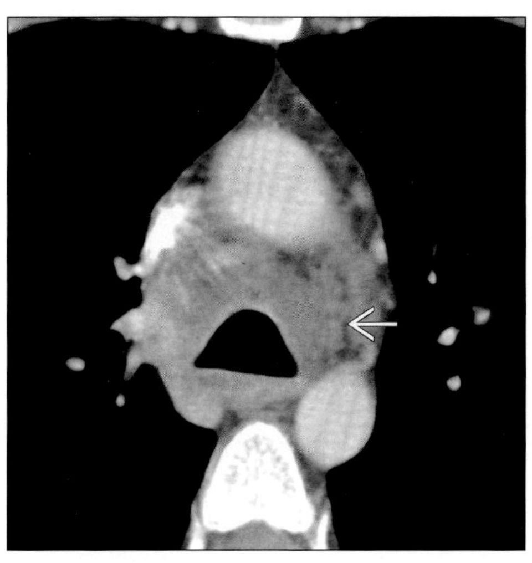

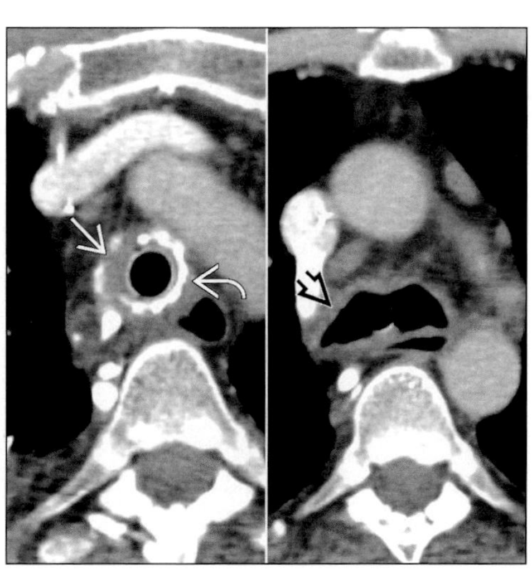

(Left) *Axial CECT of a patient with mediastinal fibrosis demonstrates infiltrative mediastinal soft tissue ➡ surrounding the trachea slightly above the carina.* ***(Right)*** *Composite image with axial CECT at the level of the mid trachea (left) and at the level of the carina (right) of a patient with airway obstruction from mediastinal fibrosis shows a tracheal stent ➡, asymmetric right tracheal wall thickening ➡, and irregular thickening of the right and left main bronchi ➡ by abnormal soft tissue.*

LOCALIZED CASTLEMAN DISEASE

Key Facts

Terminology
- Castleman disease (CD)
- Benign lymphoproliferative lymph node hyperplasia

Imaging
- Location: 70% of CD occurs in thorax
  - Tracheobronchial, hilar, mediastinal lymph nodes
- Radiography
  - Smooth or lobular hilar mass most common
  - Mediastinal: Middle-posterior compartment
- CT
  - Solitary or multiple enlarged lymph nodes
  - Smooth or lobular margins
  - Intense contrast enhancement characteristic
- MR
  - T1WI: Low to intermediate signal intensity
  - T2WI: Hyperintense
  - T1WI C+: Intense enhancement

Top Differential Diagnoses
- Kaposi sarcoma
- Lymphoma & leukemia
- Metastatic lymphadenopathy
- Paraganglioma

Pathology
- Etiology unknown; several proposed theories
  - Chronic inflammation, immunodeficiency, hamartomatous process, autoimmunity
- 2 classification systems
  - Histology: Hyaline vascular, plasma cell, mixed
  - Distribution: Localized, multicentric

Clinical Issues
- Most asymptomatic; symptoms from mass effect rare
- Complete surgical excision is usually curative
- Variable response to chemotherapy & radiation

*(**Left**) PA chest radiograph of a patient with Castleman disease shows a well-marginated lobulated right paratracheal mass ➔. (**Right**) Axial CECT of the same patient shows a large, intensely enhancing right paratracheal lymph node ➔ with pretracheal extension. 70% of Castleman disease occurs within the thorax, and the most common imaging manifestation is mediastinal &/ or hilar lymphadenopathy.*

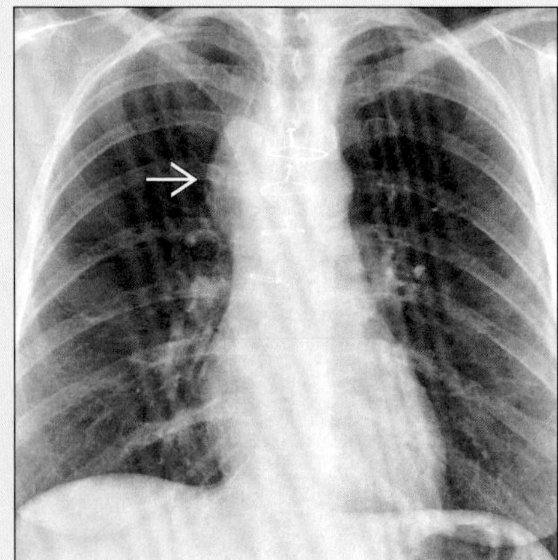

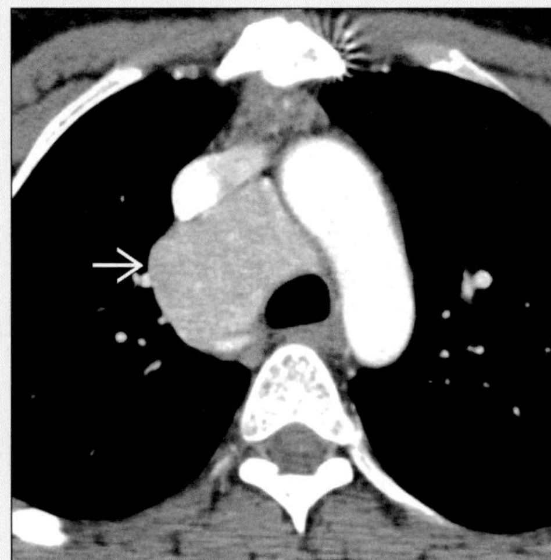

*(**Left**) Graphic demonstrates the morphologic features of Castleman disease. The affected right hilar lymph node ➔ exhibits hypervascularity, which accounts for the intense enhancement seen on contrast-enhanced CT and MR. (**Right**) Composite image with axial NECT in lung (left) and soft tissue (right) window shows a well-circumscribed right lower lobe mass ➔ that exhibits intense contrast enhancement ➔. Although pulmonary involvement by CD is rare, the intense contrast enhancement should suggest the diagnosis.*

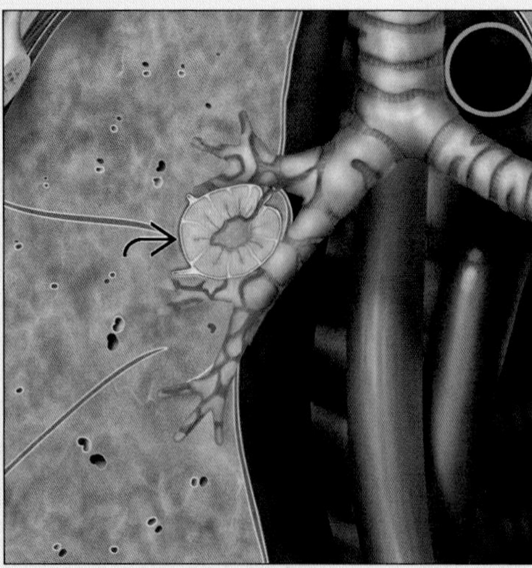

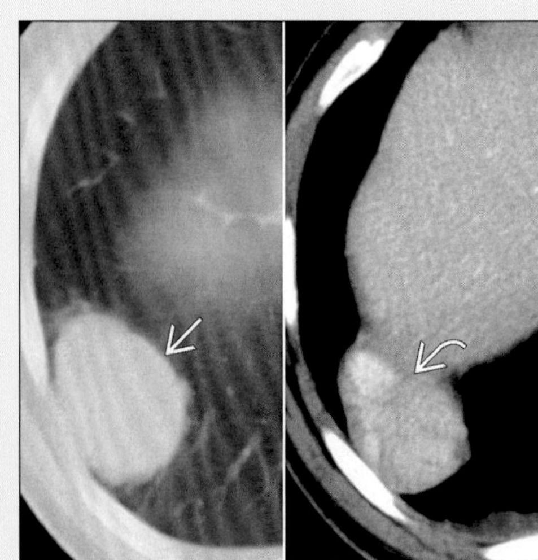

LOCALIZED CASTLEMAN DISEASE

TERMINOLOGY

Abbreviations

- **Castleman disease (CD)**

Synonyms

- Angiofollicular lymph node hyperplasia
- Giant lymph node hyperplasia

Definitions

- Benign lymphoproliferative lymph node hyperplasia

IMAGING

General Features

- Best diagnostic clue
  - Enhancing solitary or multiple lymph nodes
- Location
  - 70% occurs in thorax
  - Tracheobronchial, hilar, & mediastinal lymph nodes
  - Rare involvement of pleura, axilla, pericardium, lung
- Size
  - Variable, often between 2-6 cm

Radiographic Findings

- Smooth or lobular hilar mass most common
- Mediastinal involvement
  - Usually middle-posterior compartment

CT Findings

- CECT
  - Solitary or multiple enlarged lymph nodes
    - Smooth or lobular margins
    - Calcification in 5-10%
    - Intense contrast enhancement is characteristic
    - May demonstrate atypical enhancement patterns
      - Uniform poor enhancement from necrosis, fibrosis, degeneration
      - Peripheral rim enhancement from central necrosis
    - Nodal mass involving adjacent structures
  - Enhancing pulmonary mass is rare

MR Findings

- T1WI
  - Low to intermediate signal intensity
- T2WI
  - Hyperintense
- T1WI C+
  - Intense enhancement

Imaging Recommendations

- Best imaging tool
  - Contrast-enhanced CT is optimal imaging modality

DIFFERENTIAL DIAGNOSIS

Kaposi Sarcoma

- Kaposi & CD may coexist in HIV(+) patients
- Enlarged lymph nodes may avidly enhance

Lymphoma & Leukemia

- Lymphadenopathy ± enhancement
- Overlap of clinical & imaging features

Metastatic Lymphadenopathy

- Intense enhancement of enlarged lymph nodes
- Renal cell & thyroid carcinoma, melanoma, sarcoma

Paraganglioma

- Uncommon mediastinal neoplasm
  - Most located in paravertebral region
- Solitary mass with intense enhancement

PATHOLOGY

General Features

- Etiology
  - Etiology unknown; several proposed theories
    - Chronic inflammation
    - Immunodeficiency
    - Hamartomatous process
    - Autoimmunity

Staging, Grading, & Classification

- 2 classification systems
  - Histology: **Hyaline vascular (90%)**, plasma cell (9%), rare mixed forms
  - Distribution: Localized & multicentric

Gross Pathologic & Surgical Features

- Thick fibrous capsule in hyaline vascular type

Microscopic Features

- Hyaline vascular
  - Germinal centers with many mature lymphocytes
    - Concentric hyaline sclerosis & onion-skin lymphocyte layer
    - Prominent interfollicular capillary proliferation
  - Areas of necrosis, especially in lymph nodes > 5 cm
- Plasma cell
  - Sheets of mature plasma cells between hyperplastic germinal centers
  - Variable capillary proliferation

CLINICAL ISSUES

Presentation

- Most common signs/symptoms
  - Most asymptomatic
  - Rarely symptoms from mass effect

Demographics

- Age
  - 20-50 years
- Gender
  - M = F

Treatment

- Complete surgical excision is usually curative
- Variable results with chemotherapy & radiation

SELECTED REFERENCES

1. Cohen A et al: Kaposi's sarcoma-associated herpesvirus: clinical, diagnostic, and epidemiological aspects. Crit Rev Clin Lab Sci. 42(2):101-53, 2005
2. Ko SF et al: Imaging spectrum of Castleman's disease. AJR Am J Roentgenol. 182(3):769-75, 2004

MULTICENTRIC CASTLEMAN DISEASE

Key Facts

Terminology

- Multicentric Castleman disease (MCD)
- Rare B-cell lymphoproliferative disorder characterized by enhancing lymphadenopathy

Imaging

- Distribution of disease
  - Superficial, axillary, supraclavicular lymph nodes
  - Less common: Mediastinal, hilar lymph nodes
- Radiography
  - Axillary or supraclavicular mass(es)
  - Well-defined hilar or mediastinal mass(es)
- CT
  - Avidly enhancing lymphadenopathy; calcification in 5-10% of affected lymph nodes
  - Lung involvement rare
- PET/CT increases detection of involved lymph nodes
  - May guide biopsy planning

Top Differential Diagnoses

- Metastatic lymphadenopathy
- Tuberculosis
- Lymphoma & leukemia
- Kaposi sarcoma

Pathology

- Associated with HIV & Kaposi sarcoma

Clinical Issues

- Constitutional symptoms: Fever, weight loss, anorexia

Diagnostic Checklist

- Consider MCD in patients with multifocal enhancing lymphadenopathy, particularly in those with HIV/AIDS
- Documentation of enlarged feeding & draining vessels may be important if surgery is considered

(Left) Axial CECT of a 39-year-old man with HIV and MCD shows avidly enhancing right axillary lymphadenopathy. MCD commonly involves the superficial and axillary lymph node chains, and avid enhancement suggests the hyaline-vascular histologic subtype. (Right) Coronal CECT of the same patient shows enhancing supraclavicular ➔ and cervical ➔ lymphadenopathy. Patients with MCD are more likely to be symptomatic than those with the localized form of the disease.

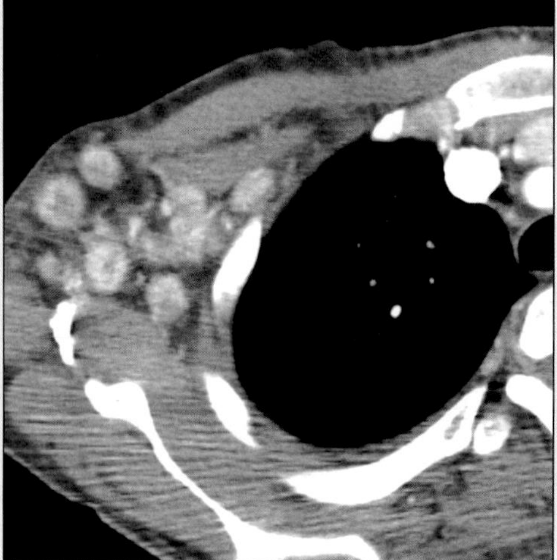

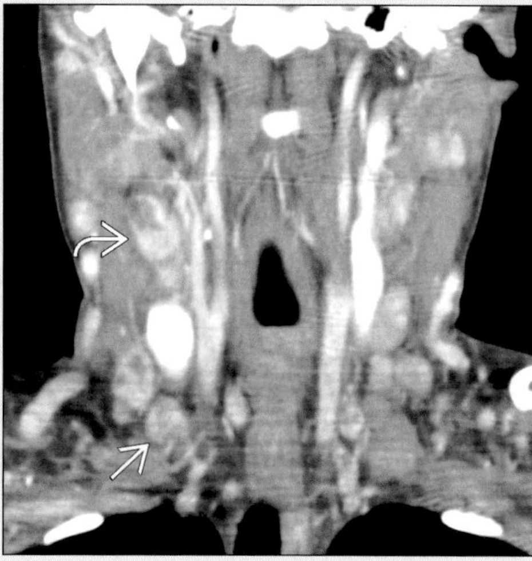

(Left) Axial CECT of a patient with multicentric Castleman disease (MCD) shows avidly enhancing mediastinal lymphadenopathy in the low paratracheal ➔ and AP window ➔ chains. Mediastinal and hilar involvement is less common than superficial disease. (Right) Axial CECT of a 56-year-old man with MCD shows enhancing mediastinal ➔ and axillary ➔ lymph nodes and bilateral pleural effusions ➔. MCD should be considered in patients with multifocal enhancing lymphadenopathy.

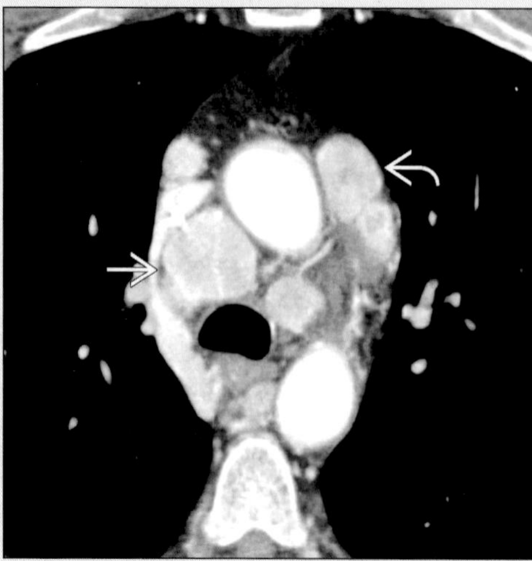

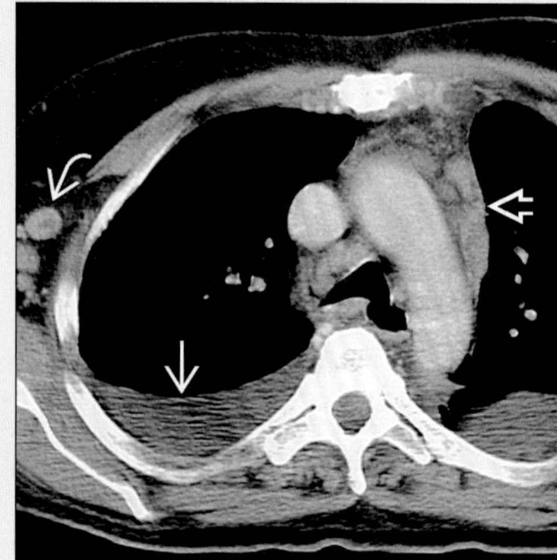

MULTICENTRIC CASTLEMAN DISEASE

TERMINOLOGY

Abbreviations

- **Multicentric Castleman disease (MCD)**

Synonyms

- Angiofollicular lymph node hyperplasia
- Giant lymph node hyperplasia

Definitions

- Rare B-cell lymphoproliferative disorder characterized by multifocal enhancing lymphadenopathy

IMAGING

General Features

- Location
  - Superficial, axillary, supraclavicular lymph nodes
  - Less common: Mediastinal, hilar lymph nodes

Radiographic Findings

- Axillary or supraclavicular mass(es)
- Well-defined hilar or mediastinal mass(es)

CT Findings

- Avidly enhancing lymphadenopathy
  - Calcification in 5-10%
  - Less common: Nonenhancing, necrotic lymph nodes
- Lung involvement rare
  - Enhancing pulmonary mass
  - Diffuse lung involvement may resemble lymphocytic interstitial pneumonia (centrilobular nodules, ground-glass opacities)

Nuclear Medicine Findings

- PET/CT
  - PET ↑ sensitivity for detection of involved sites
  - May guide biopsy planning

Imaging Recommendations

- Best imaging tool
  - CECT optimally demonstrates location & extent of lymphadenopathy & pulmonary disease
  - PET/CT may be used for disease surveillance
- Protocol advice
  - Contrast enhancement suggests hyaline-vascular histological subtype of MCD

DIFFERENTIAL DIAGNOSIS

Metastatic Lymphadenopathy

- Renal cell, thyroid cancers, melanoma, sarcoma
- Affected lymph nodes may exhibit enhancement

Tuberculosis

- Lymphadenopathy common in patients with HIV
  - May exhibit central low attenuation
- Cavitary lung disease, tree-in-bud opacities on CT

Lymphoma & Leukemia

- May resemble MCD clinically
- Enhancement rare, but seen in subtypes of non-Hodgkin lymphoma

Kaposi Sarcoma

- May coexist with MCD
- Enhancing lymphadenopathy & peribronchovascular pulmonary disease

HIV/AIDS

- Generalized HIV-related lymphadenopathy typically not avidly enhancing

PATHOLOGY

General Features

- Etiology
  - Human herpesvirus 8 (HHV-8) present in many patients with MCD
  - High levels of IL-6 in MCD
- Associated abnormalities
  - Human immunodeficiency virus & Kaposi sarcoma

Gross Pathologic & Surgical Features

- Lymph node enlargement
- Lung involvement rare

Microscopic Features

- Most MCD cases are plasma-cell subtype
  - Hyaline-vascular & mixed subtypes reported

CLINICAL ISSUES

Presentation

- Most common signs/symptoms
  - Constitutional symptoms: Fever, weight loss, anorexia
  - Hepatosplenomegaly
- Other signs/symptoms
  - Anemia, proteinuria, elevated ESR
  - Erythematous cutaneous lesions
  - Central & peripheral neurological symptoms

Natural History & Prognosis

- MCD has worse prognosis than localized disease
  - Mean survival of 24-33 months when treated
- 20% of patients with MCD develop lymphoma

Treatment

- Chemotherapy, corticosteroids, radiation therapy
- Surgical resection attempted when neurological symptoms present
- Ganciclovir & rituximab may improve outcome

DIAGNOSTIC CHECKLIST

Consider

- MCD in patients with multifocal enhancing lymphadenopathy, particularly those with HIV/AIDS

Reporting Tips

- Documentation of enlarged feeding & draining vessels may be important if surgery is considered

SELECTED REFERENCES

1. Sun X et al: The value of MDCT in diagnosis of hyaline-vascular Castleman's disease. Eur J Radiol. Epub ahead of print, 2011

BRONCHOGENIC CYST

Key Facts

Terminology

- Abnormal ventral foregut budding, thought to occur between 26th & 40th days of gestation

Imaging

- Radiography
  - Middle-posterior mediastinal mass
  - Sharply marginated spherical soft tissue lesion
- CT
  - Majority in middle-posterior mediastinum (80%)
  - Well-defined, unilocular, spherical cyst
  - Thin wall; may exhibit enhancement, calcification
  - Variable attenuation ranging from fluid to soft tissue, may contain milk of calcium
  - No enhancement of cyst contents
- MR
  - Variable signal on T1WI
  - High signal on T2WI, parallels that of CSF

Top Differential Diagnoses

- Congenital thoracic cystic lesions
  - Pericardial, thymic, esophageal duplication cyst
- Mediastinal cystic neoplasms
  - Mature teratoma, thymoma, lymphoma

Pathology

- Lined with respiratory epithelium
- Mural cartilage, smooth muscle, mucous glands

Clinical Issues

- Treatment
  - Asymptomatic cysts: Observation
  - Symptomatic cysts: Aspiration, ablation, resection

Diagnostic Checklist

- Consider bronchogenic cyst in asymptomatic patient with spherical subcarinal lesion

*(**Left**) PA chest radiograph of a patient with a bronchogenic cyst shows abnormal thickening and convexity ➔ of the right paratracheal stripe. (**Right**) Coronal CECT of the same patient shows a large right paratracheal bronchogenic cyst ➔ of homogeneous fluid attenuation and multiple unrelated hepatic cysts ⇨. Bronchogenic cysts often exhibit fluid attenuation, may have an imperceptible cyst wall (as in this case), and characteristically abut the trachea or carina.*

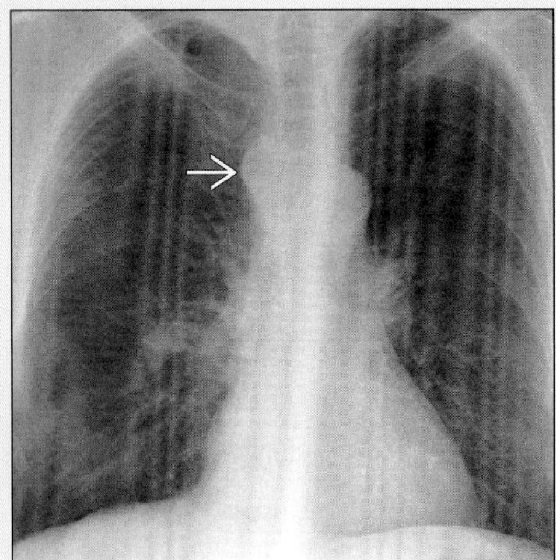

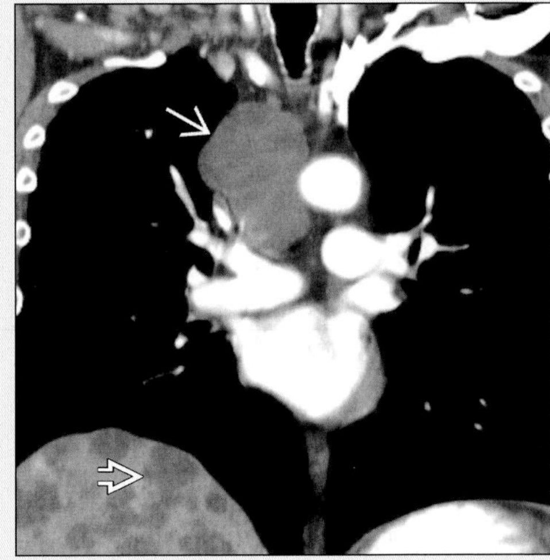

*(**Left**) Composite image with lateral chest radiograph (left) and axial CECT (right) of a patient with a bronchogenic cyst shows typical imaging features. The lesion manifests as a spherical mass ➔ in the subcarinal middle-posterior mediastinum and exhibits homogeneous water attenuation ➔ on chest CT. (**Right**) Graphic shows the classic morphologic features of bronchogenic cyst. These are thin-walled unilocular spherical cysts that typically abut the trachea &/or carina. A subcarinal location is typical.*

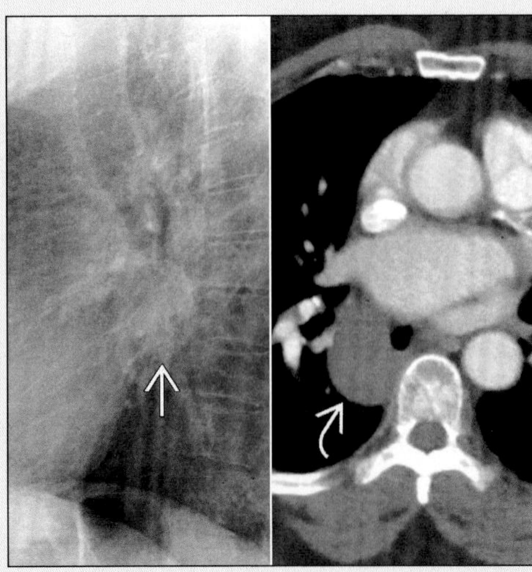

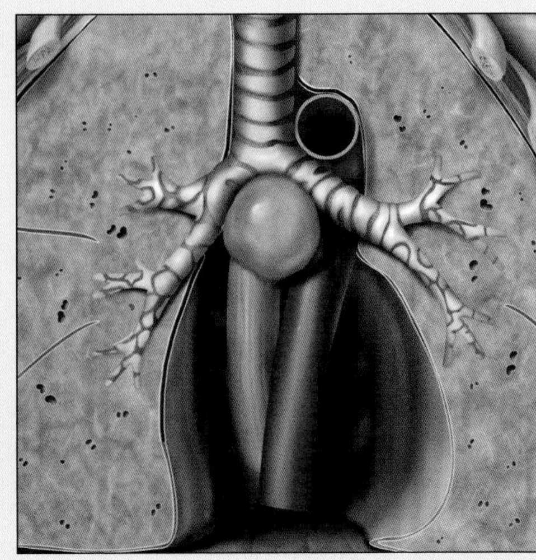

BRONCHOGENIC CYST

TERMINOLOGY

Definitions

- Bronchogenic cyst
  - Abnormal ventral foregut budding, thought to occur between 26th & 40th days of gestation
- Other foregut cysts
  - Esophageal duplication cyst, neurenteric cyst
- Other thoracic congenital cystic lesions
  - Lymphatic: Lymphangioma
  - Mesothelial: Pericardial cyst
  - Thymopharyngeal duct: Congenital thymic cyst
  - Leptomeningeal: Meningocele

IMAGING

General Features

- Best diagnostic clue
  - Spherical unilocular cyst near tracheal carina
- Location
  - Mediastinal bronchogenic cyst: Middle-posterior mediastinum
  - Pulmonary bronchogenic cyst: Medial 1/3 of lower lobe
- Size
  - Variable
  - 1.5-11 cm in diameter
- Morphology
  - Spherical, unilocular

Radiographic Findings

- **Middle-posterior mediastinal mass**
  - **Typically subcarinal**
  - Protrudes toward right hilum
  - Mass effect on medial aspect of bronchus intermedius
- Sharply marginated spherical soft tissue lesion
  - Very rarely contains air or air-fluid level
- Pulmonary bronchogenic cyst: Lower lobe, medial 1/3

Fluoroscopic Findings

- Esophagram
  - Extrinsic esophageal compression

CT Findings

- NECT
  - Well-defined spherical lesion
  - Majority in **middle-posterior mediastinum (80%)**
    - **Subcarinal, paratracheal regions**
    - Other mediastinal compartments may be involved
    - Rarely: Pleura, diaphragm, pericardium, lung
  - Thin wall: May exhibit calcification
  - Cyst content attenuation
    - Homogeneous, usually water attenuation due to serous fluid (0-20 HU)
    - High attenuation due to viscous, mucoid, hemorrhagic, or calcium-containing fluid (40%)
    - Rarely milk of calcium-fluid level
  - Soft, rarely causes obstruction
    - Mass effect on bronchi, esophagus, vessels
    - Associated atelectasis/consolidation uncommon
  - Cyst infection: Enhancing irregular wall
    - Airway communication: Air, air-fluid level
  - Pulmonary bronchogenic cyst
    - Solitary, well-defined, unilocular, spherical/ovoid
    - Usually lower lobe, rarely upper lobe
    - Medial 1/3 of lung
    - 3-5 cm in diameter
    - Homogeneous, variable attenuation (9-40 HU)
    - Infection: Irregular enhancing wall
      - May develop air-fluid level vs. entirely air-filled
    - Adjacent mosaic attenuation or linear bands
- CECT
  - **May exhibit cyst wall enhancement**
  - **Unilocular** cystic morphology
  - No enhancement of cyst content

MR Findings

- T1WI
  - Typical low signal intensity, parallels cerebrospinal fluid
  - Variable signal intensity from protein, blood, or mucous
- T2WI
  - High signal intensity, parallels cerebrospinal fluid
    - Isointense or hyperintense to CSF
  - Visualization of low signal intensity cyst wall
- T1WI C+
  - ± cyst wall enhancement; nonenhancing content

Ultrasonographic Findings

- Grayscale ultrasound
  - Transesophageal echocardiogram: Anechoic thin-walled cyst with increased through transmission

Imaging Recommendations

- Best imaging tool
  - CT is diagnostic in fluid-attenuation lesions
  - MR useful for further evaluation of indeterminate lesions

DIFFERENTIAL DIAGNOSIS

Congenital Thoracic Cystic Lesions

- Pericardial cyst
  - Usually right cardiophrenic angle, adjacent to pericardium
  - Fluid attenuation, imperceptible wall
- Thymic cyst
  - Anterior mediastinum, in region of thymus
  - Unilocular or multilocular
  - Fluid attenuation, may exhibit mural calcification
- Esophageal duplication cyst
  - Adjacent to esophagus, often right-sided
  - Mass effect on esophagus
  - Cyst wall may be thick
- Neurenteric cyst
  - Right-sided; long vertical tubular lesion
  - Associated vertebral anomalies cephalad to cyst
    - Hemivertebra, butterfly vertebra, sagittal cleft
- Lymphangioma (cystic hygroma)
  - Unilocular, multilocular; thin septa
  - May also involve neck/chest wall
  - Complications: Airway compression, infection, chylothorax, chylopericardium
- Meningocele
  - Herniation of leptomeninges through intervertebral foramen or vertebral body defect
  - Fluid attenuation/signal, continuity with thecal sac

BRONCHOGENIC CYST

Mediastinal Cystic Neoplasms

- Mature teratoma
  - Anterior mediastinal unilocular or multilocular cystic lesion
  - May contain soft tissue, fluid, fat, &/or calcium
- Thymoma
  - Anterior mediastinal cystic lesion with mural nodules
- Neurogenic neoplasm
  - Spherical paravertebral soft tissue mass
  - Pressure erosion of adjacent skeleton
  - May exhibit cystic degeneration
- Mediastinal Hodgkin lymphoma
  - Lymphadenopathy
  - Cystic degeneration may follow treatment

Pancreatic Pseudocyst

- History of pancreatitis
- Abdominal pseudocyst not always present

Mediastinal Abscess

- Signs/symptoms of infection/sepsis

Pulmonary Cystic or Cavitary Lesions

- Pulmonary airway malformation
  - Neonates & infants
  - Multilocular cystic air-filled lung lesion
- Bulla
  - Multifocal pulmonary involvement
  - May become infected & develop air-fluid level
- Pneumatocele
  - Spontaneous resolution
- Lung abscess
  - Usually develops in consolidated lung
- Lung cancer
  - Smooth thin-walled cavities uncommon
  - Image-guided biopsy for diagnosis
- Intralobar sequestration
  - Heterogeneous lesion, may exhibit cystic change
  - Systemic arterial supply

PATHOLOGY

General Features

- Etiology
  - Congenital cyst
    - Foregut malformation
    - Abnormal budding from ventral foregut
      - Precursor of trachea & major bronchi
      - Early anomalous budding = mediastinal cyst
      - Late anomalous budding = pulmonary cyst
      - Notochord adjacent to foregut may give rise to neurenteric cyst
- Associated abnormalities
  - Extralobar sequestration
  - Congenital lobar emphysema

Gross Pathologic & Surgical Features

- Bronchogenic cyst: 1/5 of mediastinal masses
  - 85% mediastinal; 15% in lung, pleura, diaphragm, or pericardium
- Unilocular cyst
- Variable cyst content
  - Clear serous fluid, thick mucoid material, purulent material, milk of calcium, hemorrhagic fluid
- Stalk or pedicle attaching cyst to adjacent mediastinal structure (50%)
- Extrathoracic extension into neck or abdomen: Dumbbell cysts

Microscopic Features

- Lined with pseudostratified columnar or cuboidal respiratory epithelium
- Mural cartilage, smooth muscle, mucous glands

CLINICAL ISSUES

Presentation

- Most common signs/symptoms
  - **Often asymptomatic**
- Other signs/symptoms
  - Chest pain, cough, dyspnea, wheezing
  - Fever, purulent sputum, dysphagia
  - Life-threatening emergency
    - Airway compression, infection, hemorrhage, rupture, pneumothorax
    - Rarely: Arrhythmia, air embolus

Demographics

- Age
  - Discovered at any age, usually < 35 years
- Gender
  - M:F = 1:1

Natural History & Prognosis

- Increasing cyst size: Consider hemorrhage, infection
- Rare malignant transformation of pulmonary congenital cystic lesions

Treatment

- Small asymptomatic lesions
  - Observation
  - Resection of selected asymptomatic cysts in young patients
    - Low surgical risk; potential for late complications, infection, hemorrhage
- Symptomatic lesions
  - Aspiration (cyst may recur), ablation
  - Surgical resection
    - Thoracotomy or video-assisted thoracoscopic surgery

DIAGNOSTIC CHECKLIST

Consider

- Bronchogenic cyst in asymptomatic patient with spherical subcarinal or paratracheal lesion

Image Interpretation Pearls

- Mediastinal bronchogenic cyst should be suspected based on morphology & location

SELECTED REFERENCES

1. Jeung MY et al: Imaging of cystic masses of the mediastinum. Radiographics. 22 Spec No:S79-93, 2002
2. McAdams HP et al: Bronchogenic cyst: imaging features with clinical and histopathologic correlation. Radiology. 217(2):441-6, 2000

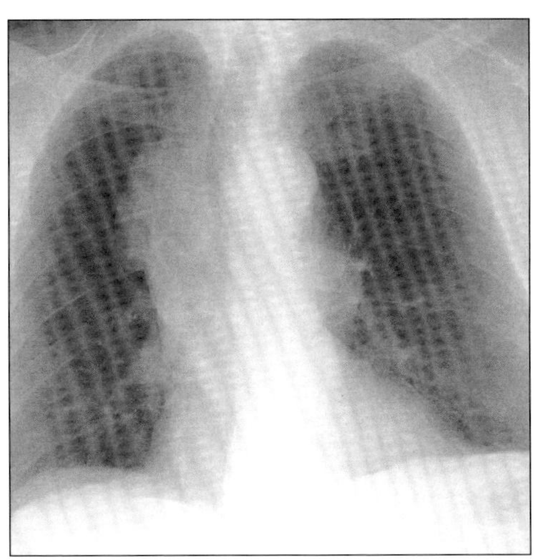

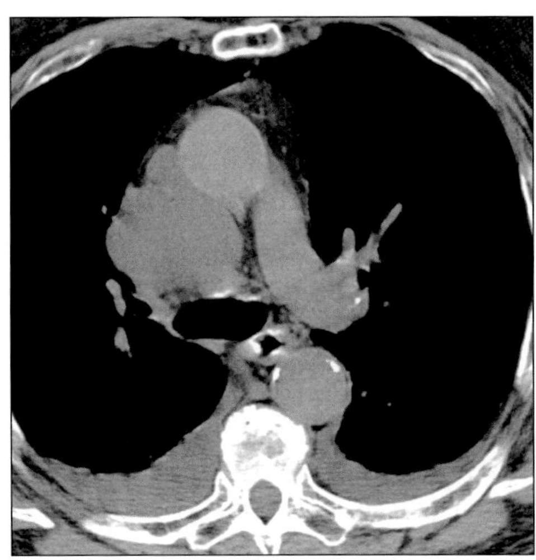

(Left) *PA chest radiograph of a symptomatic adult with a large bronchogenic cyst shows a large, well-marginated right paratracheal soft tissue mass.* ***(Right)*** *Axial NECT of the same patient shows a large fluid-attenuation lesion that extends to the precarinal region and bilateral small pleural effusions. Given progressive symptoms, the lesion was surgically excised. Bronchogenic cysts may be entirely asymptomatic, but symptomatic lesions should be treated with aspiration, ablation, or excision.*

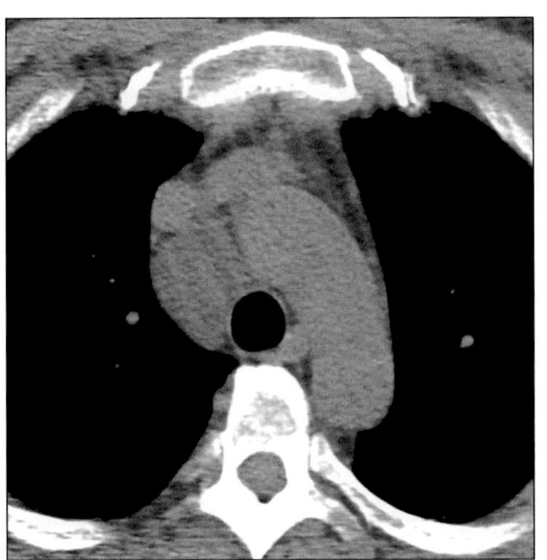

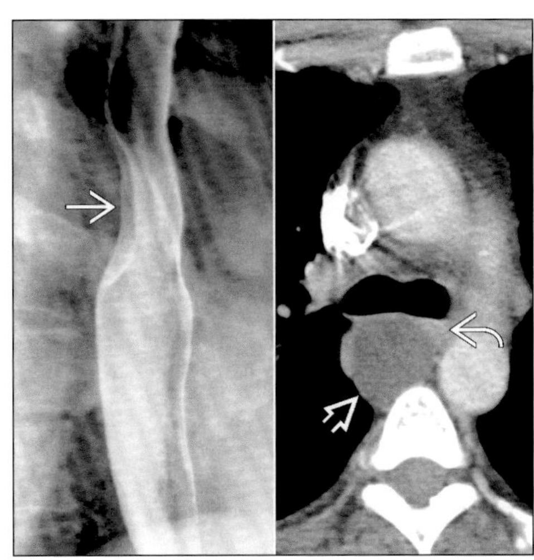

(Left) *Axial NECT of an asymptomatic patient with a bronchogenic cyst shows a right paratracheal spherical lesion of water attenuation. Note absence of mass effect on the adjacent structures.* ***(Right)*** *Composite image with esophagram (left) and axial CECT (right) of a patient with bronchogenic cyst and dysphagia shows smooth mass effect on the esophagus ➡ produced by the spherical subcarinal fluid-attenuation cyst ⮚, which is intimately related to the mid esophagus ↪.*

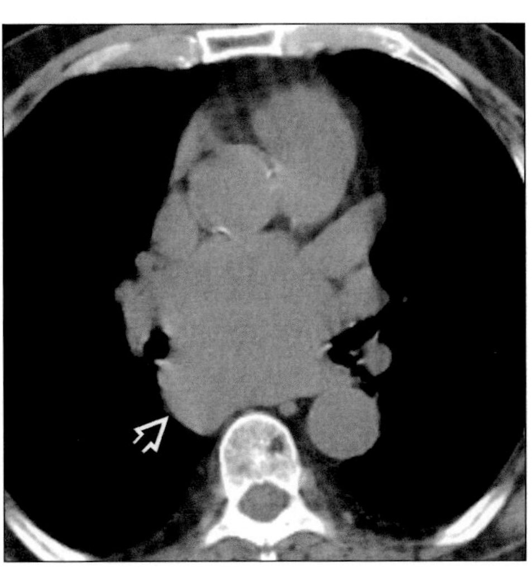

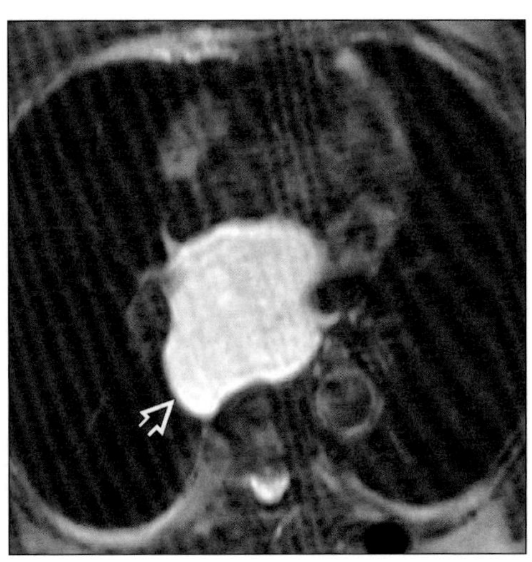

(Left) *Axial NECT of a patient with chronic renal insufficiency shows a soft tissue attenuation and roughly spherical subcarinal mass ⮚ that displaces the upper azygoesophageal recess laterally.* ***(Right)*** *Axial T2WI MR of the same patient shows that the lesion represents a large fluid-filled subcarinal unilocular cyst ⮚ with homogeneous high signal intensity content. The presumptive diagnosis of bronchogenic cyst can be made based on the location, morphology, and MR features of the lesion.*

ESOPHAGEAL DUPLICATION CYST

Key Facts

Terminology
- Abbreviations
  - Enteric cyst (EC)
  - Esophageal duplication cyst (EDC)
- Synonyms
  - Foregut or esophageal duplication cyst
  - Enterogenous cyst
- Definition; anomalous budding of dorsal foregut

Imaging
- Radiography
  - Spherical middle-posterior mediastinal mass
- CT
  - Spherical paraesophageal cystic lesion
  - Variable attenuation content
  - Unilocular cyst; enhancement of thin cyst wall
- MR
  - Variable signal on T1WI; high signal on T2WI

Top Differential Diagnoses
- Bronchogenic cyst
- Benign esophageal neoplasm
- Esophageal diverticulum
- Esophageal carcinoma
- Neurenteric cyst

Pathology
- Discrete unilocular cyst with variable fluid content
- Enteric or respiratory epithelium
- Ectopic gastric mucosa in 50%
- Cyst wall; 2 smooth muscle layers, no cartilage

Clinical Issues
- Age: 75% occur in children
- Symptoms; mass effect, dysphagia, chest pain
- Treatment is surgical excision
- Prognosis is excellent

*(**Left**) Graphic shows the characteristic anatomic location of esophageal duplication cyst ➔ in the inferior aspect of the middle-posterior mediastinum, to the right of the distal esophagus and within or adjacent to the esophageal wall. (**Right**) Axial CECT (mediastinal window) shows a unilocular EDC ➔ manifesting as a water attenuation nonenhancing ovoid lesion abutting the right wall of the distal esophagus. EDC are thought to result from anomalous development of the primitive dorsal foregut.*

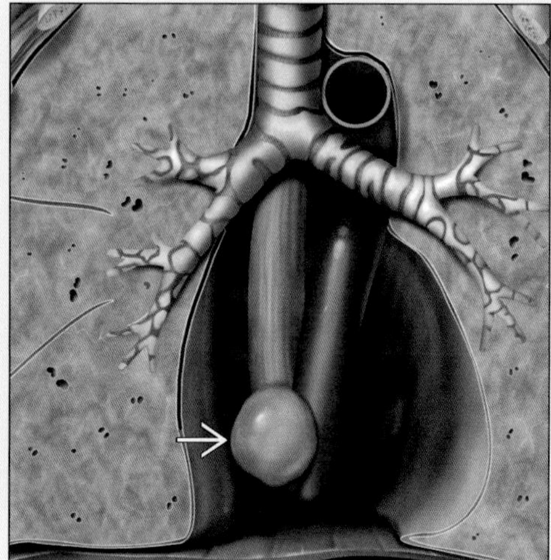

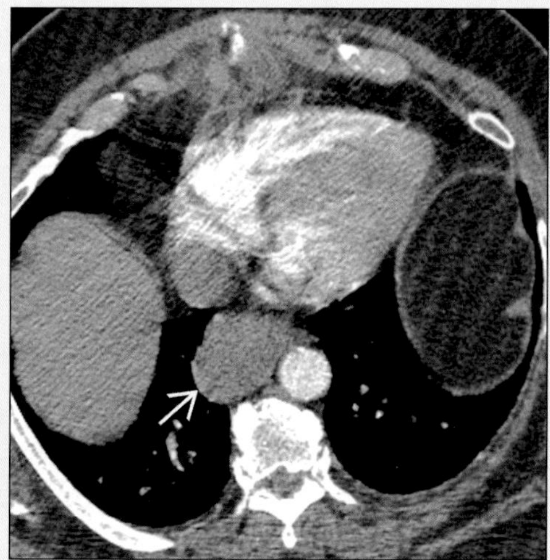

*(**Left**) Axial NECT (mediastinal window) shows an EDC manifesting as a right inferior middle-posterior mediastinal mass abutting the right distal esophagus and exhibiting an intrinsic fluid-fluid level ➔, which confirms the cystic nature of the lesion. (**Right**) Axial CECT (mediastinal window) shows a small water attenuation nonenhancing spherical EDC ➔ abutting the right posterior esophageal wall. EDC exhibit nonenhancing cyst contents of variable attenuation ranging from fluid to soft tissue.*

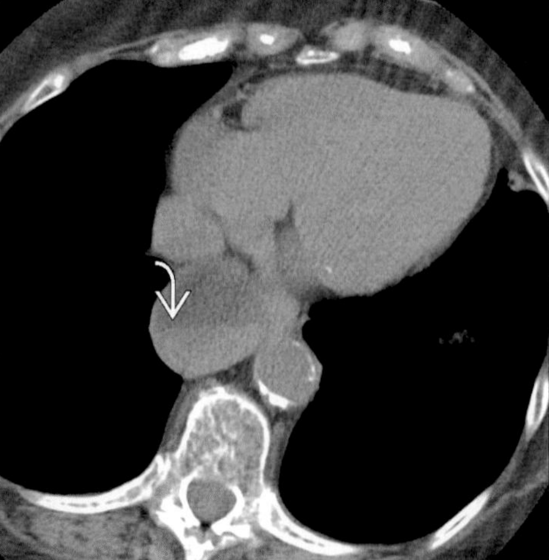

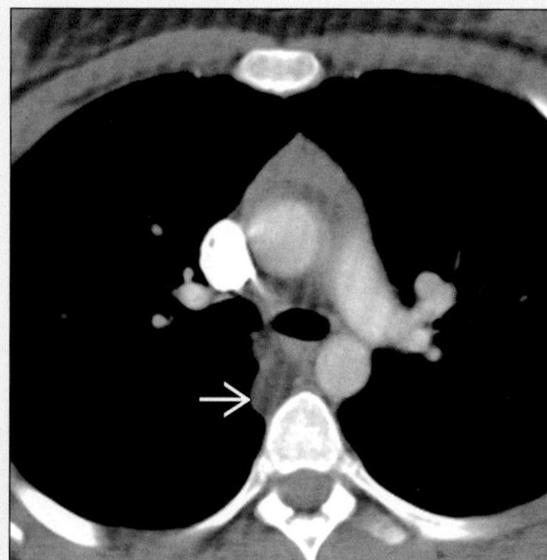

ESOPHAGEAL DUPLICATION CYST

TERMINOLOGY

Abbreviations

- **Enteric cyst (EC)**
- **Esophageal duplication cyst (EDC)**
- **Foregut duplication cyst (FDC)**

Synonyms

- Foregut or **esophageal duplication cyst**
- Enterogenous cyst

Definitions

- **FDC**: Anomalous budding of embryonic foregut
- **FDC** arises from **dorsal foregut**
  - Esophageal duplication cyst
  - Neuroenteric cyst

IMAGING

General Features

- Best diagnostic clue
  - Well-defined inferior **paraesophageal cystic lesion**
- Location
  - **Most** arise from **distal ileum** and **duodenum**
  - **10-15%** arise from esophagus
    - Typically distal 1/3, right-sided
    - May traverse diaphragm
  - May be multiple along gastrointestinal tract
- Size
  - **≤ 5 cm**
- Morphology
  - **Spherical**, ovoid, tubular; **unilocular**

Radiographic Findings

- Spherical mass or contour abnormality in **lower middle-posterior mediastinum**

CT Findings

- NECT
  - **Spherical paraesophageal** mass
  - Variable attenuation of cyst content
    - May exhibit soft tissue attenuation content
    - May exhibit intrinsic fluid-fluid level
  - May traverse the diaphragm
    - May communicate with GI tract; duodenum
- CECT
  - **Unilocular cystic paraesophageal** lesion
  - **Thin cyst** wall may enhance
  - **No enhancement of cyst content**

MR Findings

- T1WI
  - Low or high signal intensity cyst content
  - May exhibit fluid-fluid or blood-fluid levels
- T2WI FS
  - **High signal intensity** cyst content

Ultrasonographic Findings

- Discrete cystic lesion within esophageal wall
- Cyst wall muscle may be contiguous with esophageal muscle/muscularis propria

Nuclear Medicine Findings

- **Tc pertechnetate**; detection of ectopic gastric mucosa

DIFFERENTIAL DIAGNOSIS

Bronchogenic Cyst

- Identical to EDC; more common than EDC

Benign Esophageal Neoplasm

- Leiomyoma; solid esophageal mass
- Fibrovascular polyp; endoluminal, upper esophagus

Esophageal Diverticulum

- Communicates with esophageal lumen

Esophageal Carcinoma

- Esophageal mural thickening or soft tissue mass

Neurenteric Cyst

- Associated vertebral anomalies

PATHOLOGY

General Features

- Etiology
  - Primitive esophagus forms vacuoles that coalesce into patent esophageal lumen
  - Persistent isolated vacuole may give rise to EDC
- Associated abnormalities
  - EC may be multiple
  - Congenital gastrointestinal anomalies in 12%

Gross Pathologic & Surgical Features

- Mural esophageal or paraesophageal cystic lesion
- **Discrete unilocular cyst** with **variable fluid content**
  - Proteinaceous fluid, hemorrhagic fluid

Microscopic Features

- Enteric or respiratory epithelium
- Ectopic gastric mucosa in 50%; pancreatic tissue in 5%
- Cyst wall; 2 smooth muscle layers, no cartilage
- Rare malignant degeneration

CLINICAL ISSUES

Presentation

- Most common signs/symptoms
  - Mass effect, dysphagia, chest pain
    - Compression, bleeding, perforation

Demographics

- Age
  - **75% occur in children**
- Gender
  - **M = F**

Treatment

- **Surgical excision** with **excellent prognosis**

DIAGNOSTIC CHECKLIST

Consider

- EDC in distal paraesophageal unilocular cystic lesions

SELECTED REFERENCES

1. Bhutani MS et al: Endosonographic diagnosis of an esophageal duplication cyst. Endoscopy. 28(4):396-7, 1996

PERICARDIAL CYST

Key Facts

Terminology
- Common congenital mediastinal cyst
- Anomalous outpouching of parietal pericardium

Imaging
- Radiography
  - Well-defined right cardiophrenic angle mass
  - Spherical, ovoid, teardrop-shaped
- CT
  - Abuts pericardium
  - Homogeneous water attenuation
  - Imperceptible wall
- MR
  - Homogeneous high signal intensity on T2WI
  - Parallels signal intensity of CSF
- Echocardiography
  - Modality of choice for evaluation of pericardium
  - Differentiation of solid from cystic masses

Top Differential Diagnoses
- Mediastinal fat pad
- Morgagni hernia
- Bronchogenic cyst
- Thymic cyst

Pathology
- Benign congenital mediastinal cyst
- Invariably connected to pericardium
- Fibrous wall lined by mesothelium

Clinical Issues
- Asymptomatic, incidental imaging finding
- No treatment required

Diagnostic Checklist
- Imaging diagnosis of pericardial cyst is based on location, morphology, & CT/MR characteristics

*(**Left**) PA chest radiograph of an asymptomatic patient with a pericardial cyst shows a contour abnormality ➡ near the right cardiac border in the region of the right cardiophrenic angle. (**Right**) Lateral chest radiograph of the same patient shows a well-marginated teardrop-shaped lesion ➡ in the inferior aspect of the anterior mediastinum overlying the cardiac silhouette. Although radiographic findings are characteristic, further evaluation with cross-sectional imaging is typically required.*

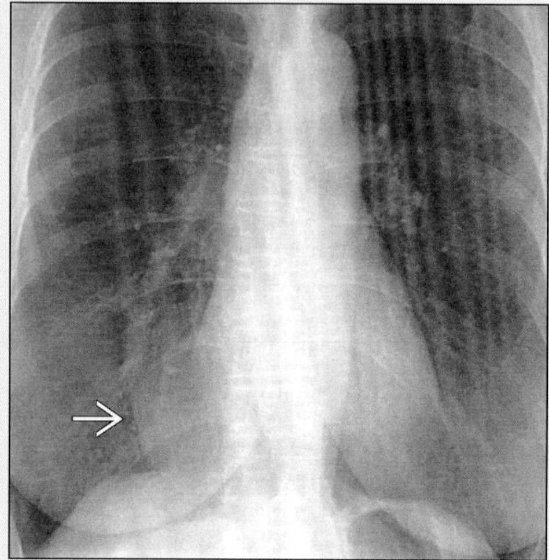

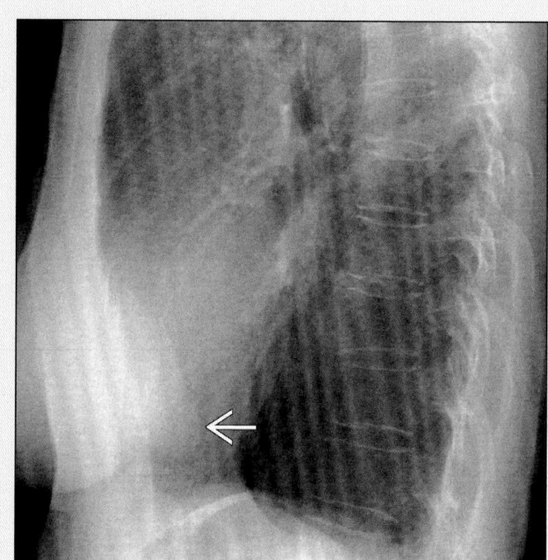

*(**Left**) Axial CECT of a patient with an incidentally discovered pericardial cyst shows a fluid attenuation lesion ➡ abutting the pericardium in the region of the right cardiophrenic angle. The lesion does not enhance with contrast and has an imperceptible wall. (**Right**) Graphic shows the characteristic morphologic features and location of pericardial cyst. The lesion abuts the pericardium, is located at the right cardiophrenic angle, and exhibits a thin wall and clear fluid content.*

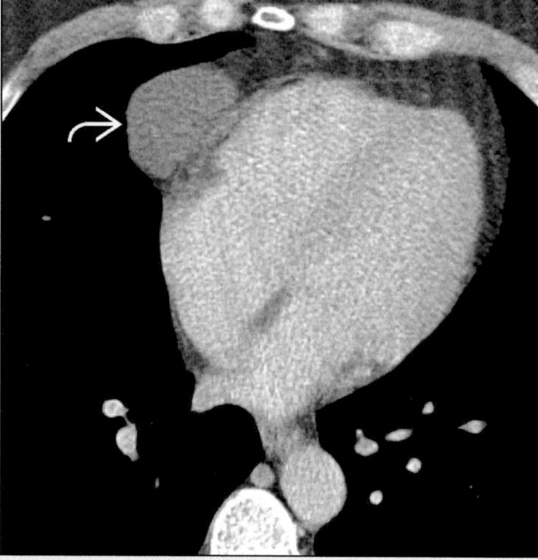

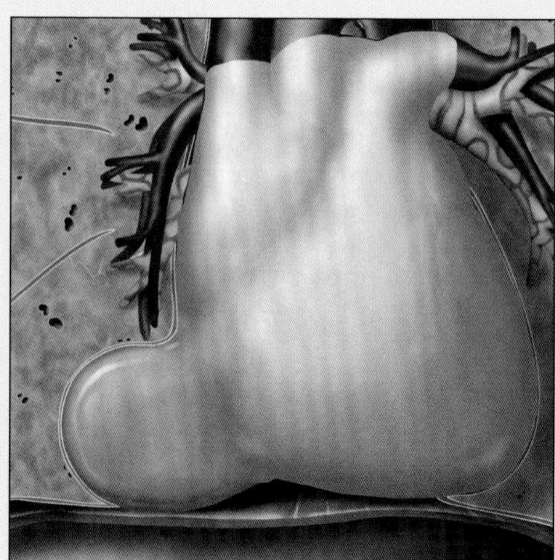

PERICARDIAL CYST

TERMINOLOGY

Definitions

- Common congenital mediastinal cyst
- Anomalous outpouching of parietal pericardium

IMAGING

General Features

- Best diagnostic clue
  - Cardiophrenic angle mass abutting heart
  - Smoothly marginated
  - Imperceptible wall
  - Water attenuation on CT
  - Fluid signal intensity on MR
- Location
  - **Cardiophrenic angle**
    - **Right (70%)**, left (10-40%)
- Size
  - Variable
  - 2-30 cm in diameter
- Morphology
  - Spherical, ovoid, teardrop-shaped
  - Unilocular (80%)
  - Multilocular (20%)

Radiographic Findings

- Radiography
  - Typically abuts pericardium
  - May occur in mediastinal location other than cardiophrenic angle
    - In such cases, difficult differentiation from other congenital mediastinal cysts
  - May exhibit change in shape with change in patient position or respiration
- PA chest radiography
  - Soft tissue mass at right cardiophrenic angle
  - Abnormal mediastinal contour near right cardiac silhouette
  - Partly spherical with sharp smooth contours
- Lateral chest radiography
  - Anterior inferior mediastinum
  - Overlying anterior inferior cardiac silhouette

CT Findings

- NECT
  - Abuts pericardium
    - Usually at cardiophrenic angle
    - Typically on right
  - Smoothly marginated
  - **Imperceptible wall**
  - **Water attenuation** (10 Hounsfield units) content
    - No mural nodules
    - May exhibit internal soft tissue septa
  - No calcification
  - No associated lymphadenopathy
- CECT
  - Homogeneous water attenuation
  - No internal enhancement
    - No mural nodules
  - No mural enhancement

MR Findings

- T1WI
  - Homogeneous signal
  - Low or intermediate signal intensity
  - May contain proteinaceous fluid & exhibit high signal intensity
- T2WI
  - Homogeneous
  - High signal intensity (follows that of water)
  - Visualization of cyst wall & septations as thin curvilinear low signal intensity structures
- T1WI C+
  - No internal enhancement
  - No enhancing mural nodules
  - No rim enhancement
- MR imaging findings are typically diagnostic, generally requiring no further intervention

Ultrasonographic Findings

- Anechoic lesion content
- Evaluation of cyst wall
- Evaluation of lesion's relationship to adjacent cardiac chambers

Imaging Recommendations

- Best imaging tool
  - Echocardiography is primary imaging modality for evaluation of pericardium
    - High sensitivity
    - Ability to differentiate solid from cystic masses
  - CT & MR
    - Allow evaluation of entire pericardium
    - Distinction of myocardial from pericardial disease
    - Further characterization of pericardial masses
  - MR may be used for further assessment of indeterminate juxtacardiac lesions found on CT
- Protocol advice
  - Limited MR protocol sufficient for diagnosis
    - Axial & coronal T1WI & T1WI C+
    - Axial & coronal T2WI
    - Coronal imaging helpful for demonstration of relationship to heart & pericardium
    - Short axis & 4-chamber imaging planes not necessary

DIFFERENTIAL DIAGNOSIS

Mediastinal Fat Pad

- May mimic pericardial cyst on radiography
- Characteristic fat attenuation on CT
- May manifest as echo-free space on echocardiography & may be difficult to distinguish from pericardial fluid

Morgagni Hernia

- Cardiophrenic angle lesion on radiography
  - Usually right-sided
  - May be indistinguishable from mediastinal fat pad or pericardial cyst
- Characteristic fat attenuation on CT
  - Contiguity of herniated fat with intraabdominal omental fat
- May contain bowel &/or abdominal viscera

Bronchogenic Cyst

- Shared imaging characteristics with pericardial cyst
- Cyst wall may exhibit enhancement &/or calcification
- Unilocular cystic lesion

PERICARDIAL CYST

- Fluid content may exhibit water or soft tissue attenuation on CT
- Characteristically located in middle-posterior mediastinum abutting trachea or carina
  - Rarely occurs in pericardium, pleura, diaphragm

Thymic Cyst

- Anterior mediastinal cystic lesion in thymic bed
  - Unilocular or multilocular
- Water attenuation on CT
- Fluid signal intensity on MR

Esophageal Duplication Cyst

- Shared imaging characteristics with pericardial cyst
- Typically within esophageal wall

Loculated Pleural Effusion

- Evaluation of ipsilateral pleural space
- History pertinent; more common postoperatively

Hematoma

- MR particularly useful
- Acute: High signal intensity on T1WI & T2WI
- Subacute: Heterogeneous signal, areas of high signal intensity on T1WI & T2WI
- Chronic: Dark peripheral rim & low signal intensity on T1WI from calcification, fibrosis, hemosiderin
- High signal intensity areas on T1WI or T2WI may correspond to hemorrhagic fluid
- No enhancement on T1WI C+

Juxtacardiac Lymphadenopathy

- Pertinent history of known lymphoma
- Mantle radiation therapy: Cardiac blockers used to protect heart, cardiophrenic angle region may be undertreated
- Recurrent lymphoma may manifest as cardiophrenic angle mass corresponding to lymphadenopathy

Pancreatic Pseudocyst

- Pertinent history of prior pancreatitis
- Usually extends through esophageal hiatus
- Associated peripancreatic inflammatory changes & fluid collections

Hydatidosis

- Cystic mass with well-defined borders
- Internal trabeculations correspond to daughter membranes
- May be pericardial or intramyocardial

PATHOLOGY

General Features

- Etiology
  - Benign congenital mediastinal cyst
  - Anomalous outpouching of parietal pericardium
  - Occurs by 4th week of gestation
  - Coalescing spaces form intraembryonic body cavity

Gross Pathologic & Surgical Features

- Invariably connected to pericardium
- Rare visible communication with pericardial space

Microscopic Features

- Fibrous tissue lined by single layer of bland mesothelium
- Differentiation from bronchogenic cyst & esophageal duplication cyst
  - Based on microscopic composition of cyst wall

CLINICAL ISSUES

Presentation

- Most common signs/symptoms
  - Typically **asymptomatic**
  - **Incidental imaging finding**
- Other signs/symptoms
  - Rarely
    - Chest pain
    - Pericardial tamponade

Natural History & Prognosis

- Benign course
- Typically remains asymptomatic

Treatment

- **No treatment required**
- Surgical excision if
  - Chest pain
  - Tamponade
  - Mistaken for malignancy
- No literature to support percutaneous drainage or fluid analysis

DIAGNOSTIC CHECKLIST

Consider

- Pericardial cyst in asymptomatic patient with homogeneous fluid attenuation cardiophrenic angle lesion

Image Interpretation Pearls

- Exclusion of cystic neoplasm in lesions with internal enhancement or mural nodules

Reporting Tips

- Pericardial cyst is typically an imaging diagnosis based on location, morphology, & CT/MR characteristics

SELECTED REFERENCES

1. Rajiah P et al: Computed tomography of the pericardium and pericardial disease. J Cardiovasc Comput Tomogr. 4(1):3-18, 2010
2. Misselt AJ et al: MR imaging of the pericardium. Magn Reson Imaging Clin N Am. 16(2):185-99, vii, 2008
3. Nijveldt R et al: Pericardial cyst. Lancet. 365(9475):1960, 2005
4. Oyama N et al: Computed tomography and magnetic resonance imaging of the pericardium: anatomy and pathology. Magn Reson Med Sci. 3(3):145-52, 2004
5. Glockner JF: Imaging of pericardial disease. Magn Reson Imaging Clin N Am. 11(1):149-62, vii, 2003

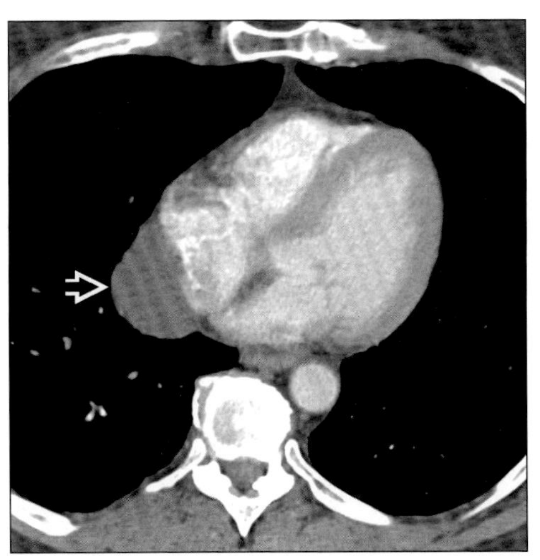

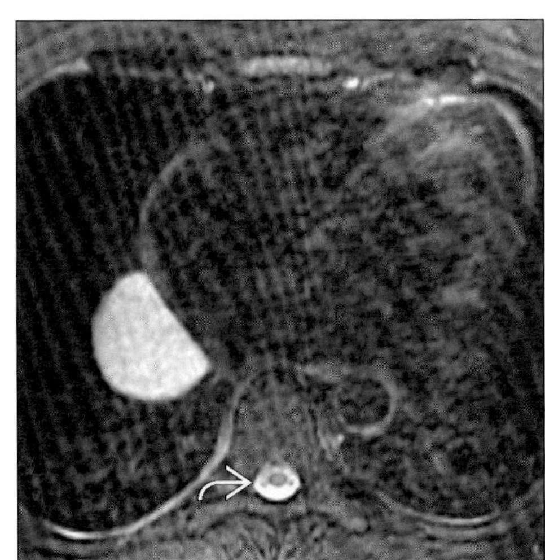

(Left) *Axial CECT of a patient with an incidentally discovered pericardial cyst shows a homogeneous water attenuation lesion ➡ with an imperceptible wall abutting the right posterior pericardium.* ***(Right)*** *T2WI MR of the same patient shows that the lesion exhibits homogeneous high signal intensity, which parallels the signal intensity of the cerebrospinal fluid ➡. Although pericardial cysts are usually located in the right cardiophrenic angle, they may occur anywhere along the pericardium.*

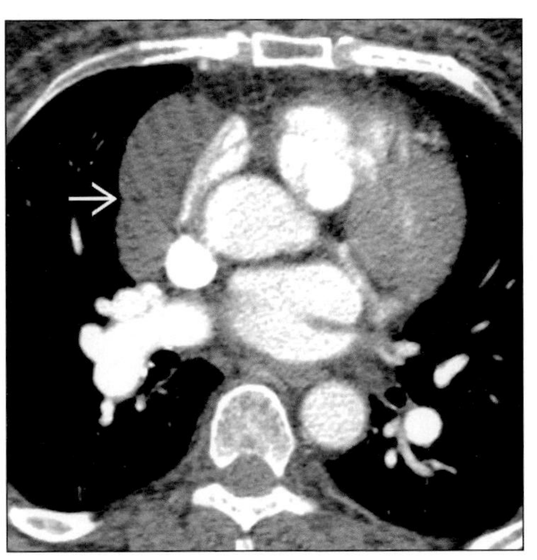

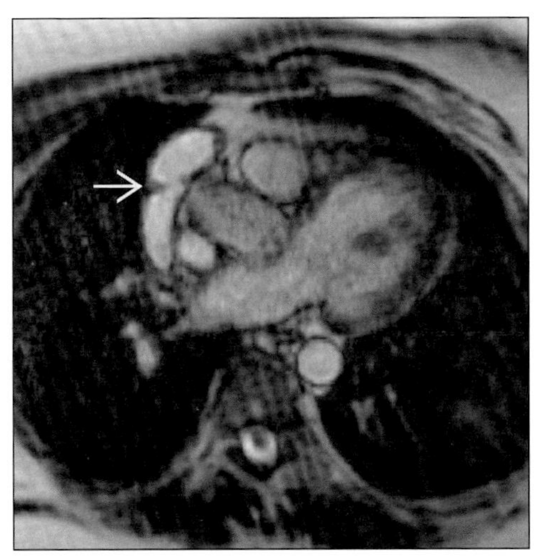

(Left) *Axial CECT of a patient with a pericardial cyst shows a water attenuation lesion in the right cardiophrenic angle. Although the cyst wall is imperceptible, there is the suggestion of a septation ➡ in the mid portion of the cyst.* ***(Right)*** *Axial T2WI MR of the same patient shows high signal intensity in the lesion paralleling that of the cerebrospinal fluid and confirms the presence of a single septation ➡ in the pericardial cyst. Note visualization of the low signal intensity cyst wall.*

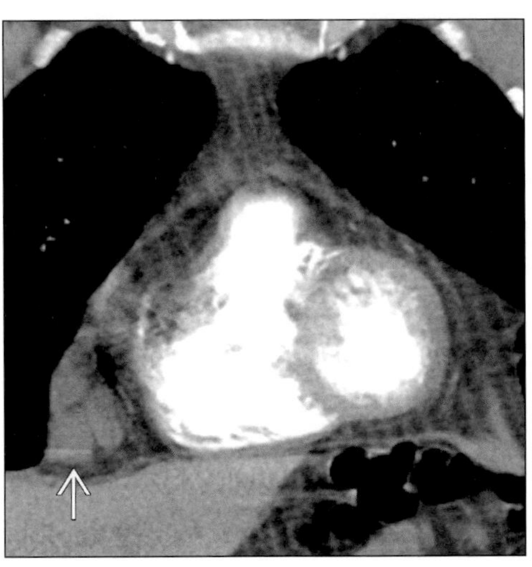

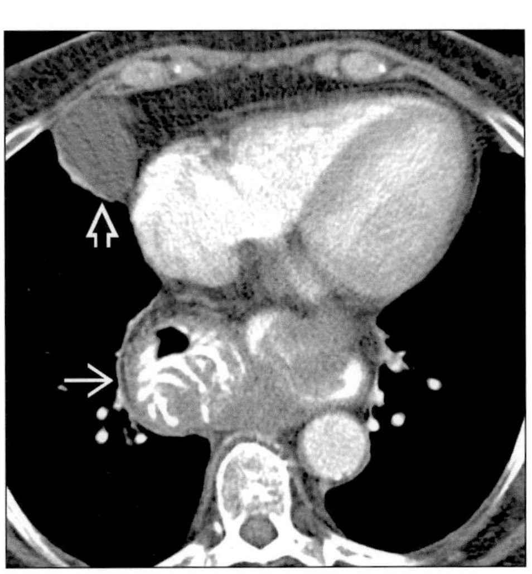

(Left) *Coronal CECT shows a multilocular pericardial cyst ➡ in the right cardiophrenic angle. While pericardial cysts are typically unilocular lesions, multilocular cysts may occur.* ***(Right)*** *Axial CECT of an asymptomatic patient with an abnormal mediastinum on radiography shows a large hiatal hernia ➡ and a right cardiophrenic angle pericardial cyst ➡. Cross-sectional imaging allows optimal evaluation of mediastinal abnormalities and in this case provides a definitive diagnosis.*

THYMIC CYST

Key Facts

Terminology

- Congenital: Thymopharyngeal duct remnant
- Acquired: Inflammation, treatment, neoplasia

Imaging

- Radiography
  - Well-defined anterior mediastinal mass
- NECT
  - Homogeneous water attenuation cyst
  - Heterogeneous/high-attenuation cyst with hemorrhage or infection
- CECT
  - Unilocular: Thin wall, water attenuation
  - Multilocular: Soft tissue attenuation components
- MR
  - T1WI: Homogeneous low signal intensity content
  - T1WI: High signal from hemorrhage or infection
  - T2WI: Homogeneous high signal intensity content

Top Differential Diagnoses

- Cystic anterior mediastinal neoplasm
  - Thymoma
  - Teratoma
  - Lymphoma
- Lymphangioma
- Pericardial cyst

Clinical Issues

- Asymptomatic, diagnosed incidentally
- Uncommon: 1% of mediastinal masses
- Treatment: Observation, drainage, excision

Diagnostic Checklist

- MR evaluation of suspected thymic cysts to exclude mural nodules
- Mural nodules in cystic mediastinal mass suggest cystic neoplasm, specifically cystic thymoma

*(**Left**) Axial CECT of a patient with a unilocular (congenital) thymic cyst shows an ovoid, water attenuation, left anterior mediastinal cyst ➔ with an imperceptible wall. Note the intact tissue plane between the cyst and the adjacent mediastinal vessels. (**Right**) Axial NECT of a patient with a multilocular (acquired) thymic cyst shows a left anterior mediastinal cyst with water attenuation contents compartmentalized by soft tissue septa ➔. Cystic neoplasm and lymphangioma should be excluded in such cases.*

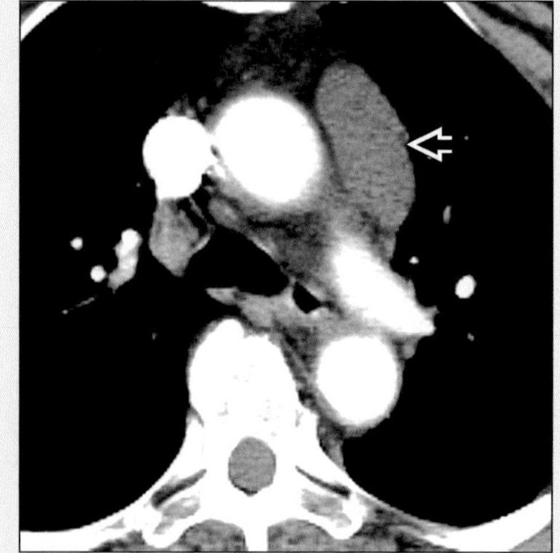

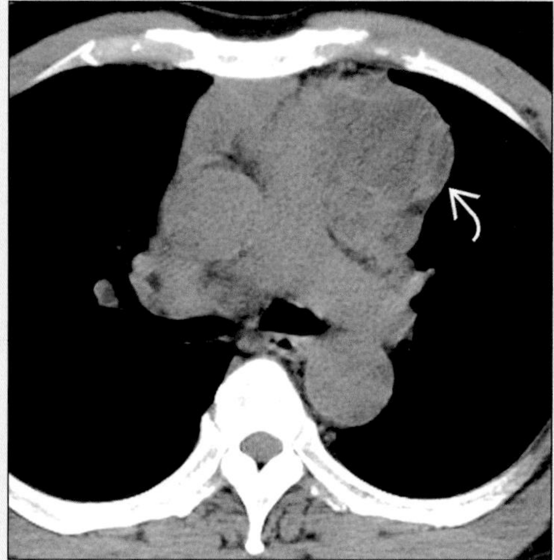

*(**Left**) Axial CECT of a patient with a unilocular thymic cyst shows a spherical left anterior mediastinal cyst with water attenuation content and calcification of the cyst wall ➔. (**Right**) Composite image with axial CECT of a child with a congenital thymic cyst involving the neck shows the cervical (left) and anterior mediastinal (right) components of the thick-walled ➔ cyst. Congenital thymic cysts may occur along the course of the thymopharyngeal duct with extramediastinal growth into the neck.*

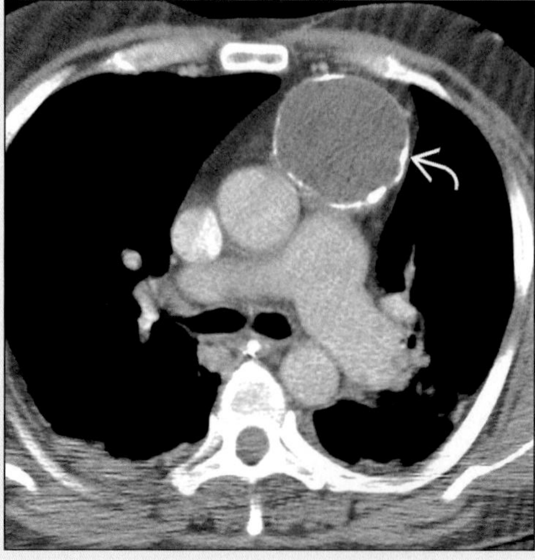

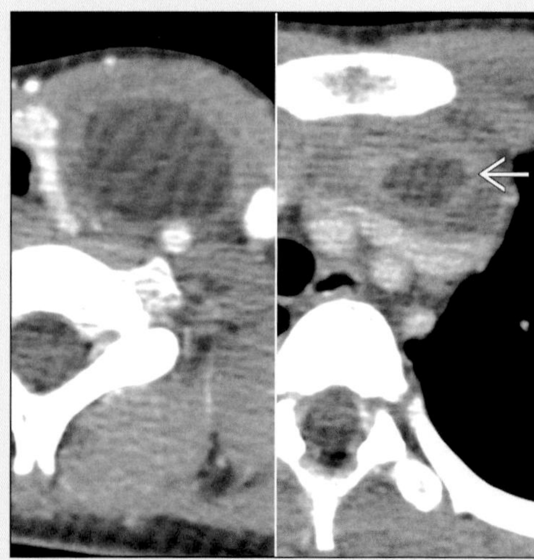

THYMIC CYST

TERMINOLOGY

Definitions

- Congenital thymic cyst: Derived from embryonic remnants of thymopharyngeal duct
- Acquired thymic cyst
  - Inflammatory process
  - Association with surgery, radiation, chemotherapy
  - Association with malignant neoplasia
  - Multilocular thymic cyst in 1% of children with HIV

IMAGING

General Features

- Best diagnostic clue
  - Well-defined mediastinal mass
- Location
  - Typically in anterior mediastinum
- Size
  - Variable: 3-17 cm
- Morphology
  - Spherical or ovoid, well-defined borders

Radiographic Findings

- Anterior mediastinal mass
  - Abnormal mediastinal contour on PA radiography
  - Anterior mediastinal location on lateral radiography
  - Rarely peripheral curvilinear calcification

CT Findings

- NECT
  - Mediastinal cyst with thin or imperceptible wall
  - Homogeneous water attenuation, may exhibit internal high attenuation from hemorrhage or infection
  - Rarely cyst wall & septal calcification
- CECT
  - Unilocular thymic cyst
    - Water attenuation anterior mediastinal cyst
    - Imperceptible or thin enhancing cyst wall
    - No soft tissue mural nodules
  - Multilocular thymic cyst
    - Heterogeneous unilocular or multilocular cyst
    - Soft tissue components, including cyst wall &/or internal septa

MR Findings

- T1WI
  - Homogeneous low signal intensity content
  - High signal content with hemorrhage or infection
- T2WI
  - Homogeneous high signal intensity content
  - Visualization of low signal cyst wall

DIFFERENTIAL DIAGNOSIS

Cystic Anterior Mediastinal Neoplasm

- Thymoma
  - May be cystic, mural nodule(s)
- Teratoma
  - Multilocular cyst, fat attenuation in 75%
- Lymphoma
  - Cyst with coalescent nodal mediastinal mass
  - Lymphadenopathy

Lymphangioma

- Multilocular cystic lesion
- Extrathoracic extension into neck, axilla, chest wall

Pericardial Cyst

- Cardiophrenic angle, water attenuation

PATHOLOGY

General Features

- Etiology
  - Congenital thymic cyst
    - Thymopharyngeal duct embryonic remnants
  - Acquired thymic cyst
    - Inflammatory, degenerative change
      - Postulated cystic dilatation, fibrosis, &/or degeneration of Hassall corpuscles
    - Neoplasia: Hodgkin lymphoma, seminoma, thymoma, thymic carcinoma

Gross Pathologic & Surgical Features

- Congenital thymic cyst: Unilocular cyst, thin wall, clear fluid content
- Acquired thymic cyst: Multilocular, thick fibrous wall, internal septa, turbid or gelatinous fluid

Microscopic Features

- Variable lining epithelium
- Thymic tissue in cyst wall
- Multilocular thymic cyst: Inflammation & fibrosis

CLINICAL ISSUES

Presentation

- Most common signs/symptoms
  - Asymptomatic, diagnosed incidentally

Demographics

- Age
  - 50% of congenital thymic cysts in 1st 2 decades
- Epidemiology
  - Uncommon
    - 1% of mediastinal masses
    - 3% of anterior mediastinal masses

Treatment

- Observation
- Drainage or excision

DIAGNOSTIC CHECKLIST

Consider

- MR of suspected thymic cyst to exclude mural nodules & cystic neoplasms

Image Interpretation Pearls

- Mural nodules in cystic mediastinal mass suggest cystic neoplasm, specifically cystic thymoma

SELECTED REFERENCES

1. Restrepo CS et al: Imaging findings of expansile lesions of the thymus. Curr Probl Diagn Radiol. 34(1):22-34, 2005
2. Jeung MY et al: Imaging of cystic masses of the mediastinum. Radiographics. 22 Spec No:S79-93, 2002

MEDIASTINAL VASCULAR MASSES

Key Facts

Terminology
- Lesions of systemic & pulmonary arteries & veins
  - 10% of mediastinal masses on radiography

Imaging
- Mediastinal mass that opacifies on CECT or CTA
- Chest radiography
  - Wide superior mediastinum
  - Middle mediastinal, paratracheal, paracardiac mass
- CT
  - Hypodense mass on NECT
  - Opacifies after contrast administration
  - Identification of parent or branch vessels
- MR: May be used as alternative to CT
- Protocol advice
  - Multiplanar reformations for lesion localization
  - Cardiac gating for evaluation of vascular lesions of cardiac origin

Top Differential Diagnoses
- Hemangioma
- Lymphangioma
- Metastatic disease
- Extracardiac mediastinal angiosarcoma
- Hemangiopericytoma

Clinical Issues
- Surgical resection or endovascular therapy
  - Lesions involving aorta & pulmonary arteries
  - Ascending aortic dissections & thoracic aortic aneurysms of certain sizes
  - Bypass graft aneurysms > 2 cm
  - Significant symptoms, mass effect, rupture

Diagnostic Checklist
- Consider a mediastinal vascular lesion when a mediastinal mass is detected on chest radiography

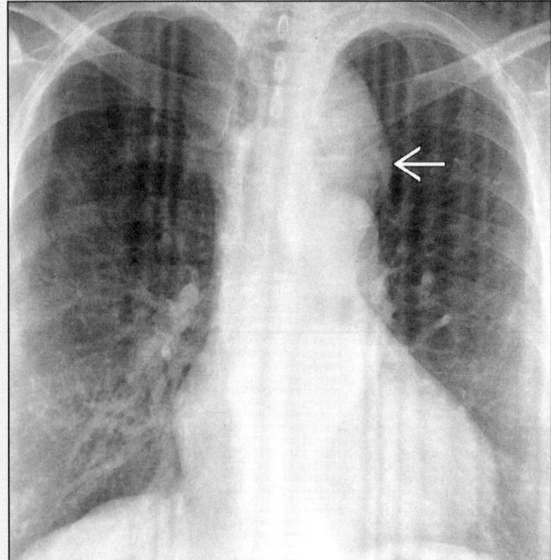

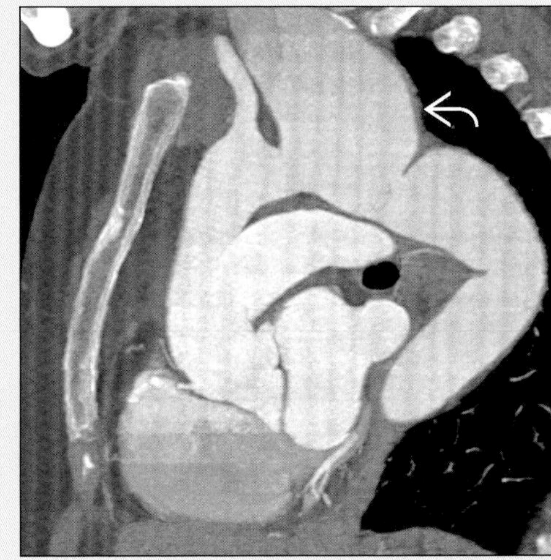

(Left) *PA chest radiograph demonstrates a left superior mediastinal mass ➡. The lesion projects above the left clavicle, indicating its middle-posterior mediastinal location.* ***(Right)*** *Sagittal CECT of the same patient shows aneurysmal dilation of the left subclavian artery ➡ at its origin from the aortic arch. Approximately 10% of mediastinal masses identified on chest radiography represent vascular lesions.*

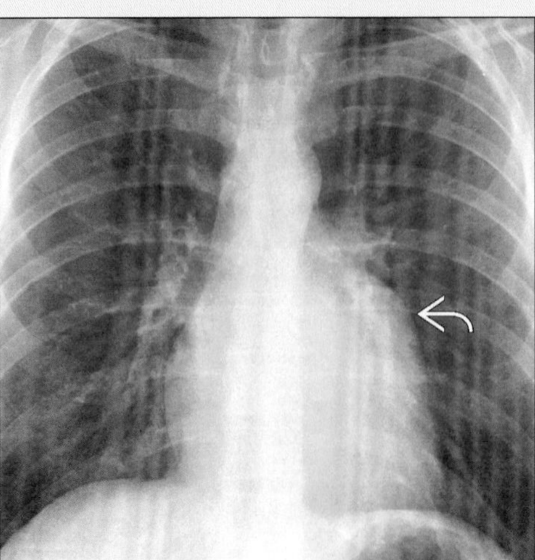

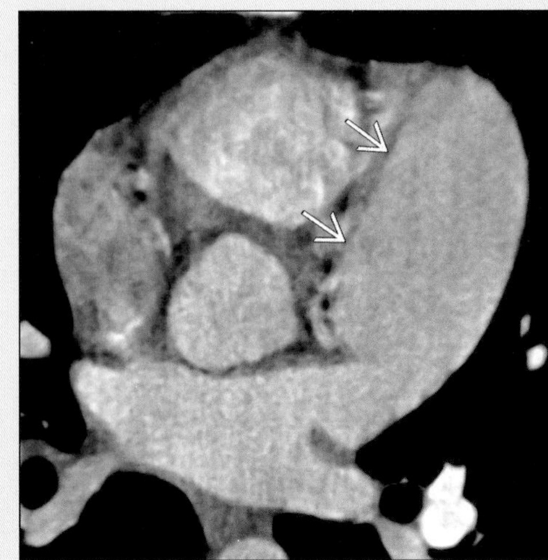

(Left) *PA chest radiograph shows a contour abnormality and increased convexity of the left cardiac border ➡.* ***(Right)*** *Axial CECT of the same patient demonstrates aneurysmal dilatation of the left atrial appendage ➡. CECT and CTA are the optimal imaging modalities for the evaluation of mediastinal vascular masses and determination of their morphology, location, size, relationship to adjacent structures, and complications.*

MEDIASTINAL VASCULAR MASSES

TERMINOLOGY

Definitions

- Lesions of systemic & pulmonary arteries & veins
  - 10% of mediastinal masses on radiography

IMAGING

General Features

- Best diagnostic clue
  - Mediastinal mass that opacifies on CECT & CTA
- Location
  - Mediastinal compartment
    - Middle-posterior > anterior
- Size
  - Variable
  - Small lesions may not be visible on radiography
  - Large lesions may mimic mediastinal neoplasms

Radiographic Findings

- Radiography
  - **Systemic arteries**
    - **Thoracic aorta**: Aneurysm & pseudoaneurysm
      - **Ascending aorta**: Convexity of right cardiomediastinal silhouette
      - **Descending aorta**: Focal mass obscuring left paraaortic interface or diffuse descending aorta enlargement & lateral displacement of left paraaortic interface
    - **Aortic dissection**
      - Most specific sign: Displacement of intimal calcification from aortic wall by > 1 cm
      - Nonspecific signs: Wide superior mediastinum, double aortic knob sign, progressive aortic enlargement, mass effect on mediastinum, apical cap, size disparity between ascending & descending aorta, cardiomegaly
    - **Coronary artery aneurysm**
      - Left or right paracardiac mass
    - Brachiocephalic artery: Tortuosity or aneurysm
      - Left or right superior mediastinal mass
    - Saphenous vein graft aneurysm
      - Paracardiac mass
    - Sinus of Valsalva aneurysm
      - May not be visible when small
      - Paracardiac mass when large
    - Left ventricular aneurysm
      - Paracardiac mass; may exhibit calcification
  - Systemic veins
    - SVC aneurysmal dilatation
      - Wide right superior mediastinum
    - Persistent left SVC
      - Wide left superior mediastinum
    - Brachiocephalic vein aneurysm
      - Appears as double aortic knob
      - May mimic aortic coarctation
    - Azygos vein
      - Enlargement: > 10 mm on upright radiography or > 15 mm on supine radiography
      - Appears as right paratracheal soft tissue
    - Hemiazygos vein
      - Wide left paravertebral stripe
    - Left superior intercostal vein
      - "Aortic nipple"
  - **Pulmonary arteries**
    - Enlargement
      - Middle mediastinal or hilar mass
    - Aberrant left pulmonary artery (pulmonary artery sling)
      - Opacity between trachea anteriorly & esophagus posteriorly
    - Ductus arteriosus aneurysm
      - Middle mediastinal mass
    - Aneurysm & pseudoaneurysm
      - Enlargement of right ventricular border
  - **Pulmonary veins**
    - Partial anomalous pulmonary venous return (PAPVR)
      - Wide left superior mediastinum
    - Pulmonary venous varix
      - Perihilar or middle mediastinal mass
    - **Pulmonary venous confluence**
      - Retrocardiac mediastinal mass
  - **Aortic arch anomalies**
    - Aneurysms & pseudoaneurysms
      - Enlargement or obscuration of aortic arch
      - Hilum overlay sign
      - Rightward tracheal deviation
    - **Right aortic arch**
      - Right paratracheal or superior mediastinal mass
    - Double aortic arch
      - Right arch appears as right paratracheal mass
    - Cervical arch
      - Superior mediastinal mass extending above superior clavicular margin
    - **Coarctation**
      - "**Figure 3" sign**: Mediastinal contour abnormality formed by dilated left subclavian artery & aorta distal to coarctation

CT Findings

- NECT
  - Vascular lesions may appear as hypodense masses
  - Communication with parent or branch vessels
- CECT
  - Vascular masses often of same density as parent or branch vessels
  - Venous lesions best seen on routine CECT
- CTA
  - Opacification of vascular lesions depends on contrast bolus timing
    - Systemic artery lesions best seen on CTA performed for detection of aortic abnormalities
    - Pulmonary artery lesions best seen on CTA performed for detection of pulmonary embolism
  - Vascular masses may be of same density as parent or branch vessels

MR Findings

- Can be used as alternative to CT
- Evaluation of lesion morphology
- Evaluation of cardiac valves & function

Imaging Recommendations

- Best imaging tool
  - CECT & CTA
    - Optimal evaluation of lesion location
    - Determination of lesion size
    - Relationship to adjacent structures & complications

MEDIASTINAL VASCULAR MASSES

- Protocol advice
  - Multiplanar reformatted images useful for lesion localization
  - Cardiac gating may be helpful for evaluation of vascular masses of cardiac origin

DIFFERENTIAL DIAGNOSIS

Hemangioma

- Rare, benign vascular tumor
- Anterior mediastinal location most common
- Well-circumscribed mass
  - Phleboliths, enhancement, & fat are characteristic

Lymphangioma

- Rare, benign tumor of lymphatic vessels
- Most commonly in superior & anterior mediastinum
- Uniform cystic mass, no contrast enhancement

Metastatic Disease

- Intense enhancement of enlarged lymph nodes
- Renal & thyroid cancer, melanoma, sarcoma

Extracardiac Mediastinal Angiosarcoma

- Anterior mediastinal location most common
- Heterogeneous attenuation on CECT
  - Hemorrhage, necrosis, & cystic change

Hemangiopericytoma

- Accounts for 1% of vascular tumors
- Intense enhancement on CECT
- Heterogeneous when complicated by hemorrhage & necrosis

PATHOLOGY

General Features

- Etiology
  - Systemic arteries
    - Thoracic aorta
      - Aneurysm & pseudoaneurysm: Atherosclerosis, cystic medial necrosis, trauma
    - Aortic dissection
      - Congenital: Marfan & Ehlers-Danlos syndromes
      - Acquired: Hypertension
    - Coronary arteries
      - Aneurysm: Atherosclerosis, infection, inflammation
      - Fistula: Congenital
    - Brachiocephalic artery
      - Atherosclerosis & hypertension
    - Bypass graft aneurysm: Degeneration
    - Sinus of Valsalva aneurysm: Congenital
    - Left ventricular aneurysm
      - Congenital & acquired (myocardial infarction)
  - Systemic veins
    - Aneurysmal SVC dilatation
      - Tricuspid valve disease & heart failure
      - SVC obstruction: Neoplasm, mediastinal fibrosis, lymphadenopathy
      - PAPVR & idiopathic (rare)
    - Left SVC: Congenital
    - Brachiocephalic vein aneurysm: Congenital, trauma, infection, inflammation, degeneration
    - Azygos & hemiazygos vein enlargement
      - Portal hypertension, vena cava & hepatic vein obstruction, cardiac disease, & azygos continuation of IVC
    - Left superior intercostal vein enlargement
      - Increased flow or pressure in thoracic veins
  - Pulmonary arteries
    - Enlargement
      - Pulmonary artery hypertension: Pre-capillary & post-capillary etiologies
      - Congenital: Valve absence or stenosis
      - Idiopathic aneurysm: Collagen vascular disease
      - Pseudoaneurysm: Infection & trauma
      - Aberrant left pulmonary artery (pulmonary artery sling): Congenital
      - Aneurysm of ductus arteriosus
  - Pulmonary veins
    - Pulmonary venous varix
      - Congenital & acquired (mitral valve disease)
    - Pulmonary venous confluence & PAPVR
  - Aortic arch
    - Aneurysm & pseudoaneurysm: Atherosclerosis, cystic medial necrosis, trauma
    - Congenital: Right aortic arch, double aortic arch, cervical arch, coarctation
- Associated abnormalities
  - SVC aneurysm associated with cystic hygroma
  - PAPVR associated with atrial septal defect
  - Congenital left ventricular aneurysm
    - Component of pentalogy of Cantrell
  - Sinus of Valsalva aneurysm associated with congenital heart defects

CLINICAL ISSUES

Treatment

- Surgical resection or endovascular therapy
  - More common for vascular lesions involving aorta & pulmonary arteries
    - Aortic dissection involving ascending aorta & thoracic aneurysms of certain sizes
  - Bypass graft aneurysm > 2 cm
  - Vascular lesions involving other vessels that result in significant symptoms, mass effect, or rupture

DIAGNOSTIC CHECKLIST

Consider

- Mediastinal vascular lesion when a mediastinal mass is detected on chest radiography

Image Interpretation Pearls

- CECT & CTA provide optimal evaluation of vascular mass morphology, location, size, relationship to adjacent structures, & complications

SELECTED REFERENCES

1. Boateng P et al: Vascular lesions of the mediastinum. Thorac Surg Clin. 19(1):91-105, 2009
2. Frazier AA et al: Coronary artery bypass grafts: assessment with multidetector CT in the early and late postoperative settings. Radiographics. 25(4):881-96, 2005
3. Demos TC et al: Venous anomalies of the thorax. AJR Am J Roentgenol. 182(5):1139-50, 2004

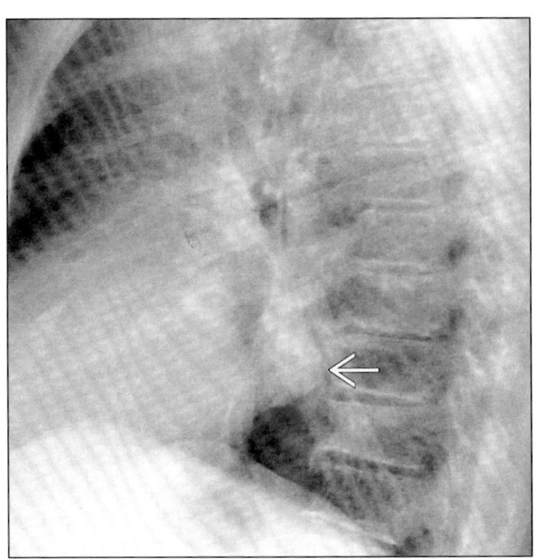

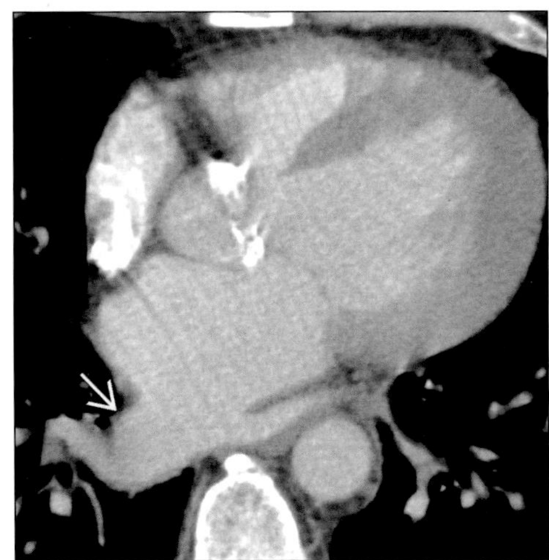

(Left) *Lateral chest radiograph shows a nodular opacity ➔ projecting over the inferior aspect of the middle-posterior mediastinum.* ***(Right)*** *Axial CECT of the same patient demonstrates that the radiographic abnormality represents enlargement of the right inferior pulmonary vein ➔ at its entry point into the left atrium. Pulmonary vein varices may be congenital or secondary to pulmonary venous hypertension in patients with mitral valve stenosis or insufficiency.*

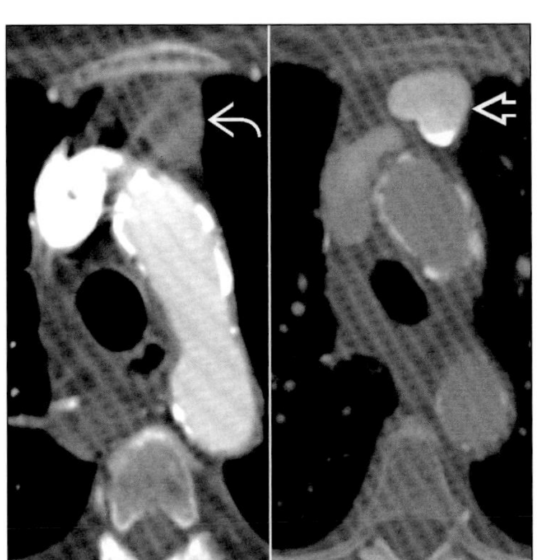

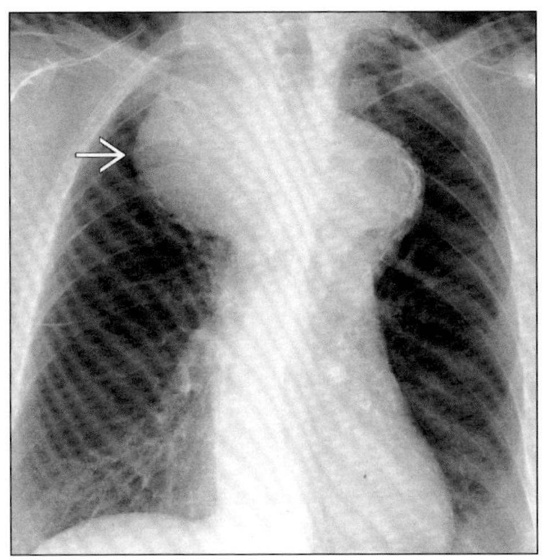

(Left) *Composite image with axial CTA (left) and axial CECT (right) of a patient with a left brachiocephalic vein aneurysm shows a hypodense left anterior mediastinal mass ➔ on the CTA that opacifies with contrast on CECT ➔. Contrast enhancement of mediastinal vascular masses is affected by the timing of the contrast bolus.* ***(Right)*** *PA chest radiograph of a patient with an aneurysmal aberrant right subclavian artery shows a large right superior mediastinal mass ➔.*

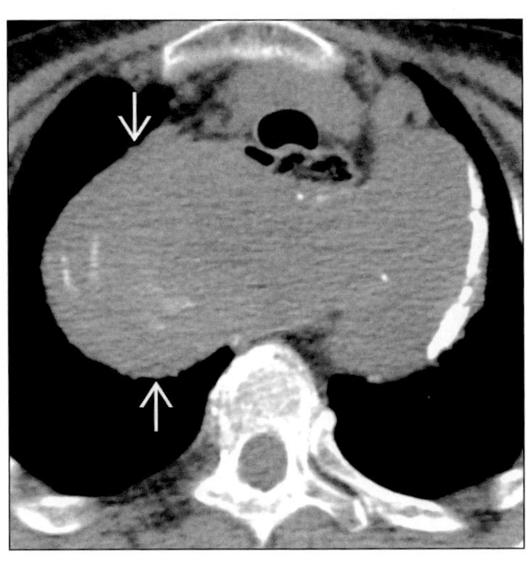

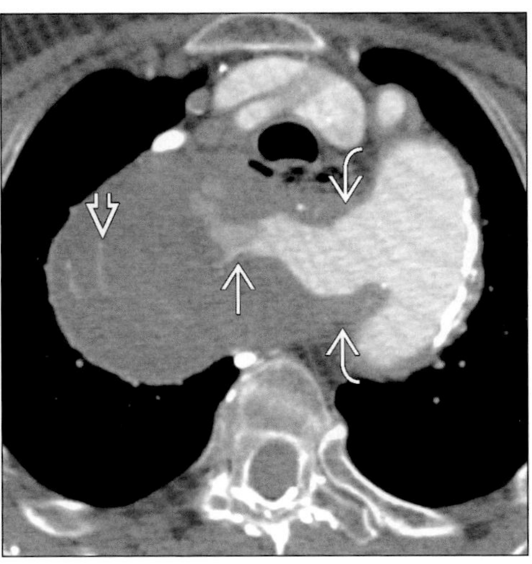

(Left) *Axial NECT of the same patient shows a soft tissue mass ➔ extending rightward from the aortic arch behind the esophagus.* ***(Right)*** *Axial CECT of the same patient shows aortic arch contrast ➔ partially opacifying the aneurysmal aberrant right subclavian artery. A large amount of hypodense thrombus is present within the aneurysm. Curvilinear hyperdense foci ➔ are consistent with displaced calcification. Note aneurysmal dilatation of the diverticulum of Kommerell ➔.*

CORONARY ARTERY ANEURYSM

Key Facts

Terminology

- Definition: Coronary artery diameter > 1.5x normal adjacent segments, involving < 50% of vessel
- Coronary artery ectasia: Diffuse coronary dilatation

Imaging

- Coronary CTA
  - Evaluation of coronary aneurysm morphology, thrombosis, dissection
  - Calcification frequently present in atherosclerosis
  - Size underestimation with mural thrombus or dissection
- MR
  - Preferred modality when surveillance required
  - Calcification difficult to detect
  - Stents & clips may degrade image quality
- Angiography: May underestimate size if mural thrombus or dissection present

Top Differential Diagnoses

- Coronary fistula
- Coronary pseudoaneurysm

Pathology

- Atherosclerosis most common cause in United States
  - Right coronary artery typically affected
- Kawasaki disease most common cause worldwide
  - Left main coronary artery most commonly affected

Clinical Issues

- Most patients asymptomatic
- Acute coronary syndrome & heart failure
- Treatment: Anticoagulants, antiplatelets, surgery

Diagnostic Checklist

- Consider coronary artery aneurysm in patients < 20 years with angina or acute myocardial infarction

*(**Left**) Axial coronary CTA of a 19-year-old woman with acute myelogenous leukemia and acute chest pain shows a focal right coronary artery aneurysm ➔ and associated hemopericardium ➔. (**Right**) Oblique CTA of the same patient shows focal disruption ➔ of the aneurysm, which had enlarged over the previous 2 days. Aneurysm rupture is a rare complication of coronary artery aneurysm. Aneurysm enlargement and rupture are indications for intervention. This patient was treated with a covered coronary stent.*

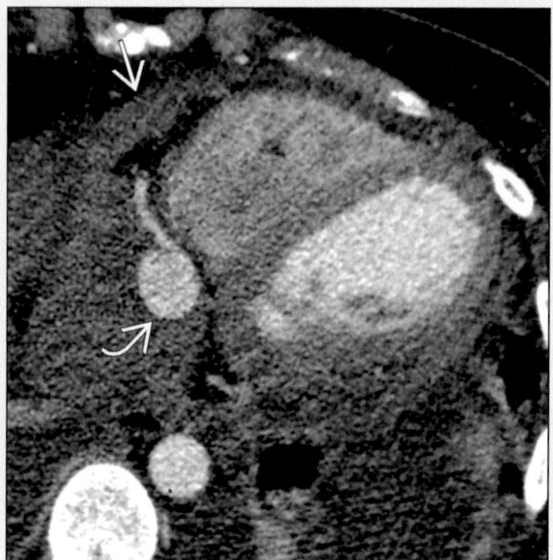

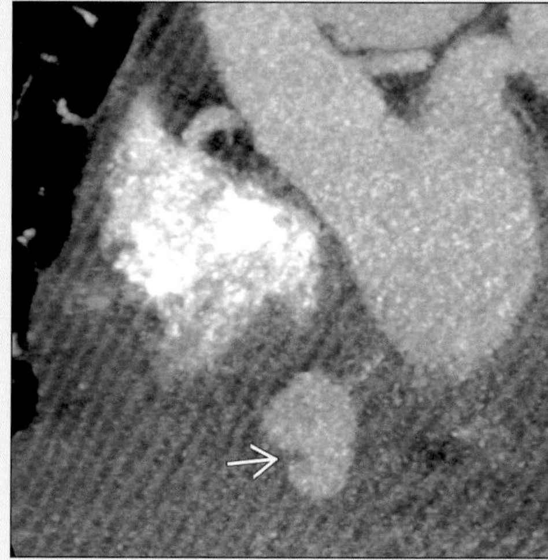

*(**Left**) Axial coronary CTA of a 26-year-old woman with Kawasaki disease shows dilatation of the right ➔ and left main ➔ coronary arteries. Note peripheral calcification of the enlarged left main coronary artery. (**Right**) 3D volume rendered image from a coronary CTA of a 42-year-old man with Kawasaki disease shows dilatation of the left anterior descending ➔ and left circumflex ➔ coronary arteries. Coronary artery aneurysms occur in 15-25% of untreated patients with Kawasaki disease.*

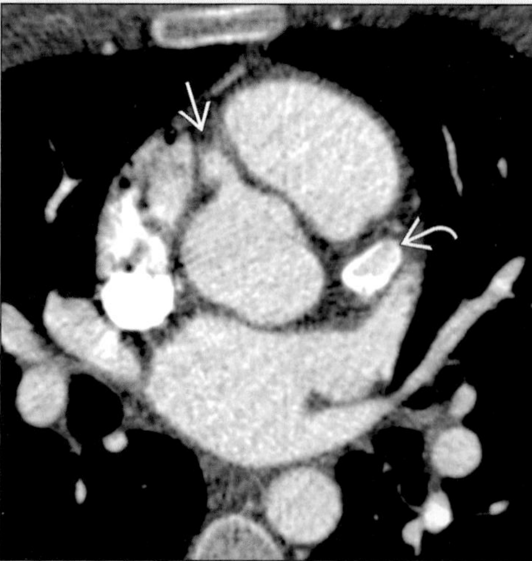

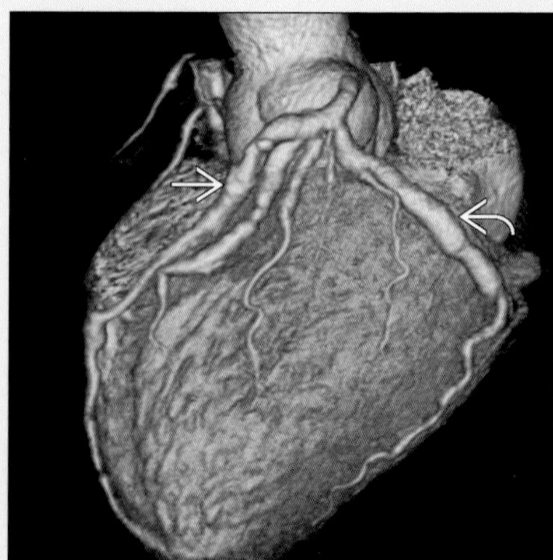

CORONARY ARTERY ANEURYSM

TERMINOLOGY

Definitions

- **Coronary artery diameter > 1.5x normal adjacent segments, involving < 50% of vessel**

IMAGING

General Features

- Best diagnostic clue
  - **Dilatation of coronary artery**
- Morphology
  - Fusiform or saccular dilatation
    - May exhibit thrombus or dissection
  - Coronary artery ectasia refers to diffuse dilation

CT Findings

- Cardiac gated CTA
  - Evaluation of coronary aneurysm morphology, thrombosis, dissection
  - Calcification frequently present in atherosclerosis

MR Findings

- Available coronary angiography sequences
  - Lumen dark on double IR FSE
  - Lumen bright on GRE or b-SSFP in absence of thrombus
- May be preferred modality when surveillance required
- Calcification difficult to detect
- Stents & clips may degrade image quality

Echocardiographic Findings

- Echocardiogram
  - Aneurysm detection in proximal coronary arteries

Angiographic Findings

- Fusiform & saccular dilatation of coronary arteries
- May underestimate size if mural thrombus or dissection present

Imaging Recommendations

- Best imaging tool
  - Gated coronary CTA is imaging modality of choice

DIFFERENTIAL DIAGNOSIS

Coronary Fistula

- Dilated vessel associated with fistula
- Coronary ectasia proximal to fistula if large shunt or steal physiology present

Coronary Pseudoaneurysm

- Frequently secondary to chest trauma or catheter-based intervention

PATHOLOGY

General Features

- Etiology
  - **Atherosclerosis** most common cause in United States
    - **Right coronary artery most commonly affected**, followed by left anterior descending, left circumflex, & left main coronary arteries
  - **Kawasaki disease** most common cause worldwide
    - Develops in 15-25% of untreated affected children
    - May regress with treatment
    - Left main coronary artery most commonly involved
  - Takayasu arteritis (12% have coronary involvement)
  - Connective tissue disease (systemic lupus erythematosus, Marfan, Behçet)
  - Other: Congenital, trauma, catheter-based intervention, mycotic emboli, cocaine use

Staging, Grading, & Classification

- True aneurysms have 3 intact vessel wall layers
- Pseudoaneurysms have 2 or fewer intact walls
- > 20 mm diameter in adults, considered "giant"

Gross Pathologic & Surgical Features

- Dilatation of coronary artery, may contain thrombus

Microscopic Features

- Atherosclerotic coronary aneurysms may exhibit thinning or destruction of media

CLINICAL ISSUES

Presentation

- Most common signs/symptoms
  - Most patients asymptomatic
  - Acute coronary syndrome & heart failure may be caused by aneurysm or concurrent disease
- Clinical profile
  - Can result in thrombosis & myocardial infarction

Demographics

- Gender
  - More common in **men** (2.2%) than women (0.5%)
- Epidemiology
  - Present in 4.9% of angiograms, 1.5% of necropsies

Natural History & Prognosis

- Related to severity of concomitant obstructive disease in patients with atherosclerosis
- Rupture reported but rare

Treatment

- Anticoagulants, antiplatelet therapy
- **Surgical intervention if enlargement, embolization, or obstruction**
  - Bypass & exclusion of aneurysm
  - Covered stent graft
- Kawasaki disease typically treated with high-dose intravenous γ-globulin & aspirin

DIAGNOSTIC CHECKLIST

Consider

- Coronary artery aneurysm in patients < 20 years presenting with angina or acute myocardial infarction

SELECTED REFERENCES

1. Díaz-Zamudio M et al: Coronary artery aneurysms and ectasia: role of coronary CT angiography. Radiographics. 29(7):1939-54, 2009
2. Cohen P et al: Coronary artery aneurysms: a review of the natural history, pathophysiology, and management. Cardiol Rev. 16(6):301-4, 2008

PARAESOPHAGEAL VARICES

Key Facts

Terminology

- Dilated vessels within (esophageal) or adjacent to (paraesophageal) esophageal wall
- Uphill varices: Lower mediastinum, usually from portal hypertension
- Downhill varices: Upper mediastinum, typically related to superior vena cava obstruction

Imaging

- Radiography
  - Lateral displacement or obscuration of inferior azygoesophageal recess
  - Visible in ~ 50% of patients with known varices
- Esophagram: Serpiginous filling defects
- CT
  - Asymmetric apparent esophageal wall thickening
  - Dilated vessels adjacent to or in esophageal wall
  - May be unopacified on arterial phase imaging

Top Differential Diagnoses

- Hiatal hernia
- Esophageal carcinoma
- Mediastinal neoplasm

Pathology

- Uphill varices: Presinusoidal (portal vein thrombosis), sinusoidal (cirrhosis), postsinusoidal (Budd-Chiari syndrome)
- Downhill varices: Superior vena cava obstruction

Clinical Issues

- Alcoholic cirrhosis most frequent cause in USA
- Infectious cirrhosis most frequent cause worldwide

Diagnostic Checklist

- Evaluate for treatable underlying cause of varices
- Endoscopy: First-line test for esophageal varices

__(Left)__ PA chest radiograph of a patient with alcoholic cirrhosis and paraesophageal varices shows lobulated masses near the gastroesophageal junction with lateral displacement of the azygoesophageal recess ➔. __(Right)__ Graphic shows the morphologic features of paraesophageal and esophageal varices. Paraesophageal varices surround the distal esophagus. Esophageal varices are located in the submucosa of the esophagus and may manifest as serpiginous filling defects on esophagram.

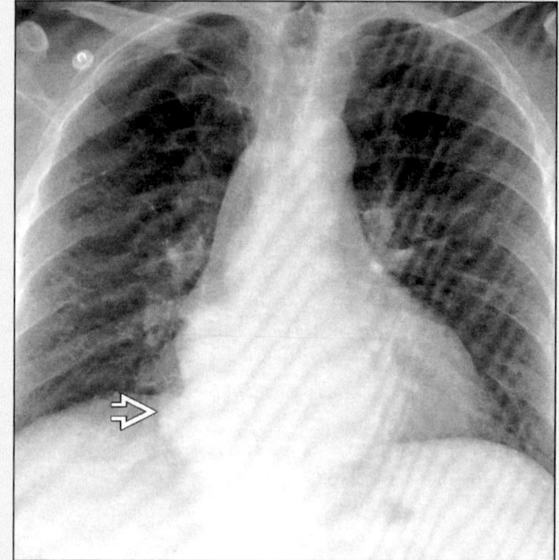

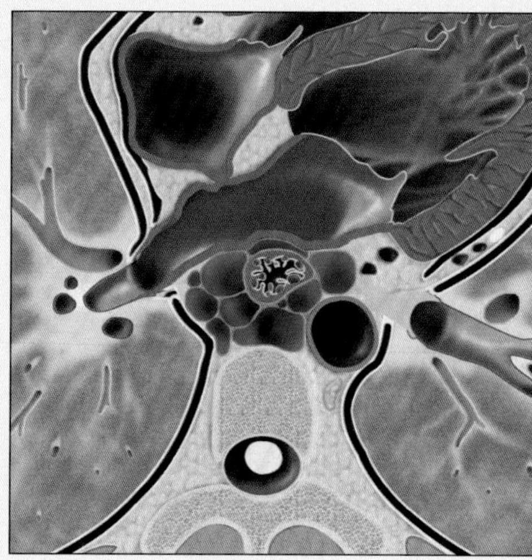

__(Left)__ Composite image with axial NECT (left) and sagittal CECT (right) shows paraesophageal varices manifesting as serpiginous soft tissue lesions ➔ surrounding the distal esophagus. These lesions exhibit intense contrast enhancement ➔ consistent with their vascular nature. __(Right)__ Composite image with axial CECT (left) and coronal volume rendered CECT (right) of a patient with catheter-associated SVC thrombosis ➔ shows extensive collateral vessels ➔ (downhill varices) in the mediastinum.

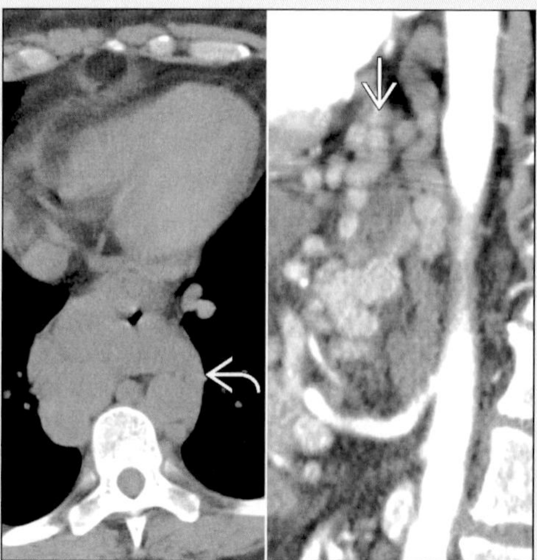

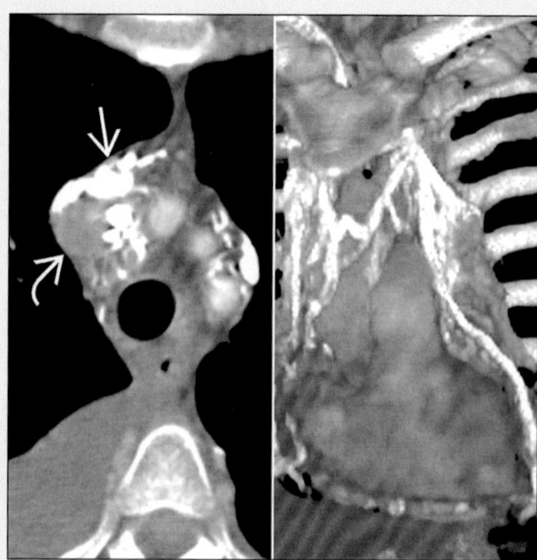

PARAESOPHAGEAL VARICES

TERMINOLOGY

Definitions

- Dilated vessels within (**esophageal**) or adjacent to (**paraesophageal**) esophageal wall
- **Uphill varices**: Lower mediastinum, usually from portal hypertension
- **Downhill varices**: Upper mediastinum related to obstruction of superior vena cava

IMAGING

General Features

- Best diagnostic clue
  - Lobular contour abnormality in lower azygoesophageal recess
  - Serpiginous vessels in or about esophageal wall
- Location
  - Most commonly at **lower 1/3 of esophagus**

Radiographic Findings

- Radiography
  - Lateral displacement or obscuration of inferior aspect of azygoesophageal recess

Fluoroscopic Findings

- Esophagram
  - Tortuous, longitudinal filling defects projecting into esophageal lumen
    - **Detection may be enhanced by Valsalva maneuver & Trendelenburg position**

CT Findings

- Asymmetric apparent esophageal wall thickening
- **Dilated vessels adjacent to or in esophageal wall**
- Increased number or tortuosity of mediastinal veins

MR Findings

- T1WI
  - Serpiginous flow voids on T1WI
    - Signal voids may be absent if slow flow
- MRV
  - **Best visualized on portal venous phase**

Ultrasonographic Findings

- Hypo-/anechoic tubular structures on endoscopic US

Angiographic Findings

- **Downhill varices**: Multiple small collateral thoracic vessels on upper extremity venography
- **Uphill varices**: May be detected during transjugular intrahepatic portosystemic shunt placement

Imaging Recommendations

- Best imaging tool
  - CECT optimal for detection & characterization
- Protocol advice
  - Imaging during portal venous phase

DIFFERENTIAL DIAGNOSIS

Hiatal Hernia

- Intrathoracic stomach, bowel, omentum

Esophageal Carcinoma

- Irregular or asymmetric esophageal wall thickening

Mediastinal Neoplasm

- Lymphadenopathy, gastrointestinal stromal tumor

PATHOLOGY

General Features

- Etiology
  - Uphill varices due to portal hypertension (hepatic venous pressure gradient > 12 mmHg)
    - Reversal of flow diverts blood through left gastric vein to esophageal venous plexus
  - Uphill varices: Presinusoidal (portal vein thrombosis), sinusoidal (cirrhosis), or postsinusoidal (Budd-Chiari syndrome)
  - Downhill varices from superior vena cava obstruction
    - May be due to obstructing mass, central venous catheter, mediastinal fibrosis
- Associated abnormalities
  - Cirrhosis, splenomegaly, recanalized umbilical vein, spleno-renal shunt

CLINICAL ISSUES

Presentation

- Most common signs/symptoms
  - Hematemesis or gastrointestinal bleeding
- Other signs/symptoms
  - Signs of cirrhosis
  - Facial or upper extremity edema due to venous obstruction in superior mediastinum
  - Arm claudication (rare) due to venous insufficiency

Demographics

- Epidemiology
  - United States: Alcoholic cirrhosis most frequent cause
  - Worldwide: Cirrhosis due to hepatitis B, hepatitis C, and schistosomiasis are most frequent causes

Natural History & Prognosis

- Hemorrhage occurs in up to 1/3 of affected patients
  - Mortality for bleeding episode approximately 30%
- Downhill varices: Prognosis based on underlying cause
  - Poor prognosis when due to obstructing neoplasm

Treatment

- Transjugular intrahepatic portosystemic shunt
- Sclerotherapy or variceal ligation

DIAGNOSTIC CHECKLIST

Consider

- Endoscopy: First-line test for esophageal varices

Image Interpretation Pearls

- Evaluate for treatable underlying cause of varices

SELECTED REFERENCES

1. Zhao LQ et al: Characteristics of paraesophageal varices: a study with 64-row multidetector computed tomography portal venography. World J Gastroenterol. 14(34):5331-5, 2008

MEDIASTINAL LYMPHANGIOMA

Key Facts

Terminology
- Synonym: Lymphatic malformation
- Rare, benign tumor of lymphatic vessels
- Often recurrent lymphangioma excised in childhood

Imaging
- Radiography
  - Well-defined smooth or lobular mediastinal mass
  - Superior anterior mediastinum in adults
  - Cervical region in children
- CT
  - Most commonly uniformly cystic mass
  - Displacement of or insinuation around vessels/ adjacent structures
- MR
  - T1WI: Hyperintense relative to muscle
  - T2WI: Typically high signal intensity
  - Visualization of cystic components & invasion

Top Differential Diagnoses
- Necrotic neoplasm
- Mature teratoma
- Thymic cyst
- Other mediastinal cyst
- Hematoma, seroma, abscess

Pathology
- Dilated vascular spaces lined by endothelium

Clinical Issues
- Asymptomatic or chest pain, cough, dyspnea
- Treatment: Complete surgical excision, percutaneous drainage & ablation

Diagnostic Checklist
- Suspect lymphangioma in adult with cystic mediastinal mass & history of childhood resection

*(**Left**) PA chest radiograph of a 53-year-old man with a mediastinal lymphangioma shows an abnormal contour of the left heart border ➔. Although most patients with lymphangioma are asymptomatic, they may also present with chest pain, cough, or dyspnea. (**Right**) Lateral chest radiograph of the same patient shows the well-defined mass ➔ overlying the cardiac silhouette. When occurring in the adult, lymphangiomas are most commonly located in the superior aspect of the anterior mediastinum.*

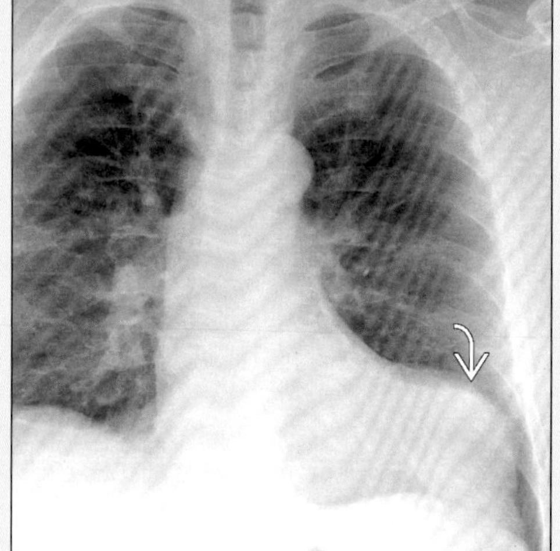

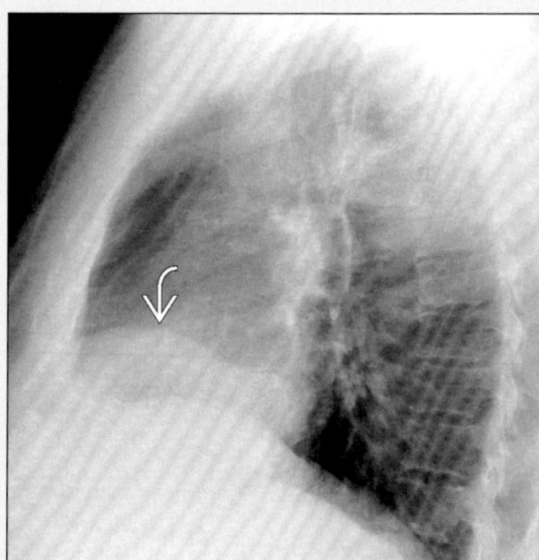

*(**Left**) Axial CECT of the same patient shows a low-attenuation, nonenhancing left anterior inferior mediastinal mass. Lymphangiomas lack definite enhancement or calcification, and local invasion is very rare. (**Right**) Composite image with axial T2W (top) and T1W post gadolinium (bottom) MR images of the same patient shows a heterogeneous mass on T1WI that is T2 hyperintense and nonenhancing. Mediastinal lymphangiomas are often treated surgically but may also be drained and ablated.*

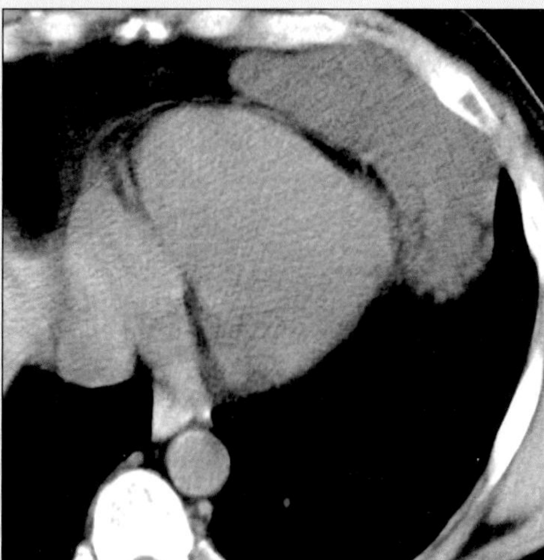

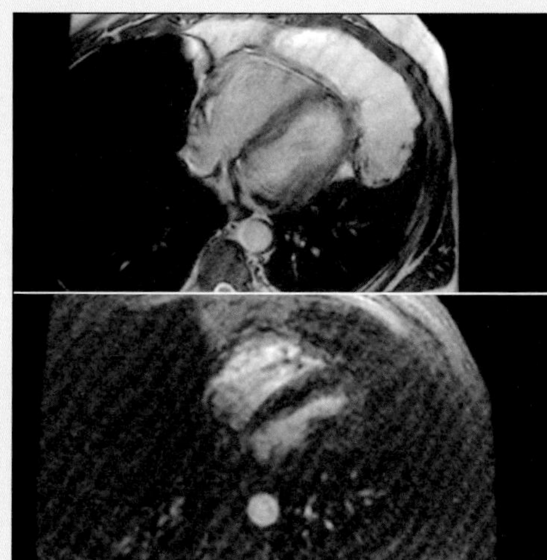

MEDIASTINAL LYMPHANGIOMA

TERMINOLOGY

Synonyms

- **Lymphatic malformation**

Definitions

- Rare, **benign tumor of lymphatic vessels**

IMAGING

General Features

- Location
  - Most common in **cervical region in children**; mediastinal extension in 10%
  - Most common in **superior aspect of anterior mediastinum in adults**
    - Recurrence of lymphangioma excised in childhood

Radiographic Findings

- Well-defined smooth or lobular mediastinal mass
- Pleural effusion, often chylous

CT Findings

- Most commonly **uniformly cystic mass**
- **Displacement of or insinuation around vessels/ adjacent structures**
- Cystic component attenuation higher than water suggests proteinaceous fluid
- Calcification rare
- Almost all lack definite enhancement
  - Hemangiomatous components or associated aneurysms may enhance

MR Findings

- T1WI
  - Hyperintense relative to muscle
- T2WI
  - Typically high signal intensity
- MR optimally depicts cystic components & invasion
- Septa may be serpentine or vessel-like

Imaging Recommendations

- Protocol advice
  - Percutaneous needle biopsy often nondiagnostic

DIFFERENTIAL DIAGNOSIS

Necrotic Neoplasm

- Metastases, thymoma, lymphoma, germ cell neoplasms
- Schwannomas may undergo cystic degeneration
- Necrosis more likely after treatment

Mature Teratoma

- Most common germ cell neoplasm
- Majority in anterior mediastinum
- Majority contain fat, calcium, fluid
  - 15% contain soft tissue & fluid

Thymic Cyst

- May be congenital or acquired
- Unilocular or multilocular
- Well-defined cystic mass with well-defined walls

Other Mediastinal Cysts

- Bronchogenic cyst: Paratracheal, subcarinal, middle-posterior mediastinum
- Pericardial cyst: Abuts pericardium
- Esophageal duplication cyst: Adjacent to or within esophageal wall
- Solitary spherical lesion; homogeneous attenuation

Hematoma, Seroma, Abscess

- Usually distinguished by clinical features
- Biopsy may be required for diagnosis in postoperative patients

PATHOLOGY

General Features

- Etiology
  - Developmental, hamartomatous, or neoplastic
    - History of childhood resection an important clue

Staging, Grading, & Classification

- **Lymphangioma** classified based on size of lymphatics: **Capillary, cavernous, cystic (hygromas)**
- **Lymphatic malformation** classified based on size of cystic spaces (for treatment purposes)
  - **Macrocystic**: > 1 cm cystic spaces
  - **Microcystic**: 0.5-10 mm cystic spaces

Microscopic Features

- Dilated vascular spaces lined by endothelium
- Some contain hemangiomas

CLINICAL ISSUES

Presentation

- Most common signs/symptoms
  - Often asymptomatic
  - Chest pain, cough, dyspnea
  - Venous compression, stridor

Demographics

- Gender
  - More common in male children
  - Adults: May be more common in women
- Epidemiology
  - More common in children < 2 years

Treatment

- Complete surgical excision recommended as tumors tend to continue to grow or recur
- Percutaneous drainage & ablation of macrocystic lesions

DIAGNOSTIC CHECKLIST

Image Interpretation Pearls

- Suspect lymphangioma in patient with cystic mediastinal mass & history of childhood resection

SELECTED REFERENCES

1. Jeung MY et al: Imaging of cystic masses of the mediastinum. Radiographics. 22 Spec No:S79-93, 2002
2. Shaffer K et al: Thoracic lymphangioma in adults: CT and MR imaging features. AJR Am J Roentgenol. 162(2):283-9, 1994

MEDIASTINAL HEMANGIOMA

Key Facts

Terminology
- Rare, benign vascular tumor

Imaging
- Radiography
  - Well-defined mediastinal soft tissue mass
  - Typically in anterior mediastinum
  - Discrete round calcifications (phleboliths) in 10%
- CT
  - Well-defined mediastinal soft tissue mass with central, peripheral, or mixed enhancement
  - Identification of phleboliths in 30%
- MR
  - Heterogeneous signal intensity on T1WI
  - Hyperintense on T2WI
  - T2WI FS high sensitivity for fat
  - Insensitive for low signal intensity phleboliths
- Image-guided needle biopsy is rarely diagnostic

Top Differential Diagnoses
- Malignant vascular neoplasms
- Germ cell neoplasms
- Lymphangioma
- Lymphoma

Pathology
- Interconnecting vascular spaces with variable stroma
- Areas of organized thrombus; may calcify

Clinical Issues
- Asymptomatic in almost 1/2 of cases
- Typically young patients, most < 35 years
- Surgical excision usually required for diagnosis

Diagnostic Checklist
- Enhancing mediastinal soft tissue mass with phleboliths is virtually diagnostic of hemangioma

(Left) PA chest radiograph of a patient with multiple peripheral hemangiomas and a mediastinal hemangioma shows a mediastinal mass ⮕ that exhibits the hilum overlay sign ⇨, which suggests an anterior mediastinal location. Phleboliths → are also present within subcutaneous hemangiomas. (Right) Lateral chest radiograph of the same patient confirms the anterior mediastinal location of the mass ⇨ as well as additional subcutaneous hemangiomas with phleboliths →.

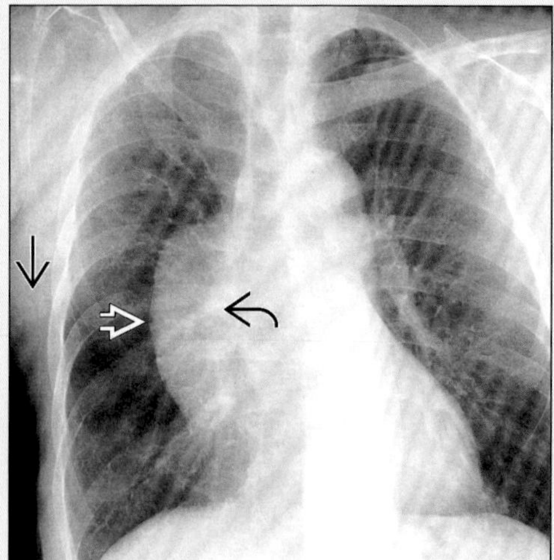

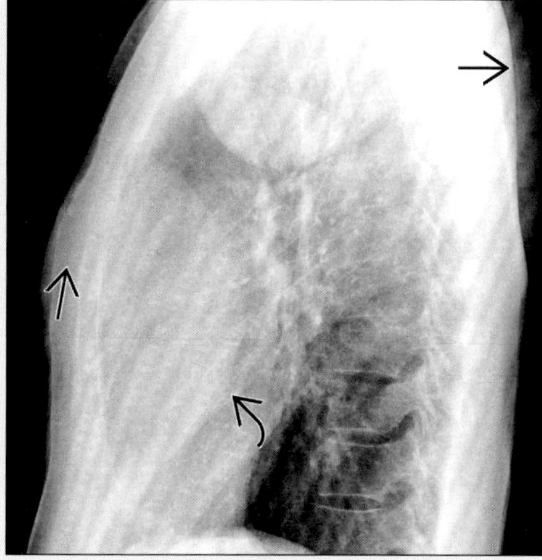

(Left) Axial CECT of the same patient shows the anterior mediastinal hemangioma as a well-defined heterogeneous mass with internal fat attenuation and central punctate calcifications ⮕. The lesion produces mass effect without evidence of invasion. Subcutaneous hemangiomas ⮕ are also present. (Right) Composite image with sagittal (left) and coronal (right) CECT of the same patient shows intratumoral vessels ⮕. Hemangiomas may exhibit central, peripheral, or mixed enhancement.

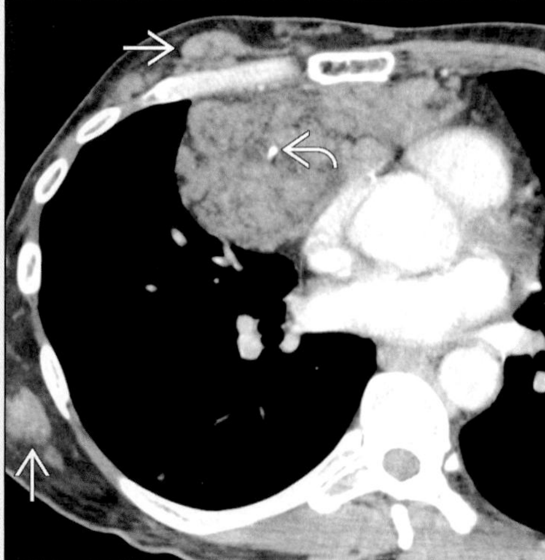

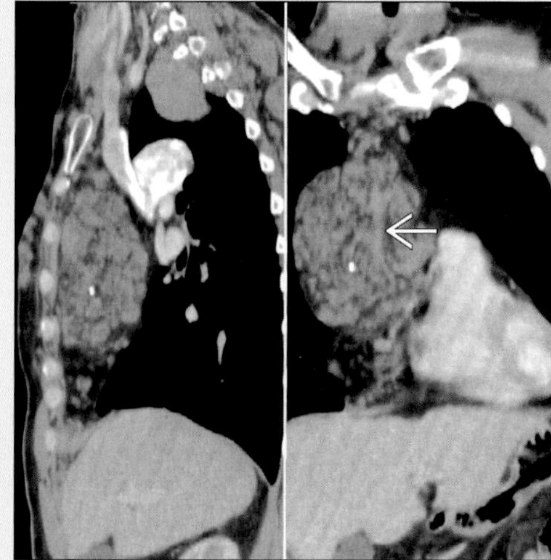

MEDIASTINAL HEMANGIOMA

TERMINOLOGY

Definitions

- Rare, benign vascular tumor

IMAGING

General Features

- Best diagnostic clue
  - Well-defined mass with contrast enhancement & punctate calcifications or phleboliths
- Location
  - Majority in anterior mediastinum
    - Uncommonly in other compartments
  - Extrathoracic extension rare, usually to neck
- Morphology
  - Well-circumscribed soft tissue mass
    - Rarely infiltrative/invasive

Radiographic Findings

- Well-defined mediastinal soft tissue mass
- Discrete round **calcifications (phleboliths) in 10%**

CT Findings

- NECT
  - Heterogeneous attenuation from intratumoral thrombus, stroma, vasculature
  - Intratumoral fat uncommon
  - Identification of **phleboliths in 30%**
- CECT
  - Enhancement: Central, peripheral, mixed
  - Large draining veins on delayed images
  - Gradually increasing enhancement on dynamic contrast-enhanced CT
- High sensitivity for calcification & phleboliths

MR Findings

- T1WI
  - Heterogeneous signal intensity: Intratumoral fat & blood products
- T2WI
  - Hyperintensity attributed to vascular spaces & myxoid components
- T2WI FS
  - More sensitive than CT for identification of fat
- MR insensitive for low signal intensity phleboliths

Imaging Recommendations

- Best imaging tool
  - CT optimally demonstrates phleboliths & extent of mediastinal neoplasm
- Protocol advice
  - Image-guided needle biopsy is rarely diagnostic

Nuclear Medicine Findings

- PET
  - Mild FDG uptake reported

DIFFERENTIAL DIAGNOSIS

Malignant Vascular Neoplasms

- Very rare
- Hemangioendothelioma, hemangiopericytoma
- Aggressive features such as invasion

Germ Cell Neoplasms

- Teratoma: Calcification, fat, & cystic spaces

Lymphangioma

- Cystic (vascular spaces); calcification is rare
- Contrast enhancement is very rare

Lymphoma

- Enlarged lymph nodes within mediastinal fat may mimic fat-containing soft tissue lesion
- Calcification exceedingly rare without treatment

PATHOLOGY

General Features

- Associated abnormalities
  - Peripheral hemangiomas
  - Hereditary hemorrhagic telangiectasia

Staging, Grading, & Classification

- Classified as **capillary**, **cavernous**, or **venous** based on size of vascular spaces

Microscopic Features

- Large interconnecting vascular spaces with variable interposed stroma
- Vascular spaces lined by flattened cuboidal epithelium
- Foci of organized thrombus, which may calcify

CLINICAL ISSUES

Presentation

- Most common signs/symptoms
  - Asymptomatic in almost 1/2 of cases
  - Cough, chest pain, dyspnea
- Other signs/symptoms
  - Rarely dysphagia, superior vena cava syndrome, neurologic symptoms

Demographics

- Age
  - Typically young patients, most < 35 years
- Epidemiology
  - Less than 0.5% of all mediastinal tumors

Treatment

- Surgical excision usually required for diagnosis
- Surgical risk of significant blood loss

DIAGNOSTIC CHECKLIST

Image Interpretation Pearls

- Enhancing mediastinal soft tissue mass with phleboliths is virtually diagnostic of hemangioma

SELECTED REFERENCES

1. Sakurai K et al: Thoracic hemangiomas: imaging via CT, MR, and PET along with pathologic correlation. J Thorac Imaging. 23(2):114-20, 2008
2. McAdams HP et al: Mediastinal hemangioma: radiographic and CT features in 14 patients. Radiology. 193(2):399-402, 1994

THYMIC HYPERPLASIA

Key Facts

Terminology

- Thymic enlargement due to thymic or lymphoid hyperplasia

Imaging

- Radiography
  - Normal radiograph or mediastinal widening
- CT
  - True thymic hyperplasia: Diffuse, symmetric thymic enlargement, typically following chemotherapy
  - Lymphoid hyperplasia: Normal thymus, enlarged thymus, focal thymic mass
  - Enhancement similar to that of normal thymus
  - Heterogeneous enhancement suggests thymic neoplasm
- MR: ↓ signal on opposed-phase gradient-echo T1WI
- FDG PET: SUV = 2.0-2.8

Top Differential Diagnoses

- Thymoma
- Recurrent or metastatic malignancy
- Lymphoma

Pathology

- True thymic hyperplasia: Secondary to recent stress, microscopically normal thymus
- Lymphoid hyperplasia: Association with myasthenia gravis, thymic lymphoid follicles

Clinical Issues

- Asymptomatic; typically no treatment required

Diagnostic Checklist

- Consider thymic hyperplasia in patient on chemotherapy with enlarging thymus
- Consider lymphoid hyperplasia in patients with myasthenia gravis

*(**Left**) Graphic shows the axial anatomy of the anterior mediastinum. The thymus is surrounded by fat, bound posteriorly by the superior vena cava and ascending aorta and anteriorly by the sternum. (**Right**) Graphic illustrates the method for measuring the thymus on CT. The AP diameter (W) and thickness of each lobe (T) are measured as shown. Thymic thickness is the most frequently used measurement and should be correlated with the patient's age.*

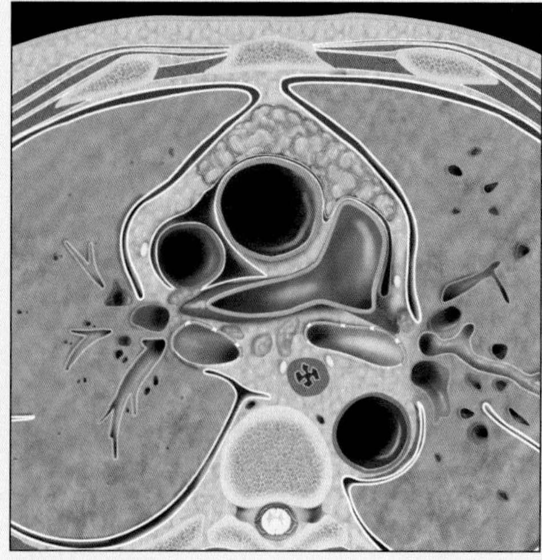

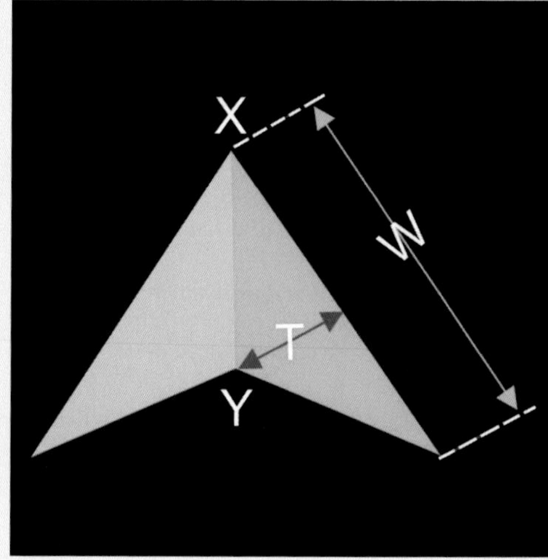

*(**Left**) AP chest radiograph of a newborn infant shows a characteristic appearance of the normal thymus ➔, the so-called sail sign, seen in approximately 10% of newborn chest radiographs. (**Right**) Composite image shows the appearance of the normal thymus in different age groups (clockwise from the top left): Ultrasound of the normal echogenic thymus ➔ anterior to the aorta and pulmonary trunk, the CT appearance of the normal thymus at ages 9, 28, and 50 years (the latter showing fatty involution).*

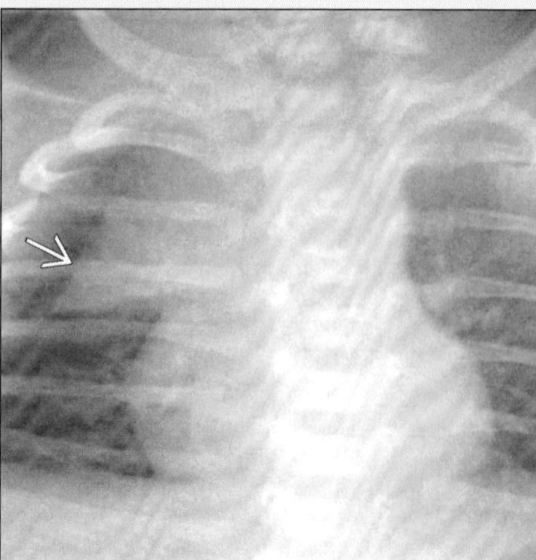

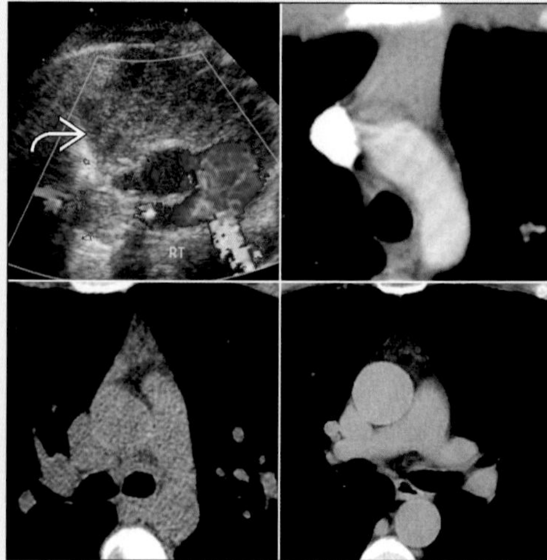

THYMIC HYPERPLASIA

TERMINOLOGY

Synonyms

- **Thymic rebound**

Definitions

- Thymic enlargement due to thymic or lymphoid hyperplasia

IMAGING

General Features

- Best diagnostic clue
  - Diffuse, nonlobular symmetric thymic enlargement
  - Thymic hyperplasia exhibits homogeneously decreased signal on opposed-phase gradient-echo T1WI MR
- Location
  - Anterior mediastinum: Anterior to ascending aorta, right ventricular outflow tract, & superior vena cava
- Size
  - Measurement: Anteroposterior, transverse, thickness
  - Normal thymic thickness on CT
    - 6-19 years
      - Right lobe 1.0 cm ± 0.39; left lobe 1.1 cm ± 0.4
    - 20-29 years
      - Right lobe 0.7 cm ± 0.24; left lobe 0.8 cm ± 0.14
    - 30-39 years
      - Right lobe 0.5 cm ± 0.14; left lobe 0.7 cm ± 0.21
    - 40-49 years
      - Right lobe 0.6 cm ± 0.23; left lobe 0.6 cm ± 0.2
    - > 50 years
      - Right lobe 0.5 cm ± 0.15; left lobe 0.5 cm ± 0.27
  - Normal thymic thickness on MR
    - Thymus appears 30-50% larger than on CT
- Normal thymus on CT
  - Age < 10 years: Extremely variable, quadrilateral shape
  - Puberty: Triangular, bilobed, or arrowhead morphology
  - After puberty: Triangular or bilobed
  - Normal margins: Straight or concave
  - Multilobular morphology at any age suggests neoplastic involvement
  - CT attenuation
    - Age < 20 years: Soft tissue (100%), homogeneous
    - 20-50 years: Homogeneous or heterogeneous from progressive fatty infiltration
    - > 50 years: Fat attenuation (90%)
    - Variable but homogeneous contrast enhancement
- Normal thymus on MR
  - Homogeneous signal intensity
  - T1WI: Higher signal intensity than that of muscle
  - T2WI: Signal intensity approaches that of fat
- Normal thymus on PET
  - Physiologic FDG uptake
    - Typically low: SUV = 1.0-1.8
    - Children
    - Young adults
    - Sporadically in older adults
- Normal thymus on ultrasound
  - Seen in > 90% of subjects aged 2-8 years
    - Approach: Intercostal imaging to left & right of sternum
    - Sharply marginated, smooth borders, molded to underlying structures
    - Echogenicity: Similar to that of liver parenchyma, linear or branching echogenic foci
    - Pliable, without mass effect (compression or displacement) on adjacent structures (as opposed to thymic neoplasms)
    - Longitudinal & AP dimensions
      - Right lobe (longitudinal): 1.54-4.02 cm (mean: 2.5 cm)
      - Right lobe (AP): 0.81-2.35 cm (mean: 1.4 cm)
      - Left lobe (longitudinal): 1.79-4.1 cm (mean: 2.9 cm)
      - Left lobe (AP): 0.78-2.47 cm (mean: 1.4 cm)

Radiographic Findings

- Typically normal chest radiograph
- Occasional mediastinal widening

CT Findings

- NECT
  - **True thymic hyperplasia**
    - **Diffuse, nonlobular symmetric thymic enlargement**
    - **Same attenuation as normal thymus** (according to age)
    - Calcification exceedingly rare
    - Thymic enlargement **following chemotherapy**
      - Follow-up imaging to document stability or resolution
      - Progressive enlargement suggests neoplasia & may require biopsy for confirmation
  - **Lymphoid hyperplasia**
    - Normal thymic size (45%)
    - Enlarged thymus (35%)
    - Focal thymic mass (20%)
- CECT
  - Enhancement similar to that of normal thymus
  - Heterogeneous enhancement suggests thymic neoplasm

MR Findings

- Chemical-shift MR imaging
  - **Thymic hyperplasia**: Homogeneously decreased signal on opposed-phase gradient-echo T1WI
  - **Thymic malignancy**: No drop in signal on opposed-phase gradient-echo T1WI

Nuclear Medicine Findings

- PET
  - Thymic hyperplasia: Standardized uptake value (SUV) = 2.0-2.8
  - SUV > 4.0 suggests malignancy
  - Benign thymic uptake has significant overlap with malignancy
- Octreoscan (indium-111-DTPA-octreotide scintigraphy)
  - Thymic hyperplasia
    - No radiotracer uptake
  - Radiotracer uptake in primary &/or metastatic thymic neoplasms

Imaging Recommendations

- Best imaging tool
  - CT is most frequently used imaging modality to detect thymic hyperplasia

- Chemical-shift MR is optimal imaging modality to differentiate thymic hyperplasia from thymic neoplasm
- Protocol advice
  - Chemical-shift MR (including in- & out-of-phase imaging)

DIFFERENTIAL DIAGNOSIS

Normal Thymus

- Borderline thymic enlargement in young subjects
- Correlation of thymic size with patient age

Thymoma

- Focal mass
- No decrease in lesion signal on opposed-phase gradient-echo T1WI MR

Recurrent or Metastatic Malignancy

- Nodular contour, necrosis, calcification, heterogeneous enhancement
- No decrease in lesion signal on opposed-phase gradient-echo imaging T1WI MR

Lymphoma

- Hodgkin more common than non-Hodgkin
- Homogeneous thymic enlargement, mediastinal &/or hilar lymphadenopathy

Thymic Cyst

- Thin wall, unilocular or multilocular
- No solid component
- No contrast enhancement

Ectopic Thyroid

- Heterogeneous lesion: Cysts & calcifications
- Uptake on thyroid scintigraphy

PATHOLOGY

General Features

- Etiology
  - **True thymic hyperplasia**
    - Usually acquired
    - Recent stress
      - e.g., chemotherapy, corticosteroid therapy, radiotherapy, Cushing syndrome treatment, bone marrow transplantation, thermal burns
    - Other causes: Hyperthyroidism, sarcoidosis, red blood cell aplasia
    - Initial thymic atrophy (approximately 40% of original size)
    - After chemotherapy
      - Thymic atrophy in 90%; minimal volume coincides with maximal myelosuppression
      - Rebound thymic hyperplasia in 10-25%
  - **Lymphoid hyperplasia**
    - Most commonly associated with myasthenia gravis
    - Other autoimmune diseases: Systemic lupus erythematosus, rheumatoid arthritis, scleroderma, vasculitis, thyrotoxicosis, Graves disease, Addison disease, polyarteritis nodosa, Behçet disease

Gross Pathologic & Surgical Features

- Weight
  - Under 30 years: > 50 g
  - 30-60 years: > 30 g

Microscopic Features

- **True thymic hyperplasia**
  - Microscopically normal thymus
  - Size &/or weight exceed upper limits of normal for age
- **Lymphoid hyperplasia**
  - Abundant medullary secondary lymphoid follicles with germinal centers; expansion of thymic medulla
  - Compression atrophy of thymic cortex
  - Independent of size & weight (often normal)
  - Few or no germinal centers correlates with rapid remission; many germinal centers favor slow remission

CLINICAL ISSUES

Presentation

- Most common signs/symptoms
  - Usually asymptomatic

Demographics

- Epidemiology
  - **True thymic hyperplasia** post chemotherapy
    - Initial thymic atrophy
    - Thymic growth to original size (within 9 months) after cessation of stress
    - Thymic growth to 50% larger than original size (rebound phenomenon)
    - Thymic rebound occurs within 2 years of chemotherapy initiation
  - **Lymphoid hyperplasia**
    - Found in ~ 65% of patients with myasthenia gravis

Treatment

- Generally not required

DIAGNOSTIC CHECKLIST

Consider

- Thymic hyperplasia in patient with enlarging nonlobular thymus undergoing chemotherapy or in patient with myasthenia gravis

SELECTED REFERENCES

1. Nasseri F et al: Clinical and radiologic review of the normal and abnormal thymus: pearls and pitfalls. Radiographics. 30(2):413-28, 2010
2. Inaoka T et al: Thymic hyperplasia and thymus gland tumors: differentiation with chemical shift MR imaging. Radiology. 243(3):869-76, 2007
3. Nishino M et al: The thymus: a comprehensive review. Radiographics. 26(2):335-48, 2006

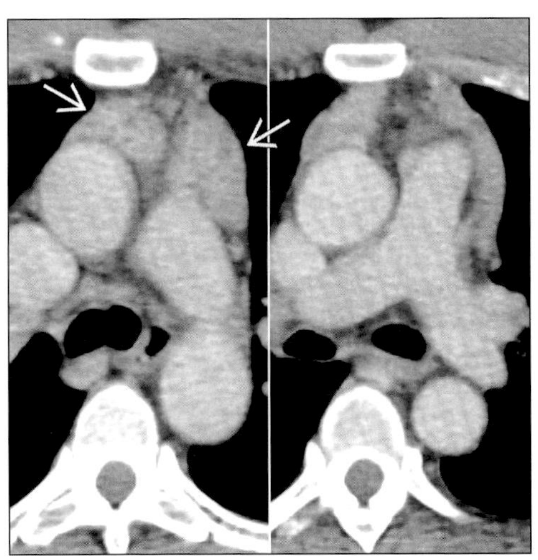

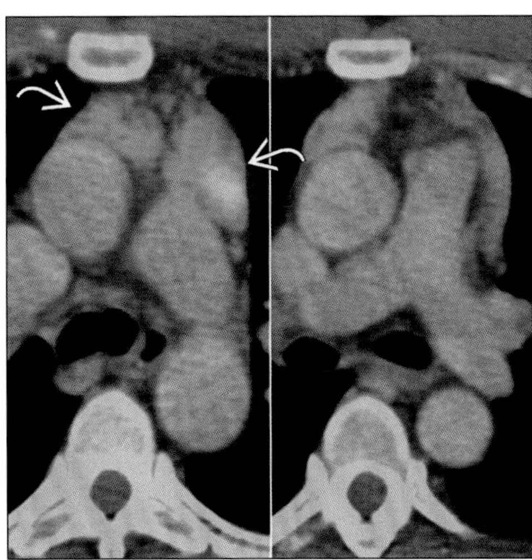

(Left) *Axial CECT of a patient who developed thymic hyperplasia after chemotherapy for lymphoma shows thymic enlargement ➔ manifesting as anterior mediastinal soft tissue with preserved lobar anatomy surrounded by fat.* ***(Right)*** *Axial fused PET/CT of the same patient shows mild FDG thymic uptake ➔. Thymic hyperplasia often exhibits little to mild FDG uptake, typically below 3.0 standard uptake value (SUV). SUV above 4.0 is characteristically seen in the setting of malignancy.*

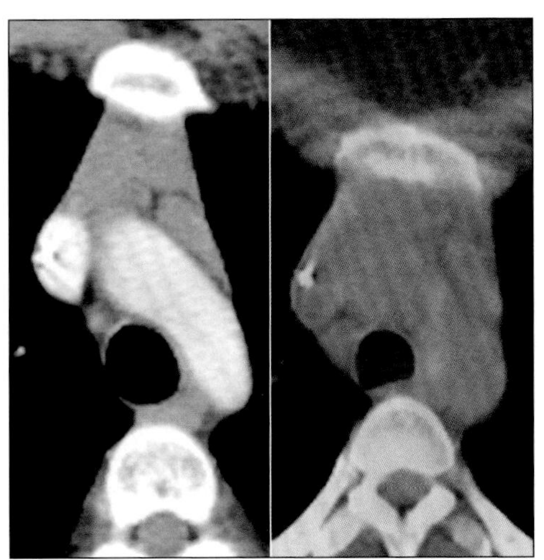

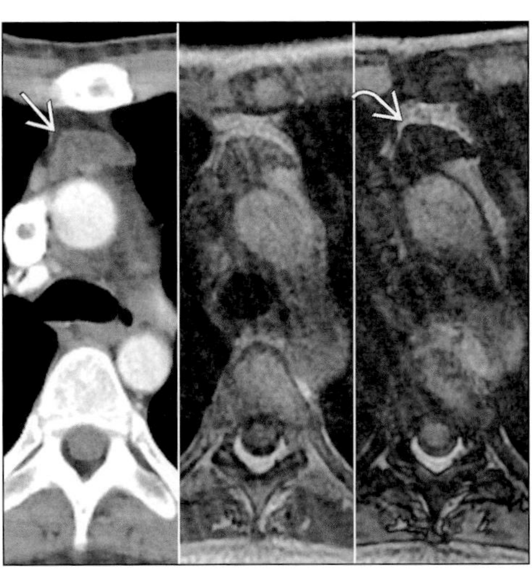

(Left) *Composite image with axial CECT (left) and FDG PET/CT (right) shows thymic hyperplasia after chemotherapy for Hodgkin lymphoma that manifests as thymic enlargement with mild FDG accumulation (below 2.0 SUV).* ***(Right)*** *Composite image with axial CECT (left) and in- (center) and out-of-phase (right) MR of a patient with pharyngeal carcinoma treated with chemotherapy shows an anterior mediastinal soft tissue mass ➔ that exhibits characteristic signal dropout ➔ on out-of-phase MR imaging.*

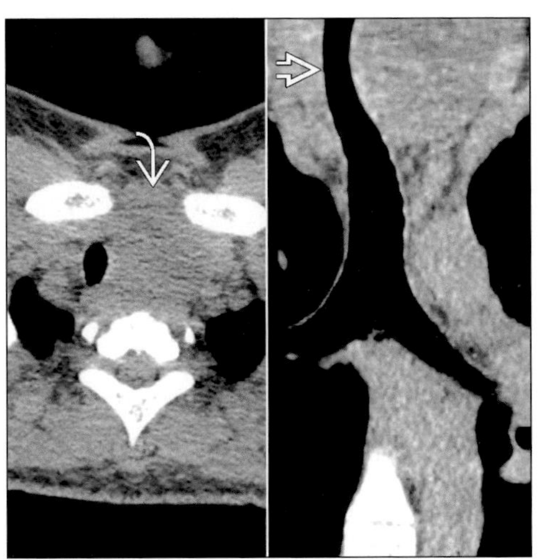

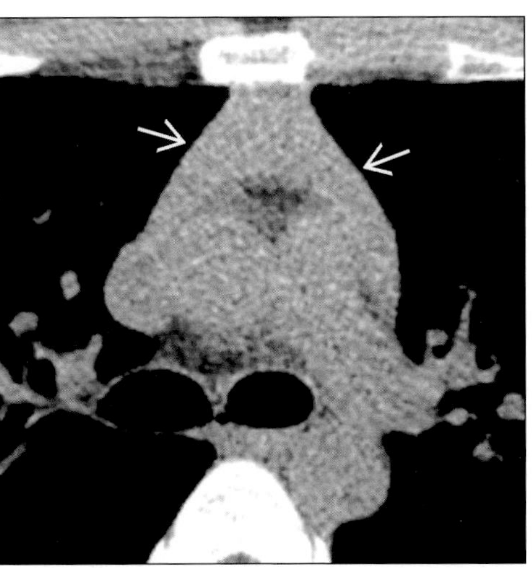

(Left) *Composite image with axial (left) and coronal (right) NECT of a patient with thyrotoxicosis and lymphoid thymic hyperplasia shows an enlarged heterogeneous thyroid ➔ with mass effect on the upper trachea ➔.* ***(Right)*** *Axial NECT of the same patient shows a diffusely enlarged homogeneous thymus ➔ with slightly convex borders. While most cases of thymic lymphoid hyperplasia relate to myasthenia gravis, other autoimmune processes, such as thyrotoxicosis, can be associated with it.*

GOITER

Key Facts

Terminology

- Goiter: Enlarged thyroid
- Retrosternal/substernal goiter: Extension into surgical superior/anterior mediastinum
- Mediastinal goiter: Extension into retroesophageal mediastinum

Imaging

- Radiography: Tracheal displacement, often beginning at laryngeal level, may extend below thoracic inlet
- CT
  - Sharply demarcated heterogeneous mass in continuity with cervical goiter
  - High attenuation given intrinsic iodine content
  - Intense, sustained contrast enhancement
  - Calcifications: Punctate, coarse (> 3 mm), ring-like
  - Cystic changes

Top Differential Diagnoses

- Thymoma
- Germ cell neoplasms
- Lymphoma
- Lymphangioma
- Congenital cysts

Pathology

- Etiology: Multinodular goiter, follicular adenoma
  - Rarely carcinoma or lymphoma

Clinical Issues

- Symptoms/signs: Asymptomatic, dyspnea, wheezing
- Treatment: Surgery is only definitive treatment

Diagnostic Checklist

- Consider goiter in differential diagnosis of asymptomatic tracheal deviation

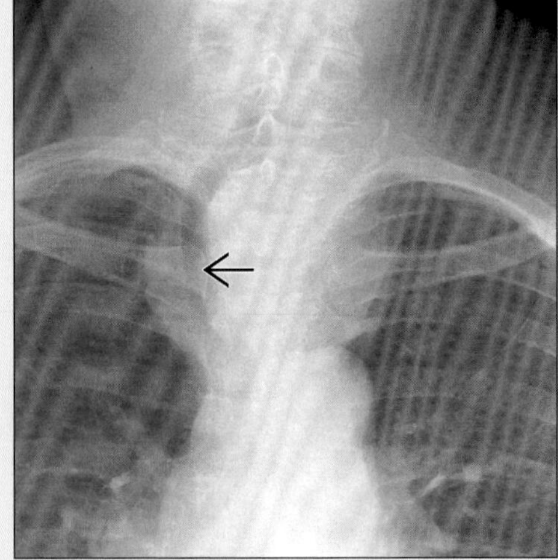

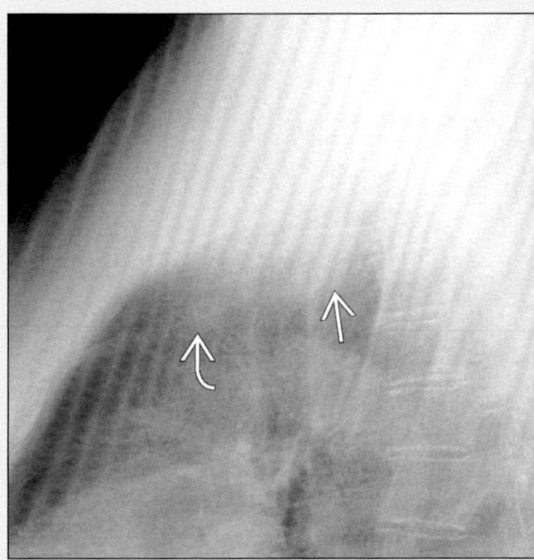

(Left) *PA chest radiograph of a patient with thyroid goiter predominantly located in the anterior mediastinum shows marked tracheal compression and displacement to the right ⇒.* ***(Right)*** *Lateral chest radiograph of the same patient shows the mass, which appears less conspicuous and mostly projects over the anterior mediastinum ➡. The posterior component of the lesion ➡ does not produce mass effect on the posterior tracheal wall, a feature typically seen in retrotracheal/retroesophageal extension.*

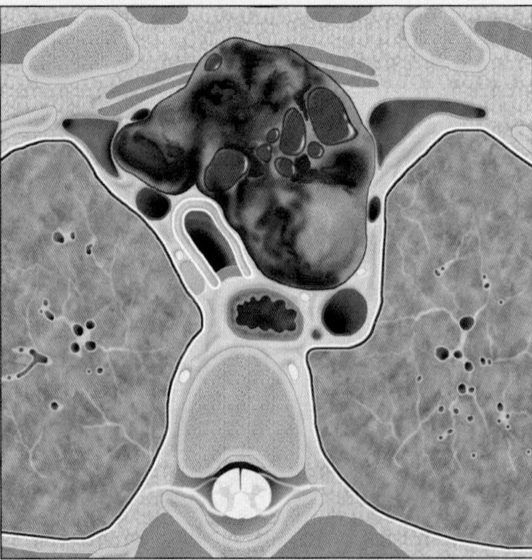

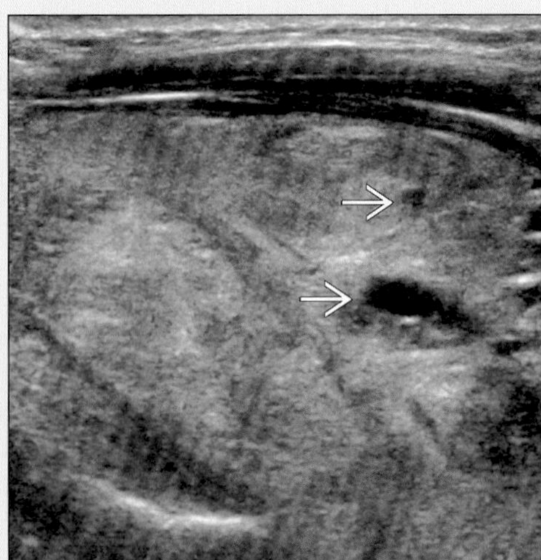

(Left) *Graphic shows the characteristic morphologic features of anterior mediastinal multinodular goiter with internal cystic and solid areas. Goiters often displace and compress mediastinal structures, including the trachea and esophagus.* ***(Right)*** *Sagittal thyroid ultrasound of a patient with multinodular goiter shows a large, heterogeneous mass with solid and cystic ➡ areas. Ultrasound is not useful in the assessment of retrosternal lesions, a well-known limitation of this imaging modality.*

GOITER

TERMINOLOGY

Definitions

- **Goiter**: Enlarged thyroid gland
- **Cervical goiter**: Completely within neck
- **Retrosternal/substernal goiter**: Extension into surgical superior or anterior mediastinum
- **Mediastinal goiter**: Extension into retrotracheal/ retroesophageal mediastinum
- **Primary goiter**
  - Origin in ectopic thyroid tissue
  - Blood supply from intrathoracic vessels
- **Secondary goiter**
  - Origin in cervical thyroid
  - Primary blood supply from neck vessels

IMAGING

General Features

- Best diagnostic clue
  - Tracheal deviation at thoracic inlet
    - Most common cause of tracheal deviation
    - Other lesions less likely to deviate trachea
- Location
  - Thyroid bed (~ 55%)
  - Mediastinal extension (~ 35%)
    - In or partially in anterior mediastinum
      - Retrosternal or substernal goiter: Exclusively in surgical superior or anterior mediastinum
    - 10-15% of mediastinal goiters exhibit retrotracheal or retroesophageal extension (mediastinal goiter)
  - Posterior or lateral to pharynx (10%)
- Size
  - Variable: Few cm to > 10 cm

Radiographic Findings

- Radiography
  - Anterior or middle-posterior mediastinal mass
  - May exhibit intrinsic calcification
  - Tracheal displacement virtually always present, often beginning at level of larynx
  - Tracheal narrowing
    - Radiography does not allow accurate evaluation of degree of narrowing
  - Lateral radiography
    - Anterior goiters fill retrosternal clear space
    - Retrotracheal goiters obscure Raider triangle, mass effect on posterior tracheal wall

Fluoroscopic Findings

- Esophagram
  - Rarely used
  - Extrinsic compression of upper esophagus
  - Upward goiter displacement on deglutition (84%)

CT Findings

- NECT
  - Sharply demarcated heterogeneous mass in continuity with cervical goiter
  - Anterior mediastinal goiter: Left side predominant, rightward tracheal deviation & compression
  - Retroesophageal goiter: Right side predominant, leftward tracheal & esophageal deviation/ compression
  - **High attenuation (70-85 HU)**, due to intrinsic iodine content
  - **Calcification**: Amorphous, irregular, ring-like, punctate, coarse (> 3 mm)
  - **Cystic changes**
    - Areas of low attenuation
    - High attenuation often due to hemorrhage
  - Goiter descends 1.0-3.0 cm when patient imaged with arms overhead
  - Ancillary findings
    - Pericardial effusion due to severe hypothyroidism & myxedema
    - Tracheomalacia due to tracheal compression
    - Lymphadenopathy (> 10 mm short axis) with discrete calcification, central necrosis, & cyst formation suggests coexistent thyroid malignancy
- CECT
  - **Prolonged & sustained enhancement** after IV contrast (> 25 HU)
  - Cystic areas do not enhance
  - Avoid contrast in patients with hyperthyroidism to prevent thyrotoxicosis & in candidates for radioiodine therapy
  - Lymphadenopathy with marked homogeneous enhancement suggests coexistent metastatic thyroid carcinoma

MR Findings

- T1WI
  - Intermediate signal, slightly higher than muscle
  - Heterogeneous signal
  - Cysts may exhibit high signal due to hemorrhage or proteinaceous material
- T2WI
  - Slightly higher signal than surrounding structures
  - Heterogeneous signal
  - Variable signal in cysts depending on contents & age of hemorrhage
- Optimal estimation of thyroid volume, better accuracy for substernal goiters

Ultrasonographic Findings

- Substernal component often difficult to assess
- Useful for evaluation of cervical goiter
- Heterogeneous echotexture often with multiple nodules of varying size
  - Uniformly hypoechoic cysts
  - Echogenic foci with posterior shadowing due to calcifications
- Image-guided biopsy of suspicious lesions

Nuclear Medicine Findings

- I-123 & I-131 diagnostic but often unnecessary
  - ↑ uptake in hyperthyroid patients
  - Absence of uptake does not exclude goiter
- Technetium pertechnetate not used due to high blood pool mediastinal activity

Imaging Recommendations

- Best imaging tool
  - Chest radiographic findings often characteristic
  - CT for definitive diagnosis & surgical planning
- Protocol advice
  - Include CT imaging of neck in patients with suspected mediastinal goiter to document connection to thyroid

GOITER

DIFFERENTIAL DIAGNOSIS

Thymoma

- May exhibit solid & cystic areas with calcification
- Absence of continuity with cervical thyroid

Germ Cell Neoplasms

- May exhibit solid & cystic areas with calcification
- Absence of continuity with cervical thyroid

Lymphoma

- Rarely calcifies before treatment
- Multicentric lymphadenopathy, nodal coalescence

Lymphangioma

- Conforms to or envelops rather than displaces structures
- Calcification is rare

Congenital Cysts

- May be hyperdense due to protein & calcium content
- Absence of continuity with cervical thyroid

PATHOLOGY

General Features

- Etiology
  - Multinodular goiter (51%): Hyperplasia resulting from increased thyrotrophin-stimulating hormone (TSH) in setting of decreased thyroid hormone
  - Follicular adenoma (44%)
  - Chronic autoimmune thyroiditis (5%)
  - Other (rare): Carcinoma, amyloid, lymphoma

Gross Pathologic & Surgical Features

- Enlarged, heterogeneous thyroid
- Cystic degeneration
- Areas or hemorrhage
- Calcification

Microscopic Features

- Irregularly enlarged follicles with flattened epithelium & abundant colloid
- Microscopic nests of cancer in 5-15%
  - Psammomatous calcification: Punctate calcifications 5-100 μm, associated with malignancy

CLINICAL ISSUES

Presentation

- Most common signs/symptoms
  - Asymptomatic mass (most common)
  - Dyspnea, wheezing
  - Cough
- Other signs/symptoms
  - Dysphagia, hoarseness, phrenic paralysis, Horner syndrome, jugular vein compression/thrombosis, cerebrovascular steal syndrome, superior vena cava syndrome, hyperthyroidism
    - Pemberton sign: Neck vein distention with upper extremity elevation due to venous obstruction
    - Thyrotoxicity due to autonomous functioning nodule, iodide ingestion, or iodinated contrast material
    - Plummer disease (toxic multinodular goiter): Development of autonomous functioning nodule leading to hyperthyroidism

Demographics

- Age
  - Increasing frequency with advancing age
- Gender
  - M:F = 1:3
- Epidemiology
  - Affects 5% of people worldwide
    - Up to 20% descend into mediastinum
    - 2-21% of patients undergoing thyroidectomy have substernal thyroid component
  - Represents up to 7% of mediastinal tumors
  - Frequency of large goiters declining

Natural History & Prognosis

- Patients with goiter should undergo thyroid function tests
- Slow growth unless underlying cause is corrected; usually asymptomatic

Treatment

- Surgery is only definitive treatment
  - Considered when patient condition allows
  - 25% of asymptomatic patients develop acute respiratory distress
  - Cervicotomy for retrosternal/substernal goiter
  - Combined cervicotomy & transthoracic approach for mediastinal goiter
    - Imaging findings that suggest need for combined approach: Inferior displacement of left brachiocephalic vein, 70% of mass below thoracic inlet, inferior border below aortic arch
- Observation considered in small lesions & elderly patients

DIAGNOSTIC CHECKLIST

Consider

- Goiter in differential diagnosis of asymptomatic tracheal deviation

Image Interpretation Pearls

- Mediastinal mass in continuity with cervical thyroid is likely to represent mediastinal goiter

SELECTED REFERENCES

1. Batori M et al: Surgical treatment of retrosternal goiter. Eur Rev Med Pharmacol Sci. 11(4):265-8, 2007
2. Chin SC et al: Spread of goiters outside the thyroid bed: a review of 190 cases and an analysis of the incidence of the various extensions. Arch Otolaryngol Head Neck Surg. 129(11):1198-202, 2003
3. Hedayati N et al: The clinical presentation and operative management of nodular and diffuse substernal thyroid disease. Am Surg. 68(3):245-51; discussion 251-2, 2002
4. Jennings A: Evaluation of substernal goiters using computed tomography and MR imaging. Endocrinol Metab Clin North Am. 30(2):401-14, ix, 2001

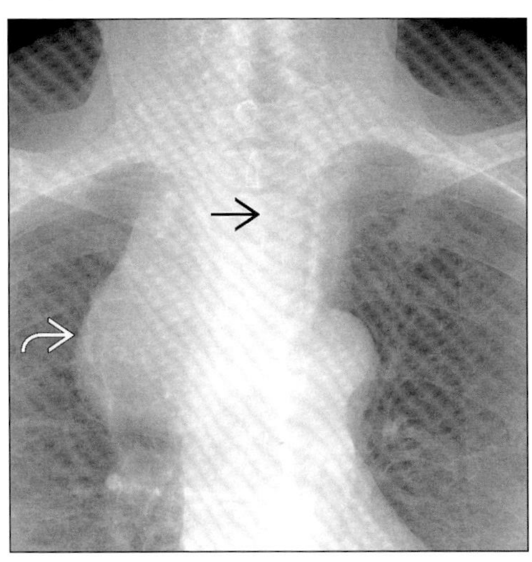

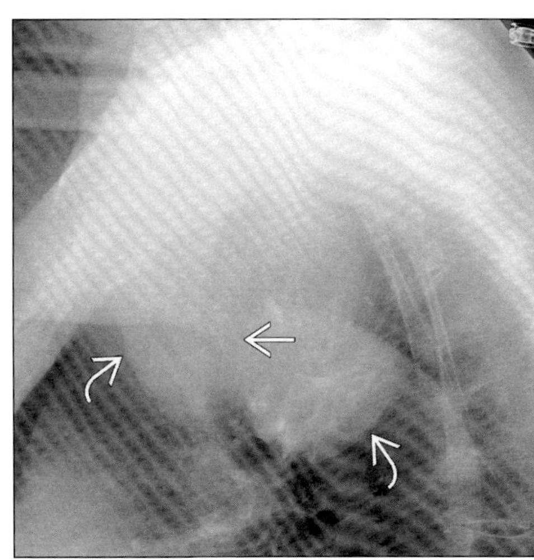

(Left) *PA chest radiograph of a patient with a large goiter shows a large mediastinal mass displacing the trachea to the left. Retroesophageal mediastinal goiters are typically right-sided and displace the trachea and esophagus to the left.* ***(Right)*** *Lateral chest radiograph of the same patient shows a large, well-defined mass displacing and bowing the posterior tracheal wall. Mass effect on the posterior trachea is a typical feature of goiters in this location.*

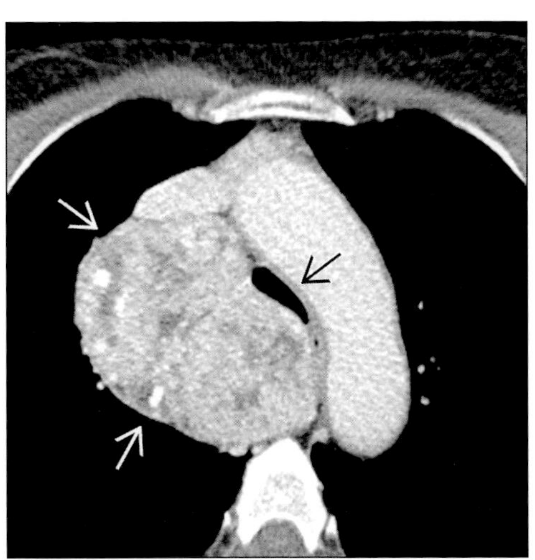

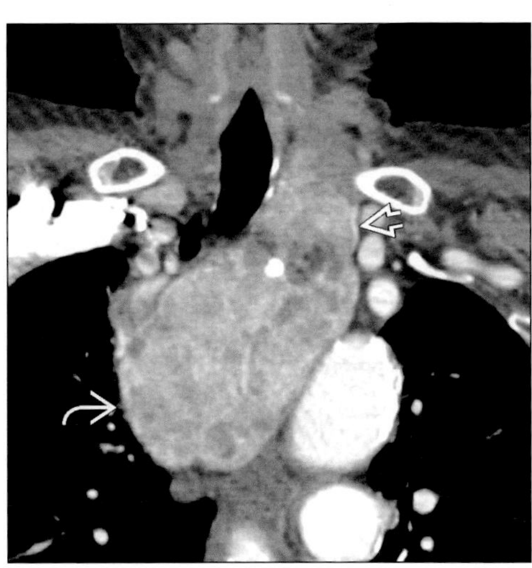

(Left) *Axial CECT of the same patient shows a large, heterogeneously enhancing mass in the right paratracheal and retrotracheal/retroesophageal regions with marked compression of the tracheal lumen and esophagus.* ***(Right)*** *Curved MPR CECT of the same patient shows continuity between the mediastinal mass and the cervical goiter. This feature allows characterization of the mediastinal mass as originating from the thyroid and is considered diagnostic of mediastinal goiter.*

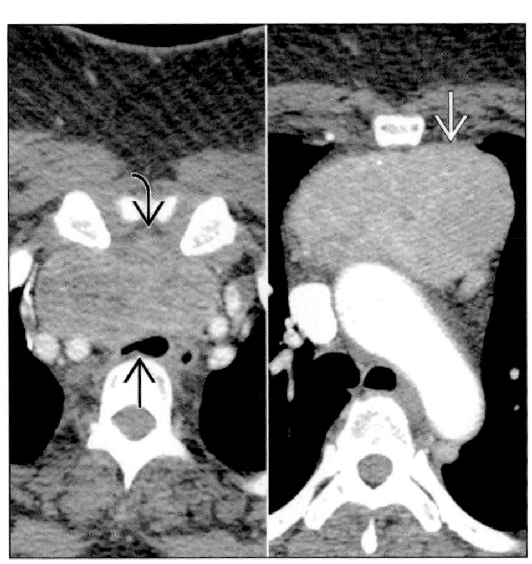

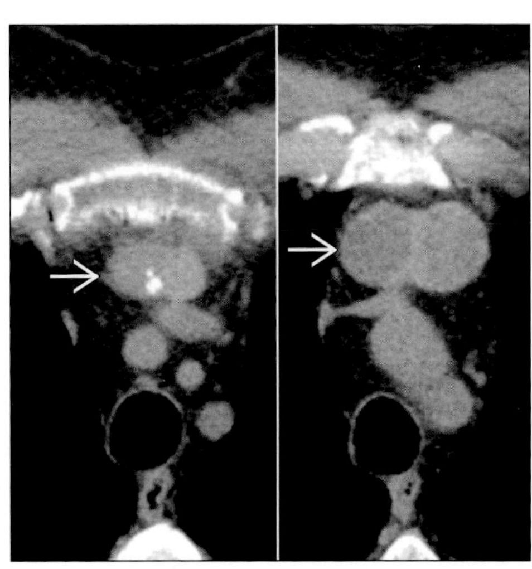

(Left) *Axial CECT of a patient with an anterior mediastinal goiter that contained a small intrinsic focus of papillary carcinoma shows a large mass in the superior and anterior mediastinum with associated tracheal compression. Occult thyroid malignancy may occur in 15% of goiters.* ***(Right)*** *Axial NECT of a patient with a mediastinal goiter originating in ectopic anterior mediastinal thyroid tissue shows a heterogeneous mass with cystic components and intrinsic calcification.*

ACHALASIA

Key Facts

Terminology

- Achalasia: Esophageal motility disorder & dilatation
- Pseudoachalasia: Involvement of gastroesophageal junction by other abnormalities

Imaging

- Radiography
  - Markedly dilated esophagus
  - Retrotracheal air-fluid level
  - Small or absent gastric air bubble
- Esophagram
  - Dilated esophagus, heterogeneous content
  - Absence of primary peristalsis
  - "Bird-beak" deformity of distal esophagus
- CT
  - Esophageal dilatation with air-fluid level
  - Abrupt, smooth narrowing of distal esophagus
  - Normal esophageal wall thickness

Top Differential Diagnoses

- Scleroderma
- Esophageal carcinoma

Pathology

- Myenteric plexus neuropathy with incomplete relaxation of lower esophageal sphincter

Clinical Issues

- Dysphagia (90%)
- Recurrent aspiration pneumonia
- Complications
  - Esophageal squamous cell carcinoma
  - Iatrogenic perforation

Diagnostic Checklist

- Importance of differentiation of achalasia from pseudoachalasia

__(Left)__ PA chest radiograph of a patient with achalasia shows marked dilatation of the entire esophagus ➡, lateral displacement of the azygoesophageal recess ➡, and an esophageal air-fluid level ⇨. __(Right)__ Lateral chest radiograph of the same patient confirms esophageal dilatation ➡ and shows a distal esophageal air-fluid level ⇨. Esophagram is the imaging study of choice for evaluation of esophageal dilatation detected on chest radiography.

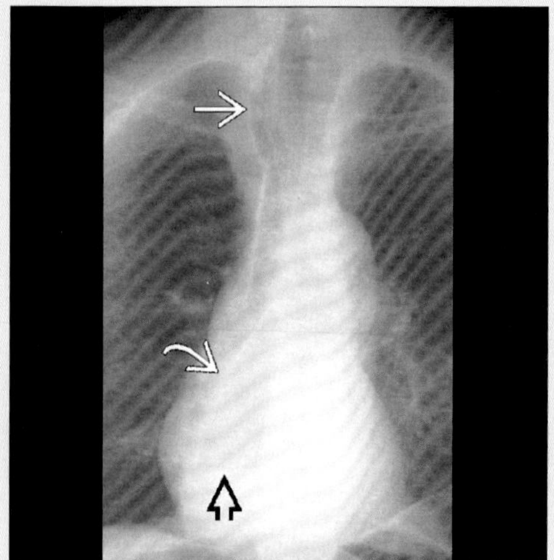

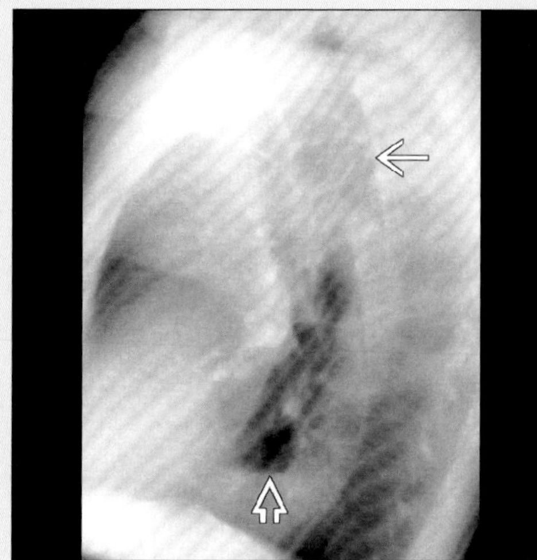

__(Left)__ Coronal NECT of the same patient shows marked esophageal dilatation ➡, a distal esophageal "bird beak" deformity ➡, and right lower lobe bronchiectasis with mucoid impaction ➡. CT is useful in the evaluation of achalasia and its complications. __(Right)__ Graphic shows the morphologic features of achalasia characterized by marked esophageal dilatation with an air-fluid level, retained food particles, and a distal esophageal "bird-beak" deformity ➡.

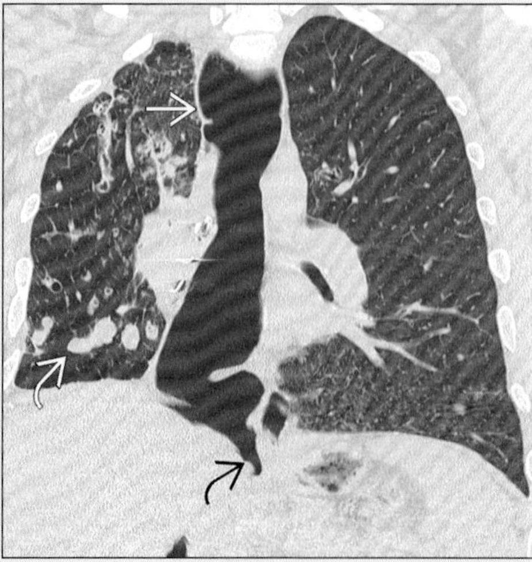

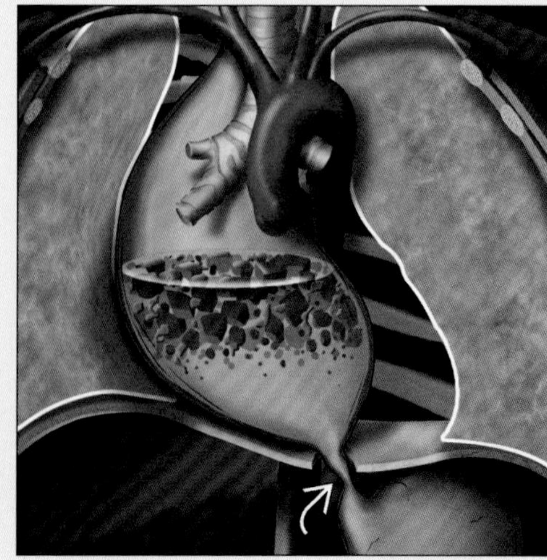

ACHALASIA

TERMINOLOGY

Definitions

- **Achalasia**: Motility disorder resulting in esophageal dilatation
  - Failure of relaxation of lower esophageal sphincter
- **Pseudoachalasia**: Involvement of gastroesophageal junction by other abnormalities
  - Reflux esophagitis
  - Chagas disease
  - Malignant neoplasm

IMAGING

General Features

- Best diagnostic clue
  - Smooth esophageal dilatation
  - "Bird-beak" configuration of esophagogastric junction on esophagram

Radiographic Findings

- Radiography
  - Mediastinal widening (double contour)
  - Markedly dilated esophagus
  - Anterior tracheal bowing
  - Thickened tracheoesophageal stripe
  - Retrotracheal air-fluid level, retained food particles
  - Small or absent gastric air bubble
- Esophagram
  - Markedly dilated esophagus, heterogeneous content
  - Absence of primary peristalsis
  - "Bird-beak" deformity of distal esophagus

CT Findings

- NECT
  - Esophageal dilatation with air-fluid level, heterogeneous esophageal content
  - Normal esophageal wall thickness
  - Abrupt, smooth narrowing of distal esophagus
  - Evaluation of complications
    - Esophageal squamous cell carcinoma (longstanding achalasia)
      - Irregular wall thickening
      - Mediastinal lymphadenopathy
    - Aspiration pneumonia
      - Focal/multifocal airspace disease
      - Tree-in-bud opacities
    - Iatrogenic perforation
      - Imaging findings of acute mediastinitis

Imaging Recommendations

- Best imaging tool
  - Esophagram is imaging study of choice
    - Evaluation of esophageal motility, reflux, aspiration
  - CT
    - Evaluation of other esophageal diseases including superimposed benign or malignant processes

DIFFERENTIAL DIAGNOSIS

Scleroderma

- Dysmotility, dilated esophagus
- Air-fluid level in stomach

Esophageal Carcinoma

- Esophagus minimally dilated
- Focal mass/mural thickening at site of tumor

PATHOLOGY

General Features

- Etiology
  - Unknown
    - Myenteric plexus neuropathy with incomplete relaxation of lower esophageal sphincter

Microscopic Features

- Decreased number of ganglion cells in myenteric esophageal plexus

CLINICAL ISSUES

Presentation

- Most common signs/symptoms
  - Dysphagia (90%)
  - Halitosis
  - Recurrent aspiration pneumonia

Demographics

- Age
  - Achalasia: Younger patients (30-50 years)
  - Pseudoachalasia: Older patients
- Gender
  - M = F

Natural History & Prognosis

- Esophageal carcinoma (2-7%)
- Aspiration pneumonia (recurrent)

Treatment

- Smooth muscle relaxants
- Pneumatic dilatation (risk of perforation)
- Heller myotomy (longitudinal incision of lower esophageal sphincter)

DIAGNOSTIC CHECKLIST

Consider

- Importance of differentiating achalasia from pseudoachalasia

Image Interpretation Pearls

- Suspect achalasia in patients with esophageal dilatation & small or absent gastric bubble on radiography
- CT used for exclusion of other diseases &/or complications

SELECTED REFERENCES

1. Ba-Ssalamah A et al: Dedicated multi-detector CT of the esophagus: spectrum of diseases. Abdom Imaging. 34(1):3-18, 2009

ESOPHAGEAL DIVERTICULUM

Key Facts

Terminology

- Esophageal saccular protrusion or outpouching
- Pulsion diverticulum: Mucosa & submucosa without muscular layer
- Traction diverticulum: All esophageal wall layers

Imaging

- Air-fluid level in superior mediastinum (Zenker) or mid-esophagus (traction)
- Barium esophagram
  - Pulsion diverticulum: Barium-filled sac; rounded
  - Traction diverticulum: Barium-filled tented or triangular outpouching
- Radiography
  - Mediastinal air-fluid level in region of esophagus
- CT
  - Incidental finding
  - Air-, water-, or contrast-filled esophageal outpouch

Top Differential Diagnoses

- Pseudodiverticulosis
- Esophageal ulcer
- Phrenic ampulla
- Esophageal perforation

Pathology

- Zenker: Mucosal herniation through anatomic weakness in region of cricopharyngeal muscle
- Traction: Common in areas of endemic tuberculosis & histoplasmosis

Clinical Issues

- Pulsion diverticulum (Zenker)
  - Upper esophageal dysphagia
  - Regurgitation & aspiration of undigested food
  - Halitosis; hoarseness; neck mass
- Traction diverticulum: Erosion, perforation

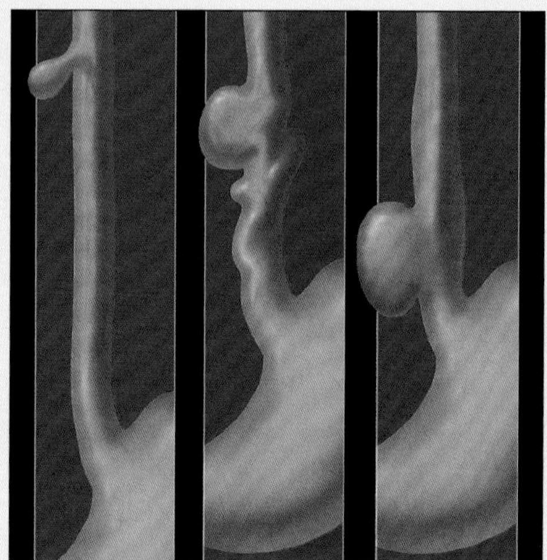

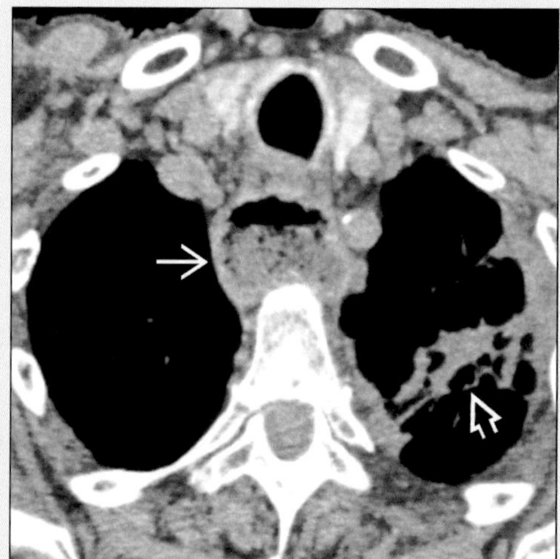

(Left) *Graphic shows the different types of esophageal diverticula: Zenker (left), traction (middle), and epiphrenic (right).* ***(Right)*** *Axial NECT shows a large posterior hypopharyngeal pulsion (Zenker) diverticulum ➔ containing retained food and an air-fluid level. Note healed tuberculosis ➲ in the left lung apex. Aspiration pneumonia may be a complication of Zenker diverticulum.*

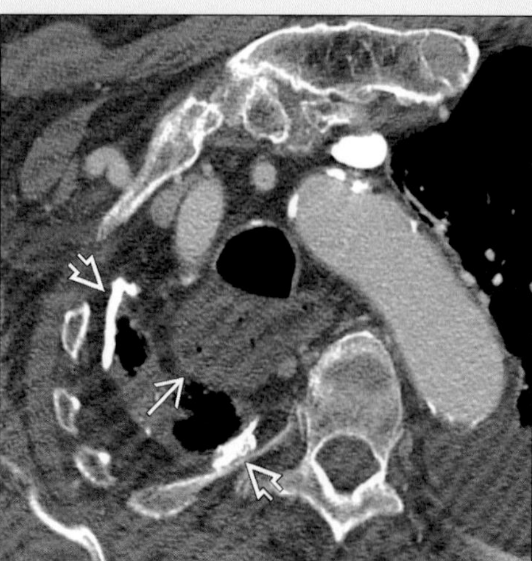

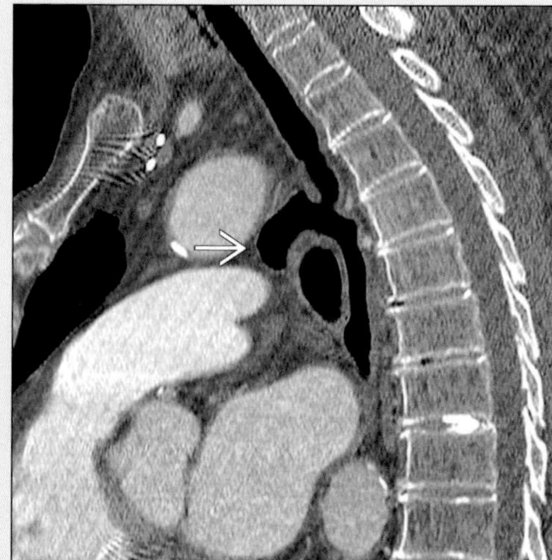

(Left) *Axial CECT of a patient with traction diverticulum shows a large outpouching ➔ from the upper esophagus and calcified right pleural plaques ➲. Traction diverticula are associated with previous tuberculosis, sarcoidosis, and histoplasmosis.* ***(Right)*** *Sagittal CECT shows a large air-distended mid-esophageal saccular outpouching ➔ filling the aorticopulmonary window. Differentiation of mid-esophageal pulsion diverticula from traction diverticula is sometimes difficult.*

ESOPHAGEAL DIVERTICULUM

TERMINOLOGY

Definitions

- **Esophageal saccular protrusion or outpouching**
- **Pulsion diverticulum**
  - Mucosa & submucosa without muscular layer (Zenker, epiphrenic)
- **Traction diverticulum**
  - All esophageal wall layers
  - Fibrosis in adjacent periesophageal tissues & granulomatous inflammation

IMAGING

General Features

- Best diagnostic clue
  - Air-fluid level in superior mediastinum (Zenker) or mid-esophagus (traction)
  - Barium esophagram
    - **Pulsion diverticulum**: Barium-filled sac, rounded contour
    - **Traction diverticulum**: Barium-filled tented or triangular outpouching
- Location
  - Pharyngoesophageal junction: **Pulsion (Zenker)**
  - Mid-esophagus: **Traction**
  - Distal esophagus: **Epiphrenic**
- Size
  - Variable: Zenker size range (0.5-8 cm)
- Morphology
  - Pulsion: Rounded or saccular
  - Traction: Triangular

Radiographic Findings

- Mediastinal air-fluid level in region of esophagus

CT Findings

- Incidental finding
  - Air-, water-, or contrast-filled outpouching

Imaging Recommendations

- Best imaging tool
  - Esophagram: Visualization of esophageal diverticula

DIFFERENTIAL DIAGNOSIS

Pseudodiverticulosis

- Diffuse (50%) or segmental tiny outpouchings in long rows parallel to esophageal long axis

Esophageal Ulcer

- Solitary ring-like/stellate ulcer with edema halo

Phrenic Ampulla

- 2-4 cm luminal dilation between "A" & "B" rings

Esophageal Perforation

- Iatrogenic, Boerhaave syndrome

PATHOLOGY

General Features

- Etiology
  - **Zenker**: Mucosal herniation through anatomic weakness in region of cricopharyngeal muscle
  - **Traction**
    - Common in areas of endemic tuberculosis & histoplasmosis

Gross Pathologic & Surgical Features

- Posterior hypopharyngeal saccular outpouching with broad or narrow neck (Zenker)

CLINICAL ISSUES

Presentation

- Most common signs/symptoms
  - **Pulsion diverticulum**
    - **Zenker diverticulum**
      - Upper esophageal dysphagia
      - Regurgitation & aspiration of undigested food
      - Halitosis, hoarseness, neck mass
  - **Traction diverticulum**
    - Dysphagia

Demographics

- Age
  - Zenker diverticulum
    - 50% of patients in 7th-8th decades
  - Traction diverticulum
    - Usually seen in elderly patients
- Gender
  - Zenker diverticulum
    - M > F
  - Traction diverticulum
    - M = F
- Epidemiology
  - Traction diverticulum
    - Previous history of granulomatous disease

Natural History & Prognosis

- Complications
  - Pulsion (Zenker)
    - Aspiration pneumonia
    - Bronchitis, bronchiectasis
    - Risk of perforation after endoscopy or enteric tube placement
  - Traction
    - Erosion, inflammation
    - Perforation, fistula

Treatment

- Asymptomatic: No treatment
- Large or symptomatic: Surgical diverticulectomy or endoscopic repair

DIAGNOSTIC CHECKLIST

Image Interpretation Pearls

- Traction diverticula tend to empty when esophagus is collapsed

SELECTED REFERENCES

1. Ba-Ssalamah A et al: Dedicated multi-detector CT of the esophagus: spectrum of diseases. Abdom Imaging. 34(1):3-18, 2009

ESOPHAGEAL STRICTURE

Key Facts

Terminology

- Acquired narrowing of esophageal lumen

Imaging

- Esophagram
  - Single-contrast: Optimal esophageal distention & stricture detection
  - Double-contrast: Optimal mucosal evaluation
  - Barium is preferred contrast medium
  - Water-soluble contrast for suspected perforation
  - Assessment of stricture location & morphology
- Radiography
  - Identification of radiopaque foreign bodies
  - Initial assessment of perforation & mediastinitis
- CT
  - Assessment of esophageal perforation/mediastinitis
  - Assessment of sequela of aspiration: Ranges from bronchiolitis to pneumonia

Top Differential Diagnoses

- Achalasia
- Vascular anomalies (rings)
- Esophageal carcinoma

Pathology

- Gastroesophageal reflux-induced (75%)
- Unrelated to gastroesophageal reflux (25%)
  - Radiation, sclerotherapy, caustic ingestion, surgical anastomosis, dermatologic disease, extrinsic compression, esophagitis, foreign bodies, infection

Clinical Issues

- Dysphagia
  - Benign: Longstanding, intermittent
  - Malignant: Recent onset, rapid progression
- Aspiration: Productive cough, wheezing, dyspnea
- Treatment: Balloon dilatation

(Left) Oblique esophagram obtained several weeks after ingestion of paint thinner demonstrates a long segment stenosis of the proximal esophagus associated with proximal esophageal dilatation ⇨. (Right) Composite image with axial CECT of the same patient shows right lower lobe tree-in-bud opacities from aspiration (left) and a fluid-filled, dilated, thick-walled esophagus ➔ (right). Esophageal stricture can result in aspiration bronchiolitis. (Courtesy K. Andresen, MD.)

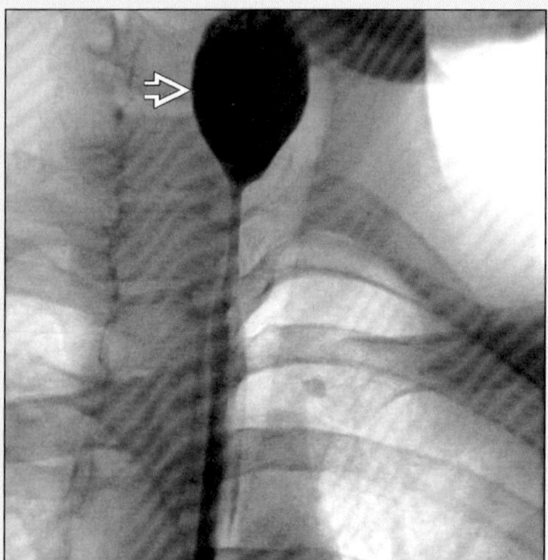

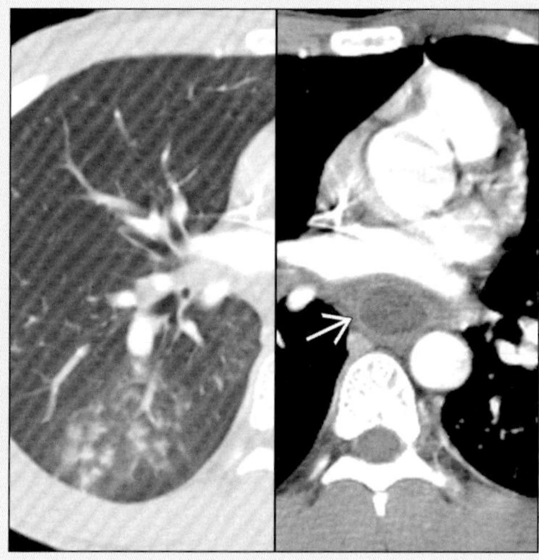

(Left) Composite image with axial CECT (left) and esophagram (right) of a patient who ingested alkaline declogger shows diffuse esophageal wall thickening ➔, which is usually evident during the acute phase of the disease. Long segment esophageal stricture ⇨ developed after several weeks. (Right) Oblique esophagram of a patient with dysphagia status post Nissen fundoplication shows a tight distal esophageal stricture ➔. Postsurgical stricture is a relatively common complication of esophageal surgery.

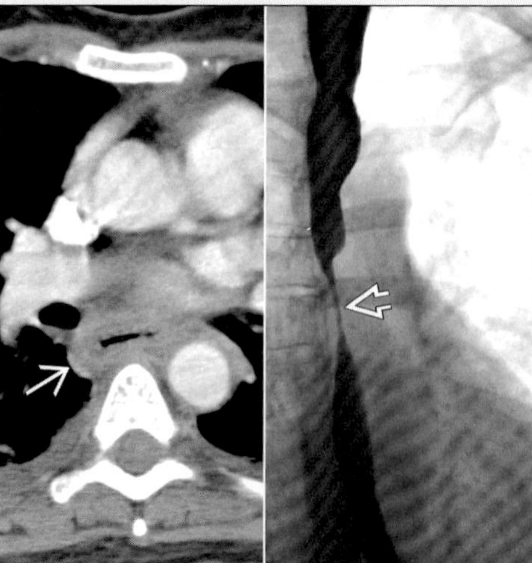

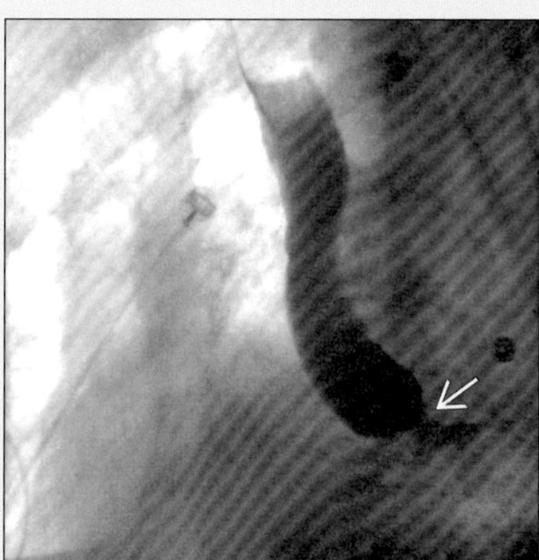

ESOPHAGEAL STRICTURE

TERMINOLOGY

Definitions

- **Acquired narrowing of esophageal lumen**

IMAGING

Radiographic Findings

- Chest radiography useful for identification of **radiopaque foreign bodies**
- Initial assessment of **complications: Perforation & mediastinitis**
  - Pneumothorax, pleural effusion, mediastinal widening, pneumomediastinum, tracheal displacement/compression, subcutaneous gas

CT Findings

- CECT
  - **Assessment of complications**
    - **Mediastinitis, esophageal perforation**
    - **Abscess formation** secondary to primary or iatrogenic perforation (esophageal dilatation)
    - Evaluation of **aspiration**: Ranges from bronchiolitis (tree-in-bud opacities) to pneumonia (consolidation)

Fluoroscopic Findings

- **Distal esophageal stricture**
  - **Gastroesophageal reflux-induced** ("peptic" stricture)
    - **Classic**: 1-4 cm in length, distal esophagus, smooth tapered concentric narrowing, associated hiatal hernia
    - **Atypical**: Sacculations, "step-ladder" appearance, ring-like narrowing
  - Scleroderma: Distal esophagus, patulous esophagus, long segment stricture
  - Stricture after esophageal tube: Distal esophagus, increasing length & severity over time, follows prolonged intubation
  - Zollinger-Ellison: Distal esophagus, long strictures
- **Upper and mid esophagus strictures**
  - Barrett esophagus: Peptic stricture, most are distal but some affect mid esophagus, ring-like stricture, reticular appearance distal to stricture
  - Radiation: Smooth long segment concentric stricture within radiation port
  - Caustic ingestion: 1-3 months after ingestion, ≥ 1 segment, may be diffuse, increased risk of malignancy
  - Drug ingestion: Upper or mid esophagus, concentric narrowing
  - Congenital esophageal stenosis: Mid esophagus, stenosis with ring-like indentations
  - Skin diseases: Upper or mid esophagus, concentric or asymmetric narrowing, ≥ 1 segment
- **Ancillary findings**
  - Esophageal intramural pseudodiverticulosis & tracking
    - Short or long segment, flask-shaped contrast-filled outpouchings outside esophageal wall, no direct communication with lumen

Imaging Recommendations

- Best imaging tool
  - **Esophagram**
    - **Single-contrast**: Optimizes esophagus distension & stricture detection
    - Biphasic esophagram (double-contrast): Use of effervescent & barium, optimizes mucosal evaluation
    - **Barium is preferred contrast medium**
    - **Water-soluble contrast** used for **suspected perforation or leak** (e.g., caustic ingestion)

DIFFERENTIAL DIAGNOSIS

Achalasia

- Failure of relaxation of lower esophageal sphincter
- Dilated esophagus with air-fluid level on upright radiograph

Vascular Anomalies (Rings)

- Extrinsic compression by anomalous vessels
- Classic esophagram findings

Esophageal Carcinoma

- Asymmetric esophageal narrowing, mass
- Local invasion, lymphadenopathy

PATHOLOGY

General Features

- Etiology
  - **Gastroesophageal reflux-induced (75%)**
    - Primary
    - Secondary to scleroderma, Zollinger-Ellison syndrome, nasogastric intubation, alkaline reflux esophagitis
  - **Unrelated to gastroesophageal reflux (25%)**
    - Radiation, esophageal sclerotherapy, caustic ingestion, surgical anastomosis, dermatologic disease (e.g., epidermolysis bullosa dystrophica), extrinsic compression (e.g., mediastinal fibrosis), eosinophilic esophagitis, foreign bodies, infection

CLINICAL ISSUES

Presentation

- Most common signs/symptoms
  - **Dysphagia**
    - Benign: Longstanding, intermittent, nonprogressive
    - Malignant: Recent onset, fast progression, weight loss
  - **Aspiration**: Productive cough, wheezing, dyspnea

Natural History & Prognosis

- Strictures may recur after treatment

Treatment

- Balloon dilatation: May be complicated by esophageal perforation & mediastinitis

SELECTED REFERENCES

1. Luedtke P et al: Radiologic diagnosis of benign esophageal strictures: a pattern approach. Radiographics. 23(4):897-909, 2003

ESOPHAGEAL CARCINOMA

Key Facts

Terminology

- Squamous cell carcinoma (SCC)
- Esophageal malignancy including squamous cell carcinoma & adenocarcinoma

Imaging

- Radiography
  - Focal mediastinal mass
  - Displacement of azygoesophageal recess
  - Dilatation of esophagus ± air-fluid level
- CT
  - Asymmetric thickening of esophageal wall
  - Local invasion (T4): Obliteration of fat planes, evaluation of esophago-airway fistula
- Endoscopic ultrasound
  - Optimal for determining depth of wall invasion
- PET or PET/CT
  - Detection of distant metastases, restaging

Top Differential Diagnoses

- Esophageal stromal tumor
  - Leiomyoma, leiomyosarcoma
- Esophageal metastases

Pathology

- Squamous cell carcinoma: Proximal 2/3 of esophagus
  - Risk factors: Smoking, alcohol
- Adenocarcinoma: Distal 2/3 of esophagus
  - Risk factors: Reflux, obesity, smoking

Clinical Issues

- Symptoms: Dysphagia, weight loss
- Average age: 65-70 years; M > F
- Treatment
  - Endoscopic therapy or surgery
  - Neoadjuvant chemoradiation followed by surgery
  - M1: Chemotherapy ± radiation

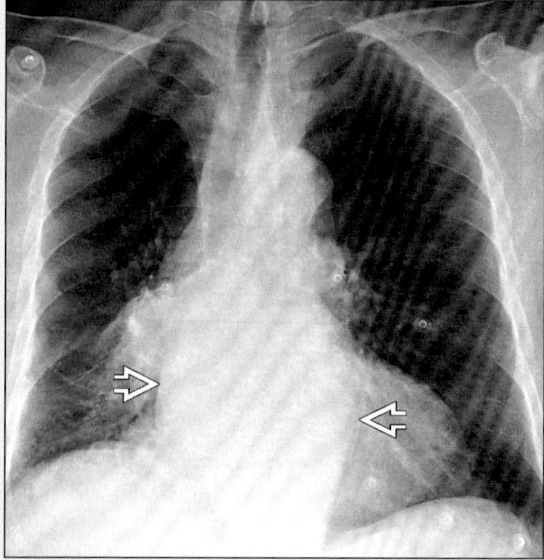

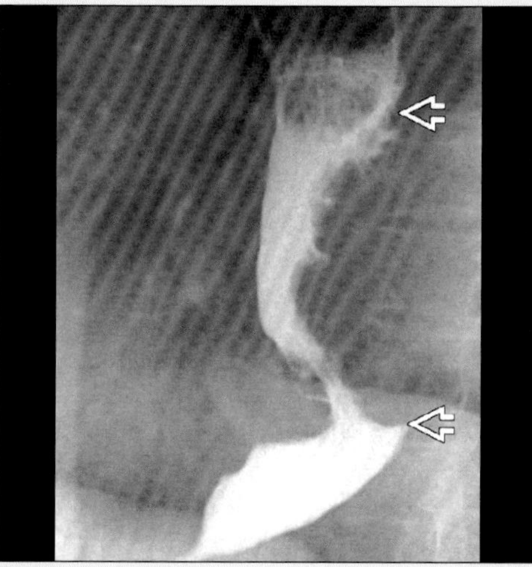

(Left) *PA chest radiograph of a patient with esophageal carcinoma who presented with dysphagia shows a lower mediastinal mass ➡ that obscures the azygoesophageal recess and the left paraaortic interface.* ***(Right)*** *Lateral esophagram of the same patient shows distention of the proximal esophagus and marked irregularity of the esophageal mucosa with irregular luminal narrowing and abrupt proximal and distal borders ➡, consistent with an intraluminal mass.*

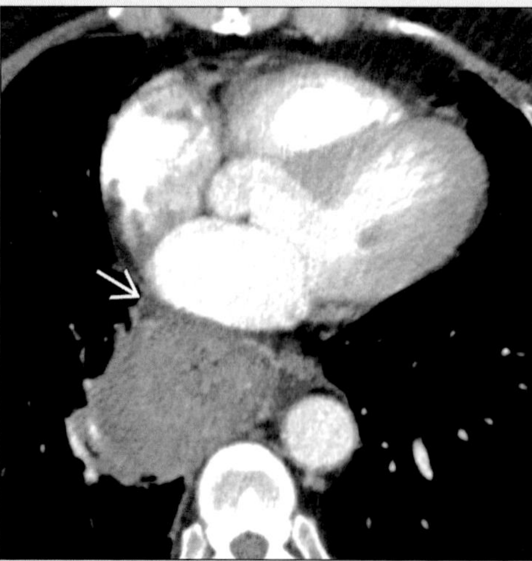

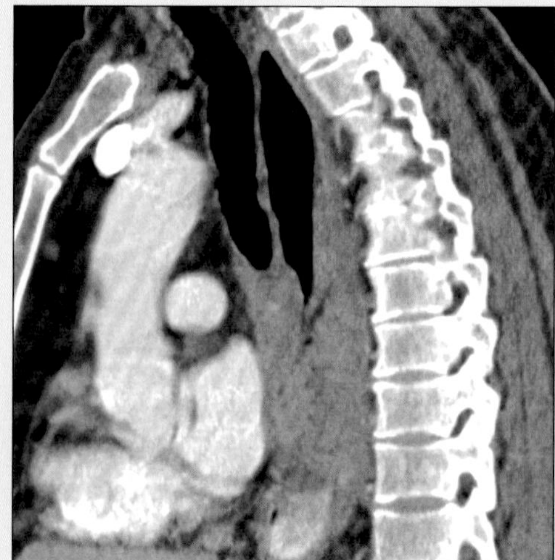

(Left) *Axial CECT of the same patient shows a large distal esophageal mass with no visible fat plane between it and the adjacent pericardium ➡, suggestive of mediastinal invasion or T4 status.* ***(Right)*** *Sagittal CECT of the same patient shows the craniocaudal extent of the mass to better advantage. Endoscopic biopsy confirmed SCC. CT is vital in detecting mediastinal invasion and delineating tumor extent when marked luminal narrowing prevents passage of the endoscope.*

ESOPHAGEAL CARCINOMA

TERMINOLOGY

Abbreviations

- **Squamous cell carcinoma (SCC)**

Definitions

- Esophageal malignancy
  - Squamous cell carcinoma
  - Adenocarcinoma

IMAGING

General Features

- Location
  - Esophagus divided into 4 regions by American Joint Committee on Cancer (AJCC) for classification & staging of esophageal cancer
    - **Cervical esophagus**: Cricoid cartilage to thoracic inlet (suprasternal notch)
    - **Upper thoracic esophagus**: Thoracic inlet to carina
    - **Mid-thoracic esophagus**: Carina to diaphragm
    - **Lower thoracic/abdominal esophagus**: Diaphragm to gastroesophageal junction (GEJ)
- Size
  - Variable: Ranges from small mucosal lesions to large masses
- Morphology
  - Focal mass
  - Esophageal wall thickening
  - Esophageal stricture
- Characteristics of esophageal carcinoma
  - Absence of esophageal wall serosa → malignancy easily spreads to adjacent structures (trachea, thyroid, aorta, etc.)
  - Interconnection & bidirectional flow of esophageal lymphatic plexuses → lymphatic spread superior or inferior to tumor
  - Hematogenous metastases to liver, lung, bone, adrenal gland, kidney, brain

Radiographic Findings

- **Focal mediastinal mass**
  - Displacement or abnormal convex contour of azygoesophageal recess
  - Thickening of posterior tracheal stripe on lateral chest radiography
  - Anterior displacement of trachea related to
    - Proximal esophageal tumor
    - Paraesophageal lymphadenopathy
    - Retained esophageal endoluminal debris due to distal obstruction by tumor
- **Dilatation of esophagus ± air-fluid level**
- Double-contrast esophagram
  - Focal mucosal irregularity, nodularity, or ulceration
  - Localized area of wall flattening & stiffening
  - Irregular luminal narrowing with abrupt proximal & distal borders
  - Large lobulated intraluminal mass

CT Findings

- **Asymmetric thickening of esophageal wall**
  - Inability to differentiate among T1, T2, & T3 disease
  - Preserved fat planes between esophageal cancer & adjacent mediastinal structures excludes T4 disease
- **Local invasion (T4)**
  - Obliteration of fat between esophagus & aorta &/or spine
  - Tracheo- or bronchoesophageal fistula
  - Displacement, indentation of, or growth into airway
  - Pericardial thickening, pericardial effusion, loss of fat plane between pericardium & esophagus/tumor
  - Contact of ≥ 90° of aortic wall circumference
- Multiplanar reformatted images help delineate craniocaudal extent of tumor for surgical or radiation treatment planning
- **Lymphadenopathy**
  - Intrathoracic & abdominal lymph nodes > 1 cm in short axis
  - Supraclavicular lymph nodes > 5 mm in short axis
  - CT not sensitive or specific

Ultrasonographic Findings

- Endoscopic ultrasound (EUS)
  - Identification of 5 esophageal wall layers of different echogenicity
    - Useful landmarks for assessment of depth of tumor invasion
    - Superior to CT for determining T1, T2, & T3 disease
    - Also used to guide fine needle aspiration of lymph nodes
  - Limitation: Large tumors may cause severe luminal narrowing, preventing passage of endoscope through site of stenosis

Imaging Recommendations

- Best imaging tool
  - EUS is modality of choice to determine T status & regional lymph node involvement
  - CT after initial diagnosis to evaluate for unresectable T4 or metastatic disease
  - PET or PET/CT for distant metastases & restaging after neoadjuvant therapy

Nuclear Medicine Findings

- PET
  - Intense uptake by primary tumor often limits evaluation of adjacent regional lymph nodes
  - Identification of previously occult distant metastases in 5-40% of patients
  - Early differentiation of "responders" from "nonresponders" undergoing neoadjuvant therapy
- PET/CT
  - Improves regional lymph node staging accuracy by delineating location of FDG uptake in vicinity of primary tumor

DIFFERENTIAL DIAGNOSIS

Esophageal Stromal Tumor: Leiomyoma, Leiomyosarcoma

- Intramural extramucosal mass
- May reach large sizes without producing proximal esophageal dilatation
- Leiomyoma: Smooth, homogeneous CT attenuation
- Leiomyosarcoma: Heterogeneous CT attenuation

Esophageal Metastases

- Typically patients with known primary cancer
  - Breast, lung, gastric cancers

ESOPHAGEAL CARCINOMA

PATHOLOGY

General Features

- Etiology
  - SCC: Most commonly in proximal 2/3 of esophagus
    - Risk factors
      - Tobacco use
      - Alcohol consumption
      - Nitrosamines in cured or pickled foods
      - Plummer-Vinson syndrome: Dysphagia (esophageal web), atrophic glossitis, iron-deficiency anemia
      - Achalasia
      - Caustic burn injury
      - Longstanding esophagitis
    - Predominant esophageal cancer worldwide
    - Incidence declining in Western countries; becoming less common than adenocarcinoma in United States
  - Adenocarcinoma: Most commonly in distal 2/3 of esophagus
    - Risk factors
      - Gastroesophageal reflux & Barrett metaplasia
      - Smoking
      - Obesity
    - Incidence increasing rapidly in Western countries

Staging, Grading, & Classification

- TNM staging developed by AJCC
  - Tumor (T) status: Depth of esophageal wall invasion
    - **Tis**: High-grade dysplasia
    - **T1**: Confined to mucosa, lamina propria, or submucosa
    - **T2**: Invasion of muscularis propria
    - **T3**: Invasion of adventitia
    - **T4a**: Resectable cancers invading adjacent structures (pleura, pericardium, diaphragm)
    - **T4b**: Unresectable cancer invading adjacent structures (aorta, vertebral body, trachea)
  - Nodal (N) status: Regional lymph nodes, any paraesophageal lymph nodes from cervical to celiac nodes
    - **N0**: No regional lymph node metastases
    - **N1**: 1-2 positive regional lymph nodes
    - **N2**: 3-6 positive regional lymph nodes
    - **N3**: ≥ 7 positive lymph nodes
  - Metastasis (M) status
    - **M0**: No distant metastasis
    - **M1**: Distant metastases
- Histologic grade (G)
  - **G1**: Well differentiated
  - **G2**: Moderately differentiated
  - **G3**: Poorly differentiated
  - **G4**: Undifferentiated
- Separate stage grouping based on T, N, M, G for SCC & adenocarcinoma
  - **SCC**: Tumor location (upper, mid, lower thoracic) also included in stage grouping

Gross Pathologic & Surgical Features

- **SCC**
  - Small, gray-white, plaque-like mucosal thickening in early stage
  - Polypoid fungating intraluminal mass
  - Necrotizing ulcerations ± erosion into airway, aorta
  - Diffuse esophageal wall thickening & rigidity
- **Adenocarcinoma**
  - Flat or raised patches in early stage
  - Nodular masses

CLINICAL ISSUES

Presentation

- Most common signs/symptoms
  - **Dysphagia**
  - **Weight loss**
- Other signs/symptoms
  - Odynophagia
  - Hematemesis
  - Recurrent pneumonia: Aspiration or tracheoesophageal fistula
  - Hoarseness: Invasion of recurrent laryngeal nerve

Demographics

- Age
  - Average: 65-70 years
- Gender
  - Men > women

Natural History & Prognosis

- 24% confined to esophagus at diagnosis
- 30% with distant metastases at diagnosis
- Overall 5-year survival for adenocarcinoma < 15%, worse for SCC

Treatment

- T1 N0 M0 disease: Endoscopic therapy or surgery
- M0 disease with deeper extent of tumor or regional lymph nodes: Neoadjuvant chemoradiation followed by surgery
- M1: Chemotherapy ± radiation
- Endoscopic procedures: Early intramucosal tumor or palliation
  - Laser therapy
  - Photodynamic therapy
  - Brachytherapy
  - Radiofrequency ablation
  - Esophageal stent placement

DIAGNOSTIC CHECKLIST

Image Interpretation Pearls

- Proximal esophageal dilatation should prompt assessment of distal esophagus for exclusion of wall thickening or mass

SELECTED REFERENCES

1. Rice TW et al: 7th edition of the AJCC Cancer Staging Manual: esophagus and esophagogastric junction. Ann Surg Oncol. 17(7):1721-4, 2010
2. Kim TJ et al: Multimodality assessment of esophageal cancer: preoperative staging and monitoring of response to therapy. Radiographics. 29(2):403-21, 2009

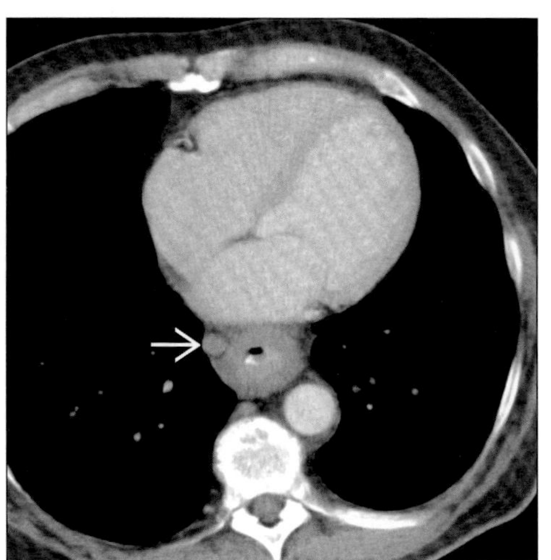

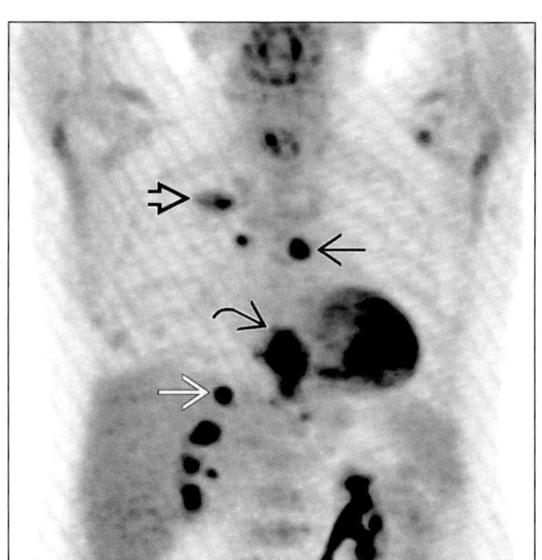

(Left) *Axial CECT of a patient with esophageal adenocarcinoma shows circumferential thickening of the distal esophageal wall and an enlarged right paraesophageal lymph node* ➔. ***(Right)*** *Coronal PET of the same patient demonstrates intense uptake of the primary tumor* ↪, *which is difficult to separate from the adjacent paraesophageal lymph node. Bilateral paratracheal lymphadenopathy* →, *right posterior rib* ⇨, *and right adrenal* ➔ *metastases are also demonstrated.*

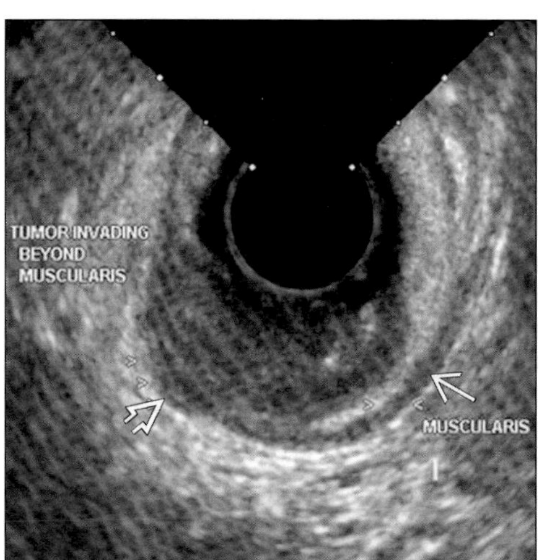

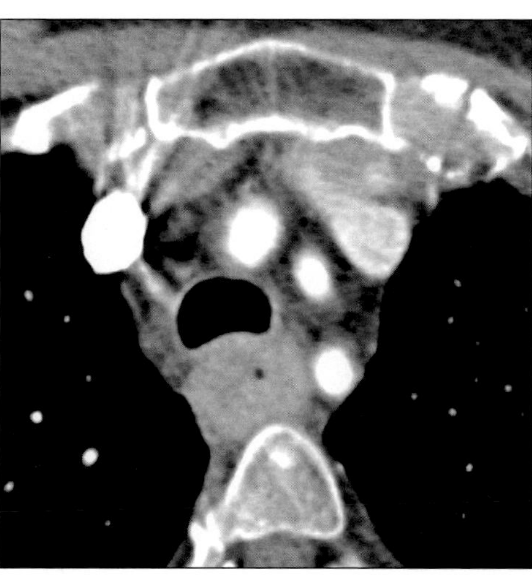

(Left) *Axial EUS shows the muscularis as a hypoechoic layer* ➔. *The hypoechoic esophageal mass* ⇨ *extends beyond the muscularis into the adventitia, consistent with T3 disease. EUS is the modality of choice to determine the T status of esophageal carcinoma.* ***(Right)*** *Axial CECT of a patient with SCC shows esophageal thickening with indentation of the posterior tracheal wall that suggests airway invasion. Bronchoscopy is usually performed to exclude airway invasion in such cases.*

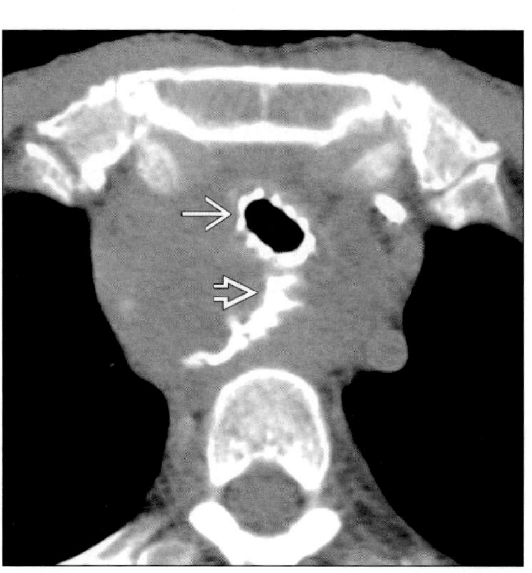

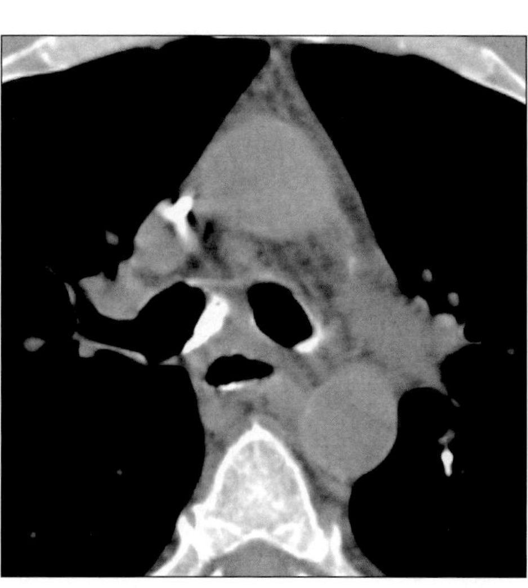

(Left) *Axial NECT with oral contrast of a patient with a large upper thoracic esophageal SCC shows a tracheoesophageal fistula* ⇨. *A tracheal stent* ➔ *was placed to keep the airway patent and exclude the airway from the fistula.* ***(Right)*** *Axial NECT of the same patient shows aspiration of oral contrast into the bilateral mainstem bronchi despite the tracheal stent. Esophageal cancer is a major cause of tracheoesophageal fistula, which can occur spontaneously or after radiation treatment.*

MEDIASTINAL LIPOMATOSIS

Key Facts

Terminology
- Excessive unencapsulated fat deposition in mediastinum

Imaging
- Radiography
  - Smooth symmetric superior mediastinum widening without tracheal narrowing or displacement
  - Symmetric increased opacity at bilateral cardiophrenic angles
  - Extrapleural fat deposition with smooth margins
- CT
  - Homogeneous fat attenuation: -130 to -70 HU
  - No compression or invasion of adjacent structures
  - Absence of dominant soft tissue components
- MR
  - High signal intensity on T1WI & T2WI
  - Isointense to subcutaneous fat

Top Differential Diagnoses
- Fat-containing mediastinal mass
- Mediastinal lymphadenopathy
- Mediastinitis

Pathology
- Etiology: Obesity, Cushing syndrome
- Diffuse adipose tissue without surrounding capsule
- Mature adipocytes and cellular hyperplasia

Clinical Issues
- Asymptomatic; incidental imaging finding
- Chest pain, dyspnea, cough

Diagnostic Checklist
- Mediastinal fat should be homogeneous on CT; dominant soft tissue or mass effect suggests neoplasia
- Consider exclusion of adrenal neoplasm in affected patients

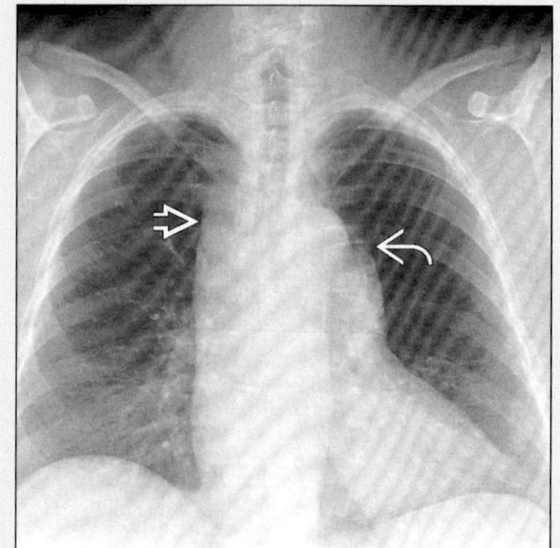

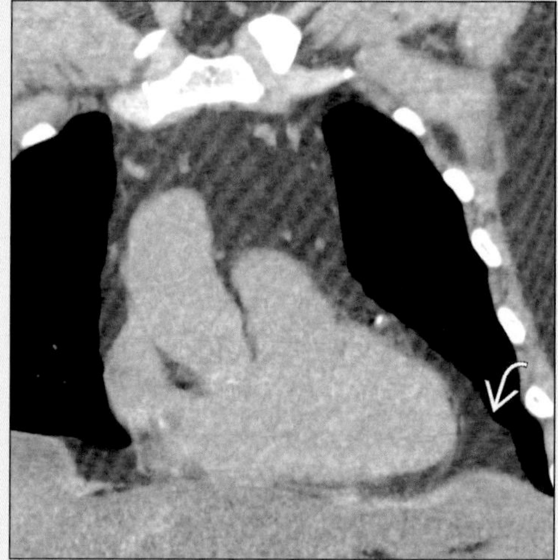

(Left) *PA chest radiograph of a patient with mediastinal lipomatosis shows smooth superior mediastinal widening ➔ and aortopulmonary window fullness ➔ without mass effect on the mediastinal structures.* ***(Right)*** *Coronal NECT of the same patient shows fat attenuation tissue affecting the superior mediastinum preferentially but also the left cardiophrenic region ➔. CT allows confident diagnosis of mediastinal lipomatosis and exclusion of underlying lymphadenopathy or mass.*

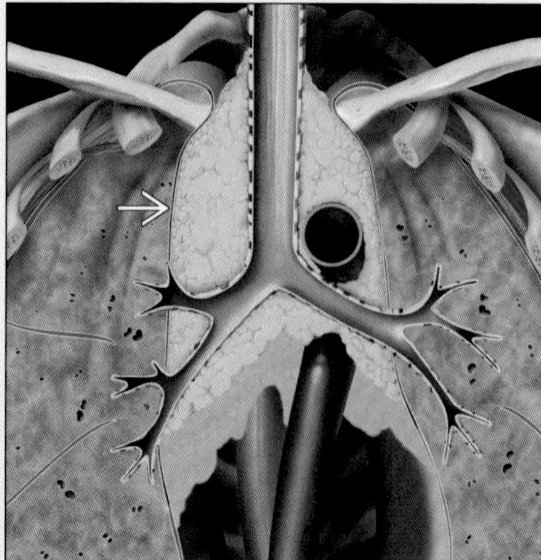

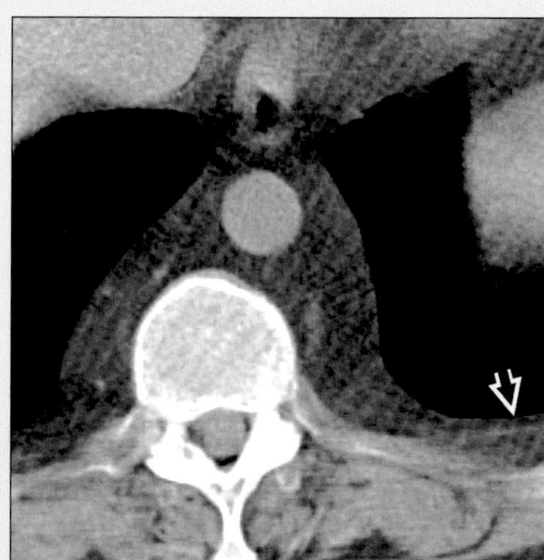

(Left) *Graphic demonstrates the morphologic features of mediastinal lipomatosis. Unencapsulated mediastinal adipose tissue ➔ surrounds the normal mediastinal structures without obstruction or mass effect.* ***(Right)*** *Axial NECT of a patient on corticosteroids shows extensive periaortic, paravertebral, and extrapleural ➔ fat deposition. Homogeneous fat attenuation is characteristic. Although mediastinal lipomatosis may be secondary to obesity, conditions with excess ACTH production should be excluded.*

MEDIASTINAL LIPOMATOSIS

TERMINOLOGY

Definitions

- Excessive unencapsulated fat deposition in mediastinum

IMAGING

General Features

- Best diagnostic clue
  - **Wide mediastinum with fat attenuation**
- Location
  - **Most frequent: Superior mediastinum**
  - Juxtacardiac mediastinum
  - May be associated with extensive extrapleural fat
- Morphology
  - Surrounds normal structures without invasion or mass effect

Radiographic Findings

- Radiography
  - Smooth symmetric superior mediastinal widening without tracheal narrowing or displacement
  - Symmetric increased opacity at bilateral cardiophrenic angles
  - Extrapleural fat deposition: Smoothly marginated, mimics pleural thickening

CT Findings

- **Homogeneous fat attenuation: -130 to -70 HU**
- No compression or invasion of adjacent structures
- Absence of dominant soft tissue components

MR Findings

- High signal intensity on T1WI & T2WI
- Isointense to subcutaneous fat
- Signal dropout with fat suppression

Imaging Recommendations

- Best imaging tool
  - CT confirms homogeneous fat attenuation when radiographic appearance is not characteristic

DIFFERENTIAL DIAGNOSIS

Fat-Containing Mediastinal Mass

- Distinction from lipomatosis: Identification of dominant soft tissue elements & mass effect
- Mature teratoma: Anterior mediastinal cystic mass; may exhibit calcification &/or fat attenuation
- Thymolipoma: Conforms to shape of adjacent structures (heart, hemidiaphragm)
- Liposarcoma: Soft tissue components; mass effect
- Lipoblastoma: Chest wall lesion; infants < 3 years
- Hibernoma: Rare benign tumor of brown fat

Mediastinal Lymphadenopathy

- Typically lobular or laterally convex contours
- Lipomatosis may mimic lymphadenopathy on radiography

Mediastinitis

- May produce mediastinal widening on radiography
- Hazy infiltration of fat, discrete fluid collections ± intrinsic gas

PATHOLOGY

General Features

- Etiology
  - Obesity
  - **Cushing syndrome**: Hypercortisolism
    - **Exogenous steroids**: Treatment of asthma, chronic obstructive pulmonary disease (COPD), connective tissue disease, or immune suppression after organ transplantation
    - **Excessive corticosteroid production by adrenal neoplasm**
    - **Cushing disease**: Excessive adrenocorticotrophic hormone (ACTH) secreted by pituitary neoplasm
    - **Ectopic production of ACTH as paraneoplastic syndrome**: Small cell lung cancer, thymic carcinoid, islet cell tumor of pancreas

Gross Pathologic & Surgical Features

- Diffuse adipose tissue without surrounding capsule

Microscopic Features

- Mature adipocytes and cellular hyperplasia

CLINICAL ISSUES

Presentation

- Most common signs/symptoms
  - **Asymptomatic**; incidental imaging finding
- Other signs/symptoms
  - Chest pain
  - Dyspnea
  - Cough

Natural History & Prognosis

- Incidentally detected lipomatosis often follows a benign indolent course

Treatment

- None necessary
- Treatment of underlying condition may cause regression

DIAGNOSTIC CHECKLIST

Consider

- Mediastinal lipomatosis as cause of mediastinal widening in patients on corticosteroids
- Exclusion of adrenal neoplasm in affected patients

Image Interpretation Pearls

- When mediastinal lipomatosis is suspected radiographically, look for other clues of excess adipose tissue
- Mediastinal fat should be homogeneous on CT; dominant soft tissue components or mass effect suggests neoplasia

SELECTED REFERENCES

1. Boiselle PM et al: Fat attenuation lesions of the mediastinum. J Comput Assist Tomogr. 25(6):881-9, 2001
2. Nguyen KQ et al: Mediastinal lipomatosis. South Med J. 91(12):1169-72, 1998

MEDIASTINITIS

Key Facts

Terminology

- Acute descending necrotizing mediastinitis (ADNM)
- Acute mediastinitis: Potentially life-threatening focal or diffuse mediastinal inflammation usually caused by infection

Imaging

- Radiography
  - Mediastinal widening
  - Pneumomediastinum
  - Mediastinal air-fluid level
- CT
  - Increased attenuation of mediastinal fat
  - Localized fluid collection ± peripheral enhancement
  - Free gas bubbles, pneumomediastinum
  - Pericardial effusion
  - Pleural effusion

Top Differential Diagnoses

- Postoperative seroma
- Fibrosing mediastinitis
- Mediastinal hematoma/hemorrhage

Pathology

- 90% of acute mediastinitis is secondary to esophageal perforation or rupture
- Median sternotomy also important etiology

Clinical Issues

- Symptoms: Fever, chills, retrosternal pain
- High mortality: 5-50%

Diagnostic Checklist

- Careful evaluation of entire thorax for exclusion of associated aspiration pneumonia, empyema, osteomyelitis

*(**Left**) PA chest radiograph of a patient who presented with neck and chest pain 3 days after a dental procedure shows abnormal soft tissue in the right paratracheal ➡ and AP window ➡ regions. (**Right**) Axial CECT shows stranding of mediastinal fat, a right paratracheal fluid collection ➡, and extensive mediastinal air pockets ➡, consistent with ADNM. The radiographic finding of widened mediastinum in the clinical setting of fever and chest pain should prompt consideration of mediastinitis.*

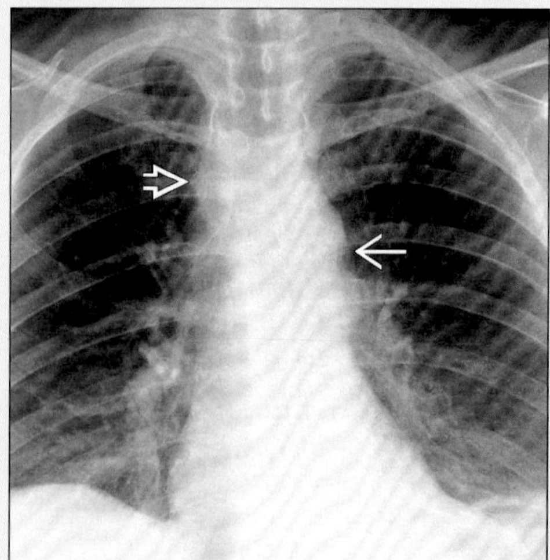

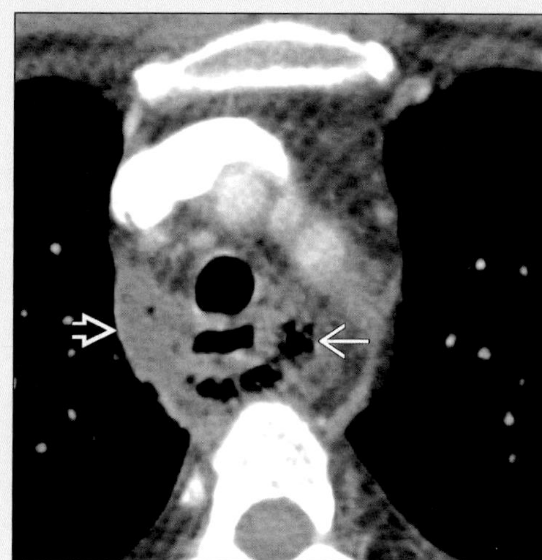

*(**Left**) Sagittal CECT of the same patient shows direct extension of extraluminal air ➡ from the neck into the retroesophageal mediastinum. (**Right**) Axial CECT of a patient who sustained a hypopharyngeal perforation during intubation shows increased attenuation of the mediastinal fat, a right paratracheal fluid collection ➡, bilateral pleural effusions, and a mediastinal drainage tube ➡. ADNM is an uncommon but potentially life-threatening condition.*

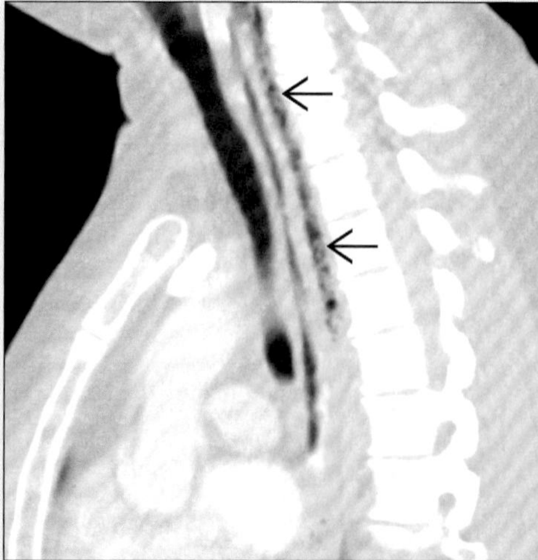

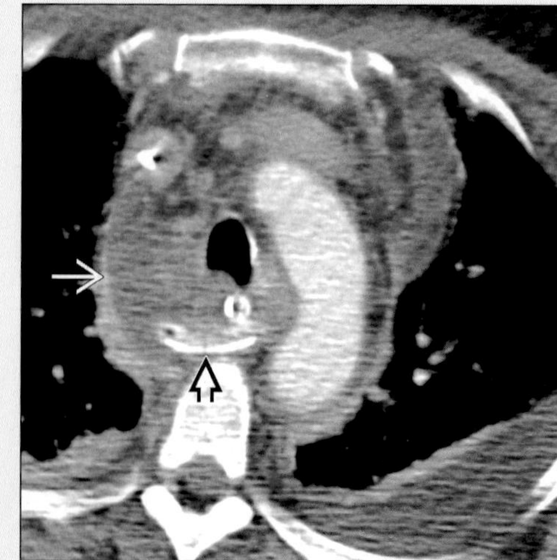

MEDIASTINITIS

TERMINOLOGY

Abbreviations

- **Acute descending necrotizing mediastinitis (ADNM)**

Definitions

- **Acute mediastinitis:** Potentially life-threatening focal or diffuse mediastinal inflammation usually caused by infection

IMAGING

General Features

- Best diagnostic clue
  - Wide mediastinum: Fluid collections ± air/air-fluid levels
- Location
  - Mediastinum
- Size
  - Variable

Radiographic Findings

- **Mediastinal widening**
- **Pneumomediastinum**
- Mediastinal air-fluid level
- Pleural effusion
- Displacement or change in alignment of sternal wires in post-sternotomy mediastinitis

CT Findings

- **Increased attenuation of mediastinal fat**
- **Localized fluid collection** ± peripheral enhancement
- Free gas, air bubbles, pneumomediastinum
- Mediastinal lymphadenopathy
- Pericardial effusion
- Pleural effusion
  - Empyema
    - Loculated pleural fluid
    - Bronchopleural fistula: Intrinsic air or air-fluid levels
- Pulmonary opacities
- Pleuromediastinal fistula
- **Post-cardiac surgery**
  - CT appearance of postsurgical mediastinum similar to mediastinitis during 1st 2-3 weeks post surgery
  - Increased attenuation of mediastinal fat
    - Nonspecific finding
    - May relate to postsurgical hemorrhage or edema
  - Gas bubbles & mediastinal fluid collection: Normal up to 21 days after surgery
  - **Diagnostic yield of CT improves after postoperative day 14**
  - New or increasing mediastinal air &/or fluid is highly suspicious for mediastinitis
  - Cortical erosion of sternum suggests osteomyelitis
  - Dehiscence of sternotomy site
- **Esophageal perforation**
  - **Leak of ingested contrast** material into mediastinum &/or pleural space
  - **Extraluminal air**
  - Pneumothorax
  - Hydropneumothorax
  - Subcutaneous gas
  - Esophageal wall thickening
  - Pleural effusion
    - Right-sided with iatrogenic, mid esophageal perforation
    - Left-sided with spontaneous, distal esophageal perforation
- ADNM
  - **Direct extension of cervical infection into mediastinum**
  - Jugular vein thrombosis
  - Demonstration of contiguity of mediastinal fluid collection with fluid collections in neck
- **Direct extension from chest wall infection**
  - Destruction of articular surface (usually at sternoclavicular joint)
  - Joint space widening
  - Adjacent chest wall air & fluid collections
  - Obliteration of fat planes around brachiocephalic vessels

Imaging Recommendations

- Best imaging tool
  - CT for evaluation of site & extent of mediastinitis & identification of drainable fluid collection
    - High sensitivity
    - Allows prompt diagnosis & treatment
    - Useful for monitoring treatment response
  - **Esophagogram with water-soluble contrast in patients with suspected esophageal perforation**
    - Contrast esophagogram: **False-negative in 10% of patients**
    - May follow with barium esophagram
- Protocol advice
  - Contrast-enhanced chest CT for optimal visualization of loculated fluid collections

MR Findings

- T1 hypointensity & T2 hyperintensity within mediastinal fat
- Enhancement of mediastinal fat
- Peripheral enhancement surrounding fluid collection

DIFFERENTIAL DIAGNOSIS

Postoperative Seroma

- Difficult to distinguish from mediastinitis within 2-3 weeks post surgery
- Must correlate imaging findings with clinical scenario
- Needle aspiration of fluid collections may be necessary to distinguish seroma from abscess

Fibrosing Mediastinitis

- Subacute or chronic (instead of acute) presentation
- Mediastinal soft tissue or calcification without pneumomediastinum or fluid collection

Mediastinal Hematoma/Hemorrhage

- Typically history of trauma, surgery, central line placement
- Hyperattenuating hematoma helpful for diagnosis when present
- Exclusion of findings of vascular injury
  - Pseudoaneurysm, dissection, contrast extravasation

MEDIASTINITIS

PATHOLOGY

General Features

- Etiology
  - **90%** of acute mediastinitis related to iatrogenic or spontaneous **esophageal perforation**
    - Dilatation of stricture or achalasia
    - Endoscopy
    - Esophageal tube/stent placement
    - Necrotic esophageal tumor
    - Ulceration of hiatal hernia
    - Esophagitis
    - Boerhaave syndrome
      - Spontaneous esophageal perforation associated with forceful vomiting
    - Ingestion of sharp foreign body or erosive chemical
  - **Postoperative acute mediastinitis** (median sternotomy)
    - 0.5-5% of cardiac surgery patients
    - Risk factors
      - Lengthy cardiopulmonary bypass time
      - Diabetes
      - Obesity
      - Tracheostomy
      - Use of bilateral internal mammary arteries for coronary artery bypass graft (CABG) surgery
  - **ADNM**
    - Anatomical continuity of fascial spaces allows spread of infection from neck to mediastinum
      - Contributing factors: Gravity & negative intrathoracic pressure during inspiration
      - Routes of spread: Carotid space (skull base to aortic arch), prevertebral space (skull base to T3)
      - Danger space: Retropharyngeal/retroesophageal space from skull base to diaphragm
    - Common causes
      - Odontogenic infection
      - Suppurative tonsillitis
      - Retropharyngeal abscess
  - Direct spread from osteomyelitis or septic joint (sternoclavicular joint)
    - Risk factors
      - Intravenous drug use
      - Diabetes
      - Rheumatoid arthritis
  - Airway perforation
    - Penetrating or blunt trauma
    - Intubation
    - Bronchoscopic procedures
    - Bronchogenic carcinoma

Gross Pathologic & Surgical Features

- Mediastinal inflammation/infection ± abscess formation

Microscopic Features

- ADNM & esophageal perforation
  - Mixed aerobic & anaerobic organisms
- Post-sternotomy & septic joint-related mediastinitis
  - Gram-positive cocci (*S. aureus*) & gram-negative bacilli (*Pseudomonas*)

CLINICAL ISSUES

Presentation

- Most common signs/symptoms
  - **Fever, chills**
  - **Retrosternal pain**
- Other signs/symptoms
  - Tachycardia
  - Dyspnea
  - Dysphagia, odynophagia
  - Subcutaneous air
  - Sepsis
  - Neck swelling in patients with ADNM
  - Purulent discharge from sternal wound in patients with post-sternotomy mediastinitis

Demographics

- Age
  - Any age group can be affected

Natural History & Prognosis

- **5-50% mortality**
  - Highest mortality rate for ADNM: 30-50%
- Mortality increases with delay in diagnosis

Treatment

- **Intravenous broad-spectrum antibiotics** as soon as possible in all cases
- CT-guided **percutaneous aspiration or drainage** of fluid collections
- Surgical irrigation & drain placement often needed
  - Esophageal perforation: Primary closure within 24 hours
  - Postoperative mediastinitis & chest wall infection
    - May require resection of involved skeletal structure(s)

DIAGNOSTIC CHECKLIST

Consider

- Acute mediastinitis in patients with widened mediastinum in the setting of fever & chest pain

Image Interpretation Pearls

- Careful evaluation of entire thorax for exclusion of associated aspiration pneumonia, empyema, osteomyelitis
- Difficult diagnosis of mediastinitis in immediate postoperative period

SELECTED REFERENCES

1. Athanassiadi KA: Infections of the mediastinum. Thorac Surg Clin. 19(1):37-45, vi, 2009
2. Restrepo CS et al: Imaging appearances of the sternum and sternoclavicular joints. Radiographics. 29(3):839-59, 2009
3. Pinto A et al: Infections of the neck leading to descending necrotizing mediastinitis: Role of multi-detector row computed tomography. Eur J Radiol. 65(3):389-94, 2008
4. Exarhos DN et al: Acute mediastinitis: spectrum of computed tomography findings. Eur Radiol. 15(8):1569-74, 2005
5. Akman C et al: Imaging in mediastinitis: a systematic review based on aetiology. Clin Radiol. 59(7):573-85, 2004

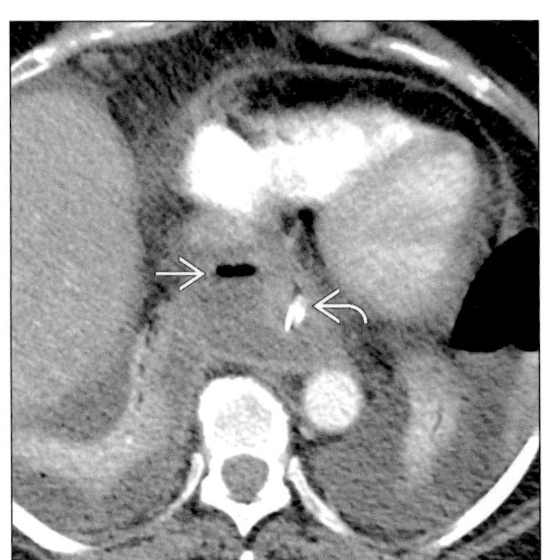

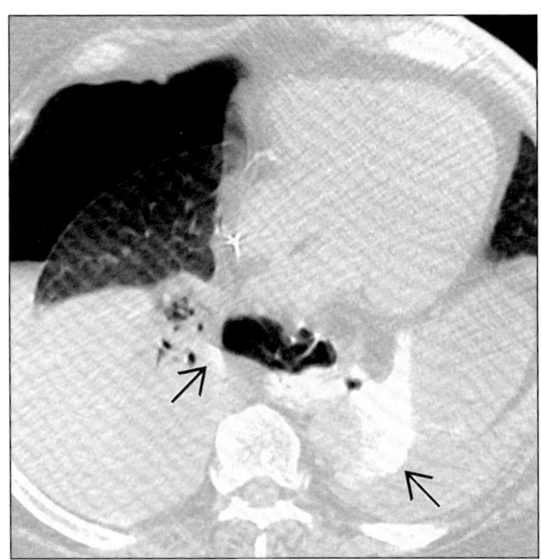

*(**Left**) Axial CECT of a patient with Boerhaave syndrome shows a right paraesophageal collection containing fluid and air ➡, as well as bilateral pleural effusions. The enteric tube ➡ shows the location of the distal esophagus. (**Right**) Axial CECT of a patient with esophageal perforation from enteric tube placement shows pneumomediastinum, a right hydropneumothorax, and extraluminal oral contrast ➡ in the bilateral pleural spaces. Esophageal perforation is the most common cause of mediastinitis.*

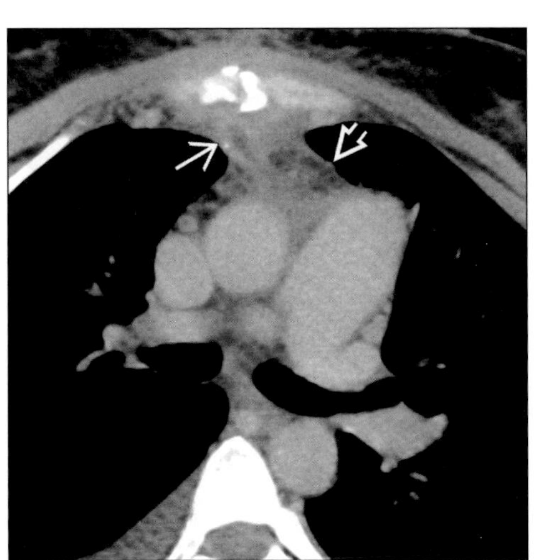

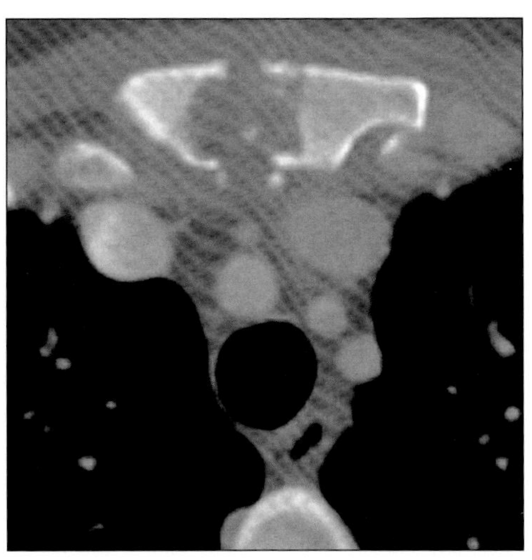

*(**Left**) Axial CECT of a patient with persistent sternal wound drainage 5 weeks post cardiac surgery shows a small thick-walled fluid collection in the anterior mediastinum ➡ and increased attenuation of the mediastinal fat ➡, consistent with mediastinitis. (**Right**) Axial CECT of the same patient shows dehiscence and lysis at the sternotomy site, consistent with osteomyelitis. When evaluating patients for post-sternotomy mediastinitis, carefully evaluate the sternum for evidence of osteomyelitis.*

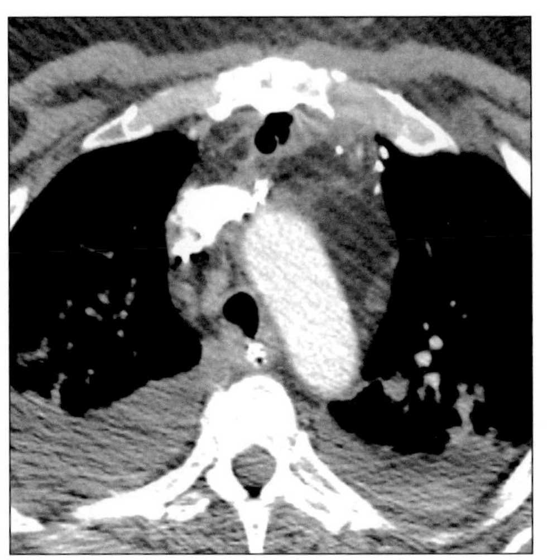

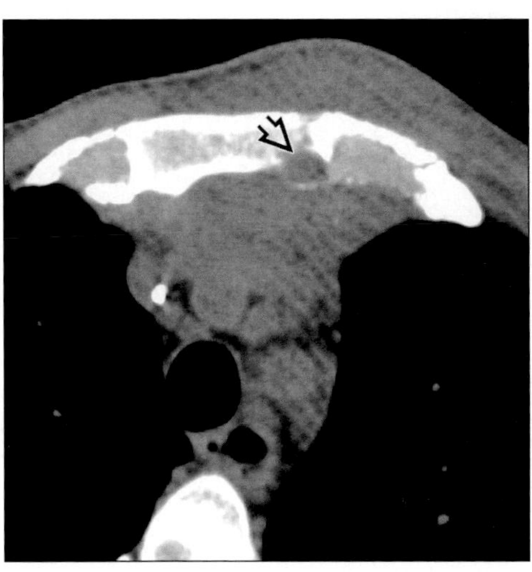

*(**Left**) Axial CECT of a patient with fever and chest pain 4 weeks after CABG shows pleural effusions and anterior mediastinal air and fluid, consistent with mediastinitis. These findings are abnormal after the 3rd postoperative week. (**Right**) Axial NECT of an IV drug user with a septic joint shows erosion of the left sternal cortex ➡, increased attenuation of the anterior mediastinal fat, and obliteration of tissue planes. Direct extension of anterior chest wall infection is an unusual cause of mediastinitis.*

EXTRAMEDULLARY HEMATOPOIESIS

Key Facts

Terminology
- Proliferation of hematopoietic cells outside bone marrow when marrow hematopoiesis fails

Imaging
- Radiography
  - Well-defined unilateral/bilateral paravertebral mass
  - No osseous erosion or calcification; rib expansion
- CT
  - Paravertebral, well-marginated soft tissue mass(es)
  - Typical location along costovertebral junctions
  - Fatty degeneration indicates old burned-out lesions
- MR
  - Fat replacement: Hyperintense on T1WI & T2WI
  - Iron deposition: Hypointense on T1WI & T2WI
- Nuclear medicine
  - May exhibit uptake of Tc-99m sulfur colloid

Top Differential Diagnoses
- Neurogenic neoplasm
- Paraesophageal varices
- Pleural/chest wall metastases
- Lateral thoracic meningocele
- Lymphadenopathy

Pathology
- Associations: Myelofibrosis, β-thalassemia, hereditary spherocytosis, hemolytic anemia, sickle cell anemia

Clinical Issues
- Often asymptomatic, incidental finding
- Rarely cord compression: Intraspinal involvement

Diagnostic Checklist
- Consider extramedullary hematopoiesis in patients with chronic anemia & paravertebral mass(es)

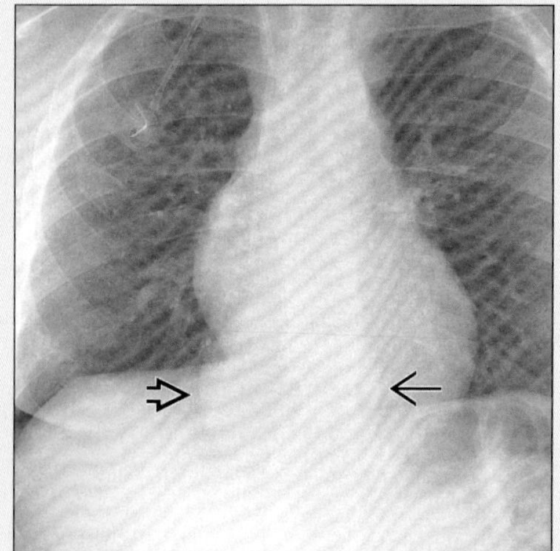

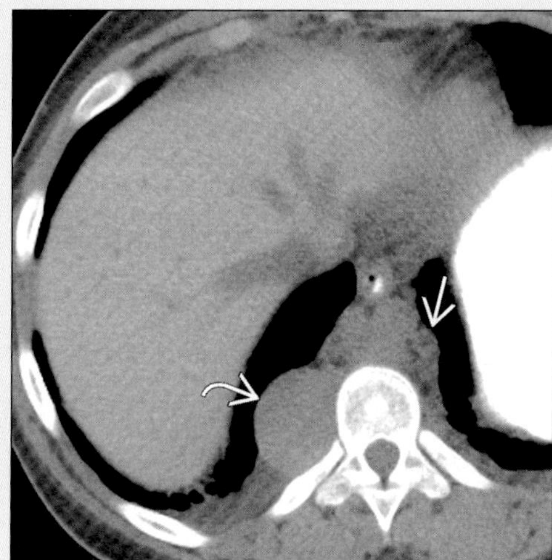

(Left) *PA chest radiograph of a patient with sickle cell anemia and extramedullary hematopoiesis shows mild cardiomegaly and bilateral lower thoracic paraspinal masses that exhibit lateral displacement of the right ⇨ and left → paravertebral stripes.* ***(Right)*** *Axial NECT of the same patient shows a well-defined right paravertebral soft tissue mass ➡ and smaller left paraaortic/paravertebral soft tissue nodules ➡. Thoracic extramedullary hematopoiesis typically affects the paravertebral regions.*

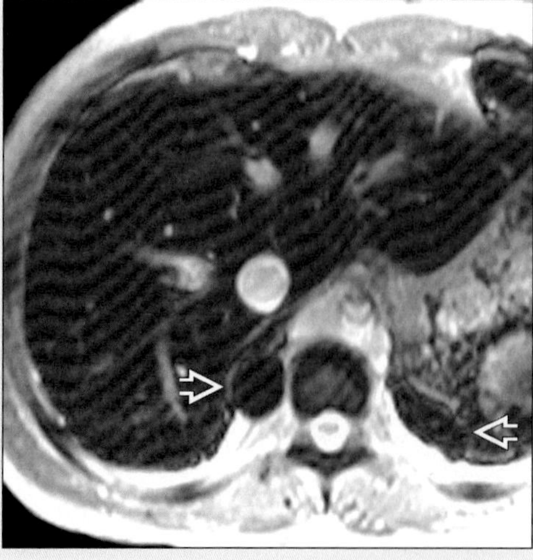

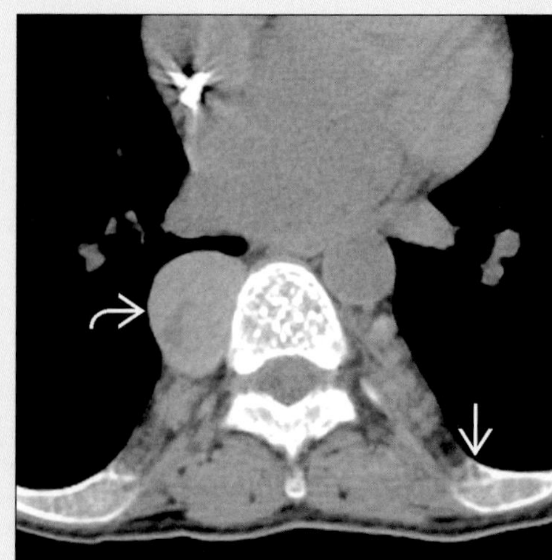

(Left) *Axial FISP MR of the same patient demonstrates marked hypointensity of the liver and bilateral paravertebral masses ➡, which indicates iron deposition.* ***(Right)*** *Axial NECT of a patient with β-thalassemia shows a well-defined, high-attenuation right paravertebral mass ➡ with intrinsic low attenuation that could represent fat and marrow expansion ➡ of the bilateral posterior ribs. Fatty degeneration &/or iron deposition are often seen in burned-out extramedullary hematopoietic lesions.*

EXTRAMEDULLARY HEMATOPOIESIS

TERMINOLOGY

Definitions

- Proliferation of hematopoietic cells outside bone marrow when marrow hematopoiesis fails

IMAGING

General Features

- Best diagnostic clue
  - **Paravertebral mass or masses** with rib expansion
- Location
  - Paravertebral region caudal to 6th thoracic vertebra
- Size: 5 mm to > 5 cm

Radiographic Findings

- Radiography
  - **Paravertebral mass**
    - Well-defined borders
    - Unilateral or bilateral; single or multiple
    - Separate or contiguous masses
    - No osseous erosion or calcifications
    - Very slow growth
  - Ribs
    - Rib expansion, conspicuous trabeculae
    - Most evident at costovertebral articulations
    - Adjacent ribs may be normal

CT Findings

- NECT
  - Paravertebral, well-marginated soft tissue mass(es)
  - Typically along costovertebral junctions
  - Fatty degeneration indicates old burned-out lesions
- CECT
  - Mild contrast enhancement; may be heterogeneous

MR Findings

- Fat replacement: Hyperintense on T1WI & T2WI
- Iron deposition: Hypointense on T1WI & T2WI
- Assessment of intraspinal extension in patients with neurologic symptoms

Nuclear Medicine Findings

- May exhibit uptake of Tc-99m sulfur colloid
- Radionuclide scans may be normal

DIFFERENTIAL DIAGNOSIS

Neurogenic Neoplasm

- Paravertebral neoplasms of peripheral nerve or sympathetic ganglion origin
- Benign pressure skeletal erosion; no osseous expansion

Paraesophageal Varices

- Serpiginous enhancing mediastinal vessels
- Ancillary findings of chronic liver disease
- No osseous expansion

Pleural/Chest Wall Metastases

- History of primary malignancy
- Bone destruction of ribs or vertebrae

Lateral Thoracic Meningocele

- Unilateral fluid attenuation paravertebral mass
- Enlarged neural foramen, scoliosis

Lymphadenopathy

- Rarely limited to paravertebral regions
- Metastatic disease, lymphoma

PATHOLOGY

General Features

- Associated abnormalities
  - Common: Myelofibrosis, β-thalassemia, hereditary spherocytosis, congenital hemolytic anemia, sickle cell anemia
  - Less common: Lymphoma/leukemia, Gaucher disease, Paget disease, rickets, hyperparathyroidism, pernicious anemia

Gross Pathologic & Surgical Features

- **Paravertebral masses of hematopoietic marrow**
- Other sites of extramedullary hematopoiesis
  - Liver, spleen, lymph nodes, retroperitoneum, kidneys, adrenal glands, breast, thymus, prostate, spinal cord, pericardium, intracranial dura matter

CLINICAL ISSUES

Presentation

- Most common signs/symptoms
  - **Often asymptomatic**, incidental finding
  - Symptoms may relate to mass effect
  - Rarely cord compression: Intraspinal growth of paravertebral mass or intraspinal hematopoiesis

Demographics

- Age
  - Clinical presentation in **3rd to 5th decades**
- Ethnicity
  - Thalassemia most common in Mediterranean countries
  - Sickle cell disease most common in African-Americans
- Epidemiology
  - Splenectomy might predispose to extramedullary hematopoiesis

Natural History & Prognosis

- Complications
  - Hemothorax, may be massive (uncommon)
  - Spinal compression (uncommon)

Treatment

- No treatment if asymptomatic
- Transfusion, hydroxyurea
- Splenectomy in hereditary spherocytosis
- Small doses of radiation in spinal cord compression

DIAGNOSTIC CHECKLIST

Consider

- Extramedullary hematopoiesis in patients with chronic anemia & unexplained paravertebral mass(es)

SELECTED REFERENCES

1. Berkmen YM et al: Case 126: extramedullary hematopoiesis. Radiology. 245(3):905-8, 2007

HIATAL AND PARAESOPHAGEAL HERNIA

Key Facts

Terminology

- Hiatal hernia, hiatus hernia (HH)
- Herniation through esophageal hiatus
- Sliding HH: Intrathoracic herniation of gastroesophageal (GE) junction & gastric cardia
- Paraesophageal hernia: Normal position of GE junction & intrathoracic gastric herniation

Imaging

- Radiography
  - Well-marginated retrocardiac soft tissue mass
  - May contain air &/or air-fluid level
  - Laterally displaced inferior azygoesophageal recess
- CT
  - Direct visualization of HH & its contents
  - Identification of GE junction in relation to herniated stomach
  - Evaluation of lung in cases of aspiration
- UGI/esophagram is imaging study of choice

Top Differential Diagnoses

- Epiphrenic diverticulum
- Esophagectomy

Clinical Issues

- Sliding HH > 90%
- Paraesophageal hernia < 10%
- Sliding HH
  - Asymptomatic; incidental finding on imaging
  - Symptoms of GE reflux disease (GERD)
  - Regurgitation, dysphagia, hoarseness
- Paraesophageal hernia
  - Ranges from asymptomatic to life-threatening emergency
- Treatment
  - Medical treatment
  - Surgery for symptomatic hernia
  - Prophylactic surgery for paraesophageal hernia

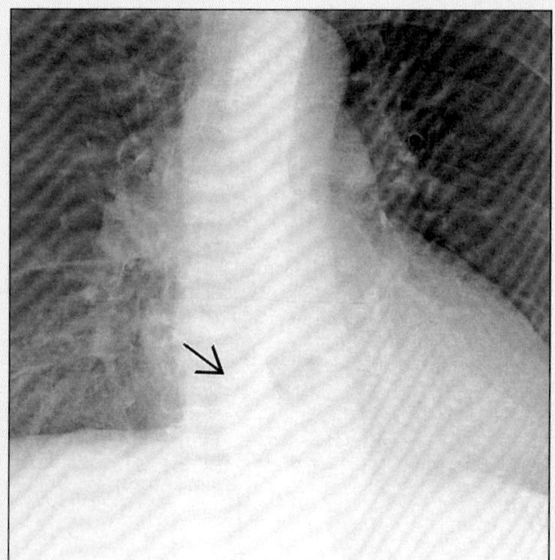

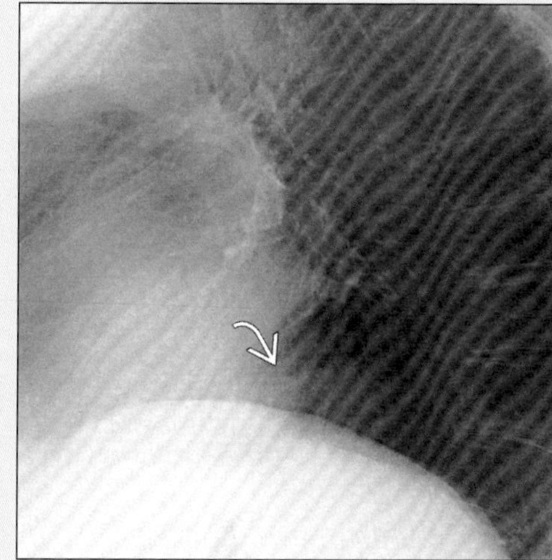

__(Left)__ PA chest radiograph of a 77-year-old woman with an asymptomatic small sliding hiatal hernia ➙ shows lateral displacement of the distal azygoesophageal recess produced by a well-defined soft tissue structure containing gas, which is the hiatal hernia. __(Right)__ Lateral chest radiograph of the same patient shows a heterogeneous retrocardiac opacity with an air-fluid level ➙, consistent with a hiatal hernia. Hiatal hernias typically affect elderly patients. Small hernias may be subtle on radiography.

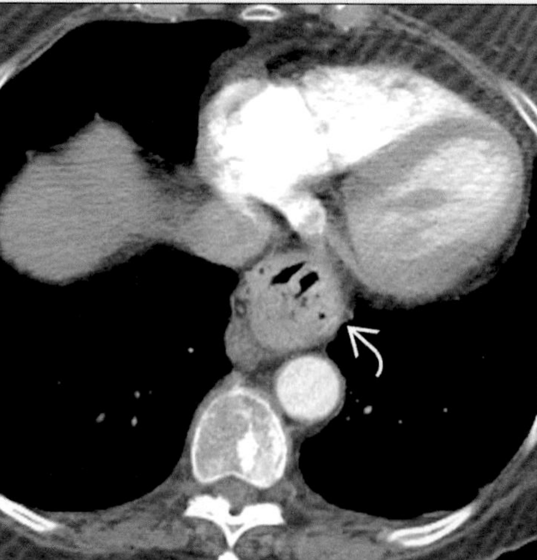

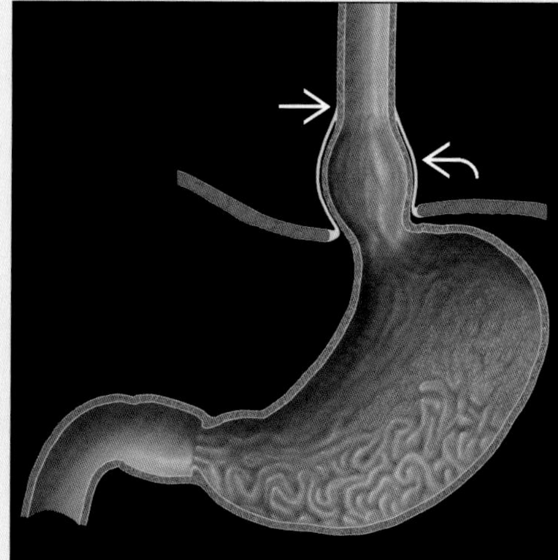

__(Left)__ Axial CECT of the same patient shows a small portion of the stomach ➙ herniating into the thorax through the esophageal hiatus. Identification of intrathoracic gastric folds allows CT diagnosis of small hiatal hernias. __(Right)__ Graphic illustrates the anatomy of sliding (type I) hiatal hernia in which both the gastroesophageal junction ➙ and gastric cardia ➙ herniate into the thorax through the esophageal hiatus. Sliding hiatal hernia is the most common type of hiatal hernia.

HIATAL AND PARAESOPHAGEAL HERNIA

TERMINOLOGY

Abbreviations

- **Hiatal hernia, hiatus hernia** (HH)

Definitions

- **Herniation through esophageal hiatus**
- **Sliding HH**: Intrathoracic herniation of gastroesophageal (GE) junction & gastric cardia
- **Paraesophageal hernia**: Normal position of GE junction & intrathoracic gastric herniation along distal esophagus

IMAGING

General Features

- Best diagnostic clue
  - Air-containing well-defined retrocardiac mass
- Size
  - Range from small HH to intrathoracic stomach

Radiographic Findings

- Well-marginated retrocardiac soft tissue mass
  - May contain air &/or air-fluid level
- May extend to left, right, or bilaterally
- Laterally displaced inferior azygoesophageal recess
- Difficult radiographic diagnosis of paraesophageal hernia or gastric volvulus; requires high index of suspicion

Fluoroscopic Findings

- Esophagram
  - Lower esophageal mucosal "B" ring observed ≥ 2 cm above diaphragmatic hiatus
  - Gastric folds within herniated stomach
  - Sensitivity with single-contrast esophagram: 100%

CT Findings

- Wide esophageal hiatus
- Direct visualization of HH & its contents
  - Stomach, omentum, other abdominal organs
- Identification of GE junction in relation to herniated stomach for diagnosis of paraesophageal hernia
  - Multiplanar reformations may be helpful
- Evaluation of lung parenchyma in cases of aspiration

Imaging Recommendations

- Best imaging tool
  - **UGI/esophagram** is imaging study of choice
  - Esophagram provides optimal mucosal evaluation
    - Evaluation of esophagitis, ulcer, stricture
    - Assessment of suspected gastric volvulus
- Protocol advice
  - CT multiplanar reformations for anatomic analysis

DIFFERENTIAL DIAGNOSIS

Epiphrenic Diverticulum

- Acquired distal esophageal diverticulum
- Association with motility disorders

Esophagectomy

- Protrusion of dilated neoesophagus to right of midline
- Appropriate history, surgical changes

PATHOLOGY

General Features

- Etiology
  - Enlarged esophageal hiatus from increased intraabdominal pressure: Obesity, pregnancy, aging

Staging, Grading, & Classification

- Surgical classification
  - **Type I**: Intrathoracic GE junction & gastric cardia (sliding HH); > **90%**
  - **Type II**: Normal GE junction, intrathoracic gastric fundus (paraesophageal hernia); very rare
  - **Type III**: Intrathoracic GE junction & fundus (paraesophageal hernia); **2nd most common type**
  - **Type IV**: Intrathoracic GE junction & stomach ± volvulus (paraesophageal hernia)

Gross Pathologic & Surgical Features

- **Sliding hiatal hernia**
  - Weakening of phrenoesophageal membrane
  - Intrathoracic GE junction & stomach
  - May spontaneously reduce in erect position
- **Paraesophageal hernia**
  - Normal GE junction location, gastric herniation
  - Herniation of GE junction & stomach
  - Typically nonreducible
  - May be complicated by gastric volvulus

CLINICAL ISSUES

Presentation

- Most common signs/symptoms
  - Sliding HH
    - Asymptomatic; incidental finding on imaging
    - Symptoms of GE reflux disease (GERD)
    - Regurgitation, dysphagia, hoarseness
    - Upper GI bleeding
    - Mass effect on tracheobronchial tree, aspiration
    - Chest pain; may mimic heart disease
  - Paraesophageal hernia: Ranges from asymptomatic to life-threatening emergency

Demographics

- Age
  - Prevalence increases with age
- Gender
  - F > M
- Epidemiology
  - Sliding HH > 90%; paraesophageal hernia < 10%

Natural History & Prognosis

- Acute gastric volvulus: Near 50% mortality

Treatment

- Medical treatment
- Surgery for symptomatic disease
- Prophylactic surgery for paraesophageal hernia

SELECTED REFERENCES

1. Gourgiotis S et al: Acute gastric volvulus: diagnosis and management over 10 years. Dig Surg. 23(3):169-72, 2006
2. Eren S et al: Diaphragmatic hernia: diagnostic approaches with review of the literature. Eur J Radiol. 54(3):448-59, 2005

HIATAL AND PARAESOPHAGEAL HERNIA

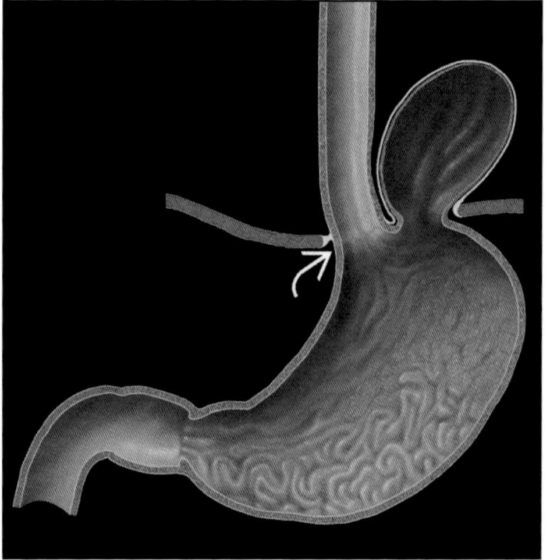

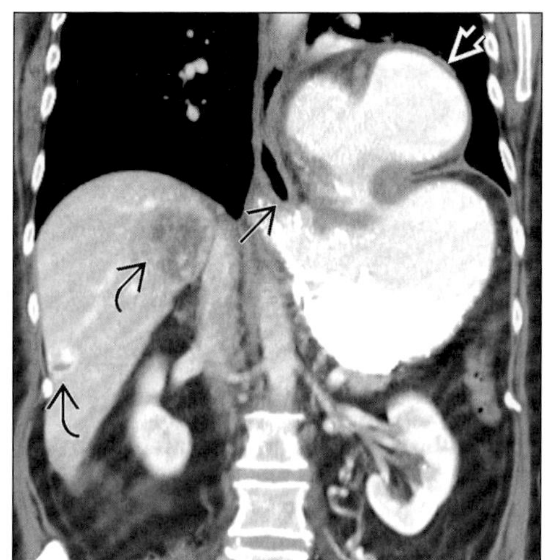

(Left) *Graphic illustrates a type II paraesophageal hernia. The gastroesophageal junction ➔ is in a normal location, and a portion of the stomach herniates into the thorax alongside the distal esophagus.* ***(Right)*** *Coronal CECT of a patient with a moderate type II paraesophageal hernia shows the normal position of the distal esophagus ➔ and gastroesophageal junction. The gastric fundus ➔ herniates into the thorax in a paraesophageal location. Note incidental hepatic hemangiomas ➔.*

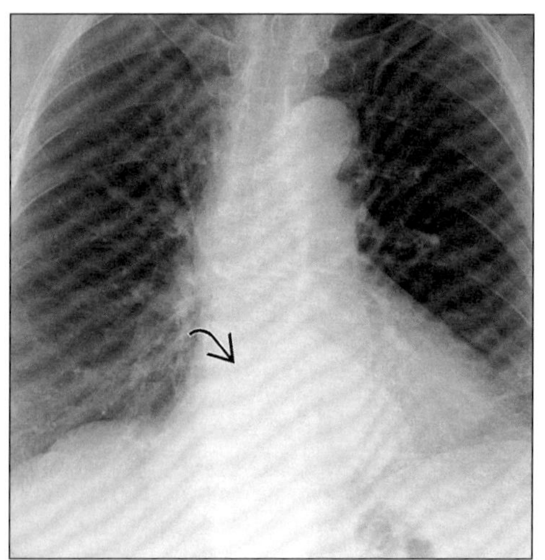

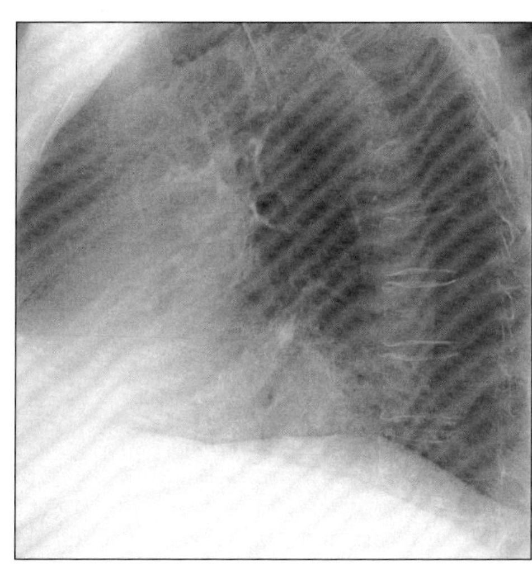

(Left) *PA chest radiograph of an asymptomatic elderly woman with a moderate hiatal hernia shows a retrocardiac mass producing lateral displacement of the inferior aspect of the azygoesophageal recess ➔. Although the lesion does not contain gas, the morphologic features are characteristic of hiatal hernia.* ***(Right)*** *Lateral chest radiograph of the same patient shows a retrocardiac soft tissue mass with a small intrinsic air bubble representing gas within the herniated stomach.*

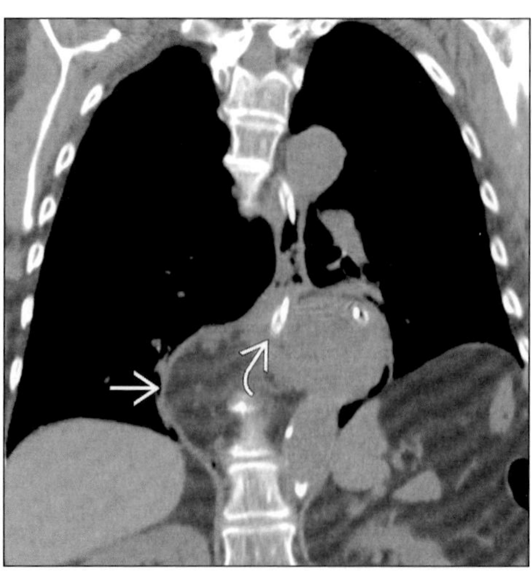

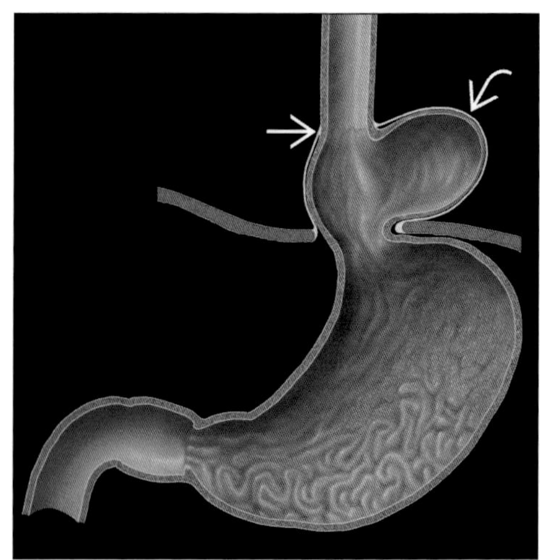

(Left) *Coronal NECT of the same patient shows an enteric tube that demonstrates the intrathoracic location of the gastroesophageal junction ➔ in this type III paraesophageal hernia. Intrathoracic omental fat produces lateral displacement of the inferior azygoesophageal recess ➔.* ***(Right)*** *Graphic demonstrates the anatomy of type III paraesophageal hernia in which both the gastroesophageal junction ➔ and a portion of the stomach ➔ herniate into the thorax through the esophageal hiatus.*

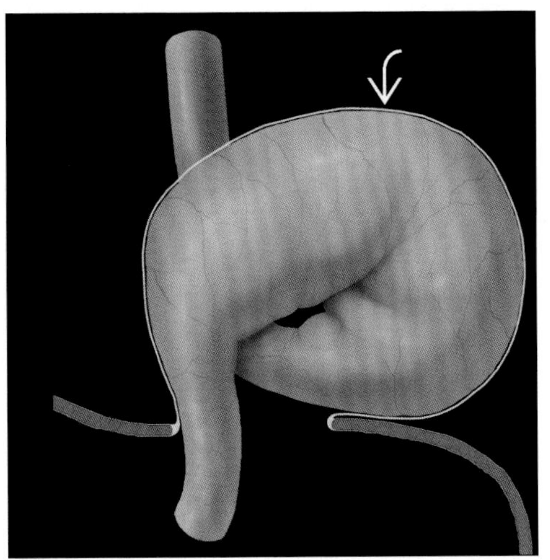

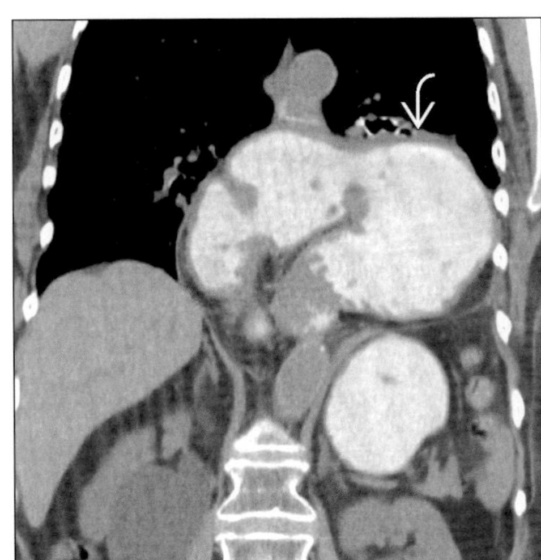

(Left) *Graphic demonstrates the morphologic features of type IV paraesophageal hernia with an intrathoracic stomach, an organoaxial gastric volvulus, and a cranial location of the greater curvature* ➔ *of the stomach.* ***(Right)*** *Coronal CECT of an asymptomatic elderly woman with a large type IV paraesophageal hernia shows a completely intrathoracic stomach with organoaxial morphology and cranial location of the greater curvature of the stomach* ➔*.*

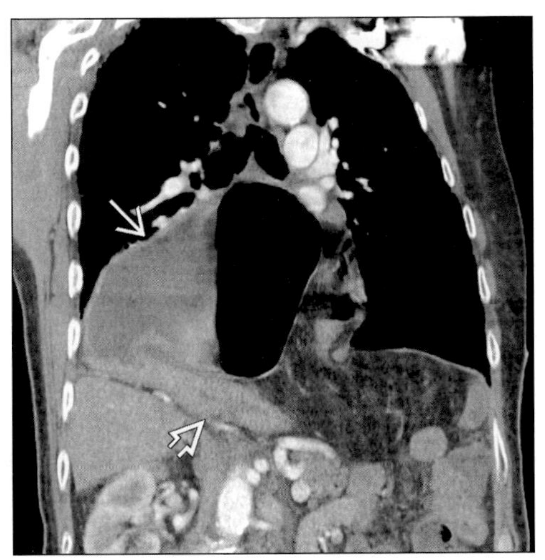

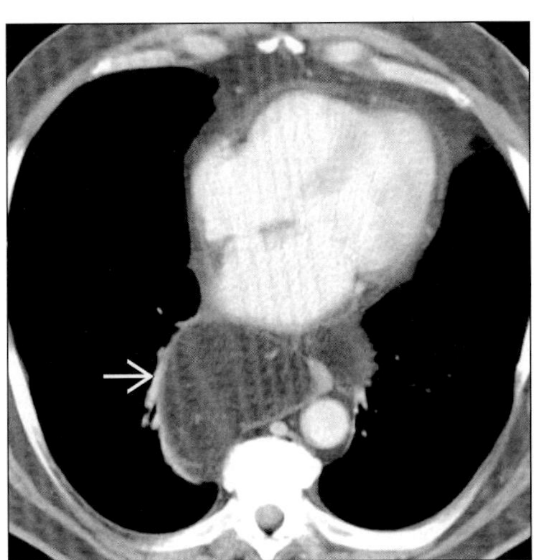

(Left) *Coronal CECT of a patient with a large strangulated type IV paraesophageal hernia shows a dilated fluid-filled proximal stomach* ➔ *and a collapsed distal stomach* ➔ *due to obstruction.* ***(Right)*** *Axial CECT of an asymptomatic patient with hiatal hernia shows herniation of omental fat* ➔ *through the esophageal hiatus. Hiatal hernia results from weakness of the gastrophrenoesophageal membrane and may result in herniation of fat &/or bowel.*

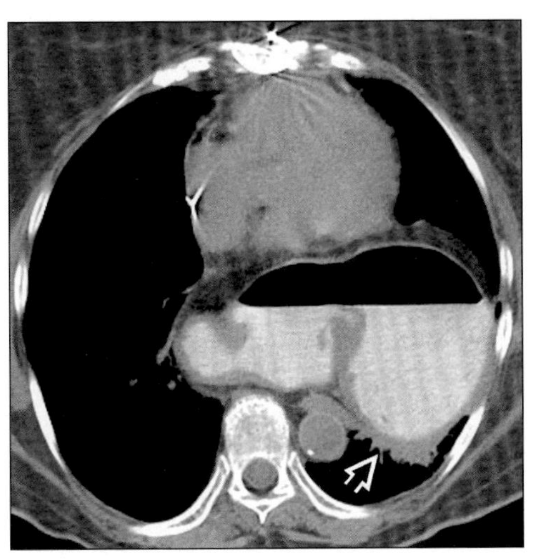

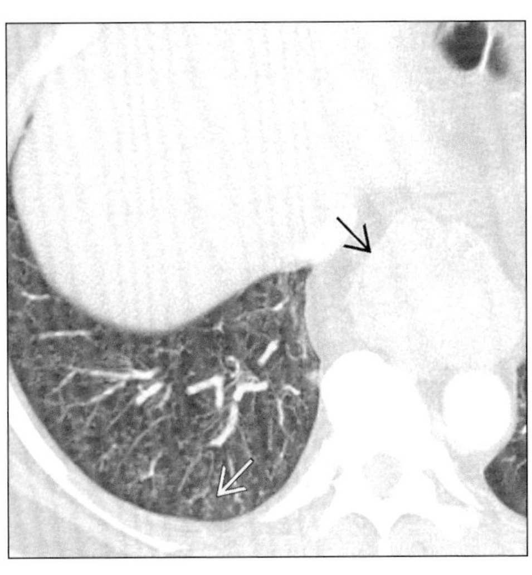

(Left) *Axial CECT of a patient with a large intrathoracic stomach shows marked gastric distention that produces mass effect on the heart and compressive atelectasis* ➔ *of the basal segments of the left lower lobe.* ***(Right)*** *Axial CECT of a patient with a moderately sized hiatal hernia* ➔ *shows profuse right lower lobe tree-in-bud opacities* ➔*, consistent with cellular bronchiolitis from chronic aspiration. Hiatal hernias may produce pulmonary abnormalities related to mass effect or aspiration.*

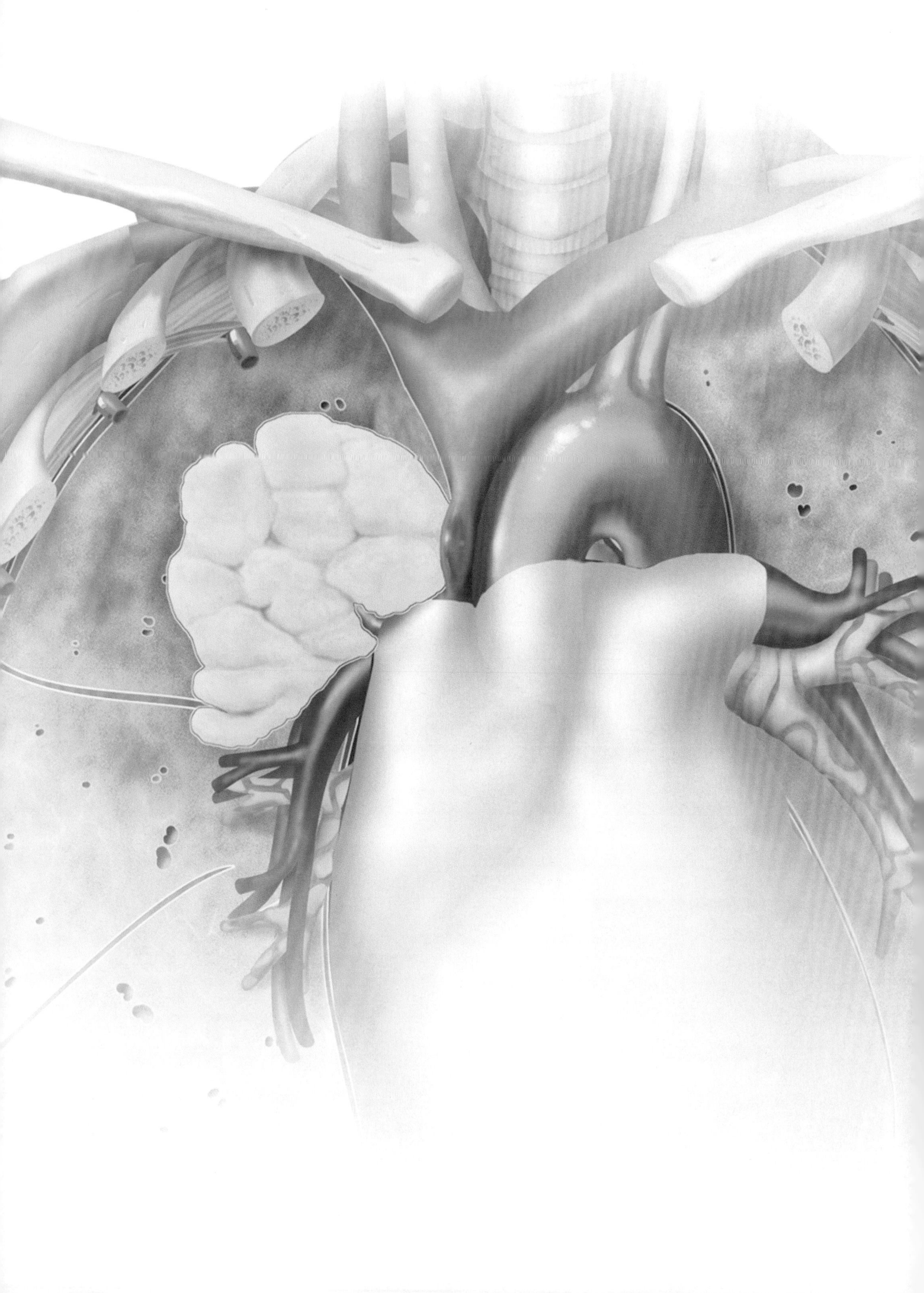

SECTION 9
Cardiovascular Disorders

Introduction and Overview

Diseases of the Aorta and Great Vessels

Pulmonary Edema

Pulmonary Hypertension and Thromboembolic Disease

Diseases of the Heart and Pericardium

Cardiovascular Neoplasms

APPROACH TO CARDIOVASCULAR DISORDERS

Introduction

The chest contains a large number of complex organs and systems. The cardiovascular system is a significant component of the thorax and may exhibit a variety of disease processes. Among these, coronary artery disease carries the highest mortality in the United States. While many cardiothoracic pathologies are well understood by practitioners of cardiothoracic and general radiology, many cardiovascular diseases have been historically considered entities outside the realm of thoracic radiology and are often evaluated and managed by nonradiologists, specifically cardiologists.

Many factors contribute to the lack of understanding of cardiovascular disorders among radiologists. While chest radiography is an excellent first imaging study for the assessment of cardiovascular disease, it often lacks sufficient sensitivity for definitive diagnosis. For example, although chest radiography can provide indirect evidence of coronary artery disease, the findings are often nonspecific (e.g., cardiomegaly, pulmonary venous hypertension). Direct evidence of critical abnormalities such as hemodynamically significant coronary artery atherosclerotic plaques is not visible on radiography and requires advanced techniques for diagnosis.

Historically, assessment of many cardiovascular disorders was performed outside the radiology department over a period of time when other imaging techniques were more appropriate (e.g., coronary angiography). It was not until multidetector CT was commercially introduced in the late 1990s that radiologists became involved in the diagnosis of many cardiovascular disorders. This noninvasive technology provides exquisite anatomic detail similar to that provided by conventional angiography. Simultaneous with the development of multidetector computed tomography, a tremendous evolution of MR technology took place, placing the comprehensive assessment of cardiovascular disorders within the realm of diagnostic radiology.

The boom of these technologies has had such an impact that today, cardiovascular imaging is an integral part of cardiothoracic radiology, and in some institutions it is even a separate subspecialty of radiology. Because the heart and great vessels are anatomically and functionally integrated to the rest of the organs and structures in the thorax, separate imaging assessment is not logical. The reintegration of cardiac and thoracic imaging and an increased understanding of cardiovascular disease can only have a positive impact on advancing and optimizing patient care.

Acute Aortic Syndrome (AAS) and Thoracic Aortic Aneurysms

The term **AAS** refers to a heterogeneous group of disorders that manifest with chest pain and share a common risk factor: Arterial hypertension. The AAS concept was introduced in an attempt to clarify the pathophysiology of **penetrating aortic ulcers** and **intramural hematomas** and their relationship with **aortic dissection**, as both lesions can result in dissection. However, although penetrating aortic ulcers can progress to intramural hematoma, the reverse is not the case. The various pathophysiologic pathways seen in AAS and the various terms used to describe the component lesions of the syndrome often create confusion. Furthermore, **complicated thoracic aortic aneurysms** also frequently manifest with chest pain and hypertension and can be clinically identical to AAS. Therefore, although complicated aortic aneurysms are not strictly included in the definition of AAS, they need to be considered when discussing AAS. It should be noted that statistically more patients presenting with chest pain have **coronary syndrome** than either AAS or complicated aortic aneurysm. The differentiation can frequently be made based on clinical grounds and laboratory findings, but this may not be the case for every patient. Finally, and to complicate matters further, coronary syndrome may coexist with AAS and complicated aortic aneurysm.

The imaging evaluation of hypertensive patients with acute chest pain begins with chest radiography. Although chest radiography is considered insensitive as a negative chest radiograph does not exclude aortic pathology, radiography can be very helpful. For example, when serial studies are available, important interval changes can be documented. These include highly suggestive findings of aortic pathology such as interval aortic enlargement, new aortic contour abnormality, and pathologic displacement of aortic intimal calcifications. In patients with contained aortic rupture of any etiology, chest radiography may demonstrate indirect signs of acute aortic bleeding such as mediastinal widening, displacement of mediastinal structures, and pleural effusion.

CT and MR remain the cornerstones of definitive diagnosis of AAS. Both techniques are equivalent in their ability to demonstrate acute aortic pathology and its complications. CT is generally considered more widely available and is more practical than MR for imaging acutely ill subjects since image acquisition takes only a few seconds. Optimal CT evaluation of AAS requires the performance of unenhanced CT (NECT) prior to performing contrast-enhanced CT (CECT). For example, intramural hematoma can only be diagnosed with certainty on NECT, and there are pitfalls related to CECT that mimic extravasation and can be easily verified only if NECT is available. Intramural hematoma manifests as a crescentic hyperdensity of the thoracic aortic wall. Penetrating aortic ulcer often manifests as a focal outpouching of contrast that extends beyond the expected aortic confines. Aortic dissection classically exhibits an endoluminal intimal flap. Finally, thoracic aortic aneurysms manifest with fusiform, saccular, irregular, or diffuse dilatations of the aorta. All these aortic disorders can be associated with aortic rupture, which often results in sudden death shortly after symptom onset. The few patients that reach the hospital often have a contained aortic rupture or slow aortic bleeding. CT often depicts the site of rupture and a variety of other findings, including mediastinal hematoma, hemothorax, and contrast extravasation in the mediastinum, pericardium, &/or pleura.

Nonacute Aortic Pathology

Several chronic disorders may also affect the thoracic aorta. An understanding of the pathophysiology and imaging features of these entities is important as they may simulate acute aortic pathology or AAS. Nonacute aortic disorders include vasculitis and neoplasia. **Takayasu arteritis** and **giant cell arteritis** are the most common vasculitides that affect the aorta. Both CT and MR are equivalent in their ability to demonstrate imaging abnormalities consistent with vasculitis, including vessel wall thickening and luminal stenosis or dilatation. Neoplastic processes of the aorta are rather rare, but when present are almost always malignant. The most common malignant neoplasm of the aorta is angiosarcoma. It should be noted that primary aortic malignancy may be difficult to differentiate from intraluminal thrombus. In these cases, contrast-enhanced MR can be helpful.

Pulmonary Thromboembolic Disease (Pulmonary Embolism [PE])

It is difficult to summarize current concepts related to imaging of thromboembolic disease since the amount of medical literature on this subject is overwhelming. Nevertheless, it is important to emphasize several generally accepted concepts. CTA of the pulmonary arteries remains the cornerstone for the diagnosis of PE. Ventilation-perfusion scintigraphy (VQ scan) is as good as CTA, but the latter provides the advantage of simultaneous evaluation of the entire thorax for other causes of chest pain. The PIOPED II investigation showed that combining CTA with venous-phase imaging (CTA-CTV) (i.e., from the inferior vena cava confluence through the popliteal veins) results in a higher sensitivity for diagnosis with similar specificity. However, this is not a protocol used in general practice given the fact that compression Doppler lower extremity sonography is as effective as CTV in the diagnosis of venous thrombosis.

It is generally accepted that CTA is overused in the evaluation of thromboembolic disease since the positivity rate remains very low. In addition, CTA delivers a not negligible dose of ionizing radiation. The problem may relate to inconsistent or suboptimal use of clinical criteria for the diagnosis of PE and the subjective overestimation of the probability of PE. Future research on this subject will likely focus on establishing better patient selection criteria that will hopefully allow a more rational use of this excellent imaging technique.

During the last decade, concerns have been raised regarding the amount of ionizing radiation associated with CT scanning and its deleterious effects. An increased radiation dose is associated with an increased risk of carcinogenesis. Children and young women (particularly pregnant women) are among the groups at higher risk. One of the most serious concerns is the development of breast carcinoma in association with radiation delivered to the breast during CTA. Several measures have been adopted to decrease this risk. Bismuth breast shields, which decrease the radiation dose to the breast without qualitative or quantitative changes in image quality, are increasingly employed. Another strategy is to perform a VQ scan in patients with suspected PE, particularly if the chest radiograph is normal. While the amount of radiation may be similar with both techniques, the amount of radiation delivered to the breast during scintigraphy is likely much less than that associated with CTA.

Cardiac Valvular Disease

The accurate assessment of cardiac valvular disease is an excellent example of the impact of new technology in cardiothoracic diagnosis. Although several radiographic abnormalities related to valvular disease are extensively described in the classic imaging literature, it was not until echocardiography and MR became widely available that objective information was extracted from imaging evaluations. These technologies allowed quantitative and qualitative evaluation of cardiovascular disorders. Such quantitative information allows identification of disease progression and helps establish management strategies for patients with valvular disease. While color Doppler echocardiography continues to be the overall imaging modality of choice, several technical limitations are recognized (e.g., poor acoustic windows, complex anatomy) including its inability to fully quantify valvular regurgitation. For this reason, MR has emerged as an excellent noninvasive diagnostic tool capable of fully quantifying all parameters needed to monitor valvular disease and plan surgery when needed. While currently the role of MR is yet to be officially defined, it is well recognized to be an invaluable tool when echocardiography is inconclusive. Finally, with the advent of coronary CTA within the last decade, some early reports on the assessment of valvular function have shown promise.

Cardiac and Pericardial Masses

In general, cardiac and pericardial masses are uncommon. **Metastatic disease** is the most common neoplastic process affecting the heart and pericardium. Less common pericardial tumors include benign neoplasms (e.g., teratoma, solitary fibrous tumor, hemangioma) and primary malignancies (e.g., mesothelioma). On the other hand, less common cardiac masses include benign lesions (e.g., myxoma, papillary fibroelastoma, cardiac rhabdomyoma, fibroma, lipoma, lipomatous hypertrophy of the interatrial septum, paraganglioma, hemangioma, lymphangioma) and malignancies (e.g., angiosarcoma, leiomyosarcoma, rhabdomyosarcoma, lymphoma).

Echocardiography and MR continue to be the mainstay of cardiac imaging diagnosis. Echocardiography is readily available, portable, fast, and inexpensive. However it has limitations such as poor acoustic windows in patients with large body habitus or in the presence of calcification. An important advantage of multidetector CT over other modalities is its consistent capability to demonstrate calcification. However, acquisition of cardiac images results in significant radiation to the chest and often requires the use of iodinated contrast. MR is considered the gold standard for the evaluation of pericardial and cardiac masses. Although the main advantage of MR is its superior tissue characterization, it also has other advantages, including no limitations regarding acoustic windows, absence of ionizing radiation, and the use of a safer contrast medium (i.e., gadolinium).

Selected References

1. Revel MP et al: Pulmonary embolism during pregnancy: diagnosis with lung scintigraphy or CT angiography? Radiology. 258(2):590-8, 2011
2. Vilacosta I et al: Acute aortic syndrome: a new look at an old conundrum. Postgrad Med J. 86(1011):52-61, 2010
3. Lohan DG et al: MR imaging of the thoracic aorta. Magn Reson Imaging Clin N Am. 16(2):213-34, viii, 2008
4. Stein PD et al: Multidetector computed tomography for acute pulmonary embolism. N Engl J Med. 354(22):2317-27, 2006

(Left) Axial CECT of a patient with type A aortic dissection shows intimal flaps in the ascending ➔ and descending aorta ➔. *(Right)* Composite image with axial (left) and oblique coronal (right) CECT shows a contrast outpouching ➔ extending beyond the confines of the aortic wall, consistent with a penetrating aortic ulcer. Penetrating aortic ulcers may remain stable or grow and may be associated with intramural hematoma, aortic dissection, or aortic pseudoaneurysm (contained aortic rupture).

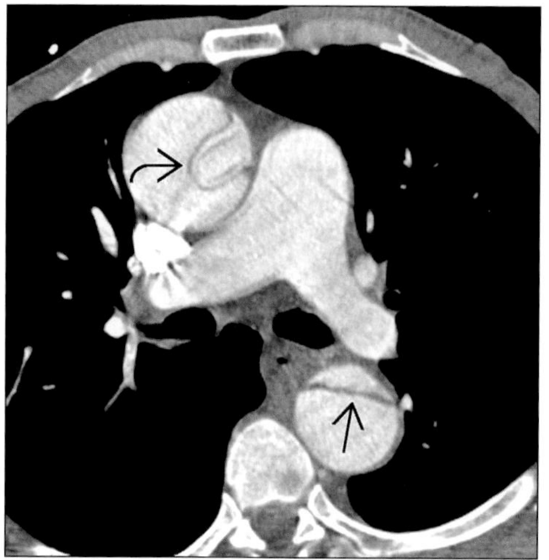

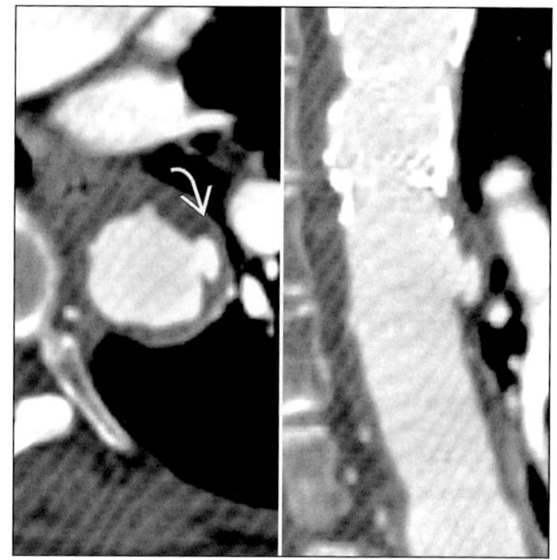

(Left) Composite image with axial NECT (left) and CECT (right) shows a type A intramural hematoma manifesting with crescentic high attenuation ➔ that mimics wall thickening ➔ on CECT. A descending aorta penetrating ulcer ➔ is associated with extraluminal crescentic hyperdensity ➔ representing a contained rupture. *(Right)* Composite image with axial NECT (left) and CECT (right) shows a saddle embolus ➔ in the pulmonary trunk. Central pulmonary emboli are rarely visible on NECT.

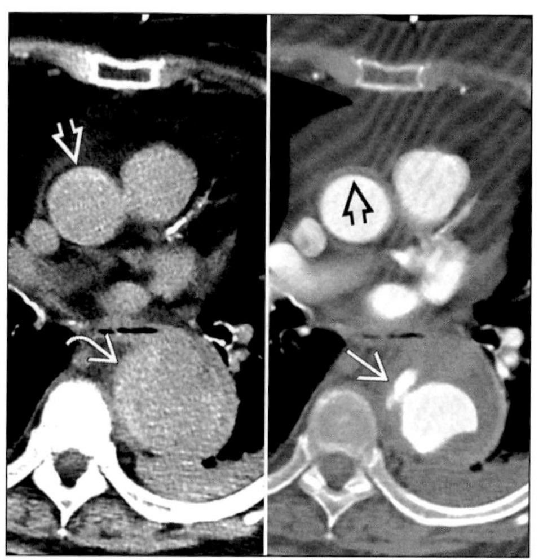

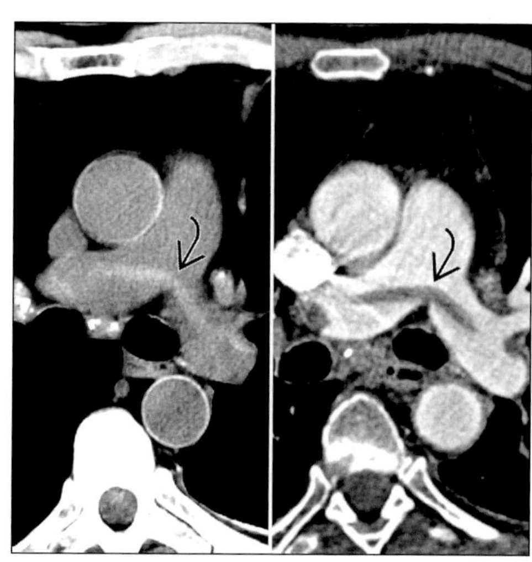

(Left) Axial CECT demonstrates bilateral pulmonary emboli ➔ with marked right atrial and right ventricular enlargement. The right ventricle ➔ is at least twice as wide as the left ventricle, consistent with right ventricular strain. *(Right)* Composite image with axial CECT (left) and pulmonary artery DSA (right) shows an intimal pulmonary artery angiosarcoma manifesting with a pulmonary artery filling defect ➔ on CT and DSA with obliteration of the right lower lobe pulmonary artery.

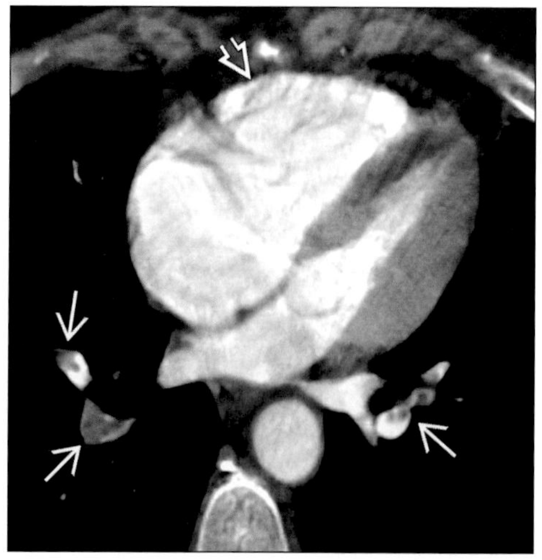

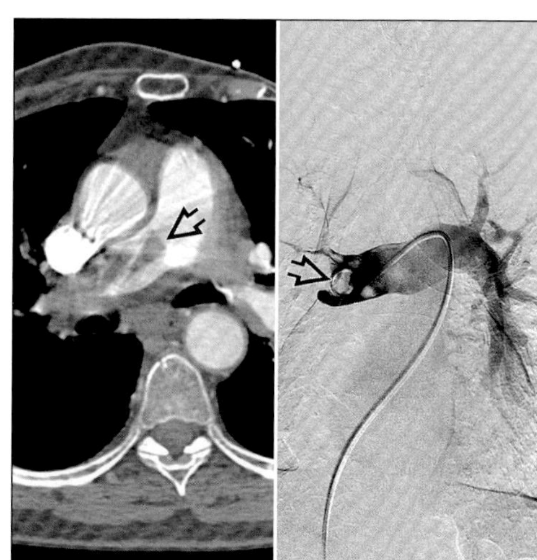

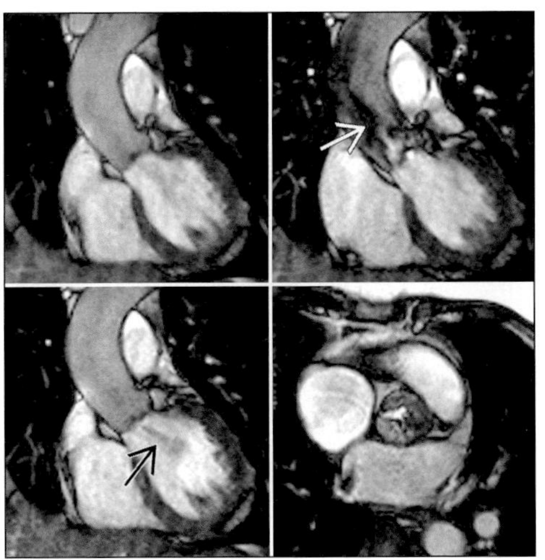
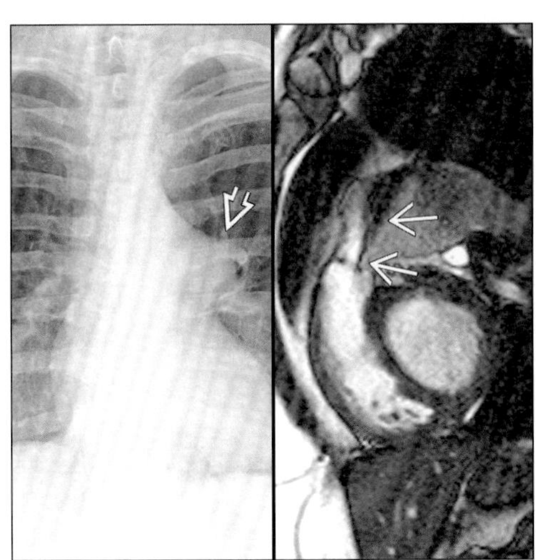

(Left) *Composite image with coronal and axial cine MR of a patient with aortic stenosis shows (clockwise from bottom left) diastolic regurgitation →, the coapted aortic valve, a systolic ejection jet ➡, and axial MR of the aortic valve showing limited aperture due to partially fused leaflets.* ***(Right)*** *Composite image with PA chest radiograph (left) and cine MR (right) of a patient with pulmonic stenosis shows an enlarged pulmonary trunk ➡ and a systolic pulmonic ejection jet ➡ on SSFP MR.*

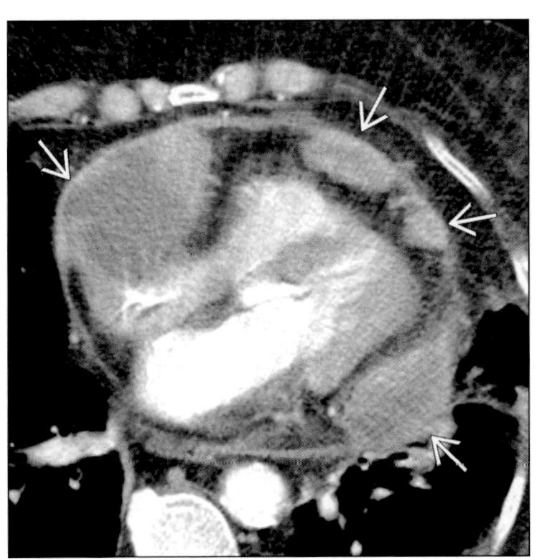
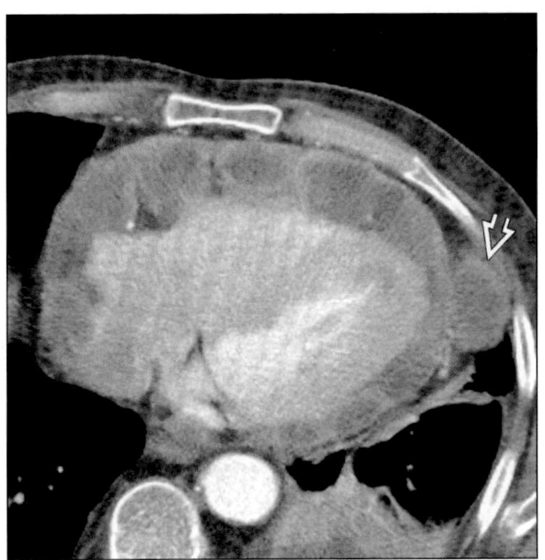

(Left) *Axial CECT of a patient with metastatic lung cancer shows heterogeneously enhancing nodules and masses ➡ of the parietal pericardium, consistent with pericardial metastases.* ***(Right)*** *Axial CECT of a patient with pericardial tamponade physiology from pericardial mesothelioma shows heterogeneously enhancing, likely necrotic, pericardial nodules and necrotic juxtacardiac lymphadenopathy ➡, which was biopsied percutaneously for histologic diagnosis.*

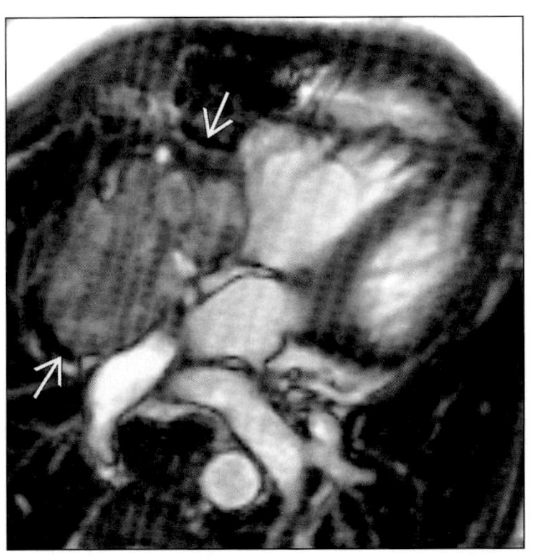
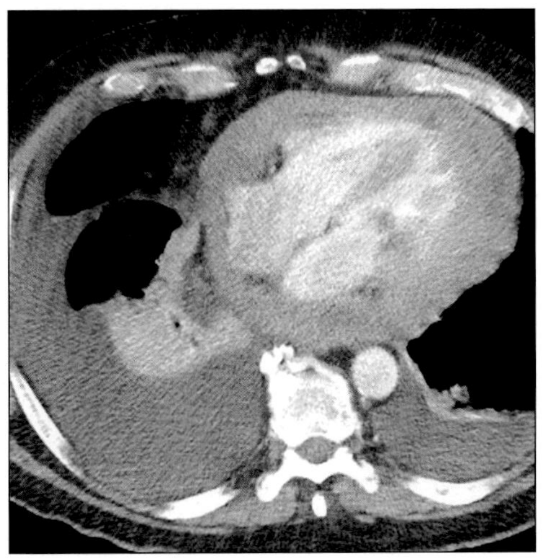

(Left) *Axial oblique SSFP MR of a patient with a right atrial angiosarcoma shows a heterogeneous mass ➡ that obliterates the right atrial lumen.* ***(Right)*** *Axial CECT of a patient with cardiac rhabdomyosarcoma shows soft tissue encasing the heart and bilateral pleural effusions. While metastases are the most common cardiac and pericardial malignancies, mesothelioma and angiosarcoma are the most common primary malignancies of the pericardium and heart, respectively.*

ATHEROSCLEROSIS

Key Facts

Terminology

- Lipid deposition on arterial walls leading to thickening, hardening, & occlusion

Imaging

- Affects medium-sized & large arteries
- Most common in descending aorta
- Predilection for vessel branch points
- Radiography
  - Vessel wall calcification
- NECT
  - Calcified atherosclerotic plaques
  - Penetrating ulcer; soft tissue beyond aortic wall
  - Hyperdense crescentic wall thickening: Intramural hematoma (IMH)
- CTA
  - Noncalcified (> 4 mm) & calcified plaques
  - Aneurysm: Often related to atherosclerosis
  - Penetrating ulcer vs. ulcerated plaque
- MR
  - Plaque characterization: Lipid hyperintense on T1WI, hypointense on T2WI
  - Equivalent to CECT for complication assessment

Top Differential Diagnoses

- Acute aortic syndrome (AAS)
- Thoracic aortic aneurysm
- Takayasu & giant cell arteritis
- Aortic sarcoma or metastases

Clinical Issues

- Asymptomatic
- Acute aortic syndrome: Chest pain from penetrating ulcer, IMH, aortic dissection
- Visceral/extremity ischemia; branch stenoses, emboli
- Treatment: Risk factor modification, medical or surgical therapy for complications

*(**Left**) Graphic demonstrates the morphologic features of aortic atherosclerosis. Deposition of fat, cholesterol, and other substances produces irregular plaque on the aortic intima, which can result in thrombus and ulceration with or without intramural hematoma. (**Right**) Macroscopic cut section of the thoracic aorta shows an irregular intimal surface. Lipid and cholesterol deposition result in irregular plaque and ulceration ➙. In turn, ulceration can lead to intramural hematoma. (Courtesy A. Burke, MD.)*

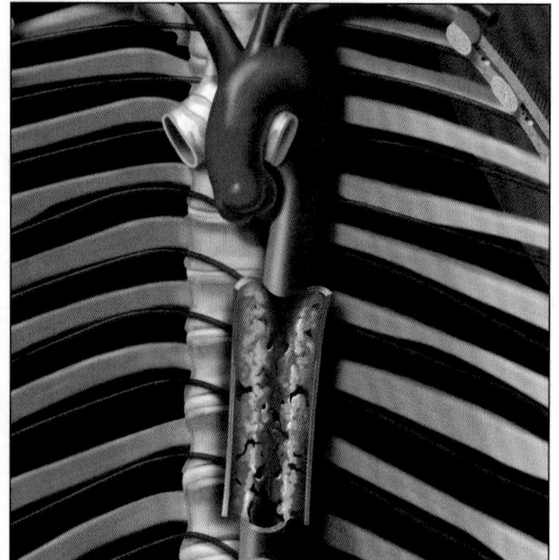

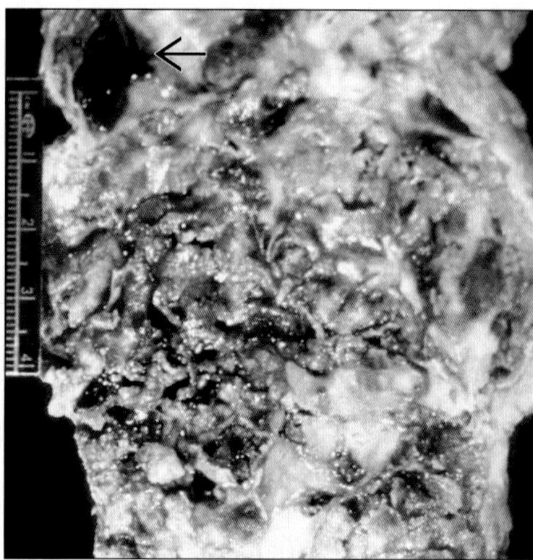

*(**Left**) PA chest radiograph of a patient with atherosclerosis shows intimal calcification ➦ of the aortic arch and descending aorta, which increases the risk of ischemic stroke. (**Right**) Lateral chest radiograph of the same patient shows extensive aortic intimal calcification ➔ secondary to calcified atherosclerotic plaques. Calcified plaque is the most common manifestation of atherosclerosis on radiography and is often associated with atherosclerosis elsewhere, including the coronary arteries.*

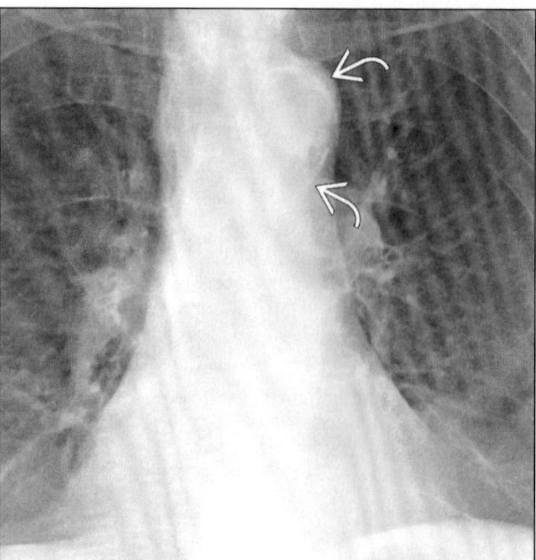

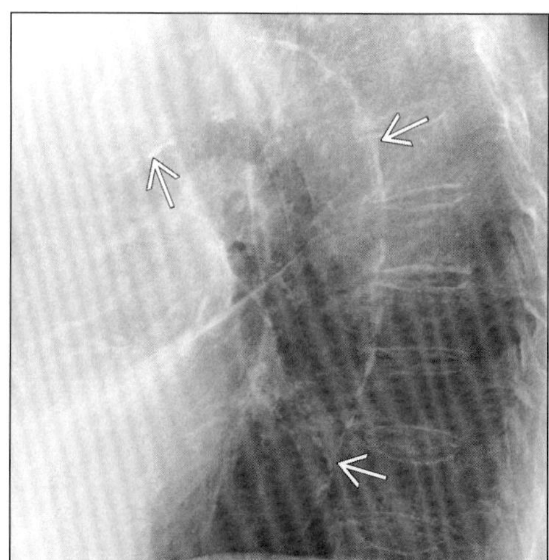

ATHEROSCLEROSIS

TERMINOLOGY

Synonyms

- **Arteriosclerosis**

Definitions

- Lipid deposition on arterial walls leading to thickening, hardening, & occlusion

IMAGING

General Features

- Location
  - Affects **medium-sized & large arteries**
  - **Most common in descending aorta**
  - Predilection for vessel branch points
  - Ascending aorta more often involved in diabetes & familial hypercholesterolemia
  - Aortic root may be involved in familial hypercholesterolemia
  - Syphilis causes ascending aortic atherosclerosis

Radiographic Findings

- Radiography
  - Visualization of **vessel wall calcification**
  - Pseudoaneurysm from penetrating aortic ulcer > 2-3 cm; may manifest as focal mass or focal aortic dilatation
  - **Coronary atherosclerosis**
    - Calcified coronary plaques occasionally visible
    - Coronary plaques imply higher risk of hemodynamically significant stenosis
  - Calcified atherosclerotic plaques along central pulmonary arteries
    - Longstanding severe pulmonary hypertension
    - Eisenmenger syndrome
    - Chronic thromboembolic pulmonary hypertension
    - ASD association

CT Findings

- NECT
  - **Calcified atherosclerotic plaques**
    - **Coronary artery calcium** (CAC)
      - Marker of atherosclerotic burden
      - CAC associated with ↑ risk of stroke, myocardial infarction, revascularization & death
      - Absence of CAC: High negative predictive value for occurrence of future events, does not exclude coronary stenosis
  - Penetrating ulcer suggested by soft tissue extending beyond presumed aortic wall
  - Hyperdense crescentic wall thickening indicates coexistent intramural hematoma (IMH)
- CTA
  - Noncalcified (> 4 mm) & calcified plaques
  - **Aneurysm**: Often related to atherosclerosis, dilatation > 50% of normal vessel diameter
  - **Penetrating aortic ulcer**
    - Contrast extends beyond aortic wall confines
    - Adjacent soft tissue often related to contained rupture (pseudoaneurysm)
    - Penetrating aortic ulcer may be associated with IMH; crescentic or concentric aortic wall thickening
  - **Ulcerated plaque**: Contrast does not extend beyond aortic wall confines
- Cardiac gated CTA
  - Does not replace diagnostic coronary angiography but is as sensitive as conventional angiography
  - Exclusion of stenoses in patients with low pretest probability of significant disease
  - Presence & extent of coronary artery disease on coronary CTA; strong, independent predictors of cardiovascular events
  - Patients with low-attenuation plaques (< 30 HU) & positive vessel remodeling (outward expansion) are at higher risk of acute coronary syndrome
    - Plaque consistency: Lipid core (11 ± 12 HU), fibrous plaque (78 ± 21 HU), calcified plaque (516 ± 198 HU)
    - Positive vessel remodeling: Enlarged coronary diameter in relation to plaque area

MR Findings

- Plaque characterization
  - **Lipid component**
    - Hyperintense on T1WI, hypointense on T2WI
    - Lipid-rich plaques tend to be more inflamed
  - **Fibrocellular components**
    - Hyperintense on T1WI & T2WI
  - **Calcium deposits**
    - Hypointense on T1WI & T2WI
- MR equivalent to CECT for complication assessment

Ultrasonographic Findings

- Intravascular ultrasonography
  - High spatial resolution for assessment of atherosclerotic plaque, its components & vascular remodeling
  - Supportive technique during conventional angiography
  - Used to follow plaque progression

Angiographic Findings

- Plaques: Filling defects or irregular luminal surface
- Penetrating ulcer: Focal contrast collection outside aortic wall confines
- Often required before therapeutic stenting or endarterectomy

Nuclear Medicine Findings

- PET/CT
  - Symptomatic & unstable plaques more FDG avid

DIFFERENTIAL DIAGNOSIS

Acute Aortic Syndrome (AAS)

- Classic aortic dissection, incomplete dissection, penetrating aortic ulcer, intramural hematoma
- May lead to aortic rupture
- Aortic dissection
  - Intimomedial flap separates true & false lumina
  - Intimal calcification displaced from aortic wall
  - Blood flow within false lumen in most cases
- Intramural hematoma (IMH)
  - Smoothly marginated high-attenuation crescentic or circumferential aortic wall thickening with variable longitudinal extension on NECT
  - Penetrating aortic ulcer with IMH often coexists with diffuse aortic atherosclerosis

ATHEROSCLEROSIS

Thoracic Aortic Aneurysm

- Saccular aortic aneurysm may be indistinguishable from pseudoaneurysm due to penetrating aortic ulcer
- Acute penetrating aortic ulcer with contained rupture (pseudoaneurysm) appears as focal peripheral crescentic hemorrhage on NECT
- Predisposing conditions: Atherosclerosis, trauma, infectious aortitis, cystic medial necrosis, bicuspid aortic valve, hypertension, smoking

Takayasu & Giant Cell Arteritis

- Concentric or circumferential wall thickening of large & medium-sized arteries with or without aneurysm
- Scattered areas of vascular stenoses
- May simulate IMH on CECT
- Aortic wall thickening not hyperdense on NECT

Aortic Sarcoma or Metastases

- Extremely rare; difficult to differentiate from exophytic atherosclerotic plaque
- Noncalcified discrete aortic wall soft tissue mass
- Frequent hematogenous metastases

PATHOLOGY

General Features

- Etiology
  - Plaque results from build up of lipid, cholesterol, & other substances on vessel walls
  - Plaques narrow & stiffen arteries, resulting in blood flow obstruction
  - Plaques may break off, embolize to smaller vessels & produce tissue damage or death (e.g., myocardial infarction, stroke)
  - Plaques may tear with clot formation that may block blood flow & produce tissue damage (e.g., myocardial infarction, stroke) or death
  - Plaques weaken vessel wall, may result in aneurysm
  - Complicated atherosclerotic plaque may lead to aortic ulceration ± intramural hematoma
- Genetics
  - Familial hypercholesteremia is major risk factor

Gross Pathologic & Surgical Features

- **Aneurysm**: Dilatation in setting of type IV, V, or VI lesions, layered luminal thrombi fill aneurysm to approximate original lumen diameter

Microscopic Features

- Precursors of symptomatic atherosclerosis
  - **Type I (initial lesion)**: Microscopic; isolated foamy macrophages, minimal intimal changes, most frequent in infants & children
  - **Type II (fatty streaks)**: Macroscopic; stratified layers of foamy macrophages, primarily contain cholesterol, more frequent in children
  - **Type III (preatheroma)**: Extracellular lipid droplets & particles form among smooth muscle cells
- Atherosclerosis
  - **Type IV (atheroma)**: Macroscopic; dense accumulation of extracellular lipid (lipid core), does not narrow vascular lumen, may develop fissures, hematoma, &/or thrombus
  - **Type V (fibroatheroma, calcific lesion, fibrotic lesion)**: Prominent fibrous connective tissue, may develop fissures, hematoma, &/or thrombus
  - **Type VI (complicated lesion or plaque)**: Type IV & type V lesions with disruption of lesion surface, hematoma or hemorrhage, & thrombotic deposits

CLINICAL ISSUES

Presentation

- Most common signs/symptoms
  - Asymptomatic
- Other signs/symptoms
  - Acute aortic syndrome: Chest pain from penetrating ulcer, IMH, incomplete dissection, classic dissection
  - Visceral or extremity ischemia from branch stenoses or emboli
- Clinical profile
  - Risk factors: Diabetes mellitus, heavy alcohol use, high blood pressure, hypercholesterolemia, high fat diet, increasing age, obesity, personal or family history of heart disease, smoking

Demographics

- Age
  - Correlates with advancing age; very common in elderly
- Gender
  - M > F
- Epidemiology
  - Common in Western cultures
  - Less common in Asia & Africa: Dietary or genetic factors may play a role

Natural History & Prognosis

- Atherosclerosis progresses with age
- Natural history & prognosis related to onset of complications

Treatment

- Modification of risk factors
- Medical or surgical therapy for complications

DIAGNOSTIC CHECKLIST

Consider

- Coronary artery disease in setting of substantial aortic atherosclerotic disease

SELECTED REFERENCES

1. Achenbach S: Computed tomography coronary angiography. J Am Coll Cardiol. 48(10):1919-28, 2006
2. Raggi P et al: Atherosclerotic plaque imaging: contemporary role in preventive cardiology. Arch Intern Med. 165(20):2345-53, 2005
3. Fayad ZA et al: Magnetic resonance imaging and computed tomography in assessment of atherosclerotic plaque. Curr Atheroscler Rep. 6(3):232-42, 2004
4. Macura KJ et al: Pathogenesis in acute aortic syndromes: aortic dissection, intramural hematoma, and penetrating atherosclerotic aortic ulcer. AJR Am J Roentgenol. 181(2):309-16, 2003

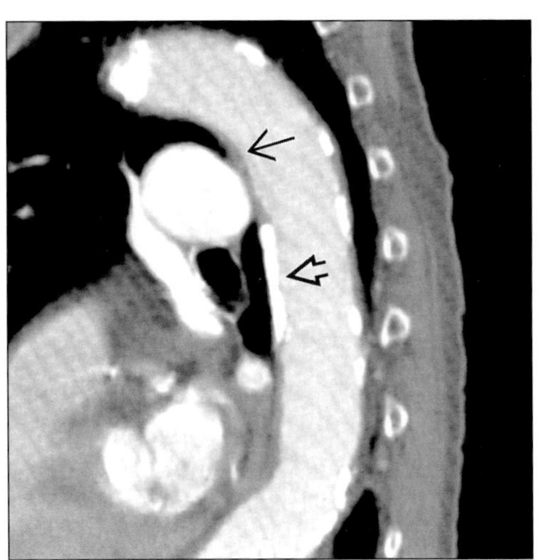

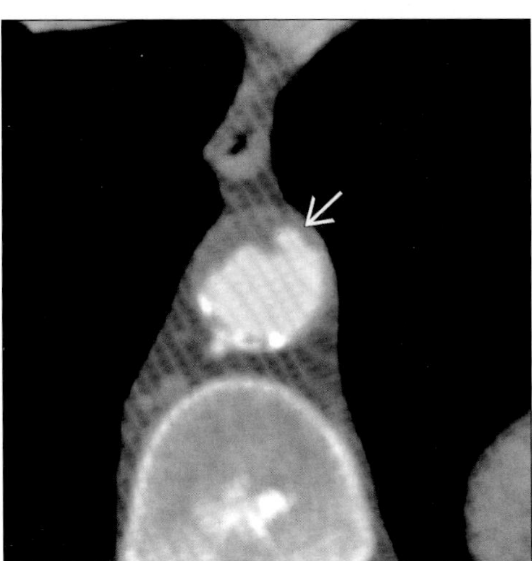

(Left) *Sagittal oblique reformatted CTA of a patient with aortic atherosclerosis demonstrates calcified ➩ and noncalcified → atherosclerotic plaques along the tortuous descending thoracic aorta.* **(Right)** *Axial CTA of a patient with atherosclerosis shows a large soft tissue atherosclerotic plaque of the descending aorta and a focal area of ulcerated plaque ➡. Ulcerated plaque differs from a penetrating aortic ulcer in that the former does not extend beyond the confines of the aortic wall.*

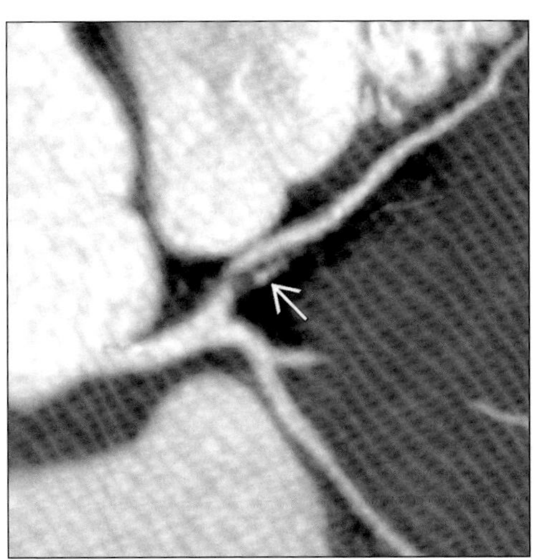

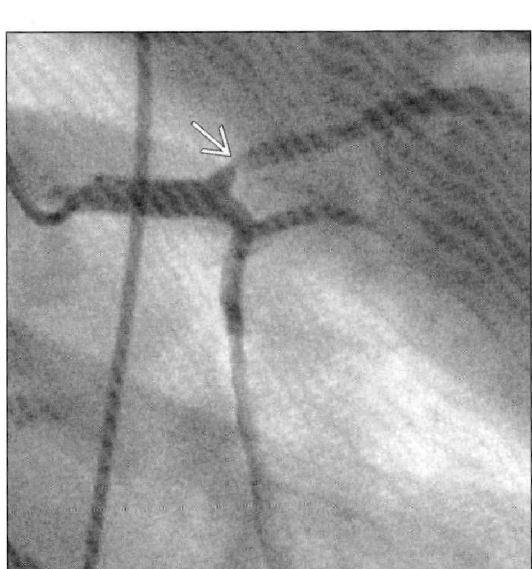

(Left) *Oblique axial reformatted coronary CTA demonstrates a mixed plaque ➡ along the proximal left anterior descending (LAD) coronary artery that reduces the lumen by more than 75% of the vessel diameter, corresponding to hemodynamically significant coronary artery obstruction.* **(Right)** *Right anterior oblique coronary angiography of the same patient demonstrates a 90% stenosis ➡ of the proximal LAD coronary artery. Coronary artery disease frequently coexists with aortic atherosclerosis.*

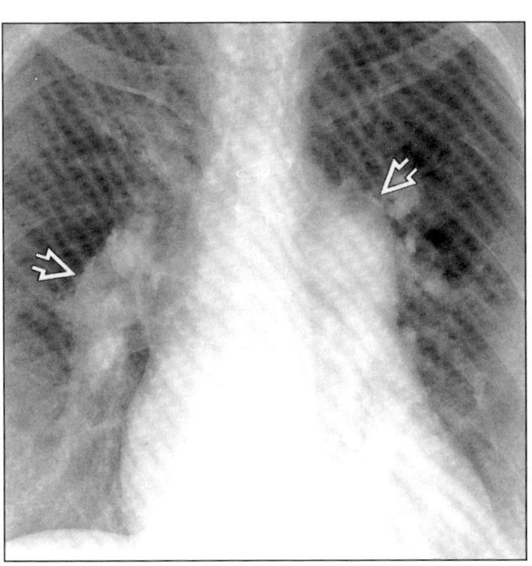

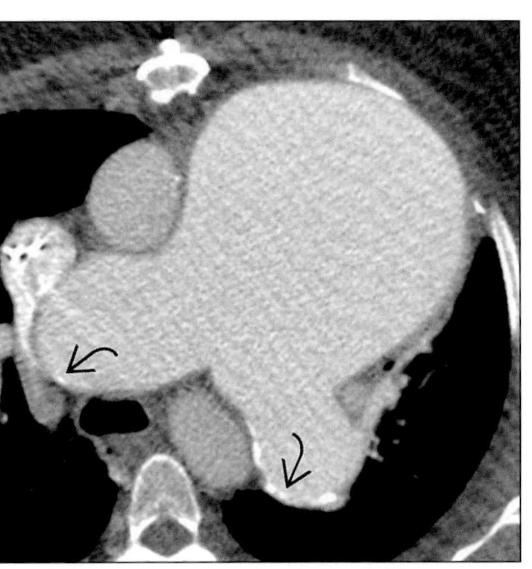

(Left) *PA chest radiograph of a patient with longstanding rheumatic heart disease and pulmonary arterial hypertension shows enlarged central pulmonary arteries with intimal calcification ➡.* **(Right)** *Axial CECT of the same patient shows massive enlargement of the pulmonary trunk and central pulmonary arteries with scattered calcified plaques ↪. Calcified plaques can occur in the setting of longstanding severe pulmonary hypertension, Eisenmenger syndrome, and chronic pulmonary embolus.*

AORTIC ANEURYSM

Key Facts

Terminology
- Aortic dilatation > 50% of normal diameter

Imaging
- Radiography
  - Ascending aortic aneurysm: Often not visible
  - Aortic arch aneurysm: Enlarged/obscured aortic arch
  - Descending aorta aneurysm: Focal or diffuse abnormality of left paraaortic interface
  - Peripheral curvilinear calcification
  - Rupture: Wide mediastinum, left pleural effusion
- CT
  - Curvilinear mural calcification
  - Crescentic mural high attenuation indicates contained/impending rupture
  - Hematoma: Hemothorax, hemopericardium, hemomediastinum

Top Differential Diagnoses
- Tortuosity (aging) of the aorta
- Mediastinal mass

Pathology
- Atherosclerotic aortic aneurysm
- Infectious (mycotic) aneurysm
- Cystic medial necrosis

Clinical Issues
- Atherosclerotic aneurysm: Most are asymptomatic
- Infectious (mycotic) aneurysm: Fever, leukocytosis

Diagnostic Checklist
- Consider ruptured aneurysm: Acute chest pain, wide mediastinum, and pleural effusion on radiography
- Normal radiography does not exclude aneurysm or dissection; cross-sectional imaging for diagnosis

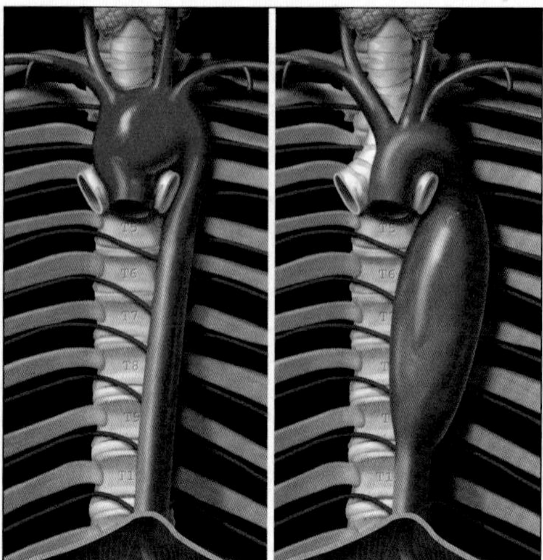

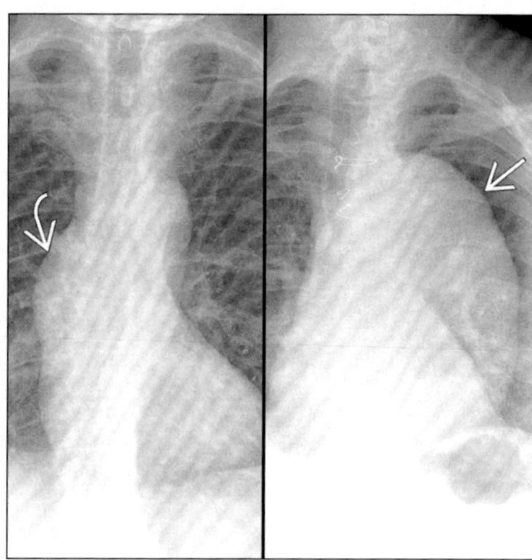

(Left) *Graphic shows the morphologic features of saccular and fusiform aortic aneurysms. Saccular aneurysms (left) are focal and mass-like. Fusiform aneurysms (right) are elongate.* ***(Right)*** *Composite image shows PA chest radiographs of 2 patients with ascending (left) and descending (right) aortic aneurysms. A focal aortic aneurysm exhibits right superior cardiomediastinal convexity and the hilum overlay sign. A fusiform aneurysm involves the entire descending aorta.*

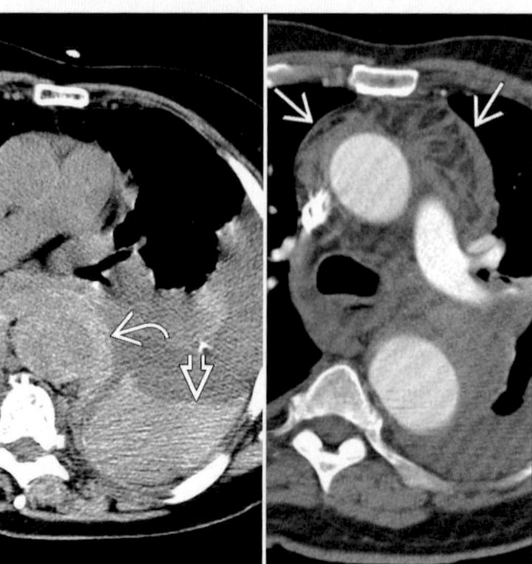

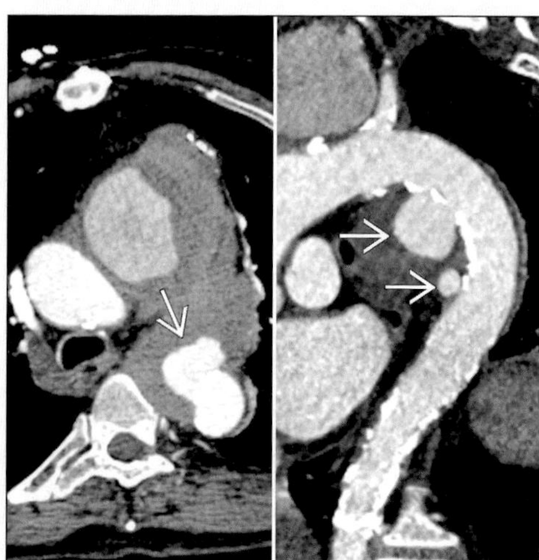

(Left) *Composite image shows axial NECT (left) and CECT (right) of 2 patients with ruptured aortic aneurysms. Signs of rupture include crescent sign, hemothorax, and mediastinal hematoma.* ***(Right)*** *Composite image with axial (left) and sagittal CTA (right) of a patient with mycotic aortic aneurysms secondary to S. aureus aortic valve endocarditis shows saccular aneurysms near the aortic isthmus. Infectious or mycotic aneurysms are typically secondary to S. aureus and Salmonella spp.*

AORTIC ANEURYSM

TERMINOLOGY

Definitions

- Aortic dilatation > **50% of normal diameter**

IMAGING

Radiographic Findings

- **Ascending aorta aneurysm**
  - Often not visible
  - Convexity of right superior cardiomediastinal silhouette
- **Aortic arch aneurysm**
  - Enlargement or obscuration of aortic arch
  - Hilum overlay sign
  - Rightward tracheal deviation
- **Descending aorta aneurysm**
  - Focal mass obscuring the left paraaortic interface
  - Diffuse enlargement of descending aorta with lateral displacement of left paraaortic interface
- **Peripheral curvilinear calcification**
- Ruptured aneurysm
  - Mediastinal widening compared to prior studies
  - Left pleural effusion

CT Findings

- NECT
  - **Curvilinear mural calcification**: Common in atherosclerotic, absent in mycotic aneurysms
  - **Crescent sign**: Crescentic mural high attenuation indicates contained/impending rupture
  - **Hematoma**: Hemothorax, hemopericardium, hemomediastinum
- CTA
  - Blunting of sinotubular junction (annuloaortic ectasia)
  - Crescent-shaped intraluminal thrombus
  - Intimomedial flap (dissection)
  - Rupture: Active extravasation (uncommon)

MR Findings

- Similar sensitivity to CT but not often used in the acute setting
- Assessment of aortic valve and cardiac function

Imaging Recommendations

- Best imaging tool
  - CECT for optimal evaluation of aneurysm location and size, relationship to major branch vessels, complications (e.g., dissection, mural thrombus, intramural hematoma, free rupture)
- Protocol advice
  - Cardiac gating for anatomic and functional aortic valve assessment

DIFFERENTIAL DIAGNOSIS

Tortuosity (Aging) of the Aorta

- Diffuse aortic dilatation

Mediastinal Mass

- Hilum overlay sign; anterior mediastinal masses
- Curvilinear calcification typical of vascular lesions
- CT differentiation of neoplasm from vascular lesion

PATHOLOGY

General Features

- **True aneurysm**: Contains all 3 aortic wall layers
- **Atherosclerotic aortic aneurysm**
  - Degenerative process, most common (75%)
  - Shape: Fusiform (most common), saccular
  - Location: Arch > descending > ascending
  - Significantly increased risk of rupture
    - Ascending aorta diameter > 5.5 cm
    - Descending aorta diameter > 6.5 cm
- **Infectious (mycotic) aneurysm**
  - Predisposing causes: IV drug abuse, valvular disease, congenital aortic/cardiac disease, prior aortic/cardiac surgery, adjacent pyogenic infection, immunocompromise
  - Most common pathogens: *Salmonella* species and *Staphylococcus aureus*
  - Shape: Saccular
  - Any location
- **Cystic medial necrosis**
  - Hypertension (more common), bicuspid aortic valve, Marfan syndrome (more severe)
  - Shape: Fusiform
  - Location: Ascending aorta, aortic annulus (annuloaortic ectasia); aortic regurgitation

Gross Pathologic & Surgical Features

- **Saccular**: Focal mass-like aortic dilatation
- **Fusiform**: Diffuse elongate aortic dilatation

CLINICAL ISSUES

Presentation

- Most common signs/symptoms
  - Atherosclerotic aortic aneurysm: Asymptomatic (most common), chest pain, compression (hoarseness, dysphagia, atelectasis, SVC syndrome)
  - Infectious (mycotic) aneurysm: Fever, leukocytosis
  - Acute chest pain: Rupture dissection

Demographics

- Gender
  - Men > women
- Epidemiology
  - Prevalence of 3-4% in patients over 65 years

Treatment

- Risk reduction: Hypertension control, smoking cessation
- Indications for surgery
  - Size criteria
    - **Ascending aorta > 5.5 cm** (5 cm for familial or Marfan syndrome and bicuspid aortic valve)
    - **Descending aorta > 6.5 cm**
  - **Growth rate > 1 cm per year**
  - Symptomatic patients

SELECTED REFERENCES

1. Posniak HV et al: CT of thoracic aortic aneurysms. Radiographics. 10(5):839-55, 1990
2. Feigl D et al: Mycotic aneurysms of the aortic root. A pathologic study of 20 cases. Chest. 90(4):553-7, 1986

ACUTE AORTIC SYNDROMES

Key Facts

Terminology

- Rhexis: Rupture of vasa vasorum leading to IMH
- Acute aortic syndrome (AAS): Aortic dissection, incomplete dissection, penetrating aortic ulcer, intramural hematoma
- Aortic dissection (AD) or class 1 dissection
  - Separation of aortic media by intimomedial flap; separates false channel from aortic lumen
  - Entrance & reentrance tears
- Intramural hematoma (IMH) or class 2 dissection
  - Aortic media hemorrhage from spontaneous rhexis of vasa vasorum
  - Absent or small entrance/re-entrance tear
- Penetrating aortic ulcer (PAU) or class 4 dissection
  - Ulceration of atherosclerotic lesion that penetrates internal elastic lamina
  - Variable amount of intramural hemorrhage

Imaging

- AD: Aortic (intimomedial flap) on CTA
- IMH: Circular or crescentic aortic wall hyperdensity on NECT
- PAU: Contrast outpouching beyond aortic wall

Pathology

- Stanford classification for AD, ID, & IMH
  - Type A: Involves ascending aorta
  - Type B: Involves only descending aorta

Clinical Issues

- Treatment of AD and IMH
  - Stanford type A: Surgical reconstruction
  - Stanford type B: Medical treatment
- Treatment of PAU: Close follow-up, medical treatment; endovascular therapy or surgery if progression or complications

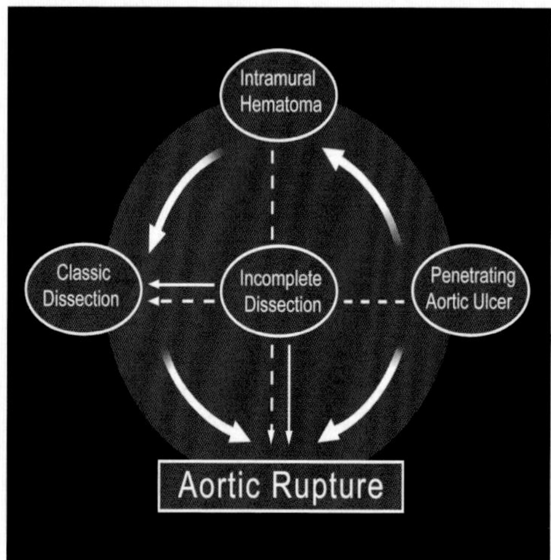

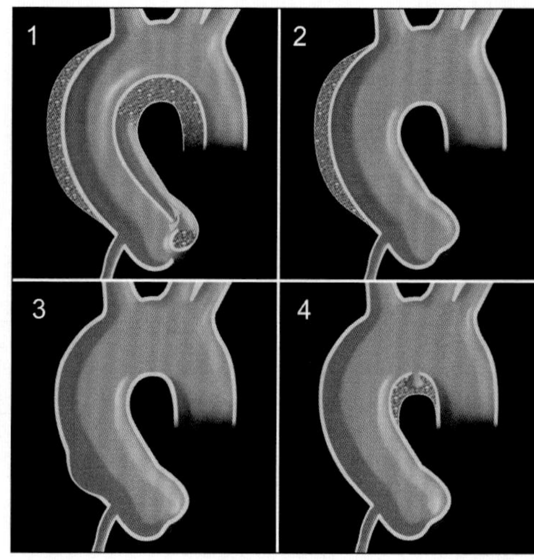

(Left) *Graphic shows the relationship between various AAS entities and their progression patterns (arrows). Classic dissection does not evolve to penetrating aortic ulcer (PAU), but the opposite may occur. All entities can result in aortic rupture, a life-threatening complication.* ***(Right)*** *Graphic shows the Svensson classification and the morphology of specific AAS entities that likely represent aortic dissection subtypes. Class 1 is a classic dissection; class 2 is an IMH; class 3 is a focal intimal tear; and class 4 is a PAU.*

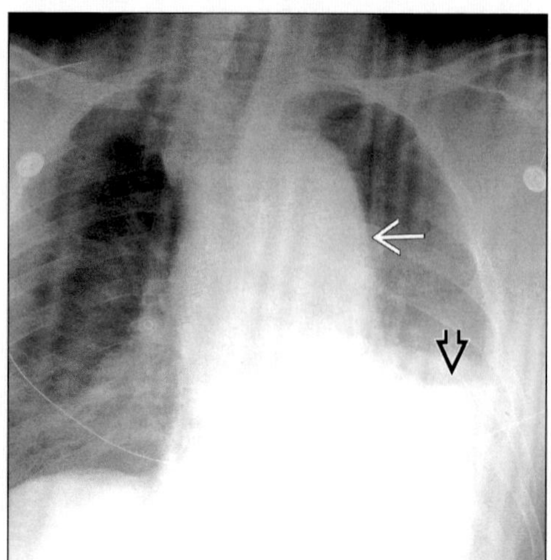

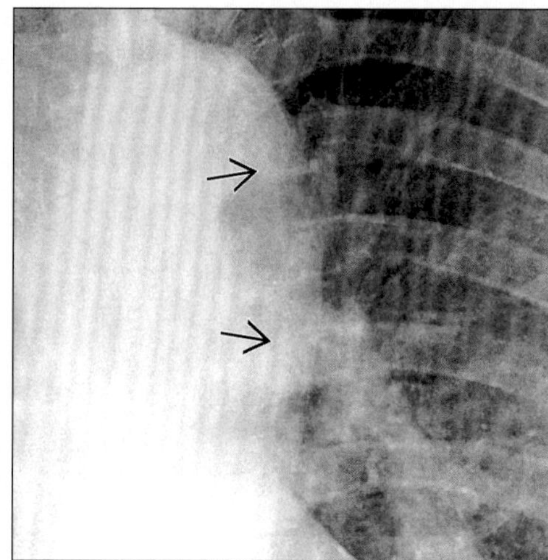

(Left) *PA chest radiograph of a patient with ruptured type B aortic dissection demonstrates mediastinal widening ➔ and a left pleural effusion ⊳ due to hemorrhage.* ***(Right)*** *PA chest radiograph of a patient with type B aortic dissection shows a double contour of the aortic arch and descending aorta. The internal contour ➔ represents the displaced intimal calcification. While chest radiography is often insensitive for diagnosing dissection, this sign is highly specific when present.*

ACUTE AORTIC SYNDROMES

TERMINOLOGY

Abbreviations

- **Acute aortic syndrome** (AAS)

Definitions

- **Acute aortic syndrome (AAS)**: Aortic dissection, incomplete dissection, penetrating aortic ulcer, intramural hematoma
  - **Aortic dissection (AD)** or class 1 dissection
    - Separation of aortic media by intimomedial flap that separates false channel from aortic lumen
    - Entrance & re-entrance tears (occasionally several communications)
  - **Intramural hematoma (IMH)** or class 2 dissection
    - Aortic media hemorrhage from spontaneous vasa vasorum rhexis (occasionally trauma)
    - Absent entrance tear (or very small) and re-entrance tear
  - **Penetrating aortic ulcer (PAU)** or class 4 dissection
    - Ulcerated atherosclerotic lesion that penetrates internal elastic lamina
    - Associated with variable amounts of intramural hemorrhage
  - **Incomplete aortic dissection (ID)** or class 3 dissection
    - Entrance tear (intimal laceration) with no flap or intramural hematoma
    - If only contained by adventitia (contained aortic rupture) appears as subadventitial hematoma
    - Better outcome compared to classic dissection (lower operative mortality, shorter hospital stay, less frequent transfusions)
- **Rhexis**: Rupture of vasa vasorum leading to IMH

IMAGING

General Features

- Best diagnostic clue
  - **AD**: Aortic (intimomedial flap) on CTA
  - **IMH**: Circular or crescentic aortic wall hyperdensity on NECT
  - **PAU**: Contrast outpouching extending beyond aortic wall confines
- Location
  - **AD**: Entrance tear more common in right lateral ascending aorta & proximal descending aorta
  - **IMH**: Descending aorta more common than ascending aorta
  - **PAU**: Descending aorta

Radiographic Findings

- Normal radiograph does not exclude diagnosis
- **AD**: Displaced intimal calcifications (rare)
- Aortic rupture (contained): Mediastinal widening, pleural effusion, mass effect from pseudoaneurysm

CT Findings

- NECT
  - **AD**: Aortic intimomedial flap can be inferred if intimal calcification is present
  - **IMH**: Hyperdense circular or crescentic appearance of aortic wall with variable extension
  - **PAU**: Aortic outpouching
  - Aortic (contained) rupture: **Crescent sign**
- CTA
  - **AD**
    - Aortic (intimomedial) flap & fenestrations
    - Differentiation of true lumen from false channel
      - True lumen: Tends to be the smaller, increases during systole, does not undergo thrombosis, exhibits laminar flow during early systole
      - False lumen: Tends to be the larger, decreases during systole, thrombosis can occur, swirling or turbulent flow during late systole, **beak sign** (acute angle between false lumen and aortic flap), **cobweb sign** (strand-like filling defects in false lumen)
      - Collapse of true lumen: Slit-like, C-shaped true lumen configuration, dismal prognosis with high mortality due to organ or limb ischemia
    - ECG-gated CTA: Useful in assessment of ascending aorta (degraded by pulsation artifact in nongated studies), relationship with coronary ostia
  - **IMH**: Circular or crescentic aortic wall thickening
  - Coexistence of IMH (on NECT) & aortic dissection (on CTA) at different levels
  - **PAU**
    - Contrast-filled outpouching surrounded by IMH, pseudoaneurysm or rupture
  - **ID**
    - No aortic flap identified
    - When associated with subadventitial hematoma often indistinguishable from IMH
    - Diagnosis suggested on aortography; sometimes on CTA, MR, or transesophageal echocardiography (TEE) by subtle eccentric bulge at tear site & aortic regurgitation
    - Other nonspecific features to differentiate from IMH: Normal aortic diameter (IMH with decreased diameter of aortic lumen), periaortic fluid
  - **Aortic rupture**: Indirect signs (mediastinal hematoma, pleural effusion, pericardial effusion) more common than direct signs (frank contrast extravasation)

MR Findings

- **AD**
  - Sensitivity & specificity as good as CTA
  - Spin echo techniques demonstrate flap & fenestration as well as periaortic hematoma & hemopericardium
  - Gradient echo (GRE): Thrombosed aortic dissection is hyperintense
  - ECG-gated steady-state free precession (SSFP): Useful in assessment of ascending aorta (degraded by pulsation artifact in nongated studies), relationship with coronary ostia
  - Cine-SSFP: Useful in assessment of aortic valve regurgitation seen as proximal signal dephasing; dephasing signal may be seen at entry & re-entry sites
  - Phase-contrast: Allows quantification of flow in false lumen & quantification of aortic valve regurgitation
  - 3D-MRA with gadolinium: Gold standard MR technique, determines flap extent & location, relationship to & patency of vital aortic branches
- **IMH**
  - T1WI: Acute IMH is isointense, subacute IMH is hyperintense
  - Phase-contrast MR very sensitive for differentiation of slow flow in dissection from no flow in IMH

ACUTE AORTIC SYNDROMES

- T2WI
  - Acute IMH is hyperintense
  - After 1 to 5 days, IMH has lower intensity
- GRE
  - IMH is hyperintense
- **PAU**
  - T1 spin echo techniques: Optimal to characterize ulceration
  - T1 & T2 spin echo: Show mural crater with adjacent iso or hyperintensity (blood products)
  - 3D-MRA: Shows mural crater

Echocardiographic Findings

- TEE is equivalent to CT & MR imaging

DIFFERENTIAL DIAGNOSIS

Acute Coronary Syndrome (ACS)

- Negative EKG & cardiac enzymes in AAS with definitive imaging findings; AAS & ACS can coexist

Aortitis (Takayasu & Giant Cell Arteritis)

- Concentric or circumferential wall thickening of large & medium sized arteries with or without aneurysm
- Scattered areas of vascular stenosis
- Can simulate IMH on CTA
- Thickened wall is not hyperdense on NECT
- Mural contrast enhancement on MR

Aortic Sarcoma

- Extremely rare, difficult to differentiate from exophytic atherosclerotic plaque
- Noncalcified discrete aortic wall mass

PATHOLOGY

General Features

- Etiology
  - **AD**: Cystic medial degeneration
  - **IMH**: Vasa vasorum rhexis, rarely blunt chest trauma
  - **PAU**: Atherosclerotic lesion ulceration

Staging, Grading, & Classification

- Acute Aortic Syndromes
  - **AAS**: Groups all 4 entities based on similar clinical presentation, risk factors, & shared pathophysiologic features
  - **AAS**: Useful concept for understanding PAU & IMH as well as their relationship with aortic dissection
- **Stanford classification** for **AD**, **ID**, & **IMH**
  - Type A: Involves ascending aorta with or without extension to descending aorta
  - Type B: Involves only descending aorta

CLINICAL ISSUES

Presentation

- Most common signs/symptoms
  - Chest (back) pain
  - History of chronic severe arterial hypertension
- Other signs/symptoms
  - D-dimer may be elevated; negative test helps exclude AAS

Natural History & Prognosis

- Patterns of evolution
  - **AD**
    - False lumen thrombosis; tends to be smaller than true lumen with early thrombosis (rare); larger than true lumen when thrombosis occurs late
    - Early false lumen rupture; if in ascending aorta, hemopericardium & tamponade often result
    - Periaortic hematoma (crescent sign); impending/ contained rupture
  - **IMH**
    - Aortic rupture with hemopericardium (tamponade), hemothorax & mediastinal hemorrhage
    - Localized communicating dissection; IMH & aortic dissection may coexist at different aortic levels
    - Growth & progression of IMH
    - Spontaneous resolution; common in distal IMH
    - Stability over time; infrequent
    - Predictors of progression to complications: Ascending aorta involvement, maximum aortic diameter (> 5 cm), large intimal erosions (> 2 cm)
  - **PAU**
    - Aneurysm formation; slow progression
    - Pseudoaneurysm (contained rupture) contained by adventitia
    - Aortic dissection; entrance tear is ulcer crater
  - **ID**
    - Contained aortic rupture
    - Classic dissection

Treatment

- **AD** & **IMH**
  - Stanford type A: Surgical reconstruction
  - Stanford type B: Medical treatment; endovascular therapy &/or surgery if progression or complications
- **PAU**: Close follow-up, medical treatment; endovascular therapy or surgery if progression or complications

SELECTED REFERENCES

1. Vilacosta I et al: Acute aortic syndrome: a new look at an old conundrum. Postgrad Med J. 86(1011):52-61, 2010
2. Lohan DG et al: MR imaging of the thoracic aorta. Magn Reson Imaging Clin N Am. 16(2):213-34, viii, 2008
3. Smith AD et al: CT imaging for acute aortic syndrome. Cleve Clin J Med. 75(1):7-9, 12, 15-7 passim, 2008
4. Svensson LG et al: Intimal tear without hematoma: an important variant of aortic dissection that can elude current imaging techniques. Circulation. 99(10):1331-6, 1999

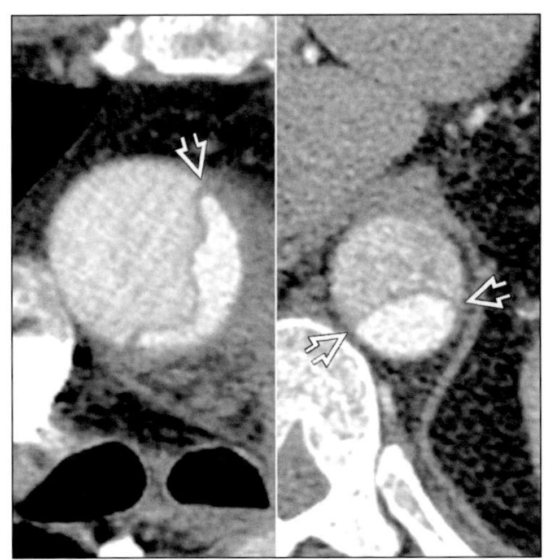

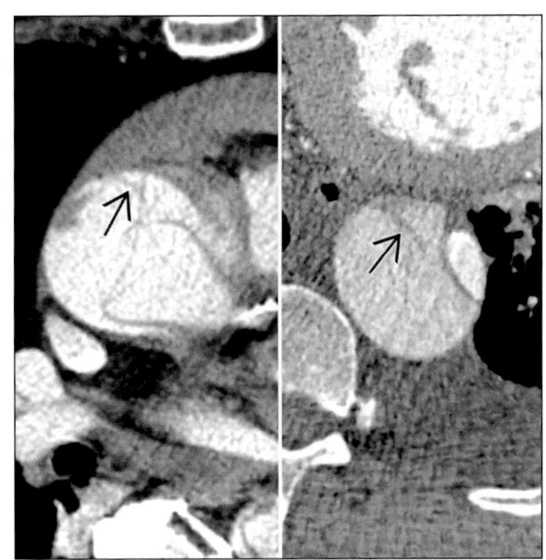

(Left) *Composite image with axial CTA of 2 patients with type A (left) and type B (right) aortic dissection shows the beak sign ➡, an acute angle between the flap and the false lumen.* ***(Right)*** *Composite image with axial CTA of 2 patients with type A (left) and type B (right) aortic dissections shows the cobweb sign ➡, manifesting with subtle linear filling defects representing strands of media in the false lumen. Both signs are important for differentiating the true lumen from the false.*

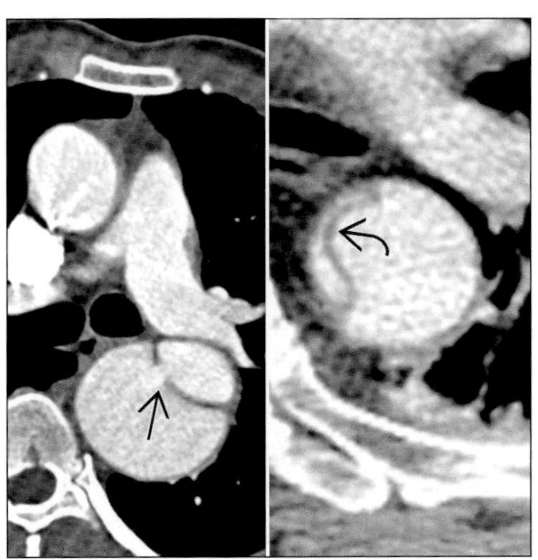

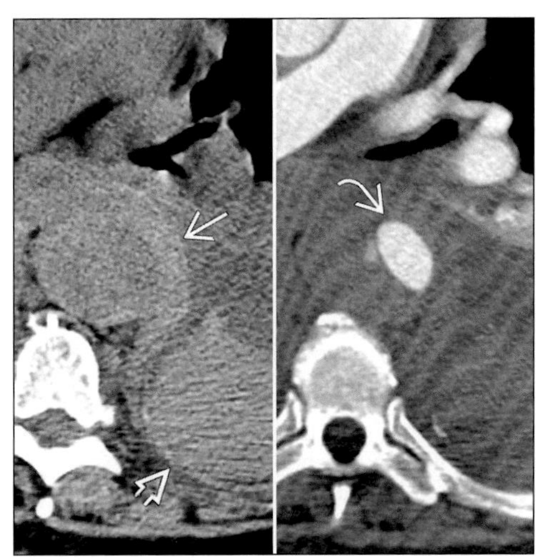

(Left) *Composite image with axial CTA shows a fenestration ➡ (left) and dynamic compression ➡ (right) of the true lumen. Dynamic compression often implies a poor prognosis with higher mortality rates due to organ or limb ischemia.* ***(Right)*** *Composite image with axial NECT (left) and CTA (right) of a patient with a ruptured type B aortic dissection shows a high-attenuation aortic hematoma ➡ producing a crescent sign, a left hemothorax ➡, and opacification of the true lumen ➡ on CTA.*

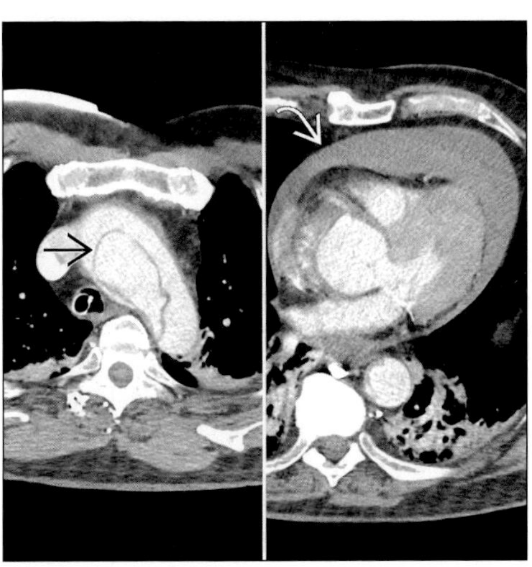

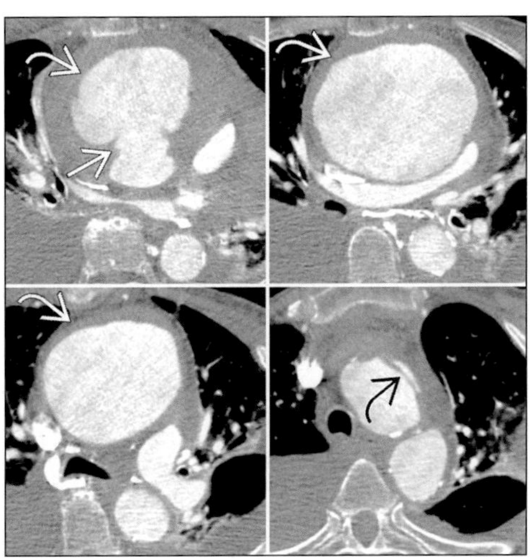

(Left) *Composite image with axial CECT of a patient with type A aortic dissection shows an aortic arch intimomedial flap ➡ and hemopericardium ➡ from rupture into the pericardial space, which often results in pericardial tamponade. Surgery is indicated in type A and in ruptured or complicated type B dissections.* ***(Right)*** *Composite image with axial CTA shows a type A aortic dissection ➡ with rupture ➡ of the false lumen resulting in a large pseudoaneurysm ➡.*

Key Facts

Terminology
- Congenital systemic connective tissue disorder; skeletal, cardiovascular, and ocular abnormalities

Imaging
- Radiography
  - Ascending aortic aneurysm
  - Cardiomegaly
  - Pectus deformity, scoliosis, scalloped vertebrae
  - Pneumothorax; apical bullae
- CT
  - Annuloaortic ectasia, aneurysm
  - Aortic rupture: Crescent sign, hematoma
  - Dissection: Intimal flap, true/false lumen
- Echocardiography
  - At diagnosis to assess ascending aorta & 6 months thereafter to determine rate of enlargement
- MR: Similar to CT in sensitivity

Top Differential Diagnoses
- Familial thoracic aortic aneurysm
- Ehlers-Danlos syndrome
- Bicuspid aortic valve

Pathology
- Mutation in *FBN1* gene encoding for fibrillin 1
- Autosomal dominant; 25% de novo mutations
- Microscopy: Cystic medial necrosis

Clinical Issues
- Cardiac/vascular abnormalities
- Pulmonary abnormalities
- Thoracic skeletal abnormalities

Diagnostic Checklist
- Consider Marfan syndrome in young patients with ascending aortic aneurysm and/or aortic dissection

__(Left)__ Composite image with coronal oblique CTA of a normal patient (left) and a patient with Marfan syndrome (right) shows a transition ➔ between the aortic root and the tubular ascending aorta, the sinotubular junction. This normal transition is absent in the patient with Marfan syndrome, a characteristic feature of this disorder. __(Right)__ Composite image with axial CTA of 2 patients with Marfan syndrome shows marked aortic root dilatation ➔ and ascending aortic dissection ➔.

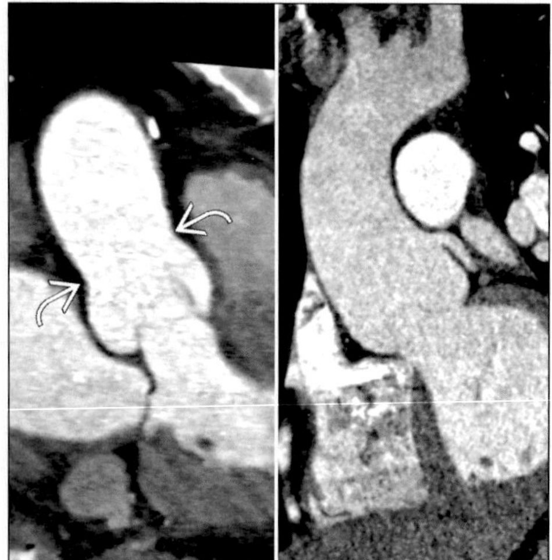

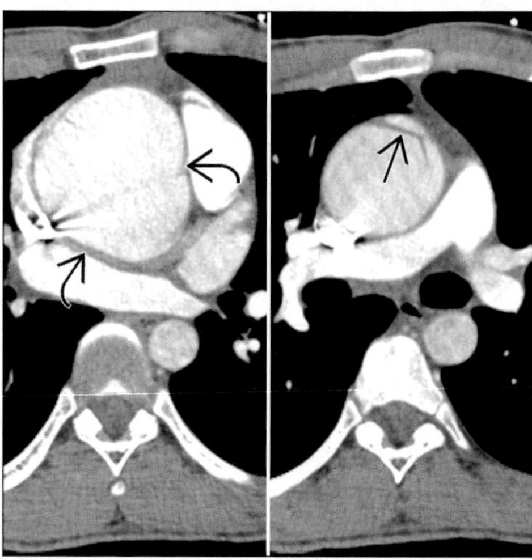

__(Left)__ Axial CTA of a patient with Marfan syndrome shows marked dilatation of the aortic root ➔ and pectus excavatum deformity ➔. These are major diagnostic criteria for Marfan syndrome. (Courtesy L. Heyneman, MD.) __(Right)__ Axial NECT of the same patient shows bilateral apical bullae ➔. Although this is a minor diagnostic criterion, it is an important abnormality that may lead to secondary spontaneous pneumothorax in patients with Marfan syndrome. (Courtesy L. Heyneman, MD.)

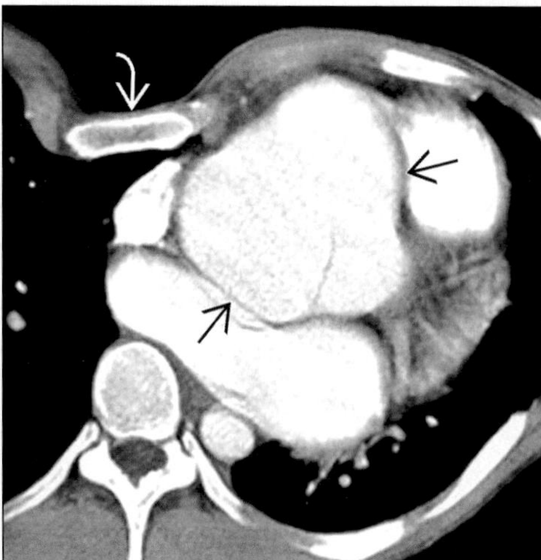

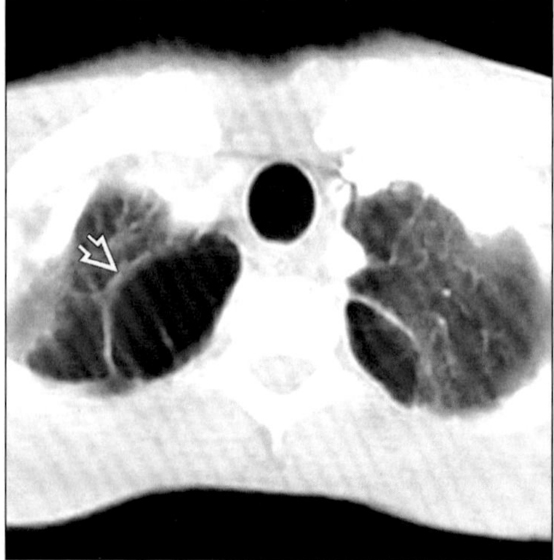

MARFAN SYNDROME

TERMINOLOGY

Definitions

- Congenital systemic connective tissue disorder characterized by **skeletal**, **cardiovascular**, and **ocular** abnormalities

IMAGING

Radiographic Findings

- **Ascending aortic aneurysm**: Mediastinal widening, right superior cardiomediastinal contour abnormality
- **Cardiomegaly**: Aortic/mitral regurgitation, cardiomyopathy
- Pectus deformity (excavatum, carinatum), scoliosis, scalloped vertebral bodies
- Pneumothorax; apical bullae

CT Findings

- NECT
  - **Annuloaortic ectasia/aneurysm**: Effacement of sinotubular junction (60-80% of patients)
    - Lack of normal transition between aortic root and tubular portion of ascending aorta
  - **Aortic rupture**, often contained
    - **Crescent sign**: Crescentic eccentric aortic high attenuation area
    - **Hematoma**: Mediastinal high attenuation, hemothorax, hemopericardium
- CTA
  - More sensitive than radiography
  - Direct visualization
    - Dissection: Intimal flap, true/false lumen
    - Rupture: Active extravasation

MR Findings

- Similar to CT in sensitivity
- Direct visualization of aortic dissection
- Optimal valve assessment: Aortic &/or mitral regurgitation

Echocardiographic Findings

- Initial assessment of aortic size and 6 months thereafter to determine rate of enlargement

Imaging Recommendations

- Protocol advice
  - Annual imaging recommended after initial echocardiography
  - Consider more frequent imaging if aortic diameter ≥ 4.5 cm or significant growth from baseline

DIFFERENTIAL DIAGNOSIS

Familial Thoracic Aortic Aneurysm

- Sinus of Valsalva aortic aneurysm

Ehlers-Danlos Syndrome

- Aneurysm/rupture: Medium/large muscular arteries
- Systemic: Joint hypermobility, atrophic scars, easy bruising, hernias, hollow organ rupture

Bicuspid Aortic Valve

- Ascending aortic aneurysm; bicuspid aortic valve

PATHOLOGY

General Features

- Etiology
  - Mutation in *FBN1* **gene** encoding for **fibrillin 1**
- Genetics
  - Autosomal dominant; 25% de novo mutations

Microscopic Features

- **Cystic medial necrosis**

CLINICAL ISSUES

Presentation

- Clinical profile
  - **Cardiac abnormalities**
    - **Mitral valve regurgitation**
      - > 50% auscultatory/echocardiographic evidence of mitral valve dysfunction, typically prolapse
      - Progression of mitral valve prolapse to mitral regurgitation by adulthood
    - **Aortic valve regurgitation**: Late occurrence from aortic annulus stretching
    - Tricuspid valve prolapse
    - Dilated cardiomyopathy (uncommon)
  - **Vascular abnormalities**: Most common life-threatening manifestations
    - **Annuloaortic ectasia** and aortic **aneurysm**
    - **Aortic dissection**
      - Often **type A**; ± propagation to descending aorta
      - Acute onset heart failure typically from severe aortic insufficiency
      - Extension to coronary arteries; myocardial infarction or sudden cardiac death
      - Dilatation/dissection of descending thoracic/abdominal aorta
    - Dilatation of pulmonary trunk
  - Pulmonary abnormalities
    - Bullae: Predisposed to spontaneous pneumothorax
  - **Thoracic skeletal abnormalities**
    - Pectus deformity; can contribute to restrictive lung disease

Demographics

- Gender
  - Males & females equally affected
- Epidemiology
  - Incidence: **2-3/10,000 individuals**

Natural History & Prognosis

- Improved prognosis with annual imaging, medical/surgical intervention
- Higher aortic dissection risk in pregnancy

Treatment

- **B-adrenergic receptor blockade:** Standard of care
- Surgical reconstruction: Elective according to aortic diameter, dissection, rupture

SELECTED REFERENCES

1. Ha HI et al: Imaging of Marfan syndrome: multisystemic manifestations. Radiographics. 27(4):989-1004, 2007

TAKAYASU ARTERITIS

Key Facts

Terminology

- Takayasu arteritis (TA)
- Pulseless disease
- Chronic granulomatous vasculitis of large vessels

Imaging

- Best diagnostic clue: Wall thickening of large vessels
  - Thoracic aorta & branches
  - Pulmonary artery involvement less common
- NECT: Aortic wall thickening
- CECT: Aortic wall thickening & enhancement
  - Stenosis, occlusion, aneurysm
- MRA: Aortic narrowing, dilatation
- Angiography: 4 types classified by location
- PET/CT used for treatment monitoring
- Complications
  - Stenosis > occlusion
  - Aneurysm
  - Dissection

Top Differential Diagnoses

- Giant cell arteritis
- Aortic coarctation

Pathology

- Autoimmune etiology suspected
- Specific types of HLA common among patients

Clinical Issues

- Disease stages
  - Early or prepulseless phase
  - Vascular inflammatory phase
  - Late quiescent occlusive or pulseless phase
  - Triphasic disease in minority of patients
- F:M = 8:1
- Heart failure most common cause of death
- Treatment
  - Corticosteroids, angioplasty, surgical bypass

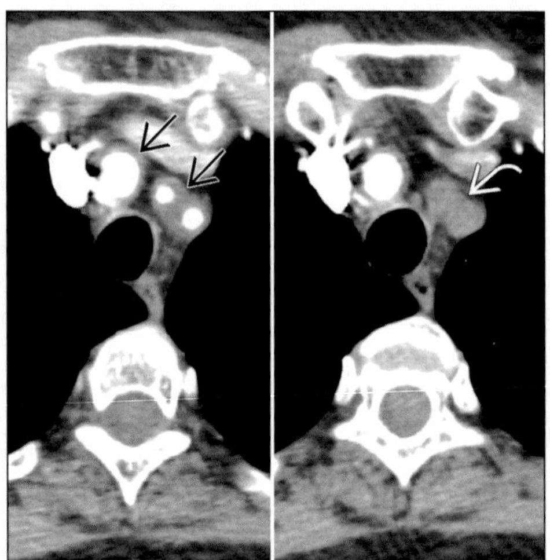
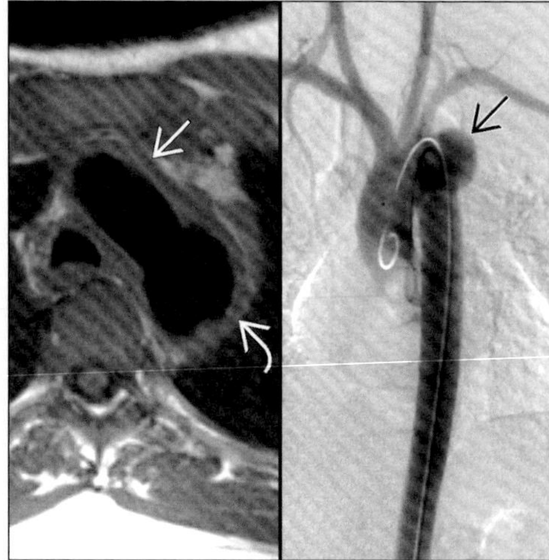

(Left) *Composite image with axial CECT shows wall thickening ➩ of the proximal right brachiocephalic, left common carotid, and left subclavian arteries. There is also occlusion ➦ of the left common carotid and left subclavian arteries. The left subclavian artery is the most common branch vessel affected in patients with TA.* ***(Right)*** *Composite image with axial T1WI MR (left) and DSA (right) shows aortic wall thickening ➔ and a focal aneurysm ➦ confirmed on subtraction aortic DSA ➩.*

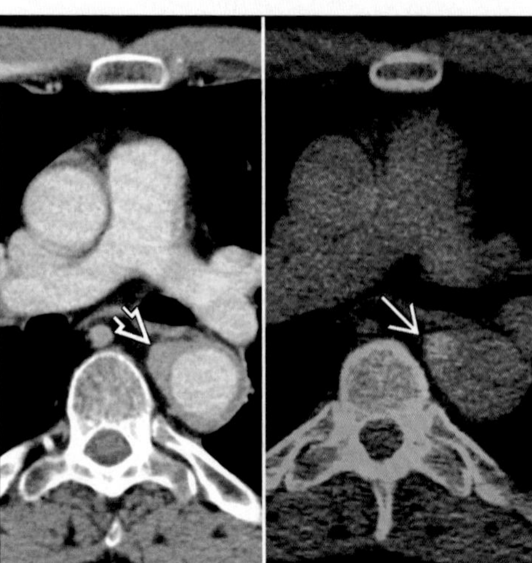
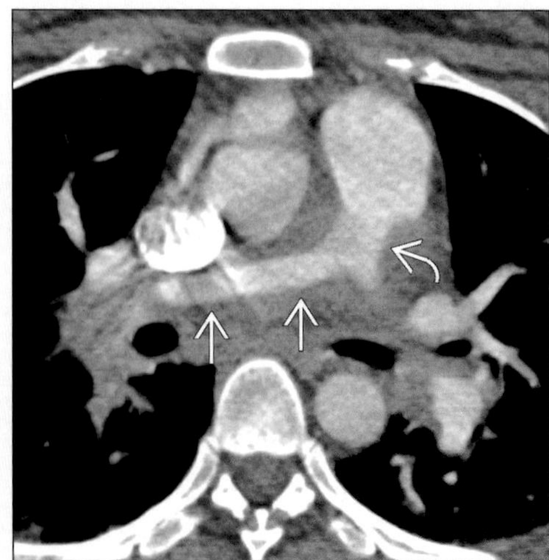

(Left) *Composite image with axial CECT (left) and axial fused PET/CT (right) shows soft tissue thickening of the wall of the descending aorta ➩ that exhibits FDG uptake ➔, consistent with active TA. PET/CT can be used to monitor treatment response in patients with TA.* ***(Right)*** *Axial CECT demonstrates diffuse soft tissue encasing the pulmonary trunk and the left and right pulmonary arteries with resultant pulmonary trunk stenosis ➦ and long segment narrowing ➔ of the right pulmonary artery.*

TAKAYASU ARTERITIS

TERMINOLOGY

Abbreviations

- **Takayasu arteritis** (TA)

Synonyms

- **Pulseless disease**

Definitions

- Chronic granulomatous vasculitis of large vessels

IMAGING

General Features

- Best diagnostic clue
  - **Wall thickening of large vessels**
- Location
  - **Thoracic aorta & branches**
    - **Left subclavian artery** most commonly affected
  - Pulmonary artery involvement less common

Radiographic Findings

- Radiography
  - Irregular or dilated descending thoracic aorta
  - Diminished pulmonary vessels & rib notching

CT Findings

- NECT
  - Vessel wall thickening, iso-/hyperdense to muscle
- CECT
  - **Vessel wall thickening & enhancement**
  - **Stenosis, occlusion, aneurysm**

MR Findings

- T1WI
  - **Wall thickening: Aorta & branches**
- T1WI C+
  - **Enhancement of thickened vessel wall**
- MRA
  - Focal/diffuse narrowing of aorta & branches
  - Aortic dilatation (ascending > descending)
  - Stenosis > occlusion
  - Aortic regurgitation, dissection, aneurysm

Angiographic Findings

- Early: Aortic wall thickening, rarely stenosis
- Late: Stenosis, occlusion, aneurysm; 4 types
  - Type I: Branches of aortic arch
  - Type II: Aorta & branch vessels
  - Type III: Aorta, coarctation may result
  - Type IV: Aortic dilation

Nuclear Medicine Findings

- PET
  - FDG uptake; may be low grade to intense
  - Treatment monitoring

Imaging Recommendations

- Protocol advice
  - Multiplanar reconstructions for stenosis

DIFFERENTIAL DIAGNOSIS

Giant Cell Arteritis

- Affects large vessels in older patients

Aortic Coarctation

- Aortic narrowing, rib notching
- More common in males

PATHOLOGY

General Features

- Etiology
  - Autoimmune etiology suspected
- Genetics
  - Specific types of HLA common among patients

Gross Pathologic & Surgical Features

- Wall thickening of large vessels

Microscopic Features

- Granulomatous inflammation of arterial wall
  - Intimal proliferation, fibrosis of media & adventitia

CLINICAL ISSUES

Presentation

- Most common signs/symptoms
  - **Early or prepulseless phase**
    - Low-grade fever, malaise, weight loss, fatigue
  - **Vascular inflammatory phase**
    - Vascular insufficiency
    - Symptoms minimized by collateral formation
  - **Late quiescent occlusive or pulseless phase**
    - Diminished/absent pulses, vascular bruits
    - Hypertension, aortic regurgitation
    - Neurologic symptoms (dizziness, seizures)
  - Triphasic pattern seen in minority of patients
    - Disease usually recurrent → phases may coexist
    - Interval between early & late phases variable
- Other signs/symptoms
  - Pulmonary hypertension when PA involved

Demographics

- Age
  - Most common in 2nd & 3rd decades of life
- Gender
  - F:M = 8:1
- Epidemiology
  - Most common in Asia
  - Affects 6/1,000 persons worldwide

Natural History & Prognosis

- Congestive heart failure most common cause of death
- Hypertension poor prognostic factor

Treatment

- Corticosteroids first-line treatment
  - Cyclophosphamide & methotrexate second-line treatment
- Angioplasty, surgical bypass, or stent placement for stenosis & occlusion

SELECTED REFERENCES

1. Khandelwal N et al: Multidetector CT angiography in Takayasu arteritis. Eur J Radiol. 77(2):369-74, 2011
2. Restrepo CS et al: Aortitis: imaging spectrum of the infectious and inflammatory conditions of the aorta. Radiographics. 31(2):435-51, 2011

SUPERIOR VENA CAVA OBSTRUCTION

Key Facts

Terminology
- Superior vena cava (SVC)
- SVC obstruction by intraluminal, intramural, or extrinsic disease
- Impaired venous return from head, neck, upper extremities, & trunk to right atrium

Imaging
- Radiography
  - May be normal
  - Mediastinal widening
  - Mediastinal/paramediastinal mass
- CT & MR
  - Nonopacification of SVC on CT & MR
  - Extrinsic compression by mass or lymphadenopathy
  - Intraluminal filling defect
  - Multiple collateral vessels

Top Differential Diagnoses
- Thoracic outlet syndrome
- Brachiocephalic vein occlusion or stenosis
- Thrombosis, stenosis, or occlusion of deep upper extremity veins
- Persistent left SVC with absent right SVC

Pathology
- Malignant etiologies (80-90%): Lung cancer, metastatic disease, lymphadenopathy, lymphoma
- Benign etiologies (10-20%): Granulomatous disease, iatrogenic, previous radiation therapy

Clinical Issues
- Face, neck, upper trunk, & upper extremity edema

Diagnostic Checklist
- Consider SVC obstruction when patient with known malignancy develops typical signs & symptoms

(Left) Graphic illustrates superior vena cava (SVC) obstruction ➡ secondary to mediastinal invasion by a lung tumor ➡ with resultant brachiocephalic vein ➡ and right intercostal collateral vessel ➡ distention. (Right) Axial CECT shows SVC obstruction by small cell lung cancer ➡ invading the mediastinum and multiple distended mediastinal collateral vessels ➡. Lung cancer is the most common cause of malignant SVC obstruction, and small cell carcinoma is the most frequent cell type.

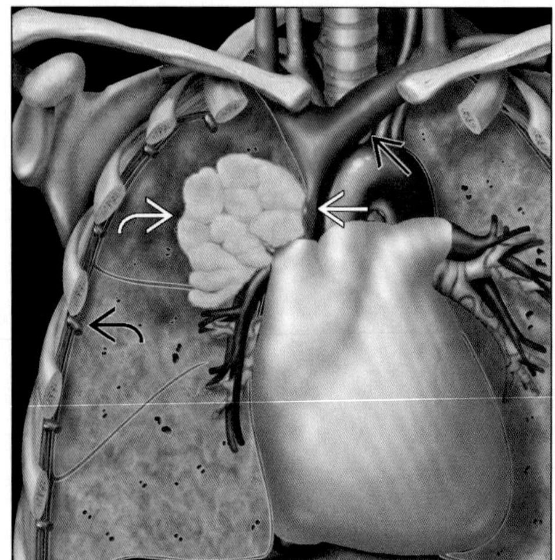

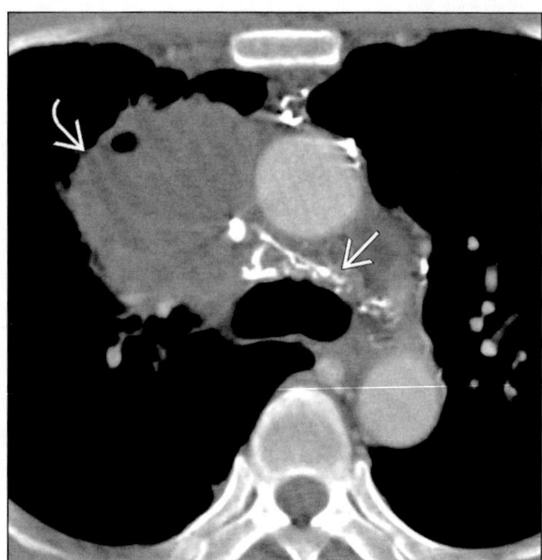

(Left) Composite image with PA chest radiograph (left) and axial CECT (right) of a patient with metastatic lung cancer manifesting with a right paratracheal mass ➡ that occludes the SVC ➡ and posterior chest wall collateral vessels ➡. (Right) Coronal CECT shows an SVC stent without apparent opacification of the stent lumen ➡ although the SVC caudal to the stent is patent ➡. Vascular stents may be used to treat SVC obstruction from benign and malignant etiologies.

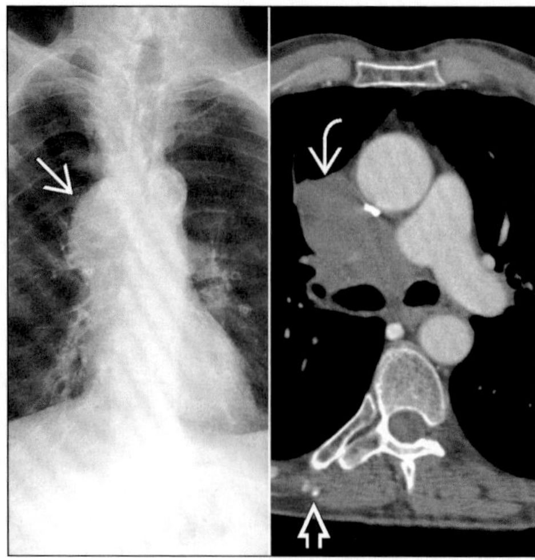

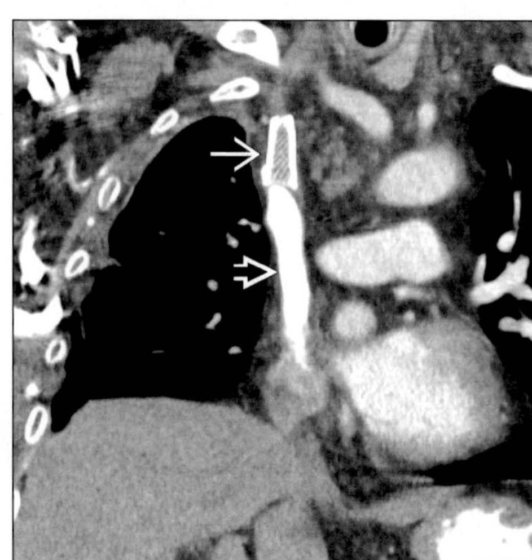

SUPERIOR VENA CAVA OBSTRUCTION

TERMINOLOGY

Synonyms

- **Superior vena cava (SVC) syndrome**

Definitions

- Obstruction of SVC due to intraluminal, intramural, or extrinsic disease
  - Impaired venous return from head, neck, upper extremities, & trunk to right atrium

IMAGING

General Features

- Best diagnostic clue
  - **Nonopacification of SVC**
  - **Multiple collateral vessels**

Radiographic Findings

- Radiography
  - May be **normal**
    - Most common in mediastinal fibrosis
    - Iatrogenic SVC obstruction
  - **Widened mediastinum**
    - Dilated SVC
    - Mediastinal mass or lymphadenopathy
  - **Right hilar or paramediastinal mass**
    - Lung cancer
    - Metastatic disease
    - Lymphadenopathy of other etiology
  - Enlarged azygos arch & vein

CT Findings

- CECT
  - **Nonopacification of SVC**
    - Obstruction
      - Extrinsic compression by mass or lymphadenopathy
      - Intraluminal thrombus
  - **Multiple collateral vessels**
    - Neck, chest wall, mediastinum
  - **Enlarged mediastinal vessels**
    - Azygos arch & vein
    - Superior intercostal veins
    - Brachiocephalic veins
  - Inflow of contrast-enhanced blood into IVC
    - Intense hepatic enhancement in quadrate lobe

MR Findings

- T1WI C+
  - Evaluation of adjacent structures & causes of external SVC compression
- MRV
  - **Nonopacification of SVC**
  - Enlarged azygos arch & vein
  - Multiple collateral vessels
    - Neck, chest wall, mediastinum

Ultrasonographic Findings

- Grayscale ultrasound
  - **Dilatation of visualized SVC**
    - Stable lumen size with respiration or cardiac cycle
  - Echogenic intraluminal thrombus
  - Distended subclavian, brachiocephalic, & jugular veins
- Pulsed Doppler
  - Altered spectral waveforms when evaluating subclavian veins
  - Absent normal transmission of atrial waveform, respiratory phasicity, or response to provocative maneuvers
    - Monophasic antegrade flow
    - Low-velocity flow
- Color Doppler
  - Sluggish or absent blood flow

Angiographic Findings

- DSA
  - Venography performed when cross-sectional imaging is nondiagnostic
    - Performed superior or peripheral to obstruction
    - Stasis or retrograde flow in subclavian or brachiocephalic veins
      - May mimic subclavian or brachiocephalic vein occlusion
  - Extrinsic compression by mass or lymphadenopathy
    - Effacement of SVC
  - Indwelling catheters & pacemaker leads
    - Long, smooth narrowing
  - Intraluminal filling defect representing thrombus
  - No intraluminal contrast = occlusion
  - Multiple collateral vessels
  - Azygos arch & vein enlargement

Nuclear Medicine Findings

- Radionuclide uptake in liver: **Hot quadrate sign**
- Radionuclide venography with Tc-99m-MAA
  - Generated time-activity curves can show evidence of SVC obstruction
  - Multiple collateral vessels

Imaging Recommendations

- Best imaging tool
  - CT & MR for optimal demonstration of nonopacification of SVC
    - Evaluation of adjacent mediastinal structures
  - Venography useful for planning endovascular or surgical procedures
- Protocol advice
  - Coronal & sagittal reformations to visualize site and extent of obstruction

DIFFERENTIAL DIAGNOSIS

Thoracic Outlet Syndrome

- Multiple collateral vessels in neck & upper chest
- Focal narrowing at junction of clavicle & 1st rib
- SVC patent on contrast-enhanced imaging studies

Brachiocephalic Vein Occlusion or Stenosis

- Multiple collateral vessels in neck & upper chest
- Stenosis or occlusion of brachiocephalic vein
- SVC patent on contrast-enhanced imaging studies

Thrombosis, Stenosis, or Occlusion of Deep Upper Extremity Veins

- Usually secondary to indwelling catheters or pacemaker leads
- Multiple collateral vessels
- Upper extremity swelling may mimic SVC obstruction

SUPERIOR VENA CAVA OBSTRUCTION

- SVC & central veins patent on contrast-enhanced imaging studies

Persistent Left Superior Vena Cava with Absent Right Superior Vena Cava

- No collateral vessels
- No SVC in right superior mediastinum on imaging studies
- Aberrant course of catheters & pacemaker leads
  - Course along left mediastinum
- Opacified venous structure in left superior mediastinum on imaging studies
  - Terminates within coronary sinus
- Dilated coronary sinus

PATHOLOGY

General Features

- Etiology
  - **Intrathoracic malignancy**
    - Lung cancer most common
    - Metastatic disease
      - Breast, renal, & testicular cancers most common
    - Mediastinal lymphadenopathy & lymphoma
    - Primary mediastinal mass
  - **Granulomatous disease**
    - Infection
      - Tuberculosis
      - Histoplasmosis
    - Sarcoidosis
    - Silicosis
  - **Iatrogenic**
    - Indwelling catheters & pacemaker leads
  - Previous radiation therapy
  - Pyogenic infection
  - Compression by mediastinal vascular lesion

CLINICAL ISSUES

Presentation

- Most common signs/symptoms
  - Edema
    - Face, neck, upper trunk, & upper extremities
  - Headaches
  - Dyspnea, dysphagia, hoarseness
  - Palpable subcutaneous collateral vessels
    - Neck & chest wall
- Other signs/symptoms
  - Syncope, seizures, visual changes
  - Coma in severe cases
- Clinical profile
  - **SVC obstruction is a clinical diagnosis**
    - Patients with well-compensated stenosis or occlusion may be asymptomatic

Demographics

- Age
  - Age range: 18-76 years
    - Mean: 54 years
  - Malignant etiologies: Older, 40-60 years
  - Benign etiologies: Younger, 30-40 years
- Gender
  - Malignant etiologies: M > F
  - Benign etiologies: M = F
- Epidemiology
  - **Malignancy: Etiology in 80-90%**
  - **Benign causes: Etiology in 10-20%**
    - 50% due to mediastinal fibrosis
    - Recent increase in iatrogenic etiologies
      - Most common benign cause in cancer patients

Natural History & Prognosis

- Gradual, progressive obstruction of SVC
  - Insidious onset of symptoms
- Survival depends on course of underlying disease
- Benign etiologies
  - Rarely fatal
- Malignant etiologies
  - Usually not cause of death
  - Most die from metastatic malignancy
    - Survival correlates with tumor histology

Treatment

- Malignant etiologies
  - Radiation therapy
  - Chemotherapy targeted toward type of neoplasm
- Anticoagulation
- Endovascular therapy
  - Catheter-directed thrombolysis
  - Endovascular stent placement
- Surgical therapy
  - Venous bypass
  - Venous transposition

DIAGNOSTIC CHECKLIST

Consider

- SVC obstruction when patient with known malignancy develops typical signs & symptoms

Image Interpretation Pearls

- Nonopacification of SVC
- Multiple collateral vessels in neck, chest wall, & mediastinum

SELECTED REFERENCES

1. Eren S et al: The superior vena cava syndrome caused by malignant disease. Imaging with multi-detector row CT. Eur J Radiol. 59(1):93-103, 2006
2. Kalra M et al: Open surgical and endovascular treatment of superior vena cava syndrome caused by nonmalignant disease. J Vasc Surg. 38(2):215-23, 2003
3. Kim HJ et al: CT diagnosis of superior vena cava syndrome: importance of collateral vessels. AJR Am J Roentgenol. 161(3):539-42, 1993
4. Parish JM et al: Etiologic considerations in superior vena cava syndrome. Mayo Clin Proc. 56(7):407-13, 1981
5. Webb WR et al: Catheter venography in the superior vena cava syndrome. AJR Am J Roentgenol. 129(1):146-8, 1977

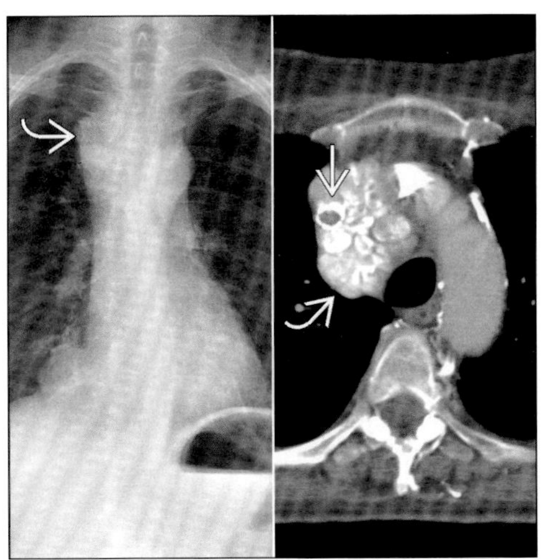

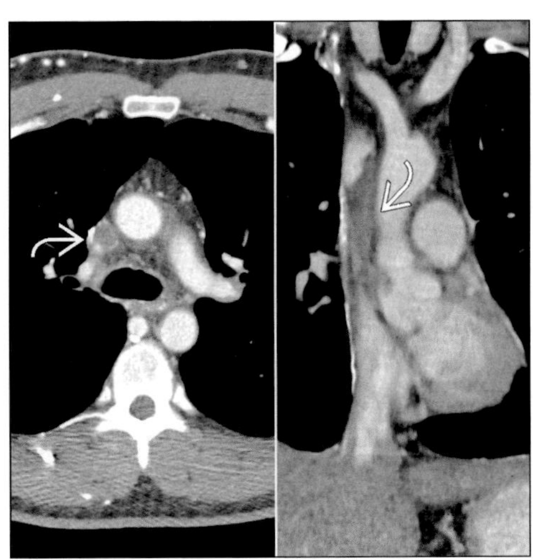

(Left) *Composite image with PA chest radiograph (left) and axial CECT (right) shows metastatic mucinous ovarian cancer manifesting with a conglomerate mass of calcified right paratracheal lymphadenopathy ➚ that obstructs the SVC. A metallic stent ➡ is demonstrated in the nonopacified SVC.* ***(Right)*** *Composite image with axial (left) and coronal (right) CECT of a patient with a history of previous indwelling central venous catheter shows a hypodense thrombus ➚ occluding the SVC.*

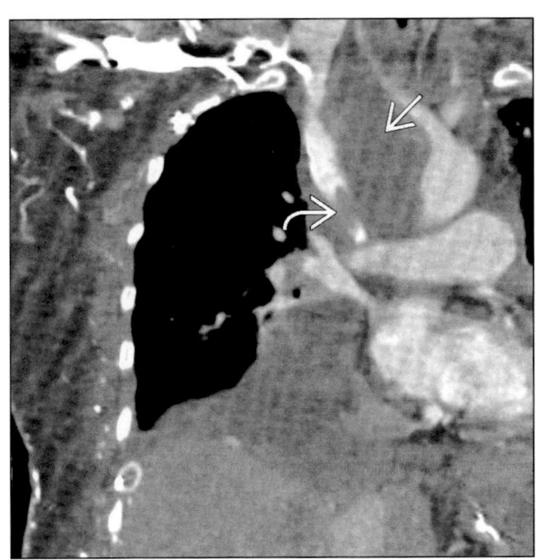

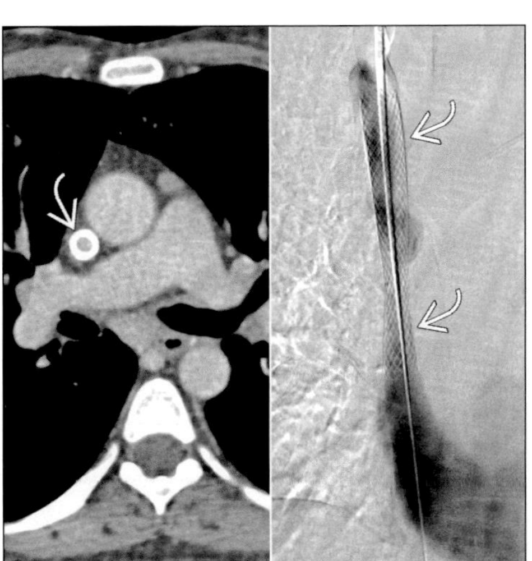

(Left) *Coronal CECT of a patient with metastatic breast cancer shows an intraluminal filling defect in the SVC ➚ and adjacent mediastinal lymphadenopathy ➡.* ***(Right)*** *Composite image with axial CECT (left) and digital subtraction angiography (right) of a patient who developed SVC obstruction after a longstanding indwelling central catheter shows an SVC vascular stent ➚ that restored flow through the SVC.*

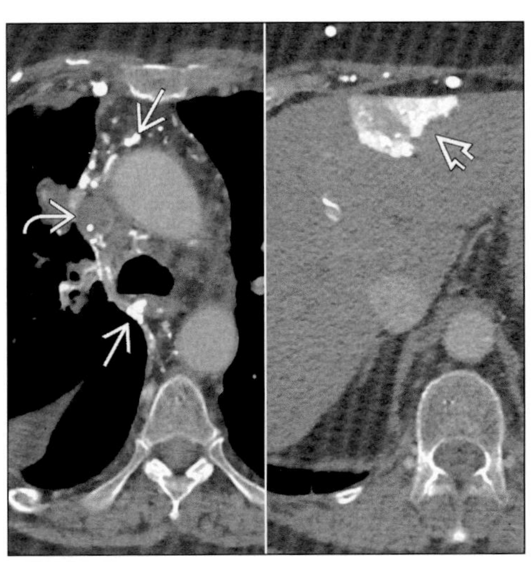

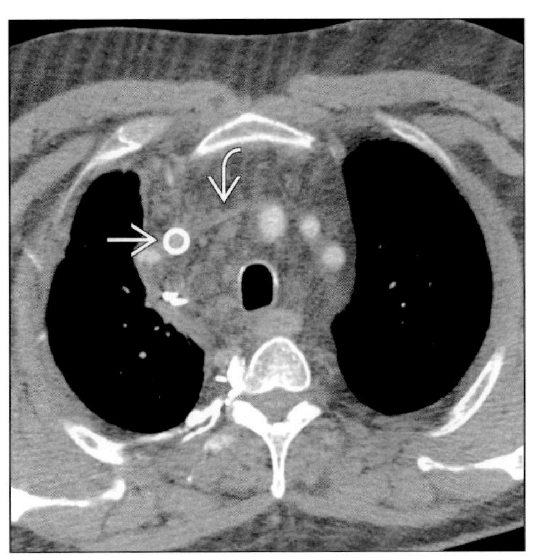

(Left) *Composite image with axial CECT of the chest (left) and abdomen (right) shows SVC occlusion ➚ and multiple mediastinal collateral vessels ➡. Intense enhancement of the medial segment of the left hepatic lobe results from collateral flow ⇨ and is an indirect sign of SVC obstruction.* ***(Right)*** *Axial CECT of a patient with mediastinal fibrosis shows an occluded SVC stent ➡ and mediastinal fat stranding ➚. Mediastinal fibrosis is the most common benign etiology of SVC obstruction.*

CARDIOGENIC PULMONARY EDEMA

Key Facts

Imaging

- Radiography
  - Perihilar haze; vascular indistinctness
  - Subpleural edema; fissural pleural thickening
  - Peribronchial thickening or cuffing
  - Interlobular septal thickening; Kerley B lines
  - Alveolar edema; consolidation
  - Cardiomegaly
  - Pleural effusion
- CT
  - Smooth thickening of interlobular septa
  - Fissural pleural thickening
  - Peribronchovascular thickening
  - Centrilobular, lobular, acinar ground-glass
  - Consolidation
  - Cardiomegaly; pleural effusion
  - Mediastinal lymph node enlargement
  - Increased attenuation of mediastinal fat

Top Differential Diagnoses

- Interstitial edema: Lymphangitic carcinomatosis
- Alveolar edema: Pneumonia, hemorrhage
- Interstitial & alveolar edema: Alveolar proteinosis

Pathology

- Increased capillary hydrostatic pressure
- Decreased intravascular plasma oncotic pressure

Clinical Issues

- Dyspnea; orthopnea; paroxysmal nocturnal dyspnea
- B-type natriuretic peptide (BNP); 90% accuracy
- Cardiogenic edema: PCWP > 18 mmHg

Diagnostic Checklist

- Chest radiography is imaging study of choice; prior studies helpful in detection of early findings
- Recognition of characteristic early CT findings

*(**Left**) PA chest radiograph of a patient with mitral valve disease shows pulmonary venous hypertension manifesting with vascular redistribution. The upper lung zone vessels ➡ are larger than those in the lower lung. (**Right**) PA chest radiograph of a patient with chronic left ventricular failure shows severe pulmonary venous hypertension manifesting with marked enlargement of upper lobe pulmonary vessels ➡. Upper lobe arteries and veins are much larger than adjacent bronchi.*

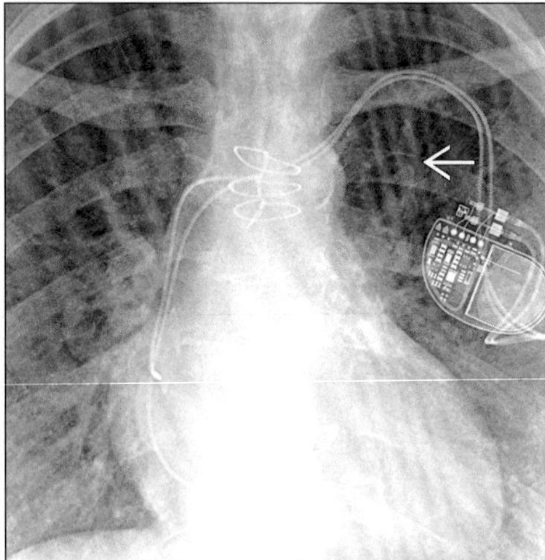

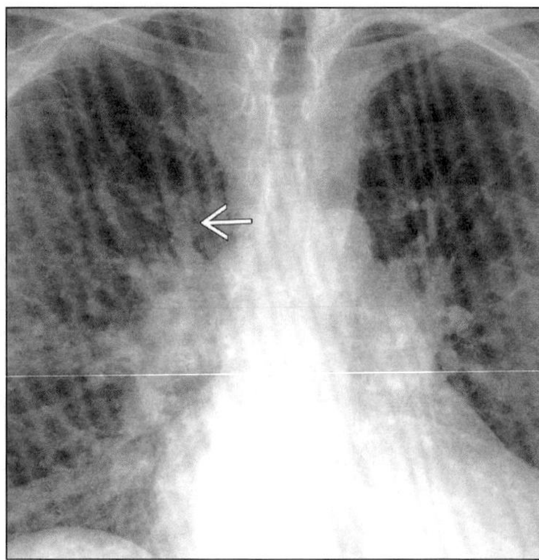

*(**Left**) PA chest radiograph of a patient with interstitial edema shows cardiomegaly and right perihilar haze, which manifests with right lower lobe ground-glass opacity and indistinct right interlobar pulmonary artery margins. (**Right**) PA chest radiograph of the same patient following treatment shows decreasing heart size as well as markedly improved visualization of the lateral border of the right interlobar pulmonary artery ➡. Perihilar haze may be the earliest manifestation of interstitial edema.*

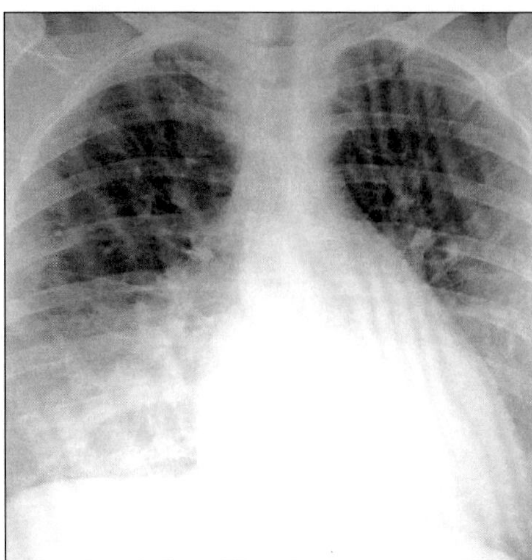

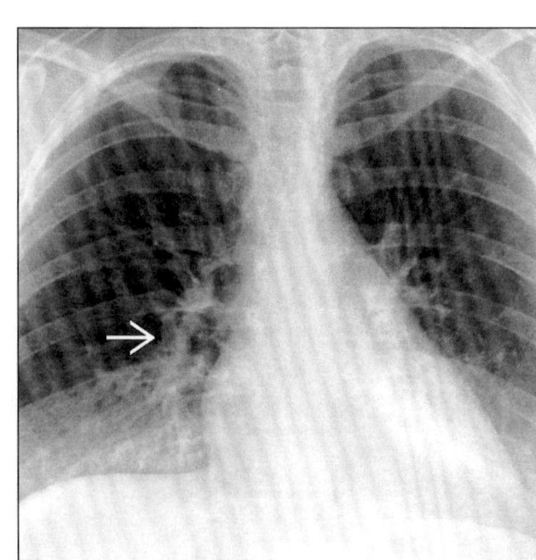

CARDIOGENIC PULMONARY EDEMA

TERMINOLOGY

Synonyms

- **Hydrostatic edema**

Definitions

- **Pulmonary edema** = abnormal **extravascular lung water accumulation**
- **Cardiogenic edema** = **elevated pulmonary capillary pressure**

IMAGING

General Features

- Best diagnostic clue
  - Cardiomegaly; wide vascular pedicle
  - Pulmonary venous hypertension
  - Interstitial edema
  - Alveolar edema
  - Pleural effusion

Radiographic Findings

- **Pulmonary venous hypertension**
  - **Chronic** elevation of left atrial pressure
    - Mitral stenosis
    - Left ventricular failure
  - **Vascular redistribution** or cephalization
    - Increased size of upper lobe pulmonary vessels
    - Evaluated on upright frontal chest radiography
    - May occur normally in supine position
    - Abnormal upper lung bronchoarterial ratios
      - Upper lobe anterior segment artery:bronchus
- **Interstitial edema**
  - **Perihilar haze** or **vascular indistinctness**
    - **Earliest manifestation** of interstitial edema
    - Blurred or indistinct vessel wall margins
    - Best evaluated in lower lobe central arteries
  - **Subpleural edema**
    - Fluid in peripheral subpleural interstitium
    - Thick interlobar fissures
      - Not related to pleural effusion
    - May precede septal thickening and peribronchial cuffing
  - **Peribronchial thickening or cuffing**
    - Fluid in axial bronchoarterial interstitium
    - Thick central bronchial walls on frontal chest radiography
  - **Septal thickening**
    - Fluid in peripheral subpleural interstitium
      - Interlobular septa
    - **Kerley B lines**
      - Common finding in interstitial edema
      - **Basilar peripheral horizontal thin lines**; perpendicular to pleura
      - 1-2 cm in length
    - **Kerley A lines**
      - Central perihilar oblique thin lines
      - Longer than Kerley B lines
    - **Kerley C lines**
      - Basilar Kerley B lines seen en face
      - Basilar reticular opacities
- **Alveolar edema**
  - Affected by gravitational effects, changes slowly
  - Appearance affected by underlying lung disease
  - **Consolidation**; poorly marginated airspace disease
    - Obscuration of underlying structures
    - Predilection for right lung
  - **Bat wing edema**
    - Central nongravitational pulmonary edema
      - Perihilar distribution
    - Rapid onset of severe heart failure
    - < 10% of cases
  - **Asymmetric alveolar edema**
    - Affected by patient position; preferential involvement of dependent lung
    - Acute mitral insufficiency from papillary muscle rupture; preferential right upper lobe involvement
- Associated findings
  - **Cardiomegaly**
    - Transverse cardiac diameter > 1/2 transverse thoracic diameter
    - Characteristic of chronic cardiogenic edema
    - Typically absent in acute edema & COPD
  - **Pleural effusion**
    - Often bilateral, larger on right
    - Rarely unilateral on left
    - Meniscus sign formed by interface of pleural fluid & adjacent aerated lung
    - Blunt costophrenic angle
    - Subpulmonic pleural effusion
      - May not blunt costophrenic angle
      - Lateral displacement of apex of pseudohemidiaphragm
    - Fissural mass-like pleural fluid or **pseudotumor**
      - Typical of pleural effusion in heart failure
  - **Wide vascular pedicle**
    - Width of superior mediastinal vascular structures
    - Marker of **increased central venous pressure** & circulating blood volume
      - Volume overload, renal failure, chronic heart failure, venous thrombosis
    - Variable size; affected by mediastinal fat
    - Useful when comparison studies available
    - Vascular pedicle width measurement
      - Right margin; superior vena cava interface where it crosses right main stem bronchus
      - Left margin; interface of proximal left subclavian artery
      - Vascular pedicle width = horizontal distance between right and left margins
      - Varies with body habitus
      - Measures **up to 58 mm in normal subjects**
- Temporal relationship of cardiogenic edema
  - Unpredictable sequence of findings
    - Interstitial edema may not follow pulmonary venous hypertension
    - Alveolar edema may not follow interstitial edema
  - Imaging findings may predate clinical signs
  - Interstitial edema resolves in hours to days
  - Radiographic improvement lags behind clinical course

CT Findings

- **Interstitial edema**
  - **Septal thickening**
    - Visualization of **interlobular septa**
    - Smooth linear opacities outlining secondary pulmonary lobule
    - Crazy paving; interstitial & alveolar edema
  - **Subpleural edema**

  - Thickened interlobar fissures
- **Peribronchovascular thickening**
  - Thickened bronchial walls
- **Vascular redistribution**
  - Enlarged central pulmonary arteries with respect to adjacent bronchi
- Distribution
  - Uniform, nongravitational
- **Alveolar edema**
  - Ground-glass opacity
  - Centrilobular ground-glass nodules
  - Lobular & acinar ground-glass opacities
  - Consolidation
  - Distribution
    - Diffuse or patchy
    - Dependent (gravitational)
    - Central & perihilar in bat wing edema
- Combined interstitial & alveolar edema
- Associated findings
  - **Pleural effusion**
    - Bilateral or unilateral
  - **Cardiomegaly**
  - Mediastinal lymph node enlargement
  - Increased attenuation of mediastinal fat

Imaging Recommendations

- Best imaging tool
  - Chest radiography; prior studies helpful in detection of early findings

DIFFERENTIAL DIAGNOSIS

Interstitial Edema

- Lymphangitic carcinomatosis
  - Known malignancy
  - Nodular interlobular septal thickening
  - Patchy distribution
  - Associated lymphadenopathy & pleural effusion
- Erdheim-Chester disease
  - Rare disease
  - Severe thickening of interlobular septa, pleura, & interlobar fissures
  - Sclerotic skeletal lesions

Alveolar Edema

- *Pneumocystis jiroveci* pneumonia
  - Severely immunocompromised patient
  - Ground-glass opacity
  - Cystic changes
- Pneumonia
  - Signs & symptoms of infection
  - Focal or multifocal consolidation
  - Parapneumonic pleural effusion
- Pulmonary hemorrhage
  - Ground-glass opacities
  - Centrilobular nodules

Interstitial and Alveolar Edema

- Pulmonary alveolar proteinosis
  - Patients may be minimally symptomatic
  - Crazy-paving pattern on CT
  - No cardiomegaly or pleural effusion

PATHOLOGY

General Features

- Etiology
  - **Increased capillary hydrostatic pressure**
    - Left heart failure
    - Left atrial/pulmonary vein obstruction
    - Volume overload; overhydration
  - **Decreased intravascular oncotic pressure**
    - Hypoalbuminemia
    - Hepatic/renal failure

Microscopic Features

- Lymphatic dilatation
- Interstitial and alveolar edema
- Hypertrophic muscularized arterioles & veins
- Hemosiderosis

CLINICAL ISSUES

Presentation

- Most common signs/symptoms
  - **Dyspnea**; orthopnea; paroxysmal nocturnal dyspnea
  - Frothy, blood-tinged sputum
  - Sweating, anxiety, pallor
  - End-expiratory crackles
  - **3rd heart sound** (S_3) (ventricular filling gallop)
- Clinical profile
  - **B-type natriuretic peptide (BNP)**
    - Used for diagnosing congestive heart failure
    - Produced as response to ventricular stretch/strain
    - 80-90% accuracy; 96% negative predictive value
  - **Pulmonary capillary wedge pressure (PCWP)**
    - Evolving role for use of pulmonary artery catheterization
      - Rate of adverse complications: 5-10%
    - > 18 mmHg; cardiogenic edema/volume overload

Natural History & Prognosis

- Acute or insidious course
- Prognosis depends on severity & reversibility of underlying hemodynamic dysfunction

Treatment

- Diuretics & afterload reduction

DIAGNOSTIC CHECKLIST

Consider

- Appearance of cardiogenic edema is affected by anatomic abnormalities, especially emphysema

SELECTED REFERENCES

1. Evans DC et al: Complications associated with pulmonary artery catheters: a comprehensive clinical review. Scand J Surg. 98(4):199-208, 2009
2. Gehlbach BK et al: The pulmonary manifestations of left heart failure. Chest. 125(2):669-82, 2004
3. Woolley K et al: Pulmonary parenchymal manifestations of mitral valve disease. Radiographics. 19(4):965-72, 1999
4. Ketai LH et al: A new view of pulmonary edema and acute respiratory distress syndrome. J Thorac Imaging. 13(3):147-71, 1998

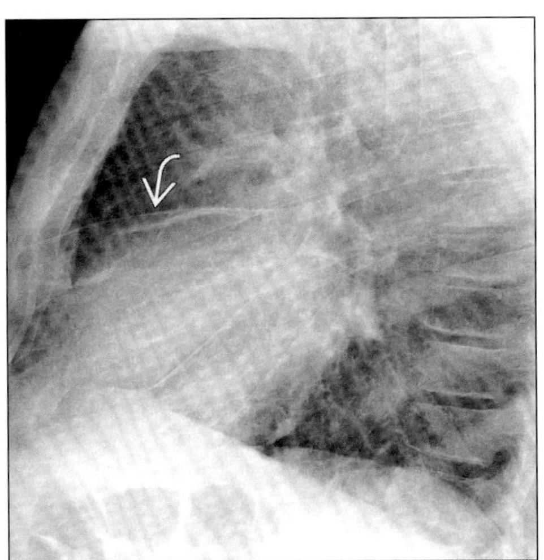

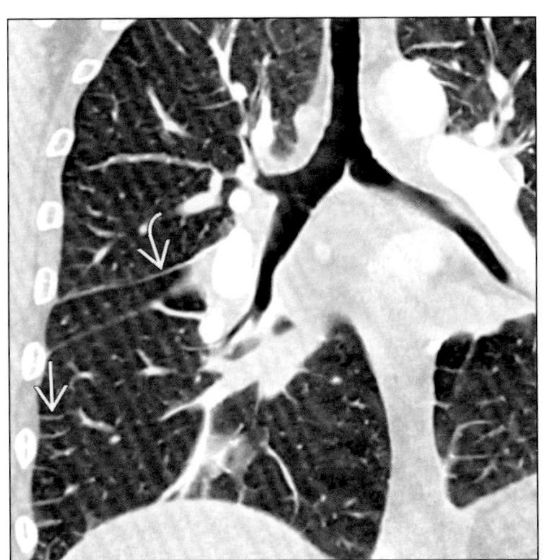

(Left) *Coned-down lateral chest radiograph of a patient with interstitial edema shows subpleural edema manifesting as thickening of the interlobar fissures ➦ in the absence of pleural effusions.* ***(Right)*** *Coronal CECT of a patient with interstitial edema demonstrates thick interlobular septa ➡ and thick interlobar fissures ➦ secondary to edema of the peripheral subpleural interstitium. Subpleural edema may precede septal thickening and peribronchial cuffing as a manifestation of interstitial edema.*

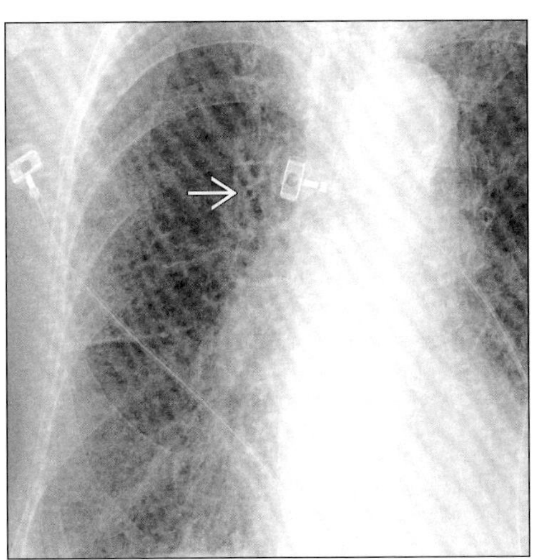

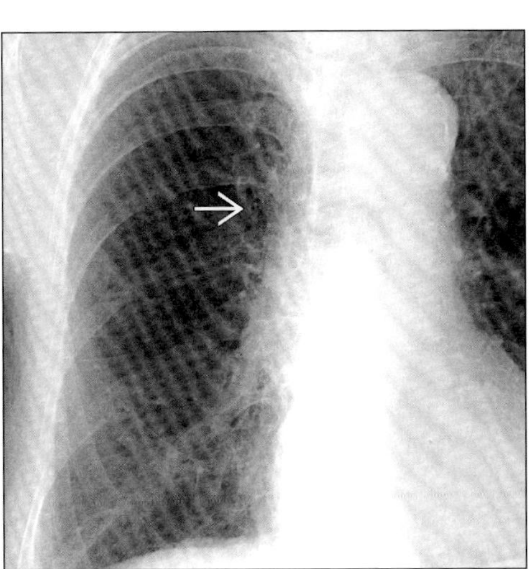

(Left) *PA chest radiograph of a patient with interstitial edema demonstrates profuse reticular opacities and peribronchial cuffing. The latter represents thickening of the peribronchial interstitium and is best appreciated around bronchi seen end-on ➡.* ***(Right)*** *PA chest radiograph of the same patient after treatment shows resolution of peribronchial cuffing and nearly imperceptible bronchial walls ➡. Peribronchial cuffing represents extravascular fluid in the axial bronchoarterial interstitium.*

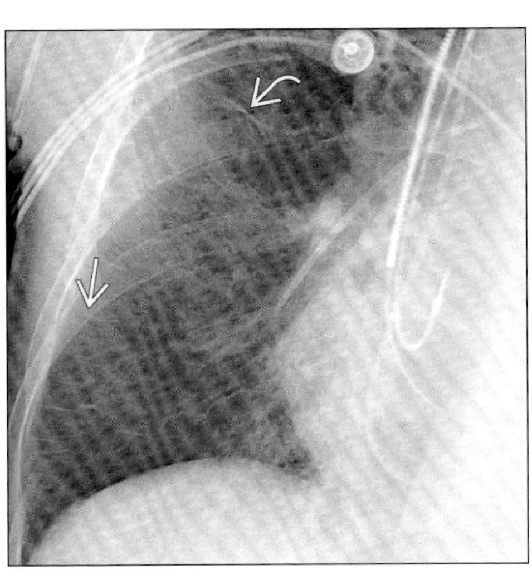

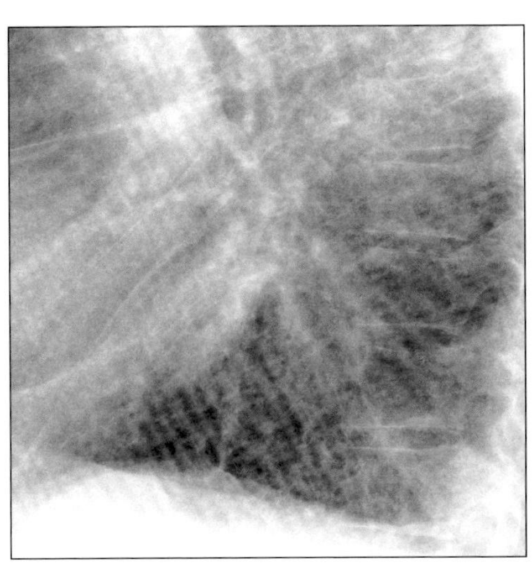

(Left) *Coned-down AP chest radiograph of a patient with interstitial edema shows Kerley B lines ➡ manifesting as short thin lines perpendicular to the lateral pleura. Longer oblique lines represent Kerley A lines ➦.* ***(Right)*** *Coned-down lateral chest radiograph of a patient with interstitial edema shows a basilar network of reticular opacities representing Kerley C lines, which are thought to represent Kerley B lines seen en face. All Kerley lines represent fluid in the interlobular septa.*

*(**Left**) Coned-down PA chest radiograph shows the method used to measure the vascular pedicle, which is the horizontal distance between the superior vena cava interface as it crosses the right main stem bronchus and the origin of the left subclavian artery. (**Right**) Composite image shows frontal radiographs of a patient with interstitial edema before (left) and after treatment (right) with resultant decreasing width of the vascular pedicle. A normal vascular pedicle may measure up to 58 mm.*

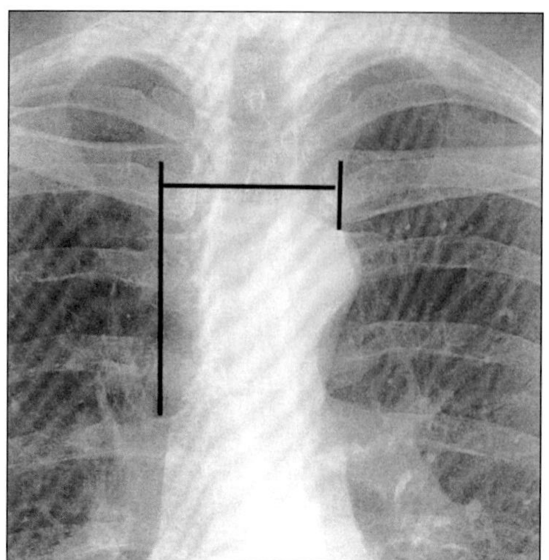

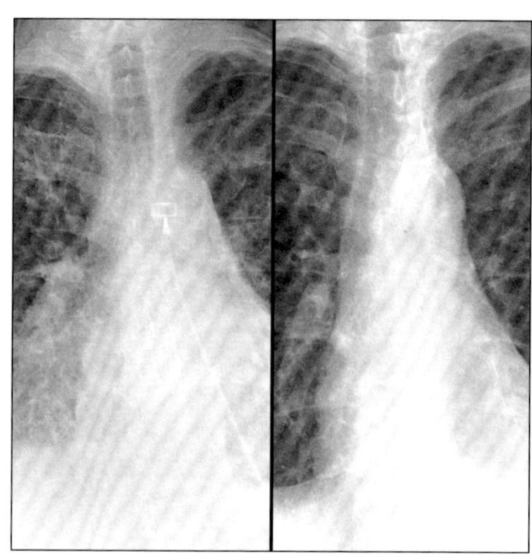

*(**Left**) AP chest radiograph shows asymmetric alveolar edema manifesting as bilateral perihilar haze and consolidation, most pronounced on the right. Note peribronchial cuffing ➔, fissural pleural thickening ➔ (subpleural edema), and bilateral pleural effusions. (**Right**) Frontal chest radiograph of a patient with interstitial and alveolar edema shows cardiomegaly, bilateral pleural effusions, profuse fine reticular opacities, and asymmetric perihilar haze and consolidations.*

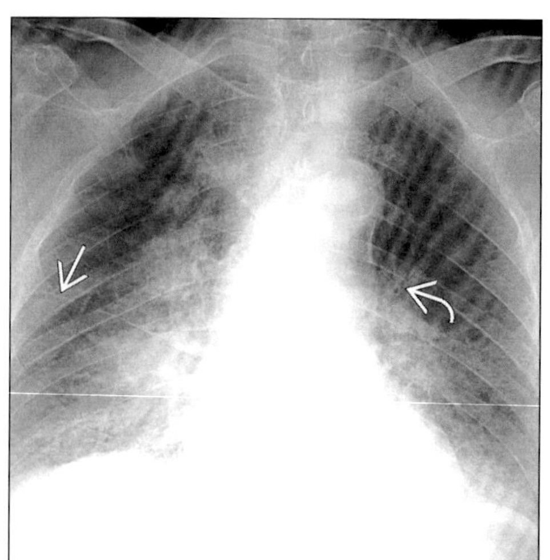

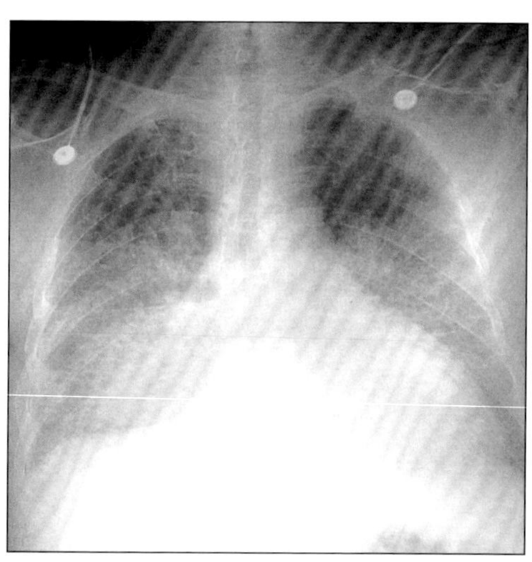

*(**Left**) Axial CECT of a patient with interstitial edema shows smooth thickening of the interlobular septa visible as linear opacities ➔ that form central polygonal arcades ➔. (**Right**) Composite image shows a normal right lower lobe on CT (left) compared to CT findings of interstitial edema (right) manifesting with peribronchial thickening ➔, patchy ground-glass opacities, and a small right pleural effusion ➔. CT optimally demonstrates the early manifestations of interstitial edema.*

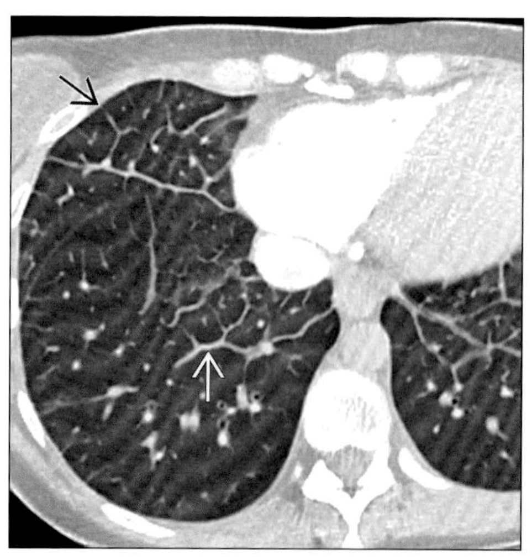

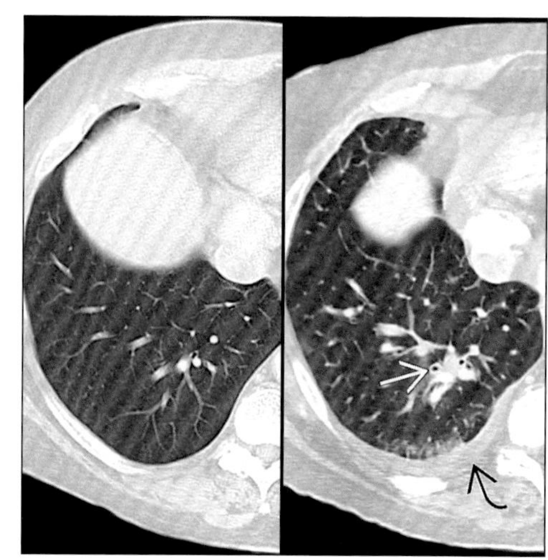

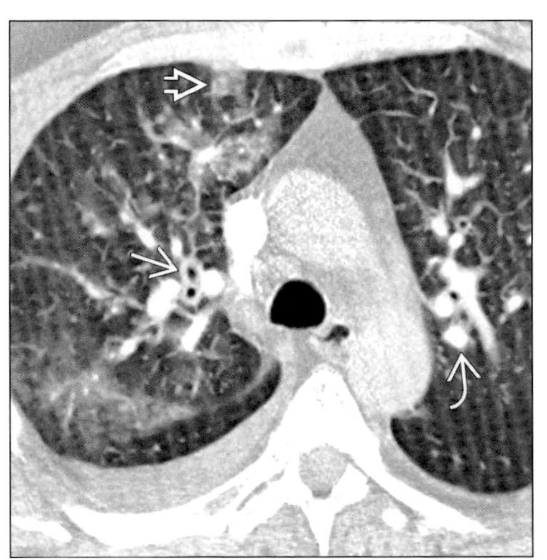

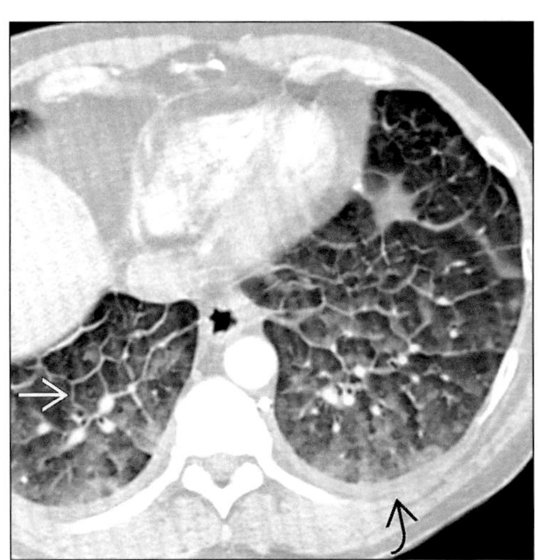

(Left) *Axial CECT shows interstitial and alveolar edema and small bilateral pleural effusions. Note abnormal upper lobe bronchoarterial ratios ➔, bronchial wall thickening ➔, and asymmetric alveolar edema ➔.* ***(Right)*** *Axial CECT of a patient with alveolar and interstitial edema shows patchy ground-glass opacities, smooth interlobular septal thickening ➔, and small bilateral pleural effusions ➔. Central thick interlobular septa form polygonal arcades on CT.*

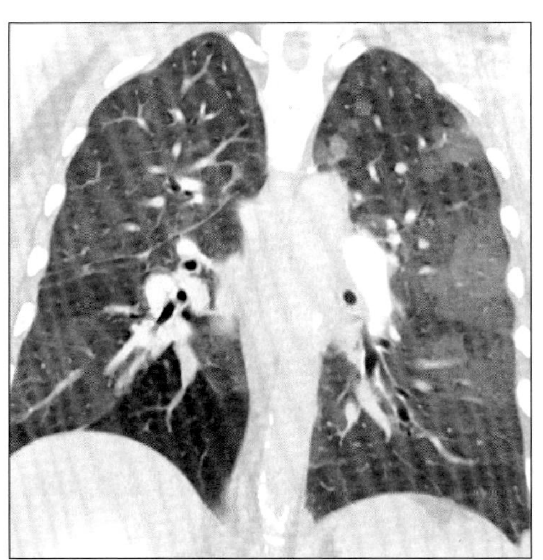

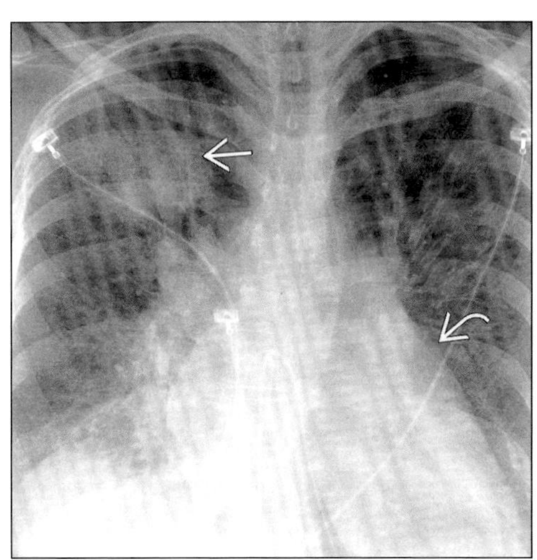

(Left) *Coronal CECT of a patient with alveolar edema shows patchy confluent, lobular, and acinar ground-glass opacities without obvious interlobular septal thickening.* ***(Right)*** *AP chest radiograph of a patient with acute mitral insufficiency shows asymmetric alveolar edema preferentially affecting the right upper lobe ➔ due to the direction of regurgitant blood flow across an incompetent mitral valve. Note cardiomegaly, left atrial appendage enlargement ➔, and right pleural effusion.*

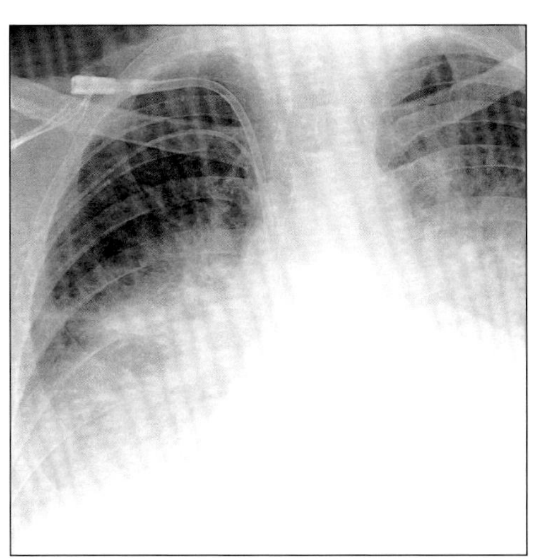

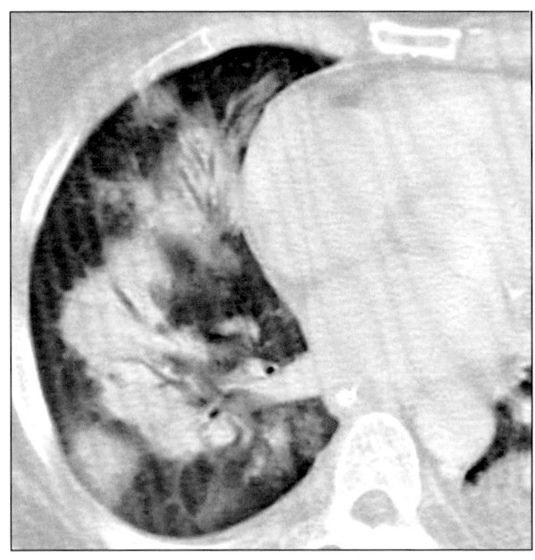

(Left) *AP chest radiograph of a patient with central or bat wing pulmonary edema shows bilateral perihilar haze and consolidations representing alveolar edema with relative sparing of the lung periphery.* ***(Right)*** *Axial NECT of a patient with bat wing pulmonary edema shows central perihilar consolidations with air bronchograms and sparing of the lung periphery. Bat wing edema occurs in < 10% of patients with pulmonary edema and is associated with rapid onset of severe heart failure.*

NONCARDIOGENIC PULMONARY EDEMA

Key Facts

Terminology
- Diffuse alveolar damage (DAD)
- Noncardiogenic edema: Increased permeability of alveolar-capillary barrier
  - Permeability edema with DAD
  - Permeability edema without DAD
  - Mixed edema

Imaging
- Radiography: Diffuse bilateral airspace opacities, normal heart size
- CT: Typical pattern
  - Ground-glass opacity & normal aerated lung
  - Dense consolidation in dependent lung
- CT: Atypical pattern
  - Ground-glass opacity & normal aerated lung
  - Dense consolidation in nondependent lung
  - Multiple thin-walled cysts

Top Differential Diagnoses
- Cardiogenic edema
- Diffuse pulmonary hemorrhage
- Pulmonary infection

Clinical Issues
- Symptoms/signs
  - Shortness of breath, tachypnea, & dry cough
- 75 cases/100,000 persons/year
- Prognosis
  - Mortality rate: 30-40%
  - 10% develop pulmonary fibrosis
- Treatment
  - Mechanical ventilation; moderate to high PEEP

Diagnostic Checklist
- Consider noncardiogenic edema in intubated patients with diffuse bilateral airspace opacities

__(Left)__ PA chest radiograph of a patient with neurogenic pulmonary edema secondary to intracranial hemorrhage demonstrates appropriately positioned endotracheal and enteric tubes and diffuse, symmetric, bilateral airspace disease. __(Right)__ Axial CECT of a patient with a history of recent smoke inhalation shows patchy ground-glass opacity and consolidations in the anterior aspects of both lungs ➦, dense bilateral posterior lower lobe consolidations ➔, and small bilateral pleural effusions.

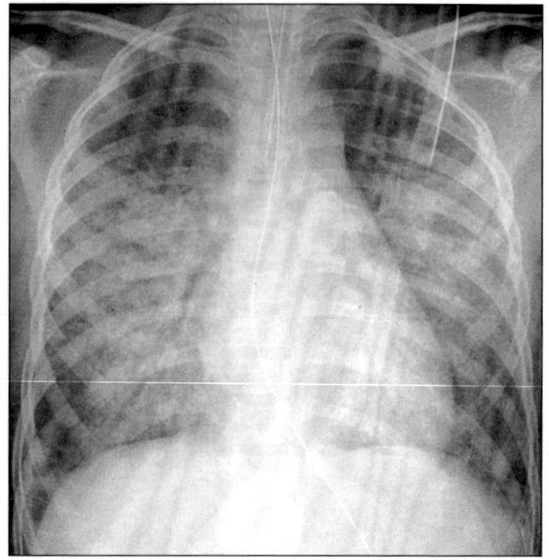

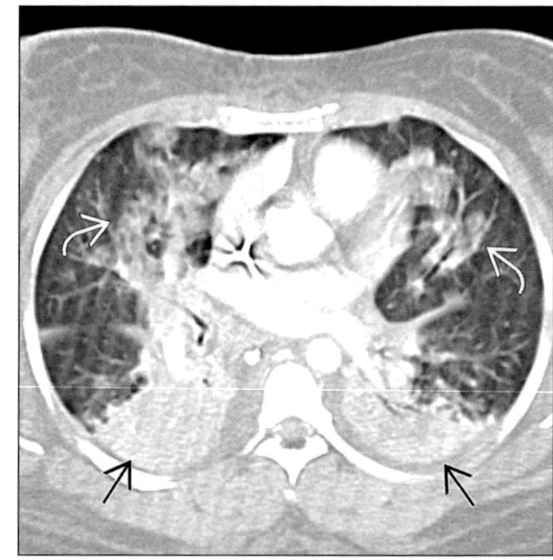

__(Left)__ Axial CECT of a patient with noncardiogenic pulmonary edema secondary to illicit drug use shows diffuse, bilateral symmetric central ground-glass opacities ➦ without interlobular septal thickening, peribronchial cuffing, or pleural effusions and a pneumomediastinum secondary to barotrauma. __(Right)__ Coronal CECT of a skier with high-altitude pulmonary edema shows bilateral, upper lobe predominant, patchy ground-glass opacities and small nodular foci of consolidation ➦.

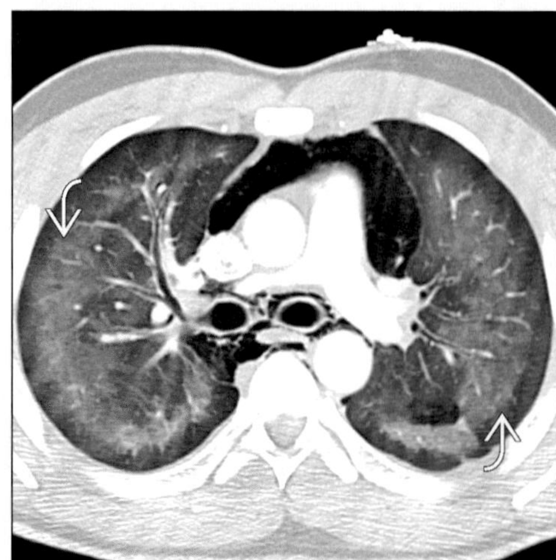

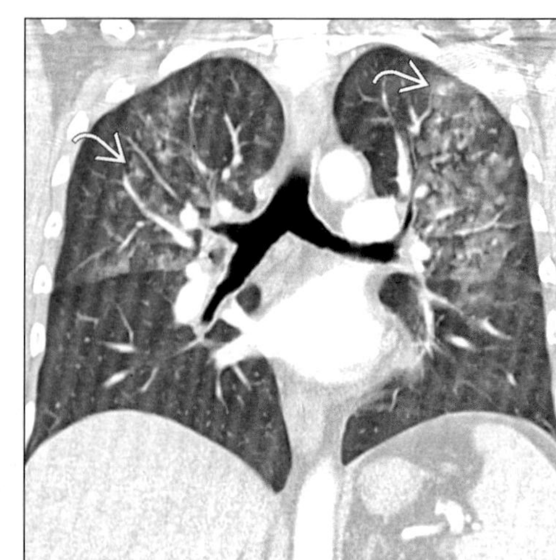

NONCARDIOGENIC PULMONARY EDEMA

TERMINOLOGY

Abbreviations

- **Adult respiratory distress syndrome (ARDS)**
- **Diffuse alveolar damage (DAD)**

Definitions

- **Noncardiogenic edema**: Increased permeability of alveolar-capillary barrier
  - Permeability edema with DAD
  - Permeability edema without DAD
  - Mixed edema
- **ARDS**: Increased permeability edema with alveolar-capillary damage
- **DAD**: Nonspecific reaction to agents that damage alveolar-capillary membrane

IMAGING

General Features

- Best diagnostic clue
  - Diffuse bilateral airspace opacities in intubated patient
- Location
  - Peripheral > central

Radiographic Findings

- Radiography
  - **Diffuse bilateral airspace disease**
    - **Peripheral** > central lung; usually **symmetric**
    - Kerley B lines, peribronchial cuffing, & pleural effusions less common than in cardiogenic edema
  - **Normal heart size**

CT Findings

- Typical pattern; more common in secondary injury
  - Mixture of ground-glass opacity & normal aerated lung
  - Dense consolidation in dependent lung
- Atypical pattern; more common in primary injury
  - Mixture of ground-glass opacity & normal aerated lung
  - Dense consolidation
    - More common in nondependent lung
    - Less common in dependent lung
  - Multiple thin-walled cysts

Imaging Recommendations

- Best imaging tool
  - Chest radiography adequate for monitoring course
  - CT used as problem solving tool

DIFFERENTIAL DIAGNOSIS

Cardiogenic Edema

- Central > peripheral opacities (bat-wing distribution)
- Kerley B lines, peribronchial cuffing, & pleural effusions
- Increased heart size

Diffuse Pulmonary Hemorrhage

- Anemia & hemoptysis
- Diffuse bilateral pulmonary opacities
- Normal heart size

Pulmonary Infection

- Fever & elevated white blood cell count
- May result in ARDS

PATHOLOGY

General Features

- Etiology
  - Permeability edema with DAD
    - Primary injury: Exposure to chemicals, gastric contents, toxic gases, & infectious organisms
    - Secondary injury: Sepsis, severe trauma, pancreatitis, & blood transfusion
  - Permeability edema without DAD
    - Illicit drug-induced pulmonary edema
      - Heroin, cocaine, & "crack"
    - High-altitude pulmonary edema
  - Mixed edema
    - Neurogenic pulmonary edema
      - Traumatic brain injury, stroke, & subarachnoid hemorrhage
    - Reperfusion pulmonary edema
      - Pulmonary thromboendarterectomy
    - Following lung transplantation or pneumonectomy
    - Reexpansion pulmonary edema

Microscopic Features

- DAD: 3 stages
  - Exudative phase (stage 1)
  - Proliferative phase (stage 2)
  - Fibrotic phase (stage 3)
- Mixed stages in different areas of lung are typical

CLINICAL ISSUES

Presentation

- Most common signs/symptoms
  - Shortness of breath, tachypnea, & dry cough

Demographics

- Epidemiology
  - 75 cases/100,000 persons/year

Natural History & Prognosis

- **Mortality rate: 30-40%**
- **10% develop pulmonary fibrosis**
- Restrictive or obstructive deficits in survivors

Treatment

- Mechanical ventilation & moderate/high PEEP

DIAGNOSTIC CHECKLIST

Consider

- Noncardiogenic pulmonary edema in intubated patients with diffuse bilateral airspace opacities

SELECTED REFERENCES

1. Rubenfeld GD et al: Epidemiology and outcomes of acute lung injury. Chest. 131(2):554-62, 2007
2. Dueck R: Alveolar recruitment versus hyperinflation: A balancing act. Curr Opin Anaesthesiol. 19(6):650-4, 2006

PULMONARY ARTERY HYPERTENSION

Key Facts

Terminology

- Pulmonary artery hypertension (PAH)
- Mean pulmonary artery pressure > 25 mmHg at rest
  - > 30 mmHg during exercise
- Mean capillary wedge pressure & left ventricular end-diastolic pressure typically < 15 mmHg

Imaging

- Radiography
  - Enlarged pulmonary trunk & central pulmonary arteries
- HRCT
  - Pre-capillary etiologies: Emphysema, fibrosis, honeycomb lung
  - Post-capillary etiologies: Centrilobular ground-glass nodules, pulmonary edema, pleural effusions
  - Chronic PAH: Patchy ground-glass opacity
- CTA: Enlargement of pulmonary trunk > 30 mm

Top Differential Diagnoses

- Congenital pulmonic valvular stenosis
- Idiopathic dilatation of pulmonary trunk
- Hilar lymphadenopathy

Pathology

- Pre-capillary etiologies: Chronic pulmonary emboli, congenital left-to-right shunts, lung disease, idiopathic PAH
- Post-capillary etiologies: Left heart failure & mitral stenosis

Clinical Issues

- Poor prognosis
- Treatment
  - Medical therapy: Calcium channel blockers
  - Idiopathic PAH: Prostaglandin I2 (epoprostenol)
  - Lung ± heart transplant

*(**Left**) PA chest radiograph of a patient with pulmonary artery hypertension shows enlargement of the pulmonary trunk ➡, left ➦ and right ➦ pulmonary arteries, and abrupt narrowing ("pruning") of the peripheral pulmonary arteries. (**Right**) Lateral chest radiograph of the same patient shows bilateral hilar masses representing pulmonary artery enlargement ➡. The patient has a patent ductus arteriosus (a left-to-right shunt that represents a pre-capillary etiology of PAH).*

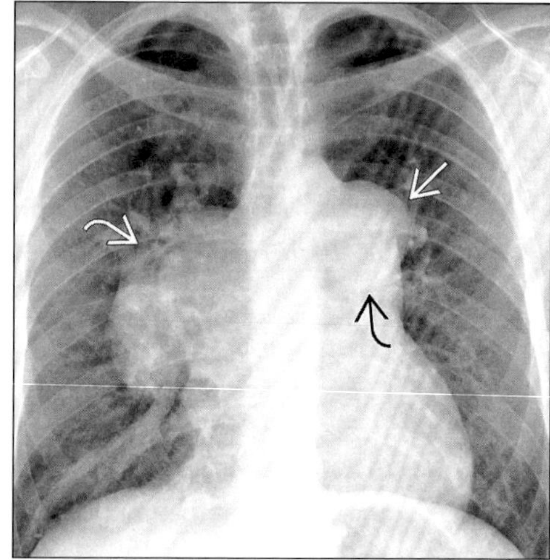

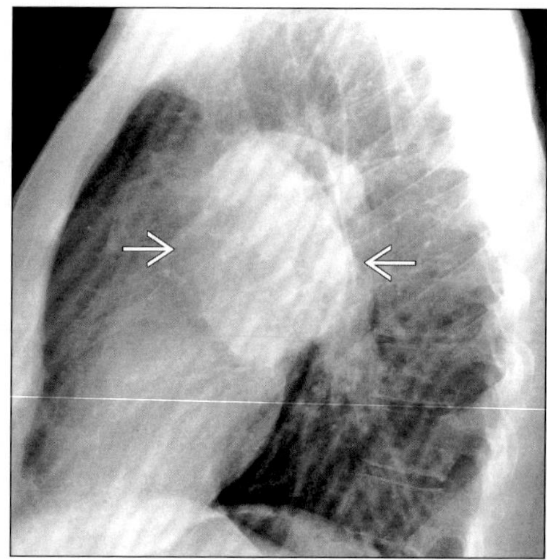

*(**Left**) Axial NECT of a patient with longstanding PAH shows marked enlargement of the right ➡ and left ➦ pulmonary arteries and intimal pulmonary artery calcification ➡. The pulmonary trunk ➡ is also enlarged. (**Right**) Phase-contrast sagittal MR shows an enlarged pulmonary trunk ➦ and enlarged proximal left and right pulmonary arteries ➡. Phase-contrast MR is useful for evaluating pulmonary artery morphology and determining the direction and velocities of blood flow.*

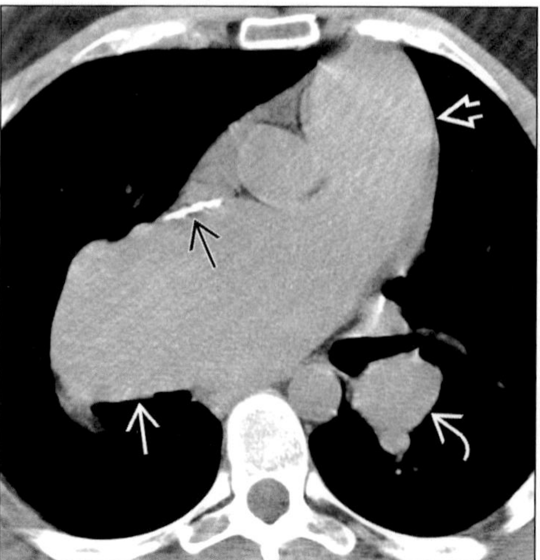

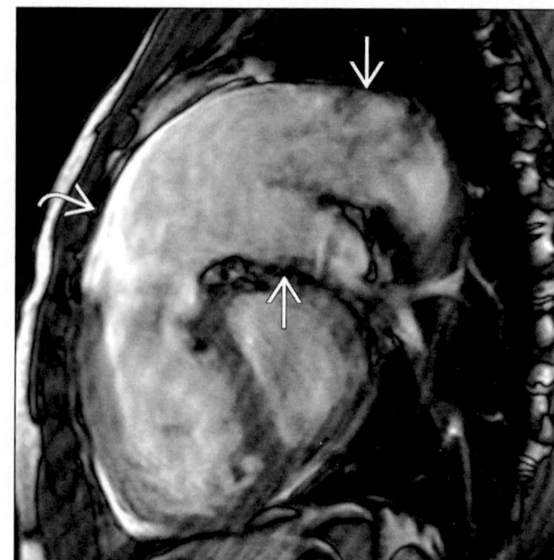

PULMONARY ARTERY HYPERTENSION

TERMINOLOGY

Abbreviations

- **Pulmonary artery hypertension (PAH)**

Definitions

- Mean pulmonary artery pressure > 25 mmHg at rest
  - > 30 mmHg during exercise
- Mean capillary wedge pressure & left ventricular end-diastolic pressure typically < 15 mmHg

IMAGING

General Features

- Best diagnostic clue
  - Enlarged pulmonary trunk
    - Variable enlargement of left & right pulmonary arteries (PA)

Radiographic Findings

- Radiography
  - General
    - **Enlargement of pulmonary trunk**
      - Left superior mediastinal convexity on frontal radiography
    - Pruning of peripheral PA branches
    - Cardiac silhouette
      - Early: Normal
      - Late: Enlargement of right atrium & ventricle
    - Chronic PAH
      - Intimal calcification of PA wall
  - Lung parenchyma
    - Pre-capillary etiologies
      - Emphysema, fibrosis, honeycomb lung
    - Post-capillary etiologies
      - Pulmonary edema & pleural effusions

CT Findings

- HRCT
  - **Pre-capillary etiologies**
    - Emphysema, fibrosis, honeycomb lung
  - **Post-capillary etiologies**
    - Centrilobular ground-glass nodules
      - Hemorrhagic foci
      - Cholesterol granulomas
    - Pulmonary edema
    - Pleural & pericardial effusions
    - Mediastinal lymphadenopathy
  - **Chronic PAH**
    - Mosaic attenuation
    - Differential perfusion
    - Diminished vascularity in regions of decreased lung attenuation
    - Ground-glass opacity less well defined than in small airways disease
- CTA
  - General
    - Enlargement of PAs
    - Pulmonary trunk > 30 mm
    - Right interlobar PA > 16 mm in men; > 14 mm in women
  - Normal PAs
    - Pulmonary trunk: 28.6 mm
      - Smaller than adjacent ascending aorta
    - Left PA: 28 mm; right PA: 24.3 mm
  - **Chronic pulmonary emboli**
    - Band-like peripheral endoluminal hypoattenuation foci
  - Schistosomiasis
    - Cirrhosis & portal hypertension
  - Chronic PAH
    - Intimal calcification of PA wall
- Cardiac gated CTA
  - Decreased distensibility of PA wall

MR Findings

- Less sensitive & specific than CT
- More difficult to perform in dyspneic patients
- Phase-contrast MR
  - Morphology of PAs
  - Direction & velocities of blood flow
  - Resistance to flow
  - Regurgitant fraction
  - PA strain

Angiographic Findings

- Most reliable means of diagnosis
- Direct measurement of right-sided pressures

Nuclear Medicine Findings

- Ventilation-perfusion scintigraphy
  - Scans usually low probability for PE
  - High probability scans with chronic thromboemboli
  - Reduced quantity of particles necessary
    - Risk of acute right heart failure from occlusion of capillary bed

Imaging Recommendations

- Best imaging tool
  - CECT
    - Quantify PA enlargement
    - Determine etiology
      - Filling defects in PAs (thromboemboli)
      - Parenchymal abnormalities
      - Cardiac morphology
- Protocol advice
  - Multiplanar imaging for accurate measurements

Echocardiographic Findings

- Echocardiogram
  - Right ventricular pressure overload
    - Enlarged right atrium & ventricle
    - Right ventricular hypertrophy
    - Reduced global right ventricular function
    - Interventricular septum
      - Increased thickness
      - Systolic flattening
      - IV septum: Posterior LV wall ratio > 1

DIFFERENTIAL DIAGNOSIS

Congenital Pulmonic Valvular Stenosis

- Enlargement of pulmonary trunk & left PA
- Thickening & calcification of pulmonic valve leaflets may be present

Idiopathic Dilatation of Pulmonary Trunk

- Enlargement of pulmonary trunk ± left & right PAs
- Diagnosis of exclusion
  - Normal right-sided pressures

PULMONARY ARTERY HYPERTENSION

Hilar Lymphadenopathy

- Enlargement of hila
- Sarcoidosis, lymphoma, metastatic disease

PATHOLOGY

General Features

- Etiology
  - Pre-capillary & post-capillary etiologies
  - Pre-capillary
    - Chronic pulmonary emboli
    - Congenital left-to-right shunts
      - Atrial & ventricular septal defects
      - Patent ductus arteriosus
    - Lung disease
      - Emphysema, fibrosis, honeycomb lung
    - Idiopathic PAH
    - Infection: Schistosomiasis & HIV
    - Drugs & toxins
    - Portal hypertension
  - Post-capillary
    - Left heart failure
    - Mitral stenosis
    - Mediastinal fibrosis
    - Pulmonary veno-occlusive disease

Staging, Grading, & Classification

- **Heath-Edwards microscopic grading**
  - Grade I: Muscularization of pulmonary arteries
  - Grade II: Intimal proliferation
  - Grade III: Subendothelial fibrosis
  - Grade IV: Plexiform lesions
  - Grade V: Rupture of dilated vessels
  - Grade VI: Necrotizing arteritis
- **WHO Classification**
  - WHO Group I: PAH
  - WHO Group II: PAH associated with left heart disease
  - WHO Group III: PAH associated with lung disease &/or hypoxemia
  - WHO Group IV: PAH due to chronic thrombotic &/or embolic disease

Microscopic Features

- **Idiopathic PAH**
  - Plexogenic pulmonary arteriopathy
    - Medial hypertrophy
    - Intimal proliferation
    - Necrotizing arteritis
- **Pulmonary veno-occlusive disease (PVOD)**
  - Microscopic findings of capillary hemangiomatosis
  - Intimal fibrosis of pulmonary veins
  - Recanalized thrombi & webs
- Centrilobular cholesterol granulomas in 25% of cases

CLINICAL ISSUES

Presentation

- Most common signs/symptoms
  - Dyspnea on exertion
- Other signs/symptoms
  - Fatigue, syncope, chest pain
  - PVOD may be preceded by flu-like illness

Demographics

- Age
  - Idiopathic PAH: 3rd decade of life
- Gender
  - Idiopathic PAH: M:F = 1:3
- Epidemiology
  - Schistosomiasis most common cause worldwide
  - Pulmonary veno-occlusive disease: 1/3 children
  - Prevalence in men
    - 10% above age 35; 25% above age 65
  - 1% of cases of acute thromboemboli become chronic thromboemboli

Natural History & Prognosis

- Diagnosis
  - Swan-Ganz catheterization
    - Normal resting mean PA pressure < 20 mmHg
  - Pre-capillary
    - Elevated mean PA pressure & increased resistance
    - Normal pulmonary capillary wedge pressure (PCWP)
  - Post-capillary
    - Elevated mean PA pressure & increased resistance
    - Elevated PCWP
- Poor prognosis

Treatment

- Medical therapy
  - 30% response
  - Calcium channel blockers
- Pulmonary thromboemboli
  - Anticoagulation
  - Inferior vena cava filter
  - Selective thromboendarterectomy
- Idiopathic PAH
  - Prostaglandin I2 (epoprostenol)
    - Vasodilator
    - Poor prognostic indicators on pre-treatment CT
      - Centrilobular ground-glass nodules
      - Interlobular septal thickening
      - Pleural & pericardial effusions
      - Lymphadenopathy
- Lung ± heart transplant

DIAGNOSTIC CHECKLIST

Consider

- PAH when imaging studies demonstrate pulmonary trunk size > 30 mm

Image Interpretation Pearls

- Evaluate mediastinum & lung parenchyma for possible etiologies

SELECTED REFERENCES

1. Badesch DB et al: Pulmonary arterial hypertension: baseline characteristics from the REVEAL Registry. Chest. 137(2):376-87, 2010
2. Sanz J et al: Pulmonary arterial hypertension: noninvasive detection with phase-contrast MR imaging. Radiology. 243(1):70-9, 2007
3. Frazier AA et al: From the archives of the AFIP: pulmonary vasculature: hypertension and infarction. Radiographics. 20(2):491-524; quiz 530-1, 532, 2000

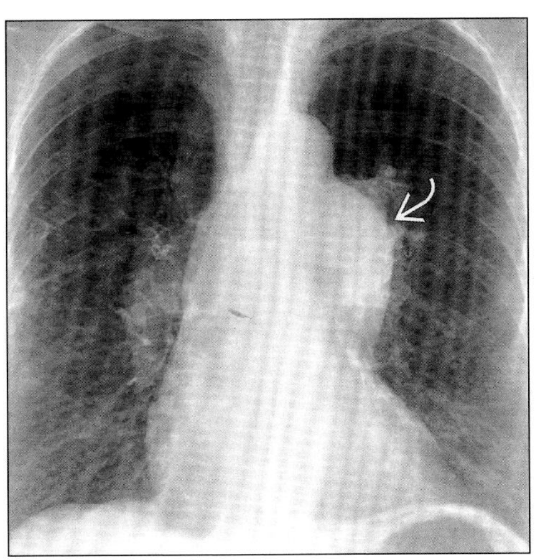

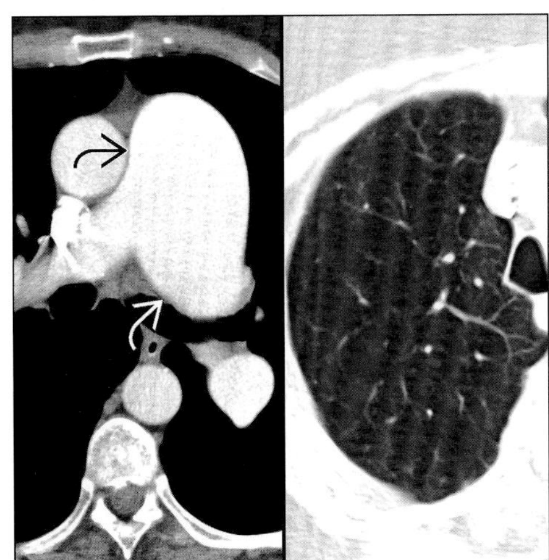

(Left) *PA chest radiograph of a patient with emphysema shows enlargement of the pulmonary trunk ➡ and the central pulmonary arteries.* **(Right)** *Composite image with axial CECT in soft tissue (left) and lung (right) window of the same patient shows enlargement of the pulmonary trunk ➡ and left ➡ pulmonary artery, and emphysema. Pulmonary abnormalities, including emphysema, pulmonary fibrosis, and end-stage honeycomb lung, are common pre-capillary etiologies of PAH.*

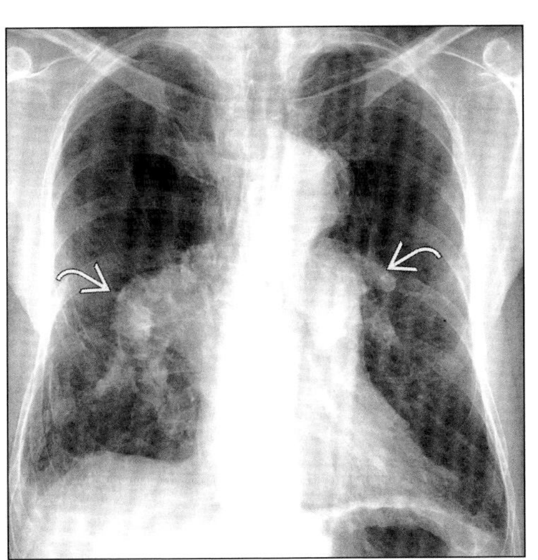

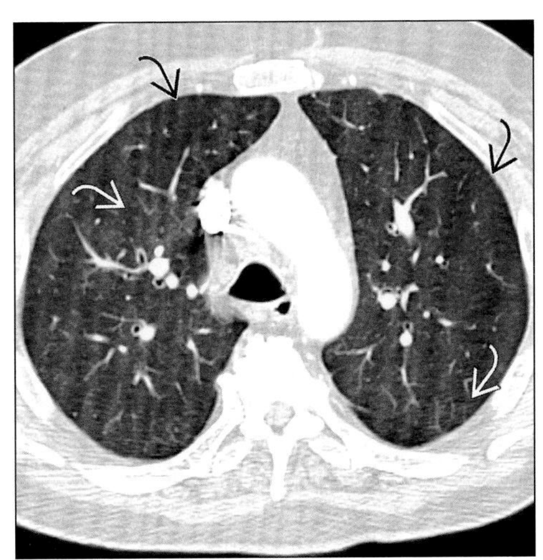

(Left) *PA chest radiograph of a patient with idiopathic pulmonary hypertension shows enlarged pulmonary arteries ➡. The imaging manifestations of idiopathic pulmonary arterial hypertension are indistinguishable from those found in cases with known etiologies.* **(Right)** *Axial CECT of a patient with chronic pulmonary artery hypertension shows bilateral patchy ground-glass opacities ➡ and scattered areas of diminished lung vascularity manifesting as low-attenuation regions ➡.*

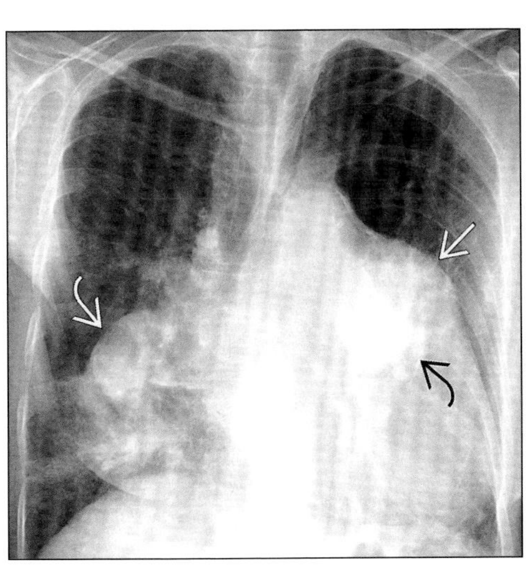

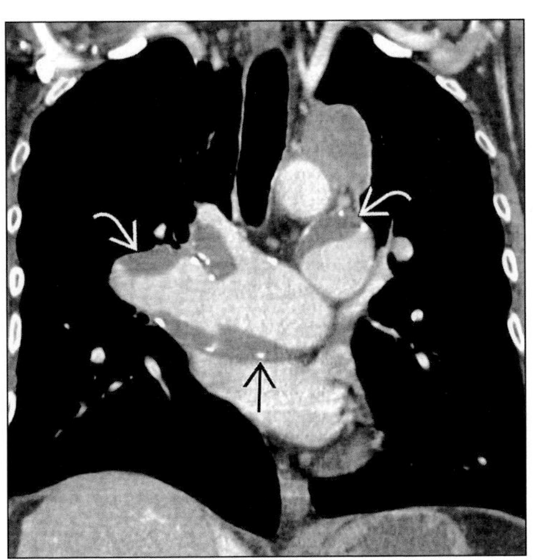

(Left) *PA chest radiograph demonstrates cardiomegaly & marked enlargement of the pulmonary trunk ➡ and left ➡ and right ➡ pulmonary arteries.* **(Right)** *Coronal CECT of the same patient shows enlarged pulmonary arteries with peripheral endoluminal band-like areas of soft tissue attenuation, consistent with chronic pulmonary thromboemboli ➡. Intimal calcification ➡ is consistent with longstanding PAH. Chronic pulmonary thromboembolic disease is a common pre-capillary cause of PAH.*

PULMONARY CAPILLARY HEMANGIOMATOSIS

Key Facts

Terminology
- Pulmonary capillary hemangiomatosis (PCH)
- Rare idiopathic disorder resulting in pulmonary arterial hypertension

Imaging
- Radiography
  - Enlarged pulmonary arteries (100%)
  - Cardiomegaly (90%)
  - Pleural effusion, often small (75%)
- CT
  - Ground-glass opacities (85%); centrilobular or diffuse
  - Thick interlobular septa (60%); smooth or nodular
  - Pericardial effusion (75%)
  - Mild lymphadenopathy, average size 12 mm (70%)
- HRCT important in differentiating PCH from primary pulmonary hypertension

Top Differential Diagnoses
- Pulmonary veno-occlusive disease (PVOD)
- Primary pulmonary hypertension (PPH)
- Chronic pulmonary thromboemboli

Pathology
- Proliferation of thin-walled capillaries in alveolar walls; venule obstruction causes pulmonary hypertension

Clinical Issues
- Progressive dyspnea & fatigue
- Elevated pulmonary artery pressure; normal or low capillary wedge pressure
- Median survival: 3 years from diagnosis

Diagnostic Checklist
- Consider HRCT in patients with newly diagnosed pulmonary artery hypertension to exclude PPH

*(**Left**) Coronal CECT of a 30-year-old man with progressive dyspnea, fatigue, and pulmonary artery hypertension shows diffuse bilateral ill-defined ground-glass nodules ➔. (**Right**) Axial CECT of the same patient shows enlargement of the pulmonary trunk ➔, which measured 4 cm in width. Notice that the width of the pulmonary trunk is much larger than that of the adjacent ascending aorta. Biopsy confirmed pulmonary capillary hemangiomatosis.*

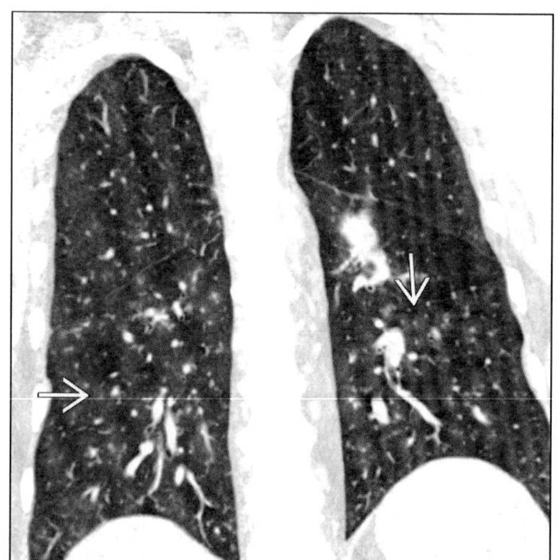

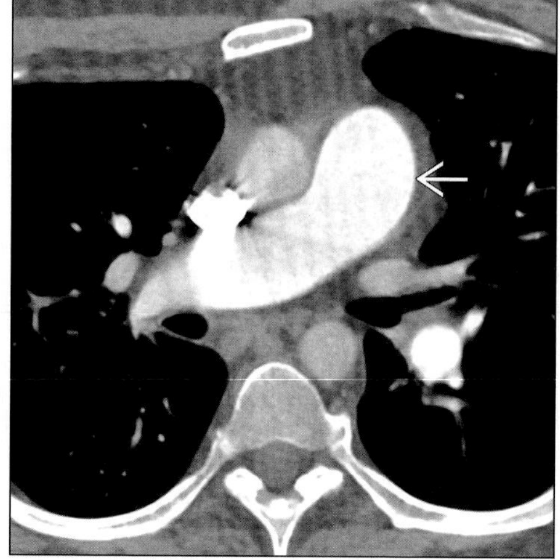

*(**Left**) Coronal NECT of a 40-year-old man who presented with hemoptysis shows enlargement of the pulmonary trunk ➔, smooth interlobular septal thickening ➔, and diffuse bilateral ground-glass opacities. (**Right**) Axial NECT of the same patient shows an enlarged pulmonary trunk ➔ and bilateral pleural effusions ➔. These findings should raise suspicion for PCH or PVOD in a patient with pulmonary artery hypertension as treatment differs from that of primary pulmonary hypertension.*

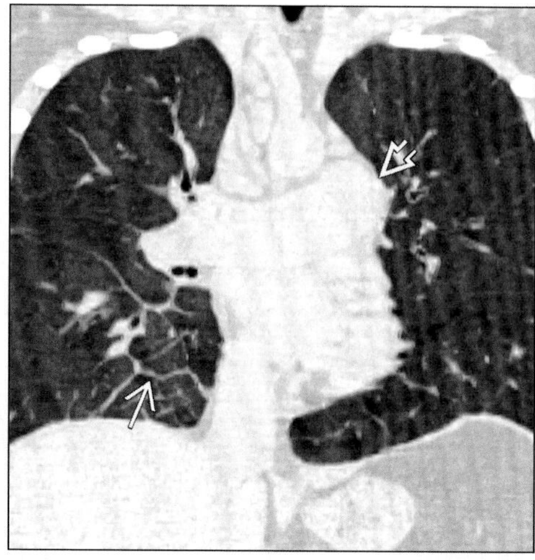

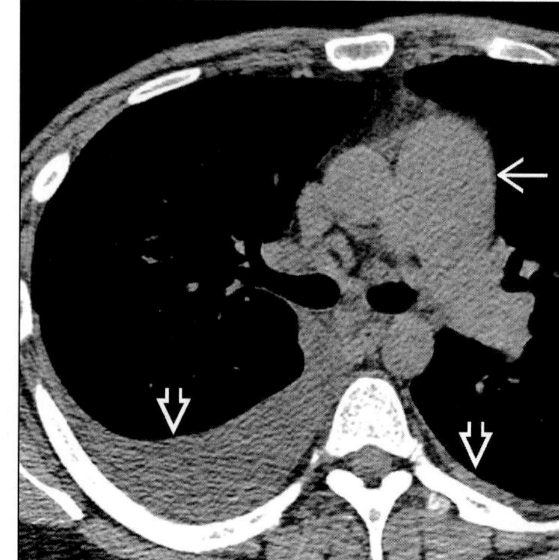

PULMONARY CAPILLARY HEMANGIOMATOSIS

TERMINOLOGY

Abbreviations

- **Pulmonary capillary hemangiomatosis (PCH)**

Definitions

- Described in 1978 by Wagenvoort
- Rare idiopathic disorder resulting in pulmonary arterial hypertension due to interstitial invasion by proliferation of thin-walled alveolar capillaries

IMAGING

General Features

- Best diagnostic clue
  - **Enlarged pulmonary arteries** & diffuse **centrilobular ground-glass nodules**
- Location
  - Diffuse involvement without zonal predominance

Radiographic Findings

- Radiography
  - **Enlarged pulmonary arteries (100%)**
  - **Cardiomegaly (90%)**
  - **Pleural effusion, often small (75%)**
  - Nonspecific basilar reticular opacities

CT Findings

- HRCT
  - **Ground-glass opacities (85%)**
    - Poorly defined **centrilobular ground-glass nodular opacities** (70%)
  - **Thick interlobular septa** (60%), may be smooth or nodular
  - **Pericardial effusion (75%)**
  - Mild lymphadenopathy, average size 12 mm (70%)

Imaging Recommendations

- Best imaging tool
  - HRCT important in differentiating PCH from primary pulmonary hypertension

Nuclear Medicine Findings

- V/Q scan
  - Not useful; results range from normal to high probability

DIFFERENTIAL DIAGNOSIS

Pulmonary Veno-occlusive Disease (PVOD)

- Similar imaging findings; some investigators view PCH as sequela of PVOD
- Lacks capillary invasion

Primary Pulmonary Hypertension (PPH)

- Primarily young women
- Findings portending poor response to epoprostenol (prostacyclin) therapy
  - Centrilobular ground-glass opacities, septal lines, pleural effusions, lymphadenopathy, pericardial effusion

Chronic Pulmonary Thromboemboli

- Identification & characterization on CTA
- Centrilobular nodules, septal lines, pleural effusions less common

PATHOLOGY

General Features

- Etiology
  - Idiopathic; also reported in scleroderma, lupus, Kartagener syndrome, Takayasu arteritis, & hypertropic cardiomyopathy
  - Viral & autosomal recessive hereditary associations also reported
- Associated abnormalities
  - Secondary hemothorax

Microscopic Features

- Proliferation of thin-walled capillaries in alveolar walls
- Secondary obstruction of pulmonary venules causing pulmonary hypertension
- Often difficult to differentiate from pulmonary veno-occlusive disease

CLINICAL ISSUES

Presentation

- Most common signs/symptoms
  - Progressive dyspnea & fatigue
- Other signs/symptoms
  - Chronic cough, chest pain, syncope
  - Stigmata of pulmonary hypertension
  - Hemoptysis (30%)
- Elevated pulmonary artery pressure; normal or low capillary wedge pressure

Demographics

- Age
  - Range: 2-71 years; mean: 30 years
- Gender
  - No gender predominance
- Epidemiology
  - Extremely rare

Natural History & Prognosis

- Typically progressive pulmonary hypertension
- Patients succumb to respiratory failure or hemoptysis
- Median survival: 3 years from diagnosis

Treatment

- Steroids; cytotoxic agents not effective
- α-interferon may be useful in some cases
- Lung transplantation
  - Recurrence in transplanted lung reported
- Vasodilators may induce fatal pulmonary edema

DIAGNOSTIC CHECKLIST

Consider

- HRCT in patients with newly diagnosed pulmonary artery hypertension to exclude PPH

SELECTED REFERENCES

1. Frazier AA et al: From the Archives of the AFIP: pulmonary veno-occlusive disease and pulmonary capillary hemangiomatosis. Radiographics. 27(3):867-82, 2007
2. Lawler LP et al: Pulmonary capillary hemangiomatosis: multidetector row CT findings and clinico-pathologic correlation. J Thorac Imaging. 20(1):61-3, 2005

PULMONARY VENOOCCLUSIVE DISEASE

Key Facts

Terminology
- Pulmonary venoocclusive disease (PVOD)
- Rare cause of pulmonary hypertension resulting from occlusion of small pulmonary veins

Imaging
- Radiography
  - Enlarged pulmonary arteries
  - Findings of lung edema
  - Cardiomegaly (90%)
  - Small pleural effusions
- HRCT
  - Centrilobular ground-glass nodules (85%)
  - Smooth or nodular thick interlobular septa (60%)
  - Right ventricular enlargement
  - Normal-sized left atrium
  - Pericardial effusion (75%)
  - Mild mediastinal lymphadenopathy (variable)

Top Differential Diagnoses
- Pulmonary capillary hemangiomatosis
  - Identical radiographic findings
- Mediastinal fibrosis
  - Pulmonary vein obstruction by calcified mass
- Pulmonary hypertension

Pathology
- Insult that causes thrombosis of pulmonary veins
- Etiologies: Viral infection, chemotherapeutic drugs, autoimmune diseases, pregnancy, bone marrow transplantation

Clinical Issues
- Any age, most < 50 years
- Dyspnea, lethargy, & nonproductive cough
- Very poor prognosis
  - Most patients die within 2 years of diagnosis

__(Left)__ AP chest radiograph shows pulmonary trunk enlargement → and diffuse bilateral septal thickening →. PVOD should be suspected in patients with findings of pulmonary hypertension and septal lines. Pulmonary capillary wedge pressures may be normal or mildly elevated. __(Right)__ Axial HRCT of a patient with PVOD shows interlobular septal thickening →, ground-glass opacities →, and a small right pleural effusion →. Pleural effusions are common in PVOD and are typically small.

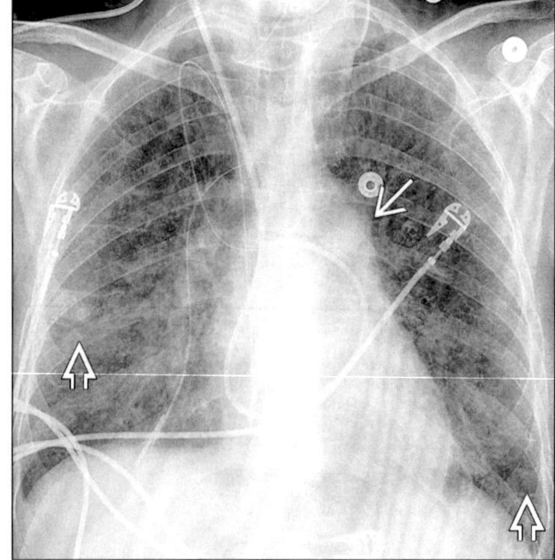

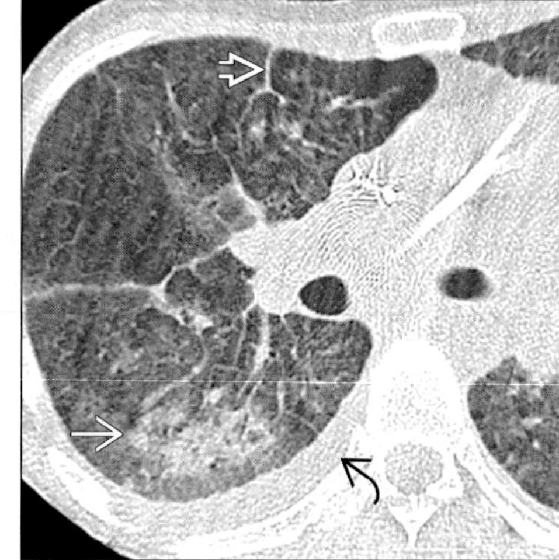

__(Left)__ Axial HRCT of a patient with PVOD shows bilateral nondependent interlobular septal thickening →, ground-glass opacities →, and pulmonary trunk enlargement →. __(Right)__ Axial HRCT of a patient with PVOD shows interlobular septal thickening →, ground-glass opacities →, and intralobular lines →. HRCT findings of PVOD are similar to those of other causes of lung edema. However, findings of pulmonary hypertension, such as pulmonary artery and right heart enlargement, are present in PVOD.

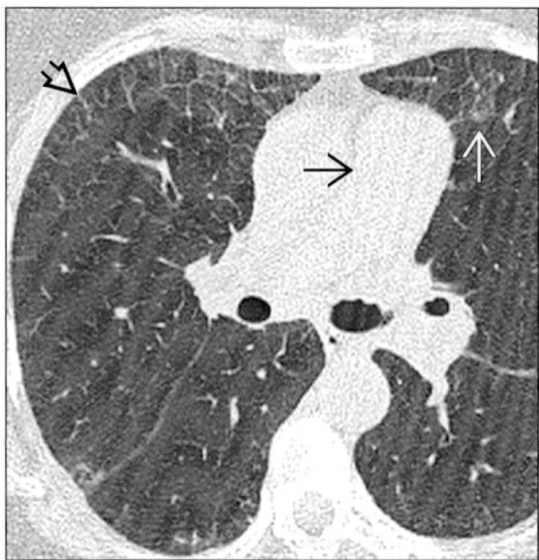

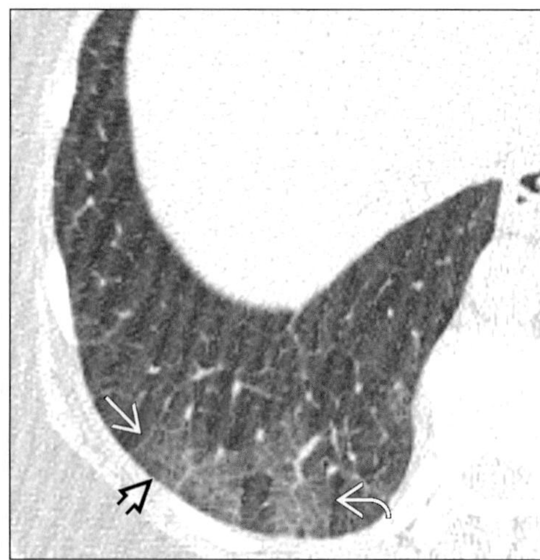

PULMONARY VENOOCCLUSIVE DISEASE

TERMINOLOGY

Abbreviations

- **Pulmonary venoocclusive disease (PVOD)**

Synonyms

- Pulmonary vasoocclusive disease
- Isolated pulmonary venous sclerosis
- Obstructive disease of pulmonary veins
- Venous form of primary pulmonary hypertension

Definitions

- Rare cause of pulmonary hypertension resulting from occlusion of small pulmonary veins

IMAGING

General Features

- Best diagnostic clue
  - Pulmonary hypertension & septal lines

Radiographic Findings

- **Enlarged pulmonary arteries** (100%)
- Findings of **lung edema**
  - Basilar interlobular septal thickening
  - Patchy opacities, often perihilar
- **Cardiomegaly** (90%)
- **Pleural effusions**, small (75%)

CT Findings

- HRCT
  - **Centrilobular ground-glass nodules** (85%)
  - Smooth or nodular **thick interlobular septa** (60%)
  - **Right ventricular enlargement**
  - Normal-sized left atrium
  - **Pericardial effusion** (75%)
  - Mild mediastinal lymphadenopathy (variable)

Imaging Recommendations

- Best imaging tool
  - HRCT useful for distinction of PVOD from primary pulmonary hypertension (PPH)

DIFFERENTIAL DIAGNOSIS

Pulmonary Capillary Hemangiomatosis (PCH)

- Identical radiographic findings
- PCH may be a sequela of PVOD

Mediastinal Fibrosis

- Major pulmonary veins obstructed by partially calcified mediastinal mass
- Central pulmonary arteries & bronchi may be affected

Pulmonary Hypertension

- Pre-capillary: PPH (young women); secondary: Chronic thromboembolism
- Findings portending poor response to epoprostenol (prostacyclin) therapy (more suggestive of PVOD or PCH)
  - Centrilobular ground-glass opacities, septal lines, pleural effusions, lymphadenopathy, pericardial effusion

PATHOLOGY

General Features

- Etiology
  - Insult that causes thrombosis of pulmonary veins
    - Etiologies: Viral infection, chemotherapeutic drugs, autoimmune diseases, pregnancy, bone marrow transplantation

Gross Pathologic & Surgical Features

- Pathologic hallmark: Extensive occlusion of pulmonary veins by fibrous tissue

Microscopic Features

- Eccentric intimal thickening of small veins within interlobular septa; recanalization of occluded veins over time
- Proliferation of thin-walled capillaries → capillary hemangiomatosis

CLINICAL ISSUES

Presentation

- Most common signs/symptoms
  - Progressive dyspnea, lethargy, & nonproductive cough
  - Occasionally preceded by flu-like illness
  - Normal to mildly elevated pulmonary capillary wedge pressure

Demographics

- Age
  - Any age; most < 50 years
- Gender
  - M:F = 2:1 in adults, but equal in children
- Epidemiology
  - Unknown incidence: PVOD may account for up to 10% of cases of PPH

Natural History & Prognosis

- Very poor prognosis: Most patients die within 2 years of diagnosis

Treatment

- Single or double lung transplantation is only therapy that significantly prolongs life in PVOD
- Vasodilators, immunosuppressive agents, & anticoagulants ineffective

SELECTED REFERENCES

1. Montani D et al: Pulmonary veno-occlusive disease. Eur Respir J. 33(1):189-200, 2009
2. Resten A et al: CT imaging of peripheral pulmonary vessel disease. Eur Radiol. 15(10):2045-56, 2005
3. Resten A et al: Pulmonary hypertension: CT of the chest in pulmonary venoocclusive disease. AJR Am J Roentgenol. 183(1):65-70, 2004
4. Swensen SJ et al: Pulmonary venoocclusive disease: CT findings in eight patients. AJR Am J Roentgenol. 167(4):937-40, 1996
5. Hasleton PS et al: Pulmonary veno-occlusive disease. A report of four cases. Histopathology. 10(9):933-44, 1986

ACUTE PULMONARY THROMBOEMBOLIC DISEASE

Key Facts

Terminology

- Pulmonary embolism (PE)
- Thrombus embolization to pulmonary arteries, from lower extremity, abdominal/pelvic veins

Imaging

- Radiography
  - Chest radiograph nonspecific; 10% normal
  - Oligemia (Westermark sign); vascular obstruction
  - Subsegmental atelectasis (Fleischner lines)
  - Pleural effusion
  - Pulmonary infarction: Hampton hump; lower lobe
- CTA
  - Standard of care for suspected PE
  - Direct visualization of intraluminal clot
  - Right ventricular strain
  - Pulmonary hypertension
  - Subsegmental atelectasis
  - Pulmonary infarction
- CTA: Detection of disease other than PE in 70%
- V/Q scanning
  - More likely to provide diagnosis when lungs are normal

Top Differential Diagnoses

- Hilar lymph nodes
- Veins with flow-related artifact
- Mucus plugging
- Pneumonia &/or atelectasis

Pathology

- Risk factors: Immobilization, malignancy, hypercoagulable/excess estrogen state, prior PE/DVT
- Epidemiology: 3rd most common cause of death

Clinical Issues

- Outcome: Good outcome with appropriate therapy
- Mortality in untreated disease, up to 30%

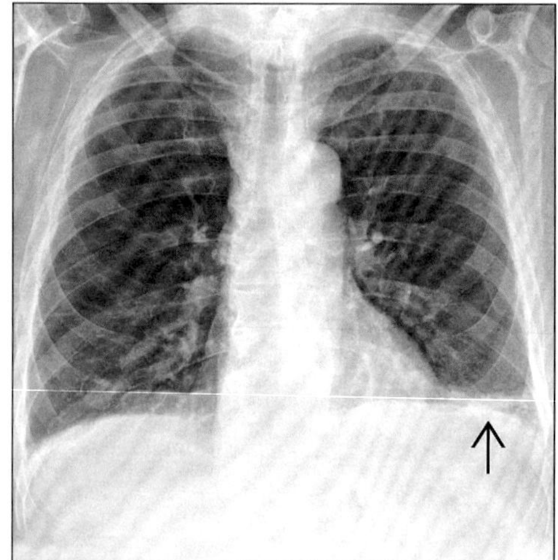

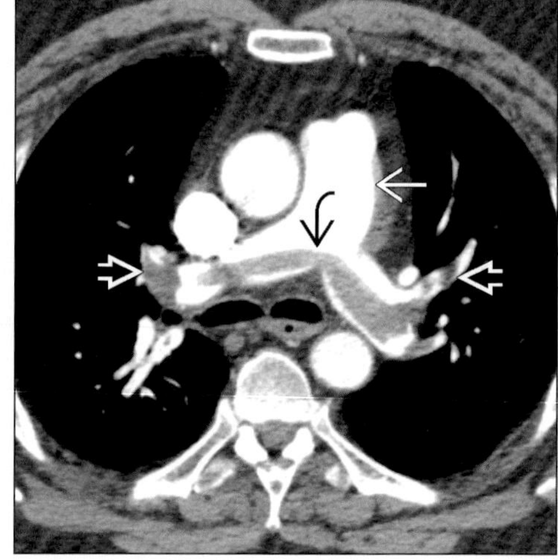

(Left) *AP chest radiograph of a patient with acute PE shows low lung volume and basilar subsegmental atelectasis ⇒. Radiographic abnormalities in acute PE are typically nonspecific.* ***(Right)*** *Axial CTA shows a saddle embolus ⇒ in the pulmonary trunk extending into the right and left pulmonary arteries, additional upper lobe emboli ⇒, and dilatation of the pulmonary trunk ⇒ from pulmonary hypertension. The tubular central embolus is a cast of the thrombosed systemic vein of origin.*

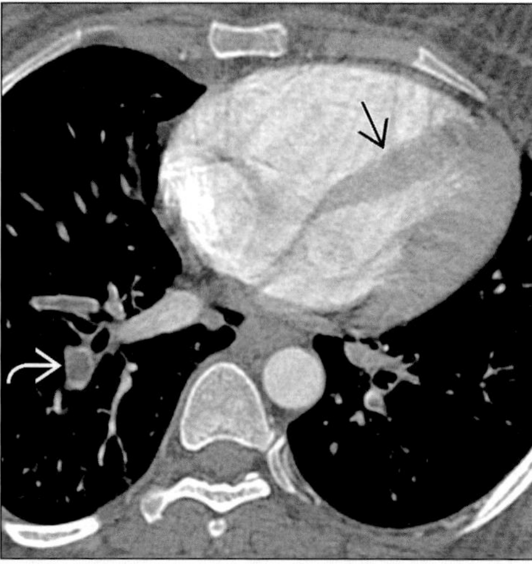

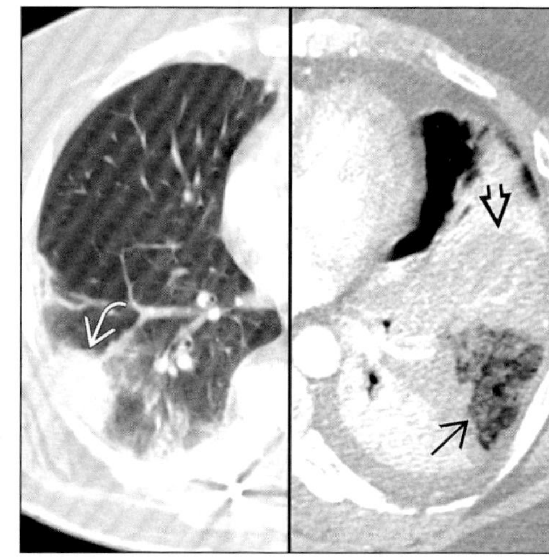

(Left) *Axial CECT of a patient with acute PE shows multiple emboli ⇒ in the bilateral lower lobe pulmonary arteries and enlargement of the right cardiac chambers with leftward bowing and flattening of the interventricular septum ⇒ from right ventricular strain.* ***(Right)*** *Composite image shows CTA features of pulmonary infarction, which may manifest with subpleural wedge-shaped consolidation ⇒ or peripheral consolidation with central lucency ⇒. Note hypoperfusion ⇒ of affected left lower lobe.*

ACUTE PULMONARY THROMBOEMBOLIC DISEASE

TERMINOLOGY

Definitions

- **Thrombus embolization to pulmonary arteries**, usually from lower extremity, abdominal/pelvic veins

IMAGING

General Features

- Best diagnostic clue
  - Intravascular filling defect(s) on CTA
- Location
  - Main, lobar, segmental, subsegmental pulmonary arteries
- Size
  - Variable
  - May occlude large central to small peripheral pulmonary arteries
- Morphology
  - Usually tubular; casts of systemic veins

Radiographic Findings

- Chest radiograph nonspecific; 10% normal
- **Vascular alteration**
  - Oligemia (**Westermark sign**); vascular obstruction
  - Enlarged central pulmonary artery (**knuckle sign**); endoluminal clot
- **Subsegmental atelectasis (Fleischner lines)**, airspace opacities, elevated hemidiaphragm(s), low volume
- **Pleural effusion**
- **Pulmonary infarcts** (uncommon); < 10% of emboli
  - **Hampton hump**: Subpleural peripheral wedge-shaped opacity, rounded apex pointing to hilum
  - Usually in **lower lungs**
  - Immediately or up to 2-3 days after embolus
  - **Melting sign**: Initial ill-defined opacity evolves to sharply defined lesion with decreasing size
  - **50% clear completely** within 3 weeks; may leave linear scars (**Fleischner lines**)
  - More common with cardiopulmonary disease

CT Findings

- NECT
  - Rarely intravascular hyperattenuation from pulmonary embolism (PE)
    - Low sensitivity, high specificity (> 90%)
    - High inter-observer agreement
- CTA
  - Standard of care for suspected PE; rapid, noninvasive, readily available
  - **Direct visualization of intraluminal clot**
    - Intraluminal filling defect
    - Partial filling defect, sharp interface, surrounded by contrast
    - Eccentric or peripheral filling defect, may form acute angles with vessel wall
    - Cutoff of vascular enhancement, arterial occlusion, may enlarge vessel caliber
  - **Right ventricular strain**/failure
    - Right ventricular dilatation
    - Left bowing/flat interventricular septum
    - Dilated IVC, contrast reflux into hepatic veins
  - **Pulmonary arterial hypertension**; enlarged pulmonary trunk
  - **Subsegmental atelectasis**
  - **Pulmonary infarction**
    - Peripheral subpleural wedge-shaped consolidation
    - No contrast enhancement
    - Consolidation with central lucency; high likelihood ratio for infarction
    - **Vessel sign**; pulmonary artery leading to consolidation
- Advantages of CTA
  - Detection of disease other than PE in 70%
    - Pneumonia, lung cancer, metastases, pneumothorax
    - Pericarditis, acute myocardial infarction, aortic dissection
- May be combined with abdomen/pelvis/lower extremity CT to exclude deep venous thrombosis (DVT)
  - Sensitivity & specificity > 90%
  - Complete, partial, or juxtamural systemic venous filling defect; venous wall enhancement
- Indeterminate or false-negative CTA
  - Poor bolus, large body habitus, image noise
  - Beam hardening, stair step, respiratory artifacts
  - **Transient contrast interruption**: Admixing of unenhanced IVC blood during inspiration
    - May be minimized by image acquisition during shallow inspiration or expiration
  - Partial volume effect; filling defect preferably seen on at least 2 sequential images
  - Failure to recognize subsegmental emboli

MR Findings

- Less available than CT; less resolution; limited role
- Gradient-recalled echo imaging with gadolinium
- Visualization of main, lobar, & segmental emboli
- Sensitivity approximately 90%, specificity 80-95%

Angiographic Findings

- Never gained widespread acceptance, not universally available
- Vascular filling defect, abrupt occlusion or pulmonary artery pruning, oligemia
- Potential to miss central & subsegmental emboli

Nuclear Medicine Findings

- **Ventilation perfusion (V/Q) scanning**: More likely to provide diagnosis when lungs are normal
  - **Normal perfusion scan excludes embolus**
  - **High probability scan diagnostic of embolus**
  - High percentage of nondiagnostic intermediate probability scans (> 60%)
  - High sensitivity; poor specificity

Ultrasonographic Findings

- Lower extremity ultrasound: Low sensitivity, high specificity
- When positive, optional pulmonary artery CTA
- 50% of patients with PE have no DVT

Imaging Recommendations

- Best imaging tool
  - CT angiography; lower extremity ultrasound
  - Pregnant patient with normal chest radiograph; consider perfusion scan only for dose reduction
- Protocol advice
  - Technique
    - ≥ 20 gauge catheter in antecubital vein; 100-150 cc contrast injection at 3-4 cc/sec

ACUTE PULMONARY THROMBOEMBOLIC DISEASE

- Bolus tracking technique; 1.25-3 mm thick slices through chest with single breath-hold
- Scan caudal to cranial; less artifact from high-density SVC contrast
- Optional: 3-4 minute delay to image abdomen/pelvis, lower extremities; ≤ 5 mm thick slices at 3 cm intervals from knees to abdomen
  - Recommendations for pregnant patients with suspected PE
    - Chest radiography as 1st radiation-associated imaging study
    - Nuclear scintigraphy if normal chest radiograph
    - CTA if abnormal chest radiograph
  - Pregnant patient: Maternal & fetal radiation reduction
    - Bismuth breast shield; lead shielding
    - Reduction in tube current & voltage

DIFFERENTIAL DIAGNOSIS

Hilar Lymph Nodes

- Reformatted images to show extraluminal location

Veins with Flow-related Artifact

- Extend toward left atrium; do not track with bronchi

Mucus Plugging

- Track with pulmonary arteries
- Originate from central bronchi

Pneumonia &/or Atelectasis

- Common in critically ill, nonspecific airspace disease
- CTA: Vessel enhancement in consolidation
- Pneumonia & edema generally "fade" away; infarcts "melt" away

Tumor Emboli

- Invasion of IVC or hepatic veins by prostate, breast, renal cell cancers, hepatocellular carcinoma
- Vascular beading, tree-in-bud appearance

Pulmonary Artery Sarcoma

- Endoluminal enhancing lobulated mass

In Situ Thrombosis

- Behçet disease: Pulmonary artery aneurysms, hemorrhage, arthritis, urogenital ulcers

Foreign Bodies: Vertebroplasty Glue

- Smaller & thinner than thrombi; metallic density

PATHOLOGY

General Features

- Etiology
  - **Risk factors for PE**
    - **Immobilization**: Hospitalized, intensive care unit, postoperative, post-trauma
    - **Malignancy**
    - **Hypercoagulable state**: Acquired, inherited
    - **Excess estrogen state**: Pregnancy, peripartum, oral contraceptives, estrogen replacement
    - **History of PE or DVT**
  - Hughes-Stovins syndrome
    - Multiple pulmonary artery aneurysms & peripheral venous thromboses
  - Epidemiology
    - Common, considered **3rd most common cause of death**
    - Found in 15% of autopsies; cause of death in 9% of autopsies
    - PE in 1.5% of CECT performed for other reasons

Gross Pathologic & Surgical Features

- Deep venous clot fragments in right heart; average of 8 pulmonary vessels embolized
- Hemodynamic consequences: > 50% reduction of vascular bed, pulmonary hypertension, & right heart strain

Microscopic Features

- Intraluminal thrombus, branching lines of fibrin-platelet aggregates, surrounded by red & white blood cells

CLINICAL ISSUES

Presentation

- Most common signs/symptoms
  - Dyspnea, tachypnea, pleuritic chest pain, syncope, or asymptomatic
- Other signs/symptoms
  - No signs, symptoms, or laboratory studies that strongly suggest PE
    - D-dimer assay, high sensitivity, poor specificity

Demographics

- Age: Variable; infants to elderly
- Gender: M = F

Natural History & Prognosis

- Most pulmonary emboli resolve without sequelae
- Outcome: Good with appropriate therapy
  - Good after negative CTA (< 1% embolic rate)
- Mortality in untreated disease, up to 30%
  - Poor survival with pulmonary artery hypertension, cor pulmonale

Treatment

- Anticoagulation and fibrinolysis; hemorrhage complications in 2-15%
- IVC filter: Contraindication to anticoagulation, recurrent emboli
- Endarterectomy for chronic organizing pulmonary emboli

DIAGNOSTIC CHECKLIST

Image Interpretation Pearls

- Incidental PE found in 4% of patients with malignancy on restaging CECT

SELECTED REFERENCES

1. Henzler T et al: CT imaging of acute pulmonary embolism. J Cardiovasc Comput Tomogr. 5(1):3-11, 2011
2. Shahir K et al: Pulmonary embolism in pregnancy: CT pulmonary angiography versus perfusion scanning. AJR Am J Roentgenol. 195(3):W214-20, 2010

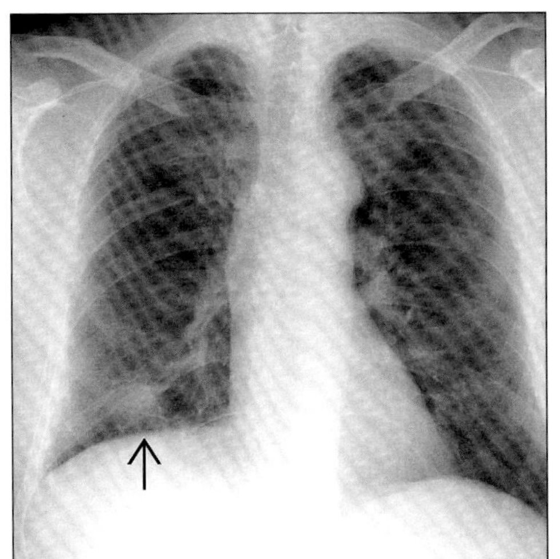

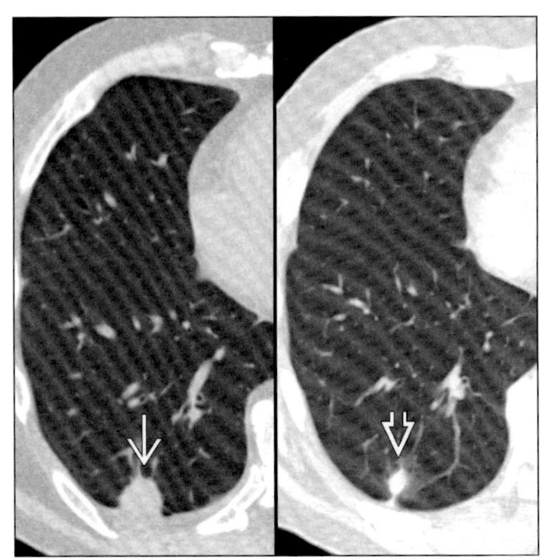

(Left) *PA chest radiograph of a patient with PE shows an indistinct right basilar nodular opacity →.* ***(Right)*** *Composite image of the same patient with axial CECT obtained 9 days (left) and 2 months (right) after acute PE shows the melting sign. The initial circumscribed peripheral subpleural right lower lobe nodule →, representing a pulmonary infarct, exhibits interval decrease in size → as it "melts" away. Opacities due to pneumonia have indistinct margins that fade and disperse over time.*

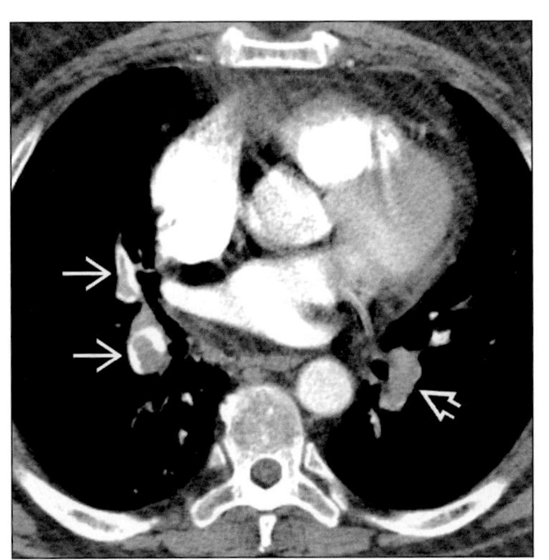

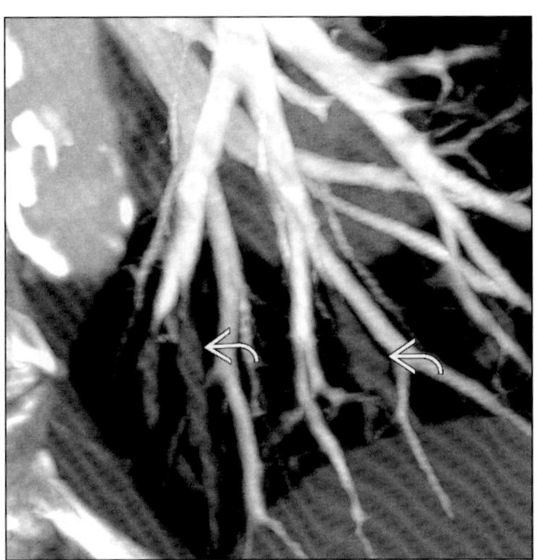

(Left) *Axial CTA of a patient with dyspnea and acute PE shows dilatation and occlusion of the left lower lobe pulmonary artery →, a CT knuckle sign. Additional emboli are noted in the right middle and lower lobe pulmonary arteries →.* ***(Right)*** *Oblique MIP image from a CTA of a patient with acute PE shows multifocal pulmonary emboli manifesting as occlusive filling defects → within several peripheral pulmonary arteries, which expand the vessel lumina resulting in a lobular tubular morphology.*

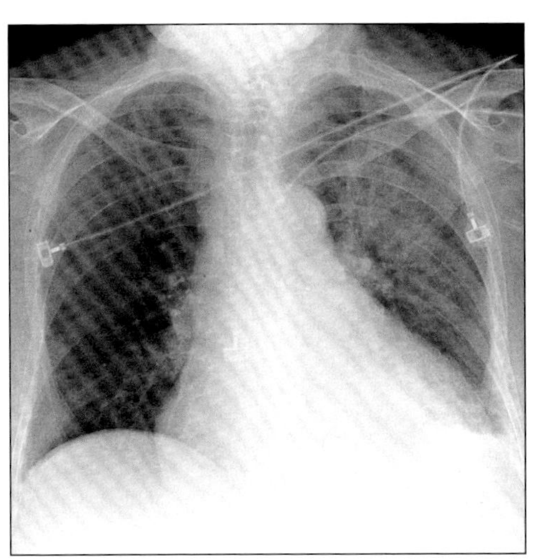

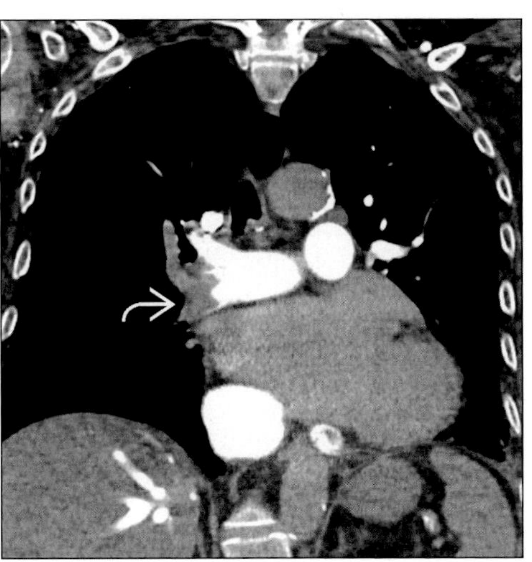

(Left) *AP chest radiograph of a patient who presented with chest pain and dyspnea shows left lower lobe airspace disease and asymmetric right lung hyperlucency and oligemia.* ***(Right)*** *Coronal CECT of the same patient shows a large PE → in the distal right pulmonary artery with extension into the right interlobar pulmonary artery and its branches. Large central pulmonary emboli can result in pulmonary oligemia and hyperlucent asymmetric lung parenchyma on CECT, known as the Westermark sign.*

CHRONIC PULMONARY THROMBOEMBOLIC DISEASE

Key Facts

Terminology
- Chronic thromboembolic pulmonary hypertension (CTEPH)
- Pulmonary embolism (PE)
- Gradual organization of thromboemboli following acute pulmonary embolism with resultant pulmonary vascular obstruction/obliteration

Imaging
- Radiography: Normal vs. findings of pulmonary arterial hypertension (PAH)
- CTA: Luminal thrombi, peripheral thrombi, pulmonary artery occlusion, webs
- Enlarged pulmonary arteries related to PAH
- Mosaic perfusion of lung parenchyma
- Cardiac chamber enlargement from PAH
- Hypertrophied bronchial arteries
- V/Q scan: Multiple mismatched defects

Top Differential Diagnoses
- Laminar flow artifact
- Pulmonary artery sarcoma
- Takayasu arteritis

Pathology
- Factor VIII, high frequency of antiphospholipid antibodies, lupus anticoagulant may be risk factors

Clinical Issues
- 5% incidence in patients with acute PE
- Symptoms: Progressive exertional dyspnea
- Treatment: IVC filter, lifetime anticoagulation, surgical thromboendarterectomy in selected patients

Diagnostic Checklist
- Consider chronic PE in patients with chronic dyspnea, PAH & eccentric or web-like thrombi or mosaic lung perfusion

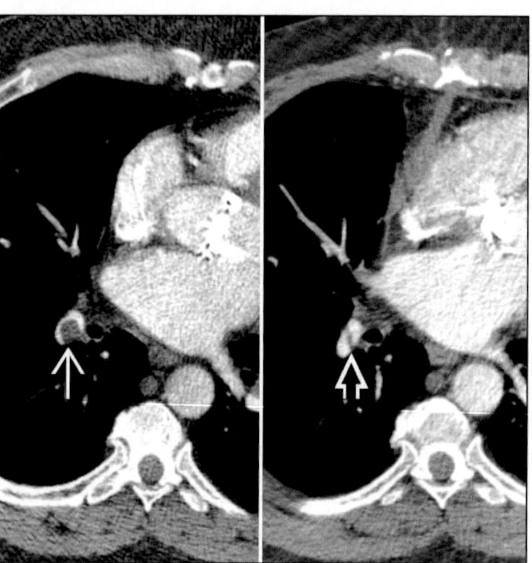
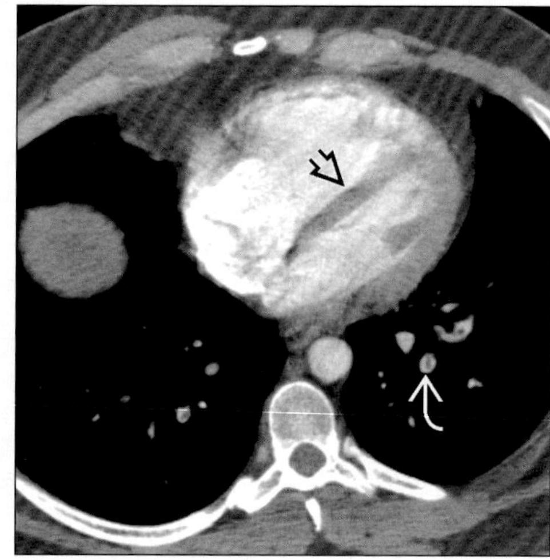

(Left) *Composite image with axial CECT (left) and axial CTA obtained 3 weeks later (right) shows a right lower lobe pulmonary embolus ➔, which manifests as a thin linear endoluminal web ⇨ on follow-up imaging.* ***(Right)*** *Axial CTA of a patient with severe pulmonary hypertension and chronic pulmonary emboli shows superimposed acute emboli in left lower lobe segmental pulmonary arteries ↷, dilatation of the right cardiac chambers, and flattening of the interventricular septum ⇨.*

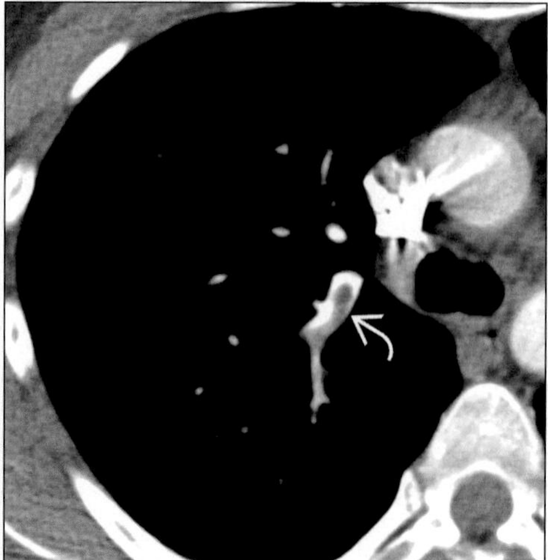
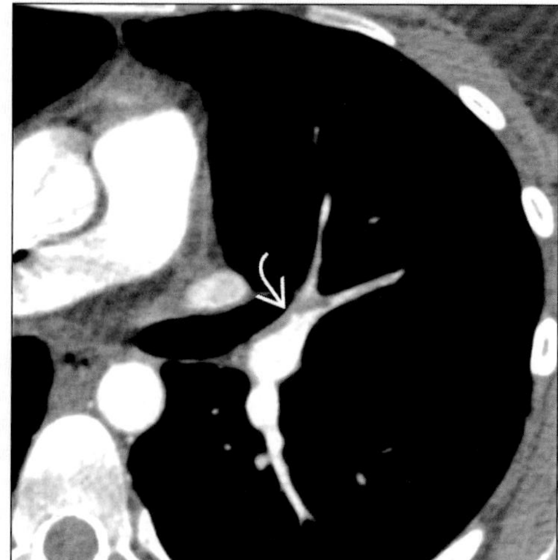

(Left) *Axial CECT of a young woman on long-term oral contraception who presented with dyspnea shows an acute right upper lobe pulmonary embolus ↷.* ***(Right)*** *Axial CECT of the same patient shows a chronic left upper lobe pulmonary embolus manifesting as a long peripheral wall-adherent filling defect ↷ in the pulmonary artery lumen. Patients with chronic pulmonary thromboembolic disease may develop acute pulmonary emboli (acute on chronic pulmonary emboli).*

CHRONIC PULMONARY THROMBOEMBOLIC DISEASE

TERMINOLOGY

Abbreviations

- **Chronic thromboembolic pulmonary hypertension (CTEPH)**
- Pulmonary embolism (PE)

Synonyms

- Chronic pulmonary arterial thromboembolic disease

Definitions

- Gradual organization of thromboemboli following acute pulmonary embolism with resultant pulmonary vascular obstruction/obliteration

IMAGING

General Features

- Best diagnostic clue
  - Eccentric, wall-adherent, low-density filling defect; dilated pulmonary artery(ies)
- Location
  - Pulmonary arteries, commonly bilateral
- Size
  - Usually smaller than acute PE

Radiographic Findings

- Radiography
  - Normal chest radiograph
  - **Findings of pulmonary arterial hypertension (PAH)**
    - Pulmonary artery enlargement, right heart enlargement
  - Subpleural opacities from prior pulmonary infarcts
  - Hypo- & hyperperfused lung regions
  - Rarely peripheral cavitary lesions; infarcts

CT Findings

- HRCT
  - **Mosaic perfusion** of pulmonary parenchyma
    - Heterogeneous lung attenuation from differential perfusion
    - Decreased attenuation from decreased perfusion; small intrinsic pulmonary arteries
  - Subpleural opacities from prior pulmonary infarcts
- CTA
  - CTA allows direct visualization of luminal thrombi, organized mural thrombi, arterial occlusion, webs
    - **Eccentric thrombi**
    - Smooth or nodular vessel wall thickening
    - Rarely eccentric wall-adherent pulmonary artery (PA) calcifications
    - **Webs**: Eccentric linear filling defects with partial intraluminal extension
    - **Abrupt vessel narrowing or occlusion**
    - "Pruning" of peripheral arteries
    - Peripheral neovascularity in longstanding PAH
  - Enlarged pulmonary arteries related to PAH
    - PA:aorta ratio > 1
    - Pulmonary trunk diameter > 29 mm
  - Cardiac chamber enlargement from PAH
    - RV enlargement: RV/LV diameter > 1 at midventricular level
    - Straight or left-bowing interventricular septum
    - D-shaped LV cavity on short axis view
  - Size & distribution of bronchial arteries & nonbronchial systemic arteries
    - Increased bronchopulmonary collaterals distinguishes CTEPH from 1° PAH
    - **Large hypertrophied bronchial arteries**
      - May complicate surgery & predict poor surgical outcome
  - Exclude alternative causes of PAH
    - Congenital cardiovascular disease: Atrial or ventricular septal defect, patent ductus arteriosus, anomalous pulmonary venous drainage
    - Other pulmonary vascular diseases: Veno-occlusive disease, capillary hemangiomatosis, vascular occlusions from mediastinal fibrosis, PA sarcoma

MR Findings

- MRA
  - Correlates well with CTA to segmental level; cannot reliably detect smaller thrombi
  - Eccentric, low signal defects along arterial wall on SSFP, MRA, & CE GRE sequences
  - Vessel occlusions, intraluminal webs & bands
  - Time-resolved MRA (TR-MRA) useful for assessment of pulmonary perfusion pattern
- MR cine
  - Allows qualitative & quantitative assessment of ventricular function
  - Phase-contrast imaging measures flow in systemic & pulmonary vessels; assessment of treatment outcomes
    - Pre- and post-pulmonary thromboendarterectomy

Echocardiographic Findings

- Evidence of pulmonary arterial hypertension
- Right atrial & ventricular enlargement/dysfunction
- Tricuspid regurgitation
- Exclusion of cardiac causes of pulmonary arterial hypertension (e.g., patent foramen ovale, septal defect)

Angiographic Findings

- Vascular occlusions, webs, stenoses, mural thrombi
- 2 orthogonal views essential for surgical planning
- Right ventricular & PA hemodynamics

Nuclear Medicine Findings

- PET
  - May aid in differentiating pulmonary arteritis (Takayasu) from chronic PE
- V/Q scan
  - Normal V/Q scan excludes chronic PE
  - Multiple mismatched segmental or larger defects
  - Magnitude of perfusion defects often underestimates degree of obstruction

Imaging Recommendations

- Best imaging tool
  - CTA is optimal imaging modality
- Protocol advice
  - Contrast bolus timing for opacification of pulmonary circulation
    - Pulmonary trunk as ROI for bolus tracking; 80-100 mL of contrast at 3 cc/sec; 1.5 mm collimation
    - ECG may be synchronized with CT scan to assess RV function; more radiation to patient
  - MR/MRA sequences: Axial SSFP, cine SSFP of heart, coronal time-resolved MRA (for perfusion), coronal CE MRA, axial & coronal post-contrast T1 GRE

CHRONIC PULMONARY THROMBOEMBOLIC DISEASE

DIFFERENTIAL DIAGNOSIS

Laminar Flow Artifact

- Inappropriate timing of contrast bolus
- Mixing of nonenhanced blood from IVC with contrast-enhanced blood
  - Inspiration during scanning increases blood return from IVC
- Linear central filling defects seen at vessel bifurcation

Pulmonary Artery Sarcoma

- Sarcoma usually irregular, lobulated, wall-adherent
- Contrast enhancement (best on MR) seen in sarcoma (vascular); not in thrombus (usually avascular)
- May involve pulmonary valve & extend retrograde into RV infundibulum; does not occur with chronic PE

Takayasu Arteritis

- Mural thickening in pulmonary vasculitis can resemble eccentric thrombus
- Other vessels involved in vasculitis (aorta)
- CT & MR may identify circumferential inflammatory mural thickening
  - MR better than CT in assessing wall enhancement; differentiates active vs. chronic vasculitis
- FDG PET shows intense uptake in active disease

PATHOLOGY

General Features

- Etiology
  - Unresolved pulmonary emboli that organize, become adherent, & incorporate into arterial wall
  - Secondary small-vessel arteriopathy in some patients
  - Proximal PA occlusion & arteriopathy contribute to elevated pulmonary vascular resistance
- Associated abnormalities
  - Patients may have **altered coagulation**
    - Factor VIII, high frequency of antiphospholipid antibodies, lupus anticoagulant may be risk factors
  - Splenectomy may increase risk of chronic thromboembolic pulmonary hypertension

Gross Pathologic & Surgical Features

- Emboli transform into fibrous tissue; incorporation into pulmonary arterial intima & media
- Small vessel vasculopathy seen in remaining open vessels, which are subjected to high flows

CLINICAL ISSUES

Presentation

- Most common signs/symptoms
  - **Progressive exertional dyspnea**
  - **Exercise intolerance**
- Other signs/symptoms
  - Exertional chest pain
  - Presyncope, syncope
  - Fatigue
  - Palpitation
  - Hemoptysis

Demographics

- Age
  - Elderly patients
- Gender
  - M = F
- Epidemiology
  - 5% incidence in patients with acute PE

Natural History & Prognosis

- 2/3 of patients may have no history of acute PE
- Often misdiagnosed with asthma, CHF, COPD, physical deconditioning, or psychogenic dyspnea
- Extent of vascular obstruction: Major determinant of development of PAH
- Low survival rate without intervention for PAH
  - 5-year survival rate of 30% with mean pulmonary artery pressure ≥ 40 mmHg
  - 5-year survival rate of 10% with mean pulmonary artery pressure ≥ 50 mmHg

Treatment

- Potentially correctable cause of PAH
- IVC filter placement
  - Lifetime anticoagulation
- Medical therapy or angioplasty for non-surgical candidates
- Surgical thromboendarterectomy in some patients
  - Location/extent of proximal thromboembolic obstructions; critical determinants of operability
  - Occluding thrombi must involve main, lobar, or proximal segmental arteries

DIAGNOSTIC CHECKLIST

Consider

- Chronic PE in a patient with chronic dyspnea, PAH, and eccentric or web-like thrombi or mosaic lung perfusion

Image Interpretation Pearls

- Eccentric web-like thrombi, differential lung perfusion, vessel calcifications, right heart strain favor chronic PE
- Intimal hyperplasia in congenital heart disease with central shunting may mimic chronic PE
  - Intravascular ultrasound helps to differentiate

SELECTED REFERENCES

1. Grosse C et al: CT findings in diseases associated with pulmonary hypertension: a current review. Radiographics. 30(7):1753-77, 2010
2. Nikolaou K et al: Diagnosing pulmonary embolism: new computed tomography applications. J Thorac Imaging. 25(2):151-60, 2010
3. Coulden R: State-of-the-art imaging techniques in chronic thromboembolic pulmonary hypertension. Proc Am Thorac Soc. 3(7):577-83, 2006
4. Hoeper MM et al: Chronic thromboembolic pulmonary hypertension. Circulation. 113(16):2011-20, 2006
5. Lang I et al: Risk factors for chronic thromboembolic pulmonary hypertension. Proc Am Thorac Soc. 3(7):568-70, 2006

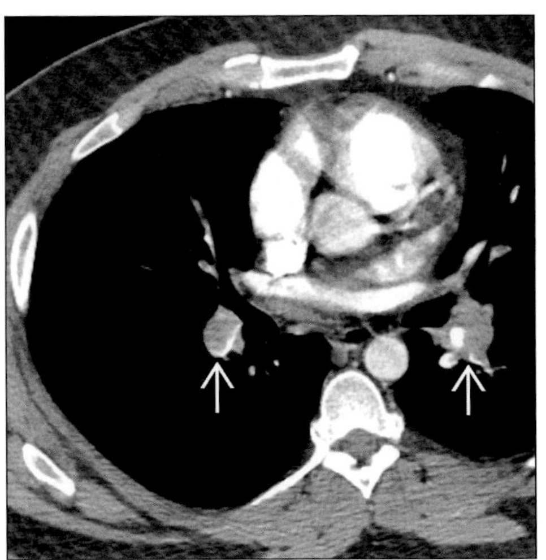

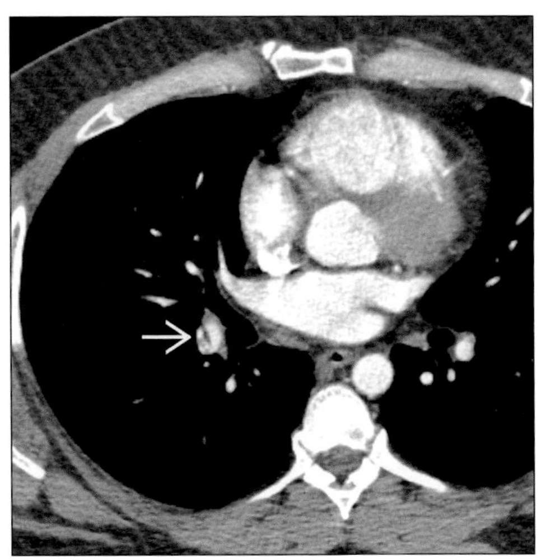

(Left) *Axial CTA of a patient with chest pain and dyspnea shows bilateral large lower lobe pulmonary emboli ➔. The right lower lobe pulmonary embolus nearly occludes the vessel lumen, while the left lower lobe embolus expands the vessel.* ***(Right)*** *Axial CTA of the same patient obtained 6 months later shows complete recanalization of the left lower lobe pulmonary artery without residual embolus and a right lower lobe pulmonary artery web ➔, consistent with chronic thromboembolic disease.*

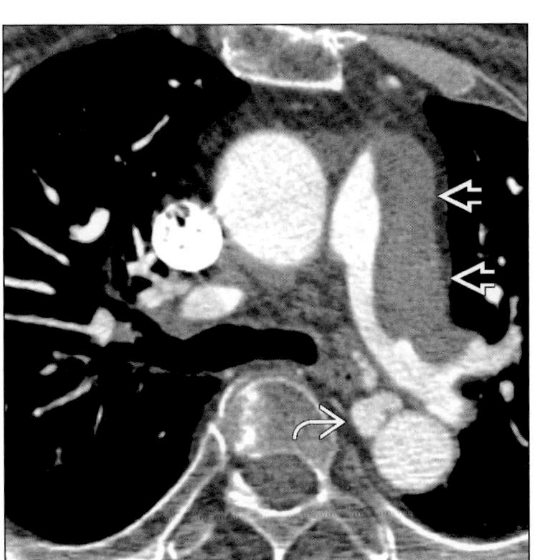

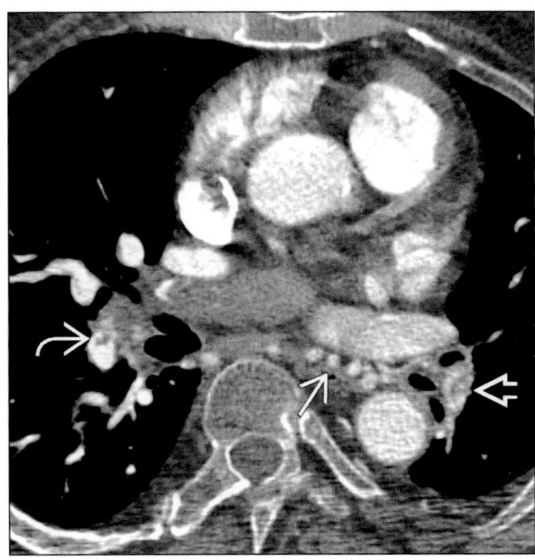

(Left) *Axial CTA of a patient with pulmonary hypertension secondary to chronic pulmonary thromboembolic disease shows a large peripheral filling defect ➔ extending from the pulmonary trunk into the enlarged left pulmonary artery. Note marked hypertrophy of bronchial arteries ➔.* ***(Right)*** *Axial CTA of the same patient shows a peripheral right lower lobe chronic pulmonary embolus ➔ and a linear left lower lobe web ➔ associated with marked bronchial artery hypertrophy ➔.*

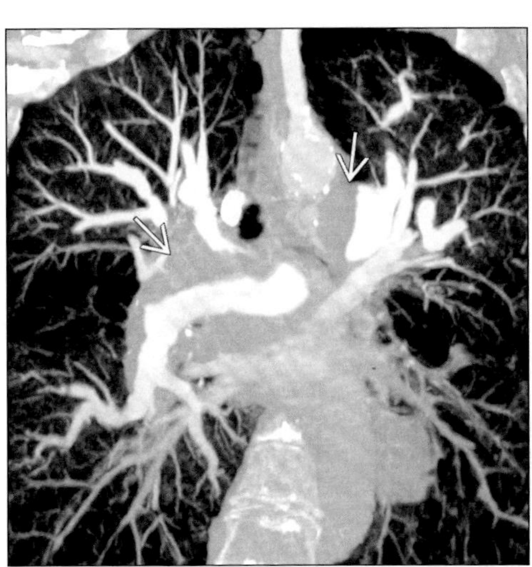

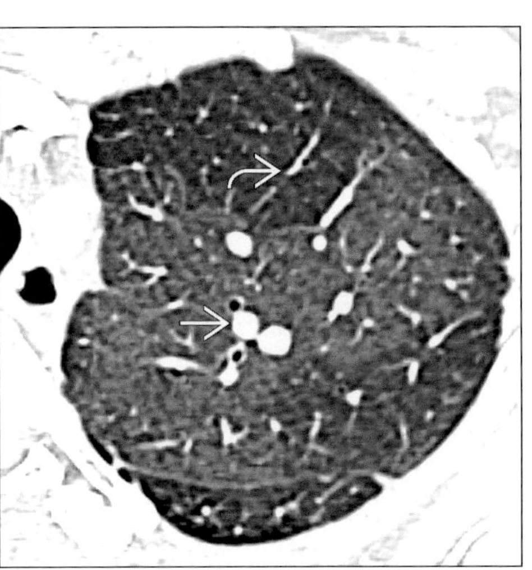

(Left) *Coronal MIP of a patient with PAH shows severe chronic pulmonary emboli manifesting as bilateral eccentric endoluminal wall-adherent soft tissue ➔ that partially encases the right pulmonary artery lumen.* ***(Right)*** *Axial CECT of a patient with PAH secondary to chronic pulmonary thromboembolic disease shows mosaic lung attenuation with differential caliber of pulmonary arteries. The pulmonary arteries in the hyperperfused lung ➔ are larger than those ➔ in the hypoperfused lung.*

SICKLE CELL DISEASE

Key Facts

Terminology

- Sickle cell disease: Abnormal hemoglobin that deforms when deoxygenated
- Acute chest syndrome: Noninfectious vasoocclusive crisis associated with chest radiographic abnormality
- Sickle cell chronic lung disease: Recurrent acute chest syndrome (ACS)

Imaging

- Best diagnostic clues: Rib expansion, H-shaped vertebrae, absent spleen
- Radiography
  - Airspace disease: Lobar, segmental, subsegmental
  - Preferential lower lobe involvement
  - Cardiomegaly
- HRCT: Mosaic perfusion; microvascular occlusion
- CECT: High osmolarity contrast contraindicated; may induce sickling

Top Differential Diagnoses

- Pulmonary edema
- Pulmonary infarction
- Bacterial pneumonia

Pathology

- Autosplenectomy: Risk of encapsulated bacteria pneumonia (*Staphylococcus, Haemophilus*)

Clinical Issues

- Wheezing, cough, & fever in patients < 10 years
- Adults: Dyspnea, arm & leg pain, frequently afebrile
- Pulmonary artery hypertension (33%)
- High output cardiac failure

Diagnostic Checklist

- Consider ACS in patients with Hb SS with chest or constitutional complaints & pulmonary opacities

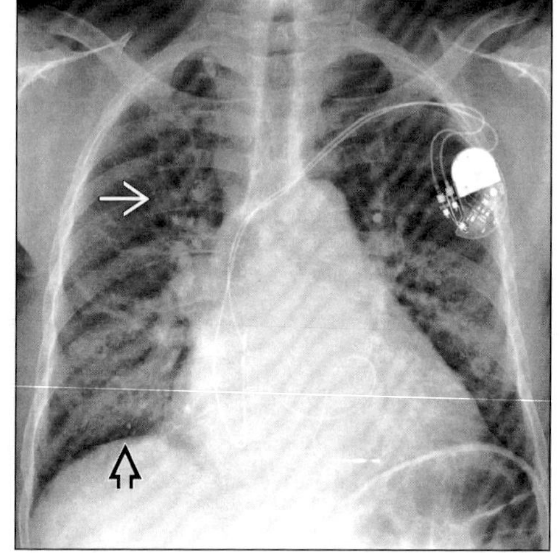

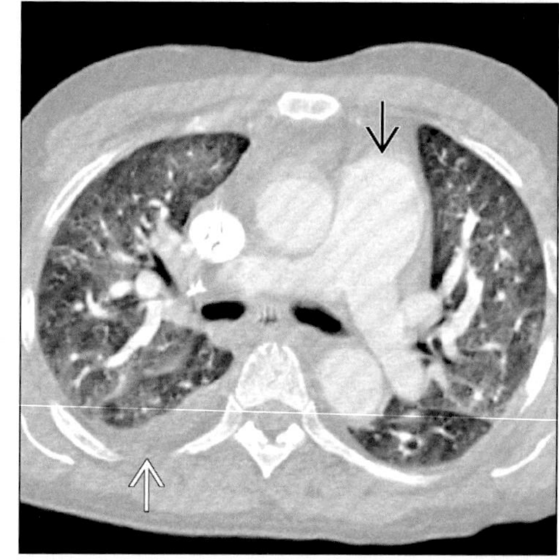

(Left) *PA chest radiograph of a 57-year-old man with sickle cell anemia shows cardiomegaly, pulmonary venous hypertension ➔, and interstitial and alveolar edema ⇨.* ***(Right)*** *Axial CECT of the same patient shows alveolar edema, enlargement of the pulmonary trunk → from pulmonary arterial hypertension, and a small right effusion ➔. Left ventricular failure in Hb SS may relate to high output failure from anemia, overhydration, or renal insufficiency. Pulmonary hypertension is a late complication.*

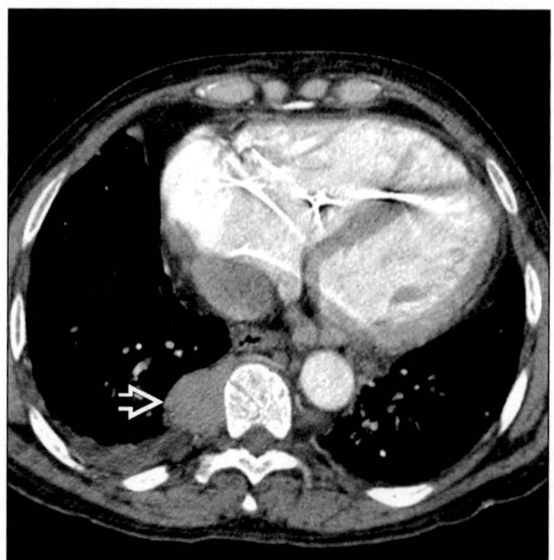

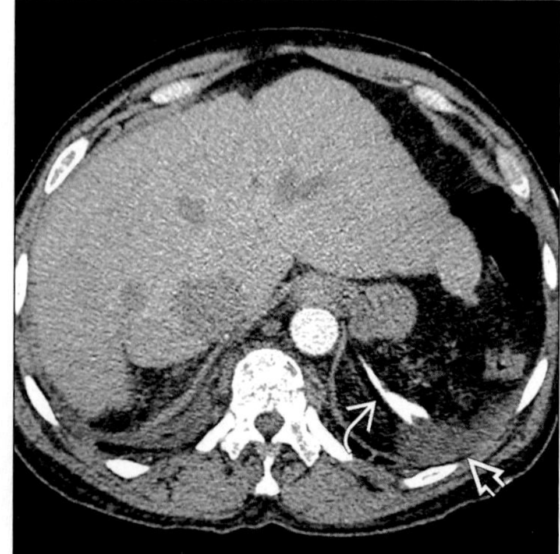

(Left) *Axial CECT of the same patient shows a right paravertebral soft tissue mass ➔ secondary to extramedullary hematopoiesis.* ***(Right)*** *Axial CECT of the same patient shows typical findings of autosplenectomy manifesting with a small calcified spleen ➔ surrounded by mild abdominal ascites ➔. Extramedullary hematopoiesis occurs in response to chronic, severe anemia. Autosplenectomy results from splenic hypoxia and repeated splenic infarctions.*

SICKLE CELL DISEASE

TERMINOLOGY

Abbreviations

- **Sickle cell disease** (Hb SS)
- **Acute chest syndrome** (ACS)

Definitions

- **Sickle cell disease**: Abnormal hemoglobin that deforms when deoxygenated
- **Acute chest syndrome**: Noninfectious vasoocclusive crisis in patients with Hb SS associated with chest radiographic abnormalities
  - Initiated by lung infection or infarction
- Sickle cell chronic lung disease: Result of recurrent acute chest syndrome

IMAGING

General Features

- Best diagnostic clue
  - Expanded ribs, H-shaped vertebrae, absent spleen
- Location
  - Lower lobe predominant opacities
- Size
  - Variable extent of pulmonary opacification
- Morphology
  - Cardiomegaly & airspace or interstitial opacities

Radiographic Findings

- Radiography
  - **Lung parenchyma**
    - Initial chest radiograph may be **normal** (50%)
    - Lobar, segmental, subsegmental opacity: Pneumonia, atelectasis, or infarct
    - Preferential **lower lobe** involvement
    - Interstitial thickening due to edema or fibrosis from prior episodes of ACS
  - **Pleura**
    - Pleural effusion: Pneumonia, infarct, left heart failure
  - **Heart**
    - **Cardiomegaly** common
      - Chronic anemia & high output heart failure
  - **Mediastinum**
    - Paravertebral mass; extramedullary hematopoiesis
      - Unilateral or bilateral, sharply marginated
  - **Skeletal**
    - **Avascular necrosis** (AVN) of humeral heads
    - **H-shaped vertebrae** (10%): Step-off deformity of superior & inferior endplates (**Reynold sign**)
    - Enlarged ribs due to marrow expansion
    - Bone sclerosis due to bone infarcts
  - Upper abdomen
    - Small or absent spleen, may be calcified (**autosplenectomy**)

CT Findings

- CT findings mirror chest radiographic findings
- Consolidation
  - Pneumonia
  - Pulmonary infarction, fat embolism
- **Mosaic perfusion** from microvascular occlusion
  - Geographic areas of hypoperfusion
    - Areas of decreased attenuation contain small vessels
  - Geographic areas of hyperperfusion
    - Areas of ground-glass opacity contain normal-sized vessels (larger than those in areas of decreased attenuation)
    - Redistribution of flow to lung with less microvascular occlusion
  - **Ground-glass opacity**: Hemorrhagic edema caused by reperfusion of ischemic lung
- CECT: High osmolarity contrast contraindicated; may induce sickling
- Acute chest syndrome sequela
  - Parenchymal bands, septal thickening, peripheral wedge-shaped opacities
  - Architectural distortion, traction bronchiectasis

Nuclear Medicine Findings

- Bone scan
  - Foci of decreased or increased radiotracer uptake in ribs from bone infarction
  - Increased skull uptake
  - Increased spleen uptake; calcification from autosplenectomy
  - Delayed renal uptake
- Tc-99m sulfur colloid
  - Uptake in extramedullary hematopoiesis
- V/Q scan
  - Limited clinical use in ACS
    - Findings mimic pulmonary embolism
    - Etiology may be sickling erythrocytes, pneumonia, or fat emboli
    - Findings resolve quickly with supportive therapy

Imaging Recommendations

- Best imaging tool
  - Chest radiographs usually provide sufficient information for evaluation & treatment
- Protocol advice
  - CT more sensitive for parenchymal abnormalities; usually not necessary; excess radiation dose in young patients

DIFFERENTIAL DIAGNOSIS

Chest Pain

- Pulmonary edema
  - Lung opacities more diffuse & bilateral
- Bacterial pneumonia
  - Clearing opacities may show decreased density & less distinct margins
- Pulmonary infarction
  - Melting sign: Clearing opacities may show decreased size & distinct margins (Hampton hump)
- Pneumothorax
  - Visceral pleural line, absent peripheral markings

PATHOLOGY

General Features

- Etiology
  - **ACS**: Multifactorial; exact cause rarely determined
    - Pneumonia &/or infarctions from thrombosis or fat emboli
    - Rib infarction → pain → splinting → linear atelectasis
    - Large vessel thrombosis possible but rare

SICKLE CELL DISEASE

- **Pneumonia**
  - Documented in 30% of ACS cases
  - More common cause of ACS in children
  - Most common pathogens: *Chlamydia pneumoniae*, *Mycoplasma pneumoniae*, respiratory syncytial virus
  - Airspace disease persists longer than in cases in which infection not documented
  - Upper lobe consolidation more likely pneumonia; oxygen tension highest in upper lung zones due to high V/Q ratio
- **Pulmonary fat embolism**
  - Emboli with fat & necrotic bone marrow in 10%
  - Bone pain, ↓ hemoglobin/platelet count, ↑ plasma free fatty acids & phospholipase A2
  - Diagnosis supported by lipid-laden macrophages in bronchoalveolar lavage fluid
- **Rib infarction**
  - High correlation between rib infarction & pulmonary opacity
  - Rib pain may result in splinting & atelectasis
  - Incentive spirometry may decrease atelectasis & prevent pulmonary complications of ACS
  - Analgesics may decrease splinting, but may cause hypoventilation
- **Left ventricular dysfunction**
  - High output failure from anemia, especially when hemoglobin ≤ 7 gm/dL
  - Overhydration with intravenous fluids
  - Fluid imbalance from renal insufficiency (from microinfarction of renal papilla)
- **Autosplenectomy**: Impaired immunity due to functional asplenia
  - Risk of pneumonia from encapsulated organisms: *Streptococcus pneumoniae*, *Haemophilus influenzae*

- Genetics
  - Valine substitution for glutamic acid in hemoglobin beta subunit (Hb S)
    - Hb S affords some protection from malaria
    - Normal hemoglobin (Hb A)
  - Sickle cell anemia
    - Exposure to low oxygen tension → Hb S becomes less soluble & forms large polymers
    - Results in distorted erythrocyte (sickle cell) → vaso-occlusion & hemolysis
  - May also occur in Hb SC, Hb SB°, Hb SB+

Microscopic Features

- Red blood cells sickle when deoxygenated

CLINICAL ISSUES

Presentation

- Most common signs/symptoms
  - **ACS**: New pulmonary opacity on chest radiograph; fever, cough, tachypnea, & chest pain
  - Difficult to distinguish infectious from noninfectious etiology
    - Wheezing, cough, & fever most common in patients < 10 years
    - Chest pain rare in pediatric age group
    - Fat embolism: Pulmonary findings preceded by bone pain
  - Adults: Dyspnea, arm & leg pain more common, frequently afebrile
- Other signs/symptoms
  - Hyperreactive airway disease, 40% of affected children

Demographics

- Epidemiology
  - Hb SS most prevalent inherited disorder among African-Americans
    - **Hb SS occurs in 0.15% of African-American population**
    - **Hb SA occurs in 8% of African-American population**
  - Average life expectancy: 42 years for men, 48 years for women
  - Lung is one of the major organs affected by Hb SS
  - ACS occurs in up to 50% of patients with Hb SS
    - Recurrent episodes in 80%
    - Children 100x more susceptible to pneumonia; recurrence rate: 30%

Natural History & Prognosis

- **ACS: Leading cause of death in Hb SS**
  - Responsible for up to **25% of deaths**
  - > 20% have fatal pulmonary complications, thromboembolus seen in 25% of autopsies
  - 2nd most common cause of hospitalization in patients with Hb SS
- Recurrent ACS long-term sequela
  - Sickle cell chronic lung disease (5%)
  - High output cardiac failure
  - Pulmonary artery hypertension (33%)
    - Late in natural history of sickle cell disease

Treatment

- **Supportive**
  - Oxygen & adequate hydration
    - Overhydration may lead to pulmonary edema
  - Pain control
  - Incentive spirometry
  - Antibiotics for presumed pneumonia
  - Bronchodilators for hyperreactive airway disease
  - Blood transfusions
- Prevention
  - Higher risk of pneumonia from encapsulated organisms; poor or absent splenic function
  - Pneumococcal & *Haemophilus influenza* vaccination

DIAGNOSTIC CHECKLIST

Consider

- ACS in patients with Hb SS presenting with chest or constitutional complaints & pulmonary opacities

SELECTED REFERENCES

1. Gladwin MT et al: Pulmonary complications of sickle cell disease. N Engl J Med. 359(21):2254-65, 2008
2. Delclaux C et al: Factors associated with dyspnea in adult patients with sickle cell disease. Chest. 128(5):3336-44, 2005
3. Maitre B et al: Acute chest syndrome in adults with sickle cell disease. Chest. 117(5):1386-92, 2000

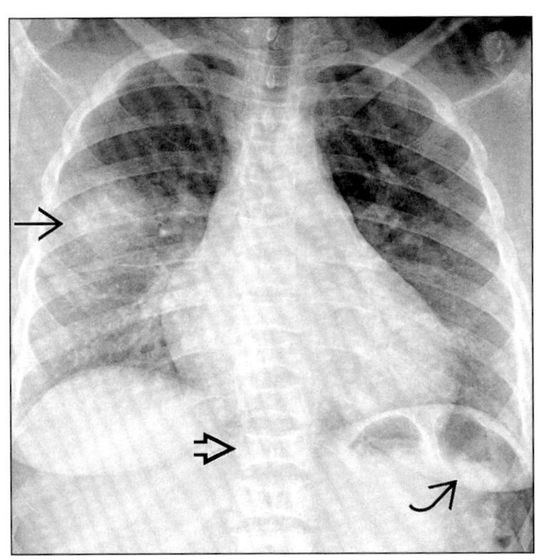

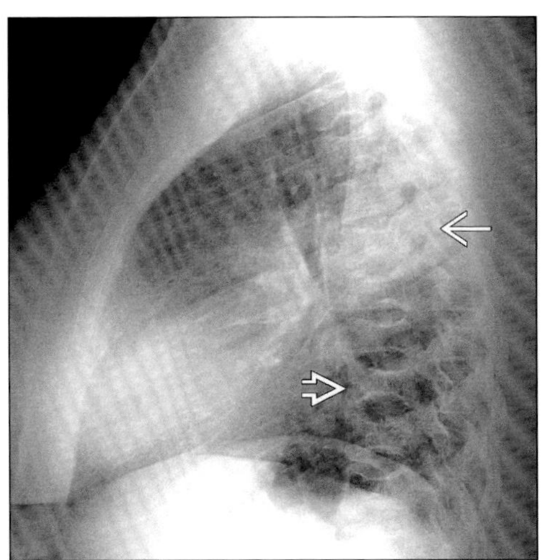

(Left) *PA chest radiograph of a 17-year-old woman with sickle cell anemia shows a right upper lobe consolidation ➔, cardiomegaly, H-shaped vertebral bodies ➲, and absence of the splenic shadow ➚, all stigmata of sickle cell disease.* ***(Right)*** *Lateral chest radiograph of the same patient shows right upper lobe pneumonia ➔ and H-shaped vertebrae ➲ from microinfarctions at vertebral endplates. Round pneumonias due to Streptococcus pneumoniae may affect patients with autosplenectomy.*

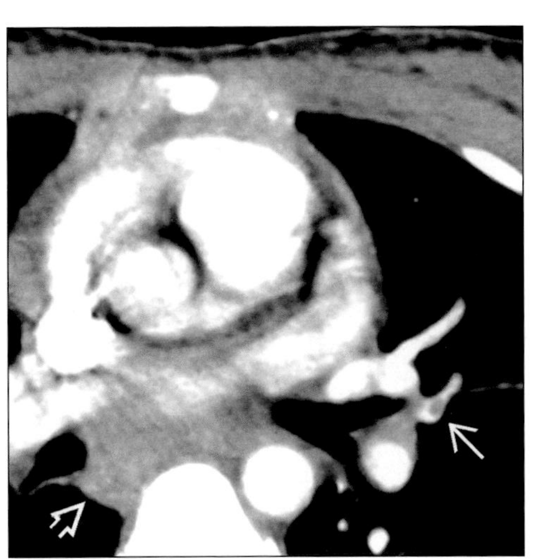

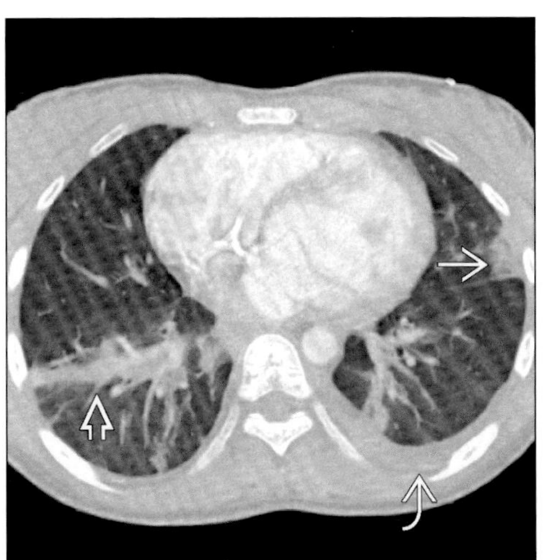

(Left) *Axial CECT of a 23-year-old woman with sickle cell anemia shows a pulmonary embolus in a lingular pulmonary artery ➔. The patient had longstanding subcarinal lymphadenopathy ➲.* ***(Right)*** *Axial CECT of the same patient shows a lingular pulmonary infarction ➔, linear subsegmental opacities ➲ in the lower lobes, and small bilateral pleural effusions ➚. Thrombosis in patients with sickle cell disease may represent venous thromboembolism or in situ thrombosis.*

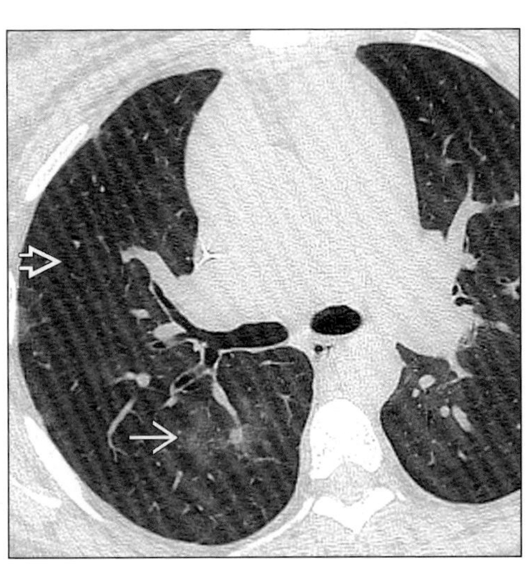

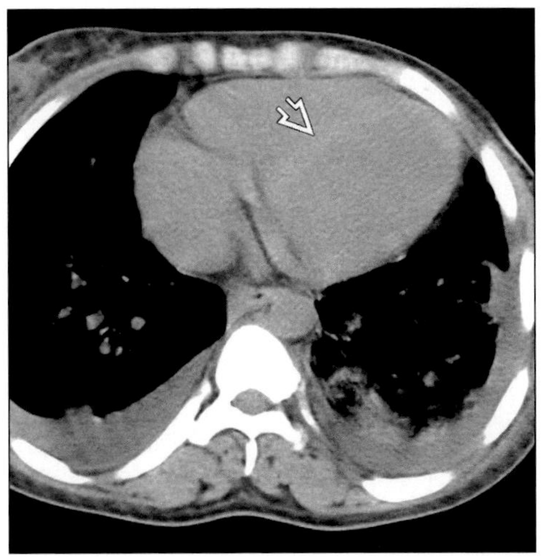

(Left) *Axial HRCT of a patient with sickle cell anemia shows mosaic attenuation. Hyperlucent hypoperfused lung ➲ results from microvascular infarction and occlusion. Hyperperfused lung ➔ results from redistributed flow to preserved microvasculature. Obliteration of pulmonary microvasculature predisposes to pulmonary artery hypertension.* ***(Right)*** *Axial NECT shows a normal density interventricular septum ➲ outlined by low-attenuation blood, consistent with anemia in sickle cell disease.*

FAT EMBOLISM

Key Facts

Terminology

- Fat embolism (FE): Release of fat globules into venous system
- Fat embolism syndrome (FES): Pulmonary, cerebral, & cutaneous manifestations

Imaging

- Best diagnostic clue: Bilateral diffuse airspace disease in trauma setting
- Radiography
  - Chest radiograph may be normal
  - Patchy or diffuse bilateral opacities
- NECT
  - Focal or diffuse consolidation ± ground-glass opacity
  - Nodules < 10 mm; centrilobular & subpleural
- CTA: Fat density endoluminal filling defect
- V/Q scan: Peripheral V/Q mismatches

Top Differential Diagnoses

- Acute respiratory distress syndrome
- Cardiogenic & noncardiogenic pulmonary edema
- Infection
- Pulmonary embolism

Clinical Issues

- FE: > 90% of patients with traumatic bone injury
- Clinical diagnosis: Gurd & Wilson criteria
  - At least 1 major & 4 minor criteria
- FE: Asymptomatic in most cases
- FES: Clinical triad of respiratory distress, cerebral dysfunction, & petechial rash
- FES develops within 1-3 days of injury
  - Mortality: 5-15%; worse in elderly & severe injuries
- Treatment: Oxygenation & hemodynamic stability
- Reduced risk: Early immobilization & stabilization

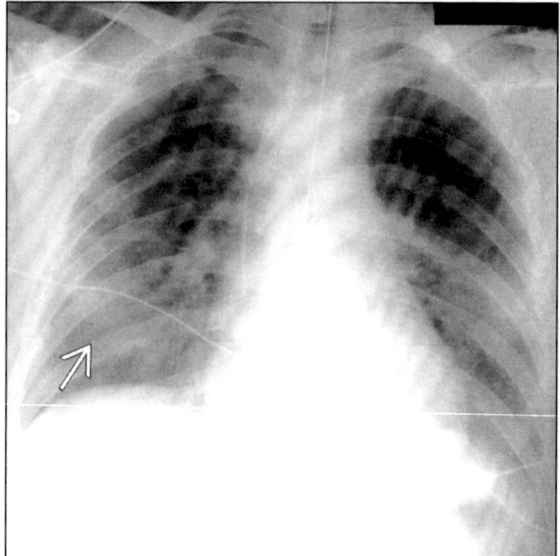

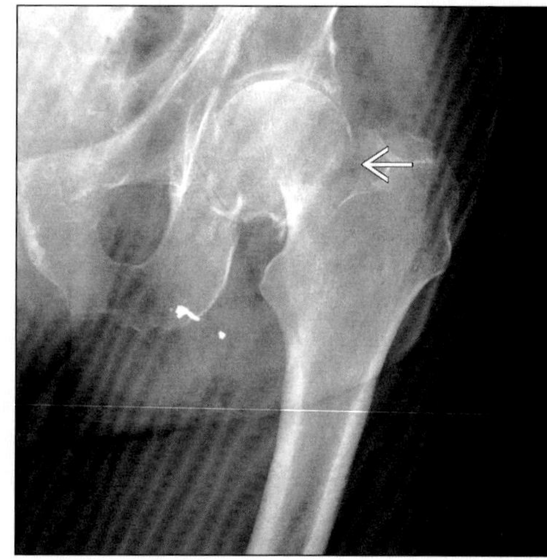

(Left) *AP chest radiograph of a patient with new onset respiratory distress after trauma shows patchy bilateral pulmonary opacities* ➔*.* ***(Right)*** *AP left hip radiograph of the same patient demonstrates a displaced left femoral fracture* ➔*. The best diagnostic clue for the presence of fat embolism and fat embolism syndrome is patchy or diffuse pulmonary opacities on chest radiography in the setting of bone trauma.*

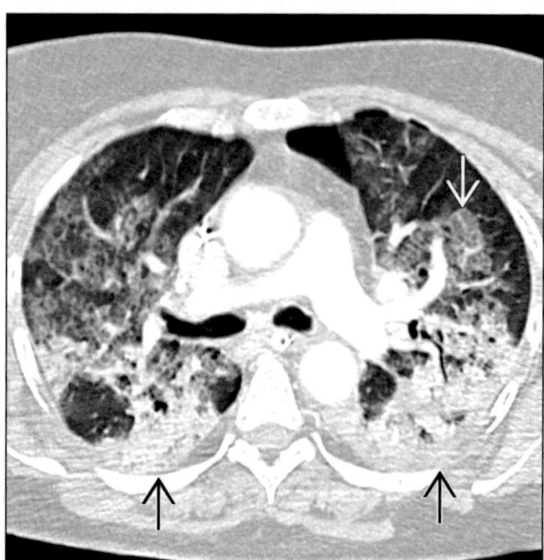

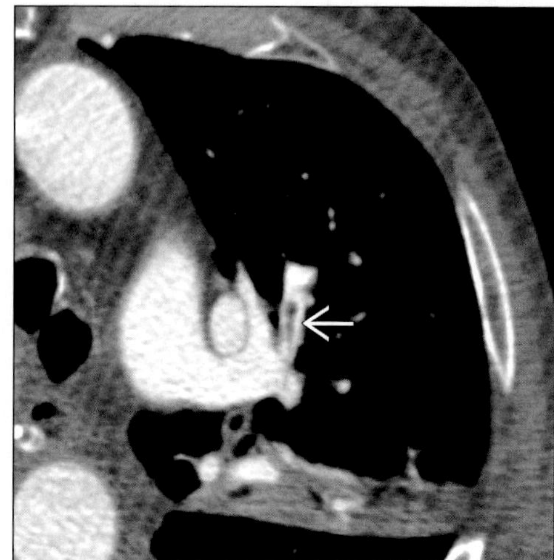

(Left) *Axial CECT of a patient with FES demonstrates bilateral consolidations* ➔ *affecting the posterior lung parenchyma. Patchy and confluent ground-glass opacities* ➔ *are located more anteriorly within the lungs. FES typically develops within 1-3 days of bone trauma.* ***(Right)*** *Axial CTA of a patient with FES shows a hypodense fat attenuation filling defect* ➔ *within a left upper lobe pulmonary artery branch. In the setting of bone trauma, this finding is consistent with FE.*

FAT EMBOLISM

TERMINOLOGY

Abbreviations

- **Fat embolism (FE)**
- **Fat embolism syndrome (FES)**

Definitions

- **Fat embolism**
  - **Release of fat globules into venous system**
  - Typically benign course
- **Fat embolism syndrome**
  - Pulmonary, cerebral, & cutaneous manifestations

IMAGING

General Features

- Best diagnostic clue
  - Bilateral airspace disease in trauma setting

Radiographic Findings

- Radiography
  - Early
    - **Chest radiograph may be normal**
  - Late
    - **Patchy or diffuse bilateral opacities**
      - Airspace, interstitial, ± nodular

CT Findings

- NECT
  - **Focal or diffuse consolidation ± ground-glass opacity**
  - **Nodules** < 10 mm
    - Centrilobular & subpleural
    - Upper lung zones
- CECT
  - **Rarely endoluminal filling defect exhibiting fat attenuation**

Nuclear Medicine Findings

- V/Q scan
  - **Peripheral V/Q mismatches**

Imaging Recommendations

- Best imaging tool
  - Chest radiography for identification & monitoring

DIFFERENTIAL DIAGNOSIS

Acute Respiratory Distress Syndrome

- Imaging & time course overlap
- Distinguish with Gurd & Wilson criteria

Cardiogenic Pulmonary Edema

- Cardiomegaly, Kerley lines, & pleural effusions

Noncardiogenic Pulmonary Edema

- Normal heart size & appropriate clinical setting

Infection

- Signs & symptoms of infection

Pulmonary Hemorrhage

- Consolidation & septal thickening

Pulmonary Embolism

- Pulmonary artery filling defects on CTA

PATHOLOGY

General Features

- Etiology
  - Intramedullary veins damaged by trauma to bone
    - Intravasation of marrow fat
    - Pulmonary microvasculature obstructed
  - Hydrolysis of fat emboli
    - Increased permeability of capillary bed
    - Delayed appearance of pulmonary failure
  - Platelet aggregation
    - Stimulated by fat globules
    - Edema, hemorrhage, & vessel disruption

Microscopic Features

- Widespread microvascular occlusion by fat emboli

CLINICAL ISSUES

Presentation

- Most common signs/symptoms
  - FE: Asymptomatic in most cases
  - FES: Clinical triad of respiratory distress, cerebral dysfunction, & petechial rash
- Clinical profile
  - Clinical diagnosis: **Gurd & Wilson criteria**
  - **At least 1 major & 4 minor criteria**
    - Major criteria
      - Hypoxemia
      - Pulmonary edema
      - Central nervous system depression
      - Petechial rash in vest distribution
    - Minor criteria
      - Tachycardia
      - Pyrexia
      - Retinal emboli
      - Jaundice
      - Sudden drop in hematocrit or platelets
      - Increasing erythrocyte sedimentation rate
      - Fat globules in sputum & urine

Demographics

- Epidemiology
  - FE: > 90% of patients with traumatic bone injury
  - FES: 3-4% of patients with FE

Natural History & Prognosis

- FES: Develops within 1-3 days of injury
- Mortality: 5-15%; worse in elderly & severe injuries

Treatment

- Adequate oxygenation & hemodynamic stability
- Reduced risk: Early immobilization & stabilization

DIAGNOSTIC CHECKLIST

Consider

- FES in a patient with an abnormal chest radiograph 1-3 days after bone trauma

SELECTED REFERENCES

1. Gallardo X et al: Nodular pattern at lung computed tomography in fat embolism syndrome: a helpful finding. J Comput Assist Tomogr. 30(2):254-7, 2006

HEPATOPULMONARY SYNDROME

Key Facts

Terminology
- Hepatopulmonary syndrome (HPS)
  - Intrapulmonary vascular dilatation
  - Increased alveolar-arterial oxygen gradient on room air
  - Liver disease

Imaging
- Radiography
  - Normal or basilar reticulonodular opacities
- CT
  - Dilated basilar lung vessels, peripheral telangiectasias, arteriovenous communications
- Tc-99m macroaggregated albumin for shunt quantification
- Pulmonary angiography
  - Documentation of arteriovenous malformations
  - May show spider-like peripheral vasculature

Top Differential Diagnoses
- Portopulmonary hypertension
- Hepatic hydrothorax
- Interstitial lung disease

Pathology
- Postulated excess circulating pulmonary vasodilators (e.g., nitric oxide)

Clinical Issues
- Symptoms/signs
  - Dyspnea, cyanosis, clubbing, hypoxemia
- HPS in 15-20% of patients with cirrhosis; increased risk of death & decreased functional status
- Orthotopic liver transplant, most effective treatment

Diagnostic Checklist
- Consider HPS in patients with cirrhosis, hypoxemia, & dilated basilar peripheral pulmonary vessels on CT

*(**Left**) PA chest radiograph of a patient with hepatic cirrhosis shows bilateral basilar reticulonodular opacities ➔. The dilated intrapulmonary vasculature and the arteriovenous communications seen in hepatopulmonary syndrome occur predominantly in the lower lobes. (**Right**) CECT of the same patient shows dilated peripheral pulmonary vessels ➔ in the lower lobes bilaterally that are approximately twice the size of the adjacent bronchi. Enlarged subpleural vessels ➔ are also present.*

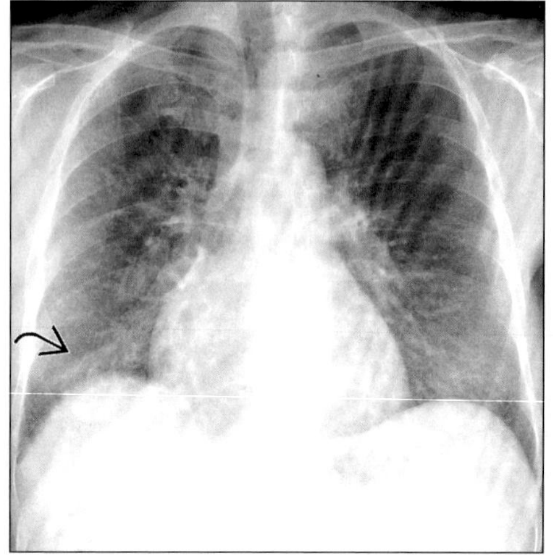

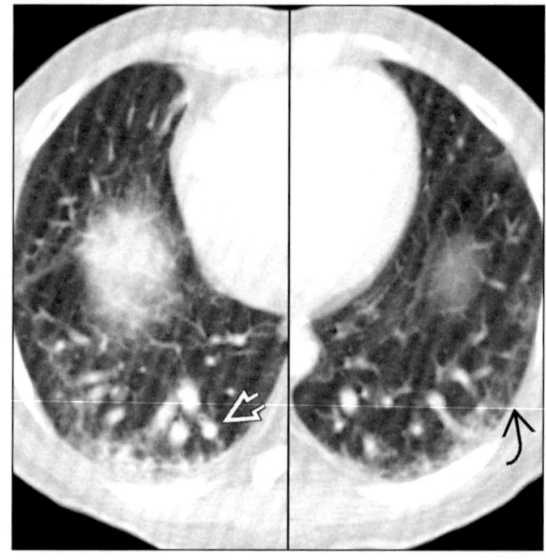

*(**Left**) Coronal CECT of the same patient shows dilated lower lobe intrapulmonary vessels with relative sparing of the upper lobe vessels. Vessel dilatation is thought to be due to increased circulating vasodilators such as nitric oxide. (**Right**) Axial CECT of a patient with cirrhosis shows abnormal communications ➔ between peripheral pulmonary arteries and veins. Such communications are not always visible on CT, but arteriovenous shunting may be demonstrated and quantified on nuclear scintigraphy.*

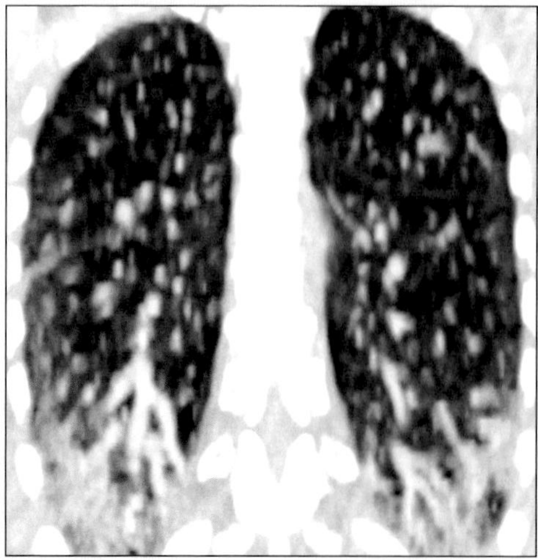

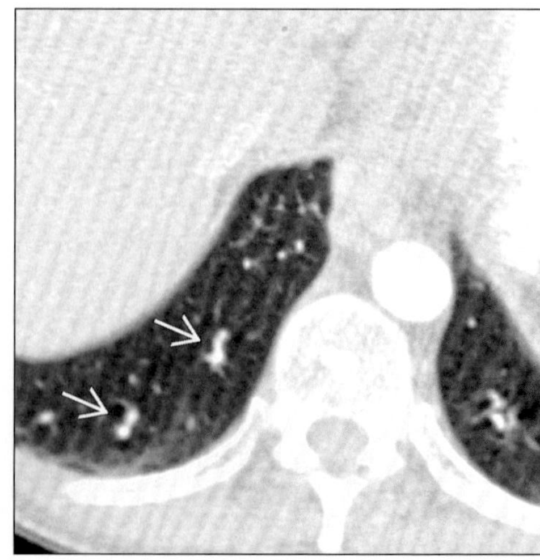

HEPATOPULMONARY SYNDROME

TERMINOLOGY

Abbreviations

- **Hepatopulmonary syndrome (HPS)**

Definitions

- Syndrome composed of the triad
  - **Intrapulmonary vascular dilation**
  - **Increased alveolar-arterial oxygen gradient** while breathing room air
  - **Liver disease**

IMAGING

General Features

- Best diagnostic clue
  - **Dilated intrapulmonary vessels, peripheral telangiectasias, & arteriovenous communications** in patients with liver cirrhosis
- Location
  - More common in **lower lobes**

Radiographic Findings

- Chest radiography may be normal
- Basilar nodular or reticulonodular opacities

CT Findings

- **Dilated subpleural vessels**; arteriovenous communications may not be visible
- **Nodular dilatation of peripheral pulmonary vessels**, representing arteriovenous communications
  - May see dilated feeding artery & draining vein

Nuclear Medicine Findings

- V/Q scan
  - Ventilation perfusion mismatch & shunt
- Tc-99m labeled macroaggregated albumin
  - Activity in brain, kidney, liver, spleen from intrapulmonary arteriovenous shunting
  - Allows shunt quantification
  - Does not differentiate intracardiac from intrapulmonary shunt

Angiographic Findings

- Pulmonary angiography can confirm arteriovenous malformation
- May demonstrate spider-like peripheral vasculature

Echocardiographic Findings

- Contrast echocardiography using microbubbles may reveal a shunt

DIFFERENTIAL DIAGNOSIS

Portopulmonary Hypertension

- Pulmonary arterial hypertension accompanying portal hypertension
- May be secondary to vasoactive substances, venous thromboembolism, or increased cardiac output
- 2-5% of patients with liver cirrhosis

Hepatic Hydrothorax

- Pleural effusion, usually right sided
- Postulated leakage of ascitic fluid into pleural space via diaphragmatic defects

Arteriovenous Malformation

- May be sporadic or familial

Interstitial Lung Disease (ILD)

- Sarcoidosis associated with interferon therapy
- Methotrexate for treatment of primary biliary cirrhosis
  - Centrilobular nodules, patchy ground-glass opacities
  - Fibrosis has been reported

Metastatic Disease

- Tumor emboli from hepatocellular carcinoma may cause dilated pulmonary vasculature

Portosystemic Collateral Vessels

- Esophageal, paraesophageal, cardiophrenic angle varices

PATHOLOGY

General Features

- Etiology
  - Postulated excess circulating **pulmonary vasodilators** (e.g., nitric oxide)

Staging, Grading, & Classification

- Type 1 (most common): Subpleural telangiectasia & peripheral vessel dilation
- Type 2: Arteriovenous communications

Microscopic Features

- Dilated precapillary arterioles & pleural vessels
- Arteriovenous communications

CLINICAL ISSUES

Presentation

- Most common signs/symptoms
  - Shortness of breath, cyanosis, clubbing
  - Cutaneous spider nevi
- Other signs/symptoms
  - Hypoxemia
  - Increased alveolar-arterial oxygen gradient
  - DLCO shows decreased diffusion capacity

Demographics

- Epidemiology
  - Occurs in 15-20% of patients with cirrhosis

Natural History & Prognosis

- HPS confers increased risk of death & decreased functional status

Treatment

- **Orthotopic liver transplant, most effective treatment**

DIAGNOSTIC CHECKLIST

Image Interpretation Pearls

- Arteriovenous communications & dilated peripheral vessels in patients with cirrhosis suggest HPS

SELECTED REFERENCES

1. Kim YK et al: Thoracic complications of liver cirrhosis: radiologic findings. Radiographics. 29(3):825-37, 2009

ILLICIT DRUG USE, PULMONARY MANIFESTATIONS

Key Facts

Terminology
- Spectrum of pulmonary complications related to abuse of inhaled or IV illicit drugs

Imaging
- Talcosis: Talc embolization to arterioles & capillaries
  - Diffuse centrilobular micronodules
  - Pulmonary arterial hypertension
  - Perihilar opacities & upper lobe volume loss
  - Hyperattenuation due to talc deposition
- Septic embolism
  - Multiple peripheral cavitary lung nodules
- Infection
  - Consolidation, ground-glass opacities, nodules
- Pulmonary edema related to cocaine, methamphetamines, heroine
- Pulmonary hemorrhage
- Emphysema

Top Differential Diagnoses
- Small nodules (< 1 cm)
  - Talcosis
  - Hypersensitivity pneumonitis
- Large nodules (1-3 cm)
  - Septic embolism
  - Fungal or mycobacterial infection
- Consolidation or ground-glass opacity
  - Infection
  - Pulmonary edema
  - Pulmonary hemorrhage

Clinical Issues
- Dyspnea, cough, wheezing, hemoptysis, chest pain

Diagnostic Checklist
- Consider illicit drug use in young adult with unexplained diffuse or focal lung disease

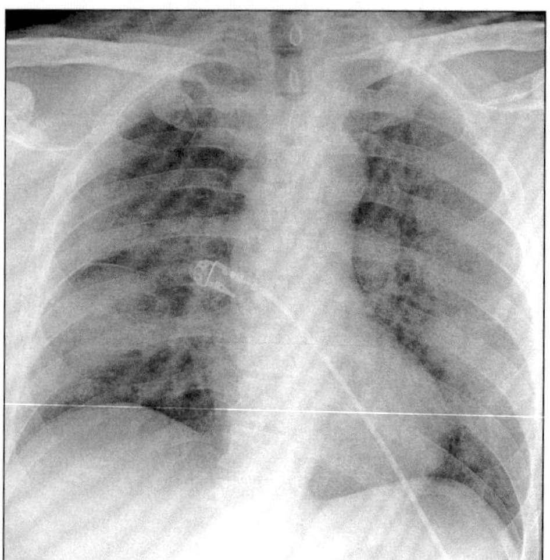
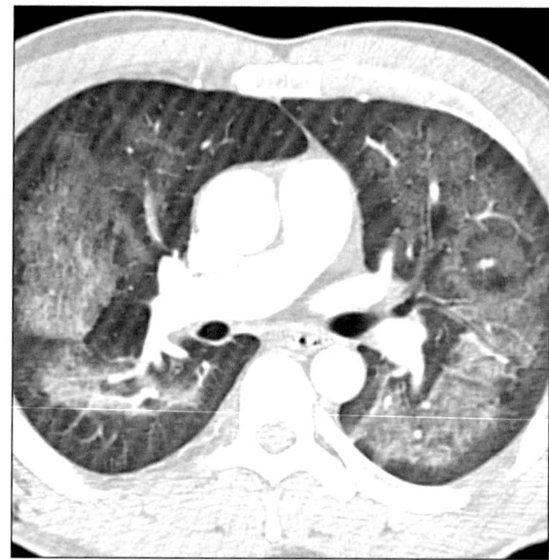

(Left) *AP chest radiograph of a crack cocaine user who presented to the emergency department with chest pain and dyspnea shows bilateral patchy ground-glass opacities.* ***(Right)*** *Axial CECT of the same patient shows bilateral perihilar ground-glass opacities and consolidations, consistent with pulmonary edema. Consider illicit drug use when pulmonary edema is seen in young patients without a history of cardiac disease.*

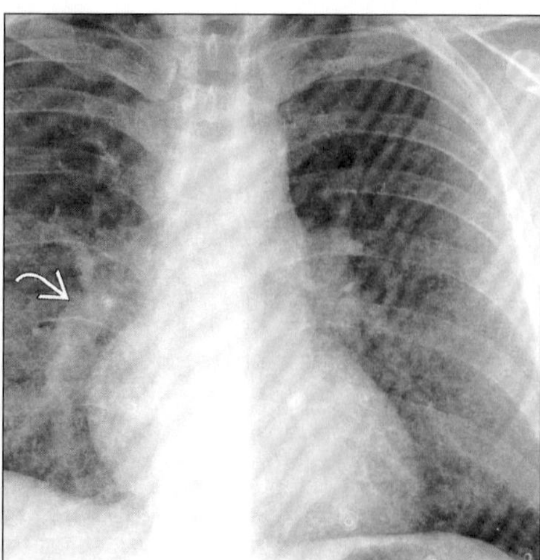
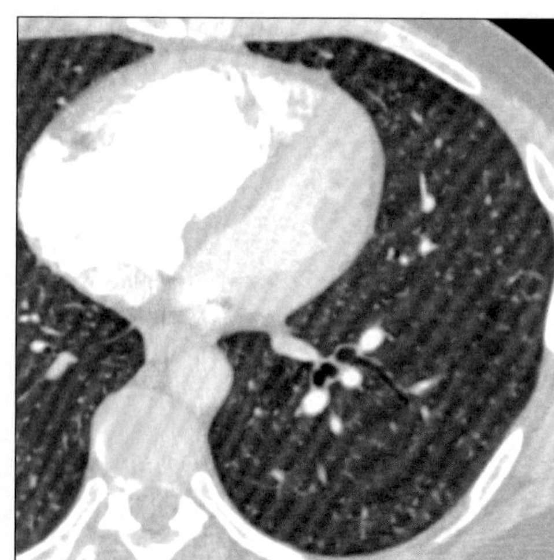

(Left) *PA chest radiograph of a patient who presented with syncope following IV injection of oxycodone shows diffuse bilateral small nodules and enlargement of the central pulmonary arteries ➔.* ***(Right)*** *Axial CTA of the same patient shows diffuse bilateral centrilobular micronodules related to impaction of talc or fillers in the pulmonary arterioles. Note also right atrial and right ventricular enlargement, consistent with right heart strain secondary to pulmonary arterial hypertension.*

ILLICIT DRUG USE, PULMONARY MANIFESTATIONS

TERMINOLOGY

Definitions

- Spectrum of pulmonary complications related to abuse of inhaled or intravenous (IV) illicit drugs
  - Typical drugs: Heroin, cocaine ("crack"), methamphetamine ("speed"), codeine, methadone, methylphenidate (Ritalin)

IMAGING

Imaging Features

- **Talcosis**: IV injection of oral medications (methylphenidate, pentazocine, cocaine, etc.)
  - Diffuse centrilobular micronodules
  - Enlarged central pulmonary arteries due to pulmonary hypertension
  - Perihilar opacities similar to progressive massive fibrosis
  - Areas of hyperattenuation due to talc deposition
- **Septic embolism**
  - Multiple angiocentric nodules with peripheral distribution, frequently cavitary
- **Infection**: Increased risk due to malnutrition, immunosuppression, or coexisting HIV infection
  - Consolidation, ground-glass opacities
  - Pulmonary nodules
- **Aspiration**: Due to altered consciousness
  - Dependent consolidation, ground-glass opacity
  - Dependent tree-in-bud opacities
- **Pulmonary edema**: Cocaine, methamphetamines, heroine
  - Bilateral perihilar consolidation or ground-glass opacities, septal thickening
  - ± pleural effusion
- **Pulmonary hemorrhage**: Multifocal, bilateral airspace disease
- **Emphysema**
  - IV injection of methylphenidate: Panacinar emphysema with lower lobe predominance
  - Marijuana & cocaine smokers: Emphysema with upper lobe predominance

CT Findings

- Optimal characterization of diffuse & multifocal lung disease
  - Distribution & morphologic features of lung nodules
  - Visualization of ground-glass opacity & consolidation
  - Visualization of interlobular septal thickening
  - Characterization & distribution of emphysema

Imaging Recommendations

- Best imaging tool
  - Chest radiographs usually suffice for detection & follow-up
  - CT more sensitive for detection & further characterization if chest radiograph does not explain clinical symptoms

DIFFERENTIAL DIAGNOSIS

Small Nodules (< 1 cm)

- Talcosis
- Hypersensitivity pneumonitis

Large Nodules (1-3 cm)

- Septic embolism
- Fungal or mycobacterial infection
- Organizing pneumonia

Consolidation or Ground-Glass Opacity

- Infection: Bacterial, viral, PCP
- Pulmonary edema
- Aspiration
- Pulmonary hemorrhage
- Organizing pneumonia
- Eosinophilic pneumonia

PATHOLOGY

General Features

- Etiology
  - **Talcosis**
    - Embolization of talc or other fillers (cornstarch, cellulose) to pulmonary arterioles & capillaries
    - Foreign body granulomatous reaction & fibrosis
  - **Septic emboli**
    - Source: Subacute bacterial endocarditis & tricuspid vegetations, septic thrombophlebitis, direct injection of infected fluid
    - *Staphylococcus* most common organism
  - **Pulmonary edema**
    - May be cardiogenic &/or related to pulmonary capillary damage with increased permeability
  - **Emphysema**
    - Damage & obliteration of capillary bed; direct drug toxicity or intermediate immune response

CLINICAL ISSUES

Presentation

- Most common signs/symptoms
  - Dyspnea, cough, wheezing
  - Hemoptysis
  - Chest pain

Demographics

- Age
  - Any; primarily 18-25 years old
- Gender
  - Males > females
- Epidemiology
  - Over 1.5 million IV drug users in North America

Natural History & Prognosis

- Mortality rate 3-4% per year

SELECTED REFERENCES

1. Nguyen ET et al: Pulmonary complications of illicit drug use: differential diagnosis based on CT findings. J Thorac Imaging. 22(2):199-206, 2007

VALVE AND ANNULAR CALCIFICATION

Key Facts

Terminology
- Calcification of valve leaflet or annulus

Imaging
- Radiography
  - Aortic stenosis: Bicuspid or degenerative; left ventricular configuration, aortic dilatation
  - Mitral stenosis: Left atrial/appendage enlargement, pulmonary venous hypertension
  - Mitral annulus calcification: Reverse C-shaped calcification
  - Pulmonic stenosis: Enlarged pulmonary trunk & left pulmonary artery
- NECT: Characterization of calcification
  - Caseous calcification of mitral annulus (CCMA): Centrally hypodense, peripheral calcification
- Echocardiography: Procedure of choice to assess valve morphology & function

Top Differential Diagnoses
- Pericardial calcification
- Ventricular calcification
- Coronary artery calcification
- Great vessel calcification

Pathology
- Aortic valve leaflets: Degenerative, congenital bicuspid aortic valve
  - Bicuspid aortic valve: 90% calcified at surgery
- Aortic annulus: Atherosclerosis
- Mitral valve leaflets: Rheumatic heart disease
- Mitral annulus: Degenerative, ESRD
- CCMA: Degenerative

Clinical Issues
- Surgical replacement of abnormal valves
- Aortic & mitral valves most commonly replaced

*(**Left**) PA chest radiograph of a patient with multiple valve replacements shows a tricuspid annuloplasty ring ➔ and artificial mitral ➔ and pulmonic ➔ valves. (**Right**) Lateral chest radiograph of the same patient shows a tricuspid annuloplasty ring ➔ and artificial mitral ➔ and pulmonic ➔ valves. Knowledge of the anatomic location of the cardiac valves allows radiographic identification of calcified valve leaflets and annuli.*

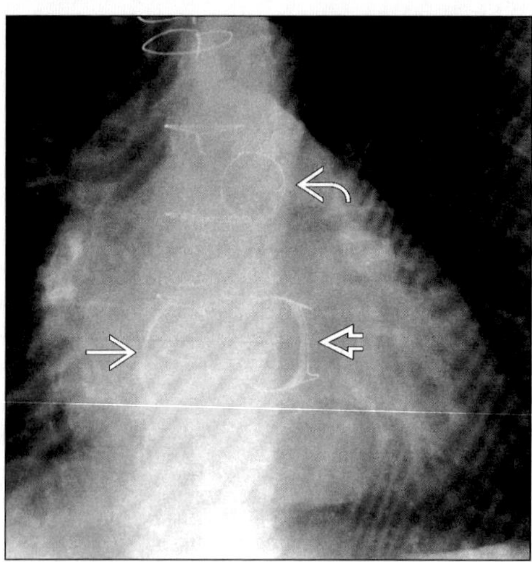

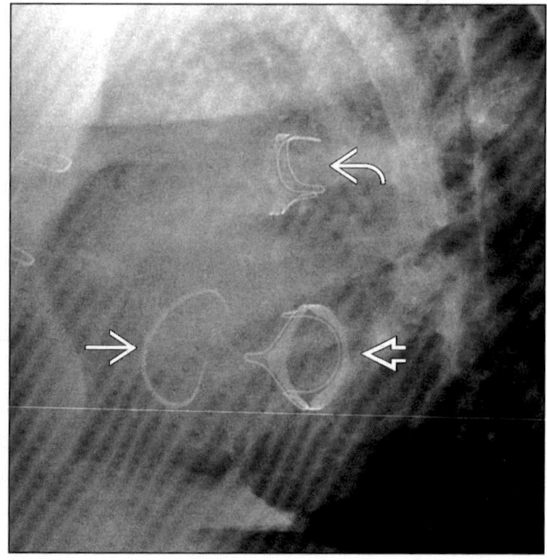

*(**Left**) Lateral chest radiograph of a patient with aortic stenosis demonstrates the complete ring pattern of aortic valve calcification ➔. (**Right**) Coronal CECT of the same patient shows calcification of the aortic valve ➔. Degenerative disease and bicuspid aortic valve morphology are the most common etiologies of aortic valve calcification. Aortic valve calcification on imaging is a strong marker for aortic valve stenosis.*

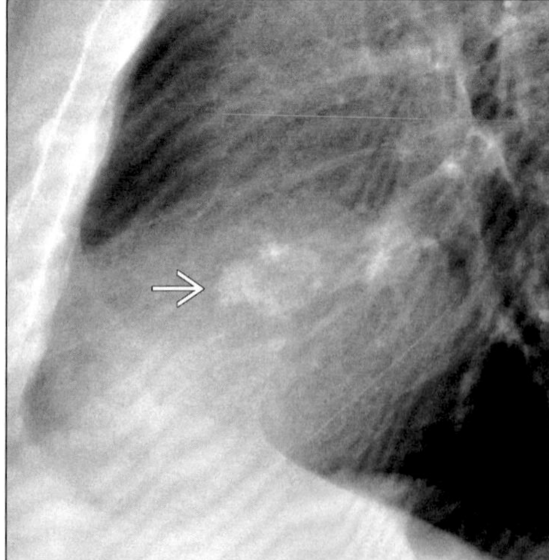

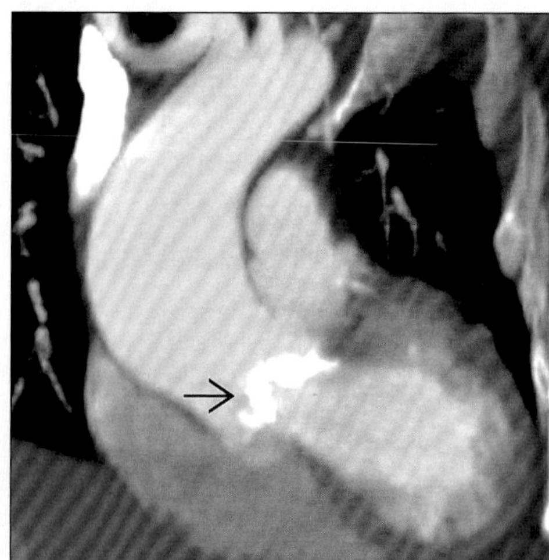

VALVE AND ANNULAR CALCIFICATION

TERMINOLOGY

Abbreviations

- **Caseous calcification of mitral annulus (CCMA)**
- **Mitral annular calcification (MAC)**

Definitions

- Calcification of valve leaflet or annulus

IMAGING

General Features

- Best diagnostic clue
  - Calcification in expected position of cardiac valve

Radiographic Findings

- **Aortic valve**
  - Frontal radiograph: Projects over spine
  - Lateral radiograph: Between anterior & posterior cardiac borders, above line from carina to sternodiaphragmatic junction
  - **3 patterns of calcification**
    - **Commissure calcification: Linear**
    - **Complete or partial ring calcification**
    - **Plaque-like calcification**
  - **Bicuspid aortic valve calcification**
    - **Circular calcification with internal linear focus (fused raphe)**
  - Strong marker for aortic stenosis
    - Secondary findings: Left ventricular configuration, poststenotic dilation of ascending aorta
- **Aortic annulus calcification**
  - Usually seen in conjunction with leaflet calcification
  - May extend into ascending aorta or interventricular septum
- **Mitral valve**
  - Frontal radiograph: Left of spine, below aortic valve
  - Lateral radiograph: Below line from carina to sternodiaphragmatic junction
  - **Mitral stenosis**
    - Left atrial enlargement
- **Double density sign**
  - Enlarged left atrial appendage
  - Pulmonary venous hypertension & edema
  - Longstanding: Hemosiderosis associated interstitial lung disease
- **MAC & CCMA**
  - Uniform, reverse C-shaped calcification
    - Junction between ventricular myocardium & posterior mitral leaflet
  - O-shaped with involvement of anterior mitral leaflet
- **Pulmonic valve**
  - Frontal radiograph: Below & medial to pulmonary trunk border, between spine & left atrial appendage
  - Lateral radiograph: Upper anterior portion of heart, behind sternum
  - Most cephalad of cardiac valves
  - Congenital pulmonic valvular stenosis
    - Enlarged pulmonary trunk & left pulmonary artery
    - Decreased pulmonary vascularity when severe
- **Tricuspid valve**
  - Below pulmonic valve
  - Separated from pulmonic valve by infundibulum of pulmonary outflow track
  - Tricuspid stenosis
    - Right heart enlargement & clockwise rotation of cardiac apex
    - Medial displacement & dilatation of SVC
    - Leftward bowing of interventricular septum
- **Tricuspid annulus calcification**
  - Mirror image of mitral annulus
  - Uniform, C-shaped calcification

CT Findings

- CECT
  - **Leaflet (central); annulus (peripheral)**
  - Quantification of aortic valve calcification with CECT not reliable
    - Contrast material may simulate calcification
    - NECT with ECG gating preferred
  - CCMA
    - Centrally hypodense mass with peripheral calcification
    - No enhancement
    - Usually involves posterior annulus; may involve entire annulus when large
- Cardiac gated CTA
  - Assessment of motion abnormalities

Echocardiographic Findings

- Calcification appears as increased echogenicity
- CCMA: Round mass with increased peripheral echogenicity, decreased central echogenicity
- Severity of stenosis determined by orifice size
- Calculation of valve jet velocities
  - Higher aortic valve calcium scores on CT correlate with higher jet velocities

Imaging Recommendations

- Best imaging tool
  - **Echocardiography**: Procedure of choice to assess valve morphology & function

DIFFERENTIAL DIAGNOSIS

Pericardial Calcification

- Focal or curvilinear calcification following cardiac contour; most commonly AV grooves
- Does not predominate at cardiac apex (unlike myocardial calcification)
- Infection, trauma, iatrogenic

Ventricular Calcification

- Thin or thick curvilinear calcification following ventricular contour
- Myocardial infarction, metastatic calcification, thrombus, tumor, aneurysms, & pseudoaneurysms

Coronary Artery Calcification

- Curvilinear or tram-track calcification
- Involvement of 1 wall may mimic calcified infarct

Great Vessel Calcification

- Rim-like aortic wall calcification
  - Atherosclerosis most common cause
- Pulmonary artery wall calcification
  - Chronic pulmonary arterial hypertension

VALVE AND ANNULAR CALCIFICATION

PATHOLOGY

General Features

- Etiology
  - Aortic valve leaflets: Degenerative, congenital bicuspid aortic valve
    - Rheumatic heart disease (RHD), syphilis, ankylosing spondylitis less common
  - Aortic annulus: Atherosclerosis
  - Mitral valve leaflets: RHD
  - Mitral annulus: Degenerative, end-stage renal disease (ESRD)
  - CCMA: Degenerative
  - Pulmonic valve leaflets: Congenital pulmonic valvular stenosis, chronic pulmonary arterial hypertension
  - Tricuspid valve leaflets: RHD, septal defects, endocarditis
  - Tricuspid annulus: RHD, congenital pulmonic valvular stenosis
- Dystrophic calcification is usually degenerative
- Calcification begins at points of maximal cusp flexion (margins of attachment)
- Calcific masses may eventually prevent cusp opening

Gross Pathologic & Surgical Features

- **Bicuspid aortic valve: 90% calcified at surgery**
- MAC: 6% at autopsy
- CCMA: 2.7% at autopsy

Microscopic Features

- CCMA: Calcium, fatty acids, cholesterol

CLINICAL ISSUES

Presentation

- Most common signs/symptoms
  - **Aortic stenosis**
    - Classic triad
      - Angina pectoris
      - Syncope
      - CHF
    - Exertional dyspnea
    - "Pulsus parvus et tardus" on physical exam
    - Crescendo-decrescendo systolic ejection murmur with paradoxical S2 split
  - **Mitral stenosis**
    - Exertional dyspnea, cough, wheezing
    - Abrupt onset atrial fibrillation
    - Stress-induced pulmonary edema
    - Loud S1 followed by S2 & "opening snap"; low-pitched, rumbling diastolic murmur
  - **CCMA**
    - Usually asymptomatic
    - Mitral stenosis if mass becomes obstructive
  - **Pulmonic stenosis**
    - Exertional dyspnea & fatigue
    - Systolic ejection click louder on expiration; ejection murmur at left upper sternal border
  - **Tricuspid stenosis**
    - Fatigue
    - Edema secondary to systemic venous congestion
    - Widely split S1 with single S2; diastolic murmur along left sternal border

Demographics

- Age
  - Aortic valve leaflets
    - < 70 years of age: Bicuspid aortic valve
      - > 90% have calcification by 40 years of age
    - > 70 years of age: Degenerative disease
  - Mitral valve leaflets: 20-30 years old
  - Mitral annulus: > 60 years old
- Gender
  - Mitral valve leaflets: M > F
  - Mitral annulus: F > M
- Epidemiology
  - Aortic valve leaflets
    - Degenerative calcification: 2-7% prevalence in patients older than 70 years
    - Bicuspid aortic valve: 2% of population
  - MAC: 6% of population
  - CCMA: 0.06-0.07% overall; 0.6% on echocardiography

Natural History & Prognosis

- Aortic annulus
  - Extension into conducting system may lead to heart block
  - High association with systemic atherosclerosis
- MAC
  - Higher incidence of new coronary events
  - Right bundle branch block
  - High association with systemic atherosclerosis
  - Associated with aortic stenosis
- CCMA
  - Usually benign
  - Rare valvular dysfunction

Treatment

- Surgical replacement of abnormal valves
  - Aortic & mitral valves most common
  - Valvuloplasty
    - Widening of stenotic valve using balloon catheter
  - Valvulotomy or commissurotomy
    - Incision of commissures
  - Valve replacement
    - Percutaneous or traditional open-heart techniques

DIAGNOSTIC CHECKLIST

Image Interpretation Pearls

- Valve & annular calcification often detected on radiography
- NECT with ECG gating best for quantifying calcification
- Echocardiography best for assessment of valve morphology & function

SELECTED REFERENCES

1. Ferguson EC et al: Cardiac and pericardial calcifications on chest radiographs. Clin Radiol. 65(9):685-94, 2010
2. Chen JJ et al: CT angiography of the cardiac valves: normal, diseased, and postoperative appearances. Radiographics. 29(5):1393-412, 2009
3. Boxt LM: CT of valvular heart disease. Int J Cardiovasc Imaging. 21(1):105-13, 2005

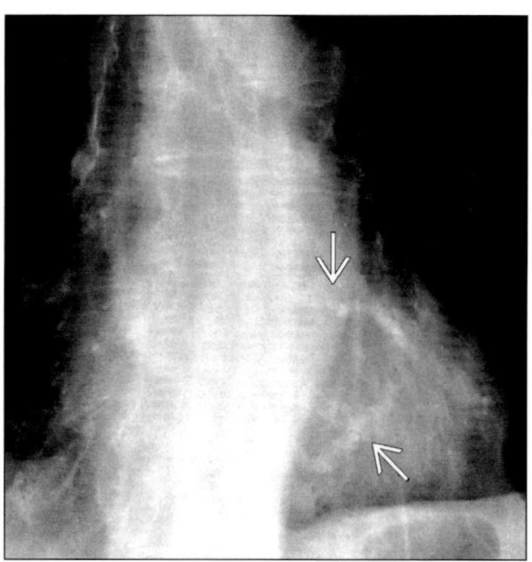

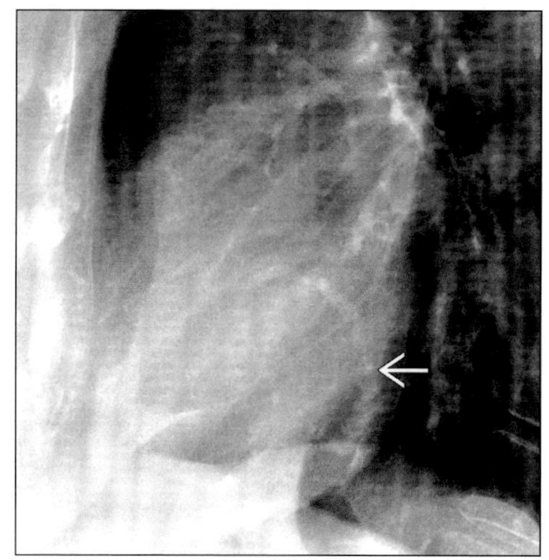

*(**Left**) PA chest radiograph of a patient with mitral annular calcification shows curvilinear calcification ➔ of the mitral annulus with the characteristic reverse C-shaped configuration. (**Right**) Lateral chest radiograph of the same patient shows curvilinear calcification ➔ most prominently involving the posterior aspect of the mitral annulus. Mitral annular calcification is more common in women than in men and is associated with end-stage renal disease.*

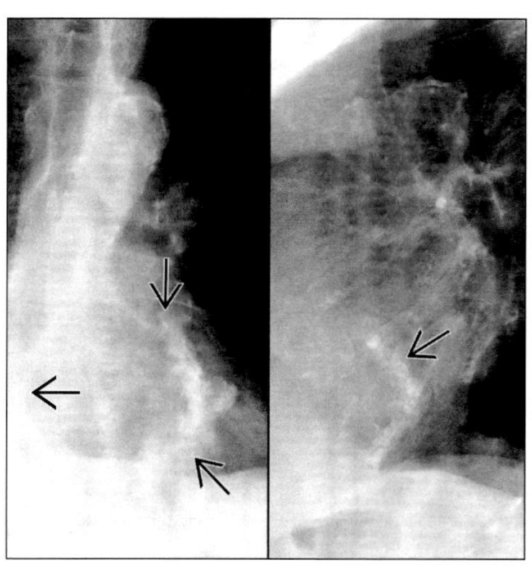

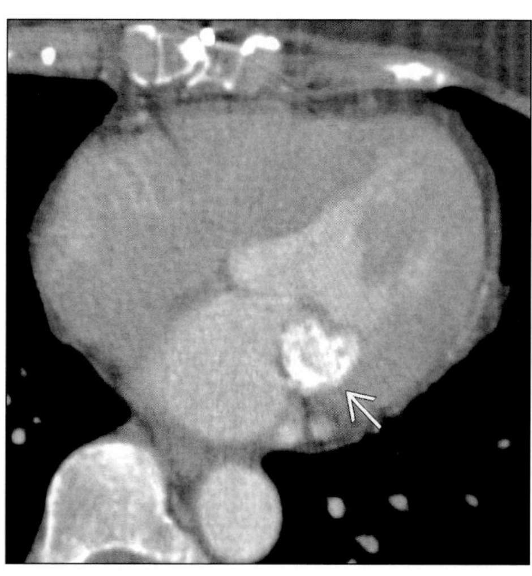

*(**Left**) Composite image with PA (left) and lateral (right) chest radiographs of a patient with end-stage renal disease shows abundant calcification → of the mitral annulus. Involvement of the anterior mitral leaflet results in an O-shaped configuration on the frontal chest radiograph. (**Right**) Axial CECT shows a heterogeneous mass ➔ along the posterior mitral annulus. The central hypodensity and peripheral calcification are characteristic of caseous calcification of the mitral annulus.*

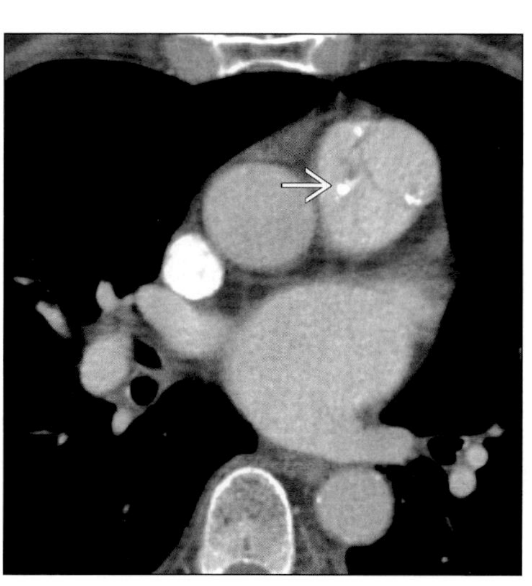

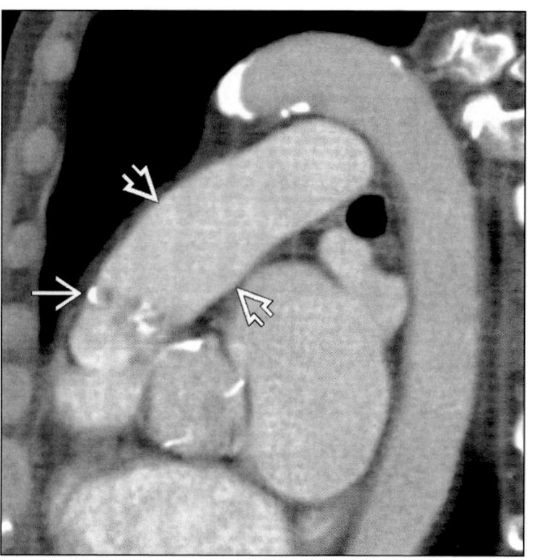

*(**Left**) Axial CECT of a patient with congenital pulmonic valve stenosis shows thickening and calcification ➔ of the pulmonic valve leaflets. (**Right**) Sagittal CECT of the same patient demonstrates pulmonic valve leaflet thickening and calcifications ➔. Note the poststenotic dilation of the pulmonary trunk ➔. Patients with pulmonic stenosis may exhibit enlargement of the pulmonary trunk and the left pulmonary artery on chest radiography. CT allows anatomic localization of valve calcification.*

AORTIC VALVE DISEASE

Key Facts

Terminology
- Aortic regurgitation (AR)
- Aortic stenosis (AS)
- Aortic valve disease: AR & AS

Imaging
- Best diagnostic clue
  - AR: Retrograde flow of blood into left ventricle on echocardiography & MR
  - AS: Systolic jet into proximal aorta on MR
- AS: Aortic valve calcification
  - Quantification of calcification on NECT
- ECG-gated CTA: Thickening & calcification of aortic valve leaflets
  - AR: Incomplete coaptation of aortic valve leaflets
  - AS: Measurement of aortic valve orifice
- MR: Volumes, velocities, & gradients quantification

Top Differential Diagnoses
- Subvalvular aortic stenosis
- Supravalvular aortic stenosis

Pathology
- Acute AR: Endocarditis, dissection, trauma
- Chronic AR: Valve disease, aortic root dilation
- AS: Degenerative, bicuspid valve, rheumatic heart disease

Clinical Issues
- AR: Chest pain, dyspnea
  - Variable progression to left ventricular failure
  - Surgery for acute AR with hypotension & pulmonary edema
- AS: Angina, syncope, dyspnea
  - Degenerative > 70 years; bicuspid valve < 70 years
  - Surgery for severe, symptomatic AS; left ventricular dysfunction; critical stenosis

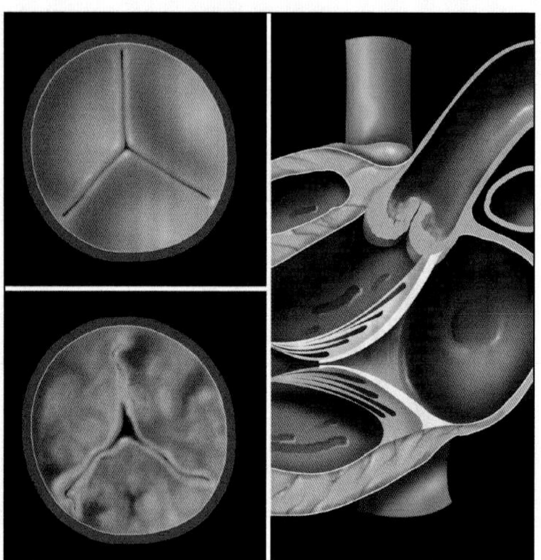

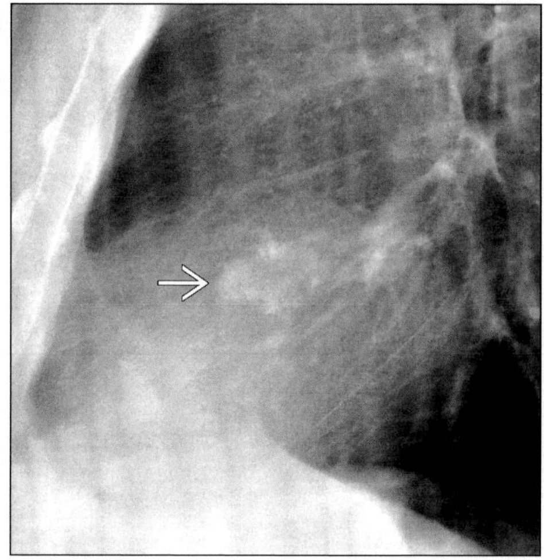

(Left) *Graphic illustrates normal and abnormal appearances of the aortic valve. Aortic valve disease secondary to degeneration and congenital bicuspid aortic valve is characterized by thickening and calcification of the valve leaflets, resulting in incomplete valve opening or closure and aortic valve dysfunction.* ***(Right)*** *Lateral chest radiograph of a patient with aortic stenosis shows calcification ➡ in the anatomic location of the aortic valve.*

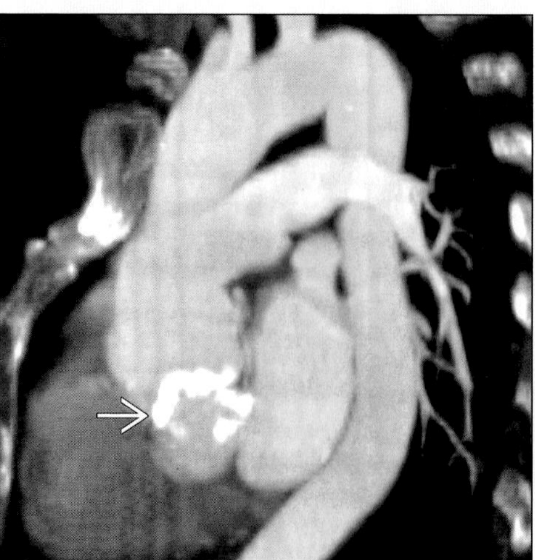

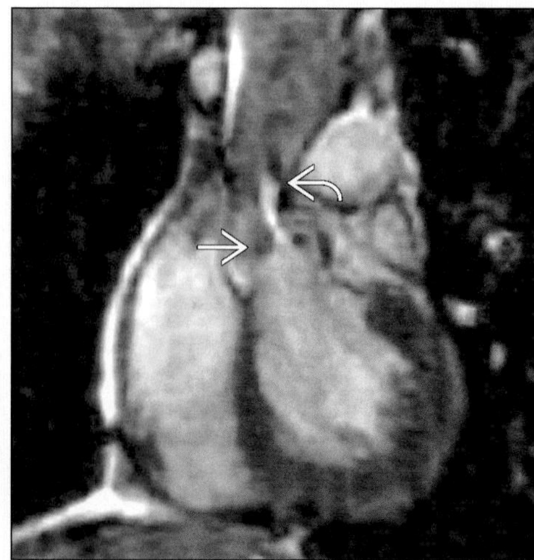

(Left) *Sagittal CECT of a patient with aortic stenosis demonstrates extensive aortic valve calcification ➡.* ***(Right)*** *Coronal MR cine of the same patient shows thickening of the aortic valve leaflets ➡ and a hyperintense systolic jet ↪ into the ascending aorta, consistent with aortic stenosis. MR cine can quantify the gradient across the stenotic aortic valve and help determine the severity of disease.*

AORTIC VALVE DISEASE

TERMINOLOGY

Definitions

- **Aortic valve disease: Aortic regurgitation (AR) & aortic stenosis (AS)**

IMAGING

General Features

- Best diagnostic clue
  - **Aortic regurgitation**
    - **Retrograde flow of blood into left ventricle** on echocardiography & MR
  - **Aortic stenosis**
    - **Systolic jet** into proximal aorta on MR
- Location
  - Aortic valve

Radiographic Findings

- Radiography
  - **Aortic regurgitation**
    - Acute: Normal heart size, pulmonary edema
    - Chronic
      - Left ventricular enlargement
      - Dilatation of aortic root ± ascending aorta
      - Pulmonary venous hypertension
  - **Aortic stenosis**
    - **Calcification** in expected position of aortic valve
      - Frontal radiograph: Projects over spine
      - Lateral radiograph: Between anterior & posterior cardiac borders, above line from carina to sternodiaphragmatic junction
    - 3 patterns of calcification
      - **Commissure calcification: Linear**
      - **Complete or partial ring calcification**
      - **Plaque-like calcification**
    - Left ventricular configuration
      - Heart size increases with AS severity
    - **Poststenotic dilation of ascending aorta**

CT Findings

- NECT
  - **Quantification of aortic valve calcification**
- CECT
  - **Aortic regurgitation**
    - Left ventricular enlargement
    - Dilatation of aortic root ± ascending aorta
    - Effacement of sinotubular junction: Annuloaortic ectasia
  - **Aortic stenosis**
    - Aortic valve calcification
      - Central location allows distinction from peripheral aortic annulus calcification
      - **Bicuspid valve**: Early thickening & calcification of valve leaflets
      - **Degenerative valve**: Greater calcification than bicuspid valve
    - Left ventricular hypertrophy
    - Poststenotic dilation of ascending aorta
- Cardiac gated CTA
  - **Aortic regurgitation**
    - Incomplete coaptation of aortic valve leaflets
      - Accurate for moderate to severe AR
      - Mild AR frequently overlooked
    - Thickening & calcification of valve leaflets
    - Left ventricular enlargement
  - **Aortic stenosis**
    - Measurement of aortic valve orifice
    - Thickening & calcification of valve leaflets

MR Findings

- MR cine
  - **Aortic regurgitation**
    - Retrograde blood flow into left ventricle in diastole on cine GRE
    - Left ventricular enlargement in chronic AR
    - Holodiastolic flow reversal highly sensitive & specific for severe AR
    - Volumes & ejection fraction quantification
    - Regurgitant fraction calculation
  - **Aortic stenosis**
    - Systolic jet into proximal aorta on bright blood sequences
    - Morphology: Bicuspid aortic valve
    - Volumes & ejection fraction quantification
    - Calculation of peak systolic velocities & gradients

Echocardiographic Findings

- Echocardiogram
  - **Aortic regurgitation**
    - Incomplete coaptation of aortic valve leaflets
    - Left ventricular enlargement in chronic AR
    - Calculation of regurgitant fraction
  - **Aortic stenosis**
    - Identification of stenotic valve & determination of etiology
    - Quantification of diastolic ± systolic dysfunction
    - Quantification of left ventricular hypertrophy
    - Assessment of coexisting disorders

Angiographic Findings

- Conventional
  - **Aortic regurgitation**
    - Regurgitant jet in left ventricle
  - **Aortic stenosis**
    - Aortic valve calcification
    - Systolic jet into aorta
    - Measurement of aortic valve orifice size
    - Quantification of gradient across stenotic valve

Imaging Recommendations

- Best imaging tool
  - Echocardiography
- Protocol advice
  - ECG-gated CTA for evaluation of leaflets, orifice, & function

DIFFERENTIAL DIAGNOSIS

Subvalvular Aortic Stenosis

- Idiopathic hypertrophic subaortic stenosis (IHSS)
- Fixed, hemodynamically significant obstruction of left ventricular outflow tract (LVOT)
- Left ventricular hypertrophy & cardiac dysfunction

Supravalvular Aortic Stenosis

- Hourglass narrowing of proximal ascending aorta above aortic valve
- Associated with Marfan & Williams syndromes

AORTIC VALVE DISEASE

PATHOLOGY

General Features

- Etiology
  - Aortic regurgitation
    - Acute: Endocarditis, dissection, trauma
    - Chronic
      - Valve disease: Degenerative, bicuspid valve, rheumatic heart disease (RHD)
      - Aortic root dilatation: Marfan, syphilis
  - Aortic stenosis
    - Degenerative, bicuspid valve, RHD
- Associated abnormalities
  - Aortic stenosis
    - Bicuspid aortic valve, aortic coarctation

Staging, Grading, & Classification

- Classification by echocardiography
- **Aortic regurgitation**
  - **Mild**: Proximal jet width < 3 mm (or < 25% of LVOT); pressure 1/2 time (PHT) > 500 ms
  - **Moderate**: Proximal jet width 3-6 mm (or 25-65% of LVOT); PHT 200-500 ms
  - **Severe**: Proximal jet width > 6 mm (or > 65% of LVOT); PHT < 200 ms
- **Aortic stenosis**
  - **Mild**: Aortic valve orifice area (AVA) > 1.5 cm^2; mean pressure gradient < 25 mmHg
  - **Moderate**: AVA 1-1.5 cm^2; transvalvular pressure gradient 25-40 mmHg
  - **Severe**: AVA < 1 cm^2; transvalvular pressure gradient > 40 mmHg
  - **Critical**: AVA < 0.7 cm^2

Gross Pathologic & Surgical Features

- Aortic regurgitation
  - Valve fibrosis & thickening in RHD
- Aortic stenosis
  - Thickening & calcification of leaflets
    - Occurs earlier in bicuspid valves
    - Calcification begins at base of cusps
  - Valve fibrosis & thickening in RHD

Microscopic Features

- Aortic stenosis
  - Accumulation of lipid & inflammatory cells

CLINICAL ISSUES

Presentation

- Most common signs/symptoms
  - Aortic regurgitation
    - Chest pain, dyspnea
    - Usually asymptomatic until valve area is reduced to 1 cm^2
  - Aortic stenosis
    - Angina, syncope, dyspnea

Demographics

- Age
  - Aortic regurgitation
    - Variable depending on etiology
  - **Aortic stenosis**
    - **< 70 years of age: Bicuspid valve**
    - **> 70 years of age: Degenerative disease**
- Gender
  - Aortic regurgitation
    - M:F = 3:1
  - Aortic stenosis
    - **Bicuspid valve: M:F = 4:1**
- Epidemiology
  - AR: Prevalence of 4.9%
  - AS: Prevalence of 2-5% > 65 years of age

Natural History & Prognosis

- Aortic regurgitation
  - Variable progression to left ventricular failure
  - Poor prognosis if valve not replaced prior to development of failure
- Aortic stenosis
  - Degenerative: Long asymptomatic period prior to development of symptoms

Treatment

- Aortic regurgitation
  - Surgery
    - Acute AR with hypotension & pulmonary edema
  - Medical management
    - Mild to moderate AR
    - Poor surgical candidates
    - Vasodilators ± inotropic agents
- Aortic stenosis
  - Surgical valve replacement
    - Severe, symptomatic AS
    - Left ventricular dysfunction
    - Critical stenosis by echocardiography
    - Coronary bypass or other valve surgery
  - Medical management
    - Endocarditis prophylaxis ± inotropic agents

DIAGNOSTIC CHECKLIST

Image Interpretation Pearls

- Echocardiography: Diagnosis & severity classification
- ECG-gated CTA: Evaluation of leaflets & orifice size
- Cine MR: Quantification of volumes, gradients, & function

SELECTED REFERENCES

1. Ferguson EC et al: Cardiac and pericardial calcifications on chest radiographs. Clin Radiol. 65(9):685-94, 2010
2. Abbara S et al: Feasibility and optimization of aortic valve planimetry with MDCT. AJR Am J Roentgenol. 188(2):356-60, 2007
3. Alkadhi H et al: Aortic regurgitation: assessment with 64-section CT. Radiology. 245(1):111-21, 2007
4. Pouleur AC et al: Aortic valve area assessment: multidetector CT compared with cine MR imaging and transthoracic and transesophageal echocardiography. Radiology. 244(3):745-54, 2007

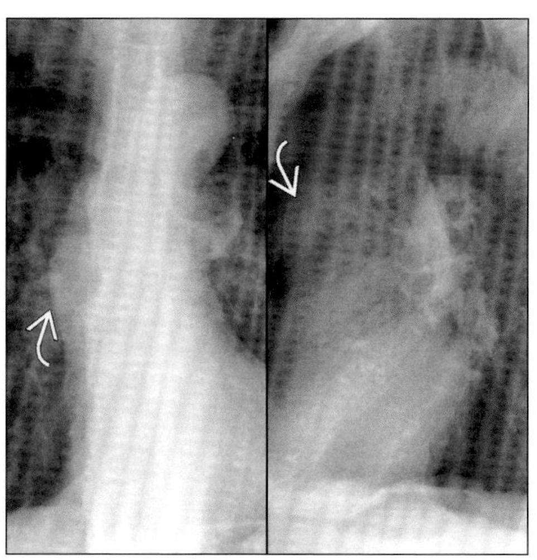

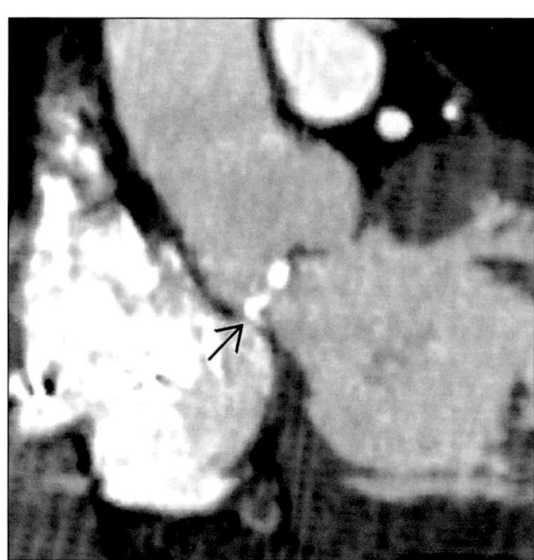

*(**Left**) Composite image with PA (left) and lateral (right) chest radiographs of a patient with aortic stenosis and regurgitation shows dilatation of the aortic root and ascending thoracic aorta ➔. (**Right**) Coronal CECT of a patient with both aortic regurgitation and stenosis shows aortic valve calcification ➔. The most common causes of aortic valve disease are degeneration and congenital bicuspid aortic valve. Rheumatic heart disease may also affect the aortic valve.*

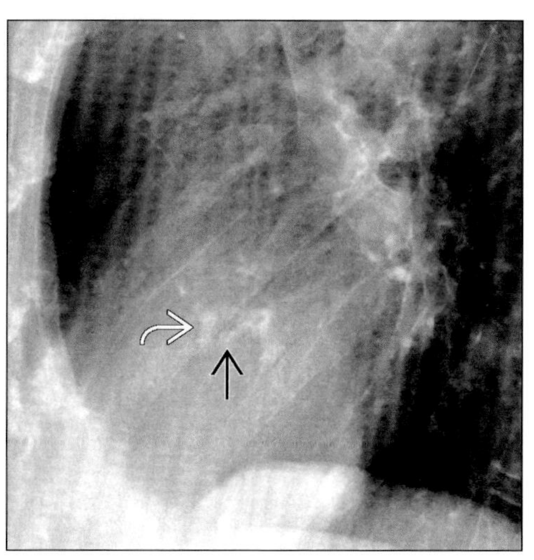

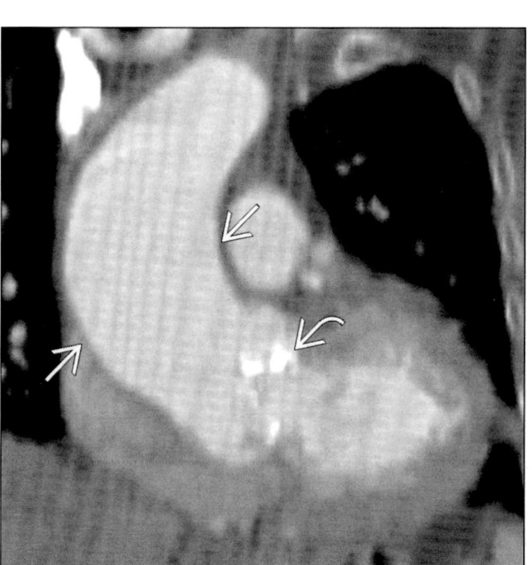

*(**Left**) Lateral chest radiograph of a patient with congenital bicuspid aortic valve and aortic stenosis shows aortic valve calcification ➔ surrounding the central calcification ➔ of the fused raphe. (**Right**) Coronal CECT of the same patient shows calcification of the aortic valve leaflets ➔ and dilatation of the aortic root and the ascending thoracic aorta ➔. Bicuspid aortic valve is more common in men than women and typically affects patients younger than 70 years old.*

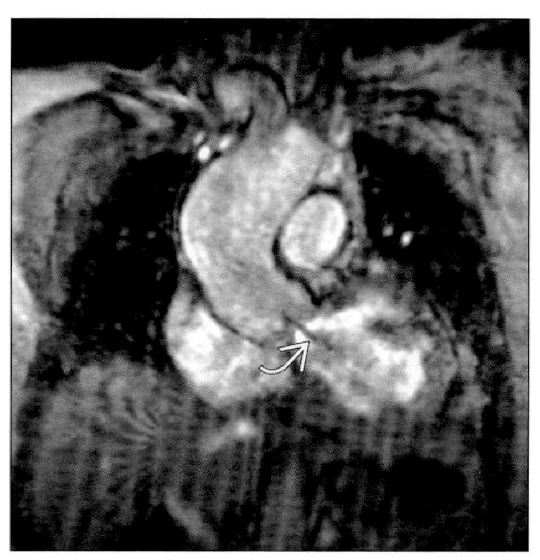

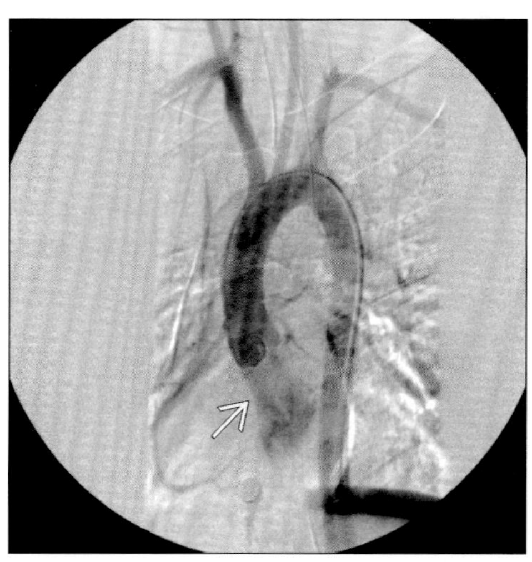

*(**Left**) Coronal MR cine demonstrates hypointense retrograde flow of blood into the left ventricle ➔, consistent with aortic regurgitation. MR cine and echocardiography allow calculation of the regurgitant fraction and help determine the severity of aortic regurgitation. (**Right**) DSA shows retrograde flow of contrast ➔ into the left ventricle in this patient with aortic regurgitation.*

MITRAL VALVE DISEASE

Key Facts

Terminology

- Mitral regurgitation (MR): Retrograde blood flow across mitral valve (MV) from left ventricle to left atrium
  - Most common valve dysfunction in USA
- Mitral valve prolapse: Protrusion of mitral valve leaflet(s) > 2 mm into left atrium
- Mitral stenosis (MS): Impaired left ventricular inflow across MV
- Mitral annular calcification (MAC): Excessive calcification of mitral annulus

Imaging

- Echocardiography is primary diagnostic tool
- MR: Left atrial enlargement
- Chronic MR: Left ventricle enlargement
- Acute MR: Localized right upper lobe asymmetric pulmonary edema
- CT & MR: Emerging roles; disease quantification, structural analysis, evaluation of surgical complications

Top Differential Diagnoses

- Mitral valve masses
- Dilated cardiomyopathy
- Ventricular septal defect (MR)
- Left atrial myxoma (MS)

Clinical Issues

- Surgical complications include paravalvular abscess, paravalvular leak, dehiscence, valve malfunction

Diagnostic Checklist

- Chronic MR causes left atrial & ventricular enlargement
- MS less common than MR & almost always secondary to rheumatic heart disease

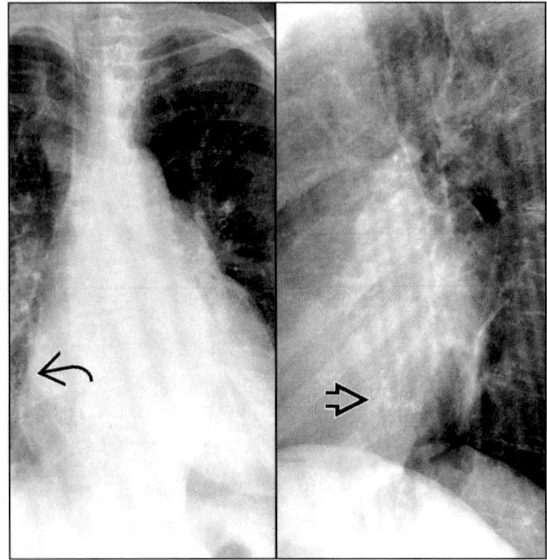

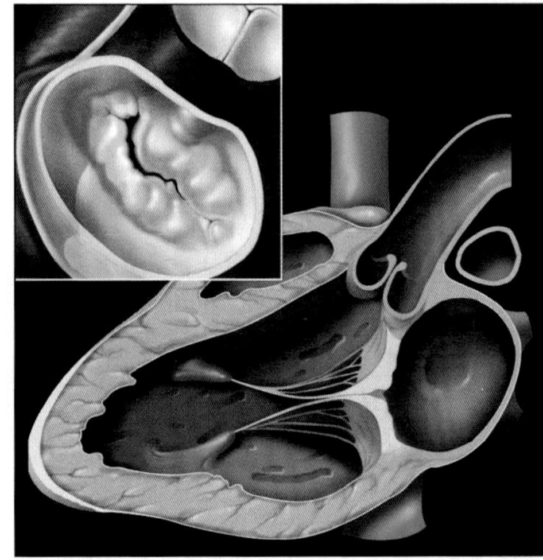

(Left) *Composite image with PA (left) and lateral (right) chest radiographs of a patient with mitral stenosis secondary to rheumatic heart disease shows left atrial enlargement manifesting with the double density sign ⮳ and mitral valve calcifications ⇨. Rheumatic heart disease is the most common cause of mitral stenosis in adults.* ***(Right)*** *Graphic shows the morphologic features of mitral stenosis. Thickening of the mitral valve results in abnormal valve leaflet motion and poor valve function.*

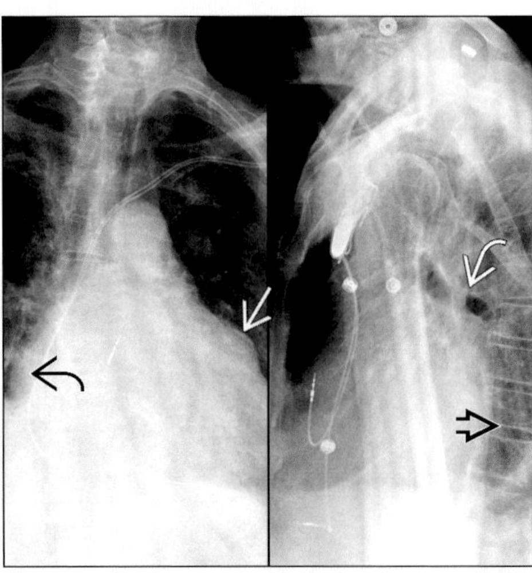

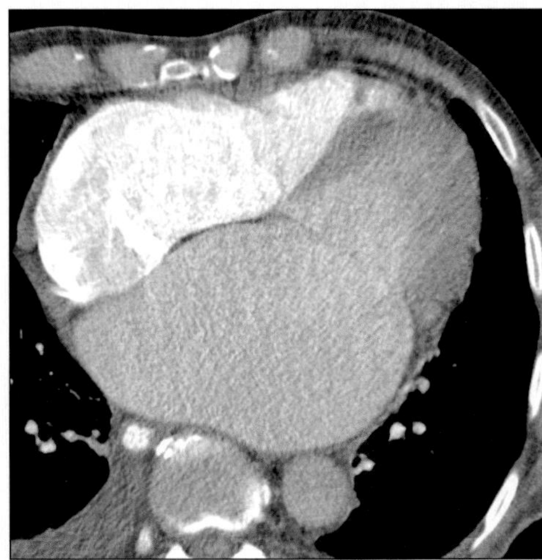

(Left) *Composite image with PA (left) and lateral (right) chest radiographs of a patient with mitral regurgitation shows the double density sign ⮳ of left atrial enlargement, carinal splaying, and left atrial appendage enlargement ➡. Note the posterior displacement of the mainstem bronchi ⮳ and carina and an edge ⇨ representing the enlarged left atrium overlying the thoracic spine.* ***(Right)*** *Axial CECT of the same patient shows left atrial enlargement, the earliest sign of mitral valve regurgitation.*

MITRAL VALVE DISEASE

TERMINOLOGY

Abbreviations

- Mitral valve (MV)

Synonyms

- Mitral insufficiency

Definitions

- **Mitral regurgitation (MR)**: Retrograde blood flow across mitral valve from left ventricle to left atrium
  - May be acute or chronic
  - Most common valve dysfunction in USA
- **Mitral valve prolapse**: Protrusion of mitral valve leaflet(s) > 2 mm into left atrium
  - Important cause of MR
- **Flail leaflet**: Systolic eversion of leaflet tip into atrium
  - Strongly associated with severe MR
- **Mitral stenosis (MS)**: Impaired left ventricular inflow across MV
- **Mitral annular calcification (MAC)**: Excessive calcification of mitral annulus
  - Central degeneration may lead to liquefaction, termed caseous MAC

IMAGING

General Features

- Best diagnostic clue
  - **Left atrial enlargement**
  - Mitral valve calcification
- Normal mitral valve morphology
  - Bicuspid valve: Anterior & posterior leaflets
  - Leaflets attached to D-shaped annulus, in fibrous continuity with aortic valve
  - Papillary muscles & chordae tendineae have no septal attachment

Radiographic Findings

- Radiography
  - Findings of left atrial enlargement
    - Frontal chest radiograph
      - **Double density** over right heart, enlarged left atrium superimposed on right heart
      - **Elevation of left main stem bronchus**
      - **Splaying of carina**
      - Convexity or straightening of left atrial appendage along left heart border
    - Lateral chest radiograph
      - Posterior convexity of left atrial silhouette
      - Posterior displacement of left main bronchus
  - Localized right upper lobe asymmetric pulmonary edema in acute MR
  - Left ventricle enlargement in chronic MR
  - Cephalization of flow due to pulmonary venous hypertension
  - MS: Enlarged central pulmonary arteries from pulmonary hypertension

CT Findings

- CECT
  - Enlargement of left atrium
  - Chronic atrial fibrillation may cause intraatrial thrombus, particularly in left atrial appendage
    - Thrombus may calcify
  - Pulmonary edema: Interlobular septal thickening, ground-glass opacity
  - Chronic MR: Left ventricular enlargement
- Cardiac gated CTA
  - Valve leaflet thickening & calcification
    - Fish-mouth deformity from commissural fusion & leaflet thickening
  - Mitral valve prolapse or flail leaflet in systole
  - Mitral valve area measured during early diastole
  - Regurgitant or stenotic contrast jet
  - Best tool to evaluate postsurgical complications

MR Findings

- T1WI
  - Left atrial enlargement
  - Chronic MR: Left ventricular enlargement
  - MS: Left atrial enlargement, pulmonary artery enlargement, right ventricular enlargement
- T2* GRE
  - MR: Regurgitant dephasing jet projects from mitral valve into left atrium during systole
  - MS: Stenotic dephasing jet projects from mitral valve into left ventricle during diastole
- SSFP white blood cine
  - Multiplanar imaging shows abnormal valve motion (MV prolapse, flail leaflet)
  - Bowing of thick anterior leaflet with "hockey stick" appearance in rheumatic MS
- Velocity-encoded phase contrast imaging used to quantify regurgitant fraction

Echocardiographic Findings

- Echocardiogram
  - Assessment of left atrial & ventricular size
  - MR: Color Doppler shows jet extending from mitral valve into left atrium during systole
  - MS: Color Doppler shows jet extending from mitral valve into left ventricle during diastole
  - Mean valve area; gradient & estimated pulmonary pressures can be calculated
  - MV prolapse well demonstrated

Angiographic Findings

- Conventional
  - MR can be quantified on 0 (none) to 4 (severe) scale
  - Calculation of regurgitant volume

Imaging Recommendations

- Best imaging tool
  - **Echocardiography primary diagnostic tool**
  - CT & MR: Emerging roles
    - Disease quantification
    - Structural analysis
    - Evaluation of surgical complications
- Protocol advice
  - 2 chamber long-axis plane perpendicular to MV; best imaging plane

DIFFERENTIAL DIAGNOSIS

Mitral Valve Masses

- Vegetations, thrombus may mimic valve thickening
- Neoplasms rare, including metastatic disease, papillary fibroelastoma, myxoma, lymphoma, sarcoma

MITRAL VALVE DISEASE

Dilated Cardiomyopathy

- Generalized cardiac enlargement
- Signs of congestive heart failure due to left ventricular dysfunction

Ventricular Septal Defect (MR)

- Left atrial enlargement
- Right ventricular enlargement; pulmonary trunk may be enlarged due to shunt vascularity

Left Atrial Myxoma (MS)

- Obstruction of mitral valve may mimic MS
- May calcify

PATHOLOGY

General Features

- Etiology
  - **Mitral regurgitation**
    - Usually caused by **myxomatous degeneration**
    - Infective endocarditis, collagen vascular disease, ischemic cardiomyopathy
    - Hypertrophic cardiomyopathy associated with systolic anterior motion of anterior mitral valve leaflet & MR
    - Papillary muscle dysfunction or rupture
  - **Mitral stenosis**
    - Almost exclusively secondary to rheumatic heart disease in adults
    - Collagen vascular disease, endocarditis
    - Substantial mitral annular calcification
  - **Mitral valve prolapse**
    - Caused by elongation/rupture of chordae tendineae
    - Connective tissue disorders, Marfan syndrome
  - Congenital mitral valve disease
    - Atrioventricular canal defects (associated with Down syndrome)
    - Parachute mitral valve (associated with Shone syndrome)
    - Double-orifice mitral valve
- Associated abnormalities
  - Rheumatic fever: Aortic & tricuspid valve involvement may also occur

Gross Pathologic & Surgical Features

- MS: Leaflets may be thickened with fused commissures

Microscopic Features

- MR: Myxomatous degeneration may be evident in mitral valve prolapse

CLINICAL ISSUES

Presentation

- Most common signs/symptoms
  - Acute MR: Sudden onset of pulmonary edema
  - Chronic MR: Shortness of breath, orthopnea, paroxysmal nocturnal dyspnea
  - MR: Holosystolic murmur
  - MS: Diastolic murmur, accentuated 1st heart sound, opening snap
- Other signs/symptoms
  - Palpitations due to atrial fibrillation
  - Atypical chest pain due to mitral valve prolapse

Demographics

- Age
  - Patients with MR from rheumatic fever; younger
  - MS: Age of symptom onset = 20-50 years
- Gender
  - MR & MS more common in women
  - **Mitral valve prolapse affects about 6% of women**
- Epidemiology
  - MR: Rheumatic fever most common in developing world; mitral valve prolapse accounts for majority of cases in developed countries
  - MS occurs early in developing world among patients with rheumatic fever

Natural History & Prognosis

- Acute MR, poorly tolerated
- Chronic MR: Volume overload may be asymptomatic for years
- 5-year survival for chronic MR: 80%
- Atrial fibrillation & heart failure may occur

Treatment

- Options, risks, complications
  - Acute MR: Treatment of pulmonary edema
  - Chronic MR: Medical treatment with diuretics & afterload-reducing agents
  - MV surgical repair or replacement indicated in severe MR with symptoms, decreased ejection fraction, or heart failure
  - Percutaneous balloon valvuloplasty in MS with heart failure or pulmonary hypertension
    - Severe calcification, fibrosis, or valve thickening are contraindications
    - Otherwise, surgical mitral valve replacement
  - Antibiotic prophylaxis in MV prolapse
  - Surgical complications include paravalvular abscess, paravalvular leak, dehiscence, valve malfunction

DIAGNOSTIC CHECKLIST

Image Interpretation Pearls

- Chronic MR causes left atrial & ventricular enlargement
- Mitral stenosis less common than regurgitation & almost always secondary to rheumatic heart disease

SELECTED REFERENCES

1. Morris MF et al: CT and MR imaging of the mitral valve: radiologic-pathologic correlation. Radiographics. 30(6):1603-20, 2010
2. Shah PM: Current concepts in mitral valve prolapse--diagnosis and management. J Cardiol. 56(2):125-33, 2010
3. Chen JJ et al: CT angiography of the cardiac valves: normal, diseased, and postoperative appearances. Radiographics. 29(5):1393-412, 2009

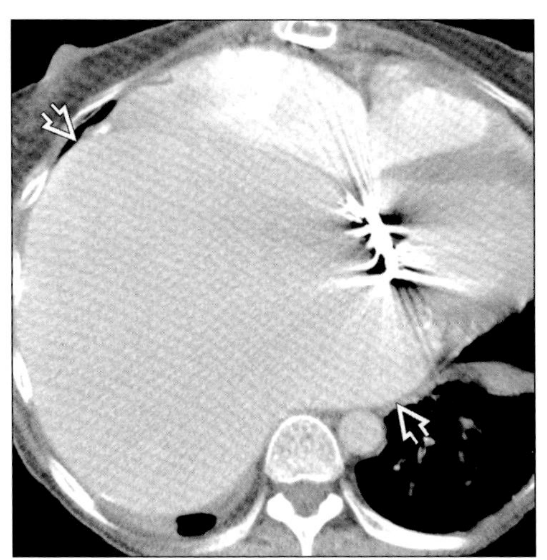

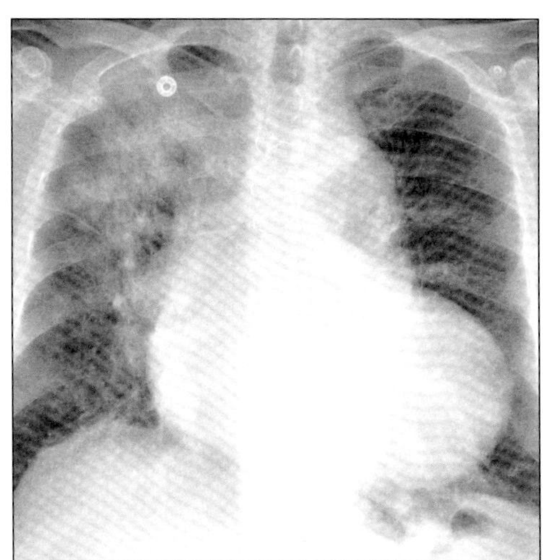

(Left) *Axial CECT of a patient with longstanding mitral stenosis status post mechanical mitral valve replacement shows massive left atrial enlargement* ⮚. ***(Right)*** *PA chest radiograph of a patient with papillary muscle rupture and acute mitral regurgitation shows marked enlargement of the cardiac silhouette and right upper lobe airspace disease, representing focal asymmetric pulmonary edema. Right upper lobe edema results from the preferential direction of the regurgitant blood flow.*

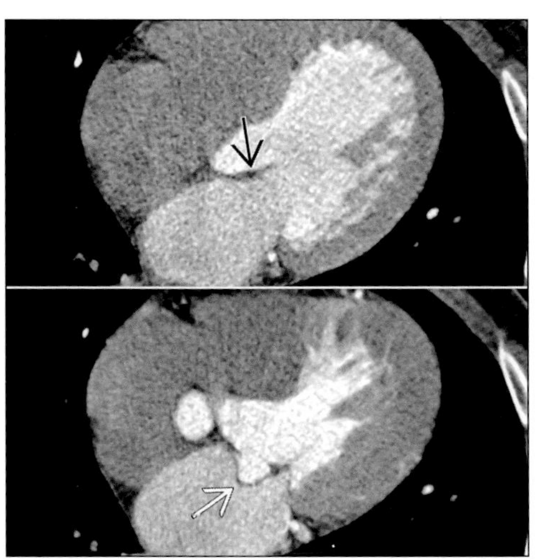

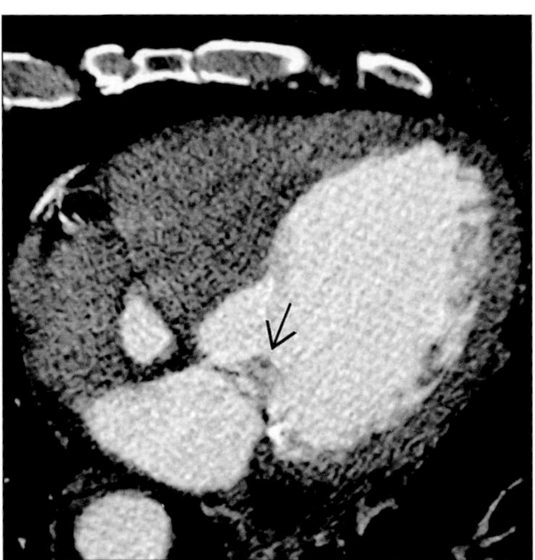

(Left) *Composite image with diastolic (top) and systolic (bottom) cardiac gated CTA of a patient with mild mitral regurgitation shows mild anterior mitral valve leaflet thickening* → *and systolic valve leaflet prolapse* → *into the left atrium.* ***(Right)*** *Axial cardiac gated CTA of a patient with endocarditis shows a low-attenuation mitral valve vegetation* →. *Vegetations and thrombus may mimic mitral valve thickening. Endocarditis may produce both mitral regurgitation and mitral stenosis.*

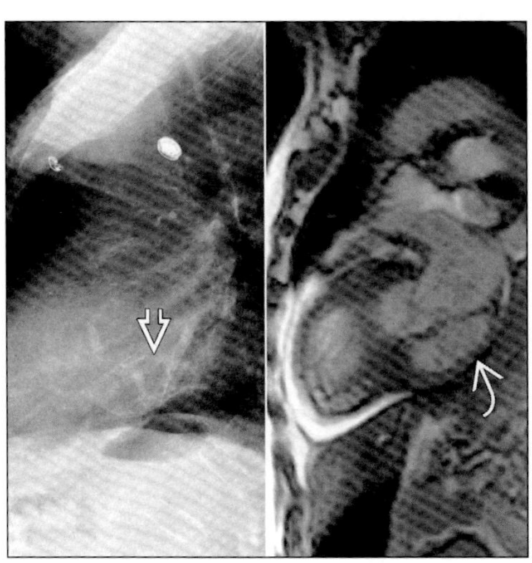

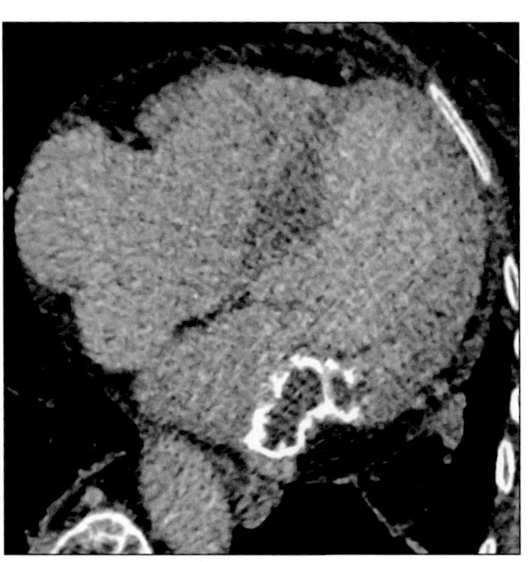

(Left) *Composite image with lateral chest radiograph (left) and sagittal SSFP MR (right) shows mitral annular calcification* ⮚ *and high signal intensity of the central substance* ↷, *consistent with caseous mitral annular calcification.* ***(Right)*** *Axial CECT of the same patient shows peripheral calcification with central low attenuation, characteristic of caseous mitral annulus calcification, which most commonly affects the posterior annulus and is reported to cause mitral stenosis when large.*

LEFT ATRIAL CALCIFICATION

Key Facts

Terminology

- Rheumatic heart disease (RHD)
- MacCallum patch: Focal calcification along posterior left atrial wall in RHD

Imaging

- Best diagnostic clue: Calcification of left atrial contour
- Atrial wall calcification: Thin, curvilinear
  - MacCallum patch
  - Left atrial appendage
- Atrial thrombus calcification: Thick, laminated
- Atrial tumor calcification: Variable
- Best imaging tool: NECT
  - More sensitive than chest radiography for detection of calcification
  - Calcification localization & characterization
  - Consider ECG-gated NECT to minimize motion

Top Differential Diagnoses

- Ventricular calcification
- Pericardial calcification
- Valve & annular calcification
- Coronary artery calcification
- Great vessel calcification

Clinical Issues

- Calcification reflects duration of untreated disease
- Symptoms/signs: Dyspnea, cough, wheezing, atrial fibrillation
- May complicate valve replacement
- Treatment: Total endoatriectomy with mitral valve replacement

Diagnostic Checklist

- Consider RHD & mitral stenosis in patients with left atrial calcification

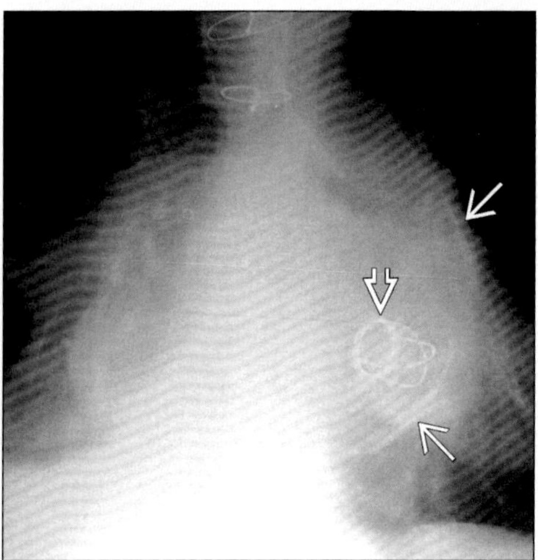

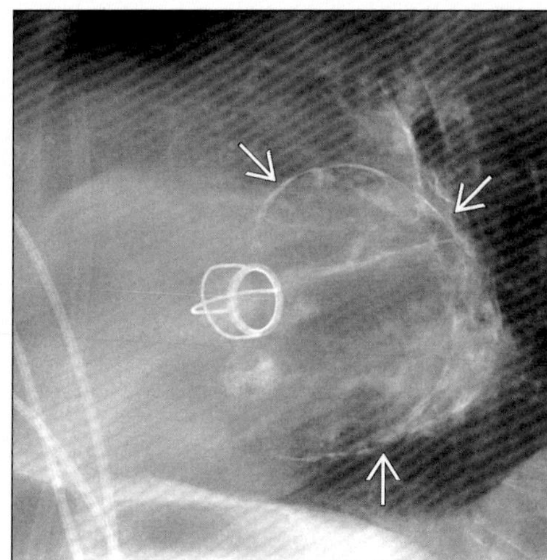

(Left) *Frontal chest radiograph of a patient with rheumatic heart disease shows curvilinear calcification ➔ following the contour of the left atrium and a mitral valve prosthesis ⇨.* ***(Right)*** *Lateral chest radiograph of the same patient demonstrates curvilinear calcification ➔ completely encircling the left atrium and findings of mitral valve replacement. Approximately 2-3% of patients with rheumatic heart disease develop left atrial calcification.*

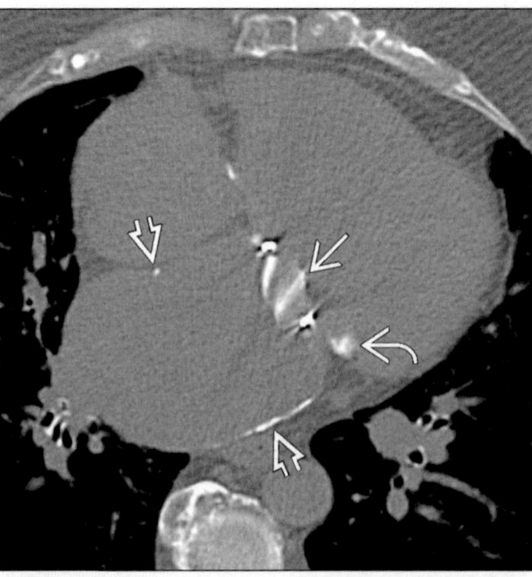

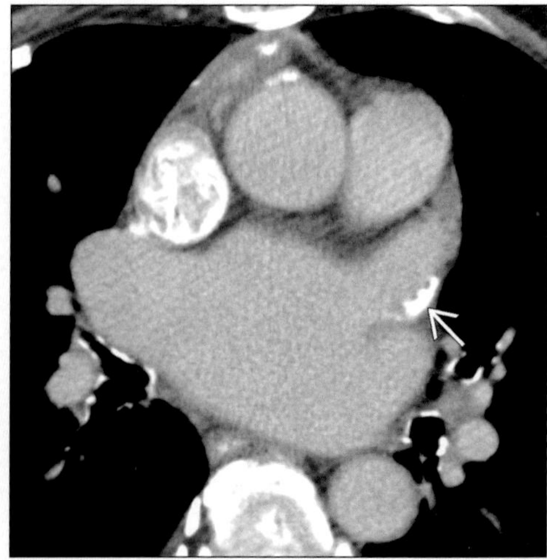

(Left) *Axial NECT of a patient with mitral stenosis treated with mitral valve replacement ➔ shows curvilinear calcification ⇨ along the walls of the left atrium. Caseous calcification of the posterior mitral annulus ↪ is partially visualized. NECT is more sensitive than chest radiography for detection of cardiac and annular calcification.* ***(Right)*** *Axial CECT of a patient with left atrial enlargement shows focal calcification of the posterolateral wall of the left atrial appendage ➔.*

LEFT ATRIAL CALCIFICATION

TERMINOLOGY

Abbreviations

- **Rheumatic heart disease (RHD)**

Synonyms

- Coconut or porcelain atrium

Definitions

- **MacCallum patch**: Focal calcification along posterior left atrial wall in RHD

IMAGING

General Features

- Best diagnostic clue
  - Calcification following left atrial contour
- Location
  - Left atrium
    - Wall
    - Chamber
    - Appendage
  - Mitral valve
- Morphology
  - Left atrial wall
    - Thin, curvilinear calcification
    - May encircle entire left atrium
    - Focal patch of isolated posterior wall calcification
  - Left atrial chamber
    - Thick, laminated layers in left atrial thrombus
    - Variable calcification in left atrial tumor

Radiographic Findings

- **Atrial wall calcification**
  - Thin, curvilinear, follows left atrial contour
  - Linear, nonlaminated
  - Posterosuperior left atrium most common
- Calcification completely encircling left atrium
  - Frontal: Ring configuration
  - Lateral: C-shaped configuration
- Isolated posterior wall calcification
  - **MacCallum patch**
- **Left atrial chamber calcification**
  - **Thrombus**
    - Thick, laminated layers; nonlinear
  - **Tumor** calcification; variable
- Left atrial appendage
  - Frontal: Calcification along left cardiac border
  - Lateral: Calcification over middle of heart

CT Findings

- NECT
  - More sensitive than chest radiography for detection of calcification
  - Calcification often more extensive than identified on radiography

Imaging Recommendations

- Best imaging tool
  - NECT for identification, localization, & characterization of left atrial calcification
- Protocol advice
  - Consider ECG-gated NECT to minimize motion

DIFFERENTIAL DIAGNOSIS

Ventricular Calcification

- Thin or thick curvilinear calcification following ventricular contour
- Myocardial infarction, metastatic calcification, thrombus, tumor, aneurysm, pseudoaneurysm

Pericardial Calcification

- Focal or curvilinear calcification following cardiac contour; most commonly AV grooves
- Infection, trauma, iatrogenic

Valve & Annular Calcification

- Aortic valve calcification
  - Marker for aortic stenosis
- Mitral calcification
  - Annular: Dense, ring-like clumps of calcium
    - F > M; common in end-stage renal disease
  - Leaflet: May be thin & delicate
    - Characteristic of rheumatic mitral stenosis

PATHOLOGY

General Features

- Etiology
  - RHD
    - Severity of inflammation & valvular damage
  - Mitral stenosis
    - Atrial wall over stretching & tissue necrosis
  - MacCallum patch: Left atrial endocardial lesion at site of mitral regurgitant flow

CLINICAL ISSUES

Presentation

- Most common signs/symptoms
  - Atrial fibrillation
  - Mitral stenosis: Exertional dyspnea, cough, wheezing

Demographics

- Age
  - 5th & 6th decades
- Gender
  - RHD: M:F = 1:3
- Epidemiology
  - 2-3% of patients with RHD; left atrial calcification

Natural History & Prognosis

- Calcification: Marker for duration of untreated disease
- May complicate valve replacement

Treatment

- Total endoatriectomy with mitral valve replacement

DIAGNOSTIC CHECKLIST

Consider

- RHD & mitral stenosis with left atrial calcification

SELECTED REFERENCES

1. Ferguson EC et al: Cardiac and pericardial calcifications on chest radiographs. Clin Radiol. 65(9):685-94, 2010

VENTRICULAR CALCIFICATION

Key Facts

Terminology
- Dystrophic, metastatic, idiopathic calcification

Imaging
- Best diagnostic clue: Calcification along ventricular contour
  - Left > right ventricle
  - Myocardium
  - Chambers
  - Aneurysms > pseudoaneurysms
- Morphology: Curvilinear, thin or thick
- NECT: Curvilinear left ventricle calcification
  - Myocardial infarction: Hypoenhancing myocardium, nonenhancing mural thrombus
  - Aneurysm: Wide neck; apical or anterolateral wall
  - Pseudoaneurysm: Narrow neck; posterior, lateral, or diaphragmatic wall
- CT: Detection & characterization of calcification

Top Differential Diagnoses
- Pericardial calcification
- Valve & annular calcification
- Coronary artery calcification
- Great vessel calcification

Pathology
- Myocardial calcification: MI, ESRD
- Cardiac chamber calcification: Tumor, thrombus
- Aneurysms & pseudoaneurysms

Clinical Issues
- MI most common > 45 years of age
- CAD: 40-70 years, M > F; > 70 years, M = F
- Calcified infarct at increased risk of sudden death
- Resection of aneurysms: CHF, arrhythmias
- Resection of pseudoaneurysms
  - Increased risk of rupture

__(Left)__ Lateral chest radiograph of a patient with prior myocardial infarction shows curvilinear calcification ➡ contouring the posterior wall of the left ventricle. __(Right)__ Axial CECT of a patient with prior myocardial infarction demonstrates calcification along the left ventricular apex ➡ and the distal interventricular septum. Ventricular calcifications typically develop 6 years after myocardial infarction and impart an increased risk of sudden death.

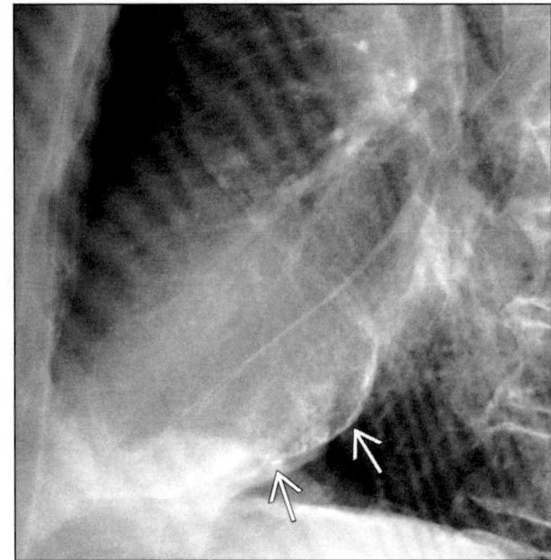

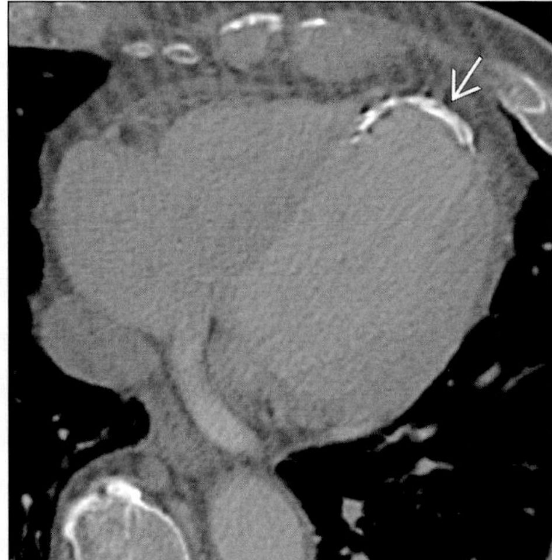

__(Left)__ Axial CECT (bone window) of a patient with end-stage renal disease shows metastatic calcification ➡ within the left ventricular myocardium. __(Right)__ Oblique sagittal CECT of a patient with prior myocardial infarction demonstrates an inferoseptal pseudoaneurysm ➡ arising from the left ventricle. Calcifications are present along the margins of the pseudoaneurysm ➡. Pseudoaneurysms are typically resected because of the increased risk of rupture.

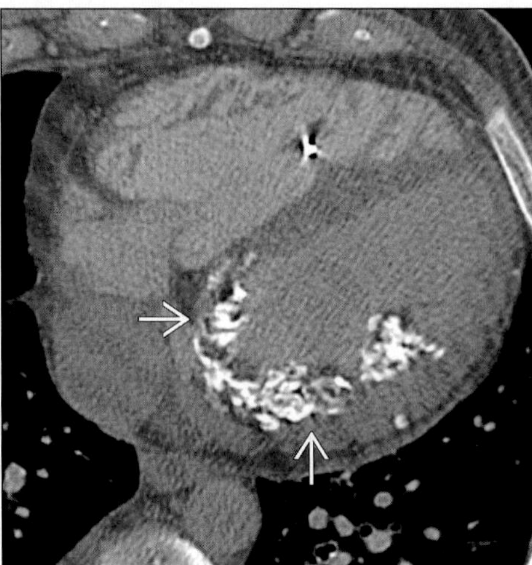

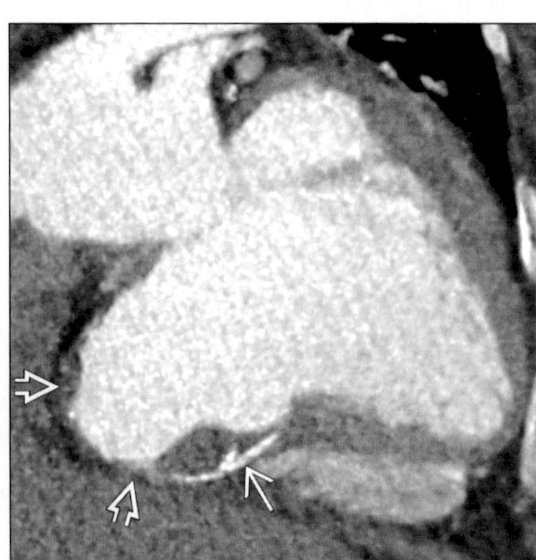

VENTRICULAR CALCIFICATION

TERMINOLOGY

Synonyms

- Dystrophic calcification
- Metastatic calcification
- Idiopathic calcification

Definitions

- **Dystrophic calcification**
  - Calcification within necrosis, hemorrhage, or fibrosis
  - Normal serum calcium & phosphorus levels
- **Metastatic calcification**
  - Calcification within normal tissue
  - Elevated calcium levels
- **Idiopathic cardiac calcification**
  - Calcification of unknown etiology

IMAGING

General Features

- Best diagnostic clue
  - Calcification following ventricular contour
- Location
  - **Left > right ventricle**
    - Myocardium
    - Chambers
    - Aneurysms > pseudoaneurysms
- Morphology
  - Curvilinear
  - Thin or thick

Radiographic Findings

- General
  - Frontal radiography: Left of midline
  - Lateral radiography: Follows left ventricular contour

CT Findings

- NECT
  - Mural curvilinear left ventricle calcification
- CECT
  - Mural curvilinear left ventricle calcification
  - Myocardial infarction (MI): Hypoenhancing myocardium, nonenhancing mural thrombus
  - **Aneurysms**: Wide neck
    - Apical or anterolateral wall
  - **Pseudoaneurysms**: Narrow neck
    - Posterior, lateral, or diaphragmatic wall

Imaging Recommendations

- Best imaging tool
  - CT for detection & characterization of calcification

DIFFERENTIAL DIAGNOSIS

Pericardial Calcification

- Focal or curvilinear calcification following cardiac contour; most commonly AV grooves
  - No preferential cardiac apex calcification (unlike myocardial calcification)
- Infection
- Trauma, iatrogenic

Valve & Annular Calcification

- Aortic valve calcification
  - Associated with aortic stenosis
- Mitral valve calcification
  - Leaflet: May be thin, delicate
    - Characteristic of rheumatic mitral stenosis
  - Annular: Dense, ring-like clumps
    - F > M; common in end-stage renal disease (ESRD)

Coronary Artery Calcification

- Curvilinear or tram-track calcification
- Involvement of 1 wall may mimic calcified infarction
- Strong correlation between calcification & atherosclerosis

Great Vessel Calcification

- Rim-like aortic wall calcification
  - Atherosclerosis most common cause
- Mural pulmonary artery calcification
  - Chronic pulmonary arterial hypertension

PATHOLOGY

General Features

- Etiology
  - Myocardial calcification
    - Calcification occurs 6 years after MI; M > F
    - Metastatic calcification in ESRD
  - **Calcification within cardiac chambers**
    - **Thrombus calcification**
      - Occurs in 20-60% of patients post MI
    - **Tumor calcification**
      - More common in left atrium
      - Myxomas most common primary cardiac tumor
      - Others include teratomas, fibromas, rhabdomyomas, carcinoid
  - **Aneurysms & pseudoaneurysms**
    - Most common after MI

CLINICAL ISSUES

Demographics

- Age
  - MI most common after 45 years
- Gender
  - Coronary artery disease (CAD)
    - 40-70 years, M > F
    - > 70 years, M = F

Natural History & Prognosis

- Calcified infarction at increased risk of sudden death
- Pseudoaneurysms at increased risk of rupture

Treatment

- Medical ± surgical therapy for CAD
- Aneurysm resection
  - Indications: CHF, arrhythmias
- Pseudoaneurysm resection

SELECTED REFERENCES

1. Ferguson EC et al: Cardiac and pericardial calcifications on chest radiographs. Clin Radiol. 65(9):685-94, 2010
2. Gowda RM et al: Calcifications of the heart. Radiol Clin North Am. 42(3):603-17, vi-vii, 2004

CORONARY ARTERY CALCIFICATION

Key Facts

Terminology

- Coronary artery calcification (CAC)
- Coronary artery disease (CAD)

Imaging

- Best diagnostic clue: Tram-track coronary calcification on radiography or CT
- Radiography: Severe calcification visible
  - Plaque or tram-track calcification
- Cardiac gated NECT more sensitive than radiography for detection of calcification
  - Scan technique: EBCT vs. MDCT
  - 3 methods for determining calcium score: Agatston, volume, & mass
- Cardiac gated CTA: Evaluation of vessel stenosis
  - Contrast administration results in underestimation of Agatston scores
- FDG uptake within coronary arteries inconsistent

Top Differential Diagnoses

- Pericardial calcification
- Ventricular calcification
- Valve & annular calcification
- Great vessel calcification

Clinical Issues

- CAC is marker for CAD
- Complications: MI, stroke, renal disease, PVD
- High Agatston score predicts significant CAD & increased cardiac risk status: > 75th percentile; 3.6% association with cardiovascular death
- Treatment: Lifestyle modification, medical, procedural therapy

Diagnostic Checklist

- Consider cardiac gated NECT in patients at intermediate risk for CAD to guide treatment

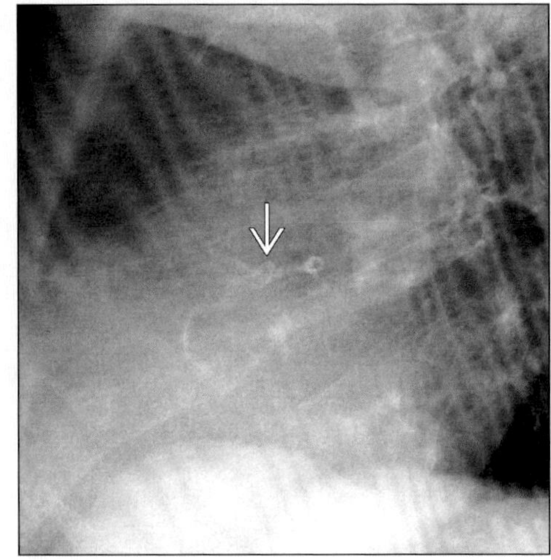

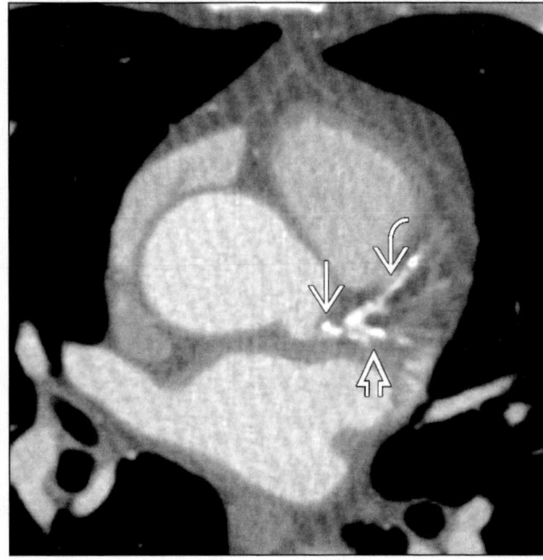

(Left) *Lateral chest radiograph shows tram-track calcification ➔ within the left anterior descending (LAD) coronary artery. Coronary artery calcification (CAC) may also manifest as focal plaques.* ***(Right)*** *Axial CECT of the same patient shows calcification in the distal left main ➔, the LAD ➔, and the ramus intermedius ➔ coronary arteries. CAC is more common in the left coronary artery than in the right coronary artery and most pronounced within the proximal aspect of the vessel.*

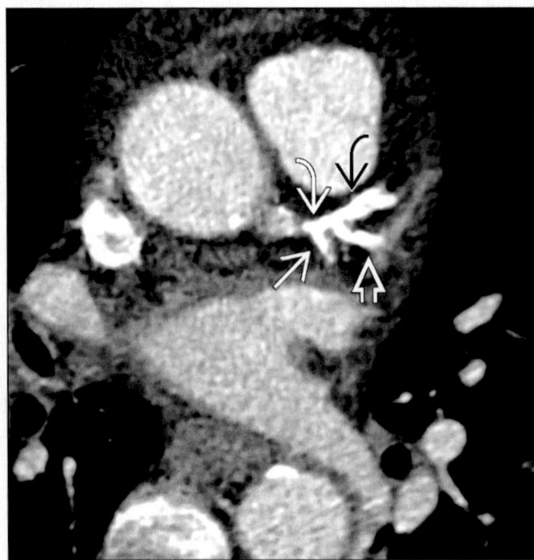

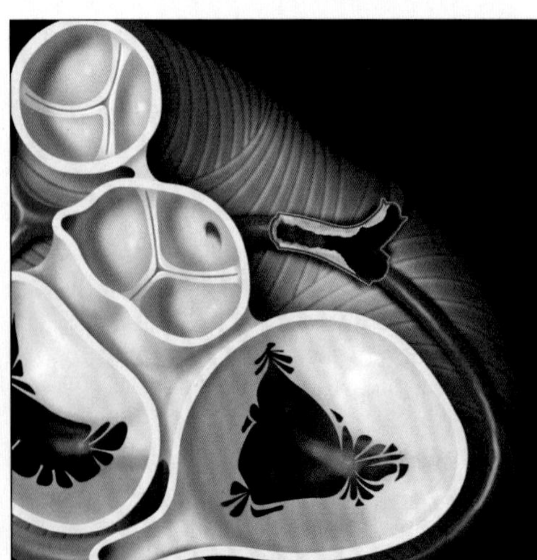

(Left) *Axial coronary CTA demonstrates calcification within the distal left main ➔, LAD ➔, ramus intermedius ➔, and left circumflex (LCx) ➔ coronary arteries. Although coronary artery CTA underestimates calcium scores, it is useful for evaluating stenosis and occlusion.* ***(Right)*** *Graphic demonstrates the morphologic features of CAC within the left main and proximal left anterior descending coronary arteries, a characteristic location for CAC.*

CORONARY ARTERY CALCIFICATION

TERMINOLOGY

Abbreviations

- **Coronary artery calcification** (CAC)

IMAGING

General Features

- Best diagnostic clue
  - Tram-track coronary calcification
- Location
  - Coronary arteries & branches
    - Left > right
    - Proximal > distal

Radiographic Findings

- General
  - CAC may not be visible on radiography
    - Small size
    - Faint
    - Obscured by overlying soft tissue & pulmonary disease
  - Severe calcification may be visible
  - Plaque or tram-track calcification
- Frontal radiography
  - **Coronary artery calcification triangle**
    - Medial to left atrial appendage
  - Left coronary artery
    - Upper left heart border
      - Left anterior descending coronary artery (LAD) & left circumflex coronary artery (LCx) branches
      - LAD: Lateral along upper left heart border
      - LCx: Medial inside cardiac border
  - Right coronary artery
    - Not usually visible
      - Obscured by overlying spine
- Lateral radiography
  - Overlies the heart
- Left anterior oblique radiograph: Optimal view

CT Findings

- NECT
  - **Cardiac gated CT**
    - More sensitive than radiography for detection of calcification
    - Scan technique: Electron beam computed tomography (EBCT) vs. multidetector computed tomography (MDCT)
      - Few comparative studies
      - General agreement in CAC scores obtained by both techniques
    - **EBCT**
      - Most literature on CAC scores based on EBCT
      - Less motion artifact
    - **MDCT**
      - Current generation of scanners are 64-slice
      - Typical scanners used in clinical practice
      - Better temporal resolution
      - Higher radiation dose
- **Quantification of calcification** = calcium score
  - 3 methods: Agatston, volume, mass
  - **Agatston score**
    - 4 main coronary arteries & branches evaluated
    - **Weighted score**: Density of CAC (Hounsfield units [HU])
      - 1: 130-199 HU
      - 2: 200-299 HU
      - 3: 300-399 HU
      - 4: ≥ 400 HU
    - **Score** = weighted score x pixels
      - 0: No plaque
      - 1-10: Minimal plaque
      - 11-100: Mild plaque
      - 101-400: Moderate plaque
      - ≥ 400: Extensive plaque
    - Percentiles normalized to age, gender, & race
    - Most commonly used in clinical practice
  - **Volume score**
    - Based on voxels above 130 HU
    - More reproducible than Agatston
    - Limited by partial volume effects
  - **Mass score**
    - Not based on HU thresholds
    - Requires calibration with phantom
  - **Nongated, low-dose chest CT**
    - Detection of CAC
    - Quantification of calcification: Ordinal scoring
      - 4 main coronary arteries evaluated
      - Absent calcification: 0
      - Mild: 1; < 1/3 length of artery with calcification
      - Moderate: 2; 1/3-2/3 of artery with calcification
      - Severe: 3; > 2/3 of artery with calcification
      - CAC scores: 0-12
- **Cardiac gated CTA**
  - Evaluation of stenosis
  - Dual-source imaging
    - Higher temporal resolution
  - Underestimates calcium scores

Nuclear Medicine Findings

- PET/CT
  - FDG uptake within coronary arteries
    - May be seen in patients with coronary artery disease (CAD)
    - Higher incidence of focal myocardial uptake & CAC
    - Inconsistent uptake within CAC
    - Uptake in segments without CAC

Imaging Recommendations

- Best imaging tool
  - Cardiac gated NECT
- Protocol advice
  - Prospective or retrospective gating

DIFFERENTIAL DIAGNOSIS

Pericardial Calcification

- Focal or curvilinear calcification following cardiac contour; most commonly in AV grooves
- Does not predominate at cardiac apex (unlike myocardial calcification)
- Infection, trauma, & iatrogenic

Ventricular Calcification

- Thin or thick curvilinear calcification following ventricular contour

CORONARY ARTERY CALCIFICATION

- Myocardial infarction (MI), metastatic calcification, thrombus, tumor, aneurysms, pseudoaneurysms

Valve & Annular Calcification

- Aortic valve calcification
  - Associated with aortic stenosis
- Mitral valve calcification
  - Leaflet: May be thin, delicate
  - Characteristic of rheumatic mitral stenosis
- Annular: Dense, ring-like clumps
  - F > M; common in end-stage renal disease

Great Vessel Calcification

- Rim-like calcification of thoracic aorta
  - Atherosclerosis most common cause
- Peripheral calcification of pulmonary arteries
  - Chronic pulmonary arterial hypertension

PATHOLOGY

General Features

- Etiology
  - Risk factors for development of CAC
    - Hypertension
    - Diabetes
    - Smoking
    - Hypercholesterolemia
    - Obesity & sedentary lifestyle
    - Family history
  - Premature development of CAC
    - Familial hypercholesterolemia
    - Pseudoxanthoma elasticum
    - Progeria
- Genetics
  - Multifactorial
  - Familial hypercholesterolemia & diabetes

Gross Pathologic & Surgical Features

- Primarily affects medium size muscular & large elastic arteries
- Deposition of lipids, platelets, fibrin, cellular debris, & calcium
- Gross findings
  - Fatty streak
  - Atheromatous plaque
  - Complicated atheroma

Microscopic Features

- Calcification; part of atheromatous plaque in atherosclerosis

CLINICAL ISSUES

Presentation

- Most common signs/symptoms
  - May be asymptomatic
  - Angina most common symptom
- Other signs/symptoms
  - Shortness of breath
  - Dyspnea on exertion
  - Decreased exercise tolerance

Demographics

- Age
  - M > 45 years, F > 55 years
- Gender
  - M > F in middle age
- Epidemiology
  - Atherosclerotic heart disease is **leading cause of death in developed world**

Natural History & Prognosis

- CAC is marker for CAD
- Complications
  - Myocardial infarction
  - Stroke
  - Renal disease
  - Peripheral vascular disease (PVD)
- Agatston score: Prediction of significant CAD (> 70% stenosis); cardiac risk status
  - 0: Low (< 5%); minimal cardiac risk
  - 1-10: Low (< 10%); low cardiac risk
  - 11-100: Mild stenosis; moderate cardiac risk
  - 101-400: Nonobstructive disease, may have stenosis; likely cardiac risk
  - > 400: High likelihood (> 90%), at least 1 stenosis; high cardiac risk
- Association with cardiovascular death
  - Incidence per Agatston score
    - > 75th percentile: 3.6%
  - Incidence per ordinal score
    - 0: 1.2%
    - 1-3: 1.8%
    - 4-6: 5%
    - 7-12: 5.3%
  - Higher CAC & risk of cardiovascular death
    - Male gender
    - Smoking

Treatment

- Lifestyle modifications
- Medical therapy
- Procedural therapy
  - Percutaneous intervention
  - Bypass grafting

DIAGNOSTIC CHECKLIST

Consider

- Cardiac gated NECT in patients at intermediate risk for CAD to guide treatment

SELECTED REFERENCES

1. Ferguson EC et al: Cardiac and pericardial calcifications on chest radiographs. Clin Radiol. 65(9):685-94, 2010
2. Shemesh J et al: Ordinal scoring of coronary artery calcifications on low-dose CT scans of the chest is predictive of death from cardiovascular disease. Radiology. 257(2):541-8, 2010
3. Mao SS et al: Comparison of coronary artery calcium scores between electron beam computed tomography and 64-multidetector computed tomographic scanner. J Comput Assist Tomogr. 33(2):175-8, 2009
4. Greenland P et al: Coronary artery calcium score combined with Framingham score for risk prediction in asymptomatic individuals. Jama. 291(2):210-5, 2004

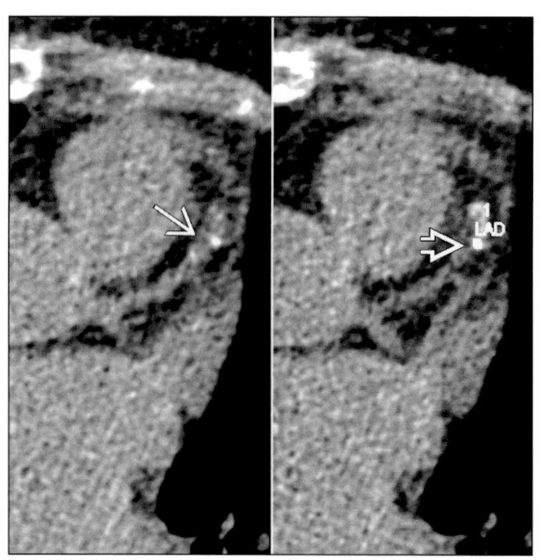

Threshold = 100 mg/cm³ CaHA (135 HU)

Artery	Number of Lesions (1)	Volume [mm³] (3)	Equiv. Mass [mg CaHA] (4)	Calcium Score (2)
LM	0	0.0	0.00	0.0
LAD	2	4.1	0.73	3.7
CX	0	0.0	0.00	0.0
RCA	0	0.0	0.00	0.0
Total	2	4.1	0.73	3.7

(1) Lesion is volume based
(2) Equivalent Agatston score
(3) Isotropic interpolated volume
(4) Calibration Factor: 0.743

(Left) *Axial cardiac gated NECT performed for calcium score quantification shows foci of hyperattenuation within the LAD, consistent with calcification. A label is placed on this calcification using software designed for calcium score calculation.* ***(Right)*** *Calcium score quantification of the same patient shown in chart format lists the total number of calcified lesions, the volume and equivalent mass of calcification, and the patient's calcium score.*

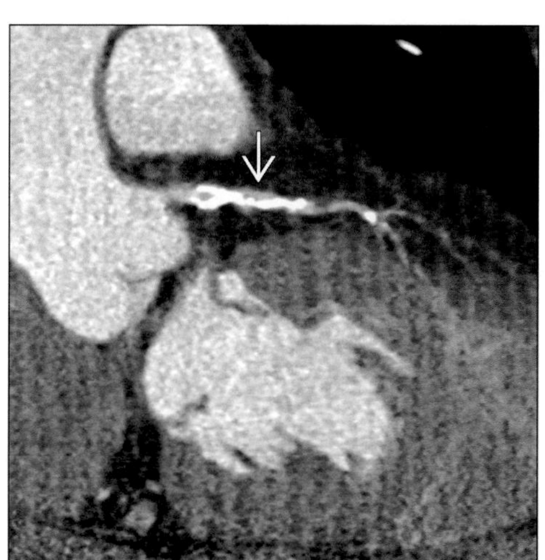

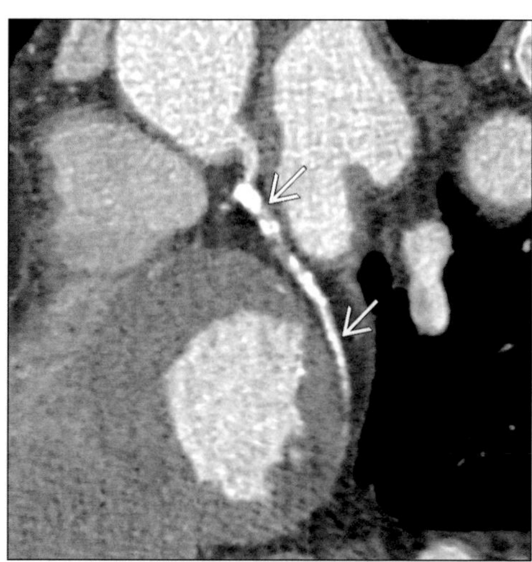

(Left) *Curved MPR coronary CTA demonstrates calcification within the LAD. Coronary CTA may be performed with prospective or retrospective ECG gating. Dual-source imaging provides higher temporal resolution relative to conventional CT scanners.* ***(Right)*** *Curved MPR coronary CTA shows calcification within the LCx coronary artery. Reformatted images allow better visualization of the coronary arteries and more precise characterization of vessel stenosis.*

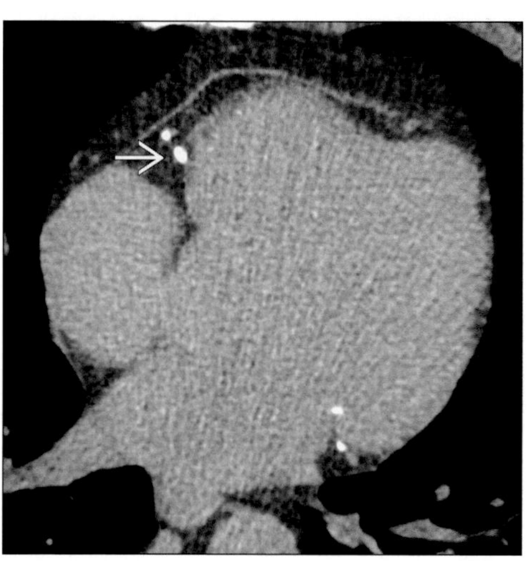

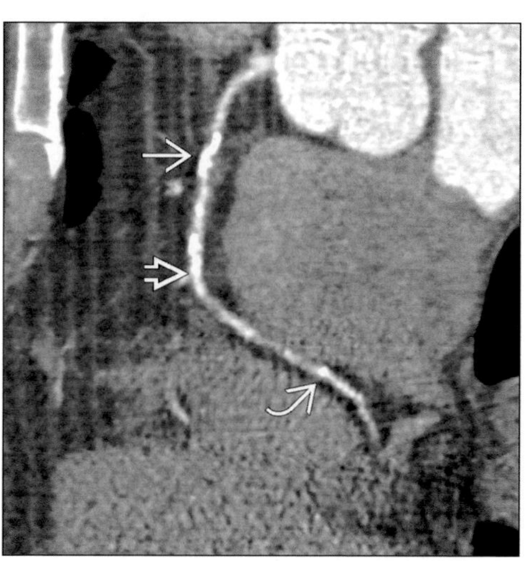

(Left) *Axial cardiac gated NECT obtained for calcium score calculation shows calcification within the right coronary artery (RCA). Cardiac gated NECT is more sensitive than radiography for detection of calcification. Higher calcium scores are associated with a higher risk of complications, such as myocardial infarction, stroke, and cardiovascular death.* ***(Right)*** *Curved MPR coronary CTA of the same patient shows calcification within the proximal, mid, and distal RCA segments.*

POST CARDIAC INJURY SYNDROME

Key Facts

Terminology

- Post cardiac injury syndrome (PCIS)
  - Post myocardial infarction syndrome (Dressler syndrome)
  - Post pericardiotomy syndrome (PPS)
- PCIS: Clinical entity characterized by inflammation of pericardium, pleura, & lung parenchyma following a variety of cardiac injuries

Imaging

- Radiography
  - Abnormal chest radiograph (95%)
  - Pleural effusion (80%)
  - Consolidation (50%)
  - Enlarged cardiac silhouette
- CT: Evaluation of heart & entire pericardial space
- Echocardiography: Primary modality of choice to evaluate pericardium

Top Differential Diagnoses

- Other cause of pericardial & pleural effusion
- Other cause of enlarged cardiac silhouette

Pathology

- Autoimmune hypersensitivity reaction

Clinical Issues

- Symptoms: Chest pain, dyspnea
- May mimic pulmonary embolism, congestive heart failure, pneumonia, myocardial infarction
- Develops 2-3 weeks after cardiac surgery; may uncommonly develop up to 6 months later
- Treatment: Anti-inflammatory agents

Diagnostic Checklist

- Consider PCIS in any patient who develops pleural or pericardial effusion after injury to the heart

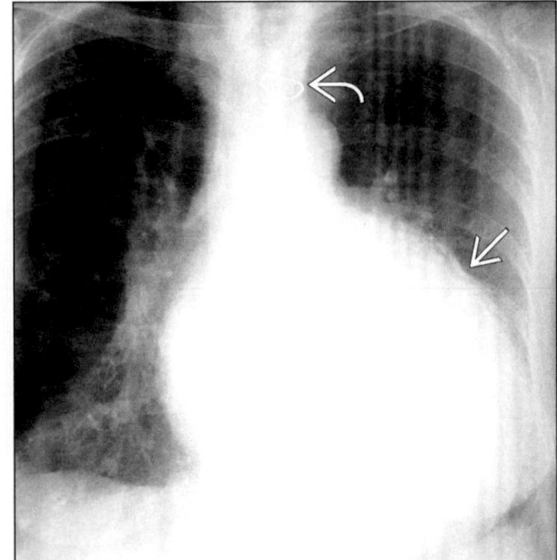

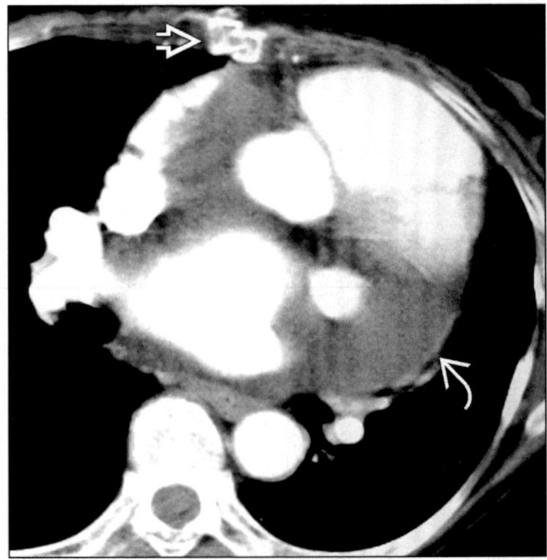

(Left) *PA chest radiograph of a patient after heart surgery shows significant cardiac silhouette enlargement ➡ and midline vertically aligned sternotomy wires ↪. The majority of patients with post cardiac injury syndrome (PCIS) have abnormal chest radiographs.* ***(Right)*** *Axial CECT of the same patient shows pericardial fluid within multiple pericardial recesses ↪ and findings of prior median sternotomy ➡. MDCT allows visualization and evaluation of the pericardium and its recesses.*

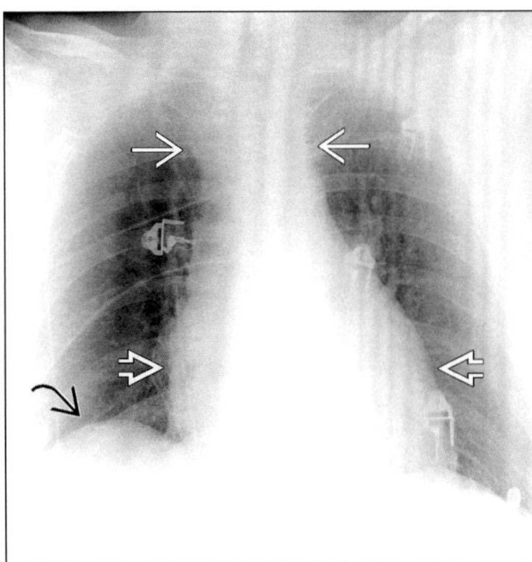

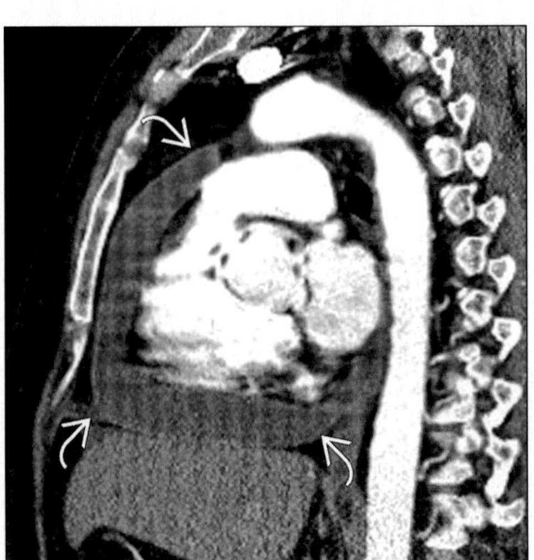

(Left) *AP chest radiograph of a patient who had a myocardial infarction shows moderate cardiac enlargement ➡, superior mediastinal widening ➡, and elevation of the right hemidiaphragm, suggestive of subpulmonic right pleural effusion ↪.* ***(Right)*** *Sagittal CTA of the same patient shows a large pericardial effusion that surrounds the heart ↪ and that mimicked cardiomegaly on radiography. Although CT is useful for pericardial assessment, the primary imaging modality of choice is echocardiography.*

POST CARDIAC INJURY SYNDROME

TERMINOLOGY

Abbreviations

- **Post cardiac injury syndrome (PCIS)**

Synonyms

- **Post myocardial infarction syndrome (Dressler syndrome)**
- **Post pericardiotomy syndrome (PPS)**

Definitions

- **PCIS**: Clinical entity characterized by inflammation of pericardium, pleura, & lung parenchyma following a variety of cardiac injuries
  - **Post myocardial infarction syndrome (Dressler syndrome)**
    - Autoimmune pericarditis following myocardial infarction or heart surgery
  - **Post pericardiotomy syndrome**
    - Autoimmune febrile pericardial & pleuropulmonary reaction after pericardiotomy

IMAGING

General Features

- Best diagnostic clue
  - Cardiac enlargement (due to pericardial effusion) & small to moderate pleural effusions following cardiac injury

Radiographic Findings

- Radiography
  - **Abnormal chest radiograph (95%)**
    - **Pleural effusion (80%)**
      - Unilateral (usually left sided)
      - Bilateral with nearly equal frequency
      - Small to moderate in size
    - **Consolidation (50%)**
      - Associated with pericardial or pleural effusion
  - **Enlarged cardiac silhouette**
    - **Pericardial effusion**
      - > 250 mL of pericardial fluid
      - Cardiac shape: Triangular, globular, flask-like
    - **Pericardial tamponade**
      - Acute tamponade: Normal heart size
      - Left ventricular failure: Pulmonary edema
      - Wide superior mediastinum: SVC dilatation

CT Findings

- CT allows evaluation of heart & entire pericardial space
- Pericardial effusion
- Pericardial tamponade findings
  - Pericardial effusion
  - Atrial dilatation
  - SVC, IVC, hepatic vein dilatation
  - Elongation of ventricles
  - Abdominal ascites

Echocardiographic Findings

- Pericardial effusion

Imaging Recommendations

- Best imaging tool
  - Echocardiography is primary imaging modality of choice to evaluate pericardium

DIFFERENTIAL DIAGNOSIS

Other Cause of Pericardial & Pleural Effusion

- Hydrostatic edema, infection, drugs, metastases, trauma, collagen-vascular disease (lupus), idiopathic

Other Cause of Enlarged Cardiac Silhouette

- Cardiac chamber enlargement
- Apparent cardiac enlargement: Projection, suboptimal inspiration, obesity, pectus excavatum, rotation
- Other: Thymolipoma, pericardial (mesothelial) cyst

PATHOLOGY

General Features

- Etiology
  - **Autoimmune hypersensitivity reaction**

Gross Pathologic & Surgical Features

- Normal pericardium contains 25-50 mL of fluid
  - Slow fluid accumulation may exceed 3 L without tamponade

CLINICAL ISSUES

Presentation

- Most common signs/symptoms
  - **Chest pain, dyspnea**
  - **Clinical differential diagnosis**
    - Pulmonary embolism, congestive heart failure, pneumonia, myocardial infarction
- Complications: **Tamponade**
  - **Beck triad:** Jugular venous distension, hypotension, muffled heart sounds

Demographics

- Age
  - Parallels prevalence of coronary artery disease in middle-aged & older adults
- Epidemiology
  - Any injury to heart or pericardium
    - Coronary artery bypass graft (CABG) surgery, temporary & permanent pacing, trauma

Natural History & Prognosis

- 2-3 weeks after cardiac surgery
- May uncommonly develop up to 6 months later

Treatment

- Anti-inflammatory agents: Aspirin, indomethacin

DIAGNOSTIC CHECKLIST

Consider

- PCIS in any patient who develops pleural or pericardial effusion after injury to the heart

SELECTED REFERENCES

1. O'Leary SM et al: Imaging the pericardium: appearances on ECG-gated 64-detector row cardiac computed tomography. Br J Radiol. 83(987):194-205, 2010

PERICARDIAL EFFUSION

Key Facts

Terminology
- Fluid in pericardial space

Imaging
- Radiography
  - Frontal: "Water bottle" sign; globular enlargement of cardiopericardial silhouette
  - Lateral: Fat pad sign; pericardial fluid outlined by surrounding fat
- CT
  - Water attenuation fluid: Uncomplicated effusion
  - High-attenuation fluid: Hemorrhage, purulent fluid, malignancy
  - Associated pericardial thickening & calcification
  - Cardiac chambers: Constriction & tamponade
- MR: Assessment of complicated effusion
  - 93% accuracy for constrictive pericarditis
- Echocardiography: Imaging modality of choice

Top Differential Diagnoses
- Pericardial cyst
- Pericardial malignancy
- Dilated cardiomyopathy

Clinical Issues
- Signs/symptoms
  - May be asymptomatic
  - Chest pain, friction rub
  - Cardiac tamponade: Rate of fluid accumulation more significant than volume or composition
- Treatment
  - Small effusions may not require treatment
  - Increased hemodialysis in chronic renal failure
  - Anti-inflammatory agents for acute idiopathic/viral pericarditis
  - Percutaneous or surgical drainage
  - Emergent management of tamponade

*(**Left**) Graphic shows features of pericardial effusion. Pericardial fluid is located in the potential space between the serous parietal ➔ and visceral pericardium or epicardium ➔. (**Right**) PA chest radiograph shows a large pericardial effusion manifesting with the "water bottle" sign, characterized by globular enlargement of the cardiopericardial silhouette and a normal superior mediastinum. Pericardial fluid may slowly accumulate and attain a large volume without producing cardiac tamponade.*

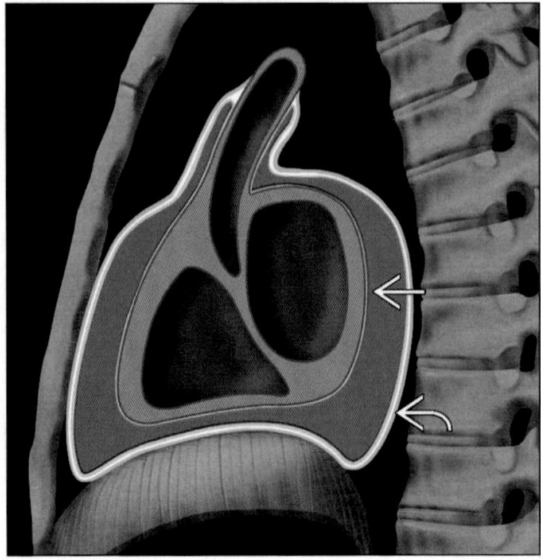

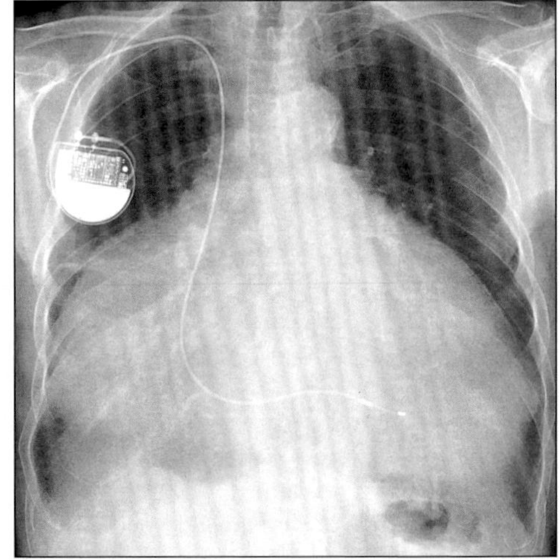

*(**Left**) Lateral chest radiograph of the same patient shows the fat pad sign. A water density stripe ➔ represents pericardial fluid visible between the retrosternal mediastinal fat ➔ and the subepicardial fat ➔. (**Right**) Graphic depicts the anatomic basis for the fat pad sign. Fluid in the pericardial space ➔ will appear as a water density stripe outlined by the fat density retrosternal mediastinal fat ➔ and the subepicardial fat ➔ located beneath the serous visceral pericardium or epicardium.*

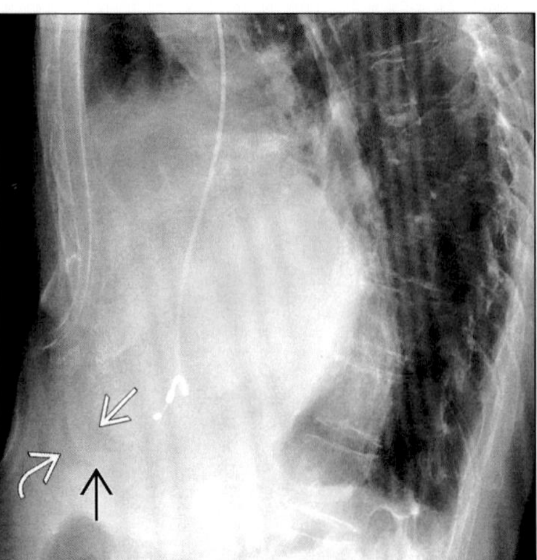

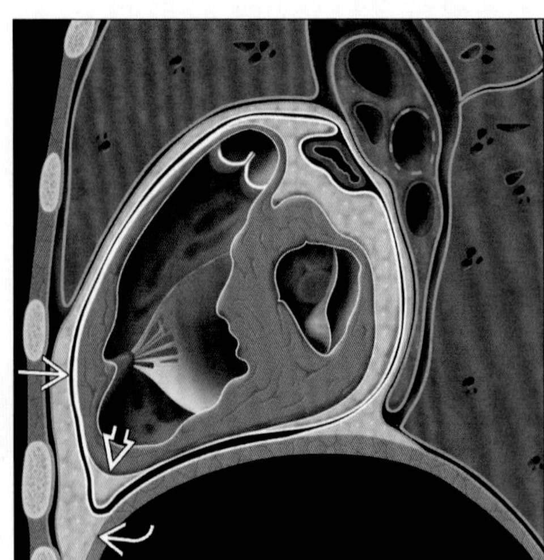

PERICARDIAL EFFUSION

TERMINOLOGY

Definitions

- **Fluid in pericardial space**
- **Cardiopericardial silhouette**: Combined pericardial and cardiac silhouette on radiography

IMAGING

General Features

- Best diagnostic clue
  - Radiography: Fat pad sign on lateral radiograph
  - CT/MR: Fluid in pericardial space
- Location
  - CT & MR
    - **Small effusion**: Posterior location; along left ventricle & left atrium
    - **Large to moderate effusion**: Anterior location; along right ventricle
    - **Very large effusion**: Surrounds heart
- Anatomic considerations
  - Pericardium surrounds heart & portions of pulmonary trunk, vena cava, & ascending aorta
  - **Fibrous pericardium**: Defines anatomic middle mediastinum
  - **Serous pericardium**: Within fibrous pericardium
    - Serous visceral pericardium: Epicardium; lines heart
    - Serous parietal pericardium: Lines fibrous pericardium
    - 2 apposed pericardial layers with intervening potential (pericardial) space
    - May contain 15-50 mL of fluid normally
- Normal pericardium
  - Radiography: Not visible
  - CT: Thin soft tissue linear structure; 0.7-2 mm thick
  - MR: Thin low signal linear structure on T1 & T2WI
  - CT & MR
    - Pericardium between retrosternal mediastinal & subepicardial fat
    - No distinction between serous & fibrous pericardial layers
    - Frequent visualization of physiologic fluid & fluid-filled pericardial sinuses & recesses

Radiographic Findings

- Frontal chest radiography
  - Small amount of pericardial fluid may be normal
  - Moderate-large (> **250 mL**) pericardial effusion
    - **"Water bottle" sign**
      - Globular symmetric enlargement of cardiopericardial silhouette
      - Normal superior mediastinum
  - Documentation of slow or rapid cardiopericardial silhouette enlargement on serial radiography
- Lateral chest radiography
  - > 2 mm water density stripe between retrosternal & subepicardial fat
  - **Fat pad sign**: Also called "Oreo cookie" sign, "sandwich" sign, & "bun" sign
- > 200 mL of fluid: Visualization of cardiopericardial silhouette enlargement

CT Findings

- NECT
  - Direct assessment of pericardial abnormalities
  - **Water attenuation pericardial fluid**
    - Heart failure, renal failure, malignancy
  - **High-attenuation pericardial fluid**
    - Hemorrhage, purulent effusion, malignancy
    - Hemopericardium: High attenuation initially; attenuation decreases over time
  - High sensitivity for associated pericardial thickening & calcification
- CECT
  - Assessment for thickening, nodules, masses
  - Enhancement of serous pericardium & pericardial thickening from inflammation
    - Associated infiltration of mediastinal fat
  - Assessment of cardiac chambers
    - Signs of constriction: Tubular ventricles, flattened/sigmoid interventricular septum
  - **Signs of cardiac tamponade**
    - Flattening of anterior heart surface, right cardiac chambers
    - Angulation or bowing of interventricular septum
    - Enlarged vena cava, periportal edema, reflux of contrast into IVC, azygos, hepatic/renal veins

MR Findings

- General
  - Uncomplicated effusion
    - T1WI: Low signal; T2WI: High signal
  - Complicated effusion: Septations, debris
  - Hemorrhagic effusion
    - T1WI: High signal; T2WI: Low signal
    - Hemopericardium
      - **Acute phase**: Homogeneous high signal
      - **Subacute phase** (1-4 weeks): Heterogeneous signal, foci of high signal on T1 & T2WI
      - **Chronic phase**: Low signal intensity foci (calcification, fibrosis), dark peripheral rim
      - No contrast enhancement
  - Assessment of pericardium & cardiac chambers to exclude constriction
    - MR: 93% accuracy for differentiation between constrictive pericarditis (pericardial thickening of > 4 mm) & restrictive cardiomyopathy

Ultrasonographic Findings

- **High sensitivity for pericardial fluid**
  - Echo-free space between pericardial layers
  - Decreased parietal pericardial motion
- Assessment of constrictive pericarditis
- Assessment of suspected tamponade
  - Mass effect
    - Diastolic compression/collapse of right heart chambers; abnormal cardiac filling
    - Compression of pulmonary trunk & thoracic IVC
  - Abnormal motion
    - Cardiac swing within pericardium
    - Doppler flow velocity paradoxus: Respiratory variation in Doppler velocities
    - Paradoxical motion of interventricular septum
    - Lack of inspiratory collapse of dilated IVC

Imaging Recommendations

- Best imaging tool
  - **Echocardiography: Modality of choice for pericardial imaging**

- CT/MR: Evaluation of complications of pericardial effusion; hemorrhage, loculation

DIFFERENTIAL DIAGNOSIS

Pericardial Cyst

- Focal water attenuation cyst abutting pericardium
- May mimic loculated pericardial effusion

Pericardial Malignancy

- 10-12% of patients with malignancy at autopsy
- 1/3 of cases: Lung cancer
- Pericardial nodular thickening, effusion, enhancement, mass

Dilated Cardiomyopathy

- Marked cardiomegaly
- May mimic pericardial effusion

PATHOLOGY

General Features

- Etiology
  - General
    - Obstruction of lymphatic or venous drainage
  - **Myocardial infarction & left ventricular failure**: Most common causes of pericardial effusion
  - **Uremic effusion**: 50% of patients with chronic renal failure
  - **Infection**
    - Acute pericarditis: 90% idiopathic or viral
    - Tuberculosis
      - Most common cause of constrictive pericarditis in developing world
      - Tamponade, frequent complication
    - Blunt/penetrating trauma
    - Thermal injury
    - Endocarditis, sepsis
  - **Cardiac surgery**: Typical spontaneous resolution
    - Up to 6% may become clinically significant; cardiac tamponade
  - **Autoimmune disease**
    - Rheumatoid arthritis: Effusion in 2-10%
    - SLE: Up to 50% with symptomatic effusion
    - Systemic sclerosis: Up to 70% with small effusion
  - **Neoplasia**
  - **Hypoalbuminemia, myxedema**
  - **Drug reaction, radiation, trauma**
  - Effusive constrictive pericarditis
    - Constrictive physiology ± associated pericardial effusion or tamponade
    - Persistent elevated right chamber pressures after pericardial fluid drainage

Pathophysiology

- Pericardial effusion: Rate of fluid accumulation
  - Gradual increase in pericardial fluid: May accommodate > 1 L without tamponade
  - Rapid increase in pericardial fluid: Cardiac tamponade; impaired cardiac filling
- Cardiac tamponade
  - ↓ intracardiac volume & ↑ diastolic filling pressures
  - ↑ intrapericardial pressure with cardiac compression
  - Rate of fluid accumulation more significant than fluid volume or composition

CLINICAL ISSUES

Presentation

- Most common signs/symptoms
  - May be asymptomatic
  - Chest pain: Worse with inspiration & supine position
  - Pericardial friction rub in acute pericarditis
- Other signs/symptoms
  - **Pericardial tamponade**
    - Anxiety, dyspnea, chest pain, jugular vein distention
    - Tachycardia, hypotension
    - Paradoxical pulse: > 10 mmHg drop in systolic arterial pressure during inspiration
    - **Beck triad**
      - Muffled heart sounds
      - Hypotension
      - Jugular vein distention

Treatment

- Small pericardial effusions may not require treatment
- Increased hemodialysis; renal failure-related effusion
- Increasing effusion or effusion > 250 mL
  - Pericardiocentesis (image guided)
    - 93% success rate
  - Surgical drainage
    - Preferred for hemopericardium, purulent effusion
    - Pericardial window, subxiphoid pericardiotomy
    - Pericardiectomy
    - Balloon pericardiotomy in recurrent tamponade
      - Emergent management of tamponade
- Anti-inflammatory agents for acute idiopathic/viral pericarditis

DIAGNOSTIC CHECKLIST

Image Interpretation Pearls

- Recognition of normal fluid-filled pericardial recesses, which may mimic lymph nodes & congenital cysts

SELECTED REFERENCES

1. O'Leary SM et al: Imaging the pericardium: appearances on ECG-gated 64-detector row cardiac computed tomography. Br J Radiol. 83(987):194-205, 2010
2. Palmer SL et al: CT-guided tube pericardiostomy: a safe and effective technique in the management of postsurgical pericardial effusion. AJR Am J Roentgenol. 193(4):W314-20, 2009
3. Parker MS et al: Radiologic signs in thoracic imaging: case-based review and self-assessment module. AJR Am J Roentgenol. 2009 Mar;192(3 Suppl):S34-48. Review. Erratum in: AJR Am J Roentgenol. 193(3 Suppl):S58, 2009
4. Little WC et al: Pericardial disease. Circulation. 2006 Mar 28;113(12):1622-32. Review. Erratum in: Circulation. 115(15):e406, 2007
5. Restrepo CS et al: Imaging findings in cardiac tamponade with emphasis on CT. Radiographics. 27(6):1595-610, 2007

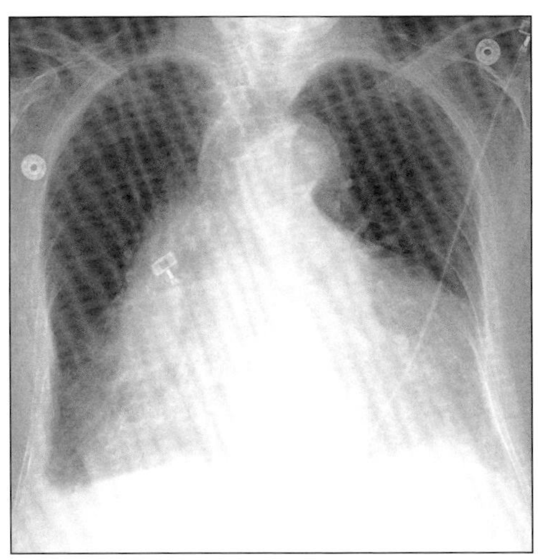

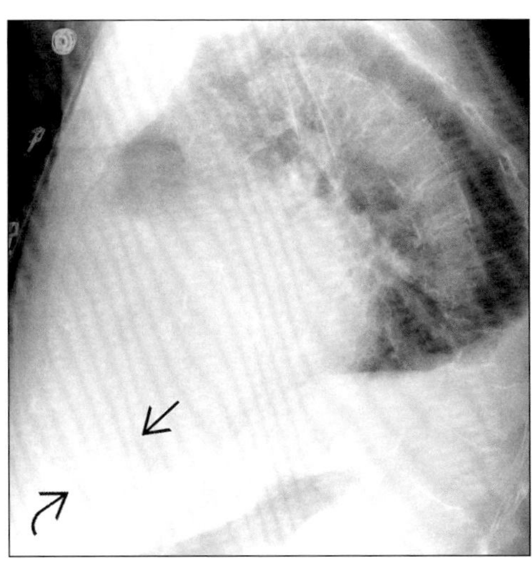

(Left) *PA chest radiograph of an elderly woman who presented with chest pain and a large pericardial effusion shows the "water bottle" sign with marked enlargement of the cardiopericardial silhouette and bilateral pleural effusions.* ***(Right)*** *Lateral chest radiograph of the same patient shows the large idiopathic pericardial effusion manifesting with the fat pad sign. A large water attenuation stripe is identified between the retrosternal mediastinal fat ⮫ and the subepicardial fat ⇨.*

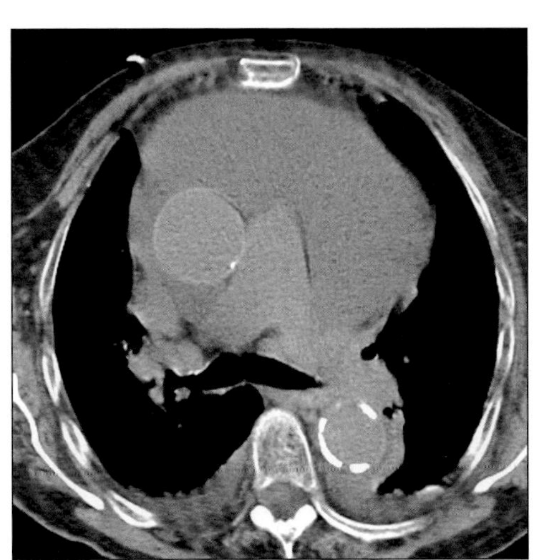

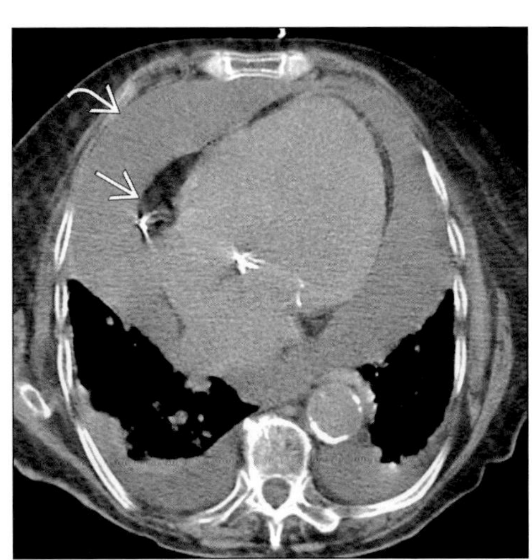

(Left) *Axial NECT of the same patient shows a large pericardial effusion manifesting as water attenuation fluid in the pericardial space. The intrapericardial ascending aorta and pulmonary trunk are also surrounded by pericardial fluid.* ***(Right)*** *Axial NECT of the same patient shows water attenuation pericardial fluid completely surrounding the heart. The serous parietal ⮫ and visceral ➡ pericardial layers are not visible, but their location is inferred by the pericardial fluid boundaries.*

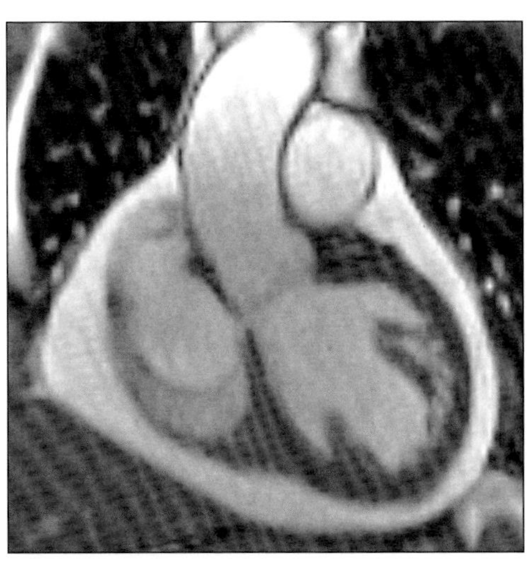

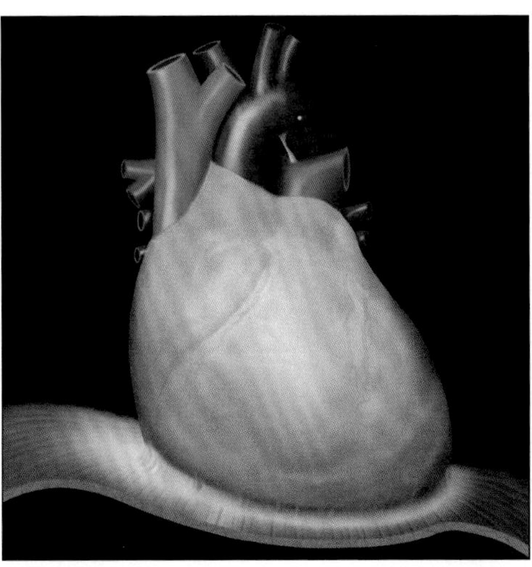

(Left) *Coronal cine MR of a patient with a pericardial effusion shows homogeneous high signal intensity fluid surrounding the heart and proximal great vessels. The pulmonary trunk and ascending aorta are intrapericardial and therefore surrounded by fluid in cases of moderate to large pericardial effusion.* ***(Right)*** *Graphic shows the anatomy of the pericardium, which envelops the heart, the distal SVC, the proximal ascending aorta, and the pulmonary trunk, forming pericardial recesses.*

*(**Left**) SSFP cine MR short axis image of a patient with a large pericardial effusion shows high signal pericardial fluid completely surrounding the heart. The combined parietal serous and fibrous pericardial layers manifest as a thin low signal linear structure surrounding the fluid. (**Right**) SSFP cine MR 4 chamber view of the same patient shows high signal pericardial fluid within the serous pericardium surrounding the heart and a visible serous visceral pericardium (a.k.a. epicardium).*

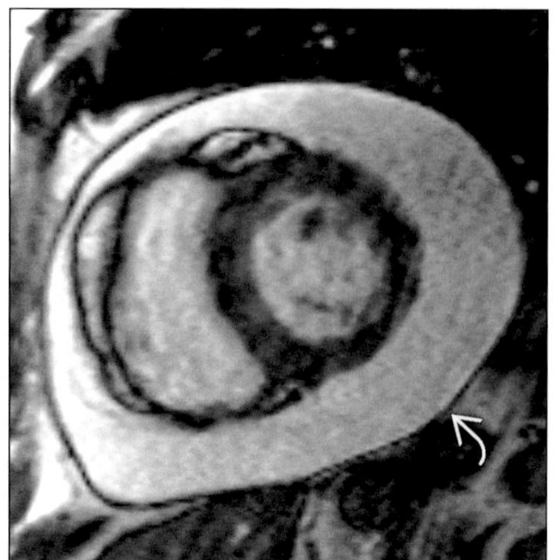

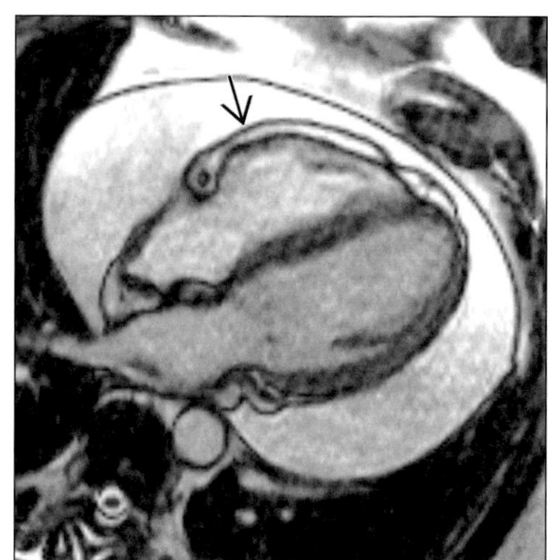

*(**Left**) Axial CECT of a patient with a loculated pericardial effusion shows a right inferior pericardial collection of water attenuation and a small component of pericardial fluid posterior to the left ventricle. (**Right**) Axial CECT of a patient with pericarditis shows enhancement of the serous pericardium. The serous parietal pericardium lines the fibrous pericardium. The serous visceral pericardium lines the heart and subepicardial fat and is also known as the epicardium.*

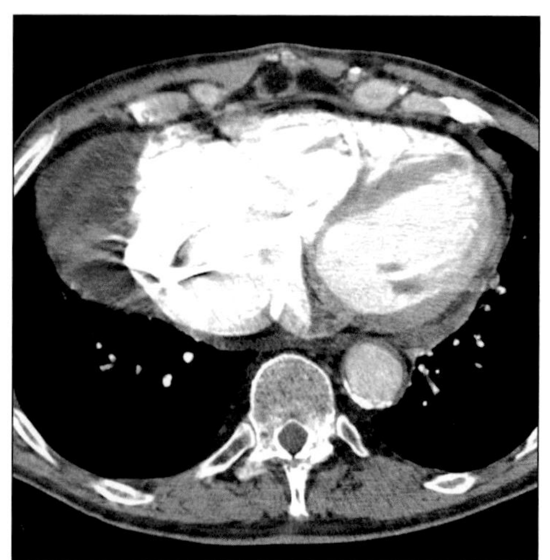

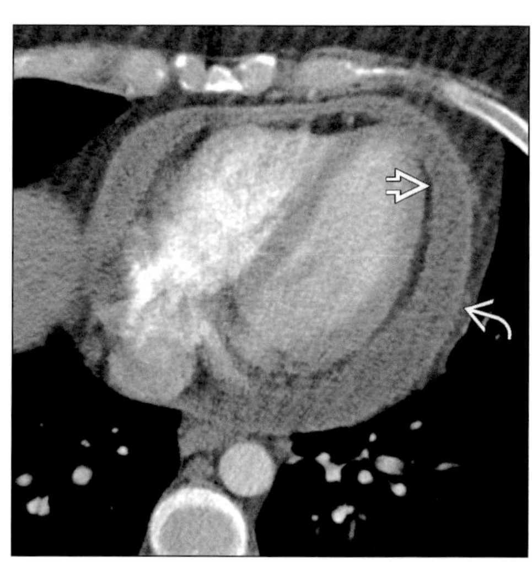

*(**Left**) Axial CECT of a patient with tuberculous pericarditis shows a water attenuation pericardial effusion, enhancement of the serous pericardium, infiltration of the adjacent mediastinal fat, right paraesophageal lymphadenopathy, and bilateral pleural effusions. (**Right**) Coronal CECT of a patient with infectious pericarditis secondary to penetrating trauma shows low-attenuation fluid and gas within the pericardial space and enhancement of the serous parietal pericardium.*

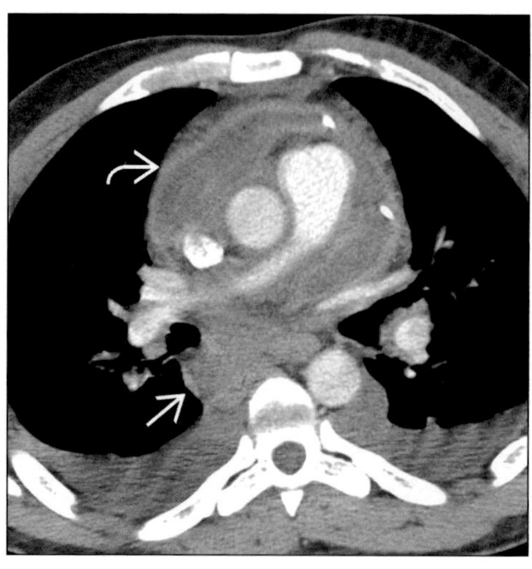

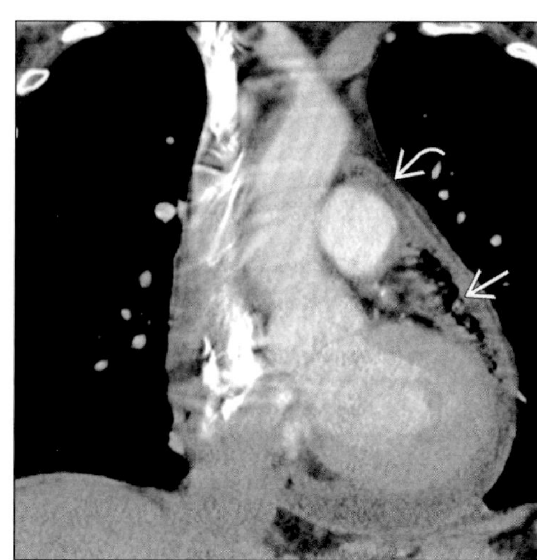

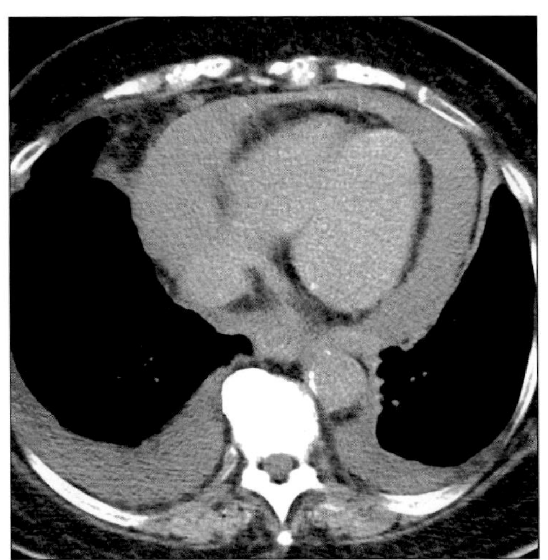

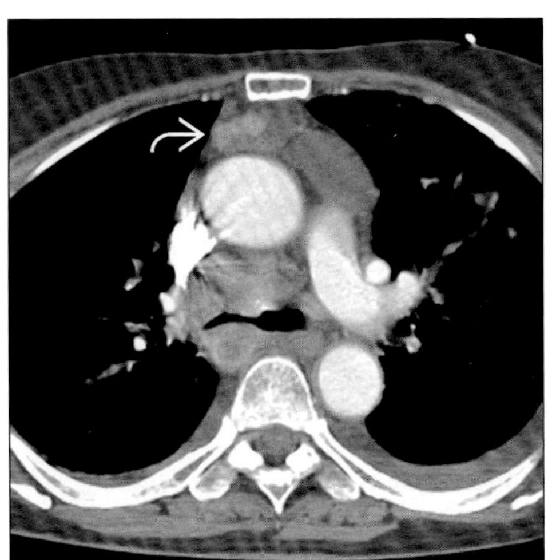

(Left) *Axial NECT of a patient with malignant pericardial effusion shows high-attenuation pericardial fluid and bilateral pleural effusions. Malignant pericardial effusion, purulent pericardial fluid, and hemopericardium may manifest with high-attenuation fluid.* ***(Right)*** *Axial CECT of a patient who presented with metastatic disease shows enhancing pericardial nodules ➔ in the superior aortic pericardial recess and mediastinal lymphadenopathy, consistent with metastases.*

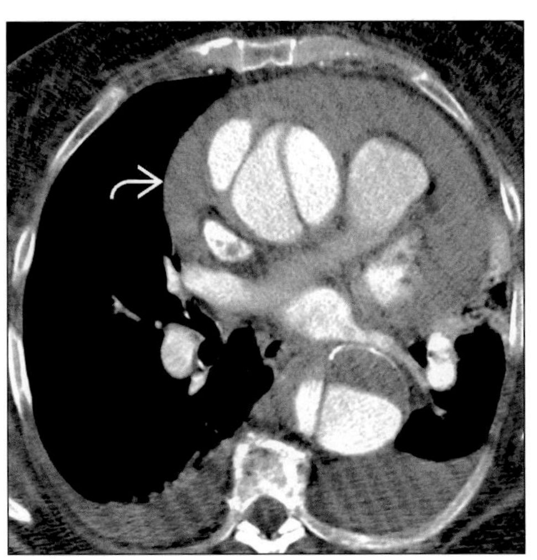

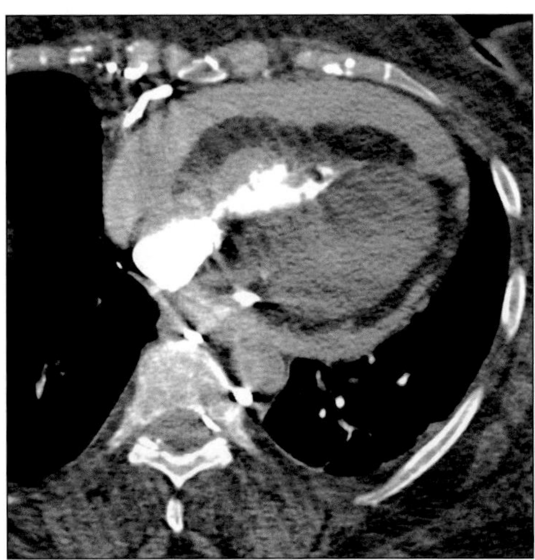

(Left) *Axial CECT of a patient with type A aortic dissection shows high-attenuation pericardial fluid ➔ secondary to hemopericardium.* ***(Right)*** *Axial CECT of a patient with pericardial tamponade after traumatic dialysis catheter placement shows high-attenuation pericardial fluid due to extravasated contrast from superior vena cava laceration and mass effect on the right ventricle. The intrapericardial location of the superior vena cava injury resulted in hemopericardium and cardiac tamponade.*

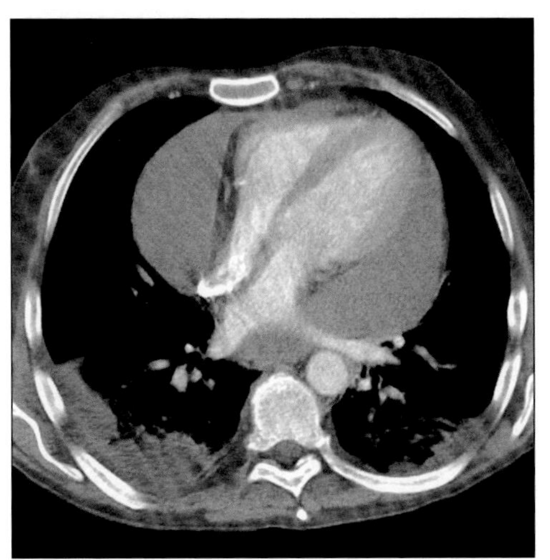

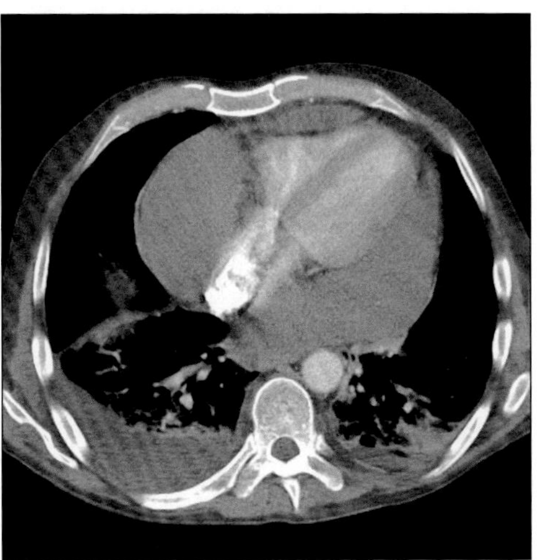

(Left) *Axial CECT of a patient with lung cancer, malignant pericardial effusion, and cardiac tamponade shows a large pericardial effusion and bilateral small pleural effusions with features of loculation. Note mass effect on the right cardiac chambers (particularly the right atrium) by the pericardial fluid.* ***(Right)*** *Axial CECT of the same patient shows pericardial fluid-producing mass effect on the right atrium and right ventricle and flattening of the interventricular septum (CT signs of tamponade).*

CONSTRICTIVE PERICARDITIS

Key Facts

Terminology

- Pericardial stiffening/adhesions with clinical hemodynamic changes & right heart failure

Imaging

- Clinical evidence of physiologic constriction
- CT
  - Normal pericardial thickness: < 3 mm
  - Pericardial thickening/calcification highly suggestive of constrictive pericarditis
  - Tubular ventricles, dilated atria
  - Waist-like narrowing of atrioventricular groove
- MR
  - Septal bounce: Paradoxical diastolic motion of interventricular septum
  - Pericardial enhancement with acute inflammation
  - More sensitive for distinction of constrictive pericarditis from restrictive cardiomyopathy

Top Differential Diagnoses

- Restrictive cardiomyopathy
- Pericarditis without constriction

Pathology

- Infectious: Viral, bacterial, mycobacterial
- Postsurgical or radiation injury
- Inflammatory: SLE, rheumatoid arthritis

Clinical Issues

- Symptoms of right heart failure
- Surgical pericardiectomy when chronic

Diagnostic Checklist

- Pericardial thickening & calcification can confirm constrictive pericarditis when clinically suspected
- Absence of pericardial thickening & calcification does not exclude constrictive physiology

*(**Left**) Lateral chest radiograph of a patient with postsurgical constrictive pericarditis shows curvilinear calcification ➔ around the heart and a pleural effusion ➔. Lateral radiography is more sensitive than frontal radiography for visualization of pericardial calcification. (**Right**) Axial NECT of a patient with constrictive pericarditis shows thick, irregular pericardial calcifications ➔ in the atrioventricular grooves causing ventricular waist-like narrowing and tubular configuration.*

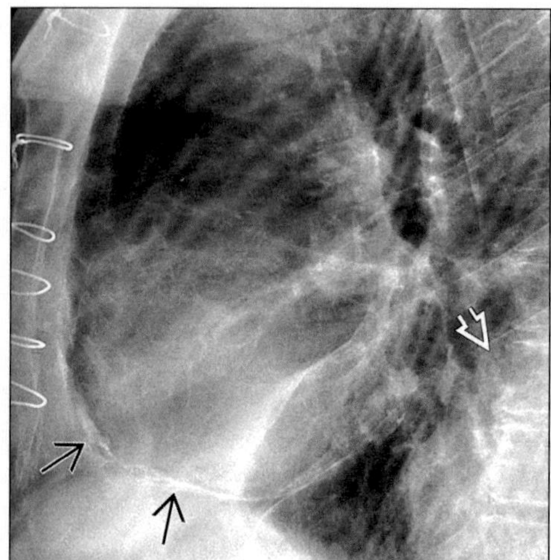

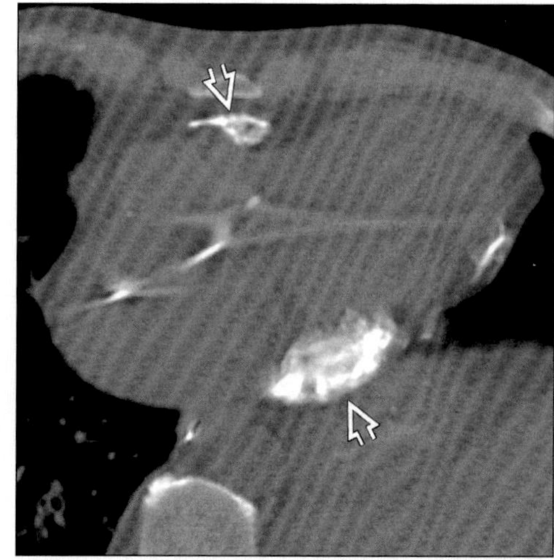

*(**Left**) Short axis T1-weighted MR shows diffuse circumferential pericardial thickening ➔, identified as a low signal intensity band between the high signal intensity mediastinal and subepicardial fat and straightening of the interventricular septum. Paradoxical motion of the interventricular septum in diastole is an important finding in constrictive pericarditis. (**Right**) Short axis T1WI C+ MR shows diffuse pericardial enhancement ➔ seen in pericardial inflammation or fibrosis.*

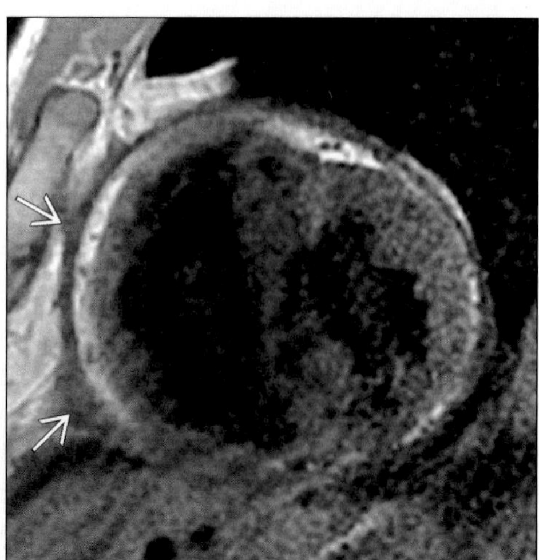

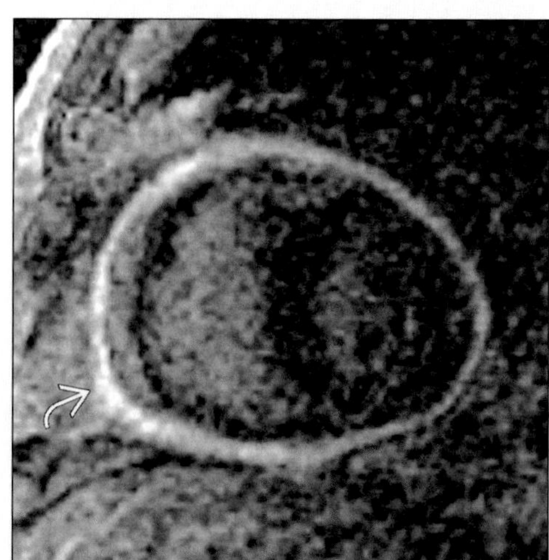

CONSTRICTIVE PERICARDITIS

TERMINOLOGY

Definitions

- Pericardial stiffening/adhesions with clinical hemodynamic changes & right heart failure

IMAGING

General Features

- Best diagnostic clue
  - Normal pericardial thickness: < 3 mm
    - Smooth linear structure between subepicardial fat & mediastinal fat
  - **Pericardial thickening/calcification** highly suggestive of constrictive pericarditis
- Morphology
  - **Atrial enlargement, tubular ventricles**
  - **Prominent leftward convexity or sigmoid shape of interventricular septum**

Radiographic Findings

- Radiography
  - **Linear or nodular calcification**, best seen on **lateral radiography**
    - Usually diffuse, right sided, along atrioventricular groove or diaphragmatic surface
  - Pleural effusion, ascites

CT Findings

- **Pericardial calcification** highly suggestive of constriction
- **Tubular ventricular configuration**, straightened or sinusoidal interventricular septum
- **Waist-like narrowing of atrioventricular groove**
- Dilated atria & vena cava
- Pleural effusions, ascites, hepatic venous congestion

MR Findings

- T1WI
  - Low signal intensity band between high signal intensity mediastinal & subepicardial fat
- T1WI C+
  - Pericardial enhancement with acute inflammatory process
- SSFP White blood cine
  - Septal bounce: Paradoxical diastolic motion of interventricular septum
- MR more sensitive in distinguishing pericardial effusion, constrictive pericarditis, & restrictive cardiomyopathy
- Myocardial tagging
  - Perturbation of magnetization marks stripes across myocardium & pericardium
  - Pericardial adhesions prevent normal stepoff or break of these stripes during cardiac cycle

Echocardiographic Findings

- **Echocardiography is primary diagnostic tool**
- Transesophageal more sensitive than transthoracic
- Can differentiate pericardial thickening from effusion
- Respirophasic changes in diastolic filling

Imaging Recommendations

- Best imaging tool
  - Imaging of patients with **clinical evidence of physiologic constriction**
  - Echocardiography primary tool to investigate pericardial effusion & cardiac hemodynamics
  - CT & MR useful to assess entire pericardium
  - CT & MR useful to distinguish myocardial from pericardial disease

DIFFERENTIAL DIAGNOSIS

Restrictive Cardiomyopathy

- Similar physiologic changes by echocardiography & cardiac catheterization
- Look for myocardial thickening or enhancement

Pericarditis without Constriction

- Distinction based on physiologic changes
- Constriction may be transient after acute pericarditis

Myocardial Calcification

- Thin, linear calcification of left ventricular wall

Pericardial Neoplasm

- Enhancing pericardium suggests metastatic disease, especially in association with known malignancy
- Primary pericardial neoplasms are rare

PATHOLOGY

General Features

- Etiology
  - Infectious: Viral (Coxsackie B, influenza), bacterial, mycobacterial
  - Postsurgical or radiation injury
  - Inflammatory: Systemic lupus erythematosus (SLE), rheumatoid arthritis
  - Metabolic: Uremia

CLINICAL ISSUES

Presentation

- Most common signs/symptoms
  - **Symptoms of right heart failure**
    - Dyspnea, orthopnea
    - May present with hepatomegaly, ascites
  - **Kussmaul sign**: Increased jugular venous pressure during inspiration

Treatment

- Medical management when subacute
- Surgical pericardiectomy when chronic
- May recur

DIAGNOSTIC CHECKLIST

Image Interpretation Pearls

- Pericardial thickening & calcification can confirm constrictive pericarditis when clinically suspected
- Absence of pericardial thickening & calcification does not exclude constrictive physiology

SELECTED REFERENCES

1. Yared K et al: Multimodality imaging of pericardial diseases. JACC Cardiovasc Imaging. 3(6):650-60, 2010
2. Bogaert J et al: Cardiovascular magnetic resonance in pericardial diseases. J Cardiovasc Magn Reson. 11:14, 2009

Key Facts

Terminology

- Metastases to heart & pericardium
  - Lymphatic spread
  - Direct extension
  - Hematogenous spread
  - Transvenous spread

Imaging

- May manifest as lung or mediastinal mass(es)
- Pericardial effusion is typical
- Mediastinal lymphadenopathy in 80%
- Pleural effusions in 50%
- Findings of metastatic disease
- MR
  - T1WI: Usually low signal intensity; melanoma/ hemorrhagic metastases may be T1 hyperintense
  - T2WI: High signal relative to myocardium
  - Most metastases enhance

Top Differential Diagnoses

- Primary cardiac tumors
- Effects of treatment
- Myopericarditis

Pathology

- Immunohistochemical markers may be needed to distinguish metastatic from primary cardiac sarcoma

Clinical Issues

- Very poor prognosis
- 1/3 die within a month of detection

Diagnostic Checklist

- Malignant pericardial effusion is often 1st sign of cardiac or pericardial metastatic disease
- Assessment for signs of cardiac tamponade & coronary artery involvement

*(**Left**) Axial CECT of a patient with metastatic melanoma shows a large enhancing soft tissue mass ➡ invading the right atrium associated with a small pericardial effusion ➡. Other metastases manifest as multiple heterogeneously enhancing subcutaneous masses, pulmonary nodules, and a small left pleural effusion with nodular pleural thickening. (**Right**) Axial CECT of the same patient shows multiple pericardial metastases ➡ as well as lung, lymph node, and subcutaneous metastases.*

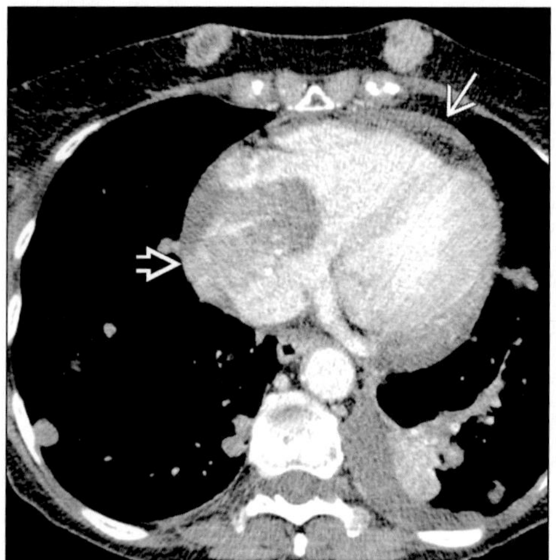

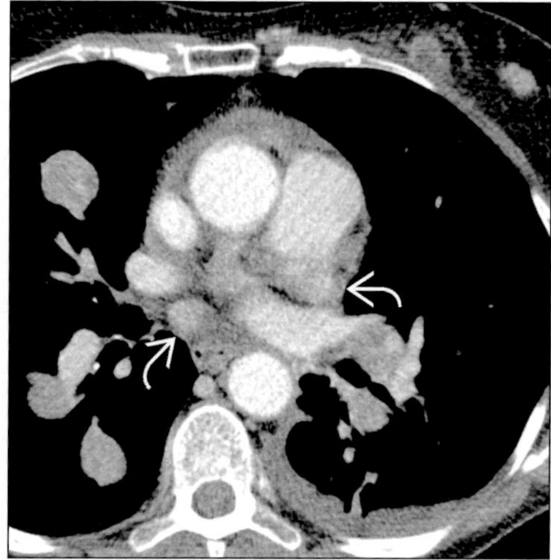

*(**Left**) Axial CECT of a patient with metastatic non-small cell lung cancer shows a large, low-attenuation mass ➡ centered in the right ventricle with extension into the pericardial space. (**Right**) Composite image with axial T2WI MR (top) and fused FDG PET-CT (bottom) of the same patient shows a heterogeneous mass ➡ in the right ventricular myocardium, which is hyperintense relative to normal myocardium. PET/CT shows marked FDG activity ➡ in this lung cancer metastasis.*

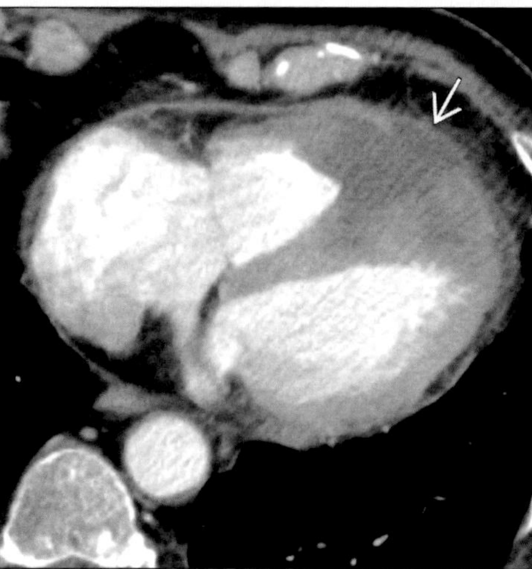

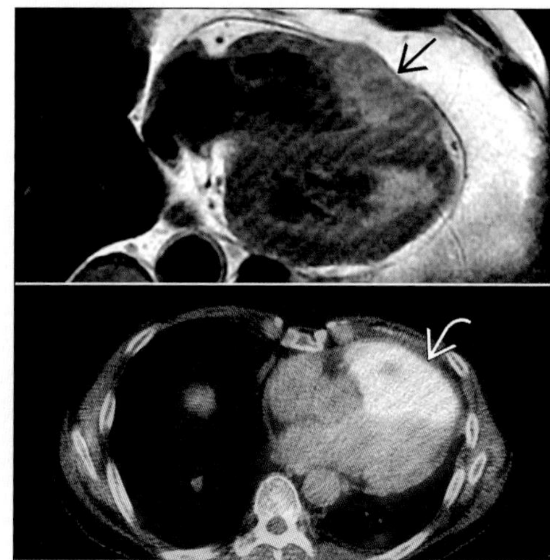

CARDIAC AND PERICARDIAL METASTASES

TERMINOLOGY

Definitions

- Metastases to heart & pericardium occur via
  - **Lymphatic spread**: Most common route; lung & breast cancer
  - **Hematogenous spread**: Typically melanoma; other sites usually involved
  - **Direct extension**: Usually lung cancer & thoracic malignancies; rarely mesothelioma
  - **Transvenous spread**
    - IVC from renal cell carcinoma, hepatocellular carcinoma, adrenal & uterine malignancies
    - Pulmonary vein from lung cancer
- About 15% of cytologically examined pericardial effusions are malignant
- In about 40% of cases, pericardial effusion is site of disease at presentation

IMAGING

General Features

- Best diagnostic clue
  - Multiple cardiac & pericardial masses
  - Associated malignant pericardial effusion
- Location
  - Pericardium may extend variable distance above aorta & pulmonary artery
  - Malignant pericardial effusion may be diffuse or loculated
  - Transvenous spread to atria
  - Hematogenous spread: Multiple, randomly distributed nodules & masses
- Morphology
  - Pericardial nodularity & thickening
  - Fluid may be of heterogeneous attenuation
  - Fluid may be loculated in irregular collections

Radiographic Findings

- Radiography
  - Initial manifestation may be lung or mediastinal mass
  - **Typical findings of pericardial effusion**
    - May simulate cardiomegaly (if quantity of fluid exceeds 250 mL)
    - **"Water-bottle" heart**, if large
    - **"Oreo cookie" sign** on lateral radiography
      - Separation of mediastinal & subepicardial fat by fluid attenuation
  - May produce unusual cardiac contour
  - **Mediastinal lymphadenopathy in 80%**
  - Pleural effusions in 50%

CT Findings

- NECT
  - Calcifications rare except in certain tumors
    - Osteosarcoma
    - Angiosarcoma
    - Tumors with psammomatous calcification
  - Associated signs of malignancy
    - Lung metastases
    - Bone metastases
    - Lymphadenopathy
    - Pleural effusion
- CECT
  - May better demonstrate solid & cystic components
  - May demonstrate associated myocardial involvement
  - Demonstration of associated lymphadenopathy
  - Visualization of central masses extending to heart via pulmonary veins

MR Findings

- T1WI
  - **Metastases are usually of low signal intensity**
  - **Melanoma & hemorrhagic metastases may be hyperintense on T1WI**
- T2WI
  - High signal intensity relative to myocardium
- T1WI C+
  - **Most metastases enhance**
  - Differentiation from thrombus (chronic thrombus may enhance peripherally)
- Better assessment of extent of disease than with CT
  - Superior contrast resolution allows better detection of myocardial metastases & pericardial disease
- Cardiac functional impairment can be detected & quantitated

Echocardiographic Findings

- Procedure of choice for initial evaluation of suspected pericardial effusion
  - Moderate effusion: Echo-free space 10-20 mm during diastole
  - Severe effusion: Echo-free space > 20 mm
- Evaluation of right & left ventricular function
- Signs of tamponade: Right ventricular or atrial diastolic collapse

Imaging Recommendations

- Best imaging tool
  - Echocardiography for initial evaluation
    - Limited evaluation of right ventricle
    - May not show entire pericardium
    - Poor demonstration of associated findings, lymphadenopathy
  - Cardiac gated MR for further evaluation

DIFFERENTIAL DIAGNOSIS

Primary Cardiac Neoplasms

- **Very rare**
- May mimic metastases with multifocal myocardial involvement or pericardial invasion
- Aggressive neoplasms
  - Sarcomas: Angiosarcoma, leiomyosarcoma, rhabdomyosarcoma
  - Primary cardiac lymphoma
- Difficult differentiation of primary cardiac sarcoma (e.g., osteosarcoma) from metastases

Effects of Treatment

- Drug- or radiation-induced myopericarditis & pericardial thickening/nodularity
  - Radiation dose usually exceeds 3,000 cGy
  - Common drugs: Doxorubicin & cyclophosphamide
- Nephrotic syndrome with pericardial effusion

Myopericarditis

- Infectious, inflammatory, or drug induced
- Enhancing, nodular pericardium & epicardial enhancement on MR may mimic metastases

CARDIAC AND PERICARDIAL METASTASES

Pericardial Cyst

- Congenital
- Homogeneous water attenuation, imperceptible wall
- Well marginated; no soft tissue components

PATHOLOGY

General Features

- Etiology
  - Most common neoplasms metastatic to heart & pericardium: **Lung, breast, melanoma, lymphoma**
  - **Metastases to heart in ~ 1% of autopsies, ~ 10% when malignant neoplasm known**
- **Malignant pericardial effusions are overwhelmingly secondary to metastases**
  - Primary cardiac neoplasms are very rare

Gross Pathologic & Surgical Features

- Over 90% are of epithelial origin (e.g., lung, breast)

Microscopic Features

- Immune markers can help discriminate among different cell types
- Psammoma bodies (lung cancer, ovarian cancer)
- Immunohistochemical markers may be needed to distinguish metastatic from primary cardiac sarcoma

CLINICAL ISSUES

Presentation

- Most common signs/symptoms
  - Asymptomatic (50%)
  - Typically related to impaired cardiac function (30%) from pericardial effusion & tamponade
    - Hypotension & tachycardia
  - Dyspnea out of proportion to radiographic abnormality
  - Chest pain, cough, peripheral edema
  - Arrhythmia common
- Other signs/symptoms
  - Signs of **cardiac tamponade**
    - **Kussmaul sign**: Increased distention of jugular veins with inspiration
    - **Friedreich sign**: Rapid diastolic descent of venous pulse
    - **Pulsus paradoxus**: Decrease of more than 10 mmHg in diastolic pressure on inspiration

Demographics

- Age
  - Age determined by incidence of malignancy
- Gender
  - Equal gender distribution
- Epidemiology
  - Melanoma has highest rate of cardiac metastases (46-71%), followed by leukemia
  - 1/3 of pericardial metastases from lung cancer
  - 1/3 of patients with lung cancer have pericardial metastases at autopsy
  - 1 in 4 patients with malignant pericardial effusion has breast cancer
  - 1 in 4 patients with breast cancer has malignant pericardial effusion at autopsy
  - 15% of pericardial metastases from hematologic malignancy
  - Other common primaries
    - Esophageal cancer; can lead to esophageal-pericardial fistula
    - Papillary thyroid carcinoma
    - Invasive thymoma
    - Renal cell carcinoma
  - Rare primaries
    - Mesothelioma
    - Endometrial cancer
    - Osteosarcoma, liposarcoma
    - Colon cancer
    - Head & neck carcinoma
    - Carcinoid

Natural History & Prognosis

- **Very poor prognosis**
- Over 80% die within 5 years of detection
  - About 1/3 die within a month of detection, usually from cardiac tamponade
  - Other causes of death: Congestive heart failure, coronary artery invasion, arrhythmia
- Cardiac tamponade from fluid accumulation in pericardial sac
  - Decreased cardiac output, progressive decrease in cardiac diastolic filling
  - **Rapid accumulation poorly tolerated**
  - Recurrent pericardial effusion in 50%

Treatment

- Surgical resection for palliation
- Treatment of cardiac tamponade from malignant pericardial effusion
  - Pericardiocentesis or pericardial window: Primary treatment choice with catheter drainage
  - Pericardial sclerosis or pericardiectomy
  - Radiation therapy

DIAGNOSTIC CHECKLIST

Image Interpretation Pearls

- Malignant pericardial effusion is often 1st sign of cardiac or pericardial metastatic disease
- **Assessment for signs of cardiac tamponade** & **coronary artery involvement**

SELECTED REFERENCES

1. Prakash P et al: Imaging findings of pericardial metastasis on chest computed tomography. J Comput Assist Tomogr. 34(4):554-8, 2010
2. Butany J et al: Cardiac tumours: diagnosis and management. Lancet Oncol. 6(4):219-28, 2005
3. González Valverde FM et al: Pericardial tamponade as initial presentation of papillary thyroid carcinoma. Eur J Surg Oncol. 31(2):205-7, 2005
4. Chiles C et al: Metastatic involvement of the heart and pericardium: CT and MR imaging. Radiographics. 21(2):439-49, 2001

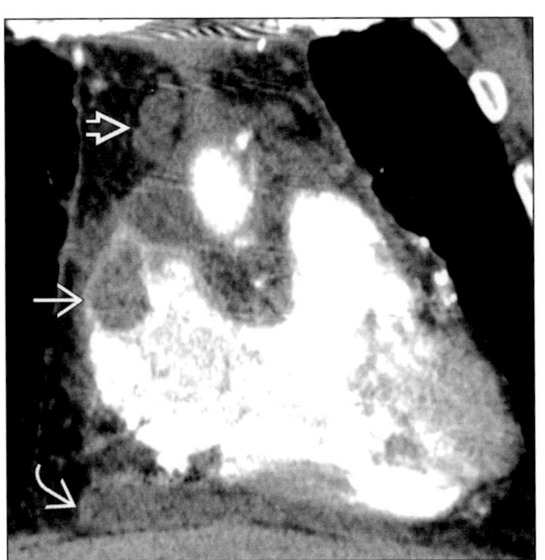

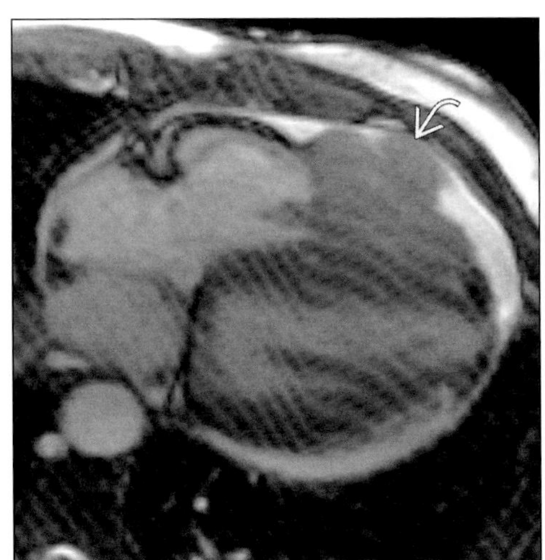

(Left) *Coronal CECT of a patient with metastatic melanoma shows an enhancing mass ➔ in the right atrium with associated pericardial effusion ➔ and enhancing mediastinal lymphadenopathy ➔.* ***(Right)*** *Cine 4 chamber MR of a patient with metastatic melanoma shows an intermediate signal intensity mass ➔ centered in the right ventricular myocardium with associated pericardial effusion. Among primary malignancies, melanoma has the highest frequency of cardiac metastases.*

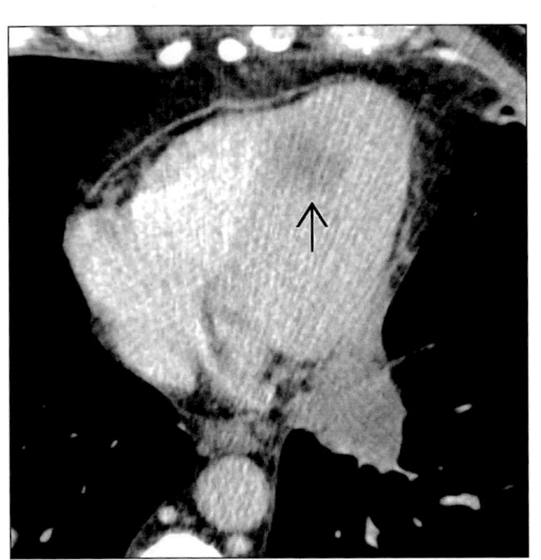

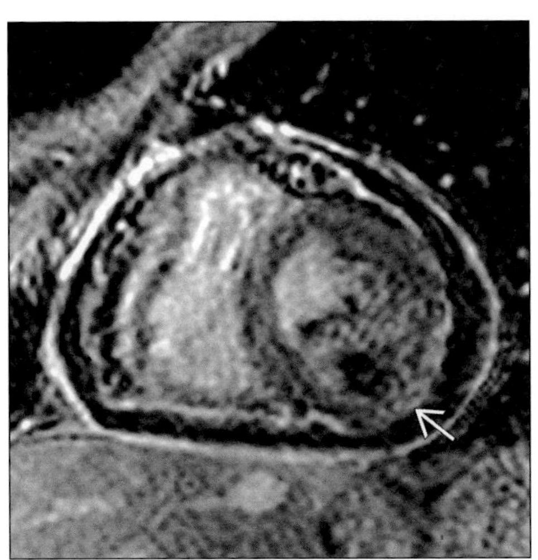

(Left) *Axial CECT of a patient with lung cancer shows a left lower lobe mass that invades the pericardium and a low-attenuation metastasis ➔ arising from the interventricular septum. Lung cancer may affect the heart and pericardium via lymphatic spread, intravascular spread, or direct invasion.* ***(Right)*** *T1WI C+ FS short axis MR of a patient with metastatic sarcoma shows a centrally necrotic, enhancing mass ➔ of the inferolateral left ventricular wall and a large pericardial effusion.*

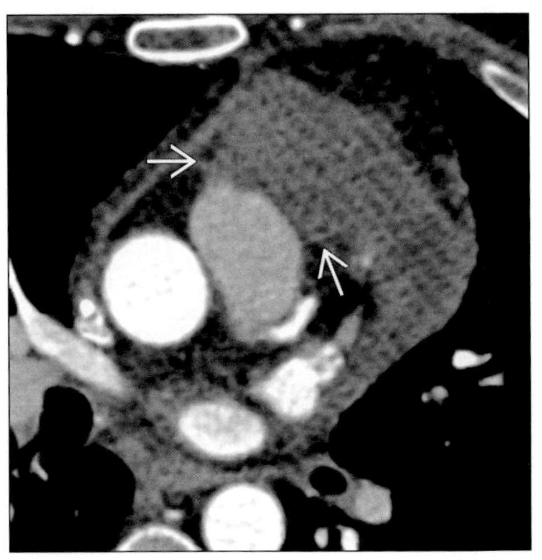

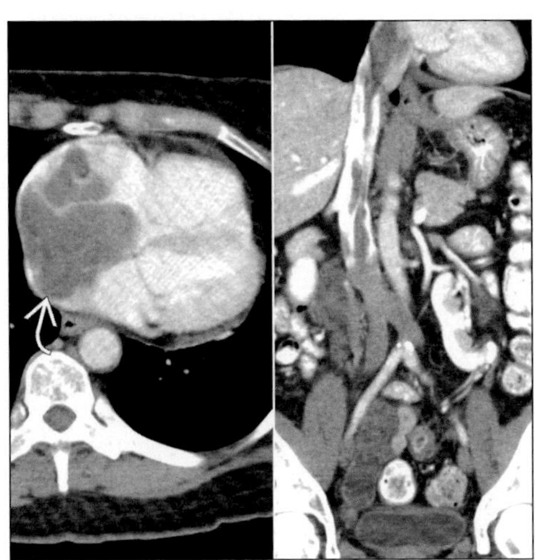

(Left) *Axial CECT of a patient with mediastinal sarcoma shows a large mediastinal mass ➔ extending through the pericardium and subepicardial fat and abutting the right ventricular outflow tract.* ***(Right)*** *Composite image with axial chest CECT (left) and coronal abdomen CECT (right) of a patient with retroperitoneal lipoleiomyoma shows a large, lobulated right atrial mass ➔ and intravascular extension of the retroperitoneal mass through the inferior vena cava into the heart.*

CARDIAC MYXOMA

Key Facts

Terminology

- Most common primary cardiac neoplasm

Imaging

- Intracavitary mass originating from interatrial septum near fossa ovalis
- Approximately 85% in left atrium; then right atrium
- CT
  - Typically low-attenuation intracavitary mass
  - Calcification in approximately 50% of right atrial myxomas
- MR
  - Heterogeneous mass, heterogeneous enhancement
  - May change position during cardiac cycle
  - May exhibit a stalk; may prolapse through or obstruct atrioventricular valve
  - Cine SSFP to evaluate mobility, valvular obstruction, & flow acceleration

Top Differential Diagnoses

- Intracardiac thrombus
- Cardiac metastases
- Cardiac lipoma
- Primary cardiac malignancy
- Papillary fibroelastoma

Clinical Issues

- Approximately 60% of affected patients are women
- Symptoms: Valvular obstruction (40%), constitutional symptoms (30%)
- Treated with surgical resection; 3-year survival > 95%

Diagnostic Checklist

- Consider cardiac myxoma in a patient with a well-defined noninvasive atrial mass
- Stalk-like connection to interatrial septum may be evident on cross-sectional imaging

*(**Left**) Composite image with PA (right) and lateral (left) chest radiographs shows an ovoid right atrial myxoma with peripheral curvilinear calcification ➔. Although more common in the left atrium, right atrial myxomas are more likely to exhibit calcification. (**Right**) Axial CECT of a patient with a left atrial myxoma shows a heterogeneous left atrial mass with smooth borders, internal vascularity, and characteristic attachment to the interatrial septum ➔ near the fossa ovalis.*

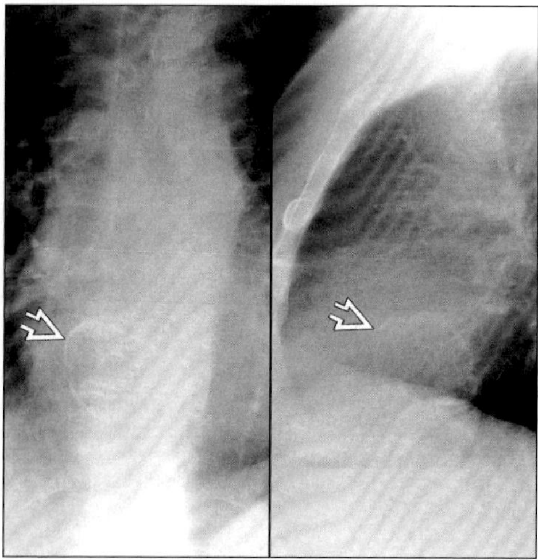

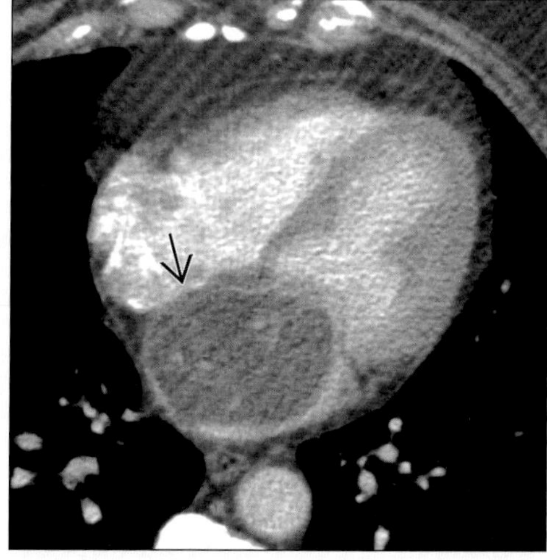

*(**Left**) Graphic shows typical morphologic features of cardiac myxoma with a thin short stalk ➔ connecting the heterogeneous left atrial mass to the interatrial septum. Large lesions may obstruct the mitral valve during systole. (**Right**) Composite image with 4 chamber cine SSFP in systole (top) and diastole (bottom) shows a large left atrial myxoma attached to the interatrial septum that prolapses through and obstructs the mitral valve ➔ during diastole, an uncommon but characteristic feature.*

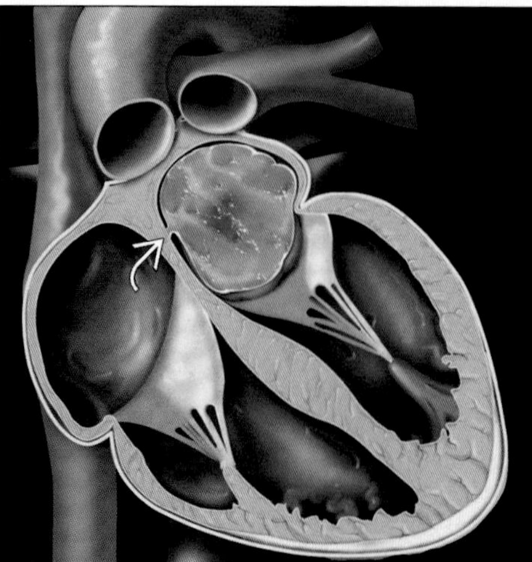

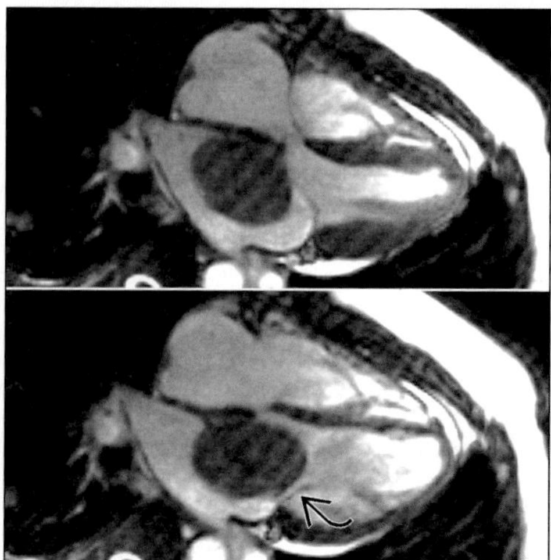

CARDIAC MYXOMA

TERMINOLOGY

Definitions

- **Most common primary cardiac neoplasm**

IMAGING

General Features

- Location
  - ~ **85% in left atrium**, followed by right atrium
  - Rare sites: Ventricle, inferior vena cava, valve
- Size
  - 1-15 cm diameter
- Morphology
  - Usually solitary; may be multiple in familial forms
  - Ovoid lesion with lobular or smooth contours

Radiographic Findings

- Rarely exhibit calcification; more frequent in right atrial myxomas
- Findings may mimic atrioventricular valve stenosis

CT Findings

- NECT
  - Low-attenuation intracavitary mass
    - Occasionally cystic
    - May change position during cardiac cycle
  - **Calcification in approximately 50% of right atrial myxomas**, rare in left atrial myxomas
- CECT
  - May exhibit heterogeneous contrast enhancement

MR Findings

- **Majority heterogeneous on MR**
  - Iso- or hypointense on T1WI
  - Usually hyperintense on T2WI
- **Heterogeneous enhancement**
- **Cine SSFP images: Evaluation of mobility, valve obstruction**, flow acceleration, stalk visualization

Echocardiographic Findings

- Tumor typically hyperechoic
- Assessment of tumor mobility & cardiac physiology

Nuclear Medicine Findings

- May be mildly FDG avid
- If very FDG avid, consider malignancy

DIFFERENTIAL DIAGNOSIS

Intracardiac Thrombus

- Common; usually in posterolateral atrium or appendage
- Associated with atrial fibrillation & mitral valve disease
- Acute thrombus does not enhance; chronic thrombus may have slight peripheral enhancement

Cardiac Metastases

- More often multiple & enhancing
- Often associated with pericardial effusion, lymphadenopathy, or other metastases

Cardiac Lipoma

- Often in interatrial septum
- Fat density on CT; fat signal on MR

Primary Cardiac Malignancy

- Most often angiosarcoma
- May exhibit pericardial effusion, metastases

Papillary Fibroelastoma

- Most common tumor of valvular epithelium
- Usually solitary, arising from aortic or mitral valve

PATHOLOGY

General Features

- Genetics
  - **90% sporadic**
  - Carney complex: Familial cardiac myxoma (< 10%)

Gross Pathologic & Surgical Features

- Usually soft gelatinous or friable frond-like tumor
- Hemorrhage, thrombus, hemosiderin (80% of cases)

Microscopic Features

- Most commonly rings & syncytial chains of myxoma cells embedded in myxomatous matrix

CLINICAL ISSUES

Presentation

- Most common signs/symptoms
  - Symptoms of valvular obstruction (40%)
  - Constitutional (30%): Fatigue, weight loss, fever
  - Arrhythmias or other electrocardiographic changes
  - Peripheral embolization (stroke, myocardial infarction)
  - May be associated with auscultation abnormalities
    - Mimics mitral valve disease
    - Tumor plop in about 15%

Demographics

- Age
  - **Mean age at presentation: 50 years**
  - Range: 1 month to 81 years
- Gender
  - Approximately **60%** of affected patients are **women**

Natural History & Prognosis

- Very slow growth, **3-year survival** > 95%

Treatment

- Surgical resection, traditionally via sternotomy
- May recur after removal in 5% of cases
- Newer minimally invasive techniques promising

DIAGNOSTIC CHECKLIST

Consider

- Cardiac myxoma in patients with well-defined noninvasive atrial mass

SELECTED REFERENCES

1. O'Donnell DH et al: Cardiac tumors: optimal cardiac MR sequences and spectrum of imaging appearances. AJR Am J Roentgenol. 193(2):377-87, 2009
2. Grebenc ML et al: Cardiac myxoma: imaging features in 83 patients. Radiographics. 22(3):673-89, 2002

CARDIAC SARCOMA

Key Facts

Terminology
- Most common primary cardiac malignancy
- Restricted to heart & pericardium

Imaging
- Best diagnostic clue: Mass involving cardiac wall &/or chamber
- Radiography may be normal or show cardiomegaly
- CECT
  - Discrete hypodense mass involving cardiac wall &/or chambers
  - Infiltration/invasion: Pericardium, myocardium, mediastinum
  - Pulmonary metastases
- MR
  - T1: Heterogeneous; necrosis & hemorrhage
  - T2: Heterogeneously hyperintense
  - T1 C+: Heterogeneous enhancement

Top Differential Diagnoses
- Cardiac metastases
- Lymphoma
- Cardiac myxoma
- Thrombus

Pathology
- Angiosarcoma most common histologic type (37%)
- Metastatic disease: 66-89% at presentation

Clinical Issues
- Dyspnea is most common symptom
- Poor prognosis
  - Mean survival: 3 months to 4 years
  - Recurrence & metastases within 1 year
- Treatment
  - Surgery: Palliative, may prolong survival
  - Palliative radiation & chemotherapy

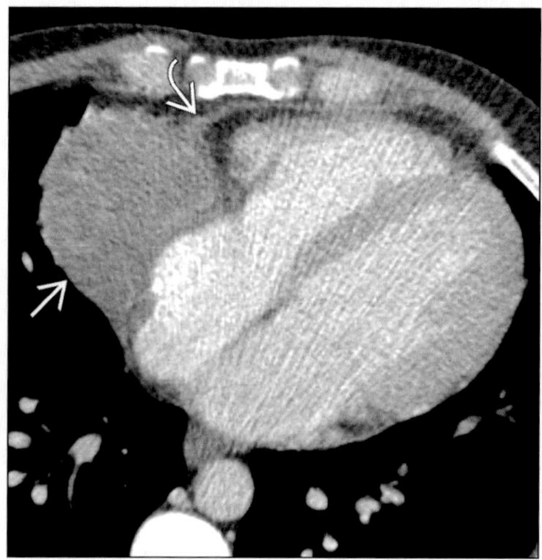

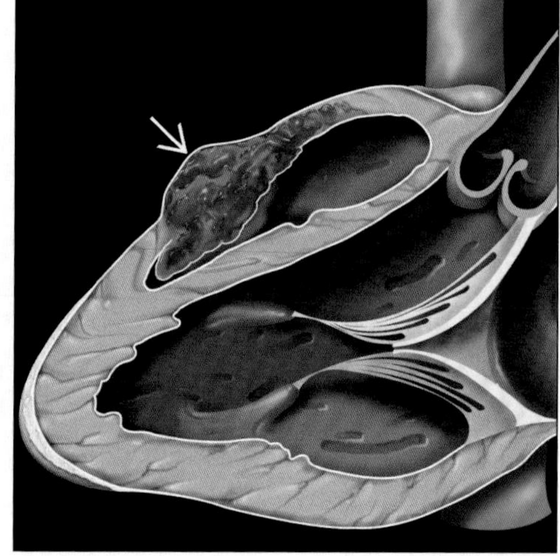

(Left) *Axial CECT of a patient with cardiac sarcoma shows a predominantly hypodense mass ➔ arising from the right atrium. Disruption and irregularity of the adjacent pericardium ➔ are consistent with local invasion. Primary cardiac sarcomas may manifest as discrete masses or as diffuse cardiac/pericardial infiltration.* ***(Right)*** *Graphic demonstrates the morphologic features of cardiac sarcomas, which are infiltrative and locally invasive cardiac neoplasms ➔ that often affect the atria.*

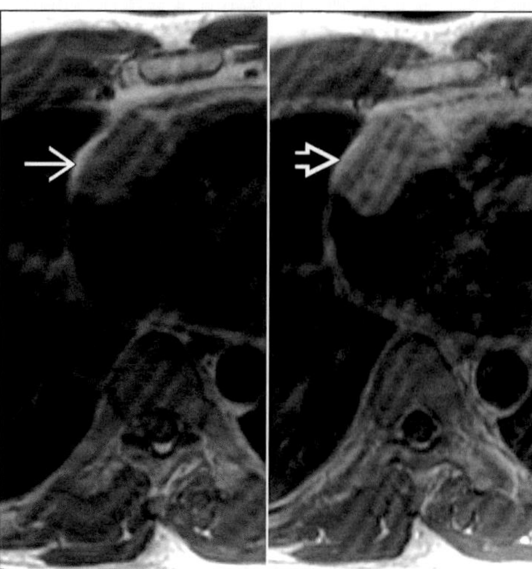

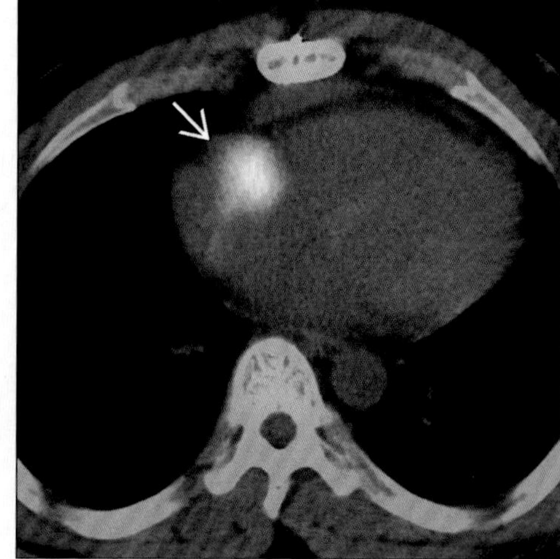

(Left) *Composite image with axial T1WI MR (left) and axial T1WI C+ MR (right) of a patient with primary cardiac angiosarcoma shows a right atrial mass ➔ that is isointense to muscle and exhibits heterogeneous contrast enhancement ➔.* ***(Right)*** *Axial fused PET/CT of a patient with angiosarcoma demonstrates FDG uptake within a right atrial mass ➔. Angiosarcomas most commonly involve the right atrium, whereas other primary cardiac sarcomas typically arise from the left atrium.*

CARDIAC SARCOMA

TERMINOLOGY

Definitions

- **Most common primary cardiac malignancy**
- Restricted to heart & pericardium

IMAGING

General Features

- Best diagnostic clue
  - Mass involving cardiac wall &/or chambers
- Location
  - **Angiosarcomas**: Right atrium > left atrium
  - Other sarcomas: Left atrium > right atrium

Radiographic Findings

- Radiography
  - Chest radiography may be normal
  - **Cardiomegaly** most common abnormality
  - Mass
  - Consolidation
  - Pericardial effusion
  - Congestive heart failure
  - Pulmonary metastases

CT Findings

- CECT
  - Discrete **hypodense mass** involving **cardiac wall & chambers**
    - Angiosarcomas are highly vascular
    - Mineralization may occur in primary osteosarcoma
  - Diffuse infiltration
  - **Pericardial invasion**
    - Pericardial thickening & nodularity
    - Disruption of pericardium
    - Hemorrhagic pericardial effusion
  - **Myocardial invasion**
    - Invasion of interatrial septum in primary osteosarcoma
  - **Mediastinal invasion**
  - Pulmonary venous extension
  - Pulmonary metastases
- Cardiac gated CTA
  - Involvement of cardiac valve

MR Findings

- T1WI
  - **Heterogeneous**
    - Hypointense: Necrosis
    - Intermediate: Viable tumor
    - Hyperintense: Hemorrhage
- T2WI
  - **Heterogeneously hyperintense**
- T1WI C+
  - **Heterogeneous enhancement**
    - Marked surface enhancement & central necrosis
  - "Sunray" appearance
    - Lines of enhancement radiating from epicardium to pericardium
    - Denotes hemorrhage within tumor

Imaging Recommendations

- Best imaging tool
  - Cardiac gated MR

DIFFERENTIAL DIAGNOSIS

Cardiac Metastases

- 20-40x more common than primary sarcoma
- Lung, breast & esophagus cancers, melanoma

Lymphoma

- More common in immunocompromised patients
- Right > left heart involvement

Cardiac Myxoma

- Endoluminal lesion without mural involvement

Thrombus

- Tumor more likely to enhance
- Acute thrombus may enhance

PATHOLOGY

Staging, Grading, & Classification

- Metastatic disease: 66-89% at presentation
  - **Lungs** > lymph nodes, bone, & liver

Gross Pathologic & Surgical Features

- Invasive mass or diffuse infiltration

Microscopic Features

- **Angiosarcoma** most common histologic type (37%)

CLINICAL ISSUES

Presentation

- Most common signs/symptoms
  - **Dyspnea**
- Other signs/symptoms
  - Chest pain, arrhythmia, peripheral edema, tamponade, & sudden death

Demographics

- Age
  - Mean age at presentation: 41 years

Natural History & Prognosis

- Poor prognosis; mean survival: 3 months to 4 years
- Better prognosis
  - Left atrial involvement
  - No metastases at diagnosis
- Recurrence & metastases within 1 year

Treatment

- Surgery: Palliative, may prolong survival
- Palliative radiation & chemotherapy

DIAGNOSTIC CHECKLIST

Consider

- Primary cardiac sarcoma in patient with locally invasive mass involving cardiac wall & chambers

SELECTED REFERENCES

1. Grebenc ML et al: Primary cardiac and pericardial neoplasms: radiologic-pathologic correlation. Radiographics. 20(4):1073-103; quiz 1110-1, 1112, 2000

PULMONARY ARTERY SARCOMA

Key Facts

Terminology
- Pulmonary artery (PA)
- Most common primary PA malignancy

Imaging
- Best diagnostic clue: Large filling defect in PA refractory to anticoagulation
- Radiography
  - Normal if intraluminal with no PA dilation
  - PA dilation: Hilar mass
  - Distal oligemia, pulmonary infarction, & extraluminal extension possible
- CECT: Filling defect in PA; may enhance
- MR: Distinction between tumor & thrombus
  - Tumor more likely to enhance
  - Acute thrombus & tumor thrombus may enhance
  - Cine MR for pulmonic valve assessment
- PET/CT: FDG uptake within tumor

Top Differential Diagnoses
- Pulmonary embolism
- Metastatic disease

Pathology
- Leiomyosarcoma most common histologic type

Clinical Issues
- Symptoms: Dyspnea, chest pain, hemoptysis
- Median age: 50 years
- Poor prognosis; mean survival: 12 months
- Treatment
  - Tumor resection, chemoradiation, palliative stenting

Diagnostic Checklist
- Consider pulmonary artery sarcoma in patient with large PA filling defect refractory to anticoagulation

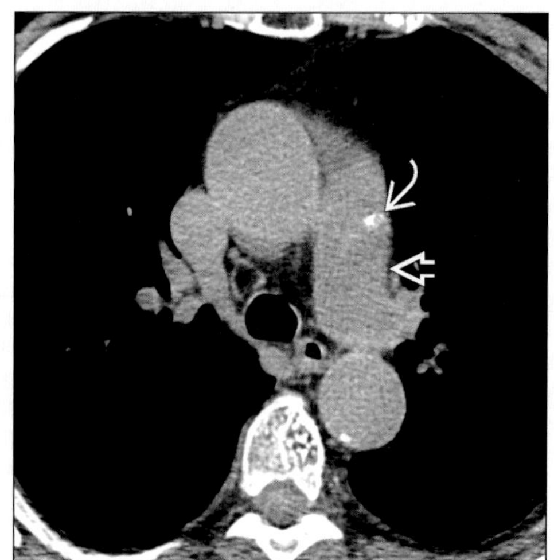

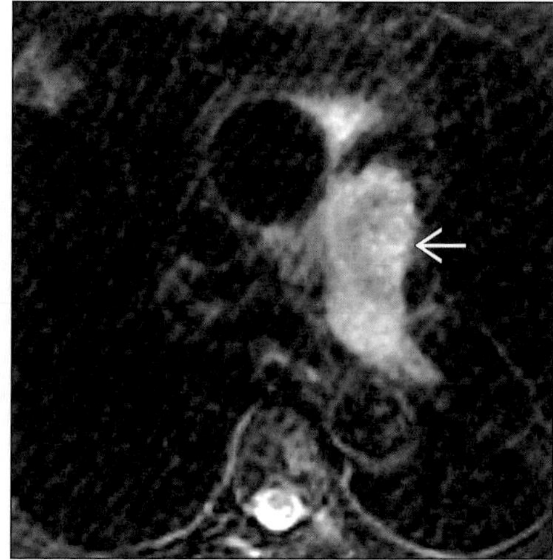

(Left) *Axial NECT shows a PA sarcoma manifesting as an ill-defined hypodense mass ➪ within the pulmonary trunk and the left pulmonary artery with a focus of intrinsic calcification ↪. The differential diagnosis includes pulmonary embolism and metastatic disease.* ***(Right)*** *Axial T2WI MR of the same patient shows an endoluminal heterogeneously hyperintense mass ➔ within the pulmonary trunk, which produces mild pulmonary artery dilatation.*

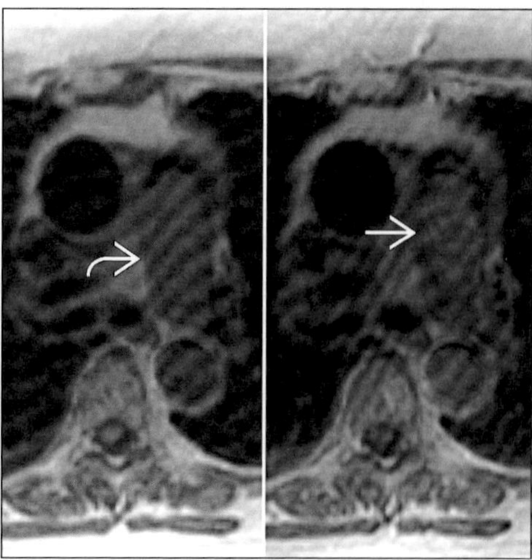

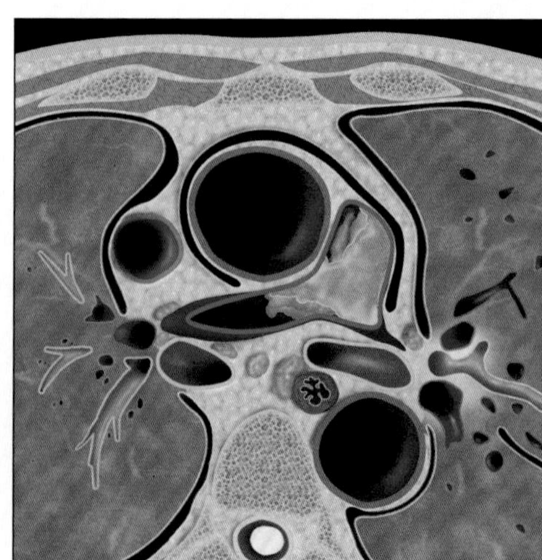

(Left) *Composite image with axial T1WI MR (left) and T1WI C+ MR (right) of the same patient shows that the mass ↪ is slightly hypointense to muscle and enhances heterogeneously ➔. Enhancement is more common in sarcomas than in pulmonary emboli, although acute thrombus and tumor thrombus may exhibit enhancement.* ***(Right)*** *Graphic shows the morphologic features of pulmonary artery sarcoma. A soft tissue mass fills the pulmonary trunk lumen and extends into the proximal right pulmonary artery.*

PULMONARY ARTERY SARCOMA

TERMINOLOGY

Abbreviations

- **Pulmonary artery (PA)**

Definitions

- Most common primary pulmonary artery malignancy

IMAGING

General Features

- Best diagnostic clue
  - Large filling defect in PA
  - Refractory to anticoagulation
- Location
  - Central PA > peripheral PA

Radiographic Findings

- Intraluminal PA sarcoma
  - **Normal chest radiograph** if PA does not dilate
  - **Hilar mass** if PA dilates
- Distal pulmonary **oligemia**
  - Hyperlucent lung
- Peripheral subpleural basilar consolidations; **pulmonary infarcts**
- Mass extension outside PA
  - **Large central mass**; mimics lung cancer
- Multifocal lung nodules; **metastases**

CT Findings

- CECT
  - **Filling defect in PA**
    - May occupy entire luminal diameter
    - PA dilatation
    - May exhibit contrast enhancement
    - May exhibit extraluminal extension
  - Mosaic lung perfusion/attenuation reported
  - Pulmonary metastases

MR Findings

- May allow differentiation between tumor & thrombus
  - **Tumor more likely to enhance**
  - Acute thrombus & tumor thrombus may enhance
- Cine MR to identify pulmonic valve involvement

Angiographic Findings

- Polypoid filling defect in PA
- Tumor & thrombus may be indistinguishable
  - Lesion movement with cardiac cycle suggests malignancy

Nuclear Medicine Findings

- PET/CT
  - **FDG uptake within tumor**

Imaging Recommendations

- Best imaging tool
  - CTA for identification of filling defect in PA
  - Contrast-enhanced MR; tumor vs. thrombus

DIFFERENTIAL DIAGNOSIS

Pulmonary Embolism

- Does not occupy entire luminal diameter
- Less commonly dilates PA
- No enhancement on CECT
- Enhancement on MR less common than in tumor
  - Acute thrombus & tumor thrombus may enhance

Metastatic Disease

- More common than primary malignancy
- Renal cell & breast cancer, melanoma

PATHOLOGY

General Features

- Etiology
  - Etiology unknown in most cases
  - Prior radiation to mediastinum
    - Long latency period

Gross Pathologic & Surgical Features

- Tumor adherent to PA

Microscopic Features

- **Leiomyosarcoma** most common histologic type
- Undifferentiated
- Malignant fibrous histiocytoma

CLINICAL ISSUES

Presentation

- Most common signs/symptoms
  - Mimics pulmonary embolism
    - Dyspnea, chest pain, & hemoptysis
  - Superior vena cava syndrome
    - Dilated superficial veins, edema, headache, & neck swelling
  - Involvement of pulmonary veins
    - Left heart failure

Demographics

- Age
  - Median age: 50 years

Natural History & Prognosis

- Poor prognosis; mean survival: 12 months

Treatment

- Tumor resection
  - Vessel wall reconstruction or conduit placement
  - May require pneumonectomy for proximal lesions
- Chemotherapy ± radiation therapy
- Palliative vascular stenting

DIAGNOSTIC CHECKLIST

Consider

- Pulmonary artery sarcoma in patients with large expansile PA filling defect refractory to anticoagulation

SELECTED REFERENCES

1. Blackmon SH et al: Management of primary pulmonary artery sarcomas. Ann Thorac Surg. 87(3):977-84, 2009
2. Yi CA et al: Computed tomography in pulmonary artery sarcoma: distinguishing features from pulmonary embolic disease. J Comput Assist Tomogr. 28(1):34-9, 2004

AORTIC SARCOMA

Key Facts

Terminology
- Primary malignant tumors of the aorta (PMTA)
- Very rare, highly aggressive class of sarcomas arising from aortic wall or intima with poor prognosis

Imaging
- Radiography
  - Lobulated mediastinal contour
  - Aortic dilatation
- CT
  - Polypoid soft tissue mass within aortic lumen, along or around aortic wall
  - Aortic aneurysm due to weakening of aortic wall by infiltrating mass
  - Stenosis of aortic lumen
  - Occlusion of aortic branches by tumor emboli
- MR
  - Enhancement & distinction from mural plaque

Top Differential Diagnoses
- Aortic aneurysm
- Severe atherosclerosis or ulcerated plaque

Pathology
- Intima: Angiosarcoma, myofibrosarcoma
- Mural: Leiomyosarcoma, malignant fibrous histiocytoma

Clinical Issues
- Progressive pain; embolic events
- May mimic aortic aneurysm ± rupture
- Treatment: En bloc resection, chemoradiation, endovascular stent graft

Diagnostic Checklist
- Consider PMTA in patients with soft tissue masses in or around aorta without evidence of atherosclerosis

(Left) *Axial CTA of a patient with acute chest pain shows aortic rupture manifesting with contrast extravasation ➡ and bilateral pleural effusions. The irregular enhancing soft tissue mass ➡ that narrows the descending aorta ➡ represents a malignant fibrous histiocytoma.* ***(Right)*** *Axial CTA shows a lobulated enhancing periaortic mass ➡ that produces irregular narrowing of the descending thoracic aorta. Aortic sarcoma characteristically manifests with a periaortic soft tissue mass.*

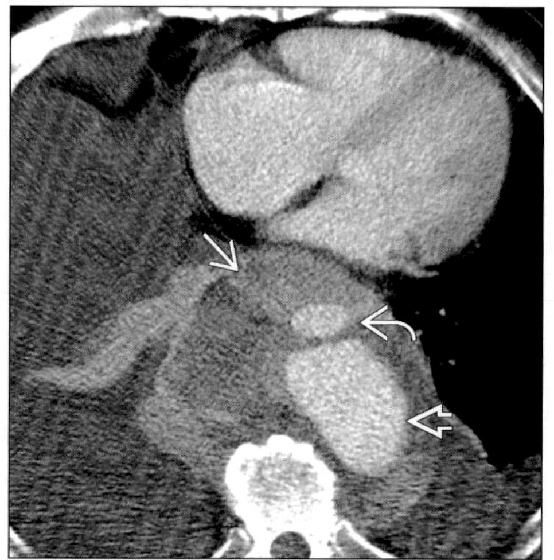

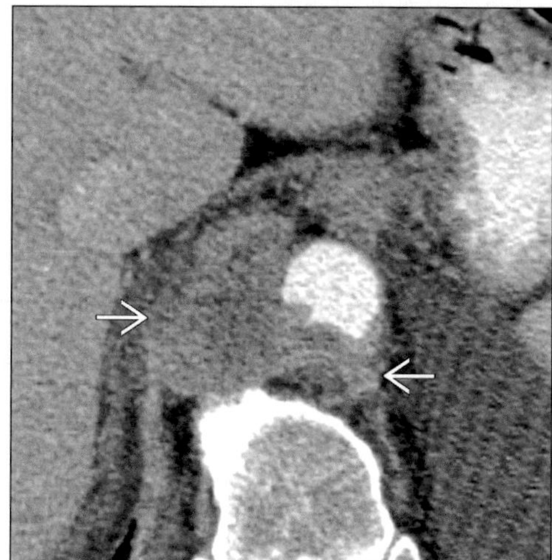

(Left) *Coronal CTA of the same patient shows an elongate periaortic soft tissue mass ➡ mimicking atherosclerotic aneurysm. Absence of calcification should prompt consideration of aortic sarcoma in such cases.* ***(Right)*** *Coronal CTA shows luminal narrowing of the distal abdominal aorta ➡, pseudoaneurysms &/ or ulcerations ➡, and left retroperitoneal hemorrhage ➡. Emergent aortic resection revealed intimal aortic sarcoma. Aortic sarcoma can mimic atherosclerotic vascular disease.*

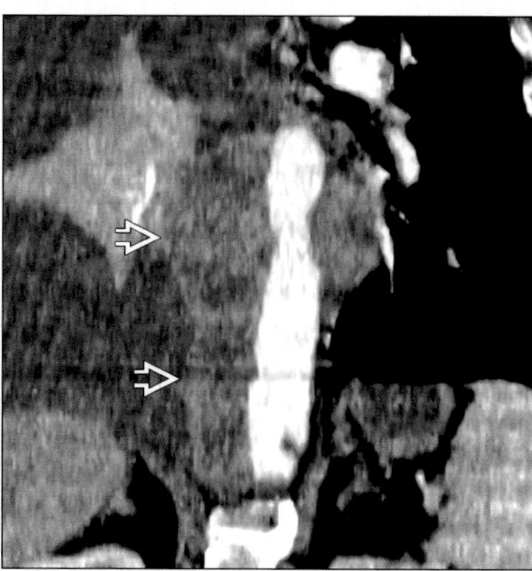

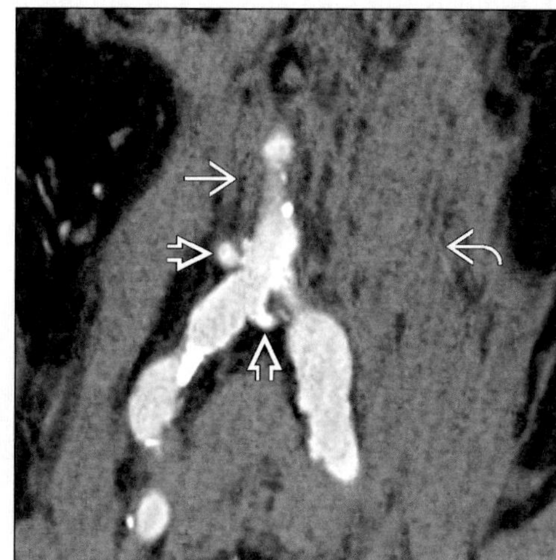

AORTIC SARCOMA

TERMINOLOGY

Synonyms

- **Primary malignant tumors of the aorta (PMTA)**

Definitions

- Very rare, highly aggressive class of sarcomas arising from aortic wall or intima with poor prognosis

IMAGING

General Features

- Best diagnostic clue
  - Soft tissue mass
    - Within aortic lumen
    - Along aortic wall
    - Surrounding aorta
- Location
  - **Descending thoracic aorta** > abdominal aorta > thoracoabdominal aorta > aortic arch

Radiographic Findings

- Abnormal, lobulated mediastinal contour
- Aortic dilatation

CT Findings

- **Polypoid soft tissue mass within aortic lumen, along or around aortic wall**
- Aortic aneurysm due to weakening of aortic wall by infiltrating mass
  - May exhibit extraluminal contrast suggestive of leakage
  - Growing periaortic soft tissue mass; may mimic expanding aneurysm
- Stenosis of aortic lumen
  - Narrowing by intraluminal mass
  - Compression by extraluminal mass
- Occlusion of aortic branch vessels by tumor emboli
  - Renal or splenic infarcts
- Metastases to liver, lungs, bone, brain, skin

MR Findings

- Endoluminal or periaortic soft tissue mass
- Enhancement more easily detected on MR
  - Enhancement allows differentiation from more prevalent, nonenhancing, aortic mural plaques or thrombi
- MR shows hepatic & osseous metastases to better advantage

Imaging Recommendations

- Best imaging tool
  - MRA
    - Superior to CT in distinguishing tumor from aortic wall plaque or thrombus
    - Less invasive than conventional angiography, which may cause iatrogenic tumor emboli

Nuclear Medicine Findings

- PET
  - Hypermetabolic foci in or around aortic wall
  - Staging; detection of unsuspected metastases

DIFFERENTIAL DIAGNOSIS

Aortic Aneurysm

- Consider PMTA if abnormal soft tissue adjacent to aortic aneurysm or rapid aneurysm growth despite exclusion by stent graft
- Consider PMTA with bone, lung, liver, brain, or skin metastases

Severe Atherosclerosis or Ulcerated Plaque

- Consider PMTA if absent calcification or absence of atherosclerosis elsewhere

PATHOLOGY

Staging, Grading, & Classification

- Intimal origin: Angiosarcoma (from endothelial cells), myofibrosarcoma (from mesenchymal cells)
- Mural origin: Leiomyosarcoma, malignant fibrous histiocytoma
- Accurate histologic diagnosis requires immunohistochemical stains

CLINICAL ISSUES

Presentation

- Most common signs/symptoms
  - **Progressive chest or abdominal pain**
  - **Embolic events** (lower extremities, abdomen)
- Other signs/symptoms
  - Aortic aneurysm ± rupture
  - Stroke
  - Intestinal angina

Demographics

- Age
  - Mean: 59 years of age
- Gender
  - Male > female
- < 200 reported cases in literature

Natural History & Prognosis

- Mean survival: 16 months

Treatment

- First line: En bloc tumor resection & graft interposition
- Alternatives
  - Endarterectomy
  - Vascular bypass
  - Chemotherapy, radiation
  - Endovascular stent graft

DIAGNOSTIC CHECKLIST

Image Interpretation Pearls

- Exclusion of metastases to bone, lung, liver, skin, or kidneys in patients with PMTA

SELECTED REFERENCES

1. Simpson WL Jr et al: Pulmonary artery and aortic sarcomas: cross-sectional imaging. J Thorac Imaging. 15(4):290-4, 2000

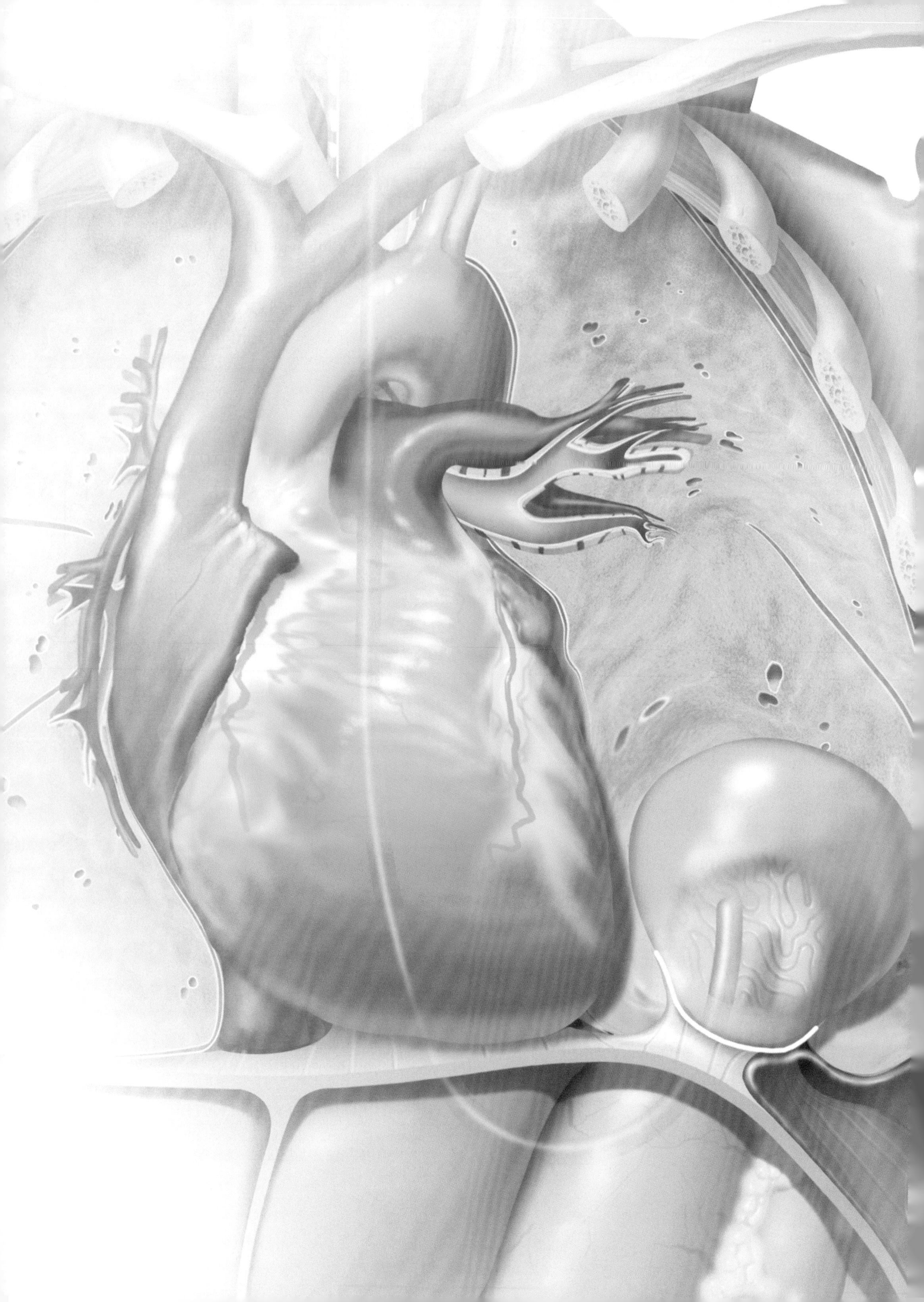

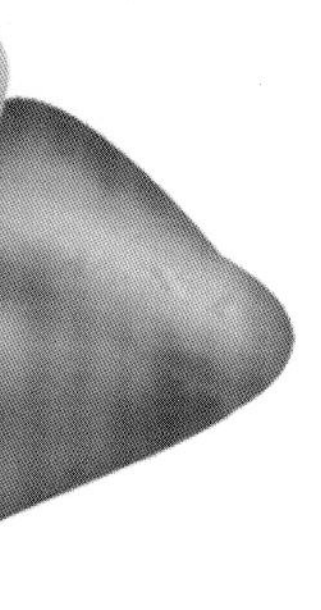

SECTION 10
Trauma

Introduction and Overview

Airways and Lung

Cardiovascular/Mediastinum

Pleura, Chest Wall, and Diaphragm

Introduction

Accidents are the fifth most common cause of death in the United States after diseases of the heart, malignant neoplasms, cerebrovascular diseases, and chronic lower respiratory diseases. Accidental deaths greatly outnumber suicides and assaults leading to homicide. Motor vehicle collisions (MVC) are an important cause of accidents and the leading cause of death among individuals aged five to thirty-four years; more than 2.3 million adults were treated in emergency departments in the United States in 2009. Several organ systems may be simultaneously affected by life-threatening injuries. Thus, evaluation of the traumatized patient requires a rapid comprehensive assessment of the head, neck, thorax, abdomen, and extremities to determine the most significant injuries, appropriately triage patients, and initiate treatment.

Chest trauma can be classified as blunt or penetrating. **Blunt injuries** are typically caused by impact or shear forces and include deceleration injuries, such as those sustained during MVCs or falls from height. **Penetrating injuries** occur when the body is pierced by an object and include low- and high-velocity types. In low-velocity penetrating trauma, such as knife wounds, injured organs are located along the path of the penetrating object. Gunshot wounds represent high-velocity penetrating injuries in which the projectile injures tissues located not only along its path but also outside its path through pressure waves that damage surrounding tissues and vascular structures that may be forcefully displaced from their normal anatomic locations. Traumatic chest injury carries a 15% mortality rate that increases to 80% with associated shock and head injury.

Imaging Modalities

Chest Radiography

Chest radiography is the initial imaging study employed in the evaluation of patients with suspected thoracic abnormalities. Ambulatory stable patients are optimally evaluated with well-positioned, well-exposed PA and lateral chest radiographs obtained at full inspiration. The superimposition of multiple structures of variable radiographic densities contributes to making the chest radiograph one of the most challenging imaging studies interpreted by radiologists.

Imaging evaluation of the chest in the traumatized patient also begins with chest radiography. However, because of the need to stabilize severely traumatized patients, supine portable or bedside chest radiography is routinely performed. Interpretation of portable chest radiographs in the setting of multiorgan trauma presents additional challenges. Overlying artifacts are frequent and include extraneous monitoring and support devices, metallic portions of the patient's clothing, and radiopaque components of the trauma board. In addition, respiratory motion and low lung volumes contribute to difficulties in interpretation. These limitations may be further augmented by obesity and lordotic &/or rotated radiographic projections. However, the portable chest radiograph expeditiously provides valuable information regarding the integrity of the various regions and organs of the thorax. In addition, suspected and unsuspected metallic foreign objects are readily identified.

Evaluation of the thorax on radiography includes **systematic assessment** of the integrity of the chest wall, pleura, lungs, airways, mediastinum, and diaphragm. Knowledge of normal anatomy and the normal appearance of the thorax allows exclusion of displaced fractures, pneumothorax, pleural effusion, lung contusion or laceration, mediastinal widening from traumatic vascular injury, pneumomediastinum secondary to airway/esophageal injury, and traumatic diaphragmatic rupture. In addition, bedside radiography allows expeditious evaluation of life-support devices for documentation of appropriate positioning.

Evaluation of the extent and location of chest radiographic abnormalities in the setting of trauma allows the radiologist to recommend and protocol the optimal follow-up imaging study or the next step in appropriate patient management. Stable patients with normal bedside chest radiographs may be brought to the radiology department for further assessment with well-positioned PA and lateral chest radiographs.

Chest CT

Multidetector CT (MDCT) and CT angiography (CTA) have revolutionized the assessment and management of the traumatized patient and are routinely employed for early diagnosis of life-threatening traumatic disorders. Short scan times enable improved blood opacification by contrast. As a result, these studies have largely supplanted conventional angiography for the diagnosis of traumatic vascular injuries and are considered valuable in planning endovascular interventional procedures and surgical therapies. The addition of post-processing techniques such as multiplanar reformatted (MPR), maximum intensity projection (MIP), shaded surface display (SSD), and volume-rendered imaging allows optimal assessment of the vascular structures of the thorax. However, it should be noted that routine use of MDCT and CTA is associated with increased radiation dose and increased incidence of finding no trauma-related injuries. On the other hand, MDCT and CTA allow direct visualization of the chest wall, pleura, lung, mediastinum, airways, and diaphragm and are reported to disclose up to 30% more unsuspected injuries that impact patient management.

Ultrasound

Ultrasound is increasingly performed in the emergency department for the prompt diagnosis of hemoperitoneum. Echocardiography is the modality of choice for evaluating the pericardium. Thoracic ultrasound can be employed for the emergent evaluation of the pleural space and exclusion of pleural effusion (hemothorax) and pneumothorax. Transesophageal ultrasonography may also be employed to assess cardiac and aortic injuries.

Angiography

With the advent of MDCT, there has been a decrease in the use of angiography to evaluate traumatic vascular injuries. However, angiography is consistently used for managing vascular injuries with endovascular stents and embolotherapy to control hemorrhage.

Magnetic Resonance Imaging

MR is not routinely used in the evaluation of acutely traumatized patients. However, it may prove useful in the evaluation of hemodynamically stable patients in whom intravenous contrast is contraindicated.

Systematic Assessment of the Thorax

Initial assessment of chest radiographs in traumatized patients requires a high index of suspicion since significant abnormalities may be obscured by respiratory motion, low lung volumes, and overlying radiopaque objects. Familiarity with normal mediastinal contours is critical in the diagnosis of subtle abnormalities produced by mediastinal hemorrhage. Supine portable chest radiographs are often compromised by lordotic projection and magnification and may erroneously suggest mediastinal widening in the absence of underlying mediastinal hemorrhage. The radiologist must promptly, carefully, and systematically assess the thorax to detect findings suggestive of life-threatening injuries to various organs and must appropriately recommend further dedicated cross-sectional imaging studies. Severely traumatized patients undergo CT imaging of the head, cervical spine, thorax, abdomen, and pelvis, yielding thousands of images that must be systematically reviewed in a variety of window settings for a comprehensive assessment of a patient's injuries.

Chest Wall

Radiographic evaluation of the chest wall involves assessment of the soft tissues and skeletal structures. Soft tissue gas may indicate penetrating injury or may result from lung &/or gastrointestinal injury. **Rib fracture** fragments may puncture the lung with resultant pneumothorax. First and second rib fractures require severe forces and are associated with increased risk of vascular injury. Inferior rib fractures are associated with injuries to the abdominal viscera. Five contiguous rib fractures or three contiguous segmental rib fractures are associated with flail chest. Fractures of the sternum and spine and sternoclavicular dislocations are difficult to diagnose on radiography but should be excluded on CT as they correlate with severity of trauma and may be associated with life-threatening vascular injury.

Pleura

Pneumothorax may be a life-threatening condition, particularly in traumatized patients supported with mechanical ventilation. Thus, the radiologist must verbally communicate the presence of an unsuspected pneumothorax to the clinical team. The classic finding of a visible apical pleural line may be absent on supine radiography, and diagnosis requires recognition of the **deep sulcus sign** secondary to anterior basilar gas in the nondependent pleural space. Although **tension pneumothorax** is considered a clinical diagnosis, the radiologist should always comment on associated mass effect on mediastinal structures.

Pleural effusion in the setting of trauma is typically the result of **hemothorax**. Large hemothoraces may be associated with hemodynamic compromise and may require surgical evacuation and repair of injured vessels.

Lungs

Airspace disease in the traumatized patient may represent pulmonary contusion or laceration. However, aspiration, infection, and atelectasis from mucus plugs or aspirated foreign bodies may also occur. CT is very sensitive in demonstrating early airspace disease and may be required for direct visualization of underlying pulmonary laceration.

Airways

Airway injuries are rare but should be suspected in patients with intractable pneumothorax or pneumomediastinum. The **fallen lung sign** is a specific but unusual radiographic finding in bronchial rupture. Although chest CT may identify the site of injury, bronchoscopy is the study of choice for diagnosis.

Mediastinum

Mediastinal hemorrhage manifests radiographically with mediastinal widening and loss of normal landmarks and should always raise suspicion for traumatic vascular injury. An abnormal mediastinum on radiography must be evaluated with emergent CTA, which allows direct visualization of traumatic partial and complete aortic injuries, traumatic dissections, and acute intramural hematomas with high sensitivity and specificity. The location of the mediastinal hematoma helps localize the site of vascular injury. Hemopericardium manifests with an enlarged cardiac silhouette on radiography and is readily confirmed with echocardiography or CT. **Pneumomediastinum** is often secondary to alveolar rupture but may also indicate traumatic aerodigestive tract disruption. Persistent pneumomediastinum should prompt evaluation of the central aerodigestive tree.

Diaphragm

Traumatic diaphragmatic rupture typically occurs posteriorly. Although left-sided tears are more common, right-sided injuries may be easily overlooked. Elevation and indistinctness of the hemidiaphragm and herniation of abdominal organs into the thorax should prompt evaluation with CT for early diagnosis.

Life Support Devices

An important role of the radiologist is the assessment of appropriate placement of life support devices. Continued reassessment of the position of these medical devices on sequential images is also required. Comparison to prior studies is crucial to identify interval changes and malpositions.

Delayed Diagnosis of Traumatic Chest Injury

Patients with polytrauma sustain multiple injuries to several organs with various degrees of severity. Emergent management of these patients requires prioritized treatment of life-threatening injuries. In some instances, severe injuries may be initially missed due to subtle imaging manifestations or failure to recognize these abnormalities in the presence of other more obvious or more serious findings. These patients may present at a later date with complaints related to remote injuries. Typical examples include delayed diagnosis of traumatic aortic pseudoaneurysm and diaphragmatic rupture. In these cases, a high index of suspicion and identification of signs of remote trauma help establish the correct diagnosis. This is of particular importance as delayed diagnosis is often associated with significant morbidity and mortality.

Selected References

1. Ho ML et al: Chest radiography in thoracic polytrauma. AJR Am J Roentgenol. 192(3):599-612, 2009
2. Scaglione M et al: Multi-detector row computed tomography and blunt chest trauma. Eur J Radiol. 65(3):377-88, 2008

(Left) *AP portable chest radiograph of a patient status post fall from a 40-foot height is limited by overlying monitoring devices and trauma board artifacts but is diagnostic for left tension pneumothorax, right pulmonary contusion, and traumatic thoracic spine dislocation ➡.* ***(Right)*** *AP portable chest radiograph of the same patient after chest tube placement shows left lung reexpansion, right lung contusion, and malpositioned endotracheal tube tip ↩ in the subglottic space.*

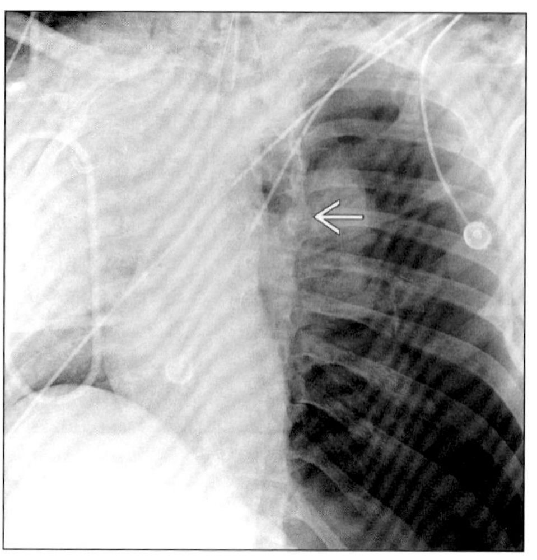

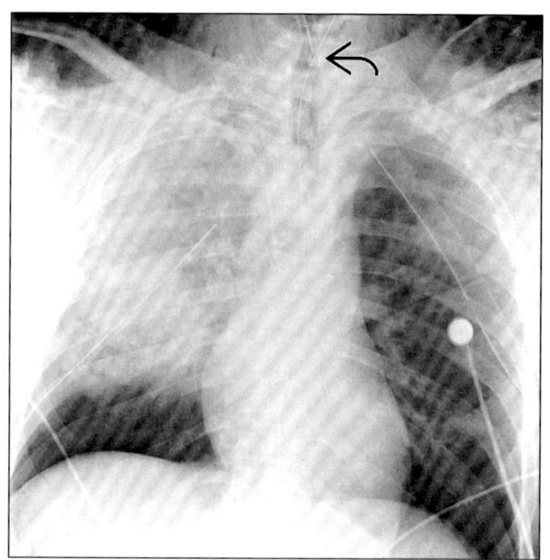

(Left) *Coronal CECT of the same patient shows discontinuity of the thoracic spine ➡ due to severe fracture dislocation and subcutaneous gas in the right supraclavicular region.* ***(Right)*** *CECT of the same patient excluded traumatic vascular injury but demonstrated bilateral pulmonary contusions ↩ with intrinsic lucencies ➡, consistent with pulmonary lacerations. Multidetector CT in the setting of chest trauma demonstrates unsuspected significant injuries in 30% of cases.*

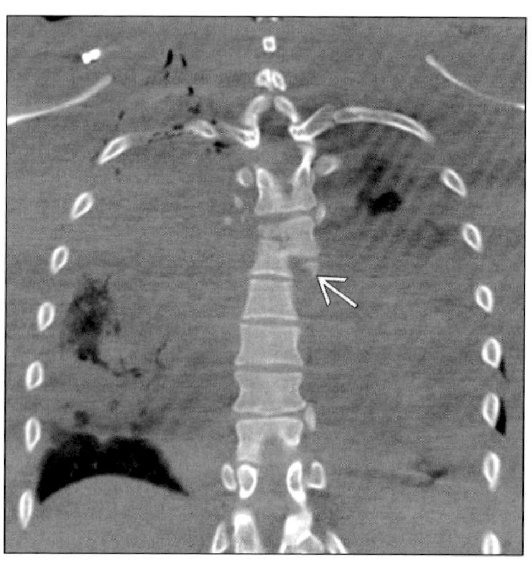

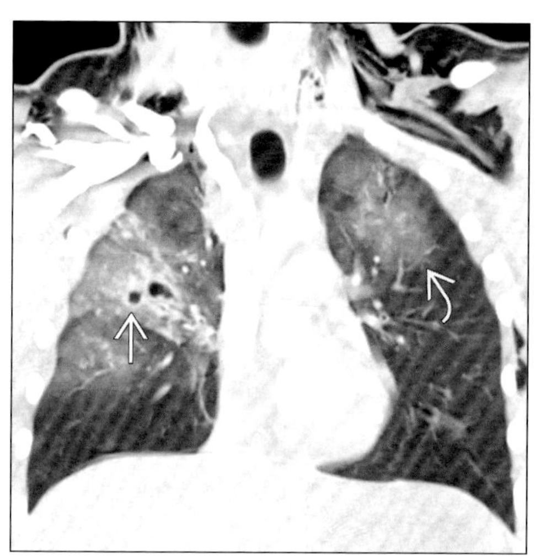

(Left) *AP portable chest radiograph of a young man post MVC shows typical limitations of radiography in trauma with exclusion of the lung bases and trauma board artifacts. However, right basilar pneumothorax and abnormal left superior mediastinal contour ➡ are evident.* ***(Right)*** *Composite image with axial (left) and coronal (right) CECT shows mediastinal hematoma ↩ surrounding an intact aortic arch. Coronal MPR shows atypical mid descending aorta traumatic injury ➡ and an intimal flap →.*

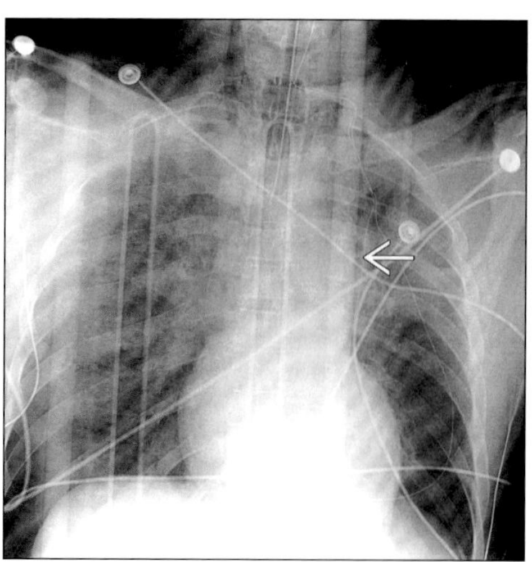

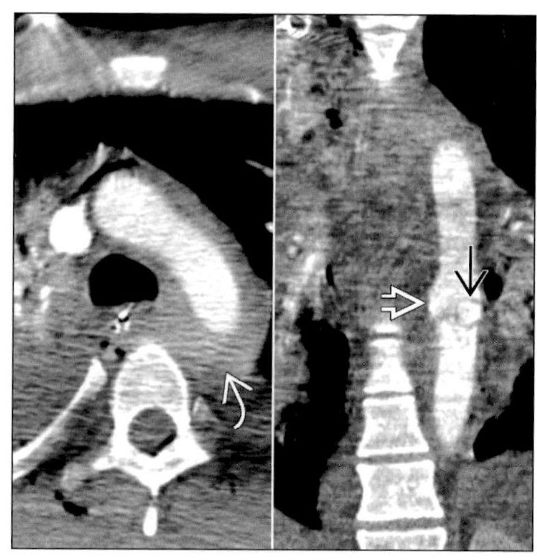

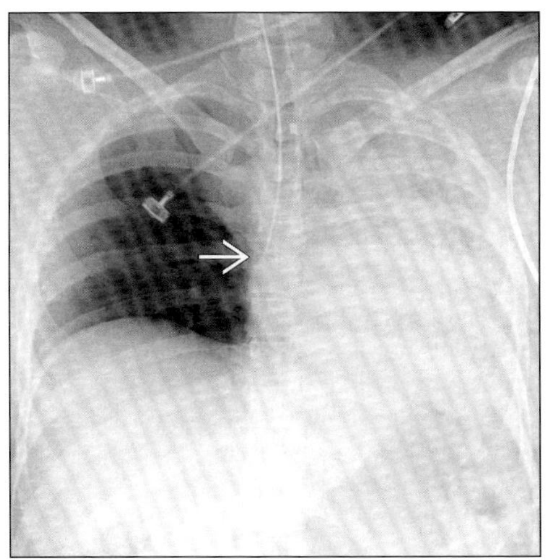

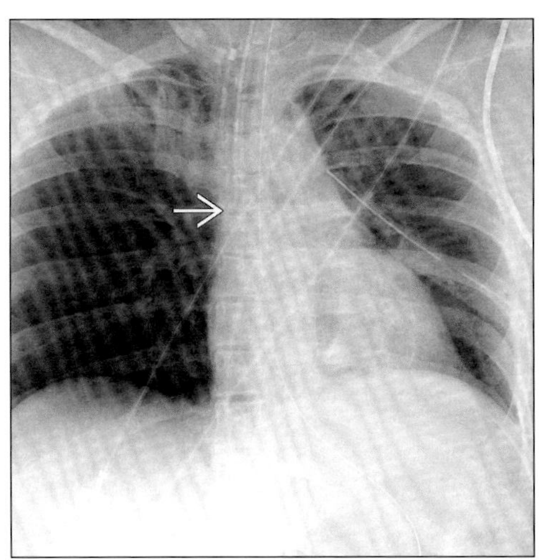

(Left) *AP portable chest radiograph of a patient status post severe motor vehicle collision shows endotracheal tube (ETT) tip ➔ in the bronchus intermedius with mediastinal shift and opaque left hemithorax from left lung atelectasis.* ***(Right)*** *AP chest radiograph of the same patient shows repositioned ETT tip ➔ in the right main bronchus, improving but persistent left lung atelectasis, and left chest tube placed for presumed hemothorax. The patient died from concurrent shock and multiorgan injury.*

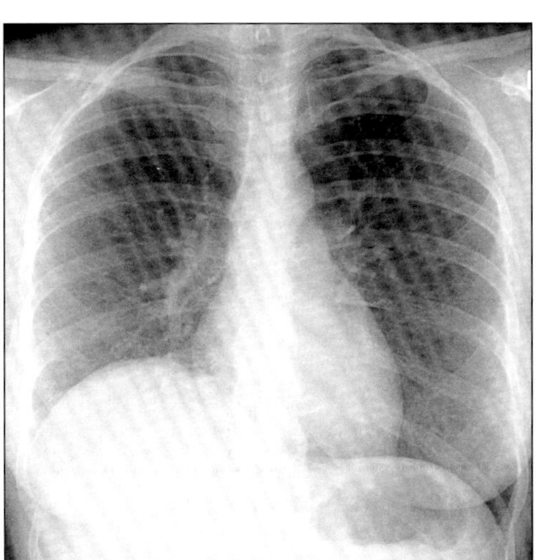

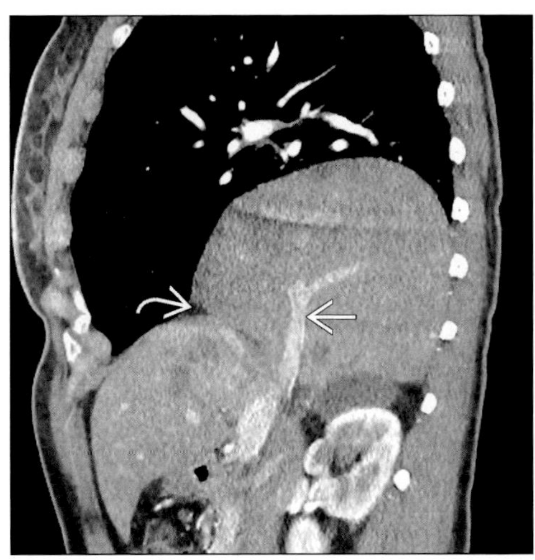

(Left) *PA chest radiograph of a young woman with remote trauma and chronic right upper quadrant pain shows right hemidiaphragm elevation.* ***(Right)*** *Sagittal CECT shows chronic right diaphragmatic rupture with intrathoracic herniation of the right hepatic lobe and the band sign ➔, representing hepatic constriction by the torn diaphragm edge. Note intrathoracic course of the right portal vein ➔. Correct imaging diagnosis prompted consideration of elective surgical repair given persistent symptoms.*

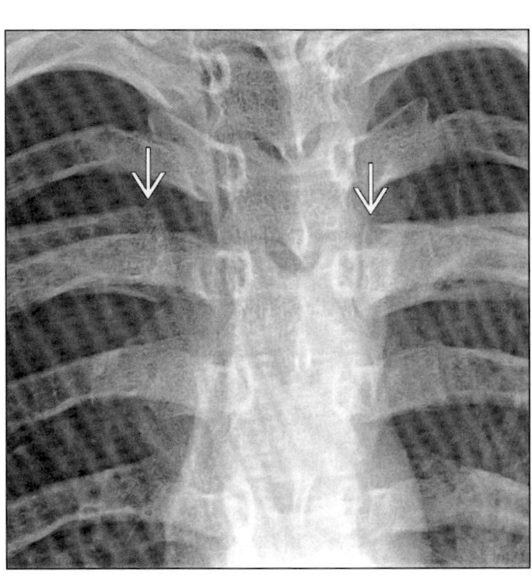

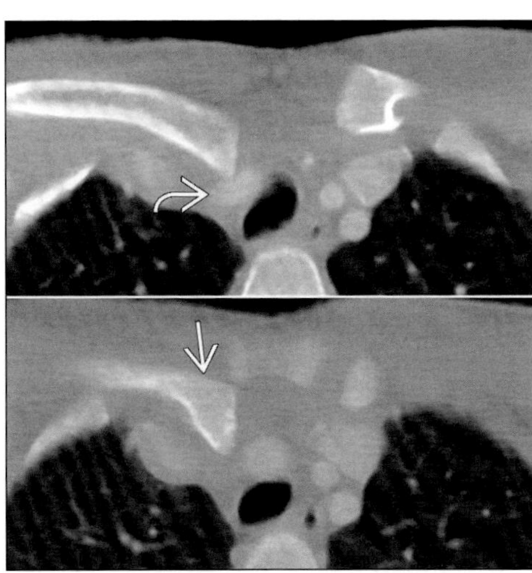

(Left) *Coned-down AP chest radiograph of a young man who sustained a blow to the right anterior chest shows subtle asymmetry of the clavicular heads ➔, with elevation of the right medial clavicle and abnormal right sternoclavicular articulation.* ***(Right)*** *Axial CECT (bone window) shows posterior right sternoclavicular dislocation with impingement on the right brachiocephalic artery ➔ by the clavicular head ➔. Radiographic findings of chest wall injuries may be subtle and easily overlooked.*

TRACHEOBRONCHIAL LACERATION

Key Facts

Terminology

- Disruption of trachea or bronchi following blunt or penetrating injury

Imaging

- Radiography
  - Pneumothorax, pneumomediastinum, subcutaneous gas; persists or progresses after chest tube placement
  - Up to 80% of patients have 1st rib fracture
  - "Fallen lung" sign
  - ETT cuff distention beyond expected location of tracheal walls; ETT cuff displacement out of trachea into neck or mediastinum
- CT
  - Direct identification of injury site in most cases
  - Chronic injury: Airway stricture ± atelectasis
  - Optimal modality for assessment of other injuries

Top Differential Diagnoses

- Pneumomediastinum
- Pneumothorax
- Esophageal rupture
- Esophageal intubation

Clinical Issues

- Signs & symptoms
  - Respiratory distress
  - Continuous air leak despite chest tube drainage
  - Extensive subcutaneous gas
- 30% of affected patients die; 50% of fatalities occur within 1 hour after trauma
- Delayed diagnosis common: 70% not identified in first 24 hours, 40% delayed more than 1 month
  - Airway stenosis, atelectasis, mediastinitis, sepsis
- Diagnosis confirmed with bronchoscopy
- Treatment: Prompt surgical repair

__(Left)__ AP chest radiograph obtained after a neck stab wound shows pneumomediastinum, subcutaneous gas, a large right pneumothorax, and right lung atelectasis with downward displacement. A tracheal laceration was found at surgery. __(Right)__ AP chest radiograph after chest trauma shows a large right pneumothorax with the atelectatic right lung "falling away" from the mediastinum secondary to a right mainstem bronchus laceration. The fallen lung sign denotes tracheobronchial injury.

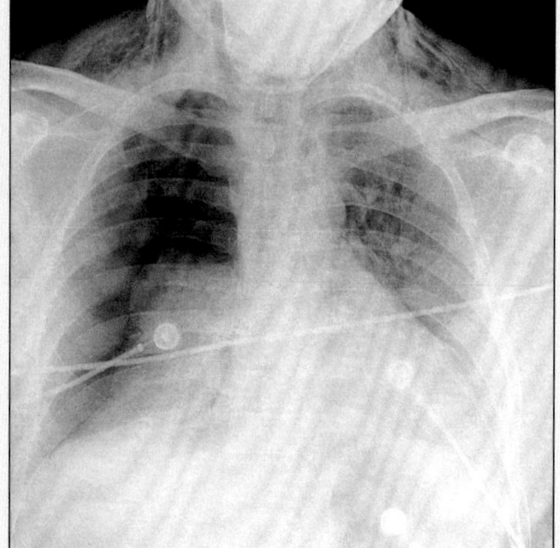

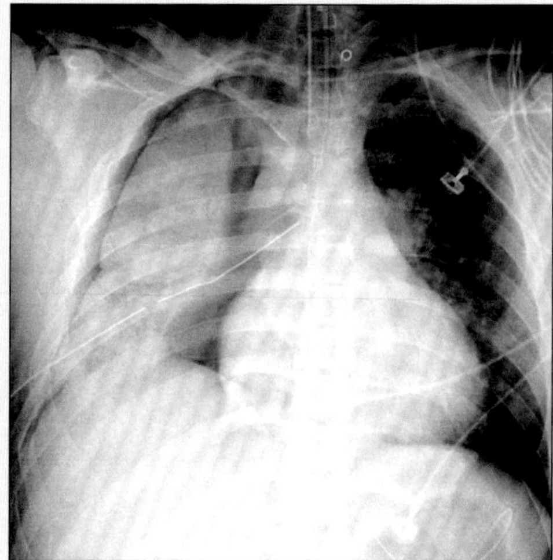

__(Left)__ Axial CECT of a 50-year-old woman involved in a motor vehicle collision shows a laceration of the posterior trachea ➔ proximal to the carina, pneumomediastinum ➔, and subcutaneous gas ➔. Tracheal injuries typically occur at the junction of the membranous and cartilaginous trachea. __(Right)__ Axial CECT (bone window) of the same patient shows a comminuted fracture of the thyroid cartilage ➔, subcutaneous gas, and gas tracking up the neck around the carotid arteries and jugular veins.

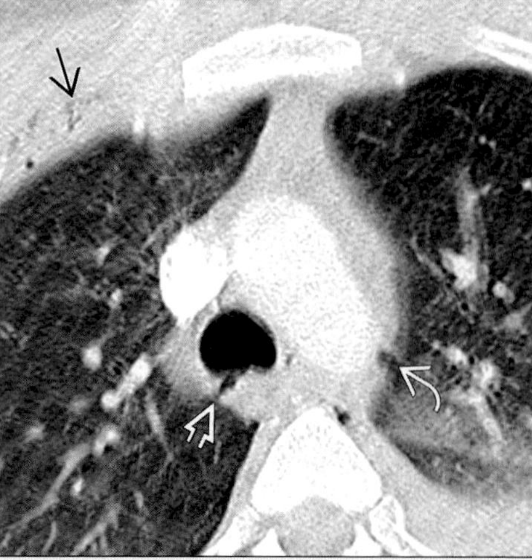

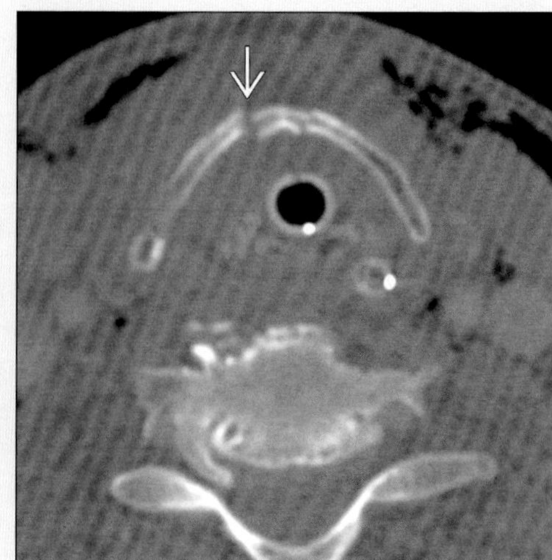

TRACHEOBRONCHIAL LACERATION

TERMINOLOGY

Synonyms

- Bronchial fracture

Definitions

- Disruption of trachea or bronchi following blunt or penetrating injury

IMAGING

General Features

- Best diagnostic clue
  - **Pneumothorax** &/or **pneumomediastinum**; persists or progresses after chest tube placement
- Location
  - Most occur **within 2.5 cm of tracheal carina**, where airway is fixed & subject to shearing injury
- Size
  - Range: Partial thickness tear to complete disruption

Radiographic Findings

- Radiography
  - Site of injury rarely visualized
  - **Subcutaneous gas**, often massive & progressive
  - **Pneumomediastinum**, large & progressive
  - **Pneumothorax**, often with tension
  - Up to **80%** of patients have **1st rib fracture**
  - **"Fallen lung" sign**
    - Lung falls away from hilum into gravitationally dependent position
  - **Endotracheal tube** (ETT)
    - Cuff distention beyond expected location of tracheal walls or cuff displacement out of trachea into neck or mediastinum

CT Findings

- CECT
  - Direct identification of site of injury in majority of cases
  - Chronic airway injury: Airway stricture ± associated lobar collapse
- CTA
  - Assessment of associated life-threatening injuries, especially traumatic aortic injury

Imaging Recommendations

- Best imaging tool
  - CT is optimal modality for identification of site of airway injury & detection of additional injuries
- Protocol advice
  - IV contrast suggested for imaging trauma patients

DIFFERENTIAL DIAGNOSIS

Pneumomediastinum

- Multiple common etiologies; rarely airway injury

Pneumothorax

- Common with trauma; often associated with rib fractures

Esophageal Rupture

- Emetic injury, blunt/penetrating trauma
- Pneumomediastinum & pneumothorax

Esophageal Intubation

- Frontal radiograph may show balloon overinflation superimposed on tracheal air column ± gaseous distention of stomach
- Lateral radiograph shows endotracheal tube posterior to trachea

PATHOLOGY

General Features

- Etiology
  - Direct compression between sternum & spine
  - Sudden deceleration of lung with fixed trachea
  - Forced expiration against closed glottis
  - Penetrating trauma: Gunshot & stab wounds
  - Iatrogenic from endotracheal tube placement
- Associated abnormalities
  - Aortic injury, esophageal injury, rib & vertebral fractures

Gross Pathologic & Surgical Features

- Tracheobronchial tears commonly occur at junction of membranous airway with cartilage rings

CLINICAL ISSUES

Presentation

- Most common signs/symptoms
  - **Respiratory distress**
  - Continuous **air leak** despite chest tube drainage
  - Extensive subcutaneous gas

Demographics

- Epidemiology
  - Uncommon; 3% of patients who die from blunt chest trauma
  - Delayed diagnosis common: 70% not identified in first 24 hours, 40% delayed more than 1 month

Natural History & Prognosis

- 30% of affected patients die; 50% of fatalities occur within 1 hour after trauma
- Delayed diagnosis
  - Airway stenosis
  - Atelectasis
  - Mediastinitis, sepsis

Treatment

- Diagnosis confirmed with **bronchoscopy**
- **Prompt surgical repair**

DIAGNOSTIC CHECKLIST

Consider

- Careful evaluation of entire thorax in trauma for detection of other life-threatening injuries

SELECTED REFERENCES

1. Scaglione M et al: Acute tracheobronchial injuries: Impact of imaging on diagnosis and management implications. Eur J Radiol. 59(3):336-43, 2006
2. Tack D et al: The CT fallen-lung sign. Eur Radiol. 10(5):719-21, 2000

PULMONARY CONTUSION/LACERATION

Key Facts

Terminology

- Injury to lung parenchyma secondary to blunt or penetrating trauma
- Contusion: Torn capillaries & small blood vessels without frank alveolar disruption
- Laceration: Disruption of alveoli leading to radial parenchymal retraction

Imaging

- Contusion: Patchy ground-glass opacity in mild injury to diffuse consolidation in severe injury
  - Typically clears within 14 days of injury
- Laceration: Cystic lung lesions; may contain air-fluid levels; surrounded by contusion & hemorrhage
  - Typically conforms to path of penetrating object
- CT: Modality of choice for initial injury assessment
- Radiography usually sufficient for follow-up

Top Differential Diagnoses

- Aspiration
- Pneumonia
- Lung abscess

Pathology

- Torn small blood vessels with sudden deceleration
- Direct lung impaction or impalement (fractured rib)

Clinical Issues

- Symptoms: Dyspnea, chest pain, hemoptysis
- Young adult men most commonly affected

Diagnostic Checklist

- CT more sensitive than radiography in detecting pulmonary contusion & laceration
- CT allows expeditious assessment of coexisting chest wall & mediastinal injuries

__(Left)__ Graphic shows the spectrum of injuries in blunt trauma, including multiple contiguous rib fractures resulting in flail chest with adjacent pulmonary contusion, hemorrhage, and associated hemopneumothorax. __(Right)__ AP chest radiograph of a 28-year-old man involved in a motor vehicle collision shows right rib fractures ➢ and adjacent right lung airspace disease that does not conform to an anatomical distribution. Pulmonary contusion is often associated with rib fractures.

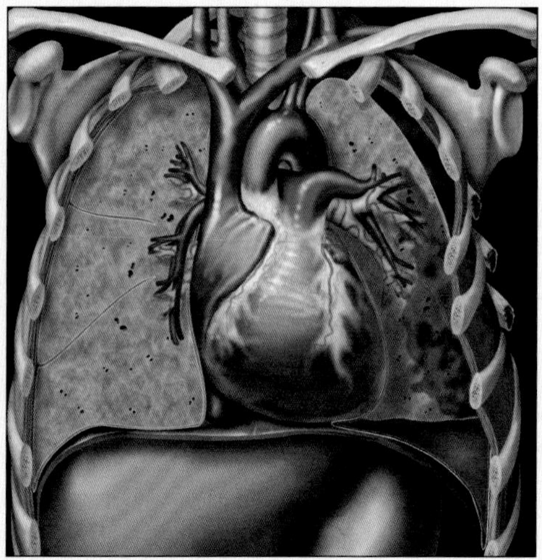

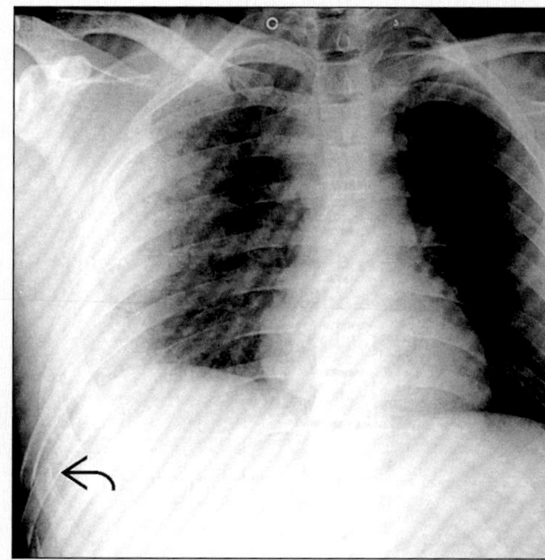

__(Left)__ Axial CECT of the same patient obtained 4 hours later shows extensive dense consolidation in the right lung and small multifocal pulmonary lacerations ➢. Note the small residual anterior pneumothorax. Pulmonary contusions often evolve for several hours following injury. __(Right)__ AP chest radiograph of a 25-year-old man involved in a motorcycle crash shows a right pneumothorax and a right lower lobe pulmonary laceration ➡ likely resulting from lung compression against adjacent vertebrae.

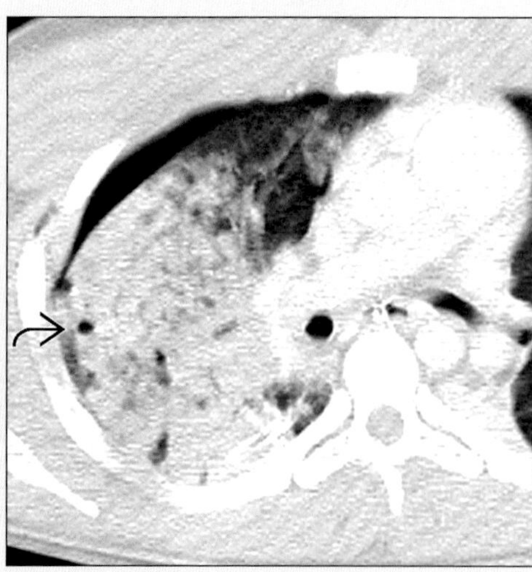

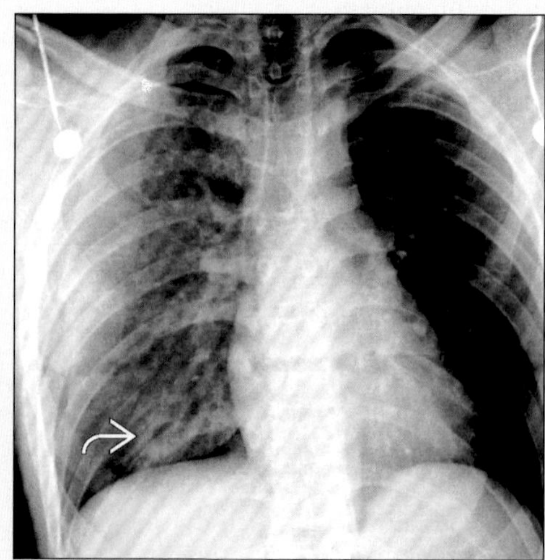

PULMONARY CONTUSION/LACERATION

TERMINOLOGY

Definitions

- Injury to lung parenchyma secondary to blunt or penetrating trauma
- Typically a combination of contusion, hemorrhage, & laceration
- **Contusion**: Torn capillaries & small blood vessels without frank disruption of alveoli
  - Marker of severe kinetic energy absorption; not simply a "lung bruise"
- **Laceration**: Disruption of alveoli leading to radial parenchymal retraction
  - **Blunt trauma**: Linear tear produces spherical hole in lung parenchyma
  - **Penetrating trauma**: Laceration conforms to path of penetrating object, commonly bullets & knives
  - Typically filled with variable amounts of air & blood
    - **Pulmonary hematoma**: Blood-filled laceration
    - **Pneumatocele**: Air-filled laceration

IMAGING

General Features

- Best diagnostic clue
  - **Contusion**: Peripheral airspace disease with adjacent acute rib fractures
    - Does not conform to normal lobar or segmental anatomic distribution
  - **Laceration**: Air-fluid level within complex cystic space surrounded by alveolar hemorrhage
- Location
  - **Contusion** occurs **at point of energy absorption**
    - Commonly peripheral lower lung, away from overlying chest wall musculature
    - Contusions do not respect anatomic boundaries such as fissures
    - Contusions do not follow bronchovascular distribution
    - Bilateral; rarely contrecoup contusions
  - **Laceration** occurs in 4 distinct locations depending on mechanism of injury
    - Laceration **conforms to track of penetrating object**
    - Small **peripheral lacerations** result from **rib fractures**
    - Large central pulmonary lacerations occur after forced chest compression against a closed glottis
    - Paravertebral lacerations occur as shearing injuries
      - Lung is squeezed over spine during anterior/ posterior compression
- Size
  - **Contusion**: Small (< 1 cm) to massive (whole lung) depending on extent of injury
    - Larger contusions can cause profound hypoxia
  - **Laceration**: Variable size; from < 1 cm up to 20 cm
    - Can be multiple & bilateral after blunt trauma
- Morphology
  - Blunt trauma: Lacerations are roughly spherical; may be multiloculated or complex in appearance
  - Penetrating trauma: Laceration conforms to path of penetrating object
  - Contusions typically involve lung periphery in a rim-like distribution

Radiographic Findings

- Radiography
  - Contusions & lacerations may be obscured by chest wall hematoma, atelectasis, pneumothorax, hemothorax
    - Become more apparent as other confounding abnormalities clear, heal, or are otherwise treated
  - Variable radiographic appearance over time
  - Initial radiographs: Usually **nonspecific patchy airspace disease**
    - History of trauma of paramount importance for accurate diagnosis
    - Usually detected within 6 hours of blunt trauma
    - Can be focal or diffuse, mimicking diffuse lung injury
  - Irregular patchy areas of airspace consolidation (mild)
  - Diffuse extensive homogeneous consolidation (severe)
  - Perihilar increased interstitial markings
    - Hemorrhage & edema in peribronchovascular interstitium
  - Contusions typically clear within 1st few days of injury
    - Complete clearance within 14 days
    - Exception is interval development of acute respiratory distress syndrome (ARDS)
    - Hematomas may appear as spiculated lung masses as they heal, mimicking malignancy
      - Sometimes called vanishing lung tumors
  - Lacerations present at time of initial injury
    - May not become apparent for hours or even days
    - May be obscured by surrounding atelectasis, contusion, & hemorrhage
    - Appearance may change over days to weeks: Initially air-filled but becoming blood-filled or vice versa
    - Heal over several weeks resulting in minimal fibrosis

CT Findings

- CECT
  - More sensitive than radiography for characterization of pulmonary parenchymal injuries & coexisting trauma to mediastinum & chest wall
  - **Contusion**: Spectrum of findings ranging from patchy ground-glass opacity in mild injury to diffuse consolidation in severe injury
  - **Laceration**: Cystic lung lesions that may contain air-fluid levels; often surrounded by contusion & hemorrhage
  - **Hematoma**
    - Slight increased attenuation centrally
    - Enhancing rim
    - May be confused with lung nodule or mass
  - Hemopneumothorax, especially from type 3 injury

Imaging Recommendations

- Best imaging tool
  - CT is imaging modality of choice for initial assessment of lung injury in trauma
  - Chest radiography usually sufficient to follow course of blunt trauma
- Protocol advice
  - IV contrast useful in trauma patients for assessment of mediastinal & vascular injury

PULMONARY CONTUSION/LACERATION

DIFFERENTIAL DIAGNOSIS

Aspiration

- May be superimposed on contusion in patients with loss of consciousness
- Follows bronchovascular distribution; perihilar predominant rather than peripheral

Pneumonia

- May mimic contusion radiographically; develops later in hospital course
- If contusion worsens after 48 hours, consider superinfection
- Lacerations rarely become secondarily infected; should not be confused with a lung abscess

Lung Abscess

- Nontraumatic clinical scenario

PATHOLOGY

General Features

- Etiology
  - Sudden deceleration results in tearing of capillaries & small blood vessels: Blood pooling & edema
  - Direct lung impaction or impalement (fractured rib)

Staging, Grading, & Classification

- CT staging of pulmonary lacerations
  - **Type 1**: Central location; shearing forces between lung & central airways (most frequent type)
  - **Type 2**: Lower lobes suddenly compressed against vertebral bodies
  - **Type 3**: Small, round, peripherally located; usually adjacent to rib fracture
  - **Type 4**: Shear forces on pleural adhesions tear lung with chest wall compression

Gross Pathologic & Surgical Features

- Airspaces filled with blood

Microscopic Features

- Tearing of capillaries without frank alveolar disruption

CLINICAL ISSUES

Presentation

- Most common signs/symptoms
  - Nonspecific dyspnea, chest pain
- Other signs/symptoms
  - Hemoptysis
  - Respiratory distress & hemodynamic instability in severe cases

Demographics

- Age
  - Young adult men suffer blunt chest trauma more commonly than other demographic groups
- Gender
  - M > F
- Epidemiology
  - Contusion: **Most common pulmonary injury** from blunt thoracic trauma
    - 30-70% of blunt chest trauma

Natural History & Prognosis

- Contusions typically clear without residua within 14 days unless there is superimposed ARDS or infection
- Lacerations take longer to clear (several weeks) & can leave residual scarring
- Extent of pulmonary parenchymal injuries plays a pivotal role in determining mortality
  - > 20% of pulmonary contusions at initial evaluation can be predicted to progress to ARDS with 90% specificity

Treatment

- Supportive therapy, surveillance for other major organ injuries or complications
- Severe contusions can lead to profound hypoxia requiring mechanical ventilation
  - Lung injury with flail chest requires prolonged mechanical ventilation
- Severe lacerations with massive hemorrhage may require lobectomy
  - Pulmonary vein laceration, potential for systemic air embolism
- Video-assisted thoracic surgery (VATS) is gaining acceptance as safe effective option to manage thoracic traumatic injuries

DIAGNOSTIC CHECKLIST

Consider

- Contusions & lacerations are common injuries following blunt & penetrating thoracic trauma

Image Interpretation Pearls

- CT more sensitive than radiography in detecting contusion & laceration
- CT allows expeditious assessment of coexisting chest wall & mediastinal injuries

Reporting Tips

- Suggest superinfection or aspiration if findings progress 2 days after trauma

SELECTED REFERENCES

1. Ahmed N et al: Role of early thoracoscopy for management of penetrating wounds of the chest. Am Surg. 76(11):1236-9, 2010
2. Nishiumi N et al: Diagnosis and treatment of deep pulmonary laceration with intrathoracic hemorrhage from blunt trauma. Ann Thorac Surg. 89(1):232-8, 2010
3. Sangster GP et al: Blunt traumatic injuries of the lung parenchyma, pleura, thoracic wall, and intrathoracic airways: multidetector computer tomography imaging findings. Emerg Radiol. 14(5):297-310, 2007
4. Mirvis SE: Diagnostic imaging of acute thoracic injury. Semin Ultrasound CT MR. 25(2):156-79, 2004
5. Mullinix AJ et al: Multidetector computed tomography and blunt thoracoabdominal trauma. J Comput Assist Tomogr. 28 Suppl 1:S20-7, 2004
6. Shanmuganathan K: Multi-detector row CT imaging of blunt abdominal trauma. Semin Ultrasound CT MR. 25(2):180-204, 2004

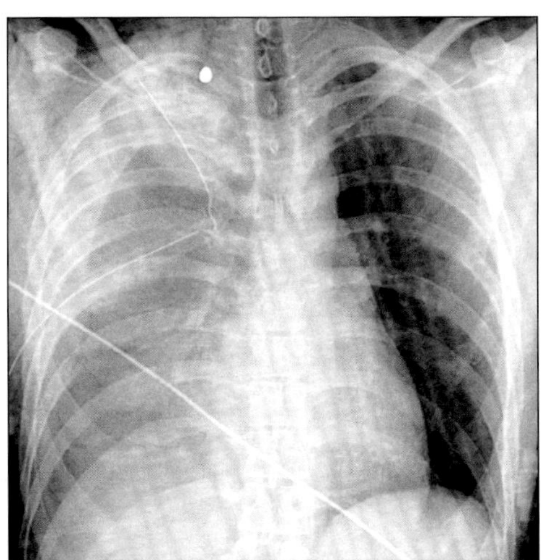

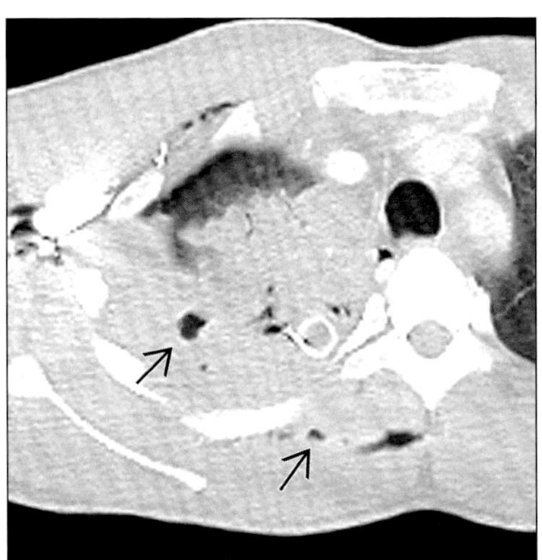

(Left) *AP chest radiograph of a 19-year-old man who sustained a gunshot wound to the chest shows a bullet overlying the right apex, a right hemothorax, and right lung airspace disease most pronounced at the right apex.* ***(Right)*** *Axial CECT of the same patient obtained 1 hour later shows diffuse pulmonary contusion in the bullet's path, which can be inferred by the tangential course of subcutaneous gas and lung laceration →. The bullet was within the right paraspinal musculature.*

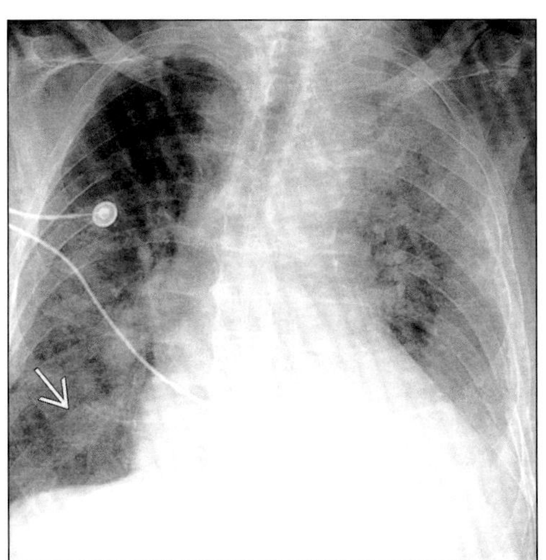

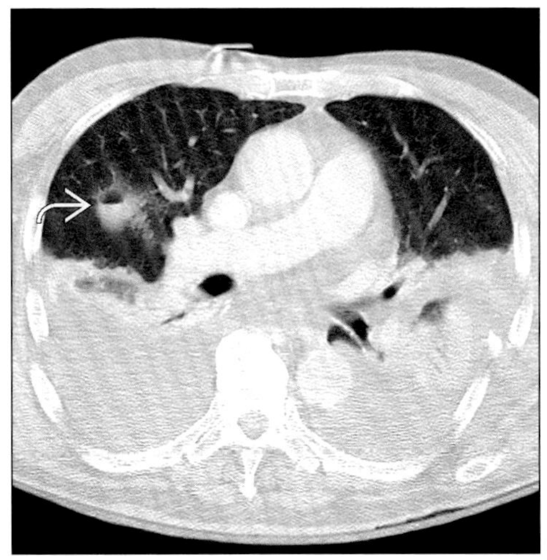

(Left) *AP chest radiograph of an 86-year-old man who sustained a fall shows a focal round opacity → in the right lower lung zone and multiple bilateral rib fractures. Note increased opacity throughout the left hemithorax, consistent with a posteriorly layering pleural effusion.* ***(Right)*** *Axial CECT of the same patient shows a right upper lobe laceration ↷ with an air-fluid level, bilateral hemothoraces, and rib fractures. The patient required mechanical ventilation and died soon after.*

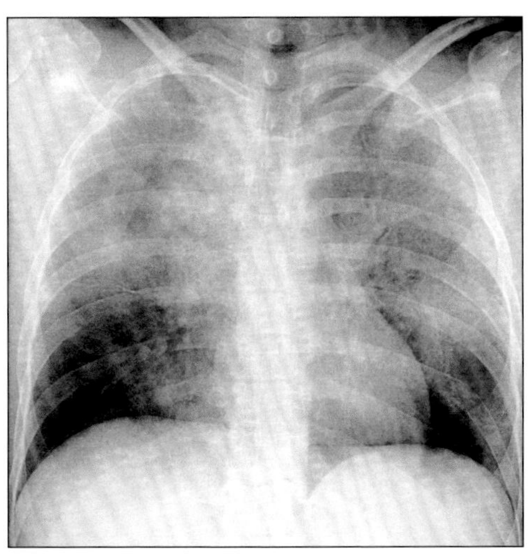

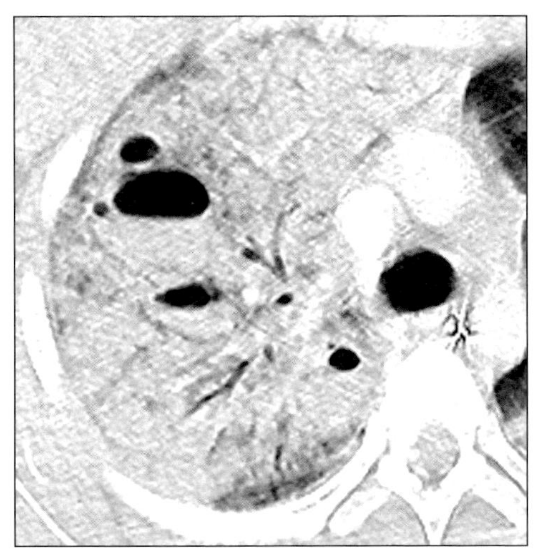

(Left) *AP chest radiograph of a 22-year-old man involved in a motorcycle crash shows bilateral patchy airspace disease involving the mid and upper lung zones.* ***(Right)*** *Axial CECT of the same patient shows diffuse right lung contusion manifesting with consolidation and several pulmonary lacerations, some of which exhibit air-fluid levels. Traumatic lung injury is often underestimated on radiography, and CT is the imaging modality of choice to determine the extent and severity of injury.*

PNEUMOMEDIASTINUM

Key Facts

Terminology
- Air within mediastinum
  - Spontaneous: Alveolar rupture and air dissection from pulmonary interstitium
  - Traumatic: Tracheobronchial/esophageal tear

Imaging
- Radiography
  - Air anterior and posterior to heart
  - Air surrounds/outlines mediastinal structures
  - Air dissects superiorly into neck subcutaneous tissues
  - Usually more conspicuous on lateral radiograph
- CT
  - More sensitive than radiography
  - Direct visualization of mediastinal air
  - Evaluation of tracheobronchial/esophageal rupture
  - Exclusion of tension pneumomediastinum

Top Differential Diagnoses
- Pneumothorax
- Pneumopericardium
- Artifact
- Air-distended esophagus
- Paratracheal air cyst
- Mediastinitis

Pathology
- High intrathoracic pressures
- Trauma; occurs in 10% of blunt chest trauma

Clinical Issues
- Signs/ symptoms
  - Chest &/or neck pain (50-90%)
  - Cough &/or dyspnea
- Pneumomediastinum is typically benign; clinical history for exclusion of occult disease/injury

__(Left)__ PA chest radiograph of a patient with spontaneous pneumomediastinum shows linear lucencies ➙ within the mediastinum and lucent lines ➙ outlining the left subclavian artery that demonstrate the tubular artery sign. __(Right)__ Lateral chest radiograph of the same patient shows air in the anterior mediastinum ➙ and surrounding the right pulmonary artery ➙, known as the ring-around-the-artery sign. Pneumomediastinum is often easier to detect on lateral chest radiography.

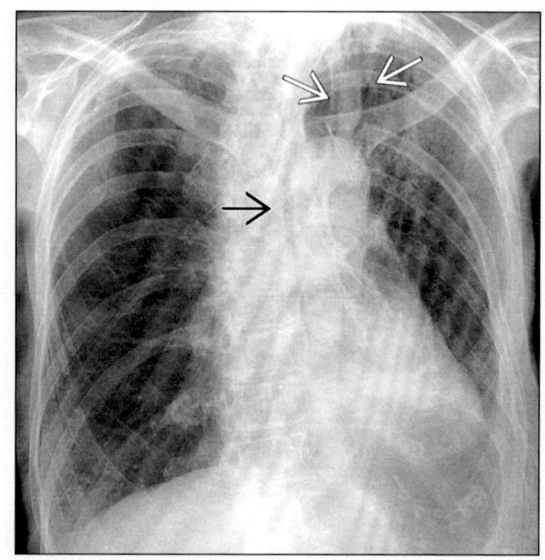

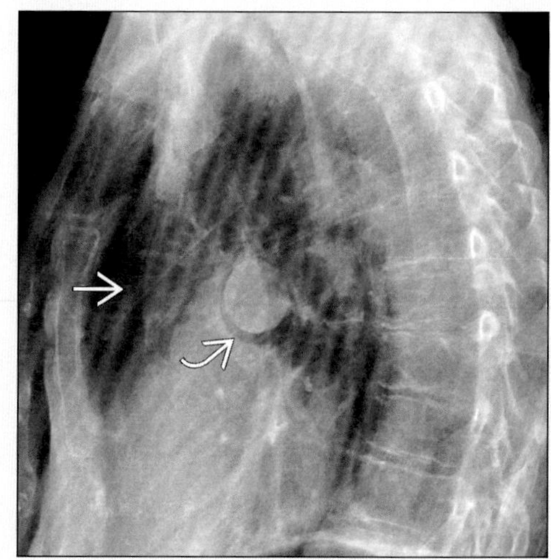

__(Left)__ Composite image with coronal (left) and sagittal (right) reformatted CT images of the same patient shows air surrounding the left subclavian artery ➙ and encircling the right pulmonary artery ➙. CT is more sensitive than radiography for detecting air within the mediastinum. __(Right)__ Axial CECT of a patient with chest trauma and bronchial injury ➙ leading to pneumomediastinum shows pulmonary interstitial emphysema ➙ and extensive chest wall subcutaneous gas.

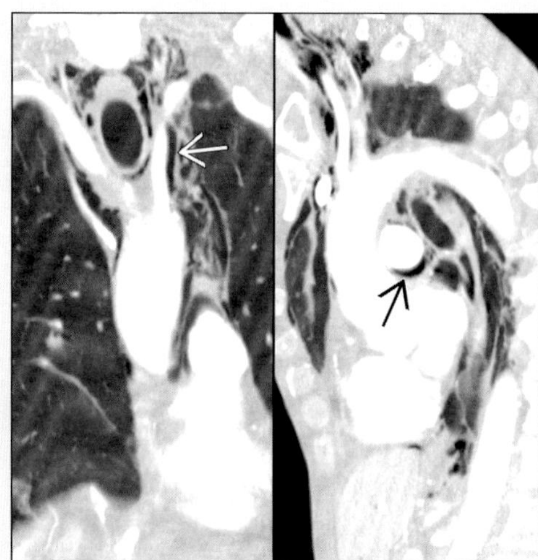

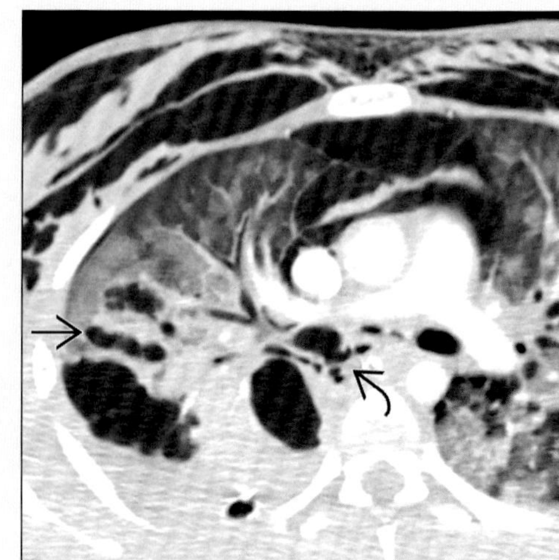

PNEUMOMEDIASTINUM

TERMINOLOGY

Synonyms

- Mediastinal "emphysema"

Definitions

- Air within mediastinum
  - **Spontaneous**: Usually secondary to **Macklin effect**
    - Alveolar rupture leads to air dissecting along axial interstitium and into mediastinum
  - **Traumatic**: Tracheobronchial/esophageal tear

IMAGING

General Features

- Best diagnostic clue
  - Air outlining heart & mediastinal structures associated with supraclavicular subcutaneous air
    - Usually more conspicuous on lateral view
- Location
  - Spontaneous: Air usually cephalad to carina
  - Esophageal tear: Air usually in paraesophageal location at level of diaphragm
- Size
  - Progressive pneumomediastinum suggests visceral injury to trachea or esophagus
- Morphology
  - Thin, linear air streaks within mediastinal contours

Radiographic Findings

- Air anterior & posterior to heart
- Air surrounds/outlines mediastinal structures
  - Aorta & major arteries
  - Trachea & central airways
  - Mediastinal parietal pleura may appear as a line
- Air dissects superiorly into neck & subcutaneous tissues, inferiorly into retroperitoneum/peritoneum
  - Air in neck soft tissues may be easier to detect than air in mediastinum
- Pulmonary interstitial emphysema (**PIE**)
  - Septal air, subtle, often unrecognized
  - Intrapulmonary or subpleural air cysts; usually < 5 mm but may also be large
  - Air cysts increase risk of pneumothorax
  - Linear nonbranching & mottled lucencies
  - Perivascular halos
- Signs of pneumomediastinum
  - **Interstitial air**
    - Double bronchial wall; air on both sides of airway wall
  - Perivascular air
    - **Ring around artery sign**; air surrounding artery or vein seen en face
    - **Tubular artery sign**; air surrounding vessel along its length
  - Subcutaneous air in neck &/or chest wall
  - **Continuous diaphragm sign**: Air outlining inferior aspect of heart above diaphragm
    - May mimic pneumoperitoneum
  - **Naclerio V sign**
    - Paravertebral air adjacent to left hemidiaphragm & descending aorta, suspicious for esophageal tear
  - **Spinnaker sail sign**
    - Elevation of thymic lobes in pediatric patients
- Signs suggestive of tracheobronchial or esophageal rupture
  - Persistent or progressive pneumomediastinum
  - Pleural effusions, rare with spontaneous pneumomediastinum
  - Esophageal tear; air preferentially collects around esophagus near diaphragm

CT Findings

- CT more sensitive than chest radiography
- Direct visualization of mediastinal air
- Pneumomediastinum
  - Air within mediastinal fat & in connective tissue sheaths around tubular structures: Trachea, pulmonary arteries, other central arteries & veins
  - Dominant paraesophageal gas at gastroesophageal junction suggests esophageal tear
- **Pulmonary interstitial emphysema (PIE)**
  - Air within pulmonary interstitium
  - Air surrounding arteries, veins, &/or airways
- Tracheobronchial or esophageal rupture site may not be visible
- Tension pneumopericardium or pneumomediastinum
  - Compression of superior vena cava, right ventricle
  - Dilatation of inferior vena cava &/or hepatic veins

Imaging Recommendations

- Best imaging tool
  - Chest radiography is usually diagnostic
    - Lateral radiograph usually more sensitive than frontal radiograph
  - CT is more sensitive than radiography
    - May be useful in evaluation of suspected tracheobronchial or esophageal tear
- Protocol advice
  - Consider esophagram to exclude clinically suspected esophageal perforation
  - Decubitus radiography: Pneumomediastinum air does not shift to nondependent position unlike in pneumothorax or pneumopericardium

DIFFERENTIAL DIAGNOSIS

Pneumothorax

- Air in pleural space; shifts on decubitus position
- Smooth pleural line; irregular pleural line in pneumomediastinum due to fascial tethering
- Apical air cap
  - Usually unilateral in pneumothorax
  - Pneumomediastinum; air may dissect extrapleurally over lung apex
    - Apical air caps from pneumomediastinum may be bilateral

Pneumopericardium

- Less common but similar pathophysiology; air tracks along pulmonary vessels into pericardium
- More common in infants than adults
- In adults, etiology is usually trauma
  - Penetrating injury, surgery, esophageal fistula, barotrauma
- Tension pneumopericardium may cause decreased cardiac output
- Key features of pneumopericardium
  - Air outlining left ventricle &/or right atrium

PNEUMOMEDIASTINUM

- Air in pericardial space; may shift on decubitus position
- Air does not extend above mid-ascending aorta
- Hydropneumopericardium may occur with concomitant pericardial effusion
- Small heart sign

Artifact

- Mach band
  - Definition: Perceived lucency at interface of soft tissue density & air density
  - Due to retinal inhibition at contrasting density interface
  - Common at heart borders & paraesophageal stripe
- Skin fold
  - Soft tissue fold may cause soft tissue edge with lucent Mach line & opposite faded margin
  - Nonanatomic course is a clue

Air-distended Esophagus

- Can mimic extraluminal mediastinal air
- Mimics of mediastinal or pericardial air
  - Achalasia, colonic interposition, hiatal hernia

Paratracheal Air Cyst

- Single or clustered small rounded air-filled cysts in right paratracheal region at thoracic inlet
- Usually not visible on radiography, but well-described appearance on CT

Mediastinitis

- Fever associated with mediastinal air raises suspicion for mediastinitis
- Low-grade fever may be present in pneumomediastinum

PATHOLOGY

General Features

- Etiology
  - High intrathoracic pressures
    - Mechanisms
      - Obstructive lung disease
      - Sustained Valsalva maneuver
      - Cough, vomiting, straining, weight lifting
      - Inhalational drug use
    - **Complicates 1-5% of asthma cases**
      - Mucous plugging & increased intra-alveolar pressure
  - Traumatic
    - Blunt chest trauma leads to pulmonary laceration & alveolar rupture
    - < 2% of cases secondary to tracheobronchial fracture
    - Esophageal rupture
    - Mechanical ventilation
  - Extrathoracic causes
    - Dental extraction, other head & neck surgeries
    - Sinus fracture
    - Pneumoperitoneum with extension into mediastinum; duodenal ulcer, diverticulitis
  - Barotrauma
  - May occur in up to 15% of patients with pulmonary fibrosis

CLINICAL ISSUES

Presentation

- Most common signs/symptoms
  - Chest &/or neck pain (50-90%)
  - Cough &/or dyspnea
  - Subcutaneous air; palpable crepitus
  - Dysphagia
  - **Hamman sign**: Precordial systolic crepitations, diminished heart sounds
  - Mill wheel murmur (bruit de moulin): Succussion splash with metallic tinkle from pneumopericardium
- Other signs/symptoms
  - Decreased cardiac output may occur in tension pneumomediastinum or pneumopericardium (rare)

Demographics

- Age
  - Peak incidence; 20-40 years
- Gender
  - Slight male predominance
- Epidemiology
  - Blunt chest trauma, 10% have pneumomediastinum
  - **1 in 30,000** emergency department visits

Natural History & Prognosis

- **Benign course**; usually resolves in 7 days (4-14 days)
- Mortality rate > 50% in esophageal rupture following vomiting (Boerhaave syndrome)
- Pneumomediastinum & PIE can lead to pneumothorax
  - Pneumothorax does not lead to PIE or pneumomediastinum

Treatment

- Spontaneous pneumomediastinum: Observation for tension or pneumothorax
- Bronchoscopy or esophagram may be required if visceral injury suspected

DIAGNOSTIC CHECKLIST

Consider

- Inhalational drug use in patients with unexplained spontaneous pneumomediastinum
- Obstructive airway disease if pneumomediastinum associated with hyperinflated lungs
- Pneumomediastinum is typically benign; clinical history important to exclude occult condition

Image Interpretation Pearls

- Lateral radiography is more sensitive than frontal radiography for visualization of pneumomediastinum

SELECTED REFERENCES

1. Sakai M et al: Frequent cause of the Macklin effect in spontaneous pneumomediastinum: demonstration by multidetector-row computed tomography. J Comput Assist Tomogr. 30(1):92-4, 2006
2. Newcomb AE et al: Spontaneous pneumomediastinum: a benign curiosity or a significant problem? Chest. 128(5):3298-302, 2005
3. Zylak CM et al: Pneumomediastinum revisited. Radiographics. 20(4):1043-57, 2000

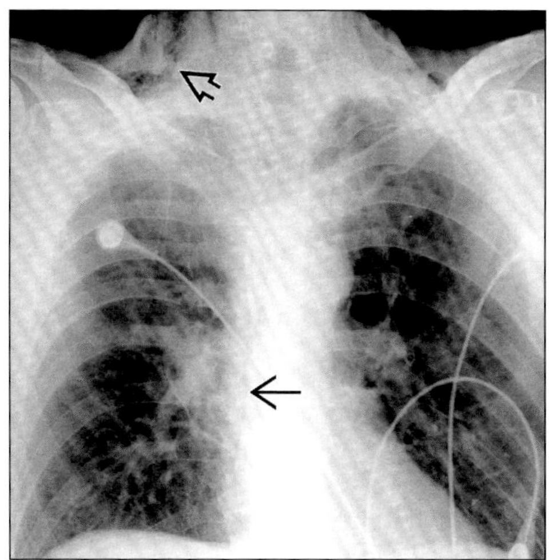

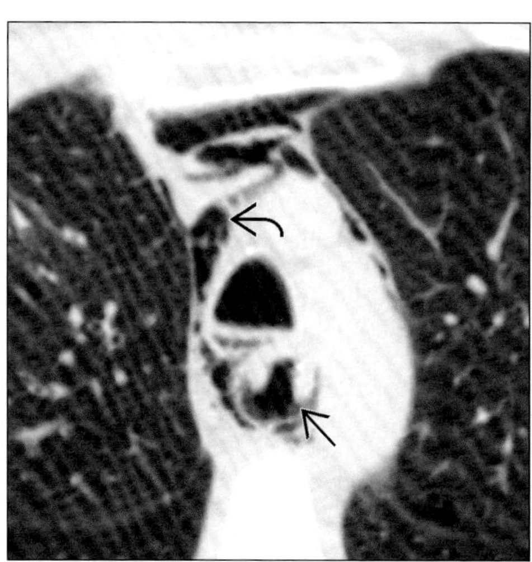

(Left) *AP chest radiograph of a patient with esophageal rupture status post esophageal dilatation for chronic stricture shows linear lucencies along the right heart border and gas within the soft tissues of the neck. Gas in the supraclavicular region is an important clue for suspecting subtle pneumomediastinum.* ***(Right)*** *Axial NECT of the same patient shows esophageal rupture and a pneumomediastinum. The esophageal defect is rarely visible on CT in patients with esophageal rupture.*

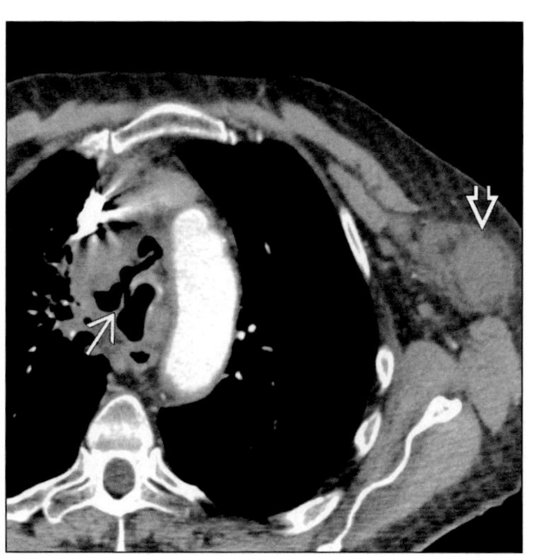

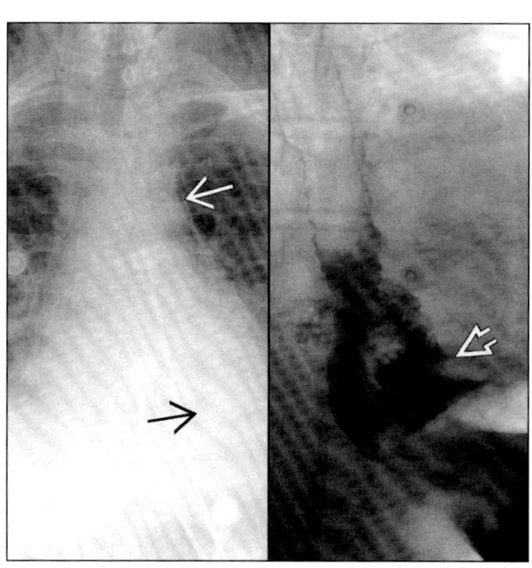

(Left) *Axial CECT of a patient with lymphoma shows a paratracheal mass eroding into the trachea, a pneumomediastinum, and a left axillary mass.* ***(Right)*** *Composite image with AP chest radiograph (left) and esophagram (right) of a patient with Boerhaave syndrome shows a pneumomediastinum manifesting with a linear lucency in the left superior mediastinum and retrocardiac gas. Esophagram confirms contrast leak.*

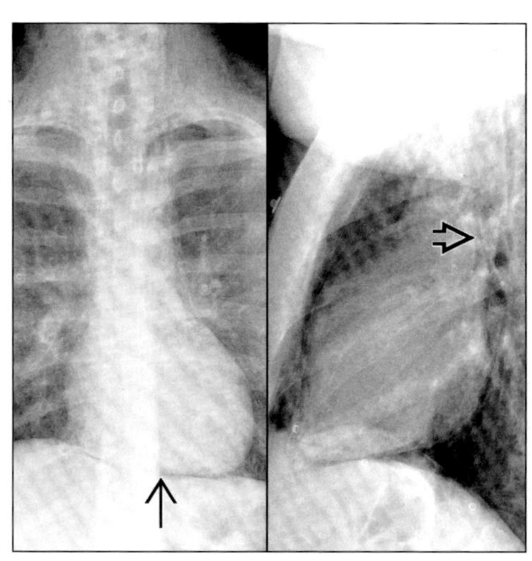

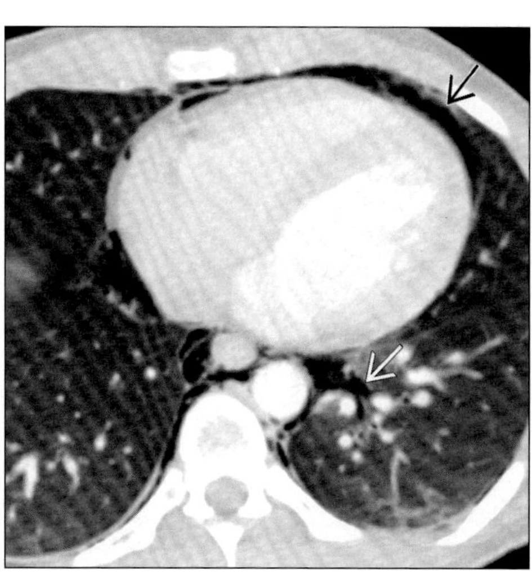

(Left) *Composite image with PA (left) and lateral (right) chest radiographs of a patient with a pneumomediastinum demonstrates lucency along the inferior mediastinum known as the continuous diaphragm sign. The lateral radiograph shows gas anterior to the trachea.* ***(Right)*** *Axial CECT of the same patient confirms a pneumomediastinum. Alveolar rupture leads to air dissection along the bronchovascular interstitium and into the mediastinum, known as the Macklin effect.*

TRAUMATIC AORTIC INJURY

Key Facts

Terminology

- Acute traumatic aortic injury (ATAI), blunt traumatic aortic rupture (BTAR), blunt aortic trauma (BAT), blunt aortic injury (BAI)
- Disruption or tear of aortic wall, usually from traumatic injury during motor vehicle collision (MVC), fall, or, less commonly, penetrating trauma

Imaging

- Radiography
  - Wide mediastinum: Hematoma, exclusion of TAI
  - 1st rib fracture: Severe trauma, possible TAI
- CTA: Imaging modality of choice
  - Aortic isthmus 90%; commonly on medial aspect
  - Aortic wall disruption or pseudoaneurysm
  - Irregular aortic contour
  - Sudden aortic caliber change
  - Sensitivity (98%), specificity (80%)

Top Differential Diagnoses

- Wide mediastinum of other etiology
- Ductus diverticulum (type III ductus)
- Fusiform enlargement proximal descending aorta
- Aortic spindle
- Atherosclerotic ulceration
- Infundibulum of bronchial-intercostal trunk

Clinical Issues

- No specific or sensitive signs or symptoms until hemodynamic instability ensues
- Urgent diagnosis; 50% die within 24 hours if untreated
- Cause of death in 20% of high-speed MVC
- Treatment
  - Surgical repair: 70-85% survival (up to 20% surgical mortality)
  - Endovascular stent graft repair gaining acceptance but limited long-term & complication data

*(**Left**) AP supine chest radiograph of a young man struck by a car while running across the highway shows widening of the superior mediastinum, a left apical cap, right tracheal/ETT and enteric tube deviation, thick paratracheal stripes, and loss of the aortic arch and the AP window. (**Right**) Axial CTA of the same patient shows active contrast extravasation ➔ from the ruptured descending aorta and a large mediastinal hematoma that produces mass effect on the esophagus, airways, and pulmonary arteries.*

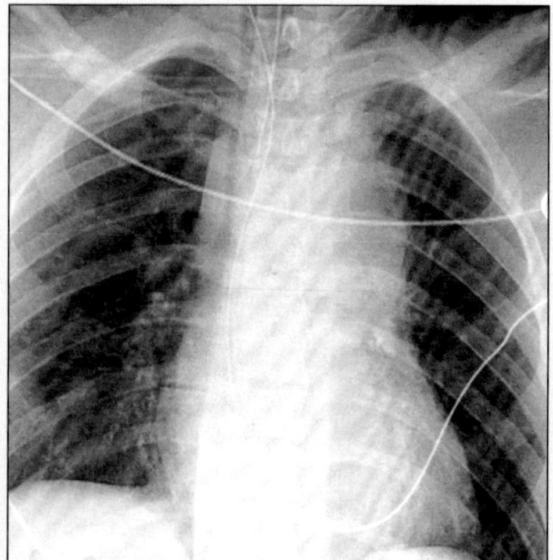

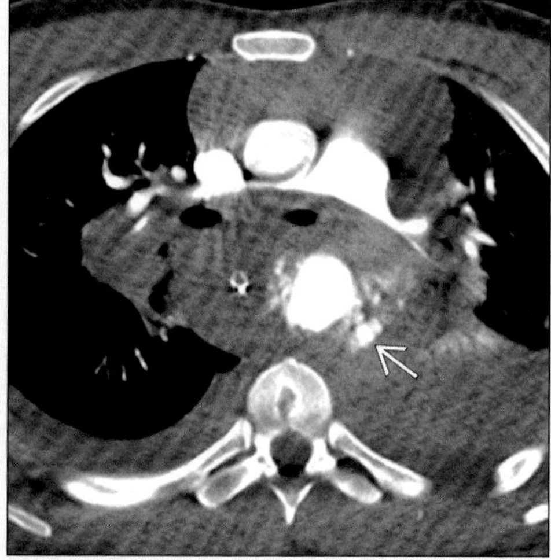

*(**Left**) Axial CTA of a 23-year-old man who sustained a stab wound to the anterior chest shows mediastinal hemorrhage and laceration ➔ of the anterior medial ascending aorta with adjacent intramural hematoma. (**Right**) Sagittal oblique aortogram following blunt chest trauma shows a large pseudoaneurysm ➔ at the aortic isthmus. CTA has largely replaced conventional angiography for the diagnosis of TAI but still plays an important role in TAI treatment with endovascular stent graft placement.*

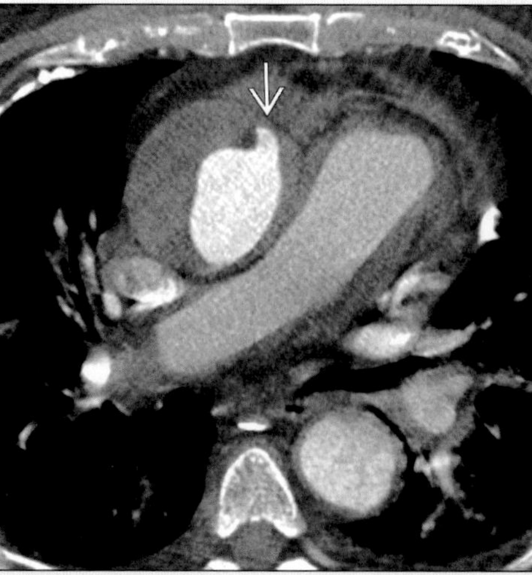

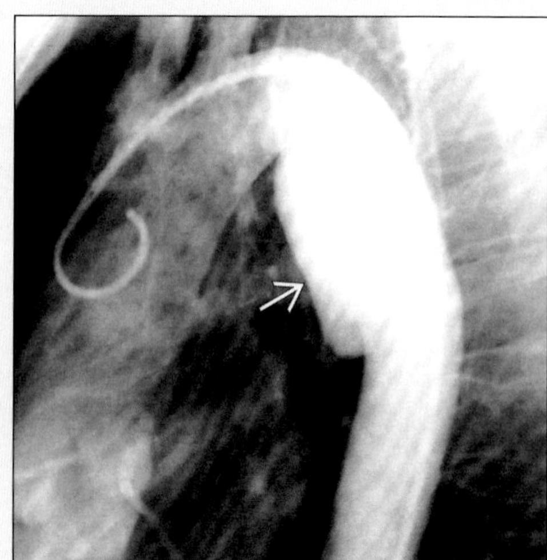

TRAUMATIC AORTIC INJURY

TERMINOLOGY

Abbreviations

- **Traumatic aortic injury (TAI)**

Synonyms

- **Acute traumatic aortic injury (ATAI)**
- Aortic transection
- **Blunt aortic injury (BAI)**
- **Blunt aortic trauma (BAT)**
- **Blunt traumatic aortic rupture (BTAR)**
- Traumatic aortic pseudoaneurysm

Definitions

- Disruption or tear of aortic wall, usually from traumatic injury during motor vehicle collision (MVC), fall, or, less commonly, penetrating trauma
  - Partial tear versus complete rupture

IMAGING

General Features

- Best diagnostic clue
  - **Widened mediastinum** on AP chest radiography
  - **Intimomedial flap** or **pseudoaneurysm** on CTA
- Location
  - **Aortic isthmus (90%)**; commonly along medial aspect at level of left pulmonary artery
  - Aortic root (5-14%); rare survival
  - Diaphragmatic hiatus (1-12%); may be associated with diaphragmatic injury
  - Multiple sites rarely affected

Radiographic Findings

- Radiography
  - Tear not visualized, identification of **indirect signs** related to mediastinal hemorrhage
  - Signs of TAI sensitive but not specific
  - Most signs present in 30-70% of patients
    - **Widened superior mediastinum** (> 8 cm or > 25% of transthoracic diameter)
    - **Abnormal aortic arch contour**
    - **Obscuration of AP window**
    - **Left apical cap**
    - **Right tracheal &/or ETT shift**
    - **Right enteric tube shift**
    - Wide paravertebral stripe
    - Wide right paratracheal stripe
    - Inferior displacement of left mainstem bronchus
  - 1st rib fracture indicates severe trauma & possibility of TAI
    - 1st rib protected by clavicle & scapula, requires considerable force to break
    - Frequency (15-30%)
  - Any of above signs requires further investigation to exclude aortic transection
  - Normal chest radiograph (7%)
  - Chronic pseudoaneurysm (2% of survivors)
    - Peripherally calcified mass at aorticopulmonary window

CT Findings

- NECT
  - Often shows mediastinal hematoma, rarely shows site of tear
- CTA
  - Imaging modality of choice
  - Direct visualization of aortic tear, markedly reducing need for aortography
  - **Direct signs**
    - **Intimomedial flap**
    - **Pseudoaneurysm or contained rupture**
    - **Irregular aortic contour**
    - **Sudden aortic caliber change**; pseudocoarctation
    - Rarely aortic dissection
    - Rarely active extravasation
  - Sensitivity (98%); specificity (80%)
  - **Indirect signs**
    - **Mediastinal hematoma**
  - **Minimal aortic injury**
    - **10%** of ATAI
    - Isolated involvement of aortic intima
    - Diagnosed with increasing frequency; likely because of improved spatial resolution of MDCT
    - May remain stable or resolve
  - Mimics of TAI
    - Pulsation or streak artifact
    - Atherosclerotic plaque
    - Ductus diverticulum
    - Opacified adjacent vessels: Bronchial artery, left superior intercostal vein, hemiazygous vein

MR Findings

- MR generally has no role in evaluation of acute trauma
  - Limited by issues related to transportation & monitoring of critically injured patients
  - Used to identify intramural hematoma in stable patients & for follow-up

Echocardiographic Findings

- Transesophageal echocardiography
  - Demonstration of intimal tear, transection
  - May be technically difficult in severely injured patients
  - Most commonly used intraoperatively when CT cannot be performed
  - Visualization of hemopericardium

Angiographic Findings

- Angiography
  - Previously considered gold standard for evaluating aorta & great vessels; sensitivity (100%), specificity (98%)
  - Using chest radiography as guide, 10 negative angiograms performed for each TAI diagnosed
  - Small risk of rupture

Imaging Recommendations

- Best imaging tool
  - **CTA is imaging modality of choice**
- Protocol advice
  - CTA with thin-section reconstructions, multiplanar reformations, and 3D volume rendering may be useful for treatment planning

DIFFERENTIAL DIAGNOSIS

Widened Mediastinum

- False-positives: Rotation, supine positioning, expiratory imaging, mediastinal fat

TRAUMATIC AORTIC INJURY

Ductus Diverticulum (Type III Ductus)

- Anteromedial outpouching of aortic isthmus
- Smooth, gently sloping shoulders
- No aortic intimomedial flap

Normal Variant: Fusiform Enlargement of Proximal Descending Aorta

- Similar to ductus diverticulum, no intimomedial flap

Atherosclerotic Ulceration

- Ulcerated plaque
- More common in older patients
- Other coexisting aortic plaques

Infundibulum of Bronchial-Intercostal Trunk

- Takeoff may show bump in aortic contour

PATHOLOGY

General Features

- Etiology: Theories of pathogenesis
  - Rapid deceleration injury with shearing forces greatest at levels of aortic immobility: Ligamentum arteriosum, aortic root, & diaphragmatic hiatus
  - Osseous pinch: Aorta compressed between anterior chest wall & spine; transverse tear at aortic isthmus
  - Water hammer effect: Marked increase in intravascular pressure during aortic compression; transverse tear at isthmus
  - Multivariate hypothesis likely: Shearing, torsion, stretching, hydrostatic forces

Gross Pathologic & Surgical Features

- 90% at aortic isthmus
  - From origin of left subclavian artery to ligamentum arteriosum, often anteromedially
- 7-8% ascending aorta; 2% descending aorta at diaphragmatic hiatus
- Ascending aortic tear: 20% of coroners' cases; rarely survive long enough to reach hospital
- Range: Intimal hemorrhage to complete transection
- Transverse tears: Segmental (55%) or circumferential (45%); partial (65%) or transmural (35%)
- Noncircumferential tears more common posteriorly
- May involve aortic layers to varying degrees
  - Survivors: Pseudoaneurysm usually contained by adventitia or, occasionally, mediastinal structures
  - Adventitial injuries occur in 40% & are almost always fatal due to rapid exsanguination

CLINICAL ISSUES

Presentation

- Most common signs/symptoms
  - No specific or sensitive signs or symptoms until hemodynamic instability ensues
  - May have chest pain or dyspnea
- Other signs/symptoms
  - Acute coarctation syndrome rare
    - Upper extremity hypertension
    - Decreased femoral pulses
- **Urgent diagnosis**, 50% expire within 24 hours if untreated
- Multiple associated injuries: Diaphragm rupture, lung contusion, rib fractures, head injury

Demographics

- Epidemiology
  - Cause of death in 20% of high-speed motor vehicle collisions

Natural History & Prognosis

- **85% die at site of trauma** (MVC)
- Survival depends on time from injury to intervention
- 2% long-term survival

Treatment

- Surgical repair
  - Delayed repair may be acceptable in many cases
  - Other injuries increase mortality of immediate repair
  - 70-85% surgical survival quoted (up to 20% surgical mortality)
  - Paraplegia 10%; directly related to cross-clamp time
    - Lower rates of paraplegia with techniques that integrate perfusion distal to clamped aorta
- Beta-adrenergic blocking agents decrease wall stress
- Endovascular stent graft repair
  - Less invasive than surgical repair
  - Feasible in patients with multiple comorbid injuries
  - Complete pseudoaneurysm resolution reported at 3 months
  - Technical success in excluding tear approaches 100%
  - Long-term efficacy & complication data are lacking
- Isolated injuries to intima (10%) may require no treatment & have been shown to resolve
  - Limited data on optimal management

DIAGNOSTIC CHECKLIST

Consider

- Careful evaluation of chest radiograph in trauma for indirect signs of aortic transection

Image Interpretation Pearls

- Consider chronic pseudoaneurysm in any patient with vascular calcification at aorticopulmonary window

SELECTED REFERENCES

1. Kaiser ML et al: Risk factors for traumatic injury findings on thoracic computed tomography among patients with blunt trauma having a normal chest radiograph. Arch Surg. 146(4):459-63, 2011
2. Berger FH et al: Acute aortic syndrome and blunt traumatic aortic injury: pictorial review of MDCT imaging. Eur J Radiol. 74(1):24-39, 2010
3. Kwolek CJ et al: Current management of traumatic thoracic aortic injury. Semin Vasc Surg. 23(4):215-20, 2010
4. Morgan TA et al: Acute traumatic aortic injuries: posttherapy multidetector CT findings. Radiographics. 30(4):851-67, 2010
5. Rojas CA et al: Mediastinal hematomas: aortic injury and beyond. J Comput Assist Tomogr. 33(2):218-24, 2009
6. Steenburg SD et al: Acute traumatic aortic injury: imaging evaluation and management. Radiology. 248(3):748-62, 2008

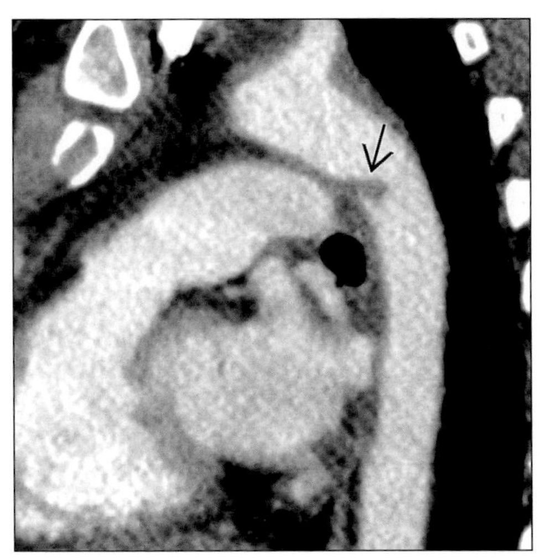

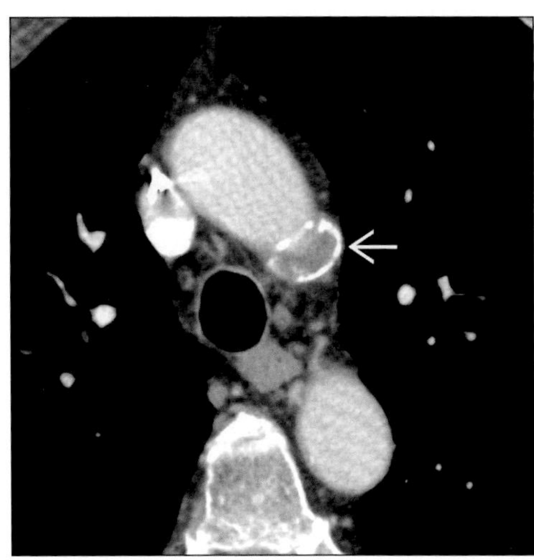

(Left) *Sagittal CECT of a patient involved in a motor vehicle collision shows a transverse segmental tear at the aortic isthmus ➡ without surrounding mediastinal hematoma. The patient had no additional chest injuries, was treated conservatively, and was followed annually with CT.* ***(Right)*** *Axial CTA of the same patient 5 years following trauma shows calcification and thrombus ➡ within a chronic posttraumatic aortic pseudoaneurysm.*

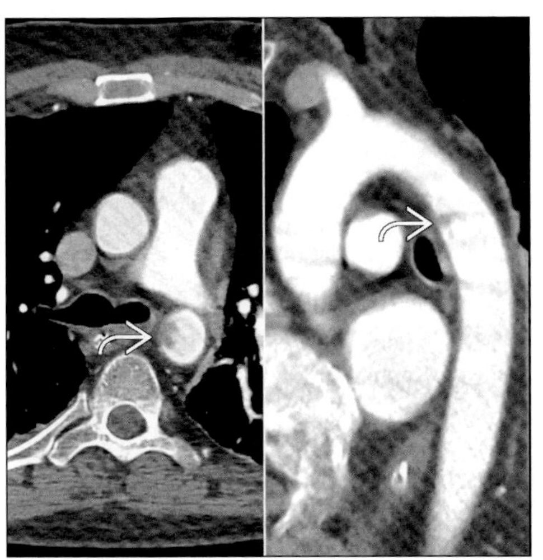

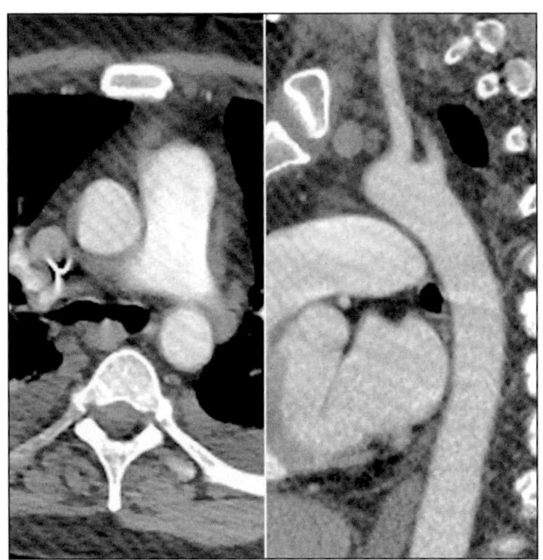

(Left) *Composite image with axial (left) and sagittal (right) CTA of a patient with blunt chest trauma shows a minimal aortic injury manifesting with a focal intimal flap ➡ in the descending aorta without mediastinal hemorrhage.* ***(Right)*** *Composite image with axial (left) and sagittal (right) CECT of the same patient 9 days later shows resolution of the aortic abnormalities. Although minimal aortic injuries are often observed and usually resolve, there is limited data on their optimal management.*

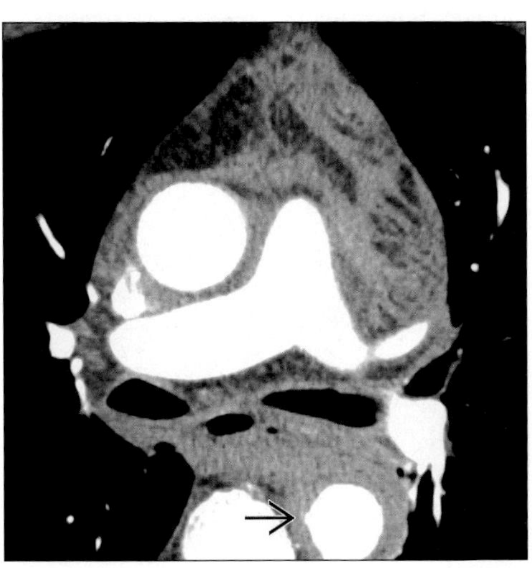

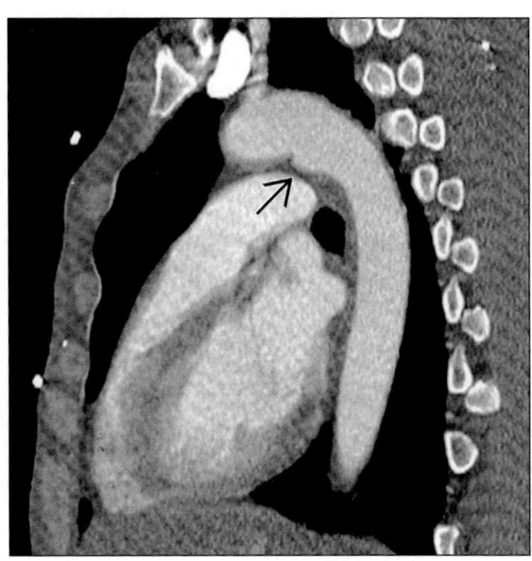

(Left) *Axial cardiac-gated CTA of an 18-year-old man following a motorcycle accident shows a mediastinal hematoma in the anterior mediastinum and around the descending thoracic aorta. Mild irregularity of the medial descending aortic wall ➡ represented a TAI.* ***(Right)*** *Sagittal NECT of a patient who sustained chest trauma shows a normal ductus bump ➡ that may mimic aortic transection. In this case there was no surrounding mediastinal hemorrhage, and there were no other significant injures.*

ESOPHAGEAL RUPTURE

Key Facts

Terminology

- Esophageal laceration/tear
- Boerhaave syndrome: Esophageal rupture after forceful emesis
- Mallory-Weiss tear: Partial thickness tear after forceful emesis

Imaging

- Radiography
  - Pneumomediastinum & subcutaneous gas (60%)
  - V sign of Naclerio: Left costovertebral angle gas
  - Bilateral pleural effusions (60%)
  - Hydropneumothorax (50%)
  - Consolidation or atelectasis adjacent to tear
- CT
  - Extraluminal oral contrast
  - Pneumomediastinum; acute mediastinitis
  - Pleural effusion or hydropneumothorax

Top Differential Diagnoses

- Mediastinal abscess
- Mediastinal hemorrhage
- Pneumomediastinum

Clinical Issues

- Sudden onset of substernal/lower thoracic chest pain
  - May mimic acute myocardial infarction, aortic dissection, perforated peptic ulcer
- Dysphagia, hemoptysis, hematemesis (50%)

Diagnostic Checklist

- Esophagography is procedure of choice for diagnosing of esophageal rupture
- Esophageal tear is often overlooked; diagnosis requires a high index of suspicion
- CT is optimal imaging modality for evaluation of mediastinal complications

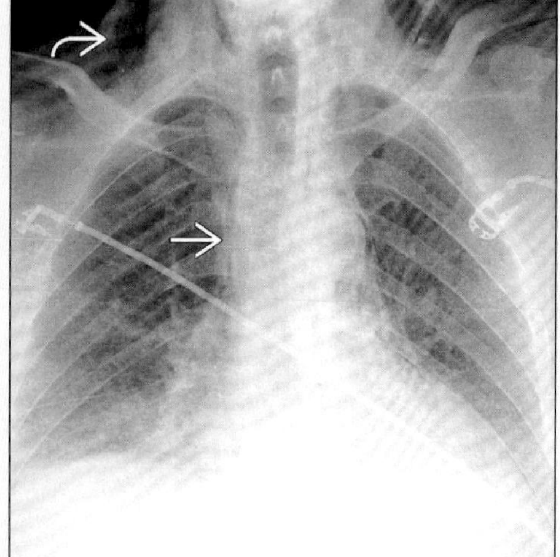

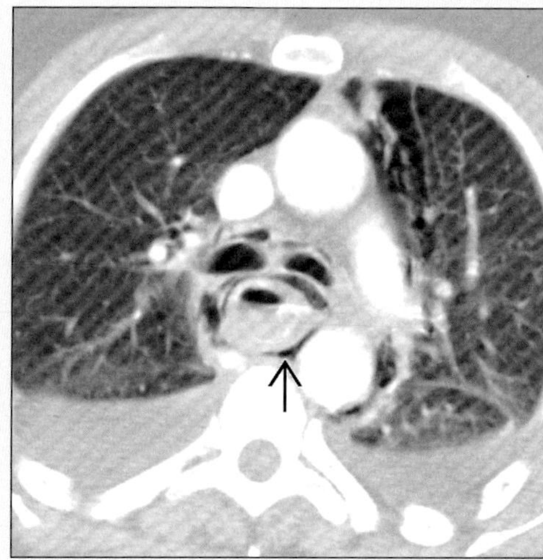

(Left) *AP chest radiograph of a patient with esophageal rupture shows pneumomediastinum ➔ and extensive subcutaneous gas ➔ in the supraclavicular regions. Note bilateral pleural effusions and associated relaxation atelectasis. The diagnosis of esophageal rupture requires a high index of suspicion.* ***(Right)*** *Axial CECT of the same patient shows pneumomediastinum with gas ➔ surrounding a dilated thickened esophagus. CT may not demonstrate the exact location of the esophageal tear.*

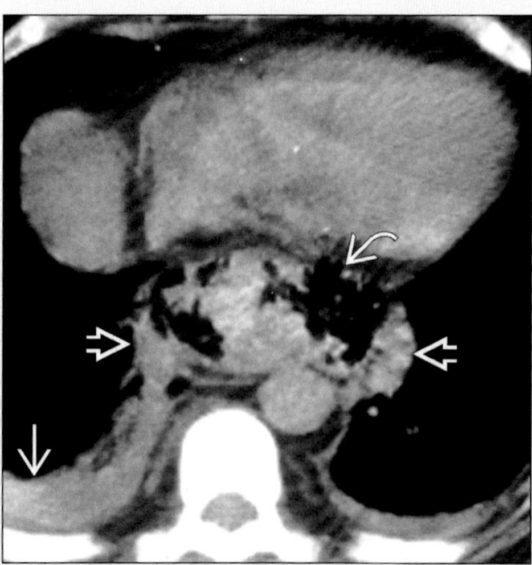

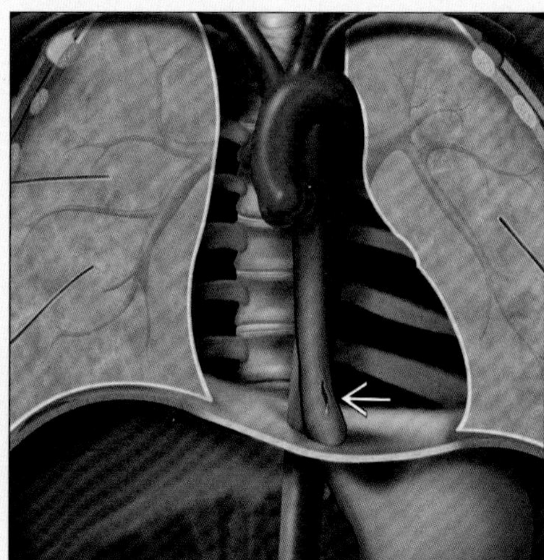

(Left) *Axial NECT of a patient with esophageal perforation after an alcoholic binge (Boerhaave syndrome) shows inferior mediastinal widening ➔, multiple extraluminal gas collections ➔, and bilateral pleural effusions ➔.* ***(Right)*** *Graphic shows the classic location of esophageal tear ➔ in Boerhaave syndrome. These vertically oriented tears are characteristically located in the left distal esophageal wall, approximately 2-3 cm proximal to the gastroesophageal (GE) junction.*

ESOPHAGEAL RUPTURE

TERMINOLOGY

Synonyms

- Esophageal tear
- Esophageal laceration

Definitions

- **Boerhaave syndrome**: Esophageal rupture after forceful emesis
- **Mallory-Weiss tear**: Partial thickness tear after forceful emesis

IMAGING

General Features

- Best diagnostic clue
  - High degree of suspicion in appropriate clinical scenario
- Morphology
  - Tear usually linear

Radiographic Findings

- Normal early (10%)
- **Pneumomediastinum** & **subcutaneous gas** (60%)
  - **V sign of Naclerio** (25%): Extraluminal air localized to left costovertebral angle
- **Bilateral pleural effusions** (60%)
- **Hydropneumothorax** (50%)
  - Mid or upper tear: Right hydropneumothorax (5%)
  - Distal tear: Left hydropneumothorax (75%)
- **Consolidation** or **atelectasis** adjacent to tear

Fluoroscopic Findings

- **Esophagram**: Detection/localization of esophageal tear
  - **Nonionic water-soluble contrast**: False-negative rate of (20%)
  - **Barium**: Improved detection of small leaks
  - **Gastrografin**: Risk of aspiration

CT Findings

- **Extraluminal oral contrast:** Does not show tear size; may not show tear site
- **Esophageal thickening:** Intramural hematoma, esophageal dissection
- **Pneumomediastinum:** Centered on esophagus (90%)
- **Acute mediastinitis:** Periesophageal fluid/gas, abscess
- **Pleural effusion/hydropneumothorax:** May progress with time

Imaging Recommendations

- Protocol advice
  - Esophagography is diagnostic procedure of choice
    - Initial assessment with nonionic water-soluble contrast
    - If no leak detected, barium esophagram
      - Barium may detect small leaks not initially visualized

DIFFERENTIAL DIAGNOSIS

Mediastinal Abscess

- Perforated esophageal neoplasm (carcinoma, lymphoma), esophagitis, foreign body, postsurgical

Mediastinal Hemorrhage

- Aortic dissection, aortic transection, blunt or penetrating trauma

Pneumomediastinum

- Bronchial fracture, esophageal fistula, asthma

CLINICAL ISSUES

Presentation

- Most common signs/symptoms
  - Sudden onset of **substernal/lower thoracic chest pain**
    - May mimic acute myocardial infarction, aortic dissection, perforated peptic ulcer
  - **Boerhaave syndrome**: Follows drinking & eating binge
    - **Mackler triad**: Vomiting, severe chest pain, subcutaneous gas (50%)
  - Dysphagia, hemoptysis, hematemesis (50%)

Demographics

- Epidemiology
  - **Iatrogenic** following endoscopic procedures
    - Esophagoscopy: 50%
    - Pneumatic dilatation (achalasia): 2-6%
  - **Postsurgical**
    - Esophageal surgery, biopsy
  - **Boerhaave syndrome**: 15% of esophageal ruptures
  - **Esophagitis**: Infectious, eosinophilic

Natural History & Prognosis

- Mortality rate directly related to time interval between perforation & treatment initiation
  - Untreated perforation, nearly 100% mortality rate (fulminant mediastinitis)
  - Intervention after 24 hours; 70% mortality rate

Treatment

- **Conservative**: Small tears
- **Surgical**: Large tears (within first 24 hours)
- **Percutaneous drainage**: Mediastinal abscess, fluid collection
- **Esophageal stent**: Used to bridge esophageal tear

DIAGNOSTIC CHECKLIST

Consider

- Esophageal rupture is often overlooked; must have high index of suspicion

Image Interpretation Pearls

- Radiographic V sign of Naclerio should prompt suspicion of esophageal tear
- CT: Not a substitute for esophagram
- CT: Optimal imaging modality for evaluation of mediastinal complications

SELECTED REFERENCES

1. Young CA et al: CT features of esophageal emergencies. Radiographics. 28(6):1541-53, 2008
2. Fadoo F et al: Helical CT esophagography for the evaluation of suspected esophageal perforation or rupture. AJR Am J Roentgenol. 182(5):1177-9, 2004

ESOPHAGEAL RUPTURE

(Left) *Axial NECT of a patient with sudden onset of chest pain and esophageal rupture demonstrates extraluminal gas surrounding the distal esophagus, bilateral pleural effusions, and a small left loculated hydropneumothorax . Left hydropneumothorax suggests a left-sided esophageal tear.* ***(Right)*** *Axial NECT of a patient with chest pain and a sticking sensation of food in the lower chest shows pneumomediastinum centered on the distal esophagus, consistent with esophageal tear or rupture.*

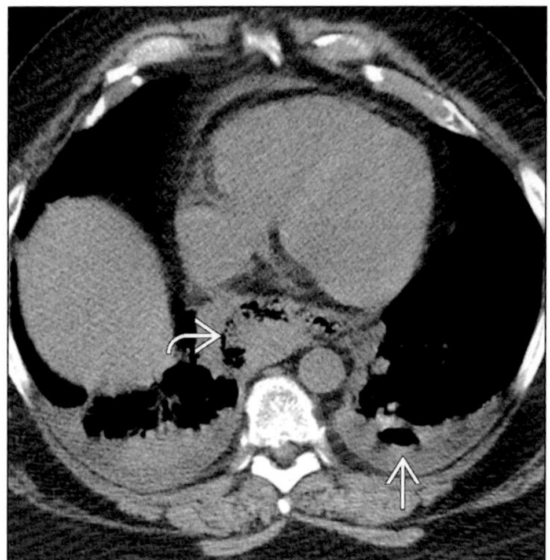

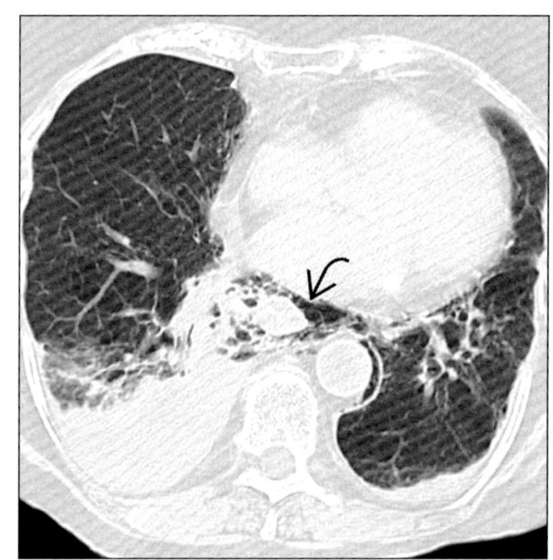

(Left) *AP chest radiograph of a patient with esophageal perforation shows a subtle pneumomediastinum and a linear gas collection at the right medial costodiaphragmatic recess. Similar extraluminal gas occurring on the left is known as the V sign of Naclerio.* ***(Right)*** *Esophagram of a patient with an iatrogenic right esophagopleural fistula shows a multilocular right basilar hydropneumothorax and extravasated contrast in the dependent right pleural space .*

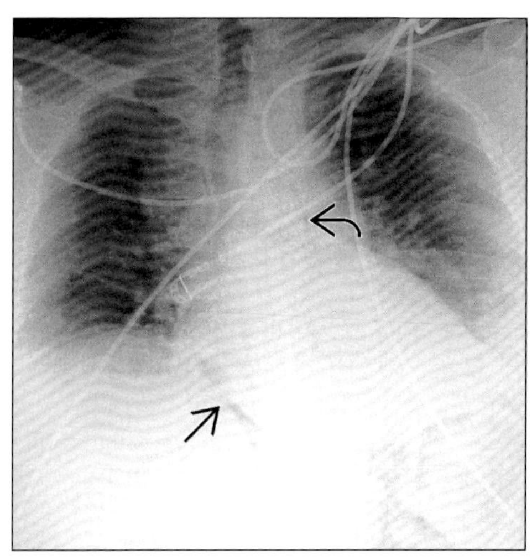

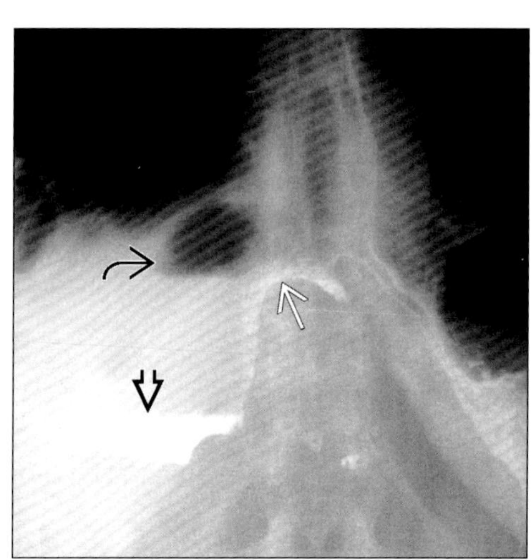

(Left) *Axial CECT of the same patient shows a multilocular right pneumothorax , right basilar relaxation atelectasis , and a communication between the mediastinum and the right pleural space .* ***(Right)*** *Axial CECT of the same patient shows a right basilar hydropneumothorax with contrast in the dependent right pleural space. Although CT is the imaging modality of choice for evaluating complications of esophageal perforation, it may not allow localization of the site of esophageal tear.*

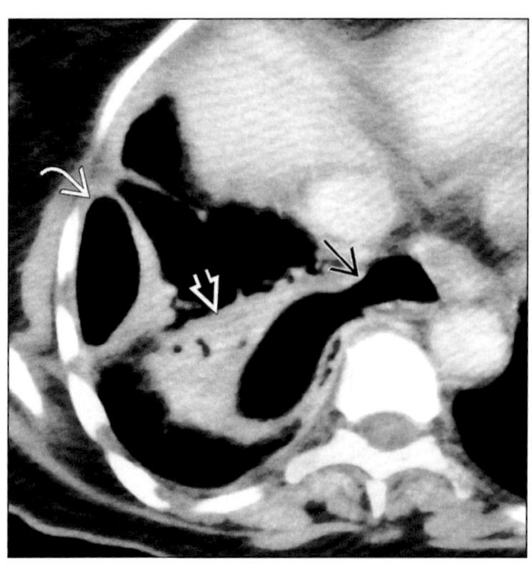

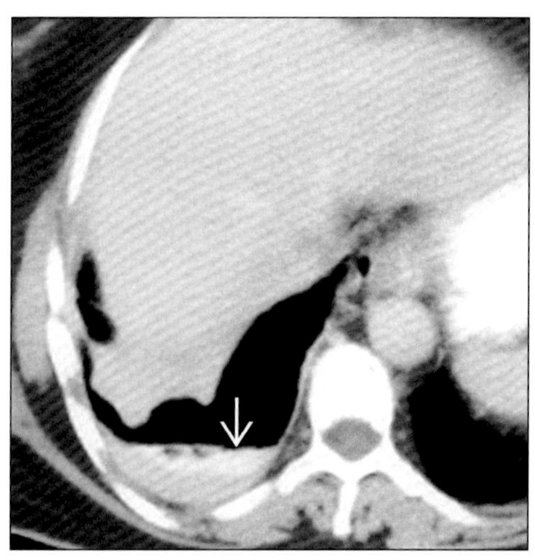

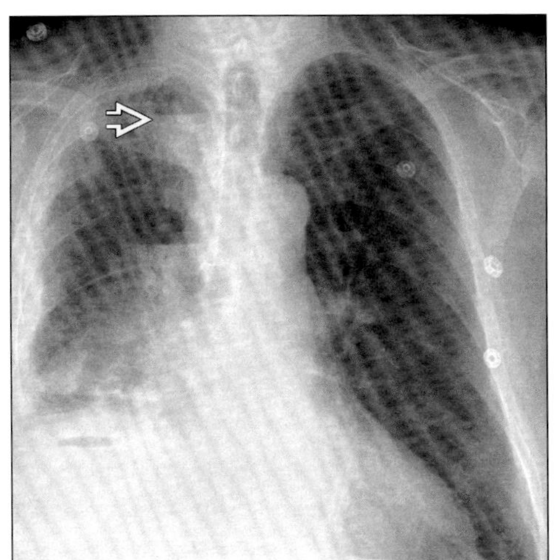

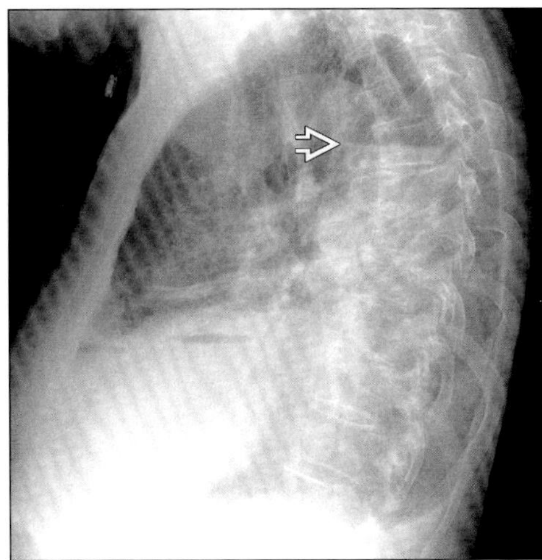

(Left) *PA chest radiograph of a patient with esophageal perforation shows a multilocular right hydropneumothorax with multiple air-fluid levels* ➲. **(Right)** *Lateral chest radiograph of the same patient shows a small left pleural effusion and multiple air-fluid levels* ➲ *associated with a loculated right pleural effusion. The findings suggest empyema with bronchopleural fistula. The diagnosis of esophageal perforation requires a high index of suspicion and careful review of the patient's history.*

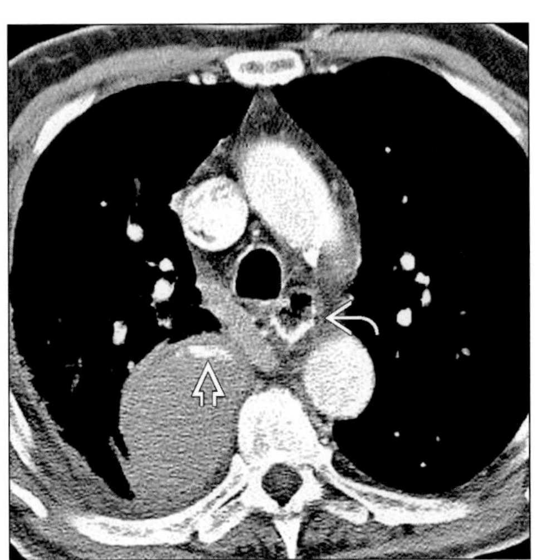

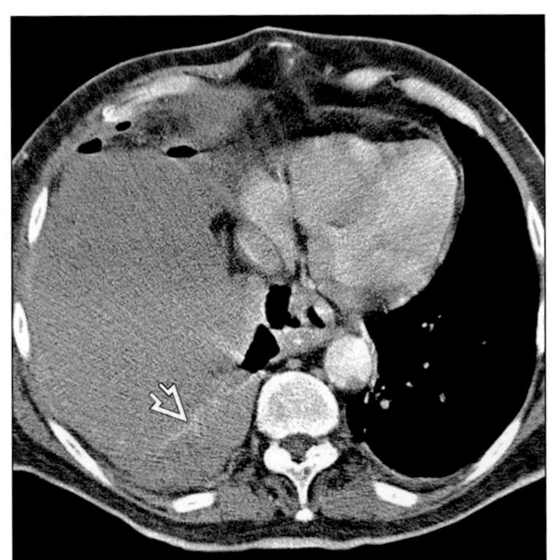

(Left) *Axial CECT of the same patient demonstrates a loculated right pleural effusion with enteric contrast* ➲ *in the pleural space and extraluminal contrast* ➲ *in the mediastinum, consistent with esophageal perforation.* **(Right)** *Axial CECT of the same patient shows the large loculated right hydropneumothorax and enteric contrast* ➲ *in the right pleural space. Pneumomediastinum centered about the right distal esophagus is consistent with esophageal tear.*

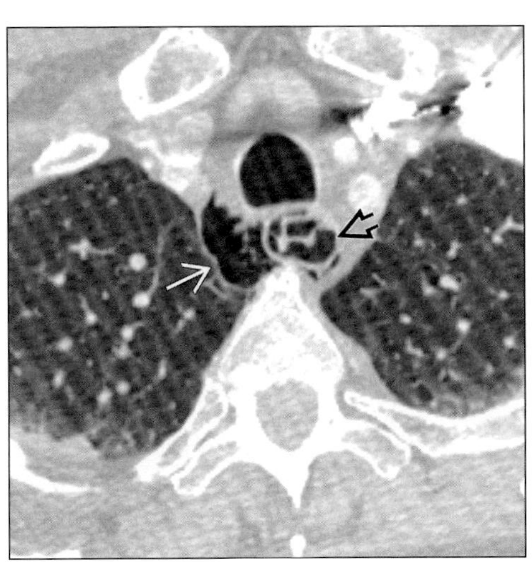

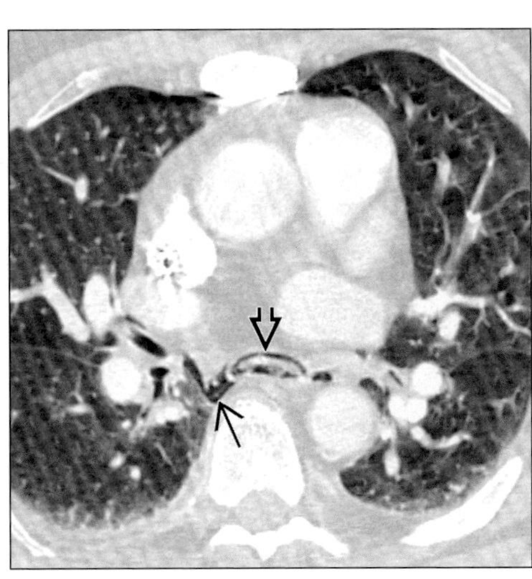

(Left) *Axial CECT of a patient with esophageal rupture shows pneumomediastinum* ➔ *and gas in the esophageal wall* ➲ *(pneumatosis).* **(Right)** *Axial CECT of the same patient shows pneumomediastinum* ➔ *and distal esophageal pneumatosis* ➲. *There are no mediastinal fluid collections or pleural effusions. Although this patient had an iatrogenic esophageal tear, she recovered with simple enteric tube drainage.*

THORACIC DUCT TEAR

Key Facts

Terminology

- Thoracic duct: Transports chyle from intestinal lacteals; typically drains into left subclavian vein
- Thoracic duct tear: Thoracic duct disruption
  - Cervical chylous fistula, chylothorax, chylopericardium, chylous ascites

Imaging

- Radiography
  - Unilateral or bilateral free pleural effusion
  - Effusion location depends on anatomic level of thoracic duct tear
  - Loculated pleural effusion
- CT
  - High sensitivity for identification of pleural fluid
  - Water attenuation; fat content obscured by high protein content of chylous effusion
- Lymphangiography; documentation of duct tear

Top Differential Diagnoses

- Other cause of chylothorax
  - Lymphangioleiomyomatosis
  - Malignancy
- Pleural effusion
- Pseudochylothorax or chyliform effusion

Pathology

- Whitish, creamy pleural fluid
- Fluid triglyceride level > 110 mg/dL
- Presence of chylomicrons
- Iatrogenic surgical injury is most common cause

Clinical Issues

- Dyspnea, nutritional deficiency
- Up to 50% mortality if untreated
- Conservative management: Drainage, low-fat diet
- High output leak: Thoracic duct ligation

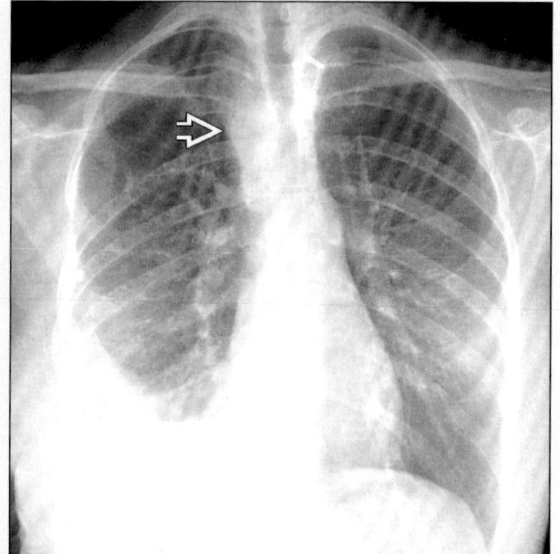

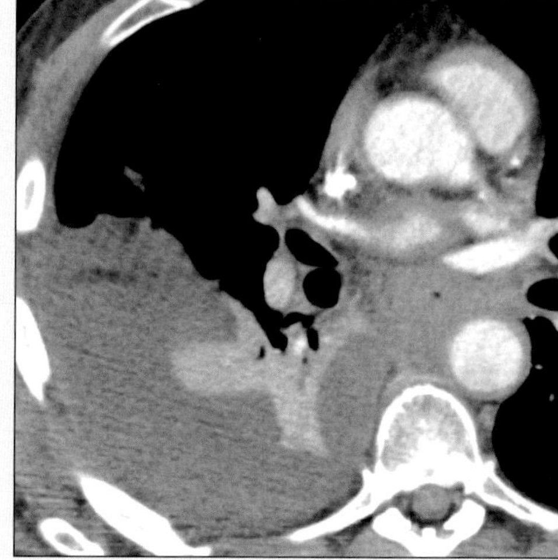

(Left) *PA chest radiograph of a patient with right-sided aortic arch ➲ and postsurgical ligation of a diverticulum of Kommerell with resultant thoracic duct injury shows a moderate right pleural effusion. Note surgical resection of right 4th rib.* ***(Right)*** *Axial CECT of a patient status post attempted esophagectomy and mediastinal lymph node dissection for esophageal cancer shows a moderate water attenuation chylous pleural effusion indistinguishable from simple pleural fluid.*

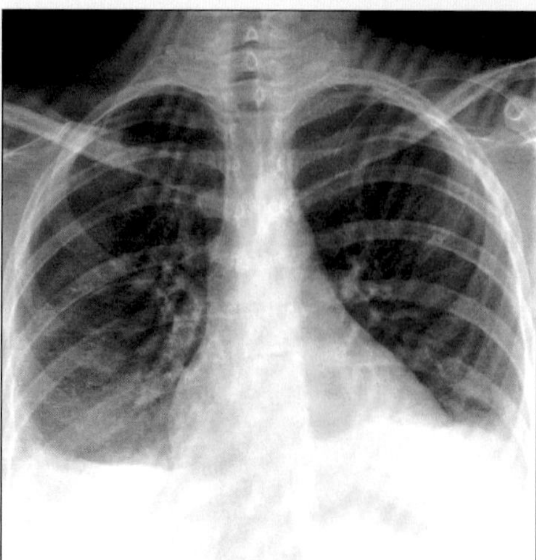

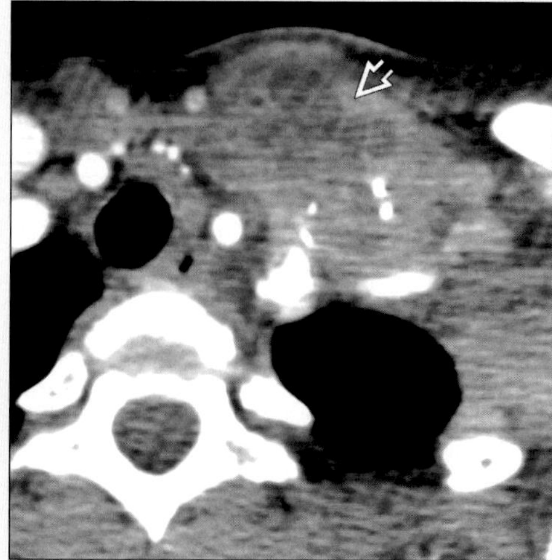

(Left) *PA chest radiograph of a patient who developed bilateral chylothoraces after surgical resection of the left 1st rib for thoracic outlet syndrome shows bilateral pleural effusions and basilar relaxation atelectasis. Chylous pleural effusions are indistinguishable from pleural effusions of other etiologies.* ***(Right)*** *Axial CECT of the same patient shows a left anterior chest wall and lower neck chyloma ➲ confirmed after fluid drainage. Thoracic duct ligation was performed.*

THORACIC DUCT TEAR

TERMINOLOGY

Definitions

- **Thoracic duct**: Transports chyle from intestinal lacteals; typically drains into left subclavian vein
- **Thoracic duct tear**: Thoracic duct disruption
  - Cervical chylous fistula, chylothorax, chylopericardium, chylous ascites

IMAGING

General Features

- Best diagnostic clue
  - **Chylous effusion** on thoracentesis
  - Milky fluid with **high triglyceride levels**
  - Recent trauma or cervical/thoracic surgery
- Location
  - Chylous effusion location depends on anatomic level of thoracic duct tear
  - **Right**
    - **Most common**
    - Thoracic duct tear in right mediastinum between hemidiaphragm & T5-T7 vertebrae
  - Left
    - Thoracic duct tear near aortic arch
  - Bilateral
    - Thoracic duct tear as it crosses midline from right to left at T5-T7 vertebrae
  - Chylous ascites
    - Injury to cisterna chyli; elongate subdiaphragmatic extension of thoracic duct in retrocrural space anterior to L1-L2 vertebrae, to right of upper abdominal aorta
- Morphology
  - Typically free pleural effusion

Radiographic Findings

- Unilateral or bilateral **free pleural effusion**
  - Blunt posterior &/or lateral costophrenic angles
  - Obscuration of ipsilateral hemidiaphragm
  - Opaque hemithorax from large pleural effusion
- Loculated pleural effusion

CT Findings

- High sensitivity for identification of pleural fluid
- Chylothorax indistinguishable from other types of pleural effusion on CT
- CT fluid attenuation
  - Low attenuation due to fat content of chylous effusion
  - Often of water attenuation; fat content obscured by high protein content of chylous effusion
- Identification & assessment of chyloma
  - Rare manifestation of thoracic duct tear
  - Complication of trauma or neck surgery
    - Most common in left neck (75%)
    - Assessment for signs of chylous fistula

Imaging Recommendations

- Best imaging tool
  - **Lymphangiography**: Documentation of duct tear; identification of exact tear location rarely necessary
  - CT useful to assess size of chylous effusion, loculation, associated spinal injury

DIFFERENTIAL DIAGNOSIS

Other Cause of Chylothorax

- Lymphangioleiomyomatosis: Diffuse thin-walled lung cysts; women of reproductive age
- Malignancy: Lymphoma, lung cancer, breast cancer

Pleural Effusion

- Indistinguishable from chylothorax based on imaging
- Requires thoracentesis for confirmation

Pseudochylothorax or Chyliform Effusion

- Chronic pleural effusion & thick/fibrotic pleura; prior tuberculosis, chronic rheumatoid pleuritis
- Production of cholesterol-rich milky pleural effusion; absence of chylomicrons

PATHOLOGY

General Features

- Etiology
  - **Thoracic duct injury: 25% of chylothoraces**
    - Iatrogenic surgical injury is most common cause
    - Complicates up to 4% of esophageal resections
    - Also: Cardiac surgery, pneumonectomy, lung transplant, spinal surgery, esophagoscopy
  - Nonsurgical causes: Trauma, childbirth, emesis
  - Thoracic duct rupture secondary to obstruction

Gross Pathologic & Surgical Features

- **Whitish, creamy pleural fluid**

Microscopic Features

- **Fluid triglyceride level > 110 mg/dL**
- **Presence of chylomicrons**
- Low serum albumin suggests malnourishment

CLINICAL ISSUES

Presentation

- Most common signs/symptoms
  - **Dyspnea, nutritional deficiency**
- Other signs/symptoms
  - Significant loss of lymphocytes & protein leads to immunosuppression

Natural History & Prognosis

- **Up to 50% mortality if untreated**

Treatment

- Conservative management: Drainage of neck wound or chylothorax; low fat diet, parenteral nutrition
- High output leak lasting > 7 days
  - Thoracic duct ligation

DIAGNOSTIC CHECKLIST

Consider

- Thoracic duct tear in patients with persistent pleural effusion following thoracic surgery

SELECTED REFERENCES

1. Euathrongchit J et al: Nonvascular mediastinal trauma. Radiol Clin North Am. 44(2):251-8, viii, 2006

TRAUMATIC PNEUMOTHORAX

Key Facts

Terminology

- Pneumothorax (PTX)
- Air in pleural space following blunt or penetrating trauma

Imaging

- Radiography
  - Visible visceral pleural line without peripheral lung markings
  - Supine radiography less sensitive, underestimates size; deep sulcus sign
  - Tension PTX: Contralateral mediastinal shift, flat ipsilateral hemidiaphragm, & hemodynamic compromise
- CT
  - Assessment of associated life-threatening injuries
  - Distinction of PTX from bullae or lung cysts

Top Differential Diagnoses

- Skin fold, scapula, hair, extraneous monitoring, or support devices
- Bullous emphysema
- Pneumomediastinum

Clinical Issues

- Chest pain, sudden dyspnea
- Tension PTX: Severe dyspnea, cyanosis, sweating, & tachycardia
- Observation & supplemental oxygen for small PTX
- Chest tube drainage for large/symptomatic PTX
- Size of PTX less important than patient's physiologic status

Diagnostic Checklist

- Report size & location of pleural separation in cases of traumatic pneumothorax

*(**Left**) PA chest radiograph of a 30-year-old man status post stab wound to the anterior left chest shows a large left pneumothorax, a moderate left pleural effusion (a presumed hemothorax), complete left lung atelectasis, and mediastinal mass effect related to tension pneumothorax. (**Right**) Lateral chest radiograph of the same patient shows a large left hemopneumothorax. After emergent chest tube placement, the patient underwent repair of a lacerated internal mammary artery.*

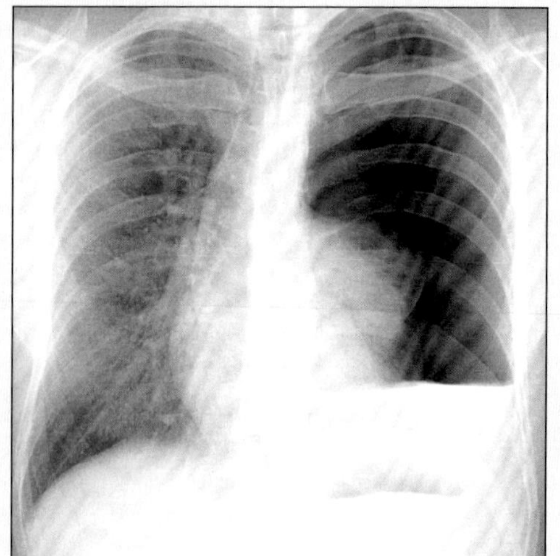

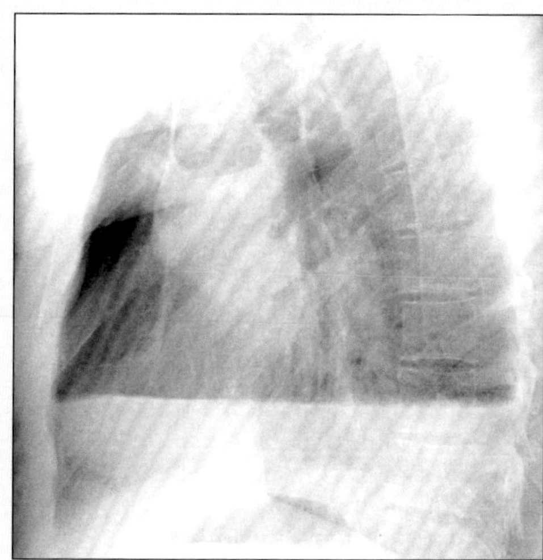

*(**Left**) Axial NECT of a patient with left chest penetrating injury shows paraseptal emphysema, left pneumothorax, pneumomediastinum, and extensive subcutaneous gas. The latter can limit radiographic visualization of pneumothorax. (**Right**) Axial NECT of a young man who sustained severe blunt chest trauma shows a right anterior pneumothorax treated with chest tube placement, right lung consolidations ➔ secondary to contusions, and cystic changes ➔ secondary to lacerations.*

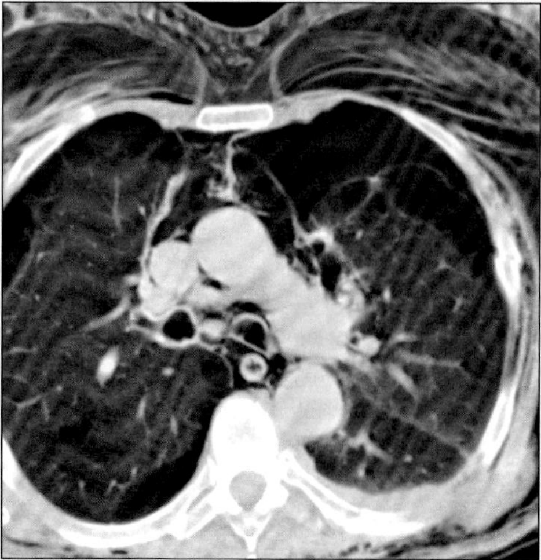

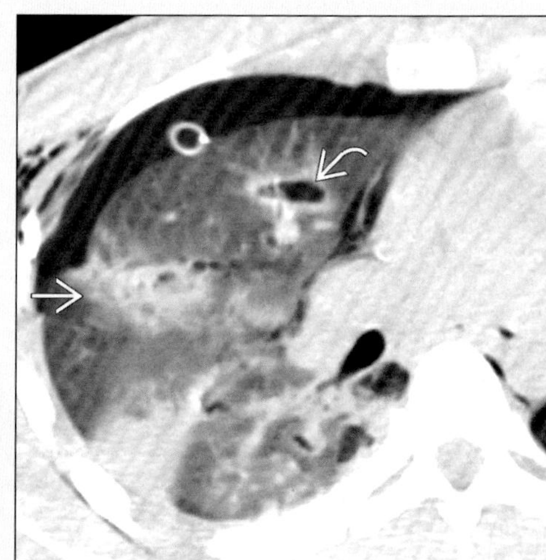

TRAUMATIC PNEUMOTHORAX

TERMINOLOGY

Abbreviations

- **Pneumothorax (PTX)**

Definitions

- Air in pleural space following blunt or penetrating trauma

IMAGING

General Features

- Best diagnostic clue
  - **Visualization of visceral pleural line** without peripheral lung markings in traumatized patient
- Location
  - Upright chest radiograph: Apical pleural space
  - Decubitus chest radiograph: Nondependent pleural space
  - Supine chest radiograph: Basilar pleural space at costophrenic sulcus
- Size
  - Small < 2 cm pleural separation
  - Large > 2 cm pleural separation

Radiographic Findings

- Visceral pleural line usually parallels adjacent chest wall
- Supine radiography; much less sensitive, underestimates size
  - **Deep sulcus sign**: Basilar pneumothorax in supine patient; pleural air results in deepening of costophrenic sulcus
  - Basilar hemithorax hyperlucency
  - Mediastinal contour, heart border, hemidiaphragm may appear sharper compared to uninvolved side
- Expiratory chest radiography
  - Not shown to be more sensitive than full inspiratory chest radiography
- **Tension pneumothorax**: Radiographic findings & hemodynamic compromise
  - Contralateral mediastinal shift
  - Ipsilateral hyperexpansion of ribs & flattening of hemidiaphragm

CT Findings

- High sensitivity for pneumothorax
- Distinction of pneumothorax from bullous emphysema or cystic lung disease
  - Important distinction prior to chest tube placement to avoid iatrogenic bronchopleural fistula
- **Assessment of associated life-threatening injuries**

Imaging Recommendations

- Best imaging tool
  - PA chest radiograph is usually sufficient for diagnosis
- Protocol advice
  - Lateral or decubitus radiographs for equivocal cases (as sensitive as CT)
  - CT assessment of chest
    - Evaluation of associated traumatic chest injuries
    - Identification of chest tube malposition
    - Evaluation of lung parenchyma to distinguish bullous lung disease from PTX

DIFFERENTIAL DIAGNOSIS

Skin Fold, Scapula, Hair, Extraneous Monitoring, or Support Devices

- Edge rather than line, often extends outside thoracic cavity

Bullous Emphysema

- Air does not change location with position

Pneumomediastinum

- Can mimic medial loculated or medially located PTX

PATHOLOGY

General Features

- Etiology
  - Penetrating trauma with laceration of visceral pleura allows air to enter pleural space
  - Blunt trauma with elevation of alveolar pressure & rupture of air into pleural space
  - Iatrogenic trauma
    - Percutaneous lung biopsy
    - Line placement: Subclavian central line, pacemaker
    - Thoracentesis

CLINICAL ISSUES

Presentation

- Most common signs/symptoms
  - Chest pain, sudden dyspnea
- Other signs/symptoms
  - Tension PTX: Severe dyspnea, cyanosis, sweating, & tachycardia

Natural History & Prognosis

- Absorption of pleural space air: 1.5% per day on room air (50-75 mL/day)
- Time for full re-expansion; mean of 3 weeks

Treatment

- Observation of small pneumothorax
  - Supplemental oxygen increases rate of absorption of pleural air by factor of 4
- Chest tube drainage for large or symptomatic pneumothorax
  - **Size of PTX less important than patient's physiologic status**
  - Small chest tubes as effective as large chest tubes

DIAGNOSTIC CHECKLIST

Image Interpretation Pearls

- Report size & location of pleural separation in cases of traumatic pneumothorax
- Assessment of associated life-threatening injuries in traumatized patients

SELECTED REFERENCES

1. Sharma A et al: Principles of diagnosis and management of traumatic pneumothorax. J Emerg Trauma Shock. 1(1):34-41, 2008

TRAUMATIC HEMOTHORAX

Key Facts

Terminology

- Blood in pleural space following blunt or penetrating trauma

Imaging

- Radiography
  - Blunt costophrenic angle on upright radiography
  - Increased density of ipsilateral lung due to layering pleural fluid on supine radiography
  - May accumulate laterally on supine radiography
  - Large hemothorax may produce contralateral mediastinal shift & "tension hemothorax"
- CT
  - Pleural fluid attenuation > 30 HU
  - Layered heterogeneous pleural fluid; "hematocrit" level
  - Exclusion of life-threatening traumatic vascular injury

Top Differential Diagnoses

- Blunt or penetrating chest injury
- Traumatic vascular injury
- Esophageal rupture
- Thoracic duct tear

Clinical Issues

- Signs & symptoms
  - Pain, dyspnea
  - Rarely isolated finding; coexisting rib fractures common
  - Associated lung contusion & pneumothorax common
  - Hemodynamic instability from intercostal or internal mammary vessel laceration
- Treatment
  - Tube thoracostomy
  - Hemothorax evacuation via VATS or thoracotomy

__(Left)__ AP supine chest radiograph of a young man post motor vehicle collision shows a large right pleural effusion ➔ and a right deep sulcus sign ➔, consistent with pneumothorax. Pleural effusion in the setting of trauma should be presumed to represent hemothorax. __(Right)__ AP supine chest radiograph of a patient post right chest stab wound shows a large right hemothorax ➔ and right lung relaxation atelectasis. The patient underwent emergent repair of a lacerated right internal mammary artery.

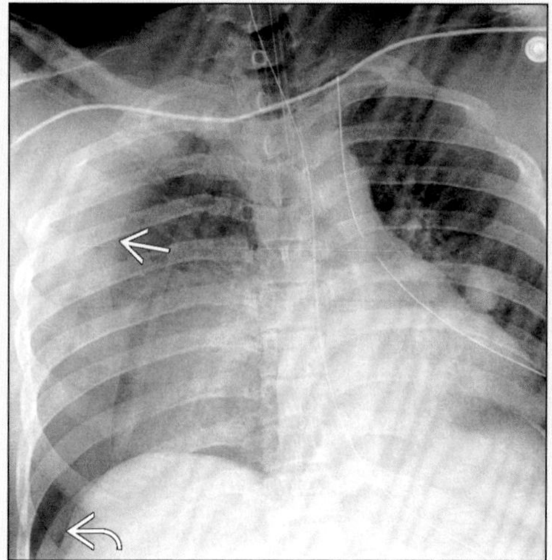

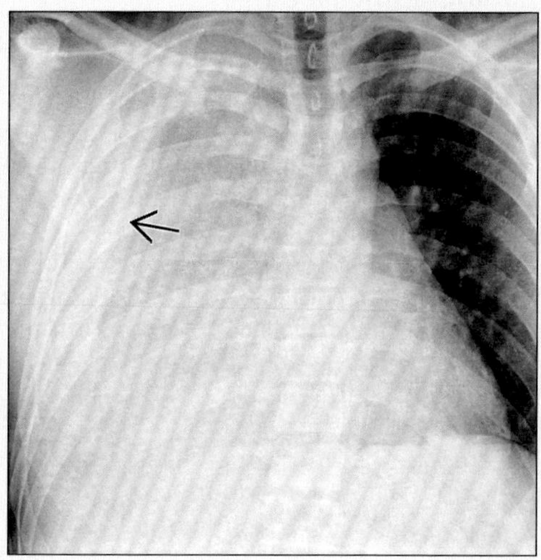

__(Left)__ Axial CECT of a 65-year-old man following a motor vehicle collision shows multiple rib fractures ➔ and a complicated right pleural fluid collection measuring 40 Hounsfield units, consistent with hemothorax. __(Right)__ Axial NECT of a patient status post motor vehicle collision shows a heterogeneous high-attenuation pleural fluid collection ➔ diagnostic of hemothorax. Hemothorax may exhibit variable CT attenuation and should be suspected in the setting of trauma.

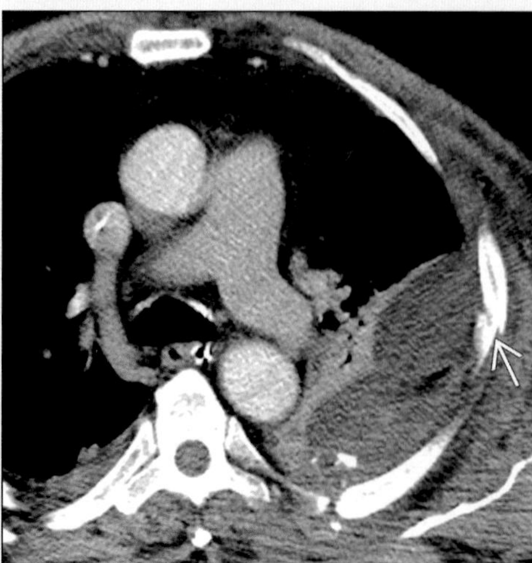

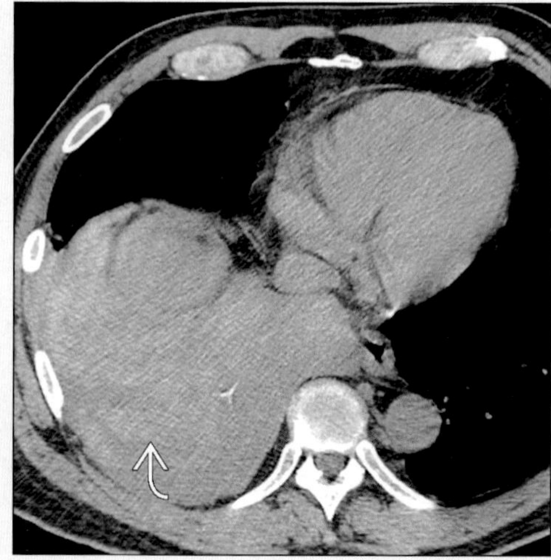

TRAUMATIC HEMOTHORAX

TERMINOLOGY

Definitions

- **Blood in pleural space following blunt or penetrating trauma**

IMAGING

General Features

- Best diagnostic clue
  - Pleural effusion in setting of trauma
- Location
  - Upright radiography: Basilar pleural fluid
  - Supine radiography
    - Hemothorax typically layers posteriorly
    - Large hemothorax may accumulate laterally, displacing adjacent lung medially
- Size
  - Variable; may be massive

Radiographic Findings

- Acute findings
  - Blunt costophrenic angle on upright radiography
  - Increased density of ipsilateral lung due to layering pleural fluid on supine radiography
  - May accumulate laterally on supine radiography
  - Large hemothorax may produce ipsilateral lung atelectasis & opaque hemithorax
  - Large hemothorax may produce contralateral mediastinal shift & "tension hemothorax"
- Subacute findings
  - Loculated pleural effusion
  - Empyema
- Chronic findings
  - Organized hemothorax may produce extensive pleural thickening with calcification
  - Fibrothorax with ipsilateral loss of lung volume

CT Findings

- Pleural fluid attenuation higher than that of simple pleural fluid (> 30 HU)
- Heterogeneous pleural fluid with layered appearance of high attenuation fluid; "hematocrit" level
- Assessment of thorax for exclusion of life-threatening traumatic vascular injury as cause of hemothorax

Imaging Recommendations

- Best imaging tool
  - Radiography is usually sufficient for diagnosis
  - Recognition of signs of hemothorax on supine radiography
  - CT for assessment of associated life-threatening injuries
- Protocol advice
  - Contrast-enhanced chest CT (CT angiography) for exclusion of traumatic vascular injury

Ultrasonographic Findings

- Emergent assessment of traumatized patients
- Rapid estimation of pleural fluid quantity in patients who cannot tolerate upright radiography

DIFFERENTIAL DIAGNOSIS

Blunt or Penetrating Chest Injury

- Motor vehicle collision is most common etiology
- Rapid bleeding typically from systemic vessel laceration
- Low-pressure bleeding from lung is usually self-limited

Traumatic Vascular Injury

- Vascular imaging with CTA for diagnosis

Esophageal Rupture

- May result in hemothorax or hemopneumothorax

Thoracic Duct Tear

- Water attenuation fluid; traumatic chylothorax

PATHOLOGY

General Features

- Etiology
  - Occurs in 30-50% of blunt thoracic trauma cases
  - Penetrating trauma
  - Iatrogenic injury, following emergent line placement
  - Laceration of intercostal/internal mammary vessels

Microscopic Features

- Pleural fluid hematocrit > 50% of serum hematocrit

CLINICAL ISSUES

Presentation

- Most common signs/symptoms
  - Pain, dyspnea
- Other signs/symptoms
  - Rarely isolated finding, coexisting rib fractures common
  - Associated lung contusion & pneumothorax common
  - Hemodynamic instability &, rarely, exsanguination from intercostal or internal mammary vessel laceration
  - Absent/diminished breath sounds, dullness to percussion

Natural History & Prognosis

- Bacterial contamination may result in empyema
- May result in fibrothorax & trapped lung

Treatment

- Tube thoracostomy
- VATS for evacuation of incompletely drained hemothorax; performed within 7 days of trauma
- Consider thoracotomy when drained blood volume > 1 L, persistent bleeding, hemodynamic instability, empyema

SELECTED REFERENCES

1. Sangster GP et al: Blunt traumatic injuries of the lung parenchyma, pleura, thoracic wall, and intrathoracic airways: multidetector computer tomography imaging findings. Emerg Radiol. 14(5):297-310, 2007

THORACIC SPLENOSIS

Key Facts

Terminology

- Autotransplantation of splenic tissue following traumatic or surgical disruption of spleen

Imaging

- Multiple left pleural nodules/masses in patient with history of trauma
- Radiography
  - Incomplete border sign: Combination of sharp & indistinct margins
  - Obtuse angles with adjacent pleura
- CT
  - Multiple left basilar pleural nodules/masses
  - Predilection for posterior inferior hemithorax
  - May exhibit contrast enhancement
  - Absence of spleen
  - Similar lesions may occur in abdomen & subcutaneous tissue

Top Differential Diagnoses

- Pleural metastases
- Asbestos-related pleural disease
- Invasive thymoma
- Malignant mesothelioma
- Localized fibrous tumor of pleura

Pathology

- Follows penetrating or blunt traumatic injury
- Transdiaphragmatic pleural tissue dissemination

Clinical Issues

- Asymptomatic; incidentally discovered on imaging
- Treatment: None

Diagnostic Checklist

- Consider splenosis in any patient with multiple left pleural nodules & absence of spleen

__(Left)__ Graphic shows the typical features of thoracic splenosis. Multiple implants of splenic tissue ➔ on the left inferior pleura are the result of prior trauma, splenic injury, and ipsilateral diaphragmatic rupture ⇨. __(Right)__ Axial CECT of a patient with prior gunshot wound to the abdomen shows multifocal left basilar pleural masses and nodules ⇨ consistent with splenosis. The spleen was surgically absent.

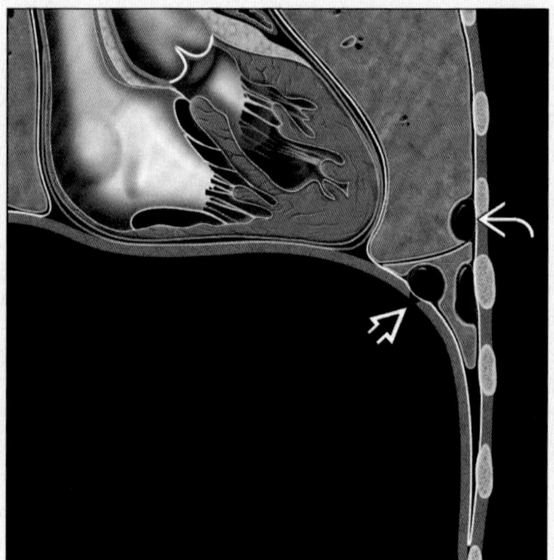

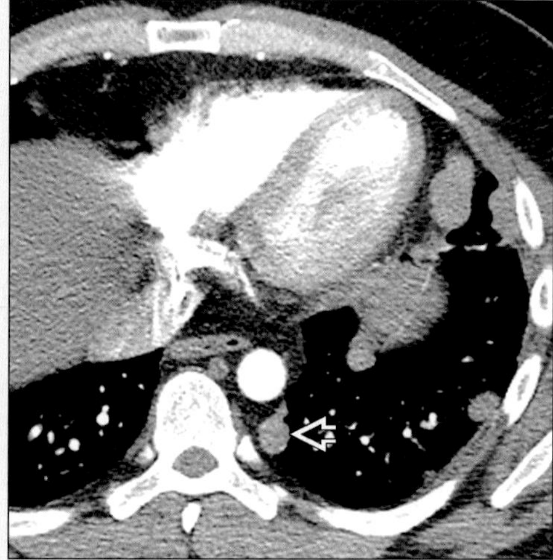

__(Left)__ Axial CECT of a patient with left thoracic splenosis shows multiple left pleural nodules ➔. Thoracic splenosis may mimic unilateral solid pleural metastases. __(Right)__ Axial CECT of a patient with prior left diaphragmatic rupture demonstrates multifocal enhancing unilateral left pleural nodules ➔. Multifocal pleural nodules in a patient with absent spleen and prior diaphragmatic injury should suggest the diagnosis of thoracic splenosis, which can be confirmed with nuclear scintigraphy.

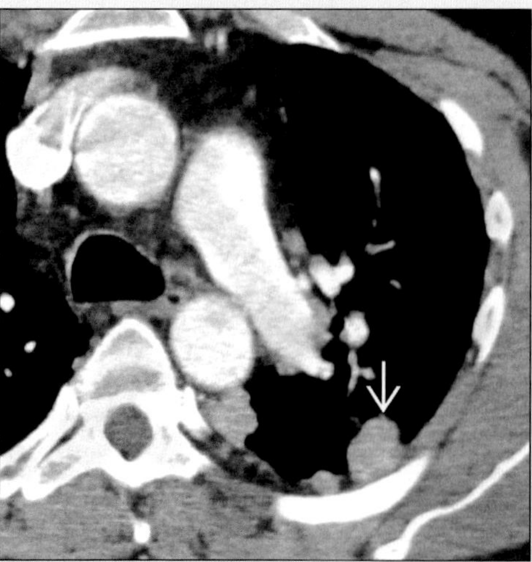

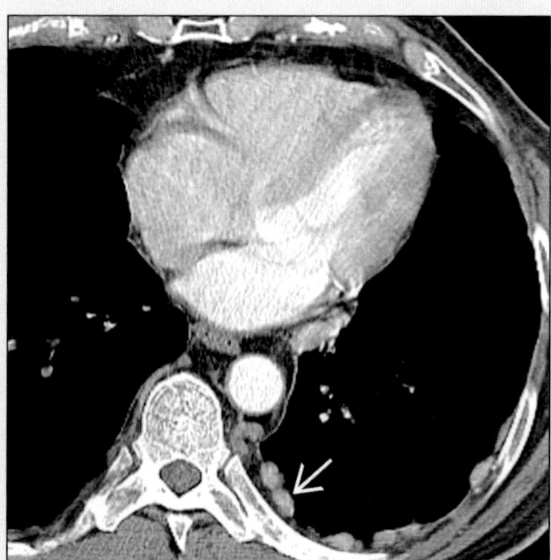

THORACIC SPLENOSIS

TERMINOLOGY

Definitions

- **Autotransplantation of splenic tissue** following traumatic or surgical disruption of spleen

IMAGING

General Features

- Best diagnostic clue
  - Multiple left pleural nodules or masses in patient with history of trauma
- Location
  - Typically abdominal, left upper quadrant
  - Thoracic splenosis; inferior posterior left pleural space
- Size
  - Typically < 3 cm in diameter

Radiographic Findings

- Radiographic features of pleural lesion
  - **Incomplete border sign**: Combination of sharp & indistinct margins
    - Sharp margin in profile
    - Indistinct margin en face
  - Obtuse angles with adjacent pleura
- **Thoracic splenosis**
  - Single or multiple left posterior basilar pleural nodules/masses
  - Most exhibit sharp borders, < 3 cm in diameter
  - Signs of remote trauma

CT Findings

- CECT
  - Multiple left basilar pleural nodules/masses
    - Predilection for posterior inferior hemithorax along costophrenic sulcus
    - Noncalcified; may exhibit contrast enhancement
    - Similar lesions may occur in abdomen & subcutaneous tissue
  - **Absence of spleen**

MR Findings

- Signal intensity comparable to normal spleen

Nuclear Medicine Findings

- Tc-99m sulfur colloid
  - Uptake in splenic tissue (reticuloendothelial tissue)
- Tc-99m labeled red cell scintigraphy
  - Uptake specific for splenic tissue
  - More sensitive than Tc-99m sulfur colloid scan

DIFFERENTIAL DIAGNOSIS

Pleural Metastases

- Circumferential nodular pleural thickening; multiple pleural masses
- Frequent associated pleural effusion
- History of known malignancy, especially adenocarcinoma

Asbestos-related Pleural Disease

- Bilateral discontinuous nodular pleural thickening; often calcified
- History of asbestos exposure

Invasive Thymoma

- Anterior mediastinal mass
- Unilateral or bilateral drop pleural metastases

Malignant Mesothelioma

- Unilateral circumferential pleural thickening; volume loss of ipsilateral hemithorax

Localized Fibrous Tumor of Pleura

- Solitary pleural nodule or mass; heterogeneous enhancement
- May be associated with hypoglycemia or hypertrophic osteoarthropathy

PATHOLOGY

General Features

- Etiology
  - Follows penetrating or less commonly blunt traumatic injury
  - Transdiaphragmatic pleural tissue dissemination; traumatic diaphragmatic injury, diaphragmatic hiatus, congenital defect

Gross Pathologic & Surgical Features

- Abdominal pleural implants: Peritoneum, omentum, serosal surfaces of bowel & liver, pelvic organs, subcutaneous tissue
- Diaphragmatic tears usually not found at surgery

CLINICAL ISSUES

Presentation

- Most common signs/symptoms
  - **Asymptomatic**; incidentally discovered on imaging

Demographics

- Epidemiology
  - May develop in up to 15% of patients with splenic trauma & diaphragmatic laceration

Natural History & Prognosis

- Interval between splenic rupture & splenosis varies from months to years

Treatment

- None; differentiation from neoplastic process

DIAGNOSTIC CHECKLIST

Consider

- Splenosis with multiple left pleural nodules/masses

Image Interpretation Pearls

- Determine presence or absence of spleen in any patient with multiple left pleural nodules/masses

SELECTED REFERENCES

1. Alaraj AM et al: Thoracic splenosis mimicking thoracic schwannoma: case report and review of the literature. Surg Neurol. 64(2):185-8; discussion 88, 2005
2. Khosravi MR et al: Consider the diagnosis of splenosis for soft tissue masses long after any splenic injury. Am Surg. 70(11):967-70, 2004

RIB FRACTURES AND FLAIL CHEST

Key Facts

Terminology

- Flail chest: ≥ 3 segmental rib fractures (≥ 2 fractures in same rib) or > 5 adjacent rib fractures
- Flail segment shows paradoxical motion with respiration

Imaging

- Radiography (specific but not sensitive)
  - Cortical break & step off
  - Ribs 4-9 most commonly fractured
  - Fractures usually multiple
  - Dedicated rib series for fracture documentation
  - Fracture visualization with healing & callus formation
  - Flail chest (up to 20% of patients with major trauma)
- CT for evaluation of underlying visceral injuries

Top Differential Diagnoses

- Pathologic rib fracture
- Thoracostomy tube

Clinical Issues

- Most common thoracic injury in blunt chest trauma
- Rib fractures common after CPR
- Cough-induced rib fractures primarily affect women
- Rib fractures in children denote significant trauma
- Treatment
  - Symptomatic pain management
  - Intubation & mechanical ventilation for flail chest

Diagnostic Checklist

- Pneumothorax & contusion more significant injuries than fractured ribs
- Lower rib fractures are markers for abdominal visceral injury

*(**Left**) Graphic shows the morphologic features of flail chest. There are 3 consecutive left rib fractures with resultant ipsilateral pneumothorax, hemothorax, and left pulmonary contusion. The presence of rib fractures should alert the radiologist to look for signs of these associated injuries in patients with chest trauma. (**Right**) AP chest radiograph shows at least 3 adjacent left posterior rib fractures, a moderate left pneumothorax ➡, and left chest wall subcutaneous gas.*

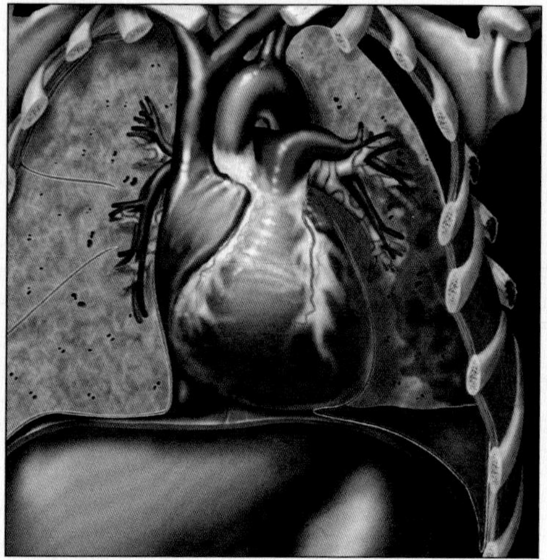

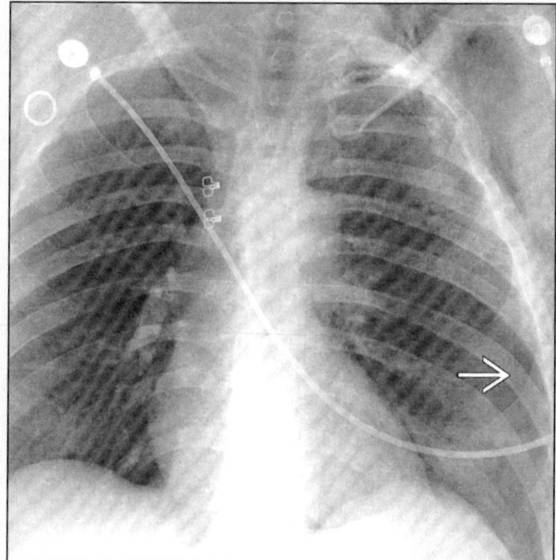

*(**Left**) AP chest radiograph of a patient status post chest trauma shows a loculated right pleural effusion ➡ and multiple right rib fractures. In such cases, the pleural effusion is presumed to represent a hemothorax. A rib corset ⇨ is present. (**Right**) Axial NECT of the same patient shows increased attenuation ➡ within the right pleural fluid (consistent with hemothorax) and a displaced right posterior rib fracture ⇨. Hemothorax often loculates as opposed to transudative pleural effusions.*

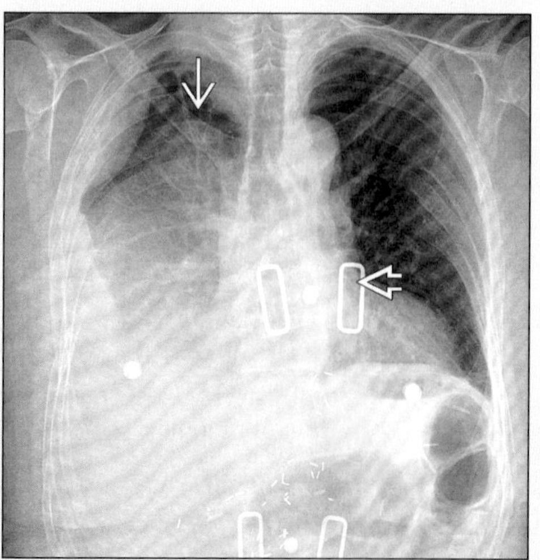

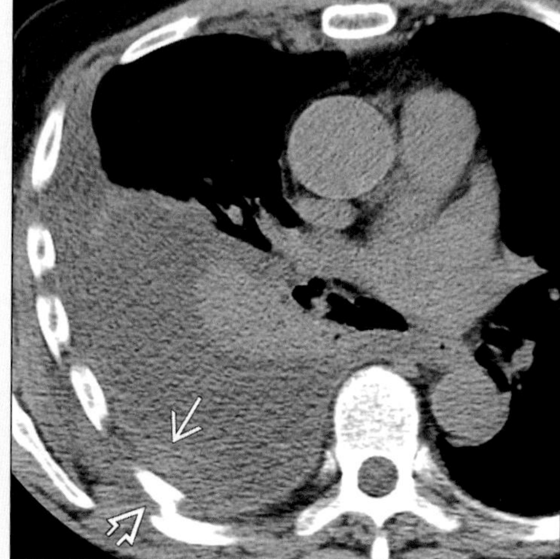

RIB FRACTURES AND FLAIL CHEST

TERMINOLOGY

Definitions

- **Rib fracture**: Displaced or non-displaced cortical break
- **Flail chest:** ≥ 3 segmental rib fractures (≥ 2 fractures in same rib) or > 5 adjacent rib fractures
  - Flail segment shows **paradoxical motion with respiration**

IMAGING

General Features

- Best diagnostic clue
  - Cortical break & step off
- Location
  - Dependent on site of energy absorption
- Morphology
  - Traumatic rib fractures; often multiple & in anatomic alignment
  - Multiple fractures of contiguous ribs typically vertically aligned

Radiographic Findings

- **Radiographs specific but not sensitive**
  - 30% sensitivity for non-displaced fracture ("normal" to miss rib fractures)
  - **Ribs 4-9** most commonly fractured
  - Fractures **usually multiple**
- Dedicated rib series occasionally helpful, especially when fracture documentation is important
  - Medical-legal cases
  - Should not substitute for chest radiography (may miss pneumothorax)
- Fractures may only become evident with healing & callus formation
  - Initial radiographs often do not show non-displaced fractures
  - Repeat radiography 4 or more days after injury usually reveals fractures
  - Early treatment for uncomplicated rib fracture identical to treatment for bruised ribs; diagnosis delay does not hinder treatment
- **Flail chest** (up to 20% of patients with major trauma)
  - ≥ 3 adjacent ribs with segmental fractures or > 5 adjacent rib fractures
  - Costal hook sign: Elephant trunk-shaped ribs (due to rotation of segmental fractures)
- Traumatic 1st rib fracture, marker of high-energy chest trauma
  - 1st rib protected by clavicle & scapula
  - Statistically: 2% associated with bronchial tear, 10% with aortic transection
    - Nontraumatic 1st rib fracture: Very low incidence of major vascular injury
- Children with nonaccidental trauma
  - 5-25% of all skeletal injuries in abused children
  - Typically fractures at costovertebral & costochondral junctions
  - Shaken baby: Fractures typically posterior near costovertebral junctions
  - 1st rib fracture virtually diagnostic of abuse

CT Findings

- More sensitive than chest radiography
- Primarily used for **evaluation of underlying visceral injuries**
- Volume rendered images significantly reduce image interpretation time for identification of rib fractures

Ultrasonographic Findings

- Ultrasound can detect rib fractures
  - Does not significantly increase detection rate
  - Too time consuming to justify routine use

Nuclear Medicine Findings

- Bone scintigraphy sensitive for detecting stress fractures, bone metastases, and fractures in suspected child abuse

Imaging Recommendations

- Best imaging tool
  - Chest radiography usually sufficient for clinically important decisions
    - Exclusion of pneumothorax, pleural effusion, pulmonary contusion
- Protocol advice
  - Routine radiographic follow-up of fractures not recommended

DIFFERENTIAL DIAGNOSIS

Pathologic Rib Fracture

- Typically not aligned or adjacent to each other
- Skeletal lesion at fracture site
- May follow minimal trauma
- Does not manifest with comorbidities such as pneumothorax

Thoracostomy Tube

- On CT, thoracostomy tubes can be confused with ribs &/or displaced rib fractures

PATHOLOGY

General Features

- Etiology
  - Rib stability
    - Maximal chest wall weakness at 60° rotation from sternum; flatter less supported ribs
    - Anterior-posterior compression: Ribs typically fracture in 2 places: 60° from sternum, and posteriorly
  - **Trauma**: Direct blow from motor vehicle collision, fall, assault, contact sports
  - **Severe coughing**
  - Stress rib fractures uncommon
    - Typical locations: Anterolateral 1st rib, lateral 4th-9th ribs, posteromedial upper ribs
    - Golfers (duffer's fracture), canoeists, rowers, swimmers, weightlifters, ballet dancers
  - Isolated 1st rib fracture
    - In proper clinical setting, may represent avulsion injury, especially from throwing motion, rowing, or related to whiplash
    - Avulsion from scalene muscle attachment

Gross Pathologic & Surgical Features

- Paradoxical flail segment motion (pendelluft breathing)

- Segment moves inward with inspiration & outward with expiration

CLINICAL ISSUES

Presentation

- Most common signs/symptoms
  - Physical exam sensitive but not specific
  - Chest wall pain, pain with deep breathing, sneezing, or coughing
  - Severe local rib tenderness, swelling &/or crepitus
- Other signs/symptoms
  - **Flail chest**
    - May not be clinically evident in 1/3 of cases
    - Clinical findings masked by positive pressure ventilation; delayed diagnosis
    - Traumatic extrathoracic intercostal lung herniation; rare extraordinary associated injury

Demographics

- Age
  - **More common with advancing age**
    - Longer duration of pain
    - Admission of elderly patients for observation & treatment of isolated rib fractures, justified & beneficial
  - Overall trauma-related mortality higher in elderly patients with multiple rib fractures than in younger patients
- Epidemiology
  - Most common thoracic injury in blunt chest trauma (10%)
  - Rib fractures ominous in children & elderly
    - Ribs difficult to fracture in children due to plasticity; fractured ribs signify significant trauma
    - Rib fractures more common in elderly due to osteoporosis & decreased muscle mass; increased morbidity & mortality
  - Rib fractures common following cardiopulmonary resuscitation (CPR)
    - Typically underreported, occur in up to 30%
  - Cough-induced rib fractures occur primarily in women with chronic cough
    - Middle ribs along lateral rib cage most commonly affected
    - Pertussis infection & post-nasal drip
  - Flail chest: Level 1 trauma center 1-2 cases/month

Natural History & Prognosis

- Typically heal with callus
  - Rarely non-union & pseudoarthrosis
- Multiple bilateral healed rib fractures common in alcoholics
- Mortality & morbidity increase with number of fractured ribs
- Location
  - Right-sided rib fractures below 8th rib: 20-50% probability of liver injury
  - Left-sided rib fractures below 8th rib: 25% probability of splenic injury
  - 1st & 2nd rib fractures not an indication for investigating aortic injury in absence of other findings of aortic transection
- Flail chest
  - Acutely, associated with mortality rates of 10-20%
  - Chronically, 25-50% have long-term disability including chronic chest wall pain & exertional dyspnea

Treatment

- Options, risks, complications
  - Atelectasis: Common sequela of rib fractures, predisposes to pneumonia
  - Often complicated by lung contusion & laceration, pneumothorax, hemothorax
  - Rarely, sharp edges of extremely displaced rib fractures may puncture or lacerate viscera
    - Diaphragm
    - Aorta
    - Airway
    - Heart
- **Symptomatic pain management**
  - Oral analgesia
  - Epidural analgesia, especially for flail chest, associated with decreased nosocomial pneumonia & shorter duration of mechanical ventilation
- **Observation** for development of delayed hemothorax
- Surgical fixation rarely necessary
- **Intubation & mechanical ventilation**
  - Need determined by underlying cardiopulmonary status, not presence or absence of flail segments

DIAGNOSTIC CHECKLIST

Consider

- Pneumothorax & contusion clinically more significant injuries than rib fractures

Image Interpretation Pearls

- Lower rib fractures are marker for abdominal visceral injury
- Dedicated rib radiographs without chest radiography may miss associated pneumothorax

SELECTED REFERENCES

1. Kamath GS et al: Isolated cervical rib fracture. Ann Thorac Surg. 89(6):e41-2, 2010
2. Peters S et al: Multidetector computed tomography-spectrum of blunt chest wall and lung injuries in polytraumatized patients. Clin Radiol. 65(4):333-8, 2010
3. Levine BD et al: CT of rib lesions. AJR Am J Roentgenol. 193(1):5-13, 2009
4. Hanak V et al: Cough-induced rib fractures. Mayo Clin Proc. 80(7):879-82, 2005
5. Bulger EM et al: Epidural analgesia improves outcome after multiple rib fractures. Surgery. 136(2):426-30, 2004
6. Hurley ME et al: Is ultrasound really helpful in the detection of rib fractures? Injury. 35(6):562-6, 2004
7. Stawicki SP et al: Rib fractures in the elderly: a marker of injury severity. J Am Geriatr Soc. 52(5):805-8, 2004
8. Holcomb JB et al: Morbidity from rib fractures increases after age 45. J Am Coll Surg. 196(4):549-55, 2003
9. Sirmali M et al: A comprehensive analysis of traumatic rib fractures: morbidity, mortality and management. Eur J Cardiothorac Surg. 24(1):133-8, 2003

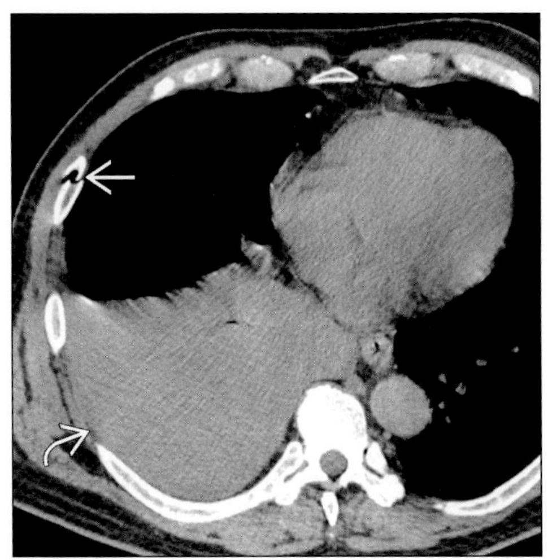

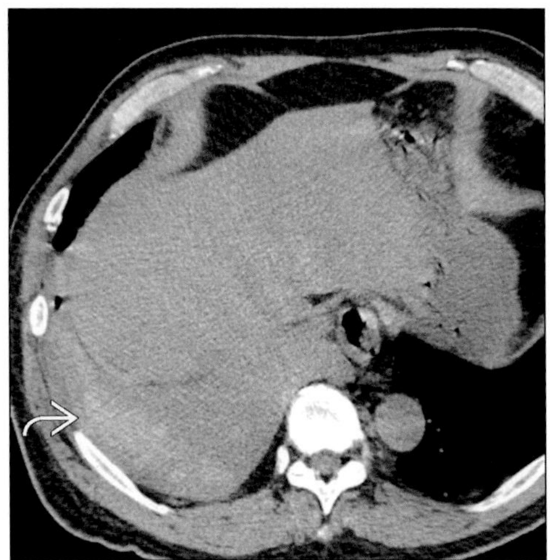

(Left) *NECT of a patient who sustained blunt chest trauma shows a right anterior rib fracture ➡ and a hyperdense right pleural effusion ➡, consistent with a hemothorax.* ***(Right)*** *Axial NECT of the same patient shows focal hyperdense clot ➡ within the high-attenuation pleural fluid collection, diagnostic of hemothorax. Although pleural effusions in the setting of trauma are often presumed to represent hemothorax, CT is useful in definitively characterizing pleural fluid as hemothorax.*

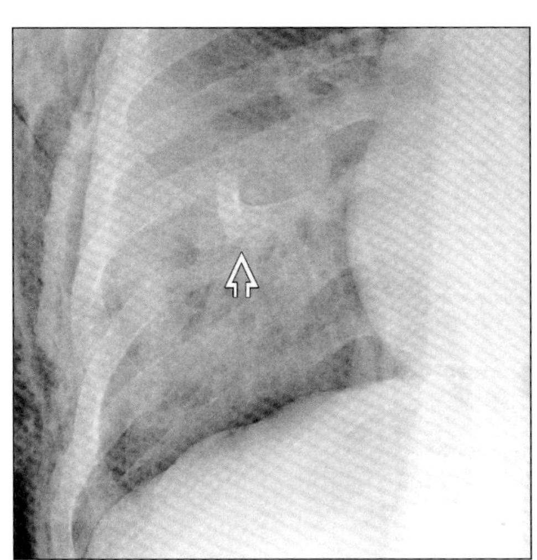

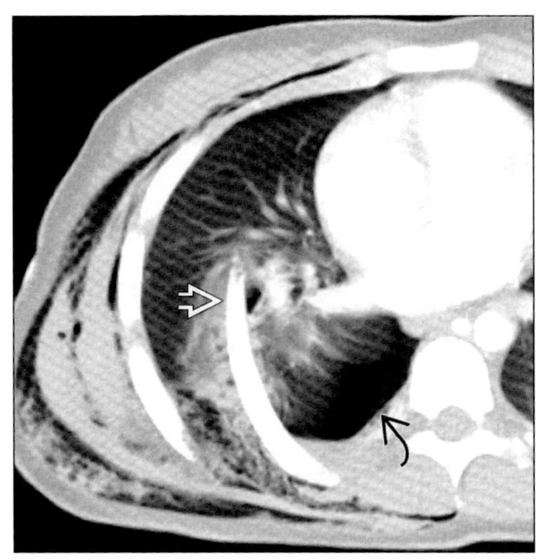

(Left) *Frontal chest radiograph coned down to the right inferior hemithorax shows an elephant trunk-shaped rib ➡ secondary to complex segmental fracture. The associated airspace disease is most consistent with pulmonary contusion and hemorrhage. There is extensive subcutaneous gas in the right chest wall.* ***(Right)*** *CECT of the same patient shows intrathoracic displacement of the fractured rib ➡ with resultant lung puncture, contusion, right pneumothorax ➡, and adjacent subcutaneous gas.*

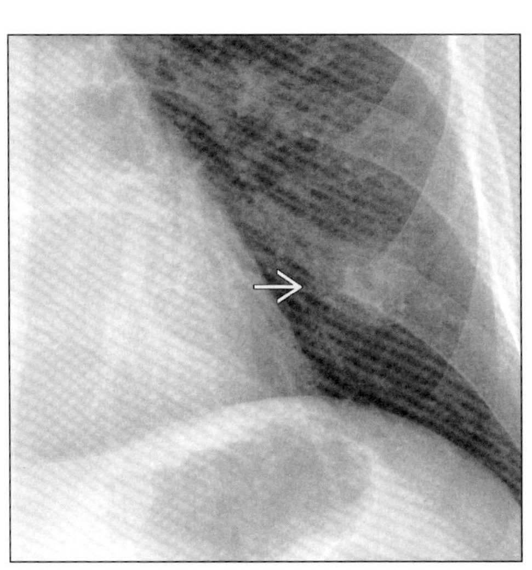

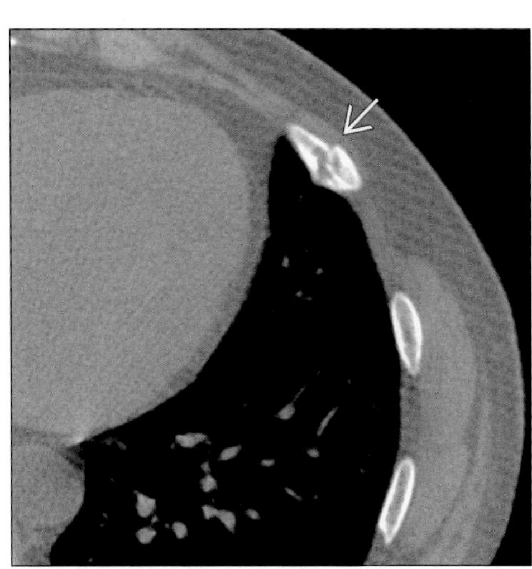

(Left) *PA chest radiograph coned down to the left inferior hemithorax shows a focal nodular opacity ➡ projecting over the left lung base; this is suspicious for a pulmonary nodule although a musculoskeletal abnormality could also have this appearance.* ***(Right)*** *NECT of the same patient confirms that the nodular opacity seen on radiography corresponds to a healing left anterior rib fracture ➡ rather than a pulmonary nodule. Rib fractures may mimic lung nodules on radiography.*

*(**Left**) AP chest radiograph of a patient with a history of blunt chest trauma shows a large left pleural effusion with partial loculation. (**Right**) CECT of the same patient shows a large pleural effusion and an extrapleural hematoma ➔ with biconvex margins. Extrapleural hematomas with biconvex margins (as opposed to those that conform to the shape of the chest wall) have a greater tendency to be hemodynamically significant due to their larger size.*

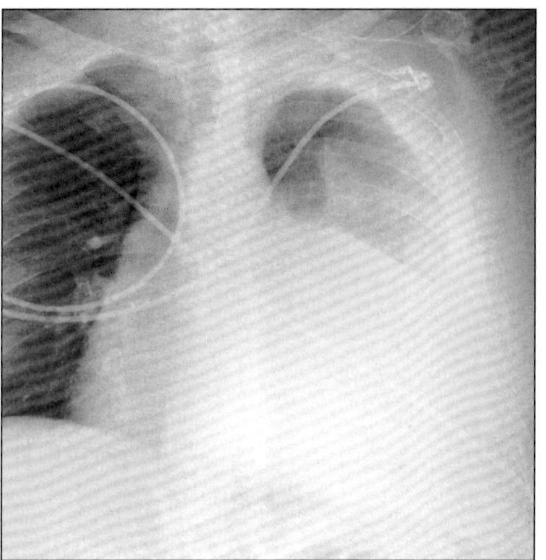

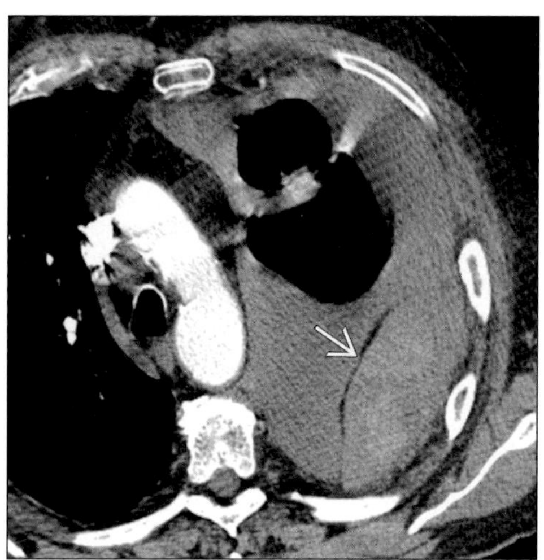

*(**Left**) Axial CECT of the same patient shows a large left pleural effusion and a mildly displaced left posterior rib fracture ➔. Note the polylobular left extrapleural hematoma ➔ with internal displacement of extrapleural fat. Extrapleural hematomas are associated with rib fractures and are likely due to intercostal vessel injury. (**Right**) 3D reformation from NECT shows multiple segmental rib fractures ➔, diagnostic of flail chest. Local paradoxical motion of the chest may be evident clinically.*

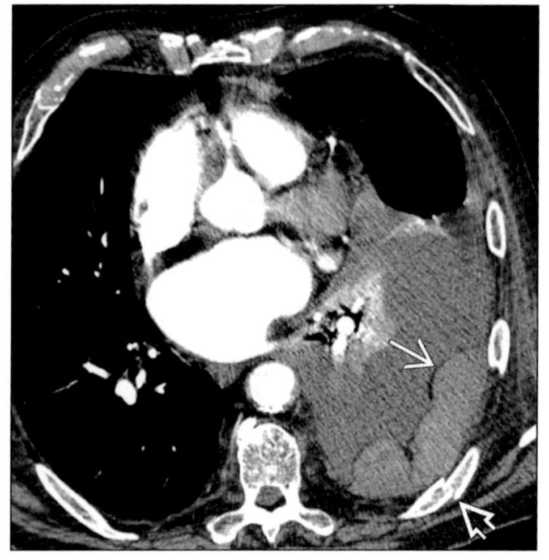

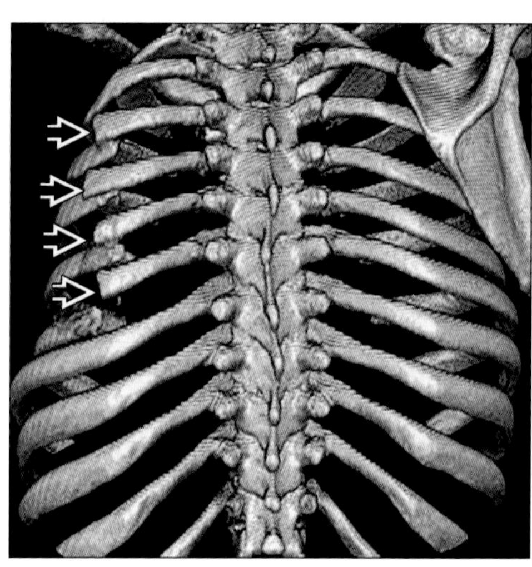

*(**Left**) Axial CECT of a patient who sustained chest trauma shows partial dislocation of the manubrioclavicular junction ➔, gas in the joint space, and right chest wall subcutaneous gas. (**Right**) Axial CECT of the same patient shows disruption of a right costochondral junction ➔, a moderate right pneumothorax, and a right hemothorax ➔. Costochondral fractures are mechanically similar to rib fractures.*

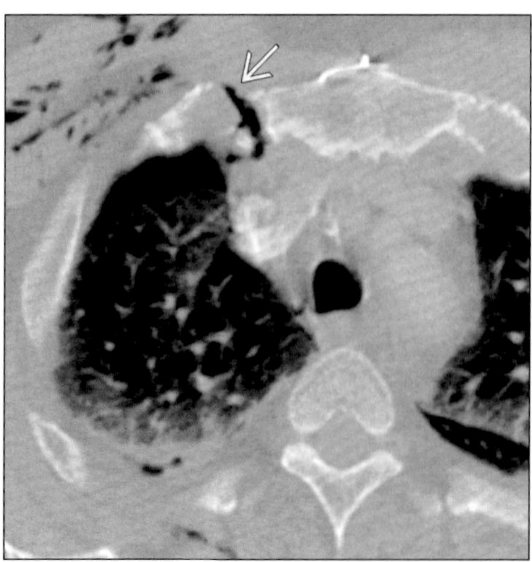

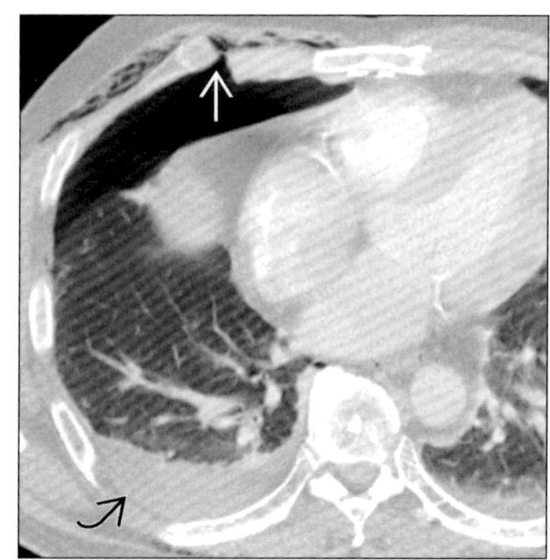

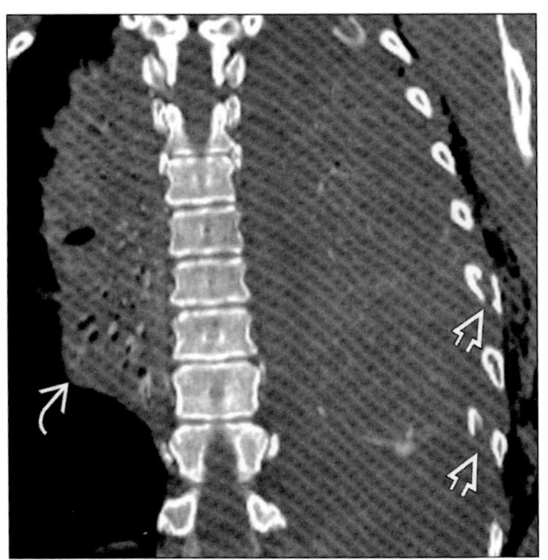

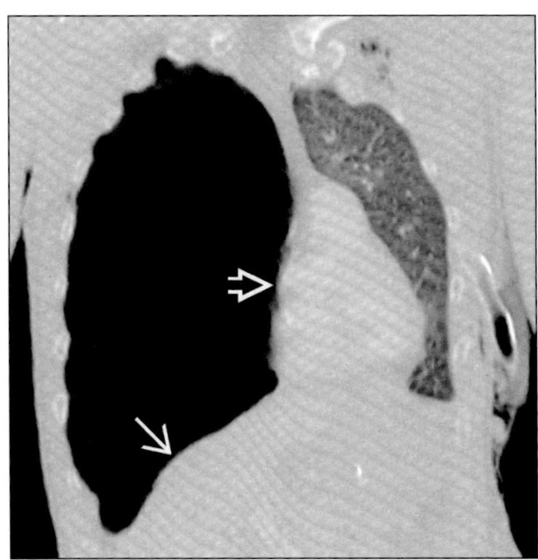

(Left) *Coronal CECT following chest trauma shows multiple left rib fractures → and a left hemothorax. Bilateral dependent consolidations → likely represent aspiration since atelectatic lung would exhibit marked contrast enhancement.* **(Right)** *Coronal CECT of the same patient shows a large right tension pneumothorax with mass effect on the right hemidiaphragm → and mediastinum →. Rib fractures are associated with pneumothorax, hemothorax, pulmonary contusions, and lacerations.*

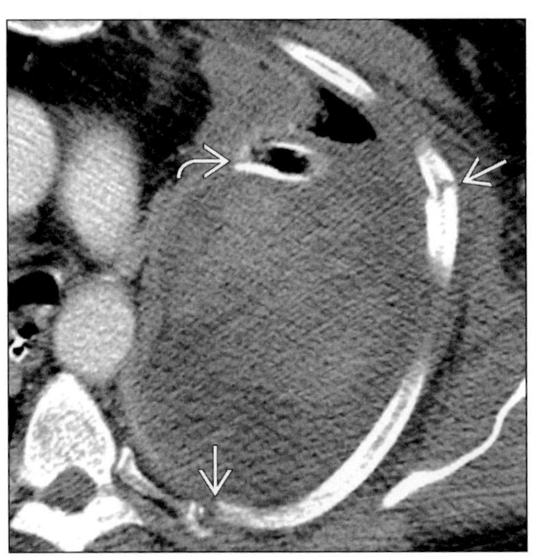

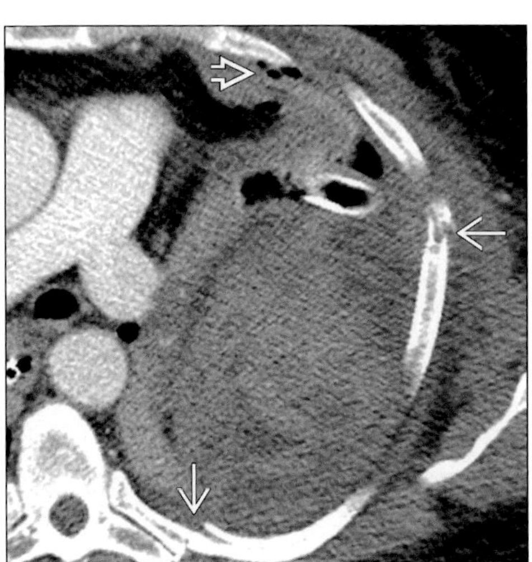

(Left) *Axial CECT of a patient with chest trauma shows multiple rib fractures →, a high-attenuation left hemothorax, and an ipsilateral chest tube →.* **(Right)** *Axial CECT of the same patient shows additional rib fractures →, a high-attenuation left hemothorax, and a tiny left pneumothorax →. Radiography is useful in identifying pleural effusions, which are likely to represent hemothorax in the setting of trauma. CT allows pleural fluid characterization as hemothorax based on attenuation.*

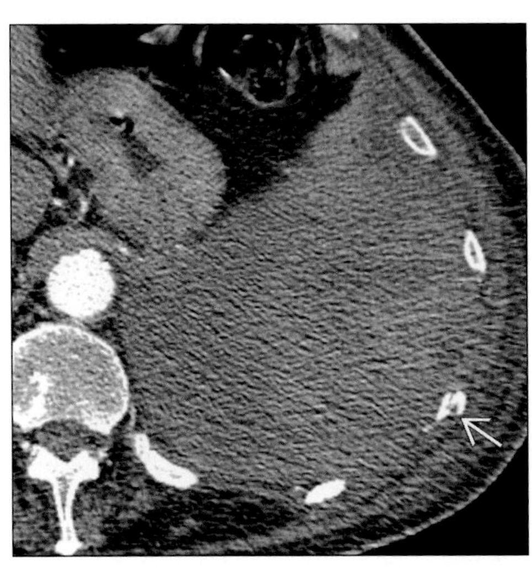

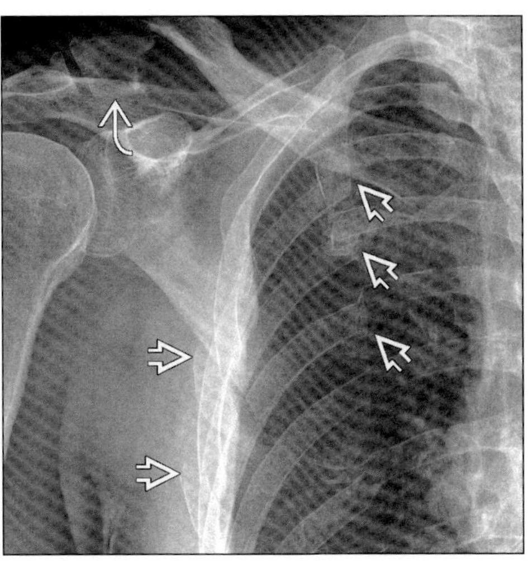

(Left) *Axial CECT shows a mildly displaced left posterior rib fracture → and a large hyperdense left pleural effusion, most consistent with hemothorax. Rib fractures may be associated with pneumothorax and hemothorax.* **(Right)** *Frontal chest radiograph shows multiple segmental rib fractures → suggestive of flail chest, a right clavicle fracture →, and a tiny right apical pneumothorax. Multifocal rib fractures are common in blunt chest trauma, particularly severe motor vehicle collisions.*

SPINAL FRACTURE

Key Facts

Imaging

- Anterior compression fracture
  - Almost always involves superior endplate
  - < 40-50% height loss with normal bone density; greater loss of height suggests Chance fracture
- Burst fracture
  - Vertebral compression on lateral radiograph
  - Wide interpedicular distance on frontal radiograph
- Flexion-distraction (Chance) fracture
  - > 40-50% vertebral body height loss
  - Focal kyphosis; separation of facet joints & increased interspinous distance
- Fracture-dislocation
  - Gross malalignment
- CT for emergent evaluation of skeletal injury & alignment
- MR for evaluation of soft tissue injury or cord contusion

Top Differential Diagnoses

- Spinal abscess
- Spinal metastasis

Pathology

- 3-column model of Davis
  - Anterior column: Anterior 2/3 of vertebral body
  - Middle column: Posterior 1/3 of vertebral body
  - Posterior column: Posterior elements
- Spinal instability if more than 2-column failure

Clinical Issues

- Signs & symptoms
  - Hypotension without tachycardia; priapism

Diagnostic Checklist

- Widened interpedicular distance suggests burst fracture & vertebral instability

__(Left)__ Graphic shows thoracolumbar fracture dislocation, a common location for spinal fractures resulting from flexion forces in blunt trauma. __(Right)__ Composite image with axial NECT (left) and sagittal volume-rendered 3D reformation (right) shows a T12 anterior column fracture ⇨. Sagittal image shows the superior endplate T12 fracture ⮫ without evidence of thoracolumbar malalignment. Given isolated single column involvement, the fracture is considered stable and is managed conservatively.

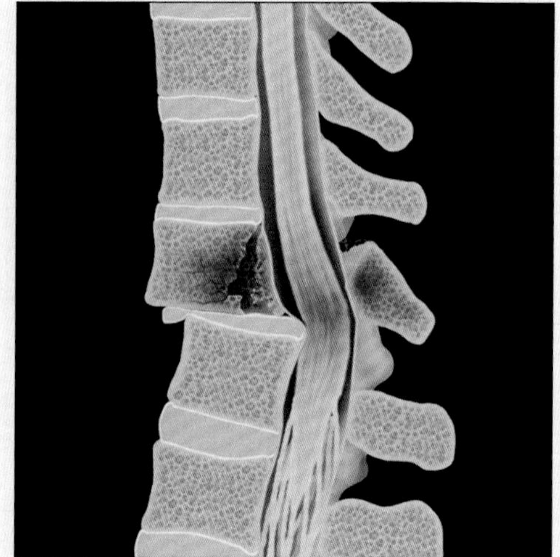

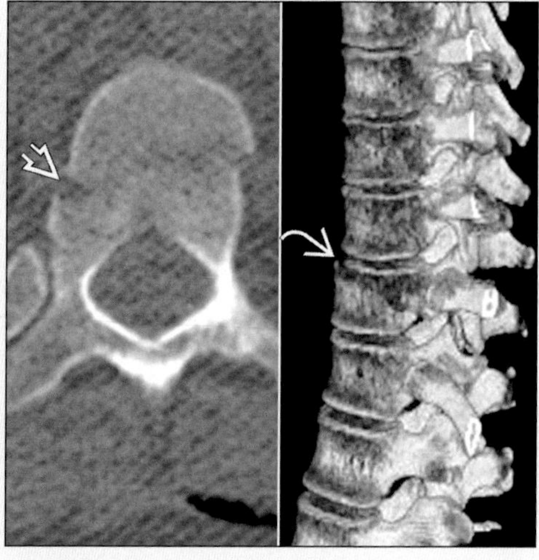

__(Left)__ Sagittal CECT shows a malaligned 3-column fracture-dislocation ➡ of the thoracic spine involving a mid-thoracic vertebral body and its posterior elements. Further evaluation is mandatory if there is concern for spinal cord injury. __(Right)__ Sagittal T2WI MR of the same patient shows increased heterogeneous signal and abnormal swelling of the thoracic spinal cord ➡, which is essentially diagnostic of cord injury (the patient was paraplegic). Adjacent paraspinal hemorrhage is also present.

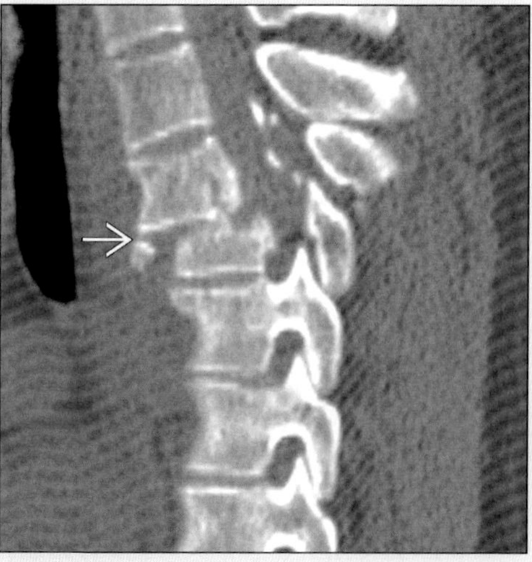

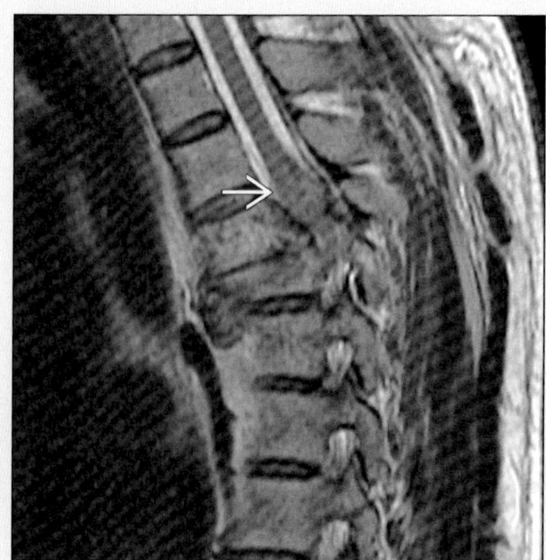

IMAGING

General Features

- Best diagnostic clue
  - **Compression fracture**
    - Most common thoracic spine fracture due to blunt trauma
    - Wedge-shaped vertebral body deformity
  - **Burst fracture**
    - Compressed thoracic vertebral body with fractured endplates & widened pedicles
  - **Flexion-distraction (Chance) fracture**
    - Anterior compression deformity with posterior distraction
  - **Fracture-dislocation**
    - Gross vertebral malalignment in association with fracture(s)
- Location
  - Thoracolumbar junction most vulnerable site

Radiographic Findings

- **Anterior compression fracture**
  - Paraspinal hematoma & kyphosis
  - Almost always involves **superior endplate**
  - < 40-50% loss of height in patients with normal bone density; if greater loss of height, probably Chance fracture
- **Burst fracture**
  - Widened interpedicular distance on AP radiograph; wedge-shaped vertebral body on lateral radiograph
  - Possible malalignment
- **Flexion-distraction (Chance) fracture**
  - Usually > 40-50% vertebral body height loss
  - Focal kyphosis; separation of facet joints & increased interspinous distance
- **Fracture-dislocation**
  - Gross malalignment

CT Findings

- Bone CT
  - **Anterior compression fracture**
    - Mild anterior wedging with associated fracture
    - Absence of posterior cortical displacement & posterior element fractures
  - **Burst fracture**
    - Stellate fracture pattern
  - **Flexion-distraction (Chance) fracture**
    - Fractured vertebral body, often comminuted
    - Separation of facet joints and increased interspinous distance
  - **Fracture-dislocation**
    - Widened, comminuted neural arch
    - Fracture through facet joints
    - Overlapping or uncovered articulating processes on axial imaging
    - Vertebral body comminution; retropulsed fracture fragments in spinal canal

MR Findings

- Burst fracture
  - May be associated with cord contusion
- Flexion-distraction (Chance) fracture
  - T2WI: Disruption of posterior longitudinal ligament, interspinous ligaments
  - Anterior longitudinal ligament usually intact but may be stripped from vertebra inferior to fracture
- Fracture-dislocation
  - Cord edema/compression, skeletal distraction

Imaging Recommendations

- Best imaging tool
  - CT is imaging modality of choice in initial evaluation of skeletal injury & alignment
  - MR for evaluation of soft tissue injury & cord contusion

DIFFERENTIAL DIAGNOSIS

Spinal Abscess

- Marrow edema in facet articular processes & adjacent laminae on MR
- Surrounding soft tissue edema/enhancement; direct visualization of abscess

Spinal Metastasis

- More likely to involve inferior cortex of vertebral body
- Involvement of posterior elements & vertebral body

PATHOLOGY

General Features

- 3-column model of Davis
  - Anterior column: Anterior 2/3 of vertebral body
  - Middle column: Posterior 1/3 of vertebral body
  - Posterior column: Posterior elements
- Spinal instability if more than 2-column failure

CLINICAL ISSUES

Presentation

- Most common signs/symptoms
  - Hypotension without tachycardia
  - Priapism

Demographics

- Epidemiology
  - 2% incidence in blunt chest trauma
  - 15% have fractures at multiple levels

Treatment

- Surgical fixation of thoracic spine fractures ± canal decompression

DIAGNOSTIC CHECKLIST

Image Interpretation Pearls

- Widened interpedicular distance suggests burst fracture & vertebral body instability
- Severe compression fracture in patient with normal bone density suggests Chance fracture
- Compression fracture of inferior endplate with normal superior endplate suspicious for pathologic fracture

SELECTED REFERENCES

1. Looby S et al: Spine trauma. Radiol Clin North Am. 49(1):129-63, 2011
2. Bernstein M: Easily missed thoracolumbar spine fractures. Eur J Radiol. 74(1):6-15, 2010

STERNAL FRACTURE

Key Facts

Imaging

- Best diagnostic clue
  - Anterior chest wall trauma; sternal tenderness
  - Direct visualization of cortical discontinuity
- Radiography
  - Lateral: Visualization of fracture line
  - Frontal: Difficult fracture visualization
  - Abnormal superior mediastinum on frontal radiography: Mediastinal hemorrhage
- CT
  - Direct visualization of sternal fracture
  - Increased sensitivity with multiplanar imaging
  - Evaluation of associated injuries
- MR
  - Useful in diagnosis of sternal stress fractures
  - T1WI: Intermediate signal intensity
  - T2-weighted fat-suppressed images: High signal intensity

Top Differential Diagnoses

- Pathologic fracture
- Osteomyelitis
- Pectus excavatum
- Ossification centers

Clinical Issues

- Mechanism of injury: Motor vehicle collision (68%)
- Symptoms
  - Localized sternal pain (98%)
  - Palpable mass with point tenderness
  - Ecchymosis (50%)
- Mortality rate (25-45%); serious intrathoracic injury

Diagnostic Checklist

- MDCT is imaging modality of choice
- Lateral radiography is useful for demonstrating fracture & degree of sternal displacement

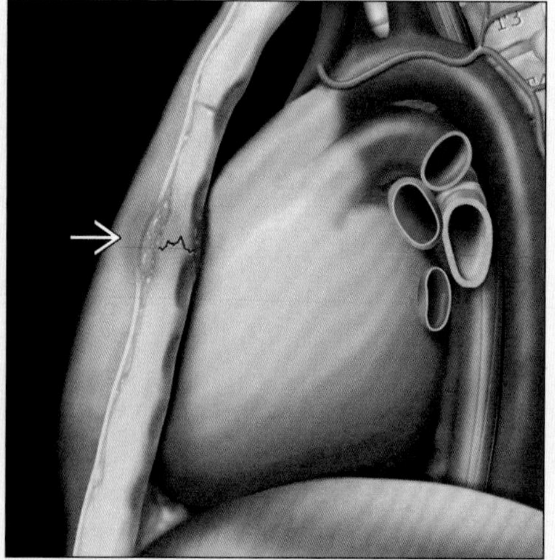

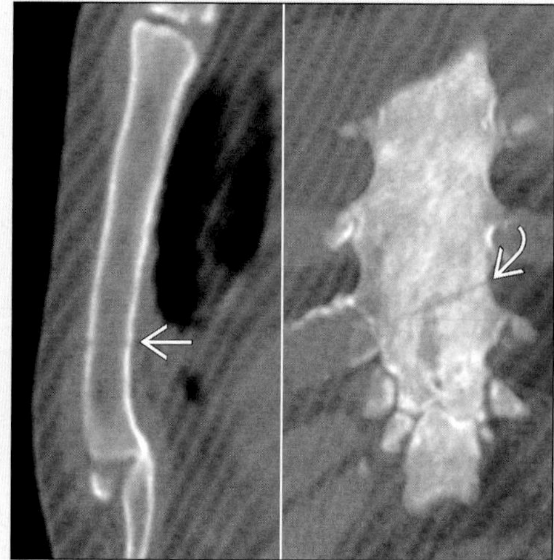

(Left) *Graphic illustrates the morphologic features of sternal fractures. These fractures are typically horizontal and may be associated with presternal ➔ and retrosternal hematoma.* ***(Right)*** *Composite image with sagittal (left) and coronal (right) CECT of a patient with a nondisplaced sternal fracture shows a minimal presternal hematoma. Sagittal CT shows a very subtle fracture line ➔, best visualized on coronal MIP ➔. Multiplanar MDCT is useful in the evaluation of sternal injuries.*

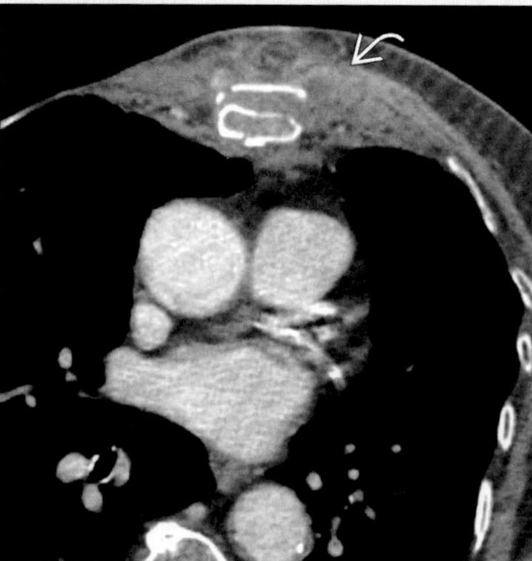

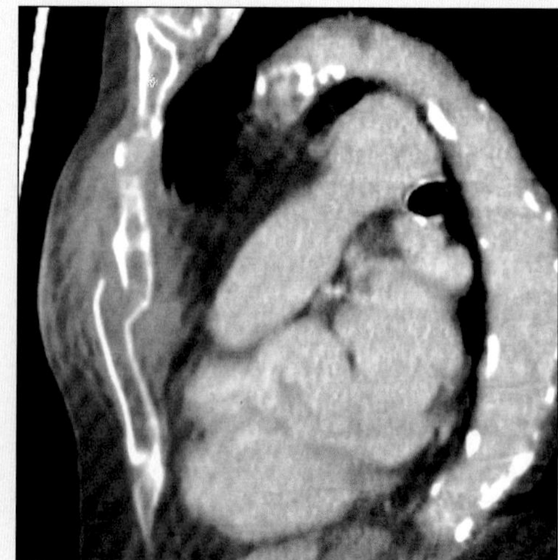

(Left) *Axial CECT of an elderly patient involved in a motor vehicle collision shows a comminuted displaced fracture through the mid sternal body with presternal ➔ and retrosternal hematoma. Note the absence of mediastinal hemorrhage or vascular injury.* ***(Right)*** *Sagittal CECT of the same patient shows a comminuted angulated fracture through the sternal body with surrounding hematoma. Sternal fracture raises suspicion for associated traumatic vascular injury, cardiac contusion, &/or vertebral fracture.*

STERNAL FRACTURE

IMAGING

General Features

- Best diagnostic clue
  - Direct visualization of sternal cortical discontinuity
  - Anterior chest wall trauma; sternal point tenderness
- Location
  - Mid sternal body, most common location
  - Sternomanubrial junction
- Morphology
  - Usually **transverse** & **nondisplaced**

Radiographic Findings

- Radiography
  - Lateral radiography
    - **Direct visualization of sternal fracture**
      - Transverse mid body (60% nondisplaced)
    - May use horizontal beam in supine patient
  - Frontal radiography
    - Difficult if not impossible visualization
  - **Abnormal superior mediastinum** on frontal radiography: More accurate terminology than "mediastinal widening"
    - Trauma
      - Normal chest radiography: 98% negative predictive value for aortic/vascular injury
      - Retrosternal or mediastinal hematoma

CT Findings

- Direct visualization & assessment of sternal fractures
- **Associated injuries**
  - **Retrosternal hematoma**: Peristernal smooth, elongated, or rounded mass (contained by pleura)
  - **Mediastinal hematoma**: Hemorrhage of sufficient magnitude; not always related to vascular injury
  - **Aortic injury**: Contrast extravasation &/or mediastinal hematoma
  - Myocardial contusion

MR Findings

- Useful in diagnosis of sternal **stress fractures**
  - T1WI: Intermediate signal intensity
  - T2-weighted fat-suppressed images: High signal intensity

Imaging Recommendations

- Best imaging tool
  - Lateral radiography; optimal projection
  - MDCT with multiplanar reformatted images improves diagnostic sensitivity
- Protocol advice
  - Sagittal & coronal reformatted images & 3D reformations improve diagnostic accuracy

DIFFERENTIAL DIAGNOSIS

Pathologic Fracture

- Underlying neoplastic lesions with bone destruction
- History of malignancy

Osteomyelitis

- Associated soft tissue mass
- Constitutional symptoms: Fever, chills, malaise
- Skeletal scintigraphy for early diagnosis

Pectus Excavatum

- No cortical discontinuity

Ossification Centers

- Nonunited ossification centers may simulate fracture

PATHOLOGY

General Features

- Etiology
  - Typically deceleration injury or direct trauma to anterior chest wall
    - **Motor vehicle crashes** (seat belt injury)
    - **Cardiopulmonary resuscitation** (CPR)
    - **Stress fractures**: Golfers, weight lifters, women with osteoporosis and kyphotic thoracic spines
- Associated abnormalities
  - Peristernal hematoma, mediastinal hematoma
  - Thoracic aortic/vascular injury
  - Pulmonary or myocardial contusion
  - Vertebral fractures in 1.4%; rib fractures

CLINICAL ISSUES

Presentation

- Most common signs/symptoms
  - **Localized sternal pain (98%)**
  - **Palpable mass with point tenderness**
  - Ecchymosis (50%)
  - Dyspnea (15-20%); painful respiration
  - Palpitations (cardiac contusion)

Demographics

- Gender
  - Elderly patients & women most commonly affected
- Epidemiology
  - Most common mechanism of injury: Motor vehicle collision (68%)

Natural History & Prognosis

- Mortality rate (25-45%); serious intrathoracic injury
  - Myocardial contusion (8%), thoracic aortic injury (4%), & heart laceration (2.5%)

Treatment

- Directed toward associated injuries
- Monitor for cardiac injury
- Analgesia with appropriate opiates or nonsteroidal anti-inflammatory drugs

DIAGNOSTIC CHECKLIST

Consider

- Evaluation of patients with sternal fracture to exclude associated serious intrathoracic injury

Image Interpretation Pearls

- No established relationship between sternal fracture & cardiac or aortic injury

SELECTED REFERENCES

1. Peters S et al: Multidetector computed tomography-spectrum of blunt chest wall and lung injuries in polytraumatized patients. Clin Radiol. 65(4):333-8, 2010

DIAPHRAGMATIC RUPTURE

Key Facts

Terminology
- Traumatic hemidiaphragm laceration; may result in intrathoracic herniation of abdominal viscera

Imaging
- Right & left sides likely equally affected
- Left visceral herniation in 70-90% of cases
- Radiography
  - Abnormal in 90% of cases; sensitivity 50% for left-sided tears & 20% for right-sided tears
  - Abnormal diaphragmatic contour
  - Intrathoracic air-filled bowel
  - Intrathoracic enteric tube
- CT
  - Dependent viscera sign: Herniated abdominal contents abut posterior ribs
  - Collar sign: Focal constriction of bowel or liver by torn diaphragm edges

Top Differential Diagnoses
- Diaphragmatic eventration
  - No dependent viscera sign
  - Hemidiaphragm intact
- Bochdalek hernia
  - More common on left
  - More common in elderly women with emphysema
- Diaphragmatic paralysis
- Pleural effusion: Subpulmonic/loculated
  - May mimic hemidiaphragm elevation

Clinical Issues
- Nonspecific complaints
- Latent: May manifest later in hospital course

Diagnostic Checklist
- Diagnosis requires high index of suspicion & careful evaluation of multiplanar reformatted images

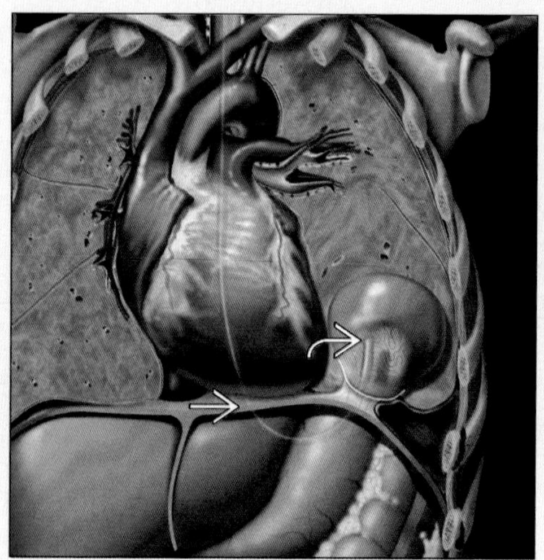

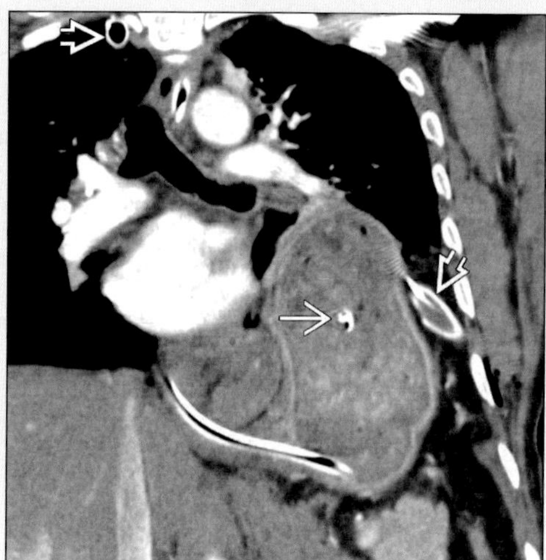

*(**Left**) Graphic depicts a left hemidiaphragmatic rupture with intrathoracic herniation of the gastric fundus through a small diaphragmatic defect. The nasogastric tube courses normally through the EG junction ➔ but terminates in the intrathoracic gastric fundus ➔. (**Right**) Coronal CECT shows intrathoracic location of the stomach consistent with a ruptured left hemidiaphragm. The nasogastric tube ➔ extends into the intrathoracic gastric fundus. Bilateral chest tubes ➔ are present.*

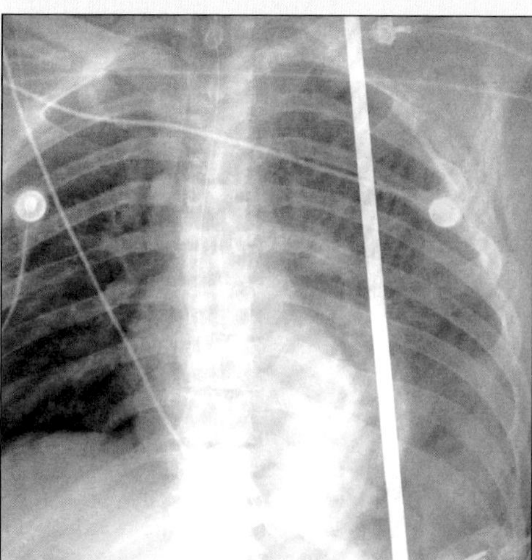

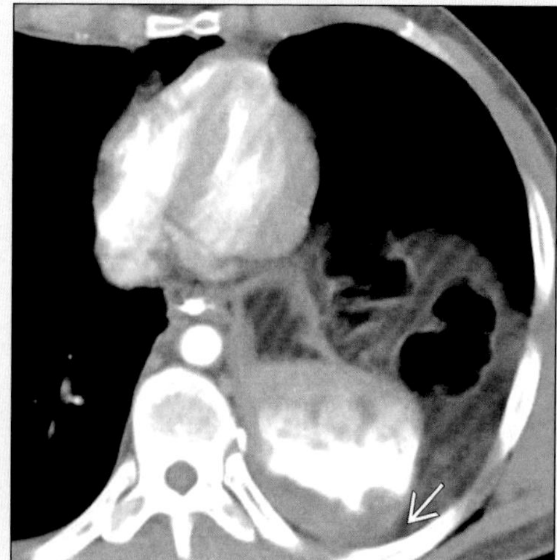

*(**Left**) AP chest radiograph of a patient who sustained severe thoracoabdominal blunt trauma shows poor visualization of the left hemidiaphragm interface and increased opacity in the left inferior hemithorax. Basilar airspace disease and pleural effusion may also obscure diaphragmatic visualization. (**Right**) Axial CECT shows intrathoracic location of the stomach, omentum, and bowel. The stomach abuts the left posterior ribs ➔ (dependent viscera sign), confirming left diaphragmatic rupture.*

DIAPHRAGMATIC RUPTURE

TERMINOLOGY

Synonyms

- Diaphragmatic tear or laceration

Definitions

- Traumatic hemidiaphragm laceration; may result in intrathoracic herniation of abdominal viscera
  - More common with blunt than penetrating trauma

IMAGING

General Features

- Best diagnostic clue
  - Air-filled bowel above hemidiaphragm
    - Increased accuracy with supradiaphragmatic enteric tube
- Location
  - Right & left sides likely equally affected
    - Visceral herniation much more common on left (70-90%)
    - Liver less likely to herniate through right-sided lacerations
- Size
  - Variable size of diaphragmatic tear: Small in penetrating trauma, large in blunt trauma
    - Prevalence of visceral herniation increases with larger tears
- Morphology
  - Blunt: Linear or radial tears typically at hemidiaphragm dome where tendon is thinnest
    - Most commonly extend posterolaterally along embryonic closure of pleuroperitoneal membrane

Radiographic Findings

- **Abnormal in 90% of cases**; sensitivity 50% for left-sided tears & 20% for right-sided tears
  - Often nonspecific because of associated lower lobe atelectasis or contusion
- **Abnormal diaphragmatic contour**
  - Hemidiaphragm elevation > 7 cm
  - Positional change of hemidiaphragm contour/shape
- **Intrathoracic air-filled bowel**
- **Intrathoracic enteric tube**
  - Tear usually spares esophageal hiatus
  - Enteric tube courses into abdomen & then courses into hemithorax
- Contralateral mediastinal shift: Visceral herniation produces mass effect
- Bowel strangulation
  - Pleural effusion suggests strangulation
  - With open communication, pleural fluid should not accumulate in pleural space
  - Omental fat may simulate pleural effusion, may layer on decubitus examination

Upper Gastrointestinal Series

- Visualization of herniated bowel
- Approximation & narrowing of afferent/efferent bowel loops (pinched limbs) through diaphragmatic defect (collar sign or kissing birds sign)

CT Findings

- **Dependent viscera sign**: Herniated bowel or viscera no longer supported posteriorly by diaphragm
  - Right: Upper 1/3 of liver contact with posterior ribs
  - Left: Stomach or bowel contact with posterior ribs
    - Stomach or bowel posterior to spleen
  - Present in 90% of cases
- **Direct visualization** of diaphragmatic discontinuity
  - Segmental absence of hemidiaphragm
  - Present in 70%
  - Potential false-positive: Normal posterolateral diaphragmatic defects in 5%
    - Diagnosis should not be based on this sign alone
- **Collar sign**: Visceral herniation with focal constriction of bowel or liver by torn diaphragm edges
  - Present in 30% on axial images; 70% on sagittal or coronal reformations
- Diaphragmatic thickening
  - Muscle retraction vs. muscular hematoma
  - Present in 30%
  - Very subjective with high proportion of false-positives
    - Normal crural thickness variation; thickness variation with age & gender
- Blunt trauma
  - Left diaphragmatic tear: Sensitivity approaching 100%, specificity 100%
  - Right diaphragmatic tear: Sensitivity 70-80%, specificity 100%
  - Coronal & sagittal reformations can increase diagnostic confidence
- Penetrating trauma
  - Same as blunt trauma but includes
    - Trajectory of missile or penetrating instrument (sensitivity 35%, specificity 100%)
    - Active extravasation of contrast (sensitivity < 10%)

MR Findings

- Similar to CT, more difficult to perform in acute traumatic setting

Nuclear Medicine Findings

- Liver-spleen colloid scans for diagnosis of right-sided diaphragmatic tear (scintigraphic collar sign)

Imaging Recommendations

- Best imaging tool
  - Diaphragmatic indistinctness/elevation on radiography should raise index of suspicion
  - CT is imaging modality of choice for global evaluation in polytrauma
- Protocol advice
  - Reformatted images increase sensitivity for diaphragmatic tears: Sagittal > coronal > axial

DIFFERENTIAL DIAGNOSIS

Diaphragmatic Eventration

- Intact hemidiaphragm
- No associated injuries
- No dependent viscera sign
- Typically elderly women without history of recent trauma
- Bowel loops not approximated in eventration
- Difficult distinction if preexisting condition in setting of recent blunt trauma

Bochdalek Hernia

- More common on left

DIAPHRAGMATIC RUPTURE

- More common in women
- Normal aging process
- More common with emphysema

Diaphragmatic Paralysis

- Paradoxical motion on fluoroscopy (sniff test)
- No recent history of trauma

Pleural Effusion: Subpulmonic/Loculated

- May mimic hemidiaphragm elevation
- No abnormally positioned air-filled bowel
- Intact diaphragm & diaphragmatic crus

Paraesophageal Hernia

- Large hernia may preferentially extend into right or left hemithorax
- Diaphragmatic contour typically intact

Esophageal Rupture

- Tear rare at esophageal hiatus

Subphrenic Abscess

- Diaphragm intact, separate from bowel
- Clinical presentation of chronic infection

PATHOLOGY

General Features

- Etiology
  - High-energy blunt thoracoabdominal trauma
    - Sudden rise in intraabdominal pressure ruptures diaphragm
    - Lateral impact distorts chest wall & shears diaphragm
  - Physiology
    - Diaphragm separates abdomen (positive intraabdominal pressure) from thorax (negative intrapleural pressure)
    - 7-20 cm H_2O pressure gradient between abdomen & pleura favors intrathoracic visceral herniation
- Associated abnormalities
  - Rib fractures 90%
  - Liver or spleen laceration 60%
  - Pelvic fractures 50%
  - Traumatic aortic injury 5%
  - High association with head injury
- Kinetic energy absorption does not respect anatomic borders
  - Multiple simultaneous injuries above & below diaphragm
- Spontaneous healing uncommon; herniated structures prevent approximation of torn edges
- Most commonly herniated organs
  - Left: Stomach > colon > spleen
  - Right: Liver
- Penetrating injuries usually smaller (< 1 cm diameter)

Gross Pathologic & Surgical Features

- Blunt: Radial tear extends from central tendon posterolaterally
  - > 2 cm long (most > 10 cm long)
- Penetrating: Any location; typically < 1 cm

CLINICAL ISSUES

Presentation

- Most common signs/symptoms
  - Nonspecific; consider in any patient with blunt thoracoabdominal injury
- Other signs/symptoms
  - Thoracic splenosis can rarely occur years after injury
  - Rupture with intrapericardial herniation occurs rarely
- Latent: May manifest later in hospital course, especially after weaning from ventilator
  - During normal respiration, pressure gradient exacerbates herniation of abdominal contents
  - High index of suspicion important
- Bowel obstruction
  - Bowel strangulation
    - 85% strangulation within 3 years (presentation may be delayed for decades)
    - Obstructive symptoms, fever, chest pain

Demographics

- Age
  - Any age but most common in young men
- Epidemiology
  - Prevalence of 5% in blunt chest trauma

Natural History & Prognosis

- Diagnosis delayed in 25%
  - Often other more compelling injuries such as aortic laceration
  - Initial nonspecific signs; injury not considered
  - Gradient for herniation dependent on normal negative pleural pressure
    - Positive pressure ventilation may delay herniation until spontaneous respiration resumes
- Morbidity & mortality higher with strangulation
  - New pleural effusion in patient with herniated bowel heralds onset of strangulation

Treatment

- Immediate surgical repair of other life-threatening injuries, such as traumatic vascular injury
- Surgical repair of torn diaphragm & reduction of herniation

DIAGNOSTIC CHECKLIST

Consider

- Diagnosis requires high index of suspicion & careful evaluation of multiplanar reformatted images

SELECTED REFERENCES

1. Losanoff JE et al: Spontaneous rupture of the diaphragm: case report and comprehensive review of the world literature. J Thorac Cardiovasc Surg. 139(6):e127-8, 2010
2. Sangster GP et al: Blunt traumatic injuries of the lung parenchyma, pleura, thoracic wall, and intrathoracic airways: multidetector computer tomography imaging findings. Emerg Radiol. 14(5):297-310, 2007
3. Eren S et al: Imaging of diaphragmatic rupture after trauma. Clin Radiol. 61(6):467-77, 2006
4. Nchimi A et al: Helical CT of blunt diaphragmatic rupture. AJR Am J Roentgenol. 184(1):24-30, 2005

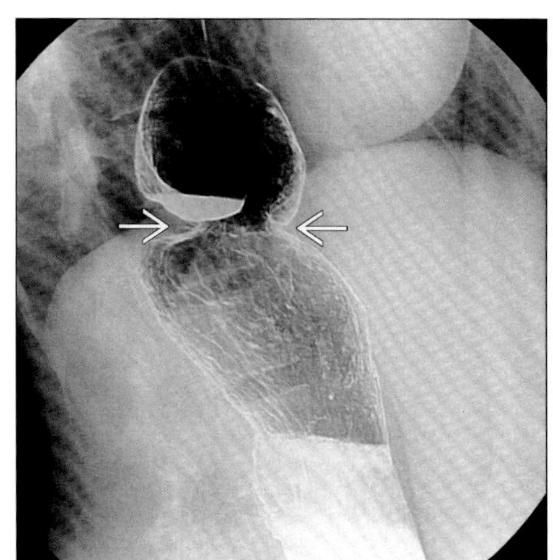

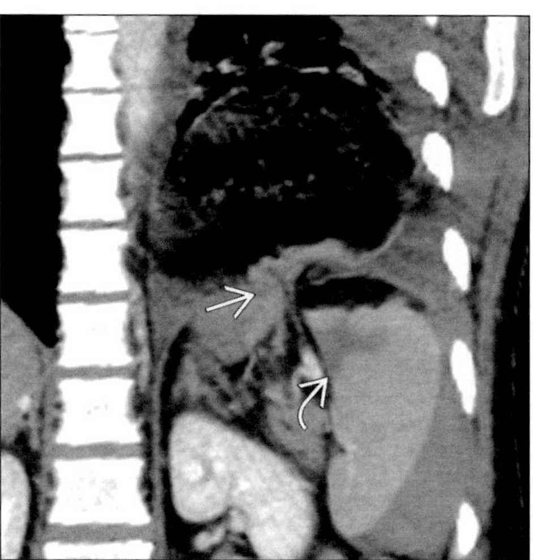

(Left) *Upper GI series of a patient with known blunt trauma shows gastric herniation through a ruptured left hemidiaphragm. The stomach is constricted ➔ by the torn diaphragm edges (the collar sign).* ***(Right)*** *Coronal CECT shows left diaphragmatic rupture with intrathoracic gastric herniation. The stomach is constricted by the edges of the torn hemidiaphragm ➔ (the collar sign). Post-traumatic splenic laceration ➔, hemoperitoneum, and hemothorax are also present.*

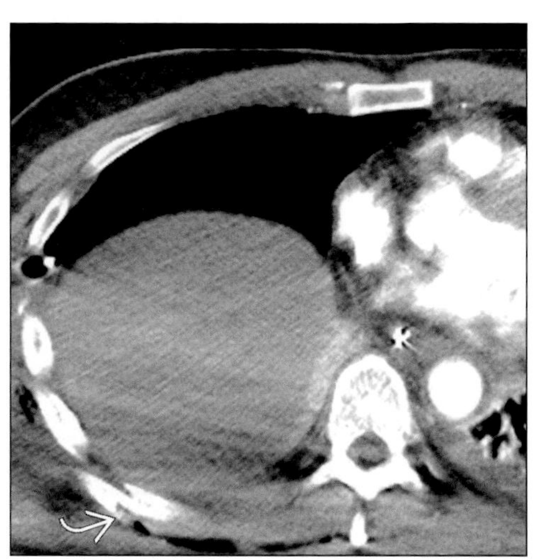

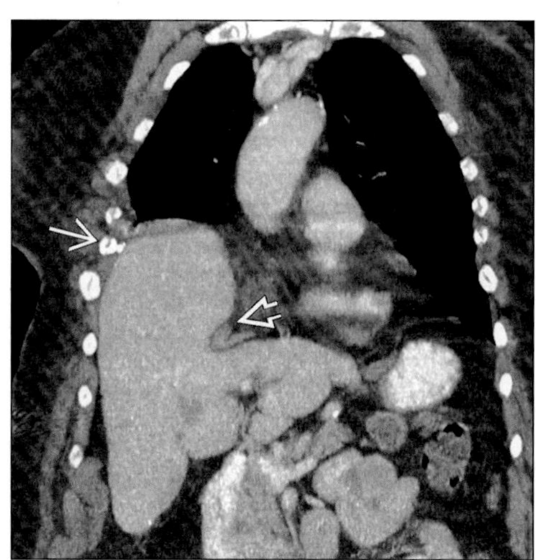

(Left) *Axial CECT of a patient who sustained blunt trauma shows the liver abutting the right posterior ribs (dependent viscera sign), one of which is fractured ➔. Note small right pleural effusion and subcutaneous gas.* ***(Right)*** *Coronal CECT of the same patient shows right diaphragmatic rupture and intrathoracic liver herniation with hepatic constriction by the torn diaphragmatic edges ➔ (the collar sign). Multiple fractured ribs ➔, a common finding in the setting of blunt trauma, were present.*

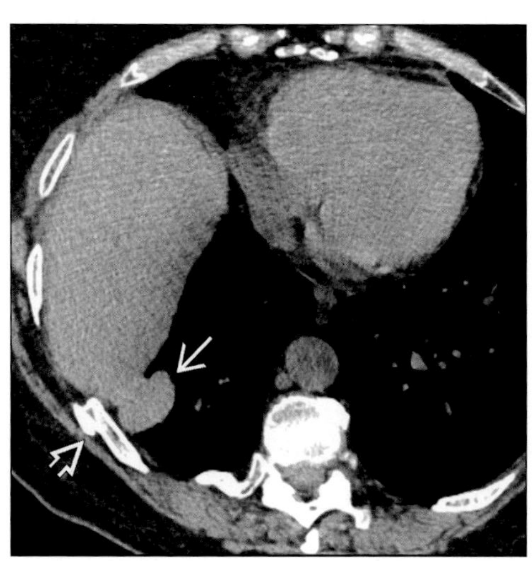

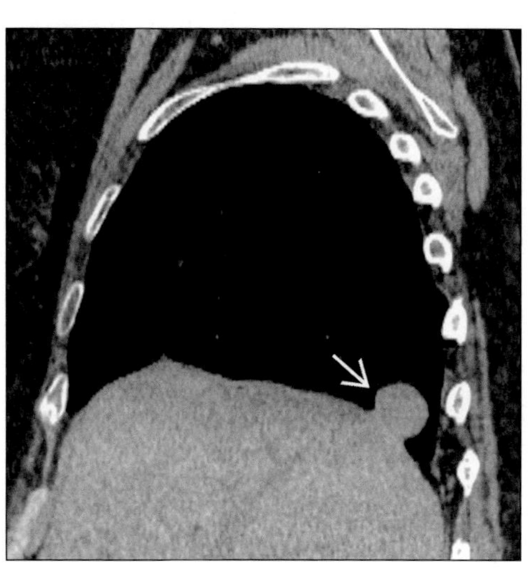

(Left) *Axial NECT of a patient with a remote history of blunt trauma shows a soft tissue mass ➔ adjacent to the right hemidiaphragm and an old right posterior rib fracture ➔.* ***(Right)*** *Sagittal NECT of the same patient shows protrusion of a small portion of the liver ➔ into the left hemithorax, consistent with small focal hemidiaphragmatic tear. The dependent viscera sign is not present due to the small and focal nature of the diaphragmatic defect and the small amount of herniated liver.*

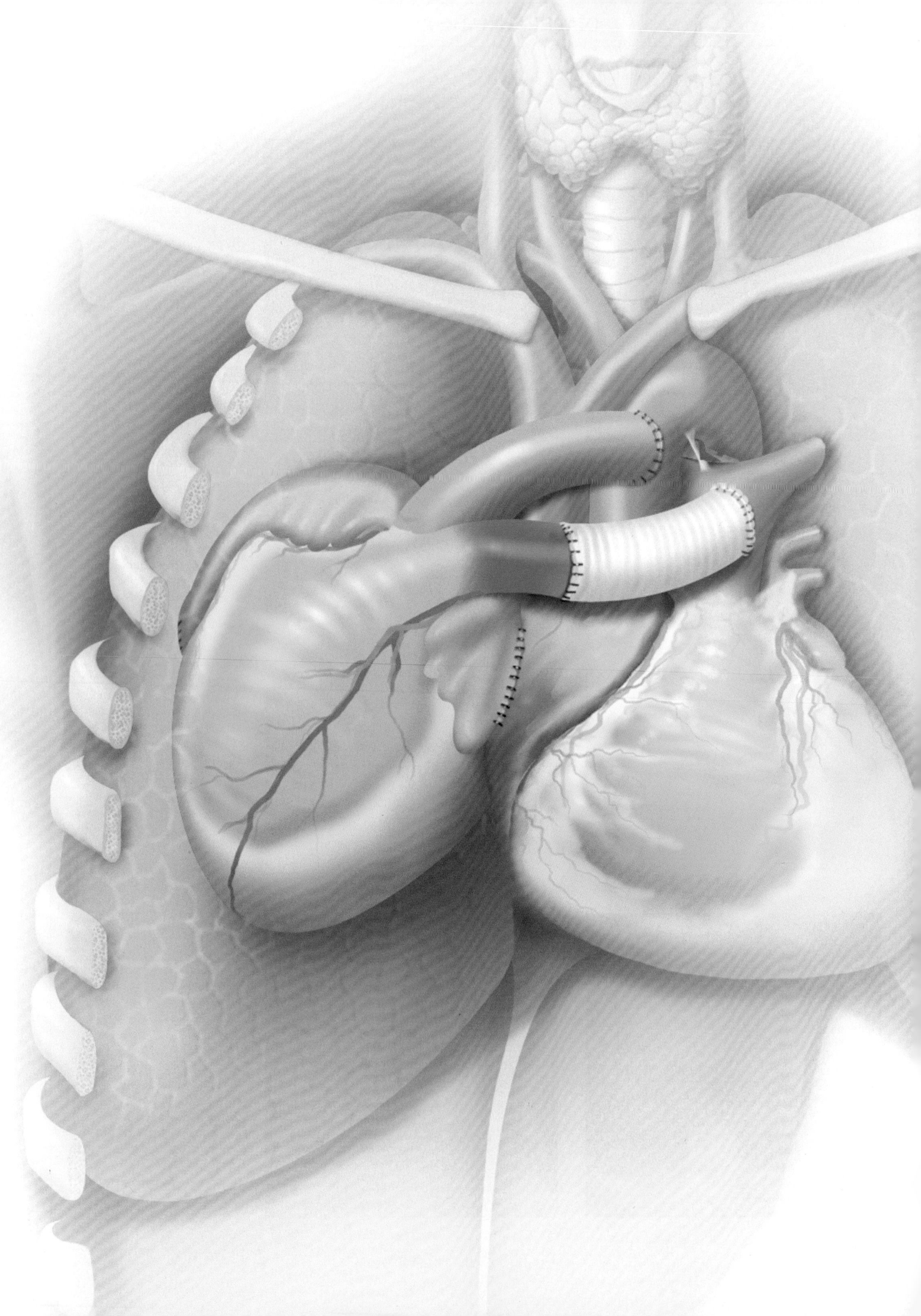

SECTION 11
Post-Treatment Chest

Introduction and Overview

Life Support Devices

Surgical Procedures and Complications

Radiation, Chemotherapy, Ablation

Introduction

A frequent challenge general and thoracic radiologists face is the imaging assessment of the chest in patients who are undergoing or have undergone treatment of thoracic and systemic conditions. Radiographic findings can often be unrevealing or nonspecific, and sometimes expected post-treatment findings can simulate pathology. An important step in the imaging assessment of the treated patient is developing an understanding of the disease process being treated and the specific treatment or treatments the patient is undergoing. Some examples include the patient's location (e.g., intensive care unit, inpatient ward, outpatient clinic), the method of treatment (e.g., surgery, ablation procedures, pleurodesis), &/or the type of medical treatment used (e.g., drugs, chemotherapy, radiotherapy).

The interpreting radiologist is provided with limited clinical information that typically consists of the indication for the specific imaging study requested. However, it is often important to gather additional relevant information via direct communication with the referring physician or the patient's nurse/nurse practitioner or by reviewing relevant entries in the patient's electronic medical record. The patient's history and physical typically list prior treatments and surgeries, current therapies, and plans for future management.

The approach to the post-treatment chest includes assessment of various medical and support devices commonly identified on radiography, evaluation of prior surgical or interventional procedures and their potential complications, monitoring response to therapy, and identification of treatment-related complications.

Tubes and Lines

A significant volume of radiographic interpretation in the inpatient setting consists of portable radiographs for assessment of medical devices, tubes, and catheters. These studies are usually performed to document the exact location of the support apparatus. Familiarity with normal imaging anatomy allows the radiologist to assess appropriate device position and alert the clinical team regarding device malpositioning and associated complications. Interpretation of portable radiographs is often challenging as radiographic technique is limited compared to conventional radiography and resultant images may be compromised by magnification, motion, body habitus, and overlying extraneous devices.

Common support devices routinely assessed with portable chest radiography include central venous catheters, peripherally inserted central catheters (PICC), pulmonary arterial catheters, endotracheal tubes, enteric tubes, intra-aortic balloon pumps (IABP), pacemakers/automated implantable cardioverter-defibrillators (AICD), ventricular assist devices (VAD), and extracorporeal membrane oxygenation (ECMO) devices.

Portable chest radiographs obtained for documentation of medical device position must be interpreted with a high index of suspicion. For example, central line placement is often initially attempted on the right side. Therefore when a left-sided catheter or line is identified, even when appropriately positioned, the entire thorax must be scrutinized to exclude contralateral pneumothorax or pleural effusion or interval mediastinal widening. These findings typically indicate a complicated line placement attempt on the right. It should be noted that radiographic abnormalities that are easily seen on conventional chest radiography may be more difficult to identify on portable radiographs. For instance, a pneumothorax on supine radiography may manifest with the "**deep sulcus**" **sign** or as a hyperlucent hemithorax rather than the apical pleural line seen on upright PA radiography. Likewise, a pleural effusion may manifest as increased haziness over the lung bases rather than the typical **meniscus sign** seen on erect radiographs.

Surgical Procedures

A variety of procedures are used in the surgical management of various thoracic diseases. These include sublobar resection, lobectomy, pneumonectomy, sternotomy, cardiac transplantation, single and double-lung transplantation, and esophagectomy. The radiologist must develop familiarity with the postoperative appearance of these procedures as well as with their known complications.

Radiographic interpretation in patients who have undergone thoracic surgical procedures can be challenging. It is usually important to review the clinical chart or consult with the clinical team to establish the nature of the surgical procedure performed. This helps avoid erroneous interpretation of expected postsurgical findings. A good example is the appearance of the pleural space following pleurodesis. Such patients characteristically develop high-attenuation nodular pleural thickening that often exhibits exuberant FDG uptake, but they occasionally develop nodular pleural thickening of soft tissue attenuation that may mimic pleural metastases. An awareness of the expected imaging manifestations of prior surgical treatments can prevent unnecessary additional imaging or tissue sampling.

Medical Treatment

Medical treatment may also produce a variety of imaging manifestations. The medical literature establishes that several drugs can produce pulmonary toxicity. The sheer number of drugs associated with pulmonary toxicity and the variable imaging manifestations of toxicity can be overwhelming. An excellent source available through the internet for public consultation can be found at www.pneumotox.com. This website provides an extensive and thorough evidence-based list of drugs producing toxicity and the specific pathologic and imaging findings of such drug reactions.

When interpreting chest imaging studies of patients undergoing drug treatment, it is important to assume that drug toxicity may be present. Knowledge of idiosyncratic manifestations, length and timeline of drug therapy, and dosage may be critical in determining whether drug-induced lung disease is more or less likely.

Selected References

1. Kim EA et al: Radiographic and CT findings in complications following pulmonary resection. Radiographics. 22(1):67-86, 2002
2. Rossi SE et al: Pulmonary drug toxicity: radiologic and pathologic manifestations. Radiographics. 20(5):1245-59, 2000
3. Aronchick JM et al: Tubes and lines in the intensive care setting. Semin Roentgenol. 32(2):102-16, 1997

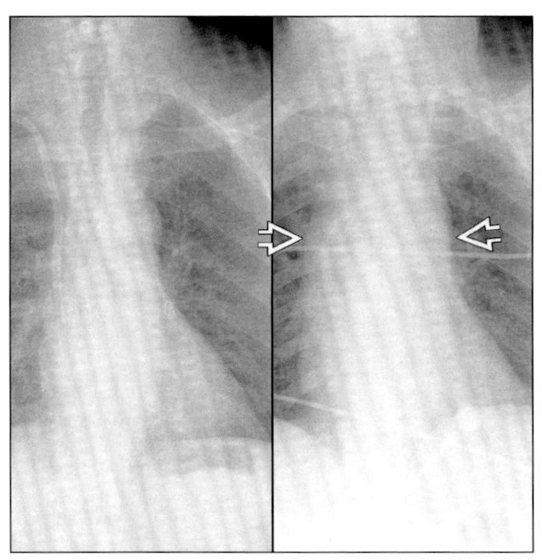

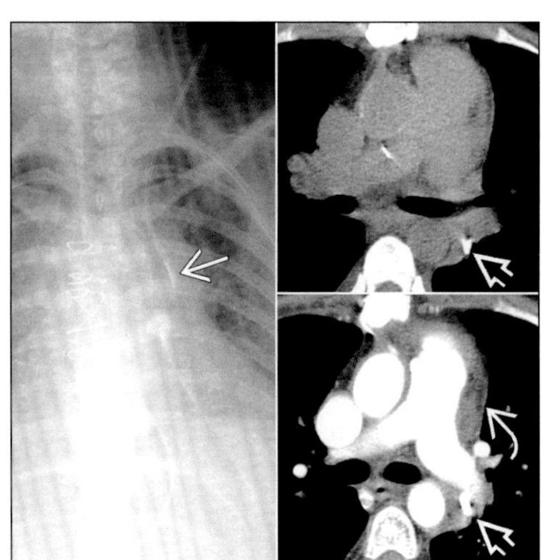

(Left) *Composite image with PA chest radiographs showing interval mediastinal widening from mediastinal hematoma after left internal jugular line placement (right) compared to prior chest radiograph (left) documenting a previously normal mediastinum.* ***(Right)*** *Composite image with PA chest radiograph (left) and axial NECT/CECT (right) shows a malpositioned left internal jugular central line that courses away from midline. CT confirms extravascular location and mediastinal hematoma.*

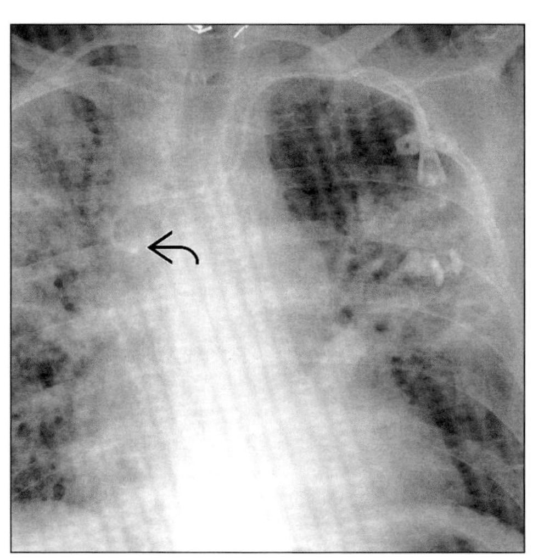

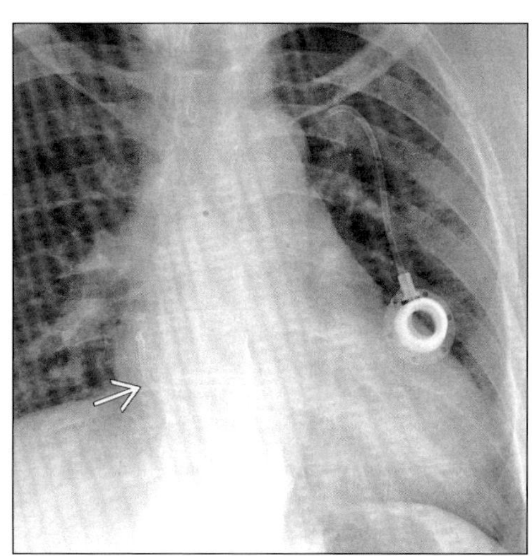

(Left) *PA chest radiograph shows a left subclavian central line with a medial curvature of its distal tip above the right mainstem bronchus terminating in the azygos arch.* ***(Right)*** *PA chest radiograph shows a left subclavian port with a short catheter segment terminating at the left clavicle and a separate catheter segment in the right atrium, consistent with embolized fractured catheter. Fractured catheter fragments can often be retrieved with endovascular interventional techniques.*

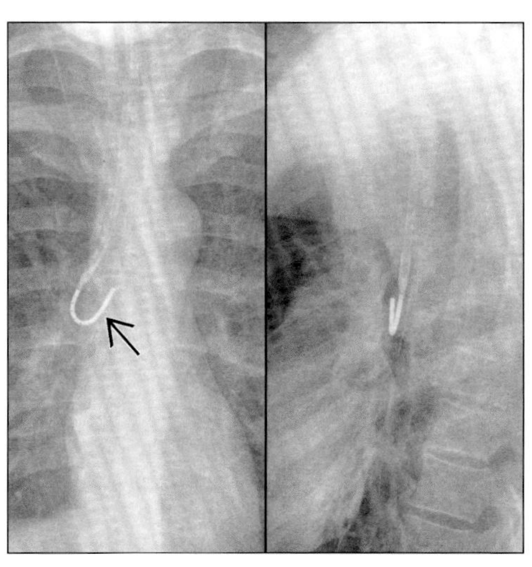

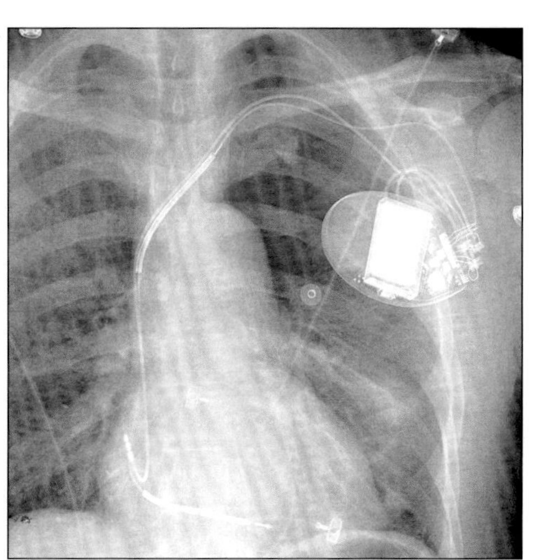

(Left) *Composite image with PA (left) and lateral (right) chest radiographs shows a feeding tube in the trachea with the tip coiled in the right mainstem bronchus. Chest radiography is performed to document appropriate position of medical devices.* ***(Right)*** *PA chest radiograph shows a moderate left pneumothorax after placement of a left pectoral AICD. Hematoma, pneumothorax, and hemothorax are known complications of line placement via subclavian approach.*

*(**Left**) Composite image with PA chest radiographs of a patient with sternal dehiscence and osteomyelitis obtained in the early postsurgical period (left) and a month later (right) shows displacement and rotation of a sternal wire ➔, two of the most common radiographic signs of dehiscence. (**Right**) Axial CECT of the same patient shows sternal dehiscence with a presternal anterior chest wall fluid collection ➔ consistent with an abscess. Note retrosternal gas ➔ abutting the anterior mediastinum.*

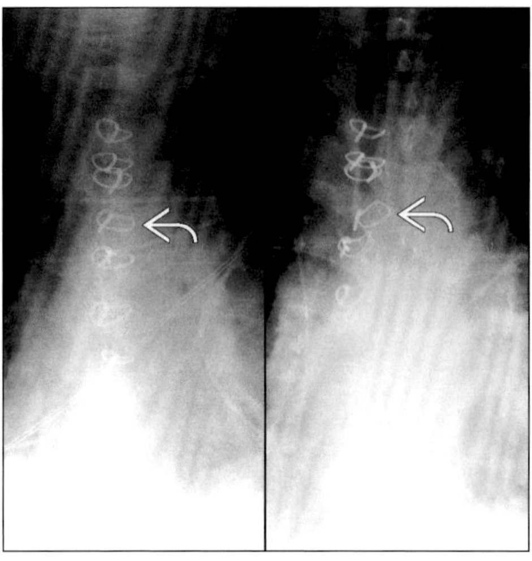

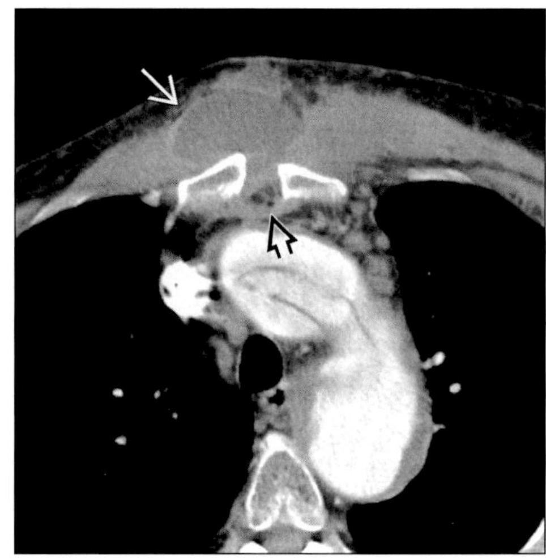

*(**Left**) Axial NECT of a patient with right upper lobectomy complicated by right lower lobe torsion shows extensive right lower lobe airspace disease. Lobar torsion is rare, but may occur spontaneously or after surgery or trauma. (**Right**) Composite image with axial NECT (left) and FDG PET (right) shows a spiculated soft tissue mass ➔ surrounding the staple line from a prior wedge resection for lung cancer. Extensive FDG uptake is consistent with recurrent tumor along the suture line ➔.*

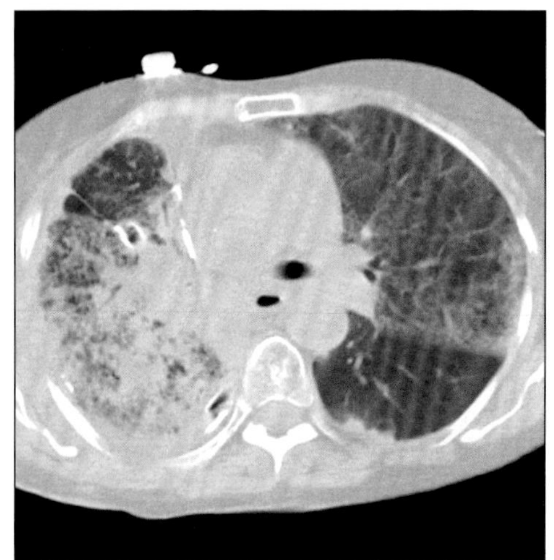

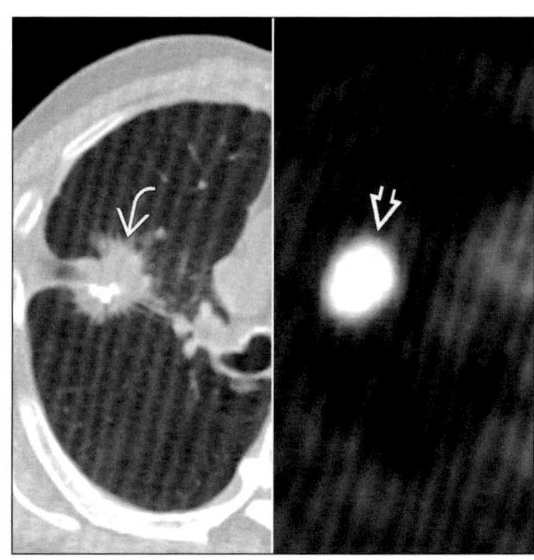

*(**Left**) Axial fused PET/CT of a patient undergoing right lung irradiation shows bilateral FDG-avid consolidations ➔. Open lung biopsy demonstrated multifocal organizing pneumonia. (**Right**) Axial NECT of a patient with single left lung transplant shows extensive right lung pulmonary fibrosis and a right lower lobe mass ➔ secondary to bronchogenic carcinoma. Primary lung cancer is a known complication in the native fibrotic lungs of patients with a prior single lung transplant.*

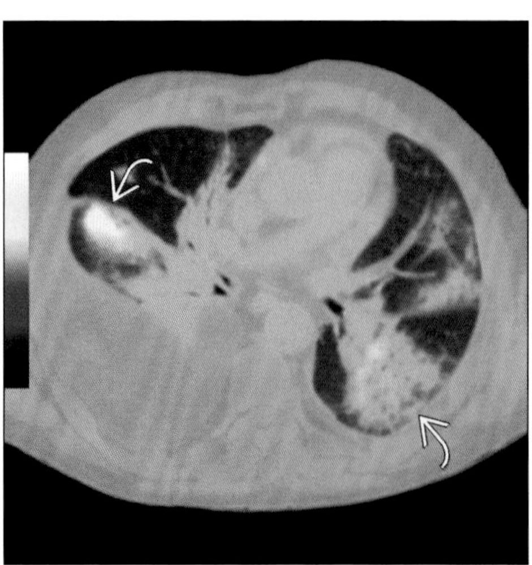

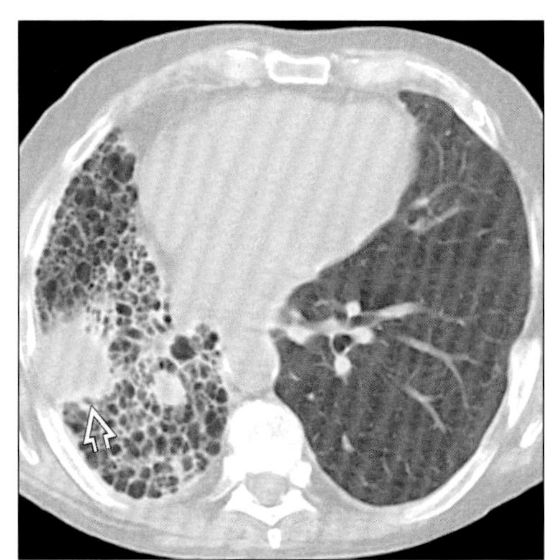

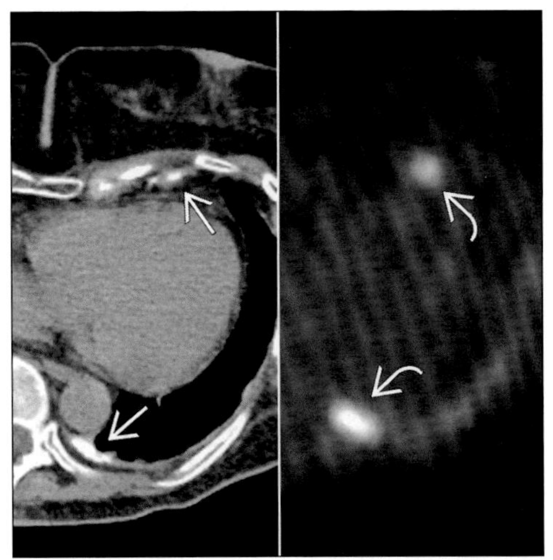

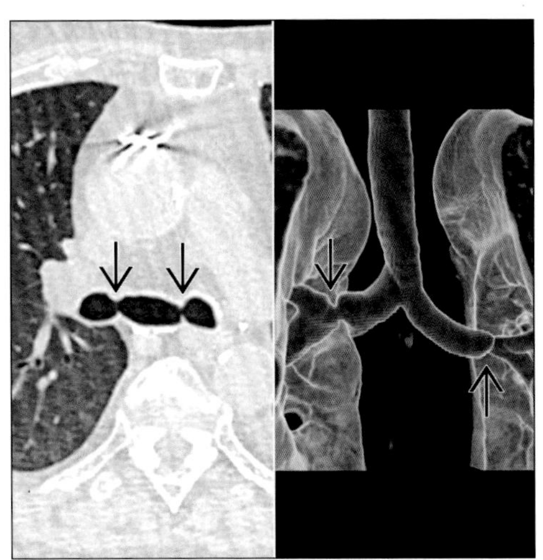

(Left) *Composite image with axial NECT (left) and FDG PET (right) of a patient with prior talc pleurodesis for malignant pleural effusion shows calcified left pleural plaques ➔. Talc elicits a pleural granulomatous reaction that is often FDG avid ➚.* **(Right)** *Composite image with axial NECT (left) and coronal 3D reformation (right) of a patient with prior bilateral lung transplant shows bilateral bronchial stenoses ➔, a common complication at the level of the bronchial anastomosis.*

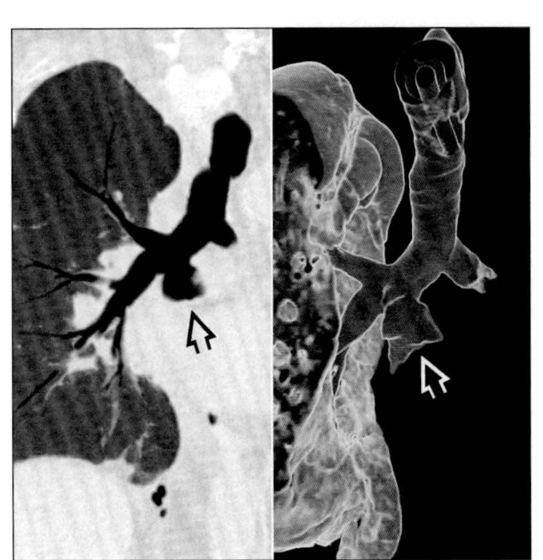

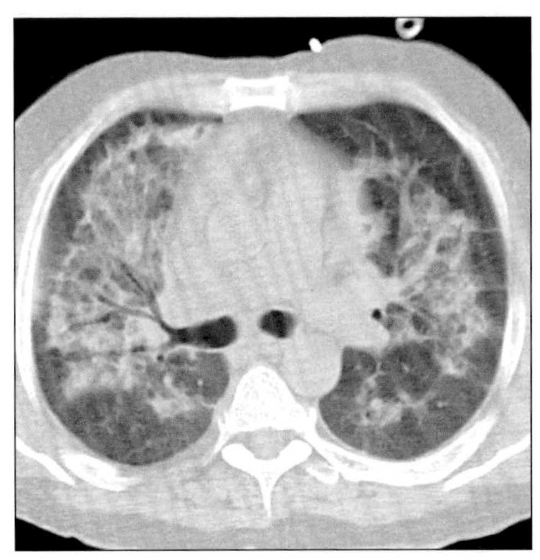

(Left) *Composite image with coronal MinIP (left) and coronal 3D reformat (right) of a patient with bilateral lung transplant shows anastomotic dehiscence manifesting with an air-filled outpouching ➢ at the right bronchial anastomosis also seen on the 3D reformatted image ➢.* **(Right)** *Axial NECT of a patient treated with busulfan shows extensive bilateral peribronchovascular heterogeneous airspace disease proven to represent organizing pneumonia on open lung biopsy.*

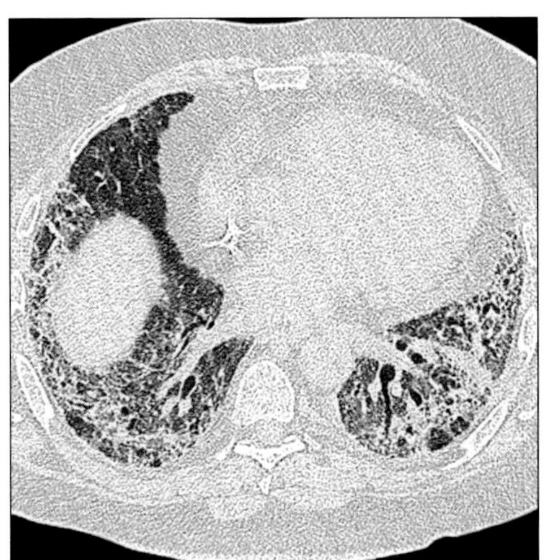

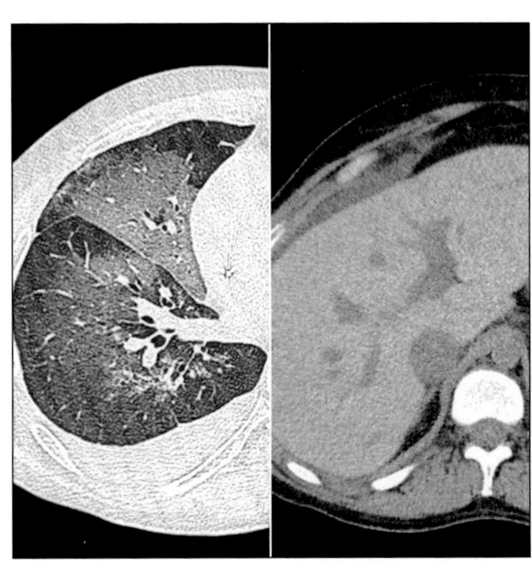

(Left) *Axial HRCT of a patient undergoing treatment with bleomycin demonstrates extensive subpleural reticular opacities, ground-glass opacities, and traction bronchiectasis secondary to pulmonary fibrosis.* **(Right)** *Composite image with axial chest (left) and abdomen (right) NECT of a patient with eosinophilia and a history of amiodarone therapy shows ground-glass opacities from eosinophilic pneumonia, pleural effusion, hyperdense liver, and mild ascites secondary to amiodarone toxicity.*

APPROPRIATELY POSITIONED TUBES AND CATHETERS

Key Facts

Imaging

- Normal & variant anatomy of accessed structure; recognition of incorrect course of lines & tubes
- ETT
  - Neutral position: Tube tip 5-7 cm from carina
  - Cervical flexion: Tube tip 3-5 cm from carina
  - Cervical extension: Tube tip 7-9 cm from carina
  - Tube width: Ideally at least 2/3 of tracheal width
- Tracheostomy tube: No mobility with cervical flexion & extension
  - Placed 1-3 weeks after endotracheal intubation
- Enteric tube: Fluid suction in supine position; tube tip in fundus
  - Air suction in supine position; tube tip in antrum
- Chest tube: Pneumothorax drainage in supine patient; tip in anterosuperior pleural space
  - Hydrothorax drainage in supine patient; tip in posteroinferior pleural space
- CVL: Ideal position, distal superior vena cava or upper right atrium
- IACPB: Ideal position, tip distal to left subclavian artery
- Pulmonary artery catheter: Ideal position, right or left pulmonary artery
- Ultrasound guidance for line/tube insertion
- Radiography always performed after insertion of tube or line to document position & identify complications
- CT rarely needed to assess tube or catheter position
- CT assessment & planning for drainage of complex pleural fluid/empyema or air collection

Clinical Issues

- Empyema: Poor or delayed drainage results in fibrothorax & requires decortication
- Pitfalls: External wires, tubes, clamps, syringes that lie on or under patient

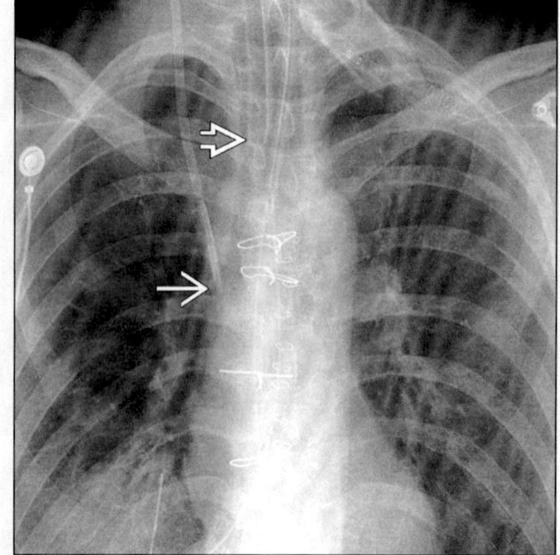

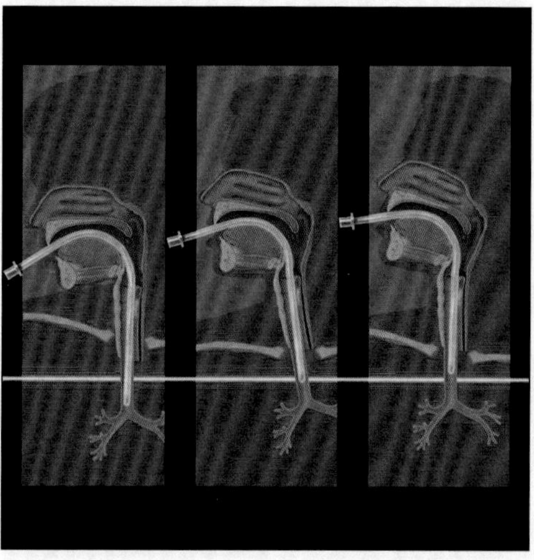

(Left) *AP chest radiograph shows a well-positioned endotracheal tube tip ⇨ approximately 5 cm above the carina. A well-positioned right internal jugular central line tip → is at the distal superior vena cava.* ***(Right)*** *Graphic shows variations in endotracheal tube tip position with neck flexion and extension. The tube tip descends with neck flexion (left) and ascends with neck extension (right). Assessment of endotracheal tube position should take into account the degree of cervical flexion or extension.*

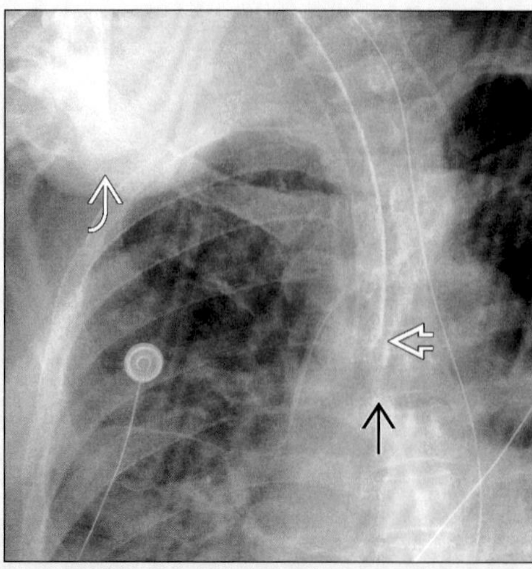

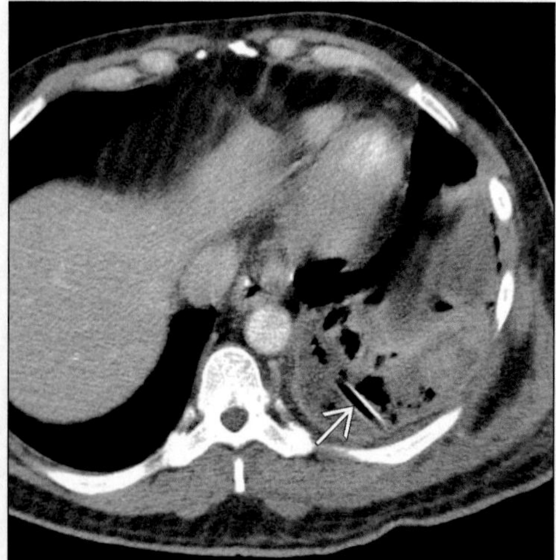

(Left) *AP chest radiograph shows an endotracheal tube tip ⇨ approximately 2 cm above the carina →. The low position results from cervical flexion as indicated by the position of the mandible ↷. The tube tip must not extend distal to the carina with cervical flexion.* ***(Right)*** *Axial CECT of a patient with left empyema shows a well-placed left chest tube → within a dependent loculated left pleural fluid collection with intrinsic air bubbles.*

APPROPRIATELY POSITIONED TUBES AND CATHETERS

TERMINOLOGY

Synonyms

- Cardiopulmonary support & monitoring devices, lines, & tubes

Definitions

- Optimal positioning of tubes, lines, & catheters

IMAGING

General Features

- Best diagnostic clue
  - Knowledge of normal & variant radiographic anatomy of accessed structure
  - Recognition of incorrect course of lines & tubes
- Location
  - Trachea, bronchi, pleura, veins, heart, aorta

Radiographic Findings

- **Endotracheal tube (ETT)**
  - **Carina is at level of T5 to T7**
  - **ETT: Neutral head & neck position**
    - **Tube tip 5-7 cm from carina**
  - **Cervical flexion**: ETT may descend 2 cm
    - Tip of mandible overlies clavicles
    - Tube tip 3-5 cm from carina
  - **Cervical extension**: ETT may ascend 2 cm
    - Tip of mandible off radiograph
    - Tube tip 7-9 cm from carina
  - Tube width: Ideally at least 2/3 of tracheal width
  - Tube cuff: Should not produce tracheal wall bulging or tube lumen narrowing
  - Double lumen endotracheal tube
    - Tube tips placed in each main stem bronchus
- **Tracheostomy tube**
  - No mobility with cervical flexion & extension
  - Tube tip several centimeters above carina
  - Tube width 1/2 to 2/3 of tracheal width
  - Cuff should not distend tracheal wall
- **Enteric or feeding tube**
  - Suction of fluid in supine position; fundus is proper tube tip location
  - Suction of air in supine position; antrum is proper tube tip location
- **Chest tube**
  - 10F-40F size, depending on viscosity of material to be drained
  - Straight, J, or pigtail catheters
  - Pneumothorax evacuation in supine patient; optimal tube tip position, anterosuperior pleural space
  - Hydrothorax evacuation in supine patient; optimal tube tip position, posteroinferior pleural space
  - Empyema & hemothorax must be drained early
- **Central venous line (CVL)**
  - Access from subclavian, internal jugular, antecubital, or femoral veins
  - Peripherally inserted central catheter (PICC), small catheter peripherally inserted at or slightly proximal to antecubital fossa
  - 1-3 lumina
  - CVL: Ideal position, distal superior vena cava or upper right atrium
- **Pulmonary artery (PA) catheter**
  - Swan-Ganz is a PA catheter
  - Access from subclavian, internal jugular, antecubital, or femoral vein
  - Ideal position: Right or left pulmonary artery with deflated balloon
  - Measurement performed with inflated balloon in lower lobe (zone 3 of West)
- **Intra-aortic counterpulsation balloon (IACPB)**
  - Access from common femoral artery
  - Long balloon (28 cm)
    - Inflates during diastole
    - Deflates during systole
  - Ideal position: Tip distal to left subclavian artery
- Surgically implanted venous catheter
  - Reservoir in infraclavicular fossa, over upper abdomen or over lower ribs
  - Catheter tip at distal superior vena cava
- Transvenous pacemaker: Permanent or temporary
  - Permanent: Pulse generator & lead wires with electrodes for contact with endocardium or myocardium
    - Pulse generator: Infraclavicular fossa
    - Single or dual leads
    - Ventricular pacer
      - Frontal radiograph: Tip at right ventricle apex
      - Lateral radiograph: Anterior course, tip 3-4 mm deep to epicardial stripe
    - Atrial pacer: Frontal radiograph, tip directed medially & superiorly to right atrial appendage
- Cardiac resynchronization therapy (CRT)
  - Right & left ventricular pacing or left ventricular pacing
  - Lead placed in coronary sinus tributary
  - Option for implantable defibrillator
- Automatic implantable cardioverter defibrillator (AICD or ICD)
  - Sensing & shocking electrodes in right atrium & right ventricle
- Diaphragmatic pacing
  - Radiofrequency receiver implanted in subcutaneous tissue
  - Electrode placed on phrenic nerve posterior to clavicle
- Polyurethane catheters
  - Stiff for percutaneous insertion
  - Soften at body temperature
  - Correctly placed catheter may normally migrate distally with softening

Fluoroscopic Findings

- Fluoroscopic guidance for insertion of lines & tubes

CT Findings

- NECT
  - NECT: Assessment & planning for drainage of complex pleural fluid/empyema or air collection
  - Demonstration of relationship between chest tube & fluid collection

Ultrasonographic Findings

- Ultrasound guidance for insertion of lines & tubes

Imaging Recommendations

- Best imaging tool
  - Radiographic assessment of tube & catheter placement
  - CT rarely needed to assess tube or catheter position
- Protocol advice

APPROPRIATELY POSITIONED TUBES AND CATHETERS

- Radiography always performed after insertion of tube or line to document position & identify complications

DIFFERENTIAL DIAGNOSIS

Pitfalls

- External wires, tubes, clamps, syringes located on or under patient
- Supporting lines & catheters without radiopaque markers

PATHOLOGY

General Features

- Etiology
  - Pulmonary &/or cardiovascular failure
  - Titration of fluid & drug administration
  - Fluid or air collection compromising respiration or cardiovascular function
- Injury of adjacent structures possible even with properly placed lines & tubes

Gross Pathologic & Surgical Features

- Airway tubes
  - Mucosal ulceration, scarring
  - Airway colonization
- Cardiovascular lines: Thrombus formation at line tip; may occlude lumen

Microscopic Features

- Line infection: Cellulitis, septic emboli
- Airway: Tracheitis, mucosal ulceration, fibrosis

CLINICAL ISSUES

Presentation

- Most common signs/symptoms
  - Endotracheal tube
    - Intubation for patients with respiratory failure
    - Double lumen endotracheal tube: Differential lung ventilation to accommodate lung compliance differences
  - Tracheostomy: For patients requiring long-term intubation
  - Enteric or feeding tube: Drainage of gastric content
    - Feeding; patients at risk for aspiration
  - Chest tube: Drainage of pneumothorax or pleural fluid/empyema
    - Treatment of malignant effusion; talc or doxycycline administration
    - Nondraining chest tube may be occluded or malpositioned
  - Infection: Infected cardiovascular lines removed & cultured
    - Systemic candidiasis in patients with CVL on broad spectrum antibiotics
  - Central venous catheters
    - Maintenance of optimal blood volume; long-term drug administration
    - Pressure monitoring
    - Drug infusion
    - Nutrition
  - Pulmonary artery catheters
    - Measurement of hemodynamic pressures & cardiac output
    - Pulmonary capillary wedge pressure reflects left atrial & left ventricular end-diastolic volume
  - IACPB
    - Improvement of coronary artery perfusion & heart function (afterload reduction)
  - Surgically implanted catheter
    - Long-term venous access
    - Instillation of fluids, drugs, chemotherapy, parenteral nutrition, blood products
    - Obtaining blood samples
  - Transvenous pacemaker
    - Treatment of heart block or bradyarrhythmias
  - CRT with implantable defibrillator
    - CRT improves ejection fraction, left ventricular size, & mitral regurgitation
    - Prophylaxis for fatal ventricular tachyarrhythmias
    - Atrial synchronized ventricular pacing to optimize atrioventricular timing
    - Biventricular pacing to promote ventricular synchrony
  - AICD or ICD
    - Patient monitoring & therapy of ventricular tachycardia or fibrillation

Demographics

- Age
  - Neonate to elderly
- Gender
  - M = F
- Epidemiology
  - Intensive care & postoperative patient: Cardiopulmonary support devices
  - Patients with arrhythmias: Pacemakers

Natural History & Prognosis

- Intubated patients with long-term mechanical ventilation requirement
  - Tracheostomy tube usually placed 1-3 weeks after endotracheal intubation
- Empyema: Poor or delayed drainage results in fibrothorax & requires decortication
- Fluoroscopy & sonography during line or tube insertion
  - Safer, faster, better than relying on anatomic landmarks
- Cardiac pacemakers improve cardiac function, reduce severity of clinical symptoms, reduce mortality & morbidity

Treatment

- None for properly placed lines & tubes

SELECTED REFERENCES

1. Burney K et al: Cardiac pacing systems and implantable cardiac defibrillators (ICDs): a radiological perspective of equipment, anatomy and complications. Clin Radiol. 59(8):699-708, 2004
2. Hunter TB et al: Medical devices of the chest. Radiographics. 24(6):1725-46, 2004

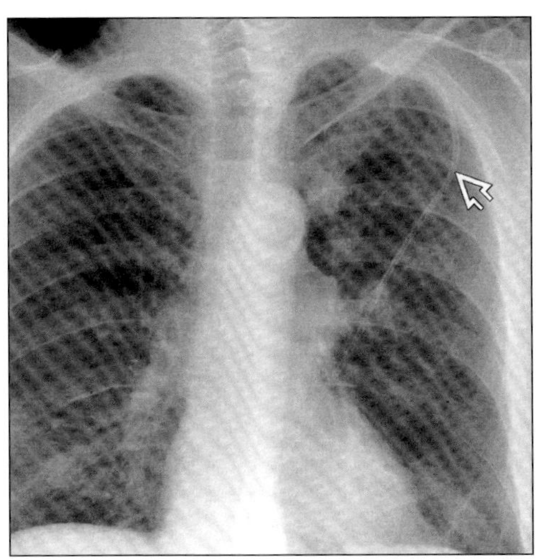

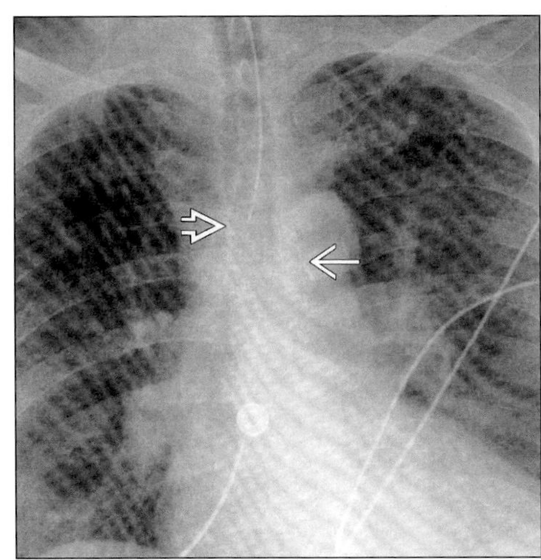

(Left) *AP chest radiograph shows a small caliber left chest tube placed for treatment of a left apical pneumothorax. No residual pneumothorax remains. The best chest tube position for pneumothorax evacuation is the anterior and superior pleural space.* ***(Right)*** *AP chest radiograph shows the marker for the aortic counterpulsation balloon device in good position distal to the origin of the left subclavian artery. The endotracheal tube tip is also in good position.*

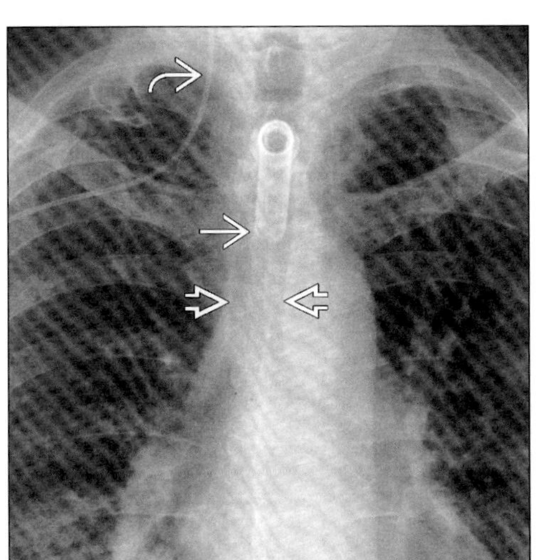

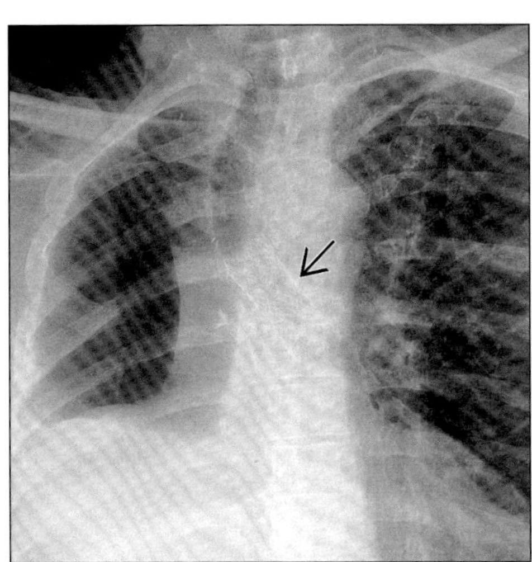

(Left) *AP chest radiograph shows an appropriately positioned tracheostomy tube. The tracheostomy tube diameter is > 50% of the diameter of the tracheal air column. The right PICC courses against blood flow into the right internal jugular vein and should be repositioned.* ***(Right)*** *PA chest radiograph of a patient with a remote right pneumonectomy and a right bronchial stump leak shows a well positioned tracheobronchial stent placed to occlude the fistula.*

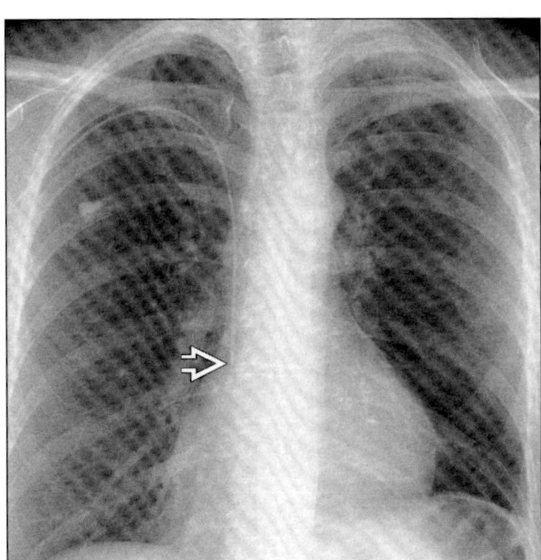

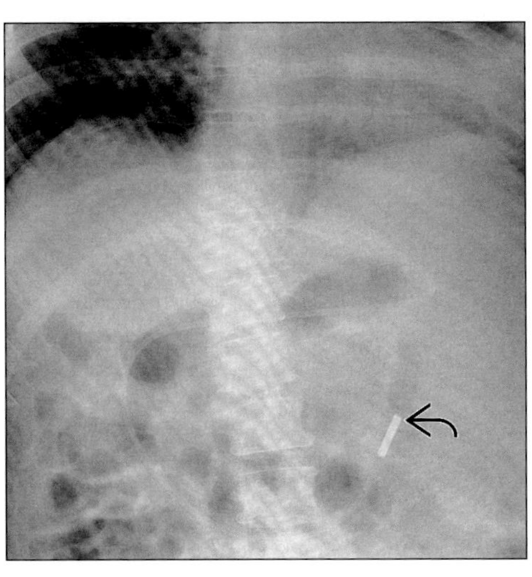

(Left) *PA chest radiograph shows a right PICC tip in good position at the superior cavoatrial junction.* ***(Right)*** *AP abdomen radiograph shows a Dobbhoff feeding tube coursing into the stomach and duodenum and terminating at the ligament of Treitz, which is a desirable feeding tube tip position.*

ABNORMALLY POSITIONED TUBES AND CATHETERS

Key Facts

Imaging

- ETT: Right mainstem bronchus intubation; left lung atelectasis, right lung hyperinflation, or pneumothorax
- ETT: Pharyngoesophageal intubation; dilated esophagus & stomach, aspiration, small lung volume
- Enteric tube: Tip in bronchus, lung, pleura; pneumothorax with lung/pleura penetration
- Chest tube: Tip impingement on mediastinum; erosion into arteries, veins, or esophagus
- CVL: Tip in right atrium, right ventricle (arrhythmias), pericardium, liver
- CVL: Assessment for pneumothorax after placement
- Pulmonary artery catheter: Lung infarction/ pulmonary artery pseudoaneurysm from wedged catheter
- IACPB: Too low, occlusion of celiac, renal, superior mesenteric arteries
- Transvenous pacemaker: Broken lead between clavicle & 1st rib "osseous pinch"
- Lines & tubes may change position over time; follow-up radiography for assessment

Clinical Issues

- CVL infection: Usually *Staphylococcus*, *Candida* in patients on broad spectrum antibiotics
- ETT: 100% inspired oxygen, immediate atelectasis from bronchial occlusion
- Fibrin sheath sign: Catheter may be flushed but not aspirated
- Tracheostenosis: At stoma, cuff, tip, or multiple foci; at tip usually 1.5 cm below stoma; circumferential stenosis, 1-4 cm long
- Tracheomalacia: At overinflated cuff site
  - Extrathoracic, airway narrowing with inspiration; intrathoracic, airway narrowing with expiration

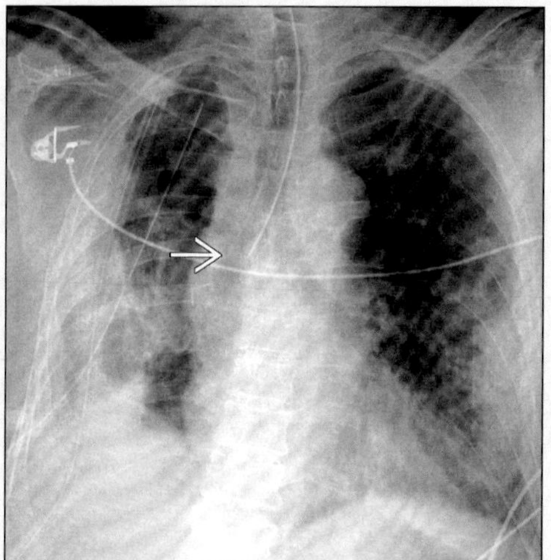
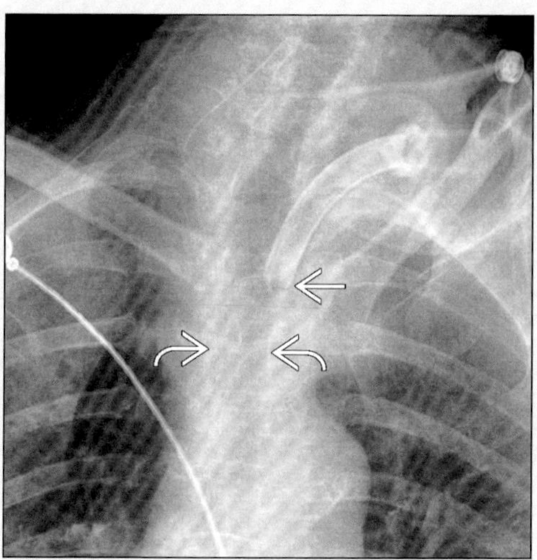

(Left) *AP chest radiograph shows a malpositioned endotracheal tube with the tip in the bronchus intermedius ➡. This type of endotracheal tube malposition often results in left lung and right upper lobe atelectasis.* ***(Right)*** *AP chest radiograph of a patient with dyspnea shows a malpositioned tracheostomy tube ➡ located to the left of the tracheal air column ➡ due to tube retraction into the soft tissues of the neck. Dyspnea resolved once the tube was appropriately positioned (not shown).*

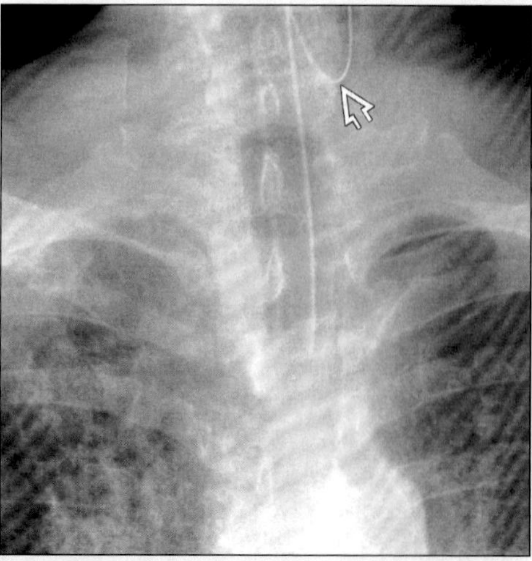
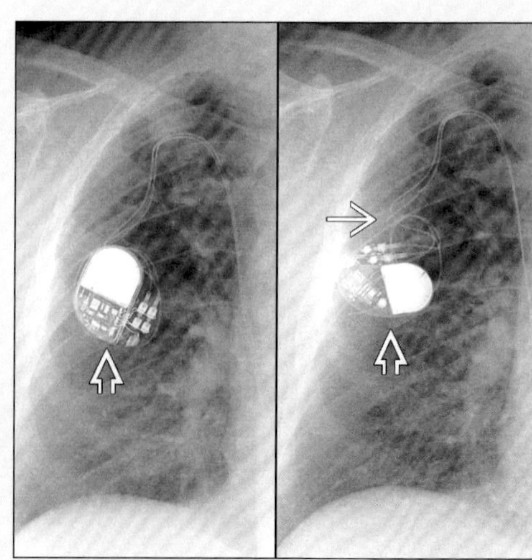

(Left) *AP chest radiograph performed to assess enteric tube position shows a portion of the enteric tube coiled in the cervical esophagus ➡.* ***(Right)*** *Composite image with PA chest radiographs (taken on separate occasions) of a patient with a right pectoral pacer shows a change in the orientation of the pacer battery pack ➡ as a result of the patient rotating or "twiddling" the battery pack within its subcutaneous space. Lead fracture ➡ resulted from increased tension on the wire.*

ABNORMALLY POSITIONED TUBES AND CATHETERS

TERMINOLOGY

Synonyms

- Cardiopulmonary support & monitoring devices, lines, tubes

Definitions

- Suboptimal positioning of tubes, lines, catheters

IMAGING

General Features

- Best diagnostic clue
  - Lines/tubes do not follow normal anatomy of catheterized or drained structure
- Location
  - Trachea, bronchi, pleura, veins, heart, aorta

Radiographic Findings

- **Endotracheal tube (ETT)**
  - **Malposition**
    - **Right mainstem bronchus intubation**
      - Left lung atelectasis, right lung hyperinflation
      - Sidehole may ventilate left lung
      - Right pneumothorax
    - **Bronchus intermedius intubation**: Left lung & right upper lobe atelectasis
    - Tip just beyond vocal cords: Vocal cord injury
    - Pharyngoesophageal intubation
      - Tube course does not conform to trachea
      - Dilated esophagus/stomach, aspiration, small lung volume
  - Overinflated cuff: Tube tip covered, pinched, or laterally deflected
  - Mucus plugging of ETT lumen
  - Tracheolaryngeal injury
    - Pyriform sinus perforation: Pneumomediastinum, subcutaneous gas, pneumothorax
    - Tracheolaryngeal laceration: Tube oriented to right, pneumomediastinum, subcutaneous gas, cuff > 2.8 cm
  - **Aspiration/pneumonia**
    - Aspirated broken teeth, fillings, denture parts during intubation
    - 5-10 mL of fluid may pool above ET cuff; subsequent cuff deflation results in aspiration
      - Suspect when air above tube cuff replaced with water density
    - Subsegmental atelectasis, dependent lung consolidation/pneumonia
  - **Barotrauma**: Overdistended alveoli may rupture from high peak pressures with mechanical ventilation
    - Interstitial emphysema; air dissects along bronchovascular connective tissue to subpleural space & mediastinum (**Macklin effect**)
    - Pneumomediastinum, pneumothorax
  - Sinusitis from nasotracheal intubation
- **Tracheostomy**
  - Perioperative
    - Hemorrhage, infection, airleak/ pneumomediastinum, pneumothorax, tube malalignment with respect to trachea
  - Overinflated cuff
    - 1.5x tracheal width at level of clavicles
    - May cover tube tip, pinch tube, or deflect tip laterally
- **Enteric or feeding tube**
  - Tube tip in bronchus, lung, pleura
    - Atelectasis with airway occlusion
    - Pneumothorax with lung/pleural penetration
  - Feeding tube tip in esophagus or gastric fundus
    - Aspiration/consolidation if fluid administered
- **Chest tube or thoracostomy tube**
  - Malposition
    - Inadequate drainage of air, fluid, or empyema
    - Tube within fissure (major or minor); tube may or may not function properly
    - Chest tube in chest wall; outer chest tube margin not visible
    - Sidehole in chest wall may lead to massive subcutaneous gas or empyema necessitatis
    - Tip impingement on mediastinum; may erode into arteries, veins, or esophagus
    - Lung penetration; bronchopleural fistula
- **Central venous line (CVL)**
  - Malposition
    - Tip in internal jugular, upper extremity, hepatic, superior intercostal, azygos, internal mammary, pericardiophrenic, or periscapular vein; subclavian artery or aorta
    - Tip perforation of vein wall, into pleura or mediastinum
    - Tip in right atrium, right ventricle (arrhythmias); tip perforation into pericardium
    - Tip in liver (hepatic veins)
  - CVL malposition: Infusion of fluid into mediastinum, heart, pericardium, liver, pleura
  - CVL placement complications: Pneumothorax
  - Mediastinal hematoma after placement
  - Catheter breakage & embolization to superior or inferior vena cava, right heart, pulmonary artery, lung
  - Aseptic or septic catheter tip thrombus with pulmonary embolization; fibrin sheath occlusion
  - Venous thrombosis
    - Directly related to catheterization duration
    - Potential source for pulmonary emboli
  - Air embolism, rare
- **Pulmonary artery catheter**
  - Arrhythmia, especially if tip in right ventricle
  - Pulmonary infarction, from wedged catheter ± clot, ± inflated balloon tip
  - Pulmonary artery pseudoaneurysm or rupture from balloon overdistention in small pulmonary artery
    - Pseudoaneurysm: Elliptical lung nodule, long axis parallel to vasculature, within 2 cm of hila, usually in right lung
  - Pulmonary hemorrhage; ruptured pseudoaneurysm
- **Intra-aortic counterpulsation balloon (IACPB)**
  - Too high; may occlude brachiocephalic arteries, may produce cerebral embolization
  - Too low; may occlude celiac, renal, or superior mesenteric arteries
  - Aortic dissection; balloon may tear intima
  - Lower extremity ischemia on side of insertion
  - Helium gas embolus from balloon rupture
- Surgically implanted catheters
  - Infection, thrombosis, septic emboli, aseptic emboli

- Torn catheter between clavicle and 1st rib "osseous pinch"; embolization of catheter fragment
- **Transvenous pacemakers**
  - Lead malposition: Unintended placement in coronary sinus (atrioventricular groove)
  - Coronary sinus: Lead points to left humeral head on frontal radiograph, posteriorly on lateral radiograph
  - Broken lead between clavicle & 1st rib "**osseous pinch**"
  - Rotation of pulse unit in soft tissues by patient; may fracture or shorten pacer lead (twiddling sign)
  - Myocardial perforation: Hemopericardium, rare

Fluoroscopic Findings

- Fluoroscopy to adjust malpositioned tubes
- Contrast injection of central line may demonstrate thrombus at line tip or occlusion

CT Findings

- NECT
  - CT to evaluate position of chest tube & relationship to air, fluid, or empyema collection
  - CT evaluation for tracheostenosis or malacia
    - Dynamic expiratory imaging to demonstrate expiratory collapse

Imaging Recommendations

- Best imaging tool
  - Chest radiography should always be performed after insertion or repositioning of a tube or line
  - Lines & tubes may change position over time; follow-up radiographs to document stability
- Protocol advice
  - CT may be helpful to evaluate desired tip location & course of line, tube, catheter

DIFFERENTIAL DIAGNOSIS

External Superimposed Tubing, Lines, Devices

- May be mistaken for intrathoracic monitoring & support devices

PATHOLOGY

General Features

- Etiology
  - Malposition: Inexperience, patient body habitus, use of anatomic landmarks for placement
  - ET/tracheostomy tubes: Overinflated cuff, low position and mobility of ETT tip
  - Infection: Immunosuppression, broad spectrum antibiotics

Gross Pathologic & Surgical Features

- Tracheal ulceration, stenosis, fistulization
- Venous thrombosis, thromboembolism, aseptic/septic embolism

Microscopic Features

- CVL tip culture may show *Staphylococcus* or *Candida*; systemic septic embolism

CLINICAL ISSUES

Presentation

- Most common signs/symptoms
  - Variable; dyspnea, wheezing, chest pain, palpitations, respiratory or cardiac failure, fever, aspiration
  - Malpositioned CVL or pulmonary artery catheter: Incorrect pressure measurements
  - **CVL infection**: Usually *Staphylococcus*; *Candida* in patients on broad spectrum antibiotics
  - Seizures in patients with air embolism
- Other signs/symptoms
  - Malpositioned ETT: Higher concentration of inspired oxygen results in more rapid atelectasis
    - **100% inspired oxygen, immediate atelectasis** with bronchial occlusion
  - **Fibrin sheath sign**: Catheter may be flushed but not aspirated

Demographics

- Age
  - Neonate to elderly
- Gender
  - M = F
- Epidemiology
  - Malposition: ETT (20%); CVL (33%)

Natural History & Prognosis

- Endotracheal or tracheostomy tubes (late sequelae)
  - ETT-related laryngeal injury: Scarring of posterior glottis, fusion of posterior commissure, arytenoid injury, subglottic stenosis
  - Fistula to adjacent structure: Artery, vein, esophagus
  - **Tracheostenosis**: At stoma, cuff, tip, or multiple foci; at tip usually 1.5 cm below stoma; circumferential stenosis, 1-4 cm long
  - **Tracheomalacia**: Overinflated cuff site
    - Extrathoracic, airway narrowing with inspiration
    - Intrathoracic, airway narrowing with expiration
- Delayed drainage of hemothorax or empyema, fibrothorax, & decortication

Treatment

- Tracheal stents or surgery for stenosis or malacia
- Infected cardiovascular line: Culture, antibiotic treatment; line may not have to be removed
- Fibrin sheath: Infusion of tissue plasminogen activator, catheter exchange if unsuccessful
- Interventional snare retrieval of embolized catheter fragments

SELECTED REFERENCES

1. Swain FR et al: Traumatic complications from placement of thoracic catheters and tubes. Emerg Radiol. 12(1-2):11-8, 2005
2. Hunter TB et al: Medical devices of the chest. Radiographics. 24(6):1725-46, 2004
3. Tseng M et al: Radiologic placement of central venous catheters: rates of success and immediate complications in 3412 cases. Can Assoc Radiol J. 52(6):379-84, 2001
4. Gayer G et al: CT diagnosis of malpositioned chest tubes. Br J Radiol. 73(871):786-90, 2000

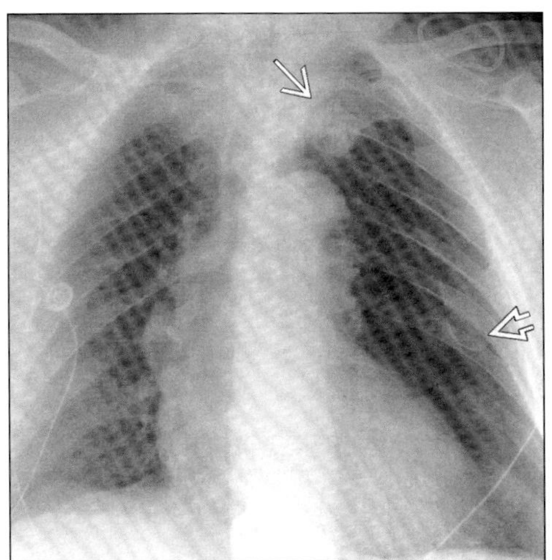

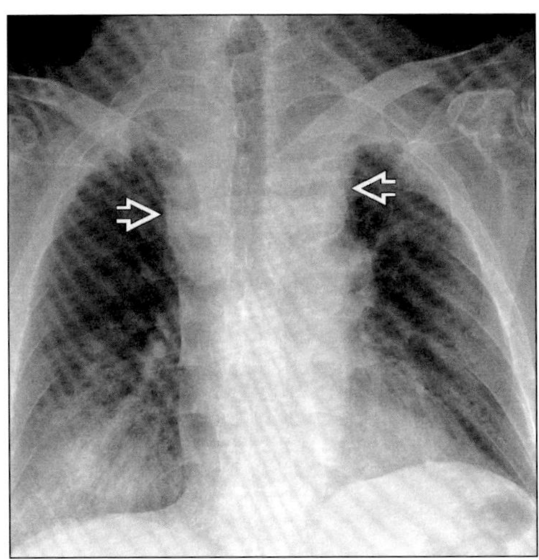

(Left) *AP chest radiograph obtained immediately after placement of a left subclavian central line ➡ shows a left pneumothorax manifesting with a visible pleural line ⇨. Chest radiography is typically obtained following central vascular line placement to document catheter position and exclude pneumothorax.* ***(Right)*** *AP chest radiograph of a patient with an attempted central vascular line placement shows a wide superior mediastinum ⇨ secondary to mediastinal hematoma.*

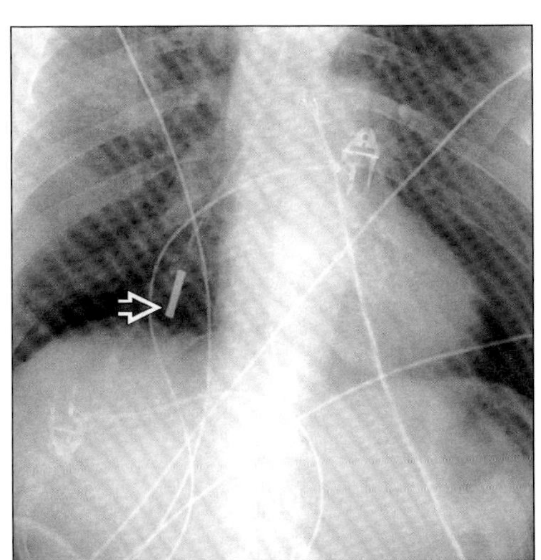

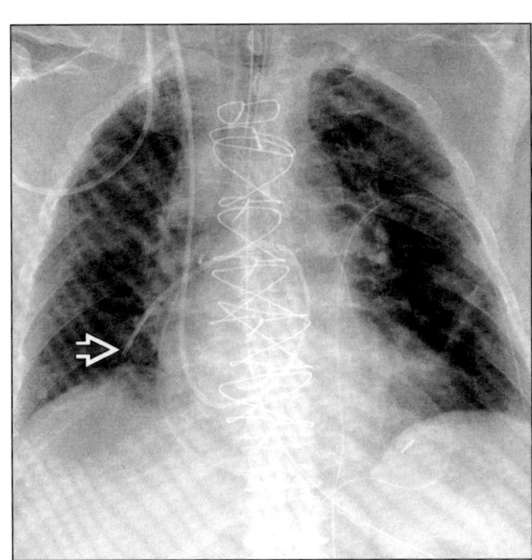

(Left) *AP chest radiograph obtained after Dobbhoff feeding tube placement shows the tube tip ⇨ within the right lower lobe bronchus. The other lines that overlie the chest are external to the patient.* ***(Right)*** *AP chest radiograph shows a pulmonary artery catheter tip wedged in a right lower lobe pulmonary artery branch ⇨. Persistence of the catheter tip in this location increases the risk of pulmonary artery pseudoaneurysm, pulmonary hemorrhage, and lung infarction.*

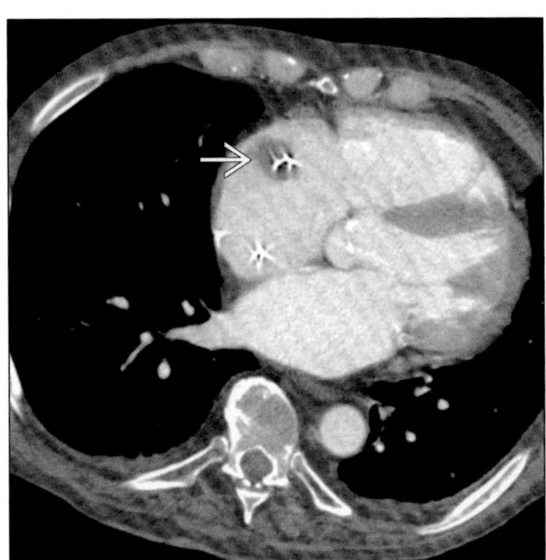

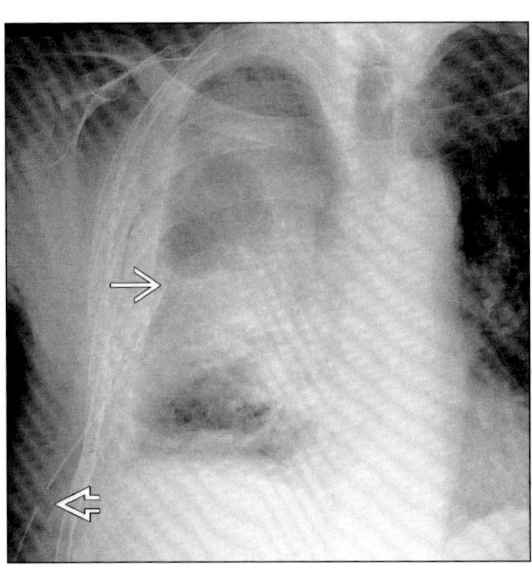

(Left) *Axial CECT shows thrombus surrounding a pacemaker lead in the right atrium ➡. Bland or septic thrombi may embolize to the lungs from central lines and pacemaker leads.* ***(Right)*** *AP chest radiograph of a patient with empyema treated with chest tube placement shows a right chest tube ➡ with its sidehole ⇨ projecting over the right chest wall soft tissues. Empyema may drain through the sidehole and infect the soft tissues, resulting in empyema necessitatis.*

PACEMAKER/AICD

Key Facts

Terminology

- Permanent cardiac pacemaker
- Cardiac resynchronization therapy (CRT)
- Automatic implantable cardioverter defibrillator (AICD)

Imaging

- Lead location variable: Right atrium, right ventricle, coronary vein via coronary sinus
- Single-chamber pacemaker
  - Single right atrial or right ventricular lead
- Dual-chamber pacemaker
  - Leads in right atrium & right ventricle
- Biventricular pacemaker
  - Dual/single chamber leads; coronary sinus lead
- Implantable cardioverter defibrillators
  - Typically 2 electrodes: SVC (defibrillator) & right ventricular apex (defibrillator & sensor)

Top Differential Diagnoses

- Other implanted pacing devices in chest wall
  - Implantable loop recorder, vagal nerve stimulator
  - Deep brain stimulator; retained leads from previously removed pacemaker

Clinical Issues

- Twiddler syndrome: Inadvertent or deliberate pacemaker unit rotation in subcutaneous pocket
- Pacemaker syndrome: Loss of atrioventricular synchrony
- Sudden cardiac arrest due to conduction disturbances related to malposition or malfunction

Diagnostic Checklist

- Frontal & lateral chest radiography for initial assessment & detection of complications
- Consider lead fracture & dislodgement in cases of pacemaker malfunction

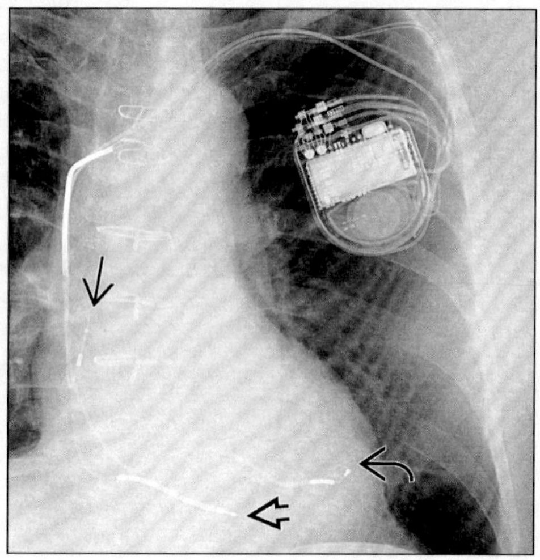

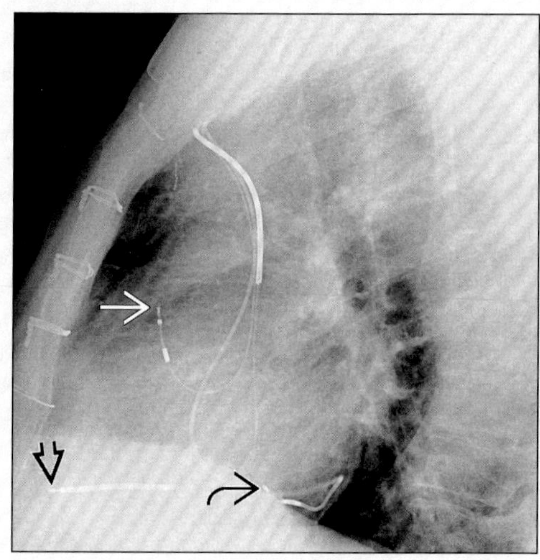

(Left) *PA chest radiograph shows normal location of a dual-chamber biventricular AICD, with leads in the right atrium ➔, right ventricle ➔, and a tributary of the coronary sinus ➔. The generator is in the left anterior chest wall, and the leads exit in a clockwise direction.* ***(Right)*** *Lateral radiograph of the same patient shows appropriate lead location in the right atrium ➔, right ventricle ➔, and a tributary of the coronary sinus ➔. The coronary sinus lead courses posteriorly.*

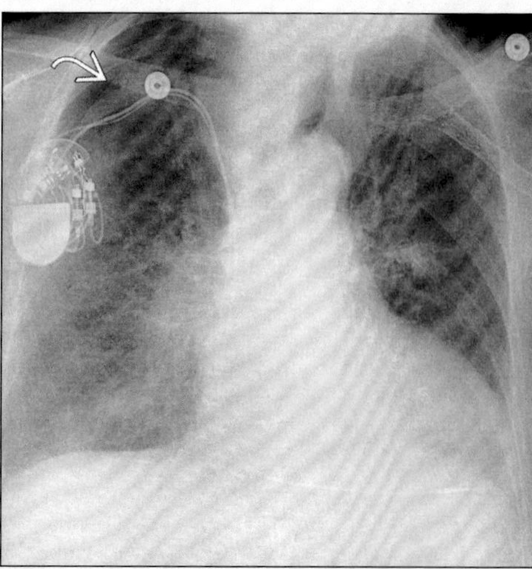

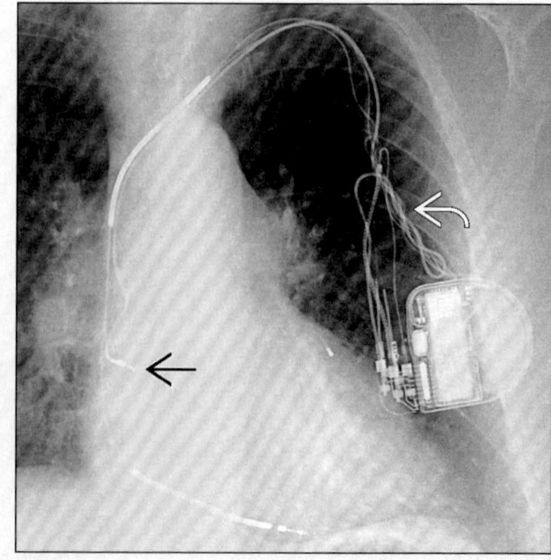

(Left) *PA chest radiograph immediately after pacemaker placement shows a right pneumothorax ➔. PA and lateral chest radiographs are routinely obtained immediately after pacemaker placement to document appropriate lead positioning and exclude complications.* ***(Right)*** *PA chest radiograph of a patient with Twiddler syndrome shows extensive coiling of the proximal leads ➔ in the chest wall. The atrial lead ➔ is retracted; the tip had previously been in the atrial appendage, directed cranially.*

TERMINOLOGY

Abbreviations

- **Automatic implantable cardioverter defibrillator (AICD)**

Synonyms

- Permanent cardiac pacemaker
- Biventricular pacemaker: **Cardiac resynchronization therapy (CRT)**

Definitions

- North American Society of Pacing and Electrophysiology generic pacemaker code
  - 1st letter denotes chamber(s) paced
    - A = atrium; V = ventricle; D = dual (both atrium & ventricle)
  - 2nd letter describes which chambers sense electrical signals
    - A = atrium; V = ventricle; D = dual
  - 3rd letter denotes response to sensed events
    - I = inhibition; T = triggering; D = dual (both inhibition & triggering)
  - 4th letter denotes activation of rate response feature (R)
  - 5th letter specifies location of multisite pacing
    - O = no multisite pacing; A = atrium; V = ventricle; D = dual (both atrium & ventricle)

IMAGING

General Features

- Best diagnostic clue
  - Lead positions with respect to cardiac chambers
- Location
  - Pacemaker unit
    - Loose subcutaneous tissue of anterior chest wall
    - May be positioned in left or right chest wall
    - Epicardial pacemaker units may be positioned in abdominal wall
  - Lead location variable: Right atrium, right ventricle, coronary vein via coronary sinus
    - Right atrium locations: Atrial appendage, sinoatrial node, atrioventricular node
    - Right ventricle locations: Right ventricle apex, right ventricle outflow tract
    - Left ventricular location: Variable epicardial location
- Size
  - Pacemaker units vary in size depending on function
  - Leads 2-3 mm in thickness
- Morphology
  - Leads may exit pacer clockwise or counterclockwise

Radiographic Findings

- **Single-chamber pacemaker**
  - Single right atrial lead near sinoatrial node, right ventricular apex, or right ventricular outflow tract
- **Dual-chamber pacemaker**
  - Leads typically positioned in right atrial appendage & right ventricular apex
- **Biventricular pacemaker**
  - Dual- or single-chamber pacemaker leads with additional lead coursing through coronary sinus
  - Coronary lead located on left ventricle surface; usually in lateral or posterolateral cardiac vein
  - Cardiac vein position confirmed by posterior location on lateral radiography
- Epicardial pacemaker
  - Pacemaker unit usually in abdominal wall with lead on cardiac surface
  - Lead usually situated on right ventricle
- **Implantable cardioverter defibrillators**
  - Typically 2 electrodes: SVC (defibrillator) & right ventricular apex (defibrillator & sensor)
  - May be a component of biventricular pacemaker
  - Leads larger; dense coiled spring appearance compared to pacemaker leads
  - Relief loop in left subclavian region often constructed to help prevent lead migration
  - Normal lucency just distal to proximal electrode, not to be confused with lead fracture
- Implantable epicardial defibrillators (anterior & posterior cardiac patches) less common
  - Patches may have crenulated appearance due to focal fibrosis or fluid collection under patch
  - Sensing unit in chest or upper abdominal wall
- Complications
  - **Early complications: 4-5%**
    - Pneumothorax: 1.5% of procedures
    - Hemothorax: Subclavian artery injury
    - Lead-related complications: Perforation, dislodgement, diaphragmatic stimulation, malposition
      - Perforation may result in cardiac tamponade
      - Dislodgement in 2-3%, usually within 24-48 hours of placement
      - Diaphragmatic stimulation due to inadvertent phrenic nerve stimulation
  - **Late complications: 3%**
    - **Twiddler syndrome**: Subconscious, inadvertent or deliberate rotation of pacemaker in its subcutaneous pocket
      - Change in orientation of pacemaker unit in pocket
      - Change in lead direction exiting pacemaker (e.g., clockwise to counterclockwise)
      - Lead retraction toward pacemaker unit
      - Increased number of wire loops around pacemaker unit
    - **Lead fracture**: May be difficult to visualize if nondisplaced
      - Usually when pinched between clavicle & 1st rib
      - Suspect when pacemaker does not capture in spite of stable lead position

Fluoroscopic Findings

- Fluoroscopy may be useful for evaluating leads for incomplete fracture or dislodgement

CT Findings

- CECT
  - Useful for detecting chamber perforation
    - Tip of lead projecting outside right ventricular myocardium
    - Exact localization may be difficult to determine due to beam-hardening artifact
    - Hemopericardium may occur; hemoperitoneum uncommon

PACEMAKER/AICD

- Detection of venous thrombus/stenosis
  - Extensive venous collateral circulation in chest wall & mediastinum

MR Findings

- MR relatively contraindicated in patients with pacemakers
  - Absolute contraindication in pacemaker-dependent patients
  - Can be performed safely in patients with demand pacemakers, particularly exams remote from chest (e.g., brain)
    - Pacemaker should be pretested outside MR suite
    - Cardiologist in attendance during procedure
    - Monitor during examination; communicate with patient between sequences
    - Post test pacemaker outside MR suite
    - Significant change in pacing thresholds in approximately 10%

Ultrasonographic Findings

- Ultrasound may be used to assess venous complications or fluid around pacemaker unit
  - Symptomatic venous thrombosis in 5%; risk increases with multiple leads

Imaging Recommendations

- Best imaging tool
  - Frontal & lateral chest radiography for initial assessment & detection of complications

DIFFERENTIAL DIAGNOSIS

Other Implanted Pacing Devices in Chest Wall

- Implantable loop recorder; long-term cardiac monitoring of patients with syncope
- Vagal nerve stimulator: Leads extend into neck, terminate in region of carotid artery
- Deep brain stimulator: Leads continue cephalad
- Retained leads from previously removed pacemaker

PATHOLOGY

General Features

- Etiology
  - Indications for pacemaker placement
    - Sinus node dysfunction: Most common indication for pacemaker insertion
    - Long-term therapy for symptomatic bradycardia
    - Neurocardiogenic syncope
    - Hypertrophic obstructive cardiomyopathy
    - Congestive heart failure; cardiac resynchronization therapy

CLINICAL ISSUES

Presentation

- Most common signs/symptoms
  - Asymptomatic with normal pacer function
- Other signs/symptoms
  - **Pacemaker syndrome**: Constellation of symptoms related to ventricular pacing
    - Congestive: Dyspnea, orthopnea, elevated neck veins, hepatomegaly, pedal edema
    - Hypotensive: Near syncope or syncope at pacing onset, decrease in systolic pressure > 20 mmHg
    - Nonspecific: Headache & fatigue
  - Atrioventricular block in single-chamber right atrial pacing
  - Sudden cardiac arrest due to conduction disturbances related to malposition or malfunction
  - Pacemaker pocket complications: Hematoma, pain, infection

Demographics

- Age
  - Variable depending on condition; majority > 50 years of age
- Gender
  - More frequently placed in men
- Epidemiology
  - > 200,000 pacemakers placed annually

Natural History & Prognosis

- Expected longevity of pacemaker: 5-10 years
- In patients with bacteremia: Risk of infected lead thrombus & subsequent septic pulmonary emboli

Treatment

- Replacement of fractured wires
- Perforation: Lead withdrawal & rescrewing into myocardium
- Surgical replacement of pacemaker unit at battery end-of-life

DIAGNOSTIC CHECKLIST

Consider

- Lead fracture & dislodgement in cases of pacemaker malfunction

Image Interpretation Pearls

- Evaluation of pacemaker should be performed with all other extraneous superficial leads removed
- Carefully evaluate pacemaker unit to look for change in orientation
- Compare direction of leads exiting pacemaker unit; prior radiographs & initial post placement radiographs

SELECTED REFERENCES

1. Mitka M: First MRI-safe pacemaker receives conditional approval from FDA. JAMA. 305(10):985-6, 2011
2. Zikria JF et al: MRI of patients with cardiac pacemakers: a review of the medical literature. AJR Am J Roentgenol. 196(2):390-401, 2011
3. Beck H et al: 50th Anniversary of the first successful permanent pacemaker implantation in the United States: historical review and future directions. Am J Cardiol. 106(6):810-8, 2010
4. Parry SW et al: Implantable loop recorders in the investigation of unexplained syncope: a state of the art review. Heart. 96(20):1611-6, 2010
5. Brown DW et al: Epidemiology of pacemaker procedures among Medicare enrollees in 1990, 1995, and 2000. Am J Cardiol. 95(3):409-11, 2005
6. Lamas GA et al: Evidence base for pacemaker mode selection: from physiology to randomized trials. Circulation. 109(4):443-51, 2004

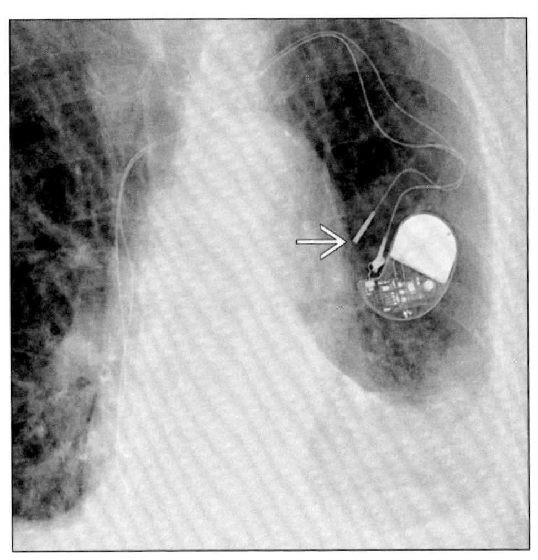

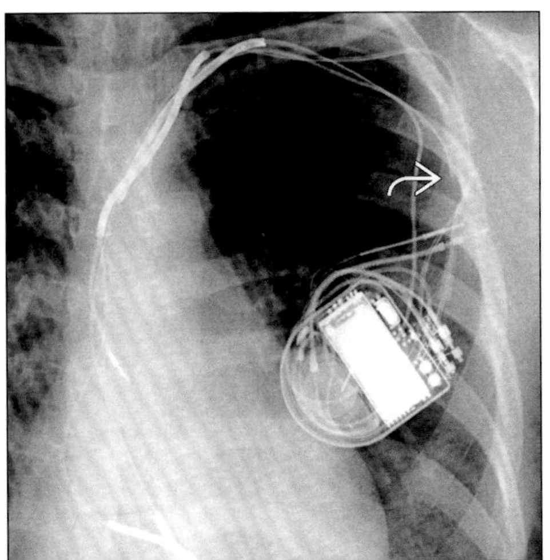

(Left) *PA chest radiograph illustrates the radiographic appearance of a disconnected proximal pacemaker lead* ➡. ***(Right)*** *PA chest radiograph shows a fracture* ➡ *within the proximal aspect of an AICD lead. Leads typically fracture between the clavicle and the 1st rib. Radiographic evaluation of patients with pacemakers and AICD devices requires assessment of the course and integrity of the pacer leads.*

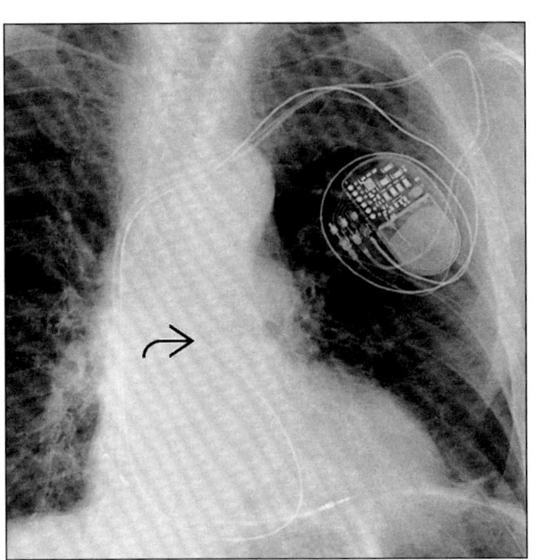

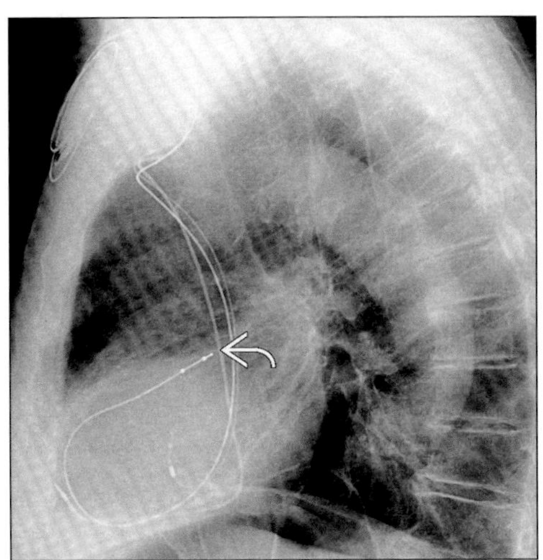

(Left) *PA chest radiograph of a 55-year-old man with syncope and previously documented appropriately positioned dual-chamber biventricular pacer shows migration of the coronary sinus lead into the right ventricle with the lead tip* ➡ *in the pulmonary outflow tract.* ***(Right)*** *Lateral chest radiograph of the same patient shows the tip of the migrated coronary sinus lead* ➡ *within the right ventricle.*

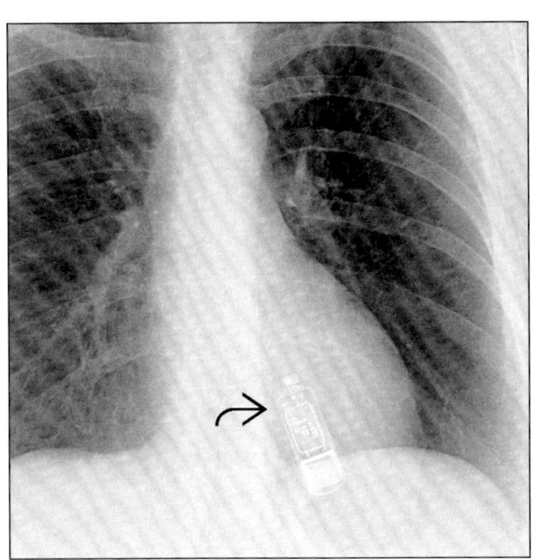

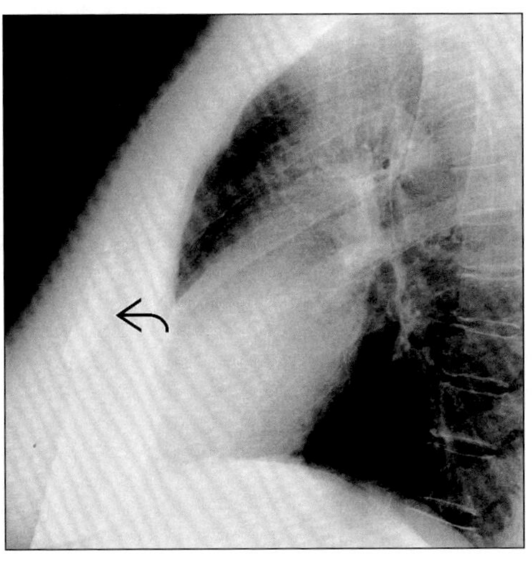

(Left) *PA chest radiograph of a 35-year-old woman with recurrent syncope shows a loop recorder* ➡ *implanted in the left anterior chest wall.* ***(Right)*** *Lateral chest radiograph of the same patient confirms the anterior chest wall location of the implantable loop recorder* ➡*. Loop recorders are placed in patients with unexplained recurrent syncope, and an arrhythmia is detected in approximately 50% of these patients, who can then be successfully treated with pacemaker placement.*

Key Facts

Terminology

- Definition: Chemical pleural sclerosis to treat pneumothorax and pleural effusion
- Pleurodesis agents and methods
  - Pure talc (hydrated magnesium silicate)
  - Bleomycin

Imaging

- Radiography
  - Focal or multifocal diffuse pleural thickening
  - Smooth or nodular pleural thickening
- CT
  - Unilateral smooth or nodular pleural thickening; posterior/basilar pleura
  - High attenuation, calcification
  - Loculated pleural fluid
- FDG PET/CT
  - FDG uptake in talc-related pleural disease

Top Differential Diagnoses

- Pleural malignancy
- Empyema
- Pleural tuberculosis
- Pleural or extrapleural hematoma
- Chest wall mass
- Mediastinal mass
- Calcified asbestos plaques

Clinical Issues

- Signs/symptoms
  - Pain & fever; fever may indicate robust inflammatory response & increased success rate
- Overall success rate (50-90%)
  - Complete drainage of pleural fluid
  - Ability of collapsed lung to reexpand
  - Absence of pleural adhesions
  - Best results with initial treatment

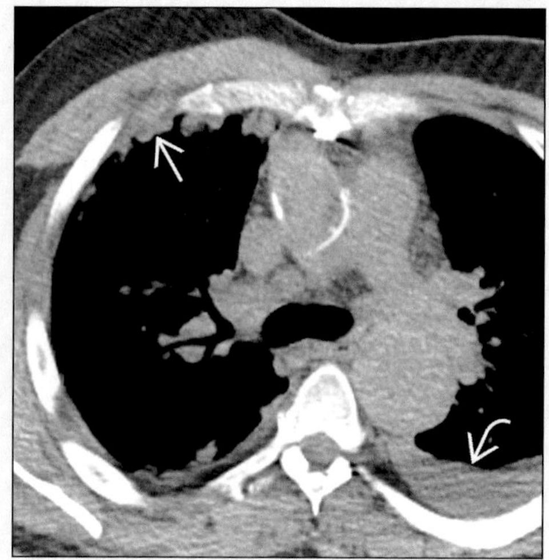

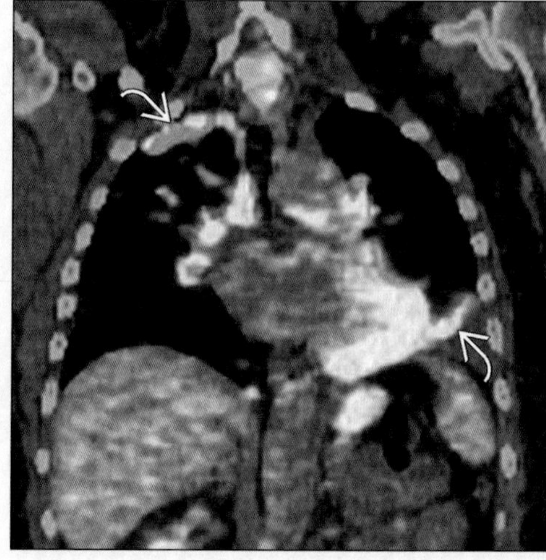

(Left) *Axial NECT after bilateral talc pleurodesis shows multifocal peripheral right-sided noncalcified pleural nodules ➔ and a small left pleural effusion ↪.* ***(Right)*** *Coronal fused PET/CT of the same patient shows increased FDG uptake in multifocal circumferential bilateral pleural nodules and masses ↪. Talc pleurodesis may result in chronic nodular pleural thickening, which may exhibit increased FDG uptake, mimicking solid pleural metastases.*

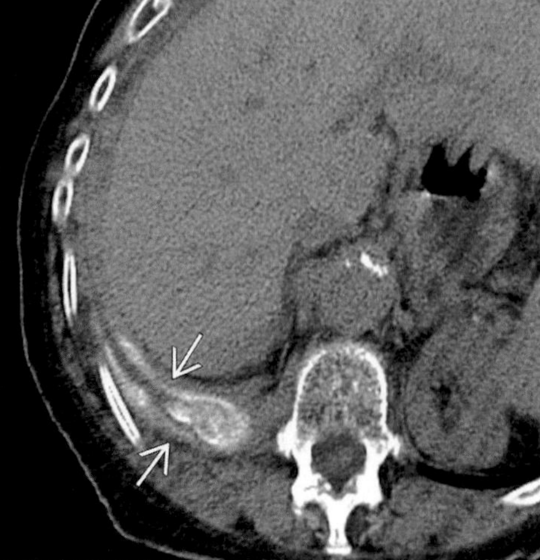

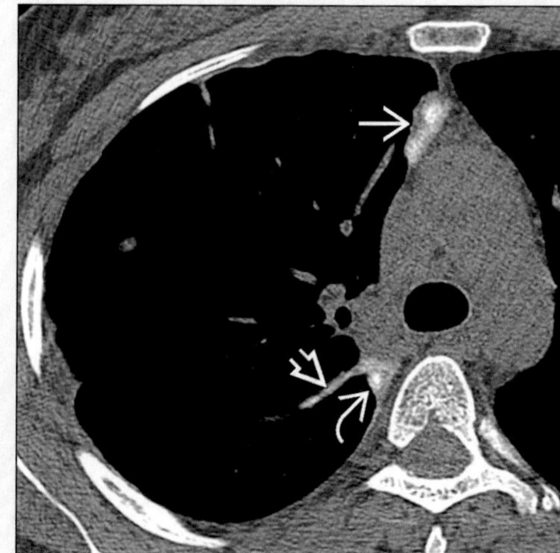

(Left) *Axial NECT after remote talc pleurodesis shows heterogeneous lenticular calcification involving the right basilar pleural surfaces ➔.* ***(Right)*** *Axial NECT of the same patient shows multifocal nodular right pleural thickening and calcification ↪ involving the major fissure ⇨ and the paramediastinal pleura ➔. Nodular pleural thickening after talc pleurodesis may mimic pleural plaques and mediastinal abnormalities.*

PLEURODESIS

TERMINOLOGY

Synonyms

- **Pleural sclerosis**
- **Talc poudrage**

Definitions

- **Chemical pleural sclerosis** to treat spontaneous **pneumothorax** and refractory **pleural effusion**
- Other indications
  - Recurrent benign effusions: Heart failure, ascites, systemic lupus erythematosus
  - Recurrent pneumothorax: COPD, lymphangioleiomyomatosis, catamenial
  - Chylothorax: Postsurgical, post-traumatic
- Contraindications
  - Infection, heart disease, coagulation disorders
- **Pleurodesis agents** & methods
  - Pure **talc** (hydrated magnesium silicate)
    - **Most frequently used**
    - Highest success rate for malignant effusion
    - 4-8% risk of respiratory failure after talc exposure
  - **Bleomycin**
    - Readily available
    - More expensive; must be used immediately
  - **Physical pleural abrasion**

IMAGING

General Features

- Best diagnostic clue
  - **High-attenuation pleural thickening**
- Location
  - **Basilar pleura**
- Size
  - Variable
- Morphology
  - Lentiform
  - Variable attenuation: Soft tissue, fluid, calcification

Radiographic Findings

- Talc pleurodesis
  - **Focal** or **multifocal diffuse pleural thickening**
  - Smooth or nodular pleural thickening
  - Blunt costophrenic angle
  - Pleural mass/talcoma, often years after procedure
  - Airspace disease; pneumonitis in 1.5%, acute respiratory distress syndrome (ARDS)

CT Findings

- **Unilateral smooth or nodular pleural thickening**; posterior/basilar pleura
- Fissural pleural thickening
- **High attenuation, calcification**
- Loculated pleural fluid

Nuclear Medicine Findings

- PET/CT
  - **FDG uptake** in talc-related pleural disease

Imaging Recommendations

- Best imaging tool
  - Chest CT for assessment of pleural abnormality & detection/characterization of calcification

DIFFERENTIAL DIAGNOSIS

Pleural Malignancy

- Lobular thickening; unilateral or bilateral

Empyema

- Unilateral noncalcified loculated pleural effusion

Pleural Tuberculosis

- Unilateral, thick pleural rind; dense calcification

Pleural or Extrapleural Hematoma

- Unilateral pleural thickening; calcification

Mediastinal Mass

- May mimic medial pleural mass or loculated fluid

Chest Wall Mass

- May mimic pleural mass

Calcified Asbestos Plaques

- Bilateral, multifocal, discontinuous ± calcification

PATHOLOGY

Gross Pathologic & Surgical Features

- Dense **pleural fibrosis**; loculated fluid

Microscopic Features

- **Dense fibrosis** from damage to mesothelium
- **Talc crystals** under polarized microscopy

CLINICAL ISSUES

Presentation

- Most common signs/symptoms
  - **Pain and fever**; fever may indicate robust inflammatory response & increased success rate
  - Reexpansion edema with rapid fluid drainage

Demographics

- Age
  - > 40 years; malignant etiologies
- Gender
  - M = F

Natural History & Prognosis

- **Overall success rate (50-90%)**
  - Optimal results
    - **Complete drainage of pleural fluid**
    - **Ability of collapsed lung to reexpand**
    - Best results with initial treatment
  - Decreased success/failure
    - Lung entrapment or long-term atelectasis
    - Steroids, NSAIDs

DIAGNOSTIC CHECKLIST

Image Interpretation Pearls

- Pleural thickening with calcification post intervention

SELECTED REFERENCES

1. Narayanaswamy S et al: CT appearances of talc pleurodesis. Clin Radiol. 62(3):233-7, 2007

SUBLOBAR RESECTION

Key Facts

Terminology

- Wedge resection
  - Partial sublobar resection not limited by segmental anatomy
  - Resection of low-stage, non-small cell lung cancer in patients with poor respiratory reserve
  - Procedure of choice for pulmonary metastasectomy
  - Used to obtain tissue for histopathological diagnosis
  - Vast majority (> 95%) performed with linear stapler
- Segmentectomy
  - Sublobar resection along segmental boundaries

Imaging

- Radiography
  - Visualization of metallic staple line
  - Associated adjacent scar or atelectasis
- CT
  - Direct visualization of staple line with adjacent architectural distortion & scar or atelectasis
  - Direct visualization of associated surgical changes
  - Surveillance of staple line on subsequent imaging to exclude recurrent neoplasm

Top Differential Diagnoses

- Segmentectomy
- Lobectomy
- Lung volume reduction surgery

Clinical Issues

- Sublobar resection of lung cancer in patients with marginal lung function
- Stage I NSCLC
  - Survival with limited resection comparable to survival with lobectomy
- Segmentectomy may decrease local rate of relapse
- Complications
  - Pneumonia, empyema, wound infection, hemorrhage, bronchopleural fistula

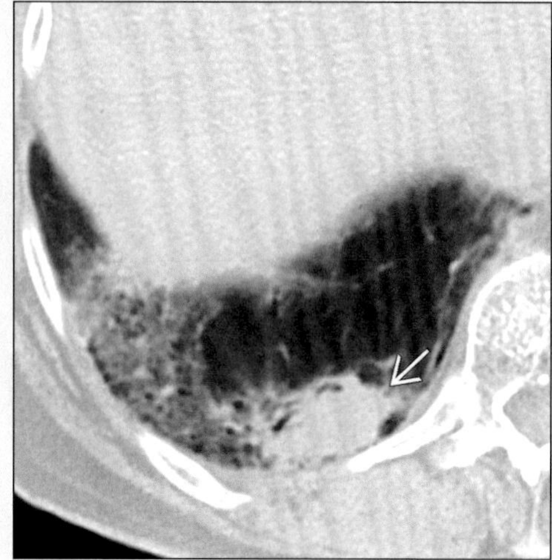

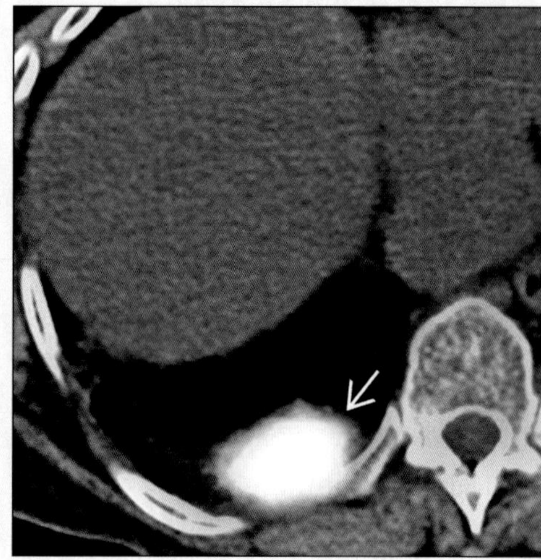

***(Left)** Axial NECT of a patient with usual interstitial pneumonia shows a right basilar lung cancer manifesting as a polylobular mass ➔ with adjacent reticulation, ground-glass opacity, and traction bronchiolectasis, consistent with pulmonary fibrosis. Pulmonary fibrosis is a risk factor for development of primary lung cancer, which tends to affect the lower lobes. **(Right)** Axial fused PET/CT of the same patient shows avid FDG uptake in the right basilar lung mass ➔.*

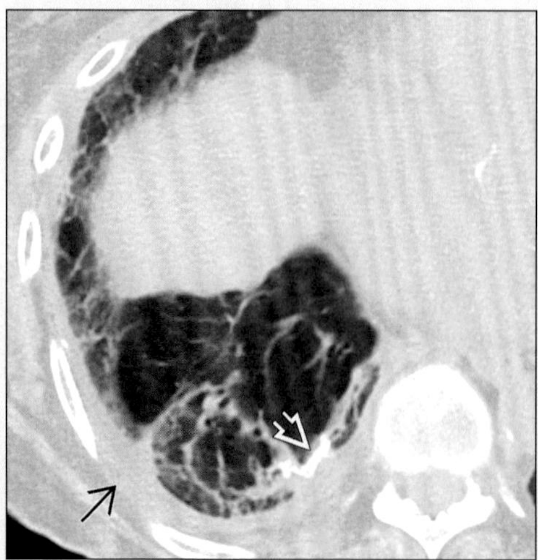

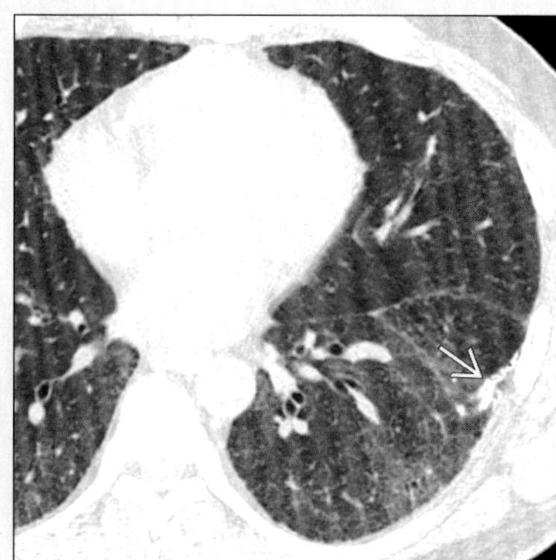

***(Left)** Axial NECT of the same patient shows a metallic staple line ➔ in the right lower lobe, consistent with wedge resection of the mass and a small ipsilateral post surgical pleural effusion ⇨. **(Right)** Axial HRCT of a patient with chronic hypersensitivity pneumonitis shows ground-glass opacity, reticulation, and peripheral traction bronchiolectasis, consistent with biopsy-proven nonspecific interstitial pneumonia (NSIP). The left lower lobe staple line ➔ is from a diagnostic wedge resection.*

SUBLOBAR RESECTION

TERMINOLOGY

Definitions

- **Wedge resection**: Partial **sublobar resection** not limited by segmental anatomy
  - Resection of low-stage, non-small cell lung cancer (NSCLC) in patients with poor respiratory reserve
  - Procedure of choice for pulmonary metastasectomy
  - Used to obtain tissue for histopathological diagnosis
  - Vast majority (> 95%) performed with linear stapler
  - Minority of wedge resections performed using Perelman procedure (precision resection)
    - Cautery or laser excision
    - Used for central benign or metastatic nodules
    - Not used for curative resection of primary lung cancer; insufficient surgical margins
- **Segmentectomy**: **Sublobar resection** along segmental boundaries

IMAGING

General Features

- Best diagnostic clue
  - Surgical staples in pulmonary lobe
  - Ipsilateral volume loss
  - Adjacent architectural distortion & scar/atelectasis
- Location
  - Most easily performed: Lesions in outer 1/3 of lung
  - Readily performed along fissures
  - Central lesions more challenging
- Size
  - Sublobar, typically subsegmental
  - Primary lung cancer, may be used for lesions < 3 cm; lung nodules

Radiographic Findings

- Radiography
  - **Visualization of metallic staple line**
  - Associated adjacent scar or atelectasis
  - Other signs of thoracotomy
    - Volume loss
    - Rib fractures
    - Chest wall deformity

CT Findings

- **Direct visualization of staple line** with adjacent architectural distortion & scar or atelectasis
  - MIP imaging for optimal staple line visualization
- Direct visualization of associated surgical changes
- Surveillance of staple line on subsequent imaging to exclude recurrent neoplasm
- Bronchogenic carcinoma
  - Low-grade NSCLC in peripheral lung: Most appropriate for sublobar wedge resection
  - Lymph node metastases; contraindication to wedge resection & segmentectomy
  - Accurate lymph node staging with CECT or PET/CT mandatory

Imaging Recommendations

- Best imaging tool
  - Surgical staples & subsegmental nature of resection best delineated with CT
  - Accurate staging of lymph node metastases in lung cancer mandatory with CECT or PET/CT
- Protocol advice
  - CECT or PET/CT for accurate staging of NSCLC

DIFFERENTIAL DIAGNOSIS

Segmentectomy

- Sublobar pulmonary resection
- Technically difficult & least commonly performed
- Theoretically superior to wedge resection in patients with lung cancer
  - Reproducible central surgical margins
  - Local lymph nodes resected along anatomic boundaries using pattern of expected nodal spread
  - More accurate staging

Lobectomy

- Standard treatment for operable lung cancer
- Abrupt termination of central lobar bronchus & ipsilateral shift of mediastinum
- Hyperinflation of other ipsilateral pulmonary lobes
- Surgical clips adjacent to bronchus of resected lobe

Lung Volume Reduction Surgery

- History of emphysema
- Usually resection of upper lung results in superior retraction of hila & tenting of hemidiaphragms

CLINICAL ISSUES

Presentation

- Clinical profile
  - Sublobar resection of lung cancer in patients with marginal lung function
    - Predicted postoperative FEV_1 close to 30%
    - Predicted postoperative DLCO close to 40% of predicted
    - Peak VO_2 of around 10 mL/kg/min
    - Upper lobe cancer & severe upper lobe emphysema; lobar resection should be considered
      - Upper lobectomy in these cases acts as lung volume reduction surgery

Natural History & Prognosis

- Usually good patient outcome in immediate postoperative period
- Long-term prognosis dependent on underlying diagnosis (lung cancer vs. benign condition)
- In stage I NSCLC, survival with limited resection comparable to survival with lobectomy
  - Segmentectomy may decrease local rate of relapse
- Complications
  - Pneumonia, empyema, wound infection, postoperative hemorrhage
  - Bronchopleural fistula, arteriovenous fistula

SELECTED REFERENCES

1. Rami-Porta R et al: Sublobar resection for lung cancer. Eur Respir J. 33(2):426-35, 2009
2. Kraev A et al: Wedge resection vs lobectomy: 10-year survival in stage I primary lung cancer. Chest. 131(1):136-40, 2007
3. Nakamura H et al: History of limited resection for non-small cell lung cancer. Ann Thorac Cardiovasc Surg. 11(6):356-62, 2005

LUNG VOLUME REDUCTION SURGERY

Key Facts

Terminology

- Lung volume reduction surgery (LVRS)
- Treatment of severe emphysema by removing approximately 20-35% of peripheral, emphysematous lung parenchyma from each lung
- LVRS decreases lung volume & improves elastic recoil of remaining lung;
- LVRS improves mechanics of diaphragm & intercostal muscles

Imaging

- Radiography
  - Reduced apical lung volume
  - Apical metallic staple line
  - Evaluation of postoperative complications
- CT pre-LVRS
  - Used for patient selection & surgical planning
  - Confirmation of emphysema as principal cause of pulmonary hyperinflation
- CT post-LVRS
  - Direct visualization of surgical site & staple line
  - May show increase in functional lung volume
- Nuclear scintigraphy
  - Evaluation of regional blood flow that reflects distribution of emphysema for surgical planning
- Combination of CT & perfusion scintigraphy superior to either study in preoperative evaluation

Top Differential Diagnoses

- Bronchoscopic lung volume reduction
- Sublobar resection or biopsy

Clinical Issues

- Best candidates for LVRS: Disabling upper lobe-predominant emphysema refractory to medical therapy
- LVRS: Overall survival advantage over best medical therapy in carefully selected patients

__(Left)__ Coronal CECT of a patient being evaluated for LVRS shows severe centrilobular emphysema with heterogeneous distribution and upper lobe predominance, features that correlate with favorable outcome of LVRS. Note flattening of the left hemidiaphragm. __(Right)__ PA chest radiograph of a patient who had bilateral lung volume reduction surgery through a median sternotomy shows faint visualization of bilateral apical staple lines ➔.

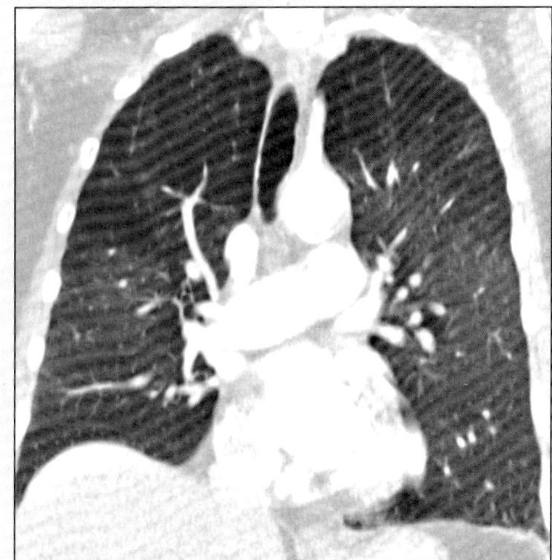

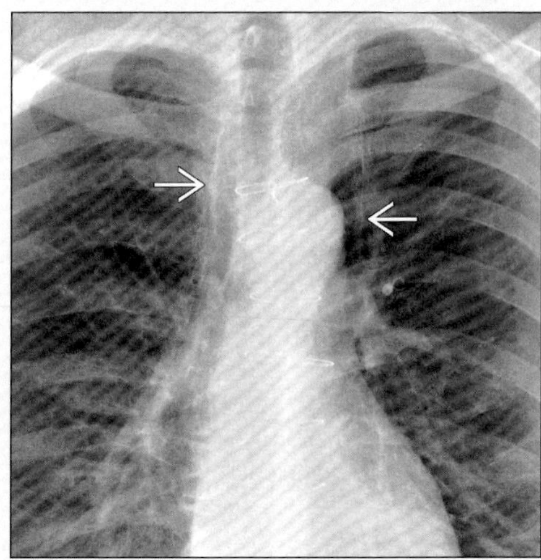

__(Left)__ Axial NECT of a patient post LVRS shows bilateral staple lines ➲ along the medial aspects of the bilateral upper lobes and severe upper lobe predominant emphysema. __(Right)__ Coronal CECT of a patient with severe upper lobe predominant emphysema who underwent a lung volume reduction procedure using bronchoscopically placed 1-way valves shows the valves ➲ in the right upper lobe segmental bronchi with associated right upper lobe volume loss and mediastinal shift to the right.

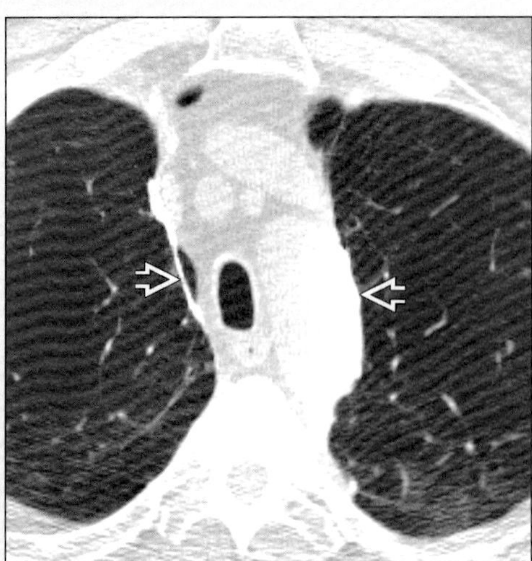

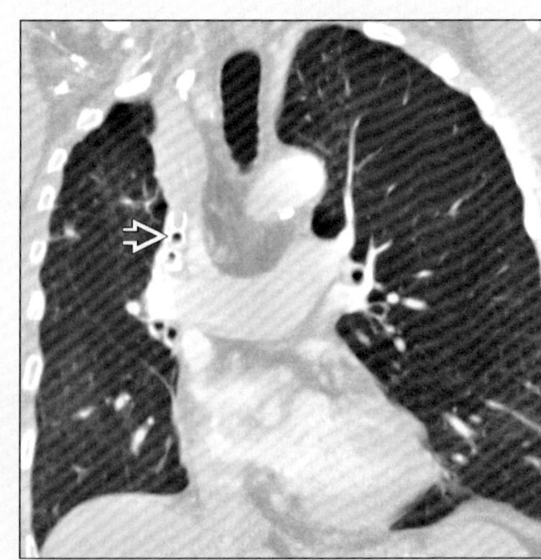

LUNG VOLUME REDUCTION SURGERY

TERMINOLOGY

Abbreviations

- **Lung volume reduction surgery (LVRS)**

Definitions

- **Treatment of severe emphysema** by removing approximately 20-35% of peripheral, emphysematous parenchyma from each lung
- **Decreases lung volume**
- **Improves elastic recoil** of remaining lung
- Improves mechanics of diaphragm & intercostal muscles

IMAGING

General Features

- Best diagnostic clue
  - Apical metallic staple line
- Location
  - Lung apex

Radiographic Findings

- Pre-LVRS
  - Large lung volume, flattening of hemidiaphragms
  - Increased AP diameter
  - Increased retrocardiac & retrosternal clear spaces
- Post-LVRS
  - Reduced apical lung volume
  - Apical metallic staple line

CT Findings

- Pre-LVRS
  - CT used for patient selection & surgical planning
  - Confirmation of emphysema as principal cause of pulmonary hyperinflation
  - Heterogeneous severe emphysema with upper lobe predominance needs to be present for LVRS to be beneficial
    - Peripheral or subpleural distribution of severe emphysema, better target for LVRS
    - Quantitative computerized densitometric analysis more reproducible than qualitative pulmonary evaluation; not proven to provide better prediction of response to LVRS
      - Most commonly used **qualitative** technique is "density mask" analysis that identifies voxels with attenuation < -900-950 HU
  - Underlying bronchiectasis, interstitial lung disease, pleural disease, infection, cancer, or cardiovascular disease may preclude LVRS
    - Resection of small indeterminate pulmonary nodules can sometimes be performed at time of LVRS
    - Approximately 3-5% of LVRS candidates have undiagnosed non-small cell lung cancer
- Post-LVRS
  - Direct visualization of surgical site & staple line
  - CT may show increase in functional lung volume

MR Findings

- Hyperpolarized helium-3 & other agents such as xenon under investigation for evaluation of extent & distribution of emphysema with MR

Nuclear Medicine Findings

- V/Q scan
  - Regional blood flow patterns reflect distribution of emphysema; useful for surgical planning
  - Combination of CT & perfusion scintigraphy superior to either study alone in preoperative evaluation

Imaging Recommendations

- Best imaging tool
  - CT useful for preoperative evaluation of severity & distribution of emphysema
  - Chest radiography helpful for evaluation of postoperative complications
    - Pneumothorax, pneumonia, hemorrhage

DIFFERENTIAL DIAGNOSIS

Bronchoscopic Lung Volume Reduction

- Instrumental obstruction of airways supplying hyperinflated lung segment or lobe
- Use of endobronchial 1-way valves; hyperdense on CT; lung collapse distal to endobronchial valve

Sublobar Resection

- Clinical history or preoperative CT most helpful
- More likely to be unilateral; LVRS more commonly bilateral

CLINICAL ISSUES

Demographics

- Patients with **disabling emphysema refractory to medical therapy**
- Patients with upper lobe-predominant emphysema & low exercise capacity most likely to benefit from LVRS

Natural History & Prognosis

- LVRS
  - Restoration of respiratory mechanics
  - Reduction of oxygen & energy consumption of respiratory muscles
  - Improvement of exercise tolerance & quality of life
- Patients with lower lobe-predominant emphysema or alpha-1 antitrypsin deficiency less likely to benefit from LVRS
- Approximately 50% of patients have prolonged air leak (> 7 days)
- Overall survival advantage over best medical therapy in carefully selected patients

Treatment

- LVRS currently most commonly performed in both lungs through video-assisted thoracoscopic surgery (VATS)
- Median sternotomy or standard thoracotomy may also be used

SELECTED REFERENCES

1. Sardenberg RA et al: Lung volume reduction surgery: an overview. Rev Assoc Med Bras. 56(6):719-23, 2010
2. Sciurba FC et al: A randomized study of endobronchial valves for advanced emphysema. N Engl J Med. 363(13):1233-44, 2010

LOBECTOMY

Key Facts

Terminology

- Lobectomy: Complete anatomic lobar resection
- Sleeve lobectomy: Resection of lobe & portion of common airway

Imaging

- Radiography
  - Postsurgical changes & ipsilateral volume loss
  - Hyperexpansion of remaining lobes
  - Analysis of hila & neofissures to determine type of lobectomy
- CT
  - Direct visualization of bronchial stump & absence of resected lobe/bronchial branches
  - Assessment of surgical staples & postoperative changes
  - Ipsilateral volume loss
  - Hyperexpansion of remaining lobes

Top Differential Diagnoses

- Lobar atelectasis
- Sublobar resection
- Pneumonectomy

Pathology

- Lung cancer
- Metastatic disease
- Bronchiectasis
- Lung abscess

Diagnostic Checklist

- Consider prior lobectomy in patients with postsurgical change & ipsilateral volume loss
- Evaluate radiographic anatomy to determine type & extent of lobar resection
- CT provides direct visualization of bronchial stump & documents absence of resected lobe

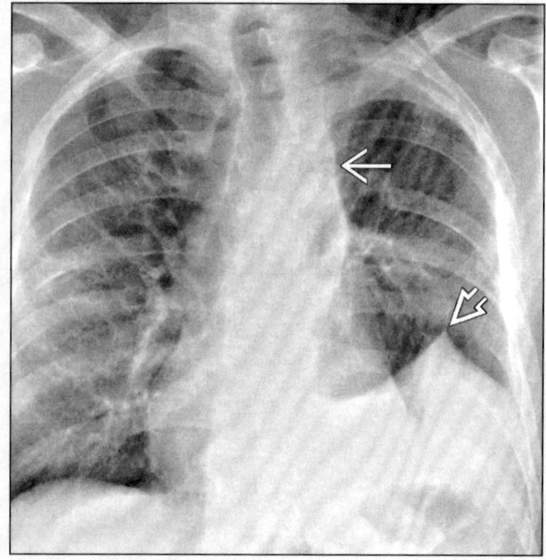
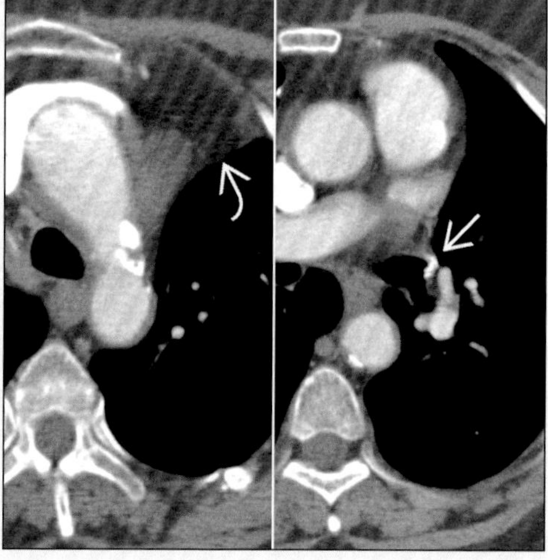

(Left) *PA chest radiograph of a patient with prior left upper lobectomy demonstrates left lung volume loss, leftward mediastinal shift ➔, and a juxtaphrenic peak of the left hemidiaphragm ➔.* ***(Right)*** *Composite image with axial CECT of the same patient shows leftward anterior mediastinal shift ➔ and surgical staples ➔ at the site of the left upper lobe bronchus resection. The best imaging clues of lobectomy are identification of the bronchial stump and absence of the resected lobe.*

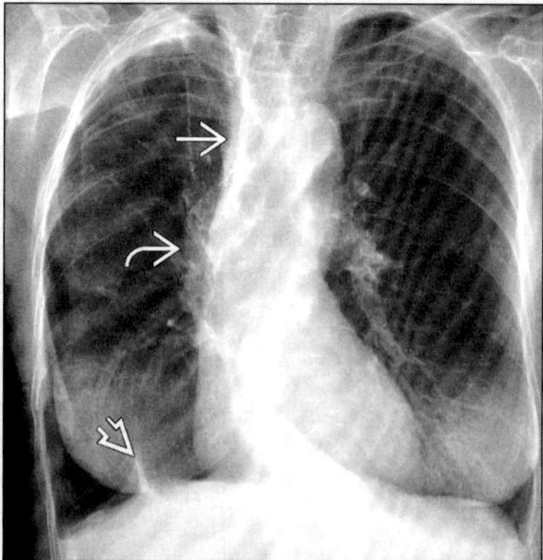
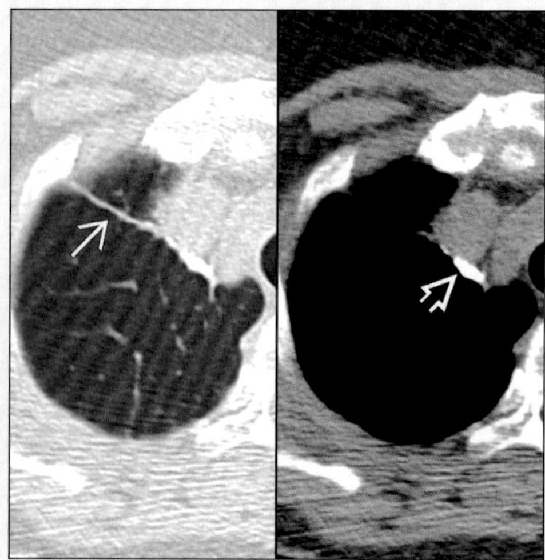

(Left) *PA chest radiograph of a patient with a history of prior right upper lobectomy shows elevation of the right hilum ➔, rightward mediastinal shift ➔, and a juxtaphrenic peak of the right hemidiaphragm ➔.* ***(Right)*** *Composite image with axial NECT of the same patient in lung (left) and soft tissue (right) window demonstrates volume loss in the right hemithorax and the presence of a neofissure ➔. Surgical staples ➔ are present adjacent to the right superior mediastinum.*

LOBECTOMY

TERMINOLOGY

Definitions

- **Lobectomy**
  - **Complete anatomic lobar resection**
  - Typically includes regional lymph node resection
- Sleeve lobectomy
  - Resection of lobe & portion of common airway

IMAGING

General Features

- Best diagnostic clue
  - CT identification of bronchial stump & absence of resected lobe/bronchial branches

Radiographic Findings

- Radiography
  - General
    - Presence of **neofissure**
      - Visceral pleural surfaces of remaining lobes
    - Signs of volume loss
    - Hyperexpansion of remaining lobes
  - Other findings
    - Surgical staples
    - Post-thoracotomy changes in chest wall
  - **Right upper lobectomy**
    - Right lung volume loss
    - Neofissure
      - Visceral pleural surfaces of right middle lobe (RML) & right lower lobe (RLL)
      - Best visualized on lateral chest radiograph
      - Follows expected course of right major fissure
      - Displaced superiorly & anteriorly
    - Decrease in tracheal bifurcation angle
    - Juxtaphrenic peak of right hemidiaphragm
    - Elevation of right hilum
      - Superior & lateral displacement of right main bronchus & bronchus intermedius
      - Superior & lateral displacement of proximal RLL pulmonary artery
  - **Right middle lobectomy**
    - Neofissure
      - Visceral pleural surfaces of right upper lobe (RUL) & RLL
      - Best visualized on lateral chest radiograph
      - Similar to course of right major fissure
    - Lateral displacement of right main bronchus & right interlobar pulmonary artery
  - **Right lower lobectomy**
    - Right lung volume loss
    - Inferior displacement of right hilum
    - **Type 1 reorientation**
      - Neofissure: Visceral pleura of RUL & RML
      - Frontal chest radiograph: Oblique orientation of neofissure with lateral aspect inferior to medial aspect
      - Lateral chest radiograph: Horizontal orientation of superior-posterior neofissure
      - Neofissure located superiorly in posterior aspect & inferiorly in anterior aspect
      - Inferior displacement of right main bronchus
      - RUL located superior & anterior to neofissure
      - RML located inferior & posterior to neofissure
      - RML expands to occupy majority of right base
    - **Type 2 reorientation**
      - Neofissure: Visceral pleura of RUL & RML
      - Neofissure best visualized on frontal chest radiograph
      - Frontal chest radiograph: Portion of neofissure in right base lower than position of type 1
      - RUL expands posteriorly & inferiorly
      - RML remains anterior
  - **Left upper lobectomy**
    - Left lung volume loss
    - No neofissure
    - Elevation of left hilum
    - Decrease in tracheal bifurcation angle
    - Leftward shift of anterior mediastinum
    - Juxtaphrenic peak of left hemidiaphragm
    - Hyperexpansion of left lower lobe (LLL)
  - **Left lower lobectomy**
    - Left lung volume loss
    - No neofissure
    - Inferior displacement of left hilum
    - Leftward shift of anterior mediastinum
    - Elevation of left hemidiaphragm
    - Hyperexpansion of left upper lobe (LUL)

CT Findings

- CECT
  - General
    - Direct visualization of bronchial stump & absence of resected lobe/bronchial branches
      - Follow bronchial tree from carina
      - Identify bronchial stump
    - Ipsilateral volume loss
    - Hyperexpansion of remaining lobes
  - Other findings
    - Surgical staples
    - Post-thoracotomy changes in chest wall
  - **Right upper lobectomy**
    - Neofissure
      - Thin line or band on CT
      - Rotates clockwise
      - Coronal orientation at level of aortic arch
      - Oblique, coronal orientation at subcarinal level
      - Coronal or sagittal orientation & anterior location at level of inferior pulmonary vein
    - Superior & lateral displacement of right main stem bronchus & bronchus intermedius
    - Superior & lateral displacement of proximal RLL pulmonary artery
  - **Right middle lobectomy**
    - Neofissure
      - Thin line or band on CT
      - Coronal orientation at all levels
      - Less vertical orientation than left major fissure
      - Inferior aspect located anterior to superior aspect
      - Anterior to left major fissure at level of inferior pulmonary vein
    - Lateral displacement of right interlobar artery
    - Inferior displacement of RUL bronchus
  - **Right lower lobectomy**
    - **Type 1 reorientation**
      - Neofissure: Thin line or band on CT
      - Absence of RLL bronchus & pulmonary artery
      - Inferior displacement of RUL bronchus

- **Type 2 reorientation**
  - Neofissure: Thin line or band on CT
  - Neofissure anterior at subcarinal level, posterior in inferior aspect
  - Absence of RLL bronchus & pulmonary artery
  - Posterior & inferior displacement of RUL bronchus
  - Hyperexpanded RUL
  - RML smaller in volume than type 1
- **Left upper lobectomy**
  - No neofissure
  - Absence of LUL artery & bronchus
  - Hyperexpansion of LLL
- **Left lower lobectomy**
  - No neofissure
  - Absence of LLL artery & bronchus
  - Hyperexpansion of LUL

Imaging Recommendations

- Best imaging tool
  - CT to identify bronchial stump & document absence of resected lobe/bronchial branches
- Protocol advice
  - Multiplanar reformatted images helpful

DIFFERENTIAL DIAGNOSIS

Lobar Atelectasis

- No neofissure
- Absence of postsurgical changes
- Tethering forces remain in place
  - Limit redistribution of lung
- Less volume loss compared to lobectomy

Sublobar Resection

- Segmentectomy & wedge resection
- Small, peripheral, & noninvasive neoplasms
- Less volume loss compared to lobectomy

Pneumonectomy

- Resection of entire lung
- Large & locally invasive tumors
- More volume loss compared to lobectomy

PATHOLOGY

General Features

- Etiology
  - **Lung cancer**
    - Leading cause of cancer-related mortality in USA
    - 5-year survival: 15.7%
      - Varies markedly with stage at diagnosis
  - Metastatic disease
  - Bronchiectasis
  - Lung abscess

Gross Pathologic & Surgical Features

- General
  - **Thoracotomy**
    - Posterolateral thoracotomy preferred
    - Anterolateral thoracotomy & muscle-sparing lateral thoracotomy
  - **Video-assisted thoracoscopic surgery**
    - Lower complication rate
    - Equivalent survival to open thoracotomy
    - Shorter hospitalization
  - RUL lobectomy most commonly performed
- **Sleeve lobectomy**
  - Alternative to pneumonectomy
  - Lesions involving main or lobar bronchi
    - Benign & low-grade malignant neoplasms
    - Airway stenosis
    - < 10% operable lung cancers
  - Impaired cardiopulmonary function
    - FEV1 < 50%
    - Maximum voluntary ventilation < 50%
  - RUL lobectomy more common than LUL lobectomy

CLINICAL ISSUES

Presentation

- Most common signs/symptoms
  - Complications
    - **Early (postoperative day 1-30)**
      - Hemorrhage, pneumonia, edema, empyema, bronchopleural fistula, dehiscence, lung herniation, & lobar torsion
    - **Late (postoperative day > 30)**
      - Bronchopleural fistula, empyema, pneumonia, recurrent neoplasm, & anastomotic stricture

Natural History & Prognosis

- Lobectomy
  - Thoracotomy
    - Complication rate: 49%
    - Mortality: 2.9%
  - Video-assisted thoracoscopic surgery
    - Complication rate: 31%
    - Mortality: 0-2%
    - Variable reports regarding recurrence rates when compared to thoracotomy
      - At least 1 meta-analysis showed reduced systemic recurrence with VATS
- Sleeve lobectomy
  - Postoperative day 1-30: Mortality 5%
  - Locoregional recurrence: 4-22%
- Prediction of postoperative lung function
  - Dynamic perfusion MR
  - Quantitative CT
  - Perfusion SPECT

Treatment

- Bronchopleural fistula
  - Completion pneumonectomy
  - Vascularized flap covering of bronchial stump
- Anastomotic stricture
  - Completion pneumonectomy

SELECTED REFERENCES

1. Yan TD et al: Systematic review and meta-analysis of randomized and nonrandomized trials on safety and efficacy of video-assisted thoracic surgery lobectomy for early-stage non-small-cell lung cancer. J Clin Oncol. 27(15):2553-62, 2009
2. Kim EA et al: Radiographic and CT findings in complications following pulmonary resection. Radiographics. 22(1):67-86, 2002
3. Seo JB et al: Neofissure after lobectomy of the right lung: radiographic and CT findings. Radiology. 201(2):475-9, 1996

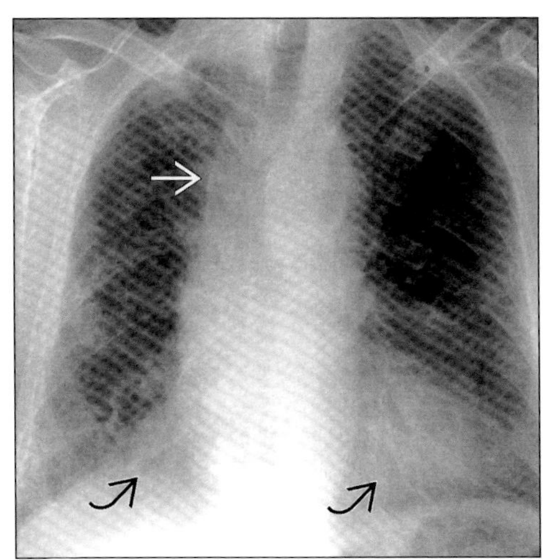

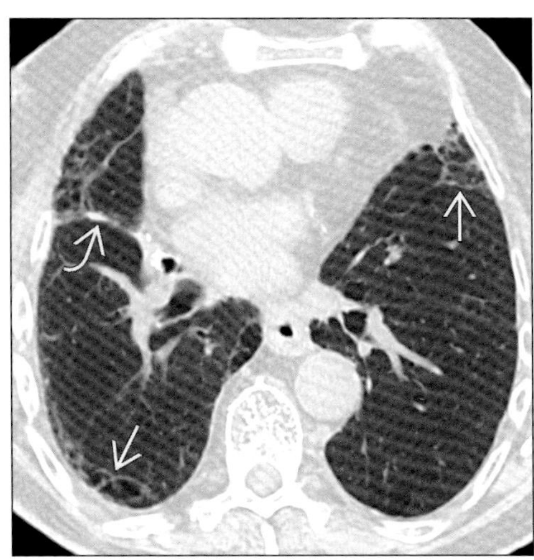

(Left) *PA chest radiograph of a patient with prior right middle lobectomy demonstrates rightward shift of the mediastinum ➔ and bilateral lower lobe reticular opacities ↗.* ***(Right)*** *Axial NECT of the same patient shows surgical staples ↗ along the neofissure. Bilateral subpleural reticular opacities represent pulmonary fibrosis ➔. Patients with pulmonary fibrosis have an increased risk of lung cancer, for which most lobectomies are performed.*

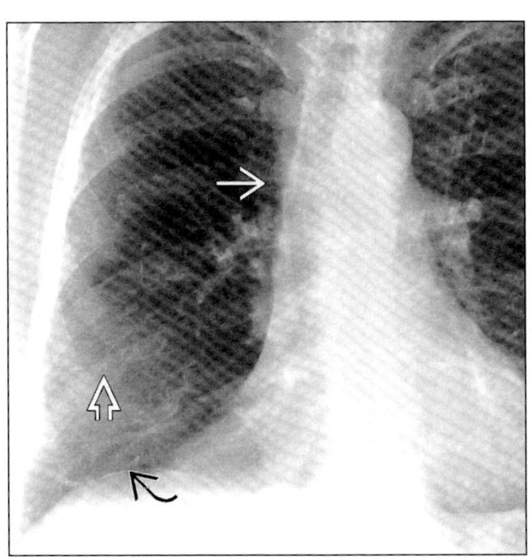

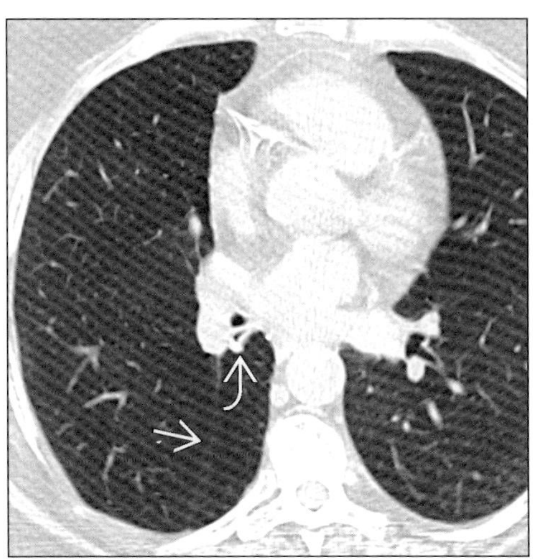

(Left) *PA chest radiograph of a patient with prior right lower lobectomy shows rightward shift of the mediastinum ➔ and surgical staples ↗ in the right lower lung zone. Note the obliquely oriented neofissure ⇨ in the right lower lung zone.* ***(Right)*** *Axial NECT of the same patient demonstrates right lung volume loss and a posteriorly located neofissure ➔. Surgical staples ↗ are present at the site of resection of the right lower lobe bronchus consistent with right lower lobectomy.*

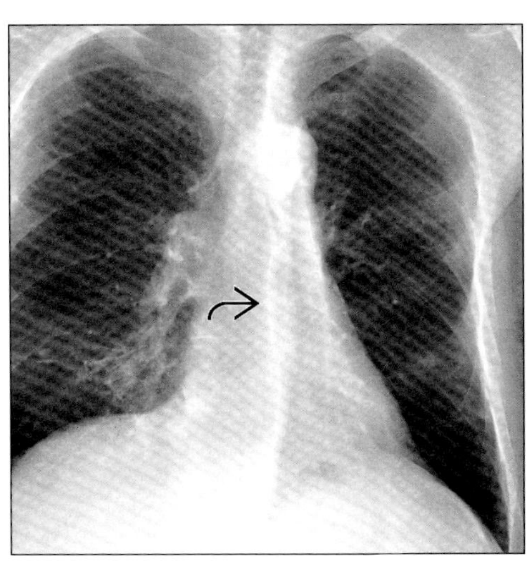

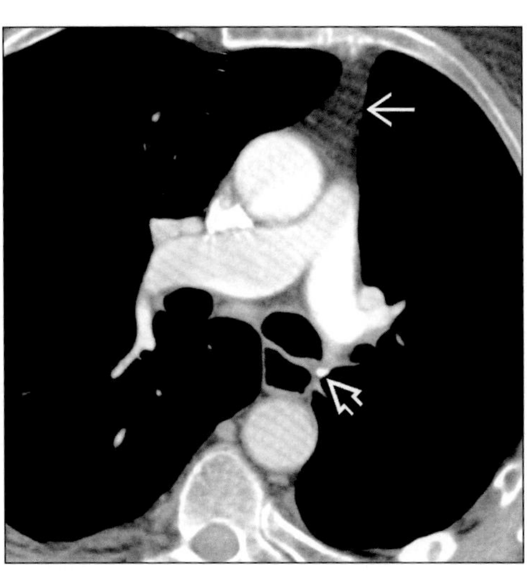

(Left) *PA chest radiograph of a patient with prior left lower lobectomy demonstrates evidence of volume loss within the left hemithorax with leftward shift of the azygoesophageal recess ↗. The left upper lobe is hyperexpanded, and the left hemithorax is more lucent than the right.* ***(Right)*** *Axial CECT of the same patient shows leftward shift of the anterior mediastinal fat ➔. Surgical staples ⇨ are present at the site of resection of the left lower lobe bronchus.*

LOBAR TORSION

Key Facts

Terminology

- Bronchovascular pedicle rotation with resultant airway obstruction, venous compromise, ischemia, infarction, and gangrene

Imaging

- Radiography
  - Reoriented major fissure may extend below hilum
  - Lobar loss of volume, subsequent volume increase
  - Abnormally located "collapsed" lobe
  - Mediastinum may shift away from affected lung
- CT
  - Tapered obliteration of proximal pulmonary artery & bronchus
  - Delayed filling of pulmonary artery with contrast
  - Bulging fissures with unusual orientation
  - Unexpected location of affected lobe
- Chest radiography usually suggests diagnosis

Top Differential Diagnoses

- Lobar atelectasis
- Pneumonia
- Infarction

Pathology

- Usually postoperative complication
- Typically follows right upper lobectomy

Clinical Issues

- Signs/symptoms
  - Rapid development shock in postoperative period
  - Sudden cessation of postoperative air leak
- High mortality if unrecognized (10-20%)

Diagnostic Checklist

- Consider lobar torsion in symptomatic patient with postsurgical findings resembling lobar atelectasis

(Left) AP chest radiograph of a patient with middle lobe torsion that developed 2 days after right upper lobectomy shows a wedge-shaped opacity ➔ overlying the right hilum and the upper medial hemithorax. The edge of the fissure ➔ extends below the right hilum. (Right) PA chest radiograph shows a large right pneumothorax and right upper lobe ➔ collapse with torsion. Lobar torsion may develop in the setting of a large pneumothorax if the interlobar fissures are complete or near complete.

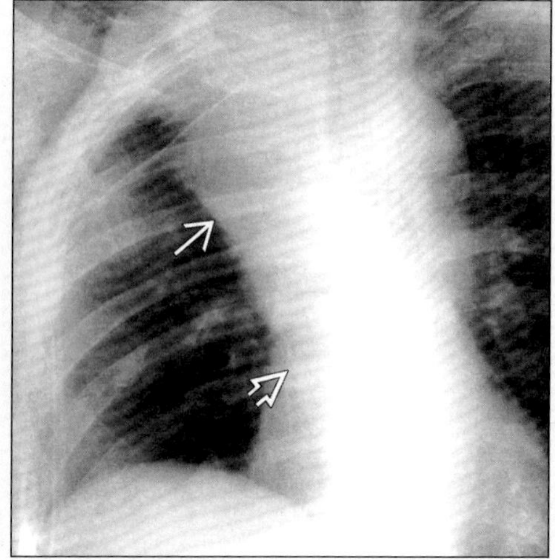

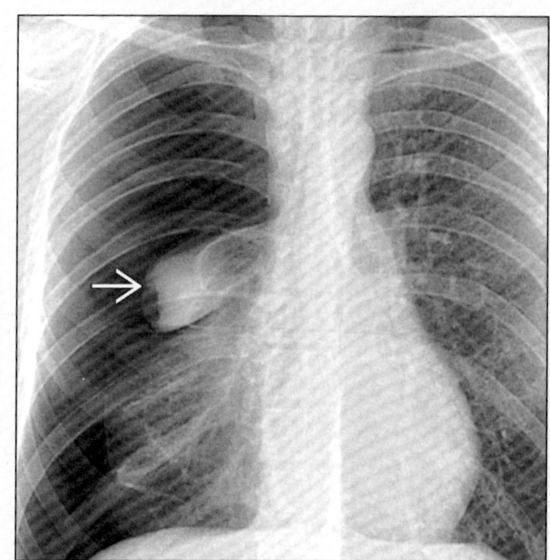

(Left) Axial HRCT of a patient with post esophagectomy torsion shows diffuse right upper lobe ground-glass opacity and septal thickening ➔ and a bulging major fissure ➔. The torsed lobe produced middle lobe atelectasis ➔, compromised the neoesophagus blood supply, and resulted in a leak ➔. (Right) Axial NECT of a patient with postoperative middle lobe torsion shows middle lobe enlargement and intrinsic hemorrhage ➔, the result of venous obstruction and hemorrhagic infarction.

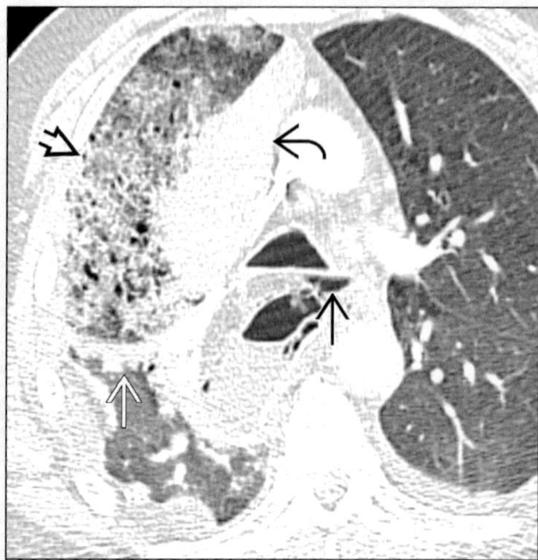

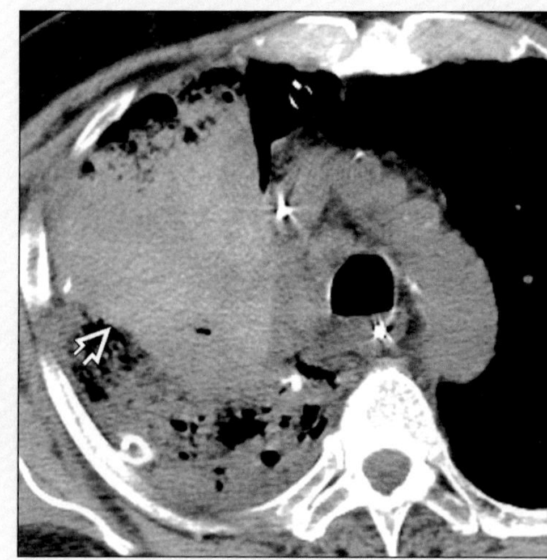

LOBAR TORSION

TERMINOLOGY

Synonyms

- **Volvulus** of a lung lobe

Definitions

- Bronchovascular pedicle rotation: Airway obstruction, venous compromise, ischemia, infarction, gangrene

IMAGING

General Features

- Best diagnostic clue
  - Post surgical rapid opacification of affected lobe
- Location
  - **Middle lobe** torsion after right upper lobectomy
- Morphology
  - Initial lobar volume loss followed by size increase

Radiographic Findings

- **Fissure**
  - **Reoriented major fissure** post right upper lobe lobectomy **may extend below hilum**
- **Lobe**
  - Lobar loss of volume, subsequent volume increase
    - Rapid postoperative lobar opacification
  - Abnormally located "collapsed" lobe
    - Lobar positional change on serial radiography
  - Lobar air trapping rare; seen in infants
- **Hilum**
  - Paradoxical displacement in relation to "atelectatic" lobe
  - Abnormal pulmonary vascular course
    - Hilar vessels course laterally and superiorly
  - Bronchial cutoff or distortion
- **Mediastinum**: May shift away from affected lung
- **Pleura**
  - New pleural effusion suggests infarction
  - May be obscured by ipsilateral pleural drain

CT Findings

- Hilum
  - Tapered obliteration of proximal pulmonary artery and bronchus
  - Delayed filling of pulmonary artery with contrast
  - Pulmonary artery acutely kinked
- Lobe
  - Volume may increase rather than decrease
  - Attenuation range from ground-glass to consolidation
  - Septal thickening from venous obstruction
  - Bulging fissures with unusual orientation
  - Unexpected location of affected lobe

Imaging Recommendations

- Best imaging tool
  - Portable chest radiography usually suffices to suggest diagnosis
    - Critical element: Awareness of radiographic signs of torsion
  - CECT may be useful in selected cases
    - Identification of hilar vessels
    - Visualization of parenchymal involvement

DIFFERENTIAL DIAGNOSIS

Lobar Atelectasis

- Most common mimic of lobar torsion
  - Common postop; retained secretions, splinting
- Torsed middle lobe may mimic atelectasis

Pneumonia

- Usually develops later in postoperative course
- Fever, ↑ white blood cell count; also occurs in torsion

Infarction

- Subacute
  - Usually later in postoperative course
  - Usually not lobar

PATHOLOGY

General Features

- Etiology
  - Usually **postoperative complication**
    - Typically follows right upper lobectomy; middle lobe torsion
    - Left lower lobe torsion following left upper lobectomy, right lower lobe torsion following right upper lobectomy

Gross Pathologic & Surgical Features

- Typically 180° of clockwise (or counterclockwise) rotation (range: 90-360°)
- Venous obstruction may lead to infarction

CLINICAL ISSUES

Presentation

- Most common signs/symptoms
  - Rapid development **shock in postoperative period**
  - Sudden cessation of postoperative air leak
- Other signs/symptoms
  - **Hemorrhagic pleural effusion**

Demographics

- Epidemiology
  - Complicates **0.1% of pulmonary resections**
  - **70% after right upper lobe lobectomy**, 15% after left upper lobe lobectomy

Natural History & Prognosis

- Diagnosis: Median 10 days after operation
- High mortality if unrecognized (10-20%)

Treatment

- Prophylactic
  - Anchoring lobes to each other after lobectomy

DIAGNOSTIC CHECKLIST

Consider

- Lobar torsion in symptomatic patient with postsurgical findings resembling lobar atelectasis

SELECTED REFERENCES

1. Kim EA et al: Radiographic and CT findings in complications following pulmonary resection. Radiographics. 22(1):67-86, 2002

PNEUMONECTOMY

Key Facts

Terminology

- Pneumonectomy
  - Lung & visceral pleural resection

Imaging

- Early
  - Air in pneumonectomy space
  - Midline trachea & mediastinum
  - Gradual fluid filling of pneumonectomy space
- Late
  - Opaque hemithorax
  - Postsurgical changes
  - Mediastinal & tracheal shift toward pneumonectomy space
- Complications
  - Pulmonary edema, pneumonia, ARDS
  - Hemothorax/chylothorax/empyema
  - Bronchopleural fistula
  - Pneumonia: Airspace disease, consolidation
- CT
  - Direct evaluation of pneumonectomy space
  - Assessment of complications
  - Incidental visualization of in situ thrombus in pulmonary artery stump

Top Differential Diagnoses

- Empyema ± bronchopleural fistula
  - Infected fluid-filled pneumonectomy space
  - Air-fluid levels with bronchopleural fistula
- Chylothorax
  - Injury to thoracic duct
  - Water attenuation fluid in pneumonectomy space

Clinical Issues

- Complications of pneumonectomy
  - Pulmonary edema; 80-100% mortality
  - Bronchopleural fistula; 16-23% mortality
  - ARDS (5% incidence); > 80% mortality

__(Left)__ AP chest radiograph on postoperative day (POD) 1 following left pneumonectomy shows air in the pneumonectomy space, right chest wall, and supraclavicular soft tissues. The trachea and mediastinum are in the midline. __(Right)__ AP chest radiograph of the same patient on POD 16 shows fluid filling approximately 50% of the pneumonectomy space with several air-fluid levels ⮫ and a midline trachea and mediastinum. Normally, the pneumonectomy space progressively fills with fluid.

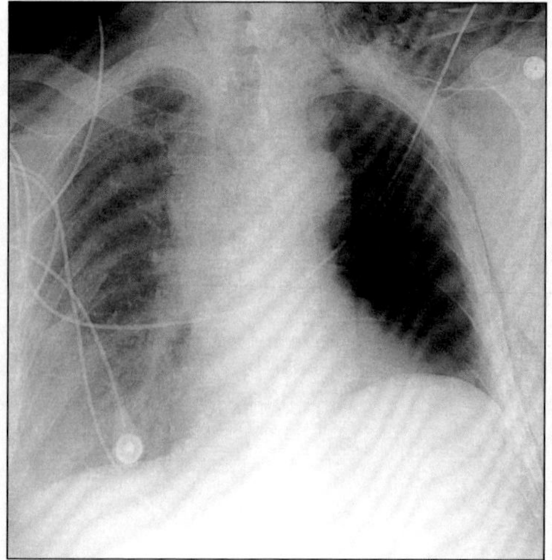

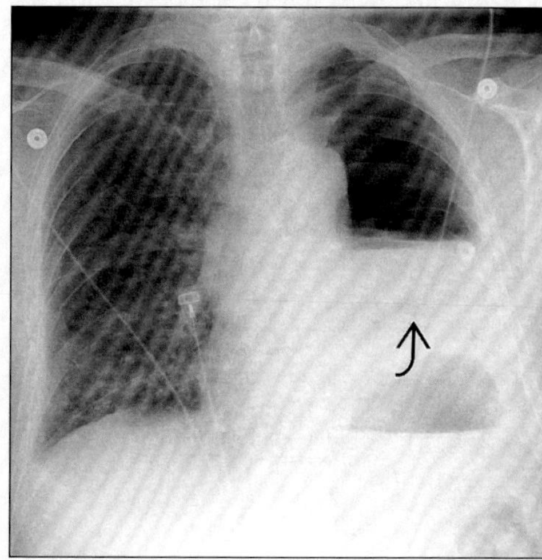

__(Left)__ PA chest radiograph of the same patient on POD 40 shows near-complete pneumonectomy space opacification with a small apical air-fluid level ⮫. Slight leftward mediastinal and tracheal shift indicate continued volume loss. Increasing gas in the pneumonectomy space should prompt exclusion of bronchopleural fistula. __(Right)__ PA chest radiograph of a patient with a remote right pneumonectomy shows marked right mediastinal and tracheal shift and rightward shift of the left upper lobe →.

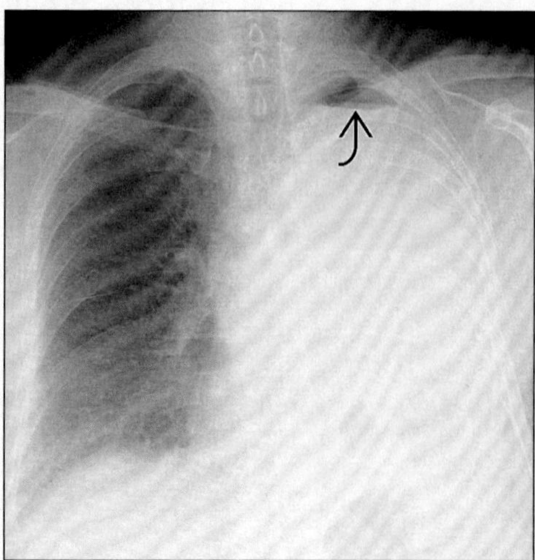

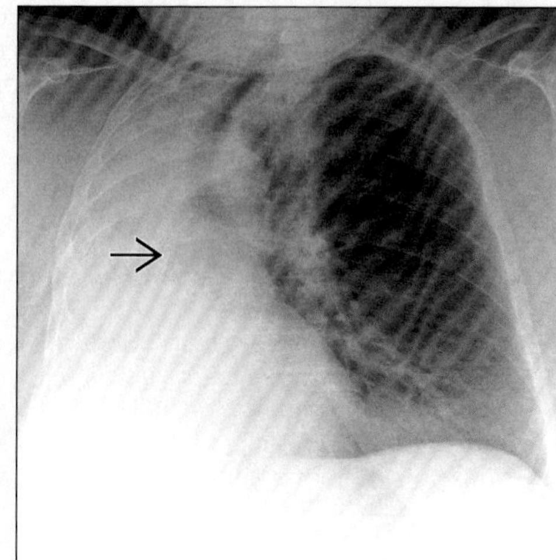

PNEUMONECTOMY

TERMINOLOGY

Synonyms

- Intrapleural pneumonectomy

Definitions

- **Pneumonectomy**: Lung & visceral pleural resection
  - Treatment of lung cancer, TB, bronchiectasis
- **Extrapleural pneumonectomy**: En block resection of lung, visceral & parietal pleura, hemidiaphragm, & pericardium
- **Intrapericardial pneumonectomy**: Pneumonectomy with intrapericardial resection of tumor
- **Sleeve pneumonectomy**: Central tumor resection; contralateral main bronchus anastomosed to trachea

IMAGING

General Features

- Best diagnostic clue
  - Opaque hemithorax & ipsilateral surgical changes

Radiographic Findings

- **Early**
  - Air in pneumonectomy space
  - Midline trachea & mediastinum
  - Gradual fluid filling of pneumonectomy space; air-fluid level on upright imaging
  - Gradual ipsilateral tracheal & mediastinal shift
- **Late**
  - Opaque hemithorax: Complete pneumonectomy space obliteration; weeks to months
  - Postsurgical changes
  - Mediastinal & tracheal shift toward pneumonectomy space
    - Heart rotates toward posterior aspect of pneumonectomy space
    - Contralateral lung shifts anteriorly
- **Postsurgical complications**
  - **Pulmonary edema, pneumonia, ARDS**
    - Airspace disease
  - **Hemothorax/chylothorax/empyema**
    - Rapid fluid filling of pneumonectomy space; mediastinal shift away from pneumonectomy
  - **Bronchopleural fistula**
    - Failure of pneumonectomy space opacification
    - Decreasing fluid & increasing air
      - ≥ 1.5 cm drop in air-fluid level
    - Mediastinal shift away from pneumonectomy
    - Increasing subcutaneous air
  - **Pneumonia**: Airspace disease, consolidation
  - Cardiac herniation
- **Late complications**
  - **Postpneumonectomy syndrome**
    - Typically with right pneumonectomy
    - Decreasing volume of pneumonectomy space
    - Increasing cardiac rotation within pneumonectomy space
    - Stretching, compression, narrowing of distal trachea/mainstem bronchus ± tracheomalacia
  - Late onset bronchopleural fistula: Infection
  - Late onset empyema: Air in pneumonectomy space; increasing size of pneumonectomy space

CT Findings

- Direct evaluation of pneumonectomy space
- Thrombus in pulmonary artery stump
  - In situ thrombus rather than pulmonary embolism
  - 12% of pneumonectomies
- Evaluation of postpneumonectomy complications
  - Localization of bronchopleural/esophagopleural fistulae
  - Empyema: Expansion of fluid-filled pneumonectomy space; coexistent fistula; thickening of residual parietal pleura
  - Hemothorax: High-attenuation fluid in pneumonectomy space, fluid-hematocrit level
  - Chylothorax: Expansion of pneumonectomy space with water attenuation fluid
  - Postpneumonectomy syndrome: Narrowing of distal trachea & mainstem bronchus; airway compression between pulmonary artery & aorta

Imaging Recommendations

- Best imaging tool
  - Radiography for postoperative follow-up
  - CECT for evaluation of complications

DIFFERENTIAL DIAGNOSIS

Empyema ± Bronchopleural Fistula

- Infected fluid-filled pneumonectomy space
- Air-fluid levels with bronchopleural fistula

Chylothorax

- Injury to thoracic duct
- Water attenuation fluid in pneumonectomy space

CLINICAL ISSUES

Presentation

- Most common signs/symptoms
  - Empyema: Chest pain, fever, hypotension
- Other signs/symptoms
  - Postpneumonectomy syndrome: Dyspnea, stridor, recurrent infection

Natural History & Prognosis

- **Complications of pneumonectomy**
  - Pulmonary edema (2.5-5% prevalence); 80-100% mortality
  - Bronchopleural fistula (0-9% incidence); 16-23% mortality
  - Empyema (< 5% incidence)
  - ARDS (5% incidence); > 80% mortality
  - Pneumonia (2-15% incidence); 25% mortality
  - Cardiac herniation (rare); 40-50% mortality

Treatment

- Management tailored to specific complications

SELECTED REFERENCES

1. Chae EJ et al: Radiographic and CT findings of thoracic complications after pneumonectomy. Radiographics. 26(5):1449-68, 2006
2. Kim SY et al: Filling defect in a pulmonary arterial stump on CT after pneumonectomy: radiologic and clinical significance. AJR Am J Roentgenol. 185(4):985-8, 2005

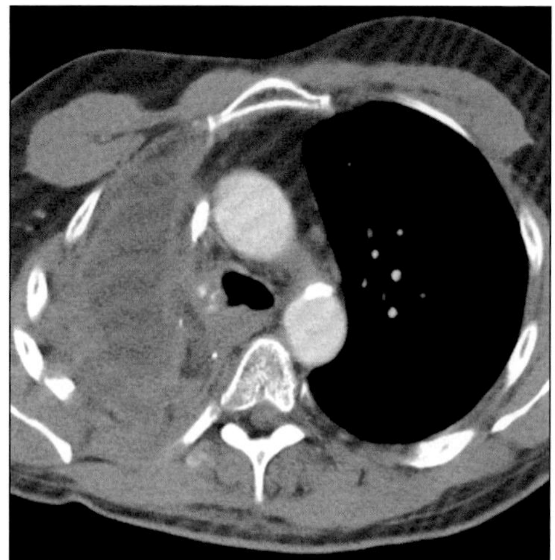
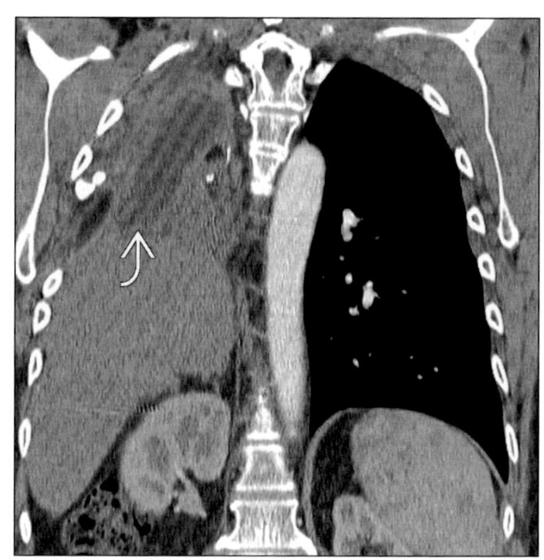

(Left) *Axial CECT of a patient status post remote right pneumonectomy shows marked volume loss in the right hemithorax, crowding of right-sided ribs, and low-attenuation material within the pneumonectomy space.* ***(Right)*** *Coronal CECT of the same patient shows marked right hemithorax volume loss and elevation of the right hemidiaphragm. Note postsurgical changes in the right chest wall. In spite of marked right hemithorax volume loss, there is little rightward mediastinal shift.*

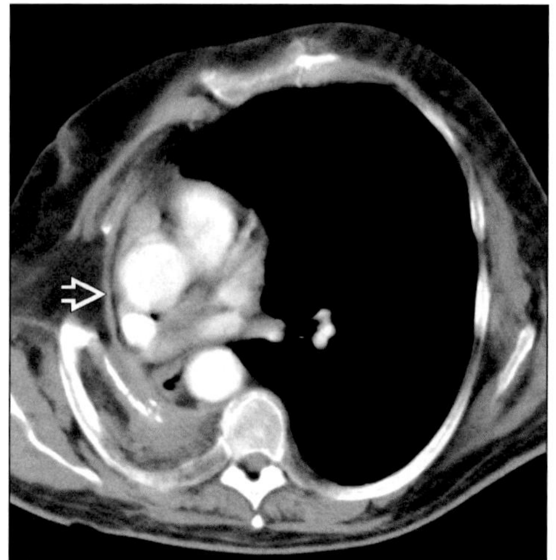
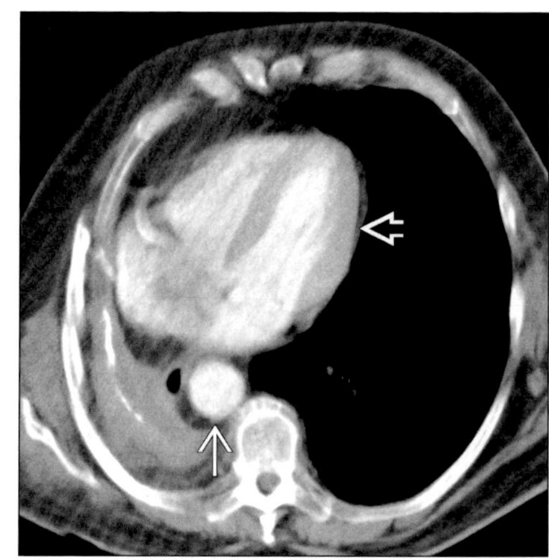

(Left) *Axial CECT of a patient status post right pneumonectomy shows severe deformity of the right hemithorax, postsurgical changes in the right chest wall, marked right hemithorax loss of volume, shift of the mediastinum to the right, and compensatory hyperexpansion of the left lung.* ***(Right)*** *Axial CECT of the same patient shows marked volume loss in the right hemithorax and right mediastinal shift. Note that the descending aorta has also shifted into the right hemithorax.*

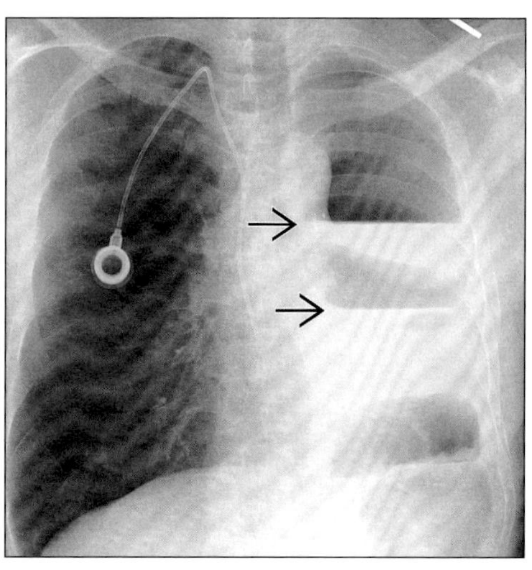
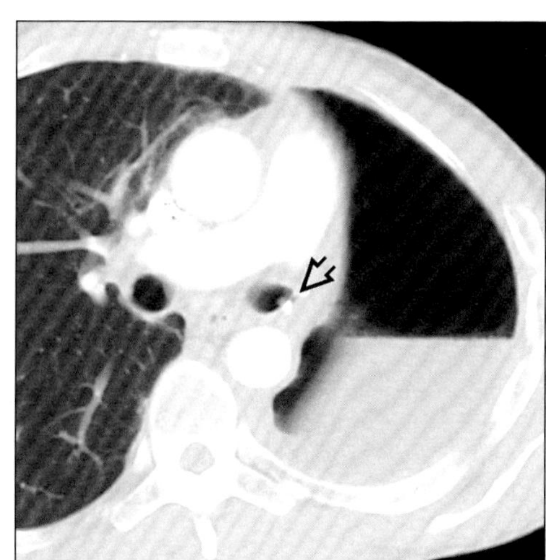

(Left) *PA chest radiograph of a patient status post left pneumonectomy complicated by bronchopleural fistula shows multiple air-fluid levels and increasing air in the pneumonectomy space since the prior study (not shown).* ***(Right)*** *Axial CECT of the same patient shows a large air-fluid level in the left pneumonectomy space and the likely site of the bronchopleural fistula, which resulted from dehiscence of the left bronchial stump.*

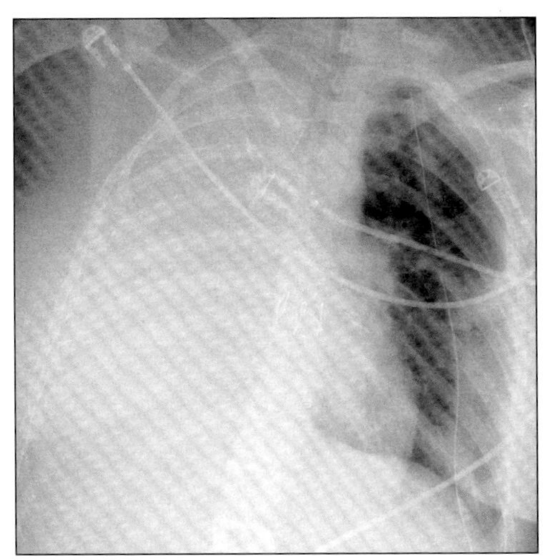

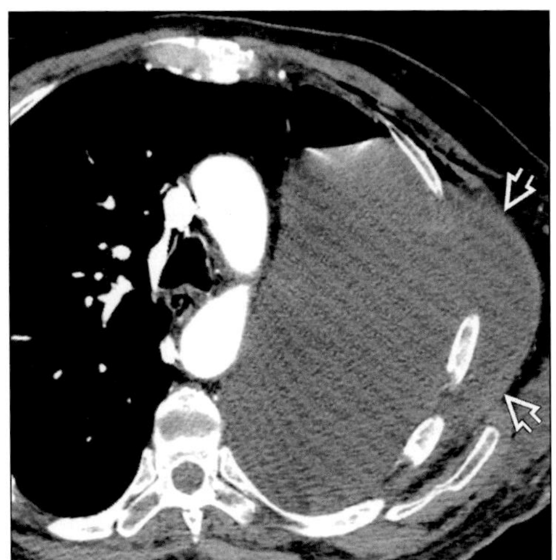

(Left) AP chest radiograph obtained 3 days after right pneumonectomy and left wedge resection shows rapid opacification of the pneumonectomy space and left mediastinal shift secondary to hemorrhage. **(Right)** Axial CECT after left pneumonectomy and rapid pneumonectomy space opacification shows a large amount of water attenuation fluid that decompresses into the left chest wall ➔ through the thoracotomy defect. Chylothorax secondary to thoracic duct injury was diagnosed at surgery.

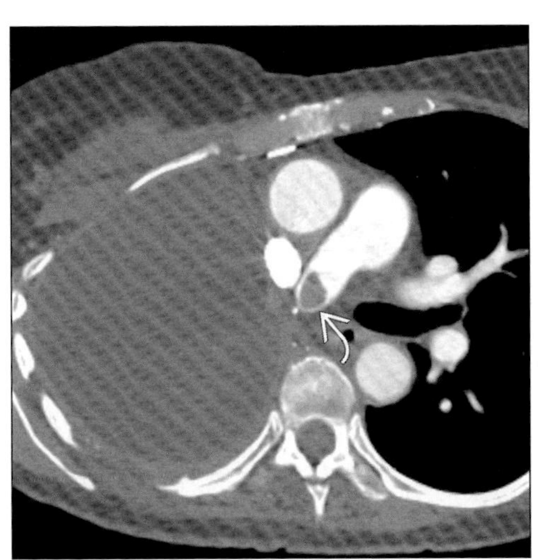

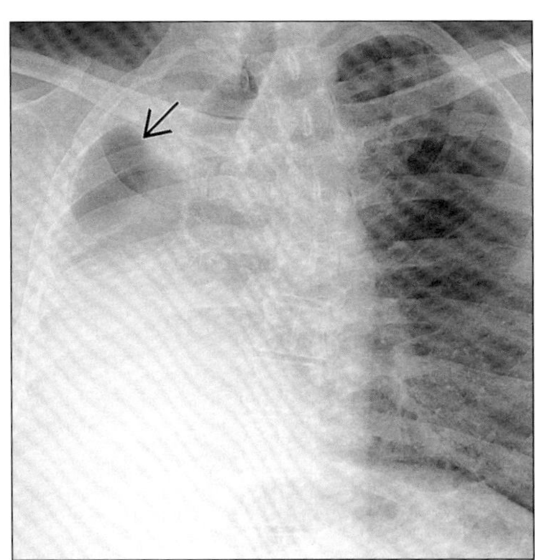

(Left) Axial CECT of a patient status post right extrapleural pneumonectomy for mesothelioma shows a distal right pulmonary artery stump thrombus ➔ thought to be secondary to in situ thrombosis rather than thromboembolic disease. (Courtesy E. Marom, MD.) **(Right)** PA chest radiograph of a patient status post right pneumonectomy complicated by postpneumonectomy syndrome shows complete right mediastinal shift, marked right tracheal deviation, and left lung shift ➔ into the right hemithorax.

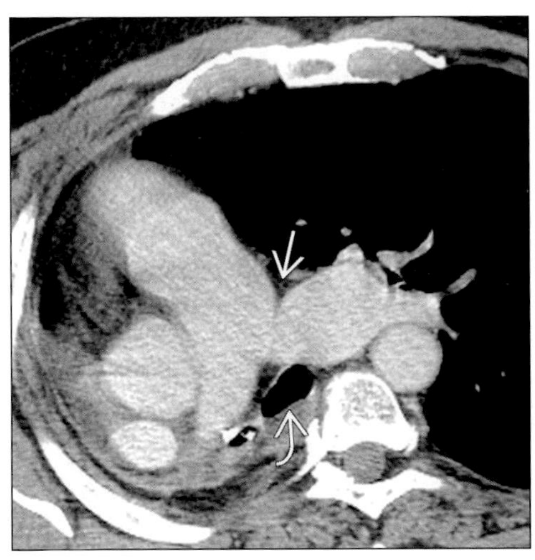

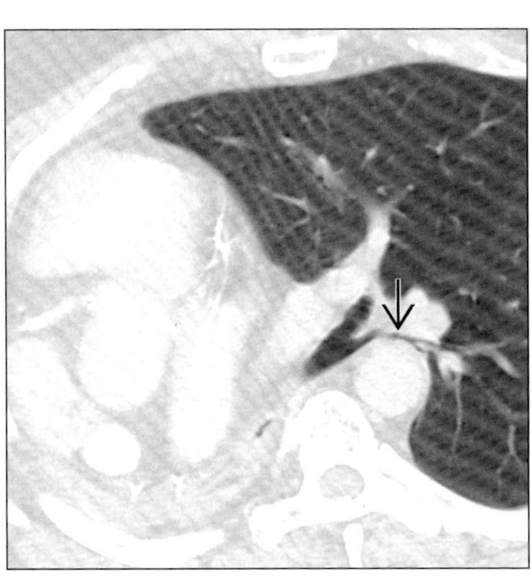

(Left) Axial CECT of the same patient shows marked rotation of mediastinal structures with displacement into the right hemithorax and shift of the left mainstem bronchus ➔ into the right hemithorax. Note kinking ➔ of the left pulmonary artery origin and enlargement of the left pulmonary artery. **(Right)** Axial CECT of the same patient shows mass effect on and narrowing of the left lower lobe superior segmental bronchus ➔ as it drapes over the descending aorta.

EXTRAPLEURAL PNEUMONECTOMY

Key Facts

Terminology
- Abbreviations
  - Extrapleural pneumonectomy (EPP)
- Definition
  - En bloc resection of parietal pleura, ipsilateral lung, pericardium, & hemidiaphragm
  - Treatment of malignant pleural mesothelioma

Imaging
- Radiography
  - Findings similar to those of postoperative intrapleural pneumonectomy
  - Early findings: Air-filled pneumonectomy space, lucent pericardial/diaphragmatic patches
  - Evolution: Fluid filling of pneumonectomy space, decreasing size
  - Late findings: Loss of volume of pneumonectomy space; ipsilateral mediastinal shift

Top Differential Diagnoses
- Empyema
- Chylothorax
- Bronchopleural fistula

Clinical Issues
- EPP used in young patients with few comorbidities & preserved functional status with curative intent
- EPP used with neoadjuvant or adjuvant chemotherapy & postoperative radiation
- Minor & major complications of EPP in 60%
  - Atrial fibrillation, epicarditis, cardiac tamponade, aspiration, ARDS, empyema, bronchopleural fistula, diaphragmatic hernia, chylothorax
- Prognosis
  - Perioperative mortality: 3-10%
  - Median survival: 16-19 months
  - 3-year survival rate: 14%

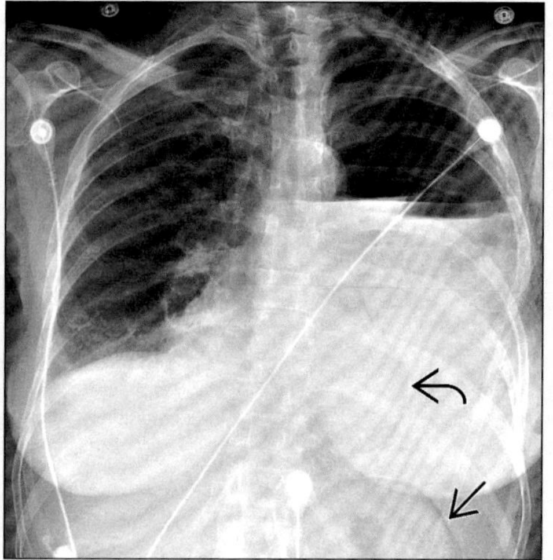
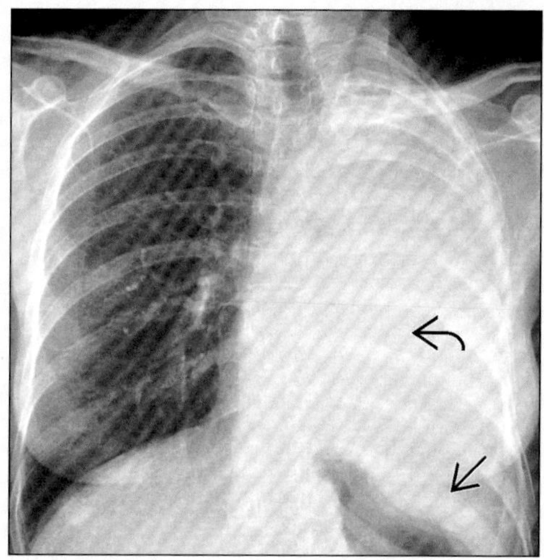

(Left) *PA chest radiograph 5 days after left EPP shows partial filling of the pneumonectomy space with fluid. Note lucent pericardial ⇨ and diaphragmatic ⇨ patches and absence of significant mediastinal shift.* ***(Right)*** *PA chest radiograph 6 months after left EPP shows a fluid-filled pneumonectomy space and left mediastinal shift. The pericardial ⇨ and diaphragmatic ⇨ patches have become more radiopaque. Gradual fluid filling of the pneumonectomy space results in an opaque hemithorax.*

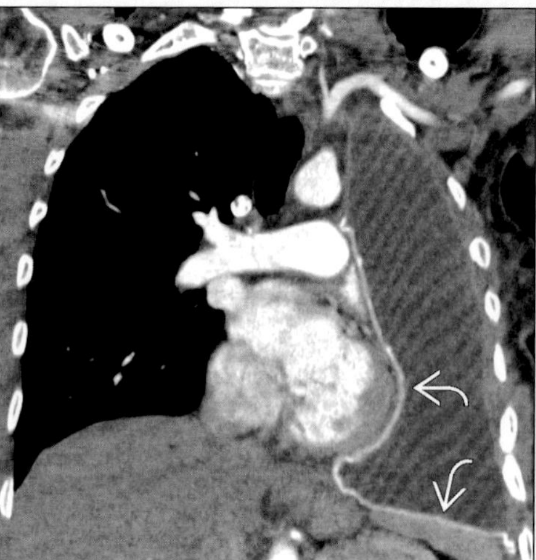
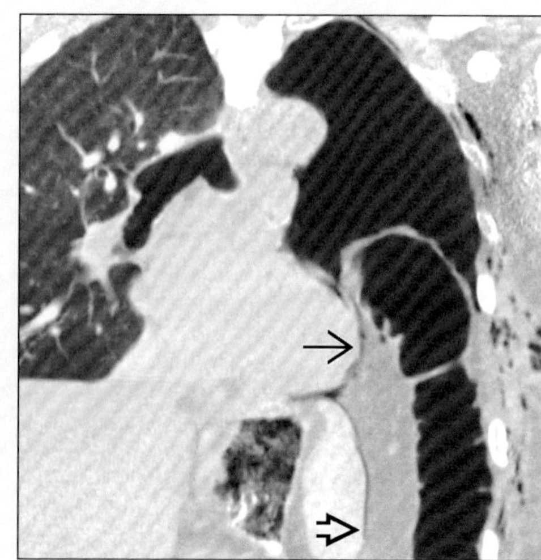

(Left) *Coronal CECT 1 year after left EPP shows a fluid-filled pneumonectomy space, left mediastinal shift, and hyperdense pericardial ➡ and diaphragmatic patches.* ***(Right)*** *Coronal NECT 2 days after left EPP shows diaphragmatic patch dehiscence ⇨ and colonic herniation into the pneumonectomy space. The pericardial ⇨ and diaphragmatic patches are relatively lucent in the early postoperative period. Visualization of pericardial and diaphragmatic patches on CT is characteristic of EPP.*

EXTRAPLEURAL PNEUMONECTOMY

TERMINOLOGY

Abbreviations

- **Extrapleural pneumonectomy (EPP)**

Definitions

- En bloc resection of parietal pleura, ipsilateral lung, pericardium, and hemidiaphragm
- Initially developed to treat tuberculous empyema; now performed almost exclusively for treatment of malignant pleural mesothelioma

IMAGING

General Features

- Best diagnostic clue
  - Opaque hemithorax with ipsilateral mediastinal shift; visible pericardial & diaphragmatic patches

Radiographic Findings

- EPP imaging findings similar to those of postoperative intrapleural pneumonectomy
- **Early** appearance of pneumonectomy space
  - Mediastinum midline or slightly shifted to pneumonectomy side
  - Air-filled pneumonectomy space
  - Enlarged ipsilateral hilum
    - When omental flap used to buttress bronchial staple line
  - Visualization of lucent pericardial/diaphragmatic patches; air interspersed within mesh material
- **Evolution** of pneumonectomy space appearance
  - Fills with fluid & decreases in size at variable rates
  - Completely fluid-filled in 2-4 months
  - Small quantity of air may persist indefinitely
  - Air bubbles may be dispersed in fluid; do not equate with empyema or fistula
  - Pericardial & diaphragmatic patches become more radiopaque
- **Late** pneumonectomy space appearance
  - Degree of mediastinal shift depends on contralateral lung compliance
  - Loss of volume on pneumonectomy side; ipsilateral mediastinal shift, approximation of ipsilateral ribs
  - Variable-sized soft tissue opacity of pneumonectomy space
- **Complications**
  - Complications of intrapleural pneumonectomy
  - **Dehiscence of pericardial patch** with cardiac herniation
    - Cardiac displacement
    - Pneumopericardium
  - **Dehiscence of diaphragmatic patch** with intrathoracic herniation of abdominal contents
    - Unusual gas patterns in ipsilateral hemithorax
  - **Tight pericardial patch**
    - Cardiac tamponade physiology; superior vena cava/azygos vein distension

CT Findings

- Absence of ipsilateral lung & tracheobronchial tree
- Variable attenuation within pneumonectomy space
- Hyperdense pericardial/diaphragmatic patch
- Increased sensitivity for detection of postoperative complications
  - Aspiration, pneumonia, ARDS, patch failure, pulmonary emboli, pericardial effusion

Imaging Recommendations

- Best imaging tool
  - Chest radiographs for postoperative surveillance
  - CT monitoring for recurrent mesothelioma; assessment of confusing radiographic abnormalities
  - PET not routinely used due to false-positive rates

DIFFERENTIAL DIAGNOSIS

Empyema

- Principal infectious complication after EPP
- Fever & leukocytosis helpful but not always present
- Difficult diagnosis based on imaging alone
- May require patch removal

Chylothorax

- Direct injury to thoracic duct at time of surgery
- Expansion of pneumonectomy space with fluid
- Thoracentesis: Cloudy fluid with elevated triglycerides
- Treatment: Fat-restricted diet, percutaneous embolization, surgical thoracic duct ligation

Bronchopleural Fistula

- Consider if increasing air in pneumonectomy space

CLINICAL ISSUES

Demographics

- EPP used in young patients with few comorbidities & preserved functional status with curative intent
- **Contraindications**: Transdiaphragmatic, mediastinal, or diffuse chest wall tumor or involvement of contralateral hemithorax

Natural History & Prognosis

- Minor & major complications of EPP in 60%
  - Atrial fibrillation, inflammatory epicarditis, cardiac tamponade, aspiration, ARDS, empyema, bronchopleural fistula, diaphragmatic hernia, chylothorax
- Perioperative mortality: 3-10%
- Median survival: 16-19 months
- 3-year survival rate: 14%

Treatment

- EPP used with neoadjuvant or adjuvant chemotherapy and postoperative radiation
- Pleurectomy & decortication are alternative treatments associated with lower complication rates but higher local recurrence rates

SELECTED REFERENCES

1. Wolf AS et al: Surgical techniques for multimodality treatment of malignant pleural mesothelioma: extrapleural pneumonectomy and pleurectomy/decortication. Semin Thorac Cardiovasc Surg. 21(2):132-48, 2009
2. Spirn PW et al: Radiology of the chest after thoracic surgery. Semin Roentgenol. 23(1):9-31, 1988

THORACOPLASTY AND APICOLYSIS

Key Facts

Terminology

- Extrapleural pneumonolysis: Plombage; oleothorax
- Extrapleural apicolysis: Pleural tent, parietal pleurolysis
- Collapse therapy: Surgical upper lobe collapse used to treat cavitary tuberculosis

Imaging

- Thoracoplasty
  - Segmental rib fractures (> 2 fractures/rib) & rib displacement into chest cavity
  - Resection of 6-7 ribs
- Extrapleural plombage
  - Extrapleural space created & enlarged with Lucite™ spheres or paraffin wax
- Lungs
  - Loss of lung volume, cicatricial atelectasis
  - Thick pleura adjacent to thoracoplasty/plombage

Top Differential Diagnoses

- Thoracoplasty or extrapleural plombage
  - Tuberculous empyema
  - Post-traumatic/postsurgical chest wall deformity
  - Malignant pleural mesothelioma
- Extrapleural apicolysis
  - Hydropneumothorax
  - Pancoast tumor

Clinical Issues

- Signs/symptoms
  - Thoracoplasty: Chronic pain, scoliosis, reduced chest wall mobility
  - Plombage: Pain uncommon, hemoptysis from vascular erosion

Diagnostic Checklist

- History of tuberculosis is helpful in recognizing imaging findings of extrapleural plombage

(Left) PA chest radiograph of a patient with surgically treated tuberculosis shows a right waterfall thoracoplasty involving ribs 1-9 ➡, right upper lobe volume loss, and right convex upper thoracic scoliosis ↪. (Right) Axial CECT of a patient with remote pleuropulmonary tuberculosis shows findings of left thoracoplasty ➡, calcified tuberculous empyema ➡, and calcified pulmonary granulomas ↪. Thoracoplasty is still used in some countries to treat drug-resistant cavitary tuberculosis.

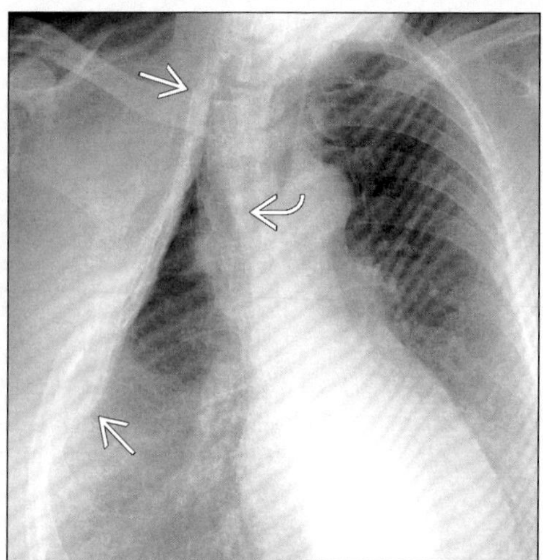

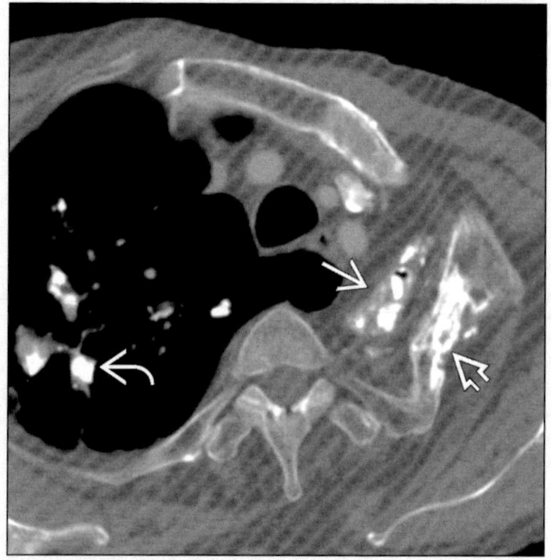

(Left) PA chest radiograph of a patient with tuberculosis treated with Lucite™ sphere plombage ➡ shows multifocal, thin-walled, air-filled spheres in the right upper hemithorax. (Right) Axial CECT of a patient with oleothorax collapse therapy for tuberculosis shows a large right extrapleural collection with predominant central low attenuation, intrinsic foci of calcification ➡, and peripheral curvilinear calcification ➡. Chronic oleothorax usually does not exhibit fat attenuation on CT.

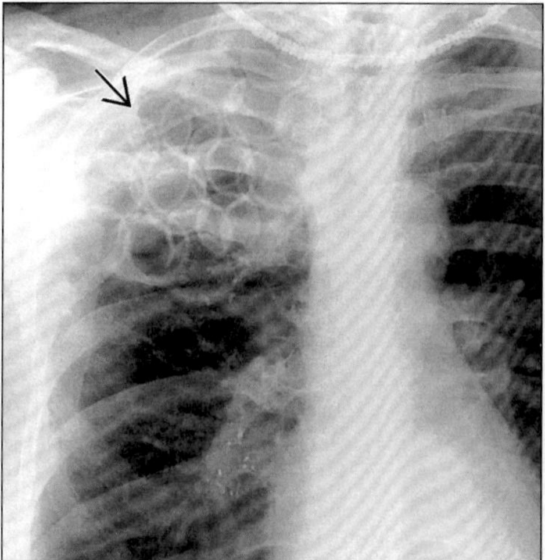

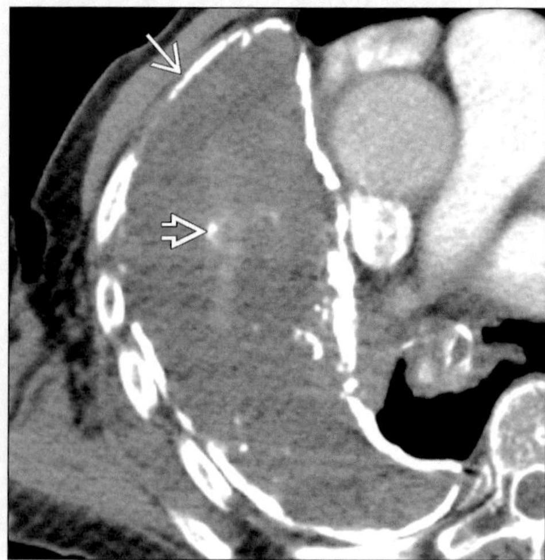

THORACOPLASTY AND APICOLYSIS

TERMINOLOGY

Synonyms

- **Extrapleural pneumonolysis**: Plombage, oleothorax
- **Extrapleural apicolysis**: Pleural tent, parietal pleurolysis

Definitions

- **Collapse therapy**
  - Surgical procedures designed to collapse upper lobe cavitary tuberculosis; used in mid 20th century before effective antituberculous drug therapy
- **Thoracoplasty**: Surgical rib removal to approximate chest wall, collapse lung, or obliterate pleural space
- **Extrapleural apicolysis** (pleural tent): Performed to reduce apical pleural dead space after upper lobectomy
  - Apical parietal pleura pulled off chest wall, creation of extrapleural space, reduced intrapleural space

IMAGING

Radiographic Findings

- **Thoracoplasty**
  - Segmental rib fractures (> 2 fractures/rib) & rib displacement into chest cavity
  - Resection of 6-7 ribs
  - Apical chest wall deformity; ribs displaced medially toward spine
- **Extrapleural plombage**
  - Extrapleural space created & enlarged with Lucite™ spheres or paraffin wax
    - Spheres initially surrounded by air, later by fluid
- Lungs
  - Loss of lung volume, calcified granulomas, cicatricial atelectasis
  - Pleural thickening adjacent to thoracoplasty or plombage
- **Thoracoplasty complications** (perioperative period)
  - Bronchopleural fistula
  - Prolonged air leak
  - Hemorrhage
  - Empyema
- **Plombage complications** (15%) (acute vs. long term)
  - Change in size, shape, appearance of previously stable plombage
    - Plombage migration
    - Erosion into major vessels or ribs
    - Dispersion of Lucite™ spheres; expanded extrapleural space
  - Acute or chronic local infection
  - Mediastinal compression by extrapleural mass
  - Secondary malignant neoplasms: Sarcoma, non-Hodgkin lymphoma, bronchogenic carcinoma
- **Extrapleural apicolysis** (pleural tent)
  - Initial: Air-containing space inseparable from air in pleural space
  - Day 2: Apical air-fluid level as fluid fills extrapleural space
  - > 30 days: Air resorption, apical cap (fluid & soft tissue), gradually diminishes in size

CT Findings

- Direct visualization of chest wall, extrapleural space, plombage; assessment of complications

Imaging Recommendations

- Best imaging tool
  - Chest radiography usually sufficient for evaluation
  - CT useful as problem-solving tool

DIFFERENTIAL DIAGNOSIS

Thoracoplasty or Extrapleural Plombage

- Tuberculous empyema
  - Focal pleural mass; variable thick peripheral calcification
  - Complications: Bronchopleural fistula, empyema necessitatis
- Post-traumatic/postsurgical chest wall deformity
- Malignant pleural mesothelioma
  - Circumferential nodular pleural thickening
  - Chest wall deformity; ipsilateral volume loss
  - Chest wall pain, weight loss, malaise

Extrapleural Apicolysis

- Hydropneumothorax
  - Loculated hydropneumothorax usually from inadequate chest tube drainage
  - May lead to empyema
- Pancoast tumor
  - Apical pleural thickening
  - Skeletal erosion
  - Pain, brachial plexus involvement, Horner syndrome

CLINICAL ISSUES

Presentation

- Most common signs/symptoms
  - **Thoracoplasty**: Chronic pain, scoliosis
- Other signs/symptoms
  - **Plombage**: Pain uncommon, hemoptysis from vascular erosion
  - **Thoracoplasty**
    - Reduced chest wall mobility, pneumonia
    - Rare right to left shunt through ipsilateral lung
  - Chronic hypoxia; pulmonary artery hypertension

Demographics

- Age
  - Elderly; thoracoplasty common in 1940s & 1950s
  - Still performed worldwide in younger individuals

Natural History & Prognosis

- Collapse therapy **curative in 75%** of tuberculosis
- Plombage complications may occur decades later

DIAGNOSTIC CHECKLIST

Image Interpretation Pearls

- History of tuberculosis is helpful in recognizing imaging findings of extrapleural plombage

SELECTED REFERENCES

1. Tezel CS et al: Plombage thoracoplasty with Lucite balls. Ann Thorac Surg. 79(3):1063, 2005
2. Weissberg D et al: Late complications of collapse therapy for pulmonary tuberculosis. Chest. 120(3):847-51, 2001

LUNG HERNIATION

Key Facts

Terminology
- Extension of lung tissue outside of thoracic cavity

Imaging
- Radiography
  - Aerated lung outside thoracic cavity when seen in profile
  - Sharply marginated focal thoracic radiolucency when seen en face
- CT
  - Direct visualization of herniated lung tissue; subsegmental lung herniation
  - Direct visualization of chest wall defect; typically intercostal defect
  - Assessment of adjacent bone & soft tissue
- Best imaging tools
  - Orthogonal chest radiographs
  - Unenhanced chest CT for indeterminate cases

Top Differential Diagnoses
- Chest wall infections
- Rib fractures & flail chest
- Thoracotomy
- Apical lung hernia

Pathology
- Thoracic surgery with failure of soft tissue closure
- Trauma
- Spontaneous
- Chronic corticosteroid use
- Congenital chest wall defect

Clinical Issues
- Most patients asymptomatic; require no treatment
- Symptomatic hernias may require treatment
  - Chest wall reconstruction, defect closure
- Strangulation rare

*(**Left**) PA chest radiograph of a patient status post left thoracotomy shows a rounded lucency with sharp lobular margins ➡ projecting over the left upper hemithorax. (**Right**) Axial NECT of the same patient shows that the lucency represents focal lung herniation ⇨ through a chest wall defect →. The herniated lung contains normal bronchovascular structures and is contiguous with the left upper lobe. CT allows a definitive diagnosis of lung herniation when chest radiography is inconclusive.*

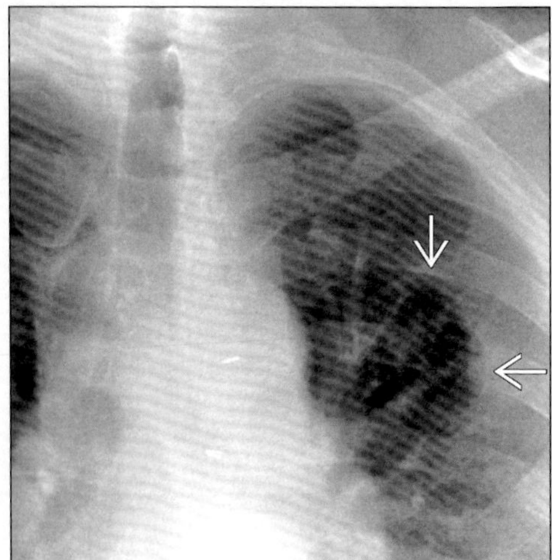

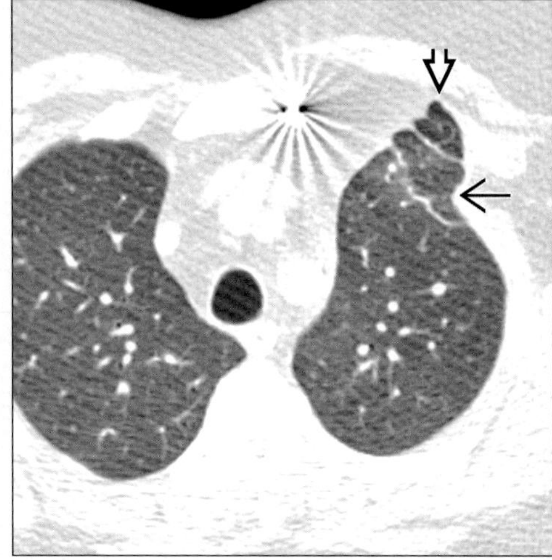

*(**Left**) AP chest radiograph obtained after thoracic surgery shows a small linear collection of extrathoracic gas adjacent to the left lateral ribs ➡. Other gas collections ➡ are noted adjacent to the left pleural drains. (**Right**) Axial NECT of the same patient shows that the linear gas collection corresponds to a left lung hernia ↗ extending through an intercostal left anterior chest wall defect →. Small air pockets ⇨ correspond to postoperative subcutaneous gas seen on chest radiography.*

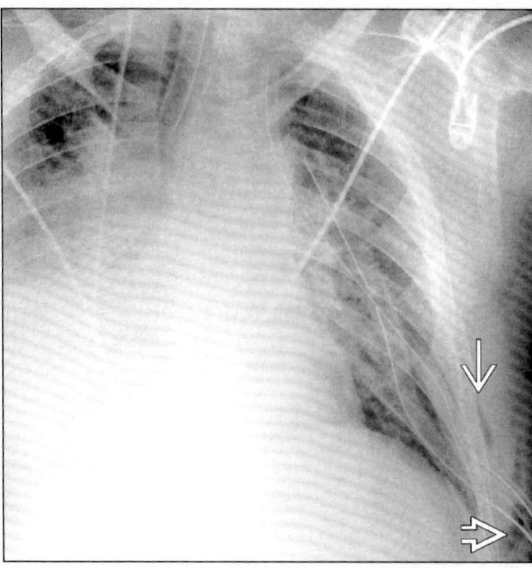

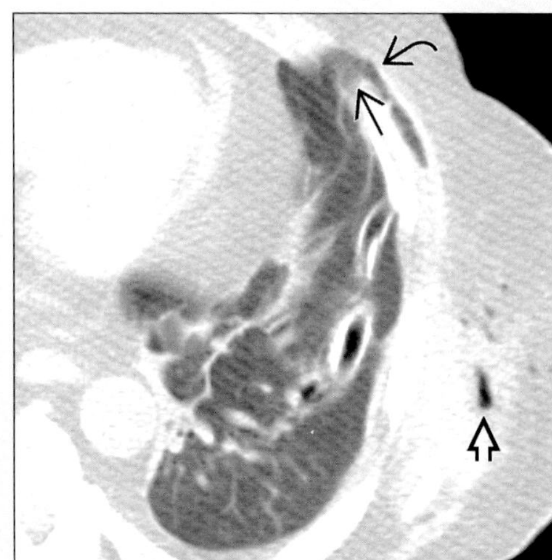

LUNG HERNIATION

TERMINOLOGY

Synonyms

- **Lung hernia**

Definitions

- **Extension of lung tissue outside thoracic cavity**

IMAGING

General Features

- Best diagnostic clue
  - Aerated lung parenchyma outside thoracic cavity
- Location
  - **Chest wall through intercostal space**
- Size
  - Usually subsegmental
- Morphology
  - Sharp peripheral margins because of overlying pleura

Radiographic Findings

- Lucency (aerated lung) outside confines of thoracic cavity when seen in profile
  - Visualization of continuity with adjacent intrathoracic lung parenchyma
- Sharply marginated focal thoracic radiolucency when seen en face

CT Findings

- Direct visualization of herniated lung tissue
  - Lung parenchyma extending through chest wall
  - Visualization of chest wall defect
  - Assessment of adjacent skeleton & soft tissues

Imaging Recommendations

- Best imaging tool
  - 2 orthogonal chest radiographs
  - Unenhanced chest CT for indeterminate cases

DIFFERENTIAL DIAGNOSIS

Chest Wall Infections

- Abscess containing loculations of gas & liquid
- Direct extension of empyema or pulmonary infection

Rib Fractures & Flail Chest

- Acute rib fractures
  - Segmental or involving large section of chest wall
- Lung remains confined within thoracic cavity
- Paradoxical motion with respiration

Thoracotomy

- Partial rib resection or osteotomy
- Lung remains confined within thoracic cavity
- Subcutaneous gas following surgery

Apical Lung Hernia

- Congenital defect
- Apical location

PATHOLOGY

General Features

- Etiology
  - Most related to **surgery**
    - Failure of soft tissue closure
      - Intercostal muscles
      - Endothoracic fascia
    - Thoracotomy, chest tube placement, minimally invasive thoracic/cardiac surgery
  - Chest trauma
  - Spontaneous
    - Rare
    - Rigorous coughing or sneezing
  - Chronic corticosteroid use
    - Muscle & connective tissue weakness
  - Congenital chest wall defect

CLINICAL ISSUES

Presentation

- Most common signs/symptoms
  - **Most patients asymptomatic**
  - Physical examination
    - Chest wall deformity
    - Palpable crepitant mass
      - Varies in size with respiration, cough, Valsalva maneuver
- Other signs/symptoms
  - Focal pain with deep inspiration
  - Dyspnea
  - Local tenderness
  - Fever

Natural History & Prognosis

- **Most require no treatment**
- Symptomatic hernias may require treatment
- Strangulation rare

Treatment

- Chest wall reconstruction
  - Primary closure
  - Mesh prosthesis

DIAGNOSTIC CHECKLIST

Consider

- Normal postoperative subcutaneous gas
- Chest wall abscess

Image Interpretation Pearls

- Herniated lung in continuity with intrathoracic lung
- Contains bronchovascular structures

Reporting Tips

- Description of hernia location, affected lobe(s), & defect size

SELECTED REFERENCES

1. Van Den Broeck S et al: Intercostal lung herniation after repeat thoracotomy. Minerva Chir. 63(4):307-10, 2008
2. Szentkereszty Z et al: Surgical treatment of intercostal hernia with implantation of polypropylene mesh. Hernia. 10(4):354-6, 2006

Key Facts

Terminology

- Median sternotomy (MS): Vertical incision through manubrium & sternum
  - Access heart, pericardium, & anterior mediastinum
  - Limited access to hila, lungs, pleura
  - Closure with cerclage or "figure 8" steel sutures
- Clamshell sternotomy (CS): Broad transverse incision across sternum & 4th anterior intercostal spaces
  - Access to both hemithoraces & mediastinum
- Indications for MS
  - CABG, valve & aortic surgery
  - Heart transplant, congenital heart disease
  - Placement of cardiac support devices
  - Anterior mediastinal mass
- Indications for CS
  - Double lung & heart-lung transplants
  - Resection of large mediastinal or cardiac mass
  - Resection of bilateral lung metastases

Imaging

- Radiography
  - Sternal wires should be aligned & intact
  - Osteotomy fragments should be fused
- CT
  - Assess for parasternal & mediastinal fluid collections/abscess & sternal dehiscence

Clinical Issues

- Most patients do well without complications or need for intervention
- Signs/symptoms of sternal infection
  - Pain ± fever, incisional drainage, crepitus
  - Osteomyelitis: Bone destruction
  - Pleural effusion, hemothorax, fibrothorax
- Treatment of sternal infection
  - Antibiotics
  - Surgical debridement

*(**Left**) Graphic shows the morphologic features of median sternotomy: A midline vertical incision through the sternal manubrium and body secured with steel wires. Sternal wires and osteotomy fragments may be diastatic or displaced due to infection, trauma, or devascularization. (**Right**) PA chest radiograph of a patient status post median sternotomy and CABG shows the sternum secured with simple cerclage ➦ and "figure 8" steel wires ➡ that are intact and aligned.*

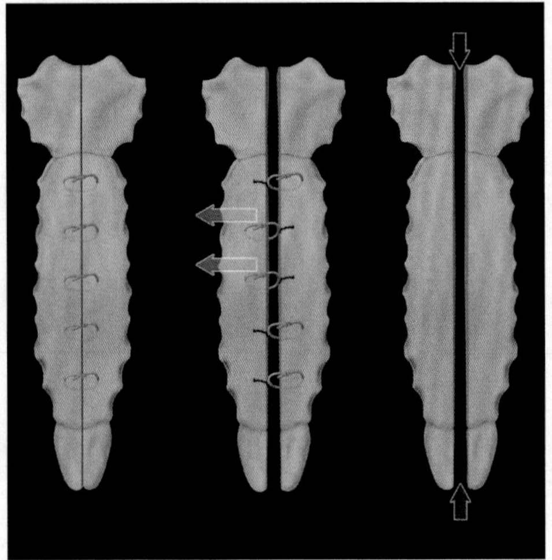

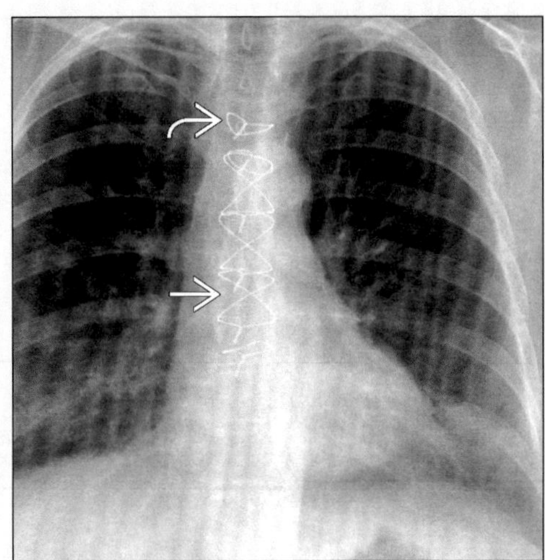

*(**Left**) AP chest radiograph of a patient status post CABG and mitral valve annuloplasty ➦ complicated by sternal dehiscence shows displaced sternotomy wires ➡, cardiomegaly, left lower lobe atelectasis, and a moderate left pleural effusion. (**Right**) Axial NECT of a patient with a sternal wound infection and mediastinitis following CABG shows diastatic osteotomy fragments ➡ and inflammatory soft tissue ⇨ infiltrating the tissue planes of the mediastinum and sternum.*

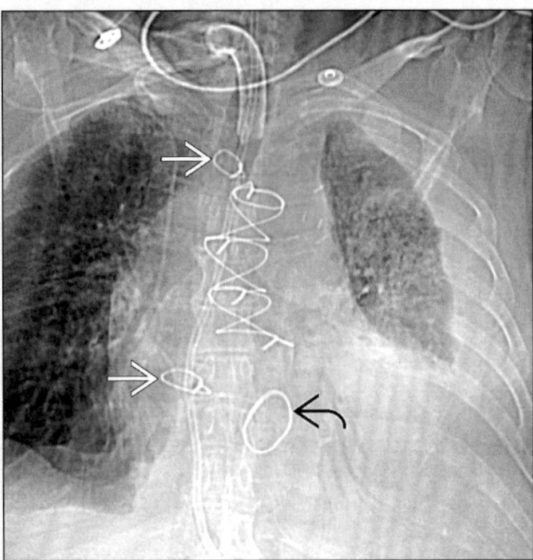

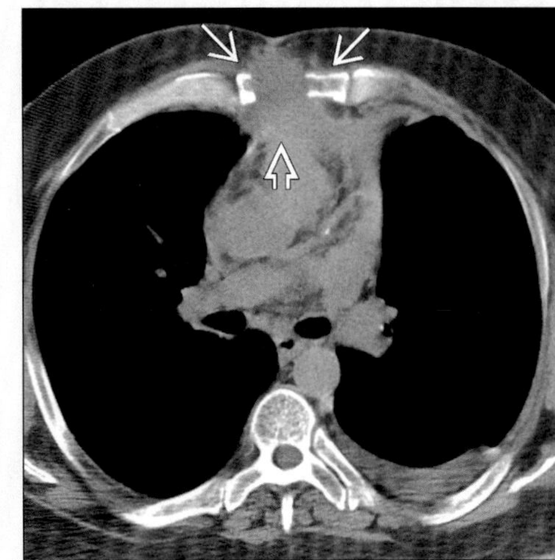

STERNOTOMY

TERMINOLOGY

Abbreviations

- **Median sternotomy (MS)**
- **Clamshell sternotomy (CS)**

Synonyms

- CS: **Transverse sternotomy**, cross-bow incision

Definitions

- MS: **Vertical incision** through manubrium & sternum
  - Access to heart & anterior mediastinum
    - Limited access to hila, lungs, pleura
  - Indications
    - Ascending aortic aneurysm or dissection
    - Coronary artery bypass graft (CABG)
    - Cardiac valve repair or replacement
    - Repair of congenital heart disease
    - Orthotopic heart transplant
    - Placement of cardiac support devices
      - Ventricular assist device
      - Extracorporeal membrane oxygenation
    - Chest trauma exploration
    - Pulmonary embolectomy
    - Resection of anterior mediastinal mass
    - Pericardial stripping
    - Double lung transplant in some cases
  - Closure with cerclage or "figure 8" steel sutures
    - 2-3 wires in manubrium, 4-5 in sternum body
    - Heals quickly with stable closure & minimal pain
- CS: **Broad transverse incision** across sternum & 4th anterior intercostal spaces
  - Excellent access to heart & both hemithoraces
    - Disrupts sternal pericardial attachments
      - Pleural spaces may communicate anteriorly
      - Chest tube may cross midline anteriorly
    - Indications
      - Double lung or heart-lung transplantation
      - Resection of large mediastinal or cardiac mass
      - Resection of bilateral lung metastases (rare)
  - Closure with steel "figure 8" sternal sutures
    - Extensive disruption of chest wall musculature
    - Increased risk of sternal complications
    - Extended painful recovery

IMAGING

General Features

- Best diagnostic clue
  - **MS: Midline sternotomy wires**
  - **CS: "Figure 8" or lower sternal cerclage wires**

Radiographic Findings

- Radiography
  - MS: Midline sternotomy wires are vertically aligned
    - Determination of type of surgery, i.e., cardiac
    - Assessment of support devices & surgical complications
    - Displaced sternal wires suggest dehiscence
    - Absent or missing wires suggest debridement
  - CS: "Figure 8" steel wires over inferior sternum
    - Determination of type of surgery, i.e., double lung transplant
    - Exclusion of sternal instability or pseudoarthrosis

CT Findings

- NECT
  - MS wires should be intact & vertically aligned
    - Sternal osteotomy fragments should be fused
      - Exclusion of diastasis, "over-ride," pseudoarthrosis
      - Exclusion of parasternal or mediastinal abscess

Imaging Recommendations

- Best imaging tool
  - CT is optimal imaging modality for evaluating complications of thoracic surgery
- Protocol advice
  - Unenhanced chest CT for assessment of osteotomy & soft tissues
  - CECT may improve detection of mediastinal abscess

CLINICAL ISSUES

Presentation

- Most common signs/symptoms
  - **Sternal infection, dehiscence, nonunion**
    - Pain ± fever, incisional drainage, crepitus
    - Osteomyelitis: Bone destruction
- Other signs/symptoms
  - Pleural & pericardial effusion, hemothorax, fibrothorax, mediastinitis

Natural History & Prognosis

- Most patients do well without complications or need for intervention

Treatment

- **Sternal infection**
  - Conservative treatment: **Antibiotics**
  - **Surgical debridement** in some cases
    - Removal of sternal wires
  - **Sternectomy in refractory cases**

DIAGNOSTIC CHECKLIST

Consider

- Evaluation of sternotomy for integrity of sternal wires & sternal fusion
- Identification of surgical indication, i.e., CABG, valve repair, tumor recurrence
- Evaluation of surgical complications & underlying disease

Image Interpretation Pearls

- Sternotomy wires should be aligned
- Evaluation for appropriate positioning of support devices

SELECTED REFERENCES

1. Losanoff JE et al: Primary closure of median sternotomy: techniques and principles. Cardiovasc Surg. 10(2):102-10, 2002
2. Macchiarini P et al: Clamshell or sternotomy for double lung or heart-lung transplantation? Eur J Cardiothorac Surg. 15(3):333-9, 1999
3. Bains MS et al: The clamshell incision: an improved approach to bilateral pulmonary and mediastinal tumor. Ann Thorac Surg. 58(1):30-2; discussion 33, 1994

*(**Left**) PA chest radiograph of a patient status post sternotomy shows multiple fractured slightly displaced sternal wires → reflecting chronic nonunion and instability of the osteotomy fragments. A fractured wire fragment ➡ has migrated into the left pectoral muscle. (**Right**) Coronal NECT MIP image of the same patient shows a smoothly marginated diastasis of the sternal fragments → and fractured and displaced sternal wires ⇨ reflecting chronic nonunion and sternal instability.*

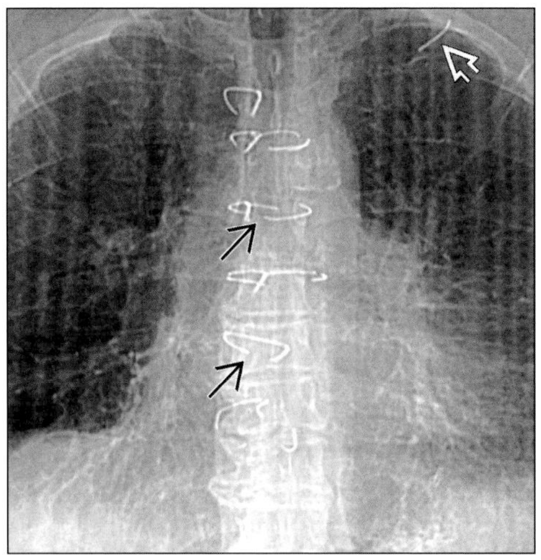

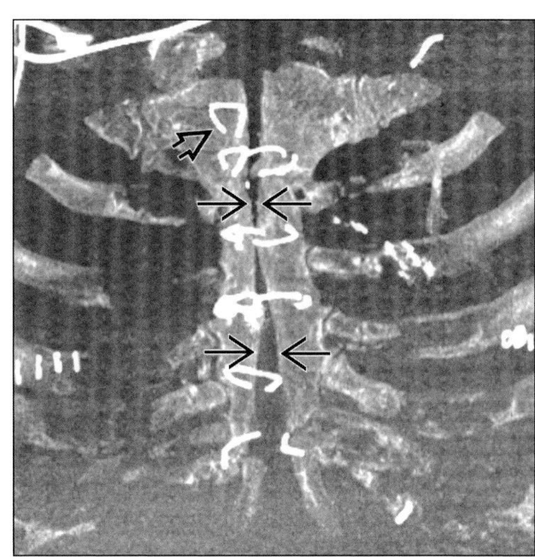

*(**Left**) AP chest radiograph of a patient with heart failure shows MS for placement of a left ventricular assist device → as a bridge to heart transplantation. An implantable cardiac defibrillator (ICD) ➡ is also present. (**Right**) PA chest radiograph of the same patient after redo MS and heart transplantation shows "figure 8" sternotomy wires →. The severed ICD lead ➡ was endothelialized in the vein and could not be removed, which provides a clue to the prior heart transplantation.*

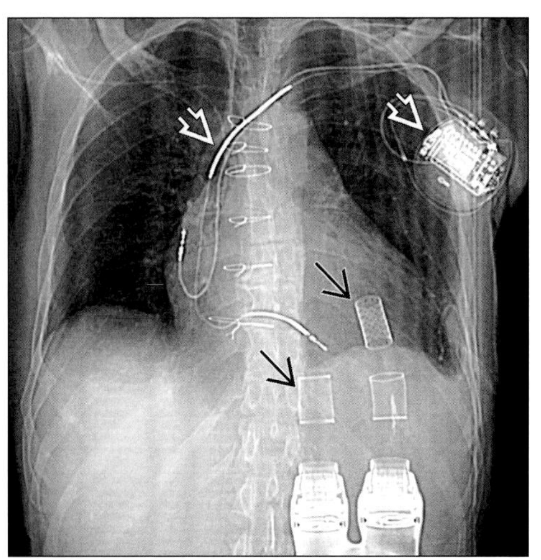

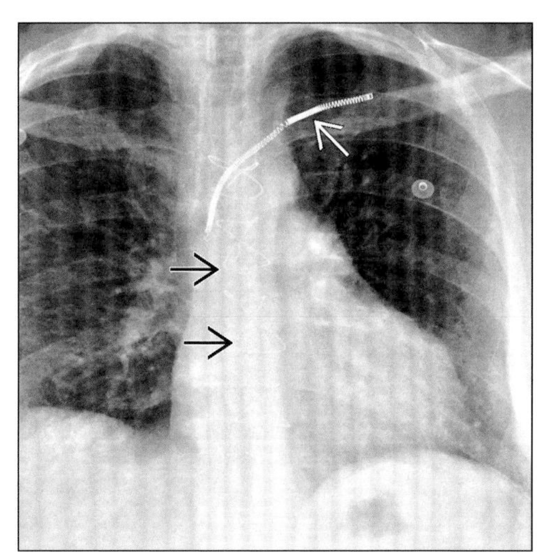

*(**Left**) PA chest radiograph of a young adult with prior surgical repair of congenital heart disease and ICD placement shows tiny pediatric sternotomy wires → that reflect sternotomy in early childhood and provide a clue to the history of congenital heart disease. (**Right**) AP chest radiograph shows a 65-year-old man who underwent left pneumonectomy via MS to resect a large central lung cancer with cardiac invasion. MS may be used to access the heart and hemithoraces in selected cases.*

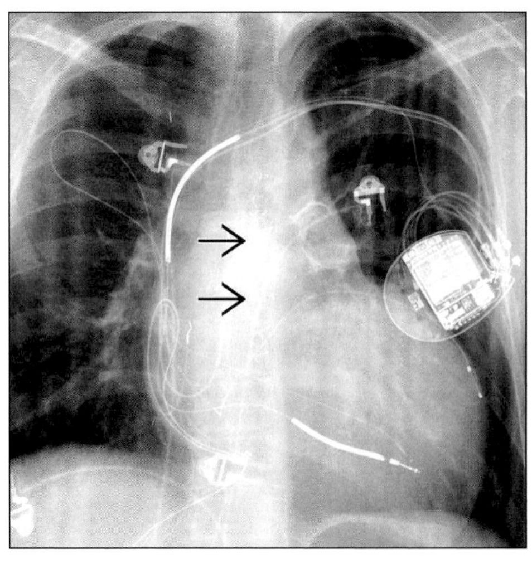

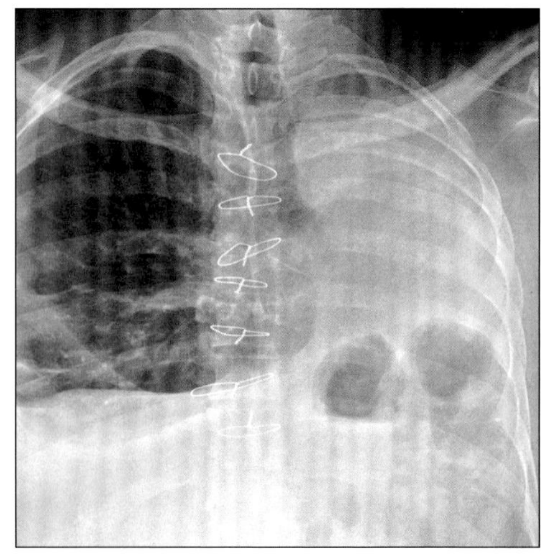

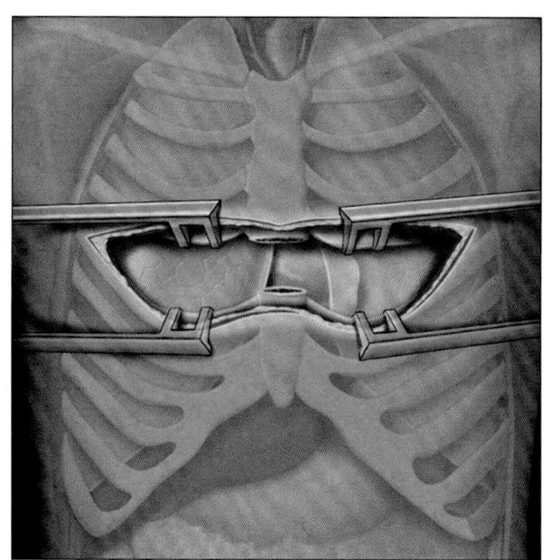

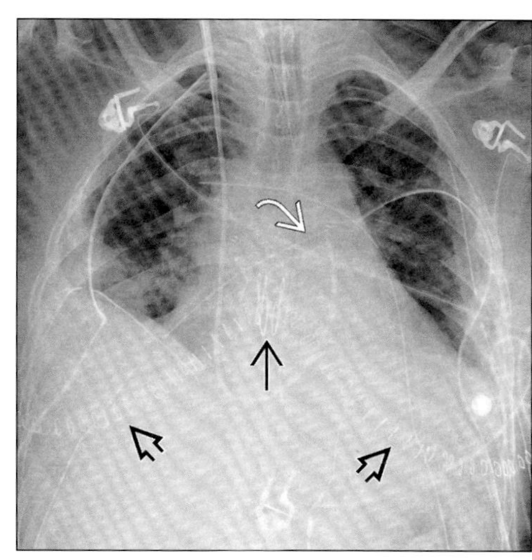

(Left) Graphic shows the clamshell sternotomy (CS), a transverse incision of the sternum that extends into both 4th intercostal spaces and allows the chest to be opened like a "clam" to access the heart and the hemithoraces. **(Right)** AP chest radiograph of a patient status post double lung transplantation via CS shows "figure 8" sternotomy wires → and skin staples ⇨ along the chest wall incision. A right chest tube ➔ crosses the midline as the pleural spaces now communicate anteriorly.

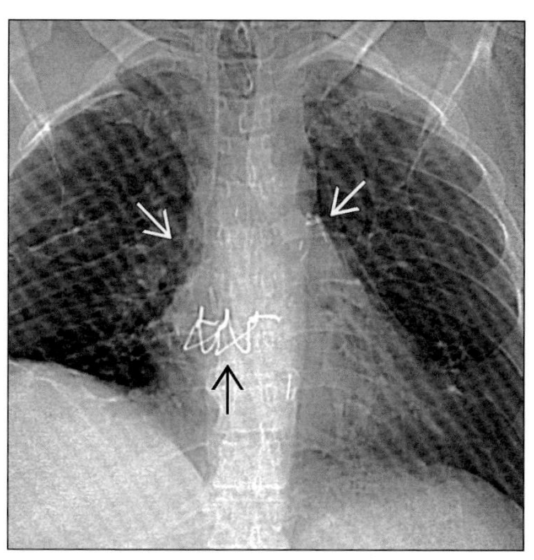

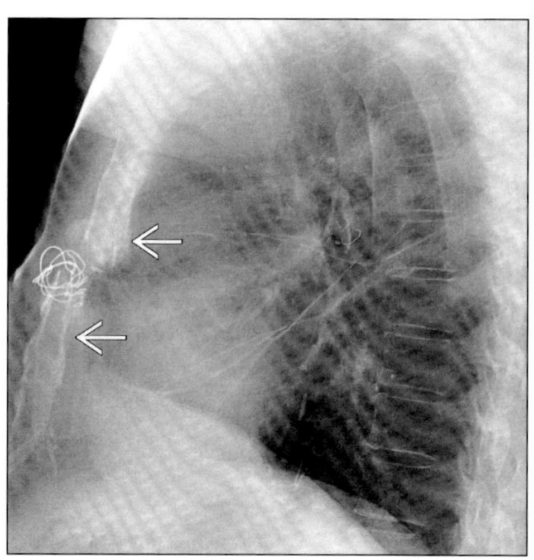

(Left) AP chest radiograph of a patient 1-year status post clamshell sternotomy for double lung transplantation shows "figure 8" cerclage wires → that secure the lower sternal incision. Bilateral hilar clips ➔ define the location of the bronchial anastomoses. **(Right)** Lateral chest radiograph of the same patient shows displaced sternal osteotomy fragments ➔ secondary to sternal nonunion and instability. Sternal complications may be difficult to detect on frontal radiography.

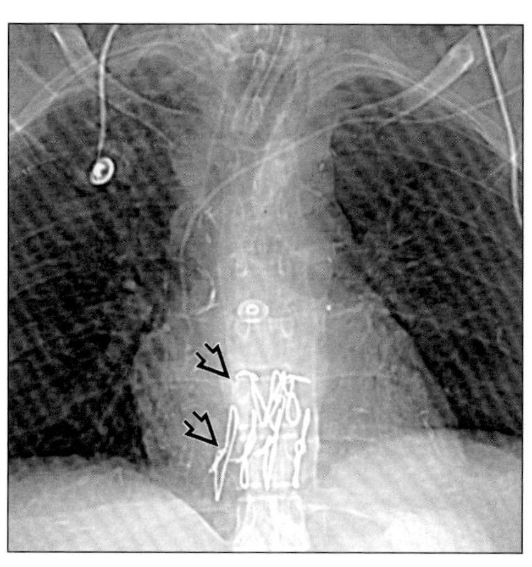

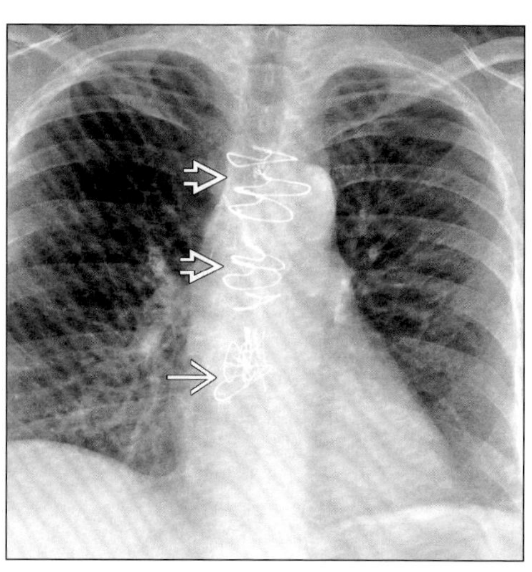

(Left) AP chest radiograph of a patient with a redo CS for double lung transplantation shows 2 sets of clamshell sternotomy wires ⇨. The initial lung transplant was performed for cystic fibrosis and repeated 5 years later for chronic rejection. **(Right)** PA chest radiograph of a patient that initially underwent MS ➔ for CABG and subsequently underwent CS ➔ and heart-lung transplantation for pulmonary hypertension. The 2 sternotomy approaches reflect sequential surgical procedures.

Key Facts

Terminology

- Treatment of end-stage congestive heart failure

Imaging

- Identification of orthotopic versus heterotopic cardiac transplant
  - Orthotopic heart transplant most common
- Cardiac MR is best imaging modality to identify transplant rejection, LV & RV failure
- Coronary CTA & IVUS are best modalities to directly visualize accelerated coronary atherosclerosis
- CTA for identification of coronary wall thickening & intimal hyperplasia characteristic of cardiac allograft vasculopathy (CAV)
- MR: Delayed hyperenhancement in myocardial necrosis (rejection) or subendocardial infarction (vasculopathy)
- Echocardiography: Monitoring of cardiac function

Top Differential Diagnoses

- Infection
- Acute allograft rejection
- Cardiac allograft vasculopathy (CAV)
- Neoplastic disease

Clinical Issues

- > 5,000 heart transplants/year performed worldwide
- Acute rejection (12%) & infection (33%) are leading causes of death in 1st year after surgery

Diagnostic Checklist

- Familiarization with imaging features of orthotopic versus heterotopic heart transplants
- Orthotopic transplantation shows enlarged atria due to anastomosis of donor heart with recipient's atria
- Imaging assessment of complications associated with cardiac transplantation

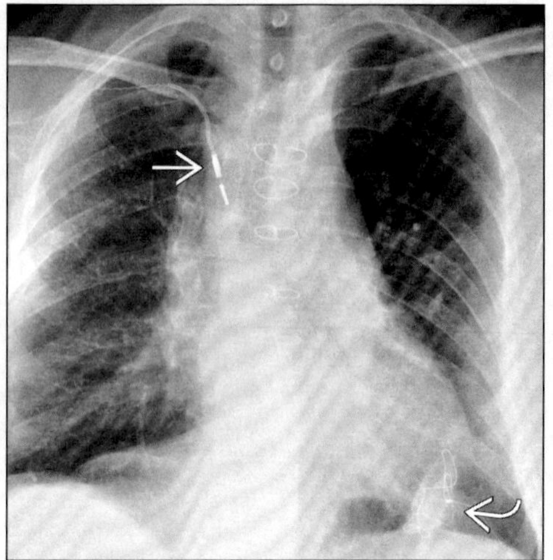
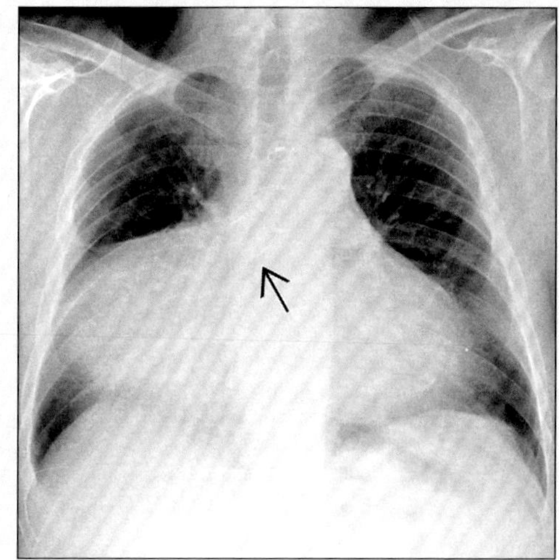

(Left) *PA chest radiograph shows a retained cardiac pacing wire ➔ in the superior vena cava and a left ventricular pacing device ➔ and sternotomy wires, clues to the history of prior orthotopic heart transplant.* ***(Right)*** *PA chest radiograph of a patient who had a heterotopic heart transplant shows abnormal contour of the right heart border and synthetic material ➔ in the pulmonary artery conduit. Heterotopic heart transplants are rare and used for recipients with pulmonary artery hypertension.*

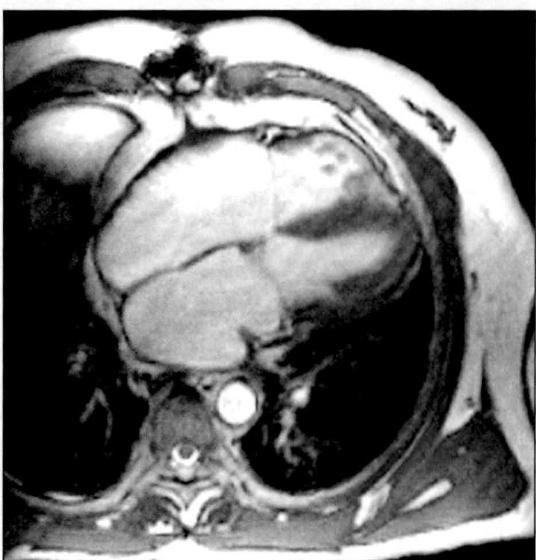
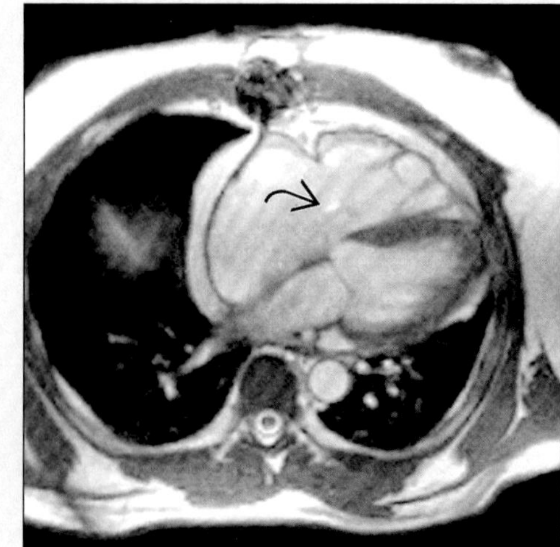

(Left) *4 chamber view cine cardiac MR of a patient with heart transplant rejection and failing right ventricular function shows an asymmetrically dilated right atrium and tricuspid regurgitation.* ***(Right)*** *4 chamber view cine cardiac MR of the same patient shows tricuspid regurgitation ➔. Rejection occurs in 30% of transplant recipients in the 1st year, usually between 2 weeks and 3 months after transplantation.*

CARDIAC TRANSPLANTATION

TERMINOLOGY

Definitions

- Most effective therapy for treatment of end-stage congestive heart failure
- Most often performed for nonischemic cardiomyopathy, followed by ischemic cardiomyopathy
- Most common complications of cardiac transplantation
  - Infection
  - Acute allograft rejection
  - Cardiac allograft vasculopathy (CAV)
  - Post-transplantation lymphoproliferative disease

IMAGING

General Features

- Best diagnostic clue
  - Cardiac allograft can be placed in orthotopic or heterotopic position
  - **Orthotopic heart transplant** is most common procedure
    - Recipient's heart removed through median sternotomy
    - Donor heart joined to recipient's atria, aorta, & pulmonary artery
  - **Heterotopic heart transplant** is rarely performed
    - Used for patients with severe pulmonary arterial hypertension
    - Used when donor heart is too small for recipient

Imaging Recommendations

- Best imaging tool
  - Cardiac MR is best imaging modality to identify transplant rejection, LV & RV failure
  - Coronary CTA & IVUS are best modalities to directly visualize accelerated coronary atherosclerosis
  - Serial echocardiograms are used to assess left & right ventricular function
  - Increased cardiac uptake on Gallium-67 scintigraphy in patients with moderate to severe transplant rejection
- Protocol advice
  - Monitoring allograft systolic function is important in suspected or known rejection
  - Delayed enhancement & T2WI should be included in cardiac MR protocol
  - Renal insufficiency is common in these patients; iodinated contrast & gadolinium should be used judiciously & with precautions
  - **Heart rate control may be challenging when performing coronary CTA**

Radiographic Findings

- Immediate postoperative findings
  - Cardiac enlargement from pericardial effusion
  - Pneumomediastinum, pneumopericardium
  - Mediastinal fluid collections
  - Pleural effusion, pneumothorax
  - Subcutaneous gas
- **Double right atrium contour** (overlap of donor & recipient right atria in orthotopic heart transplant)
- Residual cardiac pacer wire fragments in thoracic veins
- Sternotomy wires

CT Findings

- Cardiac gated CTA
  - Evaluation of coronary arteries for thickening & intimal hyperplasia characteristic of CAV
  - 64-slice MDCT provides moderate to good test characteristics for detection of CAV when compared to IVUS as reference standard
- Evaluation of aortic & pulmonary artery anastomoses
- High & redundant pulmonary trunk
- **Space between SVC & ascending aorta; increased space between aorta & pulmonary trunk**
- Atrial waist due to anastomosis of right & left donor & recipient atria
- Vertical atrioventricular groove

MR Findings

- Hyperenhancement in delayed images
  - **Myocardial necrosis indicating rejection in early postoperative period**
  - **Subendocardial enhancement indicating CAV in late postoperative period**
- T2WI can demonstrate T2 prolongation in myocardium consistent with myocardial edema
- **Abnormal T2 prolongation** is strong predictor of biopsy-defined rejection when clinically suspected
- **Spatial resolution** allows accurate measurement of ejection fractions
- Evaluation of quantitative changes in myocardial mass

Ultrasonographic Findings

- Echocardiography is primary noninvasive modality for monitoring cardiac function
- Pericardial effusion occurs frequently
- Myocardial edema may manifest as relative **increase in wall thickness**

Nuclear Medicine Findings

- Technetium-labeled agents for diagnosis of CAV
  - Sensitivity of 86%, specificity of 80%
- **Dobutamine stress test may be advantageous given inotropic response**
- Normal dobutamine stress myocardial perfusion imaging study associated with 96-98% negative predictive value for major adverse cardiac events at 2 years

DIFFERENTIAL DIAGNOSIS

Infection

- 1st month of transplantation: *Pseudomonas aeruginosa*, *Staphylococcus aureus*, *Enterococci*, & *Enterobacteriaceae*
- Later infections are commonly caused by viruses (CMV) & opportunistic fungi (*Pneumocystis*, *Candida*, *Aspergillus*)
- Aspergillus infection: Isolated pulmonary nodular disease, upper lobe predilection, cavitation
- Mediastinitis: Mediastinal fluid collections ± air, focal contrast enhancement

Acute Allograft Rejection

- T-cell mediated inflammatory response causing myocardial edema & cellular damage
- Symptoms related to LV dysfunction: Dyspnea, paroxysmal nocturnal dyspnea, orthopnea, palpitations, syncope

CARDIAC TRANSPLANTATION

- Endomyocardial biopsy may be used for surveillance or diagnosis
- Rejection occurs in 30% of transplant recipients in 1st year, usually between 2 weeks & 3 months after transplantation
- Grading system based on biopsy findings

Cardiac Allograft Vasculopathy (CAV)

- Concentric intimal hyperplasia (vs. eccentric disease in traditional coronary artery disease)
- Diffuse process; starts with small distal vessels & spreads to all coronary arteries
- Incidence of 8% at 1 year, 30% at 5 years, > 50% at 10 years
- High mortality rate: 10% of patients die within 12 months of diagnosis of CAV
- Increased risk in recipients of male allografts; risk increases with donor age
- Exacerbation of vascular disease with hyperlipidemia, hypertension, diabetes, steroid use
- Diagnosis difficult because transplanted hearts are denervated
  - Affected patients rarely present with chest pain
  - Blunted heart rate response to exercise decreases sensitivity of stress testing
- Due to lack of symptoms, surveillance coronary artery evaluation performed annually (typically cardiac catheterization with IVUS)

Neoplastic Disease

- Incidence of any malignancy is 35% by 10 years
- Most common neoplasms
  - Skin cancer most common: Squamous cell carcinoma, basal cell carcinoma, melanoma
  - Lymphoproliferative malignancies
  - Kaposi sarcoma
  - In situ carcinomas of uterine cervix
  - Anogenital cancers

PATHOLOGY

General Features

- Etiology
  - Disease processes that require transplantation
    - Nonischemic cardiomyopathy: 46%
    - Ischemic cardiomyopathy: 42%
    - Valvular disease: 3%
    - Adult congenital heart disease: 2%
    - Miscellaneous: 7%

CLINICAL ISSUES

Presentation

- Most common signs/symptoms
  - Early disease is defined as occurring < 1 year after surgery
    - Graft failure & infectious disease are leading causes of death in 1st year after surgery
    - Infectious disease accounts for almost 33% of deaths in 1st year
    - Acute rejection accounts for 12% of deaths
  - Major complications in late postoperative stage: Coronary artery disease & neoplastic disease

Demographics

- Epidemiology
  - Over 5,000 cardiac transplants performed annually worldwide
    - 1st successful heart transplant performed in 1967
  - Over 89,000 cardiac transplants reported worldwide

Natural History & Prognosis

- 1-year survival of heart transplant recipients > 80%
- 10-year survival rate approaches 50%
- Median survival (time at which 50% of recipients remain alive) for combined group of adult & pediatric heart recipients is currently 10 years
- Improvement in early survival statistics
  - Establishment of recipient selection criteria
  - Use of endomyocardial biopsy to diagnose rejection
  - Improvements in immunosuppression techniques

Treatment

- Retransplantation is required in 2% of cases
- Post-transplant immunosuppression often includes tacrolimus, mycophenolate mofetil, & prednisone

DIAGNOSTIC CHECKLIST

Consider

- Familiarization with features of orthotopic versus heterotopic transplantation
- Orthotopic transplantation shows enlarged atria due to anastomosis of donor heart with recipient's atria
- Imaging assessment of complications
  - Impaired ventricular function: Echocardiography, cardiac MR, cardiac-gated CT
  - Atherosclerotic plaque & coronary stenosis: Coronary angiography, coronary CTA, IVUS
  - Rejection: Cardiac MR; hyperenhancement in delayed images & hyperintensity on T2WI suggest myocardial necrosis/edema
  - Chest radiography & CT: Assessment of lung & mediastinal infection & tumors

SELECTED REFERENCES

1. Stehlik J et al: The Registry of the International Society for Heart and Lung Transplantation: twenty-seventh official adult heart transplant report--2010. J Heart Lung Transplant. 29(10):1089-103, 2010
2. Estep JD et al: The role of multimodality cardiac imaging in the transplanted heart. JACC Cardiovasc Imaging. 2(9):1126-40, 2009
3. Bogot NR et al: Cardiac CT of the transplanted heart: indications, technique, appearance, and complications. Radiographics. 27(5):1297-309, 2007
4. Gregory SA et al: Comparison of sixty-four-slice multidetector computed tomographic coronary angiography to coronary angiography with intravascular ultrasound for the detection of transplant vasculopathy. Am J Cardiol. 98(7):877-84, 2006

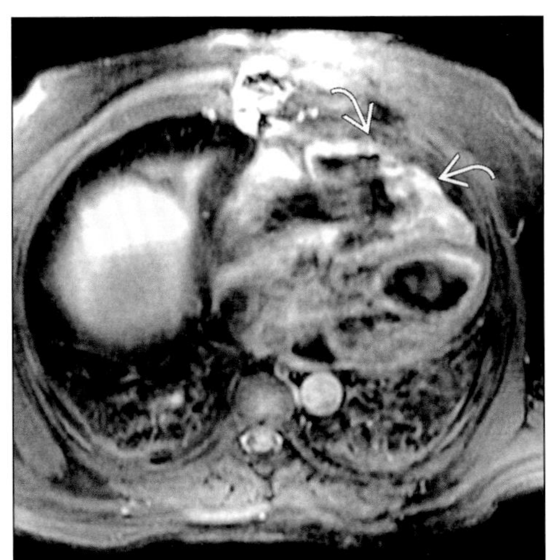

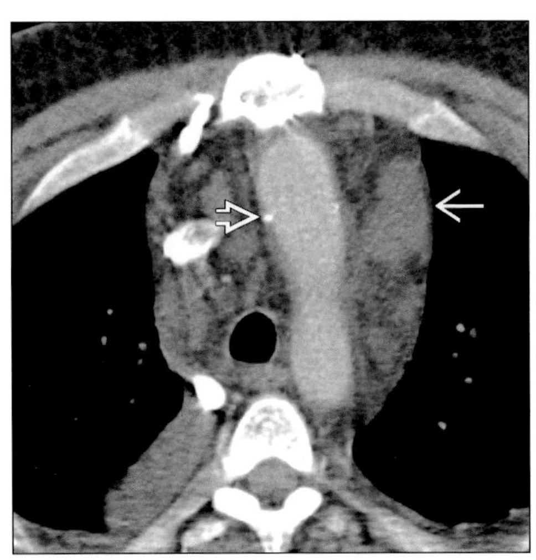

(Left) *Four chamber T2WI FS MR shows diffuse hyperintensity of the right ventricular free wall ➔, suspicious for mural edema and transplant rejection.* **(Right)** *Axial CECT of a patient with lymphoma status post heart transplant shows bulky mediastinal lymphadenopathy ➔. Suture material ➔ at the aortic anastomosis and sternotomy wires are clues to the history of prior heart transplant when clinical information is not provided.*

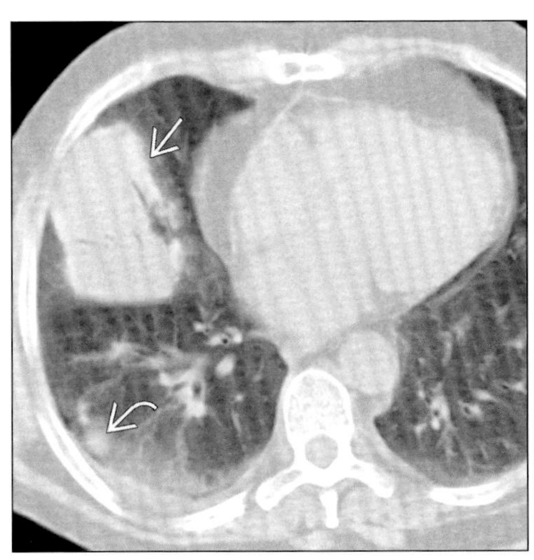

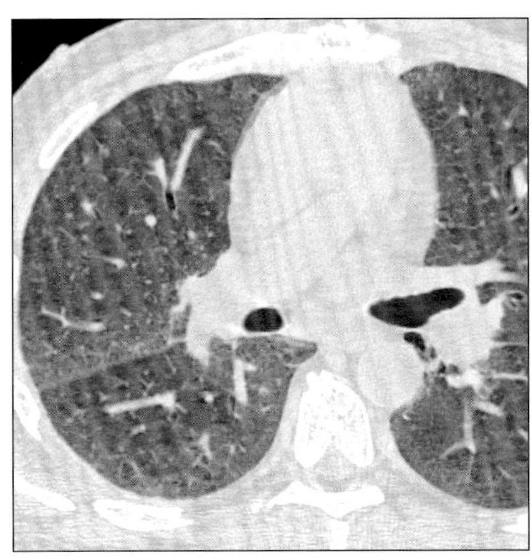

(Left) *Axial NECT of a heart transplant recipient with Cytomegalovirus (CMV) pneumonia shows middle lobe consolidation ➔ and patchy right lower lobe ground-glass opacities ➔. CMV infection is the most important infectious cause of morbidity and mortality in heart transplant recipients.* **(Right)** *Axial NECT of a heart transplant recipient with Pneumocystis pneumonia shows diffuse bilateral patchy ground-glass opacities. Pneumocystis pneumonia may superinfect patients with CMV pneumonia.*

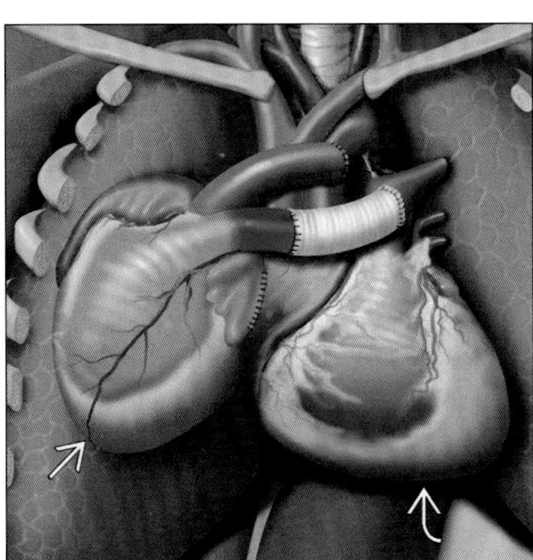

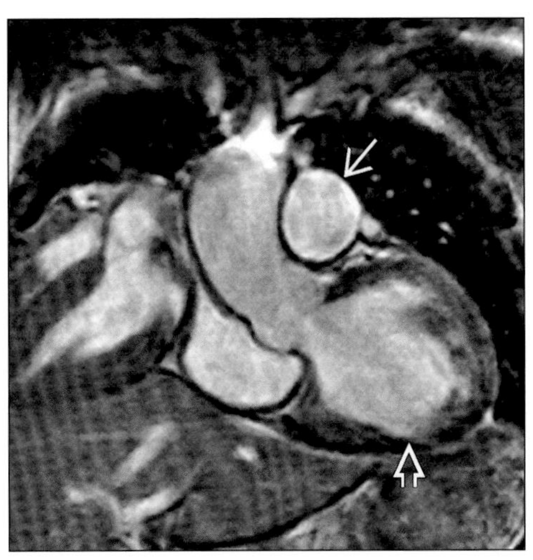

(Left) *Graphic shows heterotopic heart transplant. The donor heart ➔ supports the cardiac output while the native heart ➔ supports the pulmonary circulation in patients with pulmonary arterial hypertension. The left atria are anastomosed, and the donor superior vena cava receives blood from an anastomosis with the native right atrium (not shown).* **(Right)** *Coronal cardiac cine MR shows a heterotopic heart transplant. The native pulmonary artery ➔ and left ventricle ➔ are enlarged.*

LUNG TRANSPLANTATION

Key Facts

Terminology

- Post-transplant lymphoproliferative disorder (PTLD)
- Surgical replacement of 1 or both lungs with those from a donor, usually cadaveric

Imaging

- Radiography
  - Thoracotomy (single) or sternotomy (double)
  - Surgical clips at hilum or bilateral hila
  - Residual disease in native lung
  - Asymmetric lungs
- Immediate post-transplant complications (< 1 month)
  - Bronchial dehiscence
  - Pneumothorax
  - Pleural effusion
  - Hyperacute rejection
  - Acute rejection
  - Reimplantation response
  - Infection
- Late post-transplant complications (> 1 month)
  - Infection
  - Bronchial stenosis & bronchomalacia
  - Vascular anastomotic complication
  - Chronic rejection
  - PTLD
  - Malignancy

Diagnostic Checklist

- Consider infection & acute rejection with new lung abnormalities on imaging
- Consider reimplantation response with early radiographic abnormalities in allograft
- Consider bronchial anastomotic complication with persistent pneumothorax or pneumomediastinum
- PTLD usually occurs within first 2 years
- Expiratory CT useful for assessing air trapping associated with chronic rejection
- Lung cancer in native lung; smoking-related disease

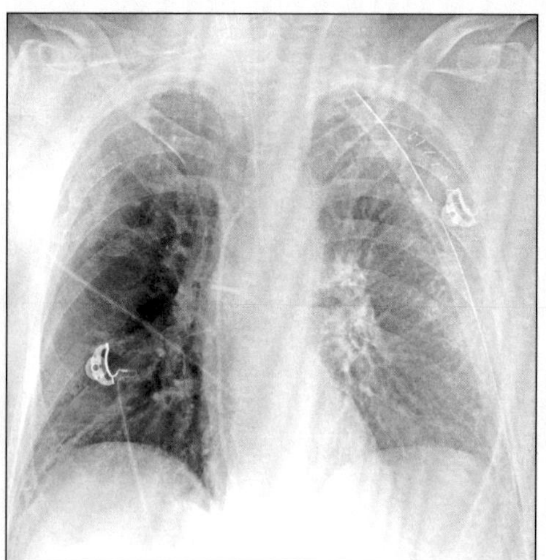

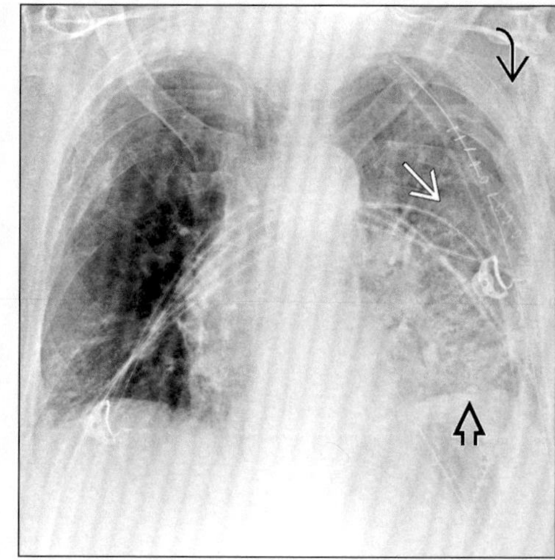

(Left) *AP chest radiograph immediately following a left lung transplant shows normal aeration of the graft. The native right lung is hyperlucent from emphysema.* ***(Right)*** *AP chest radiograph of the same patient 24 hours after transplantation shows fine linear opacities ➡ representing interstitial edema from reimplantation response, left basilar atelectasis ⇨, and mild chest wall subcutaneous gas ↗. The reimplantation response usually peaks at around 4 days and slowly resolves thereafter.*

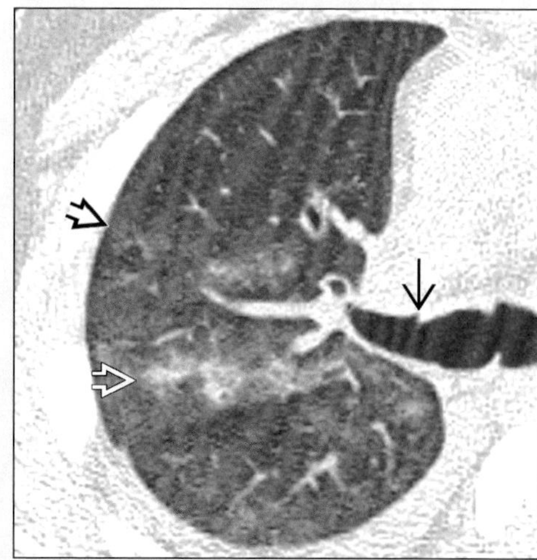

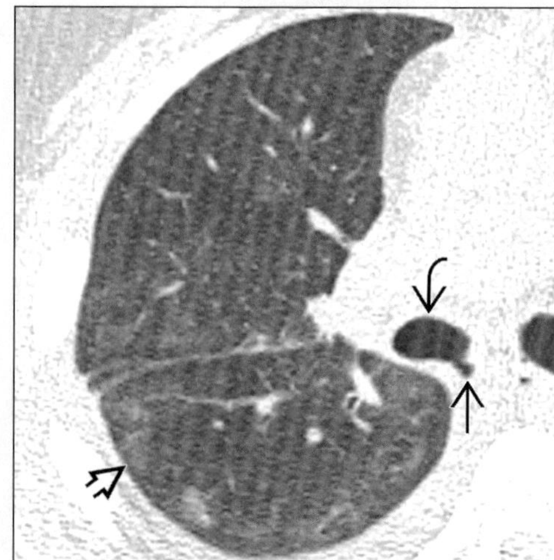

(Left) *Axial HRCT shows patchy consolidation ➡ and ground-glass opacity ⇨ in the right lung allograft resulting from acute rejection. Note the normal appearance of the telescoped bronchial anastomosis →.* ***(Right)*** *Axial HRCT shows a focal extraluminal mediastinal gas collection → that directly communicates with the right mainstem bronchus ↗, representing focal bronchial dehiscence from ischemic necrosis. Patchy ground-glass opacity ⇨ is from acute rejection.*

LUNG TRANSPLANTATION

TERMINOLOGY

Synonyms

- Lung allograft

Definitions

- Surgical replacement of 1 or both lungs with those from a donor, usually cadaveric

IMAGING

General Features

- Best diagnostic clue
  - Thoracotomy (single) or transverse sternotomy (double)
  - Surgical clips at hilum or bilateral hila
  - Residual disease in native lung; asymmetric lung parenchyma
- Location
  - Lungs
  - 1 or both lungs

Radiographic Findings

- Radiography
  - **Single lung transplant**
    - Unilateral postsurgical changes
    - Surgical clips at ipsilateral hilum
    - Asymmetric lung parenchyma
      - Abnormal lung parenchyma in native lung
  - **Double lung transplant**
    - Bilateral postsurgical changes
    - Surgical clips at bilateral hila
    - Symmetric-appearing lung parenchyma
  - Bronchial dehiscence
    - Extensive pneumomediastinum
    - Pneumothorax despite adequate pleural drainage
- Radiography of post-transplantation complications
  - **Immediate post transplant (< 1 month)**
    - Pneumothorax
      - Usually small with adequate pleural drainage
      - Enlargement or persistence suggests air leak
    - Pleural effusion
      - Common in first 2 weeks after transplant
      - Persistent effusion should be evaluated
    - Hyperacute rejection
      - Immediate acute opacification of allograft
    - Acute rejection
      - Usually within first 3 months after transplant; typically within a few days
      - Perihilar hazy opacity, septal lines
      - Radiograph may be normal
    - Reimplantation response
      - Mimics interstitial edema
      - Usually develops within 24-48 hours after surgery; peaks at around 96 hours
      - Slow resolution
    - Infection
      - Bacterial, viral, fungal
      - Nosocomial infections most common
      - Focal/multifocal consolidation/nodules
  - **Late post transplant (> 1 month)**
    - Infection
      - Community-acquired pneumonia
      - Bacterial, fungal, viral pneumonia
      - Focal/multifocal consolidation/nodules
    - Bronchial stenosis
      - Segmental or lobar atelectasis
    - Chronic rejection
      - Invariably develops
      - Manifests as constrictive bronchiolitis
      - Radiographs are usually normal in early phase
      - Vascular attenuation reflects reflex vasoconstriction from regional hypoxia
      - Hyperinflation in advanced disease
    - Post-transplant lymphoproliferative disorder (PTLD)
      - Ranges from low-grade lymphoproliferative disorder to lymphoma
      - Much more common in donors seronegative for Epstein-Barr virus antibodies
      - Multiple lung nodules & lymphadenopathy most common findings
    - Malignancy
      - Growing lung nodule
      - Most commonly affects native lung

CT Findings

- NECT
  - Direct visualization of postsurgical changes
    - Evaluation of bronchial anastomoses
  - Direct visualization of pulmonary architecture
    - Evaluation of native lung & allograft
- CECT
  - Direct visualization of postsurgical changes
    - Evaluation of vascular anastomoses
- HRCT of post-transplantation complications
  - **Immediate post transplant (< 1 month)**
    - Bronchial dehiscence
      - Small air collection adjacent to anastomosis common immediately after transplant
      - Enlargement or persistence of air collection indicates dehiscence
    - Vascular anastomotic complications
      - < 5% of patients
      - Arterial anastomosis affected more commonly than venous
      - Stenosis or kink readily visualized on CECT
      - Hypoperfusion of affected lung
      - Diffuse edema with venous stenosis
    - Infection
      - Nodules, consolidations, ground-glass opacity
      - Isolated ground-glass opacity suggests pneumocystis pneumonia, less commonly CMV pneumonia
  - **Late post transplant (> 1 month)**
    - Infection
      - Bacterial, viral, fungal
      - Consolidation, nodules, ground-glass opacity
      - Nodule predominant favors fungi
      - Lobar consolidation favors bacteria
    - Bronchial stenosis & bronchomalacia
      - Stenosis in up to 10% of patients
      - May cause obstructive atelectasis or pneumonia
      - Bronchomalacia best evaluated on expiratory CT; > 50-70% luminal collapse
    - Acute rejection
      - Nonspecific imaging findings
      - Patchy ground-glass opacity & septal lines
    - Chronic rejection

- Mosaic attenuation
- Low attenuation persists/accentuated on expiratory CT; air trapping
- Bronchial dilatation & wall thickening
- PTLD
  - Lung nodules & lymphadenopathy most common
  - Septal lines, consolidation, endobronchial lesion, thymic enlargement
  - Pericardial or pleural disease less common

Imaging Recommendations

- Best imaging tool
  - Chest radiography for surveillance
  - HRCT for problem solving or suspected lung disease with normal radiographs
- Protocol advice
  - Expiratory HRCT for suspected or known constrictive bronchiolitis

DIFFERENTIAL DIAGNOSIS

Lung Metastases

- May mimic infection or PTLD

Lobar Atelectasis

- Secondary to bronchial stricture
- Bronchogenic neoplasm
- PTLD

Eventration of Diaphragm

- May mimic phrenic nerve injury

PATHOLOGY

Microscopic Features

- Acute rejection
  - Perivascular & interstitial mononuclear infiltrates
- Chronic rejection
  - Lymphocytic infiltration of airway wall
  - Intraluminal polyps of granulation tissue
  - Advanced disease with obliteration of airway lumen by fibrosis

CLINICAL ISSUES

Presentation

- Most common signs/symptoms
  - Acute rejection
    - Fever, dyspnea, graft dysfunction
  - Bronchiolitis obliterans syndrome
    - Progressive dyspnea, airflow obstruction
  - Infection
    - Fever, cough, leukocytosis
  - Drug toxicity
    - Fever, cough, leukocytosis
  - PTLD usually within first 2 years, median 6 months
    - Viral-like illness
    - Weight loss, fatigue, night sweats
    - Symptoms related to tumor mass effect
  - Lung cancer in native lung; patients with smoking-related lung disease or fibrosis
    - Weight loss, fatigue
    - Cough
    - Paraneoplastic syndromes
    - Symptoms related to tumor mass effect

Natural History & Prognosis

- Mean survival 1 year after transplant approximately 85%-90%
  - Early death from acute graft failure or infection
- 5 years after transplant approximately 50% of patients still alive
  - Late mortality commonly related to chronic rejection

Treatment

- Acute rejection
  - Corticosteroids
  - Immunosuppression management
- Chronic rejection
  - Retransplantation for select patients
- Infection
  - Broad-spectrum antimicrobials
- Bronchial anastomotic complications
  - Dilatation, stenting, surgical repair
- PTLD
  - Reduction in immunosuppression
  - Antiviral agents
- Lung carcinoma
  - Resection, stereotactic radiation therapy, ablation

DIAGNOSTIC CHECKLIST

Consider

- Opportunistic infections & acute rejection with any new lung abnormality on imaging
  - Nodules & consolidation favor infection
- Bronchial anastomotic complication with persistent pneumothorax or pneumomediastinum despite adequate pleural drainage

Image Interpretation Pearls

- Early radiographic abnormalities in allograft usually relate to reimplantation response
  - Failure to clear should suggest infection or rejection
- Typical appearance of telescoping bronchial anastomosis should not be confused with dehiscence
  - Small curvilinear air pocket
    - Superior, anterior, &/or inferior to anastomosis
- Expiratory CT useful for assessing air-trapping associated with chronic rejection

SELECTED REFERENCES

1. Ahmad S et al: Pulmonary complications of lung transplantation. Chest. 139(2):402-11, 2011
2. Borhani AA et al: Imaging of posttransplantation lymphoproliferative disorder after solid organ transplantation. Radiographics. 29(4):981-1000; discussion 1000-2, 2009
3. Hochhegger B et al: Computed tomography findings of postoperative complications in lung transplantation. J Bras Pneumol. 35(3):266-74, 2009
4. Ng YL et al: Imaging of lung transplantation: review. AJR Am J Roentgenol. 192(3 Suppl):S1-13, quiz S14-9, 2009

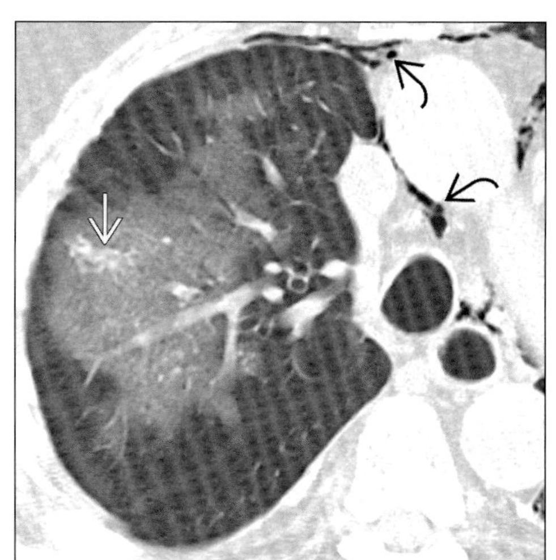
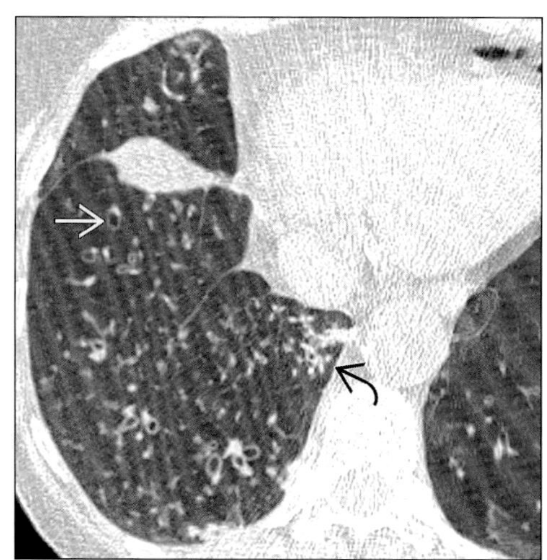

(Left) *Axial NECT shows a large area of ground-glass opacity containing a small focus of consolidation ➡ in the right lung allograft secondary to CMV pneumonia. Note extensive pneumomediastinum ↪ from a ruptured emphysematous bulla (not shown) in the native left lung.* ***(Right)*** *Axial HRCT shows numerous centrilobular nodules and tree-in-bud opacities ↪ in the right lung allograft secondary to airway aspergillosis. Note mild bronchial dilatation ➡, the sequela of chronic rejection.*

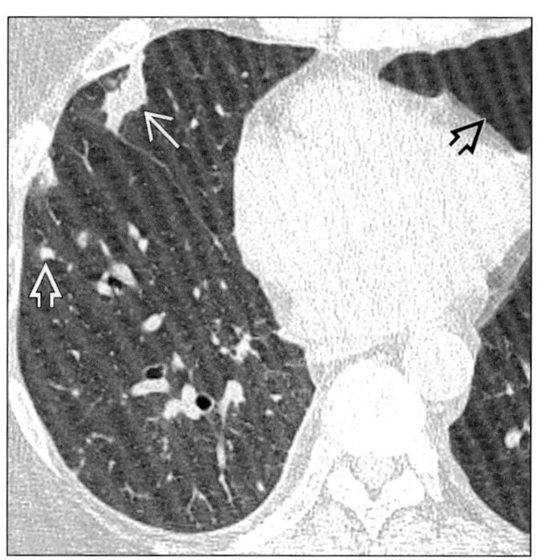
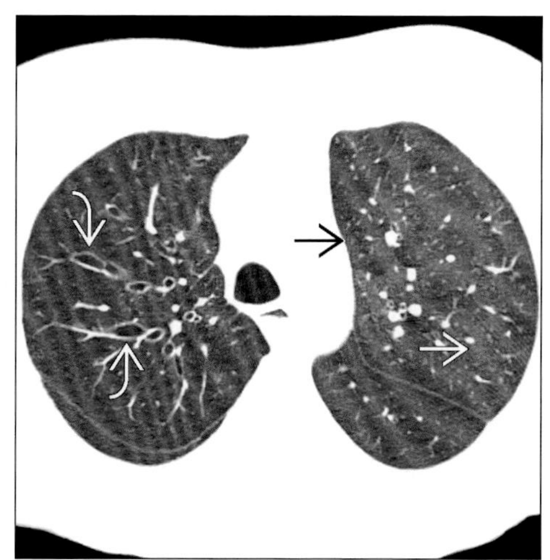

(Left) *Axial HRCT shows nodular foci of consolidation ➡ as well as smaller nodules ➡ in the right lung allograft secondary to histoplasmosis. Note severe emphysema ⇨ in the native left lung.* ***(Right)*** *Axial HRCT shows diffuse heterogeneous attenuation of the lungs from chronic rejection. Areas of apparent ground-glass opacity ➡ represent relatively spared lung, while low-attenuation areas → reflect air-trapping. Bronchiectasis ↪ commonly develops with chronic rejection.*

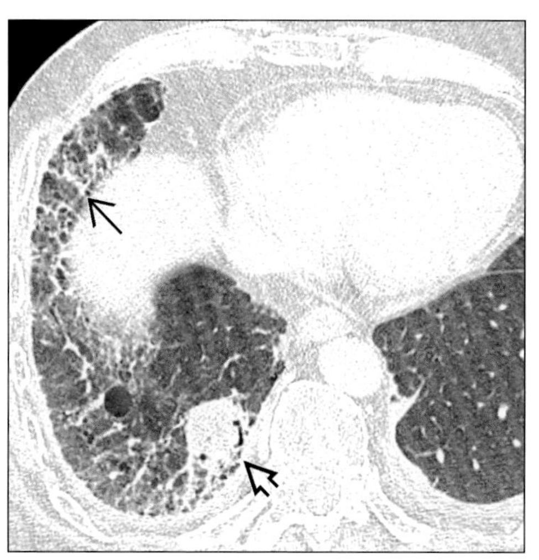
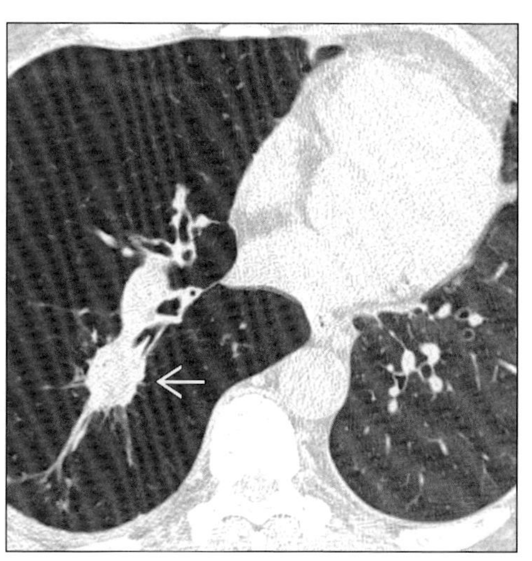

(Left) *Axial HRCT shows a round right lower lobe mass ⇨ with intrinsic air bronchograms in the fibrotic → native right lung. Biopsy showed PTLD, which can develop in the mediastinum, the native lung, or the allograft.* ***(Right)*** *Axial HRCT shows a spiculated right lower lobe mass ➡ in the emphysematous native lung. Patients with a history of tobacco abuse and emphysema are at increased risk of developing primary lung cancer in the native lung. Primary lung cancer is uncommon in the allograft.*

POST-TRANSPLANTATION AIRWAY STENOSIS

Key Facts

Terminology

- Acquired airway narrowing following lung transplantation
  - Most common at surgical anastomosis

Imaging

- Radiography
  - Post surgical changes of lung transplantation
  - Narrowing of bronchial air column
  - Post obstructive changes
- CT
  - Direct visualization & assessment of transplanted lung
  - Direct assessment of surgical site
  - Bronchial luminal narrowing; typically at site of surgical anastomosis
  - Calcification or fragmentation of bronchial cartilages
  - Lobar collapse
- Imaging recommendations
  - CT with multiplanar reformatted images is helpful for visualizing strictures or webs
  - CT is complementary to bronchoscopy; provides information on stenosis length & distal airway patency

Top Differential Diagnoses

- Airway malacia
- Telescoping bronchial anastomosis

Pathology

- Donor bronchus ischemia; suboptimal arterial supply

Clinical Issues

- Often asymptomatic
- 10% of lung transplant patients
- Treatment: Balloon dilatation, stent placement, endoscopic intervention

*(**Left**) Axial NECT of a patient with bilateral lung transplant shows marked narrowing ⇨ of the right mainstem bronchus at the anastomosis. (**Right**) Coronal NECT of the same patient shows web-like narrowing ⇨ of the right mainstem bronchus at the anastomosis, consistent with stenosis which was confirmed with bronchoscopy. Multiplanar reformatted CT is helpful for detection and characterization of post-transplantation bronchial stenosis.*

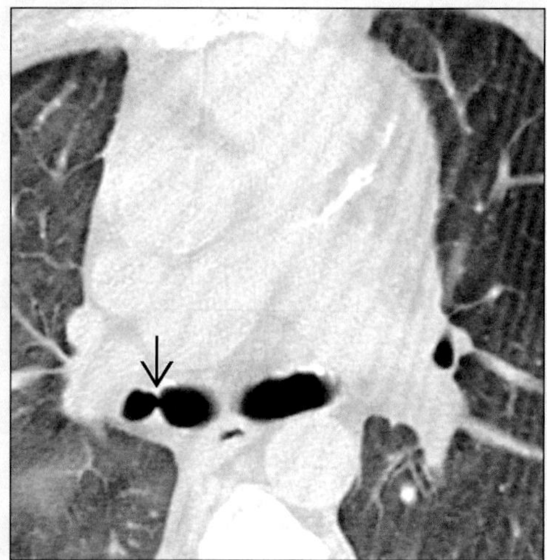

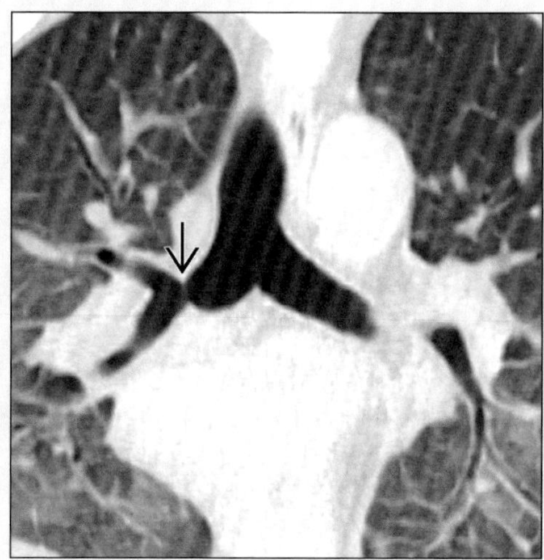

*(**Left**) Axial NECT of a patient with left mainstem bronchus stenosis post bilateral lung transplant shows a metal stent ➡ placed across the stenosis after multiple failed balloon dilatation procedures. (**Right**) Axial NECT of a patient post bilateral lung transplant shows the recipient right mainstem bronchus telescoped into the donor right bronchus at the anastomosis. This creates a flap ⇨ that can mimic focal stenosis. Note the characteristic curvilinear air density adjacent to the flap.*

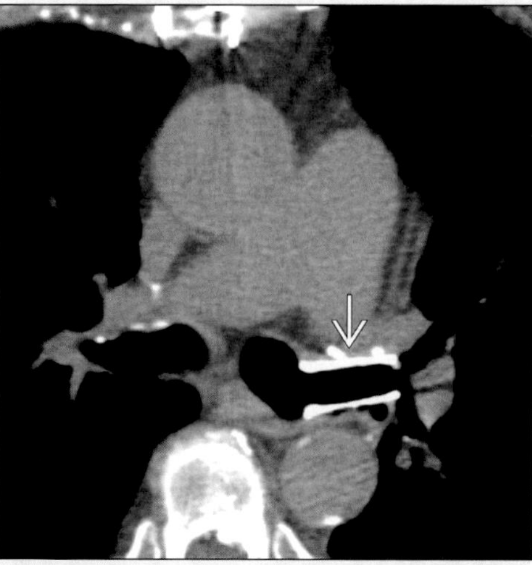

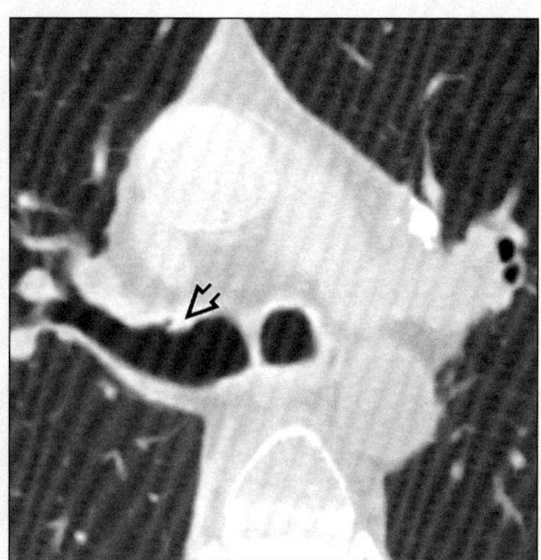

POST-TRANSPLANTATION AIRWAY STENOSIS

TERMINOLOGY

Definitions

- Acquired airway narrowing following lung transplantation

IMAGING

General Features

- Location
  - Most common at surgical anastomosis
  - Rarely segmental nonanastomotic bronchial stenosis distal to surgical anastomosis
    - Most commonly involves bronchus intermedius: Vanishing bronchus intermedius syndrome
- Size
  - Variable degree of airway stenosis
- Morphology
  - Localized airway luminal narrowing

Radiographic Findings

- Post surgical changes of lung transplantation
  - Single lung transplant
    - Surgical clips at hilum of transplanted lung
    - Ipsilateral chest wall post surgical changes
    - Asymmetric lung parenchyma
  - Double lung transplant
    - Surgical clips at bilateral hila
    - Clamshell sternotomy
- **Narrowing of bronchial air column**
- Post obstructive effects including atelectasis

CT Findings

- Direct visualization & assessment of transplanted lung
- Direct assessment of surgical site
  - Assessment of airway lumen at anastomosis
- Bronchial luminal narrowing
- Calcification or fragmentation of bronchial cartilages
- Lobar collapse

Imaging Recommendations

- Best imaging tool
  - CT assessment of extent of airway stenosis
  - CT with multiplanar reformatted images helpful for visualizing strictures or webs
  - CT complementary to bronchoscopy; provides information on stenosis length & distal airway patency

DIFFERENTIAL DIAGNOSIS

Airway Malacia

- Can occur in isolation or in association with airway stenosis
- > 50% narrowing of airway lumen on expiration

Telescoping Bronchial Anastomosis

- Invagination of smaller bronchus (donor or recipient) into larger bronchus during transplant
- Focal band-like constriction of bronchial lumen
- Small curvilinear air pocket often visible along superior, anterior, or inferior aspect of anastomosis

PATHOLOGY

General Features

- Etiology
  - Bronchial arteries are not reanastomosed during lung transplant
  - Suboptimal vascular supply leads to ischemia of donor bronchus & subsequent stricture &/or bronchomalacia

CLINICAL ISSUES

Presentation

- Most common signs/symptoms
  - **Asymptomatic**, incidental finding at surveillance bronchoscopy
  - Dyspnea
  - Cough
  - Wheezing
- Other signs/symptoms
  - Post obstructive pneumonia
  - Declining forced expiratory volume in 1 second (FEV1)

Demographics

- Epidemiology
  - **10%** of lung transplant recipients
  - Most frequent late airway complication of lung transplantation
  - Bilateral lung transplant
    - Tracheal anastomosis no longer used because of high airway complication rate (75%)
  - Risk factors
    - Long donor bronchial stump
    - Extended donor mechanical ventilation time
    - Pre- & post-transplant pulmonary infection

Natural History & Prognosis

- Occurs an average of 3 months post lung transplant

Treatment

- **Balloon dilatation**
  - Immediate improvement, but long-term success rate only approximately 50%
- **Stent placement**
  - Used after failure of balloon dilatation
  - Commonly complicated by granulation tissue formation
  - Improvement of FEV1
- **Endoscopic intervention**
  - Cryotherapy
  - Electrocautery
  - Laser therapy
  - Brachytherapy

SELECTED REFERENCES

1. Ng YL et al: Imaging of lung transplantation: review. AJR Am J Roentgenol. 192(3 Suppl):S1-13, quiz S14-9, 2009
2. Santacruz JF et al: Airway complications and management after lung transplantation: ischemia, dehiscence, and stenosis. Proc Am Thorac Soc. 6(1):79-93, 2009

ESOPHAGEAL RESECTION

Key Facts

Terminology

- Various surgical procedures for benign and malignant esophageal lesions
- Most common: Transthoracic esophagectomy through right thoracotomy (Ivor Lewis)

Imaging

- Radiography
  - Initial postoperative assessment
  - Assessment of postoperative complications
  - Right mediastinal contour abnormality produced by gastric conduit
  - Contrast studies (Gastrografin): Exclusion of anastomotic leak
- CT
  - Assessment of postoperative complications
  - Assessment of tumor recurrence
- PET/CT: Staging & post-treatment restaging

Top Differential Diagnoses

- Surgery-related complications
- Postoperative tumor recurrence

Pathology

- Stomach: Most convenient esophageal substitute
- Other: Gastric tube, colon, jejunum, free revascularized graft

Clinical Issues

- Frequent sources of morbidity: Pneumothorax, pleural effusion, pneumonia, respiratory failure
- Mediastinitis & sepsis: High morbidity/mortality

Diagnostic Checklist

- Consider Gastrografin studies for evaluation of site & size of anastomotic leaks
- CT is optimal imaging modality for evaluation of surgical complications & tumor recurrence

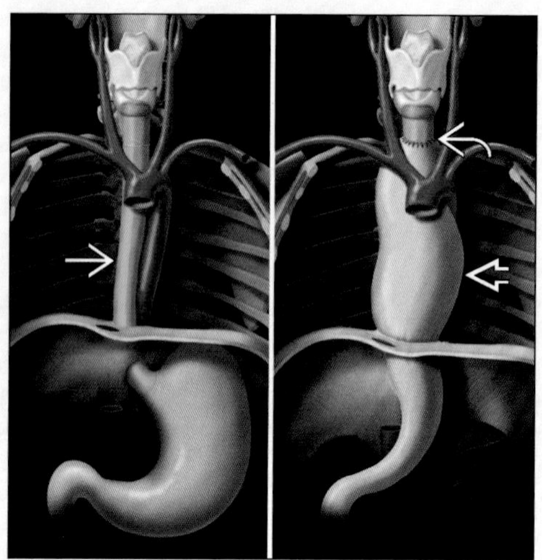

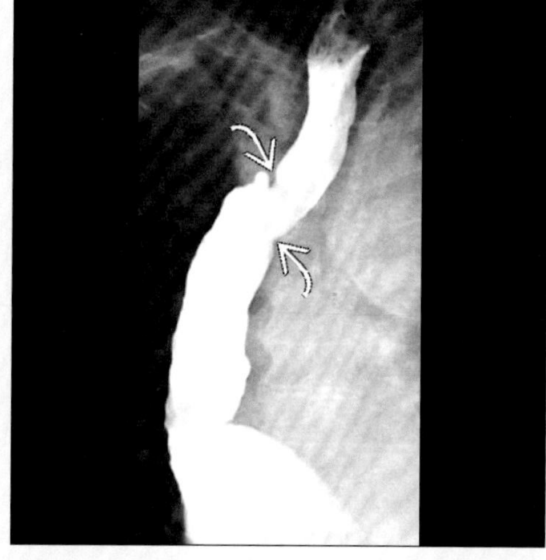

(Left) *Graphic illustrates the Ivor Lewis transthoracic esophagectomy. The native esophagus is resected, the stomach is "pulled through" into the thorax and anastomosed to the proximal esophagus.* ***(Right)*** *Oblique upper GI series shows postsurgical changes of transthoracic esophagectomy and a normal esophagogastric anastomosis. This is the preferred surgical procedure for resectable tumors located in the middle 3rd of the esophagus.*

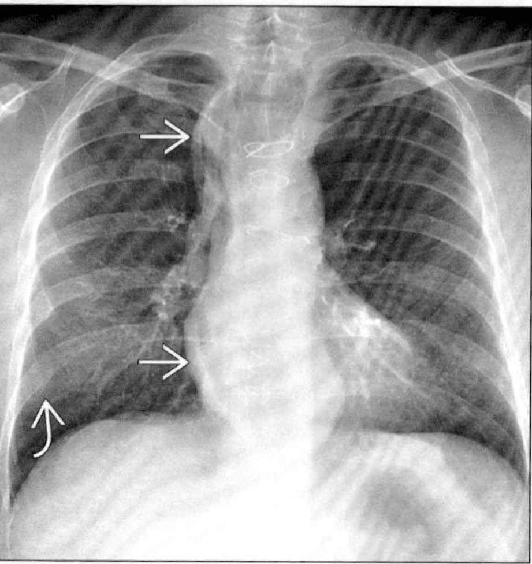

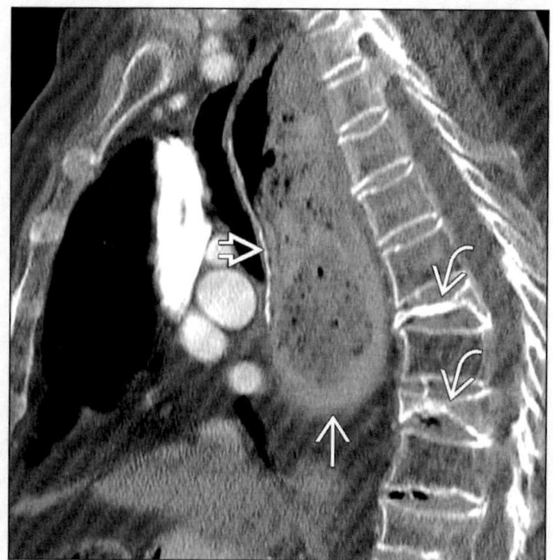

(Left) *PA chest radiograph of a patient with prior Ivor Lewis esophagectomy and CABG shows mild dilatation of the air-filled gastric conduit, which protrudes to the right of midline. Note post-surgical changes in the right chest wall.* ***(Right)*** *Sagittal CECT post esophagectomy shows a mildly dilated gastric conduit, the gastric staple line, and vertebral compression fractures. CT is the optimal imaging modality to evaluate post-surgical complications and tumor recurrence.*

ESOPHAGEAL RESECTION

TERMINOLOGY

Definitions

- Surgical procedures for benign & malignant esophageal lesions
  - Transthoracic esophagectomy through right thoracotomy (**Ivor Lewis** procedure)
    - **Most common** technique
    - Middle & lower 3rd esophageal carcinomas
  - Transhiatal esophagectomy without thoracotomy
    - Thoracic-cervicothoracic esophageal carcinoma
    - Achalasia, caustic injury
  - Transthoracic esophagectomy through left thoracotomy
    - Benign & malignant distal esophagus lesions
  - Radical en bloc esophagectomy
    - Potentially curable tumor (pre- & intraoperative staging)

IMAGING

Radiographic Findings

- Right mediastinal contour abnormality produced by gastric conduit
- Initial postoperative assessment
  - Wide mediastinum, pneumomediastinum, subcutaneous gas, pleural effusion
- Assessment of postoperative complications
  - Wide mediastinum, pneumomediastinum
  - Pleural effusion
  - Large air-fluid level in conduit
- Contrast studies (Gastrografin): Exclusion of anastomotic leak

CT Findings

- Assessment of anastomosis & suture lines
- **Mediastinitis:** Induration of mediastinal fat, fluid collections, extraluminal gas
- **Anastomotic leak:** Perianastomotic fluid/gas, mediastinal abscess; may not show leak site
- **Delayed emptying:** Dilated conduit, air-fluid level
- **Tumor recurrence**: Mass, lymphadenopathy

Ultrasonographic Findings

- Endoscopic ultrasound
  - Tumor invasion, lymphadenopathy

Nuclear Medicine Findings

- PET/CT
  - Assessment of distant metastases
  - Restaging after neoadjuvant therapy

DIFFERENTIAL DIAGNOSIS

Surgery-related Complications

- Mediastinitis
- Anastomotic ischemia
- Anastomotic leak

Postoperative Tumor Recurrence

- Local recurrence at anastomosis
- Recurrence at esophageal substitute

PATHOLOGY

General Features

- **Stomach**: Most convenient esophageal substitute
- Other: Gastric tube, colon, jejunum, free revascularized graft
- **Complications**
  - **Surgical**
    - **Anastomotic Leak:** Major complication
      - Early (2-3 days) or late (3-7 days)
      - Subclinical (50%)
      - Fistula to adjacent structures
    - **Anastomotic stricture:** Late postoperative period (exclusion of recurrence)
    - **Mediastinitis:** Life threatening; associated with high morbidity and mortality
    - **Delayed emptying:** Large mediastinal air-fluid level
      - Lack of pyloric drainage, hiatal obstruction
      - Redundant intrathoracic esophageal substitute
  - **Postoperative tumor recurrence**
    - Local tumor recurrence
    - Tumor of esophageal substitute; stomach, colon

CLINICAL ISSUES

Presentation

- Most common signs/symptoms
  - Frequent sources of morbidity
    - Pneumothorax, pleural effusion
    - Pneumonia (aspiration)
    - Respiratory failure

Natural History & Prognosis

- Mediastinitis & sepsis: High morbidity/mortality
- Mortality rate varies with tumor stage, patient condition, and surgical procedure
  - Transthoracic esophagectomy through right thoracotomy (16%)
  - Transhiatal esophagectomy without thoracotomy (11%)
  - Transthoracic esophagectomy through left thoracotomy (17%)
  - Radical en bloc esophagectomy (8%)

Treatment

- **Anastomotic leaks**: Catheter or chest tube drainage, surgical treatment

DIAGNOSTIC CHECKLIST

Consider

- Gastrografin studies for evaluation of site & size of anastomotic leaks
- CT is optimal imaging modality for evaluation of surgical complications & tumor recurrence

SELECTED REFERENCES

1. Kim TJ et al: Multimodality assessment of esophageal cancer: preoperative staging and monitoring of response to therapy. Radiographics. 29(2):403-21, 2009

RADIATION-INDUCED LUNG DISEASE

Key Facts

Terminology

- Radiation-induced lung disease (RILD)
- Radiation fibrosis

Imaging

- Radiography
  - Consolidation with sharply defined linear or curvilinear margins conforming to radiation portals
  - Progressive volume loss in irradiated lung
- CT
  - Radiation pneumonitis: Ground-glass opacity & consolidation
  - Radiation fibrosis: Architectural distortion with intrinsic traction bronchiectasis
- PET/CT
  - Radiation pneumonitis may exhibit FDG avidity
  - Detection of recurrent tumor within RILD

Top Differential Diagnoses

- Cardiogenic pulmonary edema
- Bacterial pneumonia
- Recurrent malignancy
- Drug reaction

Pathology

- COP after RT for breast cancer

Clinical Issues

- Concomitant treatment with some chemotherapeutic agents raises risk of RILD
- Subsequent treatment with chemotherapy can cause recall radiation pneumonitis
- Steroids are standard treatment for radiation pneumonitis & COP
- Sudden withdrawal of steroids puts patients at risk for recurrent radiation pneumonitis

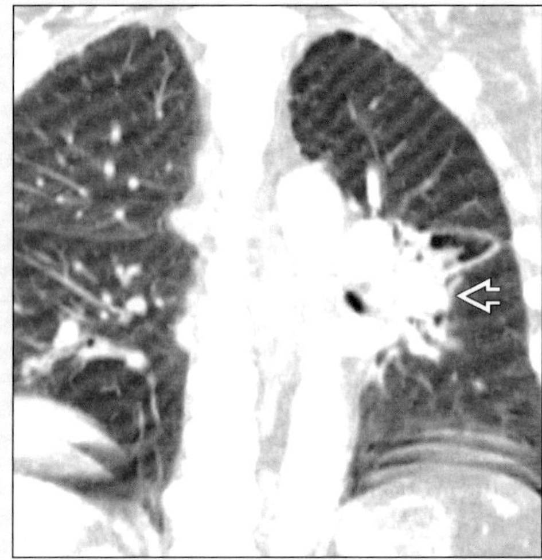

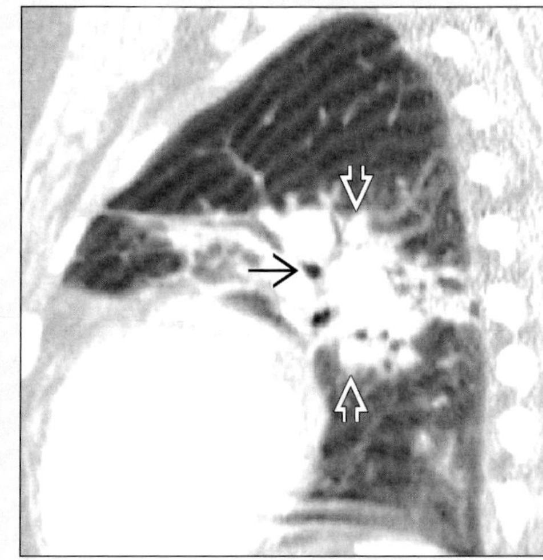

*(**Left**) Coronal NECT of a patient with left upper lobe lung cancer 17 months after completion of radiation therapy shows a left perihilar mass-like consolidation ➡ with well-defined peripheral borders that conform to the radiation portal. (**Right**) Sagittal NECT of the same patient shows radiation fibrosis ➡ with intrinsic air bronchograms ➡ involving the left upper and lower lobes. Radiation fibrosis may manifest with mass-like consolidations that do not conform to anatomic boundaries.*

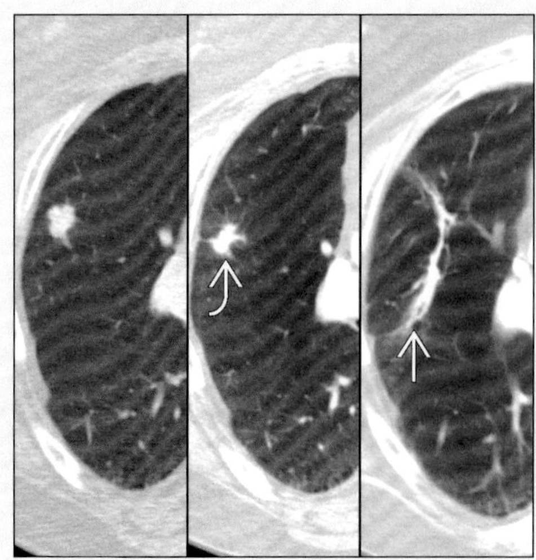

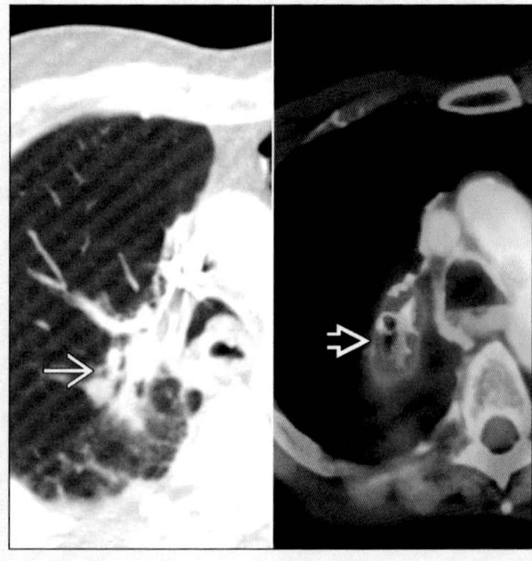

*(**Left**) Composite image with serial axial NECT images of a patient with stage IA lung cancer at diagnosis (left), 1 month (center), and 16 months (right) after stereotactic radiotherapy shows decreased tumor volume ➡ and a curvilinear scar ➡ at the completion of treatment. (**Right**) Composite image with axial CECT (left) and fused FDG PET/CT (right) shows right perihilar radiation fibrosis ➡ 3 years after treatment for lung cancer. Intrinsic FDG avidity ➡ is consistent with recurrent lung cancer.*

RADIATION-INDUCED LUNG DISEASE

TERMINOLOGY

Abbreviations

- **Radiation-induced lung disease (RILD)**

Definitions

- **Radiation pneumonitis**: Radiation-induced lung inflammation, usually from radiation therapy
- **Radiation fibrosis**: Radiation-induced lung fibrosis or scarring, usually from radiation therapy

IMAGING

General Features

- Best diagnostic clue
  - Pulmonary consolidation with **sharply defined linear or curvilinear margins**
  - **RILD does not conform to anatomic boundaries** but **conforms to radiation portals**
- Location
  - Usually **within radiation portals**
- Size
  - Extent of radiation injury varies with radiation portal size
- Morphology
  - Acute radiation pneumonitis: Diffuse alveolar damage
  - Chronic radiation fibrosis: Architectural distortion with traction bronchiectasis

Radiographic Findings

- Typical timeline (**rule of 4s**)
  - 4 weeks to complete therapy delivery; 40 Gy
  - 4 weeks after therapy completion: Earliest radiation pneumonitis; indistinct vessel margins
  - 4 months after therapy completion: Peak of radiation pneumonitis; consolidation involving irradiated lung
  - 12 (4 x 3) months after therapy completion: Following peak pneumonitis, consolidation gradually clears & evolves into scar (cicatricial atelectasis)
  - Scarring produces progressive volume loss in irradiated lung
  - 12-18 months following therapy: Cicatricial atelectasis stabilizes
  - Thereafter, changes within radiation portal likely relate to recurrent tumor or infection
  - Timeline sequence accelerates 1 week for each extra 10 Gy of therapy
- Typical patterns
  - Neck radiation: Apical consolidation with sharp inferior margins
  - Paramediastinal radiation: Medial consolidation with linear or parenthesis-shaped margins
  - Mantle radiation: Y-shaped consolidation over clavicles & along mediastinum; sharp margins
  - Tangential breast radiation: Obliquely oriented margin of subpleural consolidation along ipsilateral anterior chest wall
  - Focal radiation: Varied, related to radiation portals tailored to treat specific lesions, such as a lung mass

CT Findings

- Patterns of radiation injury following **conventional radiation therapy**
  - Homogeneous ground-glass opacities corresponding to minimal radiation pneumonitis
  - Patchy consolidation within radiation field
  - Discrete consolidation within radiation field but not totally involving it
  - Dense consolidation totally involving radiation field, corresponding to fibrosis
- Patterns of radiation fibrosis after **3-dimensional conformal radiation therapy (RT)**
  - Modified conventional fibrosis less extensive than that resulting from RT
  - Mass-like fibrosis
  - Scar-like fibrosis
- **Stereotactic body radiation therapy (SBRT)**
  - Focused high-dose radiation to localized lesions
  - Pulmonary opacities may not precisely correspond to planned target volume
  - Decreased size of tumor nodule at 1-3 months
  - Ground-glass opacities at 3-6 months
  - Consolidation at 3-8 months
  - May change shape & migrate toward hilum during 1st year
- Associated findings
  - Pleural thickening or effusion
  - Pericardial effusion
  - Calcified lymph nodes, thymic cysts
  - Bleb formation near regions of radiation fibrosis
    - Pneumothorax may result from bleb rupture
  - Uncommonly, RT to lung can induce development of cryptogenic organizing pneumonia (COP)
    - Migratory peripheral nodular opacities outside radiation portal

MR Findings

- **Acute phase** (1-3 months after irradiation)
  - Enhancement of irradiated lung with gadolinium-based contrast material is most pronounced
- **Late phase** (4 months after irradiation)
  - First pass shows decreased enhancement, but contrast material accumulates with redistribution

Nuclear Medicine Findings

- PET
  - Radiation pneumonitis may exhibit increased glucose metabolism in first few months after RT
  - PET very useful for detecting recurrent tumor within regions of radiation fibrosis
- V/Q scan
  - Radiation therapy causes ventilation/perfusion mismatch with nonsegmental distribution conforming to radiation portal
  - SPECT perfusion scans useful for assessing regional effects of lung injury from RT

Imaging Recommendations

- Best imaging tool
  - High-resolution chest CT optimally demonstrates areas of involvement & helps distinguish radiation pneumonitis from fibrosis
- Protocol advice
  - RILD is visible on conventional chest CT protocols
  - RILD often recognizable on chest radiography

RADIATION-INDUCED LUNG DISEASE

DIFFERENTIAL DIAGNOSIS

Cardiogenic Pulmonary Edema

- Interstitial edema, perihilar haze, ground-glass opacities/consolidation
- Cardiomegaly, pleural effusion

Bacterial Pneumonia

- Segmental or lobar consolidation
- Fever, elevated white blood cell count

Recurrent Malignancy

- Development of mass ± lymphadenopathy or other metastases

Lymphangitic Carcinomatosis

- Smooth or nodular thickening of interlobular septa & peribronchovascular interstitium
- Often associated with lymphadenopathy
- More frequently unilateral

Drug Reaction

- Ground-glass opacities, consolidation, fibrosis
- Often caused by chemotherapy

PATHOLOGY

General Features

- Etiology
  - **RT for carcinoma or lymphoma: Most common cause for RILD**
    - Total dose, fractionation, dose rate, type of RT, & volume of irradiated lung affect RILD
  - Lung disease outside radiation portal probably COP from lymphocyte-mediated immune reaction
- Associated abnormalities
  - COP after RT for breast cancer
    - 2.4% of women treated with surgery and RT for breast cancer
    - 2-7 months after RT
  - Cardiomyopathy
  - Pulmonary gangrene may occur

Gross Pathologic & Surgical Features

- Radiation fibrosis: Airless, firm lung with extensive scar formation

Microscopic Features

- Radiation pneumonitis: Damage to type II pneumocytes & endothelial cells, hyaline membranes

CLINICAL ISSUES

Presentation

- Most common signs/symptoms
  - Many patients asymptomatic
  - Cough, fever
  - Dyspnea
- Other signs/symptoms
  - Elevated polymorphonuclear leukocyte count
  - Elevated sedimentation rate
- Clinical profile
  - Doses < 20 Gy rarely cause radiation pneumonitis
  - Doses > 40 Gy usually cause radiation pneumonitis

Demographics

- Age
  - RT is used mostly to treat carcinoma & lymphoma, which typically affect middle-aged or elderly patients
- Gender
  - COP after RT occurs mostly in women who have received RT for breast cancer
- Epidemiology
  - Acute radiation pneumonitis develops in 5-15% of patients who receive RT

Natural History & Prognosis

- Acute: Capillary damage, edema, hyaline membranes, & mononuclear cell infiltration
- Subacute: Increased mononuclear cells & fibroblasts
- Chronic: Capillary sclerosis, alveolar & interstitial fibrosis
- Patients with preexisting pulmonary fibrosis are at greater risk for developing RILD

Treatment

- Concomitant treatment with some chemotherapeutic agents raises risk of RILD
- Subsequent treatment with chemotherapy can cause recall radiation pneumonitis
- Steroids are standard treatment for radiation pneumonitis and COP
- Sudden withdrawal of steroids puts patients at risk for recurrent radiation pneumonitis

DIAGNOSTIC CHECKLIST

Image Interpretation Pearls

- Determine stage of patient's carcinoma or lymphoma
- If standard treatment for that stage of malignancy is RT, correlate pulmonary abnormalities with radiation portals
- New soft tissue nodules or masses within RILD should be investigated with PET/CT to exclude recurrent malignancy
- If ectatic bronchi within radiation fibrosis fill in with soft tissue on follow-up CT, suspect recurrent malignancy

SELECTED REFERENCES

1. Choi YW et al: Effects of radiation therapy on the lung: radiologic appearances and differential diagnosis. Radiographics. 24(4):985-97; discussion 998, 2004
2. Miwa S et al: The incidence and clinical characteristics of bronchiolitis obliterans organizing pneumonia syndrome after radiation therapy for breast cancer. Sarcoidosis Vasc Diffuse Lung Dis. 21(3):212-8, 2004
3. Takeda T et al: Radiation injury after hypofractionated stereotactic radiotherapy for peripheral small lung tumors: serial changes on CT. AJR Am J Roentgenol. 182(5):1123-8, 2004
4. Koenig TR et al: Radiation injury of the lung after three-dimensional conformal radiation therapy. AJR Am J Roentgenol. 178(6):1383-8, 2002
5. Ogasawara N et al: Perfusion characteristics of radiation-injured lung on Gd-DTPA-enhanced dynamic magnetic resonance imaging. Invest Radiol. 37(8):448-57, 2002
6. Libshitz HI et al: Filling in of radiation therapy-induced bronchiectatic change: a reliable sign of locally recurrent lung cancer. Radiology. 210(1):25-7, 1999

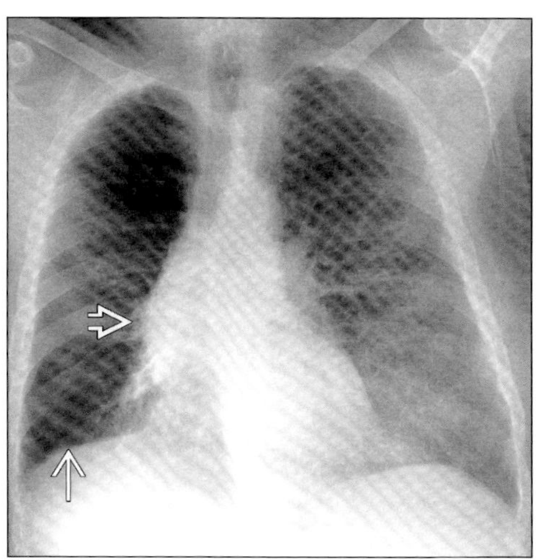

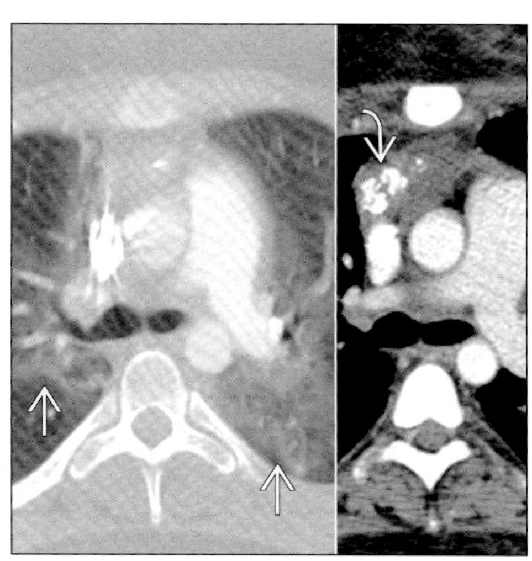

(Left) *PA chest radiograph shows post radiation mass-like fibrosis in the right hilum ➡ and right lung hyperlucency and oligemia ➡ outside the radiation portal from radiation-induced fibrosis and vascular injury.* ***(Right)*** *Composite image with axial CECT in lung (left) and soft tissue (right) window of a patient with Hodgkin disease treated with radiation shows bilateral paramediastinal ground-glass opacity ➡ from radiation pneumonitis and calcification ➡ in the treated tumor 2 years later.*

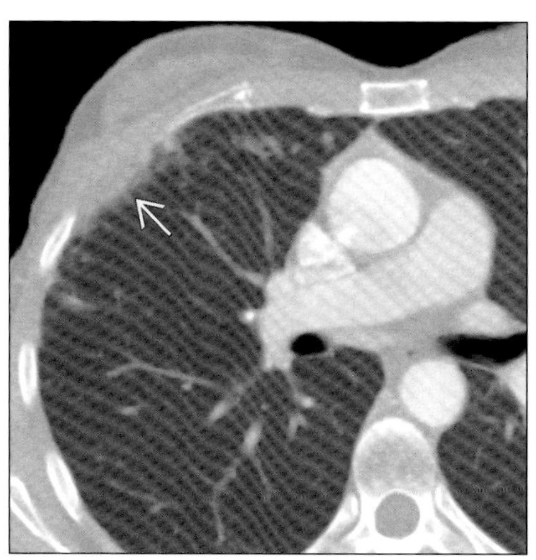

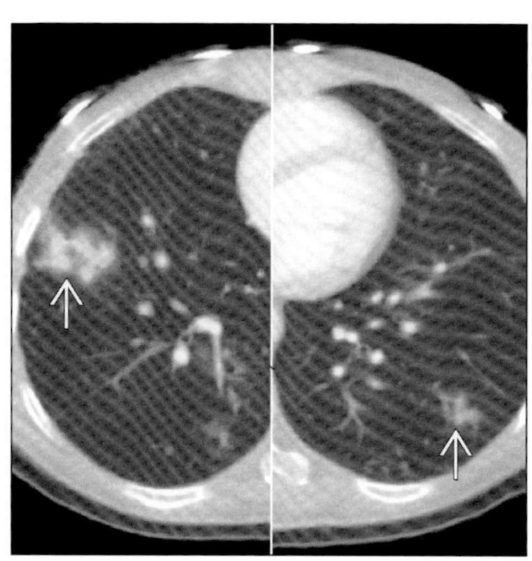

(Left) *Axial CECT of a patient with right breast cancer treated with radiation shows a tangential right upper lobe subpleural opacity ➡ that represents radiation fibrosis.* ***(Right)*** *Composite image with axial CECT of the same patient shows bilateral mixed solid and ground-glass nodules ➡ outside the radiation portal. Open lung biopsy showed cryptogenic organizing pneumonia. Nodular opacities outside the radiation portal in breast cancer patients treated with RT may represent COP.*

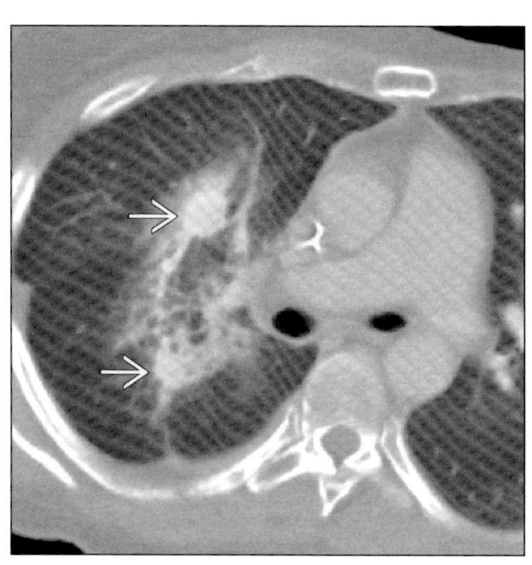

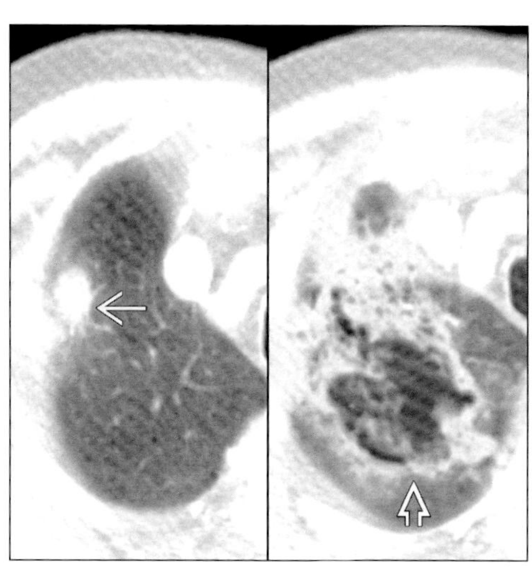

(Left) *Axial CECT of a patient with lung cancer obtained more than a year after completion of radiation therapy shows 2 new solid nodules ➡ within areas of radiation fibrosis, suspicious for tumor recurrence.* ***(Right)*** *Composite image with axial CECT of a patient with peripheral lung cancer ➡ (left) and CECT performed 2 months after radiation therapy (right) shows a large thick-walled pulmonary cavity ➡ with necrotic debris secondary to radiation-induced pulmonary gangrene.*

DRUG-INDUCED LUNG DISEASE

Key Facts

Terminology

- Drug-induced lung disease, described with > 350 drugs

Imaging

- Patterns
  - DAD: Identical to ARDS from other causes
  - Fibrosis: Traction bronchiectasis & honeycomb lung
  - Chronic interstitial lung disease: NSIP pattern
  - HP: Fleeting opacities
  - Eosinophilic pneumonia: Peripheral upper lobe homogeneous airspace disease
  - COP: Airspace disease; subpleural, peribronchial
  - Pulmonary edema: Indistinguishable from noncardiogenic or cardiogenic edema
  - DAH: Patchy or diffuse alveolar opacities
  - SLE syndrome: Pleuro-pericardial effusions
- High-attenuation lung, pleura, liver, spleen: Pathognomonic of amiodarone toxicity; drug contains 37% iodine by weight

Top Differential Diagnoses

- NSIP pattern: Collagen vascular disease
  - Scleroderma: Dilated EG junction/esophagus
  - Rheumatoid arthritis: Distal clavicle erosion
  - Inflammatory bowel disease, ulcerative colitis, Crohn disease: Bronchiectasis

Clinical Issues

- Symptoms: Dyspnea, cough, fever, eosinophilia
- Treatment: Discontinuation of drug, corticosteroids

Diagnostic Checklist

- Almost any focal or diffuse pulmonary process could potentially be secondary to drug use

*(**Left**) Axial NECT of a 77-year-old man with amiodarone toxicity shows a peripheral right upper lobe consolidation ➔, patchy ground-glass opacities ⇨, and septal thickening. (**Right**) Axial NECT of the same patient shows a high-attenuation consolidation ➔ secondary to amiodarone's iodine content. Cryptogenic organizing pneumonia, interstitial fibrosis, and pleural effusions ⇨ are also features of amiodarone toxicity confirmed with BAL findings of neutrophilic alveolitis and foamy macrophages.*

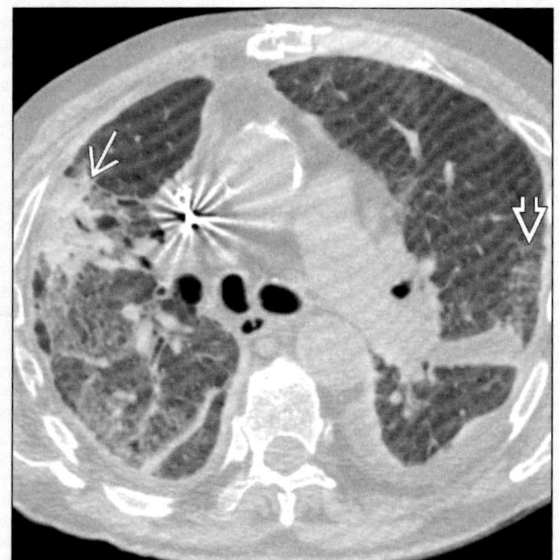

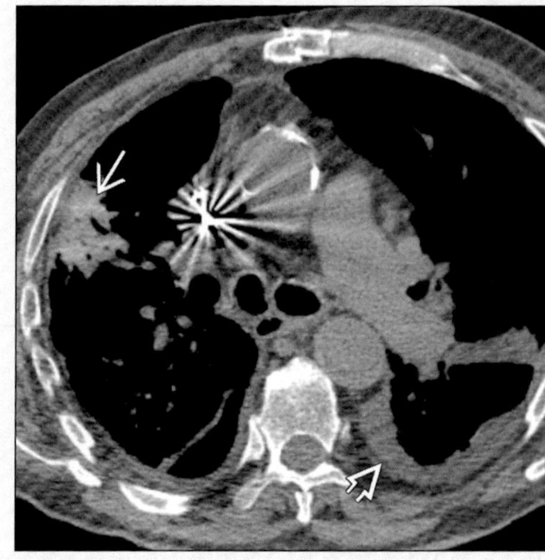

*(**Left**) AP chest radiograph of a 37-year-old woman who presented with dyspnea after smoking crack cocaine shows diffuse bilateral ground-glass opacities. (**Right**) Axial HRCT of the same patient shows diffuse bilateral ground-glass opacities with areas of subpleural sparing ⇗. Pulmonary edema and diffuse alveolar damage are associated with smoking crack cocaine.*

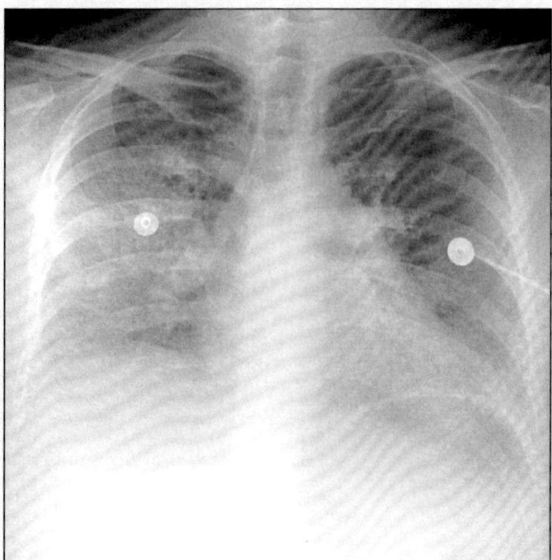

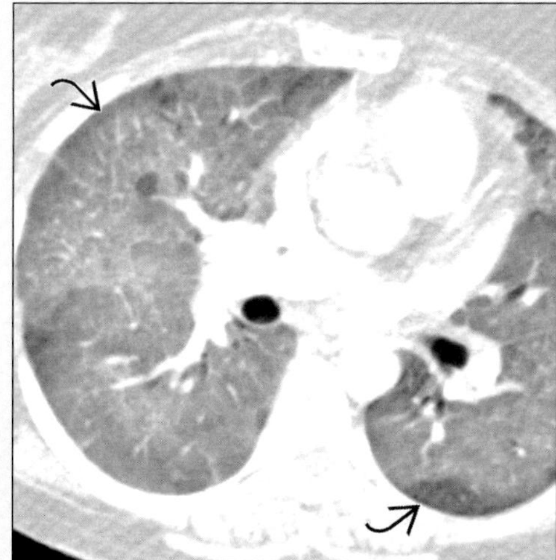

DRUG-INDUCED LUNG DISEASE

TERMINOLOGY

Definitions

- Drug-induced lung disease, described with > 350 drugs

IMAGING

General Features

- Best diagnostic clue
  - High index of suspicion for drug-related lung abnormalities
  - Diagnosis of exclusion
- Location
  - Variable
- Size
  - Variable
- Morphology
  - Variable, often nonspecific

Radiographic Findings

- Radiography
  - Radiographic abnormalities may be 1st indicator of pulmonary toxicity
- Patterns
  - **Lung abnormalities**
    - **Diffuse alveolar damage (DAD)**: Identical to acute respiratory distress syndrome (ARDS) from other causes
    - Interstitial fibrosis: Basilar subpleural interstitial thickening, traction bronchiectasis, honeycomb lung
    - **Nonspecific interstitial pneumonia (NSIP) pattern**: Basilar reticular opacities &/or patchy, peripheral ground-glass opacities
    - **Hypersensitivity pneumonitis (HP)**: May develop within hours, days or months of starting drug; opacities may be fleeting ("eosinophilic pneumonia-like")
    - **Eosinophilic pneumonia**: Peripheral upper lobe homogeneous opacities, diffuse airspace disease
    - **Cryptogenic organizing pneumonia (COP)**: Unilateral or bilateral patchy airspace opacities with subpleural & peribronchial distribution
    - **Pulmonary edema**: Indistinguishable from noncardiogenic or cardiogenic edema, diffuse mixed interstitial/alveolar pattern
    - **Diffuse alveolar hemorrhage (DAH)**: Patchy or diffuse alveolar opacities
    - **Vasculitis**: Patchy interstitial &/or airspace opacities, subsegmental, peripheral distribution, cavitation in areas of infarction
    - **Granulomas**: Conglomerate basilar chronic masses (lipoid pneumonia)
    - **Airways disease**: Hyper-reactive airways & hyperinflation from asthma; hyperinflation with bronchiolitis obliterans
    - **Pulmonary calcification**: Extremely fine, high-density deposits, upper lobe predominance
  - **Pleural abnormalities**
    - **Systemic lupus erythematosus (SLE) syndrome**: Lupus-like pleuro-pericardial effusions (common), basal interstitial opacities (uncommon)
    - **Pleural/mediastinal fibrosis**: Pleural thickening, abnormal mediastinal contours, airway constriction
    - **Air leak**: Pneumothorax/pneumomediastinum
  - **Vascular abnormalities**
    - **Thromboembolism**
    - **Pulmonary hypertension**: Enlarged pulmonary trunk & central pulmonary arteries, right or left heart failure from incompetent valves
  - **Lymphadenopathy**: Hilar, mediastinal, cervical

CT Findings

- NECT
  - Optimal assessment of early lung involvement, lymphadenopathy, pleuro-pericardial disease
  - High-attenuation lung, pleura, liver, spleen: Pathognomonic of amiodarone toxicity; drug contains 37% iodine by weight
  - Lipoid pneumonia: Low (fat) attenuation focal consolidation or mixed diffuse ground-glass & reticular opacities
  - Mediastinal fibrosis: Soft tissue encasing & sometimes obliterating arteries, veins, bronchi (rare)
- HRCT
  - Optimal characterization of ground-glass, interstitial (reticular nodular), alveolar opacities & their distribution

Nuclear Medicine Findings

- Bone scan
  - May demonstrate pulmonary activity in pulmonary metastatic calcification

Imaging Recommendations

- Best imaging tool
  - HRCT for optimal detection & characterization of ground-glass/interstitial lung disease
- Protocol advice
  - Thin slice (1-3 mm) CT at 10-15 mm intervals
  - Supine inspiratory/expiratory imaging & supine expiratory imaging

DIFFERENTIAL DIAGNOSIS

Nonspecific Interstitial Pneumonia Pattern

- Collagen vascular disease
  - **Scleroderma**: Patulous esophagogastric junction, dilated air-filled esophagus
  - **Rheumatoid arthritis**: Erosion of distal clavicles, other skeletal abnormalities
  - **Inflammatory bowel disease, ulcerative colitis, Crohn disease**: Bronchiectasis

PATHOLOGY

General Features

- Etiology
  - **DAD/interstitial fibrosis**: Amiodarone, bleomycin, cyclophosphamide, nitrofurantoin, methotrexate, gemcitabine, rituximab
  - **Chronic interstitial pneumonia/NSIP**: Amiodarone, ACE inhibitors, β-blockers, bleomycin, carmustine, methotrexate, nitrofurantoin, sulfasalazine, procarbazine
  - **Eosinophilic pneumonia**: Nonsteroidal anti-inflammatory drugs, amiodarone, antidepressants, β-blockers, captopril, nitrofurantoin, erythromycin, penicillin, isoniazid, sulfasalazine, penicillamine

DRUG-INDUCED LUNG DISEASE

  - **COP**: Amiodarone, amphotericin, bleomycin, methotrexate, cyclophosphamide, nitrofurantoin
  - **Pulmonary edema**: Aspirin, codeine, hydrochlorothiazide, interferon, heroin, cocaine, methadone, epinephrine, contrast media, tricyclic antidepressants
  - **Hemorrhage**: Anticoagulants, sirolimus, azathioprine, penicillamine, cytarabine
  - **SLE syndrome**: Procainamide, isoniazid, phenytoin, nitrofurantoin, penicillin, sulfonamides, propranolol, thiazides, penicillamine, levodopa
  - **Pleural effusions** (without SLE syndrome): Methotrexate, procarbazine, nitrofurantoin, bromocriptine, methysergide, interleukin-2, amiodarone
  - **Pleura/mediastinal fibrosis**: Methysergide, ergotamine, ergonovine
  - **Pneumothorax/pneumomediastinum**: Carmustine, cocaine
  - **Vasculitis**: Aspirin, sulfonamides, sulfasalazine, phenytoin, propylthiouracil, leukotriene receptor antagonists
  - **Granulomas**: Methotrexate, nitrofurantoin, mineral oils, talc
  - **Thromboembolism**: Oral contraceptives; oil embolism; pulmonary artery hypertension: Talc, fenfluramine; damaged heart valves: Fenfluramine
  - **Hilar/mediastinal lymphadenopathy**: Methotrexate, hydantoin
  - **Pulmonary calcification**: Vitamin D, calcium therapy
  - **Airways disease**: Hyper-reactive airways: β-blockers, aspirin, contrast media
    - **Bronchiolitis obliterans**: Penicillamine, sulfasalazine, gold
  - **Lipoid pneumonia**: Aspiration of mineral oil; drug-induced phospholipidosis: Amiodarone
- Direct **lung toxicity**: Damaged alveolar macrophages, neutrophils & lymphocytes; release of cytokines & humoral factors that may result in fibrosis
- **Hypersensitivity reaction**: Type I (immediate) & type III (immune complex) responses, eosinophilic infiltration
- **Vasculitis**: Type III & IV (cell-mediated), usually systemic, involving skin, kidneys, liver; seen with sulfonamides

Gross Pathologic & Surgical Features

- Most lung biopsies are not pathognomonic: Useful for exclusion of other diseases & documentation of injury pattern

Microscopic Features

- **Diffuse interstitial pneumonia**: DAD, usual interstitial pneumonia, desquamative interstitial pneumonia, NSIP
- **COP**: Immature fibroblasts plug respiratory bronchioles & alveolar ducts
- **Eosinophilic pneumonia**: Eosinophil, lymphocyte, plasma cell infiltration of alveolar septa

CLINICAL ISSUES

Presentation

- Most common signs/symptoms
  - **Variable presentation**: Dyspnea, cough, fever, eosinophilia; drug toxicity often overlooked as possible cause
- Onset: Variable from immediate to years after drug initiation
  - Bleomycin, < 3 months; cytosine arabinoside, < 21 days; busulfan, months to years; methotrexate, within weeks; cyclophosphamide, < 6 months to years; nitrofurantoin, 1 day to 1 month or > 6 months; hydrochlorothiazide, < hours; tricyclic antidepressants, < hours; salicylates, < hours; methysergide, 6 months to years; interleukin-2, usually < 8 days; amiodarone, approximately 6 months; hydantoin, 1 week to 30 years
- With some cytotoxic drugs (carmustine), preexisting pulmonary disease, smoking, irradiation, & combination chemotherapy increase risk of toxicity
- Mitomycin: Asthma, microangiopathy, hemolytic anemia (renal failure, thrombocytopenia, noncardiogenic edema)
- Penicillamine: Acute glomerulonephritis, pulmonary hemorrhage, identical to Goodpasture syndrome

Demographics

- Age
  - Neonate to elderly
- Gender
  - M = F

Natural History & Prognosis

- Recovery after discontinuance of drug, variable
- Methotrexate: Reinstitution of treatment without recurrent toxicity
- Mortality from respiratory failure
  - Mortality from toxicity: Nitrofurantoin 10%; amiodarone 20%; mitomycin (hemolytic-uremic syndrome) > 90%
- Malignant transformation: Hydantoin lymphadenopathy may evolve into lymphoma, Hodgkin or non-Hodgkin

Treatment

- **Discontinuation of drug, corticosteroids**

DIAGNOSTIC CHECKLIST

Consider

- Almost any focal or diffuse pulmonary process could potentially be secondary to drug use

Image Interpretation Pearls

- Differentiation requires investigation of drug history & individual drug's pattern of pulmonary injury

SELECTED REFERENCES

1. Torrisi JM et al: CT findings of chemotherapy-induced toxicity: what radiologists need to know about the clinical and radiologic manifestations of chemotherapy toxicity. Radiology. 258(1):41-56, 2011
2. Erasmus JJ et al: High-resolution CT of drug-induced lung disease. Radiol Clin North Am. 40(1):61-72, 2002

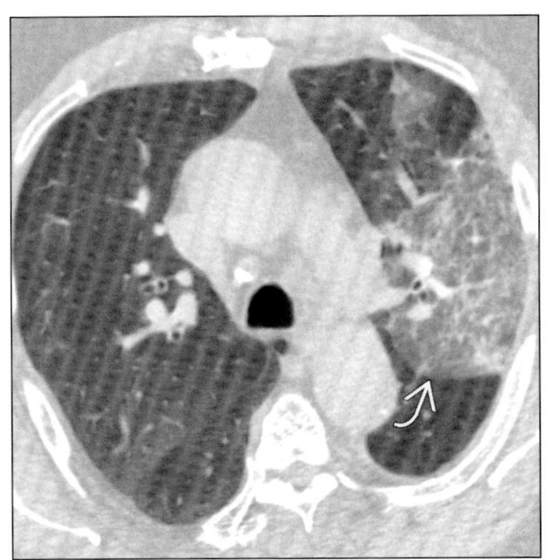

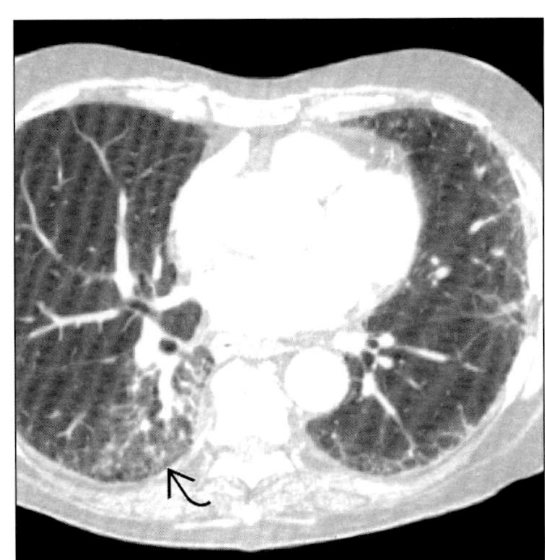

(Left) *Axial NECT of a 73-year-old patient with hemoptysis secondary to hemorrhage from excessive anticoagulation with Coumadin shows left upper lobe ground-glass opacity* ➔ *that represents alveolar hemorrhage.* ***(Right)*** *Axial NECT of an 82-year-old man who had prostate cancer, prolonged nitrofurantoin therapy for urinary tract infections, and presented with dyspnea shows peripheral subpleural ground-glass and reticular opacities* ➔*, an NSIP pattern of pulmonary involvement.*

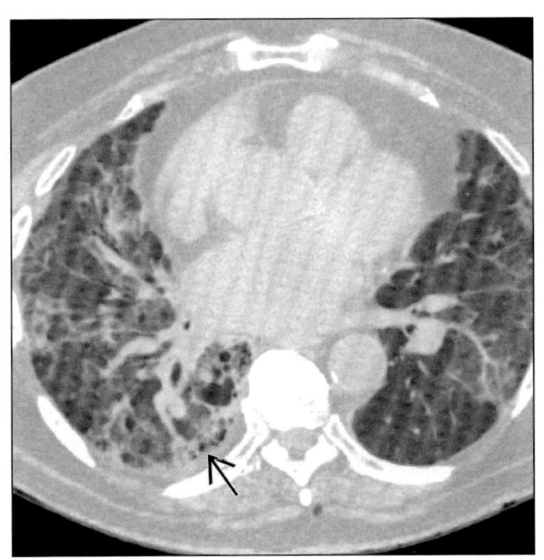

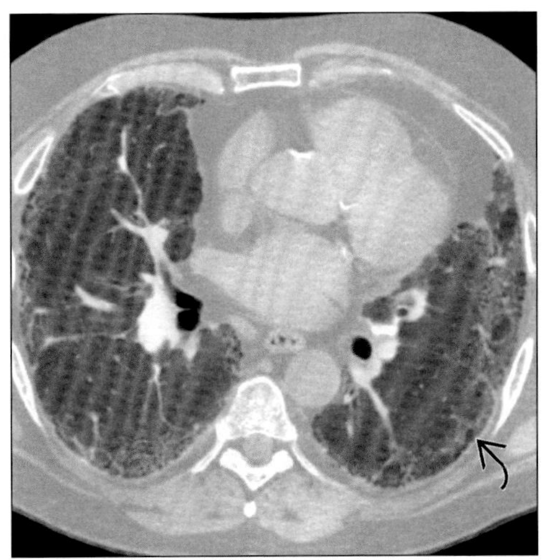

(Left) *Axial HRCT of a 73-year-old man on cyclophosphamide for Goodpasture syndrome shows reticular and ground-glass opacities* ➔*. Bronchoscopy showed neutrophilic alveolitis indicating fibrosis from cyclophosphamide toxicity.* ***(Right)*** *Axial NECT of a patient on azathioprine for Crohn disease who presented with dyspnea shows peripheral reticular opacities and honeycomb lung* ➔*. Pulmonary fibrosis may be due to Crohn disease or drug toxicity.*

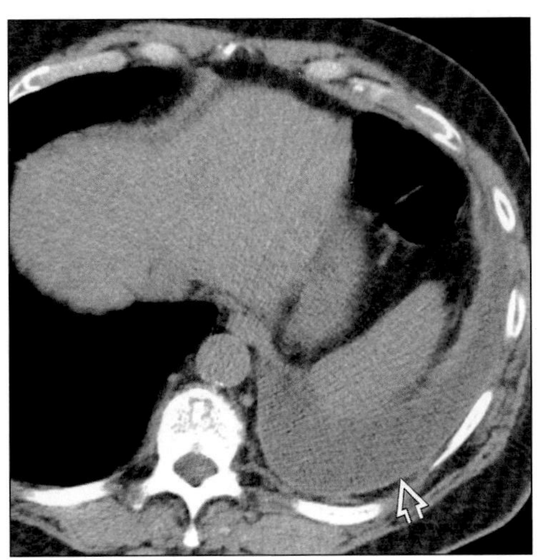

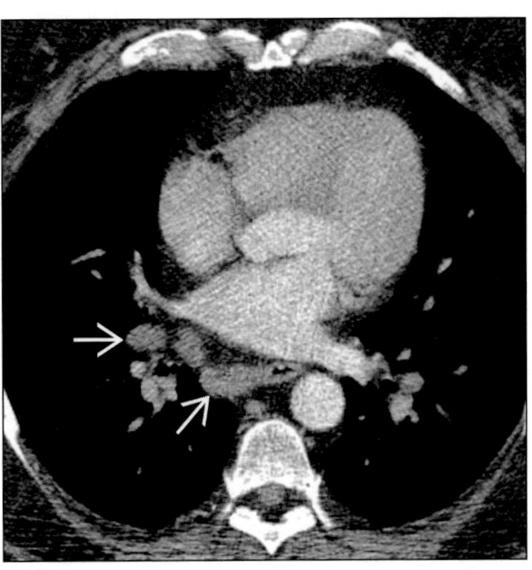

(Left) *Axial NECT of a 59-year-old man treated with propranolol for hypertension shows a moderate left pleural effusion* ➔*. Thoracentesis confirmed an exudate. Propranolol is associated with exudative pleural effusions and drug-induced SLE syndrome.* ***(Right)*** *Axial CECT of a 62-year-old man treated with carbamazepine (Tegretol) for seizures shows borderline enlarged right hilar and mediastinal lymph nodes* ➔*. Carbamazepine is associated with intrathoracic lymphadenopathy.*

AMIODARONE TOXICITY

Key Facts

Terminology

- Amiodarone = iodinated benzofuran derivative used to treat various cardiac arrhythmias

Imaging

- Consolidation
  - Peripheral, peribronchial, perilobular common
  - High-attenuation (**82-175 HU**) foci in approximately 70% of symptomatic patients
- Reticulation
  - Peripheral & basal predominant
- Pleural effusions in approximately 50% of patients
- Diffuse high attenuation in liver

Top Differential Diagnoses

- Cryptogenic organizing pneumonia
- Pneumonia
- Nonspecific interstitial pneumonia

Pathology

- Damage to lung by amiodarone & its metabolites
- Immunologic reaction
  - Organizing pneumonia
  - Nonspecific interstitial pneumonia
  - Diffuse alveolar damage

Clinical Issues

- More common with higher doses
- Toxicity in 2-5% of treated patients
- Risk of toxicity increases with age
- Toxicity more common in men
- Treatment
  - Cessation of amiodarone; corticosteroids

Diagnostic Checklist

- Consider amiodarone toxicity in treated patients with new chest imaging abnormalities

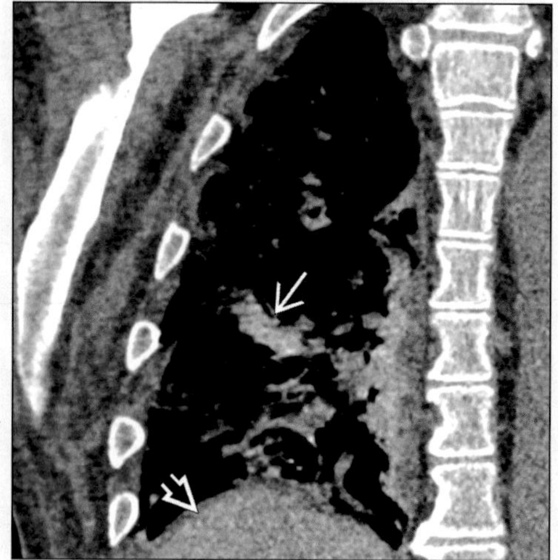

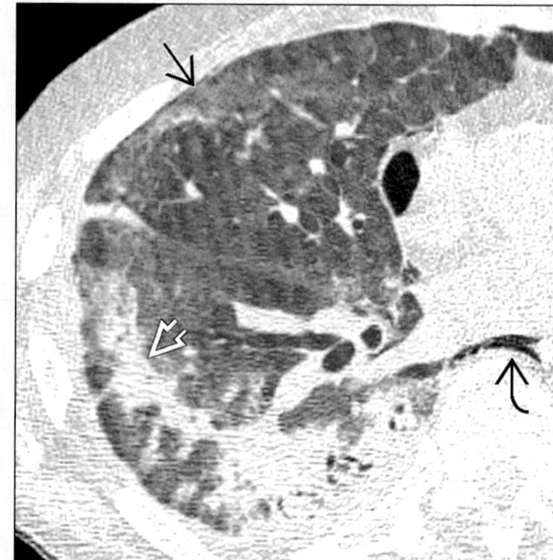

(Left) *Coronal NECT (mediastinal window) shows high-attenuation patchy right lung consolidations ➡ from amiodarone deposition as well as high attenuation in the liver ➡. These findings help suggest the diagnosis in the appropriate clinical setting.* ***(Right)*** *Axial HRCT shows patchy peripheral ground-glass opacities ➡ and peripheral perilobular consolidations ➡ in a patient with acute lung injury from amiodarone therapy. Pneumomediastinum ➡ developed as a consequence of barotrauma.*

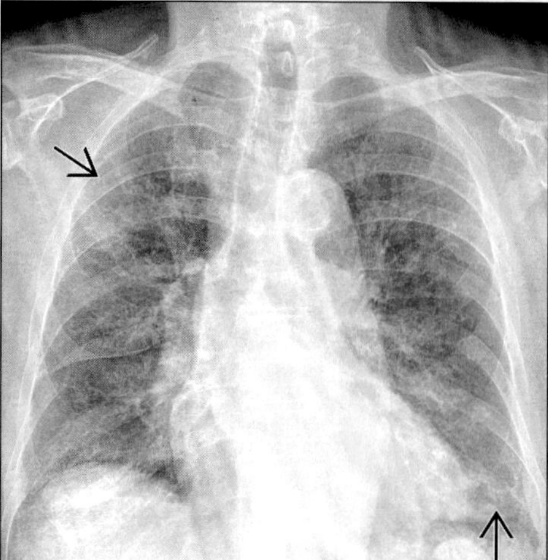

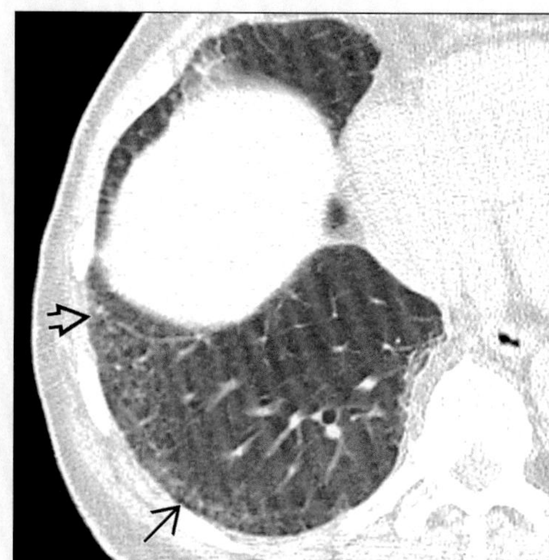

(Left) *PA chest radiograph shows patchy bilateral fine reticular opacities ➡ due to amiodarone-induced pulmonary fibrosis. Amiodarone should be discontinued in patients with early fibrosis to prevent disease progression.* ***(Right)*** *Axial HRCT shows peripheral subpleural ground-glass opacity ➡ and reticulation ➡ in the right lower lobe, suggestive of mild interstitial fibrosis. Nonspecific interstitial pneumonia (NSIP) is the most common pattern of fibrosis resulting from amiodarone.*

AMIODARONE TOXICITY

TERMINOLOGY

Synonyms

- **Amiodarone-induced lung disease**
- **Amiodarone drug reaction**

Definitions

- **Amiodarone = iodinated benzofuran derivative** used to treat various **cardiac arrhythmias**
- Lung injury by amiodarone & its metabolites either from direct cytotoxic effect or immunologic reaction
  - Concentration in the lung; long half-life

IMAGING

General Features

- Best diagnostic clue
  - **High-attenuation foci in lung**
  - **Diffuse high attenuation in liver**
- Location
  - Lungs most frequently affected
- Morphology
  - Patchy pulmonary opacities

Radiographic Findings

- Radiography
  - Diffuse or basal predominant reticular opacities
  - Patchy bilateral consolidations
    - **Peripheral & upper lobe predominant**
    - May mimic eosinophilic pneumonia
  - Focal consolidation much less common
  - Small nodules very uncommon
  - Pleural effusions in approximately 50% of patients

CT Findings

- HRCT
  - High-attenuation (82-175 HU) foci in approximately 70% of symptomatic patients
  - **Consolidation**
    - Peripheral, peribronchial, perilobular
    - Focal round consolidation less common
  - **Ground-glass opacity**
    - Basal predominant or diffuse
  - **Reticulation**
    - **Peripheral & basal predominant**
  - **Pleural effusions** in approximately **50%** of patients

Imaging Recommendations

- Best imaging tool
  - **HRCT**
- Protocol advice
  - Unenhanced thin-section CT; optimal visualization of high-attenuation foci in lung consolidations

DIFFERENTIAL DIAGNOSIS

Cryptogenic Organizing Pneumonia

- May mimic amiodarone toxicity
- High attenuation of liver suggests amiodarone toxicity

Pneumonia

- Usually has acute clinical presentation
- Lobar consolidation favors bacterial pneumonia

Nonspecific Interstitial Pneumonia

- Can be a manifestation of amiodarone toxicity
- Typically associated with connective tissue disease
- High attenuation of liver suggests amiodarone toxicity

PATHOLOGY

General Features

- Etiology
  - Lung damage by amiodarone & its metabolites
    - Direct cytotoxic effect, oxygen radical production
    - Accumulation of phospholipids in tissues
  - Immunologic reaction
    - Organizing pneumonia
    - Nonspecific interstitial pneumonia
    - Diffuse alveolar damage
    - Diffuse alveolar hemorrhage (rare)

Microscopic Features

- Chronic inflammation/fibrosis of alveolar septa

CLINICAL ISSUES

Presentation

- Most common signs/symptoms
  - Dry cough, dyspnea on exertion
- Other signs/symptoms
  - Hypoxemia, fever, inspiratory crackles

Demographics

- Age
  - Risk of toxicity increases with age
- Gender
  - Toxicity more common in men
- Epidemiology
  - Toxicity in **2-5%** of patients on amiodarone
  - More common with higher doses but may occur with any dose
  - Onset of symptoms typically months after treatment initiation

Natural History & Prognosis

- **5-10%** mortality from amiodarone toxicity

Treatment

- Cessation of amiodarone
- Corticosteroids

DIAGNOSTIC CHECKLIST

Consider

- Amiodarone toxicity in treated patients with new parenchymal abnormalities on chest imaging

Image Interpretation Pearls

- **High-attenuation liver parenchyma & lung consolidation** are highly suggestive of the diagnosis

SELECTED REFERENCES

1. Wolkove N et al: Amiodarone pulmonary toxicity. Can Respir J. 16(2):43-8, 2009
2. Camus P et al: Amiodarone pulmonary toxicity. Clin Chest Med. 25(1):65-75, 2004

ABLATION PROCEDURES

Key Facts

Terminology

- Thermal ablation: Treatment of primary or metastatic malignancies in medically inoperable patients
- Radiofrequency ablation (RFA): Use of electrical current to induce coagulative necrosis
- Microwave ablation (MWA): Use of high-frequency electromagnetic waves to induce frictional heat & coagulative necrosis
- Cryoablation = percutaneous cryotherapy (PCT): Use of compressed argon gas to induce intracellular ice formation & cellular necrosis

Imaging

- Ground-glass halo ≥ 5 mm desirable immediately after nodule ablation
- Cavitation in ablation zone & adjacent pleural thickening common up to 3 months post ablation
- Ablated nodules may "grow" in 1st 6 months; growth after 6 months suggests local tumor progression
- Focal nodular enhancement or FDG avidity any time after ablation suggests local tumor progression

Top Differential Diagnoses

- Recurrent malignancy
- Pulmonary infection

Clinical Issues

- Local recurrence typically asymptomatic
- Fever & fatigue common
  - Post ablation syndrome
- Chest pain & dyspnea may be due to delayed pneumothorax

Diagnostic Checklist

- Radiologists must differentiate normal post ablation findings from tumor progression
- Percutaneous biopsy should be considered when tumor progression suspected

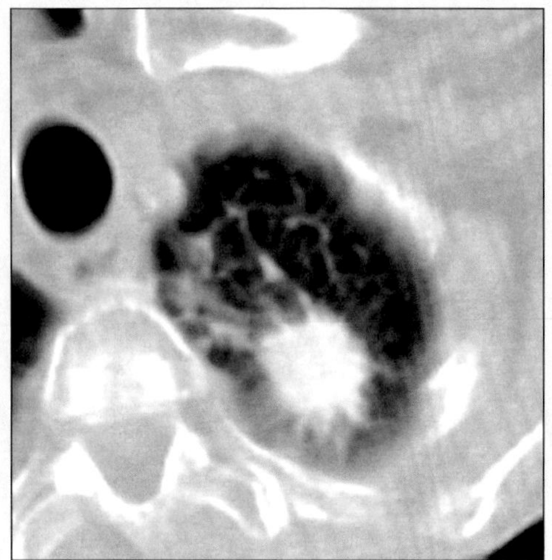

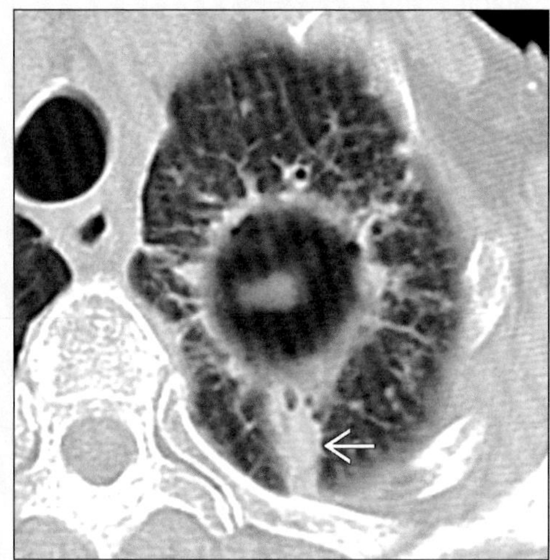

(Left) *Axial NECT of an elderly patient previously treated for lung cancer with right lower lobectomy shows a new 2.4 cm left upper lobe spiculated adenocarcinoma.* ***(Right)*** *Axial NECT of the same patient 3 months after two 12-minute RFA treatments using a cooled tip cluster electrode with a 2.5 cm active tip shows a left upper lobe cavitary lesion without focal enhancement. Thermal scarring posterior to the lesion ➡ remained stable without evidence of local recurrence on subsequent PET/CT.*

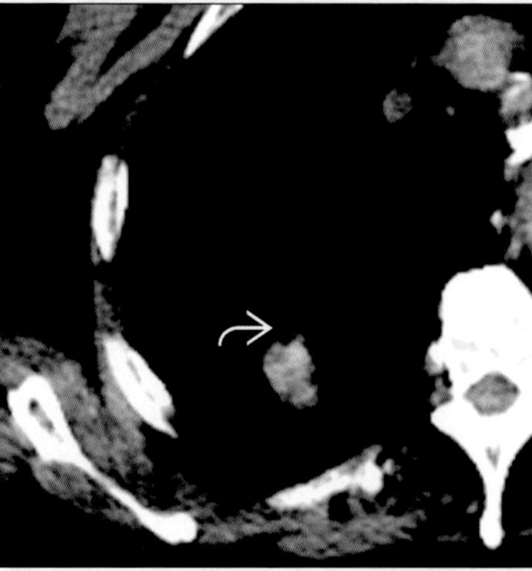

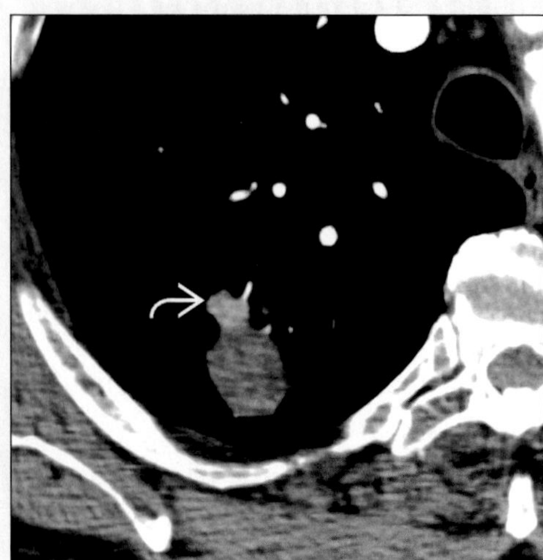

(Left) *Axial PET/CT 6 months after RFA of a 2.2 cm right upper lobe non-small cell lung cancer shows new FDG uptake ➦ at the anterior margin of the ablation scar. FDG uptake following RFA, even when subtle, is suspicious for recurrence.* ***(Right)*** *Axial CECT of the same patient 3 months after the PET/CT shows new focal nodular enhancement ➦. Biopsy confirmed recurrent lung cancer, and repeat ablation was performed. FDG uptake and contrast enhancement post ablation suggest tumor recurrence.*

ABLATION PROCEDURES

TERMINOLOGY

Abbreviations

- **Radiofrequency ablation (RFA)**
- **Microwave ablation (MWA)**
- **Cryoablation = percutaneous cryotherapy (PCT)**

Synonyms

- Thermal ablation

Definitions

- **Thermal ablation**: Used to treat primary or metastatic malignant neoplasms in medically inoperable patients; treatment probes placed percutaneously using real-time image guidance, usually CT
  - RFA uses **electrical current** to induce coagulative necrosis
    - 4 commercially available systems in USA
    - Single treatment typically lasts 10-12 minutes
  - MWA uses **high-frequency electromagnetic waves** to induce frictional heat & coagulative necrosis
    - 7 commercially available systems in USA
    - Single treatment typically lasts 10 minutes
  - PCT uses **compressed argon gas** to induce intracellular ice formation & cellular necrosis
    - 2 commercially available systems in USA
    - Single treatment usually consists of two 10-minute freeze cycles separated by an 8-minute thaw cycle
- **Heat sink effect**: Blood flowing in large vessels adjacent to tumor may dissipate heat away from tumor & compromise treatment zone

IMAGING

General Features

- Location
  - Pulmonary or chest wall masses can be treated with thermal ablation
  - Peripheral tumors are preferable
  - Tumors adjacent to large vessels or airways are more difficult to locally control due to **heat sink effect**
  - Central tumors may be difficult to access due to close proximity to critical structures
- Size
  - Nodules (< 3 cm) treated with better local control, but no definite size limitation
  - Larger tumors require several treatments; can be performed simultaneously using multiple applicators

CT Findings

- Surveillance imaging using both CT & PET/CT is common following thermal ablation
  - Some authors suggest CT with & without contrast at 1 & 3 months, PET/CT at 6 months, then alternating CT & PET/CT every 3 months for 1st 2 years after ablation
  - Beyond 2 years, imaging with CT or PET/CT every 6 months is reasonable
- Immediately after ablation of parenchymal nodule, ground-glass halo measuring at least 5 mm completely surrounding nodule is desirable
  - **Cockade phenomenon**: Appearance of concentric ring(s) surrounding nodule following ablation
- During **PCT**, **low-attenuation ice ball** can be seen surrounding probes, but iceball size underestimates lethal ablation zone
- Ground-glass halo typically resolves within 1 month post ablation
- Locoregional lymph nodes may enlarge & show FDG avidity 1 month post ablation; lymphadenopathy beyond 6 months suggests metastatic disease
- Cavitation within ablation zone & adjacent pleural thickening commonly present up to 3 months post ablation
- Nodules may "grow" within 1st 6 months; growth after 6 months suggests local tumor progression
- Focal nodular enhancement at any point after ablation is suspicious for local tumor progression

MR Findings

- MR uncommonly used to follow pulmonary ablation but has been used following chest wall ablation
  - Focal enhancement following gadolinium administration is suspicious for local tumor recurrence

Ultrasonographic Findings

- US can be used to guide thermal ablation of chest wall masses
- Does not play role in imaging follow-up

Imaging Recommendations

- Best imaging tool
  - Close imaging follow-up with both CECT & PET/CT critical for detection of tumor progression
- Protocol advice
  - Follow-up NECT & CECT suggested; enhancement > 15 HU suspicious for local tumor progression
  - PET/CT performed earlier than 6 months after ablation fraught with false positivity

Nuclear Medicine Findings

- PET/CT
  - FDG-avid foci within ablation zone & locoregional lymph nodes 6 months after ablation are highly suspicious for malignancy; pathologic correlation should be performed

Image-Guided Biopsy

- Commonly performed prior to ablation; in selected patients both procedures can be performed in 1 session with on-site cytology

DIFFERENTIAL DIAGNOSIS

Recurrent Malignancy

- Up to 43% of ablated lesions
- Typically with ablation of lesions > 3 cm
- New or growing nodules within ablated tissue
- FDG avidity &/or contrast enhancement

Pulmonary Infection

- Focal pneumonia
- Fever, leukocytosis

PATHOLOGY

General Features

- Ablation commonly used to treat primary bronchogenic neoplasms & lung metastases (most commonly from colorectal primaries)

ABLATION PROCEDURES

Staging, Grading, & Classification

- Modified RECIST (Response Evaluation Criteria in Solid Tumors) may be used to identify disease progression
  - Any 2 of the following suggest disease progression
    - 20% increase in sum length of tumor
    - Solid mass invading adjacent structures
    - Increasing FDG uptake

Gross Pathologic & Surgical Features

- Ground-glass opacity immediately following ablation corresponds to 3 histologic layers
  - **Peripheral layer**: Nonnecrotic & hemorrhagic debris containing viable cells
  - **Intermediate layer**: Fluid in alveolar spaces
  - **Central layer**: Nuclei with condensed chromatin suggesting cell death

CLINICAL ISSUES

Presentation

- Most common signs/symptoms
  - Local recurrence is typically asymptomatic
  - Chest pain & dyspnea may be due to delayed pneumothorax; a rare complication
    - Most pneumothoraces occur within 2 hours of ablation
- Other signs/symptoms
  - Fever & fatigue common; referred to as **post ablation syndrome**

Natural History & Prognosis

- RFA
  - Complications
    - Pneumothorax is most common with most studies reporting close to 30% incidence
      - More common with emphysema, centrally located tumors, multiple pleural punctures, probe placement through fissure
      - Risk factors similar for all ablation modalities
      - If large or symptomatic, will require chest tube placement
    - Pleural effusions in up to 50%
    - Post ablation syndrome (fever & flu-like symptoms) common following ablation; treated symptomatically
    - Hemoptysis in 2%; may require angiography/ embolization or surgery
    - Bronchopleural fistula: Rare complication that may require treatment with blood patch, endobronchial valves, or surgery
    - Death rarely reported
  - Local tumor progression seen in 30-43% of treated tumors; more frequent in those > 3 cm
    - Histology does not correlate with local control rate
    - Recurrent disease can be re-treated; unlike external beam radiation, there is no limit to number of ablations
  - Stage I non-small cell lung cancer overall survival
    - 78% at 1 year, 57% at 2 years, 36% at 3 years, 27% at 5 years
    - 3-year survival comparable with that of sublobar resection in high-risk patients
    - Shorter hospital stay for patients treated with ablation
- MWA
  - Less clinical data than RFA
  - Complications
    - Pneumothorax: 39%
    - Hemoptysis: 6%
  - Local control rate 67% at 1 year
    - Size of tumor not associated with local control rate
  - Cancer specific mortality yielded 83% 1-year, 73% 2-year, & 61% 3-year survival
- Cryoablation
  - Less clinical data than both RFA & MWA
  - Complications
    - Hemoptysis: Up to 62%
    - Pneumothorax: 12%
  - Limited long-term local tumor progression & outcome data
  - Comparable 3-year survival with that of sublobar resection in high-risk patients

Treatment

- Ablation is typically an outpatient procedure requiring local anesthesia & conscious sedation (rarely requires general anesthesia)
- Choice of ablation modality depends on available technology, operator experience, & local resources
  - No single ablation modality outperforms others in terms of safety or long-term survival
- Combined multimodality treatment using ablation & external beam radiation therapy advocated in small series; may provide survival benefit at increased cost

DIAGNOSTIC CHECKLIST

Consider

- Immediately following ablation, 5-10 mm ground-glass halo is desirable
- Local tumor progression is not uncommon following ablation; radiologists must be familiar with both normal post ablation findings & those that indicate disease progression
- Percutaneous biopsy should be considered when progression of disease is suspected

SELECTED REFERENCES

1. Healey TT et al: Radiofrequency ablation: a safe and effective treatment in nonoperative patients with early-stage lung cancer. Cancer J. 17(1):33-7, 2011
2. Sharma A et al: How I do it: radiofrequency ablation and cryoablation of lung tumors. J Thorac Imaging. 26(2):162-74, 2011
3. Brace CL et al: Pulmonary thermal ablation: comparison of radiofrequency and microwave devices by using gross pathologic and CT findings in a swine model. Radiology. 251(3):705-11, 2009
4. Wolf FJ et al: Microwave ablation of lung malignancies: effectiveness, CT findings, and safety in 50 patients. Radiology. 247(3):871-9, 2008

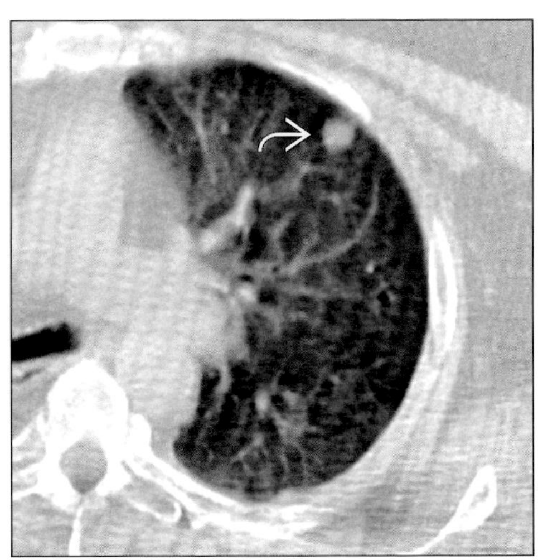

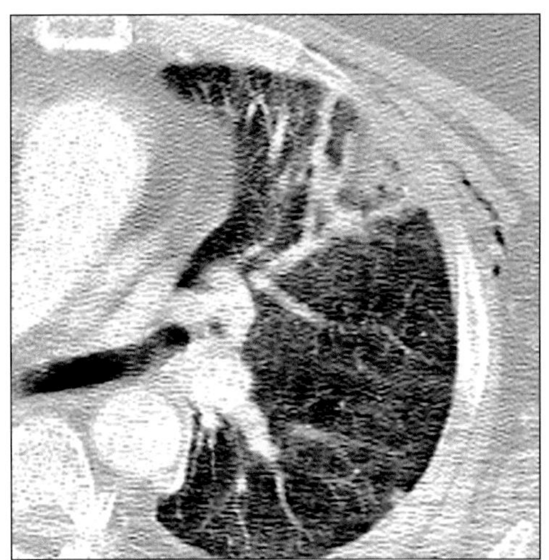

(Left) *Axial NECT shows a peripheral left upper lobe metastasis ➔ in a 65-year-old man with colorectal cancer. The patient also had an expansile right 9th rib lesion (not shown).* ***(Right)*** *Axial NECT of the same patient immediately after a 5-minute radiofrequency ablation shows a 1 cm ground-glass halo surrounding the lung nodule, suggesting adequate safety margins. Left anterior chest wall subcutaneous gas is consistent with recent intervention.*

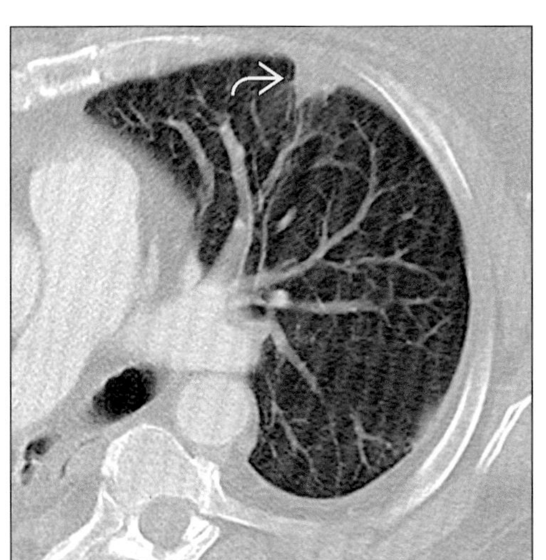

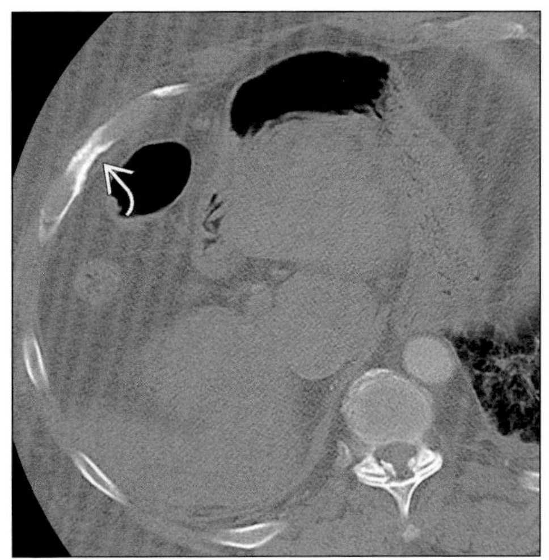

(Left) *Axial CECT of the same patient 2 years after RFA shows retraction and decreased size of the previous abnormality without focal enhancement, findings typical of an ablation scar ➔.* ***(Right)*** *Axial CECT of the same patient shows residual sclerosis in the right 9th anterior rib ➔ 2 years following cryoablation (performed on the same day as lung RFA). A 2.4 cm active tip applicator was used to deliver two 10-minute freeze cycles with an intervening 8-minute thaw cycle.*

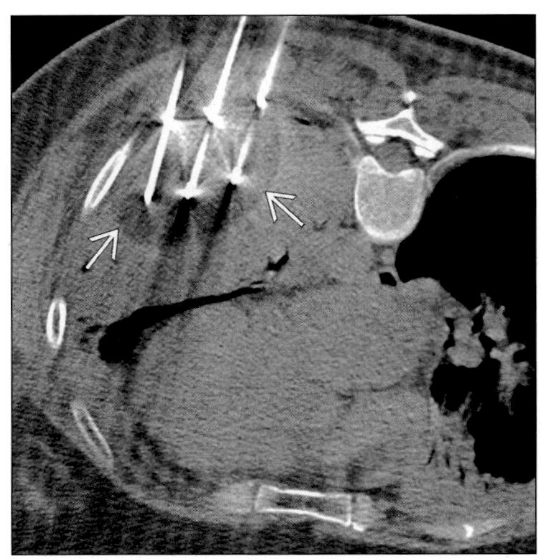

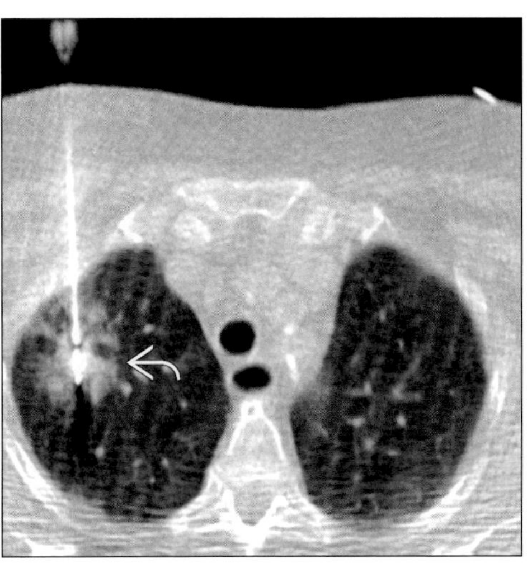

(Left) *Axial NECT of a 56-year-old woman with recurrent painful metastatic left lower lobe primitive neuroectodermal tumor during thermal ablation for palliation shows 3 applicators spaced 2 cm apart at several overlapping locations throughout the 10 cm mass. A low-attenuation iceball ➔ is easily recognized during the freeze cycle.* ***(Right)*** *Axial NECT during a MWA of a 2 cm right upper lobe lung cancer performed with CT fluoroscopy guidance shows an evolving halo of ground-glass opacity ➔.*

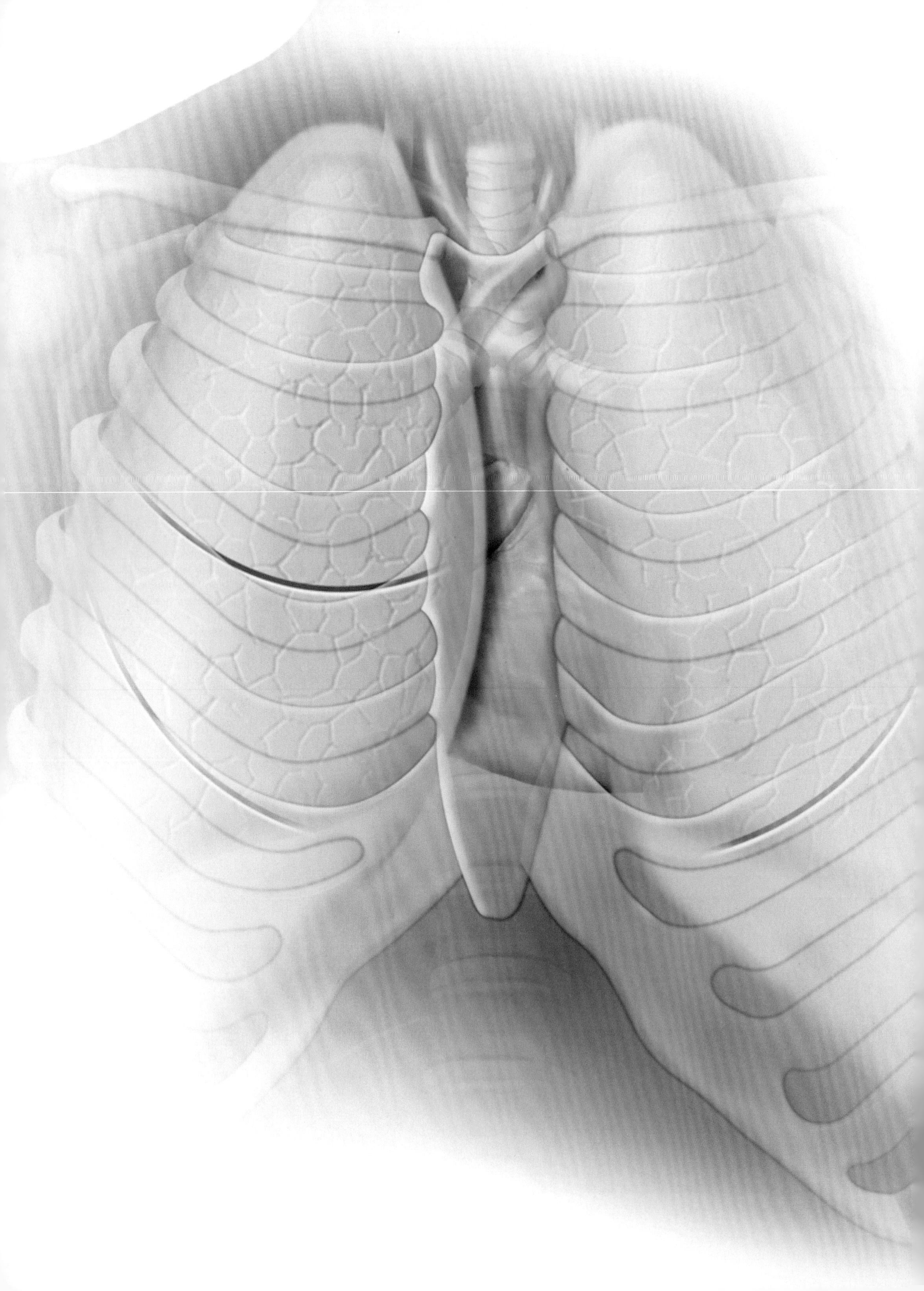

SECTION 12
Pleural Diseases

Introduction and Overview

Effusion

Pneumothorax

Pleural Thickening

Neoplasia

APPROACH TO PLEURAL DISEASES

Introduction

The imaging features of pleural disease are unique and variable, ranging from the thin visceral pleural line of a pneumothorax to pleural masses that may occupy most of a hemithorax. Because of its anatomic distribution, the imaging manifestations of pleural disease may be found from the apex to the most caudal extent of the costodiaphragmatic pleural reflection at the level of the upper abdomen.

The normal pleura is thin and discrete on imaging studies and is most often visible as the thin line of an interlobar fissure on chest radiography. On thin-section CT, the normal pleura is barely visible and may manifest as a thin (1-2 mm) soft tissue line in the intercostal regions.

Radiographic detection of abnormal fluid or air in the pleural space may require the use of decubitus or other views to maneuver the fluid or air into the most dependent or least dependent portions of the thorax, respectively.

Abnormal Air in the Pleural Space

Detection of a pneumothorax should prompt consideration of the clinical setting in which it occurs. In healthy young individuals, a primary spontaneous pneumothorax may develop in the absence of radiographically evident lung disease, most typically in healthy young men. Blunt or penetrating chest trauma may result in unilateral or bilateral pneumothoraces. Iatrogenic causes include placement of central venous catheters, thoracic biopsy procedures, and abdominal procedures at the level of the costodiaphragmatic sulcus. Patients with underlying lung disease may develop secondary spontaneous pneumothoraces, typically related to underlying cystic or infiltrative lung disease. Associated conditions include chronic obstructive lung disease (COPD), emphysema, *Pneumocystis jiroveci* pneumonia (PCP), lymphangioleiomyomatosis, Langerhans cell histiocytosis, and Marfan syndrome. In all cases of pneumothorax, it is imperative to search for imaging signs of tension, which is a medical emergency due to the potential for mediastinal displacement that may lead to fatal vascular compromise.

Abnormal Fluid in the Pleural Space

The imaging manifestations of pleural effusion vary with the size of the fluid collection. In the upright patient, the smallest pleural effusions may blunt the costophrenic sulcus, with volumes as small as 50 mL detectable on lateral chest radiography whereas 200 mL is the minimum volume detectable on frontal radiography. With increasing volume, pleural effusions may obscure the ipsilateral hemidiaphragm in upright patients or manifest as a veil-like opacity extending over the involved hemithorax in supine individuals. Less commonly, fluid may accumulate in the pleural space between the undersurface of the lung and the underlying hemidiaphragm (subpulmonic effusion) or form focal opacities within interlobar fissures (pseudotumors).

Loculated pleural effusions form opacities that are typically lenticular in shape with tapering, obtuse margins along their interface with the adjacent pleural surface; they may produce compressive atelectasis in the adjacent lung, with resultant airspace opacity that may obscure the margins of the loculated fluid collection. When an air-fluid level is detected within a loculated pleural fluid collection, it is most suggestive of an underlying bronchopleural fistula rather than infection with gas-forming microorganisms. A useful radiographic clue as to the nature of the air-fluid level is the evaluation of the length of such air-fluid levels on orthogonal (PA vs. lateral) radiographs. Air-fluid levels within loculated pleural fluid collections tend to have a disparity in their lengths when compared on PA and lateral radiographs, whereas air-fluid levels within roughly spherical lung abscesses tend to be equal on similar comparisons.

The thickened visceral and parietal pleura that surrounds a loculated pleural fluid collection is most readily demonstrated on contrast-enhanced CT. The involved pleural layers may appear to separate or split to enclose such collections and manifest as the "**split pleura" sign**, a CT finding that is suggestive, but not necessarily diagnostic, of an empyema.

The most common cause of a transudative pleural effusion is congestive heart failure (CHF). Most effusions associated with CHF are bilateral (88%), but they may be unilateral and right-sided (8%) or left-sided (4%). Because of its relatively low incidence in patients with CHF, detection of a unilateral pleural effusion should prompt consideration of other etiologies. For instance, it has been shown that 25% of patients with CHF have pleural effusions related to pneumonia or pulmonary emboli.

Parapneumonic pleural effusions occur in 44% of patients with pneumonia and may be sterile or infected. In patients with community-acquired pneumonia and pleural effusions, there is an increased relative risk of mortality, whether such effusions are unilateral (3.4x higher) or bilateral (7.0x higher). Parapneumonic pleural effusions may be free flowing or loculated.

Malignant pleural effusions are the most common thoracic manifestation of metastatic disease and are typically exudates. They occur most commonly in patients with primary malignancies of the lung and breast but may also develop in patients with any other primary malignant tumor that involves the thorax. The imaging manifestations of malignant pleural effusions are similar to those of other pleural effusions, but pleural thickening &/ or nodularity may be apparent, especially on CT imaging.

Pleural Thickening without Calcification

Pleural thickening may be focal, multifocal, or diffuse. Focal pleural thickening is most commonly related to pleural fibrosis but may also be a manifestation of pleural malignancy, whether primary (i.e., mesothelioma) or metastatic. Pleural fibrosis is the second most common pleural abnormality after pleural effusion. It may be due to a variety of etiologies but is most often a complication of inflammatory disease. It is often focal but may be diffuse and may encase the lung to the extent that functional abnormalities result. Focal pleural fibrosis represents healed pleuritis that may be related to previous bacterial or mycobacterial infection or related to trauma, including iatrogenic causes (e.g., surgery, radiation therapy). It may obscure the involved costophrenic sulcus and mimic a small pleural effusion.

Pleural plaques are benign hyalinized fibrous tissue collections that are considered a marker of previous asbestos exposure, with a latency period of 15-20 years or more. They occur as bilateral, multifocal discontinuous areas of pleural thickening that may or may not be calcified. They are typically distributed along the costal pleural surfaces posterolaterally (6th-9th ribs), the diaphragmatic pleura, and the paravertebral pleura. Electron microscopic studies demonstrate submicroscopic asbestos fibers in the majority of pleural plaques evaluated in this manner.

Pleural Thickening with Calcification

Pleural calcification may occur with pleural thickening related to pleural plaques or as a result of focal or diffuse pleural fibrosis caused by various etiologies, including pleurodesis. Calcification in pleural plaques may be focal or multifocal, punctate or extensive, and is often more easily detectable on chest radiography than its associated soft tissue components.

Incomplete Border Sign

Pleural lesions may manifest with incomplete borders on chest radiography, a finding suggestive of an extraparenchymal process (typically of pleural or chest wall origin). Subpleural parenchymal lesions and mediastinal/paravertebral masses should also be considered when the incomplete border sign is detected.

Extraparenchymal masses arising from the pleura, chest wall, or mediastinum may have tapering components that form obtuse margins along their interface with the adjacent pleural surface. Tapering and obtusely angled margins are the components of a mass most likely to lack a tangential relationship to an x-ray beam and thus produce the incomplete border sign.

Pleural lesions that produce the incomplete border sign may be neoplastic or nonneoplastic. Nonneoplastic entities include pleural plaques and loculated pleural effusion. Neoplastic entities include localized fibrous tumor, pleural metastases, and malignant mesothelioma.

Pleural Neoplasms

Pleural neoplasms manifest with a variety of imaging features, a reflection of the growth patterns that may occur with pleural tumors. Typically, a pleural mass has a lentiform shape with tapering, obtusely angled interfaces where the mass merges with the adjacent pleural surface. Tumors with such obtusely angled margins often manifest as masses with incomplete borders on chest radiographs, an imaging feature that should prompt consideration of extrapulmonary etiologies. Larger pleural tumors often overgrow those obtusely angled interfaces and manifest with acutely angled junctions at the pleural interface. Pleural masses that occur within interlobar fissures may be fusiform in configuration, with tapering margins oriented along the axis of the involved fissure.

Four CT features of pleural thickening that have been associated with pleural malignancy are **pleural thickening > 1 cm**, associated **nodularity**, **circumferential pleural thickening** within the involved hemithorax, and **involvement of the mediastinal pleura**. Detection of these CT features in cases of pleural thickening should raise the suspicion of pleural malignancy, whether each feature is present as an isolated finding or in any combination with other features. Involvement of the mediastinal pleura is a suspicious feature because benign pleural thickening (e.g., fibrothorax) spares the mediastinal pleura in 88% of cases, a significant exception being pleural thickening related to tuberculosis.

Pleural Metastases

Pleural metastases are the most common pleural malignancy and should be considered when a malignant pattern of pleural thickening is detected. Pleural metastases may be focal or multifocal, unilateral or bilateral, and more commonly involve visceral rather than parietal pleural surfaces. The presence of bilateral pleural masses is most suggestive of metastatic disease.

Mesothelioma

The imaging features of mesothelioma cannot be reliably distinguished from those of pleural metastases, and both are leading diagnostic considerations when the malignant pattern of pleural thickening is detected in adult patients. Approximately 90% of mesotheliomas are confined to one hemithorax, and, although most cases of mesothelioma can be linked to a history of asbestos exposure, only 25% of individuals with mesothelioma will also have pleural plaques as a marker of that exposure.

Mimics of Pleural Malignancy

Loculated pleural fluid may produce focal or multifocal mass-like opacities that may mimic pleural malignancy on chest radiography by manifesting with similar imaging features. CT typically reveals the fluid attenuation content of these opacities and resolves concerns for malignant pleural disease.

Victims of penetrating trauma to the left upper abdominal quadrant are susceptible to splenic disruption that may disperse fragments of spleen onto the adjacent peritoneal surface, where they may implant and flourish as peritoneal splenosis. When the left hemidiaphragm is disrupted, this process may extend into the left lower hemithorax as thoracic splenosis, with resultant nodular implants of functioning splenic tissue along the pleural surfaces. Radionuclide liver-spleen scintigraphy demonstrates activity within the implants and is diagnostic of this condition.

Prior talc pleurodesis may produce multifocal pleural nodules and areas of pleural thickening that are typically FDG-avid on PET-CT. Knowledge of the history of prior pleural intervention and high attenuation or dense calcification within the pleural abnormalities allow the formulation of a specific diagnosis.

Selected References

1. Noppen M: Spontaneous pneumothorax: epidemiology, pathophysiology and cause. Eur Respir Rev. 19(117):217-9, 2010
2. Cugell DW et al: Asbestos and the pleura: a review. Chest. 125(3):1103-17, 2004
3. Lee YC et al: Management of malignant pleural effusions. Respirology. 9(2):148-56, 2004
4. Rosado-de-Christenson ML et al: From the archives of the AFIP: Localized fibrous tumor of the pleura. Radiographics. 23(3):759-83, 2003
5. Light RW: Clinical practice. Pleural effusion. N Engl J Med. 346(25):1971-7, 2002
6. Peacock C et al: Asbestos-related benign pleural disease. Clin Radiol. 55(6):422-32, 2000
7. Leung AN et al: CT in differential diagnosis of diffuse pleural disease. AJR Am J Roentgenol. 154(3):487-92, 1990

(Left) Graphic shows the distribution of the parietal pleura (blue), including its caudal extent in the costophrenic recesses ➡. The lungs with their visceral pleural investment are visible through the parietal pleura. The interlobar fissures ↗, formed by 2 layers of visceral pleura, demarcate the pulmonary lobes. *(Right)* Coronal NECT shows visceral pleura forming the minor ➡ and right and left major fissures ➡. Fissures manifest on CT as thin linear or ground-glass opacities.

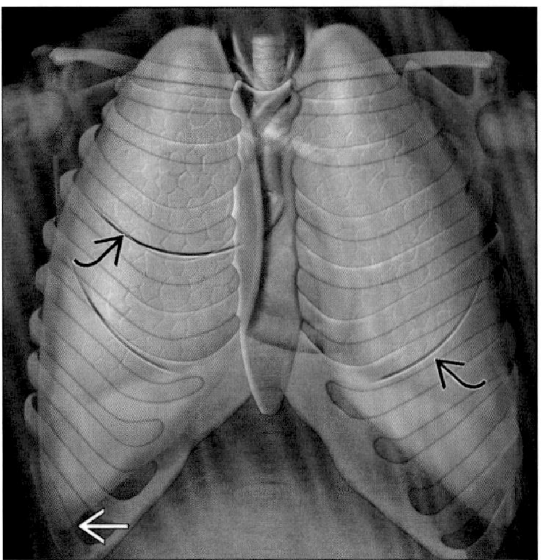

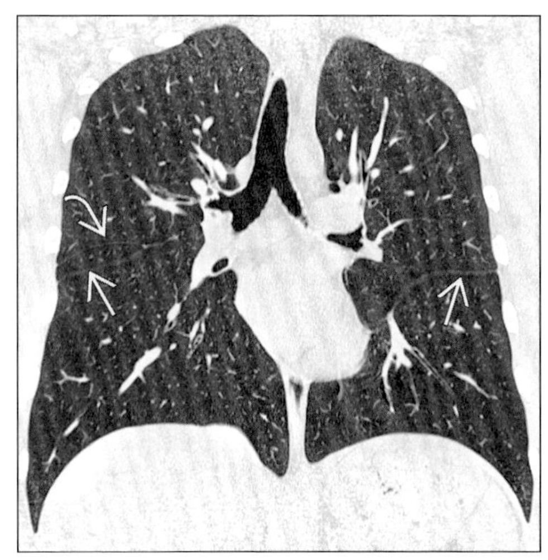

(Left) Graphic shows the caudal extent of the lateral costophrenic sulcus, formed by apposing layers of visceral pleura ➡. The recess extends inferiorly to the level of the kidney whereas the visceral pleura covering the lung ➡ has a more limited caudal extent within the costophrenic sulcus. *(Right)* Composite image with PA chest radiograph (left) and coronal MR (right) shows a costophrenic sulcus pneumothorax ↗ in a supine patient and mesothelioma in the costophrenic sulcus ➡.

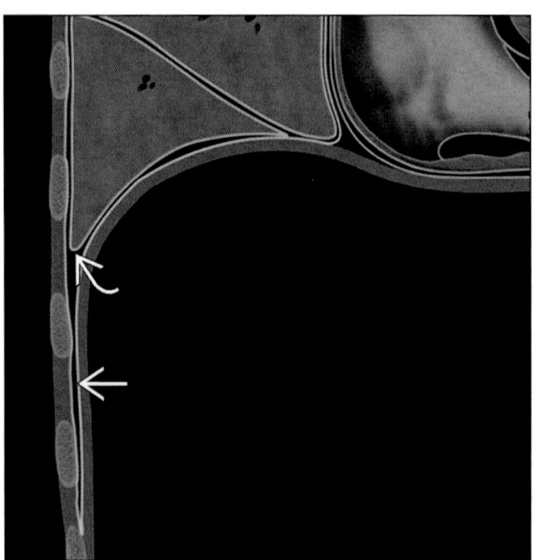

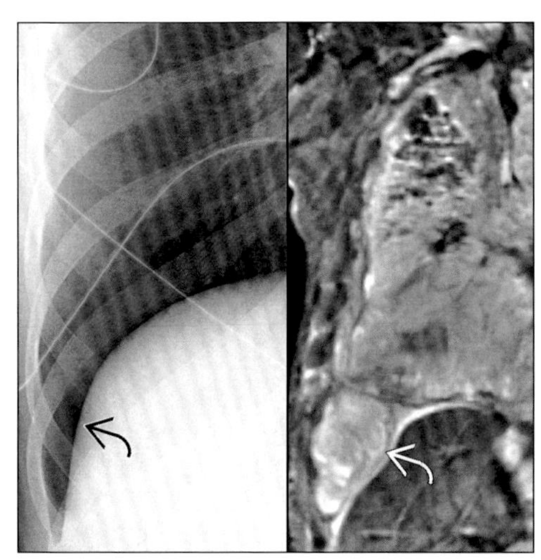

(Left) Composite image with PA chest radiographs of the right and left lungs shows a right pneumothorax manifesting with a visceral pleural line ➡. The normal apposed left visceral and parietal pleural surfaces are not apparent on radiography. *(Right)* Composite image with PA chest radiographs of small (left) and moderate (right) pleural effusions shows a meniscus-shaped opacity ↗ in the costophrenic sulcus and a moderate effusion extending into the minor ➡ and major ➡ fissures.

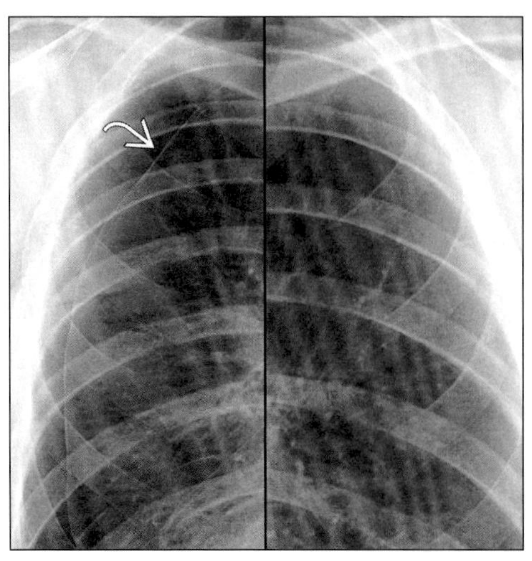

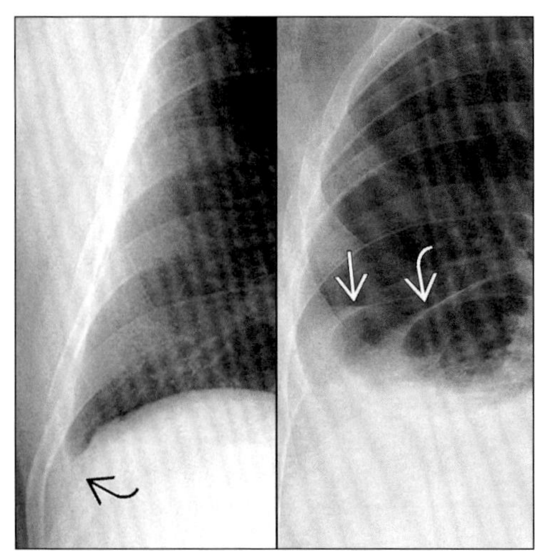

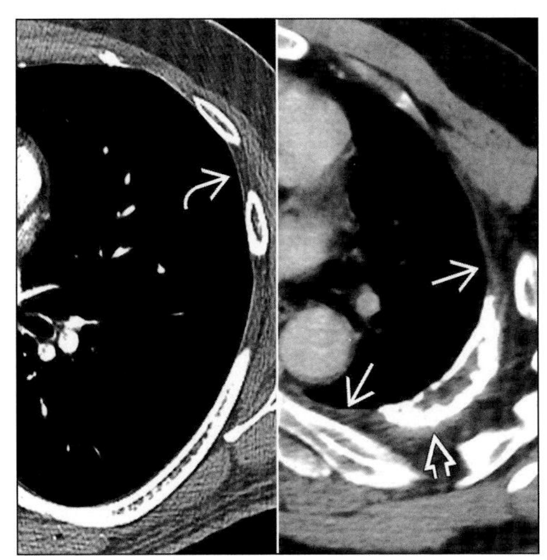

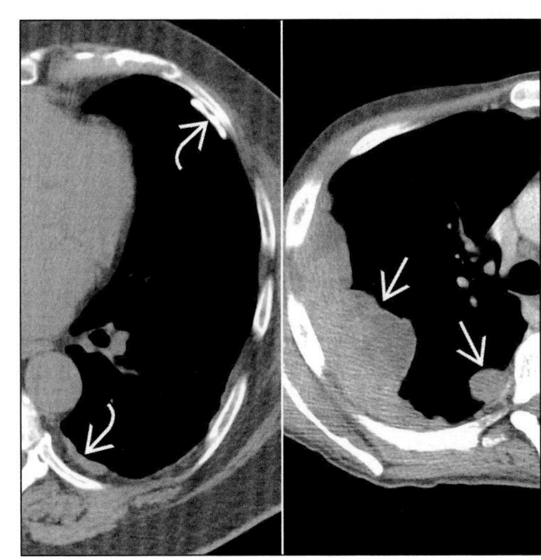

(Left) *Composite image with axial CECT of normal pleura (left) and pleural thickening (right) shows the inconspicuous CT appearance of normal pleura, seen as a 1-2 mm line , and pleural thickening manifesting as a more apparent soft tissue line/band that merges with extensive pleural calcification .* ***(Right)*** *Composite image with NECT (left) and CECT (right) shows noncalcified and calcified pleural plaques and pleural metastases manifesting as pleural thickening and nodularity .*

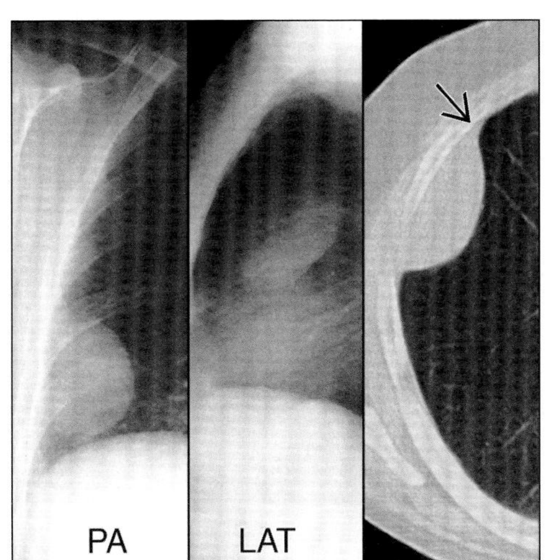

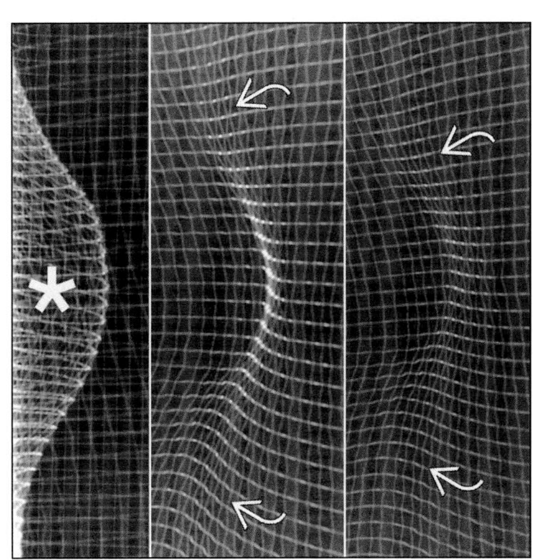

(Left) *Composite image with PA (left) and lateral (center) chest radiographs and axial NECT (right) shows the characteristic shape of a pleural mass with obtuse margins at its interface with the adjacent pleura .* ***(Right)*** *Composite radiograph of a wire-mesh model of a mass (*) was obtained with tangential x-ray beam (left) and at 30° (middle) and 60° (right). As the "mass" loses its tangential relationship to the beam, its radiographic image loses those parts of its border with obtuse margins .*

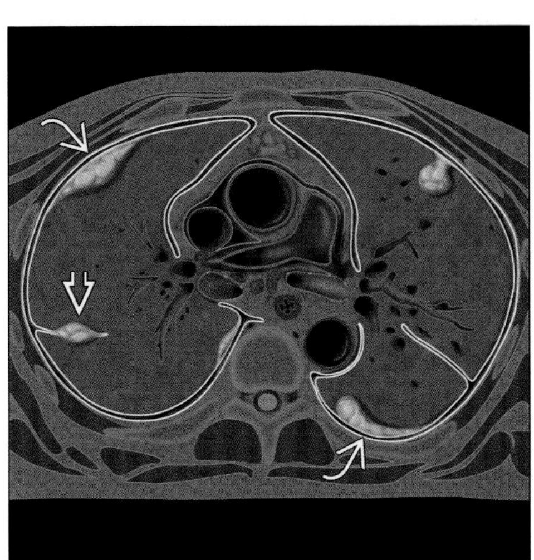

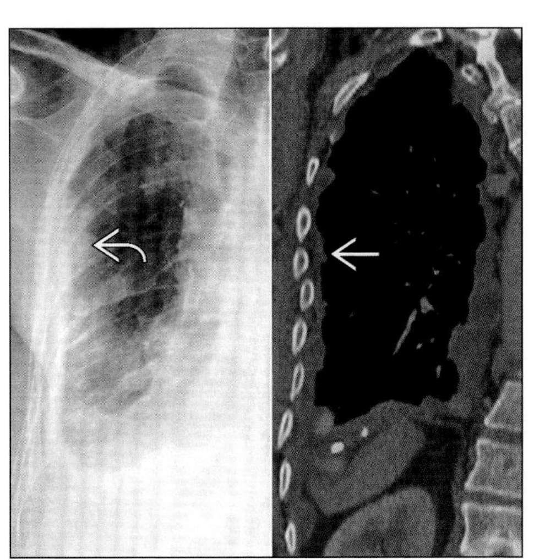

(Left) *Graphic shows the variable shapes of pleural masses. Those along fissures may be fusiform , while those along peripheral pleural surfaces may be symmetrically or asymmetrically lenticular with obtuse or acute angles at their interface with the adjacent pleura.* ***(Right)*** *Composite image with PA chest radiograph (left) and fused PET-CT (right) shows mesothelioma manifesting as circumferential nodular pleural thickening that exhibits FDG avidity .*

TRANSUDATIVE PLEURAL EFFUSION

Key Facts

Terminology
- Ultrafiltrate of plasma; low cell & protein content
- Rate of pleural fluid production exceeds reabsorption

Imaging
- Radiography
  - Blunt costophrenic sulci
  - Subpulmonic pleural effusion
  - Supine radiography: Decreased sensitivity for fluid
  - Fissural fluid: Pseudotumor
  - Mediastinal shift away from effusion; > 1,000 mL
  - Layering fluid 1 cm thick, effusion amenable to thoracentesis
- CT
  - Increased sensitivity for pleural fluid
  - No distinction between exudate & transudate
- Ultrasound: Anechoic fluid; may represent either transudate or exudate

Top Differential Diagnoses
- Exudative pleural effusion
- Elevated diaphragm
- Chronic pleural fibrosis
- Pleural mass

Pathology
- Intact pleural surfaces
- Imbalance of Starling forces
- Congestive heart failure
- Hypoalbuminemia: < 1.5 g/dL

Clinical Issues
- Signs & symptoms
  - Dyspnea, mild nonproductive cough, chest pain
- Treatment
  - Treatment of underlying condition
  - Thoracentesis, chest tube, pleurodesis

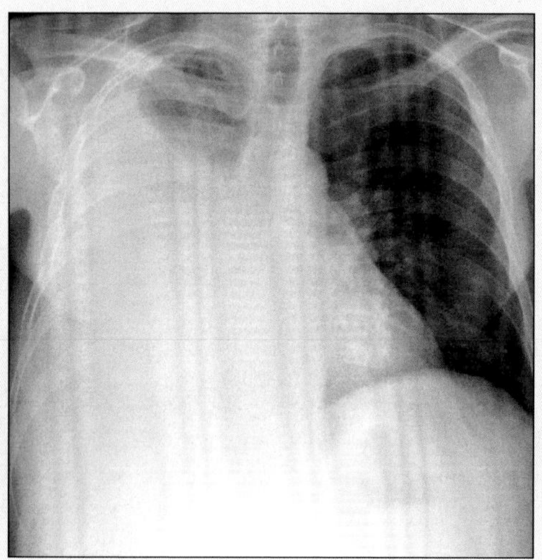

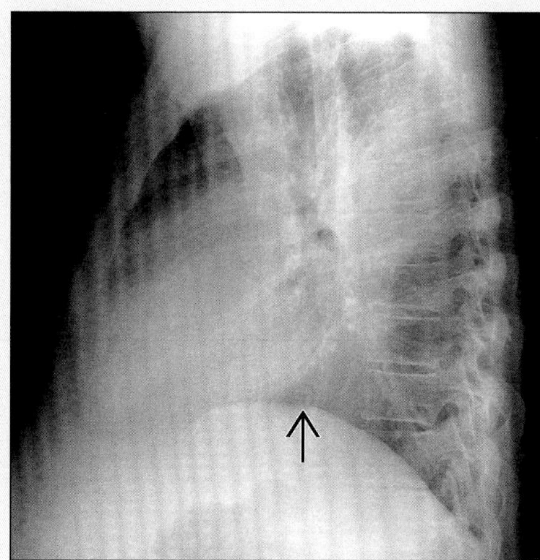

(Left) *PA chest radiograph of a 54-year-old man with dyspnea and a history of cirrhosis shows a large right pleural effusion that produces extensive right lung relaxation atelectasis and obscures the right heart border and the right hemidiaphragm. The left pleural space is normal.* ***(Right)*** *Lateral chest radiograph of the same patient shows obscuration of the right hemidiaphragm by the large right pleural effusion. Only the left hemidiaphragm ➔ is visible.*

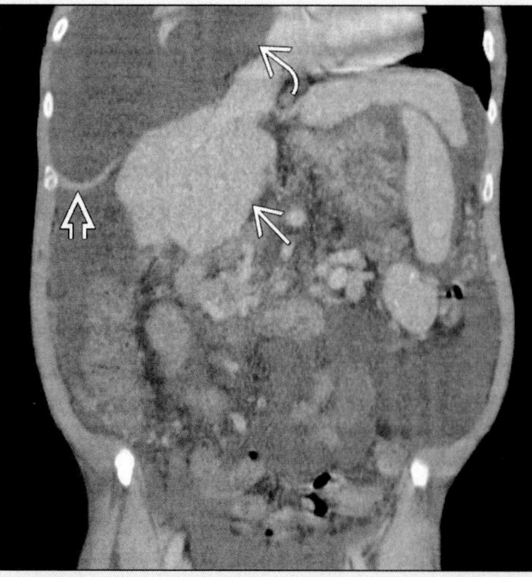

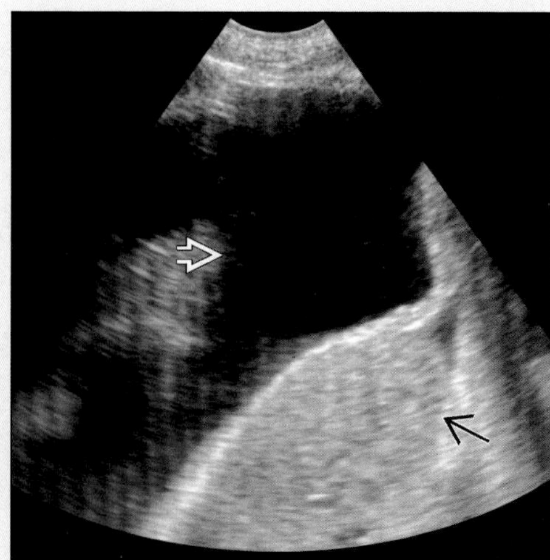

(Left) *Coronal CECT of the same patient shows a small shrunken nodular liver ➔ secondary to known cirrhosis, massive ascites, and a large right pleural effusion ➔ that produces inversion of the right hemidiaphragm ➔.* ***(Right)*** *Long axis ultrasound of the same patient was performed to evaluate the right inferior hemithorax prior to thoracentesis. It shows a large anechoic right pleural effusion ➔ that proved to be transudative and a small cirrhotic hyperechoic liver ➔.*

TRANSUDATIVE PLEURAL EFFUSION

TERMINOLOGY

Definitions

- Ultrafiltrate of plasma characterized by low cell & protein content
- **Diagnostic criteria**
  - < 1,000 cells/mm³, lymphocytes, mesothelial cells
  - Ratio of pleural fluid:serum protein < 0.5
  - Ratio of pleural fluid:serum lactate dehydrogenase (LDH) < 0.6
  - Pleural fluid LDH < 2/3 of upper limit of normal serum value
- Rate of pleural fluid production exceeds reabsorption

IMAGING

General Features

- Best diagnostic clue
  - Blunt costophrenic angle (CPA)
- Location
  - Pleural space
- Size
  - Variable: Small to massive
- Morphology
  - Variable

Radiographic Findings

- Fluid accumulation on upright radiography
  - Subpulmonic > posterior CPA > lateral CPA
- **Blunt costophrenic sulci**
  - Blunt posterior costophrenic sulcus (lateral radiograph); 50 mL of pleural fluid
  - Blunt lateral costophrenic sulcus (frontal radiograph); 200 mL of pleural fluid
- **Subpulmonic pleural effusion**
  - Interface between basilar lung & fluid: Pseudohemidiaphragm
  - Flattening & elevation of pseudohemidiaphragm
  - Lateral shift of pseudohemidiaphragm apex
  - Separation of gastric bubble from pseudohemidiaphragm (normal < 1.5 cm)
  - Pseudohemidiaphragm flat anteriorly with sharp descent at major fissure (Rock of Gibraltar sign)
- **Hemidiaphragmatic inversion**
  - Large pleural effusion: > 2,000 mL
  - Medial displacement of gastric air bubble
  - Paradoxical respiration on fluoroscopy (pendelluft)
    - Inspiration: Inverted hemidiaphragm ascends
    - Expiration: Inverted hemidiaphragm descends
- **Fissural fluid**
  - May preferentially accumulate fluid or air in COPD
  - Pseudotumor (mass-like fissural fluid) formation
  - Fluid in incomplete major fissure may mimic pneumothorax or pneumomediastinum
  - Fissural fluid exhibits curvilinear edge concave toward hilum
- Mediastinal shift away from effusion: > 1,000 mL
- Supine radiography: Decreased sensitivity for fluid
  - Sensitivity 70%, up to 500 mL for reliable detection
  - Diffuse increase in hemithorax density with visible vascular structures, meniscus often absent
  - Apical cap
    - Apex most dependent portion of pleural space in supine position
- Common associated conditions
  - **Congestive heart failure** (CHF)
    - Bilateral effusions, relatively equal size
    - Cardiomegaly, vascular indistinctness, interstitial & alveolar edema
  - **Hepatic cirrhosis**
    - Right effusion (70%); left (15%); bilateral (15%)
    - Small to massive

CT Findings

- **High sensitivity** for detection of pleural fluid
  - Visualization of effusions as small as 10 mL
- No reliable distinction between exudates & transudates
- Homogeneous pleural fluid attenuation (water)
- Smooth thin pleural surfaces, extrapleural fat attenuation
- Ex vacuo pleural effusion
  - Secondary to bronchial obstruction by neoplasm or foreign body
- Pleural effusion vs. ascites
  - Pleural fluid peripheral; ascites central
  - Pleural fluid displaces diaphragmatic crus anteriorly, posterior to bare area of liver
  - Pleural fluid interface with liver or spleen indistinct, sharp with ascites
  - Pleural fluid appears progressively smaller from cephalad to caudad
  - Pitfall: Findings reversed for inverted hemidiaphragm

Ultrasonographic Findings

- **High sensitivity** for detection of pleural fluid
- Anechoic effusions may be transudates or exudates (50%)

Imaging Recommendations

- Best imaging tool
  - Lateral decubitus radiography: Detection of as little as 5 mL of pleural fluid
    - Documentation of free pleural effusion
    - Fluid layering of 1 cm: Indicates effusion > 200 mL, amenable to thoracentesis
- CECT can provide information about pleural fluid quantity, pleural surfaces, & underlying lung
- Ultrasound useful for thoracentesis guidance
  - Can be performed at bedside; can be used for chest tube placement

DIFFERENTIAL DIAGNOSIS

Exudative Pleural Effusion

- Heterogeneous fluid attenuation
- Nodular thickened pleural surfaces

Elevated Diaphragm

- Sharp costophrenic angles, apex not shifted laterally

Chronic Pleural Fibrosis

- No fluid layering on decubitus views
- No fluid on ultrasound

Pleural Mass

- Contrast enhancement
- Solid lesion on ultrasound

TRANSUDATIVE PLEURAL EFFUSION

PATHOLOGY

General Features

- Etiology
  - Congestive heart failure
  - Cirrhosis: Associated with transdiaphragmatic movement of ascites
  - Atelectasis: Decreased pleural pressures
  - Peritoneal dialysis: Transdiaphragmatic movement of peritoneal dialysate into pleural space
  - Hypoalbuminemia: < 1.5 g/dL
  - Nephrotic syndrome: Hypoalbuminemia, hypervolemia, increased hydrostatic pressures
  - Urinothorax: Retroperitoneal urine leakage migrates to pleural space through diaphragmatic lymphatics
  - Postpartum: Hypervolemia & high intrathoracic pressures from Valsalva maneuvers
  - Central line placement in pleural space
  - Myxedema: Due to associated heart failure or pneumonia

Physiologic Features

- Pleural fluid normally formed as ultrafiltrate from parietal pleura capillaries
  - Removed by lymphatics draining lower costal, mediastinal, & diaphragmatic pleura
  - Removed by capillaries across visceral pleural mesothelium
- Starling forces: Balance between
  - Hydrostatic & oncotic forces in visceral & parietal pleural vessels
  - Lymphatic drainage
- Pleural effusions result from imbalance of Starling forces
- Specific diseases
  - Left heart failure
    - Pulmonary venous hypertension essential for pleural fluid development
    - Increased interstitial pressure in subpleural region
    - Edema fluid leaks from visceral pleura
  - Isolated right heart failure: Pleural effusion, unusual

Gross Pathologic & Surgical Features

- Normal pleural fluid volume: Approximately 5 mL total (2.5 mL/hemithorax)
- Normal pleural surface area: 2,000 cm^2, no communication between pleural spaces

Microscopic Features

- Intact visceral and parietal pleural surfaces

CLINICAL ISSUES

Presentation

- Most common signs/symptoms
  - **Dyspnea**
  - Mild nonproductive cough
  - Chest pain
  - Large effusions may invert hemidiaphragm & impair ventilation
  - Asymptomatic effusions common in CHF, postoperative and postpartum patients
- Other signs/symptoms
  - Physical findings do not usually manifest unless pleural effusions > 300 mL
  - **D'Amato sign**
    - Change in dullness to chest percussion with change in patient position due to movement of free pleural fluid
  - Patients with CHF on diuretics, effusions incorrectly diagnosed as exudative

Demographics

- Age
  - Neonatal to elderly
- Gender
  - M:F = 1:1
- Epidemiology
  - Common: **1,300,000 pleural effusions per year diagnosed in United States**
  - CHF is most common cause
    - 3/4 of patients will have effusions at some time
    - Bilateral (88%); unilateral right (8%); unilateral left (4%)

Natural History & Prognosis

- Treated CHF: Fluid resorbs in days to weeks
- Ex vacuo effusions: Resolve as lung expands

Treatment

- CHF: Diuretics, digitalis, afterload reduction
- **Thoracentesis**
  - May partially relieve symptoms
  - Fluid analysis essential to differentiate transudate from exudate
  - Blind tap safe for fluid > 1 cm thickness on lateral decubitus radiography
- Relative indications for thoracentesis
  - Unilateral effusion or effusions of disparate size
  - Absence of cardiomegaly
  - Fever, pleuritic chest pain
- Relative contraindications for thoracentesis
  - Effusions < 1 cm thickness on lateral decubitus radiography; bleeding diathesis, systemic anticoagulation
  - Mechanical ventilation; cutaneous disease over puncture site
- Complications of thoracentesis
  - Pneumothorax, hemothorax, empyema, chest wall hematoma, reexpansion pulmonary edema
- Chest tube drainage for symptomatic effusions
- Pleurodesis with doxycycline or talc for refractory large effusions
  - CHF: May result in increased contralateral effusion

DIAGNOSTIC CHECKLIST

Image Interpretation Pearls

- Pleural pseudotumor typically occurs in CHF-related pleural effusion

SELECTED REFERENCES

1. Ayres J et al: Imaging of the pleura. Semin Respir Crit Care Med. 31(6):674-88, 2010
2. Abramowitz Y et al: Pleural effusion: characterization with CT attenuation values and CT appearance. AJR Am J Roentgenol. 192(3):618-23, 2009

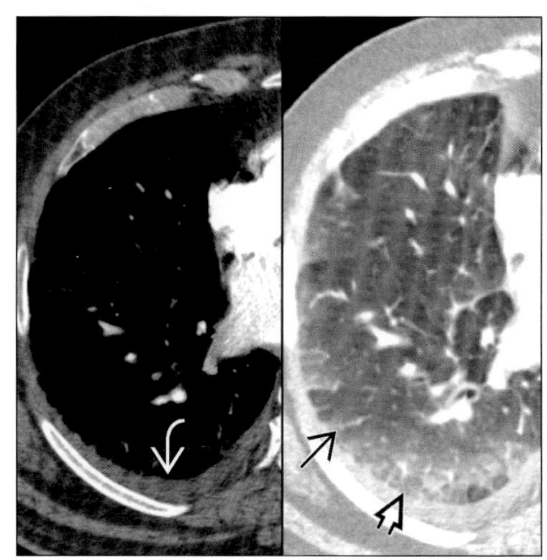

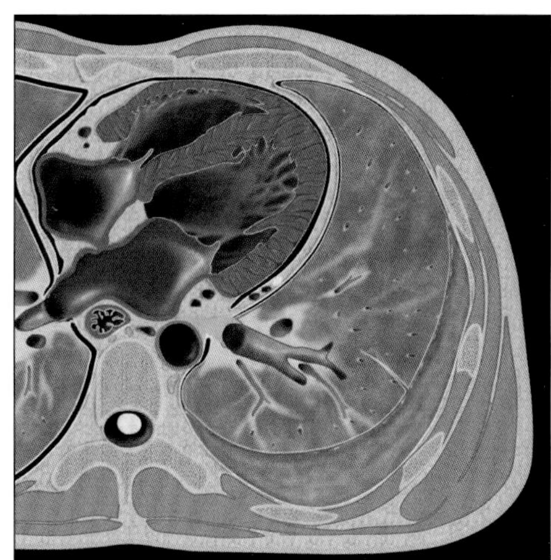

(Left) *Composite image with axial CECT in soft tissue (left) and lung (right) window of a 60-year-old man who presented with dyspnea, frothy sputum, and heart failure shows a small right pleural effusion, smooth interlobular septal thickening, and patchy ground-glass opacities, consistent with interstitial and alveolar edema.* ***(Right)*** *Graphic shows features of transudative pleural effusions, which are typically free and occur without associated pleural thickening or nodularity.*

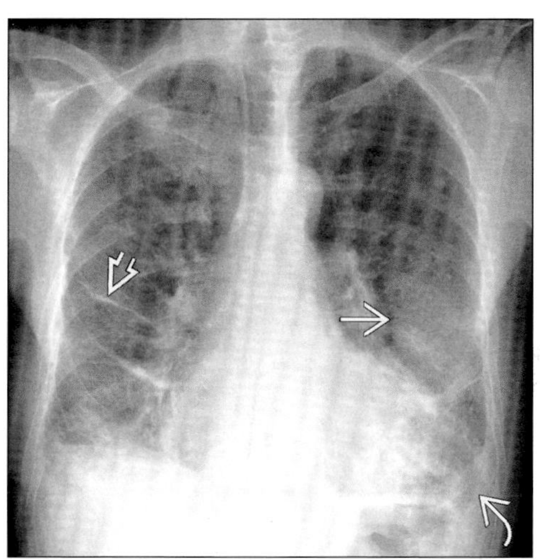

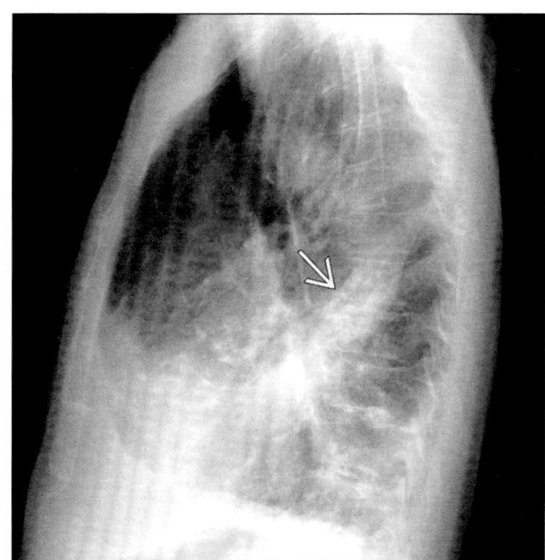

(Left) *PA chest radiograph of a 63-year-old man with heart failure shows interstitial edema manifesting with interlobular septal thickening with Kerley A and B lines and bilateral transudative pleural effusions. Loculated fluid in the major fissure results in a vague opacity in the left hemithorax.* ***(Right)*** *Lateral chest radiograph of the same patient shows pleural fluid in the left major fissure, a so-called pseudotumor. Fissural fluid is frequent in patients with heart failure.*

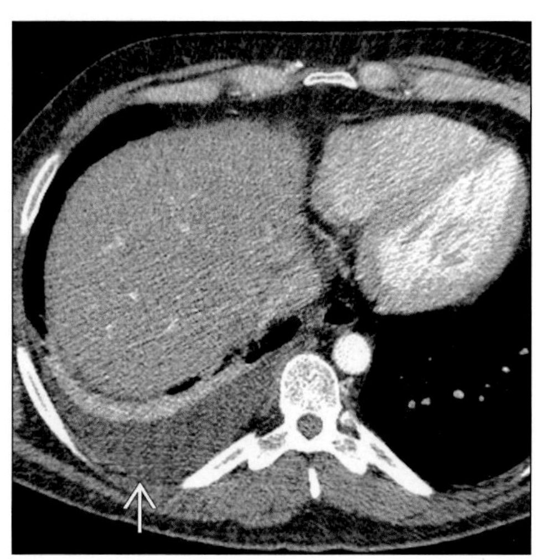

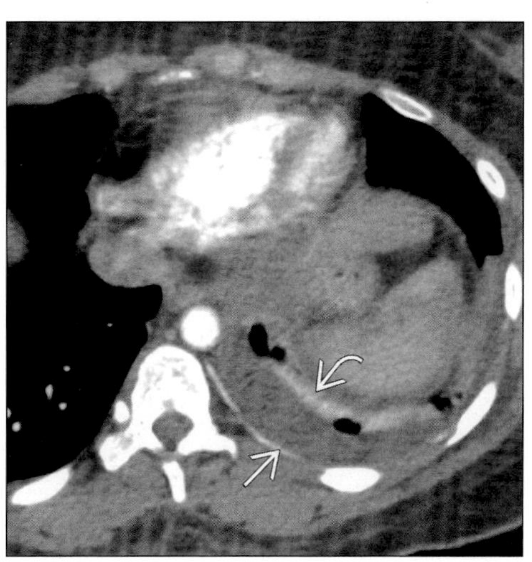

(Left) *Axial CECT of a 45-year-old man with myxedema shows a right transudative pleural effusion that resolved after 3 months of thyroid hormone replacement therapy.* ***(Right)*** *Axial CECT of a 16-year-old woman with acute nephrotic syndrome shows a transudative left pleural effusion with associated left lower lobe relaxation atelectasis. Transudative pleural effusions commonly affect patients with decreased plasma oncotic pressure due to entities such as cirrhosis and nephrotic syndrome.*

EXUDATIVE PLEURAL EFFUSION

Key Facts

Terminology

- Definition
  - Proteinaceous fluid; increased pleural permeability
  - Pleural inflammation; lymphatic obstruction
- Pleural fluid characteristics
  - Pleural fluid protein:serum protein > 0.5
  - Pleural fluid LDH:serum LDH > 0.6
  - Pleural fluid LDH > 2/3 upper limit of serum LDH

Imaging

- Radiography
  - Pleural effusion; may be loculated
  - Air-fluid level; bronchopleural fistula
- CT
  - Variable attenuation pleural fluid
  - Pleural thickening; smooth, nodular
  - Assessment of empyema
  - Air-fluid level; bronchopleural fistula
- PET: Assessment of underlying malignancy

Top Differential Diagnoses

- Transudative pleural effusion
- Empyema
- Pleural malignancy
- Pleural fibrosis & fibrothorax

Pathology

- Etiologies
  - Infection
  - Malignant neoplasms
  - Collagen vascular diseases
  - Pulmonary embolism & infarction
  - Drug induced

Clinical Issues

- Pleural fluid analysis for diagnosis
- Empyema requires early chest tube drainage

(Left) *PA chest radiograph of a 66-year-old man with chest pain shows a large right pleural effusion and adjacent right lung relaxation atelectasis.* ***(Right)*** *Axial CECT (mediastinal window) of the same patient shows enhancement of a smoothly thickened parietal pleura ⇨ and relaxation atelectasis → of the right lower lobe. Pleural fluid analysis showed a lymphocytic exudate consistent with tuberculous pleural effusion. Exudative pleural effusions are often secondary to infection or malignancy.*

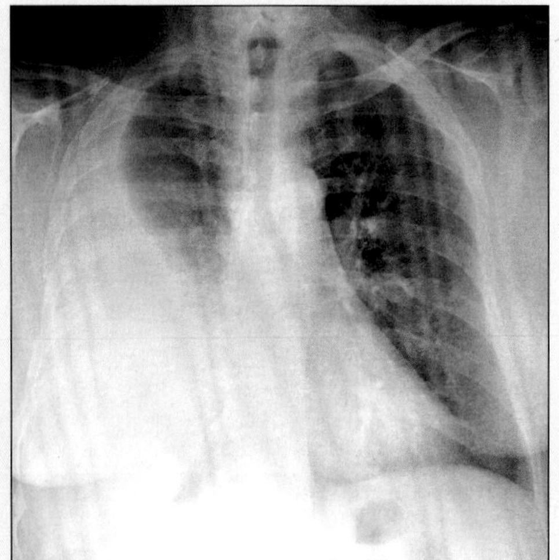

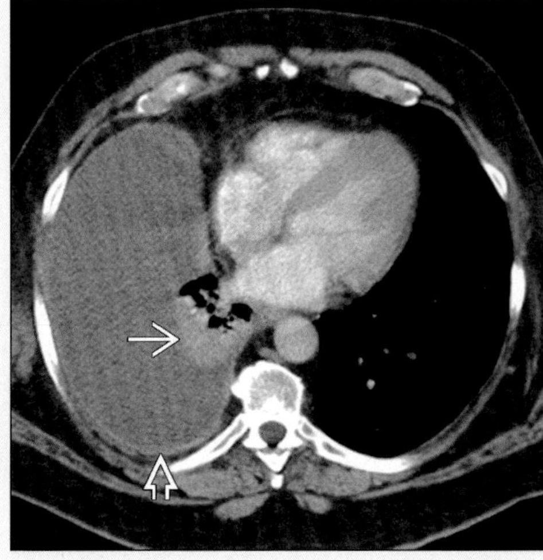

(Left) *Graphic shows features of exudative pleural effusions including smooth → and nodular ↗ thickening of the visceral and parietal pleural surfaces.* ***(Right)*** *Axial CECT of a patient with rheumatoid arthritis shows a loculated water-attenuation right pleural effusion ↗. Thoracentesis revealed turbid green fluid with low glucose, cholesterol crystals, and high rheumatoid titers, consistent with rheumatoid pleural effusion. Exudative pleural effusions may result from collagen vascular disease.*

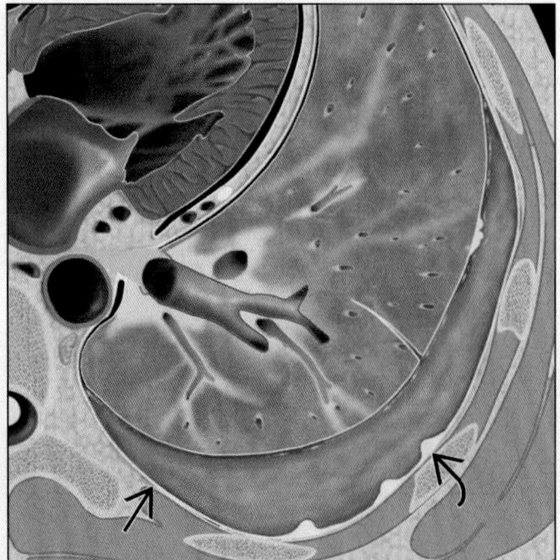

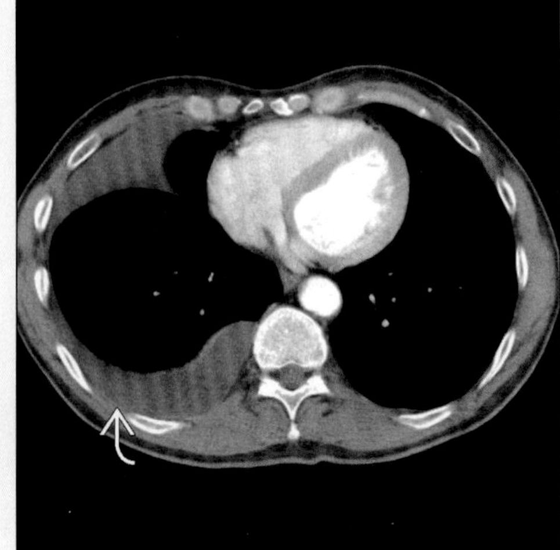

EXUDATIVE PLEURAL EFFUSION

TERMINOLOGY

Definitions

- **Proteinaceous fluid** in pleural space from **increased pleural permeability**
- Pleural inflammation &/or lymphatic obstruction
- Pleural fluid analysis
  - Pleural fluid protein:serum protein > 0.5
  - Pleural fluid LDH:serum LDH > 0.6
  - Pleural fluid LDH > 2/3 upper limit of serum LDH
- **Parapneumonic pleural effusion** refers to pleural effusion associated with pulmonary infection
  - **Empyema**: pH < 7.0; glucose < 40 mg/dL

IMAGING

General Features

- Size
  - Variable
- Morphology
  - Free pleural fluid; dependent pleural space
  - Loculated pleural fluid; peripheral, lenticular, mass-like pleural fluid collection

Radiographic Findings

- Pleural effusion, may be loculated
- Air-fluid level in pleural space; bronchopleural fistula, Boerhaave syndrome, trauma, empyema
- Decubitus radiographs: Free &/or loculated fluid

Fluoroscopic Findings

- Esophagram
  - Exclusion of esophageal perforation as possible etiology for exudative pleural effusion

CT Findings

- Pleural fluid
  - Variable attenuation: Water, high attenuation, homogeneous, heterogeneous
  - CT may not allow differentiation between transudative, exudative, & chylous effusions
  - Fluid-fluid level; **dependent high attenuation fluid** suggests acute **hemorrhage**
  - **Empyema**
    - Lenticular **loculated pleural effusion**, smooth margins, displaces lung
    - Intrinsic gas or air-fluid levels; suspect **bronchopleural fistula**
  - Benign and malignant effusions may be indistinguishable
- Pleura
  - Smooth, thin, visible pleural surface; nodular pleural thickening
  - Malignant pleural disease
    - **Circumferential nodular pleural thickening** involving mediastinal pleural surface
    - Pleural thickening > 1 cm
  - **Empyema**
    - Elliptical loculated pleural fluid collection
    - Parietal and visceral pleural surface enhancement separated by pleural fluid = **split pleura sign**
    - Smooth pleural thickening
    - Sharply defined border between empyema & lung
    - Displacement of vessels and bronchi
- Lung
  - Exclusion of abscess, tumor, pulmonary embolism
  - Abscess
    - Round, thick-walled, heterogeneous mass
    - Ill-defined borders with adjacent lung
    - Bronchi & vessels course into lesion
- Extrapleural fat
  - Empyema; thick extrapleural subcostal tissues & fat
  - Infection/tumor; soft tissue stranding/infiltration
- Mediastinum
  - Exclusion of lymphadenopathy, mediastinitis, esophageal perforation
  - Cardiac surgery or myocardial infarction
- Chest wall: Exclusion of contiguous involvement, empyema necessitatis
- Abdomen: Exclusion of subphrenic abscess, tumor, pancreatitis

Ultrasonographic Findings

- Transudate: Anechoic or echogenic
- Exudate: Echogenic loculated fluid, septations, pleural thickening

Nuclear Medicine Findings

- PET
  - High sensitivity for malignant pleural thickening

Imaging Recommendations

- Best imaging tool
  - CECT for assessment of pleural surfaces, pleural fluid, lung, mediastinum, chest wall
  - CT angiography for exclusion of pulmonary embolism

DIFFERENTIAL DIAGNOSIS

Transudative Pleural Effusion

- Free pleural effusion; smooth pleural thickening, rare nodularity

Empyema

- Loculated pleural effusion with split pleura sign

Pleural Malignancy

- Circumferential nodular pleural thickening

Pleural Fibrosis & Fibrothorax

- Pleural thickening ± calcification; no pleural fluid

PATHOLOGY

General Features

- Etiology
  - **Malignant neoplasia**
    - Metastases: Lung, breast, lymphoma, ovarian, & gastric primary cancers
    - Mesothelioma; lymphoma
  - **Infection**
    - Bacterial: Anaerobic, aerobic, mixed pathogens, actinomycosis
    - Viral; Mycoplasma
    - Tuberculosis
    - Fungal: Coccidioidomycosis, aspergillosis, mucormycosis, blastomycosis
    - Parasites: Amebiasis, hydatidosis
  - **Collagen vascular disease**; rheumatoid arthritis, systemic lupus erythematosus (SLE)

- Drug-induced SLE; hydralazine, procainamide, isoniazid, phenytoin, chlorpromazine
- Drug-induced effusion; nitrofurantoin, dantrolene, bromocriptine & other dopamine agonists, amiodarone, interleukin-2
- **Pulmonary embolism and infarction**
- Other causes
  - Benign asbestos-related pleural effusion
  - Meigs syndrome
    - Ovarian fibroma, ascites, pleural effusion
  - Injury to thoracic duct, traumatic or neoplastic (lymphoma)
  - Post cardiac surgery or myocardial infarction (Dressler syndrome)
  - Thoracic trauma with hemothorax
  - Uremic pleuritis
  - Yellow nail syndrome
    - Rhinosinusitis, pleural effusion, bronchiectasis, lymphedema, yellow nails
  - Gastrointestinal diseases
    - Perforated esophagus, pancreatic disease, subdiaphragmatic abscess

Gross Pathologic & Surgical Features

- Pleural fluid
  - Bloody: Trauma, anticoagulation, iatrogenic, metastases, uremia
  - Blood-tinged: Metastases, mesothelioma, benign asbestos effusion, pulmonary embolism, tuberculosis, pancreatitis
  - Milky: Chylous
  - Brown: Amebic abscess; black: Aspergillus
  - Yellow-green: Rheumatoid
  - Golden, iridescent: Chronic chylothorax, tuberculosis, rheumatoid
  - Opaque: Mesothelioma, chronic empyema
  - Putrid odor: Anaerobic infection

Microscopic Features

- Parapneumonic effusion, neutrophils, & bacteria; mycotic pleurisy, granulomas
- Chylothorax: High lipid content (neutral fat, fatty acids); low cholesterol
  - Sudanophilic fat droplets; triglycerides > 110 mg/dL
- Cholesterol effusion: Cholesterol crystals, up to 1 g/dL; low neutral fat & fatty acids
- Immunohistochemistry & electron microscopy to differentiate mesothelioma from adenocarcinoma

Laboratory Findings

- High amylase, red blood cell count, high LDH level, lymphocytes, neutrophils, eosinophils, plasma cells
- High antinuclear antibody, rheumatoid factor titer, cholesterol crystals
- Low glucose, pH, complement
- Exudative pleural fluid characteristics

CLINICAL ISSUES

Presentation

- Most common signs/symptoms
  - Fever, dyspnea on exertion, chest pain
  - May be asymptomatic
- Other signs/symptoms
  - Post cardiac injury syndrome (Dressler syndrome)
    - After myocardial infarction, cardiac surgery, chest trauma, pacemaker implantation, angioplasty
    - Fever, pleuropericarditis, unilateral/bilateral small to moderate effusions, lung opacities

Demographics

- Age
  - Adults
- Gender
  - Males; rheumatoid arthritis, pancreatitis
- Epidemiology
  - Pulmonary embolism: 3/4 with exudative effusion; suggests pulmonary infarction

Natural History & Prognosis

- Benign asbestos effusion; 5 to > 30 years post exposure
- Malignant pleural effusion; life expectancy 3-6 months

Diagnosis

- **Thoracentesis**
  - Exclusion of exudative pleural effusion
  - Chemical, bacteriologic, cytologic fluid analysis
- **Biopsy**
  - CT/ultrasound-guided pleural biopsy
  - Video-assisted thoracoscopic surgery (VATS)
  - Open biopsy

Treatment

- **Treatment of underlying abnormality**
  - Antibiotics, steroids, chemotherapy, surgery
- **Thoracentesis**
  - Relief of dyspnea
  - Removal of < 1,000 mL of fluid at a time
- **Thoracostomy tube**
  - Empyema, hemothorax, large malignant effusion
    - May require decortication of fibrothorax
  - Pleurodesis or fibrinolysis
    - Drainage of pleural fluid prior to instillation of sclerosing agents
- **Decortication in cases of fibrothorax**

DIAGNOSTIC CHECKLIST

Image Interpretation Pearls

- Visualization of split pleura sign does not denote empyema; may be seen with chronic pleural effusion
- Important to distinguish empyema from lung abscess
  - Empyema treated with early chest tube drainage; lung abscess treated with antibiotics
- Drainage not indicated for tuberculous effusion; drainage indicated for tuberculous empyema

SELECTED REFERENCES

1. Heffner JE et al: Diagnostic utility and clinical application of imaging for pleural space infections. Chest. 137(2):467-79, 2010
2. Mishra EK et al: Advances in the investigation and treatment of pleural effusions. Expert Rev Respir Med. 4(1):123-33, 2010
3. Abramowitz Y et al: Pleural effusion: characterization with CT attenuation values and CT appearance. AJR Am J Roentgenol. 192(3):618-23, 2009

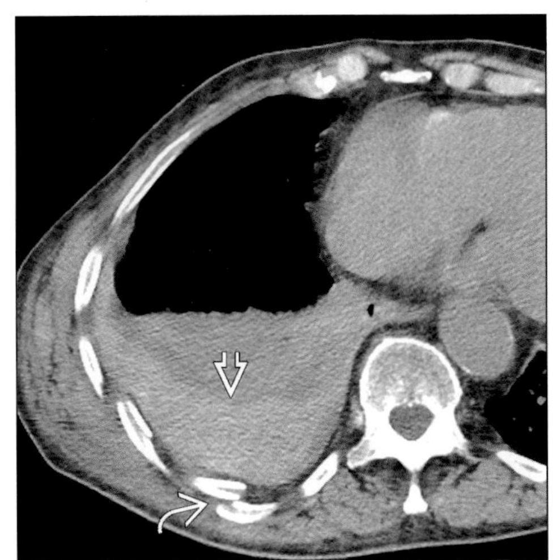

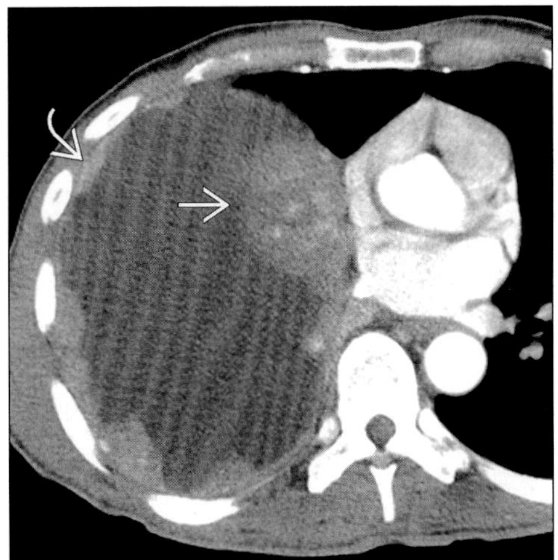

(Left) *Axial NECT of a patient with acute traumatic hemothorax shows a right pleural effusion with a fluid-fluid level and an adjacent right posterior rib fracture.* ***(Right)*** *Axial CECT of a patient with stage IV lung cancer metastatic to the right pleura shows a large loculated right pleural effusion associated with circumferential heterogeneously enhancing pleural nodules and masses. Exudative effusions may exhibit high attenuation &/or nodular pleural thickening.*

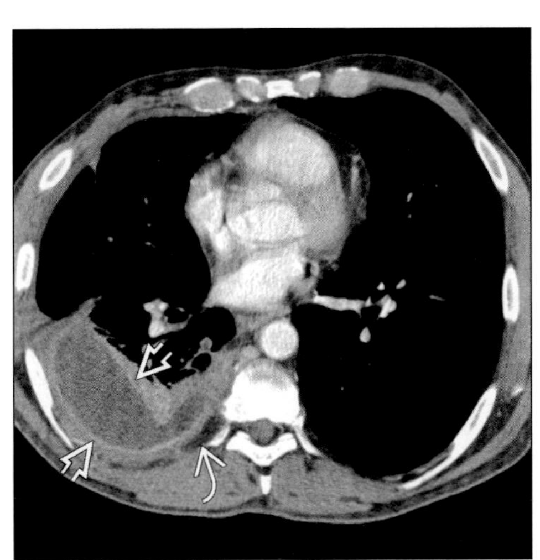

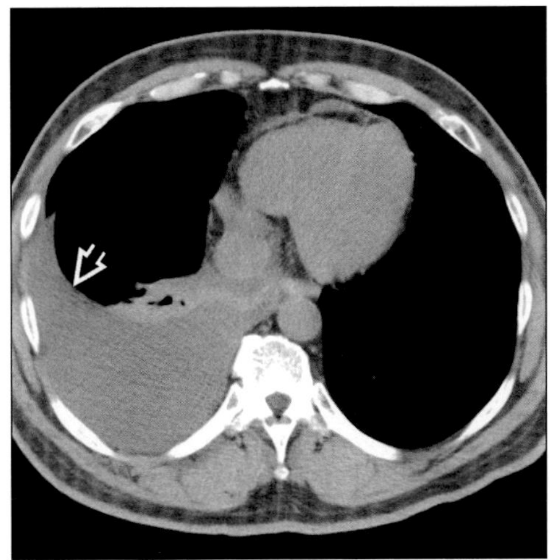

(Left) *Axial CECT of a 56-year-old man with Fusobacterium infection shows an empyema manifesting as a loculated right pleural effusion with an enhancing pleural rind, the split pleura sign. Thick extrapleural fat is consistent with the pleural inflammatory process.* ***(Right)*** *Axial NECT of a 60-year-old man on dasatinib therapy for chronic myeloid leukemia shows a moderate exudative right pleural effusion. Exudative pleural effusions may result from a variety of drug therapies.*

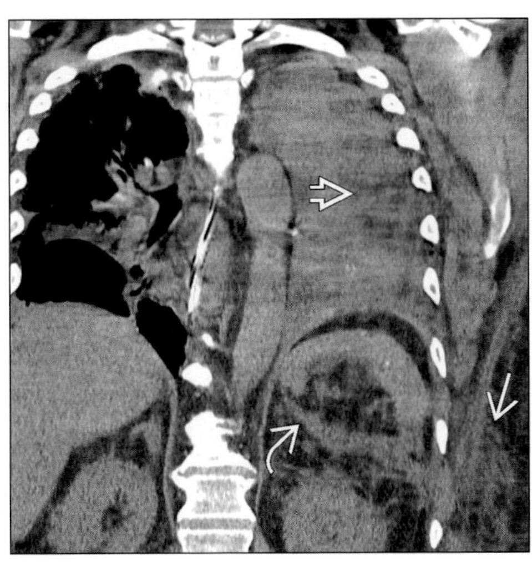

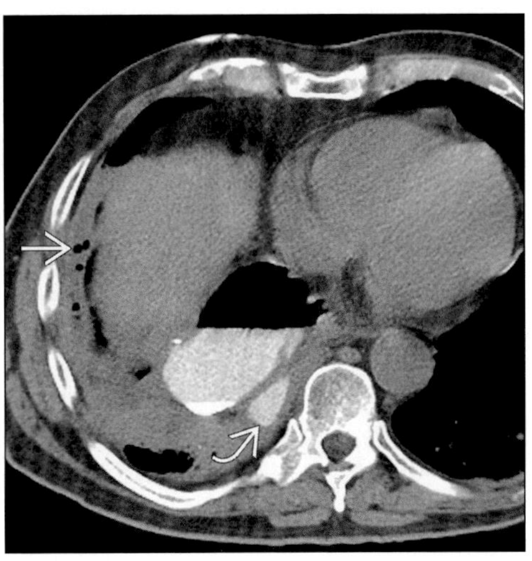

(Left) *Coronal NECT of a patient with acute pancreatitis manifesting with retroperitoneal and left chest wall soft tissue stranding shows a left exudative pleural effusion.* ***(Right)*** *Axial NECT of a patient status post esophagectomy and gastric pull-up shows contrast leakage and gas bubbles within a right exudative pleural effusion/empyema secondary to an anastomotic leak. Exudative pleural effusions may result from traumatic or inflammatory gastrointestinal disorders.*

HEMOTHORAX

Key Facts

Terminology

- Hemothorax (HTX)
- Bloody pleural effusion; hematocrit > 50% than that of peripheral blood

Imaging

- Radiography
  - Pleural effusion
  - Variable size; frequent loculation; pleural thickening
  - Chronic HTX may result in pleural calcification
- CT
  - High attenuation pleural fluid > 35 HU
  - Hematocrit effect; fluid-fluid level
  - Assessment of bleeding source
  - Chronic HTX; development of pleural calcification
- MR: Variable signal of pleural fluid depending on blood age & MR sequence

Top Differential Diagnoses

- Chest trauma
- Pulmonary embolism
- Malignant pleural effusion
- Anticoagulation
- Transudative pleural effusion; heart failure
- Exudative pleural effusion
- Chylothorax

Clinical Issues

- Symptoms: Respiratory distress, hemoptysis, hypotension
- Untreated HTX may progress to fibrothorax

Diagnostic Checklist

- Consider hemothorax in patients with high-attenuation pleural effusion; careful evaluation for identification of bleeding source

*(**Left**) AP chest radiograph of a patient who sustained blunt trauma with multiple rib fractures shows a large partially loculated right pleural effusion →. (**Right**) Axial NECT of the same patient shows a large right hemothorax →. Higher-attenuation extrapleural hemorrhage is also present and is separated from the hemothorax and contained by displaced extrapleural fat →. Displacement of extrapleural fat reflects high-pressure intercostal arterial bleeding.*

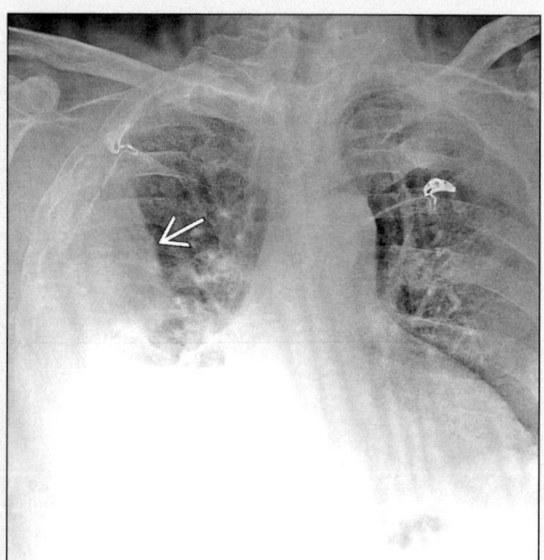

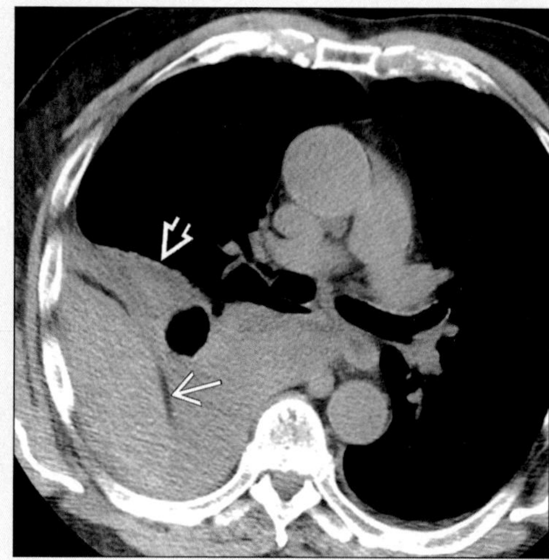

*(**Left**) Axial CECT of a patient with traumatic aortic injury → shows hemomediastinum that tracks into the dependent portion of the adjacent left pleural space, resulting in a left hemothorax → of moderately high attenuation. (**Right**) Axial NECT of a patient status post double lung transplantation shows a right fissural subacute hemothorax that exhibits a hematocrit effect →. The sedimented dependent red blood cells exhibit higher attenuation than the nondependent lower-attenuation supernatant.*

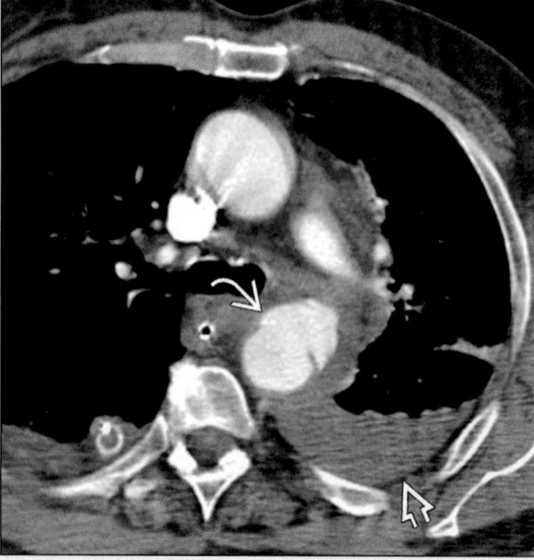

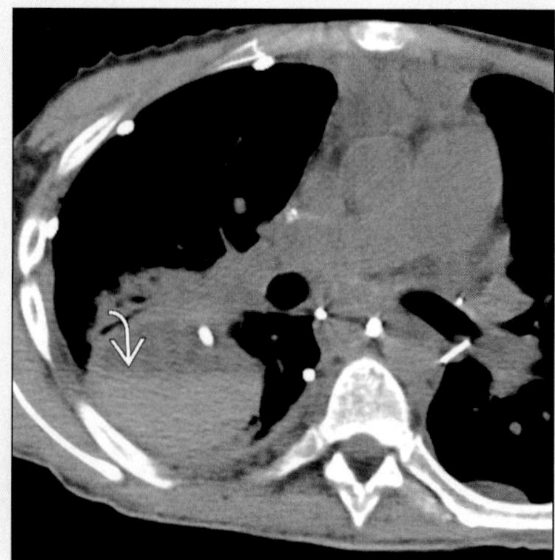

HEMOTHORAX

TERMINOLOGY

Abbreviations

- **Hemothorax (HTX)**

Definitions

- **Bloody pleural effusion**
- **Pleural fluid hematocrit > 50% than peripheral blood hematocrit**

IMAGING

General Features

- Best diagnostic clue
  - High-attenuation pleural effusion
    - Pleural thickening common
- Location
  - Bleeding source
    - Mediastinum
    - Lung
    - Chest wall
    - Diaphragm
- Size
  - Low-pressure bleeding from lung; tamponade effect of pleural fluid
  - High-pressure bleeding from systemic artery or large mediastinal vessel typically unremitting
    - Patient may exsanguinate into pleural space
- Morphology
  - Typically multilocular

Radiographic Findings

- Radiography
  - Pleural effusion
  - Variable size
    - Depends on site of hemorrhage & coagulation profile
  - Frequent loculation
  - Chronic HTX may result in pleural calcification
    - Fibrothorax, lung entrapment

CT Findings

- NECT
  - **High-attenuation pleural effusion**
    - > 35 Hounsfield units (HU) for fresh blood
    - > 70 HU for clotted blood
    - Hematocrit effect (fluid-fluid level) with layering of serum & sedimented red blood cells
    - Low-attenuation HTX in patients with anemia
  - Loculated pleural effusion; pleural thickening
  - Chronic hemothorax; development of pleural calcification
    - Assessment of fibrothorax, lung entrapment

MR Findings

- Deoxyhemoglobin in blood several hours to days old
  - Low signal on T1WI & T2WI
- Methemoglobin in blood several days to weeks old
  - Intracellular: High signal on T1WI; low signal on T2WI
  - Extracellular: High signal on T1WI & T2WI
- Hemosiderin in blood several weeks to months old
  - Low signal on T1WI & T2WI

Ultrasonographic Findings

- Multilocular complex echogenic pleural effusion

Imaging Recommendations

- Best imaging tool
  - CT assessment of pleural fluid attenuation; high attenuation in HTX depending on time frame
- Protocol advice
  - Unenhanced CT is typically diagnostic
  - Enhanced CT for assessment of bleeding source

DIFFERENTIAL DIAGNOSIS

Chest Trauma

- Aortic or large mediastinal vessel injury
- Penetrating lung injury from displaced rib fractures
  - Intercostal or internal mammary artery laceration
  - Extrapleural blood displaces subpleural fat
- Iatrogenic: Traumatic life support device placement

Pulmonary Embolism

- May induce multilocular effusion, occasional HTX

Malignant Pleural Effusion

- Pleural effusion with nodular pleural thickening

Anticoagulation

- Bleeding into pleural space from various sources

Transudative Pleural Effusion

- Heart failure; pleural fluid typically 10-20 HU

Exudative Pleural Effusion

- Variable attenuation; typically loculated fluid

CLINICAL ISSUES

Presentation

- Most common signs/symptoms
  - Respiratory distress, hemoptysis, hypotension

Natural History & Prognosis

- Untreated HTX may progress to fibrothorax & lung entrapment

Treatment

- **Tube thoracostomy** to remove blood & gas
- **Surgery**; HTX evacuation, control of bleeding site
- Blood transfusion
- Intracavitary fibrinolytic therapy
- Embolization in selected cases

DIAGNOSTIC CHECKLIST

Consider

- Hemothorax in patients with high-attenuation pleural effusion; identification of bleeding source

Reporting Tips

- Localize blood within pleural or extrapleural space

SELECTED REFERENCES

1. Abramowitz Y et al: Pleural effusion: characterization with CT attenuation values and CT appearance. AJR Am J Roentgenol. 192(3):618-23, 2009

CHYLOTHORAX

Key Facts

Terminology

- Abbreviations
  - Chylothorax (CTx)
- Synonym: Chylous pleural effusion
- Definition
  - Presence of chyle in pleural space
  - Usually from thoracic duct (TD) disruption or blockage

Imaging

- Radiography
  - Large pleural effusion, usually unilateral
  - Typically post cardiothoracic surgery or trauma
- CT
  - Large unilateral water attenuation pleural effusion
  - No pleural thickening
  - No lung entrapment
- MR: High signal intensity due to fat content

Top Differential Diagnoses

- Traumatic/iatrogenic TD disruption
- TD obstruction from lymphadenopathy
- Miscellaneous conditions
  - Lymphangioleiomyomatosis
  - Lymphangioma
  - Idiopathic chylothorax

Pathology

- Milky opaque pleural fluid with high lipid content

Clinical Issues

- Signs/symptoms
  - Dyspnea & cough
  - Pleural effusion that decreases with fasting
- Therapy: Treatment of underlying condition
  - Thoracentesis; electrolyte & fluid replacement
  - TD ligation: 90% success rate

*(**Left**) Graphic shows a right chylothorax and the thoracic duct (TD) ➔ anatomy. The TD arises from the cisterna chyli at the level of the L2 vertebra, courses along the right paravertebral region, crosses to the left at the level of the carina (T5), and drains into the left brachiocephalic vein. Unilateral TD injury may result in ipsilateral CTx. (**Right**) Axial CECT of a 60-year-old woman with left tension chylothorax after left pneumonectomy for lung cancer shows a large water-attenuation left pleural effusion.*

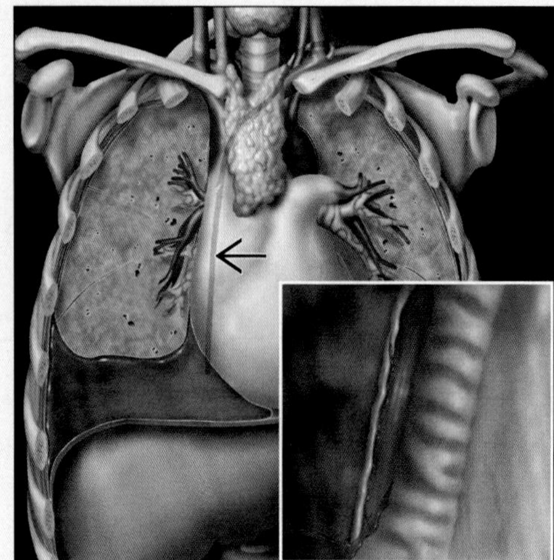

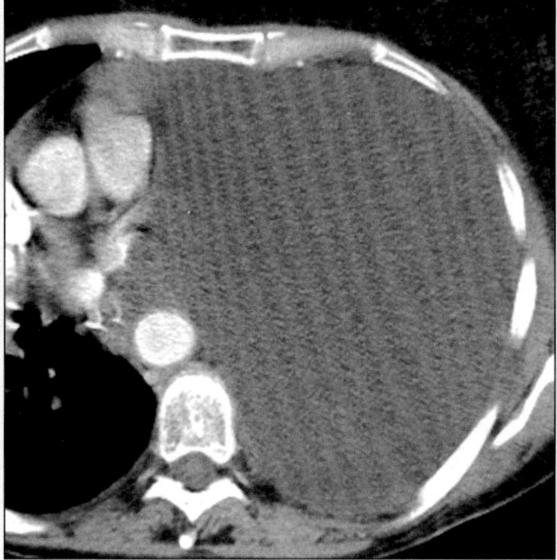

*(**Left**) Axial NECT of a patient status post resection of a T12 sarcoma who developed a right postsurgical CTx shows a moderate right pleural effusion, pleural drains ➔, and postsurgical changes in the spine ➔. This intractable CTx required ablation of the cisterna chyli. (**Right**) Axial NECT of a 40-year-old woman with lymphangioleiomyomatosis (LAM) shows a moderate right chylous pleural effusion and profuse bilateral small thin-walled pulmonary cysts. LAM is an unusual etiology of chylothorax.*

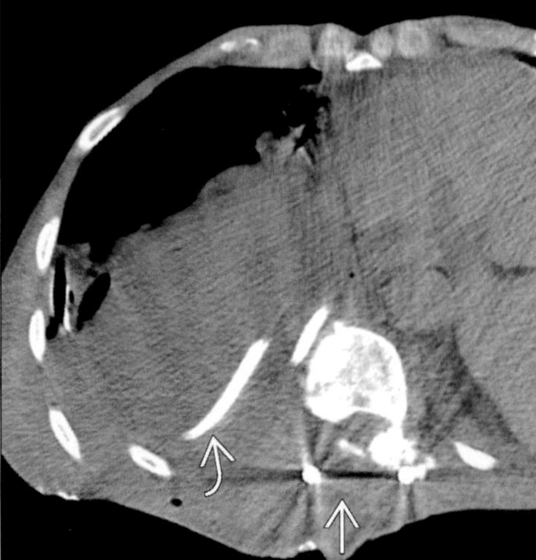

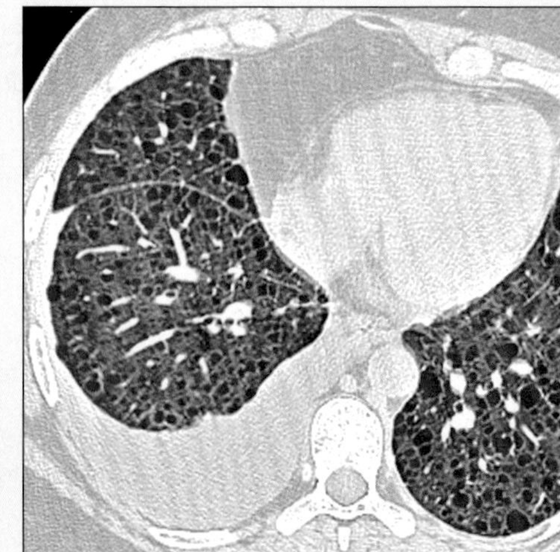

CHYLOTHORAX

TERMINOLOGY

Abbreviations

- **Chylothorax** (CTx)

Synonyms

- **Chylous pleural effusion**

Definitions

- Presence of chyle in pleural space
- Disruption or obstruction of thoracic duct (TD) or its tributaries
- **Lymphocytic exudative** pleural effusion
  - Triglyceride concentration > 110 mg/dL
  - Pleural fluid chylomicrons confirm diagnosis
  - Noninflammatory etiology of pleural effusion

IMAGING

General Features

- Best diagnostic clue
  - Large pleural effusion, usually unilateral
  - Often follows cardiothoracic surgery or trauma
- Location
  - Injury of **lower 1/3 of TD** results in **right CTx**
  - Injury of **upper 2/3 of TD** results in **left CTx**
  - Injury of TD as it crosses **midline**, **bilateral CTx**
- Size
  - Typically large
    - Production of up to 3 liters of chyle per day
    - Rapid accumulation of pleural fluid
- Morphology
  - May be loculated

Radiographic Findings

- Pleural effusion
  - Typically **unilateral**
  - Typically **large**
  - May be loculated

CT Findings

- Large pleural effusion
  - Typically unilateral
  - Characteristic **water attenuation fluid**
- Usually no pleural thickening or nodularity
- Usually no lung entrapment

MR Findings

- T1WI
  - **High signal intensity due to fat content**

Imaging Recommendations

- Best imaging tool
  - CT useful for exclusion of other etiologies of pleural effusion
  - Anatomic assessment of TD with lymphangiography or lymphoscintigraphy

Angiographic Findings

- Lymphangiography with Iodinated contrast or radionuclide
  - Localization of TD leak or obstruction

DIFFERENTIAL DIAGNOSIS

Traumatic/Iatrogenic TD Disruption

- Rapid onset of large pleural effusion

TD Obstruction from Lymphadenopathy

- Lymphoma, lung cancer
- Tuberculosis, sarcoidosis

Miscellaneous Conditions

- Lymphangioleiomyomatosis
- Lymphangioma
- Lymphangiectasis
- Idiopathic chylothorax

PATHOLOGY

Gross Pathologic & Surgical Features

- Milky opaque pleural fluid with high lipid content

CLINICAL ISSUES

Presentation

- Most common signs/symptoms
  - Dyspnea, cough
  - Large pleural effusion that decreases with fasting
    - Recurs after resuming fat intake

Natural History & Prognosis

- **50% resolve spontaneously**
- TD **ligation successful in 90%** of refractory CTx

Treatment

- Treatment of underlying condition
- **Conservative treatment**
  - **Thoracentesis**
  - **Fluid & electrolyte replacement**
  - Talc pleurodesis in some refractory cases
  - Pleuroperitoneal shunt
  - Somatostatin & octreotide
    - Reduce intestinal chyle production
- **Surgical treatment**
  - Ligation of TD & tributaries
  - Cannulation & embolization of TD

DIAGNOSTIC CHECKLIST

Consider

- Most CTx are iatrogenic or secondary to trauma
- Lymphadenopathy & lymphangioleiomyomatosis should be included in differential diagnosis
- Other etiologies of pleural effusion: Exudative effusion, empyema, hemothorax

Image Interpretation Pearls

- Rapid onset of large pleural effusion in setting of trauma or cardiothoracic surgery suggests CTx

SELECTED REFERENCES

1. Huggins JT: Chylothorax and cholesterol pleural effusion. Semin Respir Crit Care Med. 31(6):743-50, 2010
2. Skouras V et al: Chylothorax: diagnostic approach. Curr Opin Pulm Med. 16(4):387-93, 2010

EMPYEMA

Key Facts

Terminology

- Empyema: Pleural space infection; abscess
  - Typically infected parapneumonic effusion

Imaging

- Best diagnostic clue: Loculated pleural effusion in febrile patient
- Radiography
  - Loculated pleural effusion
  - Lentiform shape on lateral or frontal radiography
  - Incomplete border sign
  - May contain air, air-fluid levels; bronchopleural fistula
- CT: Most findings not specific for empyema
  - Loculated pleural fluid
  - May contain air; bronchopleural fistula
  - Split pleura sign, pleural thickening
  - Hypertrophy of extrapleural fat

Top Differential Diagnoses

- Malignant pleural effusion
- Malignant mesothelioma
- Iatrogenic pleural loculation
- Abdominal causes

Pathology

- Most often due to spread from adjacent pneumonia

Clinical Issues

- Symptoms: Chest pain, fever, rigors
- M > F; median age: 50 years
- Early diagnosis depends on high index of suspicion
- Antibiotics & drainage are first lines of therapy

Diagnostic Checklist

- Consider empyema in any febrile patient with loculated pleural effusion or unexplained pleural air

*(**Left**) Axial CECT of a patient with empyema shows a right pleural effusion with lobular borders, a probable lung abscess ➡, and enhancement of the pleural surfaces ➡. The circumferential nature of the pleural fluid collection is indicative of loculation, which would be inconsistent with a simple transudative pleural effusion. (**Right**) Coronal CECT of a patient with empyema shows a large loculated right pleural effusion ➡, pleural enhancement ➡, and a large basilar fibrin ball ➡.*

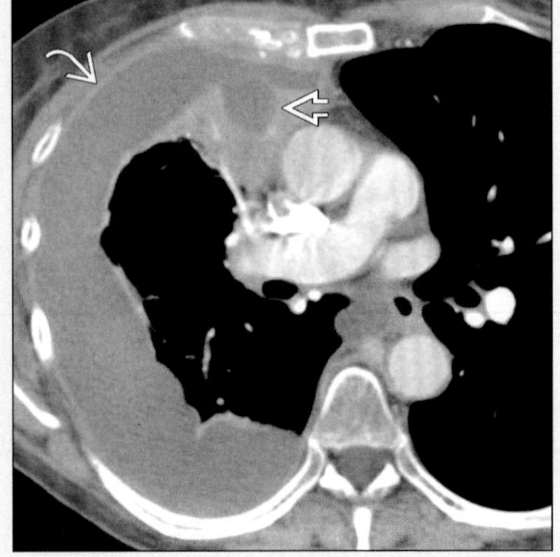

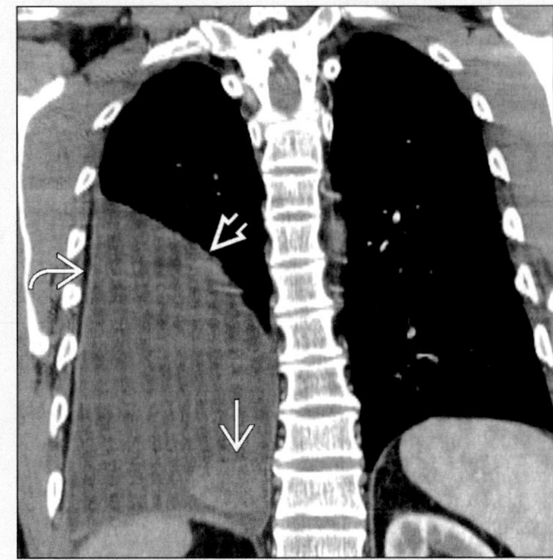

*(**Left**) Axial CECT of a patient with fever shows a loculated left pleural effusion with intrinsic air collections ➡ and enhancement of thickened left pleural surfaces ➡. In this clinical setting and in the absence of prior intervention, the findings are diagnostic of empyema with bronchopleural fistula. (**Right**) Graphic shows features of empyema, which may include loculation, mass effect on the adjacent lung parenchyma, and gas in the pleural space from associated bronchopleural fistula.*

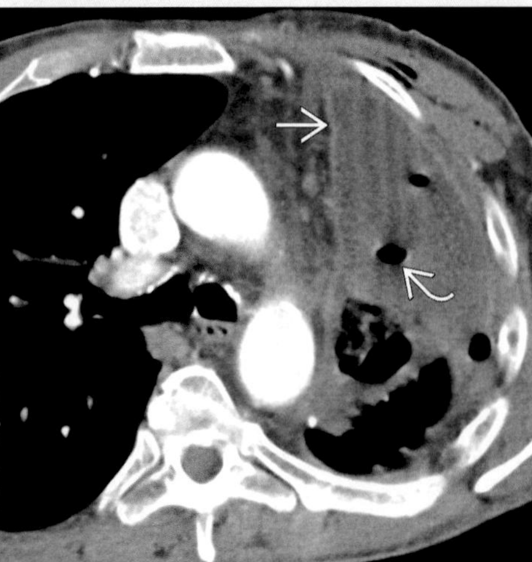

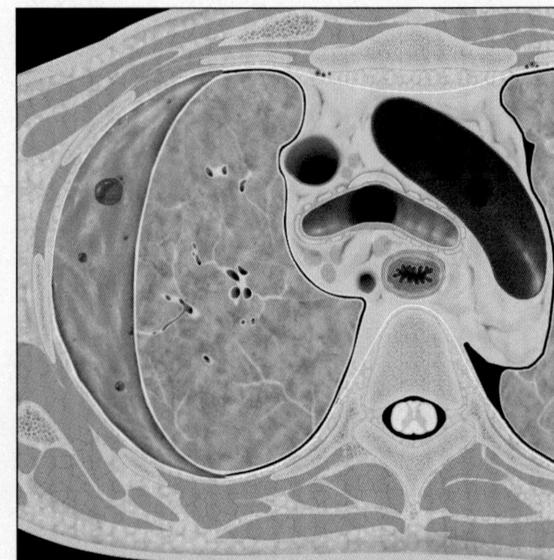

TERMINOLOGY

Definitions

- **Pleural space infection; abscess**
  - Typically infected parapneumonic effusion
  - May result from hematogenous seeding of bacteria
  - Rare but dangerous complication of chest surgery
- **Empyema necessitatis**
  - Empyema spontaneously draining to chest wall; pleurocutaneous fistula
  - Typically in empyema from tuberculosis, fungal infection, actinomycosis
  - Can involve breast, causing mastitis
- Tension empyema
  - Large or rapidly expanding pleural infection, with lung compression & mediastinal shift
  - Cardiac arrest has been reported

IMAGING

General Features

- Best diagnostic clue
  - Loculated pleural effusion in febrile patient
  - May contain air pockets
    - Suggests development of bronchopleural or esophagopleural fistula
    - Empyema may result in fistula, or fistula may precede empyema
- Location
  - Typically posterior or basal
  - May affect nondependent portions of pleural space
- Size
  - Variable
- Morphology
  - Loculation: Lentiform fluid collection, including fissural fluid (pseudotumor)

Radiographic Findings

- Blunt costophrenic angle
- **Loculated pleural effusion**
  - No fluid motion on decubitus radiography
- May contain air, air-fluid-levels; **bronchopleural fistula**
- Lentiform shape on lateral or frontal radiography
- **Incomplete border sign**
  - Sharp borders when imaged tangentially
  - Discrepant border visualization, shape, size on orthogonal views
  - Indicates loculated fluid, not specific for empyema
- Loculated fissural pleural fluid; **pseudotumor**
  - May mimic lung mass
  - Incomplete border sign
  - Conforms to anatomic location of fissures

CT Findings

- CECT
  - **Loculated pleural effusion; nonspecific finding**
    - Indistinguishable from other loculated pleural effusions
      - Primary or metastatic tumor
      - Sterile reactive collection
      - Fluid from abdominal sources
  - **Air, air-fluid level in pleural space**
    - Indicative of bronchopleural fistula in the absence of prior pleural intervention
  - **Split pleura sign**; not specific for empyema
    - Enhancement of visceral & parietal pleura
    - "Split" by intervening pleural fluid
  - **Pleural thickening**
    - May be seen in noninfected pleural effusions
    - Empyema typically thicker
  - **Hypertrophy of extrapleural fat**
    - May be seen in noninfected pleural fluid
    - Typical of tuberculous or fungal pleural effusions
  - CT essential for treatment planning
    - Location & extent of pleural fluid collection
    - Evaluation of loculation, multiple collections
  - Tuberculous pleuritis produces thick calcification, rib thickening, adjacent trapped lung

MR Findings

- MR offers no diagnostic advantages over CT in imaging of empyema

Ultrasonographic Findings

- Variable ultrasound features
  - May appear as simple, nonseptated fluid
  - Complex fluid collections, with internal echoes & septations
    - Echogenic material & septa may be seen in noninfected fluid
    - Identification of septa important for treatment planning
      - Increased likelihood that surgical intervention will be needed
  - Shadowing from gas pockets

Imaging Recommendations

- Best imaging tool
  - Chest radiography is best initial study; CT often needed to plan intervention
- Protocol advice
  - Intravenous (IV) contrast useful for demonstrating pleural enhancement but not essential

DIFFERENTIAL DIAGNOSIS

Malignant Pleural Effusion

- Most common tumors
  - Adenocarcinoma
    - Breast, ovary, lung
  - Invasive thymoma
- Pleural thickening or nodularity often absent

Malignant Mesothelioma

- Unilateral circumferential nodular pleural thickening
- Variable amount of pleural fluid
- Asbestos-related pleural plaques in 25%

Iatrogenic Pleural Loculation

- Pleurodesis; often for malignant effusions

Abdominal Causes

- Catamenial hemothorax
  - Vast majority right sided
  - Cyclic, complex cystic collections
- Pancreatic pseudocyst
  - May erode through diaphragm to reach pleural space

EMPYEMA

PATHOLOGY

General Features

- Etiology
  - Most often due to **spread from adjacent pneumonia**
    - Effusions in setting of pneumonia (parapneumonic) may be bland or infected
    - Overall, pleural effusions related to pneumonia more common in patients with diabetes mellitus
    - Bland & infected parapneumonic effusions may have similar appearances
    - Tuberculosis
      - Noninfected effusions from delayed hypersensitivity reaction to tuberculous antigens
      - Reactive effusions much more common than empyema
  - Can be **iatrogenic**
    - Overall incidence about 1% after lung resection for cancer
    - May occur early or late
    - Late cases may be due to hematogenous seeding of bland fluid collections
    - About 75% have associated bronchopleural fistula
    - May occur due to breakdown of bronchial stump
    - Organisms
      - *Staphylococcus* most common organism
      - *Streptococcus*
      - Anaerobes
      - Gram-negative rods
  - May result from fistulous connections to GI tract or skin
    - Chest wall infections, fasciitis
    - Tumor erosion from skin or esophagus
- Associated abnormalities
  - Bronchopleural fistula
    - May be related to necrotizing lung infection
    - May be related to airway invasion by tumor

Staging, Grading, & Classification

- Empyema evolves through 3 stages, none of which is distinct on imaging
  - Exudative stage
    - Sterile fluid with normal glucose & normal pH
  - Fibrinopurulent stage
    - Accumulation of neutrophils, bacteria, fibrin
    - Decreased glucose & pH
  - Chronic organizing stage
    - Pleural peel develops & encases lung
    - Exudate is thick & frankly purulent
- Evolution may take weeks or days

Gross Pathologic & Surgical Features

- Thickened pleural rind
- Often tightly adherent to underlying lung
- Purulent pleural fluid
- If underlying lung noncompliant, reexpansion after drainage may not be possible ("trapped lung")

Microscopic Features

- Fibrinous exudate
- Microbial organisms
- Associated hemorrhage

CLINICAL ISSUES

Presentation

- Most common signs/symptoms
  - **Chest pain, fever, rigors**
- Other signs/symptoms
  - Tuberculous empyemas may have fewer symptoms

Demographics

- Age
  - Median age in most series: Approximately **50 years**
  - Can affect children, mostly related to pneumonia
  - Elderly, outcome often based on concomitant illness
- Gender
  - **M > F**
  - Most published series include more men than women

Natural History & Prognosis

- Early diagnosis depends on high index of suspicion
  - Early thoracentesis essential for diagnosis
  - Imaging features & symptoms nonspecific
- In postoperative empyema, panendoscopy essential
  - Exclusion of airway/esophageal fistulae
- Median hospital stay approximately 20 days
- Mortality overall approximately 10%
  - Poorer outcome with fungal infection or afebrile patient, indicating inadequate host response

Treatment

- Antibiotics & drainage are first lines of therapy
- Tube thoracostomy
  - All loculated pockets must be drained
  - Imaging guidance to access separate areas of involvement
  - Infusion of fibrinolytic agents into pleural space
    - Break up loculations; facilitate complete drainage
    - Use has led to decreased need for surgical intervention, shorter hospital stays
- Video-assisted thoracoscopy
  - Essential in complex cases, direct pleural fluid visualization, physical disruption of loculations
- Open drainage
  - Required for complex or unresponsive cases, assessment of underlying lung
    - Drainage will not be successful if lung cannot expand to fill space
    - Thoracoplasty to eliminate potential space
    - Particularly a problem in tuberculous empyema
  - Long-term open drainage post pneumonectomy
    - Clagett thoracotomy or Eloesser flap procedure

DIAGNOSTIC CHECKLIST

Consider

- Empyema in any febrile patient with loculated pleural effusion or unexplained pleural air

SELECTED REFERENCES

1. Chae EJ et al: Radiographic and CT findings of thoracic complications after pneumonectomy. Radiographics. 26(5):1449-68, 2006
2. Qureshi NR et al: Imaging of pleural disease. Clin Chest Med. 27(2):193-213, 2006

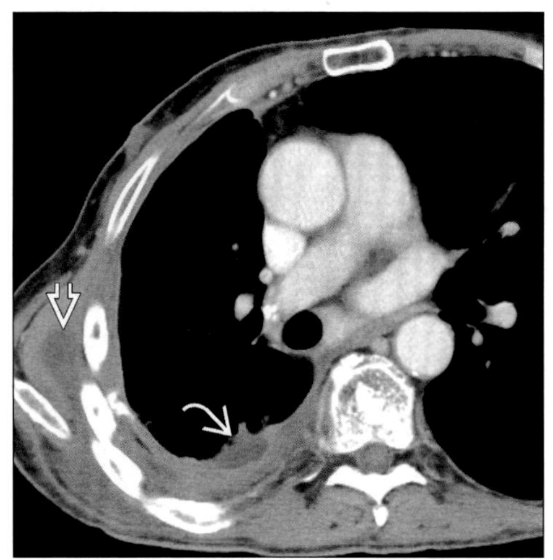

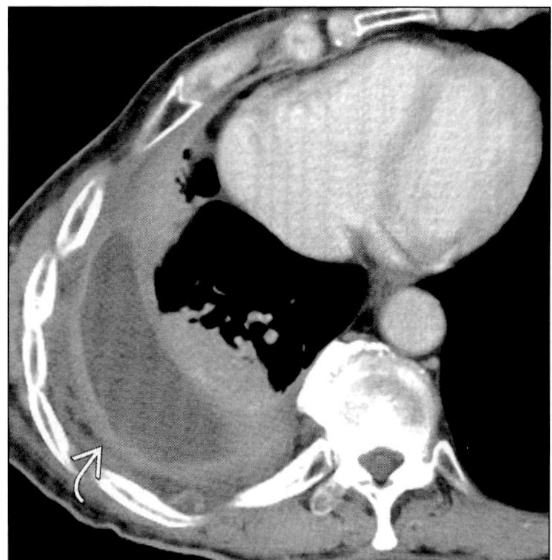

(Left) *Axial CECT of a patient with a right chronic empyema shows pleural thickening and a small right pleural effusion* ➔ *with involvement of the adjacent chest wall forming a fluid collection* ⇨*, indicative of empyema necessitatis.* ***(Right)*** *Axial CECT of the same patient shows a small right hemithorax and a loculated right pleural effusion with surrounding pleural thickening* ➔*. Adjacent atelectasis or consolidation is present and is commonly seen in association with pleural fluid collections.*

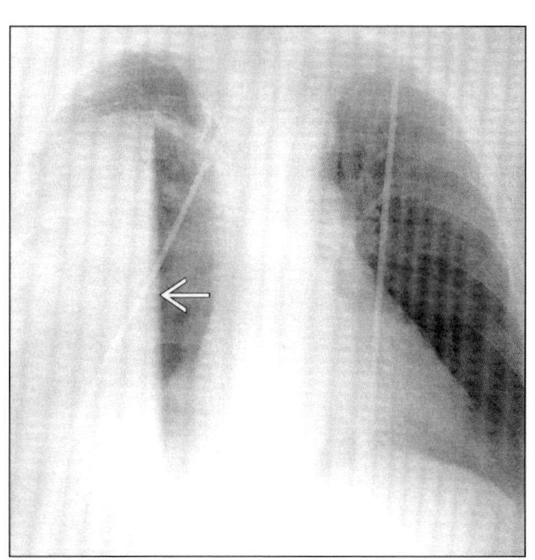

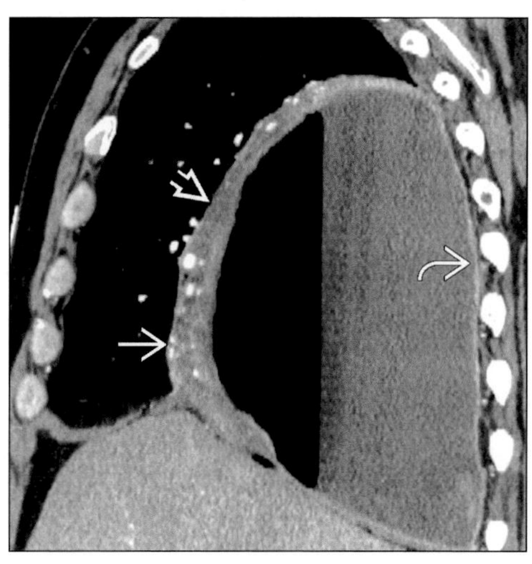

(Left) *Right lateral decubitus chest radiograph shows a large air-fluid level* ➔ *in the right hemithorax. The elongated shape of the gas-fluid collection is consistent with complicated pleural effusion rather than lung abscess.* ***(Right)*** *Sagittal CECT of the same patient shows a large empyema with pleural enhancement* ➔ *and mass effect on the adjacent lung* ➔*. Heterogeneous hypoattenuation* ⇨ *of the atelectatic lung suggests pneumonia. The air-fluid level is indicative of bronchopleural fistula.*

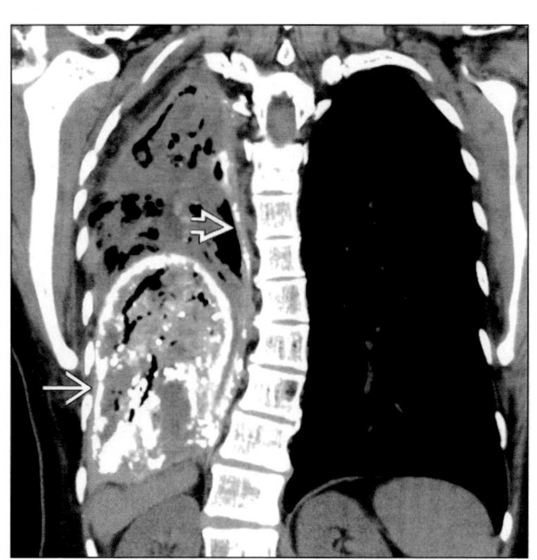

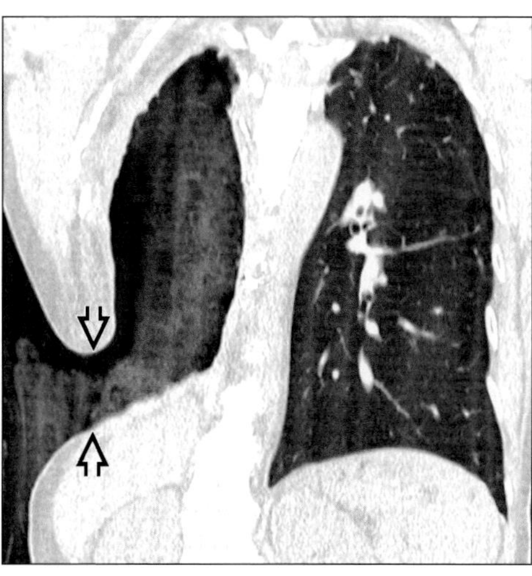

(Left) *Coronal NECT of a patient with chronic aspergillus pneumonia, empyema, and bronchopleural fistula shows right lung consolidation, a coarsely calcified right pleural collection* ➔ *with internal debris and gas, and adjacent pleural thickening and calcification* ⇨*.* ***(Right)*** *Coronal NECT of the same patient at a later date shows a right pneumonectomy and Eloesser flap* ⇨ *procedure performed for treatment of end-stage lung infection and chronic empyema/ bronchopleural fistula.*

BRONCHOPLEURAL FISTULA

Key Facts

Terminology

- Bronchopleural fistula (BPF)
  - Connection between pleura & large bronchus
- Parenchymal-pleural fistula (PPF)
  - Connection between distal airway & pleural space

Imaging

- Radiography
  - Drop (caudal migration) of gas-fluid level with increasing air in pneumonectomy space
  - Development of hydropneumothorax without pleural intervention or procedure
  - Decubitus radiography contraindicated: Infected pleural fluid may spill into contralateral lung
- CT
  - Detection of small amounts of pleural gas
  - Direct visualization of fistula

Top Differential Diagnoses

- Gas-forming infection in pleural space
- Hydropneumothorax
- Esophagopleural fistula

Pathology

- BPF: Most often due to surgery
- BPF: May complicate empyema
- PPF: COPD, necrotizing infection, neoplasm

Clinical Issues

- Signs/symptoms
  - Purulent sputum, cough, fever, chest pain
- Treatment: Pleural fluid drainage & antibiotics

Diagnostic Checklist

- Increased gas in pneumonectomy space or new gas within loculated effusion; highly suggestive of BPF

(Left) PA chest radiograph of a patient status post left pneumonectomy complicated by bronchopleural fistula shows a gas-fluid level ➡ in the previously opaque left pneumonectomy space. (Right) Subsequent PA chest radiograph of the same patient shows caudal migration of the gas-fluid level ➡ within the left pneumonectomy space in the absence of pleural intervention, consistent with bronchopleural fistula. Bronchopleural fistula resulted from dehiscence of the left bronchial stump.

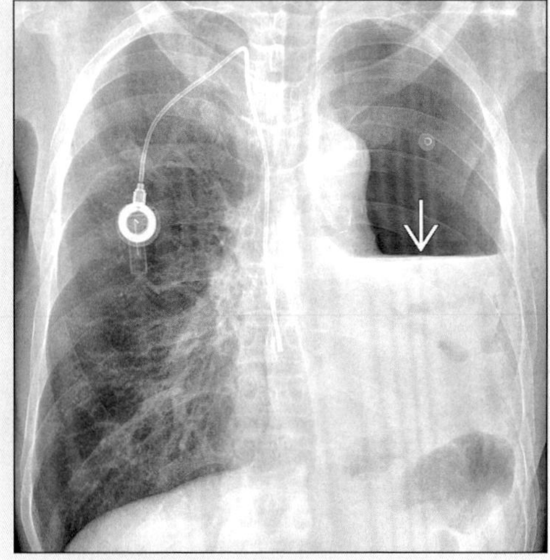

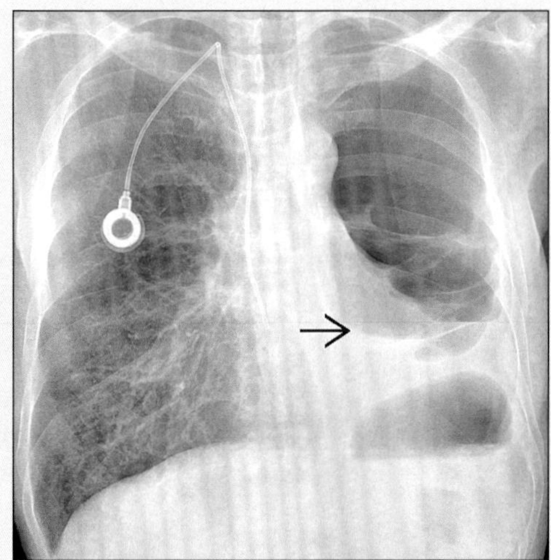

(Left) Graphic shows the features of parenchymal-pleural fistula (PPF), a complication of empyema resulting in abnormal communication between a distal airway ➡ and the pleural space characterized by pleural gas in the absence of intervention. (Right) Axial CECT of a patient with anaerobic pulmonary infection complicated by empyema shows a loculated right pleural effusion ➡ and a PPF ↪ to the fissural pleural space ⇨. BPF may complicate pleural empyema or pneumonectomy.

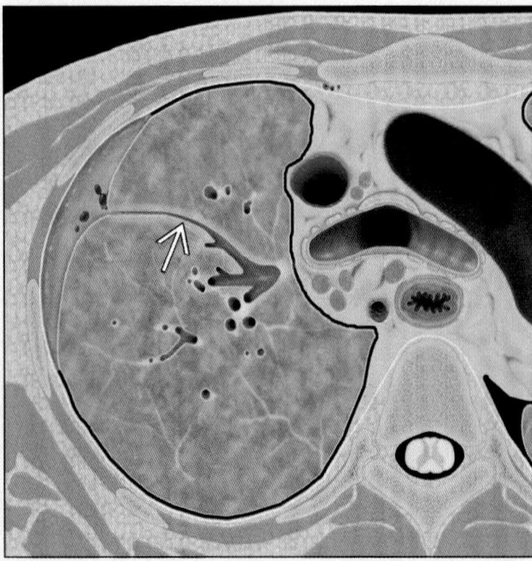

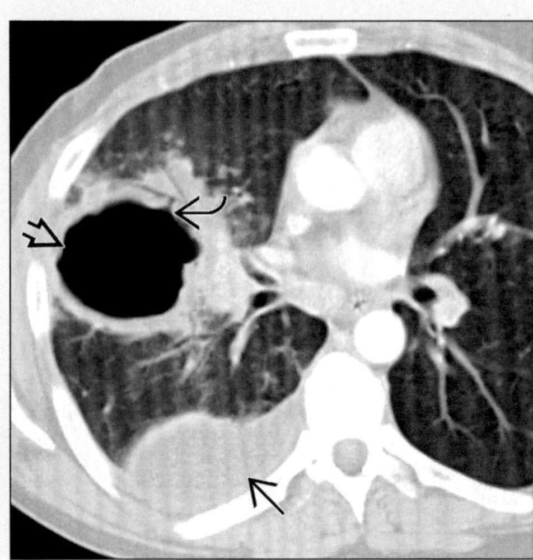

BRONCHOPLEURAL FISTULA

TERMINOLOGY

Abbreviations

- **Parenchymal-pleural fistula (PPF)**
- **Bronchopleural fistula (BPF)**

Synonyms

- **BPF = central BPF**
- **PPF = peripheral BPF**

Definitions

- **BPF**: Connection between pleura and large bronchus
- **PPF**: Connection between distal airway and pleural space

IMAGING

General Features

- Best diagnostic clue
  - Drop (caudal migration) of gas-fluid level with increasing air in pneumonectomy space
  - Development of hydropneumothorax without pleural intervention or procedure
    - Most hydropneumothoraces related to pleural tubes or thoracentesis

Radiographic Findings

- After pneumonectomy, air-fluid level expected
  - Over time, fluid should increase and air decrease
  - Air often entirely absorbed over time (2-4 months)
  - Decreased fluid/increased air indicates BPF

CT Findings

- NECT
  - Actual connection to bronchus visible in < 50%
  - Probable cause identified in majority of cases
- CECT
  - Pleural enhancement; empyema
  - Contrast introduced into pleural space via pleural tubes may be visible within airways

Ultrasonographic Findings

- Ultrasound useful for guiding intervention

Nuclear Medicine Findings

- Xe-133 or aerosolized DTPA: Accumulation of activity in affected pleural space

Imaging Recommendations

- Best imaging tool
  - Chest radiography often sufficient for diagnosis
  - Chest CT may allow direct visualization of fistula
- Protocol advice
  - IV contrast not essential
  - Contrast administered into pleural collection may be visible in airways
  - Decubitus radiographs contraindicated: Infected pleural fluid may spill into contralateral lung

DIFFERENTIAL DIAGNOSIS

Gas-forming Infection in Pleural Space

- Rare (*Clostridium perfringens* & *Bacteroides fragilis*)
- Most pleural gas is iatrogenic or fistulous

Hydropneumothorax

- Spontaneous, iatrogenic, or traumatic

Esophagopleural Fistula

- Similar imaging findings to BPF; typically occurs within 6 weeks of esophageal surgery
- Endoscopic evaluation generally required to locate esophageal tear

PATHOLOGY

General Features

- Etiology
  - BPF: Most often due to surgery
    - 6% of pneumonectomies, 4% after lung surgery
    - More common after right pneumonectomy & in patients requiring postoperative ventilation
    - Usually diagnosed within 2 weeks of surgery
    - More common in certain surgical situations
      - Preoperative radiation therapy, incomplete tumor resection, diabetes mellitus, emphysema
    - Less common causes: Necrotizing pneumonia, neoplasm, & radiation
  - BPF: May complicate empyema
  - PPF: COPD, necrotizing infection, neoplasm

CLINICAL ISSUES

Presentation

- Most common signs/symptoms
  - Expectoration of purulent sputum
  - Fever, cough, hemoptysis, chest pain
  - Large air leak from pleural drainage tubes

Demographics

- Age
  - Mean: Late 50s
- Gender
  - Male > female

Natural History & Prognosis

- Mortality rate about 25% overall
  - Higher in setting of pneumonectomy
- Up to 1/3 of BPF may close spontaneously
- Chronic empyema (> 5 years) may lead to malignancy

Treatment

- Adequate drainage of pleural fluid collections & antibiotic therapy
- Surgery usually necessary

DIAGNOSTIC CHECKLIST

Image Interpretation Pearls

- Increased gas in pneumonectomy space or new gas within loculated effusion; highly suggestive of BPF

SELECTED REFERENCES

1. Chae EJ et al: Radiographic and CT findings of thoracic complications after pneumonectomy. Radiographics. 26(5):1449-68, 2006
2. Jones NC et al: Bronchopleural fistula treated with a covered wallstent. Ann Thorac Surg. 81(1):364-6, 2006

IATROGENIC PNEUMOTHORAX

Key Facts

Terminology
- Pneumothorax from medical procedure/treatment

Imaging
- Radiography
  - Upright imaging: Visualization of curvilinear visceral pleural line
  - Supine imaging: Basilar pneumothorax, deep sulcus sign, double diaphragm sign
- CT
  - Direct visualization of pleural air
  - Air in nondependent aspect of pleural space

Top Differential Diagnoses
- Primary spontaneous pneumothorax
- Pneumothorax ex vacuo
- Skin fold
- Bullae or cysts

Pathology
- Needle biopsy, thoracentesis, subclavian puncture
- Positive pressure ventilation
- Thoracotomy, bronchoscopy
- Catheters, chest/endotracheal/feeding tubes, pacemaker electrodes

Clinical Issues
- Signs/symptoms
  - Chest pain, dyspnea
  - May be asymptomatic
- Prognosis: Generally good
- Treatment: Chest tube, supplemental oxygen

Diagnostic Checklist
- Consider tension pneumothorax in patients with contralateral mediastinal shift & depression of ipsilateral hemidiaphragm

*(**Left**) Prone axial NECT shows a moderate pneumothorax that occurred during percutaneous needle biopsy of a right lower lobe nodule ➡. A chest tube was subsequently placed. (**Right**) Supine AP chest radiograph of an intubated critically ill patient shows right basilar lucency, sharp margins of the right hemidiaphragm, and a deep sulcus sign ⇨ secondary to a right pneumothorax. Middle lobe atelectasis ➡ was also present. Iatrogenic pneumothorax may result from thoracic interventions or barotrauma.*

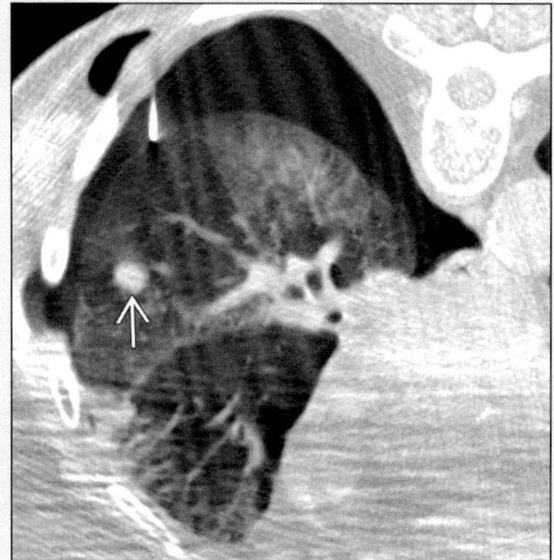

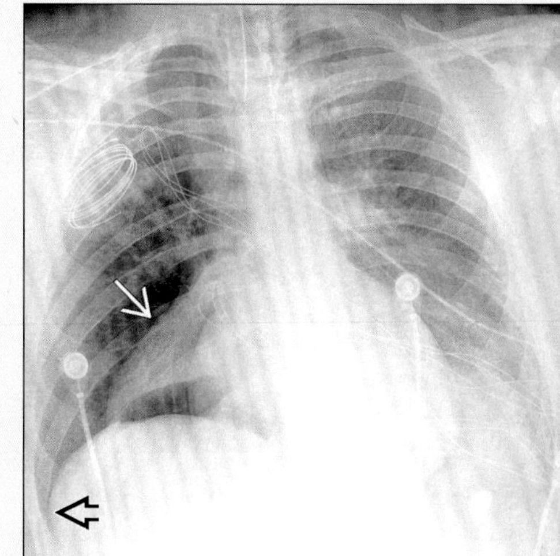

*(**Left**) AP chest radiograph of an upright patient status post thoracentesis shows a small right apical pneumothorax manifesting with a thin visceral pleural line ➡. (**Right**) PA chest radiograph of a patient with malignant pleural mesothelioma status post right thoracentesis shows a right pneumothorax ex vacuo due to failure of the right lung to reexpand because of a thickened visceral pleural surface ➡. Note multifocal right pleural masses and nodules ⇨ characteristic of mesothelioma.*

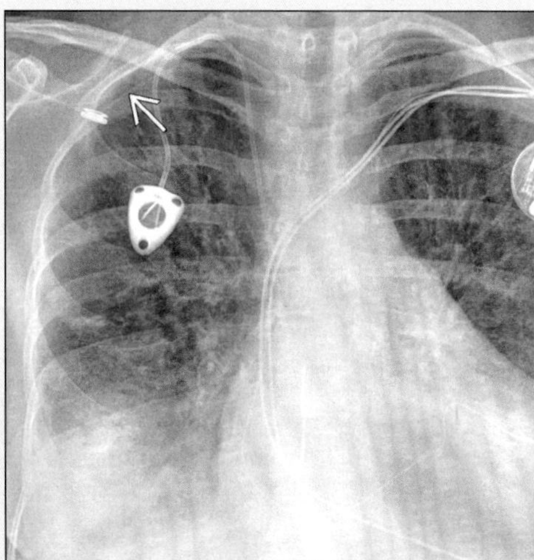

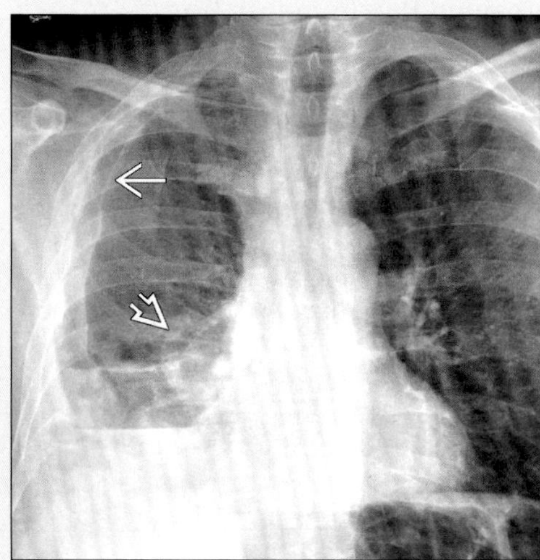

IATROGENIC PNEUMOTHORAX

TERMINOLOGY

Definitions

- Accumulation of pleural air related to medical procedures or treatments
- Outnumbers other causes of pneumothorax

IMAGING

Radiographic Findings

- Upright radiography
  - Apical lucency conforming to shape of pleural space
  - Visualization of curvilinear visceral pleural line
    - Separates vessel-containing lung from avascular air-filled pleural space
- Supine radiography
  - Increased sharpness of mediastinal/diaphragmatic margins
  - **Deep sulcus sign**: Basilar pleural air leading to larger or deeper lateral costophrenic sulcus compared to contralateral hemithorax
  - **Double diaphragm sign**: Simultaneous visualization of anterior costophrenic sulcus & diaphragmatic dome
  - Medial retraction of middle lobe with visualization of its borders
    - Upper & lower lobes maintain contact with lateral chest wall
- Visualization & evaluation of life support devices consistent with thoracic intervention or barotrauma

CT Findings

- Direct visualization of air in pleural space
- Air in nondependent aspect of pleural space
- More sensitive and specific than radiography for diagnosis of pneumothorax

Ultrasonographic Findings

- "Comet tail" artifact with reverberations extending from echogenic pleural line to edge of image
- Absence of normal lung beneath echogenic pleural line

Imaging Recommendations

- Best imaging tool
  - Upright chest radiography usually diagnostic
  - CT highly sensitive for small pneumothoraces

DIFFERENTIAL DIAGNOSIS

Primary Spontaneous Pneumothorax

- Occurs spontaneously without preceding procedures or medical treatment

Pneumothorax Ex Vacuo

- Follows drainage of pleural fluid with failure of lung reexpansion
  - Lung entrapment
  - Thick visceral pleura or obstructing central lesion
- Usually asymptomatic; chest tube placement not indicated

Skin Fold

- May extend beyond chest wall inner margin
- Thicker linear opacity with sharp outer edge

Bullae or Cysts

- Convex inner margin; does not conform to expected lung shape

PATHOLOGY

General Features

- Etiology
  - Transthoracic needle aspiration/biopsy, thoracentesis, subclavian venipuncture
  - Positive pressure ventilation
  - Thoracotomy, bronchoscopy
  - Placement of catheters, chest tubes, endotracheal tubes, feeding tubes, & pacemaker electrodes

CLINICAL ISSUES

Presentation

- Most common signs/symptoms
  - Chest pain, dyspnea
  - May be asymptomatic
- Other signs/symptoms
  - Tachypnea, tachycardia, hypotension with tension pneumothorax

Demographics

- Epidemiology
  - Transthoracic needle aspiration/biopsy; emphysema, long needle path, increased number of pleural punctures

Natural History & Prognosis

- Generally good prognosis
- Unrecognized tension pneumothorax associated with mechanical ventilation may be rapidly fatal

Treatment

- Chest tube for symptomatic, enlarging, or moderate to large iatrogenic pneumothorax
  - Reported duration of chest tube treatment of iatrogenic pneumothorax: Average of 4.7 days
- Supplemental oxygen enhances rate of pleural air absorption
- Aspiration may be sufficient for treatment of small pneumothorax secondary to needle biopsy

DIAGNOSTIC CHECKLIST

Consider

- Tension pneumothorax with contralateral mediastinal shift & depression of ipsilateral diaphragm

Image Interpretation Pearls

- In patients with mechanical ventilation, pneumothorax is more likely to be bilateral, under tension, & associated with pneumomediastinum

SELECTED REFERENCES

1. Zhan C et al: Accidental iatrogenic pneumothorax in hospitalized patients. Med Care. 44(2):182-6, 2006
2. Spillane RM et al: Radiographic aspects of pneumothorax. Am Fam Physician. 51(2):459-64, 1995
3. Despars JA et al: Significance of iatrogenic pneumothoraces. Chest. 105(4):1147-50, 1994

PRIMARY SPONTANEOUS PNEUMOTHORAX

Key Facts

Terminology
- Pneumothorax (PTX)
- Primary spontaneous pneumothorax (PSP)
  - Pneumothorax without precipitating event in otherwise healthy patient

Imaging
- Radiography
  - Visible pleural line; no peripheral lung markings
  - Apical subpleural bullae adjacent to PTX; 15%
  - Tension PTX: Mediastinal shift, tracheal deviation, ipsilateral diaphragmatic flattening & rib splaying
  - Deep sulcus sign on supine radiography
  - Decubitus radiography helpful in emphysema
  - Pleural effusion in 15%
- CT
  - Evaluation of underlying lung
  - Apical subpleural bullae/blebs

Top Differential Diagnoses
- Ruptured bleb or subpleural bulla
- Iatrogenic pneumothorax
- Traumatic pneumothorax
- Secondary spontaneous pneumothorax
- Mimics: Skin folds, life support devices

Clinical Issues
- Symptoms
  - Chest pain 90%; dyspnea 80%
- Young men; 20-40 years
- Tall, thin patients
- Treatment
  - Oxygen, chest tube, resection of bullae/blebs

Diagnostic Checklist
- Consider PSP in young, thin, tall patients presenting with acute unilateral chest pain

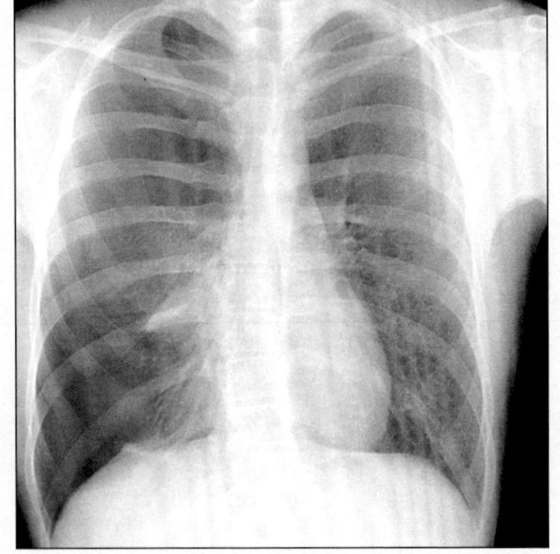

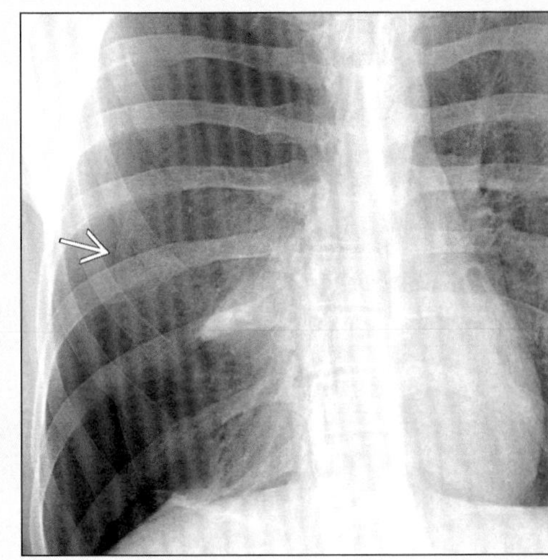

(Left) *PA chest radiograph of a 27-year-old man with a primary spontaneous pneumothorax who presented with acute right chest pain shows a large right pneumothorax and atelectatic changes in the right lung. The contralateral lung appears normal.* ***(Right)*** *Coned-down PA chest radiograph of the same patient shows the large right pneumothorax manifesting with a visible pleural line ➡ and absence of peripheral pulmonary markings. PSP affects otherwise healthy patients without precipitating events.*

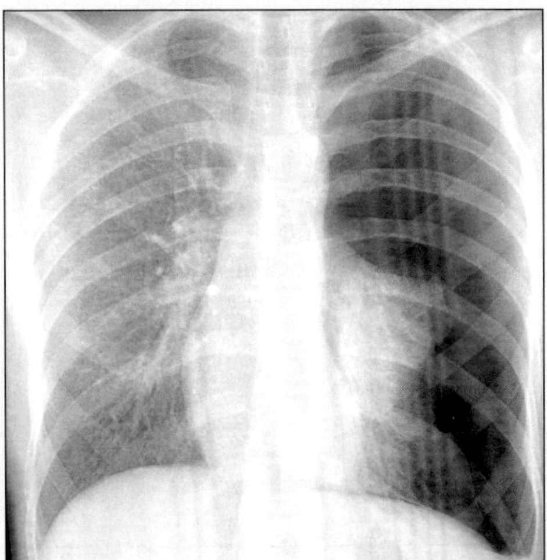

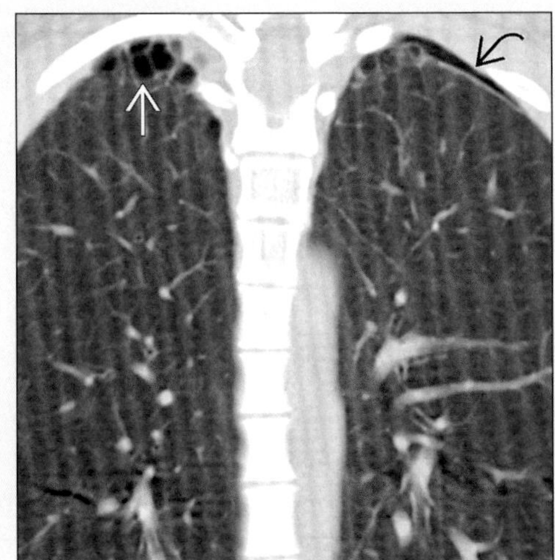

(Left) *PA chest radiograph of a 20-year-old man with a history of prior pneumothorax and new left chest pain shows a large left PTX with associated left lung atelectasis.* ***(Right)*** *Coronal NECT of the same patient after chest tube placement shows a small residual left apical PTX ↗. Note biapical bullae &/or blebs ➡ without centrilobular emphysema. Patients with recurrent spontaneous pneumothorax often have apical bullae and blebs but may also be evaluated for genetic or cystic lung diseases.*

PRIMARY SPONTANEOUS PNEUMOTHORAX

TERMINOLOGY

Abbreviations

- **Pneumothorax (PTX)**
- **Primary spontaneous pneumothorax (PSP)**

Definitions

- **PSP**: Pneumothorax occurring **without precipitating event** in an **otherwise healthy patient** without obvious evidence of underlying lung disease

IMAGING

General Features

- Best diagnostic clue
  - Visualization of **visceral pleural line** without peripheral lung markings
- Location
  - Upright radiography: Apical pleural space
  - Supine radiography: Basilar pleural space; at costophrenic angle or medially along mediastinal border
  - Slightly more common on right side
  - Rarely bilateral
- Size
  - Small: < 20% of hemithorax volume
  - Large: > 20% of hemithorax volume
- Morphology
  - May be loculated
  - May be associated with ipsilateral pleural fluid (hydropneumothorax)

Radiographic Findings

- Visualization of visceral pleural line
  - Typically apical on upright chest radiography
  - May be laterally located with apical pleural adhesions
- Visualization of **apical subpleural bullae in presence of PTX**; up to **15%**
  - Apical subpleural bullae rarely seen in absence of PTX
  - Typically normal-appearing lung
- **Pleural effusion in 15%**
- Expiratory radiography does not increase sensitivity for PTX detection
- Tension PTX: Mediastinal shift, tracheal deviation, ipsilateral diaphragmatic flattening & rib splaying
- **Deep sulcus sign**; supine radiography
  - Hyperlucent deep costophrenic angle & ipsilateral upper abdomen
  - Sharply marginated adjacent hemidiaphragm
  - Underestimates PTX size
- Decubitus radiography can be helpful in differentiating PTX from apical bullous disease
- Measurement of apical pleural separation for follow-up assessment
- Volume estimation
  - Measurement of transverse diameter of thorax, hemithorax, aerated lung
    - [Diameter of hemithorax^3-Diameter of aerated lung^3]/Diameter of hemithorax^3
    - Example of a 2 cm PTX with hemithorax diameter of 10 cm: $[10^3-8^3]/10^3=48.8\%$
  - Not often used in clinical practice

CT Findings

- Increased sensitivity for pneumothorax
- **Evaluation of underlying lung parenchyma**
- **Frequent paraseptal &/or centrilobular emphysema**
- Pleural blebs indistinguishable from subpleural bullae
- **Contralateral disease commonly identified**
  - Important for operative planning

Imaging Recommendations

- Best imaging tool
  - Upright radiography usually diagnostic
  - CT more sensitive in evaluating lung parenchyma for secondary causes of PTX & identification of contralateral disease
  - CT can be used for problem solving; particularly in severe emphysema
- Protocol advice
  - Decubitus radiography useful in differentiating PTX from apical bullae
  - Expiratory radiographs do not improve diagnostic sensitivity
  - Contrast not helpful when performing CT for evaluation of PTX

DIFFERENTIAL DIAGNOSIS

Ruptured Bleb or Subpleural Bulla

- Most common etiology

Marfan Syndrome

- Rare genetic disorder secondary to fibrillin-1 gene mutation
- Systemic abnormalities: Most commonly aortic aneurysm/dissection, scoliosis, pectus excavatum, dural ectasia, ectopia lentis, tall slender build

Ehlers-Danlos Syndrome

- Rare genetic disease resulting in skin hyperextensibility, easy bruising, joint hypermobility
- Mutation of collagen V genes

Cutis Laxa

- Rare genetic disease resulting in wrinkled & redundant skin, emphysema, hernias, diverticula of the GI & GU tracts
- Mutation to the elastin genes

Birt-Hogg-Dubé Syndrome

- Rare autosomal dominant disease: Renal cell carcinoma, cutaneous fibrofolliculoma, pulmonary cysts
- Mutation of folliculin gene

Iatrogenic Pneumothorax

- Line placement, mechanical ventilation
- Thoracentesis, biopsy, thoracotomy

Traumatic Pneumothorax

- Penetrating or blunt trauma

Secondary Spontaneous Pneumothorax

- Infection: *Staphylococcus aureus*, *Pneumocystis jiroveci*, tuberculosis
- Malignancy: Classically osteosarcoma metastases
- Cystic lung disease: Lymphangioleiomyomatosis, Langerhans cell histiocytosis
- Catamenial PTX; ectopic endometrial tissue
- Asthma, bronchiolitis, cystic fibrosis
- Cavitary lesion: Abscess, malignancy, septic emboli

PRIMARY SPONTANEOUS PNEUMOTHORAX

Mimics

- Skin fold: May extend beyond thoracic cavity; will not be seen on decubitus radiography
- External support or monitoring devices: Should be removed & radiograph repeated if diagnosis of PTX in doubt
- Pneumomediastinum: May be indistinguishable from loculated medial PTX
- Apical bullae
  - Chest tube placement into bulla can result in bronchopleural fistula

PATHOLOGY

General Features

- Etiology
  - Typically rupture of apical visceral pleural bleb or subpleural bulla
    - Surface pressure & transpulmonary pressure greatest at apices; predisposes these alveoli to become distended
      - Accentuated in tall thin individuals

Gross Pathologic & Surgical Features

- Subpleural lung bullae & visceral pleural blebs
- Frequent eosinophilic infiltrates adjacent to visceral pleural blebs
- Subpleural fibrosis with fibroblastic foci in adjacent lung parenchyma
- Buffalo chest
  - Communication between right & left pleural spaces
    - May be congenital or iatrogenic
  - Affected patients with bilateral PTX can be treated with unilateral chest tube

CLINICAL ISSUES

Presentation

- Most common signs/symptoms
  - Chest pain 90%
  - Dyspnea 80%
  - Rarely asymptomatic
- Other signs/symptoms
  - Tension PTX
    - Tachycardia, hypotension, cyanosis
- Clinical profile
  - Strong association with cigarette smoking
  - May be precipitated by coughing or sneezing
  - PSP often occurs in **winter months**

Demographics

- Age
  - **20-40 years**
- Gender
  - Men 5x more commonly affected than women
    - When controlling for height, no significant gender discrepancy
- Body habitus
  - More common in **tall, thin patients**

Natural History & Prognosis

- Pleural gas absorbed 1.5% per day on room air
  - Complete absorption & complete lung reexpansion; average of 3 weeks
  - Daily radiography of little utility in stable patients
- Recurrent spontaneous PTX in up to 50% of patients
  - Most occur within 2 years
  - Risk of additional recurrence up to 85%
  - Recurrent PTX may be contralateral to prior PTX

Treatment

- **100% oxygen**
  - Small PTX
  - Pleural gas resorbed up to 4x faster than on room air
- **Chest tube**
  - Urgent chest tube placement for tension or symptomatic PTX
  - Small chest tubes as effective as large chest tubes in treating uncomplicated PTX
  - Chest tubes managed with suction, water seal, or 1-way valve based on presence of air leak
- Open thoracotomy or video-assisted thoracoscopic surgery
  - **Resection of bullae & blebs**
  - **Talc pleurodesis**
  - Both
- Incomplete lung reexpansion may be due to malpositioned chest tube, bronchopleural fistula, or trapped lung from pleural thickening
- Patients with PSP should avoid air travel for 6 weeks & scuba diving for life

DIAGNOSTIC CHECKLIST

Consider

- PSP in young, thin, tall individuals presenting with acute onset of unilateral chest pain
- Decubitus radiography or chest CT if there is any uncertainty in the diagnosis of PTX; particularly in patients with emphysema

Image Interpretation Pearls

- Visualization of a visceral pleural line without peripheral lung markings is diagnostic of PTX

Reporting Tips

- Small: PTX < 2 cm
- Large: PTX > 2 cm

SELECTED REFERENCES

1. Haynes D et al: Management of pneumothorax. Semin Respir Crit Care Med. 31(6):769-80, 2010
2. Noppen M: Spontaneous pneumothorax: epidemiology, pathophysiology and cause. Eur Respir Rev. 19(117):217-9, 2010
3. Ha HI et al: Imaging of Marfan syndrome: multisystemic manifestations. Radiographics. 27(4):989-1004, 2007
4. Adley BP et al: Birt-Hogg-Dubé syndrome: clinicopathologic findings and genetic alterations. Arch Pathol Lab Med. 130(12):1865-70, 2006

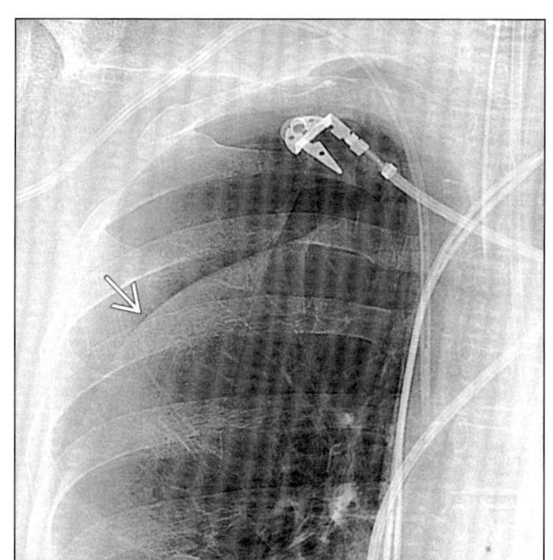

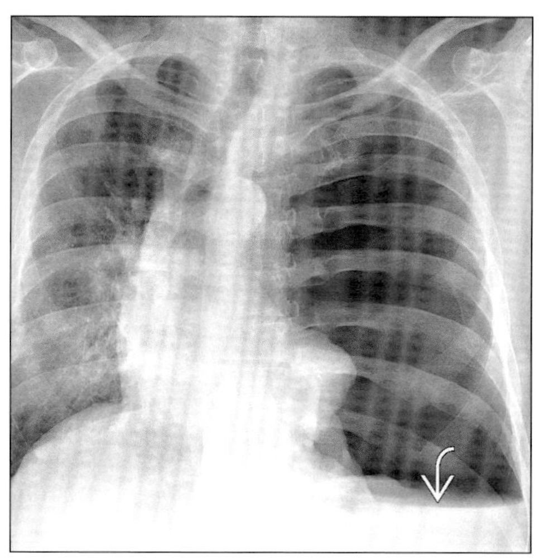

(Left) *AP portable chest radiograph of a mechanically ventilated patient shows a right apical skin fold ➡ manifesting as an edge rather than a pleural line. Note visible lung markings coursing beyond the skin fold. Skin folds may mimic PTX.* ***(Right)*** *AP chest radiograph of a patient with acute left chest pain shows a large left spontaneous tension pneumothorax and a small left pleural effusion ↪. Note complete left lung atelectasis, mediastinal shift to the right, and widened left rib interspaces.*

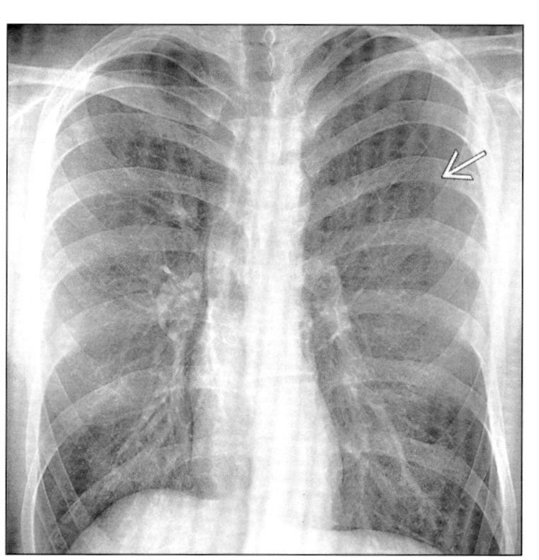

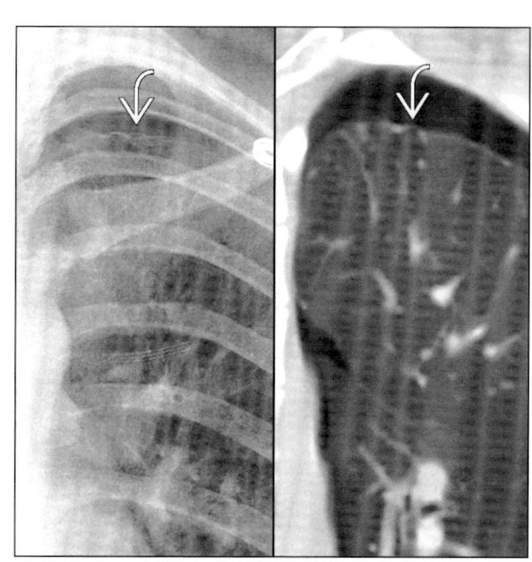

(Left) *PA chest radiograph of a young man with acute chest pain shows a left primary spontaneous pneumothorax manifesting with a visible pleural line ➡ and mild mediastinal mass effect. The lungs appear normal. The patient had the characteristic long thin body habitus seen in patients with PSP.* ***(Right)*** *Composite image with PA chest radiograph (left) and coronal NECT (right) of a young man with PSP shows a subtle tiny left apical bulla ↪ confirmed on CT and likely responsible for the PTX.*

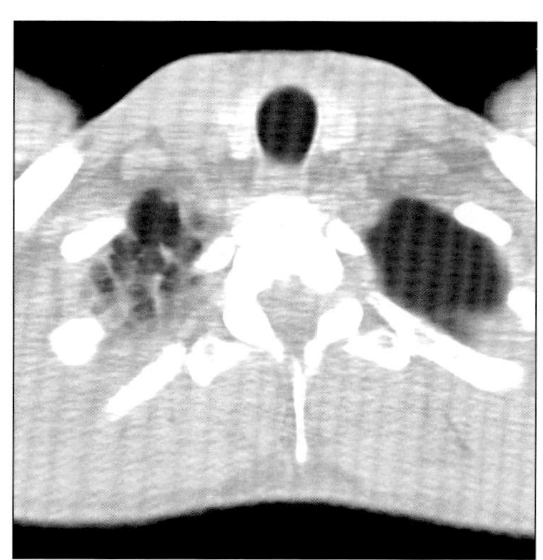

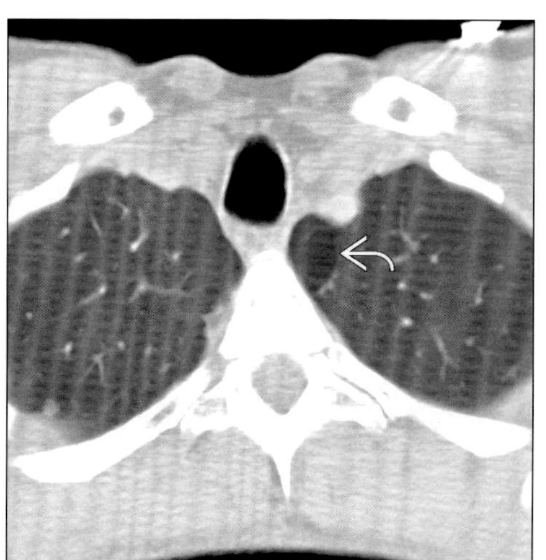

(Left) *Axial NECT of a 35-year-old man with a left primary spontaneous pneumothorax shows right apical subpleural fibrosis with probable subpleural bullae and a small left apical pneumothorax.* ***(Right)*** *Axial NECT of the same patient shows a small residual left apical pneumothorax and a dominant left apical bulla or bleb ↪, which likely caused the pneumothorax. Because patients with PSP have biapical bullous disease, recurrent pneumothorax may be ipsilateral or contralateral to the original PTX.*

SECONDARY SPONTANEOUS PNEUMOTHORAX

Key Facts

Terminology

- Secondary spontaneous pneumothorax (SSP)
- Pneumothorax associated with underlying lung disease in the absence of trauma or intervention

Imaging

- Radiography
  - Thin visceral pleural line parallel to chest wall
  - Absence of peripheral lung markings
  - Focal, diffuse, or cystic/cavitary lung disease
  - Decubitus radiography; equal or superior to upright radiography
  - Supine radiography; least sensitive
- CT
  - Gas within pleural space
  - Increased sensitivity/specificity for diagnosing SSP
  - Optimal evaluation of underlying lung disease

Top Differential Diagnoses

- Chronic obstructive pulmonary disease
  - Emphysema, cystic fibrosis, asthma
- Interstitial lung disease
  - Cystic lung disease: Lymphangioleiomyomatosis (80%), Langerhans cell histiocytosis (25%)
  - Fibrotic interstitial lung disease: Small SSP
- Neoplasm
  - Metastases, primary lung cancer, mesothelioma
- Pneumonia
  - *Pneumocystis* or *Staphylococcus* pneumatoceles

Clinical Issues

- Chest pain, sudden dyspnea

Diagnostic Checklist

- Careful assessment of the lung in spontaneous pneumothorax; exclusion of underlying lung disease

*(**Left**) PA chest radiograph shows bilateral bronchial wall thickening, bronchiectasis ➢, and basilar mucus plugs secondary to cystic fibrosis and a large left pneumothorax with visualization of the visceral pleural line ➡ and absence of peripheral lung markings. (**Right**) Lateral chest radiograph shows bronchiectasis and bronchial wall thickening ➢. The pneumothorax is less apparent. Secondary spontaneous pneumothorax occurs in association with cystic, cavitary, or infiltrative lung disease.*

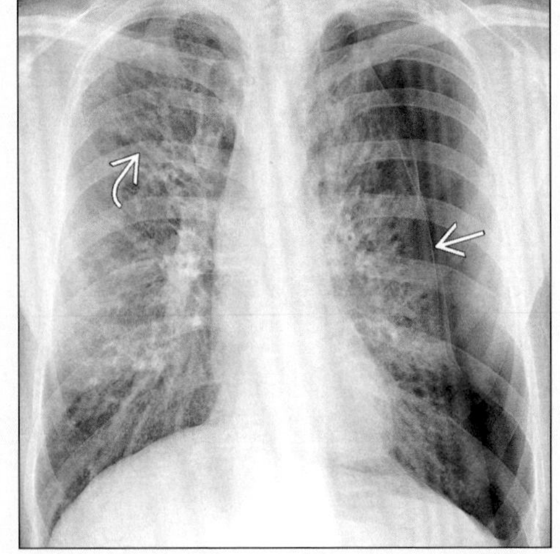

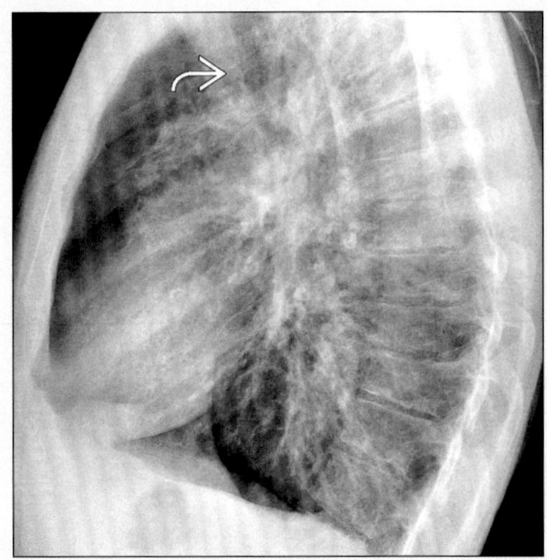

*(**Left**) Axial CECT shows severe paraseptal ➡ and centrilobular emphysema ➢. Note a small right apical pneumothorax manifesting as air within the pleural space. (**Right**) Axial CECT shows scattered foci of bilateral centrilobular emphysema ➢ and a small pneumothorax in the nondependent right anterior pleural space. CT has high sensitivity and specificity for the diagnosis of pneumothorax and allows characterization of associated pulmonary disease.*

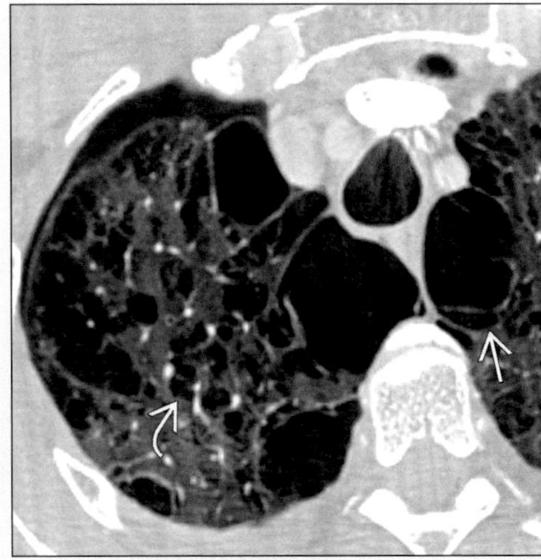

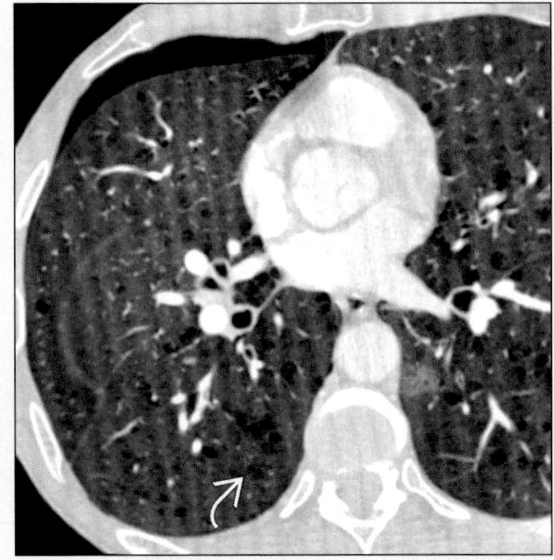

SECONDARY SPONTANEOUS PNEUMOTHORAX

TERMINOLOGY

Abbreviations

- **Secondary spontaneous pneumothorax (SSP)**

Definitions

- Pneumothorax associated with underlying lung disease in the absence of trauma or intervention

IMAGING

General Features

- Best diagnostic clue
  - Radiography: Visualization of thin visceral pleural line; absence of peripheral lung markings; evaluation of underlying lung disease
  - CT: Gas within pleural space; optimal evaluation of underlying parenchymal disease
- Location
  - Nondependent pleural space
    - Upright imaging; apical pleural space
    - Supine imaging; anterior basilar pleural space
    - Decubitus imaging; lateral nondependent pleural space
- Size
  - Variable; small, moderate, large

Radiographic Findings

- **Thin visceral pleural line** parallel to chest wall
- **Absence of peripheral lung markings**
- **Focal, diffuse, or cystic/cavitary lung disease**
- Sensitivity depends on patient position
  - Decubitus radiography; equal or superior to upright radiography
  - Supine radiography; least sensitive, inaccurate estimation of pneumothorax size
    - **Deep sulcus sign**: Gas in anterior inferior pleural space
    - ↑ sharpness of mediastinal/diaphragmatic contours
    - ↑ translucency of affected hemithorax

CT Findings

- Gas within pleural space; between chest wall & lung
- Increased sensitivity & specificity for diagnosing SSP
- Optimal evaluation of underlying pulmonary disease

Ultrasonographic Findings

- Loss of **lung sliding sign**, loss of B-lines
- Detection of A-lines, detection of "lung point"
- Sensitivity 60-100%; specificity 83-100%

Imaging Recommendations

- Best imaging tool
  - Diagnosis typically made on **upright radiography**
    - Expiratory imaging does not increase sensitivity
  - CT most sensitive & specific for diagnosis of SSP & assessment of pulmonary disease

DIFFERENTIAL DIAGNOSIS

Chronic Obstructive Pulmonary Disease

- Most common cause of SSP
- Emphysema, cystic fibrosis, asthma

Interstitial Lung Disease

- Cystic lung disease: Lymphangioleiomyomatosis (80%), Langerhans cell histiocytosis (25%)
- Fibrotic interstitial lung disease: Small SSP, often asymptomatic
- Sarcoidosis: Subpleural granulomas; bullous disease

Neoplasm

- Metastases, primary lung cancer, mesothelioma
  - Metastatic osteosarcoma; best described
- SSP may develop after induction of chemotherapy

Pneumonia

- Bronchopleural fistula from necrotizing pneumonia or septic emboli
- Pneumatoceles: *Pneumocystis* or *Staphylococcus* infection

Catamenial Pneumothorax

- SSP near time of menses; usually parous women
- Majority (90%) right-sided, small, recurrent
- Diaphragmatic defect allowing passage of peritoneal gas vs. pleural endometrial implants

Wegener Granulomatosis

- Bronchopleural fistula from cavitary lung nodules
- Pulmonary hemorrhage or consolidation ± cavitation
- Airway mural thickening; typically subglottic trachea

Collagen Vascular Disease

- Marfan syndrome: Abnormal fibrillin; pneumothorax in 4-15%, associated bullous disease
- Ehlers-Danlos syndrome: Typically type IV, associated skeletal abnormalities
- Rheumatoid arthritis: Bronchopleural fistula from subpleural necrobiotic nodules

CLINICAL ISSUES

Presentation

- Most common signs/symptoms
  - **Chest pain, sudden dyspnea**
- Other signs/symptoms
  - Cyanosis, sweats, tachycardia

Treatment

- Observation of small, minimally symptomatic SSP
- **Chest tube drainage** for large, symptomatic SSP
- Treatment of underlying lung disease

DIAGNOSTIC CHECKLIST

Consider

- Careful assessment of the lung in spontaneous pneumothorax; exclusion of underlying lung disease

Image Interpretation Pearls

- Supine radiography; underestimation of SSP size

SELECTED REFERENCES

1. Simpson G: Spontaneous pneumothorax: time for some fresh air. Intern Med J. 40(3):231-4, 2010
2. Shen KR et al: Decision making in the management of secondary spontaneous pneumothorax in patients with severe emphysema. Thorac Surg Clin. 19(2):233-8, 2009

SECONDARY SPONTANEOUS PNEUMOTHORAX

(Left) Axial CECT shows centrilobular micronodules, small lung cysts ➔, and a tiny right pneumothorax ➔ secondary to Langerhans cell histiocytosis. *(Right)* Sagittal HRCT of the same patient shows cysts ➔ and micronodules that spare the posterior lung base. A right pneumothorax ➔ is largest in the anterior inferior pleural space. Pneumothorax is typically located in the nondependent pleural space, the anterior inferior pleural space in the supine position.

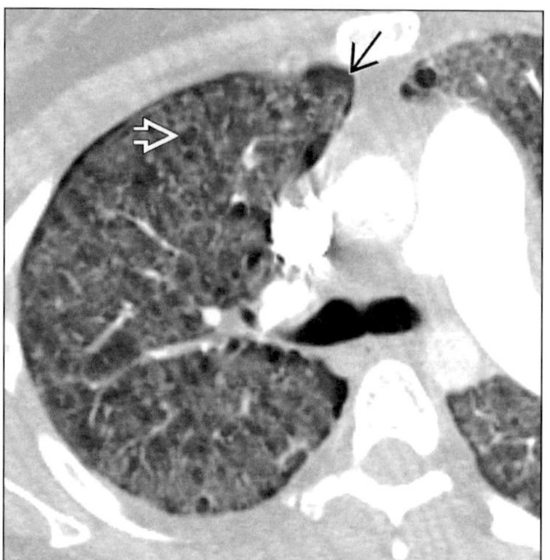

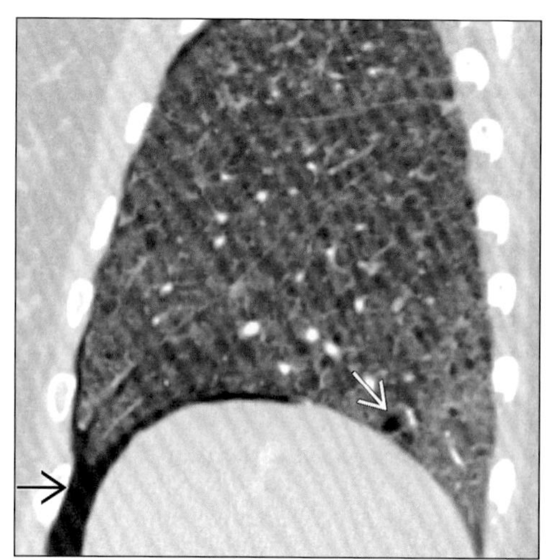

(Left) Axial NECT shows multiple thin-walled cysts ➔, subcentimeter nodules ➔, and a left pneumothorax ➔ secondary to lymphocytic interstitial pneumonia. *(Right)* Axial NECT of the same patient shows a subpleural thin-walled cyst ➔ and a moderate left pneumothorax ➔. The pulmonary cysts in lymphocytic interstitial pneumonia are often peribronchovascular and subpleural and are usually associated with ground-glass opacities and nodules.

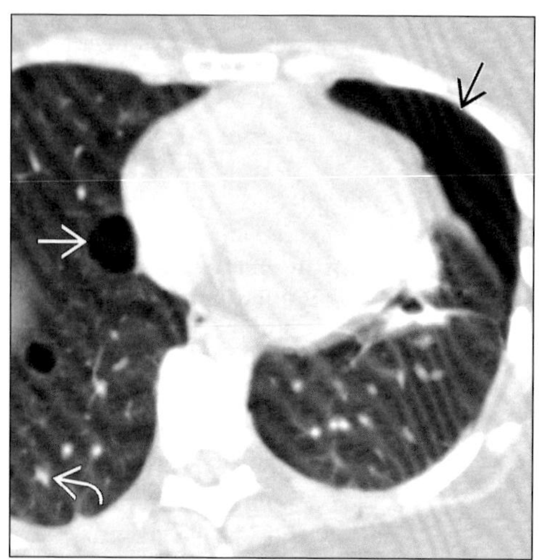

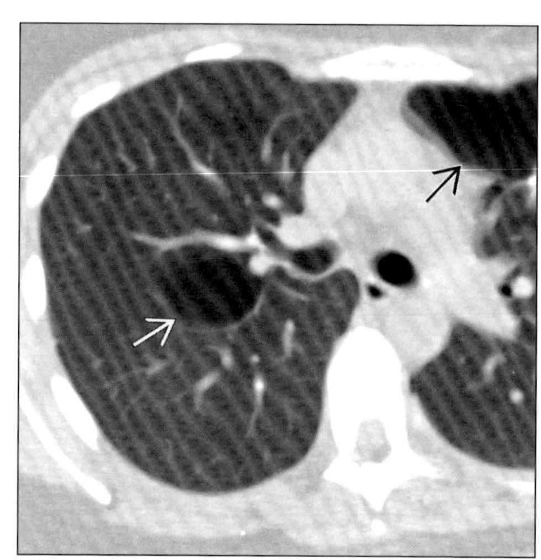

(Left) Axial CECT shows a bilobed left upper lobe nodule ➔, a small left pleural effusion ➔, and a small left pneumothorax ➔ secondary to metastatic colon cancer. *(Right)* Axial CECT shows a cavitary left lower lobe pneumonia with an air-fluid level ➔, a bronchopleural fistula ➔, and a left pneumothorax ➔. Primary and secondary lung neoplasms as well as cavitary lung lesions may produce secondary spontaneous pneumothorax.

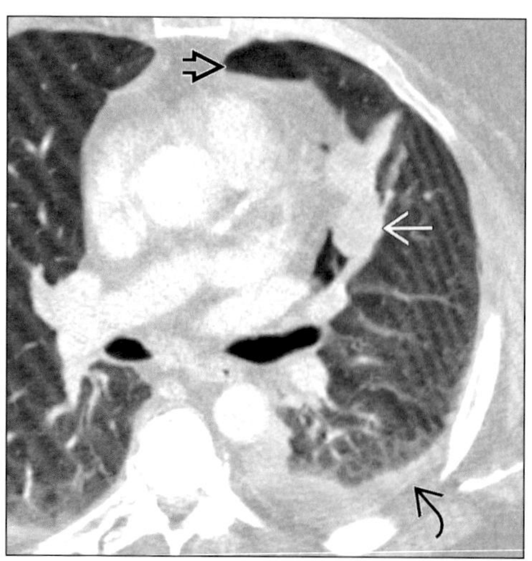

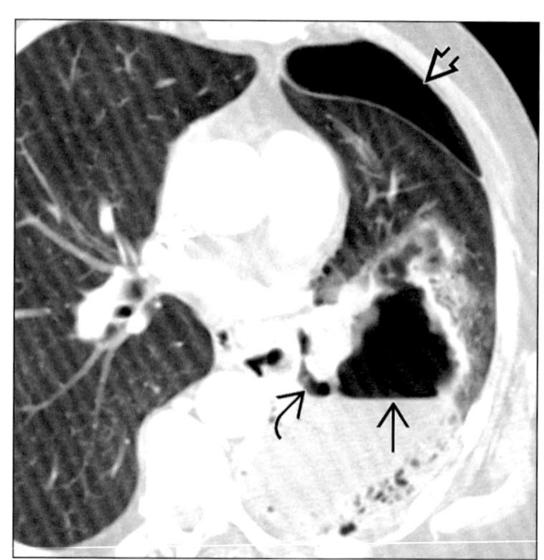

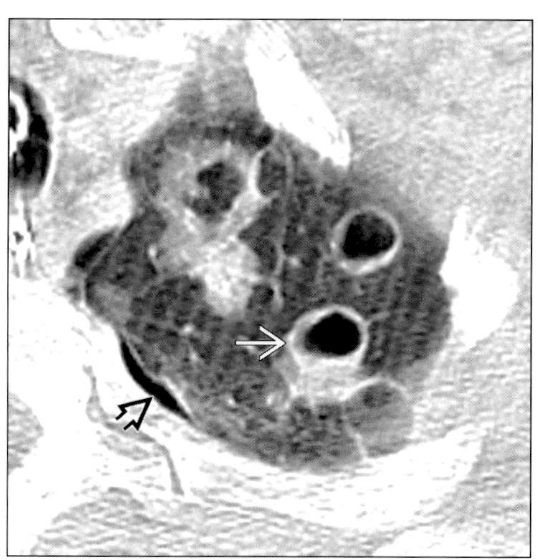

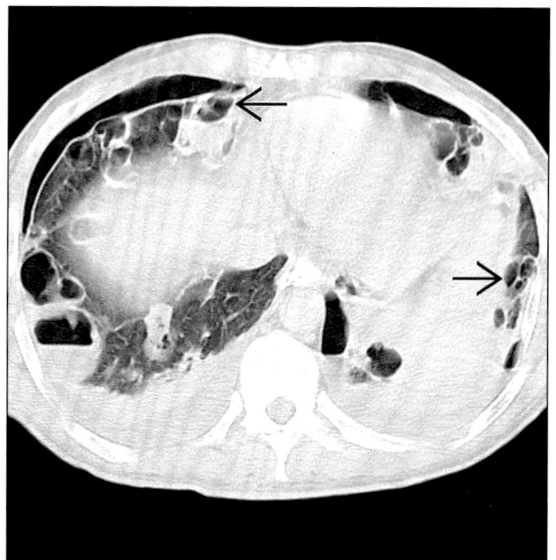

(Left) *Axial NECT of a patient with staphylococcal pneumonia shows multiple cavitary lung nodules* → *and a small left pneumothorax* →*.* ***(Right)*** *Axial NECT of the same patient shows multiple bilateral cavitary lung nodules* → *with intrinsic air-fluid levels, many of which are subpleural. Note bilateral hydropneumothoraces. Subpleural cavitary lung nodules can result in pneumothorax and bronchopleural fistula, particularly in cases of staphylococcal pneumonia.*

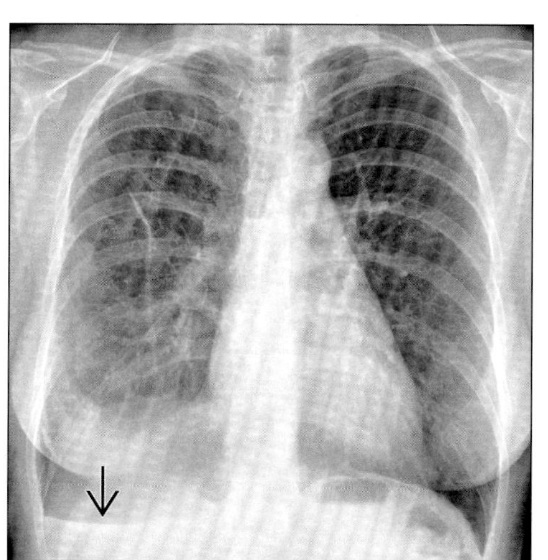

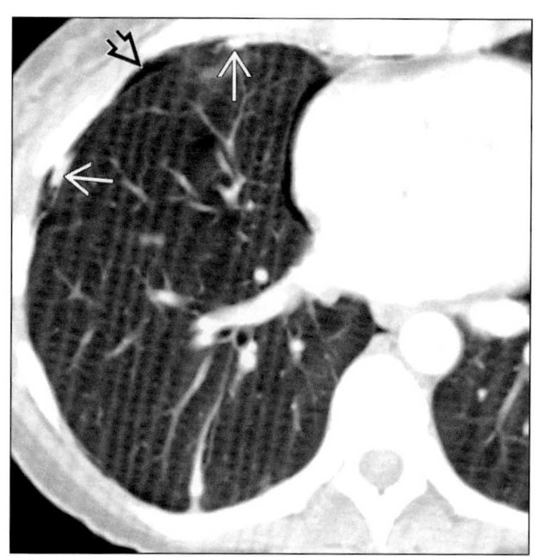

(Left) *PA chest radiograph of a patient with recurrent catamenial pneumothoraces shows a right hydropneumothorax producing an air-fluid level* → *in the right inferior pleural space.* ***(Right)*** *Axial CECT of the same patient shows a small right anterior pneumothorax* → *and pleural soft tissue nodules* → *suggestive of endometrial pleural implants. Catamenial pneumothorax is a rare form of secondary spontaneous pneumothorax.*

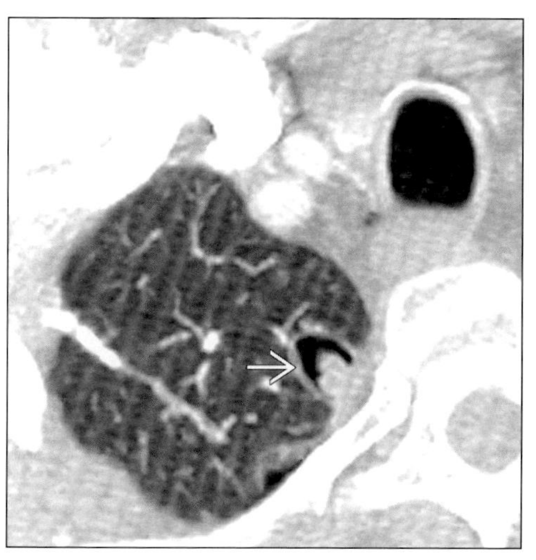

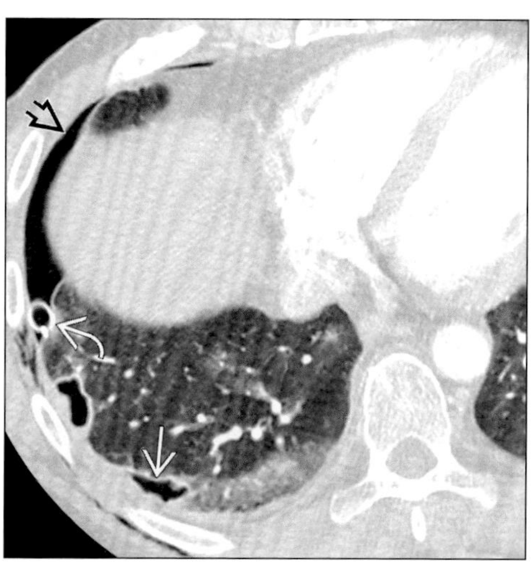

(Left) *Axial CECT of a patient with rheumatoid arthritis and necrobiotic lung nodules shows a cavitary lesion* → *with an intrinsic eccentric soft tissue nodule in the right lung apex.* ***(Right)*** *Axial CECT of the same patient shows more cavitary subpleural necrobiotic nodules* → *and a small right pneumothorax* →*. Note right pleural tube* → *and right posterior chest wall subcutaneous gas. CT allows evaluation of underlying parenchymal disease in patients with SSP.*

APICAL CAP

Key Facts

Terminology

- Synonyms
  - Apical pleural cap, apical scar
- Definition
  - Apical pleuroparenchymal thickening

Imaging

- Crescentic apical soft tissue opacity < 5 mm thick
- Sharp, smooth, or undulating margin
- Thickness usually within 5 mm of contralateral side
- Subpleural apical soft tissue on CT
- Extrapleural fat often thickened

Top Differential Diagnoses

- Pancoast tumor (superior sulcus tumor)
- Pulmonary tuberculosis
- Mediastinal hemorrhage
- Radiation fibrosis
- Extrapleural fat

Pathology

- Postulated chronic apical lung ischemia
- Pleuroparenchymal fibrosis
- Cicatricial emphysema adjacent to scar
- Peripheral pneumatocyte hyperplasia may mimic carcinoma associated with scar

Clinical Issues

- Asymptomatic radiographic abnormality
- Incidence increases with age
  - 5% at age 40; 50% at age 70

Diagnostic Checklist

- Bilateral apical caps are within 5 mm in thickness
- Consider apical cap in asymptomatic elderly patients with stable or symmetric apical thickening
- Exclude malignancy in cases of asymmetric indistinct apical caps with associated skeletal destruction

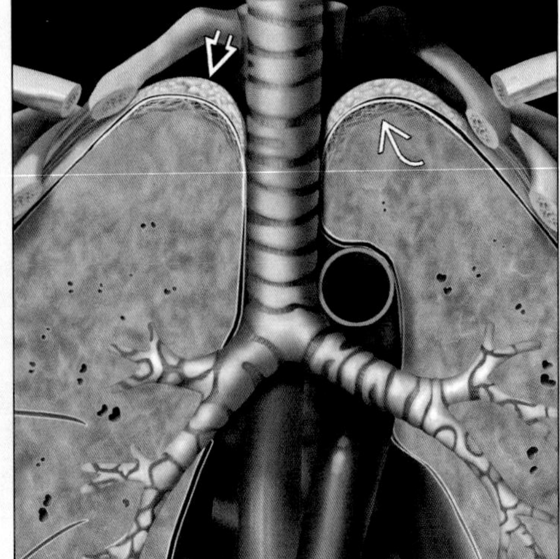

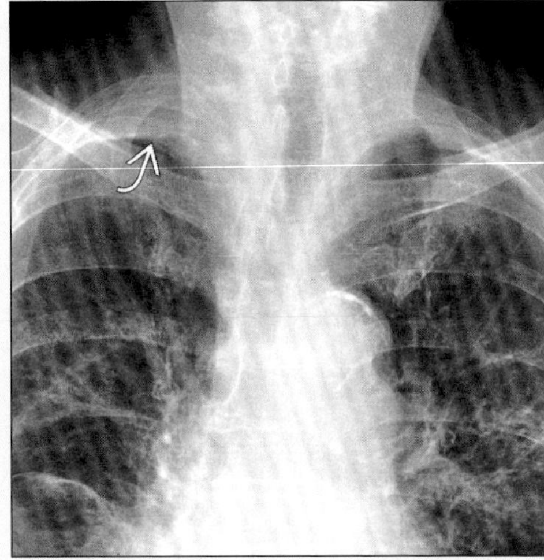

(Left) Graphic shows biapical fibrosis ➡ and extrapleural fat thickening ➡, which account for apical caps seen radiographically. (Right) PA chest radiograph shows bilateral crescentic apical opacities ➡ consistent with bilateral apical caps. A benign apical cap exhibits smooth margins and no more than 5 mm difference in thickness when compared to the contralateral side. Long-term stability in this elderly patient supports a benign etiology such as ischemia or granulomatous disease.

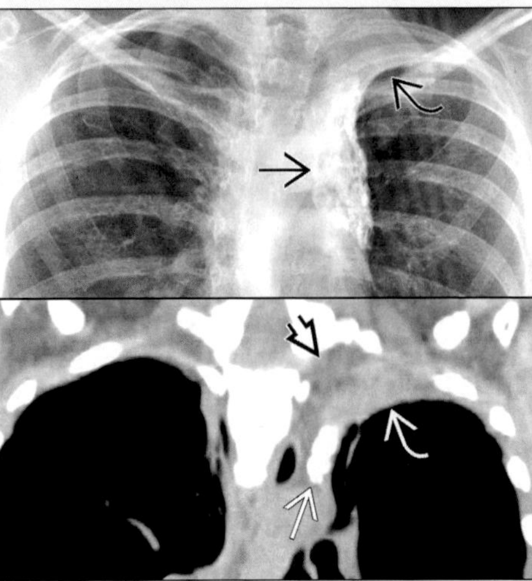

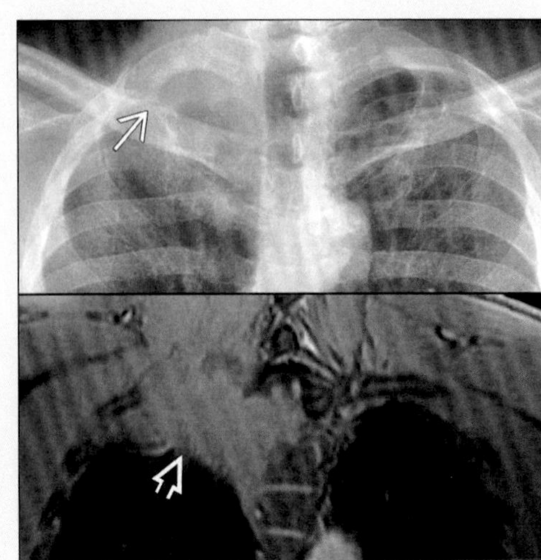

(Left) PA chest radiograph (top) shows a left apical cap ➡ and calcified mediastinal lymph nodes ➡ in a patient with lymphoma treated with radiation. Coronal NECT (bottom) shows the apical cap ➡, calcified lymph nodes ➡, and thickened extrapleural fat ➡. (Right) PA chest radiograph (top) shows an irregular right apical opacity ➡ with destruction of adjacent ribs and vertebrae. Coronal T2WI MR (bottom) confirms an invasive apical lung cancer ➡ (Pancoast tumor) with chest wall involvement.

APICAL CAP

TERMINOLOGY

Synonyms

- (Pulmonary) apical cap, apical pleural cap, apical scar

Definitions

- Apical pleuroparenchymal thickening on radiography

IMAGING

Radiographic Findings

- **Crescentic apical opacity**; usually < **5 mm thick**
- **Sharp**, **smooth**, or **undulating** margin
- **Bilateral** more common than unilateral
  - Bilateral; apical cap **within 5 mm in thickness** compared to contralateral side
  - Unilateral, more common on right

CT Findings

- Subpleural soft tissue adjacent to lung apex
- **Extrapleural fat** often **thickened**
- Adjacent **paracicatricial emphysema**

MR Findings

- **Multiplanar imaging** may help exclude apical mass

DIFFERENTIAL DIAGNOSIS

Pancoast Tumor (Superior Sulcus Tumor)

- Apical bronchogenic carcinoma
- Associated rib or vertebral body destruction
- Inferior margin may be indistinct
- Asymmetry > 5 mm suspicious for malignancy

Tuberculosis or Other Inflammatory Disease

- Apical cicatricial scar, often contains small calcified nodules, associated hilar retraction from volume loss
- Thickened extrapleural fat common on CT
- Usually irregular apical cap > 5 mm thick

Mediastinal Hemorrhage

- Extrapleural blood from great vessel injury dissecting along subclavian artery
- Unusual as isolated radiographic abnormality
- More common on left

Radiation Fibrosis

- Lung apex in radiation field for head & neck cancer, lymphoma, breast cancer (supraclavicular therapy)

Peripheral Upper Lobe Collapse

- Apical &/or posterior upper lobe segment atelectasis

Pleural Effusion (Supine)

- Lung apex most dependent portion of pleural space in supine position

Excess Extrapleural Fat

- Usually bilateral
  - May be seen in normal subjects
  - Obesity, corticosteroids, Cushing syndrome
- Fat attenuation on CT

Mesothelioma

- Typically diffuse irregular pleural thickening

Extrapleural Neoplasm

- Invasive thymoma with extrapleural involvement
- Perivascular spread of lymphoma in superior sulcus
- Paravertebral mass; neurogenic neoplasm

Vascular Abnormalities

- Dilatation/ectasia of subclavian vessels
- Post-traumatic aneurysm or arteriovenous fistula

PATHOLOGY

General Features

- Etiology
  - Postulated **chronic apical lung ischemia**
    - Histologic vascular abnormality similar to lung infarct
    - Apical lung ischemia leads to pleuroparenchymal fibrosis

Gross Pathologic & Surgical Features

- Depressed apical plaque with triangular cross-sectional morphology
- Overlying pleural thickening with sharp lateral margins

Microscopic Features

- Hyaline fibrosis of visceral pleura identical to pleural plaque in 50% of cases
- Collapsed but intact elastic framework and increased fibers
- Cicatricial emphysema adjacent to scar
- Peripheral pneumatocyte hyperplasia may mimic carcinoma associated with scar

CLINICAL ISSUES

Presentation

- Most common signs/symptoms
  - **Asymptomatic** radiographic abnormality

Demographics

- Epidemiology
  - **Incidence increases with age**
    - 5% by age 40; **50% by age 70**

Natural History & Prognosis

- Normal process of aging

DIAGNOSTIC CHECKLIST

Consider

- Benign apical cap in asymptomatic elderly patients with stable or symmetric apical thickening
- Exclusion of malignancy in cases of asymmetric indistinct apical cap with associated skeletal destruction

SELECTED REFERENCES

1. Yousem SA: Pulmonary apical cap: a distinctive but poorly recognized lesion in pulmonary surgical pathology. Am J Surg Pathol. 25(5):679-83, 2001
2. Im JG et al: Apical opacity associated with pulmonary tuberculosis: high-resolution CT findings. Radiology. 178(3):727-31, 1991

PLEURAL PLAQUES

Key Facts

Terminology

- Definition
  - Fibrohyaline acellular lesion predominantly involving parietal pleura

Imaging

- Radiography
  - Multifocal bilateral nodular discontinuous pleural thickening ± intrinsic calcification
  - Along diaphragm & adjacent to 6th-9th ribs
  - May exhibit incomplete border sign
  - Calcified plaques; "holly leaf" appearance
- CT
  - More sensitive than radiography
  - Multifocal bilateral nodular discontinuous pleural thickening
  - Calcification in 40-90% of cases
  - Assessment of associated lung abnormalities

Top Differential Diagnoses

- Extrapleural fat
- Chest wall trauma
- Pleural infection
- Pleural metastases
- Primary pleural neoplasms
  - Malignant pleural mesothelioma
  - Localized fibrous tumor of the pleura
- Talc pleurodesis

Clinical Issues

- Etiology: Occupational asbestos exposure
- Symptoms: Asymptomatic patients
- Treatment: None

Diagnostic Checklist

- Bilateral calcified pleural plaques are virtually diagnostic for asbestos-related pleural disease

*(**Left**) PA chest radiograph shows bilateral densely calcified pleural plaques that affect the anterior pleura and the central diaphragmatic pleura ➔. Pleural plaques seen en face appear less dense centrally and exhibit sharply marginated borders. The lesion morphology has been likened to the shape of a holly leaf ➔. (**Right**) Lateral chest radiograph of the same patient shows anterior calcified pleural plaques ➔ and calcified pleural plaques over the central hemidiaphragms ➔.*

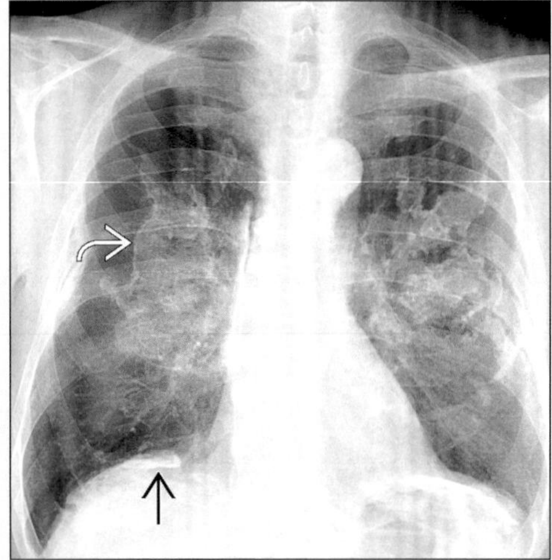

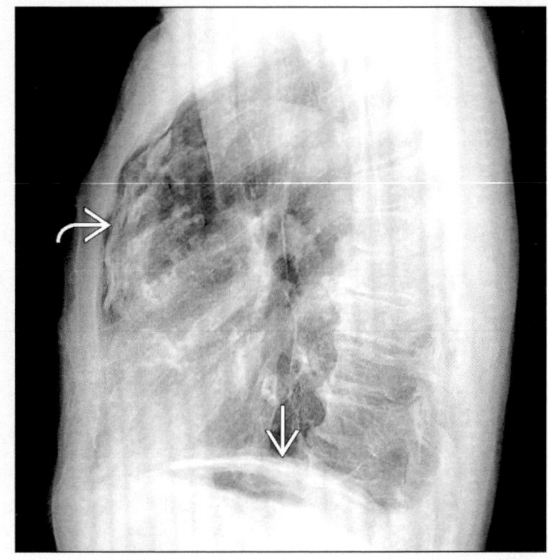

*(**Left**) Axial NECT of a patient with a history of asbestos exposure shows bilateral calcified pleural plaques. Note preferential involvement of the pleura over the central tendinous portion of the hemidiaphragm ➔ and the paravertebral regions ➔. (**Right**) Graphic shows the typical distribution of asbestos-related pleural plaques involving the parietal pleura over the central tendinous portions of the hemidiaphragms, the paravertebral regions, and the undersurfaces of the posterior ribs.*

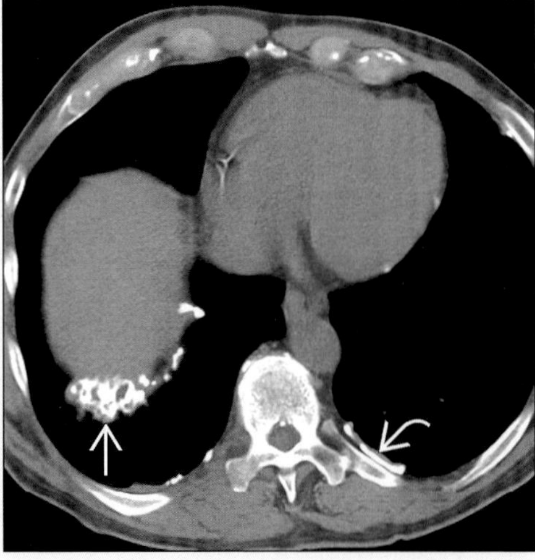

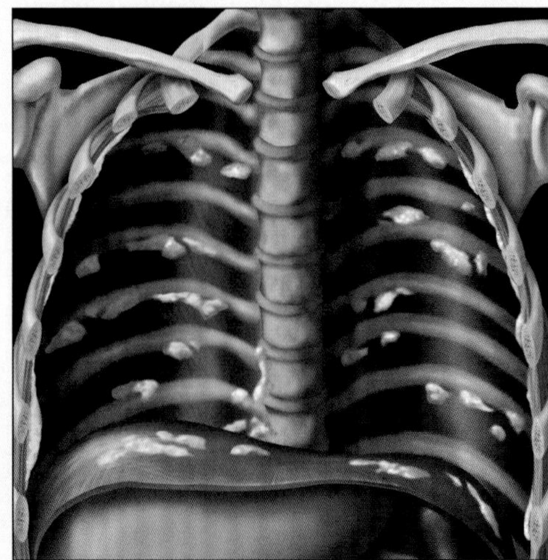

TERMINOLOGY

Definitions

- **Fibrohyaline acellular lesion** predominantly involving **parietal pleura**, often along diaphragm & beneath ribs

IMAGING

General Features

- Best diagnostic clue
  - Multifocal, bilateral pleural lesions that may exhibit calcification
- Location
  - Most common along diaphragmatic & posterolateral pleura, typically spare apical, costophrenic, & mediastinal pleura
- Size
  - Few mm to several cm in diameter
- Morphology
  - Flat or nodular soft tissue lesions; may exhibit intrinsic calcification

Radiographic Findings

- General
  - Radiography is 40% sensitive in detecting pleural plaques
  - Pleural plaques are the **most frequent radiographic manifestation of asbestos exposure**
- **Multifocal bilateral nodular discontinuous pleural thickening** ± calcifications
  - Plaques over diaphragmatic pleura are best visualized on lateral radiography
  - Plaques over posterolateral pleura adjacent to 6th-9th ribs are best visualized on oblique radiography
  - Calcified plaques over anterior or posterior pleura may exhibit a "**holly leaf**" morphology on frontal radiography
- Noncalcified plaques may exhibit smooth margins & may form obtuse angles with pleural surfaces resulting in the **incomplete border sign**
  - Cannot differentiate from other pleural lesions
  - May mimic parenchymal nodules
- Pleural plaques rarely extend over > 4 rib interspaces
- Associated findings
  - Unilateral or bilateral small pleural effusions
  - Rounded atelectasis
    - Rounded peripheral parenchymal mass
    - May mimic malignancy

CT Findings

- **CT is much more sensitive than radiography** in detecting pleural plaques
  - Pleural plaques are easily detected when adjacent to ribs or vertebral bodies
  - Noncalcified pleural plaques adjacent to intercostal muscles may be overlooked
- **Multifocal bilateral nodular discontinuous pleural thickening**
  - **Calcification in 40-90% of cases**
  - Measure from 1 mm to several cm
  - Separated from chest wall by thin layer of extrapleural fat
  - Typically affect pleura along central aspects of hemidiaphragms & adjacent to 6th-9th ribs
  - Coronal reformatted images extremely helpful in characterizing diaphragmatic pleural plaques
- Associated findings
  - Small unilateral or bilateral pleural effusions in 3% of patients with asbestos-related pleural disease
  - Rounded atelectasis in 10% of patients with asbestos-related pleural disease
    - Round peripheral lung mass adjacent to pleural thickening/plaque with volume loss & swirling bronchovascular structures; **comet tail sign**
    - Atypical findings should prompt tissue sampling
  - Usual interstitial pneumonia pattern of pulmonary fibrosis suggests asbestosis
    - Parenchymal bands, subpleural reticulation, bronchiectasis, honeycomb lung with an apical-basilar distribution gradient
  - Diffuse pleural thickening
    - Pleural thickening > 3 mm, extending > 8 cm craniocaudad, > 5 cm in length on axial CT; affecting > 25% of pleural surface along chest wall

MR Findings

- Bilateral discontinuous nodular pleural thickening with variable signal intensity on T1WI and T2WI
- May be incidentally detected on MR performed for other reasons, such as thoracic spine MR

Ultrasonographic Findings

- Grayscale ultrasound
  - Differentiation of pleural fluid from pleural plaque
  - May be used for image-guided biopsy of suspicious pleural nodules/masses or atypical pleural plaques
- Soft tissue pleural nodules; may exhibit intrinsic calcification

Imaging Recommendations

- Best imaging tool
  - CT is significantly more sensitive than radiography in detecting and characterizing pleural plaques
  - Coronal & sagittal reformatted images useful for characterization of diaphragmatic pleural plaques
- Protocol advice
  - Intravenous contrast helpful in characterizing pleural lesions, particularly if associated with pleural fluid

DIFFERENTIAL DIAGNOSIS

Extrapleural Fat

- Symmetric bilateral mid thoracic pleural thickening
- Lateral pleural thickening on frontal radiography
- CT demonstration of fat attenuation is diagnostic

Chest Wall Trauma

- Pleural thickening ± calcification adjacent to rib fractures
  - Visualization of acute or nonacute adjacent rib fractures
- Often lateral or posterior chest wall, unilateral
- Diaphragmatic pleura usually spared unless associated with hemothorax

Pleural Infection

- Chronic pleural thickening following parapneumonic effusion or empyema
  - Usually unilateral
  - Diffuse pleural thickening ± calcification

- Often associated with adjacent parenchymal scarring or bronchiectasis

Pleural Metastases

- Primary lung or chest wall malignant neoplasms may directly invade pleura
- Primary breast, renal, gastrointestinal, ovarian, thyroid, & prostate cancers may hematogenously spread to pleura
- Invasive thymoma may produce "drop" pleural metastases
- Osteosarcoma pleural metastases often calcify

Primary Pleural Neoplasms

- Malignant pleural mesothelioma
  - Circumferential nodular pleural thickening often involving fissures; associated pleural effusion & ipsilateral volume loss
  - Patients usually symptomatic
- Localized fibrous tumor of the pleura
  - Well-circumscribed focal soft tissue pleural mass; may be pedunculated
  - Small lesions may be found incidentally
  - Large lesions are usually symptomatic

Talc Pleurodesis

- Treatment of recurrent pleural effusion or pneumothorax
- High-attenuation pleural plaques
- Located posteriorly, along basilar pleural surfaces or along fissures

PATHOLOGY

General Features

- Etiology
  - Almost always related to occupational asbestos exposure
  - Typically occur **20-30 years post exposure**
  - Postulated mechanism
    - Transpleural or lymphatic migration of inhaled chrysotile asbestos fibers resulting in pleural inflammation & plaque formation
    - Crocidolite & amosite fibers usually remain within lung; more carcinogenic & fibrogenic
- Associated abnormalities
  - Pleural effusion; usually exudative, < 500 mL
    - May be initial manifestation of asbestos exposure; occur > 10 years before pleural plaques

Gross Pathologic & Surgical Features

- Hyaline fibrosis involving parietal pleura
- No evidence of malignant degeneration
- Not associated with malignant mesothelioma

Microscopic Features

- Hyalinized acellular collagen fibers in a "basketweave" pattern
- Dystrophic calcification

CLINICAL ISSUES

Presentation

- Most common signs/symptoms
  - **Asymptomatic** patients; **incidental finding**

Demographics

- Epidemiology
  - Highest incidence in patients with occupational exposure to asbestos (50-60%)
  - Incidence increases with degree of exposure

Natural History & Prognosis

- Plaques are not premalignant lesions
  - Asbestos exposure is a risk factor for lung cancer, mesothelioma, & asbestosis
- Plaques commonly enlarge or coalesce
- Dystrophic calcification develops as plaques slowly grow over time
- Diffuse pleural thickening may result in restrictive lung disease

Treatment

- None

DIAGNOSTIC CHECKLIST

Consider

- Asbestos-related pleural disease as the most common etiology of pleural plaques
- Other lesions may produce multifocal pleural calcification; clinical history is helpful in suggesting alternate diagnoses

Image Interpretation Pearls

- Bilateral calcified pleural plaques along the central hemidiaphragms are virtually diagnostic of asbestos-related pleural disease

Reporting Tips

- Patients with radiographic evidence of pleural plaques and other risk factors for lung cancer, such as cigarette smoking, may be evaluated with chest CT to exclude early occult malignancy

SELECTED REFERENCES

1. Kukkonen MK et al: Genetic susceptibility to asbestos-related fibrotic pleuropulmonary changes. Eur Respir J. 38(3):672-8, 2011
2. Larson TC et al: Workers with Libby amphibole exposure: retrospective identification and progression of radiographic changes. Radiology. 255(3):924-33, 2010
3. Paris C et al: Pleural plaques and asbestosis: dose- and time-response relationships based on HRCT data. Eur Respir J. 34(1):72-9, 2009
4. Peretz A et al: Pleural plaques related to "take-home" exposure to asbestos: An international case series. Int J Gen Med. 1:15-20, 2009
5. Greillier L et al: Mesothelioma and asbestos-related pleural diseases. Respiration. 76(1):1-15, 2008
6. Hansell DM et al: Fleischner Society: glossary of terms for thoracic imaging. Radiology. 246(3):697-722, 2008
7. Burkill GJ et al: Re: CT appearances of talc pleurodesis. Clin Radiol. 62(9):914-5, 2007
8. Clarke CC et al: Pleural plaques: a review of diagnostic issues and possible nonasbestos factors. Arch Environ Occup Health. 61(4):183-92, 2006

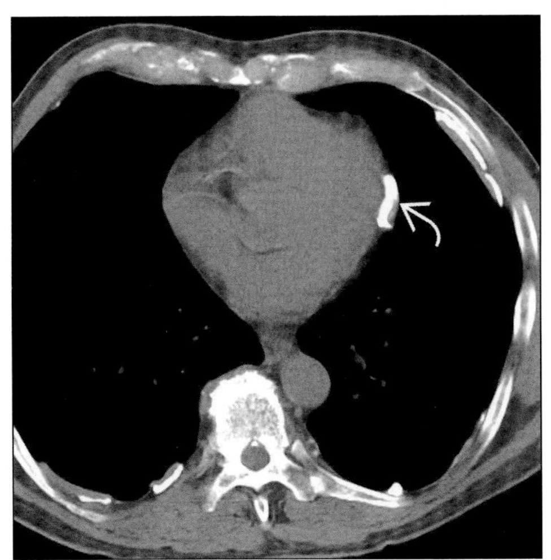

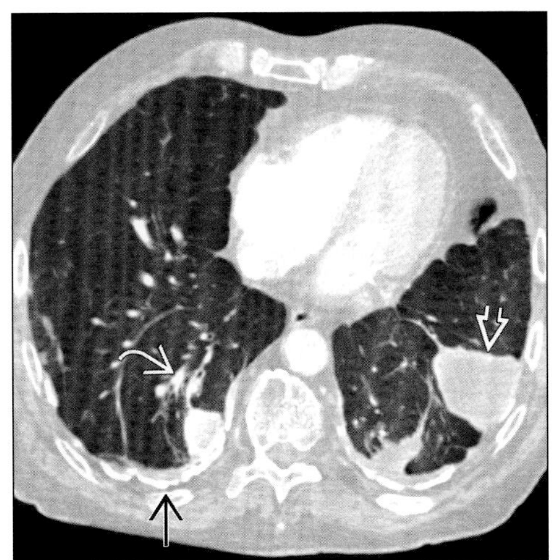

(Left) *Axial NECT of a patient with occupational asbestos exposure shows multifocal bilateral discontinuous calcified pleural plaques with left mediastinal pleural involvement ⇒.* ***(Right)*** *Axial CECT of an 82-year-old man with occupational asbestos exposure shows bilateral calcified pleural plaques → and peripheral triangular mass-like lesions ⇒ adjacent to thickened pleura. Associated volume loss and visualization of the comet tail sign ⇒ are consistent with multifocal rounded atelectasis.*

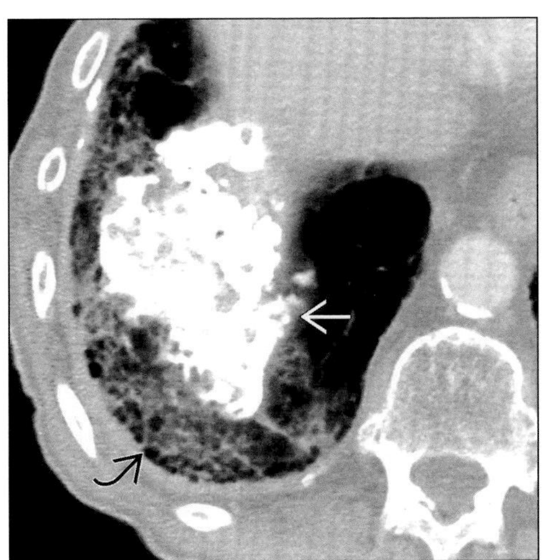

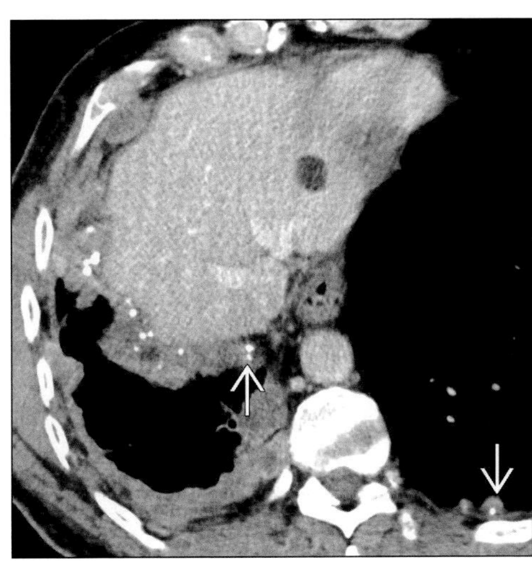

(Left) *Axial NECT of a patient with asbestos exposure and restrictive lung function shows a calcified pleural plaque ⇒ over the central right hemidiaphragm and basilar lung fibrosis manifesting with subpleural reticular opacities and cysts ⇒, consistent with asbestosis.* ***(Right)*** *Axial CECT of a patient with malignant mesothelioma shows circumferential nodular right pleural thickening and calcified pleural plaques ⇒. Pleural plaques may occur in association with other asbestos-related diseases.*

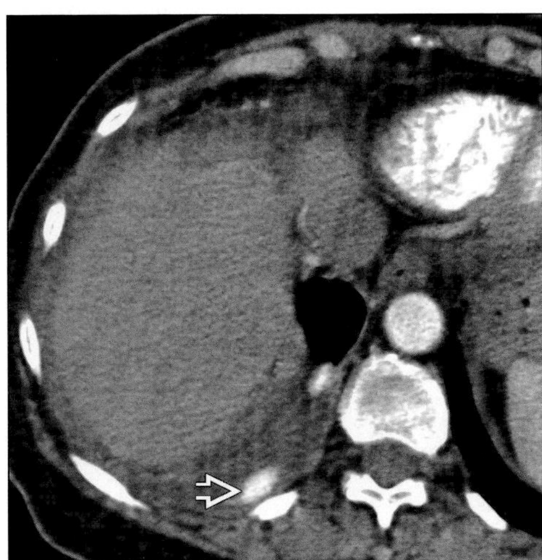

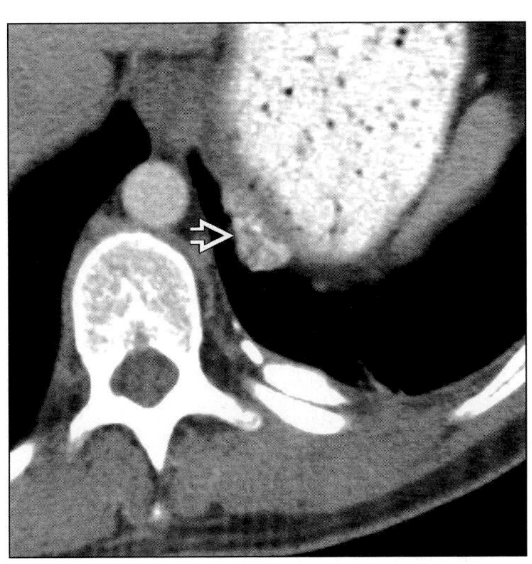

(Left) *Axial CECT of a 50-year-old man treated with talc pleurodesis for recurrent pneumothorax shows high-attenuation right pleural plaques ⇒ and a small right pleural effusion.* ***(Right)*** *Axial CECT of a 33-year-old man with pleural metastases from osteosarcoma shows densely calcified left basilar pleural lesions ⇒. The sequela of pleurodesis and bone-forming pleural malignancies may mimic asbestos-related pleural plaques. Both entities may exhibit FDG uptake on PET/CT.*

PLEURAL FIBROSIS AND FIBROTHORAX

Key Facts

Terminology

- Synonyms
  - Pleural fibrosis
  - Fibrothorax
- Definition
  - Visceral & parietal pleural thickening & calcification resulting in volume loss

Imaging

- Radiography
  - Dense circumferential pleural calcification
  - Ipsilateral volume loss
  - Narrowed intercostal spaces
  - Ipsilateral mediastinal shift
- CT
  - Coarse continuous pleural calcification
  - Pleural fluid between calcified pleural surfaces
  - Ipsilateral volume loss

Top Differential Diagnoses

- Malignant mesothelioma
- Pleural metastases
- Asbestos-related pleural disease

Pathology

- Etiology
  - Infection
  - Hemothorax

Clinical Issues

- Signs/symptoms
  - Most asymptomatic; incidental finding
  - Dyspnea, dyspnea on exertion
  - Restrictive lung disease
- Treatment
  - Decortication in carefully selected symptomatic patients without underlying lung disease

*(**Left**) PA chest radiograph of a patient with prior tuberculosis and right fibrothorax shows right volume loss, a right apical cap, elevation of the right hemidiaphragm, and narrowing of the right intercostal spaces from diffuse circumferential right pleural calcification ➔. (**Right**) Coronal NECT (bone window) of the same patient shows right pleural calcification, narrowed intercostal spaces, and low right lung volume. Fibrothorax typically manifests with diffuse unilateral pleural calcification.*

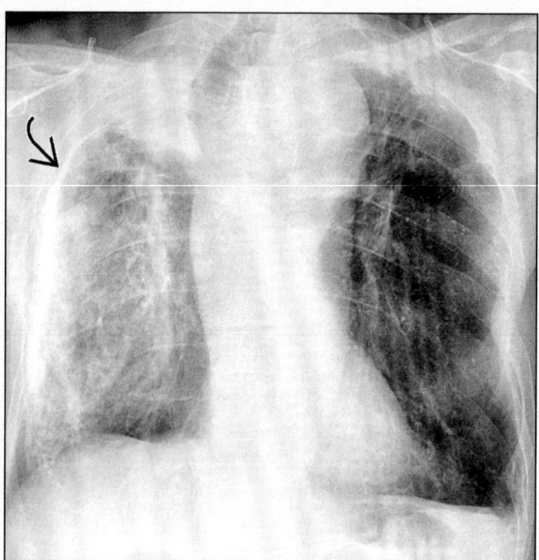

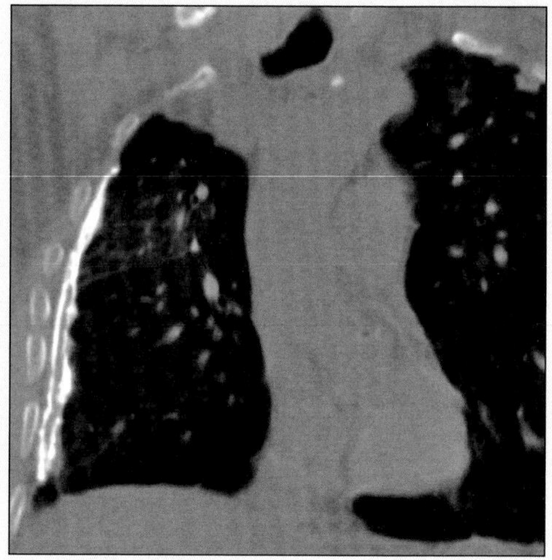

*(**Left**) Axial NECT (bone window) of a patient with bilateral fibrothoraxes from prior CABG shows heterogeneous basilar pleural thickening and calcification with associated volume loss. (**Right**) Axial NECT of a patient with remote left chest trauma and hemothorax shows dense calcification of the visceral and parietal pleural surfaces with complex central material ➔ exhibiting fluid and soft tissue attenuation. Fibrothorax may result from incompletely evacuated post-traumatic or iatrogenic hemothorax.*

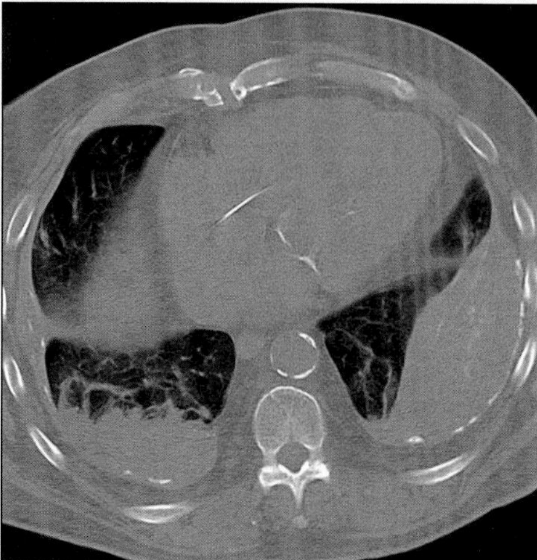

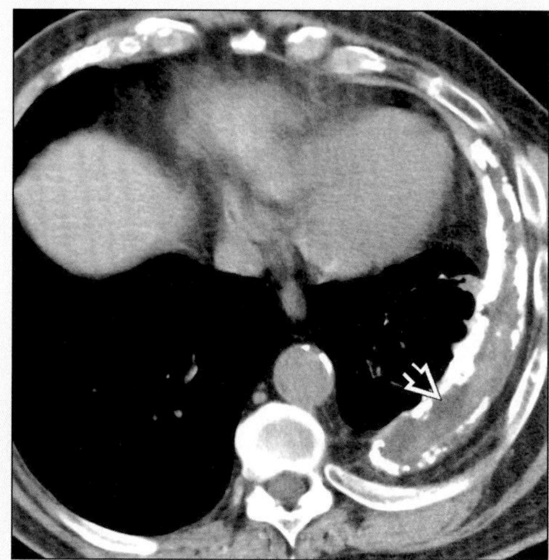

PLEURAL FIBROSIS AND FIBROTHORAX

TERMINOLOGY

Synonyms

- Pleural fibrosis
- Fibrothorax

Definitions

- Abnormal **thickening and calcification** of parietal & visceral pleural surfaces resulting in **volume loss**

IMAGING

General Features

- Best diagnostic clue
  - Unilateral diffuse pleural calcification with associated volume loss, mediastinal shift, & narrowed intercostal spaces
- Location
  - Typically unilateral; may be bilateral
- Size
  - Variable
  - May be focal or involve entire hemithorax
- Morphology
  - Thick circumferential pleural calcification

Radiographic Findings

- Dense **circumferential pleural calcification**
- Ipsilateral **volume loss**
- Narrowed intercostal spaces
- Ipsilateral mediastinal shift

CT Findings

- Coarse continuous pleural calcification
  - Often **affects > 25% of pleural surface area**
- Pleural fluid between calcified visceral pleura & parietal pleural surfaces is common
  - Variable attenuation; fluid, soft tissue
- Ipsilateral pulmonary volume loss

Imaging Recommendations

- Best imaging tool
  - CT is imaging modality of choice for assessment of pleural space & adjacent lung parenchyma
- Protocol advice
  - Intravenous contrast administration is useful in excluding enhancing soft tissue nodules that can be seen with metastases & mesothelioma

DIFFERENTIAL DIAGNOSIS

Malignant Mesothelioma

- Circumferential nodular pleural thickening
- Preferential involvement of basilar pleura
- May exhibit intrinsic calcification; calcification typically focal, not diffuse
- Pleural effusions common

Pleural Metastases

- Indistinguishable from malignant mesothelioma on imaging
- Osteosarcoma pleural metastases often calcify; typically nodular

Asbestos-related Pleural Disease

- Bilateral discontinuous multifocal nodular pleural thickening with calcification
- Parietal pleural involvement
  - Central tendinous portions of hemidiaphragms
  - Posterolateral at the level of 6th-9th ribs
- Rounded atelectasis; may occur adjacent to pleural thickening or plaques

PATHOLOGY

General Features

- Etiology
  - **Infection**
    - Tuberculosis is most common etiology
    - Bacterial empyema
  - **Hemothorax**
    - **Trauma: Penetrating or blunt injury**
    - **Iatrogenic: Most commonly following coronary artery bypass graft surgery (CABG)**
  - Immunologic disorder
    - Up to 50% of patients with rheumatoid arthritis develop pleural effusions & fibrosis
  - Uremic pleuritis
    - May occur after several years of hemodialysis
  - Drug reaction
    - Ergot derivatives, bromocriptine, cyclophosphamide
- Pathogenesis
  - Mesothelial cell inflammation with resultant release of cytokines and growth factors
  - Disordered fibrin turnover with resultant fibrosis

CLINICAL ISSUES

Presentation

- Most common signs/symptoms
  - Most are **asymptomatic**; incidental finding
  - Dyspnea, dyspnea on exertion
  - Restrictive lung disease

Natural History & Prognosis

- Stable chronic process not associated with malignant degeneration

Treatment

- Decortication in carefully selected symptomatic patients without underlying lung disease
- Steroid treatment is not effective
- Fluid aspiration does not result in lung reexpansion
  - Inability of lung to reexpand; "trapped lung"

DIAGNOSTIC CHECKLIST

Consider

- Fibrothorax in patients with unilateral diffuse pleural calcification & ipsilateral volume loss

SELECTED REFERENCES

1. Donath J et al: Restrictive chest wall disorders. Semin Respir Crit Care Med. 30(3):275-92, 2009
2. Jantz MA et al: Pleural fibrosis. Clin Chest Med. 27(2):181-91, 2006

MALIGNANT PLEURAL EFFUSION

Key Facts

Terminology
- Malignant pleural effusion (MPE)
- Exudative pleural effusion
- Contains neoplastic cells from pleural involvement by malignancy

Imaging
- Radiography
  - Typically demonstrates MPE
  - Variable size; unilateral or bilateral
- CT
  - Fluid attenuation not reliable indicator of MPE
  - Pleural effusion with nodular pleural thickening
- FDG PET
  - High metabolic activity of pleura

Top Differential Diagnoses
- Transudative pleural effusion
  - Typically associated with heart failure
- Exudative pleural effusion
  - Typically occurs in malignancy and infection
- Empyema
  - Loculated pleural effusion
  - Signs & symptoms of infection

Pathology
- Most frequent malignancies associated with MPE
  - Lung cancer (36%), breast cancer (25%)
- Diagnosis: Malignant cells in pleural fluid/tissue

Clinical Issues
- Poor prognosis
- Palliative fluid drainage for symptom relief

Diagnostic Checklist
- Consider MPE in cases of massive pleural effusions or pleural effusions with associated pleural thickening or nodularity

__(Left)__ PA chest radiograph of a patient with lung cancer shows a massive left pleural effusion with mass effect on the mediastinum. Malignant neoplasms may obstruct the airways, causing both atelectasis and MPE, with variable effects on the mediastinum. __(Right)__ Axial CECT shows a left lower lobe lung cancer →, a large pleural effusion, and focal posterior pleural thickening ↪ from metastatic disease. MPE may manifest as pleural effusion with or without associated pleural thickening or nodularity.

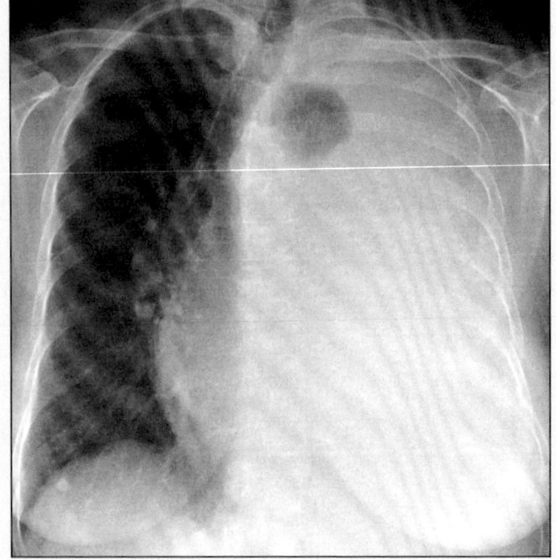

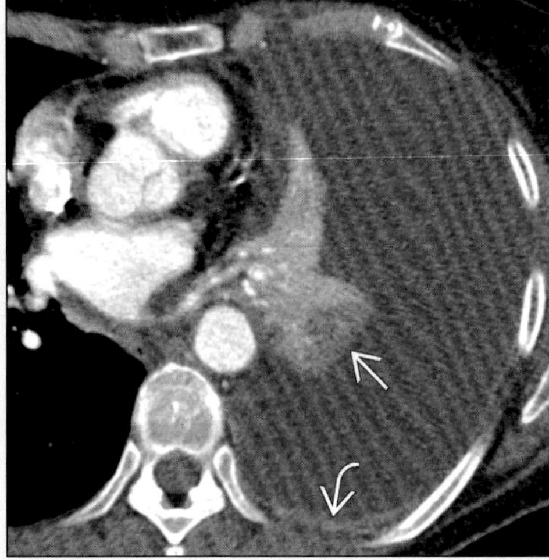

__(Left)__ Axial CECT of a patient with pancreatic cancer metastatic to the pleura shows bilateral large pleural effusions and enhancing pleural nodules ↪ on the basilar visceral pleural surfaces and the parietal pleura →. Pleural effusion with nodular pleural thickening is highly suspicious for MPE. __(Right)__ Axial fused PET/CT demonstrates FDG uptake within a left posterior pleural metastasis ↪. FDG uptake associated with pleural effusion → is consistent with MPE.

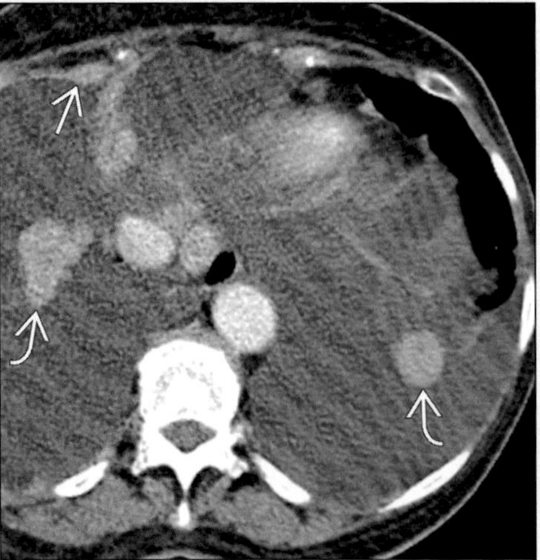

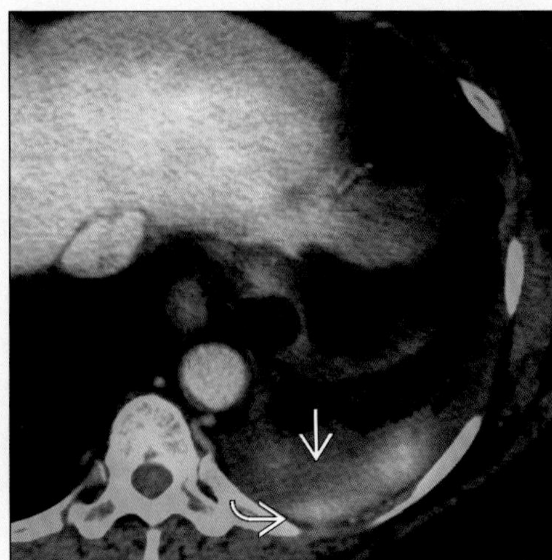

MALIGNANT PLEURAL EFFUSION

TERMINOLOGY

Abbreviations

- Malignant pleural effusion (**MPE**)

Definitions

- **Exudative pleural effusion** containing **neoplastic cells** from **pleural involvement by malignancy**
- **Paramalignant effusion**
  - Pleural effusion in setting of malignancy; no direct evidence of pleural malignancy or other etiology for the pleural effusion

IMAGING

General Features

- Best diagnostic clue
  - **Unexplained pleural effusion** in patient with **known malignancy**
  - Unexplained **massive pleural effusion**
  - Pleural effusion with **nodular pleural thickening**
- Location
  - Unilateral or bilateral
  - Nondependent fluid in loculated pleural effusion
- Size
  - Small or large
- Morphology
  - Free or loculated
  - Asymmetric or symmetric bilateral pleural effusions

Radiographic Findings

- MPE usually apparent on chest radiography; may be very large
- **Small** pleural effusion: Blunt costophrenic angle
  - Decubitus radiography for detection of small amounts of pleural fluid
- **Moderate** pleural effusion: Obscuration of hemidiaphragm; forms meniscus along chest wall
- **Moderate to large** pleural effusion: Opaque mid to inferior hemithorax
  - Frequent basilar relaxation atelectasis with moderate to large pleural effusion
- **Massive** pleural effusion: Opaque hemithorax; variable degrees of mediastinal shift
- Mass-like pleural opacity in loculated pleural effusion
- Pleural effusion with **associated smooth or nodular pleural thickening**

CT Findings

- General
  - High sensitivity for detection of pleural fluid
  - Pleural fluid attenuation not reliable indicator of malignancy
  - Direct visualization of parietal and visceral pleural surfaces
  - Separation of visceral and parietal pleural surfaces by intervening fluid; **split pleura sign**
  - Free pleural effusion of variable size
  - Loculated pleural effusion; rounded/elliptical contours, nondependent fluid
  - **CT more sensitive than radiography** for visualization of **pleural thickening/nodularity**
  - **Evaluation of adjacent structures** for evidence of malignancy; lung, mediastinum, chest wall, diaphragm, abdomen
- CECT
  - Improved visualization of pleural surfaces, atelectatic lung, lung masses
  - Improved visualization & assessment of pleural thickening &/or pleural nodules
  - **Higher sensitivity for hilar lymphadenopathy**

MR Findings

- High sensitivity for detection of pleural fluid
- Superior contrast resolution; **detection of pleural soft tissue nodules**
- T1WI
  - Variable fluid signal
- T2WI
  - High signal intensity pleural fluid
  - Pleural fluid hyperintense to or isointense with cerebrospinal fluid

Ultrasonographic Findings

- High sensitivity for detection of pleural fluid
- Evaluation of pleural thickening or nodularity
- Provides guidance for diagnostic or therapeutic thoracentesis

Nuclear Medicine Findings

- FDG PET
  - May allow **differentiation between benign & malignant pleural effusion**
  - May document high **metabolic activity of pleural thickening/nodules**
  - **May not differentiate between MPE & empyema**

Imaging Recommendations

- Best imaging tool
  - Chest radiography typically demonstrates MPE; decubitus radiography may demonstrate small MPE
  - CT most sensitive for detection of associated pleural thickening and nodularity
  - Ultrasound may help guide diagnostic/therapeutic thoracentesis
- Protocol advice
  - CECT may increase conspicuity of pleural thickening/nodularity

DIFFERENTIAL DIAGNOSIS

Transudative Pleural Effusion

- May be indistinguishable from MPE
- Usually associated with heart failure
  - Imaging findings of interstitial edema
- Pleural fluid attenuation not reliable in distinguishing transudates from exudates
- May be associated with hypoalbuminemia in patients with malignancy

Exudative Pleural Effusion

- Malignancy, infection, pulmonary infarction are most common etiologies
- May be associated with pleural thickening
- Benign exudative effusion may be seen with malignancy
  - Central neoplasm with obstructive pneumonia
  - Lymphatic/pulmonary vein obstruction by tumor
  - Systemic effects of neoplasm
  - Post-treatment adverse effects

Empyema

- Typically unilateral & loculated
- Affected patients have signs & symptoms of infection
- May be complicated by bronchopleural fistula or empyema necessitatis

PATHOLOGY

General Features

- Any malignancy may metastasize to the pleura
- Most frequent primary malignancies associated with MPE
  - **Lung cancer (36%)**
  - **Breast cancer (25%)**
  - Lymphoma (10%)
  - Ovarian cancer (5%)
  - Gastric cancer (2%)
  - Unknown primary malignancy (7%)
  - All other malignancies (14%)

Staging, Grading, & Classification

- MPE in lung cancer patients: Stage IV disease, unresectable
- MPE in breast cancer patients: Stage IV disease

Gross Pathologic & Surgical Features

- Pleural fluid in MPE may be hemorrhagic
- MPE may occur with or without pleural thickening &/ or nodularity

Microscopic Features

- Diagnosis of MPE
  - Detection of exfoliated malignant cells in pleural fluid
  - Demonstration of malignant cells in pleural tissue
- Pleural fluid cytology diagnostic in 40-60% of cases
- Increased diagnostic yield with pleural biopsy

Pleural Fluid Analysis

- High levels of protein
- Low pH
- Low levels of glucose
- High levels of lactate dehydrogenase (LDH)
- Elevated amylase in 10%; even if primary neoplasm is not in pancreas

CLINICAL ISSUES

Presentation

- Most common signs/symptoms
  - Dyspnea on exertion
  - May be asymptomatic
- Other signs/symptoms
  - Chest pain uncommon; more common in mesothelioma due to parietal pleural involvement

Natural History & Prognosis

- **Lung cancer**
  - **MPE indicates incurability**
- Breast cancer
  - Ipsilateral MPE suggests lymphatic invasion
  - Contralateral or bilateral MPE suggest hepatic metastases

Treatment

- **Observation**
  - Appropriate in asymptomatic patients with small MPE
  - Most small asymptomatic MPE progress & require treatment
- **Drainage**
  - Exudative pleural effusions in patients with cancer **often require drainage** whether malignant or not
- **Thoracentesis**
  - Relief of dyspnea
  - Variable recurrence rate
- **Chest tube drainage or thoracoscopy with talc slurry/poudrage**
  - Control of effusion in > 90% of patients without lung entrapment
- **Indwelling catheter**
  - Effective in patients with MPE with lung entrapment
- Chemotherapy may be effective in certain neoplasms
  - Small cell lung cancer
  - Breast cancer
  - Lymphoma
- Radiotherapy to mediastinum may be effective in lymphoma

DIAGNOSTIC CHECKLIST

Consider

- MPE in patients with massive pleural effusions or pleural effusions with associated pleural thickening/ nodularity
- MPE in patients with advanced lung or breast cancer with new pleural effusion
- CECT is most efficacious and sensitive imaging modality for evaluation of MPE
  - Visualization of pleural thickening as evidence of malignant nature of effusion

Image Interpretation Pearls

- 10% of malignant pleural effusions are massive
  - 70% of massive pleural effusions are malignant
- Unilateral MPE more frequently associated with lung cancer & mesothelioma

Reporting Tips

- Presence or absence of pleural thickening &/or pleural nodules should be documented, particularly for patients with pleural effusion in setting of malignancy

SELECTED REFERENCES

1. Hooper C et al: Investigation of a unilateral pleural effusion in adults: British Thoracic Society Pleural Disease Guideline 2010. Thorax. 65 Suppl 2:ii4-17, 2010
2. Heffner JE et al: Recent advances in the diagnosis and management of malignant pleural effusions. Mayo Clin Proc. 2008 Feb;83(2):235-50. Review. Erratum in: Mayo Clin Proc. 84(9):847, 2009
3. Qureshi NR et al: Thoracic ultrasound in the diagnosis of malignant pleural effusion. Thorax. 64(2):139-43, 2009
4. Qureshi NR et al: Imaging of pleural disease. Clin Chest Med. 27(2):193-213, 2006
5. McLoud TC: CT and MR in pleural disease. Clin Chest Med. 19(2):261-76, 1998

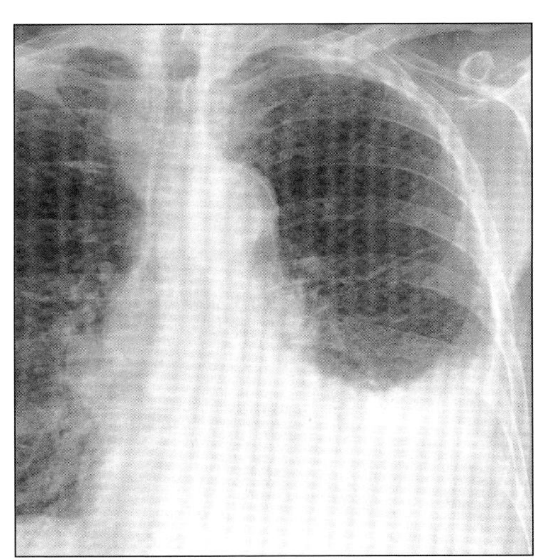

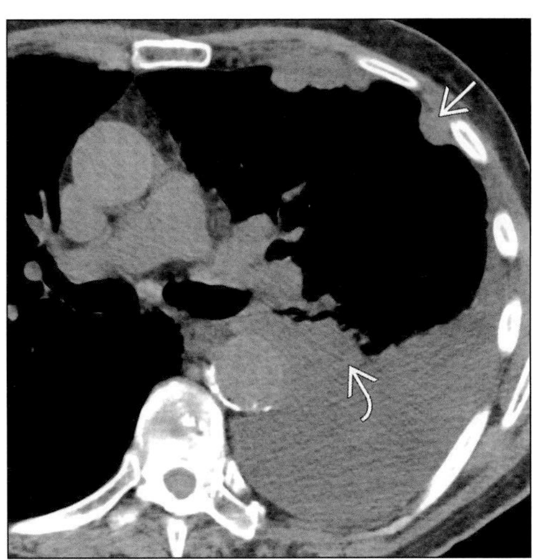

(Left) *PA chest radiograph of a patient with metastatic bladder carcinoma demonstrates a moderate left pleural effusion without apparent pleural nodularity.* ***(Right)*** *Axial NECT of the same patient shows a left pleural effusion associated with multifocal anterior pleural soft tissue nodules ➔ and left hilar lymphadenopathy ➔ representing metastatic disease. CT is more sensitive than radiography for the detection of pleural thickening and nodularity.*

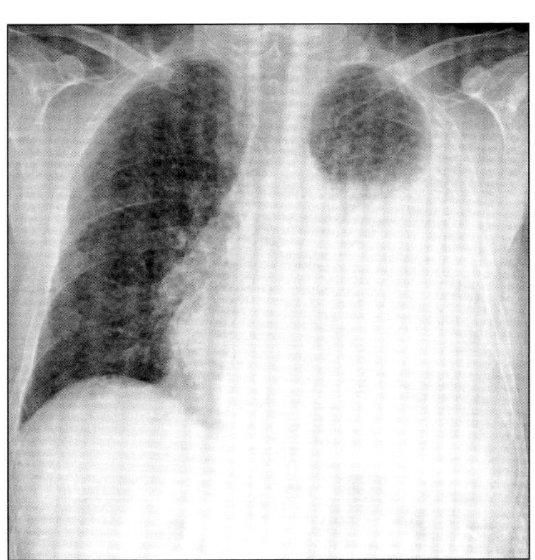

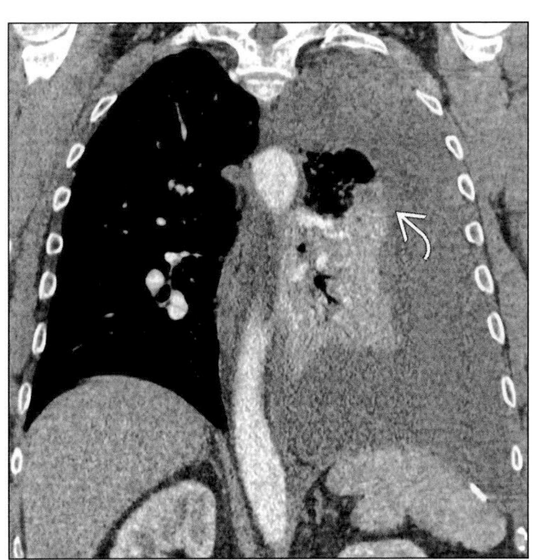

(Left) *PA chest radiograph of a patient with metastatic lung cancer shows a large left MPE. Bilateral small lung nodules represent pulmonary metastases.* ***(Right)*** *Coronal CECT of the same patient shows the large left MPE and a peripheral left upper lobe lung cancer ➔ but no apparent pleural thickening or nodularity. Lung cancer is the most common primary malignancy associated with MPE. Lung cancer (36%), breast cancer (25%), and lymphoma (10%) together account for 70% of all MPE.*

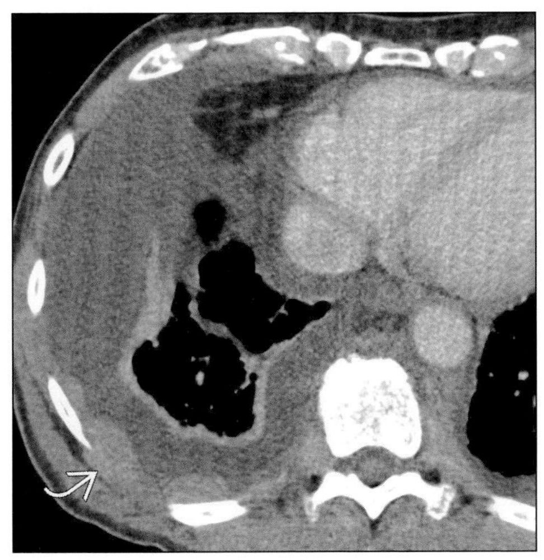

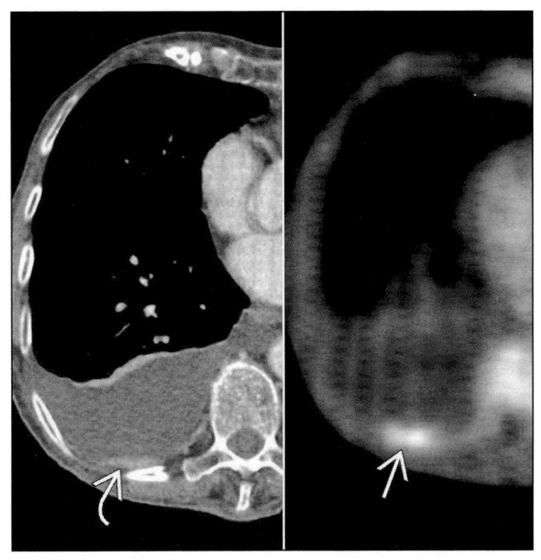

(Left) *Axial CECT of a patient with lymphoma shows a large right pleural effusion and posterior nodular pleural metastases ➔. The thickness (> 1 cm), nodularity, and circumferential growth pattern are characteristic of pleural malignancy.* ***(Right)*** *Axial CECT and correlative PET image of a patient with metastatic gastric cancer show a right pleural effusion and a band of posterior pleural thickening ➔ that demonstrates contrast enhancement on CT and matched FDG uptake ➔ on PET imaging.*

SOLID PLEURAL METASTASES

Key Facts

Terminology

- Definition
  - Secondary pleural malignancy manifesting with solid pleural nodules or masses

Imaging

- Radiography
  - Focal or multifocal pleural nodules/masses
  - Circumferential nodular pleural thickening
  - Associated pleural effusion common
- CT
  - Pleural nodules &/or masses
  - Involvement of mediastinal pleura
  - Thickness > 1 cm
  - CT may underestimate extent of disease
- MR: Hyperintense relative to muscle
- PET: FDG uptake in malignant pleural tissue/fluid
- MR & FDG-PET help delineate pleural involvement

Top Differential Diagnoses

- Malignant mesothelioma
- Localized fibrous tumor of pleura
- Pleural fibrosis & fibrothorax
- Loculated pleural effusion

Pathology

- Most common pleural malignancy
- Typically from adenocarcinomas & lung cancer
- Visceral pleura more commonly involved than parietal pleura

Clinical Issues

- Signs/symptoms
  - Dyspnea on exertion & cough
  - Asymptomatic in 25%
- Poor prognosis given advanced tumor stage
- Treatment: Periodic thoracenteses, talc pleurodesis

*(**Left**) Axial CECT of a patient with metastatic myofibroblastic sarcoma shows a focal left pleural metastasis ➡ manifesting as a heterogeneously enhancing polylobular pleural mass. (**Right**) Axial CECT of a patient with metastatic chondrosarcoma demonstrates a fusiform heterogeneously enhancing right posterior pleural metastasis ↗. Note multifocal tiny pleural nodules ➡ along the right lateral pleura. Pleural metastases may be focal or multifocal and may involve the pleura circumferentially.*

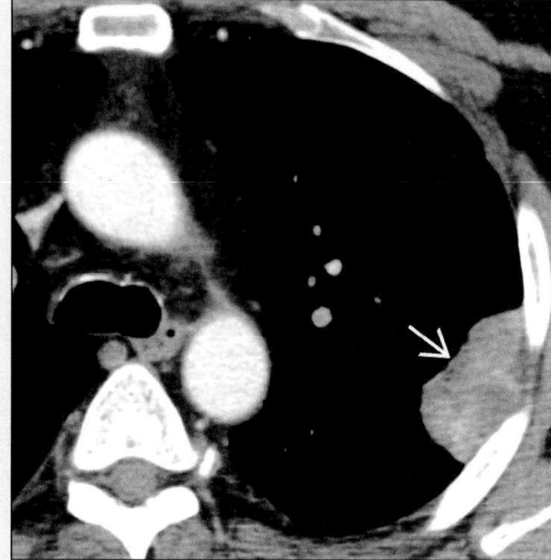

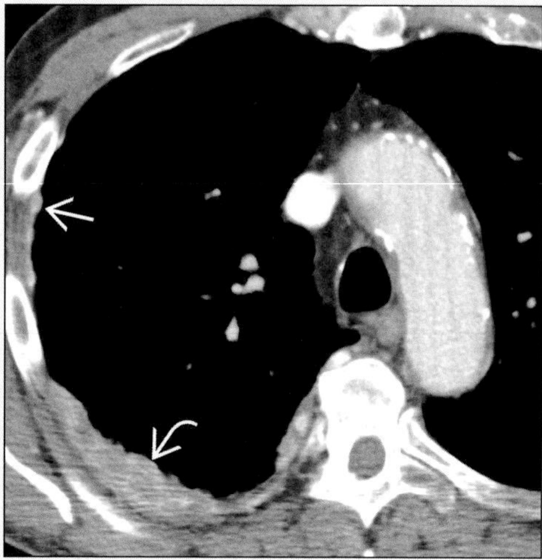

*(**Left**) Axial CECT of a patient with metastatic lung cancer shows a right pleural effusion and multiple nonenhancing nodular metastases along the right diaphragmatic ➡ and paravertebral ↗ pleural surfaces. (**Right**) Axial CECT of a patient with metastatic renal cancer shows right-sided circumferential nodular pleural thickening, right lobular pleural metastases, a left lung metastasis ➡, and a small left malignant pleural effusion ↗. Solid pleural metastases may be unilateral or bilateral.*

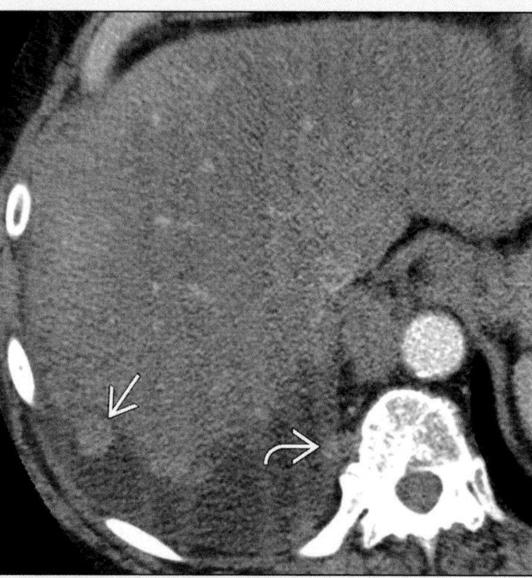

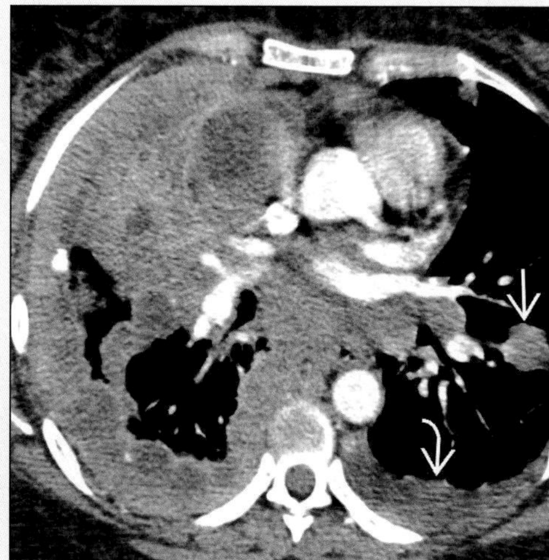

SOLID PLEURAL METASTASES

TERMINOLOGY

Definitions

- Secondary pleural malignancy manifesting with solid pleural nodules or masses
- Most common cause of malignant pleural thickening

IMAGING

General Features

- Best diagnostic clue
  - Focal or multifocal pleural nodules or masses in patient with malignancy
- Location
  - Visceral or parietal pleura
  - Unilateral or bilateral
- Morphology
  - Focal or diffuse

Radiographic Findings

- Focal or multifocal pleural nodules/masses
- **Circumferential nodular pleural thickening**
- **Associated pleural effusion** is common
  - Large effusions may obscure pleural nodules

CT Findings

- Pleural nodules &/or masses
  - Focal or multifocal; unilateral or bilateral
  - **Circumferential nodular pleural thickening**
  - May exhibit contrast enhancement
- **Involvement of mediastinal pleura**
- Fissural involvement
- Thickness > 1 cm
- Associated pleural effusion is common
- **Lung cancer**
  - Nodular pleural thickening ipsilateral to primary lung cancer; highly suggestive of metastases
  - CT may underestimate extent of pleural involvement
  - Staging
    - Visceral pleural invasion; **T2** lesion
    - Parietal/mediastinal pleural invasion; **T3** lesion
    - Malignant pleural effusion/nodules; **M1a, stage IV**
- **Breast cancer**
  - **Pleural effusion** is most common manifestation of pleural metastatic disease
    - Typically unilateral, ipsilateral to primary cancer
  - Pleural thickening, nodules, masses less common; rarely occur without pleural effusion
- **Lymphoma**
  - Typically small pleural effusion
  - May manifest as pleural plaques, nodules, masses
    - May grow along visceral pleura & involve extrapulmonary soft tissues
  - Association with mediastinal lymphadenopathy
  - Rare isolated pleural involvement
- **Invasive thymoma**
  - Pleural plaques, nodules, or masses
    - Variable association with pleural effusion
  - Unilateral disease more common than bilateral
  - Retroperitoneal extension possible
  - **Associated anterior mediastinal mass**

MR Findings

- T2WI
  - **Hyperintense** relative to intercostal muscles
- T1WI C+
  - **Hyperintense** relative to intercostal muscles
  - **Enhancement** of pleural nodules
  - Pleural fluid enhancement has been reported
- Overall: **Sensitivity 100%, specificity 93%**, positive predictive value (PPV) 96%, negative predictive value (NPV) 100%

Nuclear Medicine Findings

- PET
  - FDG uptake in malignant pleural effusions, pleural nodules, pleural masses
  - Overall: **Sensitivity 96.8%, specificity 88.5%**, PPV 93.8%, NPV 93.9%

Imaging Recommendations

- Best imaging tool
  - Radiography may show earliest abnormality
  - Chest CT is imaging modality of choice but may underestimate extent of pleural involvement
  - MR and FDG-PET may show extent of involvement
- Protocol advice
  - Multiplanar reformatted images useful for problem solving & demonstrating extent of disease

DIFFERENTIAL DIAGNOSIS

Malignant Mesothelioma

- Most common primary pleural neoplasm
- 80% occur in patients exposed to asbestos
- Pleural plaques present in 10%
- Higher association with pleural effusion (95% vs. 50%)

Localized Fibrous Tumor of Pleura

- Small lesions; homogeneous, obtuse margins
- Large lesions; heterogeneous, acute margins
- Calcification uncommon

Pleural Fibrosis and Fibrothorax

- Fibrous obliteration of pleural space
- Hemorrhagic & tuberculous effusions, empyema
- Parenchymal disease with previous TB or empyema
- Mediastinal pleura spared in 88%
- May demonstrate extensive calcification

Loculated Pleural Effusion

- Not circumferential
- Usually spares mediastinal pleura
- Adjacent smooth pleural thickening, not nodular

Asbestos-related Pleural Fibrosis

- Bilateral thickening involving 25% of chest
- Unilateral thickening involving 50% of chest
- Pleural thickening > 5 mm at any site
- Calcification rare (unlike pleural plaques)

Rounded Atelectasis

- Mass-like opacity abutting pleural surface
- Associated adjacent pleural thickening
- Associated with asbestos-related pleural disease &/or chronic pleural effusion

Pleurodesis

- Thickening of parietal and visceral pleura
- Hyperattenuation secondary to talc deposition

SOLID PLEURAL METASTASES

Splenosis

- Splenic tissue implants on peritoneum & pleura
- History of trauma or surgery
- Pleural nodules or masses; typically unilateral
- Diagnosis with Tc-99m sulfur colloid or Tc-99m damaged erythrocyte scintigraphy

Epithelioid Hemangioendothelioma

- Rare vascular tumor of lung and liver
- Pleural effusion & nodularity
- Mimics pleural metastases & mesothelioma

PATHOLOGY

General Features

- Etiology
  - **Most common pleural malignancy**
    - **Adenocarcinoma** most common cell type
    - **Lung cancer 40%**
    - **Breast cancer 20%**
    - **Lymphoma 10%**
    - Unknown primary malignancy 10%
    - Ovarian & gastric cancer 5%
  - Pleural involvement
    - Hematogenous or lymphatic spread of tumor
    - Direct pleural invasion by tumor
- Pleural space; potential space in which fluid &/or cells may accumulate
- Visceral pleura more commonly involved than parietal
- Parietal pleural metastases from lung cancer
  - Extension of tumor across pleural space from affected visceral pleura
  - Exfoliation of visceral pleura tumor cells
- Pleural metastases from breast cancer
  - Invasion of chest wall lymphatics
  - Hematogenous spread through hepatic metastases
- Pleural metastatic disease from primary malignancies below the diaphragm result from hepatic metastases

Gross Pathologic & Surgical Features

- Rich lymphatic system present in pleura
- **Visceral** pleura more commonly involved than parietal pleura
- Associated pleural effusion thought to be secondary to obstruction of pleural lymphatics by tumor
  - Serous, serosanguineous, or hemorrhagic fluid
- No relationship between extent of metastatic disease and occurrence of pleural effusion
- Pleural metastases may only be visible at surgery

Microscopic Features

- Malignant effusions; usually exudative, rarely transudative
- Diagnosed by presence of tumor cells in fluid or pleura
- Cytology is more sensitive than percutaneous pleural biopsy
- Yield from exfoliative thoracoscopy 90-95% vs. 50-60% with pleural biopsy

CLINICAL ISSUES

Presentation

- Most common signs/symptoms
  - **Dyspnea on exertion**
  - **Cough**
  - Severity relates to fluid volume & lung function
- Other signs/symptoms
  - **Weight loss and fatigue**
  - **Chest pain** from involvement of parietal pleura or chest wall
  - Lymphadenopathy in 1/3 at presentation
  - **Asymptomatic in 25%**

Natural History & Prognosis

- Generally **poor prognosis** given advanced stage
- Short survival after diagnosis, especially in lung & gastric cancers
- Longer survival with breast cancer depending on treatment
- Lung cancer; pleural metastases; **stage IV**

Treatment

- Asymptomatic patients may not need treatment immediately
- Periodic thoracenteses on outpatient or inpatient basis
- Pleurodesis with talc slurry preferred
  - Doxycycline & tetracycline alternatives
- Delayed initiation of thoracenteses may reduce efficacy of pleurodesis

DIAGNOSTIC CHECKLIST

Consider

- Video-assisted thoracoscopic surgery (VATS) enables visualization of the pleural space, diagnosis of pleural abnormalities, & cytoreduction of metastases
- Pleurodesis may be performed at time of VATS
- Preprocedural planning in multidisciplinary environment is important

Image Interpretation Pearls

- Presence of pleural effusion in patient with known malignancy should raise suspicion for pleural metastases even in absence of pleural thickening or nodularity
- CT may underestimate extent of disease
- MR and FDG-PET may serve as problem-solving tools

SELECTED REFERENCES

1. UyBico SJ et al: Lung cancer staging essentials: the new TNM staging system and potential imaging pitfalls. Radiographics. 30(5):1163-81, 2010
2. Lim MC et al: Pathological diagnosis and cytoreduction of cardiophrenic lymph node and pleural metastasis in ovarian cancer patients using video-assisted thoracic surgery. Ann Surg Oncol. 16(7):1990-6, 2009
3. Qureshi NR et al: Imaging of pleural disease. Clin Chest Med. 27(2):193-213, 2006
4. Hwang JH et al: Subtle pleural metastasis without large effusion in lung cancer patients: preoperative detection on CT. Korean J Radiol. 6(2):94-101, 2005
5. Duysinx B et al: Evaluation of pleural disease with 18-fluorodeoxyglucose positron emission tomography imaging. Chest. 125(2):489-93, 2004

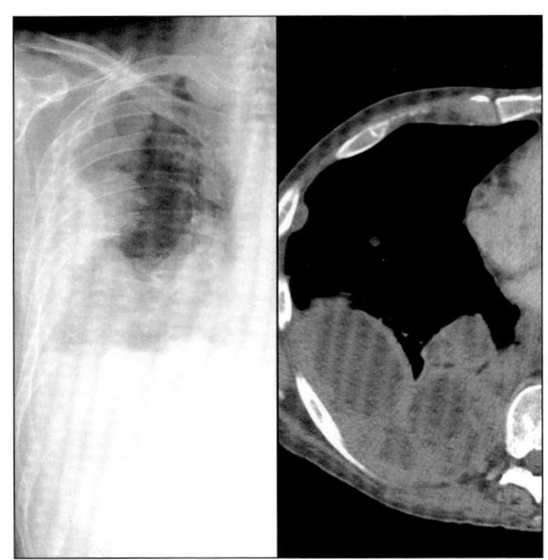

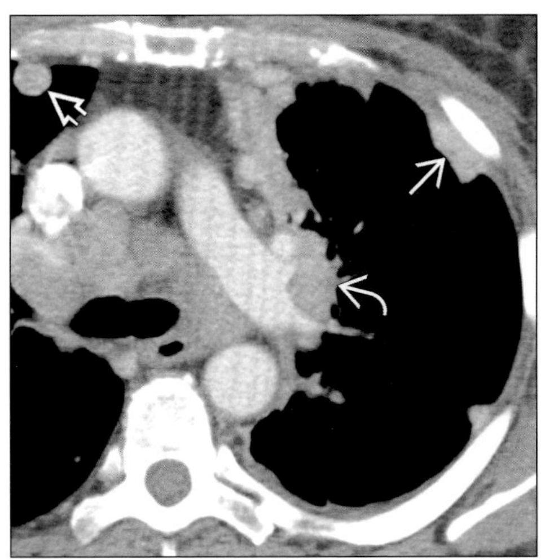

(Left) *Composite image of a frontal chest radiograph (left) and an axial CECT (right) of a patient with metastatic renal cancer shows extensive lobular right pleural thickening by heterogeneous pleural masses.* ***(Right)*** *Axial CECT of a patient with metastatic renal cancer shows multifocal nodular left pleural metastases ➔ and involvement of the mediastinal pleura ➜. Note mediastinal lymphadenopathy and a right pleural metastasis ⇨. Pleural metastases may mimic malignant pleural mesothelioma.*

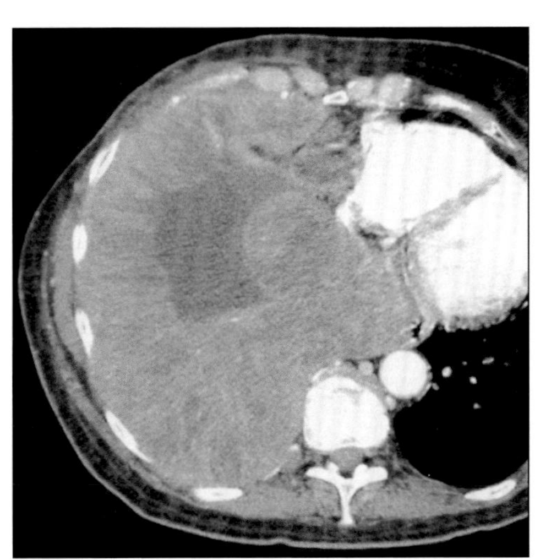

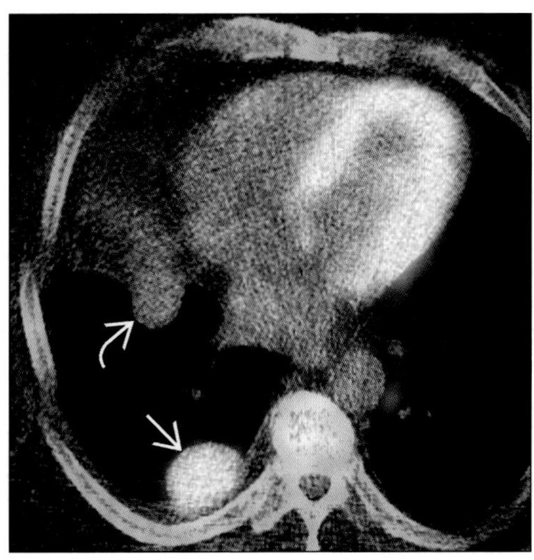

(Left) *Axial CECT of a patient with metastatic melanoma shows marked circumferential right pleural thickening by lobulated heterogeneous pleural metastases that produce mass effect on the mediastinum.* ***(Right)*** *Axial fused PET/CT of a patient with metastatic malignant fibrous histiocytoma shows intense FDG uptake in a right posterior pleural metastasis ➔. A previously treated right pleural metastasis ➜ is less FDG avid. PET demonstrates high sensitivity in the diagnosis of pleural metastases.*

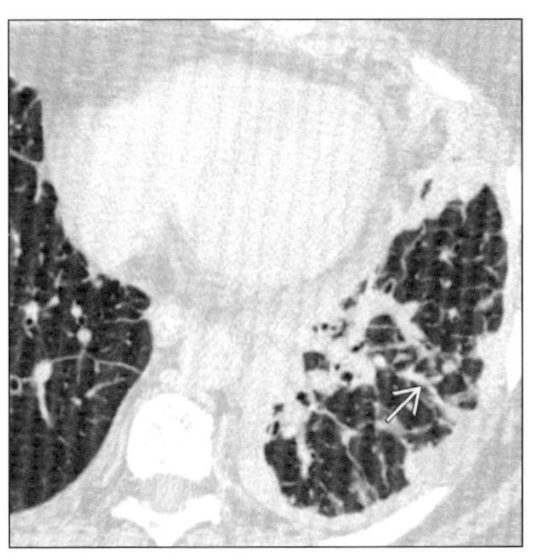

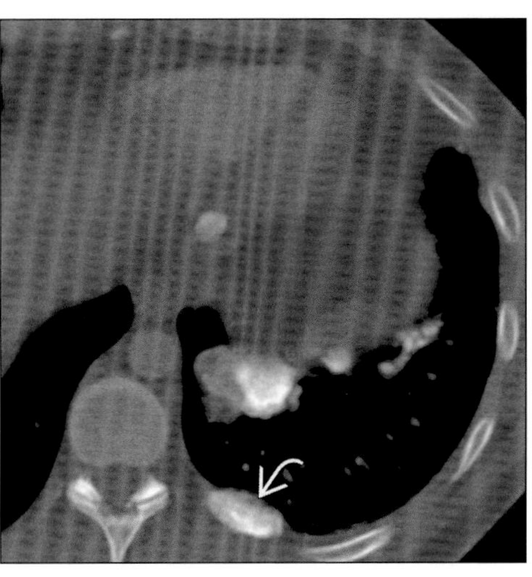

(Left) *Axial CECT of a patient with metastatic renal cancer shows left-sided circumferential nodular pleural thickening and left basilar interlobular septal thickening ➔ secondary to associated lymphangitic carcinomatosis.* ***(Right)*** *Axial CECT of a patient with metastatic osteosarcoma shows multifocal calcified left pleural metastases ➜. While most solid pleural metastases result from metastatic lung cancer and metastatic adenocarcinoma, any malignancy may metastasize to the pleura.*

MALIGNANT PLEURAL MESOTHELIOMA

Key Facts

Terminology

- Malignant pleural mesothelioma (MPM)
  - Most common primary pleural neoplasm

Imaging

- Radiography
  - Pleural effusion
  - Circumferential nodular pleural thickening
  - Loss of volume of affected hemithorax
- CT
  - Pleural effusion
  - Nodular &/or lobular pleural thickening
  - Loss of volume of affected hemithorax
  - Chest wall, mediastinal, diaphragmatic invasion
  - Mediastinal/thoracic lymphadenopathy
  - Calcified pleural plaques in 25% of cases
- MR & PET/CT more sensitive than CT for diagnosis of local invasion

Top Differential Diagnoses

- Solid pleural metastases
- Invasive thymoma
- Localized fibrous tumor of the pleura
- Pleural fibrosis and fibrothorax
- Asbestos-related diffuse pleural thickening

Pathology

- Strong association with asbestos exposure

Clinical Issues

- Symptoms: Nonpleuritic chest wall pain, dyspnea
- Prognosis: Mean survival time is 12 months

Diagnostic Checklist

- Consider MPM in differential diagnosis of symptomatic patients with unilateral circumferential nodular pleural thickening

*(**Left**) Graphic depicts features of MPM, including circumferential nodular pleural thickening and involvement of the right interlobar fissures, the right mediastinal pleura ⇨, and the right diaphragmatic pleural surfaces ➡. Note resultant right hemithorax volume loss. (**Right**) Coronal CECT of a patient with MPM shows diffuse nodular right pleural thickening involving the interlobar fissures ➡. Note involvement of the diaphragmatic pleura ➡ and invasion of the right hemidiaphragm.*

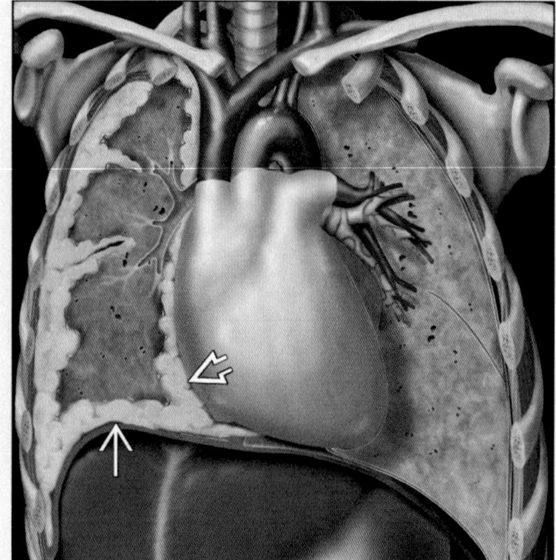

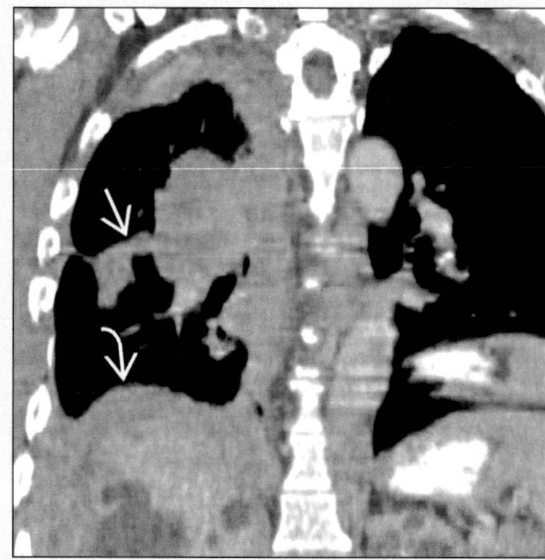

*(**Left**) Axial T2WI MR of a patient with MPM demonstrates extensive right pleural thickening ➡ that is heterogeneously hyperintense when compared to muscle. (**Right**) Axial fused PET/CT image of a patient with MPM shows intense FDG uptake within circumferential nodular right pleural thickening ➡ with involvement of the right mediastinal pleura and a right pleural effusion. MR and FDG PET/CT are more sensitive than CT in detecting chest wall, mediastinal, and diaphragmatic invasion.*

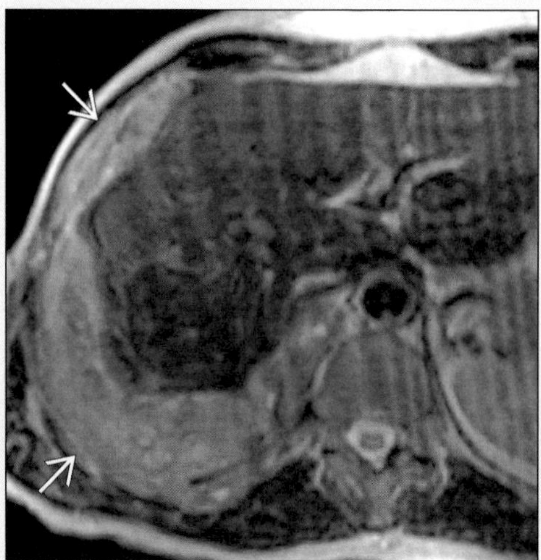

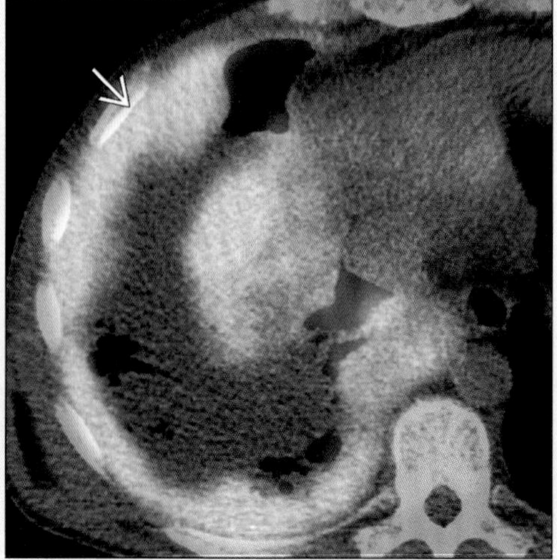

MALIGNANT PLEURAL MESOTHELIOMA

TERMINOLOGY

Abbreviations

- **Malignant pleural mesothelioma (MPM)**

Definitions

- **Most common primary pleural neoplasm**
- Strong association with **asbestos exposure**
  - Long latency period between exposure and MPM

IMAGING

General Features

- Best diagnostic clue
  - Pleural effusion ± circumferential nodular pleural thickening
- Location
  - Parietal > visceral pleura
  - Basilar pleura

Radiographic Findings

- Radiography
  - Pleural effusion
    - Unilateral > bilateral
  - **Circumferential nodular pleural thickening**
    - Fissural pleural thickening
  - Loss of volume of affected hemithorax
  - Evidence of asbestos-related pleural disease

CT Findings

- Pleural effusion
- Nodular &/or lobular pleural thickening
  - Circumferential pleural thickening
  - > 1 cm thick
- Loss of volume of affected hemithorax
- Chest wall, mediastinal, diaphragmatic invasion
- Mediastinal/thoracic lymphadenopathy
- Calcified pleural plaques in 25% of cases

MR Findings

- T1WI
  - Hyperintense to muscle
- T2WI
  - Isointense or hyperintense to muscle
- T1WI C+
  - Tumor enhances with gadolinium
- MR is more sensitive than CT for detection of local invasion

Nuclear Medicine Findings

- PET/CT
  - Intense FDG uptake within tumor & metastases
  - Sensitive for detection of local invasion and metastases

Imaging Recommendations

- Best imaging tool
  - CT is optimal modality for evaluating extent of disease
  - MR and FDG PET more sensitive than CT for evaluation of chest wall, mediastinum, & diaphragm invasion

DIFFERENTIAL DIAGNOSIS

Solid Pleural Metastases

- May be indistinguishable from MPM
- Lower association with pleural effusion
- Involvement of visceral pleura more common

Invasive Thymoma

- Obliteration of tissue planes, local invasion
- Gross or microscopic extension beyond capsule

Localized Fibrous Tumor of the Pleura

- Small lesions: Homogeneous, obtuse margins
- Large lesions: Heterogeneous, acute margins
- Calcification uncommon

Pleural Fibrosis and Fibrothorax

- Fibrous obliteration of pleural space
- Hemorrhagic & tuberculous effusions, empyema
- Parenchymal disease; previous TB or empyema
- Mediastinal pleura spared in 88%
- May demonstrate extensive calcification

Asbestos-related Diffuse Pleural Thickening

- Bilateral pleural thickening involving 25% of chest
- Unilateral thickening involving 50% of chest
- Pleural thickening > 5 mm at any site
- Calcification rare (unlike pleural plaques)

Loculated Pleural Effusion

- Not circumferential
- Usually spares mediastinal pleura
- Adjacent pleural thickening not nodular

Rounded Atelectasis

- Peripheral mass-like lesion abutting pleural surface
- Associated adjacent pleural thickening
- Associated asbestos-related plaques/effusion

Pleurodesis

- Thickening of parietal & visceral pleura
- Hyperattenuation secondary to talc deposition
- FDG avid

Splenosis

- Splenic implants on pleural & peritoneal surfaces
- History of trauma or surgery; absent spleen
- Pleural nodules or masses, typically unilateral
- Diagnosis made with Tc-99m sulfur colloid or Tc-99m damaged erythrocyte scintigraphy

Epithelioid Hemangioendothelioma

- Rare vascular tumor of lung & liver
- Pleural effusion & nodularity
- Mimics pleural metastases and MPM

PATHOLOGY

General Features

- Etiology
  - Strong association with **asbestos exposure**
    - Carcinogenicity of asbestos fibers proportional to aspect ratio (length:width) & durability in tissue
    - Higher aspect ratio, greater tumorigenicity
  - **Increased risk of MPM with duration & intensity of exposure**

Staging, Grading, & Classification

- **Tumor descriptors (T)**
  - T1: (20%)

MALIGNANT PLEURAL MESOTHELIOMA

  - T1a: Limited to ipsilateral parietal pleura (including mediastinal & diaphragmatic)
  - T2b: Ipsilateral parietal& visceral pleura
- T2: (50%)
  - Involvement of diaphragm, fissures, &/or lung
- T3: (25%)
  - Involvement of endothoracic fascia, mediastinal fat, single focus extending into chest wall &/or pericardium (nontransmural)
- T4: (< 5%)
  - Diffuse or multiple chest wall masses, transdiaphragmatic extension, &/or extension into contralateral pleura, mediastinal organs, spine, pericardium (transmural)

- **Lymph nodes (N)**
  - N0: No regional lymph node metastases
  - N1: Ipsilateral bronchopulmonary or hilar lymph nodes
  - N2: Subcarinal or ipsilateral mediastinal lymph nodes (including ipsilateral internal mammary lymph nodes)
  - N3: Contralateral mediastinal & internal mammary lymph nodes, contralateral or ipsilateral supraclavicular lymph nodes
- **Metastases (M)**
  - M0: No distant metastases
  - M1: Distant metastases
- **TNM Classification**
  - IA: T1a N0 M0
  - IB: T1b N0 M0
  - II: T2 N0 M0
  - III: Any T3 M0, N1 M0, or N2 M0
  - IV: Any T4, N3, or M1

Gross Pathologic & Surgical Features

- Parietal pleura > visceral pleura
- Right hemithorax > left hemithorax
- Tumor masses coalesce into sheet-like or confluent pleural masses
- Pleural effusion in 60% at diagnosis
- Metastases in > 50% at autopsy
- Asbestos-related pleural plaques
  - Not premalignant

Microscopic Features

- Difficult differentiation between mesothelioma, metastatic adenocarcinoma, asbestos-related pleural fibrosis, & reactive pleural hyperplasia
- MPM: Greater nuclear atypia than adenocarcinoma
- Diagnostic yield of pleural fluid cytology is low; image-guided and surgical biopsies preferred
  - Image-guided core biopsy: Sensitivity (86%), needle track seeding (4%)
  - Thoracoscopy/thoracotomy & biopsy: Sensitivity (94% & 100%); needle track seeding (22% combined)
- 3 histologic categories
  - **Epithelioid (55-65%)**
    - Uniform cuboidal cells with eosinophilic cytoplasm, central nuclei, & distinct nucleoli
    - Difficult to distinguish from lung adenocarcinoma & adenocarcinoma metastases
  - **Sarcomatoid (10-15%)**
    - Spindle cells with nuclear atypia
    - Difficult to distinguish from true sarcoma
  - **Biphasic (20-35%)**
    - Elements of epithelioid & sarcomatoid cell types
    - Intermediate transitional areas common
- **Asbestos body**: Hallmark of asbestos exposure

CLINICAL ISSUES

Presentation

- Most common signs/symptoms
  - Nonpleuritic chest wall pain, dyspnea
- Other signs/symptoms
  - Weakness, fatigue, cough, weight loss; less common
  - Dullness to percussion & decreased breath sounds

Demographics

- Age
  - 50-70 years
- Gender
  - Predominantly men (85-90%)
- Epidemiology
  - 80% of patients with MPM had asbestos exposure
    - 35-40 year latency period post exposure
  - 10% of patients exposed to asbestos develop MPM
  - Simian virus 40 (SV-40) infection of mesothelial cells possible cofactor in causation

Natural History & Prognosis

- **Mean survival time: 12 months**
- Longer survival: Disease limited to parietal pleura
- Reduced survival: Thoracic nodal & distant metastases, advanced pleural involvement
- SV-40 infection indicator of poor prognosis

Treatment

- Palliative pleurectomy to relieve chest wall pain
- Pleurectomy or pleurodesis for recurrent effusion
- Incomplete resection along mediastinal & diaphragmatic pleura frequent
- Curative extrapleural pneumonectomy in absence of lymph node & distant metastases
- Prolonged survival with combination of surgery, chemotherapy, & radiation therapy

DIAGNOSTIC CHECKLIST

Consider

- MPM in differential diagnosis of patients with unilateral circumferential nodular pleural thickening

SELECTED REFERENCES

1. Agarwal PP et al: Pleural mesothelioma: sensitivity and incidence of needle track seeding after image-guided biopsy versus surgical biopsy. Radiology. 241(2):589-94, 2006
2. Wang ZJ et al: Malignant pleural mesothelioma: evaluation with CT, MR imaging, and PET. Radiographics. 24(1):105-19, 2004

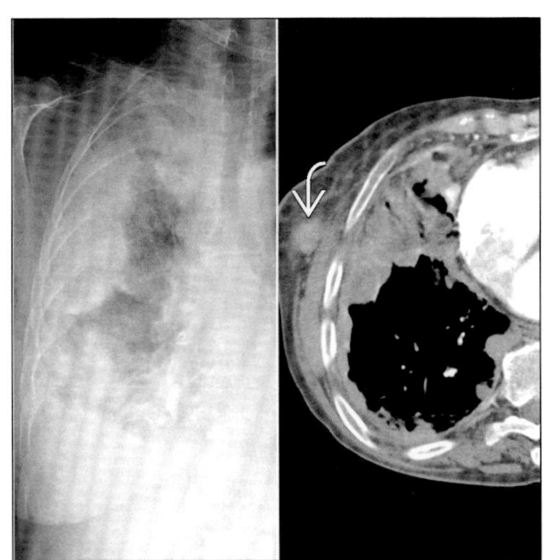

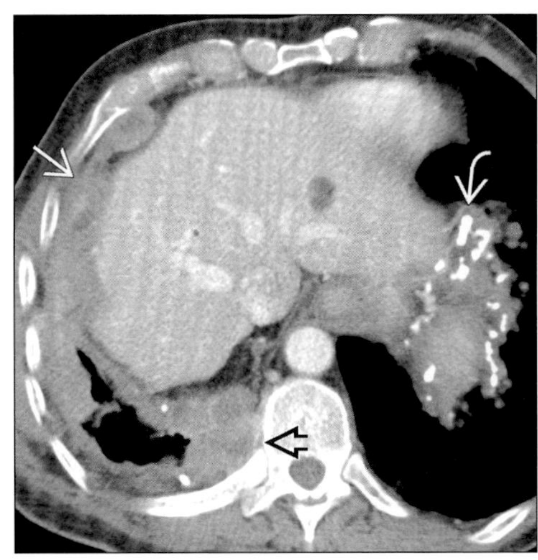

(Left) *Composite image with PA chest radiograph (left) and axial CECT (right) of a patient with MPM shows circumferential nodular right pleural thickening with right lung encasement and a right chest wall metastasis ➔.* ***(Right)*** *Axial CECT of a patient with MPM shows circumferential nodular right pleural thickening ➔ and invasion of the right paravertebral soft tissues ➔. Bilateral calcified pleural plaques ➔ are present and typically manifest 20-30 years after asbestos exposure.*

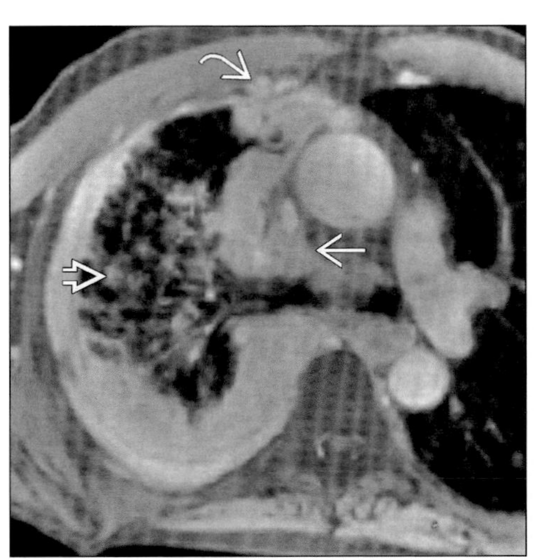

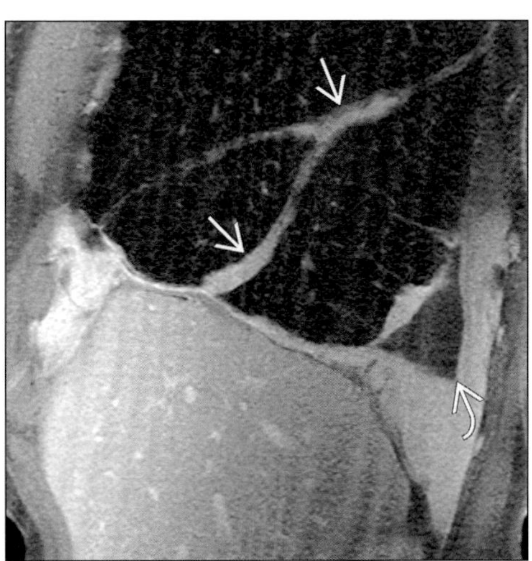

(Left) *Axial T1WI C+ FS MR of a patient with MPM shows invasion of the anterior chest wall ➔, mediastinal invasion, lymphangitic carcinomatosis ➔, and mediastinal lymphadenopathy ➔. Metastatic lymphadenopathy is present in 40-45% of cases of MPM at autopsy.* ***(Right)*** *Sagittal T1WI C+ FS MR of the same patient demonstrates tumor growth along the right interlobar fissures ➔ and a small right pleural effusion ➔. Circumferential pleural involvement is typical of MPM.*

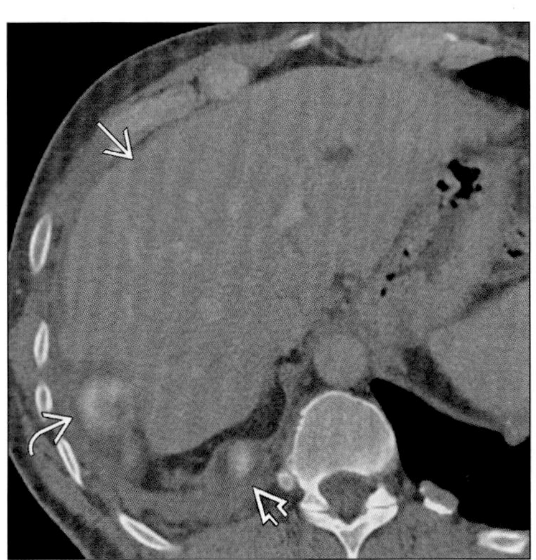

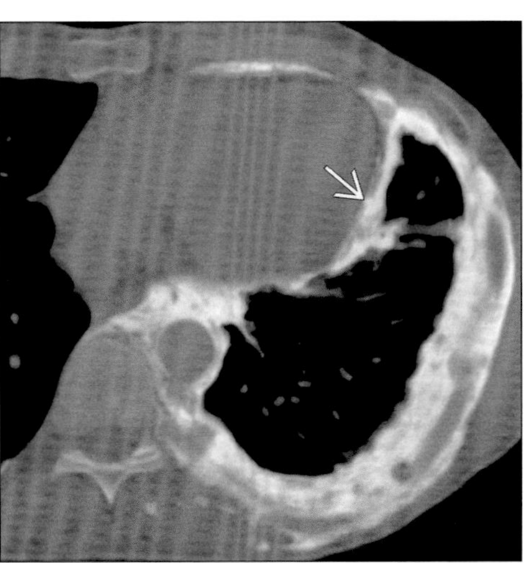

(Left) *Axial fused PET/CT of a patient with MPM shows FDG-avid tumor ➔ abutting the liver and invading the right hemidiaphragm ➔. FDG-avid metastases ➔ are present within the liver. PET/CT can differentiate between benign and malignant pleural disease with a sensitivity of 96.8% and specificity of 88.5%.* ***(Right)*** *Axial NECT of a patient with MPM shows circumferential hyperdense left pleural thickening ➔ consistent with osseous and cartilaginous differentiation of MPM.*

LOCALIZED FIBROUS TUMOR OF THE PLEURA

Key Facts

Terminology

- Localized fibrous tumor of the pleura (**LFTP**)

Imaging

- Radiography
  - Mass of variable size
  - Abuts pleura
  - Incomplete border sign
- CT
  - Well-defined lobular contours
  - Heterogeneous peripheral mass without local invasion or lymphadenopathy
  - Low attenuation; cysts, hemorrhage, necrosis
- MR
  - Exclusion of local invasion
  - Heterogeneous signal on T1WI and T2WI
  - Low signal on T2WI; fibrous septa, tumor capsule
  - High signal on T2WI; cysts, hemorrhage, necrosis

Pathology

- Origin from submesothelial connective tissue
- Most arise from visceral pleural surface
- Lobular mass with whorled fibrous appearance
- Often pedunculated (50%)
- Low-grade neoplasm; variable histologic appearance

Clinical Issues

- Wide age range; mean: 50-57 years
- Asymptomatic in up to 50% of affected patients
- Large LFTP typically symptomatic
  - Cough, dyspnea, chest pain/discomfort
  - Systemic complaints
  - Paraneoplastic syndromes
- Therapy & prognosis
  - Complete excision is typically curative
  - Favorable prognosis
  - Long-term follow-up recommended

*(**Left**) PA chest radiograph shows a right mid thoracic polylobular mass with a sharply marginated medial border and an ill-defined lateral border ➡. (**Right**) Lateral chest radiograph shows that the lesion abuts the anterior chest and exhibits a sharply marginated posterior border. The discrepant margin visualization is typical of the incomplete border sign that confirms the extrapulmonary location of this localized fibrous tumor of the pleura (LFTP).*

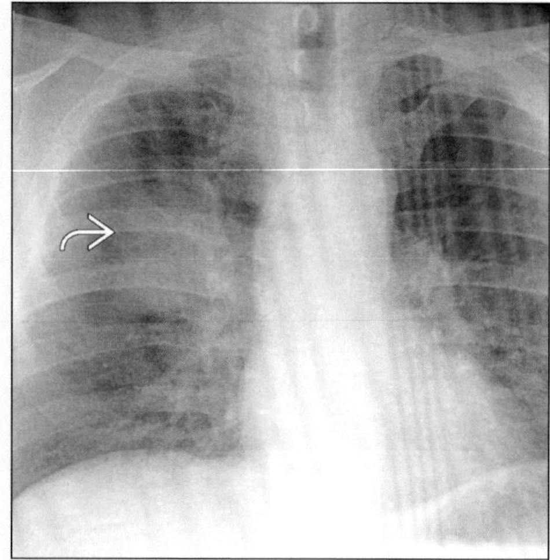

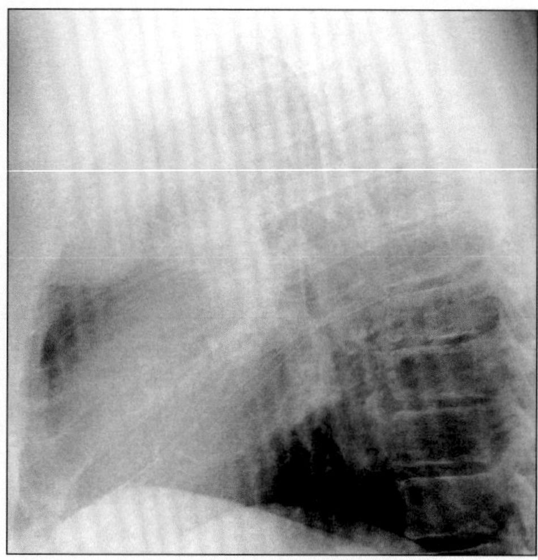

*(**Left**) Axial CECT shows a polylobular heterogeneously enhancing LFTP that forms obtuse angles ➡ with the adjacent pleural surfaces. (**Right**) Graphic depicts the gross features of LFTP. The mass is attached to the visceral pleura by a pedicle ➡ and exhibits a whorled nodular appearance and foci of necrosis on cut section. These lesions often form at least 1 acute angle ➡ with the adjacent pleural surface on cross-sectional imaging studies.*

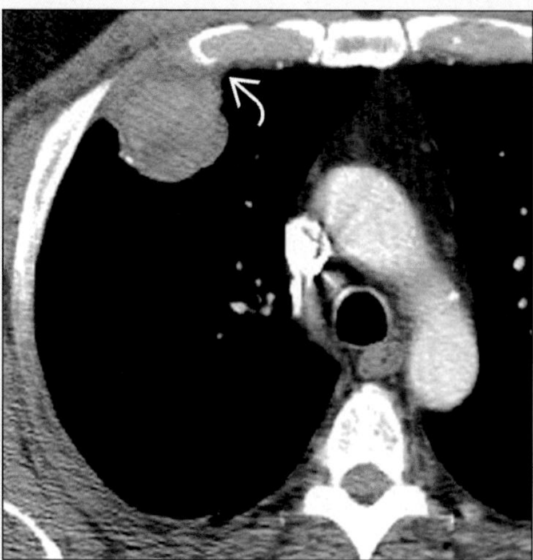

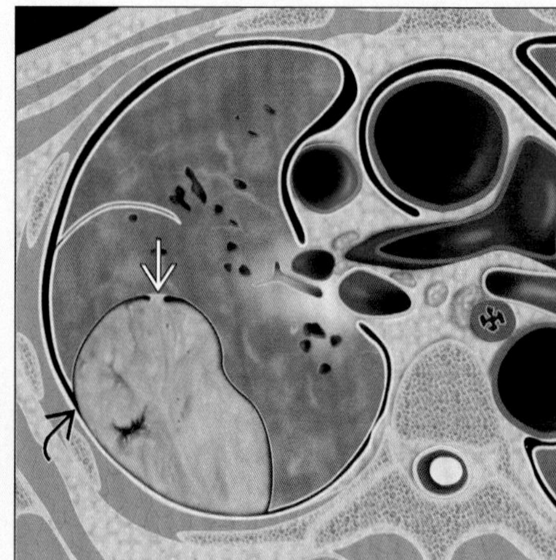

LOCALIZED FIBROUS TUMOR OF THE PLEURA

TERMINOLOGY

Abbreviations

- **Localized fibrous tumor** of the pleura (**LFTP**)

Synonyms

- Solitary fibrous tumor

Definitions

- **2nd most common primary pleural neoplasm**
- < 5% of pleural neoplasms
- **Neoplasms of similar histology** reported in lung, mediastinum, pericardium, breast, & other extrathoracic organs and locations
- Term "localized **mesothelioma**" inaccurate
  - LFTP **originates from submesothelial tissues**
- Term "**benign** fibrous tumor" is inaccurate
  - **12-37% of LFTP are malignant**

IMAGING

General Features

- Best diagnostic clue
  - Peripheral nodule/mass; **incomplete border sign**
  - No evidence of chest wall involvement
  - Fissural nodule or mass without pleural effusion
  - **Positional change** in lesion shape/location; pedicle
  - Large intrathoracic mass without local invasion or lymphadenopathy
- Location
  - Abuts pleura
  - Predilection for mid/inferior hemithorax
- Size
  - Variable size; slow growth

Radiographic Findings

- Small LFTP
  - Well-defined peripheral nodule or mass
    - Abuts pleural surface
    - **Incomplete border sign**
    - **Fissural location**
- Large LFTP
  - Pleural location may not be evident; may mimic pulmonary or mediastinal mass
  - Mass effect on adjacent structures
  - May occupy entire hemithorax
- **Pedunculated LFTP** may exhibit **positional change**
- Predilection for mid and inferior hemithorax
  - May mimic diaphragmatic elevation/eventration
- Ipsilateral pleural effusion in 20%

CT Findings

- Soft tissue nodule or mass (rarely multicentric)
  - Variable size
  - Well-defined lobular contours
  - Whorled fibrous cross-sectional appearance
  - Low attenuation; **cysts, hemorrhage, necrosis**
  - Calcification (up to 26%); punctate, linear, coarse
  - Mass effect without local invasion
  - Rare visualization of tumor pedicle
  - Although obtuse angles with adjacent pleura are considered typical, acute angles are more frequent
    - Smoothly tapered margin with adjacent pleura
    - Obtuse angles often seen in small LFTP
    - Acute angles often seen in large LFTP
  - Rarely adjacent focal skeletal sclerosis
- NECT
  - Small lesions; often with homogeneous attenuation
  - Large/malignant LFTP; heterogeneous attenuation
- CECT
  - Heterogeneous enhancement in most lesions
  - Increased conspicuity of heterogeneity and low-attenuation areas
    - Geographic, rounded, or linear
    - More frequent in malignant LFTP
    - Correspond to cysts, hemorrhage, necrosis, and myxoid degeneration
  - Visualization of enhancing intratumoral vessels
  - 3D CT angiography; evaluation of vascular supply

MR Findings

- Excellent for tissue characterization
- Documentation of intrathoracic location of juxtadiaphragmatic LFTP
- Evaluation of adjacent structures to exclude invasion, particularly with multiplanar imaging
- Heterogeneous signal intensity on T1WI & T2WI
  - Increase in signal on T2WI compared to T1WI
  - Low signal intensity fibrous elements on T2WI; fibrous septa, tumor capsule
- High signal on T2WI; cystic change, hemorrhage, necrosis, myxoid degeneration, hypercellular areas
- **Heterogeneous contrast enhancement**

Angiographic Findings

- Preoperative angiography to identify vascular supply; aorta, internal mammary, phrenic or bronchial arteries
- Preoperative embolization reported in large LFTP

Imaging Recommendations

- Best imaging tool
  - CECT considered imaging study of choice
  - Multiplanar MR for exclusion of mediastinal &/or diaphragmatic invasion by large LFTP
- Protocol advice
  - Prone imaging may document tumor mobility
  - CECT for evaluation of extent of central necrosis

DIFFERENTIAL DIAGNOSIS

Chest Wall Lipoma

- Peripheral nodule/mass with incomplete border sign
- CT/MR diagnostic; fat attenuation/signal

Pleural Metastasis

- Rarely a solitary nodule or mass
- Solid pleural nodules/masses, pleural effusion, both

Chest Wall Metastasis

- Peripheral nodule/mass with incomplete border sign
- Skeletal destruction &/or soft tissue involvement

Thymoma

- Cross-sectional imaging to document lesion localization within anterior mediastinum
- Mediastinal pleural LFT may mimic thymoma

Neurogenic Neoplasm

- Paravertebral nodule/mass with benign pressure erosion of adjacent ribs/vertebrae
- Paravertebral LFT may mimic neurogenic neoplasm

Lung Cancer

- Peripheral lung cancer may mimic LFTP
- Local invasion, lymphadenopathy, metastases

PATHOLOGY

General Features

- Etiology
  - Unknown
  - No association with exposure to asbestos, cigarette smoke, or other carcinogens

Gross Pathologic & Surgical Features

- Well-marginated lobular soft tissue mass
- Variable size, ranging from 1-39 cm
- Typically arises from **visceral pleura**
- **Frequent vascular pedicle** (up to 50%)
- Grayish-white whorled or nodular cut surface
- Necrosis, hemorrhage, cystic degeneration; typically in large or malignant tumors

Microscopic Features

- Origin from **submesothelial connective tissue**
- Low-grade neoplasm; variable histologic appearance
  - Ovoid or spindle-shaped cells, round to oval nuclei
  - Faint cytoplasm, indistinct cell borders
  - Surrounded by variable amounts of collagen
- Haphazardly arranged tumor cells ("**patternless pattern**")
- Criteria for malignancy
  - High cellularity
  - Pleomorphism
  - > 4 mitoses/10 high-power fields
- Immunoreactive with CD34 and bcl-2

CLINICAL ISSUES

Presentation

- Most common signs/symptoms
  - Up to **50% of patients asymptomatic**; small LFTP
  - Large LFTP typically symptomatic
    - Cough, dyspnea, chest pain/discomfort
- Other signs/symptoms
  - Systemic complaints
    - Chills, sweats
    - Weakness, weight loss
  - Paraneoplastic syndromes, typically with large LFTP
    - Hypoglycemia
      - Doege-Potter syndrome
      - Postulated production of insulin-like growth factor 2
    - Hypertrophic osteoarthropathy, 17-35% of cases
      - Pierre Marie-Bamberger syndrome
      - Postulated production of hyaluronic acid
    - Digital clubbing

Demographics

- Age
  - Wide age range; **mean age**: **50-57 years**
- Gender
  - Slightly more common in women

Natural History & Prognosis

- Favorable prognosis with **5-year survival rates of up to 97%**
  - Complete excision is best prognostic factor
  - Pedunculated LFTP less likely to recur
  - 12% of patients die of recurrent or unresectable LFTP
- Recurrence in up to 23%; more likely with malignant and sessile LFTP
  - Most recurrences within 24 months after resection
  - Recurrence typically in ipsilateral pleura; rarely lung
- Malignant LFTP may produce distant metastases

Treatment

- **Complete excision** typically **curative**
  - May require en bloc resection of adjacent lung, pleura, chest wall
  - Video-assisted thoracotomy for small LFTP
  - Thoracotomy for large LFTP
- Resection of recurrent LFTP
- Role of adjuvant therapy not established
  - May be used in malignant sessile LFTP

Imaging Follow-up

- Long term follow-up recommended; rate of recurrence highest within 1st 24 months
- CT follow up every 6 months for the 1st 2 years; annual follow-up thereafter

DIAGNOSTIC CHECKLIST

Consider

- LFTP in lesions exhibiting incomplete border sign
- LFTP in **large peripheral masses without local invasion or lymphadenopathy**

SELECTED REFERENCES

1. Song SW et al: Malignant solitary fibrous tumor of the pleura: computed tomography-pathological correlation and comparison with computed tomography of benign solitary fibrous tumor of the pleura. Jpn J Radiol. 28(8):602-8, 2010
2. Cardinale L et al: Fibrous tumour of the pleura (SFTP): a proteiform disease. Clinical, histological and atypical radiological patterns selected among our cases. Radiol Med. 114(2):204-15, 2009
3. Lee SC et al: Solitary fibrous tumors of the pleura: clinical, radiological, surgical and pathological evaluation. Eur J Surg Oncol. 31(1):84-7, 2005
4. Mitchell JD: Solitary fibrous tumor of the pleura. Semin Thorac Cardiovasc Surg. 15(3):305-9, 2003
5. Rosado-de-Christenson ML et al: From the archives of the AFIP: Localized fibrous tumor of the pleura. Radiographics. 23(3):759-83, 2003
6. de Perrot M et al: Solitary fibrous tumors of the pleura. Ann Thorac Surg. 74(1):285-93, 2002
7. Tateishi U et al: Solitary fibrous tumor of the pleura: MR appearance and enhancement pattern. J Comput Assist Tomogr. 26(2):174-9, 2002
8. England DM et al: Localized benign and malignant fibrous tumors of the pleura. A clinicopathologic review of 223 cases. Am J Surg Pathol. 13(8):640-58, 1989

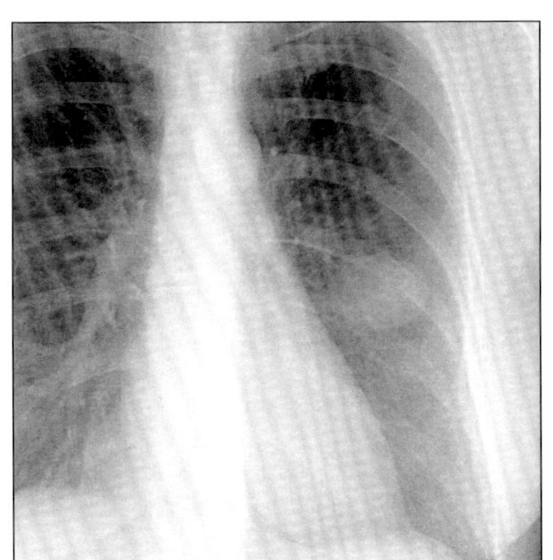

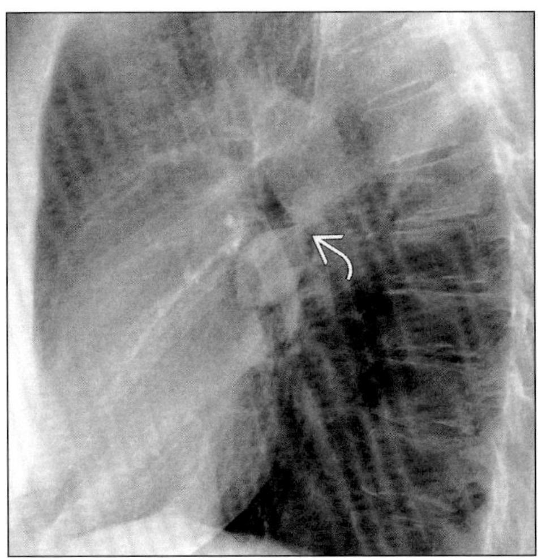

*(**Left**) PA chest radiograph shows a lobular mass in the left mid thorax with a sharply marginated lateral border and an ill-defined medial border. (**Right**) Lateral chest radiograph shows that the lesion is located in the left major fissure with a beak-like morphology of the lesion borders adjacent to the superior ➔ and inferior aspects of the fissure. Although not common, the fissural location of the lesion is highly suggestive of LFTP.*

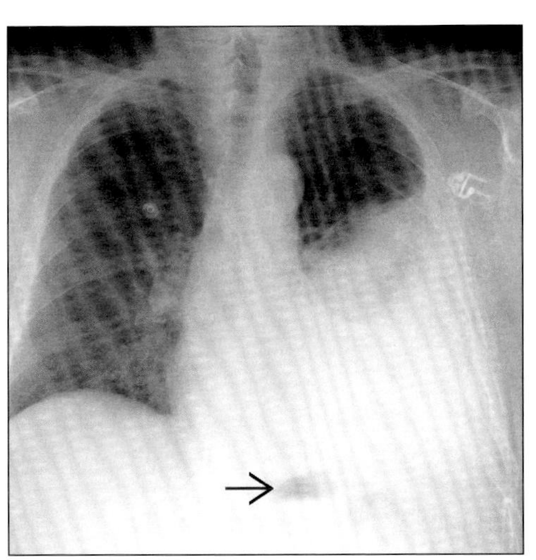

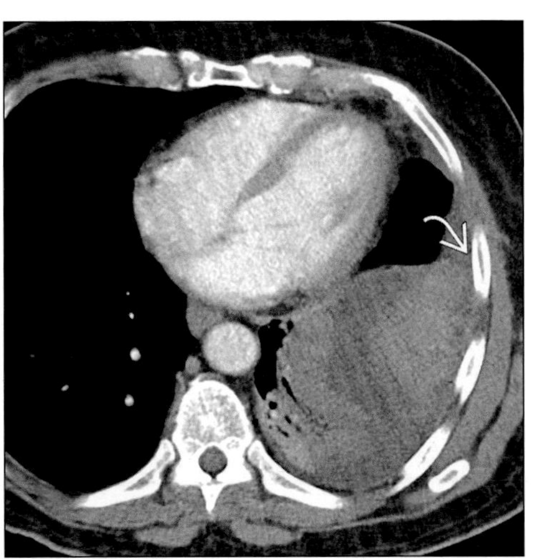

*(**Left**) PA chest radiograph shows a large LFTP occupying the left mid and inferior hemithorax with an ipsilateral pleural effusion and inversion of the left hemidiaphragm with mass effect on the gastric bubble ➔. (**Right**) Axial CECT shows a large heterogeneously enhancing LFTP with low-attenuation areas corresponding to tumor necrosis. Note mass effect on the adjacent lung and a small left pleural effusion. The tumor forms an acute angle ➔ with the adjacent pleura.*

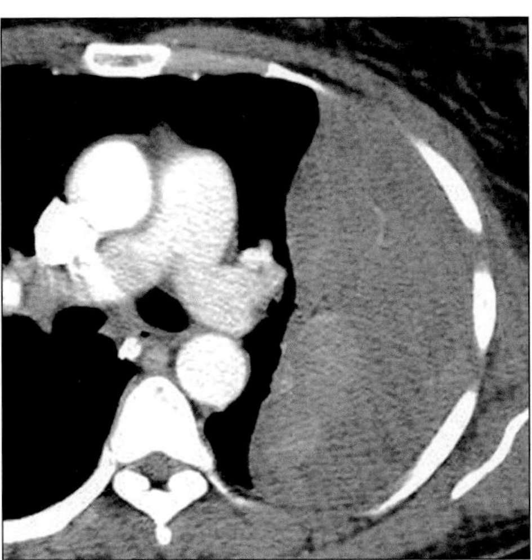

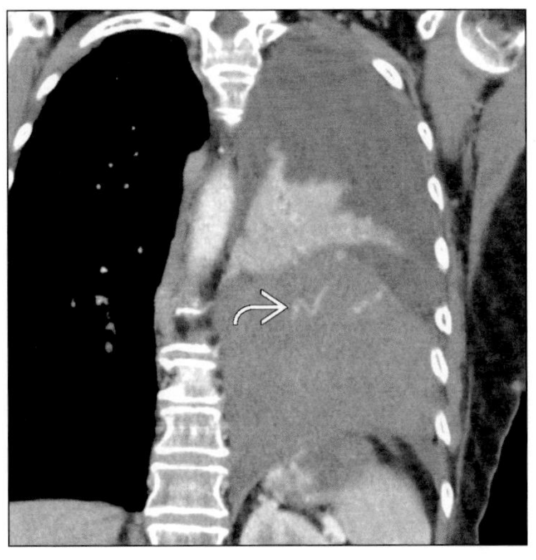

*(**Left**) Axial CECT shows a large LFTP abutting the left lateral pleural surface with heterogeneous enhancement that highlights its characteristic whorled nodular appearance. (**Right**) Coronal CECT shows a large left basilar LFTP with intrinsic enhancing vessels ➔, a large left pleural effusion, and left lung atelectasis. Multiplanar imaging allows evaluation of the adjacent hemidiaphragm and helps confirm the completely intrathoracic location of large tumors.*

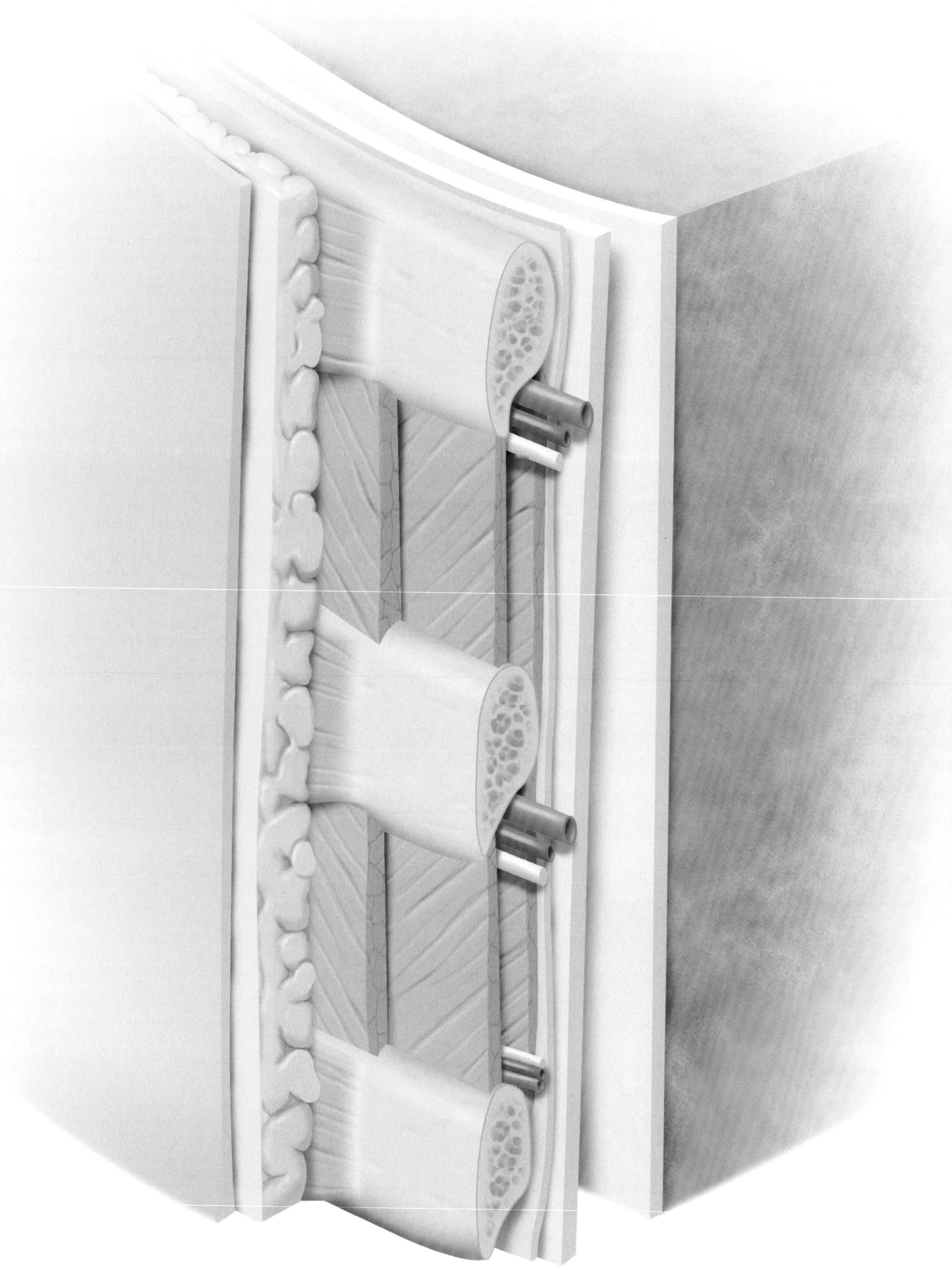

SECTION 13
Chest Wall and Diaphragm

Introduction and Overview

Chest Wall

Diaphragm

APPROACH TO CHEST WALL AND DIAPHRAGM

Introduction and Imaging Modalities

The chest wall consists of multiple tissue components (muscles, nerves, fat, bone, cartilage, and vessels) that surround the lungs and pleura and that are enveloped by the skin. These mesenchymal, vascular, osseous, and cartilaginous tissues may be affected by a wide range of disease processes, and the detection, localization, and characterization of these lesions may be challenging. Chest radiography is useful for the initial assessment of chest wall deformities, osteocartilaginous lesions, and chest wall tumors. Chest wall masses characteristically exhibit the **incomplete border sign** on radiography, which, together with radiographic documentation of skeletal &/ or soft tissue involvement, allows lesion localization in the chest wall and the formulation of an appropriate differential diagnosis. Cross-sectional imaging modalities (CT, MR) enable more precise determination of the extent of chest wall involvement and more extensive lesion characterization. In some instances, imaging studies reveal a definitive diagnosis (e.g., chest wall lipoma). CT and MR have complementary roles for imaging chest wall disorders. CT provides higher spatial resolution and shows calcification and bone erosion and destruction more readily than MR. The advantages of MR include its multiplanar capabilities, improved contrast of soft tissue structures, and the availability of flow-sensitive pulse sequences.

Image Interpretation and Chest Wall Abnormalities

The symmetric arrangement of the chest wall structures allows side-to-side comparison on radiography and cross-sectional imaging studies. Any asymmetry should prompt consideration of congenital or acquired disorders. Correlation with clinical history is vital in constructing a reasonable differential diagnosis. A history of recent trauma, for instance, should prompt consideration of acute abnormalities (e.g., fractures, dislocations) whereas a one-month history of progressive chest wall pain would suggest subacute etiologies (e.g., tumor, infection, inflammatory lesions).

Important anatomic regions of the chest wall to evaluate on CT and MR include the supraclavicular fossa, axilla, and parasternal-internal mammary zone.

Congenital and Developmental Anomalies

Congenital chest wall abnormalities may involve osseous structures (e.g., pectus and rib deformities, cleidocranial dysostosis), soft tissues (e.g., Poland syndrome), or vascular structures (e.g., hemangioma, arteriovenous malformation.) Many of these entities have characteristic radiographic features that do not require cross-sectional imaging. When a congenital vascular lesion is suspected, contrast-enhanced CT &/or MR with flow-sensitive pulse sequences are required.

Inflammatory and Infectious Diseases

Infections may reach the chest wall through hematogenous routes or by direct extension and may manifest as soft tissue &/or fluid-attenuation lesions. Associated findings of osseous destruction suggest advanced disease. Radiography and cross-sectional imaging of the chest allow evaluation of the entire thorax for exclusion of associated pulmonary, mediastinal, or pleural abnormalities.

Benign Neoplasia

Chest wall lipoma is the most common benign chest wall neoplasm; its CT features are characteristic and diagnostic. If significant soft tissue components are visible within an otherwise fatty tumor, the possibility of liposarcoma must be considered.

Other benign mesenchymal tumors may involve the chest wall, including desmoid tumors (e.g., aggressive fibromatosis), which are cytologically bland fibrous neoplasms that have a propensity to occur in the shoulder region and to recur.

Malignant Neoplasia

Metastatic disease is the most common chest wall malignancy, and chondrosarcoma is the most common primary chest wall malignant neoplasm. Other malignant chest wall tumors include myeloma, fibrosarcoma, malignant fibrous histiocytoma, and lymphoma, as well as other malignant mesenchymal neoplasms.

Osseous Changes in Chest Wall Lesions

The osseous structures of the chest wall may be abnormally expanded, smoothly eroded, or may demonstrate frank destruction. Fibrous dysplasia and enchondroma may manifest with rib expansion. Neurogenic neoplasms may produce characteristic benign pressure erosion along the rib margins. Rib destruction in an adult should prompt consideration of metastatic disease, myeloma, or chondrosarcoma as the underlying cause. Primitive neuroectodermal tumors (PNET) typically destroy ribs in adolescents and young adults.

Approach to Diaphragmatic Abnormalities

The diaphragm serves as a partition between the thoracic and abdominal cavities, and by its contraction and relaxation alters intrathoracic pressure and facilitates ventilation. In normal individuals, the diaphragm is clearly visible on orthogonal chest radiographs. Because of its dome-like configuration, it is difficult to fully assess it on axial CT and MR images, and it is optimally evaluated in the coronal &/or sagittal planes.

The diaphragm may be abnormal in its contour (e.g., eventration) and lack of excursion (e.g., paralysis), or it may be affected by blunt or penetrating trauma. Normal and abnormal apertures in the diaphragm permit a variety of herniations to occur (e.g., Bochdalek, Morgagni, hiatus hernias).

Diaphragmatic apertures enlarge in older patients and in patients with emphysema. The most common congenital diaphragmatic defects are the posterior Bochdalek hernia (posterolateral vertebrocostal triangle) and the anterior Morgagni hernia (sternocostal hiatus). Acquired hiatal hernias are common, especially in the older adult population, with widening of the esophageal hiatus.

Selected References

1. Nam SJ et al: Imaging of primary chest wall tumors with radiologic-pathologic correlation. Radiographics. 31(3):749-70, 2011
2. Kuhlman JE et al: CT and MR imaging evaluation of chest wall disorders. Radiographics. 14(3):571-95, 1994

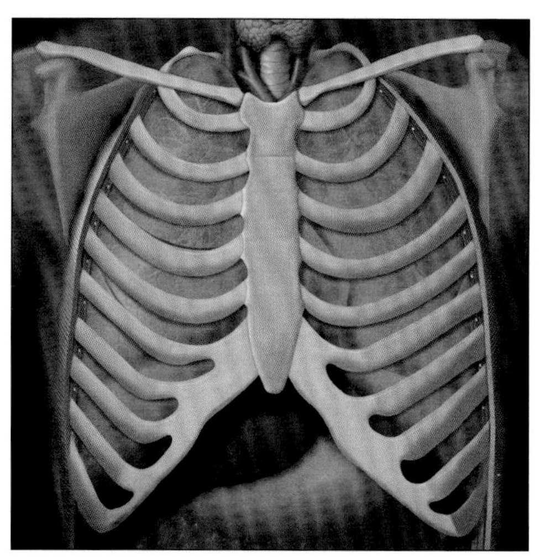

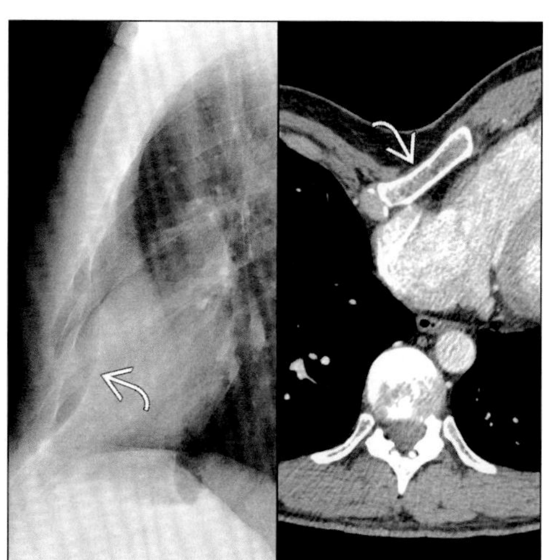

(Left) *Graphic illustrates the chest wall osseous structures, including the ribs, sternum, clavicle, and scapulae. These structures support the chest wall soft tissues, comprised of muscle, fat, and neurovascular structures. They also provide protection for the internal organs of the thorax.* ***(Right)*** *Composite image with lateral chest radiograph (left) and axial CECT (right) shows pectus excavatum with posterior displacement and rotation of the sternum ➔ and resultant compression of the right heart.*

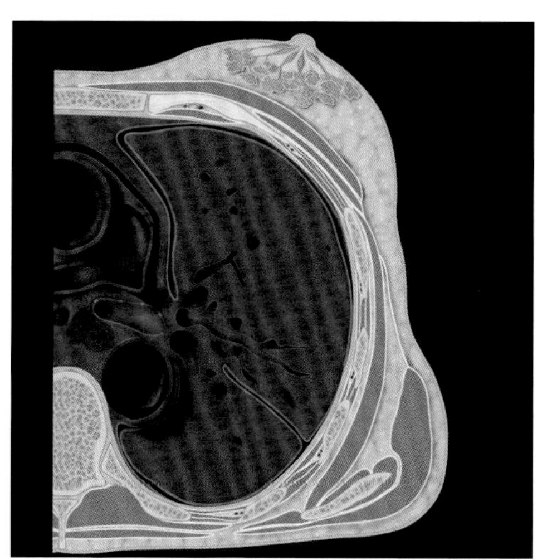

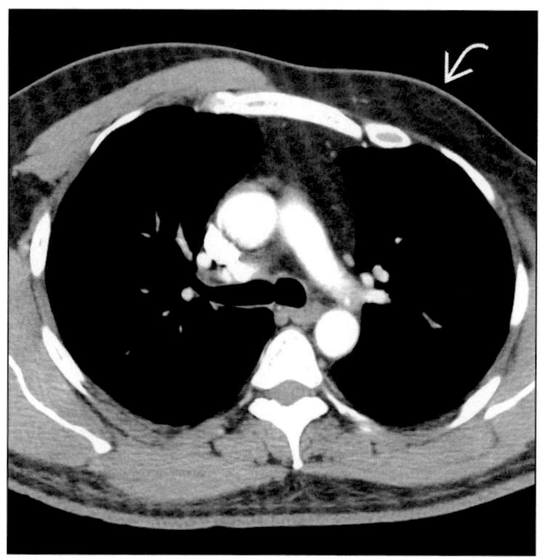

(Left) *Graphic illustrates the anatomic layers of normal chest wall soft-tissue structures, including skin, fat, muscle, and breast tissue.* ***(Right)*** *Axial CECT of a patient with Poland syndrome shows congenital absence of the left pectoralis major muscle ➔. This condition manifests as unilateral hyperlucency on chest radiography, with absence of the normal axillary fold on the affected side. Associated anomalies include rib deformities, syndactyly, and pectus excavatum.*

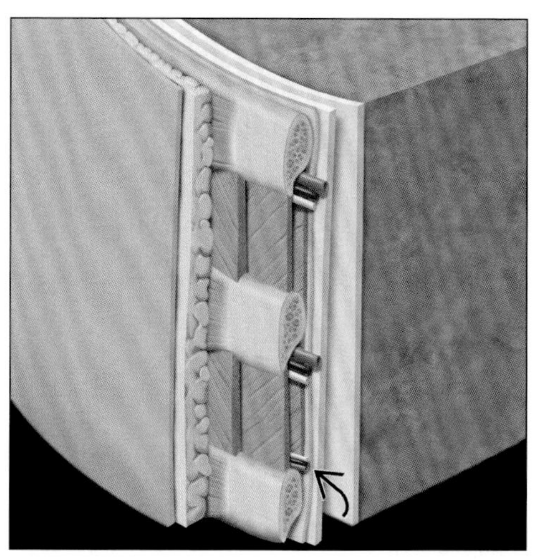

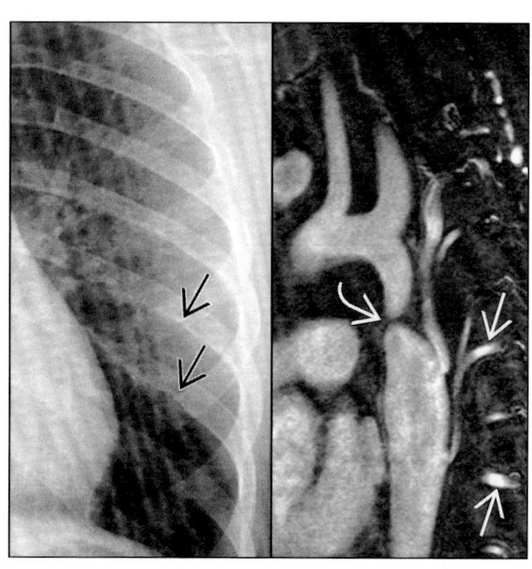

(Left) *Graphic illustrates normal layers of chest wall structures and normal neurovascular bundles ➔ along the undersurface of ribs.* ***(Right)*** *Composite image with PA chest radiograph (left) and sagittal MR image (right) demonstrates rib notching with focal areas of smooth pressure erosion along the undersurface of multiple ribs ➔. This finding results from enlarged collateral intercostal vessels ➔ secondary to aortic coarctation ➔. Rib notching may also occur with neurogenic neoplasms.*

*(**Left**) Axial CECT shows right chest wall fascitis with abnormal soft tissue thickening of the latissimus dorsi muscle ➔ and edema in the adjacent fat ➔ lateral to the infraspinatus muscle. (**Right**) Composite image with PA chest radiograph (left) and coronal NECT (right) shows a chest wall lipoma manifesting as a lenticular opacity with incomplete borders on radiography ➔ and the diagnostic CT feature of a fat-attenuation lesion ➔ with tapering obtuse margins at its pleural interface.*

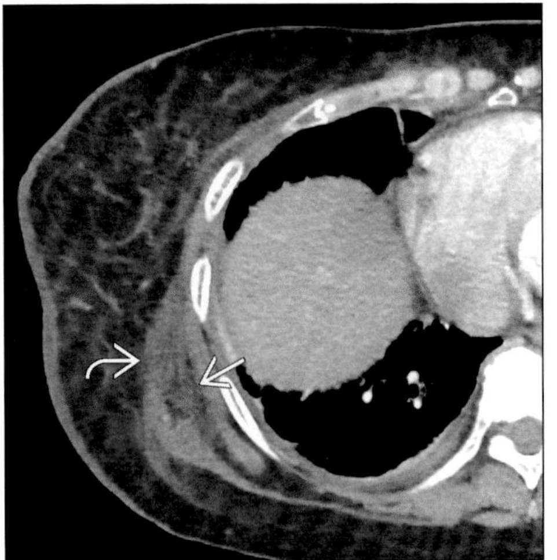

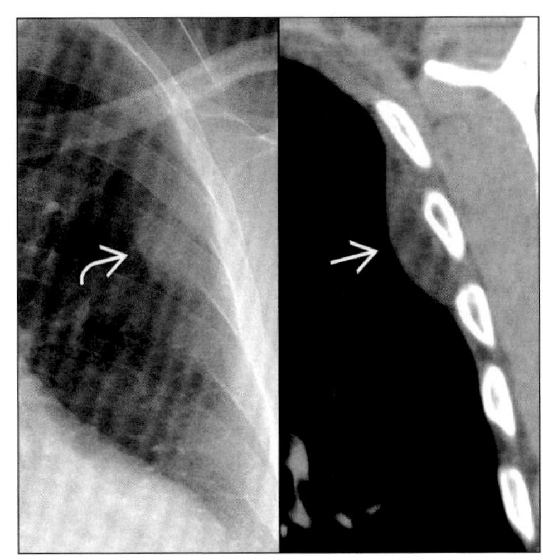

*(**Left**) Composite image with PA (left) and lateral (middle) chest radiographs and sagittal MR image (right) shows characteristic features of a chondrosarcoma of the right 6th costochondral junction. The tapering obtuse margins of the tumor ➔ manifest as incomplete borders on both orthogonal radiographs. (**Right**) Axial CECT demonstrates Hodgkin disease invading the anterior chest wall ➔, a finding that usually represents direct extension of tumor involving internal mammary lymph nodes.*

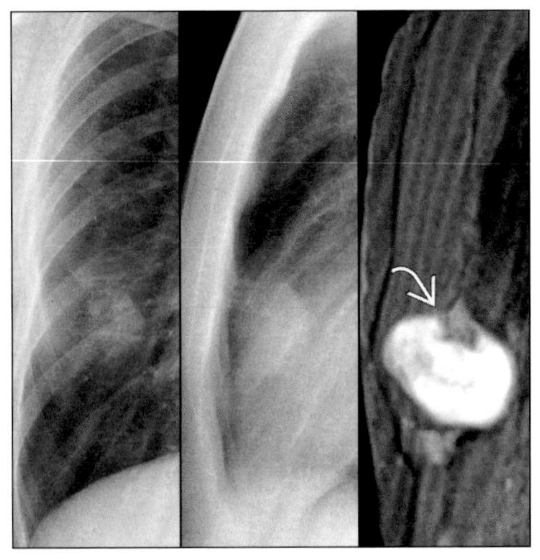

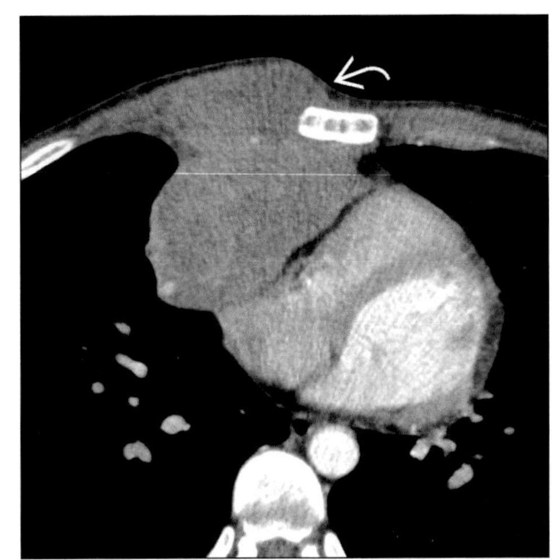

*(**Left**) Composite image with axial CECT shows a primary breast cancer (left) manifesting as a right breast polylobular mass and metastatic melanoma (right) involving the right supraclavicular, subpectoral, and axillary regions. (**Right**) Composite image with PA chest radiograph (left) and coronal NECT (right) shows metastatic renal cell carcinoma destroying the left 8th rib ➔. Rib destruction in an adult is typically caused by metastatic tumor, multiple myeloma, or chondrosarcoma.*

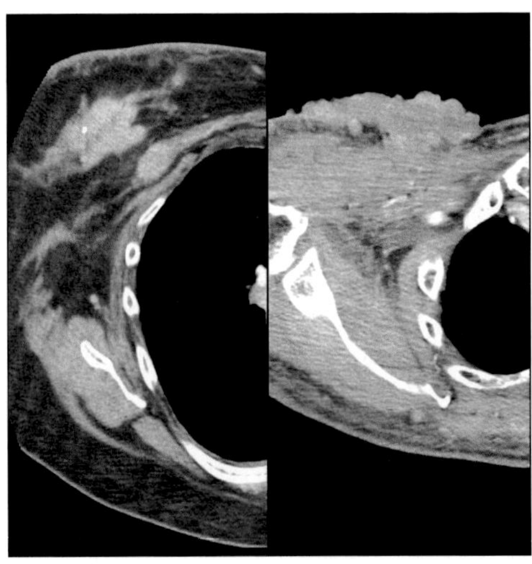

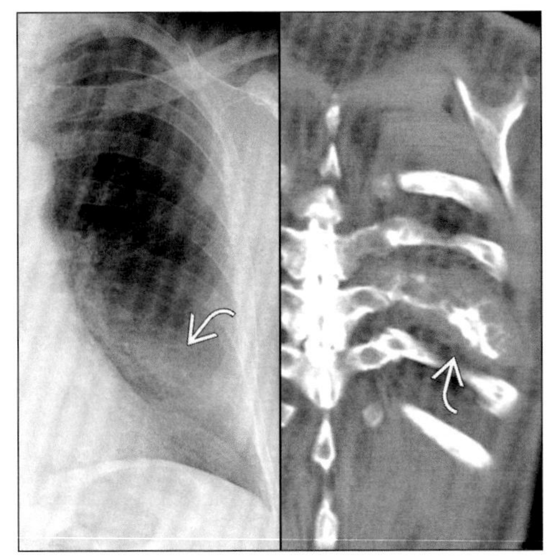

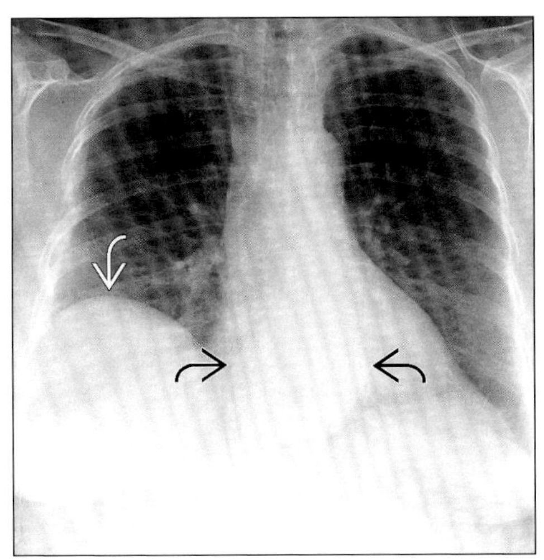

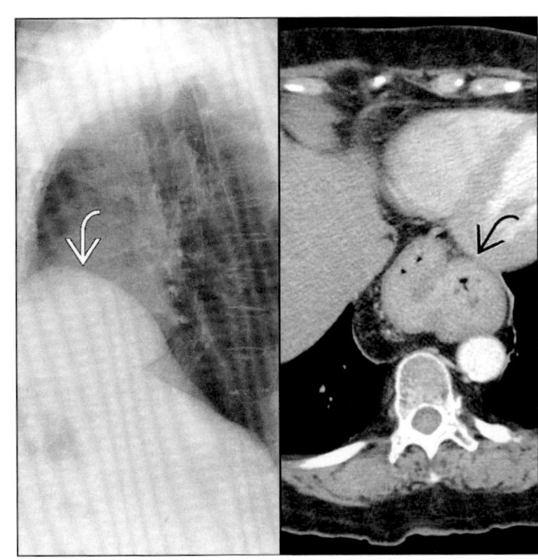

*(**Left**) PA chest radiograph demonstrates eventration of the right hemidiaphragm ➡ and a moderately sized hiatus hernia ➡. Hiatus hernias typically manifest on chest radiography as retrocardiac opacities with lateral displacement of the inferior aspect of the azygoesophageal recess. (**Right**) Composite image with lateral chest radiograph (left) and axial CECT (right) of the same patient demonstrates eventration of the right hemidiaphragm ➡ and a moderately sized hiatus hernia ➡.*

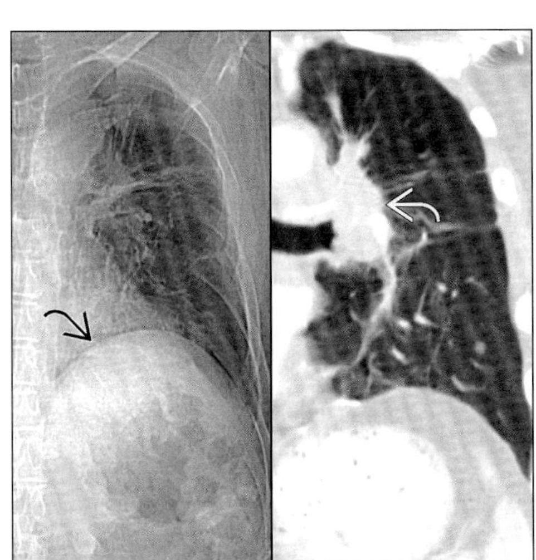

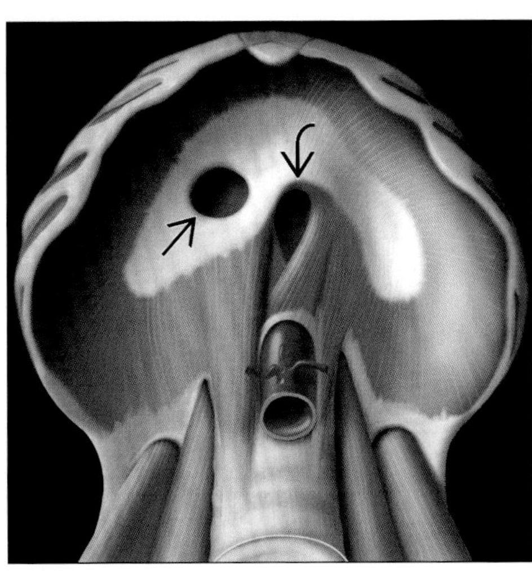

*(**Left**) Composite image with AP scout radiograph (left) and coronal CECT (right) shows elevation of a paralyzed left hemidiaphragm ➡ caused by a central lung cancer ➡ that invaded the phrenic nerve. (**Right**) Graphic shows the undersurface of the diaphragm and its origins from the sternum, costal cartilages, and lumbar vertebrae and insertion into the central tendon. The IVC hiatus ➡ passes through the central tendon. The esophageal hiatus ➡ is surrounded by the right crus.*

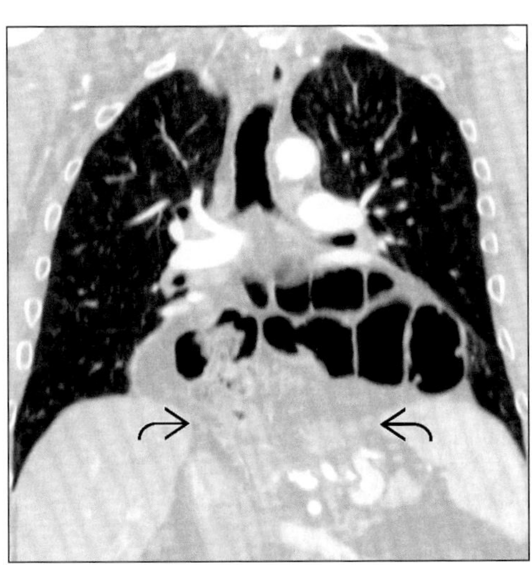

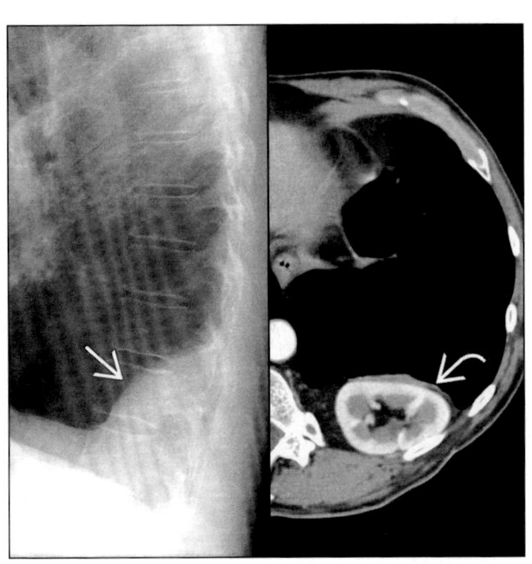

*(**Left**) Coronal CECT demonstrates herniated colon and mesentery through an enlarged diaphragmatic hiatus ➡. Hiatal hernias often manifest as air-containing bowel (typically stomach) within a retrocardiac opacity. Larger hernias may contain large &/or small bowel loops. (**Right**) Composite image with lateral chest radiograph (left) and axial CECT (right) shows a Bochdalek hernia ➡ that contains the left kidney ➡ herniating through the Bochdalek foramen.*

CHEST WALL INFECTIONS

Key Facts

Terminology

- Definition
  - Infection involving chest wall bones & soft tissues

Imaging

- Radiography
  - Lung consolidation with skeletal involvement
  - Pleural effusion
  - Subcutaneous gas; necrotizing infection or fistula
- CT
  - Lung consolidation & chest wall involvement
  - Sensitive for identification of subcutaneous gas
  - Pleural effusion; bronchopleural fistula
  - Displaced sternotomy wires suggest dehiscence
- MR
  - More sensitive than CT for early bone involvement
  - Soft tissue & fascial plane edema
  - Use of intravenous contrast to determine extent of soft tissue involvement

Top Differential Diagnoses

- Actinomycosis
- Tuberculosis
- Necrotizing soft tissue infection
- Sternotomy infection
- Chest wall malignancy

Clinical Issues

- Etiology
  - Direct extension from adjacent lung infection
  - Complication of trauma or surgery
- Symptoms/signs
  - Fever & chest wall pain
  - Palpable chest wall lesion; abscess, edema
  - Cutaneous fistulas
- Treatment
  - Abscess drainage & antimicrobic therapy
  - Surgical debridement for severe infection

*(**Left**) Axial CECT of a patient with chest tube-related Alcaligenes infection shows low-attenuation consolidated atelectatic lung, gas-containing left pleural effusion, and pleural fluid and gas in the chest wall with associated soft tissue edema. (**Right**) Axial CECT shows a tuberculous empyema manifesting with left pleural effusion, thick enhancing pleura, and posterior chest wall involvement with resultant rib and vertebral destruction.*

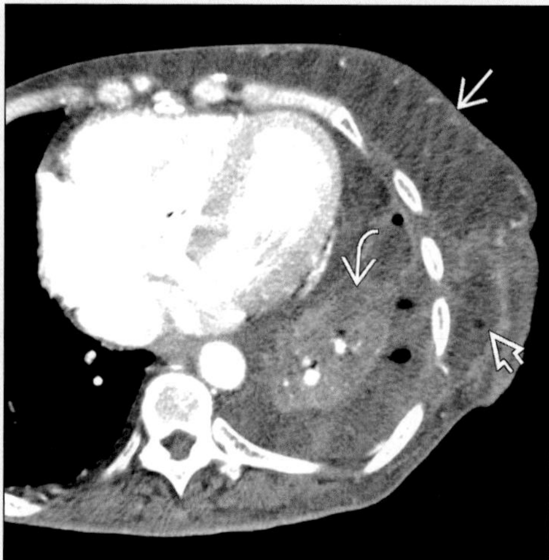

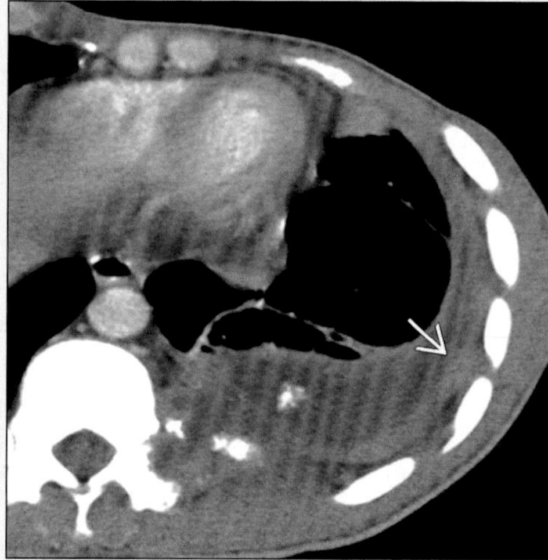

*(**Left**) Composite image with axial CECT in soft tissue (top) and lung (bottom) window of a patient with invasive aspergillosis shows an inflammatory mass with destruction of the ribs and manubrium sternum and extension into the anterior chest wall, as well as ground-glass and nodular lung opacities. (**Right**) Sagittal T1WI C+ FS MR of a patient with Streptococcus pneumonia and secondary chest wall infection shows a complex rim-enhancing mass involving lung, pleura, and chest wall.*

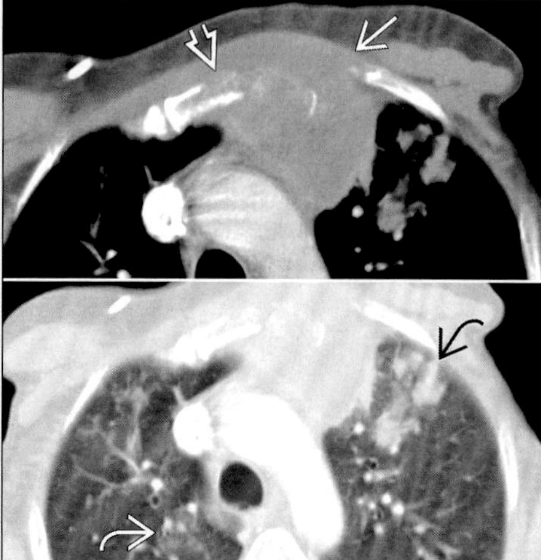

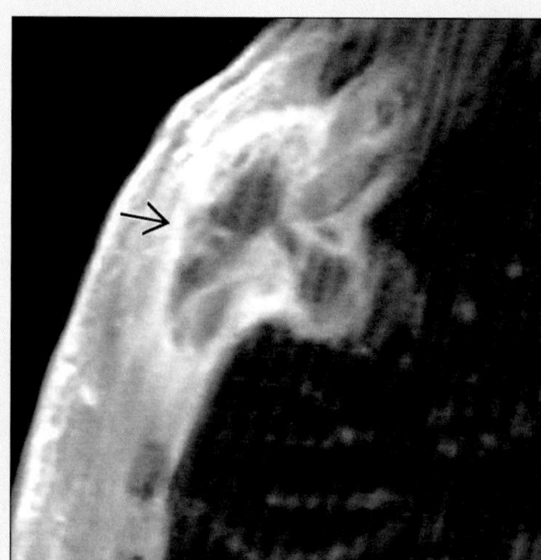

CHEST WALL INFECTIONS

TERMINOLOGY

Definitions

- **Infection involving chest wall skeletal structures & soft tissues**

IMAGING

Radiographic Findings

- **Pulmonary consolidation** with associated **skeletal involvement**; bone destruction & periosteal reaction
- Pleural effusion
- Subcutaneous gas; necrotizing infections or fistulas
- **Displaced sternotomy wires** suggest **dehiscence**

CT Findings

- Pulmonary consolidation & chest wall involvement
  - Soft tissue mass, skeletal destruction, periostitis, osteomyelitis
- Pleural effusion; bronchopleural fistula
- **Identification of subcutaneous gas**

MR Findings

- More **sensitive** than CT for early bone involvement
- Soft tissue and fascial plane edema
- Contrast enhancement; evaluation of extent of soft tissue involvement

Nuclear Medicine Findings

- **Skeletal scintigraphy: Sensitive & specific** for diagnosing **osteomyelitis**

Imaging Recommendations

- Best imaging tool
  - CT for optimal evaluation of chest wall invasion, fistulous tracks, & skeletal involvement

DIFFERENTIAL DIAGNOSIS

Actinomycosis

- Mouth flora; aspiration after dental manipulation or in patients with dental disease
- Typically lung abscess with chest wall involvement

Nocardiosis

- Gram-positive bacterium; immunocompromised hosts
- Consolidation or cavitary nodules; rare chest wall involvement

Tuberculosis

- Chest wall mass or cutaneous fistula
- Rib involvement more common in IV drug users
- Tuberculous spondylitis (Pott disease); hematogenous infection
- Extension of empyema into chest wall (empyema necessitatis)

Streptococcus Pneumonia

- Most common gram-positive pneumonia
- Chest wall invasion rare

Necrotizing Soft Tissue Infection

- Most frequent in postoperative patients
- Predisposing condition; chest wall malignancy
- High mortality; early surgical intervention required

Sternotomy Infection

- 0.3-5% of median sternotomy cases
- Mortality rates range from 14-47%
- Risk factors: Diabetes, obesity, COPD, smoking
- Most common pathogens: *Staphylococcus aureus* (29%), *S. epidermidis* (22%), and *Pseudomonas aeruginosa*

Chest Wall Malignancy

- Peripheral locally invasive lung cancers may mimic chest wall infections
- Mesothelioma may invade chest wall
- Primary chest wall neoplasms
  - Rare; chondrosarcoma, osteosarcoma, & lymphoma
- Secondary chest wall neoplasms
  - Breast, prostate, & renal cell cancer; melanoma

PATHOLOGY

General Features

- Etiology
  - **Hematogenous** dissemination of infection
  - **Direct extension** from adjacent lung infection
  - Complication of **trauma or surgery**

CLINICAL ISSUES

Presentation

- Most common signs/symptoms
  - **Fever & chest wall pain**
  - **Palpable chest wall lesion**; abscess, edema
- Other signs/symptoms
  - **Cutaneous fistulas**

Demographics

- Epidemiology
  - Incidence of mediastinal & chest wall infection after cardiac surgery ranges from 0.3-5%

Diagnosis

- Biopsy/aspiration may be warranted to exclude chest wall malignancy

Treatment

- Abscess drainage & culture-tailored antimicrobic therapy
- Necrotizing or severe chest wall infection: Early & aggressive surgical debridement

DIAGNOSTIC CHECKLIST

Consider

- Chest wall infection in febrile patients with palpable chest wall mass ± adjacent lung consolidation

Image Interpretation Pearls

- Subcutaneous gas may be absent in cases of necrotizing chest wall infection

SELECTED REFERENCES

1. Blasberg JD et al: Infections and radiation injuries involving the chest wall. Thorac Surg Clin. 20(4):487-94, 2010
2. Chelli Bouaziz M et al: Imaging of chest wall infections. Skeletal Radiol. 38(12):1127-35, 2009

DISCITIS

Key Facts

Terminology

- Definition: Disc space infection

Imaging

- Radiography
  - Disc space narrowing
  - Erosion/irregularity of adjacent vertebral endplates
  - Laterally displaced paravertebral stripes
- CT
  - Disc space narrowing (best appreciated on sagittal reformatted images)
  - Paravertebral inflammatory mass or fluid
- MR
  - Affected disc & adjacent vertebrae hypointense on T1WI, hyperintense on T2WI due to edema
  - Enhancement of disc, adjacent vertebrae, paravertebral soft tissues, epidural abscess
  - MR is highly sensitive & specific for diagnosis

Top Differential Diagnoses

- Degenerative disc disease
- Spinal metastases

Pathology

- Bacterial infection
  - Staphylococcus aureus in > 50%
- Granulomatous infection

Clinical Issues

- Focal back pain not relieved by rest
- Fever, chills, malaise
- Risk factors: Spine surgery, diabetes, bacteremia

Diagnostic Checklist

- Consider discitis in patients with back pain & signs and symptoms of infection
- Review sagittal reformatted CT images to assess disc height & adjacent endplate abnormalities

__(Left)__ Graphic shows destruction and narrowing of the intervertebral disc space with associated erosion of adjacent vertebral body endplates ⇒, consistent with discitis. Extension of infection into the epidural space ➔ and narrowing of the spinal canal are also illustrated. __(Right)__ Sagittal reformatted CECT (bone window) shows loss of disc height ➔ with associated erosion and irregularity of adjacent vertebral body endplates. Discitis characteristically affects a single disc space.

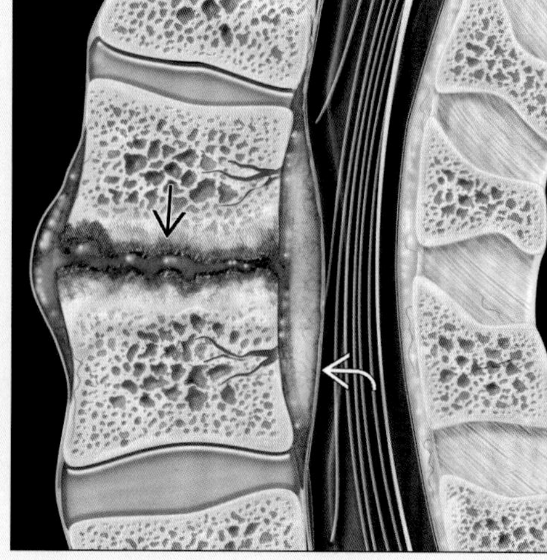

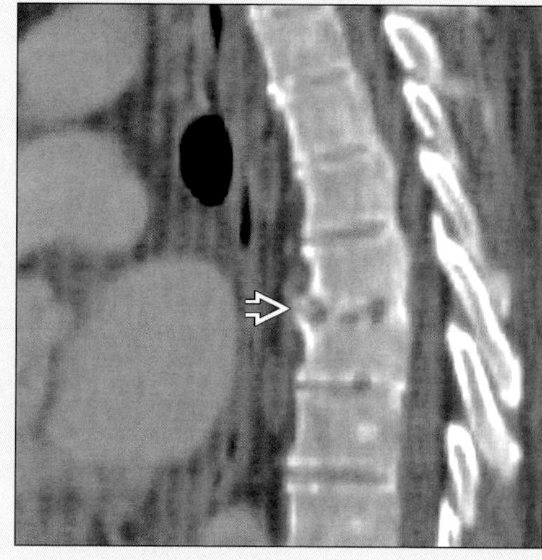

__(Left)__ Sagittal T1-weighted MR image shows hypointense signal of the affected disc ➔ and the adjacent vertebral bodies ➔ with associated loss of disc height, consistent with discitis. __(Right)__ Contrast-enhanced sagittal T1-weighted MR image with fat suppression demonstrates disc space narrowing ➔ and vertebral body enhancement, consistent with discitis. Note epidural enhancement ➔ not appreciated on unenhanced T1WI. MR optimally demonstrates epidural involvement in patients with discitis.

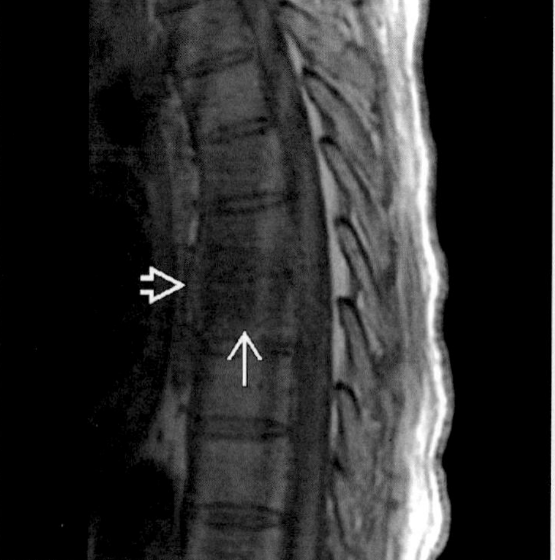

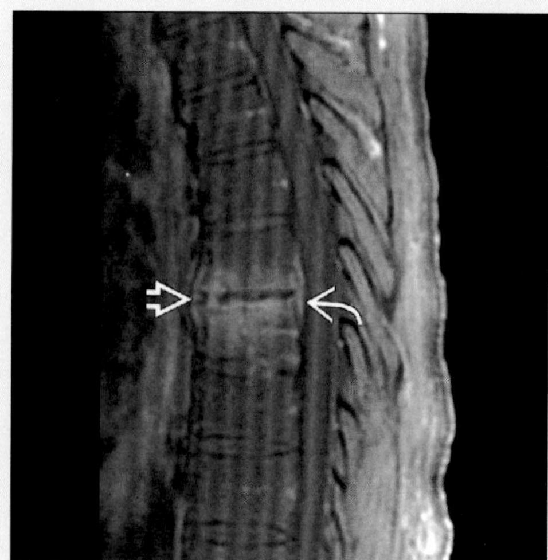

DISCITIS

TERMINOLOGY

Synonyms

- **Diskitis**

Definitions

- **Disc space infection**
- Adjacent vertebral bodies also usually involved

IMAGING

General Features

- Best diagnostic clue
  - **Disc space narrowing**
  - Erosion/irregularity of adjacent vertebral endplates
- Location
  - Lumbar spine most frequently involved, followed by thoracic spine
  - **Single disc** typically involved

Radiographic Findings

- Radiography may be normal in first 2 weeks after onset of symptoms
- Earliest finding: **Disc space narrowing**
- Indistinctness or destruction of adjacent endplates
- **Endplate sclerosis** develops after 8 weeks
- **Lateral displacement of paravertebral stripes** by adjacent soft tissue infection
- Pulmonary consolidation; pneumonia may be the source of hematogenous spread of infection

CT Findings

- **Disc space narrowing**
  - Best appreciated on sagittal reformatted images
- Irregularity or destruction of vertebral endplates
- **Endplate skeletal sclerosis**
- Paravertebral inflammatory mass or fluid collection
- Epidural involvement; difficult to appreciate on CT

MR Findings

- Early findings: Disc space narrowing, subtle endplate enhancement; may mimic degenerative disc disease
- Affected disc & adjacent vertebrae **hypointense on T1WI; hyperintense on T2WI** due to edema
- Enhancement of disc & adjacent affected vertebrae, paravertebral soft tissues, & epidural abscess

Imaging Recommendations

- Best imaging tool
  - **MR with and without contrast**; highly **sensitive** and **specific** for diagnosis
    - Allows optimal evaluation of adjacent soft tissue & epidural involvement
- Protocol advice
  - **MR T1WI** with **contrast** & **fat suppression**
  - **Sagittal** imaging for optimal visualization of disc height loss

Nuclear Medicine Findings

- Ga-67 scintigraphy
  - **Highly sensitive**
  - Assessment of response to antibiotic treatment
  - Evaluation of postoperative patients with hardware and patients in whom MR is contraindicated

DIFFERENTIAL DIAGNOSIS

Degenerative Disc Disease

- Disc space narrowing without endplate destruction or disc enhancement
- Characteristic multilevel involvement, unlike discitis

Spinal Metastases

- Involvement of multiple vertebral bodies
- Spared intervertebral disc; preserved disc height

PATHOLOGY

General Features

- Etiology
  - Bacterial infection; *Staphylococcus aureus* in > 50%
  - Granulomatous infection
    - Tuberculosis, brucellosis, fungal infection
    - Involvement of adjacent paravertebral soft tissues &/or vertebral bodies
    - Relative sparing of disc space
  - Hematogenous dissemination of infection
    - Respiratory tract, urinary tract
  - Direct inoculation of infection
    - Surgery, discography, penetrating trauma
  - Local extension of adjacent infection
    - Retroperitoneum, abdomen, thorax

CLINICAL ISSUES

Presentation

- Most common signs/symptoms
  - **Focal back pain** not relieved by rest
  - **Fever, chills, malaise**
- Other signs/symptoms
  - Neurologic compromise
  - Elevated erythrocyte sedimentation rate (ESR)

Demographics

- Epidemiology
  - Risk factors: Recent spine surgery, preceding bacteremia, immunosuppression, diabetes, intravenous drug use

Natural History & Prognosis

- **Mortality: 2-20%**

Treatment

- **Intravenous antibiotic therapy** for at least 6 weeks

DIAGNOSTIC CHECKLIST

Consider

- Discitis in patients with back pain & signs and symptoms of infection

Image Interpretation Pearls

- Review **sagittal reformatted CT images** to assess disc height & adjacent endplate abnormalities

SELECTED REFERENCES

1. Dunbar JA et al: The MRI appearances of early vertebral osteomyelitis and discitis. Clin Radiol. 65(12):974-81, 2010

EMPYEMA NECESSITATIS

Key Facts

Terminology
- Synonym
  - Empyema necessitans
- Definition
  - Chronic empyema draining into chest wall

Imaging
- Radiography
  - Chest wall soft tissue mass or asymmetry
  - Chest wall osseous involvement
  - Adjacent pleural effusion, typically loculated
- CT
  - Chest wall involvement; soft tissues, skeleton
  - Pleural effusion; loculation, split pleura sign
  - Gas within pleural space/chest wall process
  - Pleural fluid continuous with chest wall process
- MR
  - Visualization of chest wall abscess

Top Differential Diagnoses
- Chest wall infection: Necrotizing fasciitis
- Costochondritis
- Malignant neoplasms crossing tissue planes
  - Lung cancer

Pathology
- Pneumonia with secondary empyema & progression to chest wall involvement

Clinical Issues
- Diagnosis
  - Fine needle aspiration biopsy
- Treatment
  - Antibiotics; surgical drainage

Diagnostic Checklist
- Consider empyema necessitatis in patients with empyema & adjacent chest wall abnormality

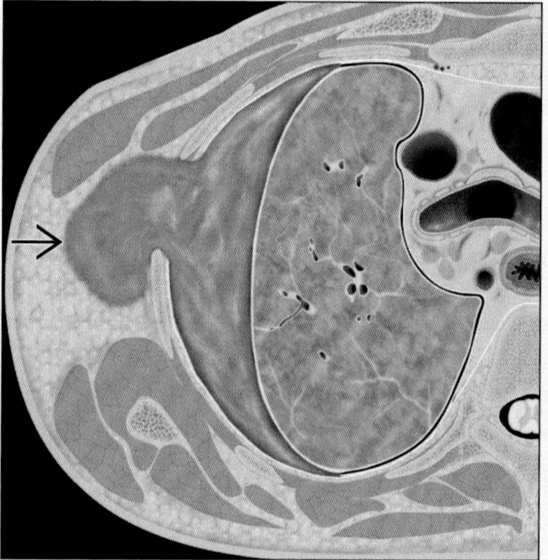

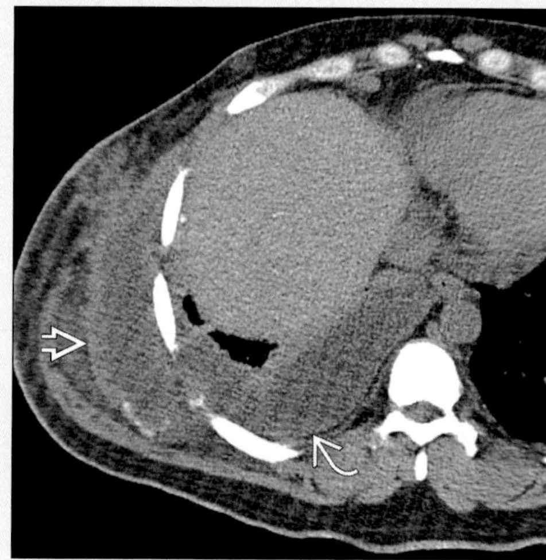

(Left) *Graphic shows the morphologic features of empyema necessitatis. Infected pleural fluid drains into the adjacent chest wall soft tissues continuous with a fluid-containing chest wall mass ⇒.* ***(Right)*** *Axial NECT of a patient with Nocardia empyema shows a loculated right pleural effusion ➡ complicated by empyema necessitatis. CT allows visualization of the extension of infected pleural fluid to the soft tissues of the adjacent chest wall ➡, resulting in a moderate fluid collection.*

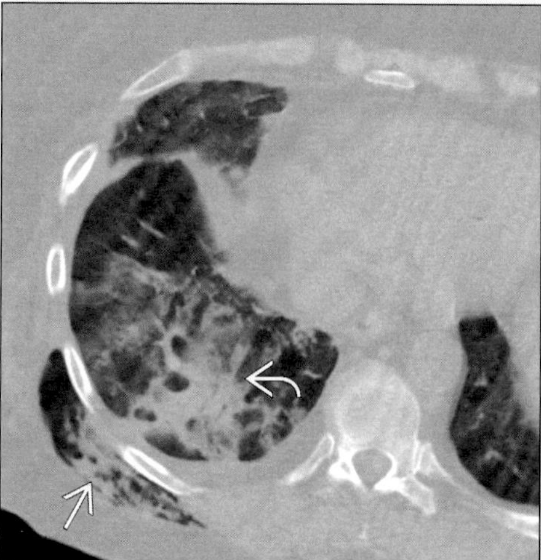

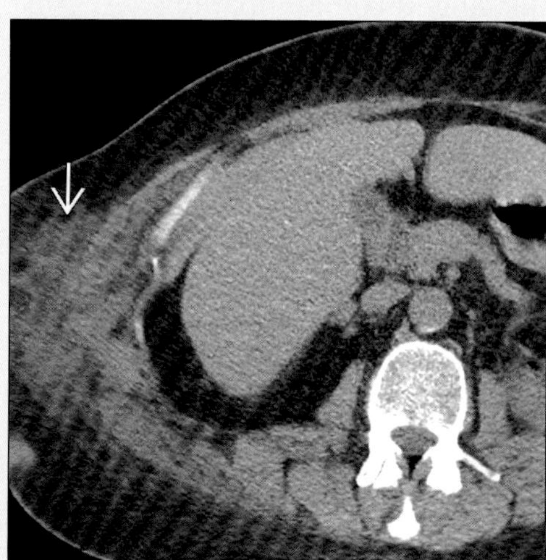

(Left) *Axial NECT of a patient status post bilateral lung transplantation complicated by invasive aspergillosis shows a right lower lobe consolidation ➡, adjacent right pleural fluid, and chest wall subcutaneous gas ➡.* ***(Right)*** *Axial NECT of the same patient shows a heterogeneous right chest wall soft tissue mass ➡. Untreated empyemas may drain into the adjacent chest wall producing an empyema necessitatis that may exhibit fluid, soft tissue, &/or air attenuation.*

EMPYEMA NECESSITATIS

TERMINOLOGY

Synonyms

- **Empyema necessitans**
- Cold abscess

Definitions

- Chronic empyema draining into chest wall

IMAGING

General Features

- Best diagnostic clue
  - Loculated pleural fluid with associated chest wall mass &/or skeletal involvement
- Location
  - Chest wall; adjacent to loculated pleural fluid
- Size
  - Variable
- Morphology
  - Asymmetry of chest wall soft tissues
  - Obscuration of fascial planes

Radiographic Findings

- Radiography
  - **Chest wall soft tissue mass** or asymmetry
    - May exhibit intrinsic gas, gas-fluid levels
  - **Chest wall osseous involvement**
    - Rib destruction, osteomyelitis, periostitis
  - Adjacent pleural effusion, typically loculated
    - Gas within free or loculated pleural fluid
      - Bronchopleural fistula
    - Calcified pleural rind in tuberculosis
  - Adjacent airspace disease
    - Consolidation
    - Lung abscess
      - Visualization of gas within lung abscess &/or adjacent chest wall

CT Findings

- CECT
  - Communication between pleural space & chest wall
  - Assessment of chest wall involvement
    - Induration of chest wall fat
    - Obliteration of chest wall tissue planes
    - Chest wall mass with soft tissue attenuation
    - Chest wall fluid collection
      - May exhibit fluid or soft tissue attenuation
      - May exhibit enhancing rim
      - May contain gas &/or gas-fluid levels
    - Skeletal involvement
      - Involvement of ribs, sternum, vertebrae
      - Skeletal destruction, osteomyelitis
      - Periostitis; may manifest with rib enlargement
  - Pleural effusion, typically loculated
    - May exhibit visceral & parietal pleural enhancement; **split pleura sign**
    - May exhibit intrinsic gas; bronchopleural fistula
  - **Tuberculosis**
    - Thick-walled, well-encapsulated pleural mass
      - Peripheral enhancement &/or calcification
      - Low-attenuation pleural content
    - Direct extension to chest &/or abdominal walls
    - Pleurocutaneous fistula, sinus tract; 25%
  - **Invasive aspergillosis**
    - Pulmonary consolidation
    - Pleural effusion
    - Chest wall mass, fistula, osteolytic rib lesions

MR Findings

- Assessment of extent of chest wall involvement
  - Soft tissue, skeletal structures
- **T1 C+ FS**: Visualization of chest wall abscess
  - Peripheral rim enhancement
  - Central low signal fluid/necrosis
- *Aspergillus* infection
  - T2WI: High signal intensity
  - T1WI: Decreased signal intensity

Ultrasonographic Findings

- Evaluation of extent & morphology of chest wall involvement
- Guidance for aspiration, biopsy, drainage

Imaging Recommendations

- Best imaging tool
  - CT is the imaging modality of choice to assess chest wall soft tissue & osseous involvement
- Protocol advice
  - CECT helpful for evaluation & characterization of pleural effusion & chest wall involvement

DIFFERENTIAL DIAGNOSIS

Chest Wall Infection: Necrotizing Fasciitis

- Infection of intermuscular fascial layers
- Spontaneous, diabetes, immunosuppression, post trauma/surgery
- *Staphylococcus aureus*, *Pseudomonas aeruginosa*, *Mycobacterium tuberculosis*
- Chest wall soft tissue mass/abscess
  - Loss of deep soft tissue planes
  - Pyogenic osteomyelitis, periostitis

Costochondritis

- Intravenous drug abusers
  - *Staphylococcus*, *Streptococcus*, *M. tuberculosis*
- Septic arthritis
  - Sternoclavicular & sternochondral joints

Malignant Neoplasms Crossing Tissue Planes

- Lung & pleura
  - Lung cancer
    - Peripheral lesion with direct chest wall invasion
    - Pancoast tumor
  - Lymphoma
    - Secondary chest wall invasion
    - May encase bones without destruction
  - Malignant mesothelioma
    - Tumor growth along biopsy or surgical sites
- Chest wall
  - Chest wall metastases
    - Lung, breast, prostate cancers
  - Multiple myeloma, plasmacytoma
    - Well-defined lytic bone lesions
    - Soft tissue masses
  - Chondrosarcoma
    - Anterior rib mass
    - Large lobular, chondroid calcifications
  - Lymphoma
  - Ewing sarcoma family of tumors

- Elastofibroma & fibromatosis
  - Often arise between scapula and ribs

PATHOLOGY

General Features

- Etiology
  - Pneumonia with secondary empyema; progression to chest wall involvement
  - Bacteria
    - *Staphylococcus aureus*, *Streptococcus pneumoniae*
      - Complication of thoracotomy, pneumonectomy, bypass surgery
    - *M. tuberculosis*
      - Acid-fast bacillus
      - Contiguous spread from infected lung or pleura
    - *Actinomyces*
      - Anaerobic bacillus; sulfur granules or grains
      - Oral colonization; caries, poor oral hygiene
      - Pleuropulmonary infection from aspiration
      - Fistulas from production of proteolytic enzymes
      - Crosses fascial planes; lung to pleura to chest wall
    - *Nocardia*
      - Weakly acid-fast bacterium
      - Typically affects immunosuppressed patients
      - May uncommonly traverse tissue planes
      - May result in central nervous system (CNS) involvement
  - Fungi
    - *Aspergillus*
      - Inhaled, dimorphic fungus
      - Invasion of vessels (angioinvasive) & adjacent tissues
      - Immunosuppressed patients; leukemia, transplant recipients, AIDS
      - Often fatal despite treatment
    - *Zygomyces*
      - Blood vessel & tissue invasion
      - Often fatal despite antibiotic treatment
    - *Blastomyces*
      - Fungus, yeast form in tissue
      - Rare pleuropulmonary disease, may involve chest wall
- Associated abnormalities
  - Rare involvement of mediastinum, retroperitoneum
  - May produce mastitis

Gross Pathologic & Surgical Features

- Infectious/inflammatory pleural process
- Spontaneous rupture into surrounding chest wall soft tissues with or without skeletal involvement
- *Actinomyces*: Sulfur granules or grains

Microscopic Features

- Tuberculous empyema necessitatis
  - Purulent fluid, white blood cells (WBC) > 100,000 cells/mL, neutrophils
  - Organism cultured in 10-47% of cases
- Actinomyces empyema necessitatis
  - Anaerobic organisms

CLINICAL ISSUES

Presentation

- Most common signs/symptoms
  - Enlarging palpable chest wall mass
    - Typically anterolateral chest wall
    - Also, breast, posterior trunk, abdominal wall, vertebral column
    - Brachial plexus involvement, cord compression
  - Chest wall sinus drainage
  - Painful or fluctuant chest wall mass
    - Tuberculous cold abscess: Absence of heat or redness
    - Pyogenic infection: Hot & red skin
- Other signs/symptoms
  - Fever, malaise, weight loss, pleuritic chest pain, night sweats
  - Immunosuppression, leukemia, transplantation
    - Fever, neutropenia
  - Actinomycosis
    - Loose teeth, gingivitis, poor oral hygiene

Demographics

- Age
  - Childhood to old age
- Gender
  - Actinomycosis: M:F = 4:1
- Epidemiology
  - Rare: Much more common in pre-antibiotic era
  - Tuberculous chest wall involvement, uncommon

Natural History & Prognosis

- Tuberculous empyema, less common than tuberculous pleuritis
  - Chronic active infection
  - Originates from pulmonary tuberculosis, lymphadenopathy, or hematogenous spread
  - Large effusion with entrapped lung
  - Complications: Bronchopleural fistula &/or empyema necessitatis

Diagnosis

- **Fine needle aspiration**
- Specimen smears; cultures for aerobic & anaerobic bacteria, fungi
- Fluid cytology

Treatment

- **Antibiotic treatment**
- **Surgical drainage**
- Tuberculous empyema & some bacterial infections require chest tube drainage

DIAGNOSTIC CHECKLIST

Consider

- Empyema necessitatis in patients with empyema/loculated effusion & adjacent chest wall abnormality

SELECTED REFERENCES

1. Heffner JE et al: Diagnostic utility and clinical application of imaging for pleural space infections. Chest. 137(2):467-79, 2010

EMPYEMA NECESSITATIS

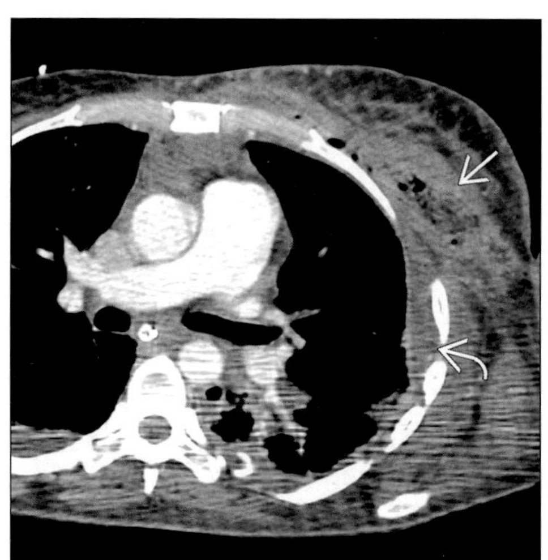

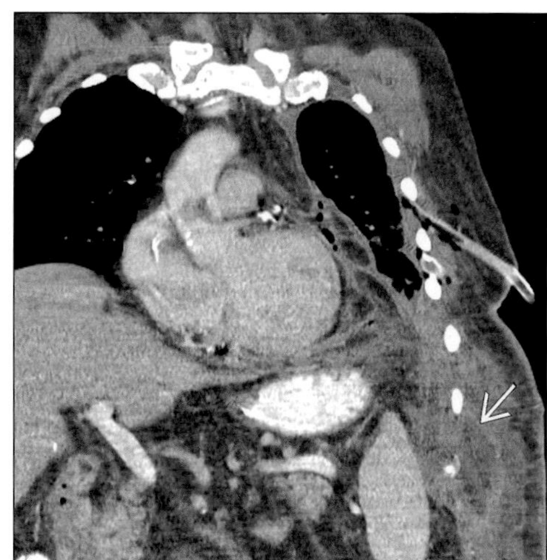

(Left) *Axial CECT of a patient with methicillin-resistant Staphylococcus aureus empyema necessitatis shows a loculated left pleural effusion and an adjacent chest wall abscess deep to the left breast. Empyema necessitatis may manifest with mastitis.* ***(Right)*** *Coronal CECT of a patient with postoperative empyema necessitatis shows heterogeneous fluid and soft tissue in the left inferior chest and upper abdominal walls. Note rim enhancement surrounding the fluid components of the lesion.*

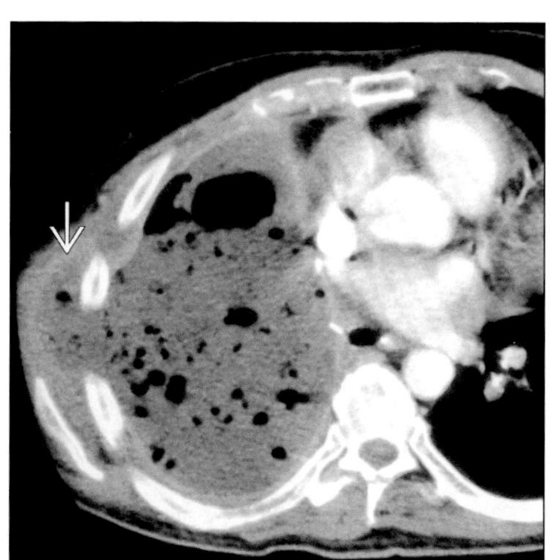

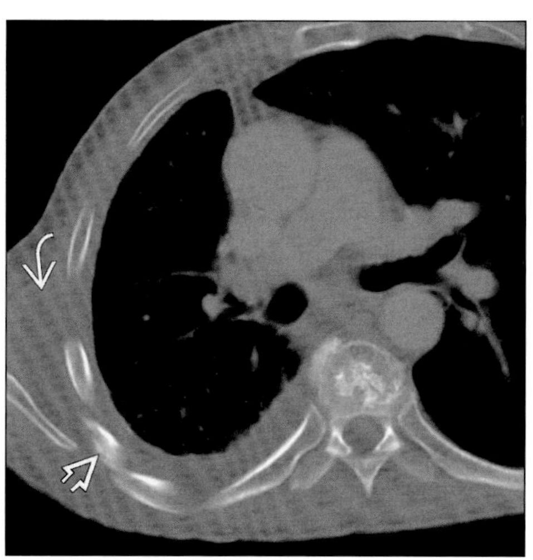

(Left) *Axial CECT of a patient with right empyema complicated by bronchopleural fistula and empyema necessitatis shows a large right pleural effusion with intrinsic gas bubbles extending into the soft tissues of the adjacent chest wall.* ***(Right)*** *Axial CECT (bone window) of a patient with empyema necessitatis demonstrates periostitis adjacent to the empyema. Skeletal involvement in empyema necessitatis may manifest with periostitis or osseous destruction.*

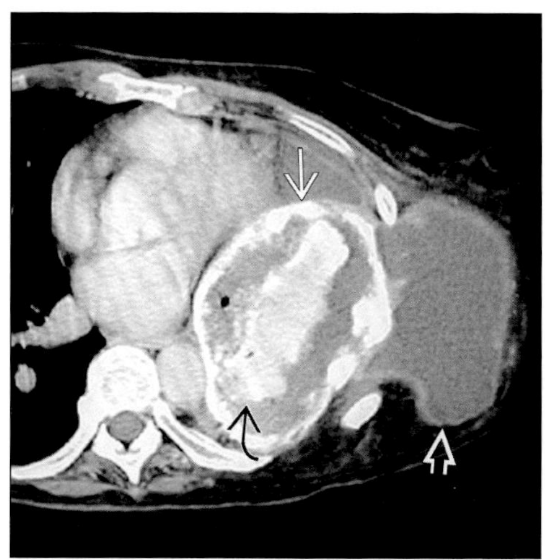

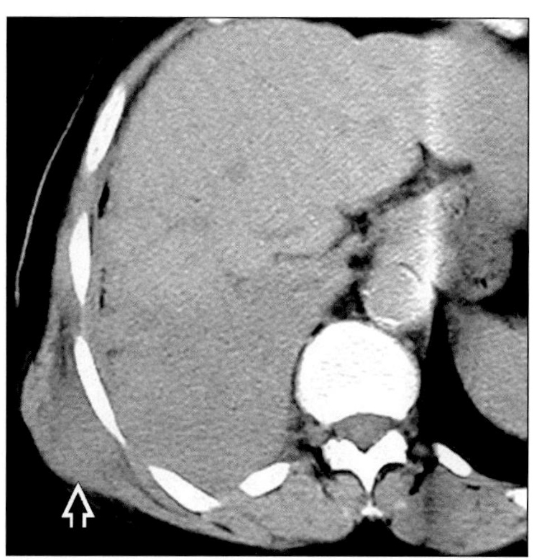

(Left) *Axial CECT of a patient with tuberculosis shows a calcified atelectatic left lung secondary to autopneumonectomy, a densely calcified pleural rind, and tuberculous empyema necessitatis manifesting as a large fluid collection in the soft tissues of the left chest wall.* ***(Right)*** *Axial NECT of a patient with poor dentition shows a right lower lobe consolidation and an adjacent right chest wall mass. Fine needle aspiration showed sulfur granules, and cultures grew Actinomyces.*

CHEST WALL LIPOMA

Key Facts

Terminology

- Abbreviations
  - Chest wall lipoma (CWL)
- Definition
  - Benign tumor composed of adipocytes

Imaging

- Radiography
  - Peripheral soft tissue mass
  - Incomplete border sign
- CT
  - Chest wall mass ± intrathoracic component
  - Fat attenuation: -50 to -100 HU
  - Thin, smooth septa < 2 mm; may enhance
- MR
  - High signal intensity on T1WI & T2WI
  - T1 signal suppresses with chemical fat saturation
  - Thin, low T1 septa may exhibit enhancement

Top Differential Diagnoses

- Liposarcoma
- Pleural lipoma
- Spindle cell lipoma

Clinical Issues

- Signs & symptoms
  - Palpable soft mobile mass
- Demographics
  - Peak incidence: 50-70 years
- Treatment
  - No treatment for small asymptomatic lesions
  - Image-guided biopsy to sample suspicious masses
  - Surgical evaluation of suspicious fatty tumors

Diagnostic Checklist

- Homogeneous chest wall mass identical to subcutaneous fat is almost certainly a benign lipoma

*(**Left**) Axial CECT (top) and FDG PET (bottom) images show a well-circumscribed, fat-attenuation chest wall lipoma (CWL) → of the upper back with thin internal soft tissue septa. FDG PET shows no FDG uptake. (**Right**) Axial T1W C+ MR (top) and T1W C+ FS MR (bottom) images show an encapsulated hyperintense right posterior CWL → that exhibits fat suppression. Note thin, smooth, hypointense septa →, some with subtle enhancement →. Most CWLs affect the back.*

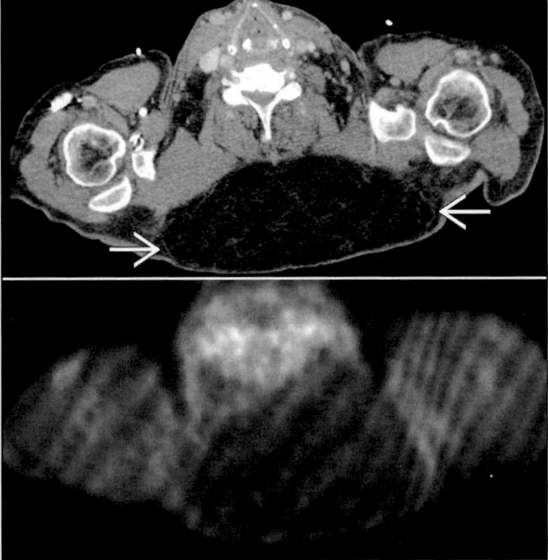

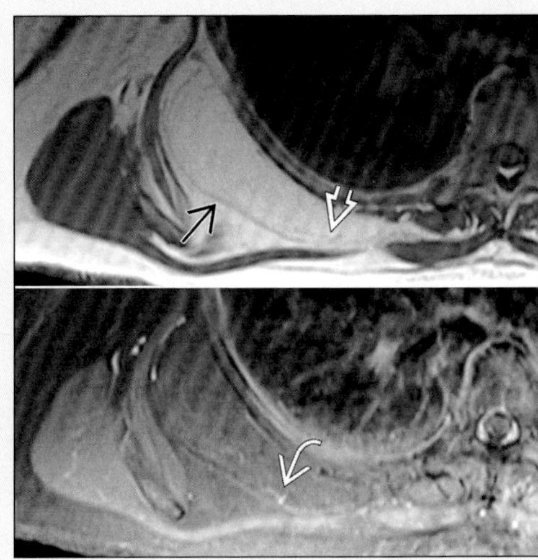

*(**Left**) PA chest radiograph (left) and axial CECT (right) images show a peripheral left upper thoracic mass with obtuse margins → relative to the chest wall. Chest CT shows a fat-attenuation mass consistent with CWL. (**Right**) Axial CECT shows an axillary liposarcoma manifesting as a mass of predominant fat attenuation with irregular soft tissue components and calcifications. Extensive soft tissue components and calcifications in chest wall fatty lesions should suggest liposarcoma rather than lipoma.*

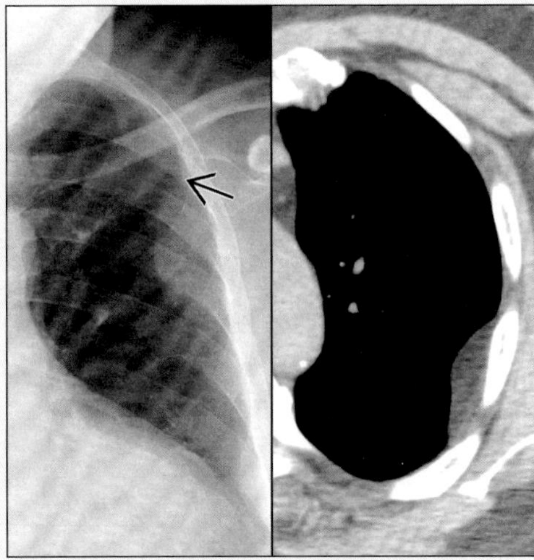

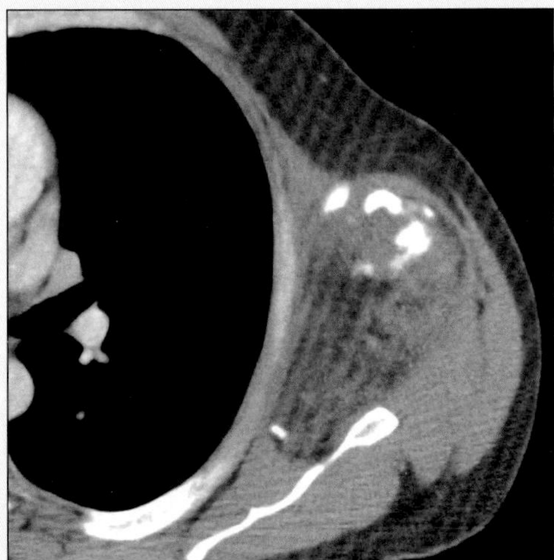

CHEST WALL LIPOMA

TERMINOLOGY

Abbreviations

- **Chest wall lipoma (CWL)**

Definitions

- **Benign tumor** composed of **adipocytes**

IMAGING

General Features

- Best diagnostic clue
  - Encapsulated mass of tissue nearly identical to subcutaneous fat
- Location
  - Back is most common chest wall location
- Size
  - Most are 1-10 cm
- Morphology
  - Usually encapsulated, sometimes infiltrating
  - Deep lipomas: Intramuscular, intermuscular, both
  - Typical
    - Smooth, sharp margins; sometimes lobulated
    - Pliable, conforming to fascial planes
    - Few or no septations

Radiographic Findings

- Peripheral soft tissue mass
- **Incomplete border sign**

CT Findings

- Chest wall mass ± variable intrathoracic component
- **Fat attenuation: -50 to -100 HU**
- Thin, smooth septa < 2 mm; may enhance

MR Findings

- High signal intensity on T1WI & T2WI
- T1 signal suppresses with chemical fat saturation
- Thin, low T1 septa may exhibit gadolinium enhancement

Nuclear Medicine Findings

- PET
  - No FDG uptake in lipomas
  - FDG uptake ratio of tumor: Normal corresponds to histological subtype of liposarcoma (LS)
  - False-positive for LS: Other sarcomas, lymphoma, inflammation
  - False-negative for LS: Well-differentiated LS

Imaging Recommendations

- Best imaging tool
  - CT
    - Excellent spatial resolution for mass characterization
    - Contrast may be warranted to characterize septa or soft tissue components
  - MR
    - Defines relationship to nerves & vessels
    - T1WI, T2WI, T2WI FS, STIR, & T1WI C+ FS sequences useful in differentiating lipomatous tumors
  - FDG PET
    - Can be helpful in evaluation of primary tumors & surveillance

DIFFERENTIAL DIAGNOSIS

Liposarcoma

- Chest wall LS make up 10% of all LS
- Suspicious features
  - Age > 70, male
  - Mass > 10 cm, septal thickness > 2 mm
  - Soft tissue components, calcification

Pleural Lipoma

- Pleural, subpleural, or diaphragmatic
- Arises from submesothelial layers of parietal pleura
- May represent CWL with intrathoracic component

Spindle Cell Lipoma

- Benign, rare; most frequent in middle-aged men
- Well-defined, complex, fatty mass
- Intense enhancement of nonadipose component

Lipoblastoma/Lipoblastomatosis

- In infants & children, indistinguishable from lipoma

PATHOLOGY

General Features

- Etiology
  - 60% of lipomas: Clonal chromosomal abnormalities
- Associated abnormalities
  - Multiple lipomas can be familial

Gross Pathologic & Surgical Features

- Soft, encapsulated, fatty, yellow to orange color

Microscopic Features

- Mature adipocytes very similar to normal fat

CLINICAL ISSUES

Presentation

- Most common signs/symptoms
  - Palpable, soft, mobile mass

Demographics

- Age
  - Peak incidence: 50-70 years
- Epidemiology
  - **Lipomas more common in obese patients**
  - Prevalence: **2% of population**

Treatment

- Image-guided biopsy to sample suspicious masses
- Surgical evaluation of suspicious fatty tumors

DIAGNOSTIC CHECKLIST

Image Interpretation Pearls

- Homogeneous mass identical to subcutaneous fat is almost certainly a benign lipoma
- CWL & LS can have similar imaging features

SELECTED REFERENCES

1. Lee TJ et al: MR imaging evaluation of disorders of the chest wall. Magn Reson Imaging Clin N Am. 16(2):355-79, x, 2008

ELASTOFIBROMA AND FIBROMATOSIS

Key Facts

Terminology
- Definition
  - Benign fibroblastic proliferations & fibroblastic soft tissue tumors
  - Elastofibroma
  - Fibromatosis (desmoid tumors)

Imaging
- Elastofibroma: CT
  - Ill-defined, lenticular, heterogeneous mass
  - Linear low-attenuation streaks from fat
  - Same attenuation as adjacent muscle
- Deep (musculoaponeurotic) fibromatosis: CT
  - Hypodense, isodense, or hyperdense to muscle
  - May exhibit contrast enhancement
- Deep (musculoaponeurotic) fibromatosis: MR
  - T1WI: Homogeneous; low to intermediate signal
  - T2WI: Heterogeneous; variable signal intensity

Top Differential Diagnoses
- Soft tissue sarcomas
- Ewing sarcoma family of tumors

Clinical Issues
- Signs/symptoms
  - Elastofibroma: > 50% asymptomatic
  - Deep fibromatosis; palpable mass
- Age
  - Elastofibroma: Elderly patients, mean age: 70 years
  - Deep fibromatosis: Puberty to 40 years
- Gender
  - Elastofibroma: F:M ratio = 5-13:1
  - Deep fibromatosis: Female predominance
- Therapy & prognosis
  - Elastofibroma: Surgery curative, rare recurrence
  - Deep fibromatosis: Wide excision, adjuvant radiation, high recurrence rate in young patients

*(**Left**) Axial CECT of a 67-year-old man with bilateral elastofibromas shows heterogeneous asymmetric soft tissue masses (left larger than right) ➔ located between the ribs and scapulae with associated rib involvement ➔. The mass on the left side displaces the left scapula. (**Right**) Axial CECT (bone window) of the same patient demonstrates bilateral rib erosion ➔ and the intrathoracic component ➔ of the left lesion. Elastofibromas affect elderly patients and may be bilateral.*

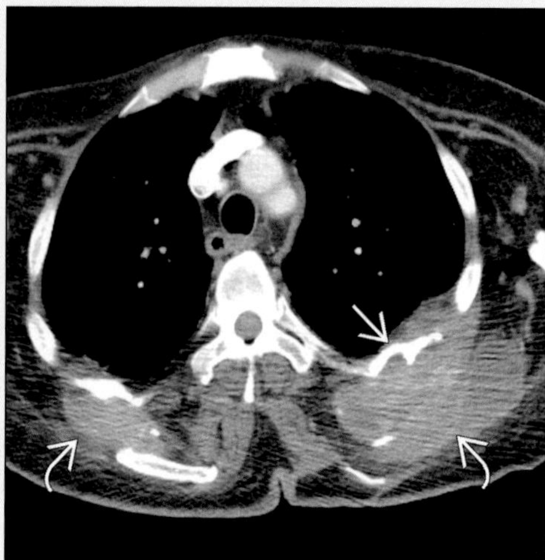

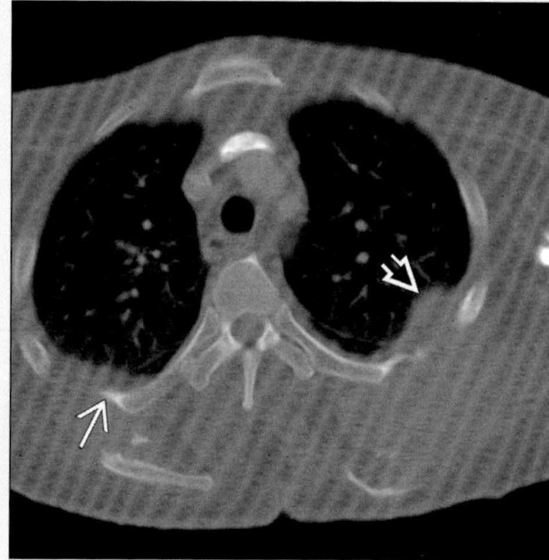

*(**Left**) Coronal T2WI MR of a 65-year-old woman with bilateral elastofibromas shows well-defined subscapular lenticular soft tissue masses ➔ with heterogeneous areas of increased and decreased signal intensity. (**Right**) Axial CECT demonstrates aggressive fibromatosis of the left inferior hemithorax manifesting as a huge heterogeneously enhancing soft tissue mass with intra- ➔ and extrathoracic ➔ components. Deep (musculoaponeurotic) fibromatosis may grow to a very large size.*

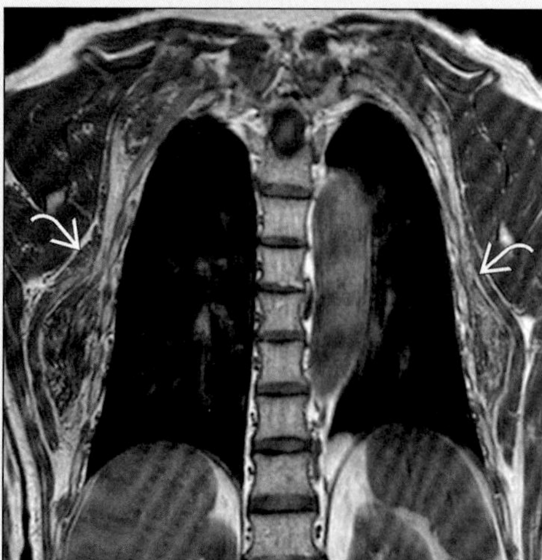

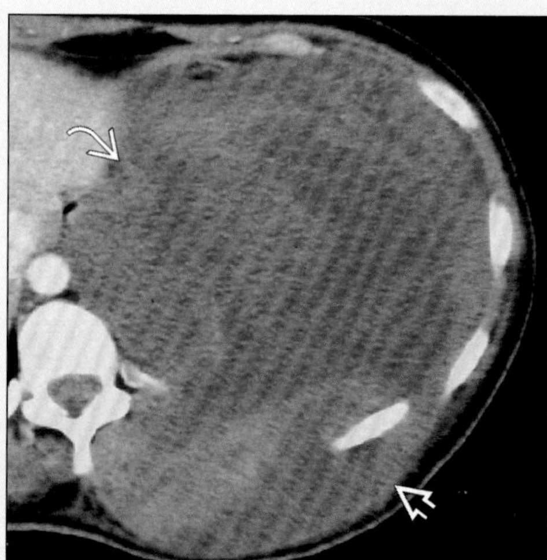

ELASTOFIBROMA AND FIBROMATOSIS

TERMINOLOGY

Synonyms

- **Benign fibroblastic proliferation**
- **Fibromatosis** (desmoid tumors)
- Elastofibroma dorsi

Definitions

- Variety of **benign fibroblastic proliferations** & fibroblastic soft tissue tumors
  - **Elastofibroma**
  - **Fibromatosis** (desmoid tumors)
    - Superficial
    - **Deep (musculoaponeurotic) fibromatosis**
      - **Extraabdominal fibromatosis**/desmoid tumor

IMAGING

General Features

- Best diagnostic clue
  - Solitary or multiple chest wall soft tissue masses
- Key concepts
  - Classification based on pathology, histology, clinical presentation, natural history, & age at presentation
  - **Elastofibroma**
    - Relatively **common fibroelastic pseudotumor** of **subscapular** region
      - 99% in subscapular region, 10-66% bilateral
  - **Deep (musculoaponeurotic) fibromatosis**
    - **Benign fibroblastic proliferation** of deep soft tissues; infiltrative, local recurrence, no metastases
    - Rare: 0.03% of all neoplasms
    - **10-28% involve the chest wall (shoulder)**

CT Findings

- **Elastofibroma**
  - CT: Pathognomonic appearance
    - Poorly defined, **lenticular, heterogeneous soft tissue mass**
    - Contains linear low-attenuation streaks from fat
    - Same attenuation as adjacent muscle
  - PET/CT
    - Mild to moderate uptake of FDG
- **Deep (musculoaponeurotic) fibromatosis**
  - CT
    - Soft tissue mass; **hypodense, isodense, or hyperdense to muscle**
    - Poorly defined margins
    - May exhibit contrast enhancement
  - PET/CT
    - Moderate to marked FDG uptake; no FDG uptake in 10%

MR Findings

- **Elastofibroma**
  - Lenticular mass, intermediate signal intensity
  - T1WI & T2WI: Foci of signal intensity similar to fat
  - Heterogeneous enhancement
- **Deep (musculoaponeurotic) fibromatosis**
  - T2WI: Heterogeneous, very low, intermediate, very high signal (proportion of collagen & spindle cells)
  - T1WI: Homogeneous low to intermediate signal

Angiographic Findings

- Extraabdominal desmoids are often hypervascular

DIFFERENTIAL DIAGNOSIS

Soft Tissue Sarcomas

- Common: Fibrosarcoma, malignant fibrohistiocytoma
- Similar CT and MR appearances

Ewing Sarcoma Family of Tumors

- Small round cells with neural differentiation
- Children or young adults
- Large chest wall mass with rib destruction, pleural thickening/effusion, lung invasion

PATHOLOGY

General Features

- Etiology
  - Elastofibroma
    - Postulated reaction to repetitive microtrauma from friction between scapula & chest wall
- Genetics
  - Deep (musculoaponeurotic) fibromatosis
    - 30% with abnormalities of chromosomes 8 (trisomy 8) or 20 (trisomy 20)

Gross Pathologic & Surgical Features

- Elastofibroma
  - Gray-white mass with entrapped adipose tissue
  - Size: 5-10 cm
- Deep (musculoaponeurotic) fibromatosis
  - May have irregular or infiltrating borders
  - White and coarsely trabeculated on cut section
  - Usually > 5 cm; may be > 15 cm

CLINICAL ISSUES

Presentation

- Most common signs/symptoms
  - **Elastofibroma: > 50% asymptomatic**
  - **Deep fibromatosis: Palpable mass**

Demographics

- Age
  - Elastofibroma: Elderly patients, mean age: 70 years
  - Deep fibromatosis: Puberty to 40 years; highest incidence 3rd-4th decades
- Gender
  - Elastofibroma: F:M = 5-13:1
  - Deep fibromatosis: Female predominance

Natural History & Prognosis

- Deep fibromatosis: High recurrence in young patients

Treatment

- **Elastofibroma**
  - Surgery curative; rare recurrence
- **Deep (musculoaponeurotic) fibromatosis**
  - Wide surgical resection and adjuvant radiation
  - Steroids, nonsteroidal anti-inflammatory drugs

SELECTED REFERENCES

1. Onishi Y et al: FDG-PET/CT imaging of elastofibroma dorsi. Skeletal Radiol. 40(7):849-53, 2011
2. Battaglia M et al: Imaging patterns in elastofibroma dorsi. Eur J Radiol. 72(1):16-21, 2009

CHEST WALL METASTASES

Key Facts

Terminology
- Metastatic disease involving chest wall
- Most common chest wall malignancy

Imaging
- Radiography
  - Incomplete border sign suggests chest wall or pleural lesion
  - Osseous destruction is most specific sign
  - Solitary or multiple chest wall masses with aggressive features
- CT: Direct chest wall evaluation for metastases
- MR
  - Typically T1 hypointense
  - Melanoma may be T1 & T2 hyperintense
- Bone scan more sensitive than radiography for bone metastases, whole body imaging
- PET/CT for staging of primary malignancies

Top Differential Diagnoses
- Chest wall infection
- Primary chest wall neoplasms
- Neurofibromatosis

Pathology
- Patterns of metastatic spread to chest wall
  - Direct extension
  - Hematogenous/lymphatic dissemination
- Common primaries: Lung, breast, prostate

Clinical Issues
- Localized pain is most frequent symptom
- Poor prognosis: Lung cancer, recurrent breast cancer

Diagnostic Checklist
- CT- or ultrasound-guided biopsy may be necessary in equivocal cases or unknown primary malignancies

*(**Left**) Composite axial CECT images of a patient with advanced right breast cancer show a large enhancing right breast mass with cutaneous, axillary, and subpectoral ➡ metastases. (**Right**) Coronal CECT of a patient with breast cancer metastatic to lymph nodes and bone shows a left breast mass ➡ with overlying skin thickening, supraclavicular lymphadenopathy, and mixed lytic and sclerotic sternal metastases. Metastatic breast cancer is a common etiology of chest wall metastases.*

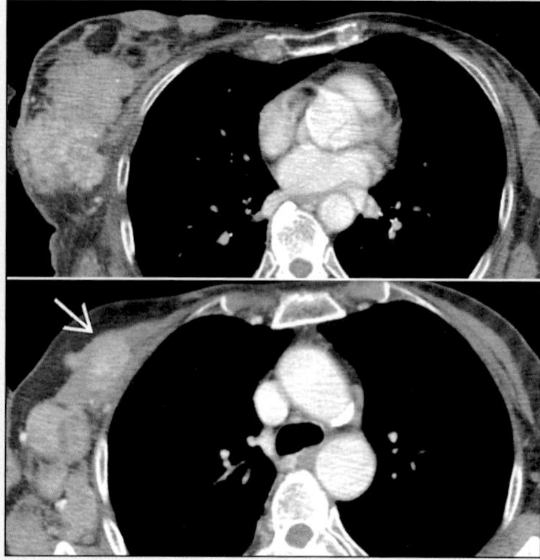

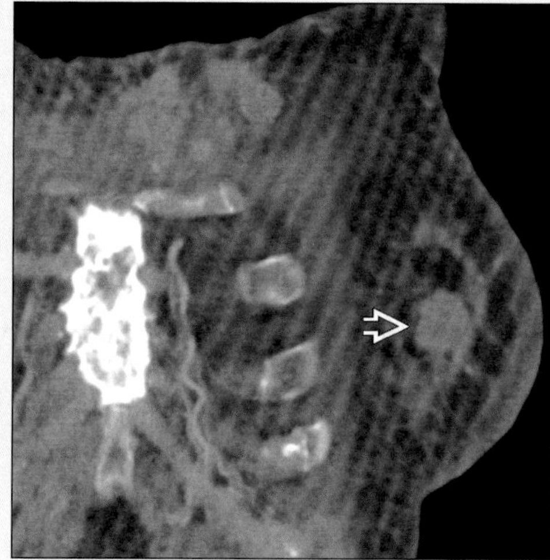

*(**Left**) Axial CECT of a patient with metastatic malignant melanoma shows a large heterogeneous cutaneous mass in the right posterior inferior chest wall. (**Right**) Composite image with axial (left) and coronal (right) NECT images of a patient with metastatic melanoma shows enhancing right chest wall masses and sclerosis of a subjacent right rib ➡. Metastatic melanoma commonly affects skin, subcutaneous fat, and muscle. Thus, these areas must be carefully evaluated on staging CT.*

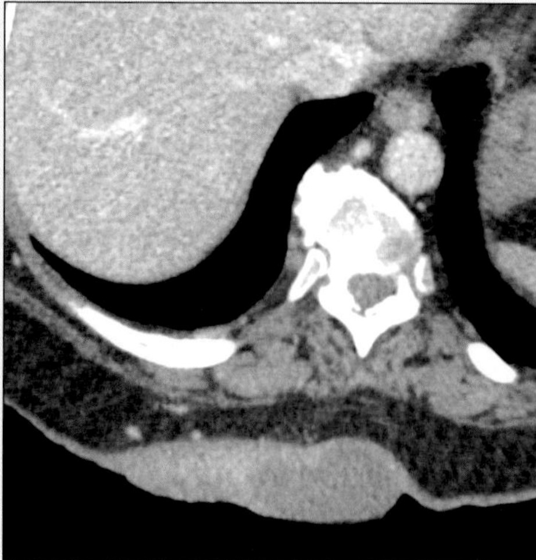

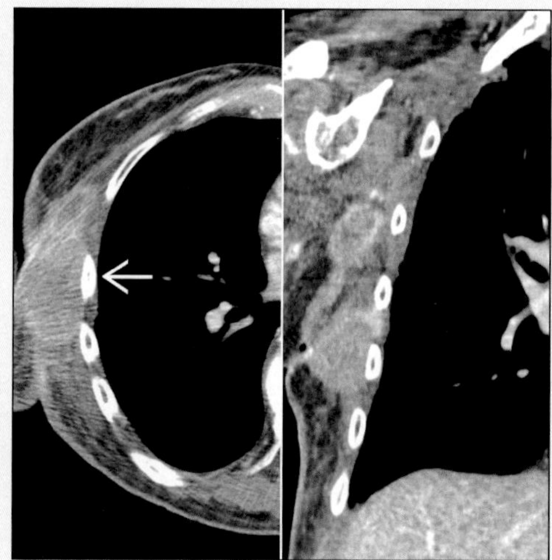

CHEST WALL METASTASES

TERMINOLOGY

Definitions

- Metastatic disease involving chest wall
- **Most common chest wall malignancy**
- Typically in terminal stages of malignancy

IMAGING

General Features

- Best diagnostic clue
  - **Rib/bone destruction most specific finding**
  - Solitary or multiple chest wall masses with aggressive features
- Location
  - Supraclavicular lymph nodes
    - Breast and lung cancer most common
    - Left-sided metastases 5x more frequent than right in abdominal/pelvic malignancies
    - High frequency in ovarian, stomach, head & neck, thyroid cancers
  - Axillary lymph nodes
    - Breast cancer & lymphoma most common
  - Skin and subcutaneous tissues
    - Chest most common site of skin metastases
    - Lung, breast, colon, melanoma most common
  - Muscle metastases rare; melanoma most common
  - Skeletal metastases from direct extension or hematogenous spread
    - Hematogenous spread most common to red marrow: Vertebrae, proximal ribs
    - Sternum: Breast & melanoma most common; renal, thyroid, gastric less common
    - Ribs: Lung, breast, prostate, thyroid most common
      - 16% of metastases involve ribs
      - Expansile lytic metastases: Renal & thyroid
      - Purely sclerotic metastases: Breast & prostate
      - Myeloma metastases may be lytic or permeative

Radiographic Findings

- **Incomplete border sign**: Discrepant size or margin visualization on orthogonal radiographs; suggests chest wall or pleural lesion
- Mass crosses anatomic lung boundaries
- **Osseous destruction most specific sign**
  - Pathologic fractures
- Solitary or multiple soft tissue masses
- Pleural effusion when pleura involved
- Calcification rare

CT Findings

- Direct chest wall visualization; evaluation of disease extent
- **Optimal evaluation of calcification & osseous destruction**
- **Most chest wall metastases enhance**, particularly melanoma & sarcoma

MR Findings

- T1WI
  - Typically T1 hypointense
  - Melanoma may be T1 hyperintense
  - Fat in liposarcoma metastases; T1 hyperintense
- T2WI
  - Typically T2 hyperintense relative to skeletal muscle
- T1WI C+
  - **Most chest wall metastases enhance**
- MR imaging
  - Useful in **evaluating direct chest wall invasion**
  - Evaluation of **extent of bone marrow involvement**
  - Multiplanar imaging for optimal evaluation of invasive superior sulcus tumors

Nuclear Medicine Findings

- Bone scan
  - **More sensitive than radiography for detecting bone metastases**
  - Extensive bony metastases may result in superscan
  - Widely available **whole body imaging** for identification of bone metastases
- PET/CT
  - Often used in staging known primary malignancies

Imaging Recommendations

- Best imaging tool
  - MR & CT complementary in evaluating direct chest wall invasion
  - PET/CT optimal for staging malignancy
- Protocol advice
  - Contrast may improve detection of small lesions

Image-Guided Biopsy

- CT- or ultrasound-guided biopsy often required to confirm diagnosis of metastatic disease

DIFFERENTIAL DIAGNOSIS

Chest Wall Infection

- Direct extension from pulmonary infection
  - Pyogenic infection, actinomycosis, nocardiosis, tuberculosis, fungal disease
  - Empyema necessitatis (73% from tuberculosis)
- Postoperative/post-traumatic
- Hematogenous seeding in bacteremia
- Primary infection in skin/chest wall

Primary Chest Wall Neoplasms

- **Rare**
- Multiple myeloma
- Chondrosarcoma, enchondroma
- Neurogenic neoplasms: Neurofibroma, schwannoma, malignant peripheral nerve sheath tumor
- Mesenchymal neoplasms: Lipoma, fibromatosis, malignant fibrous histiocytoma, fibrosarcoma
- Ewing sarcoma family of tumors

Neurofibromatosis

- Multiple masses along neurovascular bundles
- Pressure erosion of ribs/vertebrae (50%)
- Progression to malignant peripheral nerve sheath tumor

Vascular Lesions

- Arteriovenous malformation, aneurysm, hemangioma
- Dilated collateral veins

Bone Disease

- Paget disease: Ribs & clavicle least common sites involved
- Fibrous dysplasia
- Langerhans cell histiocytosis of bone

CHEST WALL METASTASES

- Metabolic bone disease
  - Hyperparathyroidism, rickets, scurvy

Chest Wall Trauma

- Healing rib fractures & hematomas may mimic malignancy

Elastofibroma Dorsi

- Benign lesion, unknown etiology
- Soft tissue mass with linear streaks of fat
- Sub or infrascapular, often bilateral

PATHOLOGY

General Features

- Calcification in metastases rare: Osteosarcoma, treated lymphoma
- Patterns of metastatic spread to chest wall
  - **Direct extension**
    - Lung cancer, inflammatory pseudotumor, carcinosarcoma
      - Pancoast tumor (superior sulcus tumor)
    - Breast cancer
    - Malignant thymic neoplasm, lymphoma, other mediastinal tumors
    - Malignant pleural mesothelioma
  - **Hematogenous spread**: Melanoma, thyroid, renal, hepatocellular cancers
  - **Lymphatic spread**: Lung cancer, breast cancer, lymphoma

Staging, Grading, & Classification

- Lung cancer
  - Direct chest wall invasion: At least T3
  - Scalene or supraclavicular lymph node metastasis: N3
  - Hematogenous chest wall metastasis: M1b
- Breast cancer patterns of chest wall metastases
  - Axillary, subpectoral, supraclavicular, internal mammary lymph node metastases
  - Direct invasion of ribs, sternum
  - Hematogenous rib, sternum, vertebral metastases
  - Local recurrence in resection margin or scar
- Melanoma metastases
  - Regional lymph nodes: 70%
  - Skin, subcutaneous fat, muscle: 70%
  - Bone: 23-49%
- Prostate cancer skeletal metastases
  - Vertebra > sternum > pelvis > ribs

CLINICAL ISSUES

Presentation

- Most common signs/symptoms
  - **Localized pain** is most frequent symptom
  - **Palpable swelling or mass**
  - Symptoms may relate to primary tumor
  - Asymptomatic in < 25%
  - Chronic skin infection or ulcerated metastases
- Other signs/symptoms
  - B symptoms in lymphoma

Demographics

- Epidemiology
  - Most common primaries: Lung, breast, prostate, renal, hepatocellular, colon cancers
    - Less common primaries: Ovarian, thyroid cancers
  - 5-8% of patients with lung cancer present with chest wall invasion
  - Seeding of biopsy tracts reported in lung cancer & malignant mesothelioma
  - Seeding of pleural drainage tracts reported in malignant pleural effusions
  - When primary unknown before biopsy, melanoma, breast, & colon cancer often implicated

Natural History & Prognosis

- Lung cancer
  - Chest wall invasion & metastasis has significant impact on 5-year survival
  - N3 disease: Approximately 9% 5-year survival
  - M1 disease: Approximately 13% 5-year survival
- Breast cancer chest wall recurrence in 5-20%
  - Chest wall recurrence is poor prognostic factor

Treatment

- Chemotherapy & radiation therapy most common
- Surgical resection may be considered
  - Isolated metastasis or locally recurrent breast cancer
  - Palliation from pain, chronic ulceration, or infection
  - Omental flaps, muscular flaps, & prosthetic material used in reconstruction
  - Resection margin, histology, smoking are important prognostic factors
    - Sarcomas & melanoma have poor prognosis after resection
- Partial or complete sternectomy in metastatic breast cancer
- Consideration of resection of involved ribs

DIAGNOSTIC CHECKLIST

Consider

- CT- or ultrasound-guided biopsy may be necessary in equivocal cases or unknown primary malignancies

Image Interpretation Pearls

- Rib/bone destruction: Most specific imaging findings of chest wall metastases
- CT & MR complementary when evaluating direct extension of malignancy

SELECTED REFERENCES

1. Hemmati SH et al: The prognostic factors of chest wall metastasis resection. Eur J Cardiothorac Surg. 40(2):328-33, 2011
2. O'Sullivan P et al: Malignant chest wall neoplasms of bone and cartilage: a pictorial review of CT and MR findings. Br J Radiol. 80(956):678-84, 2007
3. Jung JI et al: Thoracic manifestations of breast cancer and its therapy. Radiographics. 24(5):1269-85, 2004
4. Sharma A et al: Patterns of lymphadenopathy in thoracic malignancies. Radiographics. 24(2):419-34, 2004

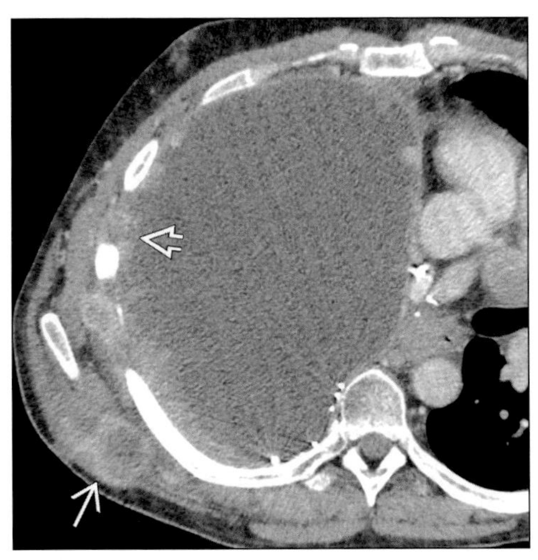

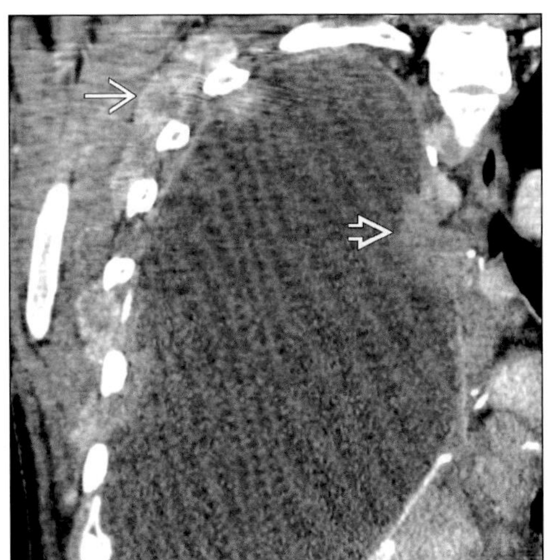

(Left) *Axial CECT of a patient with metastatic osteosarcoma treated with pneumonectomy and brachytherapy shows multiple right chest wall heterogeneously enhancing masses ➡ and tumor invasion ⇨ of the prosthetic material lining the pneumonectomy space.* **(Right)** *Coronal CECT of the same patient shows metastatic disease extending superiorly along the right chest wall ➡ and additional regions of metastatic disease invading the prosthetic material ⇨.*

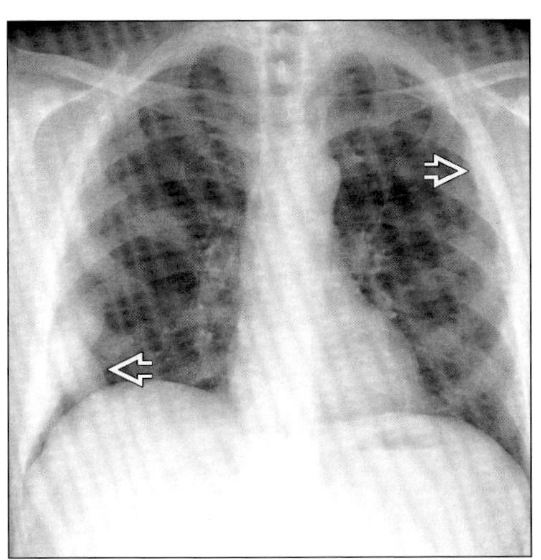

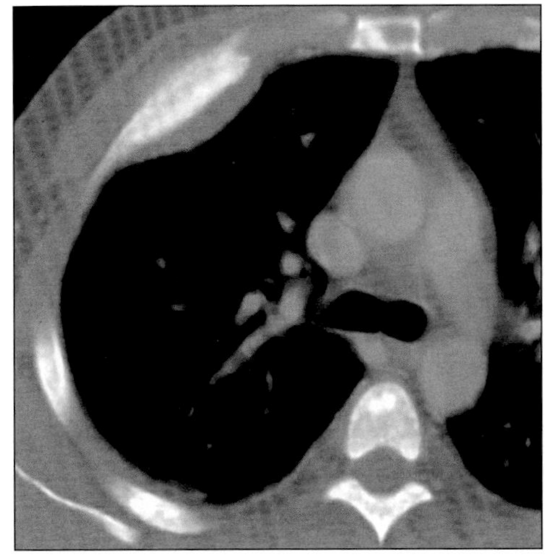

(Left) *PA chest radiograph of a patient with metastatic prostate cancer shows multiple expansile, sclerotic, bilateral rib metastases ⇨.* **(Right)** *Axial CECT (bone window) of the same patient shows sclerotic rib, vertebral, and sternal metastases. The anterior rib metastasis exhibits a soft tissue component. The ribs and vertebral bodies are the most common sites of skeletal metastases from prostate cancer. Diffuse skeletal prostate cancer metastases may produce a superscan on skeletal scintigraphy.*

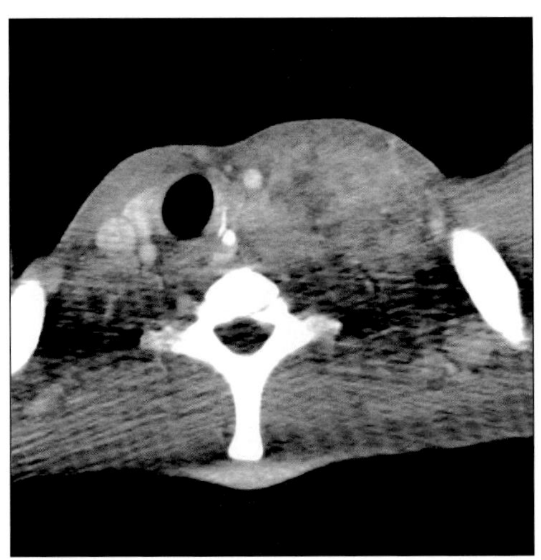

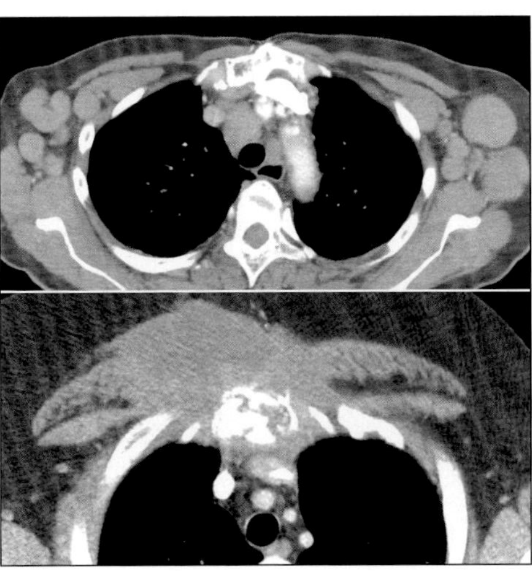

(Left) *Axial CECT of a patient with metastatic renal cell cancer shows a heterogeneous left supraclavicular metastasis. Supraclavicular metastatic lymphadenopathy from abdominal or pelvic malignancies is 5x more likely to occur on the left.* **(Right)** *Composite image with axial CECT of 2 different patients with lymphoma shows bilateral axillary and mediastinal metastases (top) and a locally invasive right anterior chest wall mass with direct sternal invasion (bottom).*

CHONDROSARCOMA

Key Facts

Terminology

- Definition: Malignant cartilaginous neoplasm

Imaging

- Radiography
  - Anterior chest wall mass
  - Incomplete border sign
  - Soft tissue cartilaginous calcifications
- CT
  - Well-circumscribed anterior chest wall mass
  - Soft tissue components, chondroid calcifications
  - Skeletal destruction
- MR
  - T1WI: Variable signal intensity
  - T2WI: High signal intensity mass, low signal intensity foci representing calcification
- Bone scan
  - > 80% of lesions show increased activity

Top Differential Diagnoses

- Chest wall metastasis
- Chest wall lipoma
- Ewing sarcoma family of tumors (Askin)
- Osteosarcoma
- Chest wall lymphoma

Pathology

- Most common primary chest wall malignancy

Clinical Issues

- Palpable painful anterior chest wall mass
- 4th-7th decades of life
- Male > female

Diagnostic Checklist

- Consider chondrosarcoma in adult with anterior chest wall mass with chondroid calcifications

__(Left)__ Axial NECT (bone window) shows a lobular right anterior chest wall soft tissue mass involving the costal cartilage with intrinsic calcified chondroid matrix. __(Right)__ Axial NECT (soft tissue window) shows a large low-attenuation mass arising from the lateral right 10th rib. The mass involves the chest wall soft tissues ➔ and produces mass effect on the liver. Note the intrinsic stippled and arc-shaped calcifications. Cartilaginous calcifications are characteristic of chest wall chondrosarcomas.

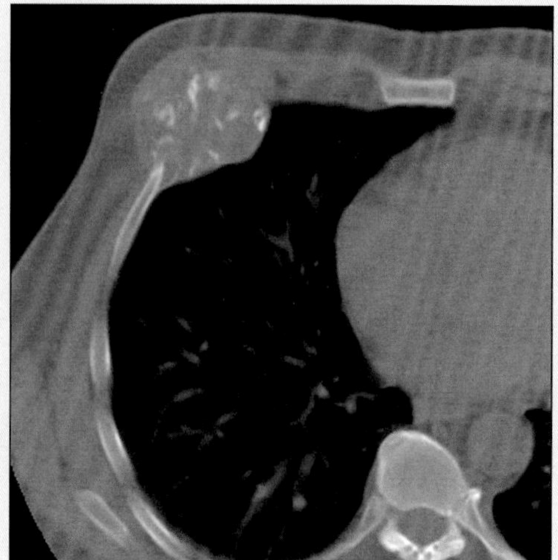

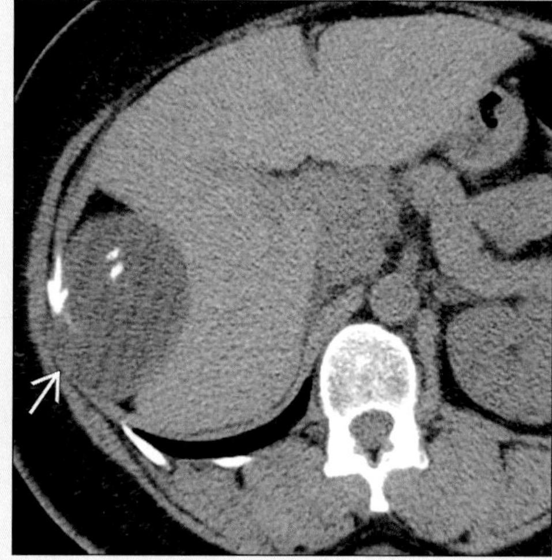

__(Left)__ Axial NECT (bone window) of a 32-year-old woman with a painful anterior chest wall mass shows a destructive sternal mass with multiple ring, arc, and stippled calcifications. __(Right)__ Oblique image from a bone scan of the same patient shows marked Tc-99m MDP activity in the manubrium sternum. Chest wall chondrosarcomas typically affect the sternum and the costochondral aspects of the ribs. Skeletal scintigraphy characteristically demonstrates increased activity within these lesions.

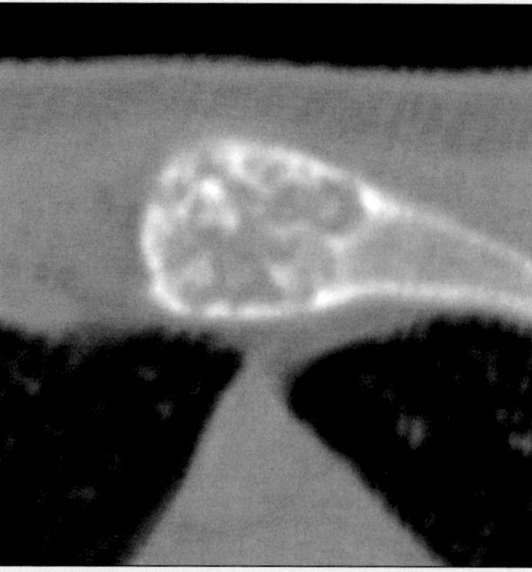

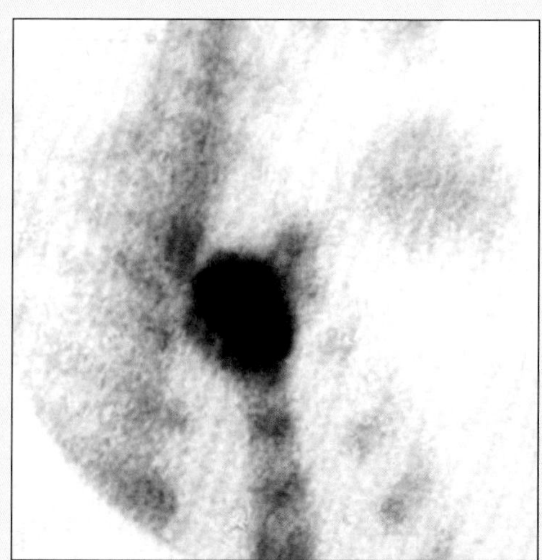

CHONDROSARCOMA

TERMINOLOGY

Definitions

- **Malignant cartilaginous neoplasm**

IMAGING

General Features

- Best diagnostic clue
  - Aggressive anterior chest wall neoplasm
  - Skeletal destruction & chondroid matrix
- Location
  - **Sternum** and **costochondral arches**
- Size
  - Variable size; often palpable
- Morphology
  - Well-circumscribed lobular soft tissue mass

Radiographic Findings

- Anterior chest wall mass
- **Incomplete border sign**
- Soft tissue **cartilaginous calcifications**

CT Findings

- NECT
  - Well-circumscribed anterior chest wall mass
    - Soft tissue components
    - Calcifications; **rings, arcs, stippled**
    - Skeletal destruction

MR Findings

- T1WI
  - Variable signal intensity
- T2WI
  - **High signal intensity mass**
  - Low signal intensity foci corresponding to chondroid calcifications

Imaging Recommendations

- Best imaging tool
  - CT is imaging **modality of choice**

Nuclear Medicine Findings

- Bone scan
  - > 80% of lesions show increased activity

DIFFERENTIAL DIAGNOSIS

Chest Wall Metastasis

- Most common malignant chest wall neoplasm
- Common primaries: Lung, breast, & prostate cancer
- Multiple myeloma with painful lytic plasmacytoma

Chest Wall Lipoma

- Mass with incomplete border sign
- Fat attenuation/signal mass with intrinsic small thin or punctate soft tissue elements

Ewing Sarcoma Family of Tumors (Askin)

- Rare malignant neoplasms in spectrum of Ewing sarcoma
- Osteolytic or osteoblastic skeletal involvement
- Frequent distant metastases

Osteosarcoma

- Rapidly enlarging painful mass
- Osteoid matrix
- Frequent distant metastases

Chest Wall Lymphoma

- Soft tissue mass
- Surrounds rather than destroys adjacent bones

PATHOLOGY

General Features

- Chondrosarcomas represent 20% of primary malignant bone neoplasms
- **Most common primary chest wall malignancy**
- **10%** of chondrosarcomas occur in **chest wall**
- Central chondrosarcomas arise in medullary cavity
- Peripheral chondrosarcomas arise from preexistent chondroma or osteochondroma

Staging, Grading, & Classification

- Histologic grades 1-3 based on mitotic activity, staining pattern, nuclear size, & cellularity

Gross Pathologic & Surgical Features

- Gray lobular mass
- Intrinsic calcification & central necrosis
- Slow growth

CLINICAL ISSUES

Presentation

- Most common signs/symptoms
  - **Palpable painful** anterior chest wall mass

Demographics

- Age
  - **4th-7th decades of life**
- Gender
  - Male > female

Natural History & Prognosis

- **10%** of patients present with **lung metastases**
- 60-90% 5-year survival rates
- Poor prognosis with high-grade tumors & metastases
- Lesion size & location do not predict outcome

Treatment

- **Complete surgical resection** with wide margins
- Refractory to chemotherapy & radiation therapy

DIAGNOSTIC CHECKLIST

Consider

- Chondrosarcoma in adult with palpable anterior chest wall mass with chondroid calcifications

SELECTED REFERENCES

1. Smith SE et al: Primary chest wall tumors. Thorac Surg Clin. 20(4):495-507, 2010
2. O'Sullivan P et al: Malignant chest wall neoplasms of bone and cartilage: a pictorial review of CT and MR findings. Br J Radiol. 80(956):678-84, 2007

PLASMACYTOMA AND MULTIPLE MYELOMA

Key Facts

Terminology
- Solitary plasmacytoma of bone (SPB)
- Extramedullary plasmacytoma (EMP)
  - Arises in soft tissues
- Multiple myeloma (MM)

Imaging
- SPB and MM: Axial skeleton
- Radiography
  - Small lesions may be occult
  - Osseous destruction
  - Lytic lesions
  - Soft tissue mass; incomplete border sign
- CT
  - SPB: Lytic bone lesion ± soft tissue mass
  - MM: Multiple lytic lesions
  - CT superior to MR for cortical destruction
  - Soft tissue attenuation similar to muscle
  - Variable enhancement of soft tissue mass
- MR
  - Untreated: T1 hypointense, T2/STIR hyperintense, diffuse enhancement
  - Treated: Variable appearance
  - No active disease: T1 hyperintense, T2/STIR hypointense, no enhancement
- PET/CT
  - Disease extent & treatment response

Top Differential Diagnoses
- Chest wall metastases
- Cartilaginous & osseous neoplasms

Clinical Issues
- SPB: Focal pain at site of lesion
- MM: Bone pain, renal failure, anemia
- Treatment
  - SPB: Lowest recurrence with surgery & radiation
  - MM: Chemotherapy, selective transplantation

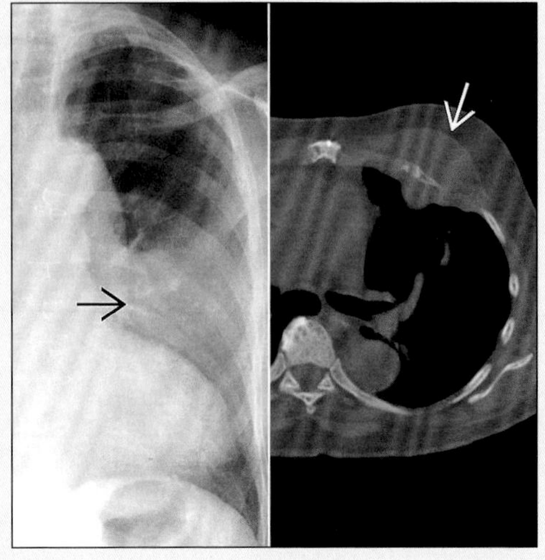

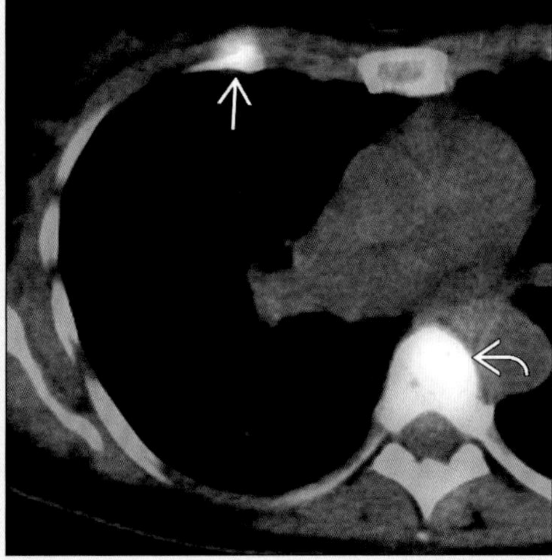

***(Left)** Composite image with PA chest radiograph (left) and axial CECT (right) of a patient with SPB shows an ill-defined opacity projecting over the left mid lung ⇨, exhibiting the incomplete border sign, and corresponding to a soft tissue mass in the left anterior chest wall with lytic rib involvement ➡. SPB more commonly affects the spine. **(Right)** Axial fused PET/CT of a patient with MM shows FDG uptake in a right anterior rib ➡ and a thoracic vertebral body ➡ at the same level. No corresponding abnormalities were present on CT.*

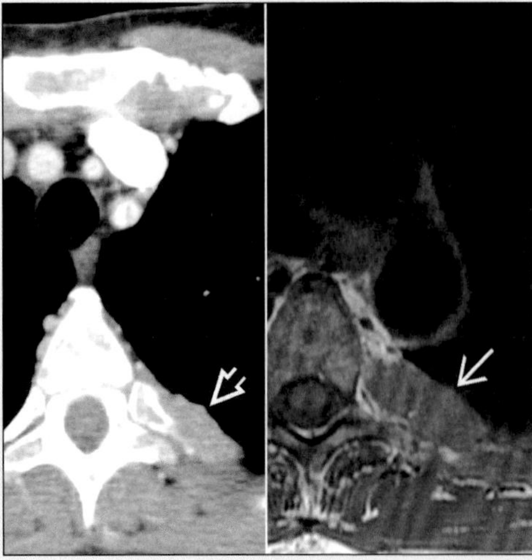

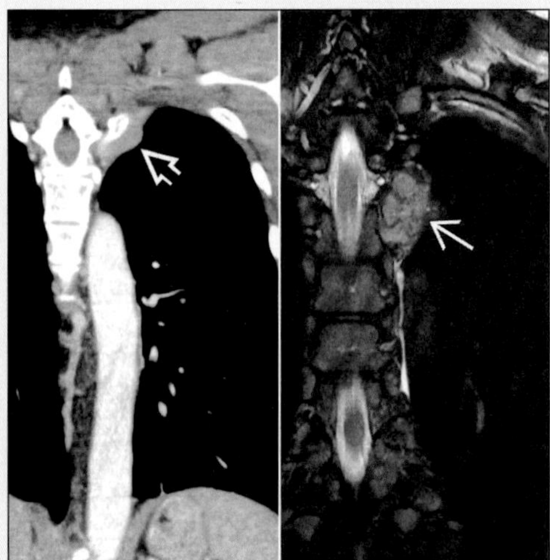

***(Left)** Composite image of a patient with MM with axial CECT (left) and axial T1WI MR (right) shows a lobular soft tissue mass of the left posterior chest wall ➡, which exhibits homogeneous hypointensity ➡ and rib invasion on MR. **(Right)** Composite image of the same patient with coronal CECT (left) and coronal T2WI MR (right) shows the left posterior chest wall soft tissue mass ➡, which exhibits hyperintensity on MR imaging ➡. MR is more sensitive than CT and FDG PET/CT in the detection of MM.*

PLASMACYTOMA AND MULTIPLE MYELOMA

TERMINOLOGY

Abbreviations

- **Solitary plasmacytoma of bone (SPB)**
- **Extramedullary plasmacytoma (EMP)**
- **Multiple myeloma (MM)**

Definitions

- **SPB: Solitary plasma cell tumor of bone**
  - No evidence of systemic disease
- **EMP: Solitary plasmacytoma** arising in **soft tissues**
- **MM: Neoplastic proliferation of plasma cells**
  - Monoclonal gammopathy
  - Multiple bone lesions

IMAGING

General Features

- Best diagnostic clue
  - Lytic bone lesion(s)
  - Soft tissue mass(es)
- Location
  - **SPB and MM**: Bones with **active hematopoiesis**
    - Skull, thoracic skeleton, vertebral bodies
    - Pelvis, proximal humeri & femora
- Size
  - Variable; may be radiographically occult

Radiographic Findings

- Radiographically occult if small
- Chest wall soft tissue mass; **incomplete border sign**
- **Osseous destruction**
  - Typically lytic skeletal lesions
  - May be advanced on skeletal surveys

CT Findings

- NECT
  - SPB: Expansile lytic bone lesion ± soft tissue mass
  - MM: Multiple lytic lesions
  - CT superior to MR for cortical destruction
- CECT
  - Variable enhancement of soft tissue component

MR Findings

- T1WI
  - Homogeneously hypointense (untreated)
  - Heterogeneous (treated)
  - Hyperintense (no active disease)
- T2WI
  - Hyperintense (untreated)
  - Heterogeneous (treated)
  - Hypointense (no active disease)
- T1WI C+
  - Diffuse enhancement (untreated)
  - Variable enhancement (treated)
  - No enhancement (no active disease)

Nuclear Medicine Findings

- PET/CT
  - Assessment of disease burden, extramedullary involvement, monitoring therapy
  - Successful treatment: Decreased or absent FDG uptake

DIFFERENTIAL DIAGNOSIS

Chest Wall Metastases

- Metastasis appearance varies according to primary
  - Sclerotic lesions: Prostate cancer, breast cancer
  - Lytic lesions: Renal cell cancer, thyroid cancer
- MR: T1 hypointense, T2 hyperintense

Cartilaginous and Osseous Neoplasms

- Chondrosarcomas: Soft tissue mass ± matrix
  - MR: T1 isointense to muscle, T2 hyperintense to fat
- Osteosarcomas: Neoplastic new bone, disorganized ossification
  - MR: T1 hyperintense, T2 iso-/hyperintense (to muscle)

PATHOLOGY

Staging, Grading, & Classification

- MM: Durie-Salmon PLUS system
  - Based on laboratory & imaging findings
    - IA: ≥ 10% plasma cells; limited disease or plasmacytoma
    - IB: IA + end organ damage; mild diffuse disease, < 5 focal lesions
    - IIA, IIB: As above; moderate diffuse disease, 5-20 focal lesions
    - IIIA, IIIB: As above; severe diffuse disease, > 20 focal lesions
- International staging system: No imaging criteria

CLINICAL ISSUES

Presentation

- Most common signs/symptoms
  - SPB: Focal pain at site of lesion
  - MM: Bone pain, renal failure, anemia

Demographics

- Age
  - SPB, EMP: 50 years; MM: 50-70 years
- Gender
  - **2/3 M**; 1/3 F
- Epidemiology
  - SPB, EMP: 5-10% of malignant plasma cell tumors
  - MM: 10% of hematologic tumors, 1% overall

Natural History & Prognosis

- Progression to MM: 50% SPB, 15% EMP
- SPB: 25-40% disease free at 10 years
- MM: Median survival 44.8 months
- Survival: EMP > SPB > MM, younger > older

Treatment

- SPB: Lowest recurrence with surgery & radiation
  - Development of MM in 3 years with radiation alone
  - Adjuvant chemotherapy delays conversion to MM
- MM: Chemotherapy, selective transplantation

SELECTED REFERENCES

1. Hanrahan CJ et al: Current concepts in the evaluation of multiple myeloma with MR imaging and FDG PET/CT. Radiographics. 30(1):127-42, 2010

EWING SARCOMA FAMILY OF TUMORS

Key Facts

Terminology
- Ewing sarcoma family of tumors (ESFT)
- Primitive neuroectodermal tumor (PNET)
- Askin tumor: Small cell cancer of thoracopulmonary region
- ESFT includes PNET & Askin tumor

Imaging
- Radiography
  - Large, unilateral, extrapulmonary mass
  - Site of origin may be difficult to determine
  - Rib destruction in 25-63% of cases
  - Pleural effusion is frequent
- CT
  - Heterogeneous soft tissue mass: Hemorrhage, necrosis, cystic change
  - Invasion of chest wall, pleura, lung, mediastinum
  - Lymphadenopathy, metastases to lung/bone

Top Differential Diagnoses
- Ewing sarcoma
- Sympathetic ganglion neoplasm
- Lymphoma
- Osteosarcoma
- Chest wall metastases

Pathology
- Arises from soft tissues of chest wall

Clinical Issues
- Signs & symptoms
  - Chest, back, shoulder pain
  - Dyspnea, cough, weight loss
- Demographics
  - 20-30 years of age; M:F = 1:1.3
- Treatment
  - Surgical excision, radiation, chemotherapy

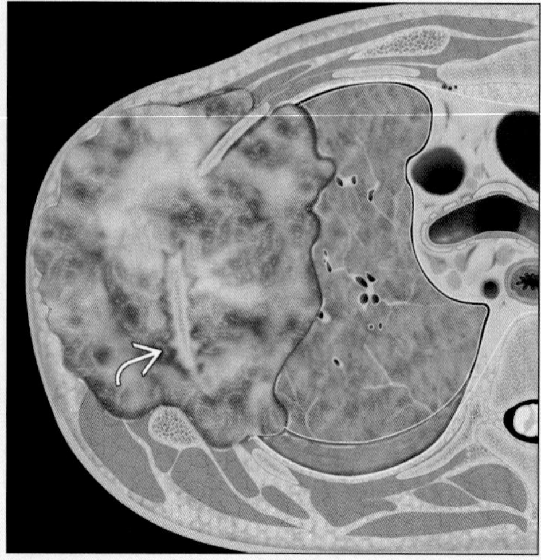

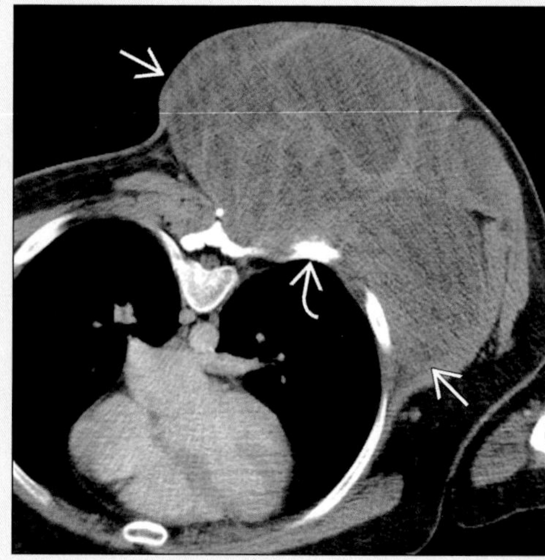

(Left) *Graphic shows the gross features of Ewing sarcoma family of tumors (ESFT) manifesting as a large heterogeneous extrapulmonary mass with chest wall invasion, skeletal periostitis, and a small right pleural effusion.* ***(Right)*** *Axial CECT (mediastinal window) shows a huge heterogeneous ESFT arising from the soft tissues of the left posterior chest wall with extensive cystic changes. Although there is periostitis of a left posterior rib, absence of skeletal destruction reflects the soft tissue origin of the neoplasm.*

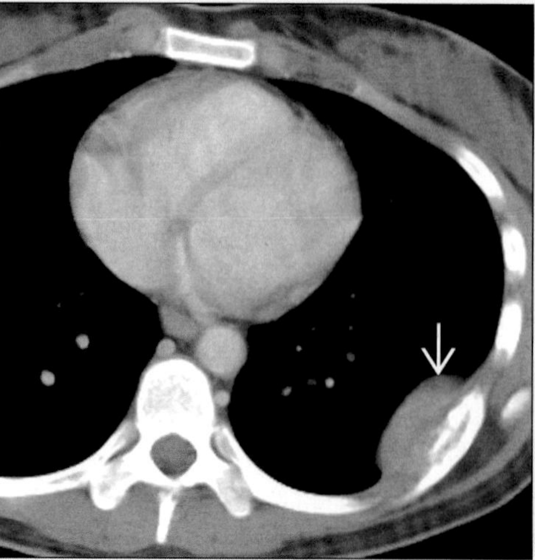

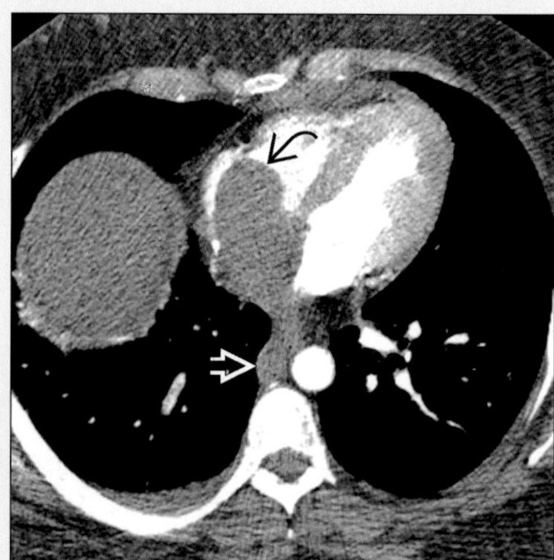

(Left) *Axial CECT (mediastinal window) shows a peripheral left intrathoracic soft tissue mass that produces skeletal destruction and aggressive periostitis of an adjacent rib.* ***(Right)*** *Axial CECT shows an aggressive abdominal ESFT with intrathoracic tumor growth via the inferior vena cava into the right atrium and involvement of the azygos vein. ESFT often exhibits extrathoracic origin and explosive tumor growth.*

EWING SARCOMA FAMILY OF TUMORS

TERMINOLOGY

Abbreviations

- Ewing sarcoma family of tumors (**ESFT**)
- Primitive neuroectodermal tumor (**PNET**)

Definitions

- **Askin tumor**: Small cell cancer of thoracopulmonary region
- **ESFT includes PNET and Askin tumor**
  - Chest wall &/or pleural sarcomas

IMAGING

General Features

- Best diagnostic clue
  - Large extrapulmonary mass in a young adult
- Location
  - Chest wall, pleura
  - Extrathoracic/extraosseous origin
- Size
  - Typically quite large; explosive growth
- Morphology
  - Soft tissue mass ± multicystic components

Radiographic Findings

- Large, unilateral, **extrapulmonary** mass
  - Site of origin may be difficult to determine
- **Rib destruction** in 25-63% of cases
- **Pleural effusion** is frequent
- Lymphadenopathy; metastases to lung &/or bone

CT Findings

- CECT
  - **Heterogeneous soft tissue mass**
    - Hemorrhage, necrosis, cystic change
    - Calcification is rare
  - Invasion of chest wall, pleura, lung, mediastinum

MR Findings

- T1WI
  - Heterogeneous mass, mixed signal intensity
- T2WI
  - Heterogeneous, intermediate/high signal intensity
- T1WI C+
  - Enhances with gadolinium

Imaging Recommendations

- Best imaging tool
  - CT: Skeletal involvement & metastatic disease
  - MR: Optimal evaluation of soft tissue involvement

DIFFERENTIAL DIAGNOSIS

Ewing Sarcoma

- Centered on bone (rib), similar imaging features

Rhabdomyosarcoma

- Thorax unlikely location but identical imaging features

Sympathetic Ganglion Neoplasm

- Elongate paravertebral mass, often with calcification
- Intraspinal extension may occur

Lymphoma

- Homogeneous mass without rib destruction

Localized Fibrous Tumor of Pleura

- Large pedunculated mass; may fill hemithorax
- Chest wall involvement rare

Osteosarcoma

- Ossifying bone malignancy of adolescents
- May originate in thoracic cage: Rib, scapula, spine

Chest Wall Metastases

- Typically from lung, breast, or prostate primaries

PATHOLOGY

General Features

- Etiology
  - Postulated origin from embryonal neural crest cells
  - May arise after radiation therapy for lymphoma
- Genetics
  - Translocation of chromosomes 11 & 22, t(11;22)
  - Related familial neuroectodermal & gastric cancers

Staging, Grading, & Classification

- Localized (80%) or metastatic (20%) at presentation

Gross Pathologic & Surgical Features

- Large, locally invasive, heterogeneous chest wall mass
- **ESFT** most commonly affects extremities and pelvis

Microscopic Features

- Undifferentiated, **small round blue cells**

CLINICAL ISSUES

Presentation

- Most common signs/symptoms
  - **Palpable mass**
  - Chest, back, shoulder pain
  - Dyspnea, cough, weight loss
  - Horner syndrome

Demographics

- Age
  - **20-30 years**
- Gender
  - **M:F = 1:1.3**
- Ethnicity
  - **9x more common** in Caucasians
- Epidemiology
  - **Rare**: 3 per 1,000,000 population per year

Natural History & Prognosis

- Poor outcomes with large tumor size, pelvic origin, & metastases

Treatment

- Based on extent of disease: Localized vs. metastatic
- Surgical excision, radiation, & chemotherapy

SELECTED REFERENCES

1. Gladish GW et al: Primary thoracic sarcomas. Radiographics. 22(3):621-37, 2002

DIAPHRAGMATIC EVENTRATION

Key Facts

Terminology
- Congenital nonparalytic weakening & thinning of anterior portion & dome of hemidiaphragm

Imaging
- Radiography
  - Diaphragmatic elevation on frontal chest radiography
  - Anterior diaphragmatic elevation on lateral chest radiography (focal eventration)
  - Preservation of anterior &/or posterior costophrenic angles: HH/APD ratio > 0.28
- Fluoroscopy
  - Eventration: Negative sniff test with inspiratory lag followed by delayed downward motion
- CT
  - Useful when radiography is inconclusive or when eventration mimics a mass

Top Differential Diagnoses
- Diaphragmatic paralysis
- Diaphragmatic tear
- Morgagni diaphragmatic hernia
- Subpulmonic pleural effusion

Pathology
- Congenital failure of fetal diaphragm to muscularize
- Thin diaphragmatic tendon & membranous muscle; decreased muscle fibers
- Permanent diaphragmatic elevation
- Usually unilateral, rarely bilateral

Clinical Issues
- Adults over 60 years of age
- Women typically affected
- Characteristic benign course with good prognosis

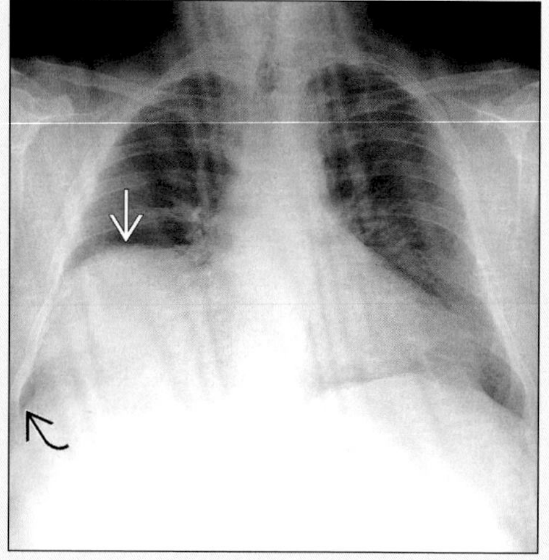

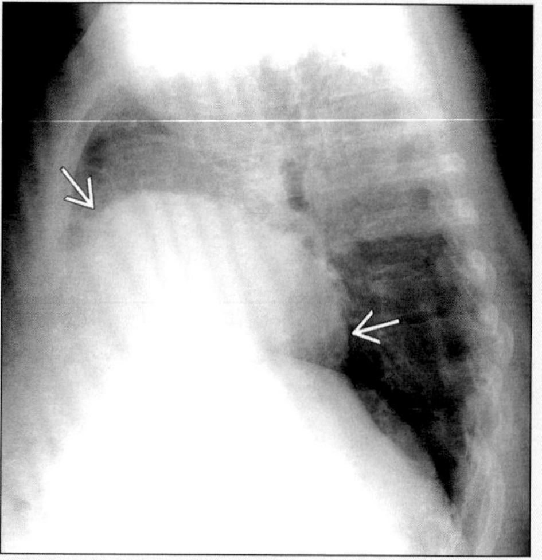

(Left) *PA chest radiograph demonstrates focal elevation and lobular contour of the right hemidiaphragm ➔. Note the normal location and morphology of the right costophrenic angle ➚.* ***(Right)*** *Lateral chest radiograph shows a hump-like morphology ➔ of the anterior portion of the right hemidiaphragm. Note normal location of the posterior costophrenic angle. Diaphragmatic eventration typically affects elderly women and characteristically occurs in the anteromedial right hemidiaphragm.*

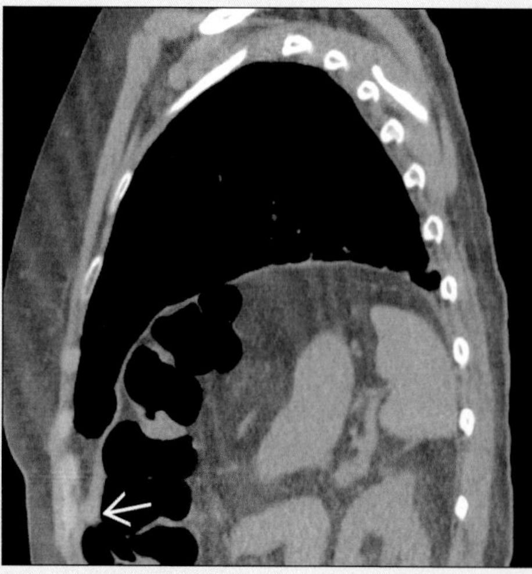

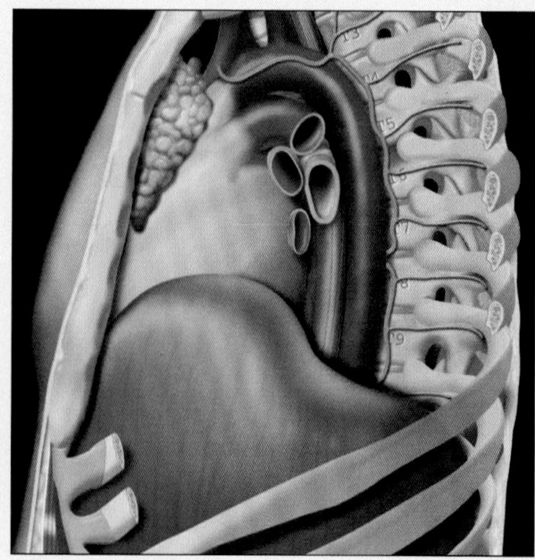

(Left) *Sagittal NECT of a patient with diaphragmatic eventration shows lobular elevation of the left hemidiaphragm. Normal location and depth of the anterior diaphragmatic attachment ➔ help differentiate diaphragmatic eventration from diaphragmatic paralysis.* ***(Right)*** *Graphic demonstrates the characteristic morphology of diaphragmatic eventration with lobular elevation of the anterior hemidiaphragm. Note that the posterior costophrenic angle is normally located.*

DIAPHRAGMATIC EVENTRATION

TERMINOLOGY

Definitions

- Congenital nonparalytic weakening & thinning of anterior portion & dome of hemidiaphragm

IMAGING

General Features

- Best diagnostic clue
  - **Lobular elevation** or smooth **hump-like morphology** of anteromedial hemidiaphragm
  - **Preservation of posterior costophrenic angle** on lateral chest radiography
- Location
  - **Right** hemidiaphragm usually affected
  - **Anteromedial** portion of hemidiaphragm

Radiographic Findings

- Radiography
  - Diaphragmatic elevation on frontal chest radiography
  - Anterior diaphragmatic elevation on lateral chest radiography (focal eventration)
  - Preservation of anterior &/or posterior costophrenic angles: **HH/APD ratio > 0.28**
    - **HH = hemidiaphragm height**
    - **APD = anteroposterior diameter**
  - May mimic an intrathoracic mass

Fluoroscopic Findings

- Chest fluoroscopy
  - **Sniff test**
    - Technique: Rapid & forced inhalation through the nose with closed mouth
    - **Normal**: Sharp brief downward displacement of both hemidiaphragms
    - **Eventration**: **Negative sniff test** with inspiratory lag followed by delayed downward motion
    - Total eventration: May be indistinguishable from diaphragmatic paralysis; false-positive sniff test

CT Findings

- Useful when radiography is inconclusive or when eventration mimics a mass
- Intact but thinned diaphragmatic muscle & tendon
- Coronal or sagittal reformations helpful to confirm diaphragmatic integrity

MR Findings

- Similar to CT findings
  - Intact but thinned diaphragmatic muscle & tendon
- Respiratory gating or real-time imaging necessary for accurate characterization

Ultrasonographic Findings

- Evaluation of real-time diaphragmatic motion
- Can be performed at bedside

Imaging Recommendations

- Best imaging tool
  - **Chest radiography** is typically **diagnostic**
  - Fluoroscopy (sniff test) or CT may be useful in problematic cases

DIFFERENTIAL DIAGNOSIS

Diaphragmatic Paralysis

- Positive sniff test
- Anterior and posterior costophrenic angles often elevated: HH/APD ratio < 0.28

Diaphragmatic Tear

- Prior high-energy blunt or penetrating chest trauma
- Associated fracture, hemothorax, pneumothorax, pulmonary contusion
- Indentation of abdominal viscera &/or bowel at site of laceration ("collar" or "waist" sign)

Morgagni Diaphragmatic Hernia

- Right cardiophrenic angle, obscures right heart border
- Contains variable amounts of omental fat & bowel

Subpulmonic Pleural Effusion

- Lateral decubitus radiography demonstrates free fluid
- Ultrasound shows subpulmonic pleural fluid

PATHOLOGY

General Features

- Etiology
  - Congenital failure of fetal diaphragm to muscularize
- Associated abnormalities
  - Usually **unilateral**, rarely bilateral
  - Rare association with Poland syndrome (ipsilateral radial ray anomalies & absent pectoral muscles)

Gross Pathologic & Surgical Features

- **Permanent diaphragmatic elevation**
- Thin diaphragmatic tendon & membranous muscle; decreased muscle fibers
- Preservation of diaphragmatic continuity & costal attachments

CLINICAL ISSUES

Presentation

- Most common signs/symptoms
  - **Adults**: Often asymptomatic
  - Children: Cardiopulmonary distress

Demographics

- Age
  - Adults **over 60 years of age**
- Gender
  - **Women** typically affected

Natural History & Prognosis

- Characteristically **benign course**; **good prognosis**

Treatment

- Asymptomatic adults do not require treatment
- Surgical repair in extreme cases; symptomatic children

SELECTED REFERENCES

1. Maish MS: The diaphragm. Surg Clin North Am. 90(5):955-68, 2010
2. Roberts HC: Imaging the diaphragm. Thorac Surg Clin. 19(4):431-50, v, 2009

DIAPHRAGMATIC PARALYSIS

Key Facts

Terminology
- Extreme form of diaphragmatic weakness
- Decreased strength of diaphragmatic musculature

Imaging
- Chest radiography
  - Diaphragmatic elevation
  - HH/APD ratio < 0.28
- Fluoroscopy (sniff test)
  - Diagnostic study of choice
  - Paralysis; absent or paradoxical upward motion
- CT
  - Diaphragmatic elevation
  - Identification of etiology of paralysis
- Ultrasound
  - Absent caudal movement on inspiration
  - Paradoxical movement on sniff test

Top Differential Diagnoses
- Diaphragmatic eventration
  - Congenital failure of muscular development
  - Negative sniff test
- Subpulmonic pleural effusion
  - May simulate diaphragmatic elevation
  - Free pleural fluid on decubitus radiography

Clinical Issues
- Signs/symptoms
  - Unilateral paralysis; asymptomatic in 50%
  - Orthopnea, tachypnea, chest pain, cough
  - Bilateral paralysis; more severe symptoms
- Treatment
  - Unilateral: Usually no treatment required
  - Bilateral: Mechanical ventilation, tracheostomy
- Prognosis
  - Poor if bilateral or associated with myopathy

*(**Left**) Anteroposterior fluoroscopic spot radiograph of the chest during inspiration demonstrates elevation of the left hemidiaphragm. (**Right**) Anteroposterior fluoroscopic spot radiograph of the chest during sniff test (expiration) shows normal excursion of the right hemidiaphragm and absence of motion of the left hemidiaphragm. The sniff test can be used to differentiate between diaphragmatic eventration and paralysis. A false-positive sniff test can occur in patients with COPD and in weak, debilitated patients.*

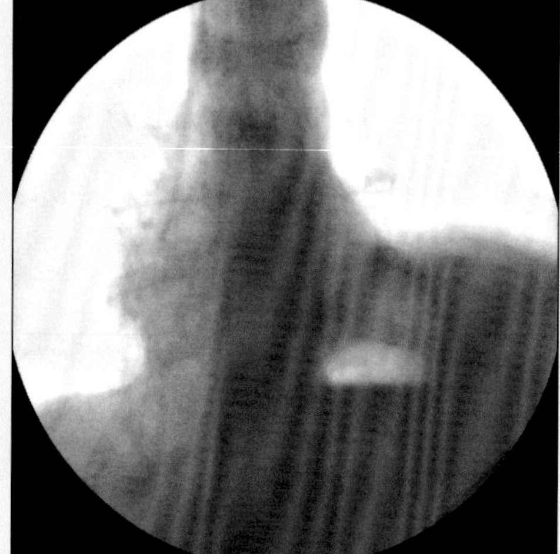

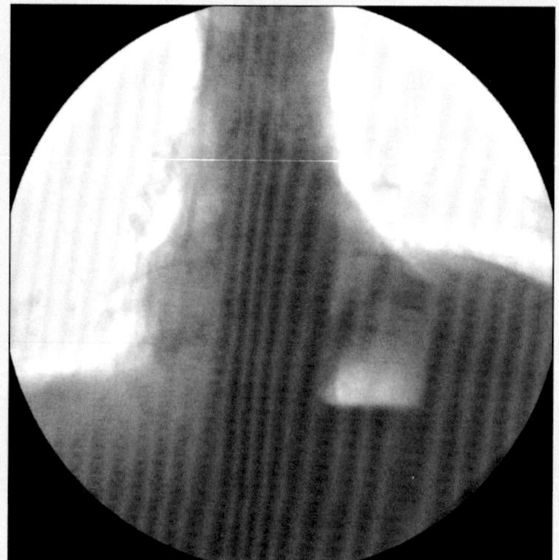

*(**Left**) PA chest radiograph of the same patient demonstrates left hemidiaphragm elevation. This finding is unreliable for diagnosing paralysis as it can also be seen in volume loss, diaphragmatic eventration, and subpulmonic pleural effusion. (**Right**) Coronal CECT shows a mass ➔ at the right lung apex with invasion of the adjacent chest wall soft tissues, which resulted in paralysis and elevation of the right hemidiaphragm ➔. CT can be useful in establishing the etiology of diaphragmatic paralysis.*

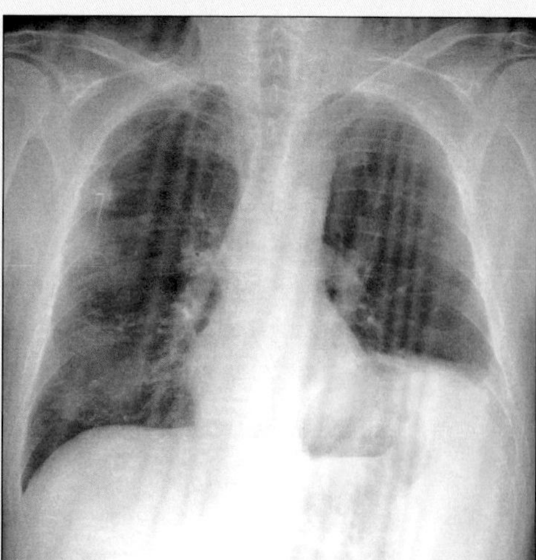

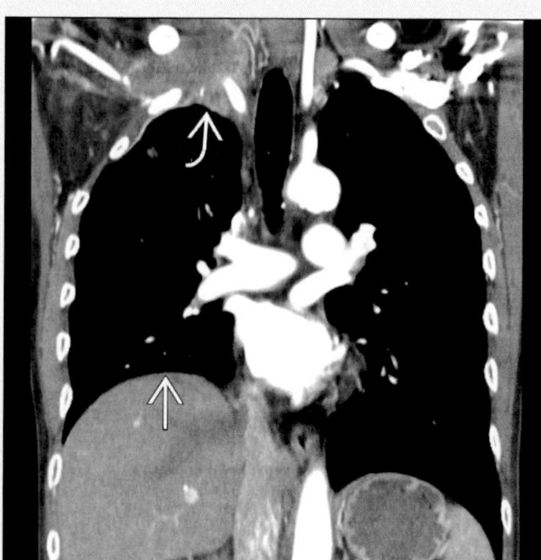

DIAPHRAGMATIC PARALYSIS

TERMINOLOGY

Synonyms

- Diaphragmatic **palsy**
- Diaphragmatic **paresis**
- Diaphragmatic weakness

Definitions

- Extreme form of diaphragmatic weakness
- Decreased strength of diaphragmatic musculature

IMAGING

General Features

- Best diagnostic clue
  - Absent or paradoxical diaphragmatic motion on chest fluoroscopy (**sniff test**)

Radiographic Findings

- Radiography
  - Normal findings
    - Right hemidiaphragm typically higher than left
    - Equal height of right & left hemidiaphragm in 9%
    - Overlap between range of motion of normal & paralyzed hemidiaphragms
  - Diaphragmatic elevation without paralysis
    - Bilateral elevation from low lung volumes
      - Pulmonary fibrosis
    - Unilateral elevation from relaxation atelectasis
  - Diaphragmatic paralysis
    - **Diaphragmatic elevation**
    - Identification of associated thoracic malignancy or thoracic infection
    - **HH/APD** = ratio of hemidiaphragm height (HH) to anteroposterior diameter (APD)
      - **APD** = distance from anterior to posterior diaphragmatic insertions on lateral radiography
      - **HH** = perpendicular height from APD to dome
      - **HH/APD < 0.28** suggests diaphragmatic paralysis

CT Findings

- Diaphragmatic elevation
- Identification of etiology of diaphragmatic paralysis

MR Findings

- Real-time diaphragm imaging; only considered when other methods are inconclusive
- May be useful for long-term follow-up & monitoring of therapeutic interventions

Ultrasonographic Findings

- Absent caudal diaphragm movement on inspiration
- Paradoxical diaphragmatic movement on sniff test during M mode (motion mode)

Imaging Recommendations

- Best imaging tool
  - **Chest fluoroscopy**
    - Normal diaphragmatic dome excursion; 3-5 cm
    - **Sniff test**
      - Technique: Rapid forced inhalation through nose with closed mouth
      - Normal: Sharp brief downward motion of both hemidiaphragms
      - Paralysis: Absent or paradoxical upward motion
      - **False-positive sniff test: COPD, weak, debilitated** patients

DIFFERENTIAL DIAGNOSIS

Diaphragmatic Eventration

- Congenital failure of diaphragm muscle development
  - Thin membranous hemidiaphragm
  - Decreased muscle fibers
- Asymptomatic adults; respiratory distress in infants
- Imaging clues
  - Negative sniff test
  - Absence of relaxation atelectasis
  - HH/APD > 0.28

Subpulmonic Pleural Effusion

- May simulate diaphragmatic elevation
- Free pleural fluid on lateral decubitus radiography
- Ultrasound demonstration of subpulmonic fluid

PATHOLOGY

General Features

- Etiology
  - Traumatic; postsurgical
  - Compression; nerve root compression, malignancy compressing or invading phrenic nerve
  - Inflammatory
  - Neuropathic
  - Idiopathic; minority of cases

CLINICAL ISSUES

Presentation

- Most common signs/symptoms
  - Unilateral paralysis; more common than bilateral
    - **Asymptomatic in 50%**
    - Orthopnea, tachypnea, chest pain, cough
    - Inward motion of abdomen during inspiration
  - Bilateral paralysis; more severe symptoms
    - Exertional dyspnea, orthopnea
    - Cor pulmonale
    - Increased incidence of pneumonia
    - Decreased oxygenation & vital capacity on supine position, worse with bilateral paralysis
  - Restrictive pattern on pulmonary function tests

Natural History & Prognosis

- Poor prognosis if bilateral when associated with myopathy, chronic demyelinating condition, or coexistent COPD or pulmonary fibrosis

Treatment

- **Unilateral**: Usually **no treatment** required; surgical plication & phrenic pacing in selected cases
- **Bilateral: Mechanical ventilation** &/or **tracheostomy**

SELECTED REFERENCES

1. Qureshi A: Diaphragm paralysis. Semin Respir Crit Care Med. 30(3):315-20, 2009
2. Roberts HC: Imaging the diaphragm. Thorac Surg Clin. 19(4):431-50, v, 2009

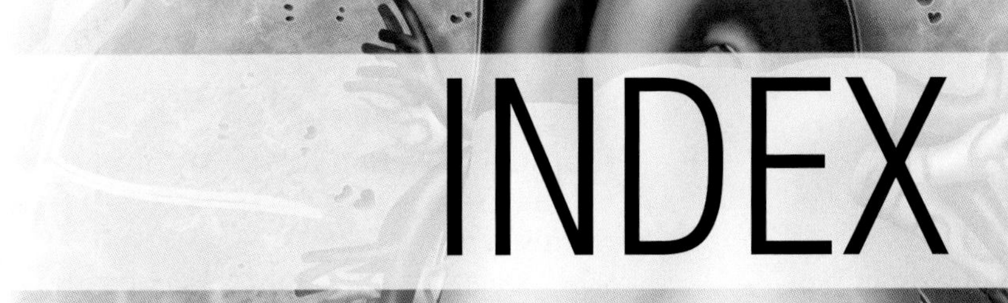

INDEX

A

INDEX

INDEX

INDEX

B

INDEX

INDEX

C

INDEX

INDEX

INDEX

INDEX

INDEX

D

INDEX

INDEX

E

INDEX

F

INDEX

G

INDEX

INDEX

I

INDEX

INDEX

INDEX

INDEX

INDEX

INDEX

INDEX

INDEX

INDEX

N

INDEX

O

P

INDEX

INDEX

INDEX

INDEX

INDEX

INDEX

INDEX

INDEX

INDEX

R

INDEX

S

INDEX

INDEX

T

INDEX

INDEX

INDEX

U

V

INDEX

INDEX

W

Y

Z